Medical-Surgical Nursing

CRITICAL THINKING
FOR COLLABORATIVE CARE

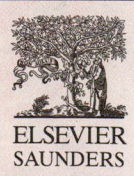

ELSEVIER
SAUNDERS

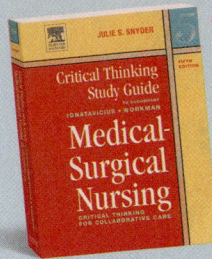
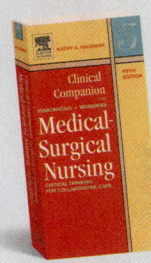
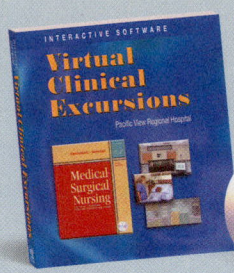
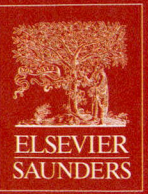

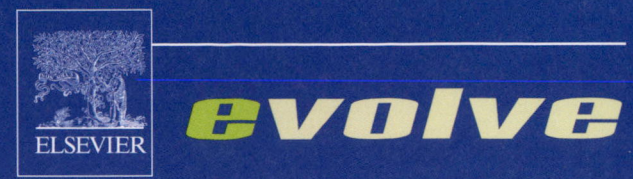

- **Integrated Management of Care Questions for the NCLEX Examination**
  Multiple-choice self-test questions are divided by chapter and focus on delegation and supervision, assignment, and prioritization/decision making. The Integrated Management of Care Questions for the NCLEX Examination help you understand and apply the material covered in the text and integrate it with material you have learned elsewhere in the curriculum—fostering the skills needed to master the NCLEX Examination.

- **Pharmacology Review Questions**
  Safe medication administration is a major theme of the NCLEX Examination. The Pharmacology Review Questions will make you more comfortable with the application of clinical drug therapy and promote readiness for safe drug administration. These questions are keyed to the text—just look for the "Evolve Pharm Review" icons.

- **Answer Guidelines—Critical Thinking Challenges and Study Guide Case Studies**
  Suggested Answer Guidelines are provided for the Critical Thinking Challenges interspersed throughout the text and for the Case Studies within the Critical Thinking Study Guide. These exercises provide a safe and effective means of practicing the on-the-spot decision making that you will face in the fast-paced world of medical-surgical nursing. The Answer Guidelines allow you to gauge your mastery of the text and readiness for your examinations.

- **WebLinks**
  An exciting resource links you to hundreds of carefully chosen websites that supplement the content of the textbook. These WebLinks are regularly updated, and new links are added as they develop.

- **Additional Resources**
  Audio Glossary, "Building" Concept Maps, Concept Map Creator, Fluid and Electrolyte Tutorial, Content Updates, Audio Clips, Video Clips, Animations, Bonus Health Assessment Images.

Medical-Surgical Nursing

CRITICAL THINKING FOR COLLABORATIVE CARE

**FIFTH
EDITION**

5

Donna D. Ignatavicius, MS, RN, C
Presenter and Consultant for Nursing Programs
President, DI Associates, Inc.
Placitas, New Mexico

M. Linda Workman, PhD, RN, FAAN
Gertrude Perkins Oliva Professor of Oncology
Frances Payne Bolton School of Nursing
Case Western Reserve University
Cleveland, Ohio

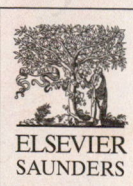

ELSEVIER
SAUNDERS

ELSEVIER
SAUNDERS

11830 Westline Industrial Drive
St. Louis, Missouri 63146

MEDICAL-SURGICAL NURSING: CRITICAL THINKING FOR
COLLABORATIVE CARE
Copyright © 2006, 2002, 1999, 1995, 1991 by Elsevier Inc.

ISBN-13: 978-0-7216-0446-6 (Single Vol.)
ISBN-10: 0-7216-0446-3 (Single Vol.)
ISBN-13: 978-0-7216-0671-2 (2-Vol. Set)
ISBN-10: 0-7216-0671-7 (2-Vol. Set)

Executive Publisher: Barbara Nelson Cullen
Editor: Lee Henderson
Developmental Editor: Laura Sieh Chu, Robin Richman
Publishing Services Manager: Deborah L. Vogel
Senior Project Manager: Jodi M. Willard
Book Designer: Teresa McBryan

Printed in United States of America

Last digit is the print number: 9 8 7 6 5 4 3 2

DEDICATION

To Charles and Stephanie
Thanks for your unending support, love, and understanding during every edition; I could
not do this without you!

Donna

To my mother, Eunice Workman, from whom I inherited the creativity and persistence to
pursue my dream of being an author.

Linda

About the Authors

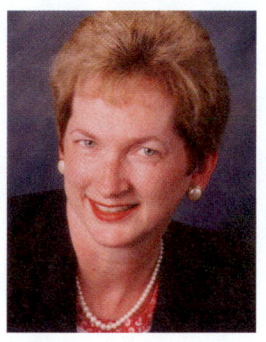

Donna D. Ignatavicius received her diploma in nursing from the Peninsula General School of Nursing in Salisbury, Maryland. After working as a staff and charge nurse in medical-surgical nursing, she became an instructor in Staff Development at the University of Maryland Medical Center. She then received her BSN from the University of Maryland School of Nursing. For 5 years she taught in several schools of nursing while working toward her MS in Nursing, which she received in 1981. Ms. Ignatavicius then taught in the BSN program at the University of Maryland for 6 years, after which she continued to pursue her interest in gerontology and accepted the position of Director of Nursing of a major skilled-nursing facility in her home state of Maryland. She has been a certified gerontologic nurse since 1989 and was certified in nursing case management by the American Nurses Credentialing Center in 1998. Recently she has taught in both diploma and associate degree nursing programs. Through her consulting and seminar business, Ms. Ignatavicius has gained national recognition in nursing education and critical thinking. She is currently the President of DI Associates, Inc. (http://www.diassociates.com/), a company dedicated to improving health care through education and consultation for both faculty and clinicians.

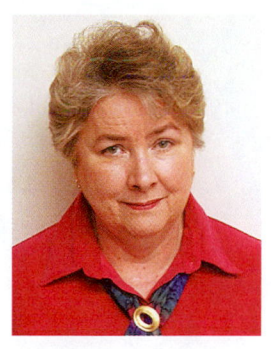

M. Linda Workman received her BSN from the University of Cincinnati College of Nursing and Health. After serving in the U.S. Army Nurse Corps and working as an Assistant Head Nurse and Head Nurse in civilian hospitals, Dr. Workman, a native of Canada, earned her MSN from the University of Cincinnati College of Nursing and Health and a PhD in Developmental Biology from the University of Cincinnati College of Arts and Sciences. Dr. Workman's 25 years of academic experience include teaching at the diploma, associate degree, baccalaureate, and master's levels. Her areas of teaching expertise include medical-surgical nursing, physiology, pathophysiology, genetics, oncology, and immunology. Dr. Workman has been recognized nationally for her teaching expertise and was inducted into the American Academy of Nursing in 1992. She received the Excellence in Teaching award at the University of Cincinnati in 2001 and at Case Western Reserve University in 2004. She is a former American Cancer Society Professor of Oncology Nursing and currently is senior faculty at the Frances Payne Bolton School of Nursing, Case Western Reserve University, where she occupies an endowed chair in oncology.

Consultants

ELAINE BISHOP KENNEDY, EdD, RN
Professor, Department of Nursing
Wor-Wic Community College
Salisbury, Maryland
Concept Maps
Plans of Care

MICHELLE M. BYRNE, PhD, RN, CNOR
Associate Professor
Department of Nursing
North Georgia College
 and State University
Dahlonega, Georgia
Culture consultant

RICHARD LINTNER, RT(R), (CV), (MR), (CT), ARRT
Program Director
School of Interventional Radiology;
 Manager
Interventional Radiology
Kansas University Medical Center
Kansas City, Kansas
Consultant for interventional radiology

Contributors

RICHARD B. ARBOUR, MSN, RN, CCRN, CNRN
Guest Lecturer, Graduate Program
LaSalle University School of Nursing;
Staff Nurse/Clinical Researcher
Albert Einstein Healthcare Network
Philadelphia, Pennsylvania

DEANNE A. BLACH, MSN, RN
Coordinator, CE Programs and Senior Health & Education
University of Arkansas for Medical Sciences
AHEC-NW at Harrison
Harrison, Arkansas

MARCIA M. BOEHMKE, DNS, RN, ANPc
Research Assistant Professor, School of Nursing
University of Buffalo, The State University of New York
Buffalo, New York

MICHELLE M. BYRNE, PhD, RN, CNOR
Associate Professor
Department of Nursing
North Georgia College and State University
Dahlonega, Georgia

LINDA J. CAPUTI, EdD, MSN, RN
Professor, Department of Nursing
College of DuPage
Glen Ellyn, Illinois

JOHN M. CLOCHESY, PhD, RN, FAAN, FCCM
Independence Foundation Professor of Nursing
 Education
Case Western Reserve University
Cleveland, Ohio

TAMMY L. COFFEE, MSN, ACNP
Acute Care Nurse Practitioner
Metro Health Medical Center
Cleveland, Ohio

JANICE CUZZELL, RN, MA, CWS
Certified Wound Specialist
Savannah, Georgia

KARRIE K. DIETZEN, MSN, RN, CGRN
Assistant Professor, Associate's of Science in Nursing
 Program
Ivy Tech State College, East Central Region
Muncie, Indiana;
PRN: Staff RN Medical/Surgical Unit & Endoscopy Lab
Community Hospital-Anderson
Anderson, Indiana

MARY R. HERON EVANS, MS, RN, ONC
Assistant Professor, School of Nursing
Gulf Coast Community College;
Staff, Gulf Coast Medical Center
Panama City, Florida

CHRISTINE A. GATES, BS, CRT
Certified Respiratory Therapist
Cincinnati, Ohio

JACQUELYN R. GIBBS, MSN, RN
Assistant Professor, Department of Nursing
Raymond Walters College, University of Cincinnati
Cincinnati, Ohio

GAYLE K. GILMORE, RN, MA, MIS, CIC
Consultant, Infection Control Education and Consultation
Duluth, Minnesota

LYNN C. HADAWAY, MEd, RNC, CRNI
President, Lynn Hadaway Associates, Inc.
Milner, Georgia

WADE HAGAN, MSN, RN, PHN, CCRN
Instructor, Nursing Department
Mt. San Jacinto Community College District
Menifee, California;
Faculty Associate
California State University
Dominguez Hills, California

KATHY A. HAUSMAN, PhD, RN, C
Assistant Professor, School of Nursing
University of Maryland
Baltimore, Maryland

MARY K. KAZANOWSKI, PhD, ARNP, CHPN, BC
Professor, Department of Nursing
Saint Anselm College;
Level III RN
VNA Hospice
Manchester, New Hampshire

ELAINE BISHOP KENNEDY, EdD, RN
Professor, Department of Nursing
Wor-Wic Community College
Salisbury, Maryland

LINDA A. LaCHARITY, PhD, RN
Assistant Professor, College of Nursing
University of Cincinnati
Cincinnati, Ohio

LINDA LASKOWSKI-JONES, RN, MS, APRN, BC, CCRN, CEN
Director, Trauma, Emergency & Aeromedical Services
Christiana Care Health System—Christiana Hospital
Newark, Delaware

RUTH LINDQUIST, PhD, RN, APRN, BC
Professor, School of Nursing;
Senior Associate Dean for Academic Affairs
   and Administration
University of Minnesota
Minneapolis, Minnesota

DEITRA LEONARD LOWDERMILK, PhD, BSN, RNC, MEd
Clinical Professor, Women's Health, School of Nursing
University of North Carolina at Chapel Hill
Chapel Hill, North Carolina

JUDY MALKIEWICZ, PhD, RN
Professor, School of Nursing
University of Northern Colorado
Greeley, Colorado

JANICE HOOT MARTIN, PhD, RN, GNP
Professor Emeritus, School of Nursing
University of Northern Colorado
Greeley, Colorado

CYNTHIA KINDLER MATZKO, MSN, RN, APRN, BC
Master's Prepared Advanced Practice Nurse;
Rheumatology Clinical Nursing Specialist
Geisinger Medical Center
Danville, Pennsylvania

LORA McGUIRE, RN, MS
Professor, Department of Nursing
Joliet Junior College
Joliet, Illinois

M. ELAINE McLEOD, MSN, APRN, BC-ADM, APRN-BC, CDE
Clinical Nurse Specialist, Diabetes
Tennessee Valley Healthcare System
Nashville, Tennessee

MADELINE B. MURPHY, MSN, NP-C
Coordinator, Adult NP Program
Breen School of Nursing
Ursuline College;
Clinical Faculty, Department of Medicine
University Hospitals of Cleveland
Cleveland, Ohio

CATHY A. MURRAY, MSN, RN, CNS, ONC
Assistant Professor, Department of Nursing
Ivy Tech State College—Community College of Indiana;
PRN Staff Nurse Orthopedics
Ball Memorial Hospital
Muncie, Indiana

FRANK EDWARDS MYERS III, MA, CIC, CPHQ
Manager of Clinical Epidemiology and Safety Systems
Scripps Mercy Hospital/Scripps Health
San Diego, California

KAREN NOVAK, MSN, RN, OCN, ACNP
Nurse Practitioner
Northwestern Medical Faculty Foundation
Chicago, Illinois

REBECCA M. PATTON, MSN, RN, CNOR
Director of Perioperative Services
EMH Regional Healthcare System
Elyria, Ohio

TOMMIE WRIGHT PNIEWSKI, MSN, RN, CNAA
Associate Professor, Department of Nursing
Hopkinsville Community College;
Education Coordinator of Special Projects
Christian Health Center/Christian Church Homes
   of Kentucky
Hopkinsville, Kentucky

SUZANNE K. POWELL, BSN, RN, MBA, CCM, CPHQ
Editor-in-Chief
*Lippincott's Case Management: The Journal for Professional
   Practice*
Lippincott, Williams & Wilkins
Philadelphia, Pennsylvania;
Director, Acute Care Quality Improvement Program
Health Services Advisory Group
Phoenix, Arizona

ANGELA SAMMARCO, PhD, RN
Assistant Professor, Department of Nursing
College of Staten Island, City University of New York
Staten Island, New York

JAMES G. SAMPSON, ND, MSN, ANP-C
Assistant Professor, Adjunct
University of Colorado School of Nursing;
Adult Nurse Practitioner
Denver Health Medical Center
Denver, Colorado

MARIAH SNYDER, PhD, FAAN
Professor Emeritus, School of Nursing
University of Minnesota
Minneapolis, Minnesota

KAREN L. TOULSON, BSN, RN, CEN
Nurse Manager, Emergency Department
Christiana Care Health Systems
Newark, Delaware

SHIRLEY E. VAN ZANDT, MS, MPH, CRNP
Instructor, School of Nursing
Johns Hopkins University
Baltimore, Maryland

CONSTANCE VISOVSKY, PhD, RN, ACNP
Assistant Professor, Frances Payne Bolton School
   of Nursing
Case Western Reserve University;
Nurse Practitioner, Ireland Cancer Center
University Hospitals of Cleveland
Cleveland, Ohio

CHRIS WINKELMAN, PhD, RN, CNP, CCRN
Assistant Professor, Frances Payne Bolton School
   of Nursing
Case Western Reserve University;
Staff Nurse, Trauma and Critical Care
MetroHealth Medical Center
Cleveland, Ohio

PAMELA C. ZICKAFOOSE, EdD, MSN, RN, CAN, BC
Instructor, Department of Nursing
Delaware Technical & Community College;
Educator
Bayhealth Medical Center
Dover, Delaware

Reviewers

JOAN P. ANDERSON, MA, RN, MALS
Suffolk County Community College
Selden, New York

MICHELE AUGUST-BRADY, DNSC, RN
Moravian College
Bethlehem, Pennsylvania

GAYLE A. BERO, MSN, RN, FNP, NCC
St. Joseph's Hospital Health Center
St. Joseph's College of Nursing
Syracuse, New York

SANDRA BRANNAN, MSN, RN
Lamar University
Beaumont, Texas

MICHELE BUNNING, MSN, RN
Good Samaritan College of Nursing and Health Science
Cincinnati, Ohio

PAMELA R. CANGELOSI, PhD, RN
George Mason University
College of Nursing and Health Science
Fairfax, Virginia

BARBARA CELIA, EdD, RN
Drexel University
College of Nursing and Health Professions
Philadelphia, Pennsylvania

CATHERINE M. CONCERT, MS, RN, APRN, BC, FNP, CGRN
Wyckoff Heights Medical Center;
Long Island University
Brooklyn, New York

PATSY ELAINE CRIHFIELD, MSN, RN, CCRN, APRN, BC, NP-C
Dyersburg State Community College
Dyersburg, Tennessee

DORIS DENISON, MSN, RN, NP, ACNP
Wayne State University
College of Nursing
Detroit, Michigan

CLAIRE P. DONAGHY, PhD, RN, APN C, CCRN, ACNP
County College of Morris
Randolph, New Jersey;
St. Clare's Health Services;
Morris Anesthesia Group
Denville, New Jersey

SHEILA A. DUNN, MSN, RN, C-ANP
St. Louis VA Medical Center
Belleville, Illinois;
St. Louis University
St. Louis, Missouri

JAYNE EDMAN, MSN, RN
Brookdale Community College
Lincroft, New Jersey

ANN E. FRONCZEK, MSN, RN, NP
Binghamton University
Decker School of Nursing
Binghamton, New York

DAVID GOEDE, MS, RN, APRN, BC
Monroe Community College;
University of Rochester
Strong Memorial Hospital
Rochester, New York

SHARRON E. GUILLETT, PhD, RN
Marymount University
Arlington, VA

ANNETTE GUNDERMAN, EdD, MSN, RN
Bloomsburg University
Bloomsburg, Pennsylvania

SUZY HARRINGTON, MS, RN, CHES
Central Colorado Area Health Education Center
Denver, Colorado

CONNIE S. HEFLIN, MSN, RN
West Kentucky Community and Technical College
Paducah, Kentucky

SARAH M. HOWELL, MSN, RN
Mississippi University for Women
Columbus, Mississippi

SUSAN J. LAMANNA, MA, MSN, RN, ANP
Onondaga Community College
Syracuse, New York

SUSAN B. LEIGHT, EdD, RNCO, CRNP
West Virginia Wesleyan College
Buckhannon, West Virginia

CAROL T. LEMAY, RN
University of Massachusetts, Amherst
Amherst, Massachusetts

JANIE LIPPS, MSN, APRN C, CDE
Vanderbilt University Medical Center
Nashville, Tennessee

JAYNE HANSCHE LOBERT, MS, RN, CS, NP
Oakland Community College
Waterford, Michigan

MARGARET A. LYNCH, MSN, FNP
The Cambridge Hospital
Cambridge, Massachusetts

CYNTHIA GLAWE MAILLOUX, PhD, RN
Pennsylvania State University, Worthington Scranton
Dunmore, Pennsylvania

DOROTHY MATHERS, MSN, RN
Pennsylvania College of Technology
Williamsport, Pennsylvania

ELIZABETH J. MILLER, MSN, MPH, APRN-BC, ABD
John Dingell Detroit VA Medical Center
Detroit, Michigan

IRIS L. MULLINS, PhD, RN
Radford University
School of Nursing
Radford, Virginia

MARIO R. ORTIZ, PhD, RN, FNP
University of Portland
School of Nursing
Portland, Oregon

AMY B. SHARRON, MS, RN, CS, GNP
United Health Care
Evercare
Auburndale, Massachusetts

MARY VIRGINIA SHINDLE, MSN, RNBC, HNC
Shepherd University
Shepherdstown, West Virginia

DARRELL R. SPURLOCK JR., MSN, RN, CCRN, CEN
Mount Carmel College of Nursing
Columbus, Ohio

PATRICIA SWEENEY, MS, APRN, BC
Pennsylvania State University, Worthington Scranton
Dunmore, Pennsylvania;
Emergency Services PC
Scranton, Pennsylvania

SUZANNE E. TATRO, MS, BSN, RN
York Technical College
Rock Hill, South Carolina

JOYCE B. VAZZANO, MSN, RN, CMSRN
John Hopkins University
School of Nursing
Baltimore, Maryland

SHARON HENRY WALICEK, MEd, MSN, RN, CCRN, CCNS, ANP-BC
Elgin Community College;
Elgin Cardiology Associates
Elgin, Illinois

COLEEN WEIL, MSN, RN, C
Wor-Wic Community College
Salisbury, Maryland

JOAN DOMIGAN WENTZ, MSN, RN
Assistant Professor
Jewish Hospital College of Nursing and Allied Health
St. Louis, Missouri

DIANE M. WHEELER, RNCS, ANP
Upper Care Internal Medicine
Falmouth, Massachusetts

CHERYLE I. WHITNEY, MSN, RN, BC
Tomball College
Tomball, Texas

CECILIA ELAINE WILSON, MS, RN, CPN
Texas Woman's University
College of Nursing
Dallas, Texas

RITA E. M. WISE, MSN, RN
Reading Hospital
School of Nursing
West Reading, Pennsylvania

Preface

The first edition of this text, entitled *Medical-Surgical Nursing: A Nursing Process Approach,* received widespread acclaim in the 1990s. The following three editions built on that achievement and further solidified the book's position as a major trendsetter for the practice of adult health nursing. Now in its fifth edition, "Iggy" charts an essential course for the future of adult nursing—a course reflected in its current title: *Medical-Surgical Nursing: Critical Thinking for Collaborative Care.*

This title was carefully chosen to emphasize the importance of developing and enhancing critical thinking skills to help today's nursing students function in interdisciplinary teams in a variety of health care settings, including both acute care and community-based settings.

KEY THEMES FOR THE 5TH EDITION

As in the extraordinarily successful fourth edition, a key theme of this edition—reflected in the book's subtitle—is critical thinking. To help achieve that emphasis on critical thinking, case-based Critical Thinking Challenges are interspersed throughout the text. These exercises provide a safe and effective means of practicing the on-the-spot decision making that students will face in the fast-paced world of medical-surgical nursing. Suggested answer guidelines for these Critical Thinking Challenges are provided on the text's Evolve website.

In addition to this key theme of critical thinking, the fifth edition also emphasizes "readiness"—readiness for the NCLEX® Examination, readiness for major emergencies such as we saw in the aftermath of the events of 9/11, readiness for safe drug administration, and readiness for the new world of genetics that is unfolding before us.

As the nursing shortage becomes more acute, it is more critical than ever that students be ready to pass the licensure exam on the first try. To help both students and faculty in reaching that goal, the fifth edition includes an innovative end-of-chapter feature called "Get Ready for the NCLEX Examination!" These unique learning aids consist of a list of Key Points *organized by NCLEX Client Needs Category* as found in the NCLEX test plan. Also included in these "Get Ready for the NCLEX Examination!" sections are highlighted reminders to go to the Student CD-ROM for "Review Questions for the NCLEX Examination" and to the Evolve website for "Integrated Management of Care Questions for the NCLEX Examination." The Review Questions for the NCLEX Examination (found on the Student CD-ROM) are keyed to the Learning Outcomes at the start of each chapter—one question per Learning Outcome. The "Integrated Management of Care Questions for the NCLEX Examination" (on the Evolve website) focus on delegation and supervision, assignment, and prioritization/decision

making. These questions are aimed at stimulating and validating critical thinking to help students understand and apply the material covered in the text and integrate it with material they have learned elsewhere in the curriculum.

To help prepare students for both common medical-surgical emergencies and mass-casualty events such as the terrorist acts and natural disasters that seem to be increasingly in the news, this edition features an entirely new unit—Unit 3 (Concepts of Emergency Nursing)—which consists of two emergency care chapters. Chapter 12 (Emergency and Mass Casualty Nursing) provides an introduction to emergency and mass casualty nursing. At the end of this chapter, the reader is "walked through" a case scenario related to bioterrorism and the response of the emergency health care team. Chapter 13 (Interventions for Clients with Common Environmental Emergencies) describes selected environmental emergencies, such as heatstroke, spider bites, and near-drowning. The first-response/emergency interventions and continuing care are discussed for each emergency.

To promote readiness for safe drug administration, the fifth edition provides Pharmacology Review Questions on the Evolve website. These questions, which are keyed to the text with distinctive "Evolve Pharm Review" icons, give students practice in concepts of safe medication administration—a major theme of the NCLEX Examination.

To promote readiness for the emerging genetic basis of many diseases and disorders, we provide a new chapter, Genetic Concepts for Medical-Surgical Nursing (Chapter 11), as well as Genetic Considerations boxes and "Etiology and Genetic Risk" headings wherever appropriate.

Additional themes carried over from the previous edition are an emphasis on women's health issues, cultural considerations, complementary and alternative therapies, and the special needs of older adults. In addition, concepts of case management and community-based care are interwoven throughout to help the reader understand these growing roles and trends.

CLINICAL CURRENCY AND ACCURACY

To ensure this text's currency and accuracy, we listened to the readers of the previous editions—their impressions of and experiences with the text. Based on this input, we formulated our revision plan. We assembled a team of clinical experts to revise, rewrite and, in some cases, draft entirely new chapters.

We also commissioned in-depth reviews of selected chapters by clinicians and instructors from across the United States and Canada and used their reviews to guide us in revising the chapters into their final form. A nursing expert in cultural issues reviewed the entire fourth edition and made recommendations for how to best present illustrations, research findings, and incidence/prevalence data. For this edition we also enlisted the assistance of an interventional radiologist to ensure the accuracy of selected diagnostic testing procedures and associated client care.

The results are reflected in the fifth edition's strong, consistent focus on critical thinking, collaborative care, pathophysiology, drug therapy, and community-based care; its foundation of relevant research; and its emphasis on the critical "need to know" information that nurses must master in order to provide safe, effective care based on solid scientific evidence. This base of scientific evidence is emphasized throughout the text and is highlighted in our Best Practice charts. In addition, our Evidence-Based Practice for Nursing boxes now designate the *level of evidence* reflected in the reported research as based on a national standard described in Chapter 1.

OUTSTANDING READABILITY

The fifth edition has been carefully revised from cover to cover for improved readability. Today's students need to be able to read information once and understand it; they do not have time to repeatedly re-read the same information. To achieve this level of readability, we took two steps: (1) We revised the text into a direct-address style, wherever appropriate, that speaks directly to the reader; and (2) we kept sentences as short as possible consistent with the complexity of the content.

Reading level is highly influenced by the length of sentences and the length of words. Thus, while we can control the length of the sentences, medical terms are often 4 to 5 syllables long and will tend to skew a chapter's reading level. Nevertheless, the result of our efforts for the fifth edition is a med-surg text of consistently outstanding readability. The average reading level is 10th-11th grade, with a few chapters above and below that threshold.

It is important to note that reducing the reading level of this edition did not reduce the quality or depth of content that students need to know. Instead, the content is clear and focused.

EASE OF ACCESS

To make the text as easy to use as possible, we have maintained the fourth edition's approach of smaller chapters of more uniform length. The fifth edition has 80 chapters.

We also have maintained the fourth edition's unit structure, with vital body systems (cardiovascular, respiratory, and neurologic) appearing earlier in the book. In these three units, we have continued to provide critical care content in separate chapters that discuss managing critically ill clients with coronary artery disease, respiratory problems, and neurologic problems.

To help break up long blocks of text and also to highlight key information, we have included numerous headings, bulleted lists, tables, charts, and in-text highlights. We end each chapter with a Selected Bibliography (with classic sources before 2000 noted with an asterisk [*]). Key Terms are in boldface type and are defined in the text to foster the learning of need-to-know vocabulary.

A COLLABORATIVE APPROACH

As in the previous four editions, we take a collaborative approach to client care. We believe that in the real world of health care, nurses, clients, and other health care providers (including physicians, advanced-practice nurses, and physician's assistants) *share* responsibility for the management of client problems. Thus we present client care in a collaborative management framework. In this framework we make no artificial distinctions between medical treatment and nursing care. Instead, under each Collaborative Management heading we cover the entire range of approaches taken by health care practitioners of all disciplines when dealing with client problems.

New to this edition are 7 additional Concept Maps (for a total of 15) that underscore this collaborative approach. Also known as *clinical correlation maps,* these Concept Maps now begin with a case scenario. They then demonstrate visually how a complex health problem is addressed. Each Concept Map spells out the steps of the nursing process and related concepts to illustrate the relationships among disease processes, medical treatments, nursing interventions, and more. Identifying these relationships not only underscores the collaborative nature of health care but also stimulates critical thinking and fosters learning.

Although our approach is collaborative, the text is first and foremost a *nursing* text. We therefore use a nursing process approach to organize discussions of client health problems and their management. Discussions of key health problems follow a full nursing process format, with the following structure:

[Health problem]
   Pathophysiology
      Etiology and Genetic Risk
      Incidence/Prevalence
   Collaborative Management
      Assessment
      Analysis
         Common Nursing Diagnoses and Collaborative Problems
         Additional Nursing Diagnoses and Collaborative Problems
      Planning and Implementation
         Nursing Diagnosis/Collaborative Problem
            Planning: Expected Outcomes
            Interventions
      Community-Based Care
         Health Teaching
         Home Care Management
         Health Care Resources
      Evaluation: Outcomes

The nursing diagnoses used in this edition are the 2003-2004 NANDA-approved diagnoses—the most recently approved diagnoses at the time of this revision.

Discussions of less common or less complex disorders, although not given this complete subhead structure, nonetheless follow the same basic format: a discussion of the problem itself (including pertinent information on pathophysiology) followed by a section on collaborative care of clients with the disorder. Common nursing diagnoses/collaborative problems are often identified as well.

Integral to this collaborative management approach is a clear delineation of just who is responsible for what. When a responsibility is primarily the nurse's, the text says so. When a decision must be made jointly by the client, nurse, physician, and physical therapist, for example, this is clearly stated. When different health care practitioners in different care settings might be involved in the client's care, this is stated.

To further emphasize the nurse's role, we have integrated pertinent components of the Nursing Interventions Classification (NIC) system and the Nursing Outcomes Classification (NOC) system. These systems were developed by the Center for Nursing Classification to standardize nursing interventions and outcomes and the terminology used to describe them. Where appropriate for health problems that receive full nursing process coverage, NIC interventions are clearly identified with a NIC symbol NIC. Selected activities associated with each identified intervention are listed in NIC Intervention Activities charts.

The expected outcomes for client care in this edition are consistent with the NOC system. However, NOC continues to be developed and refined to ensure that outcomes are evidence-based. We have therefore included NOC outcomes and specified indicators when appropriate, as well as other outcome statements validated empirically by clinical practice. Those statements that are particularly consistent with NOC language are identified with a NOC symbol *NOC*.

ORGANIZATION

The 80 chapters of *Medical-Surgical Nursing: Critical Thinking for Collaborative Care* are grouped into 17 units. Unit 1, Health Promotion and Illness, lays the foundation for the health care concepts incorporated throughout the text. Unit 2 covers important biopsychosocial concepts related to health care, including pain and rehabilitation. Chapter 11 is a new chapter in this unit and introduces the major concepts of genetics and related nursing implications for client care. A new unit, Unit 3, consists of two emergency care chapters as previously described.

Unit 4 consists of six chapters on the management of clients with fluid, electrolyte, and acid-base imbalances. This unit includes an expanded chapter on infusion therapy (Chapter 17) and is supplemented with an online fluid and electrolyte tutorial on the companion Evolve website.

Unit 5 presents the perioperative nursing content that medical-surgical nurses need to know. This content provides a solid foundation to help the student better understand the specific surgeries covered throughout the remainder of the text.

Unit 6 provides core content on health problems related to immune system function. This content includes normal inflammation and the immune response, altered cell growth and cancer development, and interventions for clients with connective tissue disease, HIV infection, and other immunologic disorders, cancers, and infections.

The remaining 11 units cover medical-surgical content by body system. Each of these units begins with an Assessment chapter and continues with one or more Interventions chapters for clients with specific health problems in that body system.

MULTINATIONAL, MULTICULTURAL, MULTIGENERATIONAL FOCUS

To reflect the increasing diversity of our society, *Medical-Surgical Nursing: Critical Thinking for Collaborative Care* takes a multinational, multicultural, and multigenerational focus. Addressing the needs of both U.S. and Canadian readers, we have included examples of trade names of drugs available in the United States and those available in Canada. Drugs that are available only in Canada are designated with a ✱ symbol.

To help nurses provide quality care for clients whose cultural background may differ from their own, numerous Cultural Considerations boxes highlight important aspects of culturally competent care throughout the text. A revised cultural health chapter (Chapter 6) is also included in this edition. Located inside the back cover is an innovative Communication Quick Reference for Spanish-Speaking Clients. This Quick Reference helps ensure clear communication between native English speakers and the rapidly growing population who speak Spanish as a first language.

Increases in life expectancy and the "graying" of the baby-boom generation add up to a steadily increasing older adult population. To help equip nurses for this challenge, the fifth edition continues to feature expanded coverage of the care of older adults. It includes a greater number of Nursing Focus on the Older Adult charts and highlights laboratory values and drug dosages typical for older clients. Charts specifying normal physiologic changes to expect in the older population are included in each Assessment chapter. In addition, Considerations for Older Adults boxes are included throughout the text to emphasize key points to keep in mind when caring for these clients.

Also appearing throughout the text is an increased number of Women's Health Considerations boxes, which address topics of concern to women and their health care providers. These in-text highlights alert the reader to gender-related differences in assessment parameters and in the incidence, severity, and treatment of common health problems.

ADDITIONAL LEARNING RESOURCES

As in previous editions, the fifth edition continues to include a rich array of "andragogic" learning aids—learning aids geared toward adult learners—to help students quickly identify and understand key information and to serve as study aids. Several of these features are new to this edition.

- Written in "client-friendly" language, Client Education Guide charts provide the types of instructions that nurses must learn to provide to clients and their families to help them cope with life changes caused by illness.
- Laboratory Profile charts summarize important information on laboratory tests commonly ordered to evaluate health problems. Information typically includes normal ranges of laboratory values (including differences for older adults, when appropriate) and the possible significance of abnormal findings.
- Drug Therapy charts summarize important information about commonly used drugs. These charts include both U.S. and Canadian trade names for typically used drugs, usual dosages (including dosages for older clients, as

appropriate), and nursing interventions with rationales. In addition, "Med Error Alerts" have been added for this edition where common mistakes could be made in medication administration. Medication errors are a major health problem in health care today, and our goal with this new feature is to help students administer drugs safely.

- Key Features charts highlight the clinical manifestations of important health problems.
- Evidence-Based Practice for Nursing boxes, provided in nearly every chapter, give synopses of recent nursing research articles and other scientific articles applicable to nursing. Each box provides a summary of the article, a brief critique, the level of evidence (new to this edition), and a summary of implications for nursing practice. The goal of this feature is to help students identify the strengths and weaknesses of the research and see how research can help guide nursing practice.
- Nursing care plans remain significant tools with which the nursing student must be familiar. The fifth edition therefore includes selected examples of these care-planning tools. It has been retitled "Plan of Care" and incorporates NIC and NOC language. Nursing Plans of Care continue to include a distinctive icon (**D**) to designate interventions that can be delegated to assistive nursing personnel.
- New to this edition, Home Care Assessment charts serve as a convenient summary of essential assessment points for clients who need follow-up home health nursing care.
- Assessment Using Gordon's Functional Health Patterns charts provide a convenient one-stop list of relevant questions to ask clients regarding the impact of health conditions on everyday function.
- Meeting *Healthy People 2010* Objectives boxes suggest specific activities that nurses can undertake to promote achievement of the specific numbered objectives of the *Healthy People 2010* program.
- Resource Management boxes (formerly "Cost of Care" boxes) provide an important financial/resource context for medical-surgical nurses when managing resources for client care. Nurses must increasingly understand cost and other resource factors in order to help clients work toward wellness.
- Legal/Ethical Issues boxes introduce students to some of the dilemmas they will face in the increasingly high-tech world of medical-surgical nursing.

AN INTEGRATED MULTIMEDIA RESOURCE BASED ON PROVEN LEARNING STRATEGIES

Medical-Surgical Nursing: Critical Thinking for Collaborative Care, 5th edition, is the hub of a comprehensive package of electronic and print publications that break new ground in the application of proven learning strategies and evidence-based educational practice. This integrated multimedia resource actively engages the student in problem solving and critical thinking. Every effort has been made to correlate content among the text and its companion publications. Unlike many textbook authors, we have personally been in-

volved in the development of most of the companion publications to ensure consistency and cohesion between the textbook and the companion publications.

RESOURCES FOR INSTRUCTORS

Resources for instructors include a printed Instructor's Resource Manual, an Instructor's Electronic Resource CD-ROM/DVD, and Evolve Learning Resources for faculty.

The printed Instructor's Resource Manual, written by Susan Behmke and Sharon Souter, along with contributions from four expert authors, continues to serve as a touchstone for new and seasoned faculty alike. The IRM for the 5th edition features a simplified new format as well as four new introductory chapters. The introductory chapters cover evaluation of critical thinking, test construction, incorporation of technology into the classroom, and teaching strategies for students with a variety of learning styles. IRM chapters now correspond directly to textbook chapters and feature Concept Map Case Studies that correspond to the 15 Concept Maps in the text.

The Instructor's Electronic Resource CD-ROM/DVD consists of a Test Bank, Image Collection, Lecture Slides, ready-to-use narrated PowerPoint Lectures, and a Faculty Development Video.

- The Test Bank is a robust 2500-item bank that includes both traditional and NCLEX Examination "alternate" item types, and each question is coded for correct answer, rationale, cognitive type, nursing process step, and NCLEX Client Needs Category. The Test Bank is provided in ExamView, Blackboard, and ParTest formats.
- The expanded Image Collection now consists of 700 images from the text and are delivered in a format that makes incorporation into lectures and presentations easier than ever.
- The Lecture Slides (formerly "LectureView") are a collection of 1200 text slides developed to correspond to each chapter in the text.
- The new, ready-to-use PowerPoint Lectures are narrated lectures by co-author Linda Workman on topics that faculty find particularly challenging.
- The new Faculty Development Video, delivered on DVD-ROM as part of the Instructor's Electronic Resource, is a 60-minute video by Donna Ignatavicius that addresses the implications of changes in the NCLEX Examination for faculty. Excerpted from one of Donna Ignatavicius's popular seminars, this DVD is a unique resource for faculty.

For the convenience of faculty, all of these resources except the Faculty Development Video are also available online on a secure instructor area of the Evolve website entitled Evolve Learning Resources.

RESOURCES FOR STUDENTS

Resources for students include a free Student CD-ROM, a thoroughly revised and updated Critical Thinking Study Guide, a Clinical Companion, a Virtual Clinical Excursions workbook/CD-ROM, and Evolve Learning Resources.

The new Student CD-ROM features Review Questions for the NCLEX Examination—one for each Learning Outcome at the beginning of the chapter. Also included on the

Student CD-ROM are animations and video clips (each keyed to the text by a distinctive "clapboard" icon, as well as a new Audio Glossary. The Audio Glossary includes the definitions of all Key Terms from the text, along with audio files for difficult pronunciations. The Student CD-ROM also includes Audio Clips that allow students to hear key sounds in health assessment.

The *Critical Thinking Study Guide* has been carefully revised and updated under the authorship of Julie S. Snyder for an increased emphasis on critical thinking and rigorous accuracy. The Study Guide features a simplified format and a greater variety of question types. Multiple-choice questions are now written in NCLEX format and emphasize the NCLEX priorities of delegation, management of care, and pharmacology. The use of Case Studies is expanded in this edition, and a new chapter on study tips is included.

The pocket-sized *Clinical Companion,* authored by Kathy A. Hausman, retains the alphabetical organization and streamlined format that made it so popular in previous editions. The new edition is printed in color and in a smaller page size for easier portability, and it includes a quick reference to nursing care after incidents of chemical terrorism and bioterrorism. The *Clinical Companion* is a pocket-sized "Iggy" for students going into clinicals and is written by an author who actively supervises clinicals and who knows firsthand what students in clinicals are being asked to know about their clients.

The *Virtual Clinical Excursions* workbook/CD-ROM package, featuring an updated and easy-to-navigate "virtual" clinical setting, will once again be available for the fifth edition. This unique learning tool guides the student through a virtual clinical environment and helps the student apply textbook content in a "safe" context. The clinical simulations and workbook represent the next generation of research-based learning tools to promote critical thinking and meaningful learning.

Also available for students in a dynamic collection of Evolve Learning Resources, available at http://evolve. elsevier.com/Iggy/. Evolve resources include the following:

- Pharmacology Review Questions (keyed to icons in the textbook)
- Integrated Management of Care Questions for the NCLEX Examination
- Answer Guidelines for Critical Thinking Challenges
- Answer Guidelines for Study Guide Case Studies
- "Building" Concept Maps ("building" versions of the 15 Concept Maps from the text)
- Concept Map Creator (a handy tool for creating customized Concept Maps)
- Fluid & Electrolyte Tutorial (a complete self-paced tutorial on this perennially difficult content)
- WebLinks (a dynamic library of Internet links, updated regularly for currency)
- Content Updates
- Health Assessment Image Collection (supplemental images of common assessment findings)
- The Audio Glossary, Audio Clips, Animations, and Video Clips from the Student CD-ROM.

For more information on any of these innovative companion publications, contact your Elsevier sales representative, visit http://www.us.elsevierhealth.com/, or contact Elsevier Faculty Support at 1-800-222-9570 or sales.inquiry@elsevier.com.

• • •

In summary, *Medical-Surgical Nursing: Critical Thinking for Collaborative Care,* 5th edition, together with its fully integrated multimedia ancillary package, provides the tools you will need to meet the challenge of nursing in the first decade of the 21st century and beyond. The only elements that remain to be added to this package are those that you alone can provide—your diligence, your commitment, your innovation, *your nursing care.*

Donna D. Ignatavicius
M. Linda Workman

Acknowledgments

Publishing a textbook and ancillary package of this depth and breadth would not be possible without the combined efforts of many people. Our contributing authors once again provided consistently excellent manuscripts in a timely fashion. Special thanks to Elaine Kennedy, who developed all of our new case-study-based Concept Maps. Our reviewers—expert clinicians and instructors from around the United States and Canada—provided invaluable suggestions and encouragement throughout the book's development.

The staff of W.B. Saunders/Elsevier once again provided us with crucial guidance and support throughout the planning, writing, revision, and production of the fifth edition. In particular, Executive Publisher Barbara Nelson Cullen and Editor Lee Henderson worked closely with us from the early stages of this edition to help us hone and focus our revision plan, and Lee oversaw the project from start to finish. Developmental Editor Laura Sieh Chu and Managing Editor Robin Richman then worked with us step-by-step to bring the fifth edition from vision to publication. Maureen Iannuzzi held the reins of our complex ancillary package and worked with a gifted group of writers and content experts to provide an outstanding library of resources to complement and enhance the text. Special thanks to Senior Editor's Assistant Marie Thomas, who handled the countless administrative details associated with a project of this size. She is without peer among editorial assistants.

Senior Project Manager Jodi Willard was once again a joy to work with. If, as is said, the mark of a good copy editor is that her work is invisible to the reader, then Jodi is the consummate copy editor. Her unwavering attention to detail, flexibility, and conscientiousness not only helped to make this edition the most consistently readable ever, but also made the entire production process incredibly smooth and headache-free.

Special thanks also to Publishing Services Manager Debbie Vogel. For two editions now, Debbie has worked quietly behind the scenes to help bring the book to publication precisely on schedule and with a very high level of quality.

Designer Teresa McBryan is responsible for the beautiful cover and interior design of the fifth edition. The praise of a book designer's work is often unsung, but Teresa's work on this edition has cast important features in exactly the right light, with neither too much nor too little emphasis, making this edition not only practical and easy to read, but beautiful.

Our acknowledgments would not be complete without recognizing Karen McKie, Bob Boehringer, Jo Beth Griffin, our dedicated team of sales representatives, and other key members of the Sales and Marketing staff who helped to put this book into your hands.

Finally, we wish to thank Executive Vice President, Nursing and Health Professions, Sally Schrefer. Sally's personal leadership style continues to create a unique publishing environment in which authors and editors have the freedom to interact creatively to produce the best books in the field.

Donna D. Ignatavicius
M. Linda Workman

Contents

UNIT TWO

BIOPSYCHOSOCIAL CONCEPTS RELATED to HEALTH CARE

UNIT **THREE**

CONCEPTS of EMERGENCY NURSING

CHAPTER **12**

Emergency and Mass Casualty Nursing, 156

LINDA LASKOWSKI-JONES • KAREN L. TOULSON

CHAPTER **13**

Interventions for Clients with Common Environmental Emergencies, 173

LINDA LASKOWSKI-JONES

UNIT FOUR

MANAGEMENT of CLIENTS with FLUID, ELECTROLYTE, and ACID-BASE IMBALANCES

UNIT SEVEN

PROBLEMS of OXYGENATION

Management of Clients with Problems of the Respiratory Tract

UNIT EIGHT

PROBLEMS of CARDIAC OUTPUT and TISSUE PERFUSION

Management of Clients with Problems of the Cardiovascular System

UNIT NINE

PROBLEMS of TISSUE PERFUSION
Management of Clients with Problems of the Hematologic System

UNIT TEN

PROBLEMS of MOBILITY, SENSATION, and COGNITION
Management of Clients with Problems of the Nervous System

UNIT ELEVEN

PROBLEMS of SENSATION
Management of Clients with Problems of the Sensory System

UNIT THIRTEEN

PROBLEMS of DIGESTION, NUTRITION, and ELIMINATION

Management of Clients with Problems of the Gastrointestinal System

UNIT FOURTEEN

PROBLEMS of REGULATION and METABOLISM

Management of Clients with Problems of the Endocrine System

UNIT FIFTEEN

PROBLEMS of PROTECTION

Management of Clients with Problems of the Skin, Hair, and Nails

UNIT SIXTEEN

PROBLEMS of EXCRETION

Management of Clients with Problems of the Renal/Urinary System

UNIT SEVENTEEN

PROBLEMS of REPRODUCTION

Management of Clients with Problems of the Reproductive System

Guide to Special Features

BEST PRACTICE for EMERGENCY CARE

CLIENT EDUCATION GUIDE

CONCEPT MAPS

DRUG THERAPY

EVIDENCE-BASED PRACTICE for Nursing

FOCUSED ASSESSMENT

HOME CARE ASSESSMENT

KEY FEATURES

LABORATORY PROFILE

LEGAL/ETHICAL ISSUES

Meeting HEALTHY PEOPLE 2010 Objectives

NIC INTERVENTION ACTIVITIES

NURSING FOCUS on the OLDER ADULT

PLAN of CARE

RESOURCE MANAGEMENT

Reference Guide for Student CD-ROM

The Student CD-ROM provided with this text contains the following features: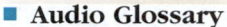

- Review Questions for the NCLEX Examination
- Health Assessment Audio Clips
- Health Assessment Images
- Audio Glossary
- Health Assessment Video Clips
- Animations

 Look for this multimedia icon in the margins of the text. This icon highlights related animations and health assessment video clips on your Student CD-ROM.

HEALTH ASSESSMENT AUDIO CLIPS

UNIT SIX MANAGEMENT OF CLIENTS WITH PROBLEMS OF THE IMMUNE RESPONSE
CHAPTER 26

Stridor

UNIT SEVEN MANAGEMENT OF CLIENTS WITH PROBLEMS OF THE RESPIRATORY TRACT
CHAPTER 30

Bronchial breath sounds
Bronchovesicular breath sounds
Vesicular breath sounds
High-pitched crackles
Low-pitched crackles
High-pitched wheeze
Low-pitched wheeze
Pleural friction rub

UNIT EIGHT MANAGEMENT OF CLIENTS WITH PROBLEMS OF THE CARDIOVASCULAR SYSTEM
CHAPTER 36

Single S1
S1 at various locations
Single S2
S2 at various locations
The fourth heart sound (S4)
The third heart sound (S3)
Murmurs: High, medium, and low
Murmurs: Blowing, harsh or rough, and rumble
Systolic murmur
Diastolic murmur
Pericardial friction rub

HEALTH ASSESSMENT VIDEO CLIPS

UNIT SEVEN MANAGEMENT OF CLIENTS WITH PROBLEMS OF THE RESPIRATORY TRACT
CHAPTER 30

Inspection: Nose (adult female)
Inspection and palpation: Breathing and respiratory excursion, anterior chest (adult male)
Inspection and palpation: Respirations, respiratory excursion, and tactile fremitus, posterior chest (adult male)
Palpation: Tactile fremitus, posterior chest (adult female)
Inspection and percussion: Diaphragmatic excursion (adult male)
Percussion: Anterior thorax (adult male)

UNIT EIGHT MANAGEMENT OF CLIENTS WITH PROBLEMS OF THE CARDIOVASCULAR SYSTEM
CHAPTER 36

Inspection and palpation: Cardiac, anterior chest (adult female)
Inspection and palpation: Cardiac, auscultatory landmarks (adult male)
Auscultation: Cardiac, with diaphragm (adult male)
Auscultation: Cardiac, with bell (adult male)
Auscultation: Cardiac, with diaphragm and bell (adult female)
Auscultation: Carotid artery (adult male)
Inspection and palpation: Pulses, lower extremities (adult female)

UNIT TEN MANAGEMENT OF CLIENTS WITH PROBLEMS OF THE NERVOUS SYSTEM
CHAPTER 44

Evaluation: Smell, cranial nerve I—olfactory nerve (adult male)
Evaluation: Central vision and visual acuity, cranial nerve II—optic nerve (adult male)
Evaluation: Pupil responses, direct and accommodation, cranial nerves III, IV, and VI—oculomotor, trochlear, and abducens nerves (adult male)
Evaluation: Sensory, light touch; face, upper, and lower extremities, cranial nerve V—trigeminal nerve (older adult female)
Inspection: Fine motor coordination, upper extremities (older adult male)
Inspection: Fine motor coordination, lower extremities (older adult female)
Evaluation: Sensory, face, and upper extremities
Evaluation: Deep tendon reflex, patellar tendon (adult male)

UNIT ELEVEN MANAGEMENT OF CLIENTS WITH PROBLEMS OF THE SENSORY SYSTEM
CHAPTER 49

Inspection and palpation: External eye (adult male)
Evaluation: Central vision and visual acuity (adult male)
Evaluation: Pupil responses, direct and consensual (older adult female)

CHAPTER 51

Inspection and palpation: External ear (older adult male)
Inspection: Ear canal (adult male)

PROBLEMS of MOBILITY, SENSATION, and COGNITION

*Management of Clients
with Problems of the
Nervous System*

Assessment of the Nervous System

KATHY A. HAUSMAN

LEARNING OUTCOMES

After studying this chapter, you should be able to:

1. Compare the functions of the major divisions of the nervous system.
2. Describe the mechanisms of nerve impulse transmission.
3. Identify the structure and function of different areas of the central and peripheral nervous system.
4. Identify common physiologic changes associated with aging that affect the nervous system.
5. Perform a neurologic history.
6. Perform a comprehensive neurologic physical assessment.
7. Perform a rapid neurologic assessment and interpret findings.
8. Interpret results of cerebrospinal fluid analysis.
9. Plan and implement pretest and follow-up care for clients undergoing common neurologic diagnostic tests.

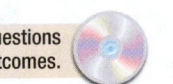

Go to your Student CD-ROM for Review Questions for the NCLEX Examination keyed to these Learning Outcomes.

The nervous system is the center of thinking, memory, judgment, sensation, movement, cognition, communication, behavior, and personality. In addition to its direct control over many processes, the nervous system innervates many other body systems and thus indirectly influences their functions. For example, damage to the spinal nerves that innervate the diaphragm may result in respiratory arrest.

Refer to current anatomy, physiology, pathophysiology, and assessment books for complete information about the nervous system and neurologic assessment. A brief review is presented in this chapter.

ANATOMY AND PHYSIOLOGY REVIEW

The major divisions of the nervous system are the central nervous system (CNS) and the peripheral nervous system (PNS).

The brain and spinal cord are the major components of the CNS. The PNS is composed of 12 pairs of cranial nerves, 31 pairs of spinal nerves, and the autonomic nervous system. The autonomic nervous system is further subdivided into sympathetic and parasympathetic fibers.

The nervous system contains two types of cells: neurons, which transmit or conduct nerve impulses, and neuroglial cells, which have an interdependent role with the neuron.

Nervous System Cells

NEURONS

Structure

The basic unit of the nervous system, the neuron, transmits impulses. Some neurons are **motor** (facilitating movement), and some are **sensory** (facilitating sensation). Some process information, and some retain information. When a neuron receives an impulse from another neuron, the effect may be excitation or inhibition as well as conduction of the impulse. Each neuron has a cell body, or soma; short, branching processes called a dendrite; and a single axon (Figure 44-1).

Dendrites may have many branches or few. Each dendrite synapses with another cell body, axon, or dendrite and brings information to the cell body from other neurons. The dendritic process is described as an afferent pathway. The axonal process, called the efferent pathway, transmits impulses from its cell body to other neurons. Although only one axon extends from each neuron, it may extend long distances.

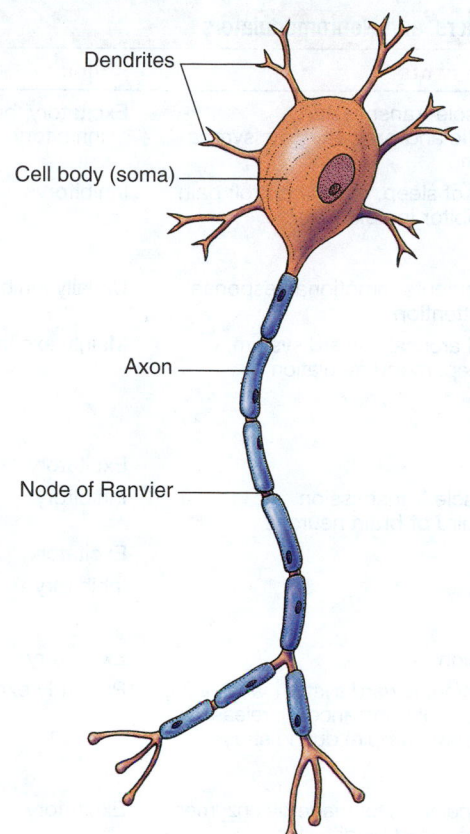

Figure 44-1 ■ The structure of a typical neuron.

Labels: Dendrites, Cell body (soma), Axon, Node of Ranvier

Many (but not all) axons are covered by a myelin sheath, a white, lipid covering. Myelinated axons appear whitish and therefore are also called white matter. Nonmyelinated axons have a grayish cast and are called gray matter. Myelinated axons have gaps in the myelin called nodes of Ranvier. The nodes of Ranvier play a major role in impulse conduction (see Figure 44-1). The enlarged, distal end of each axon is called the synaptic, or terminal, knob. Within the synaptic knobs are the mechanisms for manufacturing, storing, and releasing a transmitter substance. Each neuron produces a specific transmitter substance (e.g., acetylcholine or serotonin) that is capable of either enhancing or inhibiting the impulse, but not both.

Mechanism for Nerve Impulse Conduction

Sodium (Na$^+$) and chloride (Cl$^-$) ions are heavily concentrated in the area outside of the cell (interstitial space). Potassium ions (K$^+$) and other organic material are present within the cell (intracellular space). The inside of the cell is negatively charged compared with the interstitial space. Because of the different concentration of Na$^+$ and K$^+$, a neuron is constantly charged, even at rest.

When a stimulus is strong enough, the permeability of the cell membrane to Na$^+$ and K$^+$ is changed, and **depolarization** (impulse conduction) begins. Certain proteins within the membrane function as gates, or channels, that open for either sodium or potassium. With depolarization, sodium diffuses through the membrane first. It is believed that calcium plays a part in controlling the amount of

sodium that diffuses through the membrane by controlling the gates. After sodium has entered the cell, potassium begins to leave the cell. Sodium is actively pumped out of the cell, and **repolarization** (return to baseline) occurs in preparation for another impulse. As an action potential or impulse occurs at one point on the cell membrane, the impulse excites adjacent cells so the impulse is conducted all along the nerve fiber membrane. If the impulse is not of sufficient strength, there will be no action potential.

Synapses

Impulses are transmitted to their eventual destination through **synapses**. There are two distinct types of synapses: *neuron to neuron* and *neuron to muscle* (or gland). Between the terminal knob and the next cell is a small space called the synaptic cleft. The knob, the cleft, and the portion of the cell to which the impulse is being transmitted constitute the synapse.

Factors Affecting Transmission

Several factors affect the transmission of an impulse. Distance is one of the established factors. Synapses on or near the body of the cell have greater influence than those farther along the dendrite. The strength of the stimulus can also be influenced by other mechanisms, such as inhibition by another neuron, inadequate supply of transmitter substance, and extracellular fluid (ECF) changes. Lack of oxygen or the effects of hypnotics and anesthetics can quickly depress nerve cell activity.

Changes in the pH of ECF also affect neuron transmission. For example, acidosis depresses nerve cell activity. Alkalosis, on the other hand, excites nerve cells. Increased nerve cell activity occurs with the use of some drugs, such as caffeine (in coffee), theophylline (in tea and asthma drugs), and theobromine (in cocoa).

Neurotransmitters

Neurotransmitters are chemical substances that enhance or inhibit nerve impulses. Other substances, although not specifically identified as transmitters, are considered probable transmitters. Table 44-1 summarizes what is currently known about them.

NEUROGLIAL CELLS

Neuroglial cells, which vary in size and shape, provide protection, structure, and nutrition for the neurons. There are 5 to 10 times more neuroglial cells than neurons in the central nervous system (CNS), and they account for 40% of the CNS cell mass. Neuroglial cells are classified into four types: astroglial cells, ependymal cells, oligodendrocytes, and microglial cells. Microglial cells play a scavenger role by responding to infection in or trauma to the CNS. Astroglial (star-shaped) cells provide the physical support for the neurons, regulate the chemical environment, and nourish the neurons. Oligodendrocytes form myelin sheaths around the axons. Ependymal cells form the lining of ventricles and the central canal of the spinal cord. They are also part of the blood-brain barrier and help regulate the composition of cerebrospinal fluid (CSF).

Central Nervous System

The central nervous system (CNS) is composed of the brain, which directs the regulation and function of the nervous system and all other systems of the body, and the spinal

TABLE 44-1 Sites, Functions, and Actions of Transmitters, Probable Transmitters, and Neuromodulators

Transmitter Substance	Site	Function/Comments	Action
Acetylcholine	Brain, brainstem, basal ganglia, autonomic nervous system	Nerve and muscle transmission Parasympathetic and preganglionic sympathetic system	Excitatory, but some inhibitory
Serotonin	Medial brainstem, hypothalamus, dorsal horn of spinal cord	Possible onset of sleep, mood control; pain pathway inhibitor in spinal cord	Inhibitory
Catecholamines			
Dopamine	Substantia nigra to basal ganglia	Complex movements, emotional response regulation, attention	Usually inhibitory
Norepinephrine (epinephrine parallels)	Hypothalamus, brainstem, reticular formation, cerebellum, sympathetic nervous system	Maintenance of arousal, reward system, dreaming sleep, mood regulation	Mainly excitatory
Amino Acids			
Aspartate	Brain, spinal cord interneurons	Sensation	Excitatory
Gamma-aminobutyric acid (GABA)	Brain, brainstem, basal ganglia, autonomic nervous system	Nerve and muscle transmission Possibly one third of brain neurons	Inhibitory
Glutamate	Sensory pathways	Sensation	Excitatory
Glycine	Spinal cord interneurons	Muscle control	Inhibitory
Peptides*			
Substance P	Brain, neurons in spinal cord	Pain transmission	Excitatory
Endorphins, enkephalins	Thalamus, hypothalamus, spinal cord, pituitary	Pleasure sensation, reward system, analgesia, (inhibits release of substance P), released with ACTH (corticotropin) during stress	Probably excitatory
Gases			
Nitric acid	Neurons	Not stored in specific site; made by enzymes as needed; released by diffusion	Excitatory
Carbon monoxide	Neurons	Function not well understood	Questionable

*Other peptides under investigation as probable transmitters are vasopressin (ADH), gastrin, cholecystokinin, glucagon, insulin, somatostatin, angiotensin, melanocyte-stimulating hormone (MSH), luteinizing hormone–releasing hormone (LH-RH), and thyrotropin-releasing hormone (TRH). Prostaglandins, also under investigation, are thought to be modulators.

cord, which initiates reflex activity and transmits impulses to and from the brain.

BONE

The brain and spinal cord are encased in the cranium and vertebral column, respectively. For the most part, they are well protected. However, there are some areas of vulnerability, such as the nasal sinuses, the palate of the throat, the ears, and the cervical spine. The upright position of humans creates additional strain on the vertebrae and musculature. Although there are some differences in structure, all of the vertebrae protect the spinal cord and give structure to the body.

BRAIN
Meninges

The **meninges** form the immediate protective covering of the brain and the spinal cord:

Situated between the arachnoid and pia mater is the subarachnoid space, where CSF circulates. The subdural space is located between the inner dura and the arachnoid. A *potential* space, referred to as the epidural space, is located between the skull and the outer layer of the dura. This area also extends down the spinal cord and is important in the delivery of epidural analgesia.

Between the two layers of dura are the venous sinuses. The inner layer of dura dips down between the two hemispheres and is called the falx. The dura also lies between the cerebral hemispheres and the cerebellum and is called the tentorium. The falx and the tentorium decrease or prevent the transmission of force from one hemisphere to another and protect the lower brainstem. Clinical references may be made to a lesion (e.g., a tumor) as being **supratentorial** (above the tentorium) or **infratentorial** (below the tentorium).

Cerebrum

The right and left hemispheres of the cerebrum are joined by the corpus callosum. The *left* hemisphere is the dominant hemisphere in most people (even in many left-handed people). Within the deeper structures of the cerebrum are the right and left lateral ventricles. At the base of the cerebrum near the ventricles is a group of neurons called the basal ganglia that regulate movement and body tone.

The motor cortex, located anterior to the central fissure of Rolando of the cerebrum, controls voluntary movement. Corticospinal tracts, also called pyramidal tracts, begin in the motor cortex and travel through the internal capsule and diencephalons and cross at the decussation of the pyramids in the medulla. Nerve fibers continue to the target muscle to initiate movement on each side of the body. The crossing of the fibers in the medulla (decussation of the pyramids) is responsible for the contralateral control of motor movement. In the motor cortex, the motor homunculus is the spatial arrangement of motor nuclei controlling voluntary muscles of the body. The cerebrum is divided into

Animation: Functional Brain Areas

TABLE 44-2   Brain Lobe Functions

Frontal Lobe
- The primary motor area (also known as the motor "strip" or cortex)
- Broca's speech center on the dominant side
- Voluntary eye movement
- Access to current sensory data
- Access to past information or experience
- Affective response to a situation
- Regulates behavior based on judgment and foresight
- Judgment
- Ability to develop long-term goals
- Reasoning, concentration, abstraction

Parietal Lobe
- Understand sensation, texture, size, shape, and spatial relationships
- Three-dimensional (spatial) perception
- Important for singing, playing musical instruments, and processing nonverbal visual experiences
- Perception of body parts and body position awareness
- Taste impulses for interpretation

Temporal Lobe
- Auditory center for sound interpretation
- Complicated memory patterns
- Wernicke's area for speech

Occipital Lobe
- Primary visual center

Limbic Lobe
- Emotional and visceral patterns connected with survival
- Learning and memory

TABLE 44-3   Diencephalon Functions

Thalamus
- All sensation except smell
- Sensation perceived at the thalamic level is crude and cannot be localized or quantified

Hypothalamus
- Regulates water metabolism, appetite, sleep-wake cycle, temperature control, and thirst
- Hormonal activity
- Posterior pituitary hormones, such as vasopressin and oxytocin
- Anterior pituitary hormone excretion
- Growth, thyrotropin, and follicle-stimulating hormones; prolactin and corticotropin
- Regulates emotions and controls basic drive for self-preservation

Epithalamus
- Often calcified by young adulthood and is radiopaque
- Used as a point of reference on an x-ray film or a computed tomography scan

Subthalamus
- Contains sensory tracts
- Connections to basal ganglia

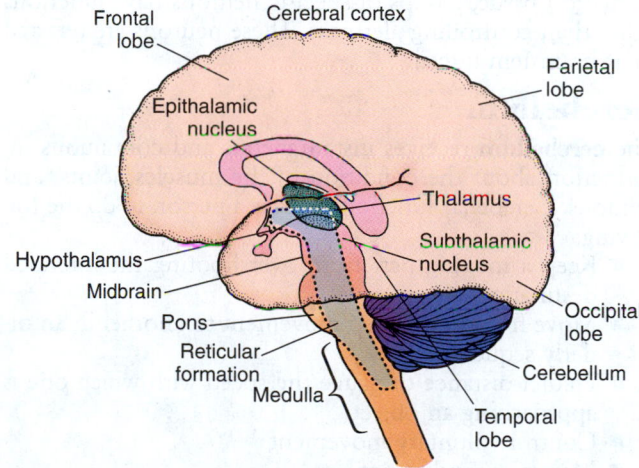

Figure 44-2 ■ The structures of the brainstem and diencephalons.

lobes by sulci (fissures). Except for the limbic lobes, these are given the same name as the overlying bone. The name and function of each lobe is listed in Table 44-2.

Two important speech areas of the cerebrum are Broca's area and Wernicke's area. **Broca's area**, located in the frontal lobe, is composed of neurons responsible for the formation of words, or speech. This requires respiratory activation of the vocal cords, which must occur at the same time as tongue and mouth movements. This association area, **Wernicke's area**, is located in the temporal lobe and plays a significant role in higher-level brain function. It enables processing of words into coherent thought and recognition of the idea behind written or printed words (language).

The general interpretive area, which is located where the temporal, parietal, and occipital lobes meet at the junction of the lateral fissure, enables a person to process complex thoughts, remember the notes of music, recite a speech heard or read long ago, recall childhood experiences, and so forth. Damage to this area on the dominant side after 5 years of age is catastrophic.

Diencephalon

The diencephalon, which lies below the cerebrum, includes the thalamus, hypothalamus, and epithalamus (Figure 44-2).

The **thalamus** is the major "relay station," or "central switchboard," for the CNS. The **hypothalamus** is an integral part of the autonomic nervous system control (controlling temperature and other functions), and plays an essential role in intellectual function. The epithalamus contains the roof of the third ventricle and the pineal gland. See Table 44-3 for additional information concerning the diencephalon.

Hypophysis (Pituitary Gland)

The **hypophysis (pituitary gland)** is situated in the sella turcica of the ethmoid bone and is connected to the hypothalamus by tissue called the hypophyseal stalk. It has two lobes, each releasing specific hormones into the circulation under the regulation of the hypothalamus. The pituitary is often referred to as the "master gland" because of its control of numerous hormonal functions.

Brainstem

The brainstem (see Figure 44-2) includes the midbrain, pons, and medulla. The functions of these structures are presented in Table 44-4.

Throughout the brainstem are special cells that constitute the **reticular activating system (RAS)**, which controls awareness and alertness. For example, this tissue awakens a person from sleep when presented with a noxious stimuli,

---

TABLE 44-4 Brainstem Structure Functions

Medulla
- Cardiac-slowing center
- Respiratory center
- Cranial nerves IX (glossopharyngeal), X (vagus), XI (accessory), and XII (hypoglossal) emerge from the medulla, as do portions of cranial nerves VII (facial) and VIII (acoustic)

Pons
- Cardiac acceleration and vasoconstriction centers
- Pneumotaxic center helps control respiratory pattern and rate
- Four cranial nerves originate from the pons: V (trigeminal), VI (abducens), VII (facial), and VIII (acoustic)

Midbrain
- Contains the cerebral aqueduct or aqueduct of Sylvius
- Location of periaqueductal gray, which may abolish pain when stimulated
- Cranial nerve nuclei III (oculomotor) and IV (trochlear) located here

---

when there is pain, or when it is time to rise. Many sensory fibers branch and terminate here. The reticular formation area has abundant connections with the cerebrum, the rest of the brainstem, and the cerebellum. Within the reticular formation tissue, groups of specific neurons have functions other than controlling alertness. These neurons are referred to as brainstem nuclei.

Cerebellum

The **cerebellum** receives instantaneous and continuous information about the condition of the muscles, joints, and tendons. Cerebellar function enables a person to do the following:

- Keep a moving part from overshooting the intended destination
- Move from one skilled movement to another in an orderly sequence
- Predict distance or gauge the speed with which one is approaching an object
- Control voluntary movement
- Maintain equilibrium

Cerebellar control of the body is **ipsilateral** (situated on the same side). The right side of the cerebellum controls the right side of the body, and the left cerebellum controls the left side of the body.

Cerebral Circulation

Circulation in the brain originates from the carotid and vertebral arteries (Figure 44-3). The internal carotid arteries branch into the anterior cerebral artery (ACA) and middle cerebral arteries (MCA). The two posterior vertebral arteries become the basilar artery, which then divides into two posterior cerebral arteries. The anterior, middle, and posterior cerebral arteries are joined together by small communicating arteries to form a ring at the base of the brain known as the **circle of Willis.**

The circle of Willis is located at about the level of the pons, or the general level of the upper nose and lower border of the eye. The middle cerebral artery supplies the lateral surface of the cerebrum from about the mid-temporal lobe upward (i.e., the area for hearing and upper body motor and sensory neurons). The anterior cerebral artery supplies the midline, or medial, aspect of the same area (i.e., the

lower body motor and sensory neurons). The posterior cerebral arteries supply the area from the mid-temporal region down and posteriorly (occipital lobe), as well as much of the brainstem.

Venous drainage occurs through the cerebral veins into the dural sinuses, which are large venous reservoirs between the inner and outer dura mater. From the dural sinuses, the blood drains into the jugular vein and then into the superior vena cava. Because cerebral veins have no valves, intracranial pressure (ICP) can be affected by central venous pressure (CVP).

Two sinuses are of particular importance: the superior sagittal sinus (SSS) and the cavernous sinus. The superior sagittal sinus receives cerebrospinal fluid (CSF) after it circulates through the ventricular system. The cavernous sinus is located near the eye and receives venous blood from the eye. In addition, the carotid artery passes through the cavernous sinus (the only place in the body where an artery passes through a vein); thus the potential exists for development of a fistula between an artery and a vein (usually from trauma).

Blood-Brain Barrier

The **blood-brain barrier (BBB)** seems to exist because the endothelial cells of the cerebral capillaries (along with ependymal cells) are joined tightly together. This keeps some substances in the plasma out of the cerebrospinal circulation and out of brain tissue. Substances that can pass through the blood-brain barrier include oxygen, glucose, carbon dioxide, alcohol, anesthetics, and water. Large molecules such as albumin, any substance bound to albumin, and many antibiotics are prevented from crossing the blood-brain barrier.

Cerebrospinal Fluid Circulation

Cerebrospinal fluid (CSF) surrounds and cushions the brain and spinal cord. While circulating through the subarachnoid space, the fluid is continuously produced by the choroid plexus, reabsorbed by the arachnoid villi, and then channeled into the superior sagittal sinus (Figure 44-4). Expanded areas of subarachnoid space, where there are large amounts of CSF, are called *cisterns.* The largest cistern is the lumbar cistern, the site of lumbar puncture, from the level of the second lumbar vertebra to the second sacral vertebra (L2-S2).

SPINAL CORD

The spinal cord controls body movement; regulates visceral function; processes sensory information from the extremities, trunk, and many internal organs; and transmits information to and from the brain. It contains H-shaped **gray matter** (neuron cell bodies) that is surrounded by **white matter** (myelinated axons). The white matter is divided into posterior, lateral, and anterior columns. Groups of cells in the white matter (ascending and descending tracts) have been fairly well identified (Figure 44-5). The gray matter divisions are posterior, intermediolateral, and anterior.

Ascending Tracts

As a general rule, **ascending tracts** originate in the spinal cord and end in the brain. Three ascending tracts are important for understanding the client with neurologic problems: spinothalamic tracts, spinocerebellar tracts, and fasciculi gracilis and cuneatus (posterior white columns).

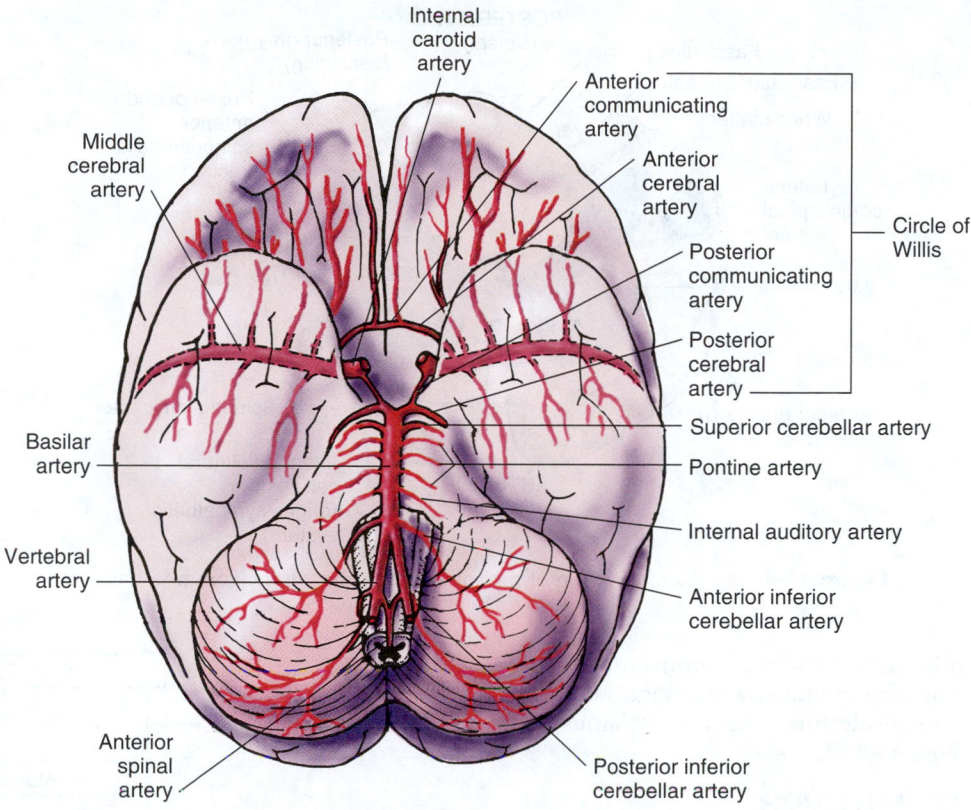

Figure 44-3 ■ Cerebral circulation and the circle of Willis at the base of the brain.

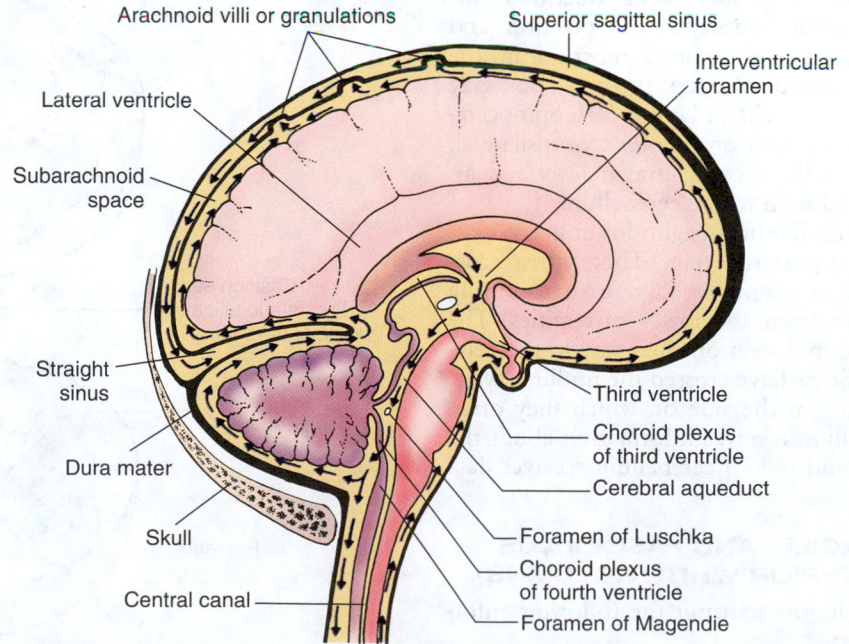

Figure 44-4 ■ Circulation of cerebrospinal fluid. Note that the fluid also extends down into the spinal column.

SPINOTHALAMIC TRACTS

As the name indicates, spinothalamic tracts begin in the spinal cord and end primarily in the thalamus. These tracts carry sensations of pain, temperature, light touch, and pressure. The axon fibers from the cells decussate (cross) the anterior white and gray commissures to the opposite side and become the contralateral (situated on the opposite side) spinothalamic tract. These fibers continue up to the thalamus. Some branches terminate in the reticular formation of the medulla and pons.

A pain or temperature impulse enters the posterior horn on the same side on which the sensation occurs. It

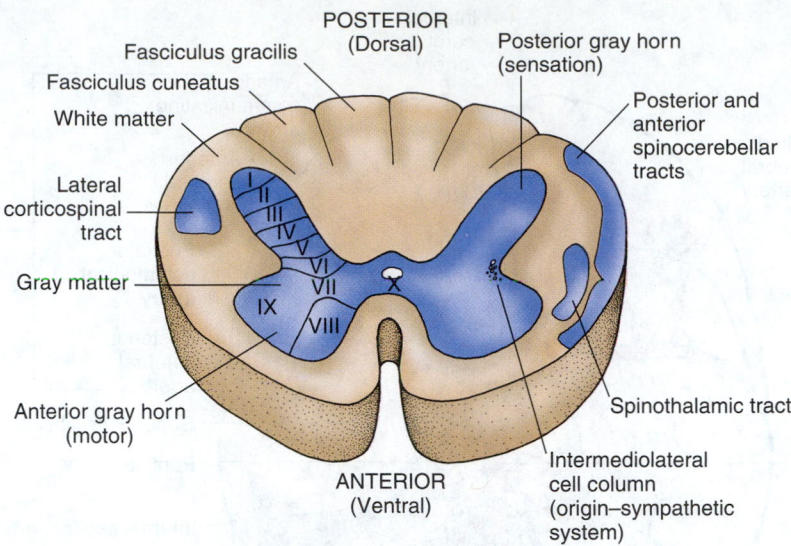

Figure 44-5 ■ A cross section of the spinal cord showing the common tracts.

is transmitted to other cells in several laminae, is further propelled to the opposite spinothalamic tract, and continues up to its ultimate destinations—the thalamus and the parietal lobe (Figure 44-6).

POSTERIOR AND ANTERIOR SPINOCEREBELLAR TRACTS

Spinocerebellar tracts begin in the spinal cord and end in the cerebellum. The *posterior* spinocerebellar tract transmits impulses of proprioception (awareness of position and movements of body parts) or kinesthesia, mostly from the lower extremities. The impulses enter the posterior gray horn and synapse with tract cells in lamina VII. Spinocerebellar axons then form the tract on the *same,* or ipsilateral, side. This tract begins at the second lumbar level and ascends to the medulla and then to the cerebellum.

The *anterior* spinocerebellar tract begins lower in the lumbar spine than does the posterior tract. These fibers cross immediately and ascend as a contralateral tract, transmitting proprioceptive impulses from the lower extremities. The fibers cross again in the midbrain on their way to the cerebellum. Because these fibers have crossed the midline twice, the sensations terminate on the side on which they originated. The *right* cerebellum receives information about the *right* side of the body, and the *left* cerebellum receives data about the *left* side.

FASCICULUS GRACILIS AND FASCICULUS CUNEATUS (POSTERIOR WHITE COLUMNS)

The posterior white columns transmit the following information to the thalamus:

- The sensation of proprioception from muscles, joints, and tendons
- Vibratory sense
- Light touch from the skin
- Discrete localization
- Two-point discrimination

Most of the fibers ascend on the *same* side as their origin to the medulla, where they cross and then synapse in the thalamus, with termination in the parietal lobe. This tract en-

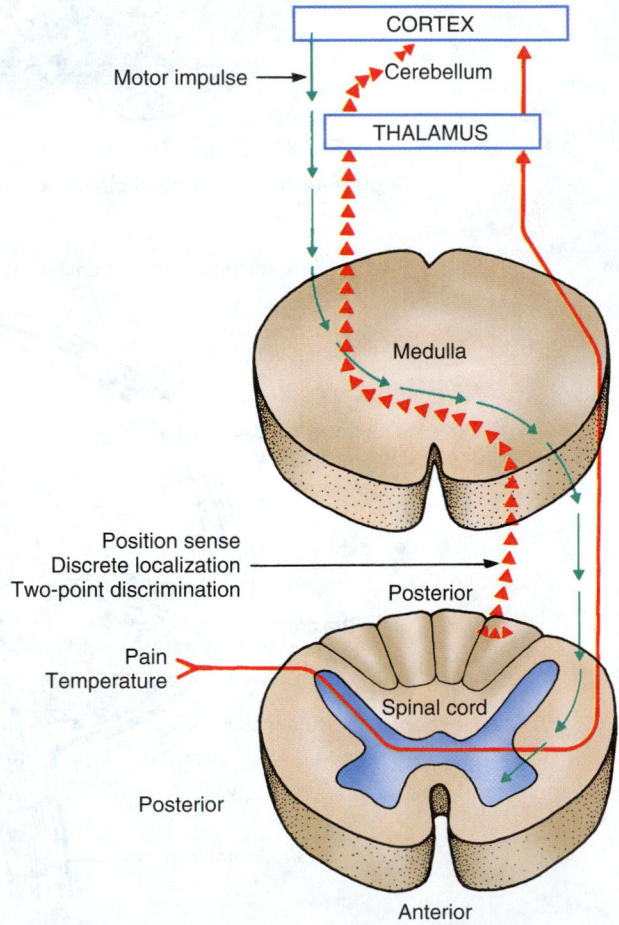

Figure 44-6 ■ Examples of common spinal tract pathways.

ables identification of the exact point of pressure on the skin. Recognition of pressure includes the shape of an object (with eyes closed), movement across the skin (a number being written), and acknowledgment of two points of touch close together.

Descending Tracts

Descending tracts *begin* in the brain and *end* in the spinal cord. The major descending tract of importance for understanding neurologic problems is the lateral corticospinal, or pyramidal, tract. The corticospinal tract originates in the motor cortex of the frontal lobe and portions of the parietal lobe. The lateral tract fibers cross to the opposite side at the level of the medulla. After crossing, the fibers descend to a predetermined level and synapse with interneurons of the gray matter. A few fibers connect directly with lower motor neurons (LMNs). The cervical area has a high concentration of fibers synapsing with interneurons, which possibly reflects the complexity of hand and finger movements.

The motor neurons of the other descending tracts and the basal ganglia used to be referred to as an extrapyramidal system. It was thought that pyramidal neurons initiated voluntary muscle activity and that extrapyramidal neurons initiated automatic or nonvoluntary muscle action. The descending tracts and the basal ganglia are necessary for the smooth function of all motor activity. The term *extrapyramidal* is still often used clinically to connote the origin of abnormal spontaneous movement.

Spinal Cord Circulation

The blood supply for the spinal cord comes from three main arteries. The anterior spinal artery originates from a branch of the vertebral arteries. The two posterior spinal arteries originate from either the vertebral or posterior inferior cerebellar artery. Additional circulation is supplied by branches of the descending aorta.

Peripheral Nervous System

The peripheral nervous system (PNS) is composed of the spinal nerves, cranial nerves, and autonomic nervous system.

SPINAL NERVES

There are 31 pairs of spinal nerves (8 cervical, 12 thoracic, 5 lumbar, 5 sacral, and 1 coccygeal) exiting from the spinal cord. Each of the nerves has a posterior and an anterior branch. The posterior branch carries sensory information to the cord (**afferent pathway**). The anterior branch transmits motor impulses to the muscles of the body (**efferent pathway**).

Each spinal nerve is responsible for the muscle innervation and sensory reception of a given area of the body. The cervical and thoracic spinal nerves are relatively close to their areas of responsibility, whereas the lumbar and sacral spinal nerves are some distance from theirs. Because the spinal cord ends between L1 and L2, the axons of the lumbar and sacral cord extend downward before exiting the appropriate intervertebral foramen. The area controlled by each spinal nerve is roughly reflected in the dermatomes. **Dermatomes** represent sensory input from spinal nerves to specific areas of the skin (Figure 44-7). For example, the client with an injury to cervical spinal nerve root C6 and C7 exhibits sensory changes in the thumb, index finger, middle finger, middle of the palm, and back of the hand.

SENSORY RECEPTORS

Sensory receptors throughout the body monitor and transmit impulses of pain, temperature, touch, vibration, pressure, visceral sensation, and proprioception. Sensory receptors also monitor and transmit the sensations of the special senses—vision, taste, smell, and hearing.

LOWER MOTOR NEURONS AND PLEXUSES

The cell bodies of the anterior spinal nerves are located in the anterior gray matter (anterior horn) of each level in the spinal cord. The anterior motor neurons are also referred to as lower motor neurons. As each nerve axon leaves the spinal cord, it joins other spinal nerves to form **plexuses** (clusters of nerves). Plexuses continue as trunks, divisions, and cords and finally branch into individual peripheral nerves.

The major plexuses are cervical, brachial, lumbar, and sacral. The latter two plexuses are also referred to as lumbosacral. An awareness of the location of the plexuses is helpful because a major concentration of nerves is present. In addition, the nerves of each plexus pass through or are surrounded by bone. Injury to the area or entrapment of a nerve by bone can cause multiple problems.

REFLEXES

Reflexes consist of sensory input from the following (Figure 44-8):
- The muscles, tendons, skin, organs, and special senses
- Small cells in the spinal cord lying between the posterior and anterior gray matter (interneurons)
- The anterior motor neurons, along with the muscles they innervate

Sensory data from a specific peripheral location account for a change in the motor impulses going to that location. This closed circuit, which requires no mediation in the cerebral cortex, is called the reflex arc.

Muscle tone is achieved by special fibers in the middle of the muscle. These special fibers, called muscle spindles or intrafusal fibers, are attached to the surrounding muscle and are able to contract only at their ends. The contractible ends are innervated by special motor fibers from the anterior horn. The middle portion of the intrafusal fibers contains special receptors that measure the degree of stretch of the muscle.

CRANIAL NERVES

There are 12 cranial nerves. The name, number, origin, type, and function of the cranial nerves are summarized in Table 44-5.

Autonomic Nervous System

The **autonomic nervous system (ANS)** is composed of two parts: the sympathetic nervous system (SNS) and the parasympathetic nervous system (PNS). Through the use of biofeedback and other mechanisms, some ANS functions can be brought under conscious control.

SYMPATHETIC NERVOUS SYSTEM

The cells of origin for the SNS are located in the gray matter of the spinal cord from T1 and through L2 or L3. This part of the ANS is considered *thoracolumbar* because of its anatomic location.

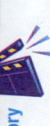
Animation: Sensory Pathways

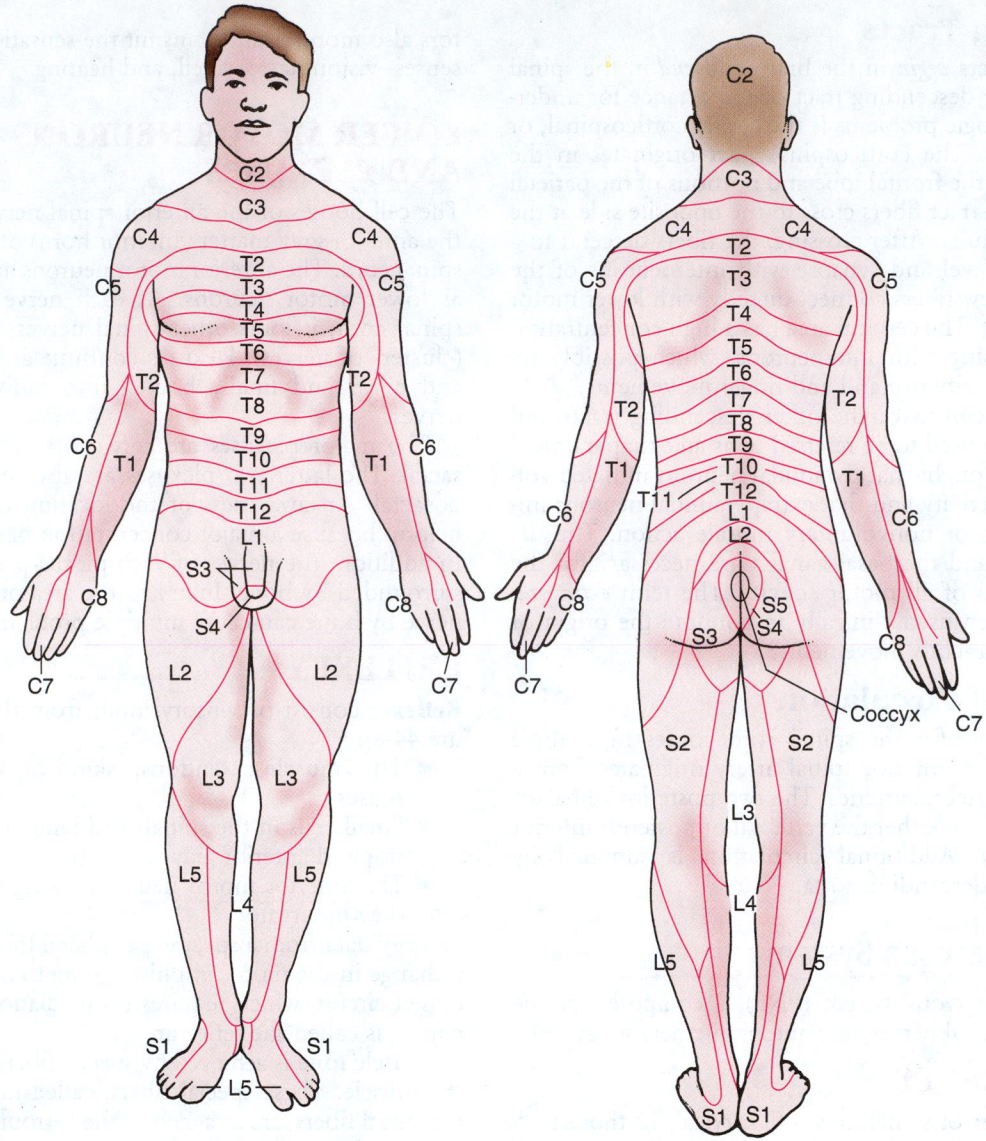

Figure 44-7 ■ Dermatomes (cutaneous innervation of spinal nerves)

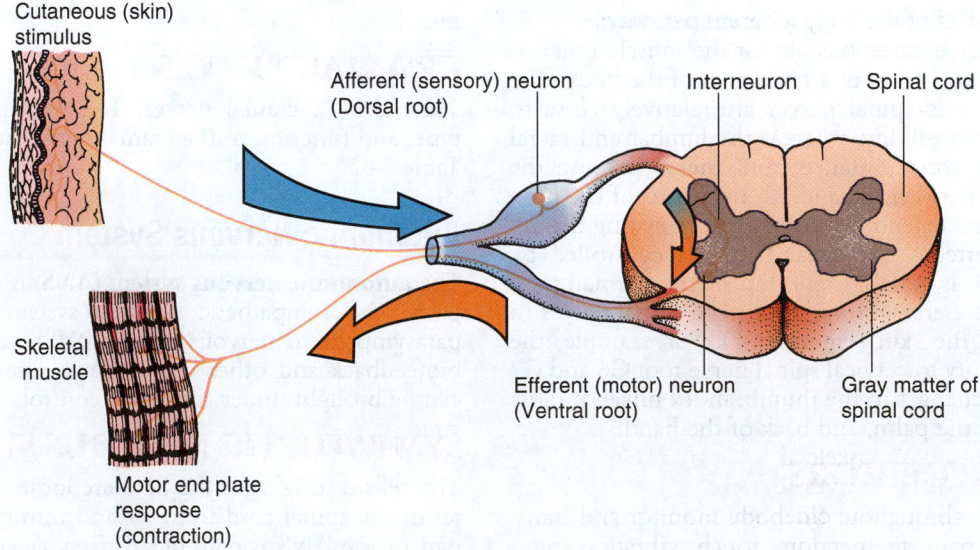

Figure 44-8 ■ An example of reflex activity. Stimulation of skin results in involuntary muscle contraction (reflex arc).

TABLE 44-5 Origins, Types, and Functions of the Cranial Nerves

Cranial Nerve	Origin	Type	Function
I: Olfactory	Olfactory bulb	Sensory	Smell
II: Optic	Midbrain	Sensory	Vision
III: Oculomotor	Midbrain	Motor to eye muscles	Eye movement via medial and lateral rectus and inferior oblique and superior rectus muscles; lid elevation via the levator muscle
		Parasympathetic-motor	Pupil constriction; ciliary muscles
IV: Trochlear	Lower midbrain	Motor	Eye movement via superior oblique muscles
V: Trigeminal	Pons	Sensory	Sensation from skin of face and scalp and mucous membranes of mouth and nose
		Motor	Muscles of mastication (chewing)
VI: Abducens	Inferior pons	Motor	Eye movement via lateral rectus muscles
VII: Facial	Inferior pons	Sensory	Pain and temperature from ear area; deep sensations from the face; taste from anterior two thirds of the tongue
		Motor	Muscles of the face and scalp
		Parasympathetic-motor	Lacrimal, submandibular, and sublingual salivary glands
VIII: Vestibulocochlear	Pons-medulla junction	Sensory	Hearing Equilibrium
IX: Glossopharyngeal	Medulla	Sensory	Pain and temperature from ear; taste and sensations from posterior one third of tongue and pharynx
		Motor	Skeletal muscles of the throat
		Parasympathetic-motor	Parotid glands
X: Vagus	Medulla	Sensory	Pain and temperature from ear; sensations from pharynx, larynx, thoracic and abdominal viscera
		Motor	Muscles of the soft palate, larynx, and pharynx
		Parasympathetic-motor	Thoracic and abdominal viscera; cells of secretory glands; cardiac and smooth muscle innervation to the level of the splenic flexure
XI: Accessory	Medulla (anterior gray horn of the cervical spine)	Motor	Skeletal muscles of the pharynx and larynx and sternocleidomastoid and trapezius muscles
XII: Hypoglossal	Medulla	Motor	Skeletal muscles of the tongue

PARASYMPATHETIC NERVOUS SYSTEM

The cells of origin for the PNS are located in the gray matter of the sacral area of the spinal cord (from S2 to S4) plus portions of cranial nerves III, VII, IX, and X (*craniosacral*). The PNS conserves the body's resources.

Parasympathetic fibers to the viscera have some sensory ability in addition to motor function. Sensations of irritation, stretching of an organ, or a decrease in tissue oxygen are transmitted to the thalamus through pathways not yet fully understood. Because pain from internal organs is often felt below the body wall innervated by the spinal nerve, it is presumed that there are connections between the viscera and body structure that relay pain sensations. Table 44-6 compares the action of sympathetic and parasympathetic systems in the body.

Neurologic Changes Associated with Aging

MOTOR/SENSORY ABILITY

Motor changes in late adulthood are interrelated with sensory function and musculoskeletal status (Chart 44-1). Any problems that affect the nerves, bones, muscles, or joints also affect motor ability. The older adult may have tremors without rigidity, and deep tendon reflexes may be hypoactive. Balance and coordination may be impaired as a result.

Sensory changes in older adults can affect their daily activities. Pupils decrease in size, which restricts the amount of light entering the eye. The pupils also adapt more slowly. Touch sensation decreases, which may precipitate falls because the older person may not feel pebbles or small objects underfoot. Vibration sense may be lost in the ankles and feet. (See also the discussion on fall prevention in Chapter 5.) Hearing also decreases, especially for high-pitched sounds (**presbycusis**).

MENTAL STATUS

Intellect does not decline as a result of aging; however, a person with certain pathologic conditions may experience a decrease in intellectual level caused by drug interactions or an insufficient oxygen supply to the brain. Some older adults may need more time than a younger person to process questions, learn new information, solve problems, or complete analogies.

Subtle memory changes are typical for many older people. Long-term memory seems better than recall (recent) or immediate (registration) memory. Older adults may need more time to retrieve information. These changes may be partly due to the loss of cerebral neurons, which is associated with the aging process.

Insomnia, anxiety, and depression in late adulthood may cause some changes in mental status. Circadian rhythm disorders may lead to wakefulness until later at night, with

TABLE 44-6 Effects of the Autonomic Nervous System on Various Organs of the Body

Organ	Effect of Sympathetic Stimulation	Effect of Parasympathetic Stimulation
Eye		
Pupil	Dilated	Constricted
Ciliary muscle	Slight relaxation	Constricted
Glands	Vasoconstriction and slight secretion	Stimulation of copious (except pancreas) secretion (containing many enzymes for enzyme-secreting glands)
Nasal		
Lacrimal		
Parotid		
Submandibular		
Gastric		
Pancreatic		
Sweat glands	Copious sweating (cholinergic)	Sweating of the palms of the hands
Apocrine glands	Thick, odoriferous secretion	None
Heart		
Muscle	Increased rate Increased force of contraction	Slowed rate Decreased force of contraction
Coronary arteries	Dilated (beta$_2$); constricted (alpha)	Dilated
Lungs		
Bronchi	Dilated	Constricted
Blood vessels	Mildly constricted	? Dilated
Gut		
Lumen	Decreased peristalsis and tone	Increased peristalsis and tone
Sphincter	Increased tone (most times)	Relaxed (most times)
Liver	Glucose released	Slight glycogen synthesis
Gallbladder and bile ducts	Relaxed	Contracted
Kidney	Decreased output and renin secretion	None
Bladder		
Detrusor	Relaxed (slight)	Excited
Trigone	Contracted	Relaxed
Penis	Ejaculation	Erection
Systemic arterioles		
Abdominal	Constricted	None
Muscle	Constricted (alpha-adrenergic) Dilated (beta$_2$-adrenergic) Dilated (cholinergic)	None
Skin	Constricted	None
Blood		
Coagulation	Increased	None
Glucose	Increased	None
Lipids	Increased	None
Basal metabolism	Increased up to 100%	None
Adrenal medullary secretion	Increased	None
Mental activity	Increased	None
Piloerector muscles	Contracted	None
Skeletal muscle	Increased glycogenolysis Increased strength	None
Fat cells	Lipolysis	None

From Guyton, A.C. (1991). *Textbook of medical physiology* (8th ed.). Philadelphia: W.B. Saunders.

extended sleeping in the morning (a pattern opposite that of most health care facility routines). Many older adults require less sleep than do their younger counterparts.

Mental status may also be compromised as the result of infection. Many times this change in mental status is a key early sign of an infectious process in the older client.

ASSESSMENT TECHNIQUES

History

The neurologic history and assessment begin the moment the nurse first meets the client. During the introduction, note the client's appearance and assess his or her speech, affect, and motor function. If the client appears to have cognitive deficits or has trouble speaking or hearing, ask a family member or significant other to stay during the history taking to help secure accurate information. Charts 44-2 and 44-3 elaborate on the information that should be obtained from the client or family.

FAMILY HISTORY AND GENETIC RISK

Ask the client questions about family history such as a history of stroke or heart attack. Ethnic and cultural background may influence the development of a neurologic disorder. For example, it has been long established that Huntington disease is

CHART 44-1

NURSING FOCUS on the OLDER ADULT
Changes in the Nervous System Related to Aging

Physiologic Changes	Nursing Implications	Rationales
Recent memory loss	Reinforce teaching by repetition and written teaching aids.	Intellect is not impaired, but the learning process is slowed. Repetition helps the client learn new information and recall it when needed.
Decreased touch sensation	Remind the client to look where his or her feet are placed when walking. Instruct the client to wear shoes that provide good support when walking. If the client is unable, change his or her position frequently (every hour) while he or she is in bed or the chair.	Decreased sensation may cause the client to fall.
Change in perception of pain	Ask the client to describe the nature and specific characteristics of pain. Monitor additional assessment variables to detect possible health problems.	Accurate and complete nursing assessment ensures that the interventions will be appropriate for the older adult (see Chapter 7).
Change in sleep patterns	Ascertain sleep patterns and preferences. Adjust the client's daily schedule to his or her sleep pattern and preference as much as possible (e.g., evening versus morning bath).	Most older adults require less sleep than do younger adults. However, frequent rest periods are needed.
Altered balance and/or decreased coordination	Instruct the client to move slowly when changing positions. If needed, advise the client to hold on to handrails when ambulating. Assess the need for an ambulatory aid, such as a cane.	The client may fall if moving too quickly. Assistive and adaptive aids provide support and prevent falls.

inherited. With the advent of the Human Genome Project and intensive research, several other neurologic diseases have been found to have a genetic basis, and the list is expanding. Neuromuscular disorders, movement disorders, migraine headaches, and epilepsy have been determined to be caused by inherited mutations of ion channels (Kullman & Hanna, 2002). Other disorders related to genetic factors include Alzheimer's disease and multiple sclerosis. Neurofilament mutations have now been associated with Parkinson disease and amyotrophic lateral sclerosis (Al-Chalabi & Miller, 2003).

PERSONAL HISTORY

Questions about the client's medical history and dietary history are necessary for any bearing they might have on the present problem. Questions about the client's level of activities of daily living (ADLs) may highlight subtle changes in neurologic function. Knowing the level of daily activity also helps establish a baseline for later comparison with changes resulting from improving or worsening neurologic function. Ask whether the client is right-handed or left-handed. This information is important for several reasons:

- The client may be somewhat stronger on the dominant side, which is expected.
- The effects of cerebral injury or disease are more pronounced if the dominant hemisphere is involved.

CURRENT HEALTH PROBLEMS AND SOCIAL HISTORY

Obtain information from the client as outlined in Charts 44-2 and 44-3.

CHART 44-2

BEST PRACTICE for
Establishing a Nursing Database: History

Demographic Data
Age
Gender

Past Medical History
Client's medical history
Family's medical history
Previous injuries or congenital problems
Chronic diseases
- Hypertension
- Diabetes mellitus
- Lung disease
Previous neurologic problems
- Headaches
- Seizures
- Head or spine trauma
- Eye problems

Current History
Current symptoms
- Blurred vision
- Headache
- Speech or swallowing difficulty
- Numbness, tingling
- Weakness, clumsiness
- Bowel or bladder difficulties
- Nausea or vomiting
- Personality seizures

Allergies
- Food
- Medications
- Environment
Pain tolerance
- Medications taken for pain
- Behaviors to reduce pain
Medications
- Prescribed
- Illicit
- Over-the-counter
Activities of daily living

Social History
Usual recreational activities
Level of physical activity each day
Hobbies
Alcohol consumption and use of recreational drugs
Smoking, use of any tobacco products
Sleep habits
- Changes in pattern, duration, or intensity
Work history
- Exposure to toxic agents
Ethnic and cultural background
Handedness (right or left)
Educational background

CHART 44-3

Neurologic Assessment
USING GORDON'S FUNCTIONAL HEALTH PATTERNS

Health Perception–Health Management Pattern
- How would you describe your general health?
- Has your health changed significantly over the past few weeks or months?
- Have you had to miss any work because of changes in your health?

Cognitive-Perceptual Pattern
- Have you noticed any changes in your vision? Hearing? Memory?
- Do you feel you are having any difficulty in making decisions? In learning?
- Are you experiencing any discomfort? Pain? Weakness?

Activity-Exercise Pattern
- Do you have enough energy for your activities?
- What is your perceived ability for the following (code for level according to key below):

Feeding?	Level 0: Full self-care
Bathing?	Level I: Requires use of equipment
Toileting?	or device
Bed mobility?	Level II: Requires assistance or
Dressing?	supervision of another person
Grooming?	Level III: Requires assistance or
General mobility?	supervision of another person
Cooking?	and equipment or device
Home maintenance?	Level IV: Is dependent and does
Shopping?	not participate

Based on Gordon, M. (2002). *Manual of nursing diagnosis* (10th ed.). St. Louis: Mosby.

Physical Assessment

Perform a focused assessment based on the client's presenting symptoms or diagnosis. The establishment of baseline data is important. Make comparisons with each assessment (e.g., to findings 5 minutes or an hour earlier, to the client's baseline, between the right and left sides, between upper and lower extremities, and to the expected progression for the client). Much of the assessment can be performed with the client sitting or lying down. Two types of neurologic assessments may be performed—a complete assessment and a "rapid" assessment. The method chosen depends upon the information needed, the time available with your client, and your skill level. Advanced practice nurses (APNs) and other health care providers usually perform the complete assessment, although parts of it can be done by any health care professional. It is important that you understand each component of the assessment and what the results might indicate. The complete assessment is described first.

ASSESSMENT OF MENTAL STATUS

While collecting the history data, make observations about the client's mental status, speech, and behavior as noted in Chart 44-4. An organized head-to-toe physical assessment begins with the mental status. It is better to start with this part of the assessment, especially when neurologic problems have been noted. For example, if the client is confused, you need to differentiate the cause of the confusion. It may be related to hypoxia rather than the immediate neurologic problem. In older adults, acute confusion may be indicative of a urinary tract infection or other health problem.

CHART 44-4

BEST PRACTICE for
Assessment of Mental Status

- Are the client's answers appropriate?
- Is the client's behavior and facial expression appropriate?
- Is the speech pattern of normal tone, rate, rhythm, and volume?
- Are the answers complete?
- Is the client's appearance neat or untidy; appropriate for age and weather conditions?
- Is the client cooperative, euphoric, hostile, anxious, withdrawn, or guarded?
- Is the client experiencing hallucinations or delusions?
- Is the client's posture and hygiene appropriate for the situation?

Level of Consciousness and Orientation

Determine **level of consciousness (LOC)** by observing the client's level of responsiveness to the environment. *A change in LOC is the **first** indication that central neurologic function has declined!* The client who is **alert** is awake and responsive. Clients who are less than alert are labeled lethargic, stuporous, or comatose. To better identify the client's level of cognitive function or exact state of consciousness, describe behavior in response to stimulation. Ask the client questions that indicate **orientation** to *person, place,* and *time.* Varying the sequence of questioning on repeated assessments prevents the client from memorizing the answers. During the history taking, responses that indicate orientation to person, place, and time include the following:

- The client's ability to relate the onset of symptoms
- The name of his or her physician/nurse practitioner/nurse
- The year and month
- His or her address
- The name of the referring physician or health care agency

Advanced age, time of day, medications, and the need for sleep may affect client responses.

Memory

Memory is one of the most important criteria for neurologic assessment. If the client cannot remember, most of the verbal assessment tests are either not feasible or are at best unreliable. Loss of memory, especially recent memory, tends to be an *early* sign of neurologic problems. Three facets of memory are tested: long-term (remote) memory, recall (recent) memory, and immediate memory.

Remote, or long-term, **memory** can be tested by asking clients about their birth date, schools attended, the city of birth, or anything from the past that can be verified. Nurses often ask the maiden name of the client's mother; this is sometimes listed on the admission form and can be checked.

Recall (recent) **memory** can be tested fairly well during the history taking by assessing the following:

- The accuracy of the medical history
- Dates of clinic or physician appointments
- The time of admission
- Health care providers seen within the past few days
- Mode of transportation to the hospital or clinic

Immediate (new) **memory** is tested by giving the client two or three unrelated words, such as "apple," "street," and "chair," and asking him or her to repeat the words to make sure they were heard. After about 5 minutes, while continuing with the examination, ask the client to repeat the words. A person normally should be able to do this correctly. An alternative to this method is to give a three-step command and observe whether it is carried out correctly.

Attention

To assess attention, ask the client to repeat a series of three numbers, such as 4, 7, and 3. The series is increased by one number with each successful repetition until seven or eight digits are achieved. If the client has difficulty at any level (cannot repeat the series), repeat the numbers. If the client cannot repeat, stop the procedure. Next, ask the client to repeat the numbers backward, starting again with three digits and increasing by one each time. Normally, a person should be able to repeat five to eight digits forward and four to six backward. Education, occupation, interest, culture, anxiety, and depression affect mental status, and what is considered normal may not be so for a particular client.

The serial seven test to determine attention may also be used. The client is asked to count backward from 100 by 7 (the examiner stops when the client reaches 65 successfully). Depending on education and other factors, it may be better to ask the person to subtract by three or to add forward by five. Use judgment and assessment skills in deciding which of these tests to use.

Language and Copying

If desired, most language and copying skills can be assessed during the initial interview. The client demonstrates language comprehension by following directions on admission (e.g., getting undressed and providing a urine specimen). If there is hesitancy in speech, indicating that the client groped for words, point to items and ask the client to name them, such as a drinking glass, the door, or the bed.

The advanced practice nurse or speech-language pathologist tests reading comprehension by writing a simple command and giving it to the client (e.g., "close your eyes"). Writing can be tested by asking the client to write a sentence. The practitioner must remember that some clients are not able to read or write and modify the examination accordingly. The practitioner usually tests copying ability by having the client copy something the nurse has drawn, such as a cross, circle, diamond, or square.

Cognition

Higher intellectual functions are assessed by asking about favorite hobbies, current events, the names of the last few presidents, or the meaning of a statement. Abstract reasoning can be evaluated by asking the meaning of proverbs (e.g., "A stitch in time saves nine" or "A rolling stone gathers no moss"). The client's judgment can be assessed, at least partially, during the interview. Did he or she make rational decisions in dealing with his or her symptoms? Ask questions such as, "What would you do if stopped for speeding?" and "What would you do if there was a fire in the wastepaper basket?" Remember that testing of cognition (general knowledge, abstraction, and judgment) is influenced by culture.

ASSESSMENT OF CRANIAL NERVES

Cranial nerves are typically tested to establish a baseline from which to compare progress or deterioration. However, they are not routinely tested unless the client has a sus-

pected problem affecting one or more of the cranial nerves (see Table 44-5). The testing of cranial nerve III is usually a part of the rapid neurologic assessment described on p. 938. Adding the specific cranial nerves to be tested on the flowsheet of a client with a problem affecting the cranial nerves helps ensure continued comparison and evaluation.

ASSESSMENT OF SENSORY FUNCTION

For the most part, the assessment of sensory function is reserved for clients with problems affecting the spinal cord or spinal nerves, such as trauma, intervertebral disk disease, Guillain Barré syndrome (GBS), neoplasm, infection, stenosis, or transverse myelitis. Components of the sensory assessment include pain, superficial and deep sensation, light touch, and proprioception. Pain and light touch are the most commonly assessed component of sensory function. Sensory assessment of the face may be completed with testing of the trigeminal nerve.

The acuity level of the client will determine the frequency of the sensory assessment and the targeted sensory parameter. Clients with acute spinal cord trauma or GBS should be assessed every hour until stable, then every 4 hours. As the condition improves, sensory assessment may be needed only once each shift. Findings of the sensory assessment are documented according to agency protocol. A special spinal cord assessment flowsheet may be used to document sensory and/or motor findings for the client with a spinal cord injury.

Pain and Temperature

Pain and temperature sensations are transmitted by the same nerve endings. Therefore if one sensation is tested and found to be intact, it can safely be assumed that the other is intact. Testing temperature sensation can usually be accomplished using a cold reflex hammer and the warm touch of the hand for clients with known or suspected spinal problems. Testing pain sensation is relatively easy and more reliable.

Assess for pain sensation with any object perceived as being sharp or dull. A cotton-tipped applicator or paper clip has a sharp end and a dull end. Instruct the client to keep eyes closed and to indicate whether the touch is sharp or dull. It is necessary to demonstrate what will be done while the client's eyes are open. The sharp and dull stimuli should be interchanged at random so the client does not anticipate the type of the next stimulus. Not all areas need to be tested unless he or she has suffered a spinal cord injury. If testing begins on the hands and feet, there is no need to test the more proximal parts of the extremities because the tracts transmitting pain and temperature sensations are intact. Compare reactions on each side. A sensation reported as dull when the stimulus was actually sharp necessitates more finite testing. A client with sensory loss as a result of diabetes mellitus or peripheral vascular disease may or may not be aware of the loss until tested. Some clients may in fact point out their sensory losses to the nurse.

Touch

Light touch discrimination is likely to be normal if pain and temperature sensations are intact. Touch discrimination and two-point discrimination are performed as part of a complete neurologic examination by the health care provider.

For testing **touch discrimination,** the client closes his or her eyes. The practitioner touches him or her with a finger and asks that he or she point to the area touched. This procedure is repeated on each extremity at random rather than at sequential points. Next, the practitioner touches the client on each side of the body on corresponding sites at the same time. The client should be able to point to both sites. An inability to sense touch on one side is called the extinction phenomenon and is a subtle test for sensory loss.

The practitioner then touches the client in two places on the same extremity with two objects, such as cotton-tipped applicators. A person can normally identify two points fairly close together depending on the location of the stimuli. The more nerve innervation in an area, the closer the two-point discrimination.

Abnormal Sensory Findings

Abnormal sensory findings may have a peripheral nervous system (PNS) or a central nervous system (CNS) cause. The neuropathies of diabetes, malnutrition, and vascular problems are due to a PNS cause and generally involve the entire extremity or both extremities. Damage to a specific spinal nerve may not result in significant sensory loss because the spinal nerves overlap. Injury to several adjacent spinal nerves is manifested as decreased or absent sensation in the dermatomes of those nerves.

CNS problems can occur within the spinal cord, the brainstem, the cerebellum, and the cerebral cortex. Sensory deficits from spinal cord damage vary with the location of the damage. Involvement of only the posterior column leads to lost **proprioception** (position sense) below the level of the damage on the same side or on both sides (if both the right and left posterior columns are involved). A lesion involving only the right spinothalamic tract results in a loss of pain and temperature sensation below the lesion on the *left* side. Problems in the brainstem, thalamus, and cortex generally result in loss of sensation on the **contralateral** (opposite) side of the body. Cerebellar lesions affect sensation on the *same* side of the body.

ASSESSMENT OF MOTOR FUNCTION

Throughout the physical assessment, observe the client for involuntary tremors or movements. Such movements need to be characterized as accurately as possible, such as "pill rolling with the thumbs and fingers at rest" or "intention tremors of both hands" (tremors that occur when the client tries to do something).

Muscle Strength

Measure hand strength by asking the client to grasp and squeeze two fingers of each of your hands. Then compare the grasps for equality of strength. As another means of evaluating strength, try to withdraw the fingers from the client's grasp and compare the ease or difficulty. He or she should release the grasps on command—another assessment of consciousness and the ability to follow commands.

To test the client's strength against resistance, ask him or her to resist your bending or straightening of the arm, hand, leg, or foot being tested (Figure 44-9). A five-point rating scale is commonly used (see Chapter 53, Table 53-1). Test results are sometimes recorded as 5/5, 3/5, and so forth, indicating the criteria that were used and the status of the client at that testing. Always evaluate and compare strength on each side. Later testing results are compared with previous results to indicate progress or regression.

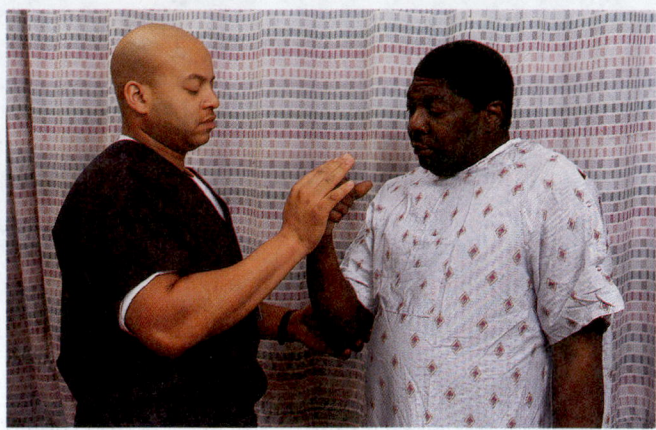

Figure 44-9 ■ Testing for strength against resistance.

Cerebral/Brainstem Integrity

Cerebral motor or brainstem integrity may also be assessed. Ask the client to close his or her eyes and hold the arms perpendicular to the body with the palms up for 15 to 30 seconds. If there is a cerebral or brainstem reason for muscle weakness, the arm on the weak side will start to fall, or "drift," with the palm pronating (turning inward). This is called a **pronator drift**. The same can be done for the lower extremities, with the client lying on his or her stomach with the legs bent upward at the knees. However, it is easier for most clients to sit on the side of the bed and extend the legs outward.

Abnormal Motor Findings

Peripheral motor problems are caused by injury, neuropathies, vascular problems, or a localized lesion in the opposite motor cortex. Tremors, unintentional movements, and changes in gait or posture represent problems in the basal ganglia or specialized nuclei of the brainstem or cerebellum. Motor cortex lesions, such as strokes, cause weakness or paralysis on the contralateral side of the body.

ASSESSMENT OF CEREBELLAR FUNCTION

Coordination

Most of the assessment of cerebellar function can be performed with the client sitting on the side of the bed or examining table. Fine coordination of muscle activity is tested. Ask the client to perform the following with his or her eyes closed:

- Run the heel of one foot down the shin of the other leg, and repeat with the other leg (the client should be able to do this smoothly and keep the heel on the shin).
- Place the hands palm-up and then palm-down on each thigh, repeating as fast as possible (this can normally be done rapidly).
- With arms out at the side, touch the finger to the nose two or three times, with eyes open and then with eyes closed (this can be done with alternating arms or with each arm individually).

Gait and Equilibrium

For the last part of the cerebellar assessment, the ambulatory client stands for testing of gait and equilibrium. Gait and equilibrium are usually tested at the end of the entire neurologic assessment. Ask the client to walk across the room,

Video Clips: Fine Motor Coordination

turn, and return. Observe for inequality in steps, difficulty maneuvering, and so forth. To evaluate balance, the client is asked to stand on one foot and then on the other. Tiptoe walking and heel-to-toe walking can also demonstrate gait problems.

To test equilibrium, ask the client to stand with arms at the sides, feet and knees close together, and eyes open. Check for swaying and then ask the client to close his or her eyes and maintain position. The examiner should be close enough to prevent falling if the client cannot stay erect. If he or she sways with the eyes closed but not when the eyes are open (the **Romberg sign**), the problem is probably **proprioceptive** (awareness of body position). If the client sways with the eyes both open and closed, the neurologic disturbance is probably *cerebellar* in origin.

If the client is not able to perform any of these activities smoothly, the problem is manifested on the same side as the cerebellar lesion. If both lobes of the cerebellum are involved, the incoordination is bilateral.

ASSESSMENT OF REFLEX ACTIVITY
Procedure

Video Clip: Deep Tendon Reflex ▶

The health care provider assesses deep tendon reflexes (DTRs) and superficial (cutaneous) reflexes. The **deep tendon reflexes** of the biceps, triceps, brachioradialis, and quadriceps muscles and of the Achilles tendon can be tested as part of the routine neurologic assessment. Striking the tendon with the hammer should cause contraction of the muscle (Figure 44-10). The appropriate muscle contraction indicates an intact reflex arc. The tendon is tapped quickly but not with too much force. If the client is tensing the muscle, the reflexes cannot be elicited. Having the client interlock his or her hands and pull outward will help to decrease muscle tensing so the reflex can be tested.

The **cutaneous (superficial) reflexes** usually tested are the plantar reflexes and sometimes the abdominal reflexes. The plantar reflex is tested with a pointed (but not sharp) object, such as the handle end of the reflex hammer or the rounded end of bandage scissors. The normal response is plantar flexion of all toes. Dorsiflexion of the great toe and fanning of the other toes (**Babinski's sign**) is abnormal in anyone older than 2 years and represents the presence of central nervous system (CNS) disease. The term "positive Babinski's sign" (abnormal response) and "negative Babinski's sign" (normal response) are clinically used terms but are not correct. **Babinski's sign** is a pathologic, or abnormal, reflex. Health care providers may also use the terms "upgoing" or "downgoing" to refer to the toes of the stimulated foot. "Upgoing" toes is an abnormal response that indicates the presence of pathology in the CNS. Babinski's sign can occur with drug and alcohol intoxication or after a seizure.

To test the abdominal reflex, stroke the client's abdomen in all four quadrants diagonally toward the umbilicus. The umbilicus should deviate toward the stimulus, but obesity may mask the reflex. The abdominal reflex can be absent in both upper and lower motor neuron disease.

Abnormal Reflex Findings

Hyperactive reflexes indicate possible upper motor neuron disease, tetanus, or hypocalcemia. Hypoactive reflexes may result from lower motor neuron disease (damage to the spinal cord), disease of the neuromuscular junction, muscle disease, or metabolic diseases such as diabetes mellitus, hypothyroidism, or hypokalemia.

Although people can display hyperactive, hypoactive, or even absent reflexes, *asymmetry* is an important finding because it probably indicates a disease process. The results of reflex testing are recorded by the use of a stick figure and a scale of 0 to 4 (Figure 44-11). A score of 2 is considered normal, although scores of 1 (hypoactive) or 3 (stronger than normal) may be normal for a particular client. **Clonus** is the sudden, brief, jerking contraction of a muscle or muscle group often seen in seizures.

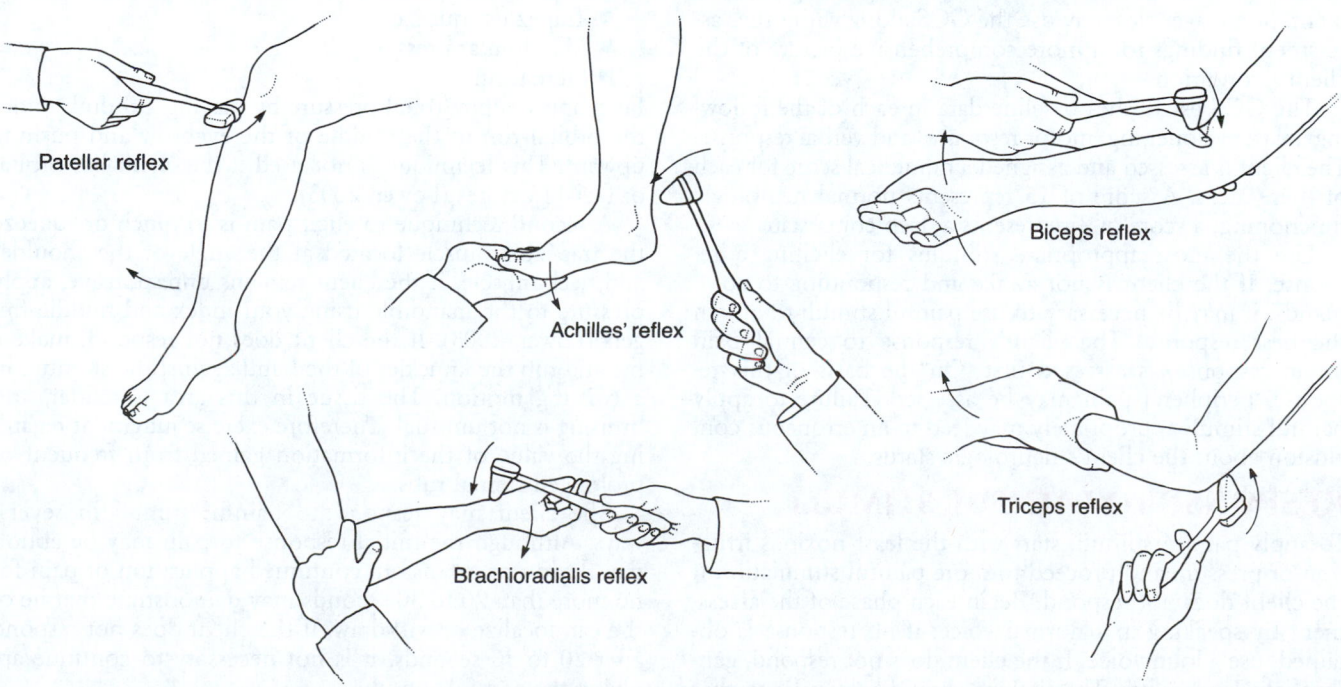

Patellar reflex

Achilles' reflex

Brachioradialis reflex

Biceps reflex

Triceps reflex

Figure 44-10 ■ Procedures for testing deep tendon reflexes.

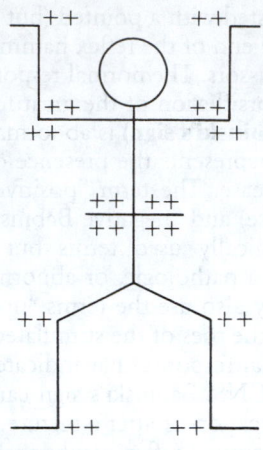

0   Absent, no response
1 (+)   Weaker than normal, hypoactive
2 (++)   Normal
3 (+++)   Stronger or more brisk than normal
4 (++++)   Hyperactive
           (Note: 1 and 3 may be normal for some individuals)

Figure 44-11 ■ A stick figure and scale for recording reflex activity.

GLASGOW COMA SCALE*	
Eye Opening	
Spontaneous	4
To sound	3
To pain	2
Never	1
Motor Response	
Obeys commands	6
Localizes pain	5
Normal flexion (withdrawal)	4
Abnormal flexion	3
Extension	2
None	1
Verbal Response	
Oriented	5
Confused conversation	4
Inappropriate words	3
Incomprehensible sounds	2
None	1
* The highest possible score is 15	

Figure 44-12 ■ The Glasgow Coma Scale. The highest possible score is 15.

Rapid Neurologic Assessment

A rapid neurologic assessment is completed when the client is admitted to a health care facility on an emergent basis, or as part of the client's routine or ongoing assessment or in the event of a sudden change in neurologic status. This is the most common type of neurologic assessment you will perform when caring for adult clients.

GLASGOW COMA SCALE

A form of the **Glasgow Coma Scale** (GCS) (Figure 44-12) is used in many health care agencies. This tool has been shown to be reliable as one measure of neurologic assessment. Some agencies may use the GCS along with other assessment findings for a more comprehensive picture of the client's condition.

The GCS establishes baseline data in each of the following areas: eye opening, motor response, and verbal response. The client is assessed and assigned a numerical score for each of these areas. A score of 15 represents normal neurologic functioning; a score of 3 represents a deep coma state.

Use the most appropriate stimulus for eliciting a response. If the client is not awake and responding to commands, it may be necessary to use painful stimuli to obtain the best response. The client's response to central pain (brain response) is assessed first. On the basis of this response, peripheral pain may be assessed. Failure to apply painful stimuli appropriately may lead to an erroneous conclusion about the client's neurologic status.

RESPONSE TO PAINFUL STIMULI

To apply painful stimuli, start with the least noxious irritation or pressure and proceed to more painful stimulation if the client does not respond. Begin each phase of the assessment by speaking in a normal voice; if no response is obtained, use a loud voice. If the client does not respond, gently shake him or her. The shaking should be similar to that used in attempting to wake up a child. If that is unsuccessful, painful stimuli are applied using one of the following methods:

- Supraorbital pressure
- Trapezius squeeze
- Mandibular pressure
- Sternal rub

First, apply supraorbital pressure by placing a thumb under the orbital rim in the middle of the eyebrow and pushing upward. This technique is not used if the client has orbital or facial fractures (Lower, 2003).

A second technique to elicit pain is to pinch or squeeze the trapezius muscle located at the angle of the shoulder and neck muscle. If the client remains unresponsive, apply pressure to the mandible using your index and middle fingers (Lower, 2003). If the client does not respond, make a fist and rub the knuckles of the hand against the sternum in a twisting motion. The tissue in this area is tender, and bruising is not unusual. Therefore exercise judgment regarding the value of the information gained from frequent or prolonged sternal rubs.

The client may respond to painful stimuli in several ways. Although the initial response to pain may be abnormal flexion or extension, continued application of pain for no more than 20 to 30 seconds may demonstrate that he or she can localize or withdraw. If the client does not respond after 20 to 30 seconds, it is not necessary to continue applying the painful stimulus.

Figure 44-13 ■ Posturing. **A,** Decorticate posturing. **B,** Decerebrate posturing.

If the client responds by moving, but not all extremities move, assess the peripheral response to pain. Place a pen or pencil on top of the client's nail bed at the base of the cuticle and apply pressure. This maneuver is performed only on the extremity that did not move.

LEVEL OF CONSCIOUSNESS

In addition to using the Glasgow Coma Scale, assess the client's level of consciousness (LOC). This area of the assessment must be meticulously recorded and described as a change in LOC. *Even a subtle change is the **first** indicator of a decline in neurologic status!* These changes include complaints of headache; restlessness, irritability, or being unusually quiet; slurred speech; and a change in the level of orientation.

Decerebrate or decorticate posturing, as well as pinpoint or dilated and nonreactive pupils, is a late sign of deterioration. The physician should be notified immediately of any change in the client's status. **Decortication** is abnormal posturing seen in the client with lesions that interrupt the corticospinal pathways (Figure 44-13, *A*). The client's arms, wrists, and fingers are flexed with internal rotation and plantar flexion of the legs. **Decerebration** is abnormal posturing and rigidity characterized by extension of the arms and legs, pronation of the arms, plantar flexion, and opisthotonos (Figure 44-13, *B*). Decerebration is usually associated with dysfunction in the brainstem area.

PUPIL ASSESSMENT

The pupils are assessed as part of ongoing "neuro" checks. Pupil constriction is a function of cranial nerve III. *P*upils should be *e*qual in size, *r*ound and *r*egular in shape, and react to *l*ight and *a*ccommodation **(PERRLA).** Estimate the size of both pupils using a millimeter ruler. Clients who have had eye surgery for cataracts or glaucoma often have irregularly shaped pupils. Clients using eyedrops for either cataracts or glaucoma may have unequal pupils if only one eye is being treated, and the pupillary response may be altered.

To test for pupil constriction, the client should be asked to close his or her eyes. Bring a penlight in from the side of the client's head and shine the light in the eye being tested as soon as the client opens his or her eyes. The pupil should constrict **(direct response)**; the other eye should also con-

strict slightly **(consensual response).** To test accommodation, the client focuses on a distant object and then immediately focuses on an object 4 to 5 inches from the nose. The eyes should converge, and the pupils should constrict.

Diagnostic Assessment
LABORATORY TESTS

For clients with a neurologic problem resulting from or concomitant with systemic infection, blood cultures are necessary to identify the causative agent of the infection. Although the cause of infection must be determined for any client, this is especially true for those with central nervous system (CNS) disease. The blood-brain barrier is often not intact in neurologic disease, and the client is more susceptible to infection of the nervous system, such as meningitis or encephalitis.

RADIOGRAPHIC EXAMINATIONS
X-ray Examinations of the Skull and Spine

Plain x-rays of the skull and spine are used to determine bony fractures, curvatures, bone erosion, bone dislocation, and possible calcification of soft tissue, which can damage the nervous system.

Several views are taken—anteroposterior, lateral, oblique, and, when necessary, special views of the facial bones. In head trauma and multiple injuries, one of the first priorities is to rule out cervical fracture by radiography.

Explain that the x-ray procedure for the skull and spine is similar to that for a chest x-ray procedure, that he or she will need to remain still during the procedure, and that the exposure to radiation is minimal. If the client is in traction and a portable x-ray unit is not available, the nurse may need to accompany him or her to assist with positioning. Any client who cannot walk from a wheelchair to the x-ray table should go to the radiology department on a stretcher. The client is positioned for each of the desired views and is asked not to move just before each x-ray. Follow-up care is not required.

Cerebral Angiography

Cerebral angiography (arteriography) is done to visualize the cerebral circulation (carotid and vertebral arteries). A contrast medium is injected into an artery (usually the femoral) to identify aneurysms, traumatic injuries, strictures/occlusions, tumors, and arteriovenous malformations.

CLIENT PREPARATION. Determine whether the client is allergic to iodinated contrast agents (Chart 44-5). The procedure is initially explained to the client by the person obtaining the written consent, usually the radiologist. Clarify the explanation by answering questions and reinforcing the following important points:
- The necessity for not moving during the procedure
- The necessity for immobilization of the head

The client is allowed nothing by mouth for 4 to 6 hours before the test. Most hospitals require that the nurse complete a preoperative checklist. Be sure to:
- Remove the client's hairpins and jewelry.
- Record neurologic and vital signs.
- Ask the client to empty his or her bladder before the procedure.

Video Clip: Pupil Responses

CHART 44-5

BEST PRACTICE for
Studies Involving the Injection of Contrast Agent

Special precautions are taken for clients who will receive a contrast agent as part of their diagnostic test. These measures include the following:

- Following institutional guidelines regarding informed consent
- Determining whether the client has any food or fluid restriction before the test
- Asking the client about allergies to contrast agents, shellfish, or iodine.
- Determining risk factors for contrast-induced nephropathy (renal damage)
  Pre-existing renal disease
  Diabetic nephropathy
  Heart failure
  Dehydration
  Medications that interfere with renal perfusion, such as metformin (Diabetic clients on the metformin require preprocedure and postprocedure changes in their medication regimen.)
- Notifying the health care provider if the client has reported a risk factor
- Checking the client's creatinine level (Clients with a level greater than 1.5 mg/dL are more at risk for contrast-induced nephropathy.)

PROCEDURE. The client is placed on an examining table and made as comfortable as possible. At this time, dentures and hearing aids must be removed. The client's head is placed in a positioning headrest or sponge. He or she is then connected to cardiac monitoring throughout the procedure. Many institutions avoid sedating these clients because sedation may mask neurologic changes.

The radiologist numbs an area at the groin and inserts a needle into the femoral artery. A soft-tip guiding wire goes through the needle and into the aorta. A thin catheter is inserted into the artery over the wire. Under fluoroscopic guidance, the catheter is advanced into a carotid or vertebral artery. Then, the physician injects 6-8 mL of iodinated contrast material into each vessel several times while recording images from different angles over the head and neck. The newest radiographic systems come with software to create three-dimensional images that can be rotated to reveal overlapping anatomic structures.

After all the vessels have been imaged, the radiologist reviews all the images and consults with the referring physician to decide whether the client could benefit from any therapeutic radiologic procedure to treat the problem. It is common to use an arterial closure device to seal the artery and prevent bleeding.

Prior to the mid-1980s, images were taken by film. Imaging now is done almost exclusively by digital means (without film). The new equipment couples x-ray machines with a digital camera and computer. The x-ray images are stored on a computer. These systems could display the so-called "subtracted image," made from two images—one just before the contrast was injected and one with the contrast in the artery. Technologic improvements allow high-resolution images and three-dimensional rotational imaging, especially useful in cerebral studies.

The risks for the procedure are contrast reaction, thrombosis (clotting), vasospasm, and bleeding from the entry site. Clients with known contrast sensitivity are pre-treated with steroids. The overall risk for complications is less than 1%.

FOLLOW-UP CARE. Obtain vital signs, "neuro" signs, and neurovascular checks according to the written physician orders. Compare these findings with the pre-angiography signs. The client is usually restricted to bedrest for several hours. The extremity into which the contrast medium was injected is kept straight and immobilized for the duration of bedrest. Check the extremity for adequate circulation, which is demonstrated by the following:

- Skin color and temperature
- Pulses distal to the injection site
- Capillary refill

Inspect the injection site frequently for evidence of bleeding. If bleeding is noted, maintain manual pressure on the site and notify the radiologic immediately. If fluids are not contraindicated, oral or IV fluid intake is increased to help the client excrete the contrast material, which takes about 24 hours.

Computed Tomography

Computed tomography (CT) scanning is relatively accurate and is the quickest, easiest, and least expensive method of diagnosing neurologic problems. With the aid of a computer, pictures are taken at many horizontal levels, or slices, of the brain or spinal cord. The cross-sectional slices build up three-dimensional pictures of the brain or spinal cord. A contrast medium may be used to enhance the image. CT scans distinguish bone, soft tissue (e.g., the brain, vascular system, and ventricular system), and fluids such as cerebrospinal fluid (CSF) or blood. Tumors, infarctions, hemorrhage, hydrocephalus, and bone malformations can be identified. A CT scan may also be performed after a myelogram (see Chapter 53 for brief discussion of this test).

CLIENT PREPARATION. Follow the guidelines listed in Chart 44-5 if a contrast agent is to be given. If a contrast medium is used, food is withheld for 4 to 6 hours before the test. Fluids are generally not withheld. Instruct the client to remove hairpins, hairpieces, or wigs.

PROCEDURE. The client is placed on a movable table. His or her head is positioned in a head-holding device. The client must remain completely still during the test, which may be difficult. The table is positioned in the machine, a large donut-shaped structure. Some clients are fearful of the machine or of being confined in a small space. A noncontrast series of pictures is taken first. Then, if needed, the client is withdrawn from the scanner and given an injection of the iodinated contrast medium. The scan is then repeated. Each set of head scans takes less than 5 minutes in newer scanners. Spine studies take about 10 minutes per body section (cervical, thoracic, lumbar) and are less likely to require contrast injection.

Most clients with new neurologic symptoms get both the precontrast and postcontrast study of the head. Contrast-enhanced CT is especially useful in locating and identifying tumor types and abscesses. For situations in which bleeding is the only concern (e.g., in trauma clients), contrast scans are not usually required.

New CT scanners can provide CT-angiography (CTA) images. Computer software can assemble three-dimensional reconstruction of the blood vessels of the neck or brain. These images are not yet as detailed as angiographic images, but are faster, cheaper, and less invasive than angiography.

FOLLOW-UP CARE. Check for a delayed allergic response to the contrast medium if it was used. If a contrast medium was used, the resultant diuresis may require the administration of replacement fluids.

Positron Emission Tomography

Positron emission tomography (PET) is a diagnostic tool that is becoming available to more medical centers. Its benefit over a computed tomography (CT) scan or magnetic resonance imaging (MRI) is that it provides information about the *function* of the brain, specifically glucose and oxygen metabolism and cerebral blood flow. Current CT scanners provide information about the *structure* of the central nervous system (CNS). Some research centers have functional magnetic resonance imaging (fMRI).

The physician or nuclear medicine technologist injects the client with the molecule deoxyglucose, which is tagged to an isotope. The isotope emits activity in the form of positrons, which are scanned and converted into a color image by computer. The more active a given part of the brain, the greater the glucose uptake. This test is used to evaluate drug metabolism and detect areas of metabolic alteration that occur in dementia, epilepsy, psychiatric and degenerative disorders, neoplasms, and Alzheimer's disease. The level of radiation is equivalent to that of five or six x-rays but much less than exposure during CT. Recently, the half-life of these isotopes has increased and more centers are able to offer this test. Regional cyclotrons can now provide isotopes for medical centers within two hours of the generator.

CLIENT PREPARATION. Explain the test and instruct the client to withhold caffeine, alcohol, and tobacco for 24 hours before the test, according to agency policy. The client is on NPO status (nothing by mouth) for 6 to 12 hours before the procedure (if the client is diabetic, no insulin is given before the test). Do not give any glucose solutions and any other drugs that alter glucose metabolism.

PROCEDURE. The client is placed on a stretcher. An IV line is started to inject the isotope. An arterial line may be used to obtain blood samples. The client may be blindfolded and have earplugs inserted for all or part of the test. The total procedure takes 2 to 3 hours. The client is asked to perform certain mental functions to activate different areas of the brain.

FOLLOW-UP CARE. The radioisotope is eliminated in the urine and requires no special precautions. However, encourage the client to increase fluid intake. Follow-up care is not required.

Single-Photon Emission Computed Tomography

The limitation of PET may be overcome through the use of **single-photon emission computed tomography (SPECT).** With SPECT, a radiopharmaceutical, an agent that enables radioisotopes to cross the blood-brain barrier is administered by IV injection. Gamma-emitting radionuclides have longer half-lives, therefore eliminating the need for a cyclotron near the scanner. Although SPECT is less expensive than PET, the resolution of the images is limited. SPECT is particularly useful in studying the following:

- Cerebral blood flow
- Stroke
- Dementia
- Acquired immunodeficiency syndrome (AIDS)
- Amnesia
- Neoplasms
- Head trauma
- Seizures
- Persistent vegetative state
- Brain death
- Psychiatric disorders

SPECT is contraindicated in pregnant women or women who are breastfeeding.

CLIENT PREPARATION. Client preparation is similar to that for PET. Determine whether the client has recently had other nuclear medicine screenings which may leave traces of the radiopharmaceutical agent in the client. Recent scanning may interfere with test results. As with other tests that involve the injection of contrast material, determine whether the client has renal disease or has had a reaction to dye in the past.

PROCEDURE. The client is injected with the material about 1 hour before the actual scan by the radiologist, certified nuclear medicine technologist, or specially trained RN.

He or she is positioned on an x-ray table in a quiet dark room for the actual scans. Several gamma cameras scan the client's head. When completed, the images are downloaded to a computer.

FOLLOW UP CARE. The client can return to his or her previous activity level. There are no food or fluid restrictions as a result of the test.

OTHER DIAGNOSTIC TESTS

Magnetic Resonance Imaging

Magnetic resonance imaging (MRI) produces images considered superior to the CT scan. It does not use ionizing radiation but instead relies on magnetic fields. Special precautions must be taken when entering the MRI procedure room. Images may be enhanced with the use of gadolinium, a non–iodine-based contrast. MRIs of the spine have replaced CT scans and myelography in most instances (see Chapter 53).

Two newer uses for MRI are **magnetic resonance angiography (MRA)** and **magnetic resonance spectroscopy (MRS).** MRA is used to identify arterial blockages, intracranial aneurysms, and arteriovenous malformations. MRS is used to detect abnormalities in the brain's biochemical processes, such as that which occurs in Alzheimer's disease and brain attack (Pagana & Pagana, 2002).

CLIENT PREPARATION. A signed consent form is obtained; no food or fluid restrictions are necessary. Tell the client that the procedure is noisy and that earplugs are available. In addition, the client should know that he or she will lie on a hard surface inside a hollow tube. If the client is claustrophobic, a mild sedative may be prescribed before the procedure.

Newer, open-sided units ("open MRI") now produce adequate images for those clients who do not wish to be sedated for standard long-bore MRI scanners. MRI is contraindicated for clients with cardiac pacemakers, other implanted pumps or devices, and ferromagnetic aneurysm clips. Other implanted devices, such as vascular stents, intravascular catheter (IVC) filters, and metal vascular embolic devices may be scanned immediately or after a certain period of time, depending on manufacturers' recommendations. MRI may also be contraindicated in clients who are confused, pregnant, or agitated; have unstable vital signs; are on continuous life support; or have tattoos. New physiologic monitoring systems made specifically for MRI allow some clients who are unstable to be scanned. A comprehensive online list of medical devices tested for MRI safety and compatibility can be found at http://www.mrisafety.com (Carr, 2002). Medical personnel must remove any medical devices they are carrying or wearing, and ensure that only approved devices are allowed in the MRI room.

PROCEDURE. MRI uses a powerful magnet to align hydrogen nuclei (usually) in the plane of the magnetic field. The scanner emits a radio frequency (RF) pulse, which is transmitted to change the hydrogen alignment. Between RF pulses, the hydrogen realigns with the magnet and nuclei transmit an RF signal back to the scanner. This signal is then converted to an image that locates hydrogen on the body. Multiple sets of images are taken that are used to determine normal and abnormal anatomy.

FOLLOW-UP CARE. No special post-procedure or follow-up care is required.

Statscan Critical Imaging System

The Statscan was first used in the United States in the Shock Trauma Center at the University of Maryland in Baltimore. This low-dose digital imaging system, small enough to fit into an average-sized trauma room, can take full-body images. In just 13 seconds, the trauma team has information about fractures and other injuries that may not be readily apparent on the initial trauma survey. No special preparation or care is needed.

Lumbar Puncture

Lumbar puncture (spinal tap) is the insertion of a spinal needle into the subarachnoid space between the third and fourth (sometimes the fourth and fifth) lumbar vertebrae. A lumbar puncture is used to do the following:

- Obtain pressure readings with a manometer
- Obtain cerebrospinal fluid (CSF) for analysis
- Check for spinal blockage attributable to a spinal cord lesion
- Inject contrast medium or air for diagnostic study
- Inject spinal anesthetics
- Inject certain medications
- Reduce mild to moderate increased intracranial pressure (ICP) in certain conditions

Because of the danger of sudden release of CSF pressure, a lumbar puncture is contraindicated in clients with symptoms suggestive of increased ICP. The procedure is also contraindicated in clients with skin infections at or near the puncture site because of the danger of introducing infective organisms into the CSF.

CLIENT PREPARATION. A consent form is signed by the client. Explain the procedure, noting that some discomfort may be felt when the local anesthetic is injected. Some clients experience pain in the leg when the spinal needle is inserted. Ask the client to empty his or her bladder as a comfort measure. Position the client on whichever side he or she is most comfortable, with his or her back close to the edge of the bed or examining table. When the health care provider is ready, ask the client to bring the knees up as close as possible to the trunk and to assume a "fetal" position (using the arms to hold the knees in place) with the head bent forward. Some clients need help in achieving and maintaining this position. To help maintain the position, grasp the client behind the knees and the back of the lower neck. A pillow under the head and between the knees aids body alignment.

PROCEDURE. The health care provider cleans the skin site thoroughly. The injection site is determined, and the local anesthetic is injected. In a few minutes, the health care provider inserts a spinal needle between the third and fourth lumbar vertebrae. Instruct the client to inform the provider if there is shooting pain or a tingling sensation. After determining proper placement in the subarachnoid space by removing the stylet and seeing CSF, the client is asked to relax a little so the pressure reading will be more accurate. Opening and closing pressure readings are taken and recorded. Three to five test tubes of CSF are usually collected and numbered sequentially. After specimen collection, the needle is withdrawn, slight pressure is applied, and an adhesive bandage strip is placed over the insertion site. The nurse may or may not be able to help with the collection and numbering of the specimens, depending on the client's ability to remain quiet. If the client is restless or unable to cooperate, two people may need to assist instead of one. Consider this possibility before beginning the procedure.

Examination of CSF has been a useful diagnostic tool for some time, and recent technical advances are increasing the number of analyses that can be done on CSF. The normal characteristics of CSF and some of the more common abnormalities are given in Table 44-7. Gram stain smears can test for particular types of meningitis, such as tubercular meningitis. CSF can be cultured, and sensitivity studies determine the best choice of antibiotic if an infection is diagnosed. A specific test for neurosyphilis is the fluorescent treponemal antibody absorption (FTA-ABS) test. Cytologic studies of CSF can identify tumor cells.

FOLLOW-UP CARE. After a lumbar puncture (LP), the client is generally restricted to bedrest in a flat position for 4 to 8 hours as prescribed by the physician or as determined by hospital policy. This prevents CSF leakage from the puncture site. However, a report by the Therapeutics and Assessment Subcommittee of the American Academy of Neurology found that the duration of bedrest does not influence the occurrence of post-LP headache (Evans et al., 2000). Instruct the client to increase fluid intake (to 3000 mL unless contraindicated) for 24 to 48 hours to facilitate CSF production, although research has not supported or refuted this practice.

A decrease in CSF may cause a severe, throbbing headache (also called a **spinal headache**). Administer analgesics as prescribed for headache if it occurs. If the lumbar puncture was done to reduce intracranial pressure, perform a rapid neurologic assessment (especially level of consciousness) more frequently until stability is ensured. Complications of lumbar puncture, although uncommon, include infection, CSF leakage, and hematoma formation.

Electroencephalography

Electroencephalography (EEG) records the electrical activity of the cerebral hemispheres. Each graphic recording represents the voltage changes in various areas of the brain (determined by recording the difference between two electrodes). The EEG may be normal even when a pathologic condition is present. The test is performed to:

- Determine the general activity of the cerebral hemispheres
- Determine the origin of seizure activity (epilepsy)

TABLE 44-7 Significance of Cerebrospinal Fluid Findings

Findings	Significance
Pressure	
Less than 20 cm H$_2$O	Normal range
Color/Appearance	
Clear, colorless	Normal
Pink-red to orange	Red blood cells present
Yellow	Bilirubin present owing to hemolysis of red blood cells; possible causes include subarachnoid hemorrhage, jaundice, increased cerebrospinal fluid (CSF) protein, hypercarotenemia, or hemoglobinemia
Brown	Methemoglobin present, indicating previous meningeal hemorrhage
Unclear or hazy	Cell count is elevated
Cells	
0-5 small lymphocytes/mm^3	Normal
More than 5 lymphocytes/mm^3	Reaction to infection, tumor, chemical substance, or blood
Proteins	
Total	
15-45 mg/dL	Normal
45-100 mg/dL	Paraventricular tumor
50-200 mg/dL	Viral infection
More than 500 mg/dL	Bacterial infection, Guillain-Barré syndrome
Less than 15 mg/dL	Meningismus, pseudotumor cerebri, hyperthyroidism, normal finding after lumbar puncture
Immune Gamma Globulin (IgG, the most important protein)	
3%-12% of total protein	Normal
More than 3%-12% of total protein	Multiple sclerosis, neurosyphilis, or viral infection
Albumin/Globulin Ratio	
8:1	Normal
Glucose	
50-75 mg/dL or 60%-70% of blood glucose level	Normal
Less than 50 mg/dL (usually accompanied by the presence of pathologic organisms)	Bacterial, fungal, or viral meningitis; central nervous system (CNS) leukemia; or cancer
Other Characteristics	
Lactic Acid	
10-25 mg/dL	Normal
More than 10-25 mg/dL	Systemic acidosis or increased CSF glucose metabolism
Glutamine	
Less than 20 mg/dL	Normal
More than 20 mg/dL	Hepatic coma or cirrhosis of liver
Lactate Dehydrogenase	
10% of serum level or 2.0-7.2 units/mL	Normal
More than 10% of serum level	Bacterial meningitis, inflammatory diseases of CNS

- Determine cerebral function in pathologic conditions other than epilepsy, such as tumors, abscesses, cerebrovascular disease, hematomas, injury, metabolic diseases, degenerative brain disease, and drug intoxication
- Differentiate between organic and hysterical or feigned blindness or deafness
- Monitor cerebral activity during surgical anesthesia
- Diagnose sleep disorders (all-night EEG)
- Determine brain death

CLIENT PREPARATION. This test is done on an ambulatory care basis. Chart 44-6 lists instructions for the client preparing to have an EEG.

Explain the purpose of and procedure for the test. If the EEG is ordered with the client "sleep deprived," he or she should be kept awake from about 2 to 3 AM through the rest of the night. CNS depressants and stimulants are usually not given for 24 hours before the test. The health care provider indicates whether anticonvulsants are to be withheld. If anticonvulsants are withheld, monitor the client for signs of seizure activity. Remind the client to avoid coffee, tea, and other stimulants. Food and other fluids may be consumed because hypoglycemia (low blood glucose) affects brain activity. The client's hair should be shampooed, clean, and free from hairpins, sprays, or oils.

BEST PRACTICE for
The Client Having an Electroencephalogram

- Thoroughly explain the procedure to the client.
- If the order is for the client to be "sleep deprived," tell the client to awaken about 2 to 3 AM and to stay awake for the rest of the night.
- Instruct the client to avoid central nervous system depressants or stimulants; withhold anticonvulsants only if instructed by the physician.
- Tell the client not to drink caffeine-containing fluids, such as coffee or tea, on the day of the test.
- Reassure the client that the test is not dangerous or uncomfortable.
- Ask the client to wash his or her hair on the morning of the test and to remove all hairpins, sprays, or oils.
- Inform the client that the hair will need to be washed again after the test to remove the electrode glue.

PROCEDURE. The client is placed on a reclining chair or bed. According to an internationally accepted procedure, 16 to 24 electrodes are usually attached to the scalp with a jelly-like substance and connected to the machine. The physician or EEG technician places glue over the electrodes to prevent slippage. The client must lie still with his or her eyes closed during the initial recording. The rest of the test engages the client in certain activities: hyperventilation, photic stimulation, and sleep. A portable EEG may be performed at the bedside if necessary, but the preference is for the EEG to be done in a room devoid of stimuli.

Hyperventilation produces cerebral vasoconstriction and alkalosis, which increases the likelihood of seizure activity. The client is asked to breathe deeply 20 to 30 times for 3 minutes.

In *photic stimulation,* a strobe light (bright light) is placed in front of the client. Frequencies of 1 to 20 flashes per second are used with the client's eyes open and then closed. If the client's seizures are photosensitive in origin, the EEG will show waves corresponding to each flash of light or waves indicating seizure activity.

Sleep is either natural or induced by an oral or IV sedative. EEG waves indicative of temporal lobe epilepsy can be demonstrated best during sleep.

Throughout the test, which takes 40 to 60 minutes, the technician watches the client closely and records any movement. These movements alter the record and must be labeled as artifacts. Examples of artifacts are tongue movement, eye blinking, muscle tenseness, and nervousness.

FOLLOW-UP CARE. If not removed in the EEG laboratory, the client removes the jelly-like substance and glue from the scalp and hair with acetone and then with shampoo. Any medications that were withheld are reinstituted. The client may need a nap if he or she was deprived of sleep before the test.

Electromyography

Electromyography (EMG) records the electrical activity of peripheral nerves by testing muscle activity (see Chapter 53 for a description of client preparation, procedure, and follow-up care). Electromyography and **electroneurography** or nerve conduction velocity studies (NCVS) are usually used together and are referred to as **electromyoneurography.**

Cerebral Blood Flow Evaluation

Cerebral blood flow (CBF) can be measured in many areas of the brain with the use of radioactive substances. It is particularly useful in evaluating cerebral vasospasm. Explain the test and, if drugs have previously been prescribed, withhold central nervous system (CNS) depressants and stimulants for 24 hours before the test.

Because xenon readily diffuses into brain tissue, it is the most common choice as an inhaled or injected tracer. The xenon travels through the vasculature to the brain, where it is detected by external scintillation counters placed on the skull. Normal CBF is 50 to 55 mm/min/100 g of cerebral tissue. The client receives various stimuli during the test. Increases in local blood flow can be seen with any neuronal activity, such as reading, hand movement, seizures, and temperature elevation (up to 107.6° F [42° C]). Local blood flow decreases with degenerative disease, comas of metabolic origin, increased intracranial pressure (ICP), or subarachnoid hemorrhage. Follow-up care for this test is not required.

Brain Scan

The **brain scan** is a radionuclide imaging study. A radioactive substance is injected to detect certain pathologic conditions. The test is especially useful in evaluating vascular abnormalities such as aneurysms and in locating tumors, hematomas, and abscesses. As technologic advances in diagnostic testing continue, this test is being performed less frequently.

Explain the test and ask the client to empty the bladder as a comfort measure immediately before the test is done. A signed consent form may be necessary, depending on agency policy.

During the procedure, the physician injects the client with a radioactive isotope, usually technetium (Tc 99m). There is a delay in the test of up to 2 hours while the brain absorbs the isotope. The client is placed on a table and must remain still with the hands at his or her side for the duration of the test. The test takes 1 to 2 hours, depending on the number of scannings used.

For follow-up care, teach the client to increase fluids to promote elimination of the isotope (urine does not need special handling).

Transcranial Doppler

Intracranial hemodynamics can be evaluated through the use of the **transcranial Doppler (TCD).** TCD does not measure cerebral blood flow or visualize the vessels, but it does measure the time needed for pulse waves to travel a specific depth and return to the skull's surface. It is particularly valuable in evaluating cerebral vasospasm. TCD is safe and repeatable and is an inexpensive alternative to angiography.

GET READY for the NCLEX Examination!

KEY POINTS

Safe Effective Care Environment

- When caring for older adults, remind them to move slowly and use caution when ambulating; older adults have an altered balance and decreased coordination.

- For tests that use contrast media, use precautions as listed in Chart 44-5.
- Check for bleeding after clients have an angiography; if bleeding is observed, call the radiologist immediately.
- Before MRI, check for ferromagnetic devices, such as pacemakers, vascular stents, and implanted pumps.

Health Promotion and Maintenance

- Reinforce teaching and use teaching aids for older adults who typically have recent memory loss.
- Explain what clients should expect before diagnostic testing for neurologic structure and function.
- Encourage clients who receive contrast media or isotopes to push fluids to increase elimination of the material.
- Teach clients having an EEG to follow the precautions listed in Chart 44-6.

Psychosocial Integrity

- Assess the mental status of clients as part of the neurologic assessment, including orientation.
- Remember that a change in level of consciousness (LOC) is the first indicator of neurologic decline.
- Assess the client's memory because loss of memory, especially recent memory, tends to be an early sign of neurologic problems.

Physiological Integrity

- Evaluate the client's sensory and motor abilities, as well as gait, balance, and coordination.
- Use the Glasgow Coma Scale as one measure of neurologic functioning; the lower the score, the poorer the function.
- Check pupils for size, shape, and reaction; pupils should be equal in size, round and regular in shape, and reactive to light and accommodation.
- Be aware that decerebrate or decorticate posturing, and pinpoint or dilated nonreactive pupils are late signs of neurologic deterioration.
- Assist with client positioning during a lumbar puncture (fetal position preferred).
- Recall that normal cerebrospinal fluid (CSF) is clear and colorless with few cells.

ADDITIONAL STUDY RESOURCES

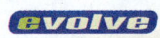 Go to your Student CD-ROM for Review Questions for the NCLEX Examination.

evolve Go to http://evolve.elsevier.com/Iggy/ for Integrated Management of Care Questions for the NCLEX Examination.

SELECTED BIBLIOGRAPHY

Al-Chalabi, A., & Miller, C.C. (2003). Neurofilaments and neurological disease. *Bioessays, 25*(4), 346-355.

Altizer, L. (2002). Orthopaedic essentials. Neurovascular assessment. *Orthopaedic Nursing, 21*(4), 48-50.

Barker, E. (2003). *Neuroscience nursing: A spectrum of care* (2nd ed.). St. Louis: Mosby.

Brenner, Z.R., & Myers, S.A. (2003). Acetylcysteine and nephropathy. *American Journal of Nursing, 103*(3), 64AA-64EE.

Carr, M.W., & Grey, M.L. (2002). Magnetic resonance imaging. *American Journal of Nursing, 102*(12), 26-32.

Chaudhuri, A. (2002). The role of neurodiagnostics in functional disorders. *Physical Medicine & Rehabilitation: State of the Art Reviews, 16*(1), 63-75.

Evans, R.W. (2003). *Saunders manual of neurological practice*. Philadelphia: W.B. Saunders.

Evans, R.W., et al. (2000). Assessment: Prevention of post-lumbar puncture headaches: Report of the Therapeutics and Technology Assessment Subcommittee of the American Academy of Neurology. *Neurology, 55*(7), 909-911.

Gambrell, M., & Flynn, N. (2004). Seizures 101. *Nursing 2004, 34*(8), 36-41.

Goetz, C.G. (2003). *Textbook of Clinical Neurology* (2nd ed.). Philadelphia: W.B. Saunders.

Hickey, J. (2002). The clinical practice of neurological and neurosurgical nursing. Philadelphia: J.B. Lippincott.

Hinkle, J. (2002). SPECT: A powerful imaging tool. *American Journal of Nursing* (March), *102*(3), 24A-24G.

Huether, S.E., & McCance, K.L. (2004). *Understanding pathophysiology* (3rd ed.). St. Louis: Mosby.

Jarvis, C. (2003). *Physical examination and health assessment* (4th ed.). Philadelphia: W.B. Saunders.

Kullman, D.M., & Hanna, M.G. (2002). Neurological disorders caused by inherited ion-channel mutations. *Lancet: Neurology, 1*(3), 157-166.

Lower, J. (2002). Facing neuro assessment fearlessly. *Nursing, 32*(2), 58-65.

Lower, J. (2003). Using pain to assess neurologic response. *Nursing 2003, 33*(6), 56-57.

Pagana, K.D., & Pagana, T.J. (2002). *Mosby's manual of diagnostic and laboratory tests* (2nd ed.). St. Louis: Mosby.

Solomon, E.P. (2003). *Introduction to human anatomy and physiology* (2nd ed.). Philadelphia: W.B. Saunders.

Interventions for Clients with Problems of the Central Nervous System
The Brain

KATHY A. HAUSMAN

LEARNING OUTCOMES

After studying this chapter, you should be able to:

1. Compare the assessment findings of migraine, cluster and tension headaches.
2. Develop a teaching plan for a client diagnosed with migraine headaches.
3. Differentiate the common types of seizures, including presenting clinical manifestations.
4. Identify collaborative management options for treating clients diagnosed with epilepsy.
5. Explain the nursing interventions required when providing care for a client having a seizure.
6. Outline the priorities for care of clients with meningitis and encephalitis.
7. Describe the pathophysiology of Parkinson disease.
8. Develop a community-based plan of care for a client with Parkinson disease.
9. Identify nursing implications related to giving medications for Parkinson disease.
10. Identify the roles of the interdisciplinary health care team and family in developing a comprehensive individualized treatment plan for the client with Alzheimer's disease.
11. Explain the use of drug therapy for clients with Alzheimer's disease.
12. Prioritize care for clients with Alzheimer's disease.
13. Develop a teaching plan for caregivers of clients with Alzheimer's disease.
14. Analyze legal/ethical concerns related to genetic counseling of clients with Huntington disease.

Go to your Student CD-ROM for Review Questions
for the NCLEX Examination keyed to these Learning Outcomes.
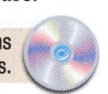

Dysfunction of the brain may be a mild disorder that a person can learn to live with or a devastating disorder that drastically affects the client and the family. With newer diagnostic tools and treatment methods, the rate and the quality of recovery and rehabilitation are improving steadily. Neurologic impairment tends to involve many aspects of the person's life:

- The neurologic problem itself
- Family life alteration or disruption
- Occupational changes
- Body image
- Self-worth conflicts
- The realization of a continuous need for numerous resources

HEADACHES

Headaches are a common symptom of a variety of neurologic and non-neurologic disorders. The challenge to the health care provider is to determine the cause of the headache so appropriate treatment may begin. To assist the health care provider in this endeavor, the International Headache Society developed a classification and diagnostic criteria of all headache disorders. This system, which identifies common terminology, has gained acceptance as a common standard throughout the world (Evans & Olesen, 2003). Three of the most common types of headaches are migraine headaches, cluster headaches, and tension headaches. Clients are managed in the ambulatory care setting by the primary health care provider.

Clients with headaches are encouraged to keep a headache diary, which may help identify the type of headache they are experiencing. They need to understand the importance of notifying their health care provider if the severity, intensity, or nature of the headache increases or changes. Clients also need to report whether the headache is associated with unusual visual changes and whether the prescribed medication is no longer effective.

Migraine Headache

PATHOPHYSIOLOGY

A **migraine headache** is an episodic familial disorder manifested by unilateral, frontotemporal, throbbing pain in the head, which is often worse behind one eye or ear. It is often accompanied by a sensitive scalp, anorexia, **photophobia** (sensitivity to light), and nausea with or without vomiting. Clients tend to have the same clinical manifestations each time they have a migraine headache. Some may have to refrain from regular activities for several days if they cannot control or relieve the pain in its early stage.

Several theories have emerged regarding the causes of migraines, which involve vascular, genetic, neurologic (central neuronal hyperexcitability) and chemical factors. It is generally agreed that migraine headaches are mediated via the trigeminal vascular system and its central projections (Welch, Cutrer, & Peter, 2003). Blood vessels in the brain overreact to a triggering event, causing spasm in the arteries at the base of the brain. This response is followed by arterial constriction and a decrease in cerebral blood flow; cerebral hypoxia may occur. Platelets clump together and serotonin, a vasoconstrictor, is released. Other arteries dilate, which triggers the release of **prostaglandins,** chemicals that cause inflammation and swelling, and substances that increase sensitivity to pain. This theory is supported by the success of medications that affect 5-HT (serotonin) in the brain.

◆COLLABORATIVE MANAGEMENT
◆Assessment

Migraines fall into three categories: migraines with aura, migraines without aura, and atypical migraines. An **aura** is a sensation that signals the onset of a headache or seizure. In a migraine, the aura occurs immediately before the migraine episode. Most headaches are migraines without aura. The signs and symptoms of both migraines with aura and those without are listed in Chart 45-1. **Atypical migraines** are less common and include menstrual and cluster migraines. Kolb-Lucas describes the stages of migraine as:

- Prodrome phase, in which the client has specific symptoms such as food cravings or mood changes
- Aura phase (if present), which generally involves visual changes, flashing lights, or **diplopia** (double vision)
- Headache phase, which may last a few hours to a few days
- Termination phase, in which the intensity of the headache decreases
- Postprodrome phase, in which the client is often fatigued, may be irritable, and has muscle pain

The diagnosis of migraine headache is based on the client's history, and physical and neurologic assessment. Neuroimaging, such as magnetic resonance imaging (MRI), may be in-

---

CHART 45-1
KEY FEATURES of
Migraine Headaches

Phases of Migraine with Aura (Classic Migraine)
First, or Prodromal, Phase
- Aura develops over a period of several minutes and lasts no more than 1 hour.
- Well-defined transient focal neurologic dysfunction exists.
- Pain may be preceded by:
  Visual disturbances
  Flashing lights
  Lines or spots
  Shimmering or zigzag lights
- Pain may be preceded by a variety of neurologic changes, including the following:
  Numbness, tingling of the lips or tongue
  Acute confusional state
  Aphasia
  Vertigo
  Unilateral weakness
  Drowsiness

Second Phase
- Headache is accompanied by nausea and vomiting.
- Pain usually begins in the temple; it increases in intensity and becomes throbbing within 1 hour.

Third Phase
- Pain changes from throbbing to dull.
- Headache, nausea, and vomiting usually last from 4 to 72 hours. (Older clients may have aura without pain, known as a visual migraine.)

Migraine without Aura (Common Migraine)
- Migraine begins without an aura before the onset of the headache.
- Pain is aggravated by performing routine physical activities.
- Pain is unilateral and pulsating.
- One of the following symptoms is present:
  Nausea and/or vomiting
  Photophobia (light sensitivity)
  Phonophobia (sound sensitivity)
- Headache lasts for 4 to 72 hours.
- Migraine often occurs in the early morning, during periods of stress, or in those with premenstrual tension or fluid retention.

Atypical Migraine
- Status migrainous
  Headache lasts longer than 72 hours.
- Migrainous infarction
  Neurologic symptoms are not completely reversible within 7 days.
  Ischemic infarct is noted on neuroimaging.
- Unclassified
  Headache does not fulfill all of the criteria to be classified a migraine.

---

dicated if the client has other neurologic findings, a history of seizures, findings not consistent with a migraine, or a change in the severity of symptoms or frequency of the attacks. Neuroimaging is recommended in clients older than 50 years of age with a new onset of headaches.

◆Common Nursing Diagnoses and Collaborative Problems

Nursing diagnoses that may apply to clients with migraine headaches include the following:

- Chronic Pain related to chronic physical disability

- Acute Pain related to biologic and chemical factors
- Anxiety related to change in or threat to health status
- Hopelessness related to deteriorating physiologic condition

◆ Interventions

The priority for interdisciplinary care of the client experiencing a migraine is pain management, which may be achieved by abortive and preventive drug therapy, as well as nondrug measures. Many of the medications have significant side effects, contraindications, and nursing implications.

Drug Therapy. Drug therapy is prescribed to manage migraine headaches. Headaches that occur more frequently than two to three times a month require preventive therapy. Mild migraine headaches may be relieved with aspirin or acetaminophen (Tylenol, Abenol✱). The health care provider must take into consideration any comorbid medical conditions when prescribing medications. In general, the client is started on a low dose of medication that is adjusted upward until the desired clinical effect is obtained.

Abortive Therapy. Abortive drug therapy is aimed at alleviating pain during the aura phase (if present) or soon after the headache has started. These medications include ergotamine derivatives, nonsteroidal anti-inflammatory drugs (NSAIDs), triptans, and isometheptene combinations. A potential side effect of these medications is rebound headache, in which another headache occurs after the medication seems effective.

Acetaminophen and NSAIDs, such as naproxen (Naprosyn, Novo-Naprox✱), are usually effective for mild migraine headaches. The health care provider may prescribe antiemetics, such as prochlorperazine (Compazine), to help control nausea and vomiting. Often, metoclopramide (Reglan, Clopra) is administered with the NSAID to promote gastric emptying and decrease vomiting.

Ergotamine tartrate (Cafergot) is given at the start of the headache; the client may take up to six tablets in 24 hours. Dihydroergotamine (DHE) may be given intravenously (IV) or intramuscularly (IM), along with an antiemetic, if satisfactory pain control and relief of nausea are not achieved with other medications. DHE should not be given within 24 hours of a triptan medication.

The triptan preparations activate the 5-HT (serotonin) receptors on the cranial arteries, the basilar artery, and the vasculature of the dura mater to produce a vasoconstrictive effect. Sumatriptan succinate (Imitrex) is given or self-administered for acute migraine relief. It is available in tablets, as a subcutaneous injection, or as a nasal spray. Examples of other drugs in this category include rizatriptan (Maxalt), naratriptan (Naramig✱), zolmitriptan (Zomig), eletriptan (Relpax), almotriptan (Axert), and frovatriptan (Frova)—all available as tablets. For many clients, these drugs are highly effective for pain, nausea, vomiting, and light and sound sensitivity, with few side effects. Most are contraindicated in clients with actual or suspected ischemic heart disease, hypertension, and peripheral vascular disease or in those with Prinzmetal's angina because of the potential of coronary vasospasm.

Teach clients taking the triptan drugs to report chest pain or tightness to their health care providers immediately. Remind them to use contraception (birth control) while taking the drug because it may not be safe for women who are pregnant. Common expected side effects include flushing, tingling, and a hot sensation. Triptan medications should not be taken with selective serotonin reuptake inhibitor (SSRI) antidepressants or St. John's wort, an herb used commonly for depression.

Preventive Therapy. Unless otherwise contraindicated, the health care provider may initially prescribe an NSAID, a beta-adrenergic blocker, or a calcium channel blocker. Propranolol (Inderal, Apo-Propranolol✱, Novopranol✱) and timolol (Blocadren, Apo-Timol✱) are the only beta blockers approved for migraine prophylaxis, but others such as atenolol are also effective. These medications lower blood pressure and decrease pulse rate. Teach the client, especially older adults, how to assess vital signs and observe for beginning clinical manifestations of heart failure.

Calcium channel blockers may be used if beta blockers are contraindicated. Although they have fewer side effects than beta blockers, they are not as effective. Other effective medications to prevent migraine headaches include tricyclic or SSRI antidepressants, antiepileptic drugs, or riboflavin (vitamin B_2). The tricyclic drugs should not be used in older adults because they have a long half-life.

Studies are ongoing concerning the use of sustained-release niacin. Low plasma levels of serotonin have been implicated in migraine pathogenesis, and niacin may act as a negative feedback regulator on the kynurenine pathway to shunt tryptophan into the serotonin pathway, thus increasing plasma serotonin levels (Velling, Dodick, & Muir, 2003).

Table 45-1 lists commonly used medications for migraine headaches. This table is not inclusive; new medications are introduced on the market regularly.

🌿 **Complementary and Alternative Therapies.** Many clients seek complementary and alternative therapies as an adjunct to their medications because medications are

---

TABLE 45-1   Commonly Used Drugs for Migraine Headache

Nonsteroidal Anti-inflammatory Drugs (NSAIDs)	Ergotamine Preparations
■ Diclofenac	■ Ergotamine with caffeine (oral or suppository)
■ Ibuprofen	■ Ergotamine metered dose inhaler (MDI) or sublingual (SL)
■ Naproxen	■ Dihydroergotamine (DHE)
■ Flurbiprofen	
Beta Blockers	**Triptan Preparations**
■ Propranolol	■ Almotriptan
■ Timolol	■ Eletriptan
■ Metoprolol	■ Frovatriptan
■ Nadolol	■ Naratriptan
■ Atenolol	■ Rizatriptan
	■ Zolmitriptan
Calcium Channel Blockers	■ Sumatriptan tablets, injection, or nasal spray
■ Verapamil	
■ Nifedipine	**Opioid Analgesic**
■ Divalproex	■ Butorphanol
	■ Hydromorphone
Antidepressants	
■ Amitriptyline	**Investigational**
■ Doxepin	■ Cyproheptadine
■ Fluoxetine	■ Droperidol
■ Imipramine	
■ Nortriptyline	
Abortive Drugs	
Analgesics	
■ Aspirin	
■ Acetaminophen	

not completely effective. Some drugs do not offer any pain relief or are associated with unpleasant side effects. Yoga, meditation, message, exercise, biofeedback, and relaxation techniques are helpful for some clients. For example, at the beginning of a migraine attack, the client may be able to alleviate pain by lying down and darkening the room. The client may want both eyes covered and a cool cloth on the forehead. If the client falls asleep, he or she should remain undisturbed until awakening.

Several small studies have found acupuncture to be effective for migraine management for some participants (Melchart et al., 2003). The studies provide suggestive, but not convincing, evidence of the efficacy of acupuncture. Further research is needed to determine the role of acupuncture in migraine treatment

There is even less scientific evidence on the efficacy of herbs and other nutritional therapies in the treatment of headaches. However, a number of herbs are also used for headaches, both for prevention and pain management. Table 45-2 describes commonly used herbs for migraines. Some clients have found that eliminating tyramine-containing products, such as pickled products, caffeine, beer, wine, preservatives, and artificial sweeteners, reduce their headaches. All herbs and nutritional remedies should be approved by the client's health care provider before they are used.

Other clients have identified specific factors that trigger an attack (Chart 45-2). Remind clients to avoid these triggers to prevent migraine episodes.

Cluster Headache

PATHOPHYSIOLOGY

The **cluster headache,** also referred to as histamine cephalalgia, is less common than the migraine headache. It occurs six times more frequently in young adult men between 20 and 50 years of age than in women. The cause and mechanism of cluster headaches are not known, but have been attributed to vasoreactivity and oxyhemoglobin desaturation. Neuroimaging studies suggest that cluster headaches are related to hypothalamic hyperactivity. In a recent study, positron emission tomography (PET) scans and magnetic resonance imaging (MRI) demonstrated an increase in neuronal hypothalamic density and hypothalamic size in clients with cluster headaches (Franzini et al., 2003). There is no genetic or family link, diet has no effect, and the disorder is unrelated to personality type.

The pain of these unilateral (one-sided), oculotemporal, or oculofrontal headaches is often described as excruciating, boring, and nonthrobbing. The intense pain is felt deep in and around the eye. The headaches occur every 8 to 12 hours and up to 24 hours daily at the same time for about 6 to 8 weeks (hence the term *cluster*), followed by a period of remission for 9 months to a year. This episodic form is the most common, although there is a chronic form in which there may not be a remission for more than a year. The average duration of each headache is 10 to 45 minutes.

The pain may radiate to the forehead, temple, or cheek. It may also radiate, but to a lesser extent, to the ear, occiput, and neck. The temporal artery may be prominent and tender. Physical activity during the attack consists of pacing, walking, or sitting and rocking. A cluster is the only headache type in which this behavior occurs. During periods of remission, alcohol does not induce a headache (as it does during the headache period). The onset of the headache is associated with relaxation, napping, or rapid eye movement (REM) sleep.

The headache is usually accompanied by **ipsilateral** (same side) tearing of the eye, **rhinorrhea** ("runny nose") or congestion, **ptosis** (drooping eyelid), eyelid edema, facial sweating, and **miosis** (abnormal constriction of pupils). The ptosis may become permanent. There may be bradycardia, flushing or pallor of the face, increased intraocular pressure, and increased skin temperature.

◆COLLABORATIVE MANAGEMENT

Question the client about prescribed and nonprescribed drugs for both the prevention and the alleviation of the headache, as well as over-the-counter (OTC) drugs he or she may be taking. Interventions used by the client may include relaxation techniques, meditation, acupuncture, or massage therapies. Ask the client to recall a typical week's activities and any recent changes in lifestyle, and specifically to identify

---

TABLE 45-2   Commonly Used Herbs to Prevent Migraine Headaches

- Feverfew (*Tanacetum parthenium*)
- Bay (*Laurus nobilis*)
- Willow (*Salix*)
- Ginger (*Zingiber officinale*)
- Red pepper (*Capsicum*)
- Lemon balm (*Melissa officinalis*)
- Purslane (*Portulaca oleracea*)

CHART 45-2

CLIENT EDUCATION GUIDE
Factors That May Trigger a Migraine Attack

Teach clients to avoid the foods, medications, and other factors that may trigger a migraine attack.
Food and beverages (tyramine-containing):
- Alcoholic drinks: beer, wine, and hard liquor
- Aged cheese
- Caffeine found in beverages such as coffee, tea, cola
- Chocolate
- Foods with yeast such as pastry and fresh breads
- Monosodium glutamate (MSG)
- Nitrates (food preservatives), pickled or fermented foods
- Nuts
- Artificial sweeteners
- Smoked fish

Medications:
- Cimetidine (Tagamet)
- Estrogens
- Nitroglycerin
- Nifedipine (Procardia, Nifed ✷)

Other factors:
- Anger, conflict
- Fatigue
- Hormonal fluctuations, such as menstruation, pregnancy, and menopause
- Light glare
- Missed meals
- Psychological stress
- Sleep problems
- Smells, such as tobacco smoke
- Travel to different altitudes

bedtimes and waking times, which helps assess changes in activity or lack of continuity in the sleep-wake cycle.

NONSURGICAL MANAGEMENT

Drug Therapy. The health care provider typically prescribes the same types of drugs used for migraines. Because an informed person is better able to comply with the therapeutic plan, instruct the client in all aspects of the drugs being taken.

Other Pain Relief Measures. During the periods of attack, teach the client to wear sunglasses and to sit facing away from the window, which helps decrease exposure to light and glare. If the health care provider prescribes oxygen, 100% oxygen via mask at 5 L/min is typically administered with the client in a sitting position. The oxygen is administered for no longer than 15 minutes and is discontinued when the headache is relieved. Oxygen reduces cerebral blood flow and inhibits activity of the carotid bodies, which are sensitive to oxygen levels in the body. To prevent future attacks brought on by precipitating factors (bursts of anger, prolonged anticipation, excessive physical activity, and excitement), discuss their relationship to the onset of cluster headaches. The necessity and importance of a consistent sleep-wake cycle should also be explained.

SURGICAL MANAGEMENT. Surgical intervention may be recommended for clients with chronic drug-resistant cluster headaches. Invasive procedures, such as radiofrequency rhizotomy and glycerol rhizolysis, have been performed with varying success rates. Findings from a small clinical trial found that long-term high frequency electrical stimulation of the posterior hypothalamus reduced or eliminated pain (Franzini et al., 2003).

Tension Headache

Tension headaches are characterized by neck and shoulder muscle tenderness and bilateral pain at the base of the skull and in the forehead. They share many of the characteristics, precipitating factors, and epidemiologic factors as migraine headaches, and distinguishing between the two is very difficult. The International Headache Society criteria define tension headaches as head pain without associated symptoms. However, the classic signs of nausea, vomiting and photophobia, phonophobia, and aggravation of the headache with activity that are part of the diagnostic criteria for migraine may also occur with a tension headache.

Treatment of tension headaches includes non-opioid analgesics, such as acetaminophen, aspirin, and nonsteroidal anti-inflammatory drugs [NSAIDs]). Muscle relaxants may be included in the treatment plan and occasionally opioids may be needed. A study by Sparano (2001) found that the combination of ibuprofen plus caffeine was more effective in relieving pain than NSAIDs alone. Prophylactic treatment is similar for migraine headaches.

SEIZURES AND EPILEPSY

PATHOPHYSIOLOGY

A **seizure** is an abnormal, sudden, excessive, uncontrolled electrical discharge of neurons within the brain that may result in alteration in consciousness, motor or sensory ability, and/or behavior. A single seizure may occur for no known reason. Seizures may be due to a pathologic condition of the brain, such as a tumor. In this case, once the underlying problem is treated, the client is often asymptomatic.

Epilepsy is a chronic disorder characterized by recurrent, unprovoked seizure activity. It may be caused by an abnormality in electrical neuronal activity, an imbalance of neurotransmitters, especially gamma aminobutyric acid (GABA), or a combination of both.

Types of Seizures

The International Classification of Epileptic Seizures recognizes three broad categories of seizure disorders: generalized seizures, partial seizures, and unclassified seizures (Table 45-3).

GENERALIZED SEIZURES

Six types of **generalized seizures** may occur and involve both cerebral hemispheres. The **tonic-clonic seizure** lasting 2 to 5 minutes begins with a tonic phase that is characterized by stiffening or rigidity of the muscles, particularly of the arms and legs, and immediate loss of consciousness. **Clonic** or rhythmic jerking of all extremities follows it. The client may bite his or her tongue and may become incontinent of urine or feces. Fatigue, confusion, and lethargy may last up to an hour after the seizure.

Occasionally, only tonic or clonic movement may occur. **Tonic seizures** are characterized by an abrupt increase in muscle tone, loss of consciousness, and loss of autonomic signs lasting from 30 seconds to several minutes. The **clonic seizure** lasts several minutes and is characterized by muscle contraction and relaxation.

The **absence seizure** is more common in children and tends to run in families. It consists of brief (often just seconds) periods of loss of consciousness and blank staring, as though the person is daydreaming. The client returns to baseline immediately after the seizure. Left undiagnosed or untreated, the seizures may occur frequently throughout the day, interfering with work or school.

The **myoclonic seizure** is characterized by a brief jerking or stiffening of the extremities, which may occur singly or in groups. Lasting for just a few seconds, the contractions may be symmetric or asymmetric.

The **atonic (akinetic) seizure** is characterized by a sudden loss of muscle tone, lasting for seconds, followed by **postictal** (after the seizure) confusion. In most cases, these seizures cause the client to fall, which may result in injury.

PARTIAL SEIZURES

Partial seizures, also called *focal* or *local* seizures, begin in a part of one cerebral hemisphere. They are further subdivided

---

TABLE 45-3 Classification of Epileptic Seizures

Generalized Seizures
- Absence (formerly petit mal)
- Generalized tonic-clonic (formerly grand mal)
- Myoclonic
- Atonic
- Clonic
- Tonic

Partial Seizures (Focal/Local Seizures)
- Simple partial
- Complex partial

Unclassified Seizures

into two main classes: complex partial seizures and simple partial seizures. In addition, some partial seizures can evolve into generalized tonic-clonic, tonic, or clonic seizures (also called "secondary generalization") (Pena, 2003). Partial seizures are most often seen in adults and generally are less responsive to medical treatment.

Complex partial seizures cause the client to lose consciousness, or "black out," for 1 to 3 minutes. Characteristic behavior known as **automatisms** (the client is not aware of the behavior) may occur, such as lip smacking, patting, picking at clothes, and so forth. In the period after the seizure, the client may experience amnesia. Because the area of the brain most often involved in this type of epilepsy is the temporal lobe, complex partial seizures are often called *psychomotor* seizures or *temporal lobe* seizures.

The client with a **simple partial seizure** remains conscious throughout the episode. He or she often reports an **aura** (unusual sensation) before the seizure takes place. This may consist of a "déjà vu" (already seen) phenomenon, perception of an offensive smell, or sudden onset of pain. During the seizure, the client may have unilateral movement of an extremity, experience unusual sensations, or have autonomic or psychic symptoms. Autonomic changes include a change in heart rate, skin flushing, and epigastric discomfort.

UNCLASSIFIED SEIZURES

Unclassified, or **idiopathic,** seizures account for about half of all seizure activity. They occur for no known reason and do not fit into the generalized or partial classifications.

Etiology and Genetic Risk

Primary or **idiopathic epilepsy** is not associated with any identifiable brain lesion. Secondary epilepsy results from an underlying brain lesion, most commonly a tumor or trauma. Seizures may also be caused by:

- Metabolic disorders
- Acute alcohol withdrawal
- Electrolyte disturbances (e.g., hyperkalemia, water intoxication, hypoglycemia)
- Heart disease.

Seizures resulting from these problems are not considered epilepsy. Certain risk factors can trigger a seizure, such as increased physical activity, emotional stress, excessive fatigue, alcohol or caffeine consumption, or certain foods or chemicals.

Several alterations in gene function that lead to seizures have been identified (Hickey, 2003):

- Defective genes for channels regulate neuronal signals or the flow of ions in and out of the cells.
- Clients with progressive myoclonus are missing the cystatin B protein.
- An abnormally active version of a gene that increases resistance to antiepileptic drugs has been identified in clients who are unable to obtain seizure control with varied and multiple drugs.
- An abnormal gene that controls neuronal migration can lead to areas of misplaced or abnormally formed neurons or dysplasia.

Incidence/Prevalence

It is estimated that 2 million people in the United States have epilepsy, 80% of whom are able to control their seizures with medications. Prevalence of epilepsy in the United States is 0.5% to 1% (Hickey, 2003).

HEALTH PROMOTION/ILLNESS PREVENTION

It is important for clients with epilepsy to take their medication as prescribed and to notify their health care provider if they are unable to take their medications. A balanced diet, proper rest, and stress reduction techniques usually minimize the risk of breakthrough seizures. Encourage the client to keep a seizure diary to determine whether there are factors that tend to be associated with seizure activity. Clients should follow state law concerning driving a motor vehicle. The client's employment may need to be modified within applicable state and federal regulations.

◆COLLABORATIVE MANAGEMENT
◆Assessment

A complete description of the type of seizure activity that occurs and events surrounding the seizure assists in determining the best treatment plan. Obtain information from the client and family or significant others regarding the presence of an aura before the seizure (**preictal phase**). Diagnosis is based on the history and physical examination. A variety of diagnostic tests are performed to rule out other causes of seizure activity and to confirm the diagnosis of epilepsy. Typical diagnostic tests include an electroencephalogram (EEG), computed tomography (CT) scan, MRI, or positron emission tomography (PET) scan. Laboratory studies are performed to identify metabolic or genetic disorders that may cause or contribute to seizure activity.

◆Common Nursing Diagnoses and Collaborative Problems

Nursing diagnoses that may apply to clients with epilepsy include the following:

- Risk for Falls related to impaired balance
- Ineffective Coping related to uncertainty and inadequate level of perception of control
- Risk for Ineffective Breathing Pattern related to neuromuscular dysfunction
- Potential for Status Epilepticus

◆Interventions

Removing or treating the underlying condition or cause of the seizure manages secondary epilepsy and seizures that are not considered epileptic. In most cases, primary epilepsy is managed through drug therapy.

NONSURGICAL MANAGEMENT. Most seizures can be completely or almost completely controlled through the administration of **antiepileptic drugs (AEDs),** sometimes referred to as anticonvulsants, for specific types of seizures.

Drug Therapy. Drug therapy is the major component of management (Chart 45-3). The health care provider introduces one drug at a time to achieve seizure control. If the chosen drug is not effective, the dosage may be increased or another drug introduced. At times, seizure control is achieved only through a combination of medications. The dosage of medications is adjusted to achieve therapeutic blood levels without causing major side effects.

Before administering an AED, the client's laboratory values are evaluated for the most current blood level of the medication, if appropriate. Be aware of drug-drug and drug-food

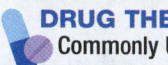

CHART 45-3

DRUG THERAPY for
Commonly Used Antiepileptic Drugs

Drug	Indication for Use	Nursing Interventions
Carbamazepine (Tegretol, Tegretol-XR, Carbatrol)	Partial, generalized tonic-clonic seizures	Monitor for headache, dizziness, diplopia or blurred vision, N/V, and leukopenia. Monitor CBC. Do not crush or chew sustained-release capsules.
Clonazepam (Klonopin)	Absence, myoclonic, and akinetic seizures	Monitor results of liver function tests.
Clorazepate dipotassium	Adjunctive management of partial seizures	Give with food; monitor blood pressure.
Diazepam (Valium, Apo-Diazepam✦), lorazepam (Ativan), Diastat (Valium rectal gel delivery system)	Status epilepticus	Monitor airway, breathing, circulation (ABCs).
Divalproex (Depakote), valproic acid (Depakene)	All types of seizures	Monitor for hair loss, tremor, increased liver enzymes, bruising, and N/V. Monitor CBC, PT, PTT, and AST.
Ethosuximide (Zarontin)	Absence seizures	Watch for N/V, skin rash, lethargy, and anorexia. Monitor CBC and liver function tests. (Drug used infrequently.)
Felbamate (Felbatol)	Adjunctive therapy for intractable complex partial seizures	Note that aplastic anemia and liver failure are major sequelae of treatment. Client must sign consent for use, acknowledging risk for aplastic anemia and liver failure. Monitor CBC. Monitor liver function tests. Watch for anorexia and weight loss.
Gabapentin (Neurontin)	Partial seizures	Watch for increased appetite and weight gain. Monitor for ataxia, irritability, dizziness, and fatigue.
Lamotrigine (Lamictal)	Partial seizures	Watch for diplopia, headaches, dizziness, drowsiness, ataxia, N/V, and life-threatening rash when given with valproic acid.
Levetiracetam (Keppra)	Adjunct management of partial seizures	Monitor renal function carefully. Notify health care provider for gait or coordination problems.
Oxcarbazepine (Trileptal)	Partial seizures	Monitor for hyponatremia.
Phenobarbital (Barbita, Luminal)	Generalized tonic-clonic seizures, partial seizures	Note that this is less desirable than other antiepileptic drugs (AEDs) because of sedation. Be aware that overdose can be fatal. Monitor for drowsiness, sleep disturbances, cognitive impairment, and depression.
Phenytoin (Dilantin), fosphenytoin (Cerebyx)	All types, except absence, myoclonic, and atonic seizures; for status epilepticus	Monitor for gastric distress, gingival hyperplasia, anemia, ataxia, and nystagmus. Check CBC and calcium levels. For IV phenytoin, flush catheter with saline before and after administration. For fosphenytoin, use phenytoin equivalent for dosing.
Primidone (Mysoline, Sertan✦)	Partial seizures, generalized tonic-clonic seizures	Monitor for vertigo and lethargy. Watch for drug interactions with phenobarbital and isoniazid.
Tiagabine (Gabitril)	Partial seizures	Monitor for dizziness, weakness, nervousness, psychomotor slowing, nystagmus, and paresthesias. Administer with food.
Topiramate (Topamax)	Adjunctive therapy for intractable partial seizures	Monitor for ataxia, confusion, dizziness, and fatigue. Be aware of increased risk for renal calculi.
Valproate (Depakote), valproate sodium injection (Depacon)	Simple and complex absence seizures Adjunct therapy for partial complex and generalized tonic-clonic seizures	Monitor for hair loss, tremor, increased liver enzymes, bruising, and N/V. Monitor CBC, PT, PTT, AST.
Zonisamide (Zonegran)	Adjunctive therapy for partial seizures	Monitor CBC, platelets, and renal function. Assess mental status, especially memory.

⚠️ *Med Error Alert! Do not confuse Keppra with Kaletra, an antiretroviral drug used to treat HIV.*

N/V, Nausea and vomiting; *CBC*, complete blood count; *PT*, prothrombin time; *PTT*, partial thromboplastin time; *AST*, aspartate aminotransferase.

CHART 45-4

CLIENT EDUCATION GUIDE
Instructions for the Client with Epilepsy

- Avoid alcohol consumption and excessive fatigue.
- Do not take any medication, including over-the-counter drugs, without asking your health care provider.
- Wear a medical alert bracelet or necklace or carry ID indicating epilepsy.
- Contact the Epilepsy Foundation of America or other organized epilepsy group.
- Investigate your local state laws covering driving and operating machinery.
- Medication information:
  Name, dosage, time of administration
  Actions to take if side effects occur
  Importance of taking as prescribed and not missing a dose
  What to do if a medication is missed or cannot be taken
  Importance of having blood drawn for therapeutic levels
- Instruct family member or significant other on care of client during and after a seizure, including when to call health care provider or emergency medical services (911).

CHART 45-5

BEST PRACTICE for
Care of the Client During a Tonic-Clonic or Complete Partial Seizure

- Protect the client from injury.
- Do not force anything into the client's mouth.
- Turn the client to the side.
- Loosen any restrictive clothing the client is wearing.
- Maintain the client's airway and suction as needed.
- Do not restrain the client; guide the client's movements if necessary.
- At the completion of the seizure:
  Take the client's vital signs.
  Perform neurologic checks.
  Keep the client on his or her side.
  Allow the client to rest.
  Document the seizure (see Chart 45-6).

interactions. Medications need to be taken on time to maintain therapeutic blood levels and maximal effectiveness. Instruct the client to avoid drugs and foods that might interfere with the absorption or metabolism of the AED. For instance, warfarin (Coumadin, Warfilone✱) should not be given with phenytoin (Dilantin). Document side and adverse effects of the prescribed medications and report to the health care provider.

Client and Family Education. An educational program must be provided for the client and family (Chart 45-4). Ask them what they understand about the disorder and correct any misinformation. As new information is presented, be sure that the client and family are able to understand it.

Emphasize that antiepileptic drugs (AEDs) must not be stopped even if the seizures have stopped. Discontinuing AEDs can lead to the recurrence of seizures or the life-threatening complication of status epilepticus (discussed later). Some clients may stop taking their medications simply because they do not have the money to purchase them. Refer limited-income clients to the social services department for financial assistance or to a case manager to locate other resources.

All states prohibit discrimination against people who have epilepsy. Clients who work in occupations in which a seizure might cause serious harm to themselves or others (e.g., construction workers, operators of dangerous equipment, pilots, railroad engineers) may need to find alternative employment. They may need to curtail or modify strenuous or potentially dangerous physical activity to avoid harm, although this varies with the individual. Various local state and federal agencies can help with finances, living arrangements, and vocational rehabilitation.

Seizure Precautions. Precautions are taken to prevent the client from injury if a seizure occurs. **Seizure precautions** vary, depending on health care agency policy. In most agencies it is recommended that oxygen and suctioning equipment with an airway be readily available. It is also appropriate to insert a saline lock in hospitalized clients who do not have an IV access and are at significant risk for generalized tonic-clonic seizures. The saline lock provides ready access if IV medication must be given to stop the seizure.

Although side rails are rarely the source of significant injury, they should be in the "up" position at all times. The use of padded side rails is controversial as to whether they maintain safety. Padded side rails may embarrass the client and the family. Keep the bed in the lowest position in case the client falls out of bed.

Padded tongue blades do not belong at the bedside and should never be inserted into the client's mouth after a seizure begins, because the jaw may clench down as soon as the seizure begins! Forcing a tongue blade or airway into the mouth is more likely to chip the teeth and increase the risk of aspiration of tooth fragments than it is to prevent the client from biting the tongue. Furthermore, improper placement of a padded tongue blade can obstruct the airway.

Seizure Management. The actions taken during a seizure should be appropriate for the type of seizure (Chart 45-5). For example, for a simple partial seizure, observe the client and document the time that the seizure lasted. Direct the client engaged in activities away from the activity to prevent injury. Turn the client on the side during a generalized tonic-clonic or complex partial seizure because he or she may lose consciousness. If possible, turn the client's head to the side to prevent aspiration and allow secretions to drain. Remove any objects that might injure the client.

It is not unusual for the client to become cyanotic during a generalized tonic-clonic seizure. The cyanosis is generally self-limiting, and no treatment is needed. Some health care providers prefer to give the high-risk client (e.g., older adult; critically ill or debilitated client) oxygen by nasal cannula or face mask during the postictal phase. He or she is not restrained, because this may cause injury and may exacerbate the situation, causing more seizure activity. However, the client with atonic seizures may benefit from wearing a protective vest to keep from falling when sitting in a chair. Follow institutional policy and procedures for use of a protective vest. For any type of seizure, careful observation of the seizure and documentation of assessment findings must be done (Chart 45-6).

Emergency Care: Acute Seizure and Status Epilepticus Management. Seizures occurring in greater intensity, number, or length than the client's usual seizures are considered **acute.** They may also appear in clusters that are different from the client's typical seizure pattern. Treatment with lorazepam (Ativan, Apo-Lorazepam✱) or diazepam (Valium, Meval✱, Vivol✱, Diastat [rectal diazepam

CHART 45-6

FOCUSED ASSESSMENT of
Seizures: Nursing Observations and Documentation

How often the seizures occur
- Date, time, and duration of the seizure

Description of each seizure
- Tonic, clonic
- Staring spells, blinking
- Automatism

Whether more than one type of seizure occurs

Sequence of seizure progression
- Where the seizure began
- Body part first involved

Observations during the seizure
- Changes in pupil size and any eye deviation
- Level of consciousness
- Presence of apnea, cyanosis, and salivation
- Incontinence of bowel or bladder during the seizure
- Eye fluttering
- Movement and progression of motor activity
- Lip smacking or other automatism
- Tongue or lip biting

How long the seizures last

When the last seizure took place

Whether the seizures are preceded by an aura
- Dizziness, numbness, or visual disturbances
- Gustatory (taste) or auditory disturbances

What the client does after the seizure
- Feels drowsy or weak
- May resume normal behavior
- May be unaware that the seizure took place

How long it takes for the client to return to preseizure status

CHART 45-7

BEST PRACTICE for
Emergency Care for the Client in Status Epilepticus

EMERGENCY CARE

- Support the ABCs (*airway*, *breathing*, and *circulation*).
- Prepare for possible intubation.
- Protect the client from injury.
- Do not force an airway into the client's mouth; provide oxygen via nasal cannula or face mask.
- Establish IV access if not already available, and begin infusion of 0.9% saline.
- Administer drugs as prescribed, and observe the client for side effects or signs of toxicity from the medications.
- Monitor vital signs and cardiac rhythm.

Medications used to treat status epilepticus include IV diazepam (Valium, Meval✶, Vivol✶), IV lorazepam (Ativan, Apo-Lorazepam✶), or diazepam rectal gel (Diastat), to stop motor movement. Lorazepam is typically the drug of choice and is given 2 to 4 mg over a 2-minute period. This procedure may be repeated, if necessary, until a total of 8 mg is reached. To prevent recurrence or arrest tonic-clonic seizures, a loading dose of phenytoin (Dilantin) or fosphenytoin (Cerebyx) is prescribed.

Initially, phenytoin is administered at no more than 50 mg/min using an infusion pump. Additional doses of 100 mg/min may be necessary. An alternative to phenytoin is fosphenytoin, a water-soluble phenytoin prodrug. Fosphenytoin can be administered IM as well as IV, and is compatible with most IV solutions. It also causes less cardiovascular complications than phenytoin and can be given in an IV dextrose solution (Pena, 2003). After administration, fosphenytoin converts to phenytoin in the body. Therefore the Food and Drug Administration (FDA) requires the dosage to be written as a phenytoin equivalent (PE); 150 mg of fosphenytoin equals 100 mg of phenytoin. Fosphenytoin may be administered at a rate of 100 to 150 mg/min IV piggyback (Pena, 2003).

Serum drug levels should be checked every 6 to 12 hours after the loading dose and then 2 weeks after oral phenytoin has started. Fosphenytoin is not available in an oral form. Teach the client about the side and adverse effects of any AED that is prescribed (see Chart 45-3).

General anesthesia may be used as a treatment of last resort to stop the seizure activity. The nurse, physician, or clinical pharmacist monitors serum drug levels closely for the first 3 days after the start of the AED and thereafter as indicated.

SURGICAL MANAGEMENT. Clients whose case cannot be managed effectively with medication may be candidates for surgery, including vagal nerve stimulation (VNS) and conventional surgical procedures. VNS is a fairly new procedure that has been very successful for many clients with epilepsy.

Vagal Nerve Stimulation. Vagal nerve stimulation (VNS) is performed for control of medically intractable simple or complex partial seizures with or without secondary generalization. Clients with multifocal or bihemisphere seizure foci, who are not candidates for surgical excision (because this may result in severe neurologic deficits), and those in whom other, less invasive treatment options are not effective may also qualify for the use of VNS. The stimulating device is surgically implanted in the left chest wall. An electrode lead is attached to the left vagus nerve,

gel]) may be given to stop the clusters to prevent the development of status epilepticus. Phenytoin or fosphenytoin may be added (Gambrell & Flynn, 2004).

Status epilepticus is characterized by prolonged seizures lasting more than 5 minutes or repeated seizures over the course of 30 minutes. It is a potential complication of all types of seizures. The usual causes of status epilepticus include the following:

- Sudden withdrawal from antiepileptic drugs
- Infections
- Acute alcohol withdrawal
- Head trauma
- Cerebral edema
- Metabolic disturbances

Convulsive status epilepticus is a neurologic emergency and must be treated promptly and aggressively! Notify the health care provider immediately if this problem occurs, and establish an airway. (Intubation by an anesthesiologist, nurse anesthetist, or respiratory therapist may be necessary.) Administer oxygen as indicated by the client's condition. If not already in place, establish IV access with a large-bore catheter, and start 0.9% sodium chloride (Chart 45-7). The client is usually placed in the intensive care unit for continuous monitoring and management for several days.

Blood is drawn to determine arterial blood gases and to identify metabolic, toxic and other causes of the uncontrolled seizure. Brain damage and death may occur in the client with tonic-clonic status epilepticus. Left untreated, metabolic changes occur, leading to hypoxia, hypotension, hypoglycemia, cardiac dysrhythmias, or lactic acidosis. Further harm to the client occurs when muscle breaks down and myoglobin accumulates in the kidneys, which can lead to renal failure and electrolyte imbalance.

tunneled under the skin, and connected to a generator. The procedure usually takes 2 hours with the client under general anesthesia. The stimulator is activated by the physician to deliver intermittent VNS. Programming is adjusted gradually over a period of time. The pattern of stimulation is individualized to the client's tolerance. A typical amount of stimulation is 30 seconds on and five minutes off, although these time frames vary among clients.

The client can activate the VNS with a handheld magnet when experiencing an aura, thus aborting the seizure. Clients experience a change in voice quality, which signifies that the vagus nerve has been stimulated. They report a relief in intensity and duration of seizures and an improved quality of life. However, the exact mechanism for how VNS works continues to be studied.

Conventional Surgical Procedures. A small percentage of clients with epilepsy cannot be fully controlled with medications or VNS. When all other medication and treatment options are exhausted, conventional surgery may be indicated to improve the quality of life.

The largest group of surgical candidates includes clients with complex partial seizures of temporal lobe origin. Partial seizures of frontal origin and from other extratemporal sites may also be treated surgically when the clinical manifestations and diagnostic studies indicate an epileptic region in a resectable area.

Preoperative care is similar to that described for clients undergoing a craniotomy (see Chapter 48). Preoperative diagnostic tests include magnetic resonance imaging (MRI) and single-photon emission computed tomography (SPECT)/positron emission tomography (PET) scans as described in Chapter 44. An intracarotid amobarbital test (Wada test) and neuropsychological testing are also done. The Wada test assesses hemispheric lateralization of language and memory after intracarotid injection of amobarbital, a short-acting anesthetic. This procedure establishes the safety of surgery in terms of language preservation and memory. Neuropsychological testing evaluates memory, visuospatial function, language function, and intelligence quotient to identify deficiencies in a restricted brain region that might correspond to areas believed to be the epileptogenic region. It is also used to compare preoperative and postoperative cognitive functioning.

Clients with seizures that do not respond to medication may benefit from surgical excision of the seizure area of the brain. The procedure involves continuous electroencephalogram (EEG) recording, close observation, and in many hospitals, video monitoring of the client at all times except during personal care activities. After the seizure area is identified, electrodes are surgically implanted into the brain tissue to identify the extent of the focal area. This step is followed by additional continuous EEG and video monitoring at all times (except during personal care), as well as close observation by the nursing staff. The area is excised if it can be safely removed without affecting vital areas of brain function.

Anterior temporal lobe resection is the safest and most effective procedure for complex partial seizures of temporal origin. Multiple suboccipital transections done over all areas of seizure foci, as well as over other stereotactic volumetric radiofrequency lesions of the intracranial structures, may be performed.

The more traditional surgical approach, the **corpuscallostomy,** is used to treat tonic-clonic or atonic seizures in clients who are not candidates for other surgical procedures.

The surgeon sections the anterior two thirds of the corpus callosum, preventing neuronal discharges from passing between the two hemispheres of the brain. This surgery usually reduces the number and severity of the seizures, making them more amenable to more conventional drug therapy.

INFECTIONS

Meningitis

PATHOPHYSIOLOGY

Meningitis is an inflammation of the arachnoid and pia mater of the brain and spinal cord and the cerebrospinal fluid (CSF). Bacterial and viral organisms are most often responsible for meningitis, although fungal meningitis and protozoal meningitis also occur. Bacterial meningitis occurs most frequently; early detection and treatment are associated with a more favorable outcome. Viral meningitis is usually self-limiting, and the client has a complete recovery. It is not considered as serious or potentially life threatening. Regardless of the causative organism, symptoms are the same.

The organisms responsible for meningitis enter the central nervous system (CNS) via the bloodstream at the blood-brain barrier. Direct routes of entry occur as a result of penetrating trauma, surgical procedures, or a ruptured cerebral abscess. **Otorrhea** (ear discharge) or **rhinorrhea** (nasal discharge, or "runny nose"), which may be caused by a basilar skull fracture, may lead to meningitis as a result of the direct communication of CSF with the environment. The invading organisms migrate throughout the CNS via the subarachnoid space. The presence of the organism in the subarachnoid space produces an inflammatory response in the pia mater, the arachnoid, the CSF, and the ventricles. The exudate formed may spread to both cranial and spinal nerves, causing further neurologic deterioration.

Viral Meningitis

Viral meningitis, the most common type, is sometimes referred to as **aseptic meningitis**. It often occurs as a sequela to a variety of viral illnesses, including measles, mumps, herpes simplex, and herpes zoster. The formation of exudate that is common in bacterial meningitis does not occur, and no organisms are obtained from the CSF. Inflammation occurs over the cerebral cortex, the white matter, and the meninges. The susceptibility of the brain tissue to the virus varies, depending on which type of cell is involved. The herpes simplex virus alters cellular metabolism, which quickly results in necrosis of the cells. The coxsackievirus and echovirus families also may cause viral meningitis. Other viruses cause an alteration in the production of enzymes or neurotransmitters, which results in dysfunction of the cells and possible neurologic defects.

Clinical manifestations of viral meningitis include fever, photophobia, headache, myalgias, and nausea. Herpes simplex type 2 may cause genital lesions. A maculopapular rash is seen when the causative organism is an enterovirus.

Treatment is symptomatic. If genital lesions are also present, acyclovir may be prescribed.

Fungal Meningitis

Cryptococcus neoformans meningitis is the most commonly seen fungal infection that affects the CNS of clients with acquired immunodeficiency syndrome (AIDS). Fulminant invasive

TABLE 45-4 Common Bacteria That Cause Meningitis

- *Neisseria meningitidis* (meningococcal)
- *Diplococcus pneumoniae* (pneumococcal)
- Streptococci, group A
- *Staphylococcus aureus*
- *Escherichia coli*
- *Klebsiella*
- *Proteus*
- *Pseudomonas*
- *Listeria monocytogenes*
- *Haemophilus influenzae* (not as common due to immunization)

CHART 45-8

KEY FEATURES of
Meningitis

Decreased (or change in) level of consciousness
Disoriented to person, place, and year
Pupil reaction and eye movements
- Photophobia
- Nystagmus
- Abnormal eye movements
Motor response
- Normal early in disease process
- Hemiparesis, hemiplegia, and decreased muscle tone possible later
- Cranial nerve dysfunction, especially CN III, IV, VI, VII, VIII
Memory changes
- Attention span (usually short)
- Personality and behavior changes
- Bewilderment
Severe, unrelenting headaches
Generalized muscle aches and pain
Nausea and vomiting
Fever and chills
Tachycardia
Red macular rash (meningococcal meningitis)

fungal sinusitis is also a recognized cause of fungal meningitis. The clinical manifestations vary because the compromised immune system affects the inflammatory response. For example, some clients have fever and others do not. Almost all clients have headache, nausea, and vomiting and show a decline in mental status. Treatment is symptomatic and includes IV antifungal agents.

Bacterial Meningitis

Bacterial meningitis is a *medical emergency* with a mortality rate of about 25%. It is seen most often in fall and winter when upper respiratory tract infections commonly occur. The most frequently involved organisms responsible for bacterial meningitis include *Streptococcus pneumoniae* (pneumococcal disease), and *Neisseria meningitidis* (Table 45-4). An estimated 17,500 cases of acute bacterial meningitis occur in the United States each year.

Meningococcal meningitis is the only type of bacterial meningitis that occurs in outbreaks, and it is most likely to occur in areas of high population density, such as college dormitories, military barracks, crowded living areas, and prisons. The number of outbreaks on college campuses has been decreasing over the past few years because many states require students to be vaccinated against meningitis. A meningitis polysaccharide vaccine (Menomune) is available to prevent infection by certain groups of meningococcal bacteria.

Most often, the client has a predisposing condition, such as otitis media, pneumonia, acute sinusitis, or sickle cell anemia that increases the likelihood of meningitis. A fractured skull or brain, or spinal surgery may also contribute to the development of meningitis. Vulnerable populations include clients who are immunosuppressed, have immunocompromised disorders, or have infections elsewhere in the body, and older adults, especially those with chronic debilitating diseases

◆COLLABORATIVE MANAGEMENT
◆Assessment

A complete neurologic and neurovascular assessment is done to detect clinical manifestations associated with a diagnosis of meningitis or suspected meningitis as outlined in Chart 45-8.

PHYSICAL ASSESSMENT/CLINICAL MANIFESTATIONS

Presenting signs and symptoms of meningitis result from meningeal irritation and include headache, nausea, vomiting, and fever. The client may also complain of photobia and have indications of increased intracranial pressure.

Although nuchal rigidity (stiff neck) and positive Kernig's and Brudzinski's signs may be positive, newer research indicates that these sign are present in only 9% of client's with a definitive diagnosis of meningitis. Seizure, decreased mental status, or focal neurologic deficits may also occur, particularly in bacterial meningitis.

Assess the client for complications that may occur, including increased intracranial pressure (ICP) resulting from the presence of exudate, which can lead to hydrocephalus and cerebral edema. Left untreated, increased ICP can lead to herniation of the brain and death (see Chapter 48).

Seizure activity may be caused by irritation of the cerebral cortex. Because of abnormal stimulation of the hypothalamic area, excessive amounts of antidiuretic hormone (ADH) (vasopressin) are produced. This results in water retention and dilution of serum sodium attributable to increased excretion of sodium by the kidneys. This syndrome of inappropriate antidiuretic hormone (SIADH) production may lead to further increases in ICP (see Chapter 48).

The client's vascular status is assessed by:
- Observing the color and temperature of the extremities
- Determining the presence of peripheral pulses
- Identifying any indicators of abnormal bleeding

Septic emboli in the blood may block circulation in the small vessels of the hands and feet, leading to gangrene. Excessive fibrinolysis that occurs in bacteremia and infections from viruses, fungi, or protozoa may lead to disseminated intravascular coagulation (DIC). Vascular involvement of the cerebral arteries, veins, and venous sinuses may lead to seizures and hemiparesis.

LABORATORY ASSESSMENT

The most significant laboratory test used in the diagnosis of meningitis is the analysis of the cerebrospinal fluid (CSF). Clients older than 60 years of age, those who are immunocompromised, or those who have signs of increased ICP usually have a CT scan preformed before the lumbar puncture. If there will be a delay in obtaining the CSF, blood is drawn for culture and sensitivity and a broad-spectrum an-

TABLE 45-5   Cerebrospinal Fluid Findings in Bacterial and Viral Meningitis

Finding	Bacterial Meningitis	Viral Meningitis
Appearance	Cloudy, turbid	Clear
White blood cells	Increased	Increased
Protein	Increased	Increased, slightly elevated
Glucose	Decreased	Normal
CSF pressure	Elevated	Varies

CHART 45-9

BEST PRACTICE for
Care of the Client with Meningitis

- Follow ABCs (airway, breathing, circulation).
- Take vital signs and perform neurologic checks every 2 to 4 hours, as required.
- Perform cranial nerve assessment, with particular attention to cranial nerves III, IV, VI, VII, and VIII, and monitor for changes.
- Manage pain through drug and nondrug methods.
- Perform vascular assessment and monitor for changes.
- Give medications and IV fluids as prescribed, and document the client's response.
- Record intake and output.
- Decrease environmental stimuli.
    Provide a quiet environment.
    Minimize exposure to bright lights from windows and overhead lights.
    Maintain bedrest with head of bed elevated 30 degrees.
- Maintain isolation precautions per hospital policy (for meningococcal meningitis).
- Monitor for and prevent complications.
    Increased intracranial pressure
    Vascular dysfunction
    Fluid and electrolyte imbalance
    Seizures
    Shock

tibiotic should be given before the lumbar puncture. The CSF is analyzed for cell count, differential count, and protein. Glucose concentrations are determined, and culture, sensitivity, and Gram stain studies are performed.

Counterimmunoelectrophoresis (CIE) may be performed to determine the presence of viruses or protozoa in the CSF. CIE is also indicated if the client has received antibiotics before the CSF was obtained. To identify a possible bacterial source of infection, specimens for culture are obtained and Gram stains of the blood, urine, throat, and nose are performed. Table 45-5 compares CSF findings in bacterial meningitis and in viral meningitis.

Polymerase chain reaction (PCR) may be used to detect viral deoxyribonucleic acid (DNA) or ribonucleic acid (RNA) in the CSF. Specificity and sensitivity in diagnosing encephalitis are excellent, especially with herpes simplex virus (HSV). The test is rapid and noninvasive, replacing the brain biopsy for diagnosis.

A complete blood count (CBC) is performed, with attention to the white blood cell (WBC) count, which is generally elevated well above the normal value. Serum electrolyte values are also assessed with attention to the sodium value. Dilutional hyponatremia may occur secondary to syndrome of inappropriate antidiuretic hormone (SIADH), a complication of bacterial meningitis. A blood culture is always performed.

OTHER DIAGNOSTIC ASSESSMENTS

X-rays of the chest, air sinuses, and mastoids are obtained to determine the presence of infection. A computed tomography (CT) or magnetic resonance imaging (MRI) scan may be performed to identify increased ICP, the presence of a brain abscess, or developing hydrocephalus.

◆ Interventions

The most important nursing intervention for clients with meningitis is the accurate monitoring and recording of their neurologic status, vital signs, and vascular assessment. Other areas of nursing care are found in Chart 45-9.

Monitoring Neurologic Status. The client's neurologic status and vital signs are assessed at least every 4 hours or more often if clinically indicated. Assess for neurologic changes indicative of cerebral complications, especially increased ICP. The health care team provides interventions for the client with increased ICP as discussed in Chapter 48. The client is at risk for seizure activity, and care should be provided as discussed under Interventions (Seizures and Epilepsy), p. 951.

Complete cranial nerve testing is included as part of the routine neurologic assessment because of possible cranial

TABLE 45-6   Anti-Infective Therapy for Meningitis

Causative Organism	Anti-Infective Agent
Staphylococcus	Vancomycin Ceftazidime
Haemophilus influenzae	Cefotaxime Ceftriaxone
Streptococcus	Third-generation cephalosporins (ceftriaxone) Rifampin Vancomycin
Neisseria meningitidis	Third-generation cephalosporins (ceftriaxone) Other cephalosporins
Fungus	Amphotericin B Flucytosine Fluconazole

nerve involvement. Particular attention is given to cranial nerves III, IV, VI, VII, and VIII (see Chapter 44). A sixth cranial nerve defect (inability to move the eyes laterally) may indicate the development of hydrocephalus. Other indicators of hydrocephalus include the usual signs of increased ICP and the presence of urinary incontinence in the previously continent client. Urinary incontinence occurs secondary to the decreasing level of consciousness (LOC).

Drug Therapy. To avoid life-threatening complications, the health care provider prescribes a broad-spectrum antibiotic until the results of the culture and Gram stain are available. After this information is available, the appropriate medication to treat the specific type of meningitis is given. Table 45-6 lists some of anti-infective medications commonly used. The medication should begin within 1 to 2 hours after it is prescribed. The client's response to the medication is monitored and documented.

The client with bacterial meningitis may experience increased ICP, and seizure activity may occur. Medications used by the physician to treat these complications include hyperosmolar agents and anticonvulsants. Controversy exists as to whether steroids have any place in the treatment of adults with meningitis. It is, however, recommended for clients with S. pneumoniae (de Gans & van de Beek, 2002). People who have been in close contact with a client with *N. meningitides* have prophylaxis treatment with rifampin, ciprofloxacin, or ceftriaxone. Prophylaxis treatment with rifampin may be prescribed for those in close contact with a client with *H. influenzae* meningitis.

Monitoring for Complications. A complete vascular assessment during each nursing shift or more often, if indicated, is performed to prevent and detect early vascular compromise from septic emboli. This severe complication is most often seen in circulation to the hand. Assess the client's temperature, color, pulses, and capillary refill. If vascular compromise is left unrecognized and untreated, gangrene can develop quickly, possibly leading to loss of the involved extremity. The health care team monitors the client for other complications, including shock, coagulation disorders, septic complications (bacterial endocarditis), and prolonged fever.

Encephalitis
PATHOPHYSIOLOGY

Encephalitis is an inflammation of the brain parenchyma (brain tissue) and often the meninges. It affects the cerebrum, the brainstem, and the cerebellum. The incidence of encephalitis is 1 in 200,000 people (Hickey, 2003). A viral agent most often causes it, although bacteria, fungi, or parasites may also be involved (e.g., malaria). Viral encephalitis is almost always preceded by a viral infection. The virus gains access to the central nervous system (CNS) via the bloodstream, along peripheral or cranial nerves, or in the meninges (e.g., varicella zoster).

After the virus invades the brain tissue, it begins to reproduce, causing an inflammatory response. Unlike in meningitis, this response does not cause exudate formation. Inflammation extends over the cerebral cortex, the white matter, and the meninges, causing degeneration of the neurons of the cortex. Demyelination of axons occurs in the involved area because the white matter is destroyed. This leads to hemorrhage, edema, necrosis, and the development of small lacunae (hollow cavities) within the cerebral hemispheres. Widespread edema can cause compression of blood vessels, leading to a further increase in intracranial pressure (ICP). Death may occur from herniation and increased ICP.

Arboviruses

Arboviruses can be transmitted to humans through the bite of an infected mosquito or tick. The most common types of encephalitis caused by arboviruses are eastern or western equine encephalitis, St. Louis encephalitis, California encephalitis, and West Nile virus.

West Nile virus has gained attention in the United States because it has spread rapidly throughout the country. This infection is generally mild and usually the client is asymptomatic. The incubation period is 3 to 12 days after being bitten by an infected mosquito. Other sources of transmission include blood products, breast milk, or an organ transplant.

In most cases the client is asymptomatic or has flu-like symptoms. Diagnostic tests to determine the presence of West Nile virus include enzyme-linked immunosorbent assay and West Nile virus–specific IgM antibody in serum or cerebrospinal fluid (CSF).

> ### CONSIDERATIONS FOR OLDER ADULTS
> Older adults are more likely to have severe infections that can result in long-term residual fatigue and weakness, as well as death. Teach older adults to avoid areas where mosquitoes or ticks are likely to be, such as near rivers and lakes. When they are near these areas, instruct the older adults to wear long-sleeved shirts and long pants and to use insect repellent.

Enteroviruses

Echovirus, coxsackievirus, poliovirus, herpes zoster, and viruses that cause mumps and chickenpox are the common enteroviruses associated with encephalitis.

Herpes Simplex Virus Type 1

Herpes simplex virus type 1 (HSV1) encephalitis is the most common nonepidemic type of encephalitis in North America. Clients with herpes encephalitis often have a history of cold sores. Mortality rates for HSV1 encephalitis can be as high as 80%, whereas mortality for the other types is much lower (Hickey, 2003).

Amebae

Amebic meningoencephalitis is caused by the amebae *Naegleria* and *Acanthamoeba*. Both are found in warm freshwater areas and can enter the nasal mucosa of people swimming in ponds or lakes. The amebae may also be found in soil and decaying vegetation. Although this infection has not often been seen in the past, the incidence in North America is increasing, perhaps because the ponds and lakes are becoming more polluted.

◆COLLABORATIVE MANAGEMENT
◆Assessment

The typical client with encephalitis has a fever and complains of nausea, vomiting, and a stiff neck. Other signs and symptoms include the following:
- Changes in the level of consciousness (LOC) and mental status
- Motor dysfunction
- Focal neurologic deficits
- Fatigue
- Symptoms of increased intracranial pressure (ICP)

Assess the client's LOC using the Glasgow Coma Scale (see Chapter 44). The client may be lethargic, stuporous, or comatose. Mental status changes include acute confusion, irritability, and personality and behavior changes (especially noted in the presence of herpes simplex). Signs of meningeal irritation include the presence of nuchal rigidity, and motor changes may vary from a mild weakness to hemiplegia. The client may have muscle tremors, spasticity, an ataxic gait (postencephalitic parkinsonism), myoclonic jerks, and increased deep tendon reflexes. Seizure activity is not uncommon. Fever, nausea, vomiting, headache, and vertigo may also occur.

Cranial nerve involvement is exhibited by ocular palsies, facial weakness, and nystagmus. The herpes zoster lesion affects cranial and spinal nerve root ganglia, which is clinically manifested by a rash, severe pain, itching, burning, or tingling in the areas innervated by these nerves.

In severe cases of encephalitis, the client may exhibit increased ICP resulting from cerebral edema, hemorrhage, and necrosis of brain tissue. Monitor vital signs for indications of a widened pulse pressure, bradycardia, and irregular respirations. The pupils become increasingly dilated and less responsive to light. Left untreated, increased ICP leads to herniation of the brain tissue and possibly death.

◆Interventions

Nursing interventions for encephalitis are similar to those for meningitis, with the exception of drug therapy. Supportive nursing care and prompt recognition and treatment of increased ICP are essential components of management. A patent airway is maintained to prevent the development of atelectasis or pneumonia, which can lead to further brain hypoxia from inadequate amounts of oxygen in the circulating blood.

Unlicensed assistive personnel help and encourage the client to turn, cough, and deep breathe at least every 2 hours. Deep tracheal suctioning may be performed, even in the presence of increased ICP, if the findings of the respiratory assessment indicate that respiratory status is compromised, possibly causing cerebral hypoxia.

Assess vital signs and neurologic signs every 2 hours or more frequently if clinically indicated. Elevate the head of the bed 30 to 45 degrees unless contraindicated (e.g., after lumbar puncture or in the client with severe hypotension).

Acyclovir (Zovirax) is the drug of choice for the treatment of herpes encephalitis and is associated with a significantly lower mortality rate than vidarabine (Vira-A). Drug therapy is most effective if begun early, before the client becomes stuporous or comatose. This usually occurs within 4 to 6 days after the appearance of the initial neurologic symptoms. No specific drug therapy is available for infection by arboviruses or enteroviruses.

If there are permanent neurologic disabilities, the client with encephalitis is usually discharged to a rehabilitation setting or a long-term care facility. The client with minimal neurologic problems is discharged to the home setting.

PARKINSON DISEASE

PATHOPHYSIOLOGY

Parkinson disease (PD), also referred to as paralysis agitans, is the third most common neurologic disorder of older adults. PD has a large economic impact in the form of direct medical costs, as well as indirect costs, such as lost wages and decreased productivity. It is a debilitating disease affecting motor ability and is characterized by four cardinal symptoms: tremor, rigidity, **akinesia** (slow movement), and postural instability.

Motor activity occurs as a result of integration of the actions of the cerebral cortex, basal ganglia, and cerebellum. The basal ganglia are a group of neurons located deep within the cerebrum at the base of the brain near the lateral ventricles. When the basal ganglia are stimulated, muscle tone in the body is inhibited and voluntary movements are refined. The secretion of two neurotransmitters accomplishes this process: dopamine and acetylcholine (ACh).

Dopamine is produced in the substantia nigra, as well as in the adrenal glands, and is transmitted to the basal ganglia along a connecting neural pathway for secretion when needed. ACh is produced and secreted by the basal ganglia, as well as in the nerve endings in the periphery of the body. ACh-producing neurons transmit excitatory messages throughout the basal ganglia. Dopamine inhibits the function of these neurons, allowing control over voluntary movement. This system of checks and balances allows for refined, coordinated movement, such as picking up a pencil and writing.

Widespread degeneration of the substantia nigra leads to a decrease in the amount of dopamine. Dopamine produced in the adrenal glands is not available, because it is quickly metabolized in the body. When dopamine levels are decreased, a person loses the ability to refine voluntary movement. The large number of excitatory ACh-secreting neurons remains active, creating an imbalance between excitatory and inhibitory neuronal activity. The resulting excessive excitation of neurons prevents a person from controlling or initiating voluntary movement.

New evidence has found that because PD involves postganglionic sympathetic noradrenergic lesions, the disease seems to be not only a movement disorder with dopamine loss in the nigrostriatal system of the brain but also a dysautonomia, with norepinephrine loss in the sympathetic nervous system of the heart. This loss results in the orthostatic hypotension frequently seen in the client with PD.

PD is separated into stages according to the symptoms and degree of disability (Table 45-7). Stage 1 is mild disease with unilateral limb involvement. Bilateral limb involvement occurs in stage 2. In stage 3, the client exhibits significant gait disturbances and moderate generalized disability. Stage 4 is characterized by severe disability, akinesia (no initiation of movement), and muscle rigidity. The client with stage 5 disease is completely dependent in all activities of daily living (ADLs). Other classifications refer simply to mild, moderate, and severe disease.

Etiology and Genetic Risk

Although the exact cause of PD is not known, evidence suggests it is due to environmental and genetic factors. Endotoxin (lipopolysaccharide [LPS]), a common airborne environmental and occupational contaminate in agriculture and other industries, may be an environmental factor in the development of PD. Other factors that increase the risk of PD include rural living, well water consumption, and living near wood pulp mills.

There is evidence of a number of inherited forms of the disease associated with gene mutation. Recently, it has been

TABLE 45-7 Stages of Parkinson Disease	
Stage 1: Initial Stage	**Stage 3: Moderate Disease**
■ Unilateral limb involvement	■ Increased gait disturbances
■ Minimal weakness	
■ Hand and arm trembling	**Stage 4: Severe Disability**
	■ Akinesia
Stage 2: Mild Stage	■ Rigidity
■ Bilateral limb involvement	
■ Masklike facies	**Stage 5: Complete Dependence**
■ Slow, shuffling gait	

found that some clients with PD have an extra copy of a normal gene (alpha-synuclein [SNCA]) that causes too much protein to build up in their brains (Guttman, Kish, & Furukawa, 2003).

Incidence/Prevalence

According to data from the National Institutes of Health, 500,000 people in the United States currently suffer from PD with some 50,000 new cases identified each year. As the population ages, the number of those affected is expected to dramatically increase. It is estimated that males are affected more often than females. Symptoms typically begin between 40 and 70 years of age with a peak onset in the 60s. However, Michael Fox, a popular actor, was diagnosed with PD in his 30s.

HEALTH PROMOTION/ILLNESS PREVENTION

There is no known way to prevent or cure PD. However, researchers from the Harvard School of Public Health have found that regular users of nonsteroidal anti-inflammatory drugs (NSAIDs) had a 45% lower risk for Parkinson disease than nonusers (Chen et al., 2003). A similar decrease in risk was observed among participants who took two or more tablets of aspirin per day compared with nonusers, but not among those taking smaller amounts of aspirin. However, because of the gastrointestinal side effects of these medications and the need for additional studies, people with PD should not take these drugs unless under the care of their health care provider.

◆COLLABORATIVE MANAGEMENT
◆Assessment

Collect data related to the time and progression of symptoms noticed by the client or the family. The older adult, who may assume that these behaviors are normal changes associated with aging, may ignore early signs and symptoms, such as fatigue, slight tremor, and problems with manual dexterity. Other signs and symptoms are listed in Chart 45-10, which summarizes the clinical manifestations of Parkinson disease. The client assessment consists of checking for evidence of **rigidity,** or resistance to passive movement of the extremities. Rigidity is classified as follows:

- Cogwheel, manifested by a rhythmic interruption of the muscle movement
- Plastic, defined as mildly restrictive movement
- Lead pipe, or total resistance to movement

Rigidity is present early in the disease process and progresses over time. Observe the client's ability to relax a muscle or move a selected muscle group.

Changes in facial expression or a masklike facies with wide-open, fixed, staring eyes are caused by rigidity of the facial muscles (Figure 45-1). This rigidity can lead to difficulties in chewing and swallowing, particularly if the pharyngeal muscles are involved. As a result, the client may have inadequate nutrition. Uncontrolled drooling may occur. Some clients develop dementia later as the disease progresses. In addition to changes in voluntary movement, many clients experience autonomic nervous system symptoms, such as excessive perspiration and orthostatic hypotension. Orthostatic hypotension was originally thought to be a side effect of levodopa therapy. Evidence suggests

---

CHART 45-10

KEY FEATURES of
Parkinson Disease

Posture
- Stooped posture
- Flexed trunk
- Fingers abducted and flexed at the metacarpophalangeal joint
- Wrist slightly dorsiflexed

Gait
- Slow and shuffling
- Short, hesitant steps
- Propulsive gait
- Difficulty stopping quickly

Motor
- Bradykinesia
- Akinesia
- Tremors
- "Pill-rolling" movement
- Masklike facies
- Difficulty chewing and swallowing
- Uncontrolled drooling, especially at night
- Fatigue
- Difficulty getting in and out of bed
- Little arm swinging when walking
- Change in handwriting (micrographia, or gets smaller)

Speech
- Soft, low-pitched voice
- **Dysarthria** (slurred speech)
- **Echolalia** (automatic repetition of what another person says) and repetition of sentences
- Change in voice volume, phonation, or articulation

Autonomic dysfunction
- Orthostatic hypotension
- Excessive perspiration
- Oily skin
- Seborrhea
- Flushing
- Changes in skin texture
- Blepharospasm (eyelid spasm)

Psychosocial assessment
- Emotionally labile
- Depression
- Paranoia
- Easily upset
- Rapid mood swings
- Cognitive impairments (i.e., dementia)
- Delayed reaction time
- Sleep disturbances

---

that it is related to baroreflex failure and loss of sympathetic innervation, most noticeably in the heart.

The diagnosis of PD is made on the basis of the clinical findings and after other neurologic diseases are eliminated as possibilities. There are no specific diagnostic tests. Analysis of cerebrospinal fluid (CSF) may show a decrease in dopamine levels, although the results of other studies are usually normal.

◆Common Nursing Diagnoses and Collaborative Problems

Nursing diagnoses that may apply to clients with Parkinson disease include the following:

- Impaired Physical Mobility related to neuromuscular impairment
- Risk for Falls related to decreased lower extremity strength and orthostatic hypotension
- Risk for Self-Care Deficit related to neuromuscular impairment

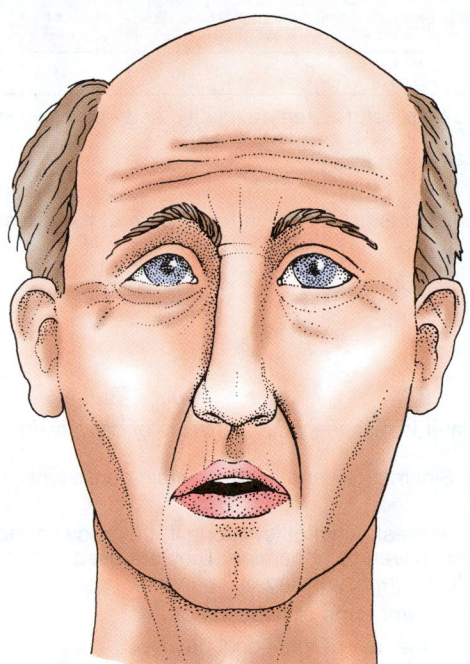

Figure 45-1 ■ The masklike facial expression typical of clients with Parkinson disease.

CHART 45-11

BEST PRACTICE for
Care of the Client with Parkinson Disease

- Administer medications promptly on schedule to maintain continuous therapeutic drug levels.
- Monitor for side effects of medications, especially orthostatic hypotension, hallucinations, and acute confusional state (delirium).
- Collaborate with physical and occupational therapists to keep the client as mobile and as independent as possible in activities of daily living (ADLs).
- Allow the client time to perform ADLs and mobility skills.
- Implement interventions to prevent complications of immobility, such as constipation, pressure ulcers, and contractures.
- Schedule appointments and activities late in the morning to prevent rushing the client, or schedule them at the time of the client's optimal level of functioning.
- Teach the client to speak slowly and clearly; use alternative communication methods, such as a communication board; refer to speech-language pathologist.
- Monitor the client's ability to eat and swallow; monitor actual food and fluid intake; collaborate with dietitian.
- Provide high-protein, high-calorie foods or supplements to maintain weight.
- Recognize that Parkinson disease affects the client's body image; focus on the client's strengths.
- Assess for depression and anxiety.

- Risk for Impaired Verbal Communication related to physiologic conditions
- Chronic Confusion related to dementia
- Risk for Imbalanced Nutrition: Less Than Body Requirements related to inability to ingest food due to biologic factors

◆Interventions

In addition to the physician and nurse practitioner, the registered nurse, physical or occupational therapist, speech-language pathologist, and social worker collaborate with the client and family to develop an interdisciplinary treatment plan. In some cases, palliative surgery may be performed to assist the client in remaining mobile for as long as possible. Chart 45-11 summarizes best practices for nursing management of the client with PD.

NONSURGICAL MANAGEMENT. Drug therapy is an essential part of management, which decreases signs and symptoms and allows the client to provide self-care and have a reasonable quality of life.

Drug Therapy. Medications are prescribed to treat the symptoms of PD with the goal of maximizing the client's functional abilities. An equally important goal is to prescribe medications with minimal long-term side effects. Many questions and controversies remain about which drugs to use, when to start therapy, and how to prevent complications. Medication administration is closely monitored, and the health care provider adjusts the dosage or changes the medication as the client's condition warrants. Teach the client and family how to monitor for and report side effects of medications. See Table 45-8 for more information on drug therapy.

Older Drugs. Anticholinergic drugs benefit the client whose primary symptom is tremor. The health care provider prescribes anticholinergic drugs less frequently to the older adult because they often cause confusion or other cognitive deficits. Amantadine (Symmetrel) may be prescribed as the first line of treatment to younger clients when tremor is the main problem (Guttman, Kish, & Furukawa, 2003). Selegiline (Carbex, Eldepryl, Novo-Selegiline✱) may be prescribed to confer mild, symptomatic benefit before initiating dopaminergics in the treatment of PD.

Dopamine agonists stimulate dopamine receptors and are typically the most effective during the first 3 to 5 years of use. The benefit of these agents is the less frequent incidents of **dyskinesias** (problems with movement) and **"wearing off" phenomenon** (loss of response to the medication), which is characterized by periods of good mobility ("on") alternating with periods of poor mobility ("off"). However, dopamine agonists are associated with side effects such as nausea, postural hypotension, hallucinations, and drowsiness.

Levodopa (Dopar, L-dopa) and its combination with carbidopa (Sinemet) is the most efficacious treatment for PD, and all clients are on it at some point in the disease process. It may be the initial drug of choice if the client's presenting symptoms are severe or interfere with work or school. Both an immediate-release (IR) and controlled-release (CR) form of Sinemet are available, although there is no difference in reducing response fluctuations. The levodopa agents are less expensive than the dopamine agonists and are better at improving motor function. Long-term use leads to dyskinesia.

When the classic dopaminergics and anticholinergics fail or are no longer effective, bromocriptine mesylate (Parlodel) or pergolide may be prescribed to activate the release of dopamine. They may be used alone or in combination with carbidopa/levodopa (Sinemet). Some providers may prescribe bromocriptine mesylate early in the course of treatment. It is especially useful in the client who has experienced side effects such as dyskinesias or orthostatic hypotension while receiving Sinemet.

Amantadine (Symmetrel) is an antiviral drug that has anti-Parkinson benefits. It may be used early in disease to

TABLE 45-8 Medications Used for Parkinson Disease

Medication	Use

Anticholinergics
  Benztropine (Cogentin)
  Procyclidine (Kemadrin)
  Trihexyphenidyl (Artane)
	Older drugs are used to help control tremor, rigidity, and excessive sweating.

Selegiline (Eldepryl)	Monoamine oxidase inhibitor is used early in the course of the disease.

Dopamine agonists (given more often to younger clients)
  Bromocriptine mesylate (Parlodel)
  Cabergoline
  Pergolide (Permax)
  Pramipexole (Mirapex)
  Ropinirole (Requip)
	These drugs mimic dopamine.
	Do not give to older adults.

Levodopa combinations
  Carbidopa/levodopa (Sinemet IR)
  Carbidopa/levodopa (Sinemet CR)
  Carbidopa/levodopa/entacapone (Stalevo)
	These drugs are used later in disease when activities of daily living (ADLs) are impaired.
	Some clients take both Sinemet CR and IR to maintain consistent therapeutic blood levels.

Catechol O-methyltransferase (COMT) inhibitors
  Tolcapone (Tasmar)
  Entacapone (Comtan)
	These inhibitors block the breakdown of levodopa in the body so more can travel to the brain and convert to dopamine. They are used in conjunction with Sinemet and help prevent "wearing off" periods.

Amantadine (Symmetrel)	This drug is given to treat symptoms of "wearing off."

Investigational
  Coenzyme Q10
  Dextromethorphan glial-derived neurotrophic factor
	Coenzyme Q10 may slow the rate of functional decline.
	This factor is administered directly into the brain.

reduce symptoms. It is also prescribed with Sinemet to reduce dyskinesias.

Newer Drugs. Catechol O-methyltransferase (COMT) inhibitors are enzymes that inactivate dopamine. Therefore COMT inhibitors block this activity, thus increasing the effectiveness of levodopa. For example, entacapone (Comtan) is used in combination with levodopa and carbidopa. Stalevo is a combination of levodopa, carbidopa, and entacapone. The benefit of these medications is that the client only needs to take one medication. However, it is not beneficial for those clients who need more specific dosages of the individual medication. Additional therapeutic strategies used for PD include the administration of monoamine oxidase (MAO) inhibitors, such as selegiline (Eldepryl), to reduce the metabolic breakdown of dopamine.

Studies are ongoing to search for more effective ways of delivering the best medications. For example, topical patches rather than pills may be available to treat PD. Neuroprotective drugs, such as coenzyme Q10, are currently in clinical trials and may replace traditional drug therapy for some clients.

Drug Toxicity. For the client on long-term drug therapy regimens, drug tolerance or drug toxicity often develops. Drug toxicity is evidenced by delirium (acute confusion), cognitive impairment, decreased effectiveness of the drug, or hallucinations. Delirium may be difficult to assess in the client who is already suffering from chronic dementia as a result of PD or another disease. If possible, compare the client's current cognitive and behavioral status with his or her baseline before drug therapy began.

When drug tolerance is reached, the drug's effects do not last as long as previously. The treatment of drug toxicity or tolerance includes the following:

- A reduction in medication dosage
- A change of medications or in the frequency of administration
- A drug holiday (particularly with levodopa therapy)

During a drug holiday, which typically lasts up to 10 days, the client receives no medications. He or she must be carefully monitored during this time.

Exercise and Ambulation. Nontraditional exercise programs, such as yoga and tai chi, may help elevate mood as well as improve mobility in the early stage of the disease. Early in the disease process, physical and occupational therapists should be consulted to plan and implement a program to keep the client mobile and flexible by incorporating active and passive range-of-motion (ROM) exercises, muscle stretching, and activity. The client is instructed to avoid watching his or her feet when walking to prevent falls.

Self-Care. The nurse and rehabilitation team encourage the client to participate as much as possible in the performance of self-care or activities of daily living (ADLs). The team makes the environment conducive to independence in activity and as stress-free and safe as possible. Occupational and physical therapists provide training in ADLs and the use of adaptive devices, if needed, to facilitate independence. The occupational therapist (OT) evaluates the client in all aspects of ADLs and determines the need for adaptive devices, for example, special utensils for eating.

Injury Prevention. Clients with PD tend to not sleep well at night. Some clients nap for short periods during the day and may not be aware that they have done so. This sleep misperception may put the client at risk for injury. For example, the client may fall asleep while driving an automobile. Therefore teach the client and family to monitor the client's sleeping pattern and discuss whether or not the client is safe to operate machinery or perform other potentially dangerous tasks.

Nutrition. A registered dietitian (RD) should see the client to evaluate his or her food intake. The client's intake of calcium, vitamin K, and other key elements is evaluated, especially in the client who is susceptible to falling or has difficulty swallowing. The RD takes into consideration the client's bowel habits and adjusts the diet if constipation occurs. If the client has trouble swallowing, a speech-language pathology consultation is made and an extensive swallowing evaluation is conducted. Based on these findings and the client interview, an individualized dietary plan is developed. Usually a soft diet or thick, cold fluids, such as milk shakes, are more easily tolerated.

Smaller, more frequent meals or a commercial powder, such as Thick-It, added to liquids may assist the client who has difficulty swallowing. The client is positioned with the head elevated to facilitate swallowing and prevent aspiration. The speech-language pathologist can be very helpful in evaluating swallowing ability and recommending specific strategies. Food intake is recorded daily or as needed. The client may experience weight loss as a result of altered food intake and the increased number of calories burned secondary to muscle rigidity. The client should be weighed once a week and adjustments made to the diet as indicated. As the disease progresses and swallowing becomes more of a problem, supplemental feedings become the main source of nutrition to maintain weight, with meals and other foods taken as the client is able to tolerate. (See Chapter 64 for additional interventions for clients with undernutrition.)

Communication. Collaborate with the speech-language pathologist if the client has speech difficulties. Together with the health care team, client, and family, a communication plan is developed. The client is taught exercises to strengthen muscles used for breathing, speech, and swallowing. The client is instructed to speak slowly and clearly and to pause and take deep breaths at appropriate intervals during each sentence. Unnecessary environmental noise should be eliminated to maximize the listener's ability to hear and understand the client. The client is asked to repeat words that the listener does not understand, and the listener watches the client's lips and nonverbal expressions for cues as to the meaning of conversation. The client is instructed to organize his or her thoughts before speaking and is encouraged to use facial expression and gestures, if possible, to assist with communication. In addition, the client should exaggerate words to increase the listener's ability to understand. If the client cannot communicate verbally, he or she must use alternative methods of communication, such as a communication board, mechanical voice synthesizer, or computer. The speech-language pathologist assesses the client's ability to use these devices before a decision is made about which method to use.

Psychosocial Support. Although not all clients with PD have dementia, impaired cognitive function and memory deficits are common. Clients may also experience changes in gait and tremors that are uncontrollable. In the late stages of the disease, they cannot move without assistance, have difficulty with articulation, have minimal facial expression, and may drool. Clients often state that they are embarrassed, and they tend to avoid social events or groups of people. They should not be forced into situations in which they feel ashamed of their appearance. They should be encouraged to undertake activities that do not require small-muscle dexterity, such as light, modified aerobic exercises.

A social worker may be able to help the family with financial and health insurance issues. The client and family may be referred to social and state agencies as well as support groups. The case manager and social workers collaborate on discharge planning issues as well as respite issues when they become necessary.

The client's abilities or strengths are emphasized and positive reinforcement is provided when he or she meets the daily goals. The client, the family or significant others, and the rehabilitation team mutually set realistic goals that can be achieved. Assisting the client with grooming and hygiene is also important in maintaining a positive body image.

The long-term management of PD presents a special challenge in the home care setting. A case manager may be required to coordinate interdisciplinary care and provide support for the client and family. Impaired mobility affects the daily lifestyle, including sexuality. The case manager or home care nurse uses a holistic approach to ensure that psychosocial, as well as physical, needs are addressed.

SURGICAL MANAGEMENT. Several options are available if surgery for the client with Parkinson disease (PD) is needed. Surgery is a last resort when drugs are ineffective in symptom management. The most common surgeries are stereotactic pallidotomy and thalamotomy, although newer surgical procedures are being tried.

Stereotactic Pallidotomy/Thalamotomy. Stereotactic pallidotomy can be a very effective treatment for controlling the symptoms associated with PD. First, the target area within the pallidum is identified via a computed tomography (CT) or magnetic resonance imaging (MRI) scan. Next, the stereotactic head frame is placed on the client. IV sedation is given, and a burr hole is made into the cranium; an electrode or cylindric rod is inserted into the target area. The target area receives a mild electrical stimulation, and the client's reaction is assessed for reduction of tremor and rigidity. If this result does not occur, or if unexpected visual, motor, or sensory symptoms appear, the probe is repositioned. When the probe is in the ideal location, a temporary lesion is made. If this is successful, the permanent lesion is made. The client is monitored in the postanesthesia care unit (PACU) for about 1 hour and is then returned to the inpatient unit for continuing postoperative care.

As an alternative to stereotactic pallidotomy, the surgeon may perform a **thalamotomy** for treatment of tremor through thermocoagulation of brain cells. This procedure is effective for a limited number of clients. Because bilateral procedures have increased surgical complication rates, only unilateral surgery is done to benefit the side of the body that is most affected by the disease.

Deep Brain Stimulation. Deep brain stimulation (DBS) is used when medications are no longer effective in controlling the client's symptoms. A thin electrode is implanted in the thalamus or subthalamus and then connected to a "pacemaker" that delivers electrical current to interfere with "tremor" cells. The electrodes are connected to an implantable pulse generator (IPG) that is placed underneath the skin in the client's chest, similar to a cardiac pacemaker. The client uses a magnet placed over the IPG to adjust the settings and to check the battery status.

Fetal Tissue Transplantation. Fetal tissue transplantation is an experimental and highly controversial procedure. Fetal substantia nigra tissue, either human or pig, is transplanted into the caudate nucleus of the brain. Preliminary reports suggest that clients show substantial clinical improvement in motor symptoms without dyskinesias after receiving the transplanted tissue. Long-term results are yet to be seen.

New therapies currently in clinical trials include the following:

- Gene therapy to replace lost gamma aminobutyric acid (GABA) inputs to the subthalamic nucleus and globus pallidus interna/substantia nigra pars reticulata
- Infusion of recombinant glial-derived neurotrophic factor directly into the brain to support at-risk nigro-striatal neurons
- Other stem cell research methods

ALZHEIMER'S DISEASE

PATHOPHYSIOLOGY

Alzheimer's disease (AD), also known as dementia, Alzheimer type (DAT), is a chronic, progressive, degenerative disease that accounts for 60% of the dementias occurring in people older than 65 years of age. It may also be seen less commonly in people in their 40s and 50s, which is referred to as early dementia, Alzheimer type, or presenile dementia, Alzheimer type. It is characterized by loss of memory, judgment, and visuospatial perception, and by a change in personality. Over time, the client becomes increasingly cognitively impaired; severe physical deterioration takes place and death occurs as a result of complications of immobility.

Structural Changes in the Brain

The brain of the older adult weighs less and occupies less space in the cranial vault than does the brain of a younger person. Other changes in the brain that occur with aging include widening of the cerebral sulci, narrowing of the gyri, and enlargement of the ventricles. In the presence of AD, these normal changes are greatly accelerated. Brain weight is reduced further, and there is marked cerebral atrophy. The cerebral sulci and fissures, as well as the ventricles, are enlarged more than those of persons of the same age without AD. The following areas of the brain are particularly affected:

- Precentral gyrus of the frontal lobe
- Superior temporal gyrus
- Hippocampus
- Substantia nigra

Microscopic changes of the brain found in people with AD include **neurofibrillary tangles,** senile or **neuritic plaques,** and granulovascular degeneration. Neurofibrillary tangles are a classic finding at autopsy in the brains of clients with AD. They consist of tangled masses of fibrous elements throughout the neurons. The same tangles and chemical changes are found in people with Down syndrome.

Senile plaques are composed of degenerating nerve terminals and are found particularly in the hippocampus, an important part of the limbic system. Deposited within the plaques are increased amounts of an abnormal protein called **beta amyloid.** Increased amounts of beta amyloid are being studied carefully for their role in the development of AD. Research is focusing on the following:

- Does beta amyloid disrupt the normal sodium, potassium, and calcium channels that are responsible for nerve function and signal transmission from one nerve cell to another?
- How does the overproduction of oxidants as a result of beta amyloid breakdown affect genetic material in the DNA of cells?

- What is the role of overproduction of immune factors in response to oxidation in the development of AD?

Although vascular degeneration occurs in the normally aging brain, its presence is significantly increased in clients with AD. Vascular degeneration accounts for at least partial loss of the ability of nerve cells to function properly. This pathologic change contributes to the mortality associated with this disorder.

Chemical Changes in the Brain

In addition to the structural changes in the brain associated with AD, abnormalities in the neurotransmitters (acetylcholine [ACh], norepinephrine, dopamine, serotonin) may occur. High levels of beta amyloid are associated with reduced ACh by as much as 75%, which leads to a decrease in the amount of acetyltransferase in the hippocampus. This loss is significant because the decrease in acetyltransferase interferes with cholinergic innervation to the cerebral cortex. This results in dysfunction of cognition, recent memory, and the ability to acquire new memories. The exact role of the reduction of neurotransmitters in the development of AD is not well understood.

Etiology and Genetic Risk

The exact cause of AD is unknown. Several theories and risk factors have been proposed: genetics, chemical imbalances, environmental agents, and immunologic changes. It is well established that age is the most important risk factor. Older adults tend to get sporadic AD rather than the familial genetic type.

There is little doubt that for many clients with AD there is a genetic predisposition to the development of the disease. The clients who seem to have this predisposition have familial AD (FAD). Studies of families are ongoing to determine the exact genetic pathway that is responsible. Most cases of early onset of AD are associated with mutations in genes (Table 45-9).

Early onset FAD seems to be related to an acceleration of beta amyloid plaque formation and apoptosis, which are caused by defective genes. Late stage AD research focuses on

---

TABLE 45-9 Alzheimer's Disease and Genetic Disposition

Generalized Seizures

Most cases of early onset of AD are associated with mutations in genes:

- Presenilin I gene on chromosome 14
- Presenilin I gene on chromosome 1
- Amyloid precursor protein on chromosome 21

Research shows an acceleration of beta amyloid plaque formation and apoptosis, a process by which cells self-destruct.

Late stage AD research focuses on the role of apolipoprotein, specifically:

- Apolipoprotein E (Apo E)-4 on chromosome 19 is a major risk factor.
  - The presence of two copies of Apo E-4 is associated with even higher risk of developing AD.
  - Some clients with Apo E-4 may not develop AD.
  - Conversely, some clients without Apo E-4 may develop AD.
- Apolipoprotein E (Apo E)-2 lowers risk of AD.

Other genetic research is focusing on the following:

- Chromosome 10 as a location for genetic factors, mutations in the proteins amyloid precursor protein (APP)
- Ubiquitin-B

the role of apolipoprotein E on chromosome 19. People with Down syndrome often develop dementia with characteristic features of AD. The importance of alpha-2 macroglobulin on chromosome 12 continues to be studied as another factor in the development of Alzheimer's disease.

Environmental agents, especially certain viruses such as herpes zoster and herpes simplex, and metal ions such as zinc and copper, have also been suggested as causes. Clients who have experienced a head injury may be more at risk for AD, and at an earlier age, than others.

Incidence/Prevalence

AD may affect anyone older than 40 years of age, although it occurs more often in those older than 65 years of age. The cost of care for clients with AD is tremendous, making it the third most expensive disease in the United States (see the Resource Management box below). Loss of wages and productivity in society adds to the increasing costs of health care.

HEALTH PROMOTION/ILLNESS PREVENTION

There are no proven ways to prevent AD. Current research activities are focusing on eating a balanced diet, eating dark-colored fruits and vegetables, using soy products and sufficient amounts of folate and vitamins B_{12}, C, and E. These substances have been associated with less risk of developing AD. Walking, swimming, and other exercise not only increase tone and muscle strength but also have been shown to decrease mental decline in AD as well as other dementias.

The use of ibuprofen and other nonsteroidal anti-inflammatory drugs (NSAIDs) has been demonstrated to reduce the risk of developing AD if taken in the years before symptoms develop (Zandi, Breitner, & Anthony, 2002). The exact mechanism of action is not fully understood. Unfortunately the long-term use of these agents, especially in the older adult, may result in significant complications such as a high risk of bleeding and gastrointestinal (GI) ulcerations. Therefore these agents should not be taken to prevent AD unless under careful health care provider supervision.

◆ COLLABORATIVE MANAGEMENT
◆ Assessment

The client with Alzheimer's disease (AD) often presents with cognitive impairment, although many other disorders, drugs, and environmental factors can cause changes in cognition as well. A thorough history and physical examination are necessary to differentiate AD from other, possibly reversible causes (Table 45-10). Obtain information from family members or significant others, as well as from the client, because the client may be unaware of the problems, denying their existence or covering them up.

The most important information to be obtained concerns the onset, duration, progression, and course of the symptoms obtained. Question the client and the family about changes in memory or increasing forgetfulness and about the ability to perform activities of daily living (ADLs). Further information obtained includes current employment status, work history, and ability to fulfill household responsibilities,

---

RESOURCE MANAGEMENT

THE CLIENT WITH ALZHEIMER'S DISEASE

Cost of Care
- Most clients live at home where care is provided by family and friends. The average out-of-pocket expenses for home care is $12,500.
- Average annual cost per client is $18,400 for clients with mild disease, $30,100 for moderate disease, and $36,100 for advanced disease, not including indirect costs such as productivity or wages.
- Overall cost of a lifetime of care for a client with Alzheimer's disease (AD) is staggering; average lifetime cost per client is more than $200,000.
- AD is the third most expensive disease in the United States, after heart disease and cancer.
- U.S. society spends at least $100 billion per year on AD.
- Lost productivity of caregivers (due to absenteeism, productivity, cost of replacement workers) averages $33 billion.
- Seven billion dollars is spent annually on health care and long-term care.
- Half of all nursing home clients suffer from AD; average cost per client for nursing home care is $42,000 per year, but cost can exceed $70,000 in some areas.
- In 1999 the federal government spent about $400 million for AD research.

Implications for Nursing
It is important for all health care providers to understand the staggering costs of caring for clients with AD, not only the monetary cost but also the psychological and emotional costs to the family and caregivers. Even with increased research funds, no cure for AD has been found. Care continues to be symptomatic; thus costs of providing care for clients increases as clients progress through the stages of the disease. Clients often require nursing home care and specialized equipment as the disease progresses.

Data from htttp://www.alzheimers.org.

TABLE 45-10 Causes of Cognitive Impairment in the Older Adult

Neurologic Causes
- Vascular insufficiency
- Infections
- Trauma
- Tumors
- Normal-pressure hydrocephalus

Cardiovascular Causes
- Myocardial infarction
- Dysrhythmias
- Heart failure
- Cardiogenic shock
- Endocarditis

Pulmonary Causes
- Infection
- Pneumonia
- Hypoventilation

Metabolic Causes
- Electrolyte imbalance
- Acidosis/alkalosis
- Hypoglycemia/ hyperglycemia
- Acute and chronic renal failure
- Fluid volume deficit
- Hepatic failure

Drug Intoxication
- Misuse of prescribed medications
- Side effects of medications
- Incorrect use of over-the-counter medications
- Ingestion of heavy metals

Nutritional Deficiencies
- B vitamins
- Vitamin C
- Hypoproteinemia

Environmental Causes
- Hypothermia/hyperthermia
- Unfamiliar environment
- Sensory deprivation/overload

Psychological Causes
- Depression
- Anxiety
- Pain
- Fatigue
- Grief
- Paranoia

KEY FEATURES of
Alzheimer's Disease

Early (Mild), or Stage I
- Forgets names; misplaces household items
- Mild memory loss
- Short attention span
- Subtle changes in personality and behavior
- No social or employment problems
- Cognitive impairment, problems with judgment
- Decreased performance, especially when stressed
- Unable to travel alone to new destinations
- Decreased knowledge of current events
- Loss of judgment
- Wandering
- Decreased sense of smell

Middle (Moderate), or Stage II
- Severe impairment of all cognitive functions
- Gross intellectual impairments
- Complete disorientation to time, place, and event
- Possible depression, agitated
- Physical impairment
- Loss of ability to care for self
- Visuospatial deficits
- Speech and language deficits
- Incontinent
- Wandering

Late (Severe), or Stage III
- Completely incapacitated
- Totally dependent in activities of daily living
- Motor and verbal skills lost
- General and focal neurologic deficits

including cleaning, grocery shopping, and preparing meals. Elicit a history concerning changes in driving ability, ability to handle routine financial transactions, and language and communication skills. In addition, document any changes in personality and behavior.

There is increasing evidence that olfactory dysfunction is associated with the development of AD (Peters et al., 2003). Therefore ask about changes in the ability to smell or changes in the sense of smell. The history taking concludes with a review of the client's medical history. Of importance is a history of head trauma, viral illness, or exposure to metal or toxic waste, as well as any family history of AD or Down syndrome.

PHYSICAL ASSESSMENT/CLINICAL MANIFESTATIONS

STAGES OF ALZHEIMER'S DISEASE. The clinical manifestations associated with AD can be grouped into three broad stages on the basis of the progress of the disease (Chart 45-12). The client does not necessarily progress from one stage to the next in an orderly fashion. A stage may be bypassed, or he or she may exhibit symptoms of one or several stages. Each client exhibits different disease stages and clinical manifestations. Consequently, some authorities now use broader terms, such as early (mild), middle (moderate), and late (severe) stages.

The primary focus of the neurologic assessment of clients with AD is to identify abnormalities in cognition, including language, personality, and behavior. Physical manifestations of neurologic impairment (seizures, tremors, or ataxia) tend to occur late in the disease process.

CHANGES IN COGNITION. Cognition refers to the ability of the brain to process, store, retrieve, and ma-

nipulate information. Therefore the client is assessed for deficits in the following abilities:

- Attention and concentration
- Judgment and perception
- Learning and memory
- Communication and language
- Speed of information processing

Typical symptoms experienced by the client include memory impairment, as well as new memory, and defects in information retrieval resulting from dysfunction in the hippocampal, frontal, or parietal region. Alterations in communication abilities, such as **apraxia** (inability to use objects appropriately), **aphasia** (inability to speak or understand), **anomia** (inability to find words), and **agnosia** (loss of sensory comprehension), are due to dysfunction of the temporal and parietal lobes. Frontal lobe impairment produces difficulties with judgment, inability to make decisions, decreased attention span, and diminished ability to concentrate. As the disease progresses, the client loses all cognitive abilities, is totally unable to communicate, and becomes less aware of the environment.

To assess the presence of cognitive impairment, the nurse or other health care provider can use one of several assessment tools. One of the most popular tools is Folstein's Mini-Mental State Examination (MMSE), also known as the "mini-mental." The MMSE assesses five major areas—orientation, registration, attention and calculation, recall, and speech-language (including reading). Figure 45-2 lists examples of the questions asked on this test. The client performs certain cognitive tasks that are scored and added together for a total score of 0 to 30. The lower the score, the greater the severity of the dementia. It is not unusual for a client with advanced AD to score below 5.

Although the MMSE is used frequently, the client must be able to read. For the client who cannot read, or for a quicker screening test, the SET test can be used, which is especially useful for the older adult. The client is asked to name 10 items in each of four categories: fruits, animals, colors, and towns (FACT). Other categories can be used, if necessary. The client receives 1 point for each item, for a possible maximum score of 40. Clients who score above 25 do not have dementia. Although this assessment is more comprehensive and easy to administer, it should not be used for clients with hearing impairments or aphasia. References describing other available tests to measure cognitive impairment may be found in the Selected Bibliography.

CHANGES IN BEHAVIOR AND PERSONALITY. One of the most difficult aspects of AD that families, significant others, and health care professionals cope with are the behavioral changes that can occur in advanced disease. The client is assessed for the following:

- Aggressiveness, especially verbal and physical abusive tendencies
- Rapid mood swings
- Increased confusion at night (**sundowning**) or in excessively fatigued clients

The client may wander and become lost or may go into other rooms to rummage through another's belongings. Hoarding objects such as washcloths is also common.

For some clients with dementia, emotional and behavioral problems accompany the primary disease. They may experience paranoia, delusions, hallucinations, and depression. These behaviors are documented, care is taken to en-

Orientation to Time
"What is the date?"

Registration
"Listen carefully, I am going to say three words. You say them back after I stop. Ready? Here they are...
HOUSE (pause), CAR (pause), LAKE (pause). Now repeat those words back to me." [Repeat up to 5 times, but score only the first trial.]

Naming
"What is this?" [Point to a pencil or pen.]

Reading
"Please read this and do what it says." [Show examinee the words on the stimulus form.]
CLOSE YOUR EYES

A

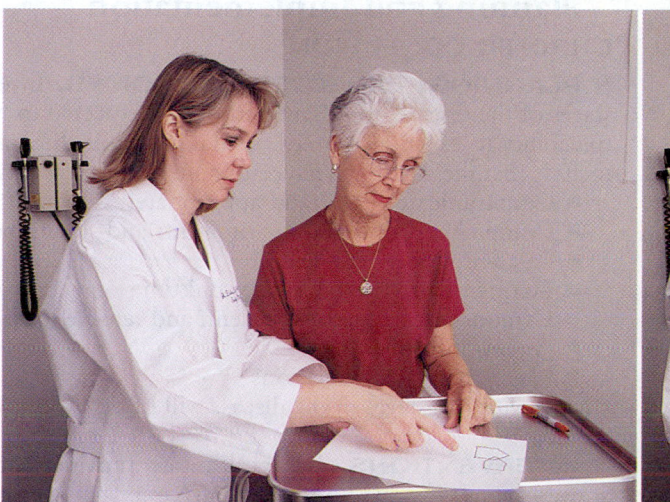
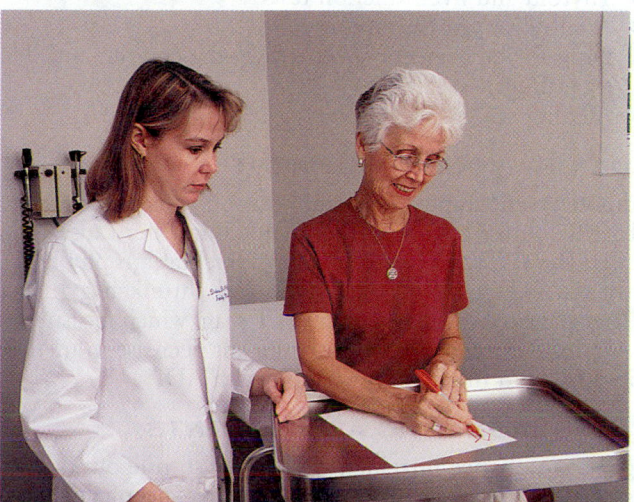

B

Figure 45-2 ■ **A,** Examples of questions that are asked on the Mini-Mental State Examination. **B,** Copying is one of the tasks on the MMSE. (**A** from Mini-Mental State Examination © 1975, 1998, 2001 by MiniMental, LLC. All rights reserved. Published 2001 by Psychological Assessment Resources, Inc. May not be reproduced in whole or in part in any form or by any means without written permission of Psychological Assessment Resources, Inc., P.O. Box 998, Odessa, FL 33556; (800) 331-8378 or (813) 968-3003. **B** from Seidel, H.M., et al. (1999). *Mosby's guide to physical examination* (4th ed.). St. Louis: Mosby.)

sure the client's safety, and the health care provider is notified. (Refer to a mental health/behavior health nursing textbook for a complete discussion of these disorders.)

Although drug therapy is not effective in treating dementia, certain drugs may help control the emotional and psychiatric manifestations, such as depression, anxiety, paranoia, and aggression associated with the primary disease.

CHANGES IN SELF-CARE SKILLS. Changes in the client's self-care skills that may be observed by the family, significant others, or nurse include the following:

- Decreased interest in personal appearance
- Selection of clothing that is inappropriate for the weather or event
- Loss of bowel and bladder control
- Decreased appetite or ability to eat

Over time, the client becomes less mobile and muscle contractures develop. He or she eventually becomes totally immobile and requires total physical care.

PSYCHOSOCIAL ASSESSMENT

In people with AD, the cognitive changes, as well as biochemical and structural dysfunctions, affect personality and behavior. In the early stage, clients often recognize that they are experiencing memory or cognitive changes and may attempt to hide the problems, deny them, or become depressed over the changes. Older clients typically attribute the changes to "old age."

As the disease progresses, clients begin to display major changes in emotional and behavioral affect. Of particular importance is the need for an assessment of the clients' reactions to changes in routine or environment. For example, a hospital admission is very traumatic for most clients with dementia. It is not unusual for them to exhibit a catastrophic response or overreact to any change by becoming excessively aggressive or abusive.

As clients become unaware of their behavior, the focus of the psychosocial assessment shifts to the family or significant others. The health care team assesses their ability to cope with the chronicity and progression of the disease and identifies possible support systems.

LABORATORY ASSESSMENT

No laboratory tests exist to confirm the diagnosis of AD. Diagnosis is made on the basis of brain tissue examination at autopsy, which confirms the presence of neurofibrillary tangles and neuritic plaques.

Genetic testing, specifically for apolipoprotein E (Apo E), may be helpful as an ancillary test (not a predictive test) for the differential diagnosis of AD. Testing for other genes that have been shown to predispose a person to AD has not become routine. A variety of laboratory tests may be performed to rule out other treatable causes of dementia or delirium, including the following:

- A complete blood count (CBC)
- Determination of serum electrolyte levels, blood urea nitrogen, and glucose
- Determination of vitamin B_{12} levels
- Determination of folate levels
- Thyroid and liver function tests
- A serologic test for syphilis
- Drug toxicity screening tests (over-the-counter and illegal drugs)
- Alcohol screening tests

RADIOGRAPHIC ASSESSMENT

Computed tomography (CT) and positron emission tomography (PET) may be performed to rule out other causes of disease. The CT scan typically shows cerebral atrophy and ventricular enlargement, wide sulci, and shrunken gyri in the later stages of the disease. The PET scan, which measures glucose in living cells, shows a significant decrease in metabolic activity in the brains of people with AD.

OTHER DIAGNOSTIC ASSESSMENTS

Magnetic resonance imaging (MRI) can also rule out other causes of neurologic disease. The electroencephalogram (EEG) shows slow-wave delta activity indicative of dementia in the second and third stages of AD.

To identify clearly the nature and extent of the client's cognitive dysfunction, the physician, usually a neurologist, administers several neuropsychological tests. The tests used depend on physician preference and the ability of the client to participate in testing. All of the tests focus on cognitive ability and may be repeated over time to measure changes.

◆ Analysis

COMMON NURSING DIAGNOSES AND COLLABORATIVE PROBLEMS

The following are priority nursing diagnoses for clients with Alzheimer's disease (AD):

1. Chronic Confusion related to Alzheimer's disease
2. Risk for Injury related to problems with orientation
3. Compromised Family Coping and Caregiver Role Strain related to the client's prolonged progression of disability and client's increasing care needs
4. Disturbed Sleep Pattern related to changes in sleep phases, anxiety, and/or depression

ADDITIONAL NURSING DIAGNOSES AND COLLABORATIVE PROBLEMS

In addition to the common nursing diagnoses, clients with AD may have one or more of the following:

- Impaired Verbal Communication related to aphasia, anomia, agnosia, and/or apraxia
- Imbalanced Nutrition: Less Than Body Requirements related to self-care deficit and/or anorexia

- Total Urinary Incontinence and Bowel Incontinence related to cognitive and self-care deficits
- Social Isolation related to personality and behavior changes
- Risk for Impaired Physical Mobility related to progression of disability
- Risk for Impaired Skin Integrity related to immobility and/or impaired nutritional status
- Self-Care Deficit (Total) related to cognitive deficit
- Risk for Other-Directed Violence and Risk for Self-Directed Violence related to behavior changes
- Hopelessness related to inability to control the progression of disease

◆ Planning and Implementation

CHRONIC CONFUSION

NOC **PLANNING: EXPECTED OUTCOMES.** In early stages of the disease, the client with AD is expected to have the ability to execute complex mental processes. Indicators include that the client will have noncompromised ability to:

- Communicate clearly and appropriately
- Comprehend the meaning of events and situations
- Be attentive and concentrate
- Be oriented to person, place, and time
- Demonstrate immediate, recent, and remote memory
- Process information
- Make appropriate decisions

Clients with late stages of the disease will cannot meet these criteria.

INTERVENTIONS. The health care provider should answer the client's questions truthfully concerning the diagnosis of AD. In this manner the client can more fully participate in the interdisciplinary treatment plan. Interventions are the same whether the client is cared for at home, in an adult day care center, in an assisted living center, or in a long-term care facility. The client with memory problems benefits from a structured and consistent environment. Many variables, including physical illness and environmental factors, can worsen or exacerbate the clinical manifestations of AD (Table 45-11). The client with AD frequently has other medical problems such as cardiovascular disease, arthritis, renal insufficiency, and pulmonary disease. Changes in vision and hearing may also be present. Treating and controlling these conditions optimize the client's functional abilities.

NIC **Cognitive Stimulation/ Memory Training.** The purpose of cognitive stimulation and memory training is to

---

TABLE 45-11 Factors That Can Worsen Alzheimer's Disease

- Stroke
- Subdural hematoma
- Space-occupying lesion
- Decrease in blood supply to the brain
- Myocardial infarction
- Dysrhythmias
- Hypoglycemia
- Impaired renal function
- Impaired hepatic function
- Infection
- Impaired vision and hearing
- Sudden changes in surroundings
- Pain and discomfort
- Drugs
- Physical restraint

reinforce or promote desirable cognitive function and facilitate memory (Chart 45-13). An individualized cognitive therapy program may provide some benefit to the client; however, reported clinical studies have not demonstrated its efficacy for early-stage AD (Clare et al., 2003).

Structuring the Environment. The health care team collaborates to identify conditions in the environment that can be modified to increase the client's ability to function. The two most important actions that are necessary for the client with AD are preventing overstimulation and providing a structured and orderly environment.

Preventing Overstimulation. Environmental distractions and noise should be kept to a minimum. The client's home (hospital or institution room) should not have pictures on the wall or other decorations that could be misinterpreted as people or animals that could harm the client. An abstract painting or wallpaper might look like a fire or an explosion and might scare the client. The room should have adequate, nonglare lighting and no potentially frightening shadows.

In addition to disturbed sleep, other negative effects of high noise levels include decreased nutritional intake, changes in blood pressure and pulse rates, and feelings of increased stress and anxiety. The client with AD is especially susceptible to these changes and needs to have as much undisturbed sleep at night as possible. Fatigue increases confusion and behavioral manifestations such as agitation and aggressiveness.

When a client is in a new setting or environment (hospital, assisted-living, or long-term care facility), the staff works with the admitting department to select a room that is in the quietest area of the unit and away from obvious exits, if possible. A private room may be needed if the client has a history of agitation or wandering. The television should remain off unless the client turns it on or requests that it be turned on.

Providing Consistency. Objects such as furniture, a hairbrush, and eyeglasses should be kept in the same place. A daily routine is established and followed as much as possible. The client's bedroom could have a communication board on which scheduled activities and other data to promote orientation are listed, such as the day of the week, the month, and the year. Pictures of people familiar to the client can be placed on this board.

Orientation and Validation Therapy. Changes in routine need to be explained to the client before the occurrence, repeating the explanation immediately before the changes take place. Clocks and single-date calendars also help the client maintain day-to-day orientation to the environment in the early stages of the disease process. For the client with early disease, **reality orientation** is usually appropriate. Family members and health care professionals should frequently reorient the client to the environment.

For the client in the later stages of AD, reality orientation is ineffective and often increases agitation. The health care team uses validation therapy for the client with moderate or severe AD. In **validation therapy,** the staff member recognizes and acknowledges the client's feelings and concerns. For example, if the client is looking for a deceased mother, ask the client to talk about what the mother looks like and what she might be wearing. This response does not refute the client, but also does not reinforce the client's belief that the mother is still living.

Promoting Independence in Activities of Daily Living. As the disease progresses, altered thought processes affect the ability to perform activities of daily living (ADLs). Encourage the client to perform as much self-care as possible and to maintain independence in daily living skills as long as possible. For example, in the home setting, complete clothing outfits that can be easily removed and put on (e.g., shirt, slacks, underwear, and socks) can be placed on a single hanger; the client selects from these groupings. When possible, the client should participate in meal preparation, grocery shopping, and other household routines.

The occupational and physical therapists provide a complete evaluation and assistance in helping the client become more independent. Adaptive devices, such as grab bars in the bathtub or shower area, an elevated commode, and adapted eating utensils, may enable the client to maintain independence in grooming, toileting, and feeding. The physical therapist prescribes an exercise program for the client to improve physical health and functionality.

Promoting Bowel and Bladder Continence. The client may remain continent of bowel and bladder for long periods if taken to the bathroom or given a bedpan or urinal every 2 hours or more often during the day, and possibly less frequently at night. The caregiver encourages the client to drink adequate fluids to promote optimal voiding. A client may refuse to drink enough fluids because of a fear of incontinence. Assure the client that he or she will be toileted on a regular schedule to prevent incontinent episodes.

When clients with AD are in the hospital or other unfamiliar place, they may get out of bed unassisted during the

---

CHART 45-13

NIC **INTERVENTION ACTIVITIES for**
The Client with Alzheimer's Disease

Cognitive Stimulation: *Promotion of awareness and comprehension of surroundings by utilization of planned stimuli*
- Offer environmental stimulation through contact with varied personnel.
- Present change gradually.
- Provide a calendar.
- Allow for rest periods.
- Use repetition to present new material.
- Present information in small, concrete portions.
- Use touch therapeutically.

Memory Training: *Facilitation of memory*
- Discuss with client/family any practical memory problems experienced.
- Stimulate memory by repeating client's last expressed thought, as appropriate.
- Reminisce about past experiences with client, as appropriate.
- Implement appropriate memory techniques such as visual imagery, mnemonic devices, memory games, memory cues, association techniques, making lists, using computers, using name tags, or rehearsing information.
- Provide for orientation training, such as client rehearsing personal information and dates, as appropriate.
- Provide for picture recognition memory, as appropriate.
- Encourage client to participate in group memory training programs, as appropriate.
- Monitor client's behavior during therapy.

NIC intervention activities selected from Dochterman, J.M., & Bulechek, G.M. (Eds.) (2004). *Nursing interventions classification (NIC)* (4th ed.). St. Louis: Mosby. No part of this work is to be altered without prior written permission from the Publisher.

night and fall while trying to locate the bathroom. In some hospitals, the side rails on beds are required to be up for all clients older than 60 or 65 years of age. However, if the client climbs over the side rail and falls, the injury is likely to be worse than if the bed had been left in the lowest position and the side rail left down (preferably the lower rail in a split rail system). Maintain an unobstructed path between the bed and bathroom at all times. For clients who are too weak to walk to the bathroom, a bedside commode may be used. (See Chapter 5 for further discussion on fall prevention.) Some clients may void in inappropriate places, such as the sink or a wastebasket. As a reminder of where they should toilet, place a picture of the commode on the bathroom door. Depending on written signs for identification is useless because most clients lose their ability to read as the disease progresses.

Assisting with Facial Recognition. As the disease progresses, the client may experience **prosopagnosia,** an inability to recognize oneself and other familiar faces. Encourage the family to provide pictures of family members and close friends that are labeled with the person's name on the picture. In addition, advise the family to reminisce with the client about pleasant experiences from the past. The nurse may also conduct reminiscence therapy while assisting the client with ADLs or performing a treatment or assessment. Referring to a personal item in the room may help the client begin to talk about its meaning in the present and in the past.

It is not unusual for the client to talk to his or her image in the mirror. This behavior should be allowed as long as it is not harmful. If the client becomes frightened by the mirror image, remove or cover the mirror. In some health care settings, a picture of the client is placed on the room door to help with facial recognition and to help the client locate his or her room. This picture also helps the staff locate the client in case of elopement (running away).

Promoting Communication. With the intervention known as **redirection,** attracting the client's attention before conversing helps with communication problems and nonlistening behaviors. The environment should be as free of distractions as possible. The caregiver speaks directly to the client in a distinct manner. Sentences should be clear and short. The client is asked to perform one task at a time, and sufficient time must be allowed for completion. It may be necessary to break each task down into many small steps.

As the disease progresses, the client is unable to perform tasks when asked. Show the client what needs to be done or provide cues to remind the client how to perform the task. When possible, explain and demonstrate the task that the client is asked to perform.

Drug Therapy. Cholinesterase inhibitors are drugs approved for symptomatic treatment of AD. These drugs improve cholinergic neurotransmission in the central nervous system (CNS) by delaying the destruction of acetylcholine (ACh) by acetylcholinesterase, thus delaying the onset of cognitive decline. None of these drugs affects the course of the disease. Examples include donepezil (Aricept), galantamine (Reminyl), and rivastigmine (Exelon).

Memantine (Namenda) is the first of a new class of medications that is a low to moderate affinity NMDA (N-methyl-D-aspartate) receptor antagonist. Overexcitation of NMDA receptors by the neurotransmitter glutamate may play a role in AD. This drug therefore blocks excess amounts of glutamate that can damage nerve cells. It is indicated for advanced AD and has been shown to slow the pace of deterioration, and it maintains functionality for a few months longer. Some clients show improved memory and thinking skills. This drug may also be given with donepezil (Aricept), a cholinesterase inhibitor.

Some clients with AD experience depression and may be treated with antidepressants. Selective serotonin reuptake inhibitors (SSRIs), such as paroxetine (Paxil) and sertraline (Zoloft), are usually prescribed. Tricyclic antidepressants, such as amitriptyline (Elavil, Levate✳), should not be used because of their anticholinergic effect.

Psychotropic drugs, also called antipsychotic and neuroleptic drugs, should be reserved for clients with emotional and behavioral health problems that sometimes accompany dementia, such as hallucinations and delusions. In clinical practice, however, these drugs are sometimes inappropriately used for agitation, combativeness, or restlessness. Psychotropic drugs are considered chemical restraints because they decrease mobility and clients' ability to care for themselves. Therefore most geriatricians recommend that these medications be used as a last resort and with caution in low doses for a specific emotional or behavioral health problem, because most clients with dementia are in late adulthood (see Chapter 5). The specific drug prescribed depends on side effects, the condition of the client, and anticipated outcomes. Institutional policy should be followed concerning the use of chemical restraints.

Complementary and Alternative Therapies. A number of complementary and alternative therapies are being researched that may prevent AD, slow its occurrence, or slow its progression in older adults. Examples of these therapies include vitamin E (antioxidants), ibuprofen, estrogen, melatonin, and nicotine patches. Art, massage, dance, and music therapy are often used in long-term care settings to minimize agitation.

RISK FOR INJURY

NOC **PLANNING: EXPECTED OUTCOMES.** The client with Alzheimer's disease (AD) is expected to remain free from physical harm and not injure anyone else. A safe home environment is also expected for those clients at home or in a homelike environment, such as assisted-living. Indicators include that there will be totally adequate:

- Provision of lighting
- Placement of handrails
- Safe storage of medications
- Provision of assistive devices in accessible locations
- Arrangement of furniture to reduce risks

INTERVENTIONS. Many clients with AD tend to wander and may easily become lost. In later stages of the disease, some clients may become severely agitated and physically or verbally abusive to others.

Coping with Restlessness and Wandering. The Alzheimer's Disease Association estimates that almost two thirds of clients will wander and become temporarily lost in the community. The client should always wear an identification badge or bracelet when at home. The badge should include how to contact the primary caregiver. In an inpatient setting, the client is checked frequently and placed in a room that can be monitored easily. The room may need to be close to the nurses' station (if the noise level in the nurses' station can be managed) and away from exits and stairs. Some health care agencies place large stop signs or red tape on the floor in front of exits. Others have installed alarm systems to indicate when a client is opening the door.

The client's family may choose to enroll in the Safe Return Program, a national, government-funded program of the Alzheimer's Association that assists in the identification and safe, timely return of individuals with Alzheimer's disease and related dementias who wander off and become lost. The program includes registration of the client and a 24-hour hotline to be called to assist in finding a lost client. If a client wanders and becomes lost, the family (or health care institutions) should immediately notify the police department. An up-to-date picture of the client makes it easier for local authorities, the public, and neighbors to identify the missing client.

Restlessness may be decreased if the client is taken for frequent walks. If the client begins to wander, he or she is redirected. For example, if the client insists on going shopping for clothes, the client is redirected to his or her closet to select clothing that will not be recognized as his or her own. This type of activity can be repeated a number of times because the client has lost short-term memory.

In any setting, clients should be kept busy with structured activities. In a health care agency, an activity therapist or volunteer may work with clients as a group or individually to determine the type of activity that is appropriate for the stage of the disease. Puzzles, board games, and art activities are often appropriate. Music and art therapy are becoming very popular in acute and long-term care for clients with dementia.

Physical restraints, such as waist belts and geri-chairs with lapboards, should be applied only as a last resort because they often increase the restlessness and cause agitation. Federal regulations in long-term care facilities in the United States mandate that all residents have the right to be free of both physical and chemical restraints. In addition, agencies accredited by the Joint Commission on Accreditation of Healthcare Agencies (JCAHO) are required to minimize the use of restraints and use alternatives (see Chapter 5).

Ensuring Safety. Clients with AD may become injured because they cannot recognize objects or situations as harmful. All potentially dangerous objects (e.g., knives, needles, and cleaning solutions) are removed or secured. Clients are often unaware that their driving ability is impaired and usually want to continue this activity even if their driver's license has been suspended secondary to the disease. Automobile keys must be secured and the client appropriately informed.

Late in the disease process, the client may experience seizure activity. If the client is cared for at home, teach caregivers what action to take when a seizure occurs (see earlier discussion under Interventions [Seizures and Epilepsy], p. 951).

Minimizing Agitation. Talking calmly and softly and attempting to redirect the client to a more positive behavior or activity is an effective strategy when he or she is agitated. Use calm, positive statements and reassure the client that he or she is safe. Statements such as "I'm sorry that you are upset. I know it's hard. I will stay until you feel better" may help.

Actions to avoid when the client is agitated include raising the voice, confrontation, arguing, reasoning, taking of-

TABLE 45-12   Minimizing Behavioral Problems at Home
Carefully evaluate the client's environment.
■ Ensure environment is safe:
Remove throw rugs.
Consider replacing tile floors with nonslippery floors.
Arrange furniture and room decorations to maximize the client's safety when walking.
Minimize clutter in all rooms in and outside of the house.
Install night lights in client's room, bathroom, and hallway.
Install and maintain smoke alarms, fire alarms, and natural gas detectors.
■ Install safety devices for the bathroom.
■ Install alarm system or bells on outside doors; place safety locks on doors and gates.
■ Ensure that door locks cannot be easily opened by the client.
Assist the client to remain oriented as long as possible.
■ Place single-date calendars in client's room and in kitchen.
■ Use large-faced clocks with a neutral background.
Communicate with the client based on his or her ability to understand.
■ As the disease progresses, use simple language and explain activities before the client needs to carry it out.
■ Break complex tasks down to simple steps.
Encourage the client to be as independent as possible in activities of daily living.
■ Place complete outfits for the day on hangers; have the client select one to wear.
■ Develop and maintain a predictable routine (e.g., meals, bedtime, morning routine)
When a problem behavior occurs, use distraction to divert client to another activity.
Minimize excessive stimulation.
■ Take the client on outings when crowds are small.
■ If crowds cannot be avoided, minimize the amount of time the client is present in a crowd, for example, at family gatherings, provide a quiet room for the client to rest throughout the visit.
Arrange for a day care program if possible.
Register the client with the Alzheimer's Association Safe Return Program.

fense, or explaining. The caregiver should not show alarm or make sudden movements out of the person's view. If the client remains agitated, ensure the client's safety and leave the room after explaining that you will return later. Frequent visual checks must be done during this time. If the client is connected to any type of tubing or other device, he or she may try to disconnect it or pull it out. These devices should be used sparingly in the client with dementia. If IV access, for example, is needed, the catheter or cannula is placed in an area that the client cannot easily see.

Another way to manage this problem is to provide a diversion. For example, if the client is doing an activity or holding an item such as a stuffed animal or doll, he or she might be less likely to pay attention to medical devices. Additional strategies to minimize behavioral problems are listed in Table 45-12.

COMPROMISED FAMILY COPING/CAREGIVER ROLE STRAIN

NOC PLANNING: EXPECTED OUTCOMES. The family or other caregivers of the client with Alzheimer's disease (AD) are expected to have a positive perception of their health status and life circumstances. Indicators include that they will be completely satisfied with their:

- Physical health
- Psychological health

- Lifestyle
- Performance of usual roles
- Social support
- Availability of respite

INTERVENTIONS. The client with AD requires continual, 24-hour supervision and caregiving. Severe cognitive changes leave the client unable to manage finances, property, or personal care. The family needs to seek legal counsel regarding the client's competency and the need to obtain guardianship or a durable medical power of attorney when necessary. The family can be referred to the local AD support group for literature and information concerning the disease and related problems.

Family members and other caregivers must be aware of their own health and stress levels. Signs of stress include anger, social withdrawal, anxiety, depression, lack of concentration, sleepiness, irritability, and health problems. When signs of stress occur, the caregiver should be referred to their health care provider or should seek one on his or her own.

DISTURBED SLEEP PATTERN

PLANNING: EXPECTED OUTCOMES. The client with AD is expected to sleep through the night and be awake at appropriate times.

INTERVENTIONS. The client with AD often has difficulty sleeping at night but tends to nap frequently during the day. Suggest ways to enhance sleep to the family or other caregiver. One way to establish the usual day-night pattern is to keep the client very active during the day. A daily routine that consists of a balance between passive activities and those requiring more strenuous exercise, such as walking or stretching activities, usually facilitates sleep at night. The client may want to take a nap in the late afternoon, but this should be discouraged if possible. In the last stage of the disease, the client may sleep during much of the day and night.

To facilitate sleep, instruct the family to establish a before-bedtime ritual. The routine usually consists of personal hygiene activities (e.g., bathing, toileting, brushing teeth) and environmental control measures to reduce noise and eliminate distractions. A back rub or small snack may help the client prepare for sleep.

The client's treatment and medication schedule is adjusted to provide for uninterrupted sleep. If more conventional measures fail to induce sleep, the health care provider may prescribe a mild antianxiety agent or hypnotic.

◆Community-Based Care

HOME CARE MANAGEMENT

Alzheimer's disease (AD) is a chronic, progressive condition that eventually leaves the client completely disoriented and totally dependent on others for all aspects of care. In the early stages, clients may be cared for at home with little need for outside intervention. Whenever possible, the client and family should be assigned a case manager who can assess their needs for health care resources and facilitate appropriate placement throughout the continuum of care.

The client usually begins to withdraw from friends and social events as memory impairment and personality and behavior changes become more apparent. This increases the family's responsibilities to minimize the impact of social isolation and decreased activity. The family may begin to

---

CHART 45-14

BEST PRACTICE for
Reducing Caregiver Stress

- Maintain realistic expectations for the person with Alzheimer's disease (AD).
- Take each day one at a time.
- Try to find the positive aspects of each incident or situation.
- Use humor with the person who has AD.
- Use the resources of the Alzheimer's Association, including attending local support group meetings.
- Explore alternative care settings early in the disease process for possible use later.
- Establish advance directives with the AD client early in the disease process.
- Set aside time each day for rest or recreation away from the client, if possible.
- Seek respite care periodically for longer periods of time.
- Take care of yourself by watching your diet, exercising, and getting plenty of rest.
- Be realistic about what you or they can do, and accept help from family, friends, and community resources.
- Use relaxation techniques.

---

decrease their own social activities as the demands of the client's care take more of their time. Emphasize to the family the importance of maintaining their own social contacts and leisure activities. Many family members experience caregiver stress, which affects their physical, mental, and emotional health. Chart 45-14 lists strategies for reducing caregiver stress. (See Chapter 5 for further discussion on caregiver role strain and interventions.)

It is now possible in most areas of the United States for the family to arrange respite care. The client may be placed in a respite facility or nursing home for the weekend or for several weeks to give the family a rest from the constant care demands. The family may also be able to obtain respite care in the home through a home care agency or the Alzheimer's Disease and Related Disorders Association (often called the Alzheimer's Association). Stress that respite care is for a short period of time; it is not a permanent placement. Some health care agencies have opened adult day care centers or specialty units for clients with AD. In the day care center, clients spend all or part of the day at the facility and participate in activities as their condition permits. Although these centers are usually open only on weekdays, this arrangement allows the caregiver to work or participate in other activities.

Teach the family how to be prepared in case the client becomes restless, agitated, abusive, or combative. In addition, the family can learn how to use reality orientation or validation therapy, depending on the stage of the disease.

HEALTH TEACHING

Usually the client with AD is cared for in the home until late in the disease process. Because health insurance coverage in the United States and family finances are usually insufficient to cover the services of a private duty nurse or home care aide, family members typically provide the care. The client care plan developed by the nurse or case manager, in conjunction with the family, must be reasonable and realistic for the family to implement.

Review how to assist with bathing, dressing, toileting, and other self-care activities. The occupational therapist teaches the family and the client how to use adaptive equipment, such as a brace, a sling, a cane, or modified eating utensils.

The client may have difficulty chewing, swallowing, or tasting foods and may not be able to eat without assistance.

The family and the dietitian should develop a diet plan to maximize the client's nutritional intake. In the late stage of AD, the client's intake often decreases, and he or she loses weight.

Provide information to the family on what to do in the event of a seizure and how to protect the client from injury. Instruct the family to notify the health care provider if the seizure is prolonged or if the client's seizure pattern changes. **DRUG THERAPY.** The name, time, and route of administration; the dosage; and the side effects of all medications are explained to the family or other caregiver. Remind the family to check with the health care provider before using any over-the-counter medications because they may interact with prescribed medication.

EXERCISE. Emphasis is placed on the need for the client to have an established exercise program to maintain mobility as long as possible, as well as to prevent complications of immobility. In collaboration with the family, the physical therapist develops an individualized exercise program. The physical therapist may continue to work with the client at home until goals are achieved, depending on the payer source.

SAFETY. Remind the family or other caregiver to take special precautions to maintain the client safely at home. The environment must be uncluttered, consistent, and structured. All hazardous items (e.g., cleaning fluids, power tools, insect spray) are removed or secured. All electrical sockets not in use should be covered with safety plugs. Handrails and grab bars should be installed in the bathroom; handrails should be along all stairways, and a guardrail should be placed around porches or open stairwells. Because the client may have a tendency to wander, especially at night, the family may want to install alarms to all outside doors, the basement, and the client's bedroom. All outside and basement doors should have deadbolt locks to prevent the client from going outside unsupervised. The temperature of the water heater should be adjusted to prevent accidental burns. Night lights should be used in the client's bedroom, hallway, and bathroom.

When the client can no longer be cared for at home, referral to an assisted-living or long-term care facility may be needed. Early in the course of the disease, advise the family that placement might be needed in the late stages of the disease. This allows the family to begin the search process for an appropriate facility before a crisis develops and immediate placement is needed. A number of facilities specialize in the care of clients with AD and other dementias. These units generally have a high staff-to-client ratio and are architecturally designed to meet the special needs of this type of client. The national office of the Alzheimer's Association publishes an outline of criteria for a dementia unit.

All families should be referred to their local chapter of the Alzheimer's Association. This organization provides information and support services to clients and their families, including seminars, audiovisual aids, and publications.

◆ Evaluation: Outcomes

Evaluate the care of the client with Alzheimer's disease (AD) on the basis of the identified nursing diagnoses. The expected outcomes include that the client will:

- Have the ability to execute complex mental processes (early AD)

- Remain free from injury and have a safe home environment
- Sleep through the night and be awake at appropriate times

The caregiver will have a positive perception of his or her health status and life circumstances. Specific indicators for these outcomes are listed for each nursing diagnosis under the Planning and Implementation section (see earlier).

HUNTINGTON DISEASE

OVERVIEW

Huntington disease (HD), formerly called Huntington chorea, is a hereditary disorder transmitted as an autosomal dominant trait at the time of conception.

Genetic Considerations

Huntington disease is a single gene disorder caused by a mutation in the HD gene located on chromosome 4. The mutation is a multiple repeat of the specific base triplet CAG, increasing the length of the gene. An autosomal dominant trait with high penetrance means that a person who inherits just one mutated allele has nearly a 100% chance of developing the disease. This gene mutation has different expressions depending on whether it is inherited from the mother or father. People who inherit the mutation from their fathers have an earlier onset and a shorter life expectancy than do those who inherit from their mothers. In addition, there is some variation in the disease depending on the size (length) of the mutation. The longer the mutation, the more severe the disease is at an earlier age.

It is estimated that 25,000 people in the United States have HD, and another 20,000 to 50,000 are thought to carry the gene. Men and women are equally affected, and symptoms begin between 35 and 50 years of age, striking at a highly productive time in life. The clinical onset of HD is gradual. The two main symptoms of the disease are progressive mental status changes, leading to dementia, and **choreiform movements** (rapid, jerky movements) in the limbs, trunk, and facial muscles. Dementia is related to the destruction of neurons within the cerebral cortex; it may also be associated with excessive amounts of dopamine found within the cerebral cortex and limbic systems of those affected. Two structures within the basal ganglia are involved in the development of HD: the caudate nucleus and the putamen. Both structures have close connections to the cerebral cortex and are closely associated with neurotransmitters. Neurotransmitters are secreted at the synapse, or junction, of one neuron with another, and it is through their specific excitation or inhibition of neurons that fine, controlled, integrated motor activity occurs.

In the presence of HD, there is a decrease in the amount of gamma-aminobutyric acid (GABA) and acetylcholine (ACh), both excitatory neurotransmitters. Dopamine is not affected. This shift in balance between dopamine (an inhibitory neurotransmitter) and GABA at the synapse leads to uninhibited motor activity. The result is brisk, jerky, purposeless movements, particularly of the hands, face, tongue, and legs, which the client is unable to stop.

There are three stages of HD, each lasting roughly 5 years, corresponding to the average 15-year course of the disease. Stage 1 is the onset of neurologic or psychological symptoms; stage 2 is characterized by an increasing dependence on others for care; stage 3 results in loss of independent function.

The diagnosis of HD is made on the basis of a family history of the disease and clinical assessment. The triad of dominant inheritance, choreoathetosis (neuromuscular symptoms), and dementia are hallmarks of the disease. The symptoms exhibited by the client vary in range and severity, age of onset, and rate of progression. Clinical manifestations include chorea, poor balance, hesitant or explosive speech, dysphagia, impaired respiration, and bowel and bladder incontinence. Mental status changes include decreased attention span, poor judgment, memory loss, personality changes, and dementia (later in the disease process).

◆ COLLABORATIVE MANAGEMENT

There is no known cure or treatment for HD. The only way to prevent transmission of the gene is for those affected to refrain from having children. Genetic counseling is important for children of clients with the disease. People at risk for the disease can be tested to determine whether or not the gene is present on chromosome 4. Before the testing procedure is undertaken, counseling is necessary to ensure that the client has voluntarily decided in favor of testing and is not being pressured by family or friends. In addition, counseling helps determine whether the benefits of knowing the results outweigh the risks of a positive result (e.g., depression or suicide).

Antipsychotic agents or monoamine-depleting agents may be used to manage movement abnormalities that interfere with ADLs or are functionally disabling. They are also used to help control agitation, hallucinations, or psychotic delusions. Medications may be use to treat other symptoms such as depression, anxiety, or obsessive-compulsive behaviors. Many of the medications used to treat HD may cause side effects that may be difficult to differentiate from signs of HD.

The care of the client with HD is managed by the collaborative efforts of the family and health care team:

- Speech-language pathologist helps with communication and swallowing.
- Registered dietitian plans meals.
- Physical and occupational therapists determine exercise conditioning and assistive devices
- Home care nurse and home health care aide give direct care and assessment of the client and assistance to the care provider.
- Case manager and social worker coordinate care and referrals to community agencies.

GET READY for the NCLEX Examination!

KEY POINTS

Safe Effective Care Environment

- For a client having a tonic-clonic or complete partial seizure, protect the client from injury. Other interventions are listed in Chart 45-5.
- For clients who have had one or more seizures, place on "seizure precautions," which includes having oxygen and suctioning emergency equipment available, starting an IV access, and putting the side rails up at all times.
- Implement interventions as summarized in Chart 45-7 for clients having status epilepticus, a life-threatening emergency.
- For clients with meningitis, carefully monitor neurologic status, including vital signs; observe for signs and symptoms of increased intracranial pressure (ICP).
- Assess level of consciousness (LOC) as a priority in clients with encephalitis.
- Monitor for drug toxicity when clients are taking medications for Parkinson disease, especially levodopa combinations, such as Sinemet. Delirium and decreased drug effectiveness are the most common indicators of toxicity.
- Observe clients with Alzheimer's disease closely because they tend to wander and make inappropriate decisions; safety is a priority for these clients.

Health Promotion and Maintenance

- Teach clients with an aura before migraine headaches the importance of taking abortive drugs to prevent a migraine episode.
- Teach clients with cluster headaches about precipitating factors, such as anger episodes, excitement, and excessive physical activity.
- In addition to prescribed drug therapy, encourage clients with headaches to use complementary and alternative therapies to help relieve pain, such as ice, darkened room, and relaxation techniques. Dietary changes help some clients by avoiding certain trigger foods (e.g., caffeine, beer, wine, pickled products).
- Teach the client with epilepsy the importance of continuing prescribed antiepileptic drugs (AEDs), even if he or she is seizure-free; additional instructions for the client and family are listed in Chart 45-4.
- If not contraindicated by other condition or age, encourage people who are in areas of high population density, such as college dormitories and crowded living areas, to become immunized against meningococcal meningitis.
- Teach people who enjoy outdoor activities to avoid areas where mosquitoes and ticks are likely to populate, especially near lakes and wooded areas. If in contact with these areas, remind them (especially older adults) to use insect repellent and keep skin exposure at a minimum.
- Teach clients and caregivers how to provide a safe home environment for clients with Parkinson or Alzheimer's disease.

Psychosocial Integrity

- Remind caregivers of clients with chronic neurologic diseases, such as Alzheimer's disease, to find ways to cope with their stress to remain physically and psychologically healthy, as suggested in Chart 45-14.
- Teach caregivers of clients with dementia to use validation therapy, rather than reality orientation; acknowledge the client's feelings and concerns.
- Be aware that clients with Parkinson disease may develop dementia as the disease progresses.

Physiological Integrity

- Assess for characteristic clinical manifestations in clients with classic migraine headaches as listed in Chart 45-1.

- Recall that the pain of cluster headaches is usually accompanied by ipsilateral (same side) eye tearing, rhinorrhea, congestion, ptosis, facial sweating, eyelid edema, and/or miosis.
- Recognize that generalized seizures, such as the tonic-clonic seizure, involve both cerebral hemispheres; partial seizures, also called focal or local seizures, usually involve only one hemisphere.
- During a seizure, document client's body movements and other assessments as described in Chart 45-6.
- Monitor for side and adverse effects of antiepileptic drugs (AEDs) as listed in Chart 45-3.
- Assess for clinical manifestations of meningitis as listed in Chart 45-8.
- Assess for key features of Parkinson disease as described in Chart 45-10.
- Collaborate with physical and occupational therapists, dietitian, and speech-language pathologist in planning and providing care for clients with Parkinson or Alzheimer's disease.
- Keep in mind that newer surgical procedures, such as deep brain stimulation, and experimental stem cell therapies are becoming available as options to control symptoms of Parkinson disease.
- Assess cognitive and functional abilities of the client with Alzheimer's disease, recognizing that it is a progressive dementia with several stages as listed in Chart 45-12.
- Recall that both familial (early onset) and late onset (advanced age) Alzheimer's disease has a genetic predisposition that continues to be researched.
- For clients with Alzheimer's disease, recall that the newer drugs seem to improve function and cognition (cholinesterase inhibitors; e.g., donepezil [Aricept]) or slow the disease process (Memantine), but they do not cure the disease.
- Administer psychotropic medications to clients with Alzheimer's disease who also have mental/behavioral health problems, such as depression and severe agitation.
- Remember that Huntington disease is a chronic, hereditary illness that is transmitted as an autosomal dominant trait at the time of conception; refer clients with the disease for genetic counseling.

ADDITIONAL STUDY RESOURCES

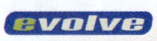 Go to your Student CD-ROM for Review Questions for the NCLEX Examination.

Go to http://evolve.elsevier.com/Iggy/ for Integrated Management of Care Questions for the NCLEX Examination.

SELECTED BIBLIOGRAPHY

Armstrong, T., Kanusky, J.T., & Gilbert, M.R. (2003). Seize the moment to learn about epilepsy in people with cancer. *Clinical Journal of Oncology Nursing, 7*(2), 163-171.

Bender, K., & Thompson, F.E. (2003). West Nile virus: A growing challenge. *American Journal of Nursing, 103*(6), 32-40.

Berg, A. (2003). How long does it take for epilepsy to become intractable? *Neurology, 60*(2), 186.

Betchen, S.A., & Kaplitt, M. (2003). Future and current surgical therapies in Parkinson's disease. *Current Opinion in Neurology, 16*(4), 487-493.

Bridy MA. (2001).The importance of quickly initiating antibiotic therapy in a 20-year-old man with bacterial meningitis. *Journal of Emergency Nursing, 27*(5), 437-439.

Burdick, W.P. (2003). Computed tomography of the head before lumbar puncture in adults with suspected meningitis. *Annals of Emergency Medicine, 41*(1), 161-162.

Chen, H., et al. (2003). Nonsteroidal anti-inflammatory drugs and the risk of Parkinson disease. *Archives of Neurology, 60*(8), 1059-1064.

Clare, L., et al. (2003). A. Cognitive rehabilitation and cognitive training for early-stage Alzheimer's disease and vascular dementia. In *The Cochrane Library*, Issue 4. Chichester, UK, John Wiley & Sons.

Clark, C.M., & Karlawish, J.H.T. (2003). Alzheimer disease: Current concepts and emerging diagnostic and therapeutic strategies. *Annals of Internal Medicine, 138*(5):400-410.

Cohen, J. (2003). Management of bacterial meningitis in adults: Algorithm from the British Infection Society represents current standard of care. *British Journal of Medicine, 326*(7397), 996-997.

Cummings, J.L., et al. (2002a). Guidelines for managing Alzheimer's disease, Part 1. *American Family Physician, 65*(11), 263-272.

Cummings, J.L., et al. (2002b). Guidelines for managing Alzheimer's disease, Part 2. *American Family Physician, 65*(12), 525-534.

de Gans, J., & van de Beek, D. (2002). Dexamethasone in adults with bacterial meningitis. *New England Journal of Medicine, 347*(20), 1549-1556, 1639-1640.

Edwards, N.E., & Scheetz, P.S. (2002). Predictors of burden for caregivers of patients with Parkinson's disease. *Journal of Neuroscience Nursing, 34*(4), 184-190.

Evans, R.W., & Olesen, J. (2003). Migraine classification, diagnostic criteria, and testing. *American Academy of Neurology, 60*(7) Supplement 2, S24-S30.

Franzini, A., et al. (2003). Stimulation of the posterior hypothalamus for treatment of chronic intractable cluster headaches. *Neurosurgery, 52*(5), 1095-1101.

Gambrell, M., & Flynn, N. (2004). Seizures 101. *Nursing 2004, 34*(8), 36-41.

Gilliam, F. (2002). Optimizing health outcomes in epilepsy. *Neurology, 8*(Supplement 5), S9-S20.

Guttman, M., Kish, S.J., & Furukawa, Y. (2003). Current concepts in the diagnosis and management of Parkinson's disease. *Canadian Medical Association Journal, 168*(3), 293-301.

Hickey, J.V. (2003). *The clinical practice of neurological and neurosurgical nursing* (5th ed.). Philadelphia: Lippincott-Raven.

Holroyd, K.A., & Mauskop, A. (2003). Complementary and alternative treatments. *Neurology, 60*(7) (Supplement 2), S58-S62.

Kolb-Lucas, K. (2003). Strategies for treating migraine. *Nursing, 33*(5), 32cc4-32cc6.

Lipton, R.B., et al. (2003). A self-administered screener for migraine in primary care. *Neurology, 61*(3), 375-382.

Lockey, A.S. (2002). Emergency department drug therapy for status epilepticus in adults. *Emergency Medicine Journal, 19*(2):96-100.

Lopez, O.L., et al. (2002). Cholinesterase inhibitor treatment alters the natural history of Alzheimer's disease. *Journal of Neurology, Neurosurgery & Psychiatry, 72*(3):310-314.

Matchar, D.B. (2003). Acute management of migraine. Highlights of the U.S. Headache Consortium. *Neurology, 60*(7) (Supplement 2), S21-S23.

McNamara, P., et al. (2003). Counterfactual cognitive deficit in persons with Parkinson's disease. *Journal of Neurology, Neurosurgery & Psychiatry, 74*(8):1065-1070.

Meador, K.J. (2002). Cognitive outcomes and predictive factors in epilepsy. Optimizing epilepsy management: Seizure control, medication tolerability, and co-morbidities. *American Academy of Neurology, 58* (Supplement 5), S21-S26.

Melchart, D., et al. (2003). Acupuncture versus placebo versus sumatriptan for early treatment of migraine attacks: A randomized controlled trial. *Journal of Internal Medicine, 253*(2), 181-188.

Miller, J.L. (2002). Parkinson's disease primer. *Geriatric Nursing, 23*(2), 69-74.

Miyasaki, J.M., et al. (2002). Practice parameter: Initiation of treatment for Parkinson's disease: An evidenced based review. *Neurology, 58*(1), 11-17.

Nussbaum, R.L., & Ellis, C.E. (2003). Alzheimer's disease and Parkinson's disease. *New England Journal of Medicine, 348*(14), 1356-1364.

Pena, C.G. (2003). Emergency: Seizure. *American Journal of Nursing, 103*(11), 73-81.

Peters, J.M., et al. (2003). Olfactory function in mild cognitive impairment and Alzheimer's disease: An investigation using psychophysical and electrophysiological techniques. *American Journal of Psychiatry, 160,* 1995-2002.

Ravina, B.M., et al. (2003). Neuroprotective agents for clinical trials in Parkinson's disease: A systematic assessment. *Neurology, 60*(8):1234-1240.

Redington, J.J., & Tyler, K.L. (2002). Viral infections of the nervous system, 2002: Update on diagnosis and treatment. *Archives of Neurology, 59,* 712-718.

Rowe, M.A. (2003). People with dementia who become lost. *American Journal of Nursing, 103*(5), 32-40.

Sheth, R. (2002). Epilepsy surgery: Presurgical evaluation. *Neurology Clinics, 20*(4), 1195.

Smith, L.P. (2003). Steady the course of Parkinson's disease. *Nursing Management, 34*(4), 35-39.

Smolowitz, J., & Waters, C. (2001). Clinical management of the adult with Parkinson's disease. *The American Journal for Nurse Practitioners, 5*(7), 9-34.

Souder, E., & Beck, C. (2004). Overview of Alzheimer's disease. *Nursing Clinics of North America, 39*(3), 545-559.

Sparano, N.I. (2001). Is the combination of ibuprofen and caffeine effective for the treatment of a tension-type headache? *Journal of Family Practice, 50*(1), 10.

Tammelleo, A.D. (2003). Was there a duty to warn nurse of meningitis risk? *Nursing Law's Regan Report, 43*(12), 1.

Thomas, E., et al. (2003). The diagnostic accuracy of Kernig's sign, Brudzinski's sign, and nuchal rigidity in adults with suspected meningitis. *Annals of Emergency Medicine, 42*(2), 311-312.

Tolosa, E. (2003). Advances in the pharmacological management of Parkinson disease. *Journal of Neural Transmission, Supplementum* (64), 65-78.

Tunkel, A.R., & Scheld, W.M. (2003). Corticosteroids for everyone with meningitis? *New England Journal of Medicine, 347*(20), 1613-1615.

United Health Care. (2002). *Clinical evidence concise.* London: BMJ Publishing Group.

Van Den Eeden, S.K, et al. (2003). Incidence of Parkinson's disease: Variation by age, gender, and race/ethnicity. *American Journal of Epidemiology, 157*(11), 1015-1022.

Vaughan, J., & Hardie, R.J. (2002). The differential diagnosis of Parkinson's disease. *Reviews in Clinical Gerontology, 12*(1):40-51.

Velling, D.A., Dodick, D.W., & Muir, J.J. (2003). Sustained-release niacin for prevention of migraine headache. *Mayo Clinic Proceedings, 78*(6), 770-771.

Welch, K.M, Cutrer, F.M., & Peter, J. (2003). Migraine pathogenesis: Neural and vascular mechanisms. *Neurology, 60*(7) (Supplement 2), S9-S14.

Zandi, P.P., Breitner, J.C., & Anthony, J.C. (2002). Is pharmacological prevention of Alzheimer's a realistic goal? *Expert Opinion on Pharmacotherapy, 3*(4), 365-380.

Zingmark, K., Sandman, P.O., & Norberg, A. (2002). Promoting a good life among people with Alzheimer's disease. *Journal of Advanced Nursing, 38*(1), 50-58.

Interventions for Clients with Problems of the Central Nervous System
The Spinal Cord

KATHY A. HAUSMAN

LEARNING OUTCOMES

After studying this chapter, you should be able to:

1. Identify risk factors that contribute to back pain.
2. Explain health promotion measures to prevent back pain.
3. Plan care for the client having a diskectomy, laminectomy, or spinal fusion.
4. Analyze the common nursing diagnoses and collaborative problems for the client with an acute spinal cord injury (SCI).
5. Describe the role of the health care team in the recognition and treatment of typical medical complications that are experienced by clients with an SCI.
6. Prioritize the nursing care of the client with an SCI.
7. Evaluate the expected outcomes for the client with an SCI.
8. Identify the clinical manifestations and treatment options associated with spinal cord tumors.
9. Explain the pathophysiology of multiple sclerosis (MS), including the six basic types.
10. Discuss the role of medications in managing clients with MS.
11. Develop a community-based teaching plan for the client with MS.
12. Compare and contrast the clinical manifestations of MS and amyotrophic lateral sclerosis.

Go to your Student CD-ROM for Review Questions
for the NCLEX Examination keyed to these Learning Outcomes.

Problems of the spinal cord may be either acute or chronic and either short term or long term. Some problems require surgery, whereas others require extensive rehabilitation. Spinal cord neurons do not regenerate, and damage to nerve fibers is permanent.

BACK PAIN

Lumbosacral Back Pain (Low Back Pain)

OVERVIEW

Back pain is one of the most common reasons for visiting a health care provider. Back problems are very costly in terms of time lost from work and medical treatment, and they are the most common cause of disability for persons younger than 43 years of age. Disabling low back pain is the single greatest cause of compensable injury in the working population. The lumbosacral (lower back) vertebrae and cervical (neck) vertebrae are most commonly affected.

PATHOPHYSIOLOGY

Lumbosacral back pain, referred to as **low back pain (LBP)**, is more common than cervical pain. Acute pain is caused by muscle strain or spasm, ligament sprain, disk degeneration, or herniation of the nucleus pulposus from the center of the disk. Herniated disks occur most often between the fourth and fifth lumbar vertebrae (L4-5) but may occur at other levels. A **herniated nucleus pulposus (HNP)** in the lumbosacral area can press on the adjacent spinal nerve (usually the sciatic nerve), causing severe burning or stabbing pain down into the leg or foot. The HNP may press on the spinal cord itself, causing leg weakness and bowel and bladder dysfunction. The specific area of pain depends on the level of herniation.

Muscle spasms of the affected leg may also occur. The pain is usually aggravated by sneezing, coughing, or straining. If LBP continues for 3 months or if repeated episodes of pain occur, the client has chronic back pain.

Etiology and Genetic Risk

Acute back pain usually results from trauma. The client typically hyperflexes or twists the back during a vehicular accident, or the injury occurs when the client lifts a heavy object. Obesity places increased stress on the back muscles and typically contributes to the occurrence or severity of back pain. Smoking has been linked to disk degeneration. Congenital spinal conditions and scoliosis can also lead to back discomfort.

CONSIDERATIONS FOR OLDER ADULTS

For older adults the cause of low back pain is usually osteoarthritis (OA), a type of arthritis seen primarily in this population. OA may be related to genetic factors, especially when the disease affects the hands and knees (Birchfield, 2001). Other factors contributing to low back pain in older adults are presented in Chart 46-1.

WOMEN'S HEALTH CONSIDERATIONS

Chronic low back pain in women often results from having poor posture or from wearing high-heeled shoes. Excessive high heels cause the body to compensate to maintain balance. The back becomes more **lordotic** (anteriorly curved), which strains back muscles.

Incidence/Prevalence

Eighty percent of the U.S. population has LBP at some time. About 85% to 90% of adults over 50 years of age have degenerative disk disease.

HEALTH PROMOTION/ILLNESS PREVENTION

Many of the problems related to acute back pain can be prevented by recognizing the cause of back pain and taking appropriate preventive measures. For example, good posture, proper lifting techniques, and exercise can significantly decrease the incidence of low back pain. Chart 46-2 summarizes ways to prevent LBP.

CHART 46-1

NURSING FOCUS on the OLDER ADULT
Factors Contributing to Low Back Pain

- Changes in support structures
    Spinal stenosis
    Hypertrophy of the intraspinal ligaments
    Arthritis
- Changes in vertebral support and malalignment
    Scoliosis
    Lordosis
- Vascular changes
    Diminished blood supply to the spinal cord or cauda equina caused by arteriosclerosis
    Blood dyscrasias
- Intervertebral disk degeneration

◆ COLLABORATIVE MANAGEMENT
◆ Assessment

PHYSICAL ASSESSMENT/CLINICAL MANIFESTATIONS

The client's *primary* complaint is continuous acute pain. Some clients have so much pain that they walk in a stiff, flexed state, or they may be unable to bend at all. The client who has low back pain (LBP) may walk with a limp, indicating possible sciatic nerve impairment. Walking on the heels or toes often causes severe pain in the affected leg, the back, or both.

Inspect the client's back for vertebral alignment and for tenderness and swelling caused by muscle spasm. Local muscle spasm in the back and affected leg is common. It is thought that a compressed nerve becomes inflamed and irritates adjacent muscle tissue. Clients complain of stabbing, continuous pain in the muscle close to the affected disk. In clients with lumbosacral involvement, pain radiates down the posterior leg. The pain usually does not extend the entire length of the limb. Clients with LBP report sharp, burning posterior thigh or calf pain that may radiate to the ankle or toes. They may also report the same type of pain in the middle of one buttock.

Ask the client whether **paresthesia** (tingling sensation) or numbness is present in the involved limb. Both extremities may be checked for sensation by using a pin or paper clip and a cotton ball for comparison of light and deep touch. The client may feel sensation in both limbs but may experience a stronger sensation on the unaffected side. The client with a severe problem may lose both bowel and bladder control from spinal nerve involvement.

If the sciatic nerve is compressed, the client reports severe pain when raising a straight leg. Foot, ankle, and leg weakness may accompany the pain. To complete the neurologic assessment, evaluate the client's muscle tone and strength. Muscles in the extremity or in the back atrophy in severe, chronic conditions. The client has difficulty with movement, and certain movements elicit more pain than others.

DIAGNOSTIC ASSESSMENT

The health care provider often orders magnetic resonance imaging (MRI) or a computed tomography (CT) scan, performed with or without contrast media enhancement, to vi-

CHART 46-2

CLIENT EDUCATION GUIDE
Prevention of Low Back Pain and Injury

- Use proper body mechanics, with specific attention to bending, lifting, and sitting.
- Assess the need for assistance with your household chores or other activities.
- Participate in a regular exercise program, especially one that promotes back strengthening, such as swimming and walking.
- Do not wear high-heeled shoes.
- Use good posture when sitting, standing, or walking.
- Avoid prolonged sitting or standing. Use a foot stool and ergonomic chairs and tables to lessen back strain.
- Keep weight within 10% of ideal body weight. Ensure adequate calcium intake.
- Stop smoking. If you are not able to stop, cut down on the number of cigarettes or decrease the use of other forms of tobacco.

sualize the herniated disk and pressure on the nerve root or spinal cord.

Electrodiagnostic testing, such as electromyography (EMG) and nerve-conduction studies, may help to differentiate motor neuron diseases, peripheral neuropathies, peripheral nerve entrapment, and radiculopathies. These are especially useful in chronic diseases because it takes at least 3 weeks for pathologic changes to produce symptoms. Chapter 44 describes these tests in more detail.

◆Interventions

Management of clients with back pain varies with the severity and chronicity of the problem. Most clients with acute low back pain (LBP) need only a short-term treatment regimen. The health care provider initially implements conservative measures; if these are unsuccessful, surgery may be indicated. Some clients experience chronic pain that must be managed for an extended period.

NONSURGICAL MANAGEMENT. Nonsurgical management of back pain may include proper positioning, exercise, anti-inflammatory analgesics, heat or ice therapy, and other pain-relief measures and preventive measures in the work setting.

Positioning. The **Williams position** is typically more comfortable and therapeutic for the client with LBP. In this position, the client lies in the semi-Fowler's position and flexes the knees to relax the muscles of the lower back and relieve pressure on the spinal nerve root.

A firm mattress or a backboard placed under a soft mattress provides back support. A flat position is particularly helpful for the client with a muscle injury. For a herniated disk causing spinal nerve root compression in the lumbar spine, a flat position may aggravate the pain. The client usually gains pain relief from reclining or sleeping in the Williams position.

Exercise. Exercises are used to strengthen the back, relieve pressure on compressed nerves, and protect the back from reinjury. A variety of exercise programs are available to treat LBP. Isometric exercises are generally the most effective.

The physical therapist (PT) works with the client to develop an individualized exercise program. The type of exercises prescribed depends on the location and nature of the injury and the type of pain. The client does not begin exercises until acute pain is reduced by other means. Several specific exercises for LBP are provided in Chart 46-3.

Drug Therapy. The health care provider often prescribes muscle relaxants, such as cyclobenzaprine hydrochloride (Flexeril) and tizanidine (Zanaflex), and nonsteroidal anti-inflammatory drugs (NSAIDs), such as naproxen (Naprosyn, Naxen❋) and ibuprofen (Motrin, Novoprofen❋). Opioid analgesics are no more effective than nonsteroidal analgesics and should be avoided if at all possible. If they must be used, the course of therapy should be short to prevent adverse side effects. An epidural or local steroid injection may also be helpful. Short-term oral steroids may be prescribed for some clients. Clients experiencing chronic back pain may require an antiepileptic drug (AED), such as gabapentin (Neurontin) and oxcarbazepine (Trileptal). For clients with chronic back problems, these drugs are used to treat neuropathic pain. Most of the drugs in this class can cause hyponatremia (low serum sodium). Older clients should be monitored very carefully for this adverse effect. Chapter 7 describes in detail the drug therapy and nursing implications for the care of clients in acute or chronic pain.

Heat and Ice Therapy. Some clients with back pain experience temporary relief from the application of heat. Heat increases blood flow to the affected area and promotes the healing of injured nerves. Moist heat in the form of heat packs or hot towels applied for 20 to 30 minutes at least four times per day may be recommended. Hot showers or baths are also often beneficial. The physical therapist (PT) may administer deep heat therapy, such as ultrasound treatments and diathermy. The PT and nurse monitor the effects of heat treatment by assessing the client's skin condition and the relief of pain.

Some clients prefer ice instead of heat to relieve pain and inflammation. Ice therapy using ice packs or ice massage may be applied over the affected area for 10 to 15 minutes every 1 to 2 hours. For some clients, a course of alternating ice and heat applications may be effective.

Diet Therapy. Weight control often helps to reduce chronic back pain by decreasing the work on the vertebrae caused by excess weight. If the client's weight exceeds the ideal by more than 10%, caloric restriction is necessary.

Health care providers must be sensitive when reinforcing the need for clients to lose weight to prevent or to lessen chronic back pain. Collaborate with the dietitian to plan and implement an appropriate calorie-restricted diet plan. Positive reinforcement and self-esteem building are integral to the diet plan.

Other Pain Relief Measures. Physical therapy with manipulation of the lower back during the first month of symptoms may be beneficial. Shoe insoles may also help to decrease pain when standing for prolonged periods. Preventive measures for the occupational setting may include a corset, supportive back belt, and ergonomic office furniture. A structured educational program about low back problems in the work setting has also been helpful in decreasing both injuries and time lost from work.

Complementary and Alternative Therapies. The client may find that other nontraditional and complementary therapies provide short-term pain relief. Distraction,

---

CHART 46-3

CLIENT EDUCATION GUIDE
Typical Exercises for Chronic or Postoperative Low Back Pain

Extension Exercises
- **Stomach lying:** Lie face down with a pillow under your chest; lift legs straight up (alternate legs).
- **Upper trunk extension:** Lie face down with your arms at your sides, and lift your head and neck.
- **Prone pushups:** Lie face down on a mat and, keeping your body stiff, and push up to extend your arms.

Flexion Exercises
- **Pelvic tilt:** Lying on your back with your knees bent, tighten your abdominal muscles to push your lower back against the mat.
- **Semi–sit-ups:** Lying on your back with your knees bent, raise your upper body at a 45-degree angle, and hold this position for 5 to 10 seconds.
- **Knee to chest:** Lying on your back with your knees bent, tighten your abdominal muscles to push your lower back against the mat. Now bring one or both knees to your chest and hold this position for 5 to 10 seconds.

imagery, magnetic-field therapy, and music therapy are examples of pain-relief therapies. Chapters 4 and 7 describe these techniques in detail.

Percutaneous Laser Disk Decompression. A nonsurgical procedure known as **percutaneous laser disk decompression (PLDD)** may relieve the pain of a herniated disk by drawing the herniated portion away from the nerve root. This treatment is performed in special spinal centers around the United States and throughout the world.

Using advanced laser technology and a local anesthetic, a thin needle is inserted under fluoroscopy. An optical fiber is placed through the needle to enable laser energy to travel and vaporize the disk nucleus. Most clients walk away from this half-hour procedure pain free and with just a small bandage. Physicians typically prescribe 24 hours of bedrest after the procedure before beginning progressive ambulation. Depending on the type of work, most clients can resume work within a week.

SURGICAL MANAGEMENT. Surgery is usually performed when conservative measures fail to relieve back pain after a month or so or if neurologic deficits progress.

Conventional Operative Procedures. The most common conventional operative procedures are diskectomy, laminectomy, and spinal fusion. These procedures involve extensive muscle and soft-tissue dissection to expose the anatomic landmarks. Major complications include nerve injuries, diskitis, and dural tears.

In a conventional **diskectomy,** the spinal nerve is usually lifted to remove the offending portion of the disk. A **laminectomy** is the removal of one or more vertebral laminae plus osteophytes, if present, and the herniated nucleus pulposus. Both procedures are performed through a 3- to 4-inch (7.5- to 10-cm) longitudinal incision. The standard hospital stay is 1 to 2 days but may be shorter or longer, depending on the client's condition and the reimbursement source.

When repeated laminectomies are performed or the spine is unstable, the surgeon may perform a **spinal fusion (arthrodesis)** to stabilize the affected area. Chips of bone are removed, typically from the iliac crest or obtained from donor bone, and are grafted between the vertebrae for support and to strengthen the back. Before closing, the surgeon may give an **intrathecal** (spinal) dose of morphine to decrease postoperative pain and respiratory complications.

An adjunct for clients for whom fusion may be difficult is the placement of an implantable **direct current stimulation (DCS)** to promote bone fusion. External bone stimulators may also be effective for healing bone fusions.

Alternative Operative Procedures. Minimally invasive lumbar procedures have the advantage of being associated with less muscle injury, decreased blood loss, and decreased postoperative pain. Three alternatives to a laminectomy that have varying degrees of popularity are percutaneous lumbar diskectomy, microdiskectomy, and laser-assisted laparoscopic lumbar diskectomy. The primary advantage of these surgical procedures is a shortened hospital stay and the possibility of an ambulatory procedure. Spinal cord complications are also less likely. New procedures for spinal fusions include laparoscopic lumbar fusion and intervertebral body fusion devices (e.g., titanium-threaded and mesh interbody cages). When possible, these procedures are preferred over conventional ones.

For a **percutaneous lumbar diskectomy,** a local anesthetic is given. The surgeon uses fluoroscopy to insert a metal cannula, or endoscope, adjacent to the affected disk. A special cutting tool is threaded through the cannula for removal of disk pieces that are compressing the nerve root. Inpatient hospitalization is not necessary.

A **microdiskectomy** involves microscopic surgery through a 1-inch incision. This procedure allows easier identification of anatomic structures, improved precision in removing small fragments, and decreased tissue trauma and pain.

Laser-assisted laparoscopic lumbar diskectomy combines a laser with modified standard disk instruments inserted periumbilically through the laparoscopic cannula. It may be used to treat herniated disks that, although bulging, have not encroached on the vertebral canal. The primary risks of this surgery are infection and nerve-root injury. The client is typically discharged in 24 to 48 hours but may be discharged the same day.

Another new treatment for herniated disks involves a hard plastic prosthesis that replaces the client's natural disk. The disk is shaped to allow full spinal movement. Recently approved for widespread use, this device could revolutionize care for clients with herniated disks.

Preoperative Care. Preoperative care of the client preparing for a lumbar laminectomy is similar to that for any client undergoing surgery (see Chapter 20). The nurse and physical therapist teach the client what to expect postoperatively and how to move in bed. The client should be warned that various sensations, such as numbness and tingling, may be experienced in the affected leg or in both legs because of the manipulation of nerves and muscles during surgery.

The client who has undergone a spinal fusion typically wears a back brace postoperatively. This brace is fitted before surgery. The nurse in the surgeon's office or clinic teaches about the importance of wearing the brace as instructed during the healing process.

The surgeon explains where the bone for grafting will be obtained. The client's own bone is used whenever possible, but supplemental bone from a bone bank may be needed. The surgeon provides verbal and written information about the type and the source of bone for surgery. The client signs an informed consent form before surgery.

Postoperative Care. Early postoperative nursing care focuses on preventing and assessing complications that might occur in the first 24 to 48 hours (Chart 46-4). As for any client undergoing surgery, take vital signs at least every 4 hours during the first 24 hours to assess for fever and for hypotension, which could indicate bleeding or severe pain. Perform a neurologic assessment every 4 hours. Of particular importance is the client's ability to move and feel sensation in the extremities.

Carefully check the client's ability to void. Pain and a flat position in bed make voiding difficult, especially for men. An inability to void may indicate damage to the sacral spinal nerves, which control the detrusor muscle in the bladder. Opioid analgesics have been associated with difficulty voiding. The client with a diskectomy or laminectomy typically gets out of bed with assistance on the evening of surgery, which may facilitate voiding.

Pain control may be achieved with patient-controlled analgesia (PCA) or intravenous (IV) medications such as

CHART 46-4

BEST PRACTICE for
Assessing and Managing the Client with Major Complications of Lumbar Spinal Surgery

Complication	Assessment/Interventions
Cerebrospinal fluid (CSF) leakage	Observe for clear fluid on or around the dressing. If CSF is present, test for glucose. (The test result is positive if glucose is present.) Report CSF leakage immediately to the surgeon. (The client is usually kept on flat bedrest for several days while the dural tear heals.)
Fluid volume deficit	Monitor intake and output; monitor drain output, which should not be more than 250 mL in 8 hr during the first 24 hr. Monitor vital signs carefully for hypotension and tachycardia.
Acute urinary retention	Assist the client to the bathroom or a bedside commode as soon as possible postoperatively. Assist male clients to stand at the bedside as soon as possible postoperatively. Give bethanechol (Urecholine) chloride as prescribed to stimulate the detrusor muscle of the bladder.
Paralytic ileus	Monitor for the return of bowel sounds. Assess for abdominal distention, nausea, and vomiting.
Fat embolism syndrome (FES) (more common in people with spinal fusion)	Observe for and report chest pain, dyspnea, anxiety, and mental status changes (particularly common in older adults). Note petechiae around the neck, upper chest, buccal membrane, and conjunctiva. Monitor arterial blood gas values for decreased Pao_2.
Persistent or progressive lumbar radiculopathy (nerve root pain)	Report pain not responsive to opioids. Document the location and nature of pain. Administer analgesics as ordered.
Infection (e.g., wound diskitis, hematoma)	Monitor the client's temperature carefully (a slight elevation is normal). Increased temperature elevation or a spike after the second postoperative day is possibly indicative of infection. Report increased pain at the wound site or in the legs. Give antibiotics as prescribed. Use sterile technique for dressing changes.

morphine. Pain medication is changed to oral administration when the client is able to take fluids. Hospital policy should be followed regarding pain management.

Inspect the surgical dressing for blood or any other type of drainage. Clear drainage may mean cerebrospinal fluid (CSF) leakage. Report such a finding to the surgeon immediately. Bulging at the incision site may be due to a CSF leak or a hematoma, both of which are reported to the surgeon.

Empty the surgical drain, usually a Jackson-Pratt or Hemovac, and record the amount of drainage every 8 hours. The surgeon usually removes the drain in 24 to 36 hours.

Correct turning of the client in bed is especially important. Teach the client to log roll every 2 hours from side to back and vice versa. In log rolling, the client turns all at once while his or her back is kept as straight as possible. A turning sheet may be used for large clients. Either turning method may require additional assistance, depending on how much the client can assist. Instruct the client to keep his or her back straight when getting out of bed. The client should sit in a straight-backed chair with the feet resting comfortably on the floor.

Teach the client to deep breathe every 2 hours to prevent atelectasis and pneumonia. Until the client can ambulate independently, he or she wears graduated compression stockings, sequential compression devices (SCDs), or pneumatic compression boots (PCBs) to prevent deep vein thrombosis (DVT) and possible pulmonary emboli. Older adults are especially susceptible to these complications of immobility.

When a spinal fusion is performed in addition to a laminectomy, more care is taken with mobility and positioning. The client usually stays in bed for 24 hours, with the nurse or assistive nursing personnel log rolling him or her every 2 hours. For the conventional fusion, inspect both the iliac and spinal incision areas for problems, as described earlier in this section. A brace or other type of thoracolumbar support is worn when the client is out of bed. Remind the client to avoid prolonged sitting or standing.

Community-Based Care

The client with back pain who does not undergo surgery is typically managed at home. If back surgery is performed, the client is usually discharged to home with support from family or significant others. For older adults without a community support system, a short-term stay in a nursing home or subacute unit may be needed. The case manager or discharge planner collaborates with the health care team, client, and family to determine the most appropriate placement.

HOME CARE MANAGEMENT

Inform the client and family members or significant other that the client should have a firm mattress to provide support for the entire vertebral column. A bed board or large piece of plywood placed under a soft mattress may suffice. After back surgery, the client may be limited in the number of times he or she is allowed to climb stairs each day. However, daily walking is encouraged. The client can usually return to work in 4 to 6 weeks, depending on the nature of the job and the extent and type of surgery. Weight that may be lifted is initially limited to 5 pounds. The amount is gradually increased as healing occurs. Driving is not permitted for several weeks until the surgeon re-evaluates the client.

HEALTH TEACHING

In collaboration with the dietitian and physical therapist, instruct the client to do the following:

- Continue with a weight-reduction diet, if needed.
- Stop smoking, if applicable.
- Use moist heat as needed.
- Perform strengthening exercises as initiated preoperatively and in the hospital setting.

The physical therapist reviews and demonstrates the principles of body mechanics and muscle-strengthening exercises. The client is then asked to demonstrate these principles (Chart 46-5).

The health care provider may want the client to continue taking medications such as anti-inflammatory drugs and muscle relaxants. The nurse reminds the client and family about the possible side effects of drugs and what to do if they occur. If the client has a conventional spinal fusion, he or she may need to wear a brace or thoracolumbar support for 3 to 6 months while the fusion heals completely. The client may not be able to return to full functioning for 6 to 12 months after a spinal fusion, depending on the type of work that is done.

The client with an acute episode of back pain typically returns to his or her usual activities but may fear a recurrence. Remind the client that he or she may never have another episode if caution is used. However, continuous or repeated

pain can be frustrating and tiring. If pain is unremitting, surgery is indicated. Encourage the client and family members to set short-term goals and to take steps toward recovering slowly.

In a few clients, back surgery is not successful. This situation, referred to as **failed back surgery syndrome (FBSS),** is a complex combination of organic, psychological, and socioeconomic factors. Repeated surgical procedures often discourage these clients, who must continue nonsurgical management of pain after multiple operations. Nerve blocks and other chronic pain-management modalities may be needed on a long-term basis (see Chapter 7).

A new drug for severe chronic pain, ziconotide (Prialt), has recently been approved for intrathecal infusion with a surgically implanted pump. Ziconotide is the first available drug in a new class called N-type calcium channel blockers (NCCBs). NCCBs seem to selectively block calcium channels on those nerves that usually transmit pain signals to the brain. Ziconotide is also used for clients with cancer, AIDS, and unremitting pain for other nervous system disorders. It can be given with opioid analgesics but should not be given to clients with severe mental health/behavioral health problems (http://www.prialt.com).

HEALTH CARE RESOURCES

Assist the client in identifying support systems (e.g., family, church groups, and clubs) after back surgery or FBSS. For example, a spouse may help the client with exercises or perform the exercises with the client. Members of a church group may help run errands and do household chores.

The client with back pain may continue physical therapy on an ambulatory basis after discharge. For unresolved pain, the client may be referred to pain specialists or clinics, which are usually found in large metropolitan hospitals. A case manager may be assigned to the client to help with resource management and utilization.

Cervical Neck Pain

PATHOPHYSIOLOGY

Cervical neck pain usually results from a herniation of the nucleus pulposus in an intervertebral disk. As seen in Figure 46-1, the herniation usually occurs laterally where the annulus fibrosus is weakest and the posterior longitudinal lig-

---

CHART 46-5

CLIENT EDUCATION GUIDE
Use of Proper Body Mechanics to Prevent Back Injury

- Size up the load to determine the number of persons needed to perform the task.
- When lifting an object, keep your back straight and do not bend at the waist; lift with your large thigh muscles.
- Push objects rather than pull them.
- Do not twist your back.
- Avoid prolonged sitting or standing. Use a footstool to lessen back strain.
- Sit in chairs with good support; sleep on a firm mattress.
- Avoid shoulder stooping; use proper posture.
- Do not walk or stand in high-heeled shoes for prolonged periods (for women).

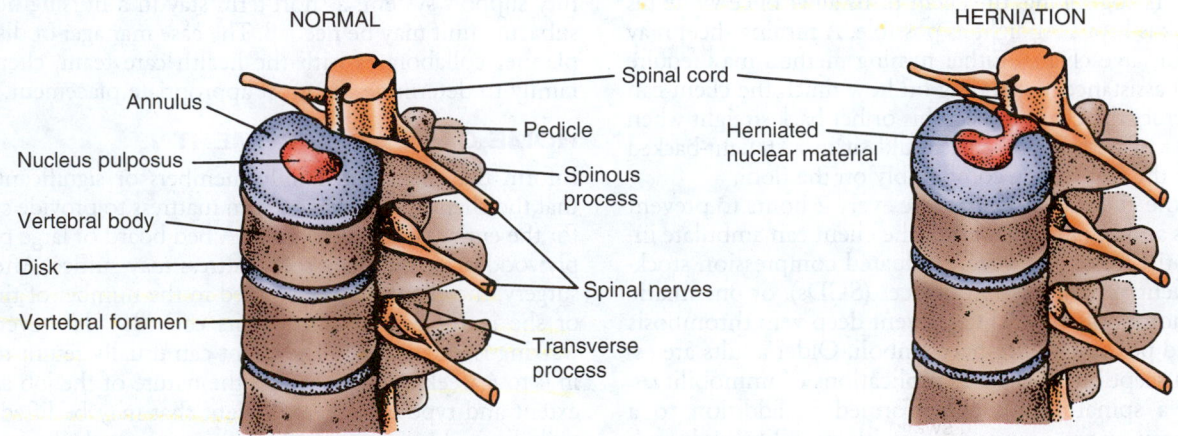

NORMAL HERNIATION

Annulus
Nucleus pulposus
Vertebral body
Disk
Vertebral foramen

Spinal cord
Pedicle
Spinous process
Spinal nerves
Transverse process

Herniated nuclear material

Figure 46-1 ■ Herniation of the nucleus pulposus.

ament is thinned. The result is spinal nerve root compression, with subsequent motor and sensory manifestations, typically in the neck and down the affected arm. The disk between the fifth and sixth cervical vertebrae (C5-6) is affected most often.

If the disk does not rupture, nerve compression may be caused by osteophyte (bony outgrowth) formation from osteoarthritis. The osteophyte presses on the intervertebral foramen, which results in a narrowing of the disk and pressure on the nerve root. A client with nerve compression may experience either continuous or intermittent chronic pain. When the disk herniates centrally, pressure on the spinal cord occurs.

Cervical pain—acute or chronic—may also occur from muscle strain, ligament sprain resulting from aging or poor posture, lifting incorrectly, tumor, or infection. The typical history of the client includes complaints of pain when moving the neck, which radiates to the scapula and down the arm. The pain may interrupt sleep and may be accompanied by a headache or numbness and tingling in the affected arm. To determine the exact cause of the pain, the health care provider orders diagnostic tests, such as computed tomography (CT) or magnetic resonance imaging (MRI), x-rays of the neck, electromyography (EMG), or a combination of these.

◆COLLABORATIVE MANAGEMENT

Conservative treatment for neck pain is the same as described for back pain except the exercises focus on the shoulders and neck. The physical therapist teaches the client the correct techniques for performing "shoulder shrug," "shoulder squeeze," and "seated rowing." If these treatments do not work, the health care provider may prescribe a soft collar, especially at night. The collar is used no longer than 10 days, or it can lead to increased pain and decreased muscle strength and range of motion.

If conservative treatment is ineffective, surgery may be required. Depending on the causative factor, either an ante-

rior or posterior approach is used. An anterior cervical diskectomy and fusion (ACDF) is commonly performed. The client requires routine preoperative and postoperative care as described in Chapters 20 and 22. Chart 46-6 summarizes best practices for postoperative care and discharge planning. Potential complications of the anterior surgical approach can be found in Chart 46-7.

? Critical Thinking Challenge

You have been assigned to a woman admitted to the medical-surgical unit following an anterior cervical diskectomy and fusion (ACDF). She is wearing a soft collar. Her diet order is clear liquids and advance as tolerated. She may ambulate with assistance. The client tells you that her pain score is 7/10; she is having difficulty swallowing, and you notice that her voice is hoarse. According to the client, no one told her she "would feel like this."

1. What is your best nursing action in response to these symptoms?
2. What would you tell the client about her symptoms?
3. What are the possible complications of an ACDF, and why might they occur?

evolve For suggested answer guidelines, go to http://evolve.elsevier.com/Iggy/.

SPINAL CORD INJURY

Despite increased awareness and the sophistication of treatment for spinal cord injury (SCI), the effects of the initial injury cannot be reversed. However, research with clients with SCI has increased, led by actor Christopher Reeve, who experienced a complete cervical spinal injury. The cost of care for clients with an SCI varies with the neurologic deficit. Clients experiencing **tetraplegia** (also called quadriplegia)—paralysis from the neck down—are the most expensive for society in terms of both health care and living expenses (see the Resource Management box on p. 984).

Loss of motor function, sensation, reflex activity, and bowel and bladder control often result from an SCI. In addition, the client may experience significant behavior and emotional problems as a result of changes in body image, role performance, and self-concept.

The SCIs are classified as complete or incomplete. A **complete** injury is one in which the spinal cord has been severed or damaged in a way that eliminates all innervation below the level of the injury. Injuries that allow some function or movement below the level of the injury are described as **incomplete.**

CHART 46-6

BEST PRACTICE for
Care of the Client Following an Anterior Cervical Diskectomy and Fusion

Postoperative Interventions
- Assess airway, breathing, and circulation (ABCs).
- Check for bleeding and drainage at the incision site.
- Monitor vital signs and neurologic status frequently.
- Check for swallowing ability.
- Monitor intake and output.
- Assess the client's ability to void (may be a problem secondary to opiates).
- Manage pain adequately.
- Assist the client with ambulation within a few hours of surgery, if he or she is able.

Discharge Teaching
- Review drug therapy.
- Teach care of the incision.
- Review activity restrictions:
  - No lifting
  - No driving until physician permission
  - No strenuous activities
- Walk every day.
- Call the surgeon if symptoms of pain, numbness, and tingling worsen or if difficulty in swallowing occurs.
- Wear collar per surgeon's orders.

CHART 46-7

KEY FEATURES of
Postoperative Complications of Cervical Diskectomy and Fusion

- Hoarseness due to laryngeal injury; may be temporary or permanent
- Temporary dysphagia; may last few days to several months; usually not severe
- Esophageal, tracheal, or vertebral artery injury
- Wound infection
- Injury to the spinal cord or nerve roots
- Dura mater tears with associated cerebrospinal fluid leaks
- Pseudoarthrosis caused by nonunion of fusion
- Graft extrusion and screw loosening if a fusion was performed.

PATHOPHYSIOLOGY
Mechanisms of Injury

When sufficient force is applied to the spinal cord, damage results in neurologic deficits. Sources of force include injury to the vertebral column (fracture, dislocation, and subluxation) or penetrating trauma (gunshot or knife wounds). Although in some cases the cord itself may remain intact, at other times the cord undergoes a destructive process caused by a contusion, compression, or concussion.

The causes of SCI can be divided into primary and secondary mechanisms of injury (Okonkwo, 2003). Four primary mechanisms may result in an SCI: hyperflexion; hyperextension; axial loading, or vertical compression; and excessive rotation. Penetrating injuries to the cord may also occur.

A **hyperflexion** injury occurs when the head is suddenly and forcefully accelerated forward, causing extreme flexion of the neck (Figure 46-2). This type of injury often occurs in head-on collisions and diving accidents. Flexion injury to the lower thoracic and lumbar spine may occur when the trunk is suddenly flexed on itself, such as occurs in a fall on the buttocks. The posterior ligaments can be stretched or torn, or the vertebrae may fracture or dislocate. Either process may disrupt the integrity of the spinal cord, causing hemorrhage, edema, and necrosis.

Hyperextension injuries occur most often in automobile accidents in which the client's vehicle is struck from behind or during falls when the client's chin is struck (Figure 46-3).

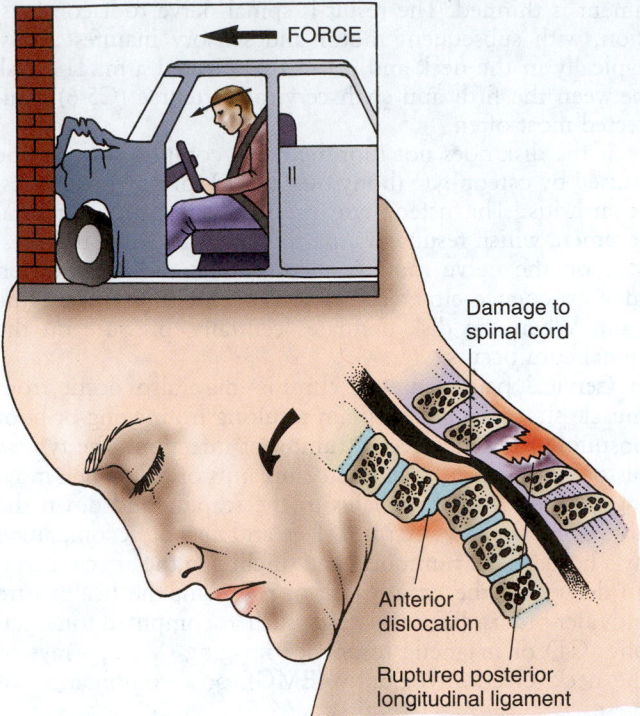

Figure 46-2 ■ Hyperflexion injury of the cervical spine.

The head is suddenly accelerated and then decelerated. This stretches or tears the anterior longitudinal ligament, fractures or subluxates the vertebrae, and perhaps ruptures an intervertebral disk. As with flexion injuries, the spinal cord may easily be damaged.

Diving accidents, falls on the buttocks, or a jump in which a person lands on the feet can cause many of the injuries attributable to **axial loading** (vertical compression) (Figure 46-4). The blow to the top of the head causes the vertebrae to shatter. Pieces of bone enter the spinal canal and damage the cord.

Rotation injuries are caused by turning the head beyond the normal range.

Penetrating injuries to the spinal cord are classified by the velocity of the vehicle (e.g., knife or bullet) causing the injury. Low-velocity or low-impact injuries cause damage directly at the site or localized damage to the spinal cord or spinal nerves. In contrast, high-velocity injuries that occur from gunshot wounds cause both direct and indirect damage.

Secondary injury exacerbates the primary injury and worsens morbidity. Secondary injuries include the following:
- Neurogenic shock
- Vascular insult
- Hemorrhage
- Ischemia
- Fluid and electrolyte imbalance

The spinal cord may be contused, lacerated, or compressed as a result of injury. Petechial hemorrhage into the central gray matter, and later into the white matter, can be caused by a contusion and laceration of the spinal cord. Spinal cord edema occurs as a result of cord compression by hemorrhage, bony fragments, or laceration. Necrosis of the spinal cord occurs from compromised capillary circulation and venous return.

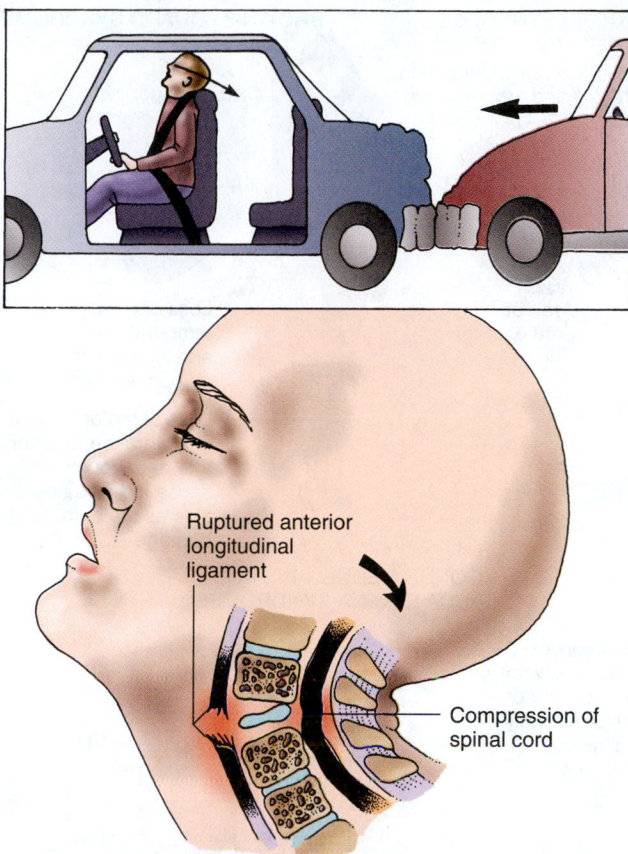

Figure 46-3 ■ Hyperextension injury of the cervical spine.

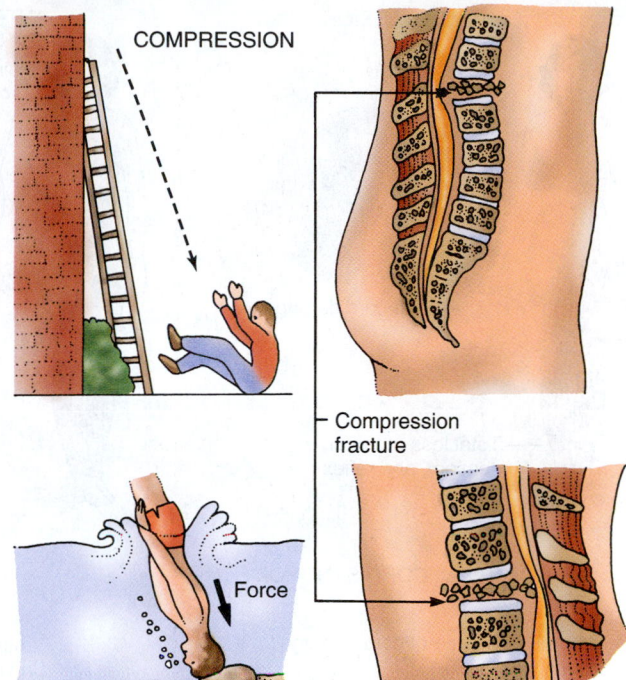

Figure 46-4 ■ Axial loading (vertical compression) injury of the cervical spine and the lumbar spine.

Extent of Injury

Incomplete SCIs are more common than complete lesions. A client experiencing an incomplete lesion typically has preservation of a mixed pattern of motor, sensory, and reflex function. Specific syndromes result from incomplete lesions (Figure 46-5). A "pure" syndrome may not be seen. Cervical injuries may produce the following:

- Anterior cord syndrome
- Posterior cord syndrome
- Brown-Séquard syndrome
- Central cord syndrome

Conus medullaris and cauda equina syndromes are associated with injuries to the lumbar and sacral cord.

CERVICAL INJURIES

Anterior cord syndrome results from damage to the anterior portion of both gray and white matter of the spinal cord, usually as a result of decreased blood supply. Although motor function and pain and temperature sensation are lost below the level of injury, the sensations of touch, position, and vibration remain intact. More than 50% of clients with this syndrome are older than 40 years, with most between 50 and 70 years. Functional motor control is recovered in 10% to 20% of clients with cervical spine injuries.

Just the opposite transpires in a rarely encountered **posterior cord lesion**, which also occurs from damage to the posterior gray and white matter of the spinal cord. Motor function remains intact, but the client experiences a loss of vibratory sense, crude touch, and position sensation.

Brown-Séquard syndrome generally results from pene-

trating injuries that cause hemisection of the spinal cord or injuries that affect half of the spinal cord. Motor function, proprioception, vibration, and deep touch sensations are lost on the same side of the body as the lesion (ipsilateral). On the opposite side of the body (contralateral) from the injury, the sensations of pain, temperature, and light touch are affected.

Lesions of the central portion of the spinal cord produce a **central cord syndrome.** Loss of motor function is more pronounced in the upper extremities than in the lower extremities. Varying degrees and patterns of sensation remain intact.

LUMBOSACRAL INJURIES

Damage to the cauda equina or conus medullaris produces a variable pattern of motor or sensory loss because the peripheral nerves have the potential for recovery and regrowth. In addition, this injury usually results in a neurogenic bowel and bladder.

Etiology

Trauma is the leading cause of spinal cord injuries (SCIs); almost 45% result from motor vehicle accidents. The second leading cause is acts of violence (24%), followed by falls (22%) and sports accidents (8%) (National Spinal Cord Injury Data Base [NSCIDB], 2001). Spinal cord damage can also result from diseases such as polio, spina bifida, and tumors.

Incidence/Prevalence

Between 250,000 and 400,000 persons in the United States have SCIs, and about 14,000 new injuries occur each year (Gibson, 2003). The client may be hospitalized for 3 months or longer, including acute care and rehabilitation. Life expectancy has increased, but it is still below that of individuals without an SCI. Clients usually die from complications of immobility or infection.

A typical client with an SCI is an unmarried man between 16 and 30 years of age. Peak incidence of injury occurs in the

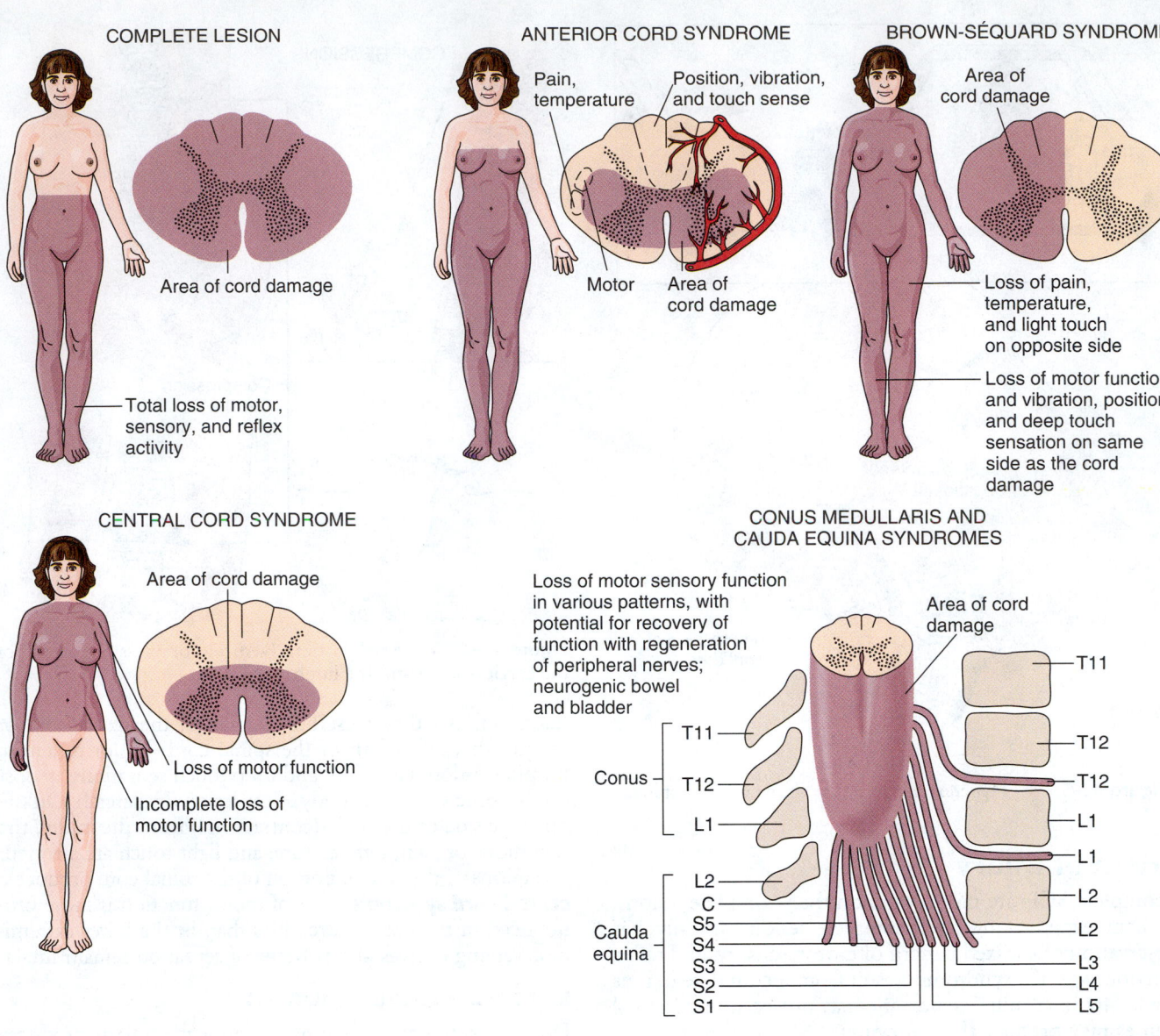

Figure 46-5 ■ Common spinal cord syndromes.

summer or warmer months. Men constitute 82% of SCI clients, and most are white. Most injuries are cervical. The percentage of persons over the age of 60 is 10% (NSCIDB, 2001).

◆COLLABORATIVE MANAGEMENT
◆Assessment

HISTORY

When obtaining a history from a client with a spinal cord injury (SCI), the nurse gathers as much data as possible about how the accident occurred and the probable mechanism of injury. Questions include the position of the client immediately after the injury, the symptoms that occurred after the injury, and the changes that have occurred since the initial appearance of signs and symptoms. If possible, pre-hospital rescue personnel are questioned about the type of immobilization devices used and whether any problems occurred during stabilization and transport to the hospital. Information is obtained about the medical treatment given at the scene of injury or in the emergency department (e.g., medications and IV fluids).

Obtain the client's medical history, including a history of arthritis of the spine, congenital deformities, osteoporosis or osteomyelitis, cancer, and previous injury or surgery of the neck or back. These health problems may cause or contribute to an SCI. A detailed history of any respiratory problems is particularly important if the client has experienced a cervical SCI.

PHYSICAL ASSESSMENT/CLINICAL MANIFESTATIONS

INITIAL ASSESSMENT. The *first priority* for the client with an SCI is assessing the respiratory pattern and ensuring an adequate airway. The client with a cervical SCI is at high risk for respiratory compromise because the cervical spinal nerves (C3-5) innervate the phrenic nerve, which controls the diaphragm. Endotracheal intubation may be necessary to prevent respiratory arrest.

The client is assessed for indications of intra-abdominal hemorrhage or hemorrhage or bleeding around fracture sites. Other indicators of hemorrhage include hypotension and tachycardia with a weak and thready pulse.

Use the Glasgow Coma Scale (see Chapter 44) to assess the client's level of consciousness (LOC). Cognitive impairment as a result of an associated traumatic brain injury (TBI) or substance abuse is seen in about half of all traumatic SCIs. A detailed assessment of the client's motor and sensory status is performed to assist in determining the level of injury and to serve as baseline data for future comparison. The level of injury is the lowest neurologic segment with intact or normal motor and sensory function. **Tetraplegia,** also called **quadriplegia** (paralysis), and **quadriparesis** (weakness) involve all four extremities, as seen with cervical cord injury. **Paraplegia** (paralysis) and **paraparesis** (weakness) involve only the lower extremities, as seen in lower thoracic and lumbosacral injuries or lesions.

Spinal shock occurs immediately after injury as a result of disruption in the communication pathways between upper motor neurons and lower motor neurons. This condition is characterized by the following:

- Flaccid paralysis
- Loss of reflex activity below the level of the lesion
- Bradycardia
- Paralytic ileus (occasionally)
- Hypotension

Spinal shock may last from a few days to several months; its reversal is indicated by the return of reflex activity.

ASSESSMENT OF SENSATION. Sensation is carried from the peripheral nerves to the spinal cord and up to the cerebral cortex via a variety of sensation-specific tracts. Injury to the spinal cord may prohibit sensory impulses from reaching the brain. To test sensory abilities, the client is asked to close his or her eyes. Touch the skin with a clean safety pin or cotton-tipped applicator and ask the client whether he or she can feel the pinprick or light touch. Bilateral responses are compared. Follow the sensory distribution of the skin dermatomes (see Figure 44-7), with the examination beginning in the area of reported loss of sensation and ending where sensation becomes normal. For example, sensation of the top of the foot and calf of the leg is spinal skin segment (dermatome) levels L3, L4, and L5. The area at the level of the umbilicus is T10, the clavicle is C3 or C4, and finger sensation is C7 and C8. The client may report a complete sensory loss, **hypoesthesia** (decreased sensation), or **hyperesthesia** (increased sensation).

The client's proprioceptive function may be assessed. Ask the client again to close his or her eyes. Next move one of his or her fingers or toes up or down. Ask the client to identify the position of the digits.

ASSESSMENT OF MOTOR ABILITY. In addition to performing a routine motor evaluation of the client, selected muscles are tested in a more systematic fashion (Chart 46-8). Many scales are available to measure motor function. The American Spinal Injury Association (ASIA) recommends a five-point grading scale, with 0 being no movement and 5 being normal strength. Ask the client to flex and extend the elbows, elevate both arms off the bed, flex and extend the wrists and fingers, and touch each finger to the thumb. Clients with spinal injuries at the fifth or sixth cervical vertebra are often able to flex but not extend

---

CHART 46-8

BEST PRACTICE for
Assessing Motor Function in the Client with a Spinal Cord Injury

- To assess C4-5, apply downward pressure while the client shrugs his or her shoulders upward.
- To assess C5-6, apply resistance while the client pulls up his or her arms.
- To assess C7, apply resistance while the client straightens his or her flexed arms.
- To assess C8, make sure the client is able to grasp an object and form a fist.
- To assess L2-4, apply resistance while the client lifts his or her legs from the bed.
- To assess L5, apply resistance while the client dorsiflexes his or her feet.
- To assess S1, apply resistance while the client plantar flexes his or her feet.

---

their arms. Observe the client's ability to move the lower extremities. Ask him or her to wiggle the toes, flex and extend the feet and knees, and move one or both hips.

The advanced practice nurse or health care provider may also test deep tendon reflexes (DTRs), including the biceps (C5), triceps (C7), patella (L3), and ankle (S1). It is not unusual for these reflexes, as well as all motor function or sensation, to be absent immediately after the injury because of spinal shock. After spinal shock has resolved, the reflexes may return if the lesion is incomplete or involves upper motor neurons.

CARDIOVASCULAR ASSESSMENT. Cardiovascular dysfunction is usually the result of disruption of the autonomic nervous system, especially if the injury is above the sixth thoracic vertebra. Bradycardia, hypotension, and hypothermia result from a loss of sympathetic input and may lead to cardiac dysrhythmias. A systolic blood pressure below 90 mm Hg requires treatment because lack of perfusion to the spinal cord would worsen the client's condition. In addition, the lack of sympathetic or hypothalamic control causes the client to lose thermoregulatory functions. As a result, the body tends to assume the temperature of the environment and attempts to compensate by increasing extracellular fluid.

EMERGENCY CARE. The client with an upper SCI must be observed for signs of **autonomic dysreflexia** (hyperreflexia). Dysreflexia is characterized by severe hypertension, bradycardia, severe headache, nasal stuffiness, and flushing (Chart 46-9). The cause of this syndrome is a noxious stimulus, most often a distended bladder or constipation. *This is a neurologic emergency and must be promptly treated to prevent a hypertensive stroke!* Chart 46-10 lists emergency care for autonomic dysreflexia.

RESPIRATORY ASSESSMENT. A client with a cervical SCI is at risk for respiratory problems resulting from immobility or from an interruption of spinal innervation to the respiratory muscles. Some clients require intubation and mechanical ventilation. A complete respiratory assessment is done in collaboration with the respiratory therapist, if available. The respiratory therapist should evaluate vital capacity and minute volume as part of the assessment. Periodic repetition of these tests should be performed as the client's clinical status indicates.

Closely monitor the client for life-threatening respiratory complications, such as an impaired gas exchange resulting

---

CHART 46-9

KEY FEATURES of
Autonomic Dysreflexia

- Sudden onset of severe, throbbing headache
- Severe, rapidly occurring hypertension
- Bradycardia
- Flushing above level of lesion (face and chest)
- Pale extremities below level of lesion
- Nasal stuffiness
- Sweating
- Nausea
- Blurred vision
- Piloerection
- Feeling of apprehension

CHART 46-10

BEST PRACTICE for
Emergency Care of the Client Experiencing Autonomic Dysreflexia:
Immediate Interventions

EMERGENCY CARE

- Place client in sitting position.
- Page/notify health care provider.
- Loosen tight clothing on the client.
- Assess for and treat the cause.
- Check the Foley catheter tubing (if present) for kinks or obstruction.
- If a Foley catheter is not present, check for bladder distention and catheterize immediately.
- Place anesthetic ointment on tip of catheter before insertion.
- Check the client for fecal impaction; if present, disimpact immediately using anesthetic ointment.
- Check the room temperature to ensure that it is not too cool or drafty.
- Monitor blood pressures every 10 to 15 minutes.
- Give nitrates or hydralazine (Apresoline, Novo-Hylazin ✱) as prescribed.

---

from pneumonia, pulmonary emboli, and atelectasis. Pneumonia and pulmonary emboli decrease the life expectancy of SCI clients and have replaced renal failure as the leading cause of death.

GASTROINTESTINAL AND GENITOURINARY ASSESSMENT. Assess the client's abdomen for indications of hemorrhage, distention, or paralytic ileus. Hemorrhage may result from the trauma, or it may occur later from a stress ulcer or the administration of steroids. Paralytic ileus may develop within 72 hours of hospital admission. During the period of spinal shock, peristalsis decreases, leading to a loss of bowel sounds and gastric distention. This lack of or interference with autonomic innervation may lead to a reflex or hypotonic bowel.

Autonomic dysfunction initially causes an areflexic bladder, which later leads to urinary retention and a neurogenic bladder. The client is at risk for urinary tract infection from an indwelling urinary catheter, from intermittent catheterizations, or from bladder distention, stasis, and overflow.

MUSCULOSKELETAL ASSESSMENT. Assess the client's muscle tone and size. Muscle wasting results from the long-term flaccid paralysis seen in clients with **lower motor neuron** (LMN) lesions. Incomplete lesions or **upper motor neuron** (UMN) lesions may cause muscle spasticity, which can lead to contractures after spinal shock has resolved.

Observe the condition of the client's skin, especially over pressure points, at least twice daily. Any reddened area is care-

fully assessed and monitored for change. A pressure-reducing mattress or special bed is used to prevent skin breakdown.

Another complication of prolonged immobility is **heterotopic ossification** (bony overgrowth, often into muscle), which occurs in 15% to 20% of all clients with spinal cord injury (SCI). It is evidenced by swelling, redness, warmth, and decreased range of motion (ROM) of the involved extremity. Changes in the bony structure are not visible until several weeks after initial symptoms appear.

PSYCHOSOCIAL ASSESSMENT

If possible, obtain information about the client's preinjury psychosocial status, usual methods of coping with illness, difficult situations, and disappointments. Determine the client's level of independence or dependence and his or her comfort level in discussing feelings and emotions with family members or close friends. Clients who are emotionally secure and have a positive self-image, supportive family, and financial and job security often adapt to their injury. Information about the client's religious beliefs or cultural background also assists the nurse in developing the plan of care. The client with an SCI must cope with changes in body image, self-esteem, independence, role relationships, and sexuality.

In addition, assess family members or significant others to determine how well they are coping with the client's injury and their role changes. The client and significant others must be prepared for extensive rehabilitation and changes in lifestyle. Financial constraints may pose additional stress.

LABORATORY ASSESSMENT

The health care provider orders routine laboratory studies for the client with an SCI to establish baseline data or to prepare for surgery. A urinalysis is used to check for the presence of blood in the urine after trauma. Arterial blood gas analysis is used to monitor the respiratory status of a client at risk for respiratory insufficiency. The findings should be within normal limits unless the client has a history of heavy smoking or preinjury pulmonary disease or is experiencing respiratory failure. Failure is indicated by decreased oxygen levels, increased carbon dioxide levels, and respiratory acidosis.

RADIOGRAPHIC AND OTHER DIAGNOSTIC ASSESSMENTS

The health care provider orders a complete radiographic series of the spine to identify vertebral fractures, subluxation, or dislocation. Computed tomography (CT) or magnetic resonance imaging (MRI) may be performed to determine the degree and extent of damage to the spinal cord and to detect the presence of blood and bone within the spinal column.

◆Analysis

COMMON NURSING DIAGNOSES AND COLLABORATIVE PROBLEMS

The following are the most common nursing diagnoses for clients with a spinal cord injury (SCI):

1. Ineffective Tissue Perfusion (Spinal Cord) related to interruption of arterial flow
2. Ineffective Airway Clearance, Ineffective Breathing Pattern, and Impaired Gas Exchange related to spinal cord injury

3. Impaired Physical Mobility or Self-Care Deficit (the level depends on the extent and level of the injury) related to decreased or absent muscle control
4. Impaired Urinary Elimination and Constipation related to sensory/motor impairment
5. Impaired Adjustment related to disability or health status change requiring change in lifestyle

ADDITIONAL NURSING DIAGNOSES AND COLLABORATIVE PROBLEMS

In addition to the common nursing diagnoses, clients with an SCI may have one or more of the following:
- Risk for Impaired Skin Integrity related to physical immobilization
- Sexual Dysfunction related to altered body function
- Acute Pain related to physical injury
- Risk for Injury related to altered mobility
- Imbalanced Nutrition: Less Than Body Requirements related to hypermetabolism or inability to absorb nutrients

Collaborative problems include the following:
- Potential for Deep Vein Thrombosis (DVT)
- Potential for Sepsis
- Potential for Hypoxemia
- Potential for Atelectasis, Pneumonia

◆Planning and Implementation

INEFFECTIVE TISSUE PERFUSION (SPINAL CORD)

PLANNING: EXPECTED OUTCOMES. The client with an SCI is expected to demonstrate adequate spinal cord tissue perfusion as evidenced by no further deterioration in neurologic status.

INTERVENTIONS. If the client has a fractured vertebra, the primary concern of the health care team is to reduce and immobilize the fracture to prevent further damage to the spinal cord from bone fragments. The health care provider typically uses nonsurgical techniques with traction or external fixation, but surgery may be necessary to stabilize the spine and prevent further spinal cord damage.

NONSURGICAL MANAGEMENT. Assess the client's vital signs and neurologic status, especially respiratory function and motor and sensory changes in the extremities every 4 hours or more often if clinically indicated. In the first 24 hours after injury, the client is at risk for **neurogenic shock** as manifested by hypotension and bradycardia. Neurogenic shock is most often associated with cervical spinal injuries and is caused by a loss of autonomic function.

NIC **Positioning: Neurologic.** Regardless of the level of SCI, keep the client in optimal body alignment to prevent further cord injury or irritability (Chart 46-11). Devices such as traction, orthoses, or collars may be used to keep the spine immobilized during healing and rehabilitation.

Immobilization for Cervical Injuries. The client with a cervical spine injury is usually placed in fixed skeletal traction to realign the vertebrae, facilitate bone healing, and prevent further injury. The most commonly used devices for immobilization are the halo fixation device and cervical tongs (Gardner-Wells, Barton, or Crutchfield tongs) (Figure 46-6). These devices may be used in conjunction with a Stryker

frame, rotational bed, or kinetic treatment table to allow frequent turning. Either device is inserted by the physician into the outer aspect of the skull. The addition of traction to the cervical tongs assists in reducing the fracture. Traction may or may not be used with the halo fixator. Traction weights may be prescribed by the physician.

The halo fixator is a static traction device (see Figure 46-6). Four pins (or screws) are inserted into the skull. The metal halo ring may be attached to a plastic vest or cast when the spine is stable, allowing increased client mobility. Never move or turn the client by holding or pulling on the halo device. Check the client's skin frequently to ensure that the jacket or cast is not causing pressure. The nurse should be able to insert one finger easily under the jacket or cast.

Monitor the client's neurologic status for changes in movement or decreased strength. The weights of the traction should hang freely at all times. Releasing the traction could cause further neurologic damage. Maintain the client in alignment, and ensure that the ropes for the traction remain within the pulley and hang freely. The insertion sites of the tongs or halo device are monitored for signs of infection. Hospital policy is followed for pin site care, which may specify the use of solutions such as hydrogen peroxide and saline.

CHART 46-11

NIC **INTERVENTION ACTIVITIES for**
The Client with a Spinal Cord Injury

Positioning: Neurologic: *Achievement of optimal, appropriate body alignment for the client experiencing or at risk for spinal cord injury or vertebral irritability.*
- Immobilize or support the affected body part, as appropriate.
- Place in the designated therapeutic position.
- Maintain proper body alignment.
- Position with head and neck in alignment.
- Turn using the log roll technique.
- Apply an orthosis collar.
- Instruct on orthosis collar care, as needed.
- Apply and maintain a splinting or bracing device.
- Monitor skin integrity under bracing device/orthosis collar.
- Instruct on pin site care, as needed.
- Monitor traction pin insertion site.
- Perform traction/orthosis device pin insertion site care.
- Monitor traction device setup.

Airway Management: *Facilitation of patency of air passages*
- Position client to maximize ventilation potential.
- Identify client requiring actual/potential airway insertion.
- Insert oral or nasopharyngeal airway, as appropriate.
- Perform chest physical therapy, as appropriate.
- Remove secretions by encouraging coughing or by suctioning.
- Encourage slow, deep breathing; turning; and coughing.
- Instruct how to cough effectively.
- Assist with incentive spirometer, as appropriate.
- Auscultate breath sounds, noting areas of decreased or absent ventilation and presence of adventitious sounds.
- Perform endotracheal or nasotracheal suctioning, as appropriate.
- Administer humidified air or oxygen, as appropriate.
- Regulate fluid intake to optimize fluid balance.
- Position to alleviate dyspnea.
- Monitor respiratory and oxygenation status, as appropriate.

NIC intervention activities selected from Dochterman, J.M., & Bulechek, G.M. (Eds.). (2004). *Nursing interventions classification (NIC)* (4th ed.). St. Louis: Mosby. No part of this work is to be altered without prior written permission from the Publisher.

Gardner-Wells tongs

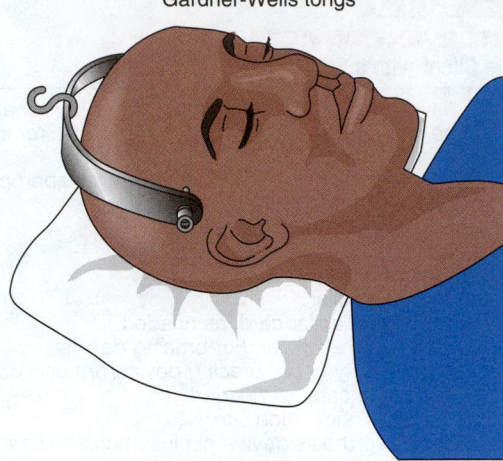

Halo fixation device with jacket

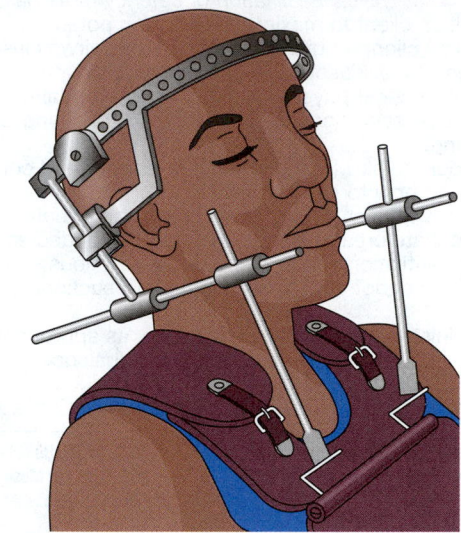

Figure 46-6 ■ Types of cervical spine traction.

Immobilization of Thoracic and Lumbar/ Sacral Injuries. The client with a thoracic injury is placed on bedrest; immobilization with a fiberglass or plastic body cast may be done (see also Chapter 55). For lumbar and sacral injuries, immobilization of the spine is typically accomplished with a brace or a corset worn when the client is out of bed. Newer lightweight, custom-fit thoracic lumbar sacral orthoses (TLSOs) are preferred over heavier braces or splints, such as the Taylor splint.

Drug Therapy. The administration of methylprednisolone (Solu-Medrol) is controversial. Previously it was thought that when given within 8 hours of injury the client showed improvement in motor and sensory function. Recent clinical trials do not support this as an evidenced-based standard of care for SCI because the adverse effects of the drug outweigh the benefits (Gibson, 2003). Dextran, a plasma expander, may be used to increase capillary blood flow within the spinal cord and to prevent or treat hypotension. Atropine sulfate is used to treat bradycardia if the pulse rate falls below 50 to 60 beats/min. Hypotension, if severe, is treated with inotropic and sympathomimetic agents such as dopamine hydrochloride (Intropin) and isoproterenol.

Research continues to explore interventions in pharmacologic and surgical management of SCIs. Naloxone (Narcan) and thyrotropin-releasing hormone (TRH) have shown promise in improving spinal cord blood flow. Sygen is being researched for use in acute SCI but may also be studied for its use for chronic SCI. Another drug, 4-AP, a potassium channel blocker, is thought to improve spinal cord conduction and remains in clinical trials for clients whose SCI is older than 18 months. Research in the areas of muscle stimulation and neural regeneration also shows promise.

Dantrolene (Dantrium) and baclofen (Lioresal) may help to control severe muscle spasticity (usually upper motor neuron [UMN] injuries). Severe spasticity may also be managed with intrathecal baclofen (ITB) therapy. The drug is administered through a programmable infusion pump and intrathecal catheter directly into the cerebrospinal fluid.

Other drugs to prevent or treat complications of immobility may be needed later during the rehabilitative phase. For example, etidronate disodium (Didronel) may be prescribed for the client with **heterotopic ossification** (bony overgrowth).

Critical Thinking Challenge

A 19-year-old college student is admitted to your neurosurgical/orthopedic unit from the neuroscience intensive care unit. He has a Halo fixator in place for an incomplete spinal cord injury following a car accident. His best friend was killed in the accident. The client has an indwelling urinary catheter and is sitting in a semi-Fowler's position when you enter his room. You notice that his face is flushed and he complains of being very hot.

1. What additional assessment data should you obtain at this time? Why?
2. Could you delegate part of the assessment to unlicensed assistive personnel? Why or why not?
3. What should you do *first* if you suspect an emergency situation? Why?

evolve For suggested answer guidelines, go to http://evolve.elsevier.com/Iggy/.

SURGICAL MANAGEMENT. Emergency surgery may be indicated if there is evidence of spinal cord compression. The procedure is usually necessary to remove bone fragments from a vertebral fracture, evacuate a hematoma, or remove penetrating objects such as a bullet. A **decompressive laminectomy** (removal of one or more laminae) allows for cord expansion from edema if more conventional measures fail to prevent neurologic deterioration. Postoperative care of clients having back surgery is discussed earlier in this chapter on p. 980.

Additional surgical procedures to stabilize and support the spine may be performed at the discretion of the physician, depending on the client's condition and the extent of the injury. Typical procedures include a spinal fusion and the insertion of metal or steel rods, such as Harrington rods, to stabilize thoracic spinal injuries. After surgery, the client usually wears a brace, a corset, or lumbosacral support (TLSO) to keep the operative area immobilized during recovery. (See also Chapter 55, Collaborative Management of Scoliosis.)

Postoperatively, assess the client's neurologic status and vital signs at least every hour for the first 4 to 6 hours after surgery and then, if the client is stable, every 4 hours. Complications of surgery, such as hematoma and edema, are manifested by a deterioration in neurologic status.

The client is also at risk for cardiovascular instability because of a loss of sympathetic innervation. In some cases the client may require a pacemaker. Log roll the client when he or she is being moved to maintain skeletal alignment or placed on a special bed such as a kinetic treatment table. Monitor the client's cardiovascular status carefully, especially with position changes. A complete discussion of postoperative nursing care is found in Chapter 22.

INEFFECTIVE AIRWAY CLEARANCE; INEFFECTIVE BREATHING PATTERN; IMPAIRED GAS EXCHANGE

NOC **PLANNING: EXPECTED OUTCOMES.** The client with an SCI is expected to have airway patency, alveolar exchange to maintain arterial blood gas (ABG) concentrations, and adequate ventilation. Indicators include that the following will not be compromised:

- Ease of breathing
- Respiratory rate and rhythm
- ABGs
- Oxygen saturation
- Auscultated breath sounds

INTERVENTIONS. Airway management is the priority for a client with spinal cord injury. Clients with injuries at or above the sixth thoracic vertebra are especially at risk for respiratory complications (e.g., pneumonia) and pulmonary embolus as a result of impaired functioning of the intercostal muscles. Depending on the level of injury, intubation or tracheotomy with mechanical ventilation may be needed.

Turn the client at least every 2 hours, and instruct him or her to breathe as deeply as possible. Assist the client who is tetraplegic to cough by placing his or her hands on either side of the rib cage or upper abdomen below the diaphragm. This technique is sometimes called "assisted coughing," "quad cough," or "**cough assist**." As the client inhales, push upward to help expand the lungs and cough.

Encourage the client to use an incentive spirometer. The nurse or respiratory therapist performs a respiratory assessment every 8 hours to determine the effectiveness of these strategies. In some cases it may be necessary to perform oral or nasal suctioning if the client cannot clear the airway of secretions effectively (see Chart 46-11).

IMPAIRED PHYSICAL MOBILITY; SELF-CARE DEFICIT

NOC **PLANNING: EXPECTED OUTCOMES.** The client with an SCI is expected to be free from complications of immobility and perform the most basic physical tasks and personal care activities as independently as possible with or without assistive/adaptive devices. Indicators include that the client will have no consequences of immobility, including the following:

- Pressure ulcers
- Venous thrombosis
- Contracted joints
- Bone fracture

Additional indicators include that the following will not be compromised:

- Transfer performance
- Wheelchair mobility
- Eating
- Dressing
- Bathing and grooming
- Oral hygiene

INTERVENTIONS. The client with an SCI is especially at risk for pressure ulcers, contractures, and deep vein thrombosis (DVT) or pulmonary emboli. Proper positioning not only helps to prevent complications but also provides alignment to prevent further spinal cord injury or irritability, as described under Positioning: Neurologic, p. 989.

Preventing Complications of Immobility. To decrease the high risk of pressure ulcers, the nurse or assistive nursing personnel turns and repositions the client in bed at least every 2 hours. When sitting in a chair, the client is repositioned or taught to reposition himself or herself more often than every 2 hours because in the sitting position most of the weight is placed on one area, the ischial tuberosities. Special pressure-relief devices, such as gel pads, may be used in the wheelchair or the bed, but these do not eliminate the need for regular turning and repositioning.

Inspect (and teach the client to inspect) the skin frequently to determine the client's tolerance for sitting and to detect reddened areas. Press on any reddened areas over the ischial tuberosities and look for blanching. If blanching does not occur, the area is vulnerable to skin breakdown.

To decrease the risk of contractures as a result of immobility, range-of-motion (ROM) exercises are performed at least once every 8 hours. The physical therapist and the occupational therapist will do the following:

- Determine the most appropriate positioning and exercise techniques
- Assess the need for hand and wrist splints
- Develop a plan to prevent footdrop (usually clients wear high-topped tennis shoes for prevention)

Assess the client's lower extremities for indications of DVT. Signs and symptoms include leg or calf pain, localized tenderness, swelling, and redness. Some clients may be totally asymptomatic. Recent guidelines for acute spinal cord injury (SCI) recommend a combination of low-molecular-weight heparin (LMWH) (e.g., enoxaparin [Lovenox]) and rotational bed, or adjusted-dose unfractionated heparin (Guides for Management of Acute Cervical Spinal Injury, 2002). Lovenox provides the same level of antithrombotic activity as heparin but may decrease the risk for hemorrhage. Graduated compression stockings (GCSs), also called sequential compression devices (SCDs), or pneumatic compression boots (PCBs) may be used with this regimen or in addition to these measures. Lovenox provides the same level of antithrombotic activity as heparin but may decrease the risk for hemorrhage (see Chapter 39 for a complete discussion of DVT prevention).

Preventing Orthostatic Hypotension. Clients with cervical cord injuries are especially at high risk for orthostatic (postural) hypotension, but any client who is immobilized may have this problem. If the client moves from a lying position to a sitting or standing position too quickly, he or she may experience hypotension, which could result in dizziness and falls. Because of interrupted autonomic innervation, the blood vessels do not constrict quickly enough to

---

CHART 46-12

BEST PRACTICE for
Care of the Client with a Spinal Cord Injury

- Assess the client's respiratory status; monitor for atelectasis, pneumonia, and pulmonary embolus.
- Take vital signs every 4 hours or more often if clinically indicated; monitor for orthostatic hypotension.
- Perform neurologic status checks every 4 hours or more often if clinically indicated.
- Notify the physician immediately of deterioration in motor status.
- Watch for and immediately treat autonomic dysreflexia.
- Give pain medication as prescribed; document the client's response.
- Prevent immobility complications.
    Have the client turn, cough, and deep breathe (TCDB) every 2 hours.
    Use pneumatic compression boots or gradated compression stockings.
    Check the skin and bony prominences for redness and breakdown.
- Assess bladder function.
    Palpate the abdomen for distention.
    Begin a bladder retraining program as appropriate.
    Assess intake and output.
- Assess bowel function.
    Auscultate bowel sounds.
    Palpate for distention.
    Chart stool frequency.
    Begin a bowel program as appropriate.
- Monitor nutritional status, including a calorie count, and collaborate with the dietitian to identify an appropriate diet.
- Assess psychological status.
    Communicate with the client.
    Answer questions honestly; refer questions that you cannot answer to someone who can.
    Assess for signs of depression or anger.

---

push blood up into the brain; this causes the dizziness or light-headedness often experienced by these clients.

Observe the client carefully for indications of orthostatic hypotension when the head of the bed is raised and when the client is permitted to dangle the legs over the side of the bed or to be up in a chair. Blood pressure is measured in each position.

To help prevent orthostatic hypotension, teach the client to change positions slowly. Some clients wear elastic corsets around the trunk to help facilitate blood flow. Thigh-high antiembolism stockings or elastic (Ace) wraps around both legs may also be used. A tilt table may be used to help the client get used to postural changes. Chart 46-12 summarizes the most important aspects of care for clients with an SCI.

Promoting Self-Care. The most important part of promoting self-care is setting realistic outcomes on the basis of the client's potential mobility and functional level. Even clients with a cervical SCI may be able to learn how to perform most activities of daily living (ADLs) independently. Collaborate with the physical therapist (PT) and occupational therapist to evaluate how the client can best transfer from a bed to the wheelchair and feed, dress, and bathe. Various assistive/adaptive devices are available to help clients regain their independence. Chapter 10 discusses self-care promotion in more detail.

Many clients with an SCI can no longer walk. They become wheelchair dependent and must learn new skills. The PT carefully measures the client and orders a custom-made

wheelchair. If the client is unable to self-propel the chair manually, electronic devices are available so he or she can use the mouth, neck, or upper arm to ambulate in the chair.

IMPAIRED URINARY ELIMINATION AND/OR CONSTIPATION

NOC **PLANNING: EXPECTED OUTCOMES.** The client with an SCI is expected to achieve control of elimination of urine and stool. Indicators include that the client will consistently demonstrate the following:

- Predictable pattern of voiding
- Voiding more than 150 mL each time
- Emptying the bladder completely
- Managing clothing independently
- No urinary incontinence
- No urinary infection
- Control of bowel movements
- Ease of stool passage

INTERVENTIONS. Clients with SCIs have reflex or neurogenic loss of bowel and bladder control. Many can become continent if they rigorously adhere to an established program. The type of program depends on the usual elimination pattern and whether the injury involved upper motor neurons (UMNs) or lower motor neurons (LMNs). A urologic evaluation may be needed to identify bladder type.

Establishing a Bladder Retraining Program. As soon as the client is medically stable, the indwelling Foley catheter is removed. Initially the physician may prescribe an intermittent catheterization program. The nurse typically catheterizes the client every 4 hours as ordered and more frequently if the urine output is greater than 500 mL. Over time the intervals between catheterizations are increased and adjusted to the client's fluid intake and sleep times. A bedside **bladder ultrasound** device is often used to measure bladder residual.

After the acute care phase has passed, the client may be able to initiate voiding by using specific techniques. Clients with UMN, or **spastic, bladder** problems (injury above the sacrum) may be able to stimulate voiding by doing the following:

- Stroking the inner thigh
- Pulling on pubic hair and hair of the upper thigh
- Pouring warm water over the perineum
- Tapping the bladder area to stimulate the detrusor muscle

Some health care providers prescribe a drug to stimulate voiding, such as bethanechol chloride (Urecholine). Bethanechol is a cholinergic agent that facilitates contraction of the detrusor muscle and is usually given two to four times daily about 1 hour before attempts to void.

Clients with injuries to the lumbosacral area usually have an LMN (flaccid) bladder. Clients with **flaccid bladders** may achieve emptying of the bladder by performing a Valsalva maneuver or tightening the abdominal muscles. These techniques are not successful for all LMN injuries. To ascertain the effectiveness of these maneuvers, catheterize the client for residual urine after voiding. Some clients rely solely on intermittent catheterization two or three times daily to empty the bladder. Obese clients and those with very high-level SCIs may need an indwelling urinary catheter (Gibson, 2003).

All clients are encouraged to drink 2000 to 2500 mL of fluid each day to prevent urinary tract infection (UTI) and calculus formation. Clients with an LMN injury may decrease fluid intake after 6 or 7 PM each evening to prevent the need for catheterization in the middle of the night.

The client with any SCI is at risk for long-term renal complications, such as hydronephrosis, renal failure, and kidney stones. UTIs are common because organisms are introduced into the urinary tract by urinary catheters. Clients with SCI may not be aware of the infection because he or she cannot perceive dysuria, urgency, or back pain. They must rely on other signs and symptoms, such as foul-smelling urine or fever.

Establishing a Bowel Retraining Program.
The following are essential elements of a bowel program:
- A consistent time for bowel elimination
- A high fluid intake (at least 2000 mL/day) unless fluid intake is restricted
- A high-fiber diet
- Rectal stimulation with or without suppositories
- If needed, stool softener medications such as docusate sodium (Colace) and docusate sodium and casanthranol (Peri-Colace)

If the client has sustained an LMN injury, the resulting flaccid large bowel may require the client to perform or undergo manual disimpaction. Additional stimuli to facilitate a bowel movement include scheduling toileting 30 minutes to 1 hour after meals to optimize the gastrocolic reflex and teaching the client to perform a Valsalva maneuver. Massaging the abdomen from right to left along the outline of the large intestine may also be helpful. Additional information about bladder and bowel retraining is provided in Chapter 10.

IMPAIRED ADJUSTMENT

NOC **PLANNING: EXPECTED OUTCOMES.** The client with an SCI is expected to develop an adaptive psychosocial response to a significant life change. Indicators include that the client will consistently demonstrate the following:
- Setting realistic goals
- Maintaining self-esteem
- Reporting feeling useful
- Verbalizing optimism about the present and future
- Identifying effective coping strategies

INTERVENTIONS. Information obtained from the psychosocial assessment is used by the interdisciplinary team to identify strategies to help the client adjust to the disability. Invite the client to ask questions, and answer them openly and honestly. Questions about prognosis and potential for complete recovery are referred to the health care provider because the timing and extent of recovery are different for each client.

Encourage the client to discuss his or her perceptions of the situation and the coping strategies that can be used. He or she should feel free to express personal feelings and emotions in an acceptable manner. The client may behave in a socially unacceptable manner (e.g., excessive anger, verbal abuse, use of illegal drugs); attempt to redirect this behavior. Begin a client education program to clarify misconceptions and provide health teaching. Referrals to clergy, rabbis, other spiritual leaders, or a psychologist or psychiatric liaison nurse may be needed to help clients adjust to their unexpected life change. Support groups are available for clients and their families.

Clients with SCIs should be referred to a social worker or financial counselor for a review of their insurance and financial status and also should be referred to the appropriate social service agencies as necessary. Many insurance policies do not provide coverage for extended rehabilitation services.

Community-Based Care

Case managers are ideal care coordinators to act as SCI client advocates. In some settings, case managers begin working with clients in the emergency department to establish a positive image of SCI rehabilitation. Rehabilitation begins in the critical care unit when clients are hemodynamically stable and spinal shock has subsided. They are usually transferred from the acute care setting to a rehabilitation setting, where they learn more about self-care, mobility skills, and bladder and bowel retraining. The length of stay in the rehabilitation hospital or unit is typically 1 to 3 months, depending on the medical complications that may occur, such as infections.

Psychosocial adaptation is one of the critical factors in determining the success of rehabilitation. The case manager or acute care nurse can help the client prepare for discharge or transfer to a rehabilitation hospital. Assist in verbalizing feelings and fears about body image, self-concept, role performance, and self-esteem. The client should be told about the expected reactions of those outside the security of the hospital environment. In the acute care setting, the nurse, family members, or friends can take the client to the hospital lobby or, if permitted, to the cafeteria or outside on the hospital grounds. Let the client know, in a tactful and nonjudgmental manner, when his or her behavior is unacceptable for the time and place in which it occurs, and encourage more positive behaviors. Role-playing or anticipating responses to potential problems is helpful. For example, the client can practice answering questions from children about why he or she is in a wheelchair or cannot move certain parts of the body.

HOME CARE MANAGEMENT

If the client is discharged home or returns home for a weekend visit from the rehabilitation setting, the environment must be assessed to ensure that it is free from hazards and can accommodate the client's special needs (e.g., a wheelchair). The occupational or physical therapist, in collaboration with rehabilitation and the home care nurse, usually assesses the client's temporary or permanent home environment. Ease of accessibility is particularly important at the entrance of the home as well as the bathroom, kitchen, and bedroom. The height of the client's bed may need to be adjusted to facilitate a smooth transfer into or out of the bed.

All adaptive devices that the client will use at home should be ordered and delivered to the rehabilitation facility. This enables the nurse and other therapists to ensure that the items fit correctly and that the client and family know how to use them correctly.

HEALTH TEACHING

The teaching plan for the client with an SCI includes the following:
- Physical mobility and activity skills (including skin care)
- Activities of daily living (ADLs) skills

CHART 46-13

CLIENT EDUCATION GUIDE
Use of a Halo Device*

- Be aware that the weight of the halo device alters balance. Be careful when leaning forward or backward.
- Wear loose clothing, preferably with hook and loop (Velcro) fasteners or large openings for head and arms.
- Bathe in the bathtub or sponge bath. (Some physicians allow showers.)
- Wash under the lamb's wool liner of the vest to prevent rashes or sores; use powders or lotions sparingly under the vest.
- Have someone change the liner if it becomes odorous.
- Support the head with a small pillow when sleeping to prevent unnecessary pressure and discomfort.
- Try to resume usual activities to the extent possible; keep as active as possible. (The weight of the device may cause fatigue or weakness.) Avoid contact sports or swimming, however.
- Do not drive because vision is impaired with the device.
- Keep straws available for drinking fluids.
- Cut meats and other food into small pieces to facilitate chewing and swallowing.
- Before going outside in cold temperatures, wrap the pins with cloth to prevent the metal from getting cold.
- Have someone clean the pin sites as recommended by physician or hospital protocol.
- Observe the pin sites daily for redness, drainage, or loosening; report changes to the physician.
- Increase fluids and fiber in the diet to prevent constipation.
- Use a position of comfort during sexual activity.

*Home care instructions may vary depending on hospital or physician preference.

CHART 46-14

NURSING FOCUS on the OLDER ADULT
What Clients Need to Know About Aging with Spinal Cord Injury

Nursing Intervention	Rationales
Get flu shots annually, tetanus shots every 10 years, and the pneumonia vaccine as required.	Respiratory complications are the most common cause of death following spinal cord injury (SCI).
For women, have annual Papanicolaou (Pap) smears and mammograms.	Limitations in movement may make breast self-examination difficult. All older women should have an annual Pap smear.
Take measures to prevent osteoporosis, such as increasing calcium intake, exercising, and avoiding caffeine and smoking.	Women over 50 years of age often lose bone density, which can result in fractures.
Practice meticulous skin care, including moisturizing and drinking plenty of water.	As a person ages, skin becomes dry and less elastic, predisposing the client to pressure ulcers.
Take measures to prevent constipation, such as drinking adequate fluids, eating a healthy diet with fiber, and exercising.	Constipation is a problem for most clients with SCI, and they are more likely to develop the problem later in life.
Modify activities if joint pain occurs; use a powered rather than a manual wheelchair. Ask the health care provider about treatment options.	Arthritis occurs in more than half of people over 65 years of age. Clients with SCI are more likely to develop arthritis as a result of added stress on the upper extremities when using a wheelchair.

- Bowel and bladder retraining program
- Medication regimen
- Sexuality education

This information should be reinforced with written handouts or other client education material that the client, family members, or significant others can use after discharge to the home.

MOBILITY AND ACTIVITIES OF DAILY LIVING. It is important that the client learn mobility skills so that he or she can negotiate movement on sidewalks, carpeting, and other flooring surfaces. The client must also be able to negotiate sidewalk curbs while walking independently with crutches or a cane or while in a wheelchair.

Some clients are discharged home or to a rehabilitation setting with a halo vest. A halo vest has a significant physical and psychological impact on clients. Physically, clients find it difficult to perform mobility skills and ADLs independently, especially dressing, bathing, and feeding. From a psychological perspective, clients perceive an altered body image. Teach the client or other caregiver going home or to a rehabilitation setting how to care for and adjust to the halo device (Chart 46-13).

The ADL training for the client with an SCI includes a structured exercise program to promote strength and endurance. The occupational therapist instructs the client in the correct use of all adaptive equipment. In collaboration with the therapists, instruct family members or the caregiver in transfer skills, feeding, bathing, dressing, positioning, and skin care as discussed previously in this chapter and in Chapter 10.

BOWEL AND BLADDER TRAINING. Collaborate with the dietitian to help the client maintain an ideal body weight and to promote bowel and bladder elimination. Re-inforce the need to follow the client's individualized bowel and bladder program, and teach the client in the procedures to follow if problems develop.

MEDICATION REGIMEN. Teach the client and his or her family or other caregiver about the name, purpose, dosage, timing of administration, and side effects of all medications. They should also understand the possible interaction of prescribed medications with over-the-counter medications or alcohol and illegal drugs.

SEXUALITY EDUCATION. The goal of sexuality education is to answer questions and correct any misinformation. Women with SCI are able to have sexual intercourse and conception, although menses may be temporarily interrupted initially. For men, SCIs often affect fertility and sexual function. Erection and ejaculation are impaired for many clients. Unless the nurse has specific training or experience in sexuality counseling of people with SCIs, detailed questions should be directed to a sexuality counselor or urologist.

CONSIDERATIONS FOR OLDER ADULTS

Many clients with SCI are living into middle and older adulthood. Thinking and planning about preventive health care for the future are important parts of health teaching. Chart 46-14 outlines important interventions for maintaining health in older adults with SCI.

HEALTH CARE RESOURCES

The nurse or case manager refers the client and family or significant others to the local, state or province, and national organizations for those with SCIs. These organizations include the National Spinal Cord Injury Association and the Spinal Cord Injury Hotline. Many consumer-oriented books, journals, and films are also available. Support groups may help the client and family adjust to a changed lifestyle and provide solutions to commonly encountered problems.

A full-time caretaker or personal assistant is usually required if the quadriplegic client returns home. The caretaker may be a family member or a nursing assistant employed to help provide care and companionship. A paraplegic client is often able to function without assistance after an appropriate rehabilitation program.

Critical Thinking Challenge

The college student with an incomplete cervical spinal cord injury will soon be discharged to home with his parents. He continues to have a Halo device but is able to void using bladder stimulation techniques rather than catheterization. The client has been reluctant to discuss the death of his friend in the car accident in which he was injured.

1. What are the priorities for discharge planning in this situation?
2. What health care resources will the client require?
3. What health teaching will he require and why?

evolve For suggested answer guidelines, go to http://evolve.elsevier.com/Iggy/.

◆ Evaluation: Outcomes

Evaluate the care of the client with an SCI on the basis of the identified nursing diagnoses and collaborative problems. The expected outcomes are that the client:

- Exhibits no deterioration in neurologic status
- Maintains a patent airway, an alveolar exchange to maintain arterial blood gas concentration, and adequate ventilation
- Is free from complications of immobility
- Performs basic activities of living as independently as possible with or without the use of assistive/adaptive devices
- Achieves control of elimination of stool and urine
- Develops an adaptive psychosocial response to a significant life change

Specific indicators for these outcomes are listed for each nursing diagnosis under the Planning and Implementation section (see earlier).

SPINAL CORD TUMORS

Spinal cord tumors occur most often in the thoracic area, followed by an almost equal distribution in the lumbar and cervical region. Signs and symptoms depend on the location of the tumor and its speed of growth.

PATHOPHYSIOLOGY

The pathologic effects of a spinal cord tumor are more often related to compression of the cord than to invasion of the spinal cord itself. As the tumor expands within the vertebral column, it compresses the cord or the spinal nerve roots. Further growth leads to displacement of the cord. In addition, a large tumor may disrupt the vascular supply to the cord by compression or obstruct the normal flow of cerebrospinal fluid (CSF). Venous occlusion by the tumor may lead to spinal cord congestion and infarction.

The appearance of neurologic signs and symptoms is related to the rate of tumor growth. The spinal cord can often accommodate a slowly growing lesion. With time, the cord may become significantly misshapen and displaced, but the client has surprisingly few symptoms. On the other hand, a rapidly growing tumor quickly leads to spinal cord compression and edema and the development of neurologic symptoms, such as numbness and paralysis.

Primary spinal cord tumors arise from the epidural vessels, spinal meninges, or glial cells of the cord. Their cause is unknown. About 20% to 30% of spinal cord tumors (called secondary tumors) develop as a consequence of metastatic tumors from the lungs, breasts, prostate, colon, and uterus.

Anatomically, spinal cord tumors may be extramedullary or intramedullary. **Intramedullary tumors** account for 10% of spinal cord tumors and are usually malignant. They originate within the spinal cord itself, in the central gray matter and the anterior commissure. **Extramedullary tumors,** representing 90% of spinal cord tumors, are found within the spinal dura but outside the cord. They are further defined anatomically as extradural and intradural tumors. Extradural or epidural tumors occur between the vertebrae and the spinal dura. They develop in the surrounding bone and cause destruction of the vertebral bodies. Intradural tumors are located within the dura and originate from the pia-arachnoid, spinal roots, or denticulate ligaments.

Spinal cord tumors account for only about 0.5% of all tumors in adults and 10% to 15% of primary central nervous system (CNS) tumors. Thoracic tumors account for 50% of all spinal cord tumors. Cervical tumors occur 30% of the time, followed by lumbosacral tumors (20%). Most of these tumors are benign. They occur equally in both men and women between 20 and 60 years of age.

◆ COLLABORATIVE MANAGEMENT
◆ Assessment

PHYSICAL ASSESSMENT/CLINICAL MANIFESTATIONS

The clinical manifestations of a spinal cord tumor depend on its location (Chart 46-15) and rate of growth. The most common complaint of the client with a spinal cord tumor is pain. Pain results from spinal cord compression, infiltration of the spinal tracts, or irritation of the spinal roots. Assess the quality, severity, and intensity of the pain. In addition, ask the client to describe factors that exacerbate and relieve the pain. **Radicular** (nerve root) pain is described as stabbing or dull, with intermittent episodes of sharp, piercing pain. The term **radiculopathy** is commonly used to refer to radicular pain. The pain may be increased during coughing, straining, or sneezing. Lying flat may increase the pain as a consequence of stretching the involved spinal nerve roots.

Involvement of the corticospinal tract may lead to motor deficits. The nurse assesses for weakness, clumsiness, spasticity, and hyperactive reflexes and compares the responses on both sides of the body. Other presenting signs include ataxia, hypotonia, and a positive Babinski's reflex. Spastic

CHART 46-15

KEY FEATURES of
Spinal Cord Tumors

General Manifestations
- Pain
- Sensory loss or impairment
- Motor loss or impairment
- Sphincter disturbance (bladder before bowel)

Cervical Manifestations
High Cervical
- Respiratory distress
- Diaphragm paralysis
- Occipital headache
- Quadriparesis
- Stiff neck
- Nystagmus
- Cranial nerve dysfunction

Low Cervical
- Pain in the arms and the shoulders
- Weakness
- Paresthesia
- Motor loss
- Horner's syndrome
- Increased reflexes

Thoracic Manifestations
- Sensory loss
- Spastic paralysis
- Positive Babinski's sign
- Bladder and bowel dysfunction
- Pain in the chest and the back
- Muscle atrophy
- Muscle weakness in the legs
- Foot drop

Lumbosacral Manifestations
- Low back pain
- Paresis
- Spastic paralysis
- Sensory loss
- Bladder and bowel dysfunction
- Sexual dysfunction
- Decreased-to-absent ankle and knee reflexes

paralysis is seen most often, although a flaccid paralysis may be seen in a tumor that affects the spinal roots, in an intramedullary tumor in the enlargements of the cervical or lumbar area, or in an extramedullary tumor complicated by spinal shock. A flaccid paralysis may also be noted in the presence of a cauda equina lesion.

Determine sensory loss on each side of the body and compare the responses. Early symptoms of sensory loss include a slowly progressive numbness or tingling, pain, and temperature loss. The sensory deficit is further marked by a decreased appreciation of touch, an inability to sense vibration, and a loss of position sense. The client often reports a tight, bandlike feeling around the trunk. Brown-Séquard syndrome or central cord syndrome may be manifested (see Extent of Injury [Spinal Cord Injury], pp. 984 and 985).

Loss of bladder control often occurs before a loss of bowel control in the client with a spinal cord tumor. Typically, bladder dysfunction is manifested by hesitancy, dribbling, incontinence, urgency, or acute retention. Bowel dysfunction is manifested by constipation. Keep in mind that the client is often embarrassed to admit to bladder or bowel dysfunction.

A lesion in the sacral area may cause a decrease in genital sensation and thus impair the client's sexual function and enjoyment. Men may be unable to have an erection or to ejaculate.

DIAGNOSTIC ASSESSMENT

Routine x-ray examinations or tomographic scans of the spine are obtained to detect a narrowing of the spinal canal, destruction of the vertebrae, or the presence of calcification. A myelogram may be useful when a block is incomplete; it indicates the level, extent, and boundaries of a tumor. This test is being performed less today due to newer imaging techniques.

A magnetic resonance imaging (MRI) scan with and without enhancement provides more detail of the pathologic condition of the spinal cord than either a computed tomography (CT) scan or myelography. EMG may help make a differential diagnosis to rule out multiple sclerosis (MS) or amyotrophic lateral sclerosis (ALS).

◆ Interventions

Nursing care of the client with a spinal cord tumor includes obtaining the vital signs and checking neurologic status at least every 4 hours and more often as clinically indicated. As for any client with a spinal cord problem, report any change in motor and sensory status immediately to the physician.

SURGICAL MANAGEMENT. The primary management of a spinal cord tumor is surgery. The goal of surgical intervention is to remove as much of the tumor as possible. Often this is not feasible, and other treatment is indicated (e.g., radiation therapy). Emergency surgery is indicated if the client experiences a rapid loss of motor and sensory function or a loss of bladder and bowel control. Surgical decompression may be performed to maintain bladder, bowel, or motor function and to preserve quality of life—even with a poor prognosis.

The neurosurgeon performs a laminectomy and surgical decompression and total or partial resection of the tumor. Depending on the extent of the tumor, a spinal fusion may be necessary. Rarely, a cordotomy or a palliative sectioning of sensory roots is done to control intractable pain. Laminectomies are discussed under Surgical Management (Back Pain), p. 980.

After surgery, assess the client's vital signs and neurologic status every 1 to 2 hours until they are stable and then every 4 hours. The client is log rolled (turned as a unit) and repositioned every 2 hours. Inspect the incision site for drainage, especially of cerebrospinal fluid (CSF), and signs of infection. The client with a cervical cord tumor must also be carefully monitored for respiratory compromise. Postoperative nursing care for a client undergoing a laminectomy is discussed under Postoperative Care (Back Pain), pp. 980 and 981.

NONSURGICAL MANAGEMENT

Radiation Therapy. Radiation therapy may be necessary, depending on the tumor type. It is usually used with low-grade malignant tumors that are not completely resected, with metastatic tumors, or with recurrent tumors when there is no other treatment option. The spinal cord cannot tolerate high doses of radiation. Overexposure to radiation may lead to radiation myelopathy, which develops over 6 to 12 months. It is manifested by progressive spinal cord degeneration and neurologic deficits such as Brown-Séquard syndrome. With time, the client experiences spastic paralysis, loss of sensation, and bowel and bladder dysfunction; death may occur. Care of the client undergoing radiation therapy is described in detail in Chapter 28.

Chemotherapy. The use of chemotherapy in the treatment of spinal cord tumors is very limited. There are no reports of clinical trials with chemotherapy for primary spinal cord tumors. However, chemotherapy may be used as an adjunctive therapy for tumors metastasized to the spinal cord from other primary sites, such as the breast. Leptomeningeal involvement may benefit from intrathecal (spinal) chemotherapy.

Pain Control. Pain control may be accomplished by pharmacologic and nonpharmacologic measures. Patient-controlled analgesia (PCA) with morphine is often used to provide immediate postoperative pain relief. The client is gradually switched to oral analgesics before discharge. As per the standard of care, assess the client's level of pain, provide appropriate pain relief medication, and document the response to the medication. If drug therapy does not provide pain relief, collaborate with the health care provider to identify a more effective medication.

Turning and proper positioning of the client often enhances pain relief. The nurse or assistive nursing personnel provides range-of-motion (ROM) exercises to prevent atrophy and contractures, which can increase pain. Hypnosis, music therapy, and imagery techniques are other methods of pain relief (see Chapters 4 and 7).

Preventing Complications of Immobility. The client who is immobilized from a spinal cord tumor or spinal surgery is especially at risk for pressure sores and deep vein thrombosis (DVT) or pulmonary emboli. The nurse or assistive nursing personnel turns the client in bed at least every 2 hours. When the client is sitting in a chair, he or she is repositioned every 30 to 60 minutes.

Inspect the client's skin frequently to determine tolerance for sitting and to detect the presence of reddened areas. Press on the reddened areas over the ischial tuberosities and look for blanching. If blanching does not occur, the area is vulnerable to skin breakdown. The physical and occupational therapists determine the most appropriate positioning and exercise techniques and assess the need for assistive devices. It may be necessary for the client to be placed on a waterbed or an air mattress to prevent or treat pressure ulcers.

Monitor the client's lower extremities for indications of DVT. Sequential compression devices may be used in place of or as an adjunct to graduated compression stockings. The health care provider may prescribe sodium heparin 5000 units subcutaneously every 12 hours, low-molecular-weight heparin (enoxaparin [Lovenox]), or sodium warfarin (Coumadin, Warfilone✱) in therapeutic dosages to help prevent DVT or embolus formation.

Bowel and Bladder Program. Ask the client about his or her normal defecation pattern. On the basis of this information, establish a bowel program. The following are the essential elements of this program:

- A consistent time for bowel elimination
- A high fluid intake (2000 mL/day) unless fluid intake is restricted
- A high-fiber diet
- Rectal stimulation with or without suppositories

- If needed, stool softener medications, such as docusate sodium (Colace) and docusate sodium and casanthranol (Peri-Colace)

Manual disimpaction may be necessary if the client has lower motor neuron (LMN) symptoms.

The client's bladder program is determined by the specific dysfunction, usually urinary retention. The nurse or assistive nursing personnel monitors the voiding pattern and strictly measures and records intake and output. Assess for suprapubic distention and other indications of retention, such as overflow and dribbling. Encourage the client to empty the bladder every 2 hours.

Community-Based Care

HOME CARE MANAGEMENT

Collaborate with the client and his or her family members or significant others to identify and suggest corrections for potential hazards in the home. If needed, make a referral to a home care nurse, social worker, or case manager to assess the need for structural alterations to the home. Structural alterations may be needed to accommodate ambulatory aids (e.g., a walker) and to enable the client to perform activities of daily living (ADLs).

Some clients may be discharged from the acute care hospital to a rehabilitation setting, where they can learn to function as independently as possible. Chapter 10 describes rehabilitation in detail.

HEALTH TEACHING

The teaching plan for the client with a spinal cord tumor depends on his or her level of dysfunction. With decompression of the tumor, the severity of the client's symptoms often lessens. Deficits that may remain include mobility and sensory loss. Learning mobility skills can enable the client to negotiate movement on sidewalks, carpeting, and other flooring surfaces. The client must also be able to negotiate sidewalk curbs independently. The physical or occupational therapist instructs the client in the correct use of all adaptive equipment. Review the individualized bowel and bladder program with the client, family member, or other caregiver.

The goal of sexuality education in the acute care setting is to answer questions and correct any misinformation. Unless the nurse has had specific training or experience in sexuality counseling of people with spinal cord tumors or injuries, more detailed questions should be directed to a sexuality counselor.

HEALTH CARE RESOURCES

The prognosis for the client with malignant tumors or secondary tumors is poor. Determine what the physician and family members have told the client about diagnosis and prognosis. Encourage the client to verbalize feelings and fears about prognosis, body image, self-concept, role performance, and self-esteem.

Clients and family members or significant others should be referred to local, state or province, and national organizations for people with spinal cord injuries, which are applicable to spinal cord tumors. These groups often have information for clients with spinal cord tumors. Refer clients with a malignancy to the American Cancer Society. Referral to support groups may also assist clients and family with adapting to lifestyle changes.

MULTIPLE SCLEROSIS

Multiple sclerosis (MS) is a chronic autoimmune disease that affects the myelin sheath and conduction pathway of the central nervous system (CNS). It is one of the leading causes of neurologic disability in persons 20 to 40 years of age.

PATHOPHYSIOLOGY

This chronic disease is characterized by periods of remission and **exacerbation** (flare). As the severity and duration of the disease progress, the periods of exacerbation become more frequent. MS has received increased public attention since actress Annette Funicello and talk show host Montel Williams were diagnosed with the disease.

Multiple sclerosis is characterized by an inflammatory response that results in random or patchy areas of plaque in the white matter of the central nervous system (CNS). When this occurs, the myelin sheath is damaged and its thickness is reduced. Myelin is responsible for the electrochemical transmission of impulses between the brain and spinal cord and the rest of the body. Impulses are still transmitted but are not as effective as before; over time they may be completely blocked. The white fiber tracts (especially the axons) that connect the neurons in the brain and spinal cord are generally involved in MS. The areas particularly affected include optic nerves, pyramidal tracts, posterior columns, brainstem nuclei, and the periventricular region of the brain. Eventually, with repeated exacerbations of the disease, damage to the axons becomes permanent.

Major types of MS include the following:
- Relapsing-remitting
- Progressive-relapsing
- Primary progressive
- Secondary progressive

The classic picture of the **relapsing-remitting** type of MS (RRMS) occurs in 85% of cases. The course of the disease may be mild or moderate, depending on the degree of disability. Relapses develop over 1 to 2 weeks and resolve over 4 to 8 months, after which the client returns to baseline. Of the 85% who start with relapsing-remitting disease, more than 50% will develop secondary progressive MS (SPMS) within 10 years; 90% develop it within 25 years (Costello & Harris, 2003).

Progressive-relapsing MS (PRMS) occurs less often, that is, in only 5% of clients with MS. It is characterized by the absence of periods of remission, and the client's condition does not return to baseline. Progressive, cumulative symptoms and deterioration occur over several years.

Primary progressive MS (PPMS) involves a steady and gradual neurologic deterioration without remission of symptoms. The client has progressive disability with no acute attacks. Clients with this type of MS tend to be between 40 and 60 years of age at onset of the disease.

Secondary progressive MS (SPMS) begins with a relapsing-remitting course that later becomes steadily progressive. Attacks and partial recoveries may continue to occur.

Etiology and Genetic Risk

The exact cause of MS remains unknown. Research continues on viral, immunologic, and genetic and environmental etiologic factors. Viruses are well recognized as causes of demyelination and inflammation; so it may be possible that a virus or other infectious agent is the triggering factor in MS. Although a number of viruses have been studied, no single virus has been identified as causing MS.

The immune theory suggests that an unidentified factor triggers an autoimmune response in the brain, spinal cord, and visual system. Both humoral and cell-mediated immune system dysfunction have been implicated. This theory is supported by research data that show elevated immunoglobulin G (IgG) and oligoclonal bands in the CSF of clients with MS (Costello & Harris, 2003).

According to the National Multiple Sclerosis Society:
- Having a first-degree relative such as a parent or sibling with MS increases an individual's risk of developing the disease.
- There is a higher prevalence of certain genes in populations with higher rates of MS.
- Common genetic factors have been found in some families in which there is more than one person with MS.
- The environment may also contribute to the development of MS. The disease is seen more often in the colder climates of the northeastern, Great Lakes, and Pacific northwestern states as well as in Canada.

Incidence/Prevalence

Multiple sclerosis (MS) usually occurs in people between the ages of 20 and 40 years, but cases may occur in those younger than 15 years and older than 50 years. It is known as the disease of young adults. Only 20% of clients with MS report that the first symptom occurred in their 40s or 50s. About 500,000 people in the United States are currently affected. Women are affected slightly more often than men (1.5:1). The incidence in first-degree relatives of persons with MS is 15 times greater than in the general population The life expectancy for those with MS is about 85% of that of the general population, or about 35 years after the onset of symptoms (Finesilver, 2003).

◆ COLLABORATIVE MANAGEMENT
◆ Assessment

HISTORY

Multiple sclerosis (MS) often mimics other neurologic diseases, which often makes the diagnosis difficult and prolonged. Therefore obtaining a thorough history is essential for accurate diagnosis. The client is queried for a history of vision changes, motor skills, and sensations, all of which are early indicators of MS. The symptoms are often vague and nonspecific in the early stages of the disease. Of significance is the client's report that symptoms were first noticed several years earlier but that medical attention was not sought because the symptoms disappeared. Other information to be obtained includes questions about the progression of symptoms, with particular attention given to determining whether the symptoms are intermittent or are becoming progressively worse. Document the date (month and year) when the client first noticed the clinical manifestations.

Next question about factors that aggravate the symptoms, such as fatigue, stress, overexertion, temperature extremes, or a hot shower or bath. Ask the client and the family about any personality or behavioral changes that have occurred (e.g., euphoria, poor judgment, inattentiveness). In addition, determine whether there is a family history of MS.

PHYSICAL ASSESSMENT/CLINICAL MANIFESTATIONS

Multiple sclerosis produces a wide variety of manifestations. Any myelinated fibers of the brain and spinal cord may be affected. To determine a client's specific manifestations, the nurse performs a complete neurologic assessment.

MOTOR ASSESSMENT. First assess the client's motor status. The client often reports increased fatigue and stiffness of the extremities, particularly the legs. Fatigue is one of the most disabling manifestations, affecting 70% to 90% of clients with MS. Unlike fatigue in others, MS fatigue is characterized by persistent sensitivity to temperature (Costello & Harris, 2003).

Flexor spasms at night may awaken the client from sleep. Further examination reveals increased, or hyperactive, deep tendon reflexes; clonus; positive Babinski's reflex; and absent abdominal reflexes. Gait may be unsteady because of leg weakness and spasticity.

Significant cerebellar findings include **intention tremor** (tremor when performing an activity), **dysmetria** (inability to direct or limit movement), and dysdiadochokinesia (inability to stop one motor impulse and substitute another). Motor movements are often clumsy; the client may lose balance easily and may exhibit signs of poor coordination.

During examination of the cranial nerves and brainstem function, the client may report tinnitus (ringing in the ears), vertigo (dizziness), and hearing loss. The client may show indications of facial weakness and have dysphagia. Speech problems include dysarthria (slurred speech), ataxia, and slow, scanning speech.

Typical clinical findings from assessment of the client's visual acuity, visual fields, and pupils include the following:

- Blurred vision
- **Diplopia** (double vision)
- Decreased visual acuity
- **Scotomas** (changes in peripheral vision)
- **Nystagmus** (involuntary, rapid eye movements)

SENSORY ASSESSMENT. Sensory findings include hypalgesia (diminished sensitivity to pain), paresthesia, facial pain, and decreased temperature perception. The client may report numbness, tingling, burning, or crawling sensations.

If demyelination of the spinal cord has occurred, the client may experience bowel and bladder dysfunctions as well as alterations in sexuality. The client may have an areflexic bladder or may experience frequency, urgency, or nocturia. Bowel problems include altered rectal tone, constipation, and incontinence. Problems with sexuality include impotence, difficulty sustaining an erection, and decreased vaginal secretion.

COGNITIVE ASSESSMENT. Finally, the client is examined for mental status changes. Cognitive changes are usually seen late in the course of the disease and include decreased short-term memory, concentration, and ability to perform calculations; inattentiveness, and impaired judgment. Chart 46-16 summarizes the common clinical manifestations of MS.

PSYCHOSOCIAL ASSESSMENT

After the initial diagnosis of MS, the client is often anxious. Apathy, emotional lability, and depression are fairly common. The client may be euphoric or giddy, either as a result of the disease itself or because of the medications used to treat the disease. The nurse assesses the client's previously used coping and stress management skills in preparing him or her for a chronic, usually debilitating disease.

CHART 46-16

KEY FEATURES of
Multiple Sclerosis

- Muscle weakness and spasticity
- Fatigue
- Intention tremors
- Dysmetria (inability to direct or limit movement)
- Numbness or tingling sensations (paresthesia)
- Hypalgesia
- Ataxia (decreased motor coordination)
- Dysarthria (slurred speech)
- Dysphagia (difficulty swallowing)
- Diplopia (double vision)
- Nystagmus (involuntary eye movements)
- Scotomas (changes in peripheral vision)
- Decreased visual and hearing acuity
- Tinnitus, vertigo (ringing in the ears, dizziness)
- Bowel and bladder dysfunction
- Alterations in sexual function, such as impotence
- Cognitive changes, such as memory loss, impaired judgment, and decreased ability to solve problems or perform calculations

---

LABORATORY ASSESSMENT

No single specific procedure is definitively diagnostic for multiple sclerosis (MS). However, the collective results of a variety of tests are usually conclusive. Changes may be evident during an acute attack. Abnormal cerebrospinal fluid (CSF) findings include an elevated protein level and a slight increase in the white blood cell count. CSF electrophoresis reveals an increase in the myelin basic protein and the presence of oligoclonal (IgG) bands. IgG bands are seen in most clients with MS.

OTHER DIAGNOSTIC ASSESSMENTS

The health care provider usually orders a computed tomography (CT) scan, which may show an increased density in the white matter and MS plaques. Magnetic resonance imaging (MRI) demonstrates the presence of plaques and is considered diagnostic for MS. A complete diagnostic evaluation is necessary to exclude other disease.

Results of visual, auditory, and brainstem-evoked potential studies are often abnormal. EMG findings may be grossly abnormal in people with advanced disease.

The diagnosis of MS is made by the exclusion of other neurologic diseases, laboratory and neuroimaging assessment, and on specific diagnostic criteria, including the presence of neurologic dysfunction that occurs over time and in more than one area of the central nervous system (CNS).

◆ Common Nursing Diagnoses and Collaborative Problems

Nursing diagnoses that may apply to clients with MS include the following:

- Fatigue related to disease state
- Activity Intolerance related to generalized weakness
- Disturbed Sensory Perception (Visual) related to altered sensory reception
- Impaired Physical Mobility related to neuromuscular impairment

- Impaired Urinary Elimination related to sensory-motor impairment
- Chronic Pain related to chronic physical disability
- Self-Care Deficit related to neuromuscular impairment
- Disturbed Thought Processes related to disease state
- Imbalanced Nutrition: Less Than Body Requirements related to difficulty swallowing
- Sexual Dysfunction related to altered body function

◆Interventions

The client with MS is often weak and easily fatigued. The Concept Map below illustrates the common problems and interventions for the client with MS. Teach the client the importance of planning activities and allowing sufficient time to complete activities. For example, the client should check that all items needed for work are gathered before leaving the house. Items used on a daily basis should be easily accessible.

Drug Therapy. A variety of medications are used to treat and control the disease, decrease specific symptoms, and attempt to slow its progression (Table 46-1).

Biological Response Modifiers. The National Multiple Sclerosis Society recommends early and continuous treatment of relapsing-remitting MS with *one* of three drugs, all classified as **biological response modifiers (BRMs) or immunomodulators**—Avonex, Betaseron, or Copaxone—the ABCs of MS therapy. As the name implies, these drugs attempt to modify the course of the disease. Interferon beta-1a

CONCEPT MAP Multiple Sclerosis

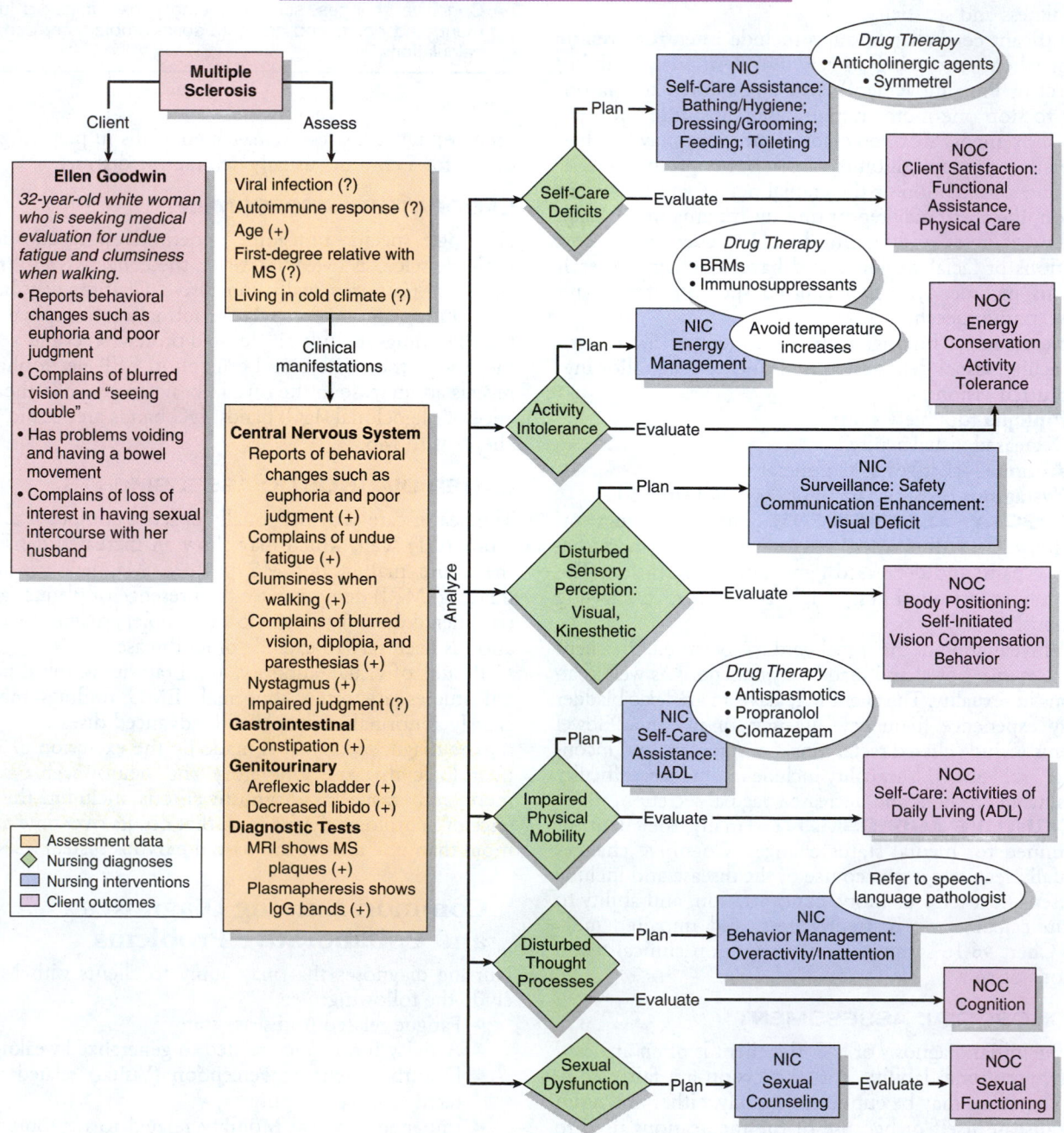

Concept Map by Elaine Bishop Kennedy, EdD, RN

(Avonex) has been approved by the Food and Drug Administration (FDA) for clients who have experienced their first episode of relapsing MS and have a magnetic resonance imaging (MRI) scan that demonstrates MS. This medication, given intramuscularly (IM) once a week, delays disability and decreases the number and severity of exacerbations. An alternative interferon beta-1a is Rebif, which is given subcutaneously three times a week (often self-administered). Interferon beta-1b (Betaseron) is administered subcutaneously every other day to reduce the frequency of exacerbations. Glatiramer acetate (Copaxone), given subcutaneously every day, decreases the clinical relapse rate and disease progression. Adherence to the self-administered daily Copaxone therapy is often difficult. Some clients feel that it is too challenging, and stop the therapy (Fraser, Hadjimichael, & Vollmer, 2001).

The interferons can cause depression, suicidal ideation, thrombocytopenia (low platelet count), leukopenia (low white blood cell count), and injection site reactions. Ice applied to the site before and after injection can help prevent redness, tenderness, or swelling. More than 20% of clients who take Copaxone experience transient chest pain.

TABLE 46-1   Commonly Used Medications for Clients with Multiple Sclerosis

Biological Response Modifiers
- Interferon beta-1a (Avonex or Rebif)
- Interferon beta-1b (Betaseron)
- Glatiramer acetate (Copaxone)

Immunosuppressive/Antineoplastic
- Cyclophosphamide (Cytoxan) and methylprednisolone combination
- Azathioprine (Imuran)
- Methotrexate
- Mitoxantrone (Novantrone)

Steroids
- Methylprednisolone (Solu-Medrol)
- IV immunoglobulin

Symptomatic Treatment of Fatigue
- Amantadine HCl (Symmetrel)
- Pemoline (Cylert)
- Methylphenidate HCl (Ritalin, Concerta, others)
- Modafinil (Provigil)

Symptomatic Treatment of Depression
- Fluoxetine HCl (Prozac)
- Sertraline HCl (Zoloft)

Symptomatic Treatment of Spasticity
- Baclofen (Lioresal)
- Tizanidine HCl (Zanaflex)
- Dantrolene sodium (Dantrium)
- Diazepam (Valium)
- Clonazepam (Klonopin)

Symptomatic Treatment of Bladder Dysfunction
- Oxybutynin chloride (Ditropan)
- Propantheline bromide (Pro-Banthine)
- Hyoscyamine sulfate (Anaspaz, Cystospaz-M)
- Desmopressin (DDA VP nasal spray)

Symptomatic Treatment of Chronic Pain
- Amitriptyline (Elavil)
- Carbamazepine (Tegretol)
- Clonazepam (Klonopin)
- Gabapentin (Neurontin)
- Nortriptyline (Pamelor)

Immunosuppressive Therapy. Mitoxantrone (Novantrone), an antineoplastic agent, has also been shown to be effective in reducing neurologic disability and the frequency of clinical relapses in clients with secondary-progressive, progressive-relapsing, or worsening relapsing-remitting MS. It is well tolerated, but its use over a long period causes cardiac problems, such as heart failure and life-threatening dysrhythmias.

Immunosuppressive therapy with a combination of cyclophosphamide (Cytoxan) and methylprednisolone (Solu-Medrol) may be used for treatment to stabilize the disease process. Methotrexate (MTX) may also have a modest benefit. Long-term side effects include sterility, mutations, and the increased risk of cancer.

Steroid Therapy. The health care provider may use methylprednisolone (Solu-Medrol) to reduce edema and the inflammatory response in acute exacerbations. One gram is administered IV daily for 3 to 14 days, depending on the provider and the extent of the client's symptoms. A course of oral prednisone 60 mg daily for 5 to 7 days may be used following the methylprednisolone. Adrenocorticotropic hormone (ACTH), 25 to 60 international units IV or IM, may be given instead of methylprednisolone and tapered gradually over 2 to 4 weeks.

Common nursing interventions while the client is receiving these medications include the following:
- Carefully monitoring fluid and electrolyte levels
- Testing the client's serum glucose concentration
- Providing dietary or supplemental potassium
- Observing for indications of gastrointestinal (GI) bleeding, such as gastric pain or blood in the stool
- Documenting any changes in personality (e.g., euphoria and insomnia)
- Minimizing the client's exposure to people with communicable or infectious diseases

Antispasmodic Therapy. The health care provider may prescribe baclofen (Lioresal), diazepam (Valium, Apo-Diazepam✦), or dantrolene sodium (Dantrium) to lessen muscle spasticity. Severe spasticity may be treated with intrathecal baclofen administered through a surgically implanted pump. A surgical tendon release may also be performed by the physician if spasms prevent the client from learning mobility and ADL skills.

Adjunctive Therapy. Paresthesia may be treated with carbamazepine (Tegretol) or tricyclic antidepressants (amitriptyline). Propranolol hydrochloride (Inderal) and clonazepam (Klonopin) have been used to treat cerebellar ataxia. If fatigue cannot be controlled through the use of nonpharmacologic measures, amantadine hydrochloride (Symmetrel) may be prescribed.

Bladder dysfunction (detrusor hyperreflexia) is treated with anticholinergic agents, including oxybutynin chloride (Ditropan) and hyoscyamine sulfate (Anaspaz, Cystospaz-M).

Pain and paresthesia are often problems for the MS client. Antispasmodics such as tizanidine (Zanaflex), antiepileptic drugs (AEDs) such as carbamazepine (Tegretol), analgesics, NSAIDs, tranquilizers, or antidepressants may be used, depending on the cause of the pain and the client's response.

Promoting Mobility and Self-Care. In collaboration with physical and occupational therapists, an exercise program is developed and includes range-of-motion (ROM) exercises and stretching and strengthening exercises. The client is encouraged to ambulate as tolerated and to use assistive ambulation devices as needed, including a cane, walker, wheelchair, or electric cart (Amigo). Additional assistive/adaptive devices may be needed to enable the client with tremor, spasticity, and weakness to remain independent in activities of daily living (ADLs). Chapter 10 describes additional interventions to increase physical mobility and promote ADL independence.

The importance of avoiding rigorous activities that increase body temperature is emphasized. Increased body temperature may lead to increased fatigue, diminished motor ability, and decreased visual acuity resulting from changes in the conduction abilities of the injured axons.

Managing Cognitive Problems. Cognitive impairment may occur early in the disease process. It is estimated that up to 65% of clients exhibit some neuropsychological dysfunction during the course of their disease (Halper et al., 2003). Areas affected include attention, memory, problem solving, visual perception, and use of speech. To assist the client with orientation, place a single date calendar in the client's room; give or encourage the client to use written lists or recorded messages. To maintain an organized environment, the client is encouraged to keep frequently used items in familiar places.

If the client experiences dysarthria, refer to the speech-language pathologist (SLP) for evaluation and treatment. It is not unusual for the client with dysarthria also to have dysphagia (difficulty swallowing). The SLP will do a swallowing evaluation. Further diagnostic testing may be indicated.

Adapting to Changes in Sexual Functioning. More than 70% of all women with MS and 90% of all men with MS report some change in their sexual life after onset of the disease (Gagliardi, 2003). Women report impaired genital sensation, diminished orgasm, and loss of sexual interest. Men most often complain of difficulty in achieving and maintaining an erection and delayed ejaculation. Many clients may be embarrassed to discuss their concerns about sexuality. Therefore, ask the client whether he or she has any concerns. The nurse with appropriate education and experience should answer the client's questions or refer the client to a therapist or urologist with experience in the field of sexuality and disability.

Managing Bladder and Bowel Problems. The client may experience a variety of bladder problems. In addition to drug therapy, other modalities include an intermittent self-catheterization program, indwelling urinary catheter, placement of a suprapubic catheter, or insertion of a bladder pacemaker. When the client activates the control on the pacemaker, the bladder is stimulated and voiding is initiated (Finesilver, 2003).

Clients with MS are at increased risk for urinary tract infections. Antibiotics may be prescribed by the health care provider. Remind the client to drink plenty of fluids unless contraindicated by other medical conditions. Teach the client procedures that stimulate bladder emptying, such as stroking the genitals and **Credé method** (applying manual pressure on the lower abdomen over the bladder to express urine). **Kegel exercises** (contracting and holding the pubococcygeal muscle) may also be helpful.

To prevent or control constipation, remind the client to increase fluid and fiber intake. If dietary control is not effective, medications such as bulk-forming agents, stool softeners, oral stimulants, mild laxatives, and suppositories or enemas may be prescribed. It is important for the client to develop a bowel program to maximize the effectiveness of dietary and medication interventions.

Treating Visual Disturbances. An eye patch that is alternated from eye to eye every few hours usually relieves **diplopia** (double vision). For peripheral visual deficits, teach scanning techniques by having the client move his or her head from side to side. Changes in visual acuity may be assisted by corrective lenses.

Complementary and Alternative Therapies. A number of complementary and alternative therapies have been reported by clients with MS to be successful in minimizing their symptoms, including beestings and nutritional supplements. These modalities continue to be researched for their efficacy.

The client may use moist, moderate heat; massage correction of posture abnormalities; exercises to increase muscle strength; and electrical stimulation of the affected area to increase their comfort level. Among other alternative treatments for pain are guided imagery, aromatherapy, and acupuncture (see Chapters 4 and 7).

> ### Critical Thinking Challenge
>
> You are a nurse in a family practice office in a small rural town. A young woman has requested a physical examination because she has "been feeling very tired lately." She has also been dropping things and has fallen twice when climbing stairs. After examination, the nurse practitioner tells her that he suspects multiple sclerosis or other neurodegenerative disease. The client begins to cry because she is planning to be married next month.
>
> 1. How should you respond to her at this time?
> 2. What diagnostic testing will most likely be prescribed for her?
> 3. What treatment options does she have?
>
> **evolve** For suggested answer guidelines, go to http://evolve.elsevier.com/Iggy/.

Community-Based Care

HOME CARE MANAGEMENT

To help the client maintain maximum strength, function, and independence, continuity of care through an interdisciplinary team in both the rehabilitation and home setting is necessary. Admission to a rehabilitation center is brief but usually provides a program to improve functional ability. In collaboration with the discharge planner and the occupational therapist, the nurse or case manager assesses the client's home for any hazards before discharge. Any items that might interfere with mobility (e.g., scatter rugs) are removed. In addition, care must be taken to prevent injury resulting from visual problems. The home environment should remain as structured and as free from clutter as possible. As the disease progresses, the home may need to be adapted for wheelchair accessibility. Any necessary assistive/adaptive device should be readily available before discharge from the hospital.

HEALTH TEACHING

The health care provider explains to the client and family the development of MS and the factors that may exacerbate the symptoms. The importance of avoiding overexertion, stress, extremes of temperatures (fever, hot baths, overheating, excessive chilling), humidity, and people with upper respiratory tract infections is emphasized. Explain all medications to be taken on discharge, including the time and route of administration, dosage, purpose, and side effects. Teach the client how to differentiate expected side effects from adverse or allergic reactions, and provide the name of a resource person to call if questions arise. Written instructions are provided as a resource to the client and caregivers at home.

The physical therapist develops an exercise program appropriate for the client's tolerance level. The client is instructed in techniques for self-care, daily living skills, and the use of required adaptive equipment, such as walkers and electric carts. The nurse should also include information on the following programs: bowel and bladder management, skin care, nutrition, and positioning techniques. Chapter 10 describes these aspects of chronic illness and rehabilitation in detail.

Instruct clients about the importance of obtaining adequate rest and avoiding undue stress. It is equally important for them to engage in regular social activities. Often clients are anxious about discharge from the hospital and worry about how long the remission will last or when the disease will progress.

Because personality changes are not unusual, teach the family or significant others strategies to enable them to cope with these changes. For example, the family may develop a nonverbal signal to alert the client to potentially inappropriate behavior (e.g., a talkative person may be reminded to be quiet if a family member displays a prearranged signal). This action avoids embarrassment for the client.

HEALTH CARE RESOURCES

The client with MS is able to live independently in the early stages of the disease. As the condition deteriorates, the assistance of a home care nurse or a family member may be required.

Stuifbergen et al. (2003) found that setting incremental health goals was a useful strategy for women with MS. Assist clients in establishing realistic short-term goals.

In severe or late disease, placement in a long-term care facility is an appropriate alternative. The population of young and middle-aged residents in nursing homes is increasing as people with chronic, disabling diseases live longer.

The nurse or case manager refers the client and family members or significant others to the local and national MS societies. Other community resources include meal delivery services (e.g., Meals on Wheels), transportation services for the disabled, and homemaker services.

AMYOTROPHIC LATERAL SCLEROSIS

PATHOPHYSIOLOGY

Amyotrophic lateral sclerosis (ALS), also known as **Lou Gehrig's disease,** is a progressive and degenerative disease that involves the motor system. It is characterized by atrophy of the hands, forearms, and legs. ALS results in paralysis and death. There is no known cause, no cure, no specific treatment, no standard pattern of progression, and no method of prevention. Unlike with many other neural degenerative diseases, the sensory and autonomic nervous systems are not involved. Mental status changes do not result from the disease.

Amyotrophic lateral sclerosis may occur at any age. The incidence in the United States is 4.6 per 100,000. The usual age of onset is between 40 and 70 years; the incidence increases with each decade of life. ALS is more prevalent in men than in women. Death typically occurs within 2 to 5 years after the onset of symptoms and is attributable to respiratory failure.

The cause of the disease is unknown. Researchers are exploring genetic, viral, and environmental factors as potential causes.

◆COLLABORATIVE MANAGEMENT
◆Assessment

The clinical manifestations of ALS include fatigue, muscle atrophy, and weakness. Early symptoms include the following:
- Fatigue while talking
- Tongue atrophy
- **Dysphagia** (difficulty swallowing)
- Weakness of the hands and arms
- **Fasciculations** (twitching) of the face
- Nasal quality of speech
- **Dysarthria** (slurred speech)

As the disease progresses, muscle atrophy, particularly of the trapezius and sternocleidomastoid muscles, develops. Muscle weakness and atrophy extend until a flaccid quadriplegia develops. Eventually the respiratory muscles become involved, leading to respiratory compromise, pneumonia, and death.

Diagnosis is based on clinical and diagnostic test findings and by ruling out other causes of the motor changes. There is no specific test to diagnose ALS, but creatine kinase (CK) is increased. The electromyogram (EMG) demonstrates fibrillations and fasciculations of the muscles. A muscle biopsy specimen typically demonstrates small, angulated, atrophic fibers. Other diagnostic studies reveal motor strength deficits in serial muscle testing; abnormal pulmonary function test results, such as a decreased vital capacity (less than 2 L); and dysphagia.

◆Interventions

There is no known cure for ALS, but an interdisciplinary approach is needed for maintaining optimum functioning. Riluzole (Rilutek) is the only drug approved by the Food and Drug Administration for use with ALS clients. It is not a cure, but it does extend survival time. The usual dose is 50 mg twice daily on an empty stomach. The client is monitored for liver toxicity from the drug by frequent measures of liver enzymes, such as alanine aminotransferase (ALT) and aspartate aminotransferase (AST). The health care provider also prescribes medication for pain, fatigue, spasticity, excessive secretions, sleep disturbances, and other complications as they occur.

The interdisciplinary health care team collaborates with the client and family to develop an individualized treatment plan. The physical therapist and occupational therapist evaluate the client's home and make recommendations for modifications as the disease progresses. An exercise and mobility program is developed and special equipment is obtained as needed to help with activities of daily living and mobility. Other interventions are directed toward preventing complications of immobility and promoting comfort.

The speech-language pathologist (SLP) evaluates the client for speech and swallowing problems, and makes recommendations as needed. The SLP teaches clients various adaptive strategies, such as techniques to help them speak louder and more clearly. He or she works with the client and family to develop a communication system to be used when the client can no longer verbally communicate.

A dietary consult is made to help with planning meals that the client can swallow. The family is taught how to ensure that the client obtains sufficient nutrients, fiber, and fluids. When the client can no longer swallow, a feeding tube is placed. The dietician can recommend the appropriate enteral feedings.

At some point the client will require respiratory support. An intermittent positive pressure ventilation [IPPV] or bi-level positive airway pressure [BIPAP]) may be used to aid breathing during sleep or full time. Mechanical ventilation enables the client to breathe and prolongs survival; it will not alter progression of the disease. For this reason, many clients elect not to be placed on a mechanical ventilator.

Refer the client to a hospice program. The hospice team works closely with the family to ensure the client's comfort. They collaborate with the health care provider to ensure that the client has the needed medication and pain control as well as quality of life for the client and family.

The hospice nurse also provides ongoing support and counseling to the client and the family as they begin to cope with the impact of this terminal disease. The client should be informed about the need for advance directives, such as a living will. Community resources include clinics and other support services run by the ALS Association or the Muscular Dystrophy Association.

GET READY for the NCLEX Examination!

KEY POINTS

Safe Effective Care Environment

- To help prevent back injury, use proper body mechanics as described in Chart 46-5.
- For clients who have back surgery, observe the incision site for bleeding and cerebrospinal leakage (clear fluid).
- Log roll clients having spinal surgery, especially those who have fusions.
- Monitor clients with cervical spinal injuries for manifestations of autonomic dysreflexia (see Chart 46-9).
- Provide emergency care for clients who experience autonomic dysreflexia as listed in Chart 46-10.
- Observe clients with spinal injuries and diseases for complications of immobility.
- Monitor respiratory status carefully in clients with amyotrophic lateral sclerosis; clients experience respiratory failure in terminal stages of the disease.

Health Promotion and Maintenance

- Teach clients who have had spinal surgery to avoid lifting and driving and to use proper body mechanics.
- Teach overweight and obese clients the importance of losing weight to reduce back pain and strain.
- Teach young adults (especially young men) to avoid potentially dangerous activities that could result in a spinal cord injury (SCI).
- Instruct clients with SCI and disease how to prevent complications of immobility (e.g., inspect skin, drink adequate fluids).

- Assess clients with spinal cord injury and disease for the need for adaptive/assistive devices to become independent in ADLs.
- Implement bowel and bladder retraining programs for clients with SCI and spinal diseases.
- Teach clients with multiple sclerosis (MS) the importance of adhering to their medication regimen.

Psychosocial Integrity

- Recognize that spinal cord injury and progressive neurologic diseases, such as MS, require the client to adjust to major life changes.
- Determine client and family coping strategies to help clients adjust to spinal trauma or disease.
- Refer clients to appropriate resources, such as a sexuality counselor or urologist for sexual dysfunction resulting from illness or disease.
- Encourage clients to share their feelings about life-altering SCI or neurodegenerative disease.
- Refer clients with spinal cord cancer to appropriate resources, such as the American Cancer Society and its support groups.

Physiological Integrity

- Assess pain level in clients with back injury, including the nature of the pain and location.
- Implement drug and nondrug interventions for back pain, including analgesics, NSAIDs, and muscle relaxants; suggest heat and ice as adjuncts to medication.
- Provide postoperative care and discharge teaching for clients having cervical neck surgery as listed in Chart 46-6.
- For clients with an SCI, assess airway *first!*
- Provide care of clients with SCI as summarized in Chart 46-12.
- Assess clients with multiple sclerosis for clinical manifestations listed in Chart 46-16; fatigue is the most common symptom.
- Assess for adverse effects of drug therapy for multiple sclerosis; drugs that are commonly used are listed in Table 46-1.
- Provide supportive care for the client with amyotrophic lateral sclerosis; refer to hospice in the terminal stage of the disease.

ADDITIONAL STUDY RESOURCES

Go to your Student CD-ROM for Review Questions for the NCLEX Examination.

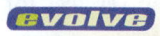
Go to http://evolve.elsevier.com/Iggy/ for Integrated Management of Care Questions for the NCLEX Examination.

SELECTED BIBLIOGRAPHY

Arce, D., Sass, P., & Abul-Khoudoud, H. (2001). Recognizing spinal cord emergencies. *American Family Physician, 64*(4), 631-638, 561-563.

Barker, E., & Saulino, M.F. (2002). First-ever guidelines for spinal cord injuries. *RN, 65*(10), 32-37.

Birchfield, P.C. (2001). Osteoarthritis overview. *Geriatric Nursing, 22*(3), 124-131.

Borasio, G.D., Voltz, R., & Miller, R.G. (2001) Palliative care in amyotrophic lateral sclerosis. *Neurologic Clinics, 19*(4), 829-847.

Charles, T., & Swash, M. (2001). Amyotrophic lateral sclerosis: current understanding. *Journal of Neuroscience Nursing, 33*(5), 245-255.

Cherry, C. (2002). Home study program. Anterior cervical discectomy and fusion for cervical disc disease. *AORN Journal, 76*(6), 996, 998-1004, 1007-1012.

Costello, K., & Harris, C. (2003). Differential diagnosis and management of fatigue in multiple sclerosis: Considerations for the nurse. *Journal of Neuroscience Nursing, 35*(3), 139-148.

Costello, K., Hill, C.A., & Tranter, M.C. (2000) Multiple sclerosis in the primary care setting: Key issues for diagnosis and management. *The American Journal for Nurse Practitioners, 4,* 9-26.

Filippi, M., et al. (2003). Evidence for widespread axonal damage at the earliest clinical stage of multiple sclerosis. *Brain, 126*(2), 433-437.

Finesilver, C. (2003). Multiple sclerosis: defenses gone awry. *RN, 66*(4):36.

Finlayson, M., VanDenend, T., & Hudson, E. (2004). Aging with multiple sclerosis. *Journal of Neuroscience Nursing, 36*(5), 245-251.

Fraser, C., Hadjimichael, O., & Vollmer, T. (2001). Predictors of adherence to Copaxone therapy in individuals with relapsing-remitting multiple sclerosis. *Journal of Neuroscience Nursing, 33*(5), 231-239.

Gagliardi, B.A. (2003) The experience of sexuality for individuals living with multiple sclerosis. *Journal of Clinical Nursing, 12*(4), 571-578.

Gibson, K.L. (2003). Caring for a patient who lives with a spinal cord injury. *Nursng 2003, 33*(7), 36-41.

Goodin, D.S., et al. (2002) Disease modifying therapies in multiple sclerosis: report of the Therapeutics and Technology Assessment Subcommittee of the American Academy of Neurology and the MS Council for Clinical Practice Guidelines. *Neurology, 58*(2): 169-178.

Guides for management of acute cervical spinal injury. (2002), *Neurosurgery, 50*(3), Suppl, S1-S84.

Grudinskas, L.V., & Nee, M.A. (2002). As assessment tool for the older person with a spinal cord injury. *SCI Nursing, 19*(2), 61-66.

Halper, J., et al. (2003) Rethinking cognitive function in multiple sclerosis: a nursing perspective. *Journal of Neuroscience Nursing, 35*(2):70-81.

Hassounch-Phillips, D.S., & McNeff, E. (2004). Understanding care-related abuse and neglect in the lives of women with SCI. *SCI Nursing, 21*(2), 75-81.

Hedger, A. (2002a). Clinical corner. Clearance of cervical spines in adult trauma patients. *Journal of Neuroscience Nursing, 34*(6), 331-335, 337.

Hedger, A. (2002b). Spinal cord injury. *Nursing 2002, 32*(12), 96.

Higo, R., et al. (2002). Videomanofluorometric study in amyotrophic lateral sclerosis. *Laryngoscope, 112*(5), 911-917.

Holland, N., et al. (2001). Adherence to disease-modifying therapy in multiple sclerosis. *Rehabilitation Nursing, 26*(5), 172-176.

Kim, J. (2003). How do I respond to autonomic dysreflexia? *Nursing 2003, 33*(2), 18.

Lassmann, H. (2003). Axonal injury in multiple sclerosis. *Journal of Neurology, Neurosurgery & Psychiatry, 74*(6), 695-697.

Linovitz, R.J., et al. (2002) Combined magnetic fields accelerate and increase spine fusion: a double-blind, randomized, placebo controlled study. *Spine, 27*(13), 1383-1389.

Lyall, R.A., et al. (2001) A prospective study of quality of life in ALS patients treated with noninvasive ventilation. *Neurology, 57*(1), 153-156.

Lysberg, K., & Seversinsson, E. (2003). Spinal cord injured women's views of sexuality: A Norwegian survey. *Rehabilitation Nursing, 28*(1), 23-26.

Massey, R., & Jedlicka, D. (2002). The Massey Bedside Swallowing Screen. *Journal of Neuroscience Nursing, 34*(5):252-253, 257-260.

Okonkwo, D.O., & Stone, J.R. (2003). Basic science of closed head injury and spinal cord injuries. *Clinics in Sports Medicine, 22*(3).

Patel, S.A., & Maragakis, N.J. (2002). Amyotrophic lateral sclerosis: pathogenesis, differential diagnoses, and potential interventions. *Journal of Spinal Cord Medicine, 25*(4), 262-273.

Rammohan, K.W. (2003). Axonal injury in multiple sclerosis. *Current Neurology & Neuroscience Reports, 3(3),* 231-237.

Richmond, T.S., & Thompson, H.J. (2002). Quality care in challenging circumstances: a patient with a spinal cord injury. *Journal of Neuroscience Nursing, 34*(1), 44-48.

Rowland, L.P., & Shneider, N.A. (2001). Medical progress: Amyotrophic lateral sclerosis. *New England Journal of Medicine, 344*(22):1688-1700.

Saal, J.S. (2002) General principles of diagnostic testing as related to painful lumbar spine disorders: a critical appraisal of current diagnostic techniques. *Spine, 27*(22), 2538-2546.

Schoeggl, A., Reddy, M., & Matula, C. (2002) Neurological outcome following laminectomy in spinal metastases. *Spinal Cord, 40*(7):363-366.

Schwendimann, R.N. (2002). A conservative approach to acute low back pain. *RN, 34*(5), 22-26, 28.

Smeltzer, S.C. (2002). Reproductive decision making in women with multiple sclerosis. *Journal of Neuroscience Nursing, 34*(3), 145-157.

Stuifbergen, A.K.,et al. (2003). The use of individualized goal setting to facilitate behavior change in women with multiple sclerosis. *Journal of Neuroscience Nursing, 35*(2), 94-99, 106.

Urban, M.K., et al. (2002). Reduction in postoperative pain after spinal fusion with instrumentation using intrathecal morphine. *Spine, 27*(5), 535-537.

Vollmer TL, et al. (2002). Disability and treatment patterns of multiple sclerosis patients in United States: a comparison of veterans and nonveterans. *Journal of Rehabilitation Research & Development, 39*(2), 163-174.

Wassem, R., & Dudley, W. (2003). Symptom management and adjustment of patients with multiple sclerosis: A 4-year longitudinal intervention study. *Clinical Nursing Research, 12*(1), 102-117.

Wilson, T.C., Morgan, P., & Blumhardt, L. (2003). Pyramidal tract mapping by diffusion tensor magnetic resonance imaging in multiple sclerosis: improving correlations with disability. *Journal of Neurology, Neurosurgery, & Psychiatry, 74*(2), 203-207.

Interventions for Clients with Problems of the Peripheral Nervous System

KATHY A. HAUSMAN

LEARNING OUTCOMES

After studying this chapter, you should be able to:

1. Compare and contrast the pathophysiology and etiology of Guillain-Barré syndrome (GBS) and myasthenia gravis (MG).
2. Analyze assessment data for a client with GBS or MG to determine common nursing diagnoses.
3. Prioritize nursing care for the client with GBS or MG.
4. Evaluate nursing care for the client with GBS or MG based on expected outcomes.
5. Differentiate between a myasthenic crisis and a cholinergic crisis.
6. Identify specific nursing actions regarding medication administration for the client with MG.
7. Develop a teaching plan for the client with peripheral neuropathy.
8. Prioritize postoperative care for the client undergoing peripheral nerve repair.
9. Compare and contrast trigeminal neuralgia and facial paralysis.
10. Discuss the role of drug therapy in managing the client with trigeminal neuralgia and facial paralysis.
11. Explain the purpose of surgery for clients with trigeminal neuralgia.

Go to your Student CD-ROM for Review Questions for the NCLEX Examination keyed to these Learning Outcomes.

Peripheral nervous system (PNS) disorders range in severity from potentially life-threatening conditions, such as Guillain-Barré syndrome, to relatively benign (but often painful) conditions, such as polyneuritis. Although hospitalization is rarely required for these less serious dysfunctions, you may encounter them as secondary disorders in hospitalized clients as well as in clients in ambulatory care, long-term care, or community settings.

GUILLAIN-BARRÉ SYNDROME

PATHOPHYSIOLOGY

Guillain-Barré syndrome (GBS) is an acute autoimmune disorder characterized by varying degrees of motor weakness and paralysis. It may be referred to by a variety of other names, such as *acute idiopathic polyneuritis* and *polyradiculoneuropathy.*

The client's life and ultimate potential for rehabilitation depend on appropriate interventions and the effectiveness of nursing care. Your expertise in providing care, monitoring for and preventing complications, and offering emotional support to the client and significant others is essential. With skilled care, the mortality rate can be very low. Mortality generally results from complications of respiratory compromise, such as pulmonary emboli or respiratory arrest.

In GBS, the immune system starts to destroy the myelin sheath that surrounds the axons. Segmental demyelination (the destruction of myelin between the nodes of Ranvier) is the major pathologic finding in GBS. This destruction affects saltatory conduction, or the leaping of impulses from node to node. The result is dispersion of impulses and slow conduction velocities or conduction block in the late stages of the disease. Although the heavily myelinated cranial and motor nerves are affected more often than are the thinly myelinated pain, touch, and temperature nerve fibers, sensory function is often affected. In addition, the brain may receive inappropriate sensory signals, resulting in tingling, "crawling skin," or pain.

On microscopic examination, aggregates of lymphocytes are seen at the points of myelin breakdown, yet the axons usually remain intact. In some instances there may be secondary damage to the cell body, the neurilemma, or the axon; this can delay recovery or result in permanent deficits.

Three stages make up the *acute* course of GBS:
- The *initial period* (1 to 4 weeks), which begins with the onset of the first definitive symptoms and ends when no further deterioration is noted
- The *plateau period* (several days to 2 weeks)
- The *recovery phase* (4 to 6 months, maybe up to 2 years), which is thought to coincide with remyelination and axonal regeneration

Chronic inflammatory demyelinating polyneuropathy (CIDP) is an unusual type of GBS that progresses over a longer period; complete recovery rarely occurs. The uncommon condition in which relapsing attacks of GBS occur is called chronic relapsing polyneuropathy.

Etiology and Genetic Risk

The cause of GBS remains obscure. Most of the evidence implicates a cell-mediated immunologic reaction. Research suggests that the humoral immune system is also involved. Defects of T-lymphocytes (T-cells) and B-lymphocytes (B-cells) of the lymphatic system may be the basis of the syndrome. T-cells are responsible for cell-mediated immunity and the phagocytosis of bacteria. B-lymphocytes produce and secrete immunoglobulin, which form the humoral part of the immune system. Normally these antibodies combine with antigens, such as viruses, and prevent the organisms from having a harmful effect. This antigen-antibody combination also induces an inflammatory reaction by attracting T-cells (Sulton, 2002).

The client with GBS often relates a history of acute illness, trauma, surgery, or immunization 1 to 3 weeks before the onset of neurologic manifestations. Other risk factors identified in epidemiologic studies include an upper respiratory tract infection or gastrointestinal (GI) illness (50% of cases) and positive antibodies to cytomegalovirus or Epstein-Barr virus (EBV). It is believed that the prodromal (earlier) event causes a limited malfunction of the immune system, which sensitizes the T-cells to the client's myelin. In response to several antigens, some clients apparently form a demyelinating antibody that has a direct toxic effect on nerves or attracts a cellular immune response; this ultimately destroys the myelin. Other factors associated with the development of Guillain-Barré syndrome (GBS) are listed in Table 47-1.

Incidence/Prevalence

The annual incidence of GBS throughout the world is about 1 to 4 cases per 100,000 population. It generally affects people between 15 and 36 and between 50 and 75 years of age.

TABLE 47-1   Factors Associated with Development of Guillain-Barré Syndrome

▪ Acute illness	▪ Vaccination
▪ Gastrointestinal illness	Flu
▪ *Campylobacter jejuni*	Group A *Streptococcus*
▪ Human immunodeficiency	Rabies
virus infection	▪ Swine flu
▪ *Mycoplasma pneumoniae*	▪ Medications
▪ Surgery	Captopril
▪ Upper respiratory infection	Danazol
▪ Virus	Penicillamine
Cytomegalovirus	Streptokinase
Epstein-Barr virus	
Varicella-zoster virus	

GBS is seen more often in clients with Hodgkin's disease, systemic lupus erythematosus, and human immunodeficiency virus (HIV) infection. In 2% to 5% of cases, a chronic or recurrent GBS develops. Mortality is estimated at 4% to 15%; generally due to autonomic instability and complications of immobility (Hughes, 2003). The mortality rate in older adults is 5% higher than in the general population secondary to dysrhythmias.

CULTURAL CONSIDERATIONS

GBS has worldwide distribution, is not seasonal, and affects people of all races and ages. Higher rates have been noted in people 45 years of age or older. The incidence of the disease is 50% higher in white individuals than in black individuals, but the cause is not known (Hughes, 2003).

HEALTH PROMOTION/ILLNESS PREVENTION

There is no way to prevent GB. Once the illness develops about 25% of those affected require mechanical ventilation for a period of time. Fatigue is a major lingering symptom in more than two thirds of those affected. The cost to treat a typical client with GB in the United States is $110,000 for acute care and results in $360,000 in lost productivity per client. Complications of GB can be minimized through meticulous nursing care.

◆COLLABORATIVE MANAGEMENT
◆Assessment

HISTORY

In addition to biographic data (e.g., age, gender, cultural background), obtain a complete medical and surgical history. Any illness (infection or other illness) 1 to 8 weeks before the onset of Guillain-Barré syndrome (GBS) should be explored. Ask the client to describe the symptoms in chronologic order, if possible.

PHYSICAL ASSESSMENT/CLINICAL MANIFESTATIONS

Manifestations of GBS depend on the degree of weakness and the progression of symptoms. Although features may vary (Chart 47-1), most people with GBS relate an abrupt onset of muscle weakness and pain. Typically, GBS does not affect level of consciousness, cerebral function, or pupillary signs.

The clinical variations of GBS reflect the areas of earliest or most severe involvement. **Ascending GBS** is the most common clinical pattern. Weakness and paresthesias begin in the lower extremities and progress upward to include the trunk and arms or affect the cranial nerves. The client may exhibit symptoms of an ascending flaccidity or weakness that evolves over hours to several days (1 to 10 days). The extent of the motor deficit ranges from mild paresis to total quadriplegia. About half of the clients with GBS experience some degree of respiratory compromise. Although they may be diminished during the initial assessment, deep tendon reflexes are absent in limbs that become paralyzed. *Pure motor GBS* is identical to the ascending variant, except sensory manifestations are absent.

The client with **descending GBS** initially experiences weakness of the face or **bulbar** muscles of the jaw, the sternocleidomastoid muscles (head rotators), and the muscles of the tongue, pharynx, and larynx. Weakness progresses downward to involve the limbs. This type of GBS may quickly affect the respiratory function. The client is monitored for breathlessness during speech, shallow respirations, dyspnea, and decreased tidal volume.

Descending GBS often includes **ophthalmoplegia** (paralysis or weakness of the eye muscles), causing diplopia. If the pupillary response to light is affected, functional blindness may result. Thus the client's visual function is assessed. Clients who experience visual problems are provided with information, explanation, and support. In this variation, numbness is more common in the hands than in the feet. Deep tendon reflexes are decreased or absent.

The **Miller Fisher variant**, a rare polyneuropathy, consists of a triad of ophthalmoplegia (paralysis of ocular [eye] muscles), areflexia (absence of reflexes), and severe ataxia (defective muscle coordination). Motor strength and sensory function are normal. The pupillary response to light is occasionally affected by the ophthalmoplegia, which results in functional blindness. Although respiratory complications are rare in clients with this variant, respiratory function is monitored frequently.

With any of the variants, *cranial nerve* involvement most often affects the facial nerve (cranial nerve VII). Involvement of the facial nerve results in the inability to smile, frown, whistle, or drink from a straw. In addition to monitoring the functions of cranial nerve VII, assess the client for dysphagia and paralysis of the larynx. Less frequently affected cranial nerves include the glossopharyngeal (IX), vagus (X), accessory (XI), and hypoglossal (XII) nerves. The client's inability to cough, gag, or swallow results from the involvement of cranial nerves IX and X. Monitor the client closely for varying blood pressure (hypertensive and hypotensive episodes or orthostatic hypotension), bradycardia, heart block, and asystole. These symptoms are characteristic of *autonomic dysfunction,* which is linked to vagus nerve (X) deficit. Cranial nerve XI (accessory) is assessed by asking the client to perform shoulder shrugs. Hypoglossal nerve (XII) deficit is evidenced by deviation or paralysis of the tongue.

Pain related to paresthesias is a commonly encountered symptom that requires aggressive management.

PSYCHOSOCIAL ASSESSMENT

In addition to determining the usual roles and responsibilities, occupation, motivation, and available support systems, the client's ability to cope with this devastating illness and the accompanying fear and anxiety is assessed. In general, GBS is self-limiting and the paralysis temporary (Gregory, 2003). It is not unusual for the client to experience depression throughout the recovery period due to a feeling of powerlessness.

LABORATORY ASSESSMENT

Although no single clinical or laboratory finding confirms the diagnosis of Guillain-Barré syndrome (GBS), the health care provider may perform a lumbar puncture (LP) to evaluate cerebrospinal fluid (CSF). An increase in CSF protein level without an increase (or only a slight to moderate increase) in cell count is a distinguishing feature of GBS. However, high protein levels may not be noted until after 1 to 2 weeks of illness, reaching a peak in 4 to 6 weeks. The CSF lymphocyte count is normal.

Peripheral blood tests may show a moderate leukocytosis early in the illness. The number of leukocytes rapidly returns to normal in the absence of complications or concurrent illness. Elevated liver function tests were found in one third of the clients in one reported study (Sharshar et al., 2003).

OTHER DIAGNOSTIC ASSESSMENTS

Electrophysiologic studies demonstrate demyelinating neuropathy. The degree of abnormality found on testing does not always correlate with clinical severity. Within 3 weeks of symptoms, nerve conduction velocities are depressed. In some cases, denervated potentials (fibrillations) develop later in the illness. Electromyographic (EMG) findings, which reflect peripheral nerve function, are normal early in the illness. Electrophysiologic changes appear only after denervation of muscle has been present for 4 weeks or longer. Nerve conduction velocity (NCV) testing is performed in conjunction with the EMG. An electrical impulse is applied to one end of a nerve in the client's arm or leg. The time it takes to reach the other end is measured. Nerve damage or disease may still exist despite normal NCV results. These tests are described in Chapter 44.

A magnetic resonance imaging (MRI) or computed tomography (CT) scan may be ordered to rule out other causes of motor weakness. Respiratory function is often compromised in clients with GBS. Vital capacity may be decreased, and arterial blood gas (ABG) values may be abnormal (decreased partial pressure of arterial oxygen [PaO_2], increased partial pressure of arterial carbon dioxide [$PaCO_2$], or increased pH).

CHART 47-1

KEY FEATURES of
Guillain-Barré Syndrome

Motor Manifestations
- Ascending symmetric muscle weakness → flaccid paralysis without muscle atrophy
- Decreased or absent deep tendon reflexes (DTRs)
- Respiratory compromise (dyspnea, diminished breath sounds, decreased tidal volume and vital capacity) and respiratory failure
- Loss of bowel and bladder control (less common)

Sensory Manifestations
- Paresthesias
- Pain (cramping)

Cranial Nerve Manifestations
- Facial weakness
- Dysphagia
- Diplopia
- Difficulty speaking

Autonomic Manifestations
- Labile blood pressure
- Cardiac dysrhythmias
- Tachycardia

Analysis

COMMON NURSING DIAGNOSES AND COLLABORATIVE PROBLEMS

The following are priority nursing diagnoses for clients with GBS:

1. Ineffective Breathing Pattern, Ineffective Airway Clearance, and Impaired Gas Exchange related to respiratory muscle weakness or paralysis, inability to cough and deep breathe effectively, and immobility
2. Acute Pain related to paresthesias
3. Impaired Physical Mobility and Self-Care Deficit related to weakness, paralysis, and ataxia
4. Impaired Verbal Communication related to intubation or paralysis of the muscles required for speech
5. Powerlessness related to the inability to perform activities of daily living (ADLs) and usual role responsibilities

ADDITIONAL NURSING DIAGNOSES AND COLLABORATIVE PROBLEMS

In addition to the common nursing diagnoses, clients with GBS may have one or more of the following:

- Risk for Impaired Skin Integrity related to altered sensation, altered nutrition, and/or immobility
- Impaired Home Maintenance related to lack of knowledge or inadequate support systems
- Disturbed Sensory Perception (Tactile, Kinesthetic, and Visual) related to paresthesias and diplopia
- Disturbed Body Image and Situational Low Self-Esteem related to loss of body function, physical changes, and dependency
- Imbalanced Nutrition: Less Than Body Requirements related to difficulty chewing, dysphagia, paralysis of the extremities, anxiety, or depression
- Risk for Aspiration related to dysphagia from motor weakness
- Risk for Deficient Fluid Volume related to cranial nerve paralysis, dysphagia, and paralysis of the extremities
- Constipation, Diarrhea, or Bowel Incontinence related to inadequate oral intake, immobility, and impaired communication
- Decreased Cardiac Output related to autonomic dysfunction

- Deficient Knowledge related to understanding the disease process and expectations

Planning and Implementation

INEFFECTIVE BREATHING PATTERN; INEFFECTIVE AIRWAY CLEARANCE; IMPAIRED GAS EXCHANGE

NOC **PLANNING: EXPECTED OUTCOMES.** The client with Guillain-Barré syndrome (GBS) is expected to have adequate ventilation, airway patency, and sufficient gas exchange in the lungs as indicated by:

- Noncompromised respiratory rate and rhythm
- Normal breath sounds
- Tidal volume and vital capacity within normal limits
- No dyspnea or cyanosis
- Arterial blood gases (ABGs) within normal limits
- Noncompromised cognitive status

INTERVENTIONS. The *priority* intervention for the client is to maintain adequate respiratory function and implement interdisciplinary actions, if necessary, to assist him or her in meeting the expected outcomes (Chart 47-2).

NIC **Respiratory Monitoring.** In the initial phase, the client is monitored closely (usually in a critical care unit) for signs of respiratory distress, such as dyspnea, air hunger, adventitious breath sounds, and cyanosis. In addition, the client's respiratory rate, rhythm, and depth are monitored every 1 to 4 hours; vital capacity is checked every 2 to 4 hours; and the lungs are auscultated at 4-hour intervals. The client's ability to cough and swallow should also be monitored for change. Assess cognitive status, especially in older adults; a decline often indicates hypoxia.

NIC **Airway Management.** The purpose of airway management is to promote airway patency and gas exchange. Elevate the head of the bed to at least 45 degrees or higher as determined by the client's response and level of dyspnea. Suctioning of the client is based on assessment data. During suctioning, the client is at risk for vagal nerve stimulation that could lead to bradycardia and cardiac arrest. Monitor the color, consistency, and amount of secretions obtained. Chest physiotherapy, performed by the respiratory therapist or nurse, and frequent position changes are combined with breathing exercises (coughing and deep breathing) to prevent pneumonia and atelectasis. Encourage the client to use the incentive spirometer to expand the lungs every few hours. Oxygen may be administered by nasal cannula at a flow rate prescribed by the health care provider.

Arterial blood gas (ABG) values are frequently monitored for acid-base abnormalities and decreasing oxygen saturation. A decrease in vital capacity to less than 15 to 20 mL/kg (or less than two thirds of the client's normal) and the inability to clear secretions may be indications for elective intubation. Keep equipment for performing an endotracheal intubation at the bedside, and keep a ventilator readily available in case of respiratory emergency. Sharshar and colleagues (2003) found the following characteristics were predictive of those clients who required intubation and mechanical ventilation:

- Rapidly progressing symptoms
- Inability to lift elbows off bed

CHART 47-2

NIC INTERVENTION ACTIVITIES for
The Client with Guillain-Barré Syndrome

Respiratory Monitoring: *Collection and analysis of client data to ensure airway patency and adequate gas exchange*
- Monitor rate, rhythm, depth, and effort of respirations.
- Monitor breathing patterns: bradypnea, tachypnea, hyperventilation, Kussmaul respirations, Cheyne-Stokes respirations, apneustic breathing, Biot's respiration, and ataxic patterns.
- Auscultate breath sounds, noting areas of decreased/absent ventilation and presence of adventitious sounds.
- Monitor PFT values, particularly vital capacity, maximal inspiratory force, forced expiratory volume in 1 second (FEV_1), and FEV_1/FVC, as available.
- Monitor mechanical ventilator readings, noting increases in inspiratory pressures and decreases in tidal volume, as appropriate.
- Monitor for increased restlessness, anxiety, and air hunger.
- Note changes in Sao_2, Svo_2, end tidal CO_2, and changes in ABG values, as appropriate.
- Monitor client's ability to cough effectively.
- Monitor for dyspnea and events that decrease and worsen it.
- Monitor chest x-ray reports.
- Place the client on side, as indicated, to prevent aspiration; log roll if cervical aspiration suspected.
- Institute respiratory therapy treatments (e.g., nebulizer), as needed.

Airway Management: *Facilitation of patency of air passages*
- Position client to maximize ventilation potential.
- Identify client requiring actual/potential airway insertion.
- Perform chest physical therapy, as appropriate.
- Remove secretions by encouraging coughing or by suctioning.
- Instruct how to cough effectively.
- Auscultate breath sounds, noting areas of decreased or absent ventilation and presence of adventitious sounds.
- Perform endotracheal or nasotracheal suctioning, as appropriate.
- Administer humidified air or oxygen, as appropriate.
- Administer aerosol treatments, as appropriate.
- Administer ultrasonic nebulizer treatments, as appropriate.
- Position to alleviate dyspnea.
- Monitor respiratory and oxygenation status, as appropriate.

NIC intervention activities selected from Dochterman, J.M., & Bulechek, G.M. (Eds.). (2004). *Nursing interventions classification (NIC)* (4th ed.). St. Louis: Mosby. No part of this work is to be altered without prior written permission from the Publisher.

PFT, Pulmonary function test; *FEV₁*, forced expiratory volume in 1 second; *FVC*, forced vital capacity; *Svo₂*, venous oxygen saturation; *Sao₂*, arterial oxygen saturation; *CO₂*, carbon dioxide; *ABG*, arterial blood gas.

- Inability to stand
- Ineffective cough
- Elevated liver enzymes
- Vital capacity less than 60% of predicted value

Interventions for Cardiac Dysfunction. Both the sympathetic and parasympathetic systems may be affected. The client is placed on a cardiac monitor because of the risk for dysrhythmias. Monitor vital signs closely. Hypertension is treated with a beta blocker or nitroprusside. Hypotension is treated with intravenous (IV) fluids and placing the client in a supine position, unless he or she is in extreme respiratory distress. Atropine may be prescribed to treat bradycardia.

Some clients experience urinary retention; maintain strict intake and output. If the client is unable to void, an indwelling urinary catheter (Foley) may be needed or an intermittent catheterization program started.

Drug Therapy/Plasmapheresis. The health care provider should follow the best practice guidelines from the American Academy of Neurology for the treatment of GBS (Hughes, 2003). These include the following recommendations:

- Treat with either plasma exchange (plasmapheresis) *or* immunoglobulin; there is no benefit to combine these treatments.
- Implement plasma exchange (PE) for nonambulatory adult clients who seek treatment within 4 weeks of the development of symptoms. It is also recommended for ambulatory clients seen within 2 weeks of onset of symptoms.
- Use IV immunoglobulin (IVIg) for ambulatory clients who seek treatment within 2 weeks of onset of symptoms.
- Do not use corticosteroids.

IV Immunoglobulin. IVIg has been shown to be as effective as plasmapheresis. It is safer and immediately available. Side effects of immunoglobulin therapy range from minor annoyances (e.g., chills, mild fever, myalgia, and headache) to major complications (e.g., anaphylaxis, aseptic meningitis, retinal necrosis, and acute renal failure). A serum IgA is drawn before administration of the medication. Infuse IVIg slowly when it is started. Observe for side and adverse effects, and report their occurrence to the health care provider. The rate of administration can be increased based on the client's tolerance.

Plasmapheresis. Plasmapheresis removes the circulating antibodies thought to be responsible for the disease. In this procedure, plasma is selectively separated from whole blood. The blood cells are returned to the client without the plasma. Plasma usually replaces itself, or the client is transfused with colloidal substitute such as albumin. Fresh frozen plasma is generally not used because of the associated risk of infection and allergic pulmonary edema (Sulton, 2002). This procedure should be started 7 to 14 days after the onset of the illness. The client usually receives three to four treatments, 1 to 2 days apart. Some clients may require a second round of treatment if they deteriorate after the first plasmapheresis.

Nursing responsibilities for the client undergoing plasmapheresis include providing information and reassurance, weighing the client before and after the procedure, and administering proper care to the shunt. Proper shunt care includes maintaining shunt patency, checking for bruits every 2 to 4 hours, keeping double bulldog clamps at the bedside, and observing the puncture site for bleeding or ecchymosis (bruising). Observe for signs of complications throughout the procedure (Chart 47-3). Atropine is prescribed in the event of bradycardia.

ACUTE PAIN

PLANNING: EXPECTED OUTCOMES. The client with Guillain-Barré syndrome (GBS) is expected to experience adequate pain control as indicated by client report and consistent demonstration of ways to manage pain.

INTERVENTIONS. Assess the severity and nature of the client's pain, which is often worse at night. The typical pain experienced is often not relieved by medication other than opiates, which can be administered via a patient-controlled analgesia (PCA) pump or continuous IV drip.

CHART 47-3

BEST PRACTICE for
Preventing and Managing Complications of Plasmapheresis

Complication	Nursing Interventions
Trauma or infection at vascular access site	Keep the site clean and dry. Monitor the site for redness, swelling, drainage, or other signs of infection.
Hypovolemia with resultant hypotension, tachycardia, dizziness, and diaphoresis	Monitor fluid and electrolyte status and vital signs. Administer fluids as prescribed. Provide an explanation of side effects, and reassure the client.
Hypokalemia and hypocalcemia	Monitor fluid and electrolyte balance. Administer replacement electrolytes, as prescribed. Observe for cardiac dysrhythmias.
Temporary circumoral and distal extremity paresthesias, muscle twitching, nausea, and vomiting related to administration of citrated plasma	Add calcium gluconate or calcium chloride to exchange fluids, as prescribed. Provide explanations, comfort measures, and reassurance.

Document the client's response to pain medication, and notify the health care provider if pain relief is not sufficient. Other pain control measures include frequent repositioning, massage, ice, heat, relaxation techniques, guided imagery, and distractions (e.g., music or visitors). Chapter 7 discusses these and other pain relief measures in detail.

IMPAIRED PHYSICAL MOBILITY AND SELF-CARE DEFICIT

NOC   PLANNING: EXPECTED OUTCOMES. The client with GBS is expected to be free of physiologic immobility consequences as indicated by *no:*

- Pressure ulcers
- Constipation, paralytic ileus, or stool impaction
- Urinary retention, calculi, or infection
- Fracture or contractures
- Venous thrombosis
- Lung congestion or pneumonia
- Orthostatic hypotension

The client is also expected to perform basic activities of daily living (ADLs) as indicated by noncompromised:

- Eating
- Toileting
- Hygiene, dressing, and grooming
- Walking or wheelchair mobility
- Self-transfer and positioning

INTERVENTIONS. The client's emotional and mental status and his or her level of acceptance of the disability is determined. The client, family, nurse, physical and occupational therapist, speech-language pathologist, and dietitian collaborate to develop interventions to prevent complications of immobility and to address deficits in self-care. Assess the client's motor (muscle) function every 2 to 4 hours as part of the neurologic assessment. The interventions prescribed for mobility and self-care and to prevent

complications depend on the degree of motor deficit experienced by the client. Assistive devices and instructions for their use are provided for the client. To ensure safety, assist the client with ambulation, transfers from bed to chair, position changes, and maintenance of proper body alignment until he or she is able to perform these activities independently. Maximal independence is always encouraged. Range-of-motion (ROM) exercises are performed actively or passively every 2 to 4 hours by the nurse or unlicensed assistive personnel (UAP). Family members may be instructed in these techniques. (See Chapter 10 for detailed discussion of ways to improve physical mobility and self-care, as well as ways to prevent immobility consequences.) Monitor the client's responses to or tolerance of activity. Provide adequate rest periods between activities and therapy sessions.

Decreased gastric motility, dysphagia, and depression can cause malnutrition. The dietitian develops an individualized nutrition plan. The client may require little assistance with feeding or may be totally dependent. If the client is unable to safely swallow food or liquids, enteral nutrition via feeding tube is prescribed. Weigh the client three times a week, and monitor serum albumin and prealbumin each week.

Malnutrition places clients at risk for pressure ulcers. Therefore special attention is paid to skin care, including interventions to prevent skin breakdown. Instruct the UAP to turn the client a minimum of every 2 hours. Assess the skin for any areas of redness that may lead to pressure ulcers. If the client's bed does not have a pressure-reducing mattress, use a mattress overlay to help prevent skin breakdown. Document changes in the client's skin condition every shift while in the acute care setting and at least daily in a subacute or rehabilitation setting. If an ulcer occurs, implement aggressive interventions to manage the wound. Chapters 10 and 70 discuss pressure ulcer care in detail.

Because pulmonary emboli and deep vein thrombosis are common complications of immobility, the health care provider may prescribe prophylactic anticoagulant therapy, such as subcutaneous heparin or Lovenox. Antiembolism stockings and sequential compression stockings may be used to promote venous return. Be sure that stockings are removed at least once every 24 hours for 15 to 30 minutes. Other prevention measures are determined by agency policy or health care provider preference. Chapter 10 describes additional interventions to prevent complications of immobility and promote self-care.

IMPAIRED VERBAL COMMUNICATION

PLANNING: EXPECTED OUTCOMES. The client with Guillain-Barré syndrome (GBS) is expected to communicate as indicated by the ability to receive, interpret, and express written and nonverbal messages to and from the staff, family, and/or significant others.

INTERVENTIONS. The client may have difficulty communicating because the muscles required for the production of speech are weak, or the client may be on a mechanical ventilator because the respiratory muscles are paralyzed. In either case, the nurse collaborates with the speech-language pathologist to develop a communication system. A simple technique involves eye blinking or moving a finger to indicate "yes" and "no." A communication board can be developed with the letters of the alphabet or a list of common requests, such as the need to be repositioned or the need for pain medication. Both the staff and the visitors must know how the client's communication system operates.

POWERLESSNESS

NOC **PLANNING: EXPECTED OUTCOMES.** The client with GBS is expected to maintain hope as indicated by consistently expressing:

- Expectation of a positive future
- Faith
- Meaning in life
- Sense of self-control
- Optimism

INTERVENTIONS. Assess the client and family or significant others for verbal and nonverbal behaviors that indicate powerlessness, anxiety, fear, and grieving. Encourage the client to verbalize feelings about the illness and its effects, if possible, while fostering hope. Previous decision-making patterns, roles, and responsibilities are examined. Ask the client and family to describe their usual lifestyles and the situations in which they coped both effectively and ineffectively to help identify factors that influence coping ability.

Refer clients who need further psychosocial support to the social worker, hospital chaplain or appropriate spiritual resource, and local support groups. If necessary, obtain a psychological consultation for further evaluation and intervention.

Community-Based Care

The severity and course of Guillain-Barré syndrome (GBS) are extremely variable, which makes it difficult to predict the prognosis. The most likely residual effects at discharge are related to motor status and mobility, self-care, and perhaps sensory alteration and disturbed self-concept. For clients who experience total quadriparesis or respiratory paralysis, the course of the rehabilitation phase is even more variable and may require weeks to years. The goal of the recovery phase is to move from dependence to independence, if possible. Cooke and Orb (2003) found that clients go through several phases during their recovery to meet that goal (see the Evidence-Based Practice for Nursing box above).

Planning for discharge begins on admission. The client may be discharged to home or to a rehabilitation unit. The nurse, discharge planner, or case manager (CM) makes appropriate referrals to a home care agency and community agencies for assistance in the home setting after discharge. Chapter 10 discusses various aspects of rehabilitation in detail.

A family member or significant other is included in the education process throughout the client's hospitalization. The client and family are given both oral and written instructions in techniques to facilitate mobility, use of adaptive-assistive devices, and prevent skin breakdown. If mobility remains markedly impaired, the physical therapist emphasizes the need for ROM exercises, positioning and frequent turning techniques, and prevention of skin breakdown.

If the client is discharged to home while still dependent on assistive devices, the interdisciplinary health care team makes certain that the necessary equipment has been delivered after evaluating the home setting. Home care management for clients with GBS is similar to that for those who have had a stroke or spinal cord injury, depending on the nature of the neurologic deficit (see Chapter 48).

EVIDENCE-BASED PRACTICE for Nursing

How do clients with Guillain-Barré syndrome gain independence during the recovery period?

Cooke, J.F., & Orb, A. (2003). The recovery phase in Guillain-Barré syndrome: Moving from dependency to independence. *Rehabilitation Nursing, 28*(4), 105-108, 130.

This small qualitative study followed five clients with Guillain-Barré syndrome (GBS) discharged from a major teaching hospital during their recovery period. Each participant was interviewed using a semistructured questionnaire to obtain data that were analyzed through a constant comparative method. Five phases were identified as these subjects progressed from dependency to independence:

- Experiencing dependency
- Encountering helplessness
- Wanting to know more about GBS
- Discovering inner strength
- Regaining independence

A central theme identified was that all clients discovered inner strengths that they did not realize they had. They also stated that when they were discharged, they had very little knowledge about their illness or prognosis.

Level of Evidence: 8—This was a very small number for subjects used for a qualitative study.

Critique. Although the sample size was very small, this study provides the groundwork for future nursing research. Qualitative research was an appropriate research method to answer the study question. This research needs to be replicated before any generalization can occur, especially focusing on themes that may emerge in varying cultural groups.

Implications for Nursing. Of particular interest are the findings related to lack of knowledge upon discharge and discovery of inner strengths. Nurses need to ensure that clients are well-informed about their health problems before hospital discharge. In collaboration with social workers, nurses should talk with clients to help them identify coping strategies and other strengths that have helped clients in other critical or stressful situations.

Self-help groups for clients with chronic illness are common. Consult with the client and the health care provider about referrals to these groups, if indicated. The Guillain-Barré Foundation provides information about local resources and information for clients and their families. The psychosocial adjustment needed may be minimal or dramatic depending on the client's residual deficit, age, gender, usual roles and responsibilities, usual coping strategies, available support systems, and occupation. Help the client identify other support systems, such as church members, social club members, or spiritual resources.

◆ Evaluation: Outcomes

Evaluate the care of the client with GBS on the basis of the identified nursing diagnoses. The expected outcomes include that the client should:

- Have adequate ventilation, airway patency, and sufficient gas exchange in the lungs
- Experience adequate pain control
- Be free of physiologic immobility consequences
- Perform basic ADLs
- Communicate with staff, family, and significant others
- Maintain hope

Specific indicators for these outcomes are listed for each nursing diagnosis under the Planning and Implementation section (see earlier).

MYASTHENIA GRAVIS

PATHOPHYSIOLOGY

Myasthenia gravis (MG) is a chronic disease characterized by fatigue and weakness primarily in muscles innervated by the cranial nerves, as well as in skeletal and respiratory muscles (Chitnis & Khoury, 2003). This autoimmune disease of the neuromuscular junction may take many forms—from mild disturbances of the ocular muscles to a rapidly developing, generalized weakness that may lead to death from respiratory failure. It is characterized by remissions and exacerbations (worsening or "flare-ups").

MG is caused by an autoantibody attack on the acetylcholine receptors (AChR) in the muscle end plate membranes (Richman & Agius, 2003). As a result, nerve impulses are not transmitted to the skeletal muscle at the neuromuscular junction.

Etiology and Genetic Risk

Although the precipitating event remains unclear, research strongly suggests that MG is caused by antibodies to the ACh receptors. Although the disease is not hereditary, there is a 5% familial incidence. Evidence also suggests a relationship between MG and hyperplasia (overgrowth) of the thymus gland. The thymus gland is often abnormal. **Thymoma** (encapsulated thymus gland tumor) occurs in about 15% of cases, and 70% of the remaining cases show hyperplasia of the thymus. There is also a very strong association between MG and hyperthyroidism. D-penicillamine, interferon-alpha, and bone marrow transplantation have been associated with drug-induced (iatrogenic) autoimmune MG (Pascuzzi, 2003).

Incidence/Prevalence

The incidence of MG in the United States is estimated to be 0.5 per 100,000 people. Although it may begin at any age, the onset of MG before 10 years of age or after 60 years of age is rare. The peak age at onset is between 20 and 30 years of age. Women are affected three times more often than are men.

◆ COLLABORATIVE MANAGEMENT
◆ Assessment

Although the onset of MG is usually insidious, some instances of fairly rapid development have been preceded by infection, emotional upset, pregnancy, or anesthesia. Thus the nurse inquires about any history of these events. A temporary increase in weakness may be noted after vaccination, menstruation, and exposure to extremes in environmental temperature.

In addition to the biographic data and history, ask the client if he or she experienced the rapid onset of fatigue. Note complaints of muscle weakness that increases on exertion or as the day wears on and improves with rest. Ask the client to describe his or her symptoms, specifically noting the affected muscle groups and any limitation or inability in performing activities of daily living (ADLs).

Additional areas of inquiry include any history of **ptosis** (drooping eyelids) or **diplopia** (double vision), difficulty chewing or swallowing (**dysphagia**), and the type of diet best tolerated. Assess the client for previous manifestations of respira-

CHART 47-4

KEY FEATURES of
Myasthenia Gravis

Motor Manifestations
- Progressive muscle weakness (proximal) that usually improves with rest
- Poor posture
- Ocular palsies
- Ptosis
- Weak or incomplete eye closure
- Diplopia
- Respiratory compromise
- Loss of bowel and bladder control
- Fatigue

Sensory Manifestations
- Muscle achiness
- Paresthesias
- Decreased smell and taste

tory difficulty, choking, or voice weakness. Other areas of assessment include asking about any difficulty holding up the head, brushing teeth, combing hair, or shaving. Inquiry is made about the presence of paresthesias or aching in weakened muscles. Finally, assess for a history of thymus gland tumor.

PHYSICAL ASSESSMENT/CLINICAL MANIFESTATIONS

MG may be diagnosed after the demonstration of *progressive* paresis of affected muscle groups that is resolved, at least in part, by rest (Chart 47-4). The most common symptoms (exhibited by more than 90% of clients) are related to involvement of the levator palpebrae or extraocular muscles. Assess for ocular palsies, ptosis, diplopia, and weak or incomplete eye closure. These symptoms may last only a few days at the onset and then resolve, only to return weeks or months later. Normal pupillary responses to light and accommodation are present.

For most clients, the muscles of facial expression, chewing, and speech are affected (**bulbar** involvement). Note the client's smile, which may be transformed into a snarl; the jaw may hang so that the client must prop it up with the hand. Chewing and swallowing difficulties, choking, and regurgitation of fluids through the nose may lead to considerable weight loss. Inquire about the client's nutritional status and any recent weight loss. It may be more difficult for the client to eat after talking. After extended conversations, the voice may become weaker or exhibit a nasal twang. In some clients, the tongue has one central and two lateral longitudinal fissures (sores or ulcers).

Less often involved are the muscles of the shoulders, the flexors of the neck, and the hip flexors. Because limb weakness is more often *proximal*, the client may have difficulty climbing stairs, lifting heavy objects, or raising the arms overhead. Neck weakness may be mild or severe enough to cause difficulty in holding the head erect. Among the trunk muscles, the erector spinae are most commonly affected. This results in difficulty sustaining a sitting or walking posture.

In the most advanced cases of MG, all muscles are weakened, including those associated with respiratory function and the control of bladder and bowel function. In these severe cases, inquire about bowel and bladder function. Assess respiratory function frequently.

Muscle atrophy, although rarely marked in degree, occurs in a small percentage of clients with myasthenia gravis (MG). The client's tendon reflexes should be assessed, but they are not often affected. Assess for pain, although this is seldom a major complaint. Some clients report aching of the weakened muscles. If present, paresthesias (painful tingling sensation) affecting the muscles of the face, hands, and thighs is not associated with any loss of sensation. Lost or decreased sensations of smell and taste have been reported. There is no alteration of consciousness.

In **Eaton-Lambert syndrome**, a form of myasthenia often observed in combination with small cell carcinoma of the lung, the muscles of the trunk and the pelvic and shoulder girdles are most commonly affected. Although weakness increases after exertion, there may be a temporary increase in muscle strength during the first few contractions, followed by rapid decline. Diagnosis is confirmed by electromyography (EMG). Management differs somewhat from other types of MG. Treatment includes removing the tumor, managing the cancer, and administering medications to release acetylcholine (ACh). Additional therapies may include plasmapheresis and immunosuppressive therapy (discussed later).

LABORATORY ASSESSMENT

In virtually all cases of MG, the diagnosis is obvious from the history and physical examination findings. MG may be immediately confirmed by the client's response to cholinergic drugs. A standard series of laboratory studies is usually performed for clients with known or suspected MG. Thyroid function should be tested because **thyrotoxicosis** (excessive thyroid hormone) is present in about 5% of myasthenic clients. Serum protein electrophoresis evaluates the client for immunologic disorders. Immunologic-based diseases, such as rheumatoid arthritis, systemic lupus erythematosus, and polymyositis, are associated with the disease.

Testing for acetylcholine receptor antibodies (AChR) has become an important diagnostic criterion, because 80% to 90% of clients with MG have elevated AChR. A positive antibody test result confirms the diagnosis, but a negative finding does not exclude the disease (Pagana & Pagana, 2002).

RADIOGRAPHIC ASSESSMENT

Some clients with MG have a thymoma, and therefore clients are assessed for this condition. The thymus, an H-shaped gland located in the upper mediastinum beneath the sternum, is one organ in which ACh receptor antibodies are formed. Although a thymoma can often be seen on routine frontal and lateral chest x-rays, special studies should be performed for any area suggestive of thymoma in the anterior mediastinum. The nurse prepares the client for these tests or for a computed tomography (CT) scan by explaining the equipment and what to expect during the tests.

OTHER DIAGNOSTIC ASSESSMENTS

TENSILON TESTING. Pharmacologic tests with the cholinesterase inhibitors edrophonium chloride (Tensilon) and neostigmine bromide (Prostigmin) have been in use since the 1950s. Tensilon is used more often because of its rapid onset and brief duration of action. This drug inhibits the breakdown of ACh at the postsynaptic membrane, which increases the availability of ACh for excitation of postsynaptic receptors. To perform the test, the physician first estimates the strength of cranial muscles. Initially, 2 mg (0.2 mL) is injected IV; if this is tolerated, an additional 8 mg (0.8 mL) is injected after 30 seconds. Within 30 to 60 seconds of the first dose, most myasthenic clients show a marked improvement in muscle tone that lasts 4 to 5 minutes. False-positive test results may be caused by increased muscle effort by the client. False-negative findings may be seen if the tested muscle is extremely weak or refractory to the drug (Pascuzzi, 2003).

Tensilon testing may also be used to help determine whether increasing weakness in the previously diagnosed myasthenic client is due to a **cholinergic crisis** (overmedication with cholinesterase inhibitors) or a **myasthenic crisis** (undermedication with cholinesterase inhibitors). In a cholinergic crisis, muscle tone does not improve after the administration of Tensilon. Instead, weakness may actually increase, and **fasciculations** (muscle twitching) may be noted around the eyes and face. The Tensilon test poses a danger of ventricular fibrillation and cardiac arrest, but these reactions rarely occur. Atropine sulfate is the antidote for Tensilon and must be available in case these complications occur.

ELECTROMYOGRAPHY. A common diagnostic test performed by the physician or technician is electromyography (EMG). Although electrical testing of the normal neuromuscular junction produces no change in the amplitude (force) of muscle contraction, the amplitude of the muscle's response diminishes with progressive stimulation. A decrease in amplitude of more than 10% between the first and fifth responses generally indicates the defective neuromuscular transmission characteristic of, but not unique to, MG. Several muscles may be tested to increase the likelihood of detecting an abnormality. Testing may be performed after exercise or exposure of the muscle to curare or to ischemia.

Single-fiber EMG is even more sensitive in detecting defects of neuromuscular transmission. This test compares the stability of the firing of one muscle fiber with that of another fiber innervated by the same motor neuron. The time interval between the two firings normally shows a minor degree of variability, called jitter. Defective transmission increases jitter or actually blocks successive discharges.

🤔 Critical Thinking Challenge

A young woman presents in the emergency department (ED) with new onset of muscle weakness in her shoulders, "droopy" eyelids, "double-vision," and extreme fatigue. During assessment, she tells you that she also has a "tingling" sensation in her hands at times. She came to the ED because her physician is out of town and she doesn't know the physician who is covering for him.

1. As her admitting ED nurse, what questions should you ask her?
2. What is the priority for care for the client at this time?
3. After physician evaluation, the probable diagnosis is myasthenia gravis. What diagnostic testing will the physician most likely prescribe and why?
4. What are the differences between Guillain-Barré syndrome and myasthenia gravis?

evolve For suggested answer guidelines, go to http://evolve.elsevier.com/Iggy/.

Common Nursing Diagnoses and Collaborative Problems

Nursing diagnoses that typically apply to clients with myasthenia gravis include the following:

- Risk for Ineffective Breathing pattern and Ineffective Airway Clearance related to intercostal muscle weakness
- Self-Care Deficit related to fatigue and muscle weakness
- Activity Intolerance related to fatigue
- Impaired Verbal Communication related to muscle weakness

Interventions

The classic presentation of MG is muscle weakness that increases when the client is fatigued and limits his or her mobility and ability to participate in activities. Management for this disease fall into two categories:

- Treatment that affects the symptoms of MG without influencing the actual course of the disease (anticholinesterases or cholinergic drugs)
- Therapeutic efforts for inducing remission, such as the administration of immunosuppressive drugs or corticosteroids, plasmapheresis, and thymectomy (removal of the thymus gland)

NONSURGICAL MANAGEMENT. Assess the client's motor strength before and after periods of activity. Provide assistance as necessary to prevent the client from becoming fatigued. He or she is scheduled for tests, treatments and other activities early in the day or during the energy peaks that follow the administration of medications. Assist the client in planning the periods of rest necessary for avoiding excess fatigue.

Providing Assistance with Activities. During periods of maximal weakness, assistance is provided for ambulation, transfers from bed to chair or toilet/commode, position changes, and maintenance of body alignment. Active or passive range-of-motion (ROM) exercises are performed every 2 to 4 hours with assistance of the nurse, unlicensed assistive personnel (UAP), or family. Assess the client's skin integrity and teach family members how to perform this skill. The client is repositioned, and bony prominences are assessed at least every 2 hours for skin breakdown and contractures. Pressure-reducing devices or mattresses are used to prevent pressure ulcers. Consult with the physical and occupational therapist to develop a program for the client to assist with mobility, self-care, and energy conservation techniques.

Drug Therapy. Two groups of drugs are typically prescribed for the treatment of myasthenia gravis (MG): anticholinesterases and immunosuppressants. These medications must be administered *on time* to maintain blood levels and thus facilitate increased muscle strength. The client's response to medications are monitored and documented. Provide information for the client and the family about the indications for, effectiveness of, and side effects of the drugs used in the treatment of MG.

Cholinesterase Inhibitor Drugs. Cholinesterase (ChE) inhibitor drugs are the *first-line* management of MG. These drugs are also referred to as anticholinesterase drugs or antimyasthenics. They enhance neuromuscular impulse transmission by preventing the decrease of ACh by the enzyme ChE, thus increasing the response of the muscles to nerve impulses and improving muscle strength. The ChE

drug of choice is pyridostigmine (Mestinon, Regonol). Expect day-to-day variations in dosage depending on the client's fluctuating symptoms.

Administer ChE medications with a small amount of food to help alleviate gastrointestinal side effects. Instruct the client to eat meals 45 minutes to 1 hour after taking these medications to avoid aspiration. This is very important if the client has bulbar involvement. Drugs containing magnesium, morphine or its derivatives, curare, quinine, quinidine, procainamide, or hypnotics or sedatives should be avoided because they may increase the client's weakness. Antibiotics such as neomycin, kanamycin, polymyxin B, and certain tetracyclines impair transmitter release and also increase myasthenic symptoms.

A potential adverse effect of these drugs is cholinergic crisis. Sudden increases in weakness and the inability to clear secretions, swallow, or breathe adequately indicate that the client is experiencing crisis. There are two types of crises:

- Myasthenic crisis—an exacerbation of the myasthenic symptoms caused by undermedication with anticholinesterase drugs
- Cholinergic crisis—an acute exacerbation of muscle weakness caused by overmedication with cholinergic (anticholinesterase) drugs

Because myasthenic and cholinergic crises have many common characteristics, the type of crisis the client is experiencing must be identified for effective treatment to be provided (Table 47-2). Monitor carefully for early detection of these emergencies.

Emergency Care: Myasthenic Crisis. Myasthenic crisis is often preceded by some type of infection. For other clients, increasing muscle weakness leads to an overdose of anticholinesterase drugs. As a result, the client may experience a *mixed* crisis. The Tensilon test (described on p. 1014), although not always conclusive, is an important procedure for differentiation. Tensilon produces a temporary improvement in myasthenic crisis, but no improvement or worsening of symptoms in cholinergic crisis.

The *priority* for nursing management of the client in myasthenic crisis is maintaining adequate respiratory function. The acutely ill client may need intensive nursing care for monitoring and maintenance of body functions. He or she may require mechanical ventilation. Cholinesterase-inhibiting drugs are withheld because they increase respiratory secretions and are usually ineffective for the first few

TABLE 47-2   Characteristics of Myasthenic and Cholinergic Crises

Myasthenic Crisis	Cholinergic Crisis	Mixed Crisis
Increased pulse and respiration	Nausea	Apprehension
Rise in blood pressure	Vomiting	Restlessness
	Diarrhea	Dyspnea
Anoxia	Abdominal cramps	Dysphagia (difficult swallowing)
Cyanosis	Blurred vision	Dysarthria (painful joints)
Bowel and bladder incontinence	Pallor	
	Facial muscle twitching	Increased lacrimation (tearing)
Decreased urine output	Pupillary miosis	Increased salivation
Absence of cough and swallow reflex	Hypotension	Diaphoresis
		Generalized weakness

days after the crisis begins. Medications are restarted gradually and at lower dosages.

Emergency Care: Cholinergic Crisis. In *cholinergic* crisis, anticholinergic drugs are withheld while the client is maintained on a ventilator. Atropine 1 mg IV may be given and repeated, if necessary. When atropine is prescribed, the nurse must observe the client carefully; secretions are thickened by the drug, which causes more difficulty with airway clearance and possibly the development of mucous plugs. Unless complications such as pneumonia or aspiration develop, the client in crisis improves rapidly after the appropriate drugs have been given. Continue to provide assistance as necessary, because the client tires easily after minimal exertion.

Immunosuppression. Immunosuppression may be accomplished with the use of corticosteroids, such as prednisone (Deltasone, Winpred✸), or with chemotherapeutic agents, such as azathioprine (Imuran), or cyclophosphamide (Cytoxan, Procytox✸). Prednisone is used initially to reduce remission and to control and improve symptoms. The drug is tapered over a period of weeks to months. Some clients may need continuous low-dose therapy because of exacerbations of symptoms. For ocular MG, corticosteroid treatment that does not cause significant systemic complications may significantly reduce the prevalence of generalized myasthenia gravis after 2 years on the medication (Kupersmith, Latkany, & Homel, 2003).

Azathioprine and cyclophosphamide are used for long-term management. Cyclophosphamide is reserved for clients who are refractory to other treatments. IV immunoglobulins (IVIg) may also be used for acute disease management or as a long-term option for disease refractory to other treatment.

Plasmapheresis. **Plasmapheresis** is a method by which antibodies are removed from the plasma. It may be used to decrease symptoms. Six exchanges occur over a 2-week period, with follow-up exchanges weekly or monthly as needed. This is usually done on an ambulatory care basis. Nursing management of the client undergoing plasmapheresis is presented in the earlier discussion of Guillain-Barré syndrome, p. 1010.

Respiratory Support. Although not all clients with MG experience respiratory compromise, ongoing assessment and maintenance of respiratory function must be done. Both myasthenic crisis (undermedication) and cholinergic crisis (overmedication) increase muscle weakness and the client's risk for respiratory compromise. The diaphragm and the respiratory and intercostal muscles may be affected, which inhibits the client's ability to maintain adequate ventilation, breathe deeply, and cough effectively. In addition, dysphagia may result in the aspiration of foods, fluids, or saliva, which compounds the respiratory problems. Because of their respiratory muscle involvement, many of these clients have an increased risk of pulmonary infections.

The client who cannot cough effectively may require oropharyngeal or nasopharyngeal suctioning. The nurse may need to teach the assisted cough technique, similar to that used by clients who are quadriplegic (see Chapter 48). Chest physiotherapy consisting of postural drainage, percussion, and vibration mobilizes secretions and helps prevent pneumonia and atelectasis. A breathing bag (e.g., Ambu), equipment for oxygen administration, and endotracheal intubation equipment are kept at the bedside in case of respiratory distress.

Because breathing difficulty or the inability to breathe easily is frightening, the nurse should be aware of the client's mental and emotional status during periods of respiratory compromise. His or her response to medications prescribed for muscle weakness, bronchodilation, and pulmonary congestion are monitored and documented.

As an alternative to mechanical ventilation, BiPAP (continuous positive airway pressure) should be tried first in clients with acute respiratory failure from MG crisis while awaiting improvement from IV immunoglobulin (IVIg) therapy or plasma exchange. Repeat arterial blood gas (ABG) measurements and clinical assessment after using the device for a few hours are used to determine its effects (Evoli et al., 2002).

Promoting Self-Care. Generalized weakness and fatigue affect the client's ability to participate in activities of daily living (ADLs). Impaired fine motor control and shoulder weakness, which result in difficulty raising the arms, often compound the problem. Self-care deficits may be complete or partial depending on the severity of the illness, the client's response to drugs, and his or her ability to tolerate activity without excessive fatigue.

To establish abilities and limitations, assess the client's ability to perform ADLs. Although the client is encouraged to perform activities as independently as possible, assistance is provided as necessary to avoid undue frustration and fatigue. For maximizing independence and making attempts at self-care successful, activities are planned to follow the administration of medication. Monitor and document the client's response to or tolerance of activity, providing alternating periods of activity and rest. Rest is critical because increased fatigue can precipitate a crisis. In addition, occupational and physical therapists evaluate the client for assistive-adaptive devices. In collaboration with the nurse, they teach the client and family energy conservation techniques and ideas for making work and self-care easier after discharge from the hospital.

Assisting with Communication. Weakness of the speech and facial muscles often results in dysarthric and nasal speech. Thus it may be difficult for myasthenic clients to make their speech understood by others.

The speech-language pathologist and nurse determine the client's ability to communicate. The client is instructed to speak slowly while the nurse attempts to lip-read. The information is repeated back to the client to verify that it is correct. Questions that can be answered with "yes" or "no" or by gestures may be used along with alternative communication systems such as eye blinking, flash cards, magic slates, notebook and pencil, and picture, letter, or word boards.

Nutritional Support. The client with myasthenia gravis (MG) may have difficulty maintaining an adequate intake of food and fluid because the muscles needed for chewing and swallowing become weakened and tire easily. In collaboration with the dietitian, occupational therapist, and speech-language pathologist, the client's nutritional status and his or her ability to receive adequate oral nutrition are evaluated. Small, frequent meals and high-calorie snacks are often well tolerated. The effectiveness of the nutrition program is monitored by recording the client's calorie counts, intake and output, serum albumin levels, and daily weights (Chart 47-5). If the client is not able to swallow, a feeding tube may be used.

Eye Protection. The client's inability to completely close the eyes may lead to corneal abrasions and further compromise vision and comfort. During the day, artificial tears are applied to keep the corneas moist and free from

CHART 47-5

BEST PRACTICE for
Improving Nutrition in Clients with Myasthenia Gravis

- Assess the client's gag reflex and ability to chew and swallow.
- Provide frequent oral hygiene as needed.
- Collaborate with the dietitian, speech-language pathologist, and occupational therapist to plan and implement meals that the client can eat and enjoy.
- Offer small, frequent meals.
- Cut food into small bites, and encourage the client to eat slowly.
- Observe client for choking, nasal regurgitation, and aspiration.
- Provide high-calorie snacks or supplements (e.g., puddings).
- Keep the head of the bed elevated during meals and for 30 to 60 minutes after the client eats.
- Avoid liquids because they can easily cause choking and aspiration; provide a soft diet.
- Monitor food intake carefully.
- Weigh the client daily.
- Monitor serum prealbumin and albumin levels.
- Administer anticholinesterase drugs, as prescribed: 45 to 60 minutes before meals.

abrasion. A lubricant gel and shield may be applied to the eye at bedtime to provide more extensive coverage. To help relieve diplopia, the eyes should be alternately covered with a patch for 2 to 3 hours at a time.

SURGICAL MANAGEMENT. For clients with MG, **thymectomy** (removal of the thymus gland) is usually performed early in the disease. The procedure is not always immediately effective, and it may take several years for remission to occur—if it occurs at all. Clients who have surgery within 2 years of the onset of myasthenic symptoms show the most improvement.

Preoperative Care. Routine preoperative care is provided as discussed in Chapter 20. Because there is no way to predict whether remission or improvement will occur, it is important to avoid making promises, although optimism is warranted. Immediately before surgery, pyridostigmine (Mestinon) may be given with a small amount of water to keep the client stable during and after surgery. If steroids have been used, they are also given before surgery and are tapered during the postoperative period. Antibiotics are administered immediately before and for several days after surgery. Plasmapheresis may be used preoperatively and postoperatively to decrease circulative antibodies more quickly.

Operative Procedures. One of two surgical approaches may be used: the transcervical incision or the sternal split. Advocates of the transcervical approach claim a lower morbidity rate and more rapid recovery with less postoperative discomfort. The client often requires only a small dressing and an IV line. However, the sternal split allows the surgeon to directly visualize the mediastinum. Because more precise and complete removal of all thymic tissue is ensured, this may be the approach of choice.

When thymoma is present, all contiguous involved structures (e.g., the pericardium, the innominate vein, a portion of the superior vena cava, and a portion of the lung) are removed. A single chest tube is placed in the anterior mediastinum. The client may be admitted to the critical care unit postoperatively. Thymoma should be considered as a potentially malignant tumor requiring prolonged follow-up. The presence of myasthenic weakness can still complicate its

management. Thymoma-related deaths are bound to outnumber those due to MG in the future.

Postoperative Care. Although clients with adequate respiratory function may be extubated immediately after the procedure, most require a gradual weaning from the ventilator. Prolonged ventilatory assistance is rare. After the client is extubated, conscientious attention is paid to pulmonary hygiene. Suctioning is performed as necessary, and the client is encouraged to turn, cough, and breathe deeply and to use incentive spirometry every 2 hours. In addition to monitoring respiratory function and providing bronchial hygiene, observe for signs of pneumothorax or hemothorax, such as the following:

- Chest pain
- Sudden shortness of breath
- Diminished or delayed chest wall expansion
- Diminished or absent breath sounds
- Restlessness or a change in vital signs (decreasing blood pressure or a weak, rapid pulse)

For the sternal surgical technique, perform chest tube care (see Chapter 35). Both surgical approaches require special wound care. Observe the client for signs of infection, such as increasing or purulent drainage; redness, warmth, or swelling around the wound; and elevated temperature. Appropriate client and family teaching is needed before discharge from the hospital.

Community-Based Care

The client with myasthenia gravis (MG) may be cared for in a variety of settings, including the home, subacute unit, rehabilitation setting, or long-term care facility. The client discharged from the hospital may be weak and may require the assistance of a family member, home care nurse, physical therapist, occupational therapist, or home care aide.

HEALTH TEACHING

The more the client and family know about the disease and the drugs used for treatment, the less likely it is that complications will develop.

Encourage the client and the family to ask questions. Discuss the episodic nature (exacerbations and remissions) of the disease, including factors that predispose the client to exacerbation, such as infection, stress, surgery, hard physical exercise, sedatives, and enemas or strong cathartics (Table 47-3). Instruct the client to collaborate with the health care team to monitor muscle strength, ability to perform activities of daily living (ADLs), and the need to adjust medications.

The importance of lifestyle adaptations such as avoiding heat (e.g., sauna, hot tubs, and sunbathing), crowds, overeating, erratic changes in sleep habits, or emotional extremes is stressed. Teach the signs of exacerbation, such as increased weakness, increased diplopia, ptosis, and problems with chewing or swallowing. Instruct the client to plan activities to allow for rest periods and to conserve energy.

Provide the medication regimen in a written format that includes the names, purposes, dosages, scheduled administration times, administrative routes, and side effects of the drugs. Explain that the drugs are normally taken before activities such as eating, participating in sports, or engaging in work. The importance of maintaining therapeutic blood levels by taking the medications on time and as prescribed and not missing or postponing doses is also stressed. In addition, inform the client of the side effects of anticholinesterase

TABLE 47-3 Factors Precipitating or Worsening Myasthenia Gravis

Various medications, including the following:
- Strong cathartics
- Antidysrhythmics
- Beta-blocking agents
- Antibiotics
- Antirheumatic drugs
- Antispasmodics
- Antihistamines
- Opioids
- Phenytoin (Dilantin)
- Antidepressants (tricyclics)

Rheumatoid arthritis
Alcohol
Hormonal changes
Stress
Infection
Seasonal temperature changes
Heat
Surgery
Enemas

CHART 47-6

CLIENT EDUCATION GUIDE
Helpful Hints for Medication Teaching of Clients with Myasthenia Gravis

- Keep medications and a glass of water at your bedside if you are weak in the morning.
- Wear a watch with an alarm function (or beeper) to remind you to take your medications.
- Post your medication schedule so others know it.
- Plan strenuous activities, when possible, when the medication peaks.
- Keep an extra supply of medications in your car or at work. Be sure they are secured.
- Do not take any over-the-counter medications without checking with your health care provider.

drugs. Advise him or her to avoid medications such as morphine, curare, quinine, quinidine, procainamide, mycin-type antibiotics, and drugs containing magnesium. These agents markedly increase muscle weakness. Additional health teachings regarding medications are listed in Chart 47-6.

In preparing the client for discharge, explain the signs and symptoms of myasthenic and cholinergic crises and the need to contact the physician or other health care professional whenever either type of crisis is suspected. Because respiratory compromise often occurs in myasthenic clients, family members are encouraged to gain skills in resuscitation procedures. A manual resuscitation bag, suctioning equipment, and oxygen should be available in the home for clients susceptible to crisis. Family members should be instructed in the proper use of equipment.

The episodic nature of MG, the potential or actual loss of independence, and body image changes (e.g., the inability to smile) affect the client's adjustment. Kittiwatanapaisan and colleagues (2003) found that fatigue was moderately correlated with depression. During discharge planning, the case manager (CM) considers factors such as age, gender, usual roles and responsibilities, available support systems, occupation, and financial status. Because the client's and family's need for psychosocial adjustment may range from minimal to dramatic, the CM remains sensitive to their needs and provides information and support. The CM encourages family members or significant others to discuss their feelings with one another.

HOME CARE MANAGEMENT

Clients with MG are usually managed at home. Hospitalization is restricted to the diagnostic and evaluation processes, myasthenic or cholinergic crisis resulting in respiratory failure, or periods of exacerbation when respiratory function is threatened.

Unless the client requires assistive devices, little preparation of the home setting is required. In consultation with physical and occupational therapists, the CM makes certain that the necessary equipment has been delivered and properly installed. In addition, the CM makes sure that the client and family members can use the equipment safely. If

the client becomes wheelchair dependent, the discharge planner or CM ensures that any necessary modifications to the home (e.g., the installation of ramps or widening of doorways) have been completed before discharge from the hospital.

HEALTH CARE RESOURCES

In consultation with the health care provider, client, and family, the staff nurse or CM may initiate referrals to home care agencies and to local self-help groups for people who have chronic illnesses and for their families. The Myasthenia Gravis Foundation, headquartered in New York City, has education and research programs and provides assistance with financial aid and community resources. The CM encourages the client to obtain and wear a medical alert (MedicAlert) bracelet or necklace and to carry identification at all times.

POLYNEURITIS AND POLYNEUROPATHY

PATHOPHYSIOLOGY

Systemic diseases, vitamin B_{12} deficiency, drug toxicity, infections, trauma, vascular or metabolic disturbances, and exogenous substances such as alcohol, medications, industrial agents, and heavy metals may damage cranial and peripheral nerves. Although the term polyneuritis implies an inflammatory process, it may also denote noninflammatory lesions. Thus the terms **polyneuritis, polyneuropathy,** and **peripheral neuropathy** may describe syndromes whose clinical hallmarks are muscle weakness with or without atrophy, pain that is described as stabbing, cutting or searing, and paresthesias or loss of sensation, impaired reflexes, autonomic manifestations, or combinations of these symptoms.

The most common type of neuropathy is a symmetric polyneuropathy in which the client experiences decreased sensation along with the feeling that an extremity is asleep. Tingling, burning, tightness, or aching sensations generally start in the feet and progress to the level of the knee before being noted in the hands (**"glove and stocking" neuropathy**). Other clients may complain of unsteadiness, clumsiness, an inability to recognize objects by feel, and injury without pain. Diabetic neuropathy is a common example, as are the neuropathies resulting from renal or hepatic failure, alcoholism, acquired immunodeficiency syndrome (AIDS),

TABLE 47-4   Factors Associated with Polyneuropathy

Diseases
- Amyloidosis
- Alcoholism
- Carcinomas
- Diabetes mellitus
- Diphtheria
- Hepatic failure
- Malabsorption or malnutrition
- Porphyria
- Renal failure (uremia)
- Vascular disease

Trauma

Vitamin Deficiencies
- Vitamin B_1 (thiamine)
- Vitamin B_6 (pyridoxine)
- Vitamin B_2 (riboflavin)
- Vitamin B_c (folic acid)
- Vitamin B_{12}
- Niacin

Drug Use
- Vincristine
- Isoniazid
- Phenytoin
- Amitriptyline
- Hydralazine

Environmental Exposures
- Heavy metals
- Industrial solvents

---

and drug or toxic exposures. Common factors associated with polyneuropathy are presented in Table 47-4.

Peripheral neuropathy is a condition that can be caused or exacerbated by the administration of certain chemotherapeutic agents. The effects of **chemotherapy-induced peripheral neuropathy (CIPN)** are dose limiting and could lead to permanent, debilitating disabilities. Oncology nurses should know the pathophysiology, pre-existing conditions contributing to an increased risk of CIPN, causative agents, and interventions used in managing CIPN. Be aware that the peripheral nervous system is divided into small fibers, large fibers, and the autonomic nervous system, which is important in the assessment, detection, and treatment of this neuropathy. Presenting symptoms are related to the specific fibers that are damaged. Because of the different mechanisms of action, symptoms vary depending on the chemotherapeutic agents used (Marrs & Newton, 2003). Early intervention and client education can have a positive effect on the quality of life for clients with this disorder.

◆COLLABORATIVE MANAGEMENT
◆Assessment

Although peripheral neuropathy rarely necessitates hospitalization, you are likely to encounter clients with this condition in a variety of settings, particularly among older adults or in clients with a related illness. Nursing assessment includes an examination of the client's sensory and motor abilities. The client can often outline a specific area of sensory deficit. Because the client may be unaware of decreased sensation, his or her distal extremities may be assessed for light touch using cotton balls or cotton-tipped applicators and for pain using a safety pin. Assess position sense, or kinesthetic sensation by gently grasping the involved digit or extremity on its sides. With the client's eyes closed, change the position of the digit or extremity, and ask the client to describe how the position was changed. The client should be able to acknowledge even slight movements. Advanced practice nurses may use a tuning fork placed on bone prominences to test for sensitivity to vibration. The examination is started at the distal sites. More proximal areas are tested only if the client fails to perceive the duration of vibration at the distal site.

The client's extremities are examined for any signs of injury of which the he or she may be unaware. Also assess the client for the following:
- Orthostatic hypotension
- Abnormal sweating
- **Miosis** (abnormal constriction of the pupil)
- Sphincter disturbances, such as loss of bowel and bladder control
- Other autonomic dysfunctions that may accompany the neuropathy

All abnormal findings are documented and brought to the health care provider's attention.

◆Interventions

Medical management of clients with peripheral neuropathy consists of the removal or treatment of the underlying cause and symptomatic therapy, including supportive care and physiotherapy. The diet is generally supplemented with vitamins, especially if vitamin deficiency is an underlying cause. However, there is no evidence that vitamins in excess of those contained in a well-balanced diet have any effect on the forms of polyneuropathy unrelated to vitamin deficiency.

With removal of the toxic agent or correction of the metabolic defects, recovery may be rapid if the continuity of the nerves has not been interrupted. If there has been axonal destruction, recovery may require several months. After severe degeneration, there may be permanent weakness, atrophy, decreased reflexes, and sensory deficits.

Extensive client teaching is essential. For clients with decreased sensation in their feet and legs, explain the importance of proper foot care (Chart 47-7). In addition, teach the client who has decreased sensation to recognize potential hazards, such as:
- Exposure to extremes of environmental temperature (e.g., frostbite)
- Bath water or dishwater that may be too hot
- Contact of the feet with heat sources (e.g., heating pads, radiators) while sleeping
- Burns associated with cooking

Smoking is discouraged because the resulting vasoconstriction may worsen the neuropathy. If needed, refer the client to a smoking cessation program. Clients with postural hypotension are taught to arise slowly and wear support or elastic stockings to minimize the pooling of blood in the legs.

Many clients, especially those with the acute forms of polyneuropathy associated with drugs or exposure to toxic substances, experience anxiety, impaired coping, and changes in family processes such as role responsibilities and sexual functioning. Thus it is vital for the health care team to establish a trusting nurse/client relationship and to provide psychosocial support. The physician, social worker, chaplain or religious leader, physical and occupational therapists, and nurse focus on the client's abilities and strengths and help identify new ways of coping, meeting needs, and restructuring activities.

Adjuvant analgesics prescribed for neuropathic pain include desipramine, nortriptyline, gabapentin, and valproic acid (Davis & Srivastava, 2003). High doses of the opioid levorphanol are more effective than low doses in reducing the intensity of chronic neuropathic pain originating in the central or peripheral nervous system. However, in many clients, pain relief is not achieved or there are intolerable side effects (Rowbotham et al., 2003).

CONSIDERATIONS FOR OLDER ADULTS

Pain management for the older adult presents unique challenges due to physiologic changes that alter the pharmacokinetics and pharmacodynamics of analgesics. The results of these changes are decreased drug effectiveness, and increased drug toxicity and drug-drug interactions.

CHART 47-7

CLIENT EDUCATION GUIDE
Peripheral Neuropathy of the Lower Extremities

- Wash your feet and legs with mild soap each day; rinse and dry them well.
- Apply lanolin or lubricating lotion to your feet and legs once or twice daily.
- Inspect your feet and legs daily; report skin changes or open areas to your physician or other health care provider.
- Wear white or colorfast stockings or socks, and change them daily.
- Check the temperature of your bath water with a thermometer before putting your feet into the water.
- Do not use heating pads or other heat sources on your feet.
- Do not use sharp devices to remove corns or calluses (use a pumice stone) or to cut nails. Seek professional podiatry care on a regular basis.
- Wear support or elastic stockings if you have orthostatic hypotension or dependent edema.
- Wear well-fitted shoes; avoid going barefoot.

PERIPHERAL NERVE TRAUMA

PATHOPHYSIOLOGY

The peripheral nerves are subject to injuries associated with mechanical or vehicular accidents, certain sports, the injection of particular drugs, military conflicts or wars, and acts of violence (e.g., knife or gunshot wounds). Specific mechanisms of injury include the following:

- Partial or complete severance of a nerve or nerves
- Contusion, stretching, constriction, or compression of a nerve or nerves
- Ischemia
- Electrical, thermal, or radiation injury

Most commonly affected are the median, ulnar, and radial nerves of the arms and the peroneal, femoral, and sciatic nerves of the legs (Figure 47-1).

After a nerve is transected, the nerve distal to the injury degenerates and retracts within 24 hours. Motor and sensory dysfunction distal to the lesion coincide with the loss of electrical excitability as the nerve fibers degenerate. Recovery occurs as Schwann cells of the neurilemma proliferate from both the proximal and distal stumps. Dividing mitotically, these cells form neurilemmal cords, which act as guidelines for the regenerating axon. Tiny unmyelinated sprouts are generated at the proximal axon and grow 1 to 4 mm each day. Some can

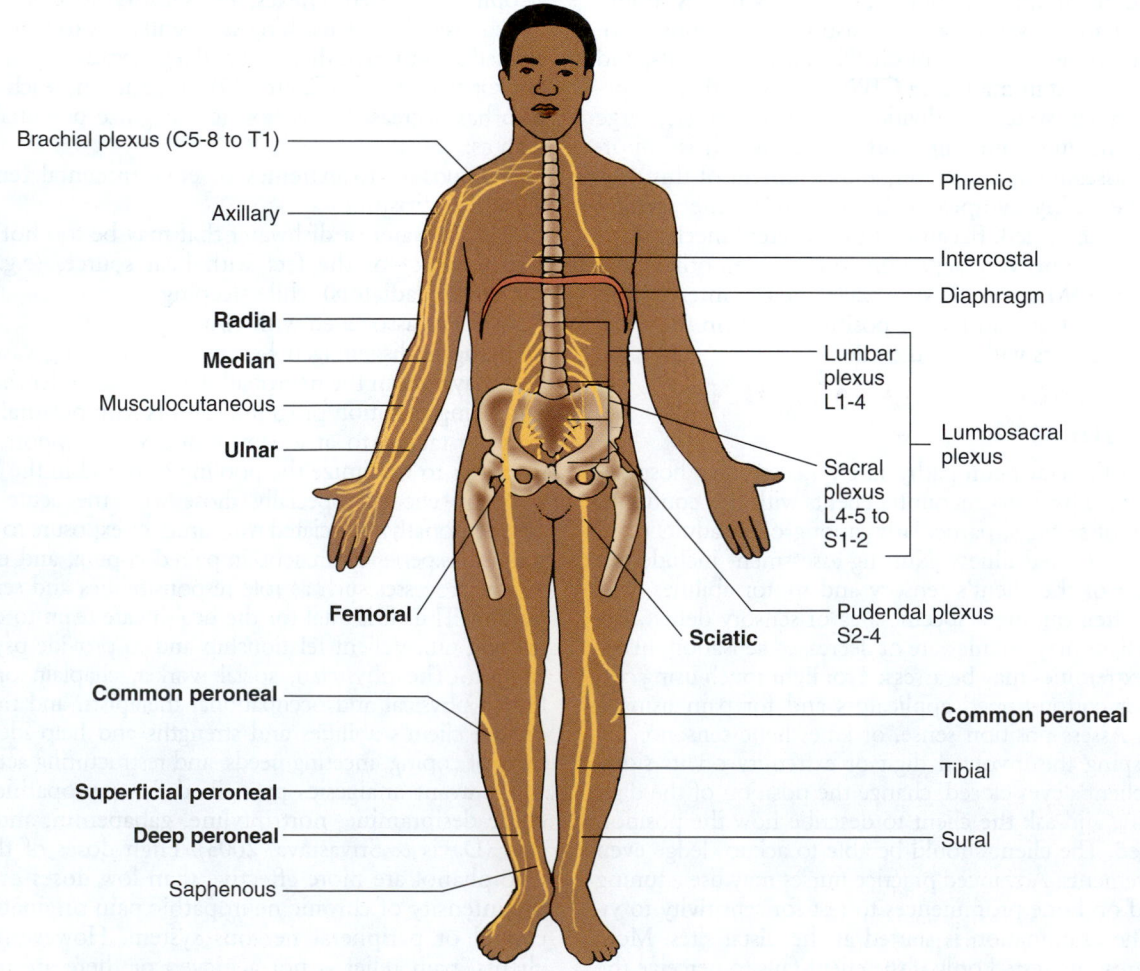

Figure 47-1 ■ Distribution of selected peripheral nerves in the body. The nerves most commonly affected by trauma are highlighted in bold type.

cross the transected gap through guidance by the neurilemma to find their way to the distal stump. The better aligned the union, the more normal the functional return (Figure 47-2).

Successfully realigned nerves remyelinate, grow to their former size, and eventually claim conduction velocities of 80% of their former capacity (Hickey, 2002). Successful reinnervation is adversely affected by the loss of anatomic continuity of the nerve, infection, and increasing age. Disorganization of the nerve or mismatched realignments may result in functional weakness, unintentional muscle movements, and poor sensory discrimination and localization of stimuli.

Some sensory function may return before the regeneration process can occur. This is because nerves proximal to the injured neurons are stimulated to produce collateral innervation to the affected areas. These collaterals provide some innervation before the axon itself has regenerated sufficiently.

◆ COLLABORATIVE MANAGEMENT
◆ Assessment

The client may relate a history of extremity or pelvic trauma, penetrating injury, recent surgery, the use of crutches, or pain after medication injections. Peripheral nerve trauma is especially common in wartime combat or other injury. In addition to weakness or flaccid paralysis, the client may complain of burning sensations distal to the trauma or pain that in-

creases with tactile or environmental stimulation. Skin and nail changes of the affected extremities may also be noted by the client.

A physical assessment is performed to determine which neurologic functions are intact. In acute trauma, the injury should first be evaluated by the physician to determine whether movement is contraindicated. If movement is not contraindicated, the client's motor function is assessed by putting the limb through the normal range of motion. Any abnormal movements, tremor, atrophy, contractions, paresis or paralysis, and weak or absent deep tendon reflexes are documented. The client is questioned about abnormal sensations.

After complete denervation, the extent of vasomotor function is reflected in skin temperature, skin color, and edema. A warm phase and a cold phase have been identified. During the **warm phase,** the extremity is warm, and the skin appears flushed or rosy. Over 2 to 3 weeks, this phase is gradually superseded by a **cold phase,** during which the skin appears cyanotic, mottled, or reddish blue and feels cool compared with the contralateral, unaffected extremity. The dorsal surface of the hand of the examiner is used to compare skin temperatures because the abundance of temperature receptors in this area facilitates more accurate assessments. Edema may be noted immediately after injury or later as a result of surgical procedures. Any evidence of trophic changes (e.g., scaling of skin, brittleness of nails, or loss of body hair) is recorded. This initial assessment serves as the baseline for comparison during subsequent examinations, which are performed every 2 to 4 hours or less frequently as the client's condition indicates.

◆ Interventions

Interventions for the client with peripheral nerve trauma depend on the location as well as the type and degree of injury. If the nerve trauma results from a primary lesion, such as a tumor, the underlying problem is addressed first.

The health care provider may prescribe immobilization of the involved area by splint, cast, or traction to provide the rest needed to limit and resolve any inflammation. The purpose of surgical management is to restore the function of the damaged nerve.

Preoperative Care. There are usually no special preoperative interventions for the client undergoing peripheral nerve repair. Chapter 20 describes the general care of the client before surgery.

Operative Procedures. If the nerve is lacerated or transected, surgery may be indicated. Restorative procedures include resecting and suturing to reapproximate the severed nerve ends, nerve grafts, and nerve and tendon transplants.

Since surgeons first began to repair injured nerves, the timing of these procedures has been controversial. In the past, a repair delay of 3 to 8 weeks after injury allowed associated injuries to heal, after which the surgeon could better assess the extent of nerve damage. Although microsurgery and the use of lasers now allow primary nerve repair at the time of injury, the physician's judgment in selecting the optimal time and surgical procedure remains crucial.

After an injury, the two severed nerve segments contract and may form scar tissue. Before surgical anastomosis, the surgeon dissects these stumps to remove any damaged nerve tissue. This further decreases the lengths of the ends to be joined. To compensate for this shortening and to avoid excessive tension on the sutured nerve, the involved extremity is positioned in exaggerated flexion. The surgeon aligns the

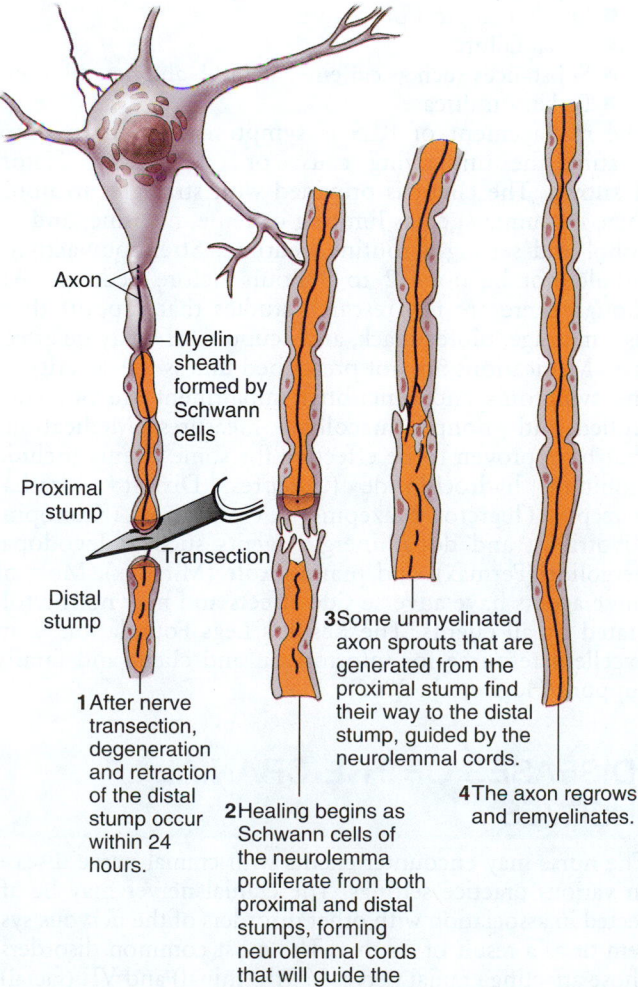

Axon

Myelin sheath formed by Schwann cells

Proximal stump

Transection

Distal stump

1 After nerve transection, degeneration and retraction of the distal stump occur within 24 hours.

2 Healing begins as Schwann cells of the neurolemma proliferate from both proximal and distal stumps, forming neurolemmal cords that will guide the regenerating axon.

3 Some unmyelinated axon sprouts that are generated from the proximal stump find their way to the distal stump, guided by the neurolemmal cords.

4 The axon regrows and remyelinates.

Figure 47-2 ■ Regeneration of peripheral nerve after injury.

segments under magnification, bringing proximal motor and sensory fibers to distal motor and sensory fibers, and then sutures the nerve tissue.

Postoperative Care. After suturing, the extremity is placed in a cast to maintain the flexed position and to avoid tension on the suture line. Ten to 14 days after nerve repair, the entire dressing is removed, the joint flexion is eased, and a new splint may be applied for an additional 2 weeks. At that time, a removable splint may be applied and physiotherapy begun. Protection of the nerve sutures is continued for a minimum of 6 weeks.

If a large segment of nerve has been damaged and direct anastomosis would be impossible without stretching the nerve more than 10% to 15% of its total length, the surgeon may interpose a nerve graft. Motor and sensory axons may regenerate through the graft, joining proximal and distal segments through the two sites of anastomosis. The amount of sensory and motor regeneration depends on the length of the graft, the type of nerve involved, the condition of the end plates, and the number of axons able to traverse the graft and suture sites. Thus the results are not usually as favorable as with direct reanastomosis. In the case of grafted nerve repairs, maintenance of the flexed position is less essential, although immobilization by splints or casts to facilitate healing of the surgical sites remains imperative.

Splints are usually held in place with elastic wrapping or hook-and-loop (Velcro) closures, which can become too tight if edema develops. Check the skin around the splints and casts frequently (hourly, initially) for tightness, warmth, and color. If the client complains of discomfort, tingling, or coolness or if the color is blanched, the cast or splint may be too tight, inform the physician. Immediately report any indication of drainage under a splint or cast.

Skin care is essential. Atrophy of the epidermis and underlying tissue causes the skin to become more fragile and more susceptible to injury and breakdown. The decreased skin nutrition and decreased vascularity associated with denervation cause delayed healing, which further compounds the problem. Thoroughly examine the skin for evidence of irritation or injury and assist or instruct the client to wash and dry the involved areas carefully. If the skin is dry, lanolin or cocoa butter may be used as a lubricant. Because sensation may be absent or inhibited, instruct the client to protect the involved areas from temperature extremes or other sources of potential trauma.

Rehabilitation. Physiotherapy is the major approach for rehabilitation after surgical repair. The nurse reinforces and helps the client perform the exercises learned in these sessions. Because the regeneration of nerves and subsequent return of sensory and motor function may be extremely slow and produce pain, the client may become discouraged and depressed. If the disability is permanent, he or she needs encouragement and assistance to cope with the changes in body image, self-esteem, and lifestyle.

RESTLESS LEGS SYNDROME

PATHOPHYSIOLOGY

Restless legs syndrome (RLS) is characterized by leg paresthesias associated with an irresistible urge to move. It affects 20 million Americans, but few health care providers

know that it exists (Cuellar, 2003). The more common type is associated with peripheral and central nerve damage in the legs and spinal cord (Kapur & Friedman, 2002). Many of those affected have a positive family history, indicating a genetic basis (Hogl et al., 2002). The incidence may be higher in nursing home and home care clients, who often have diabetes and renal failure—two very common conditions correlated with RLS. The incidence is equal in men and women. The client complains of intense burning or "crawling-type" sensations in the limbs and subsequently feels the need to move the limbs repeatedly. These symptoms are worse in the evening and at night and when the client is still for a period of time. Clients feel they need to move to relieve the symptoms. For that reason, clients with RLS often refer to themselves as "night walkers."

◆COLLABORATIVE MANAGEMENT

Diagnosis is made on the history; there is no known etiology. Potential contributing factors include the following:
- Vitamin and mineral deficiencies
- Anemias
- Polyneuropathies
- Diabetes mellitus (type II)
- Pregnancy
- Peripheral nerve disease
- Pinched nerves
- Lumbar surgical procedures
- Renal failure
- Substances such as caffeine, alcohol, and beta blockers
- Parkinson disease

The management of RLS is symptomatic and involves treating the underlying cause or contributing factor, if known. The client is provided with strategies to minimize insomnia such as limiting caffeine, nicotine, and alcohol and setting a routine bedtime. Strenuous activity should not be done 2 to 3 hours before bedtime. Although there are few research studies that support their use, massage, biofeedback, and acupuncture may be effective. Medications are not prescribed unless the severity of the symptoms and functional impairment are not controlled with nonpharmacologic measures. Medications that have proven to be effective for some clients include clonidine hydrochloride (Catapres, Dixarit✶), carbamazepine (Tegretol, Mazepine✶), clonazepam (Klonopin, Rivotril✶), and dopaminergic agents such as levodopa, pergolide (Permax), and pramipexole (Mirapex). Most of these agents have adverse side effects and may not be tolerated by all clients. The Restless Legs Foundation is an excellent resource for information and client and family support (Hogl et al., 2002).

DISEASES OF THE CRANIAL NERVES

The nurse may encounter clients with cranial nerve disease in various practice settings. The cranial nerves may be affected in association with other disorders of the nervous system or as a result of trauma. The most common disorders, those affecting cranial nerves V (trigeminal) and VII (facial), are discussed here.

Trigeminal Neuralgia

PATHOPHYSIOLOGY

Trigeminal neuralgia also known as tic douloureux:

- Is a disease that affects the trigeminal or fifth cranial nerve
- Entails a specific type of unilateral facial pain, which occurs in abrupt, intense paroxysms (spasms)
- Is usually provoked by minimal stimulation of a trigger zone
- Is unilateral and confined to the area innervated by the trigeminal nerve, most often the second and third branches (Figure 47-3)

Clients younger than 30 years of age with pain in more than one branch of the trigeminal nerve may be further evaluated to rule out the possibility of a tumor or multiple sclerosis.

> ### CONSIDERATIONS FOR OLDER ADULTS
> Trigeminal neuralgia usually appears in people older than 50 years of age. The female-to-male ratio is 2:1.

When describing the pain, clients use terms such as "excruciating," "sharp," "shooting," "piercing," "burning," and "jabbing." Between bursts of pain, which last from seconds to minutes, there is usually no pain. Often no sensory or motor deficits are found on examination, but the condition can be agonizing for the client. The fear of precipitating attacks often causes clients to avoid talking, smiling, eating, or attending to hygienic needs such as shaving, washing the face, and brushing the teeth.

The cause of trigeminal neuralgia is thought to be related to impaired inhibitory mechanisms in the brainstem caused by excessive firing of irritated fibers in the trigeminal nerve. In addition, trauma and infection of the teeth, jaw, or ear may be contributing factors.

The course of trigeminal neuralgia is characterized by bouts of pain for several weeks or months followed by spontaneous remissions. The length of these remissions may vary from days to years, but attack-free periods tend to become shorter as the client grows older. Symptoms rarely disappear permanently.

◆COLLABORATIVE MANAGEMENT

Management of the client with trigeminal neuralgia is determined by the amount of pain he or she is experiencing. Conservative measures are usually tried first.

NONSURGICAL MANAGEMENT. Medical management is accomplished with the use of drugs such as carbamazepine (Tegretol, Apo-Carbamazepine✣, Mazepine✣), phenytoin (Dilantin), baclofen (Lioresal), and occasionally amitriptyline (Elavil, Meravil✣) or diazepam (Valium, E-Pam✣). Initial therapy should always be nonsurgical, and drugs may be used singly or in combination. Surgical management may be considered if the client and the physician agree that the pain or the toxic effects of drug therapy are worse than the risk of surgery.

About 70% of clients respond to carbamazepine, 20 to 1200 mg daily, alone or in combination with phenytoin in average daily doses of 200 to 400 mg. Fosphenytoin (Cerebyx) may also be given IV to abort an acute attack. Phenytoin and fosphenytoin are anticonvulsants believed to decrease the paroxysmal afferent impulses in much the same way as when they are used to treat seizure disorders.

Injection of alcohol or phenol into the affected branch of the trigeminal nerve may relieve pain for up to 16 months. Injection into the gasserian ganglion, where sensory root fibers arise, may provide permanent pain control but carries with it a greater risk of extraocular palsies, keratitis, blindness, or masticatory paralysis. In both blocking procedures, there is complete anesthesia to the portion of the face innervated by the injected branch.

SURGICAL MANAGEMENT. Surgery is performed if the client is unable to tolerate the side effects of medications or they are ineffective in controlling pain. Surgical procedures include microvascular decompression, percutaneous balloon compression, and radiofrequency thermocoagulation.

Preoperative Care. In addition to the general preoperative care provided to all clients (see Chapter 20), the surgeon thoroughly explains the surgical benefits and any expected neurologic deficits.

Operative Procedures. In some clients, a small artery compresses the trigeminal nerve as it enters the pons. Surgical relocation of this artery (**microvascular decompression**) may relieve the pain of trigeminal neuralgia without compromising facial sensation. The surgeon carefully lifts the loop of artery off the nerve and places a small silicone (Silastic) sponge between the vessel and the nerve. Complications include aseptic meningitis, cerebrospinal fluid leak, ataxia, **ipsilateral** (same side) hearing loss, and seventh and eighth nerve defects (Filipchuk, 2003). Older adults and clients with other medical problems may not be a candidate for this procedure.

Radiofrequency thermalcoagulation may provide lasting relief of pain without compromising touch or motor function. During this procedure, the client is sedated with small doses of diazepam (Valium), midazolam hydrochloride (Versed), or fentanyl (Sublimaze) but is alert and able to follow commands in response to sensory and motor testing. The physician inserts a needle electrode and, under radiographic control, advances it to the appropriate area, where a heat lesion is made. The advantages of this procedure include long-term pain

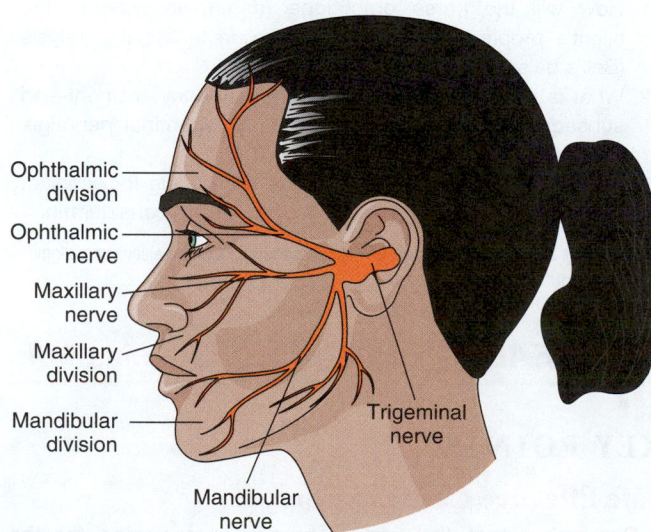

Figure 47-3 ■ Distribution of the trigeminal nerve and its three divisions: ophthalmic, maxillary, and mandibular.

Ophthalmic division
Ophthalmic nerve
Maxillary nerve
Maxillary division
Mandibular division
Trigeminal nerve
Mandibular nerve

relief, tolerance by older adults, absence of facial paralysis and preservation of the sensation of touch. The possibility of puncturing the internal carotid artery and the occurrence of anesthesia dolorosa are disadvantages (Hickey, 2002). The affected side is permanently insensitive to pain.

A **percutaneous balloon microcompression** is performed under general anesthesia. Under guided fluoroscopy, a balloon catheter is threaded through a large-bore needle and inflated, compressing the gasserian ganglion and nerve root (Filipchuk, 2003). Complications that may occur during this procedure include bradycardia and hypotension.

Unlike the other procedures, the **injection of glycerol** to destroy the myelinated fibers of the trigeminal nerve may take up to 3 weeks for pain relief to occur.

Postoperative Care. In addition to general postcraniotomy care (see Chapter 48), monitor the client for complications associated with these procedures, including headache, permanent cranial nerve dysfunction, and hemorrhage. The client's corneal reflex, extraocular muscles, and facial nerve are assessed and abnormal findings are documented and reported to the surgeon.

Apply an ice pack to the operative site on the jaw for 3 to 4 hours. A soft diet is prescribed, and the client is discouraged from chewing on the affected side until the paresthesias is abated. Instruct the client to avoid rubbing the eye on the affected side because the protective mechanism of pain will no longer warn of injury. He or she should inspect the eye daily for redness or irritation and report any change or blurred vision to the physician. Regular dental examinations are encouraged because the absence of pain may not warn the client of potential problems.

Psychosocial considerations for the client with trigeminal neuralgia include disappointment with ineffective drug protocols or surgical procedures, as well as the fear that the pain may recur with any activity. The client may fail to move the face in an attempt to prevent pain. This behavior may be misinterpreted by others as withdrawal, antisociability, or depression.

Facial Paralysis

PATHOPHYSIOLOGY

Facial paralysis, or **Bell's palsy** (acute paralysis of cranial nerve VII), was first described by Sir Charles Bell of England in 1821. The incidence is 23 persons per 100,000 population; men and women are equally affected (Hickey, 2002). Although the incidence may be slightly higher among people with diabetes, the condition occurs in all ages and at all times of the year.

The onset of Bell's palsy is acute. Maximal paralysis is attained within 48 hours in about half the clients and within 5 days in almost all clients. Pain behind the ear or on the face may precede paralysis by a few hours or days. The disorder is characterized by a drawing sensation and paralysis of all facial muscles on the affected side. The client cannot close the eye, wrinkle the forehead, smile, whistle, or grimace. The face appears masklike and sags. Taste is usually impaired to some degree, but this symptom seldom persists beyond the second week of paralysis.

Although the cause of Bell's palsy remains obscure, it may be the result of an inflammatory process. Clients with Bell's palsy are rarely hospitalized, but the nurse may en-

counter them in community-based settings such as clinics, physicians' offices, or emergency departments.

◆COLLABORATIVE MANAGEMENT

Medical management consists of the administration of prednisone (Deltasone, Winpred✱), 30 to 60 mg daily, during the first week after the onset of symptoms. Analgesics may help relieve the pain. Nursing care is directed toward managing the major neurologic deficits and providing psychosocial support. Because the eye does not close, the cornea must be protected from drying and subsequent ulceration or abrasion. Instruct the client to manually close the eyelid at intervals and to instill artificial tears four times daily. The eye may be patched or taped closed at bedtime.

The client may be unable to chew, sip fluids through a straw, or control drooling on the affected side. Thus mealtime may become a problem. Encourage the client to eat and drink using the unaffected side of the mouth. Frequent, small meals may be better tolerated, and clients may require a soft diet. Simple techniques of massage; the application of warm, moist heat; and facial exercises are explained to the client.

A facial sling may prevent drooping of the affected side. As muscle tone improves, instruct the client to grimace, wrinkle the brow, force the eyes closed, whistle, and blow air out of the cheeks three or four times daily for 5 minutes in front of a mirror.

Although most clients recover fully within a few weeks or months, about 15% to 20% experience some residual weakness; a few have permanent neurologic deficits. These clients require a great deal of support because body image and self-esteem are drastically affected. The nurse is a valuable source of both information and psychosocial support.

❓ *Critical Thinking Challenge*

An older adult in a long-term care setting complains to you that the left side of her face is very painful. She has had this problem before, but does not recall what her health care provider told her about the cause of her problem. After a thorough pain assessment, you decide to call the nurse practitioner to inform her of the client's complaint and your findings.

1. How will the nurse practitioner determine whether the client's problem is trigeminal neuralgia or facial paralysis (Bell's palsy)?
2. What is the difference between the nerve involvement and subsequent clinical manifestations of trigeminal neuralgia and Bell's palsy?
3. What options for treatment will the client have for either of these diseases, taking her advanced age into consideration?

evolve For suggested answer guidelines, go to http://evolve.elsevier.com/Iggy/.

GET READY for the NCLEX Examination!

KEY POINTS

Safe Effective Care Environment

■ Remember that the *priority* nursing intervention for the client with Guillain-Barré syndrome (GBS) is to assess for and maintain his or her respiratory function.

- Observe for and report side and adverse effects of IV immunoglobulin (IVIg), such as chills, fever, headache, and anaphylaxis; infuse the drug slowly when it is started.
- Observe for, prevent, and/or manage complications of plasmapheresis as outlined in Chart 47-3.
- Monitor clients on cholinesterase (ChE) inhibitor drugs for early manifestations of cholinergic or myasthenic crisis as listed in Table 47-2.
- Use caution when feeding clients with dysphagia to prevent aspiration, a common potential problem in clients with GBS and myasthenia gravis (MG).

Health Promotion and Maintenance

- In collaboration with the physical and occupational therapists, plan interventions to promote self-care for clients with GBS.
- Demonstrate to clients and family members basic measures to prevent complications of immobility, such as turning and repositioning, and range-of-motion exercises.
- For clients with MG, reinforce the importance of taking medications at appropriate times as listed in Chart 47-6.
- For clients with MG, teach them to rest frequently and avoid stressors that may exacerbate their illness (see Table 47-3).
- Teach care of lower extremities for clients with peripheral neuropathy, as detailed in Chart 47-7.
- Refer clients with chronic peripheral nervous system (PNS) diseases to appropriate community resources and support groups, such as the Restless Legs Foundation and Myasthenia Gravis Foundation.

Psychosocial Integrity

- Encourage clients with GBS and MG to verbalize feelings about their illness and its effects, while fostering hope and optimism.
- Assist clients with PNS diseases to identify coping strategies they have used in the past as they adapt to their health problems.
- Assess clients with PNS disease for depression; teach clients and families to notify the health care provider if changes in mental status or outlook occur.

Physiological Integrity

- Ask clients with suspected GBS about recent history of acute illness, trauma, surgery, or immunization.
- For clients with GBS, implement interventions and associated activities as listed in Chart 47-2.
- Be aware that edrophonium (Tensilon) testing is commonly used for diagnosing MG and for differentiating myasthenic (undermedication) crisis and cholinergic (overmedication) crisis.
- Evaluate clients with GBS or MG to determine whether outcomes related to adequate ventilation and airway patency were met.
- For clients having a thymectomy, maintain adequate respiratory function and observe for signs of pneumothorax or hemothorax, such as chest pain and sudden shortness of breath.
- Assess clients who have peripheral nerve injury for a warm phase (extremity is warm and skin is flushed initially) or a cold phase (extremity later becomes cold and skin is cyanotic, mottled, or reddish blue).

- Recognize that restless legs syndrome is a common, underdiagnosed disorder in which the client has leg paresthesias with urges to move the legs frequently, especially at night; pain is described as an intense burning.
- Assess clients with severe facial pain for associated clinical manifestations of trigeminal neuralgia or facial paralysis; evaluate effect of pain control measures.
- Recognize that trigeminal neuralgia is unilateral (one-sided) and usually provoked by minimal stimulation, such as talking or eating.

ADDITIONAL STUDY RESOURCES

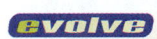 Go to your Student CD-ROM for Review Questions for the NCLEX Examination.

evolve Go to http://evolve.elsevier.com/Iggy/ for Integrated Management of Care Questions for the NCLEX Examination.

SELECTED BIBLIOGRAPHY

Chitnis, T., & Khoury, S.J. (2003). Immunological neuromuscular disorders. *Journal of Allergy and Clinical Immunology, 111,* 231-246.

Cooke, J.F., & Orb, A. (2003). The recovery phase in Guillain-Barré syndrome: Moving from dependency to independence. *Rehabilitation Nursing, 28*(4), 105-108, 130.

Cuellar, N. (2003). Restless legs syndrome: A case study. *Journal of Neuroscience Nursing, 35*(4), 193-201.

Cunning, S. (2000). When the Dx is myasthenia gravis. *RN, 63*(4), 26-30.

Davis, M.P., & Srivastava, M. (2003). Demographics, assessment and management of pain in the elderly. *Drugs & Aging, 20*(1):23-57.

Dochterman, J.M., & Bulechek, G.M. (2004). *Nursing interventions classification (NIC).* St. Louis: Mosby.

Evoli, A., et al. (2002). Thymoma in patients with MG: Characteristics and long-term outcome. *Neurology, 59*(12), 1844-1850.

Filipchuk, D. (2003). Classic trigeminal neuralgia: A surgical perspective. *Journal of Neuroscience Nursing, 35*(2), 82-86.

Gregory, R.J. (2003). Recovery from depression associated with Guillain Barré syndrome. *Issues in Mental Health Nursing, 24*(2), 129-135.

Hickey, J.V. (2002). *The clinical practice of neurological and neurosurgical nursing* (5th ed.). Philadelphia: Lippincott-Raven.

Hogl, B., et al. (2002). Transient restless legs syndrome after spinal anesthesia: A prospective study. *Neurology, 59,* 1705-1707.

Hughes, R.C., et al. (2003). Practice parameter: Immunotherapy for Guillain-Barré syndrome: Report of the Quality Standards Subcommittee of the American Academy of Neurology. *Neurology, 61,* 736-740.

Kapur, N., & Friedman, R. (2002). Oral ketamine: A promising treatment for restless legs syndrome. *Anesthesia and Analgesia, 94,* 1558-1559.

Kittiwatanapaisan, W., et al. (2003). Fatigue in myasthenia gravis patients. *Journal of Neuroscience Nursing, 35*(2), 87-93, 106.

Kupersmith, M.J., Latkany, R., & Homel, P. (2003). Development of generalized disease at 2 years in patients with ocular myasthenia gravis. *Neurology, 60*(2), 243-248.

Marrs, J, & Newton, S. (2003). Updating your peripheral neuropathy "know-how." *Clinical Journal of Oncology Nursing, 7*(3), 299-303.

Moorhead, S., Johnson, M., & Maas, M. (2004). *Nursing outcomes classification (NOC).* St. Louis: Mosby.

Pagana, K.D., & Pagana, T.J. (2002). *Mosby's manual of diagnostic and laboratory tests.* St. Louis: Mosby.

Parker, J.N., & Parker, P.M. (2002). *The official patient's source book for Guillain-Barré syndrome.* San Diego: Icon Health Publications.

Pascuzzi, R.M. (2003). The edrophonium test. *Seminars in Neurology, 23*(1), 83-88.

Rabinstein, A., & Wijdicks, E.F. (2002). BiPAP in acute respiratory failure due to myasthenic crisis may prevent intubation. *Neurology, 59*(10), 1647-1649.

Richman, D., & Agius, M. (2003). Treatment of autoimmune myasthenia gravis. *Neurology, 61*(12), 1652-1661.

Rowbotham, M.C., et al. (2003). Oral opioid therapy for chronic peripheral and central neuropathic pain. *New England Journal of Medicine, 348*(13), 1223-1232.

Sharshar, T., et al. (2003). Early predictors of mechanical ventilation in Guillain-Barré syndrome. *Critical Care Medicine, 31*(1), 278-283.

Sulton, L.L. (2002). Meeting the challenges of Guillain-Barré syndrome. *Nursing Management, 33*(7), 25-30.

Sweeney, C.W. (2002). Understanding peripheral neuropathy in patients with cancer: Background and patient assessment. *Clinical Journal of Oncology Nursing, 6*(3), 163-166.

Worsham, T.L. (2000). Easing the course of Guillain-Barré syndrome. *RN, 63*(3), 46-50.

Zimmermann, P.G. (2003). Lessons learned: On watching for zebras. *Journal of Emergency Nursing, 29*(1), 85-86.

Interventions for Critically Ill Clients with Neurologic Problems

RICHARD B. ARBOUR

LEARNING OUTCOMES

After studying this chapter, you should be able to:

1. Identify the common types of strokes.
2. Discuss risk factors that increase the likelihood of strokes.
3. Describe typical clinical manifestations associated with stroke.
4. Analyze assessment data to determine common nursing diagnoses that are pertinent to clients with strokes.
5. Identify the purpose of intracranial pressure (ICP) monitoring and signs of increasing ICP.
6. Explain the role of drug therapy in managing clients with strokes.
7. Prioritize nursing care for a client who has experienced a stroke.
8. Discuss the purpose of rehabilitation for the client who has had a stroke.
9. Develop a teaching plan for the client who has experienced a stroke.
10. Differentiate the common types of traumatic brain injury (TBI).
11. Explain the pathophysiologic changes that can result from moderate or severe TBI.
12. Describe the psychosocial and behavioral manifestations associated with TBI.
13. Prioritize nursing care for the client with TBI.
14. Explain the role of sedation and analgesia in managing the client with intracranial hypertension.
15. Describe common complications of brain tumors.
16. Develop a postoperative plan of care for a client having a craniotomy.

Go to your Student CD-ROM for Review Questions
for the NCLEX Examination keyed to these Learning Outcomes.

Certain neurologic problems can cause clients to become critically ill or die. Stroke, head injury, brain tumor, and brain abscess can cause increased intracranial pressure (ICP), a life-threatening complication that may easily compound disability and risk of death from the initial brain insult. Permanent neurologic dysfunction or death may be prevented by prompt recognition and aggressive management of this complication by the interdisciplinary health care team.

STROKE

A **stroke** is caused by a disruption in the normal blood supply to the brain. This disruption in blood supply may be in the form of an interruption in blood flow to the brain, in which case the stroke is ischemic in origin. The blood supply disruption may also take the form of bleeding within or around the brain. This is called a hemorrhagic stroke. Formerly called *cerebrovascular accident* (CVA), the National Stroke Association now uses the term *brain attack* to describe a stroke. A stroke is a *medical emergency* that strikes suddenly, and it should be treated immediately to prevent neurologic deficit and permanent disability.

Stroke is the second most common cause of death and major disability worldwide. Although the number of stroke deaths has decreased during the past several years in the United States, stroke remains the third most common cause of death and the primary cause of adult disability (Goldszmidt

& Caplan, 2003). The direct and indirect costs of stroke are more than $41 billion annually (see the Resource Management box above).

PATHOPHYSIOLOGY
Pathophysiologic Changes in the Brain

The brain is unable to store oxygen or glucose and therefore must receive a constant flow of blood to provide these substances to function normally. In addition, blood flow is important for the removal of metabolic waste, carbon dioxide, and lactic acid. If blood supply to any part of the brain is interrupted for more than a few minutes, this may lead to death of cerebral tissue. This in turn can cause death as well as varying degrees of disability, depending on the location and amount of brain tissue affected.

Through the processes of cerebral **autoregulation,** blood flow is maintained at a fairly constant rate of 1000 mL/min. Put another way, the brain receives at least 20% of the available cardiac output. To maintain stability of cerebral blood flow, the cerebral arteries dilate or constrict in response to changes in blood pressure, carbon dioxide tension, and oxygen tension. For example, with normal, intact autoregulation, low blood pressure, high arterial carbon dioxide, or low arterial oxygen tension will cause a dilation of cerebral arteries to maintain cerebral blood flow.

In an **occlusive stroke,** ischemia occurs in the brain tissue supplied by the affected artery, and brain dysfunction results. **Ischemia** leads to hypoxia or anoxia and hypoglycemia within the affected brain tissue. These processes set in motion a series of events that ultimately lead to **infarction** or death of neurons, glia, and the involved area of the brain. In addition, brain metabolism and blood flow after a stroke is affected in stroke "watershed" area as well as in the **contralateral** (opposite side) hemisphere. Effects of a stroke on the contralateral side may be due to brain swelling as well as to further changes in blood flow throughout the brain.

Small lacunar infarctions may also occur. Lacunae are small, deep cavities within the brain that result first from occlusion of a small vessel. This occlusion leads to infarct and necrosis of the area of the brain supplied by the affected vessel. Lacunar infarcts occur almost exclusively in the internal capsule, basal ganglia, and thalamus. They produce either a pure motor deficit (internal capsule) or a pure sensory deficit (thalamus). A lacunar infarct is generally regarded as a type of ischemic stroke.

Types of Strokes

Strokes are generally classified as ischemic (occlusive) or hemorrhagic. Most ischemic strokes are either thrombotic strokes or embolic strokes (Table 48-1).

ISCHEMIC STROKE

An **ischemic stroke** is caused by the occlusion of a cerebral artery by either a thrombus or an embolus. A stroke that is caused by a thrombus is referred to as a thrombotic stroke, whereas a stroke caused by an embolus is referred to as an embolic stroke. About 80% of all strokes are ischemic.

THROMBOTIC STROKE. Thrombotic strokes account for more than half of all strokes and are commonly associated with the development of atherosclerosis of the blood vessel wall. Atherosclerosis is a complex process that includes altered function of the inner lining of arterial vessels, inflammation, and increased growth of vascular smooth muscle cells. It is the process by which plaques develop on the inner wall of the affected arterial vessel.

The first step in plaque development is accumulation of low-density lipoprotein (LDL) particles within the arterial vessel wall. These may undergo chemical changes and then stimulate endothelial cells to adhere to **monocytes** (inflammatory cells) and **T-cells** (immune system cells). The endothelium produces chemical messengers, which signal the monocytes and T-cells to incorporate within the intimal layer.

The second step is maturation of monocytes into macrophages. The macrophages, in turn, ingest LDL particles.

The third step occurs when the macrophages ingest a "critical mass" of LDL particles; they are then called foam cells. These cells constitute the fatty streak on the inner arterial wall, the earliest manifestation of arterial plaque.

The fourth step is additional growth of the lesion through influence of inflammatory molecules, which also help form a fibrous cover or cap over the lipid core. This covering makes the plaque larger but also separates it from blood flow through the vessel.

The fifth step occurs with plaque rupture. Rupture of the plaque exposes foam cells to clot-promoting elements in the blood. The end result is clot formation. If the clot is of sufficient size, it may interrupt blood flow to the brain tissue supplies by the vessel, causing an occlusive stroke. This process may occur over many years because collateral circulation to the involved area develops to compensate for the occlusion.

As the artery becomes completely occluded, blood flow to the area is markedly diminished. Decreased blood flow causes transient ischemia, which progresses to complete ischemia and infarction of the brain tissue. Within 72 hours, the area is edematous and necrotic, and cavities develop. The **bifurcation** (point of division) of the common carotid artery and the vertebral arteries at their junction with the

TABLE 48-1 Differential Features of the Types of Stroke

| Feature | Ischemic | | Hemorrhagic |
	Thrombotic	Embolic	
Evolution	Intermittent or stepwise improvement between episodes of worsening Completed stroke	Abrupt development of completed stroke Steady progression	Usually abrupt onset
Onset	Daytime (10 AM to 12 PM) Gradual (minutes to hours)	Daytime Sudden	Daytime Sudden, may be gradual if caused by hypertension
Level of consciousness	Preserved (client is awake)	Preserved (client is awake)	Deepening stupor or coma
Contributing associated factors	Hypertension Atherosclerosis	Cardiac disease	Hypertension Vessel disorders
Prodromal symptoms	Transient ischemic attack		
Neurologic deficits	Deficits during the first few weeks Slight headache Speech deficits Visual problems Confusion	Maximal deficit at onset Paralysis Expressive aphasia	Focal deficits Severe, frequent
Cerebrospinal fluid	Normal; possible presence of protein	Normal	Bloody
Seizures	No	No	Usually
Duration	Improvements over weeks to months Permanent deficits possible	Rapid improvements	Variable Permanent neurologic deficits possible

basilar artery are the most common sites involved. Because of the gradual occlusion of the arteries, thrombotic strokes tend to have a *slow* onset.

A **lacunar stroke** is another type of thrombotic stroke. A lacunar stroke causes a soft area or cavity to develop in the white matter or deep gray matter of the brain. This type of stroke may result in significant neurologic dysfunction if it damages a critical area in the brain.

EMBOLIC STROKE. An **embolic stroke** is caused by an **embolus** or a group of emboli (clots) that break off from one area of the body and travel to the cerebral arteries via the carotid artery or vertebrobasilar system. The usual sources of emboli are cardiac. Emboli can occur in clients with nonvalvular atrial fibrillation, ischemic heart disease, rheumatic heart disease, and mural thrombi following a myocardial infarction (MI) or insertion of a prosthetic heart valve. Another source of emboli may be plaque that breaks off from the carotid sinus or internal carotid artery. Emboli tend to become lodged in the smaller cerebral blood vessels at their point of bifurcation or where the lumen narrows. Embolic strokes account for almost half of all strokes.

The middle cerebral artery (MCA) is most commonly involved in an embolic stroke. As the emboli occlude the vessel, ischemia develops, and the client experiences the clinical manifestations of the stroke. However, the occlusion may be temporary if the embolus breaks into smaller fragments, enters smaller blood vessels, and is absorbed. For these reasons, embolic strokes are characterized by the *sudden* development and rapid occurrence of focal neurologic deficits. The symptoms may resolve over several hours or a few days. A cerebral hemorrhage may result if significant damage to the wall of the involved vessel has occurred. Conversion of an occlusive stroke to a hemorrhagic stroke may occur because the arterial vessel wall is also vulnerable

---

CHART 48-1

KEY FEATURES of
Transient Ischemic Attack

Visual Deficits
- Blurred vision
- Diplopia (double vision)
- Blindness in one eye
- Tunnel vision

Motor Deficits
- Transient weakness (arm, hand, or leg)
- Gait disturbance (ataxic)

Sensory Deficits
- Transient numbness (face, arm, or hand)
- Vertigo

Speech Deficits
- Aphasia
- Dysarthria (slurred speech)

---

to ischemic damage from blood supply interruption. Sudden hemodynamic stress may result in vessel rupture, causing bleeding directly within the brain tissue.

TRANSIENT ISCHEMIC ATTACK AND REVERSIBLE ISCHEMIC NEUROLOGIC DEFICIT. Ischemic strokes are often preceded by warning signs, such as a **transient ischemic attack (TIA),** also called a "silent" stroke (Chart 48-1) or a **reversible ischemic neurologic deficit (RIND).** Both warning signs cause transient focal neurologic dysfunction resulting from a brief interruption in cerebral blood flow, possibly resulting from cerebral vasospasm or transient systemic arterial hypertension. The difference between a TIA and an RIND is the length of time the client is symptomatic. A TIA lasts a few minutes to fewer than 24 hours,

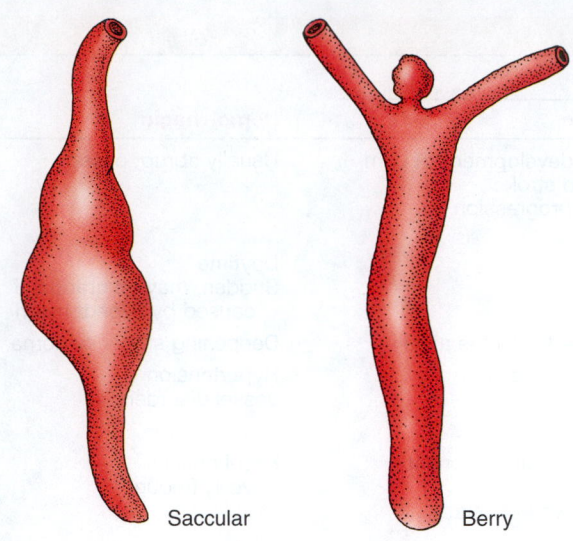

Figure 48-1 ■ Two common types of cerebral aneurysms.

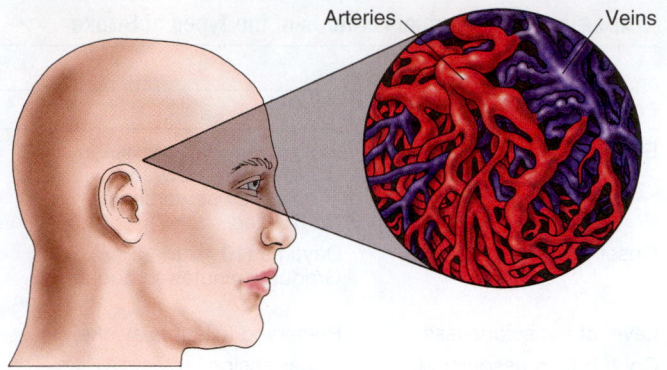

Figure 48-2 ■ Appearance of an arteriovenous malformation. Note the dilated, entangled blood vessels.

whereas RIND symptoms last longer than 24 hours but less than a week. Both TIAs and RINDs may damage the brain tissue with repeated insults, as evidenced by magnetic resonance imaging (MRI) or computed tomography (CT). Multiple TIAs indicate significant increased stroke risk.

HEMORRHAGIC STROKE

The second major classification of stroke is **hemorrhagic stroke.** In this type of stroke, vessel integrity is interrupted, and bleeding occurs into the brain tissue or into the spaces surrounding the brain (ventricular, subdural, subarachnoid). Hemorrhage into the brain tissue generally results from a ruptured aneurysm (localized weakening and distortion of vessel wall); rupture of an arteriovenous malformation; or, more commonly, severe hypertension.

ANEURYSM. A ruptured cerebral aneurysm results in hemorrhagic stroke. An **aneurysm** is an abnormal ballooning or blister on the involved artery (Figure 48-1). Aneurysms may be congenital or traumatic. A congenital aneurysm is a developmental defect in the media and elastica (adventitia or outer layer) of the vessel wall. Both etiologies weaken the vessel wall. Continued force on the weakened vessel wall from elevated blood pressure stretches and thins the vessel wall, causing the intimal or innermost vessel layer to protrude. This is the point most vulnerable to rupture. Although the rupture may occur at any time, it usually happens during activity. Aneurysms are often found at the bifurcations (branching) of major cerebral arteries.

Aneurysm rupture causes the development of an intracerebral hematoma, bleeding into the subarachnoid space, or bleeding directly into the ventricles. **Vasospasm,** a sudden and transient constriction of a cerebral artery, often occurs after a cerebral hemorrhage from aneurysm rupture. This occurs because blood is also an irritant to arterial vessels. Blood flow to distal areas of the brain supplied by the artery is markedly diminished, which leads to cerebral ischemia and infarction and further neurologic dysfunction.

ARTERIOVENOUS MALFORMATION. An **arteriovenous malformation (AVM)** is a developmental abnormality that occurs during embryonic development. It is a tangled or spaghetti-like mass of malformed, thin-walled, dilated vessels (Figure 48-2). The congenital absence of a cap-

illary network in these vessels forms an abnormal communication between the arterial and venous systems. The vessels may eventually rupture, causing bleeding into the subarachnoid space or into the intracerebral tissue. The risk of rupture and cerebral hemorrhage exists because normally the capillary network intervenes between the arterial and venous systems. In the absence of the capillary network, the thin-walled veins are subjected to arterial pressure.

HYPERTENSION. Although the exact mechanisms involved are unknown, it is hypothesized that elevated systolic and diastolic blood pressures cause changes within the arterial wall that leave it susceptible to rupture. An intracerebral hemorrhage occurs when the vessel ruptures. Damage to the brain occurs from bleeding, causing distortion or displacement. Brain tissue edema acts as a direct irritant to brain tissue. Hemorrhagic strokes may be more likely with sudden, dramatic blood pressure elevations, such as those seen with cocaine intoxication.

Etiology and Genetic Risk

Certain major risk factors increase the likelihood of strokes, especially the following:

- Hypertension
- Diabetes mellitus
- Heart disease
- Hypercholesteremia
- **Hypercoagulable** (increased clotting) state
- Illicit drug use (especially cocaine)
- Obesity
- Nonvalvular atrial fibrillation

Most of these disorders have a familial or genetic predisposition and are discussed elsewhere in this text. For example, relative stroke risk increases with a strong family history of hypertension or atherosclerotic disease. Close blood relatives of a client with an aneurysm may be at higher risk for intracranial aneurysms and are potential candidates for diagnostic testing and follow-up.

CULTURAL CONSIDERATIONS

Black individuals tend to have one of the highest rates of strokes compared with other groups, possibly because they have a high rate of hypertension and diabetes mellitus. The cause for the higher occurrence is unknown, but it might be due to dietary habits or problems with access to health care, especially in rural areas.

CHART 48-2

CLIENT EDUCATION GUIDE
Common Risk Factors for Developing a Stroke

- Atrial fibrillation or heart murmur
- Myocardial infarction
- Previous stroke or transient ischemic attack (TIA)
- Heart surgery
- Valvular heart disease
- Diabetes mellitus
- Smoking
- Substance abuse (particularly cocaine)
- Obesity
- Sedentary lifestyle
- Oral contraceptive use
- Elevated serum cholesterol, lipoprotein, triglyceride, low-density lipoprotein (LDL) and high-density lipoprotein (HDL) levels
- Previous stroke or TIA
- Heavy alcohol use
- Sudden discontinuation of antihypertensive medications (causes hemorrhagic stroke)
- Heredity/familial tendency
- Migraines
- Older age
- Male
- Black heritage
- Sickle cell anemia
- Use of phenylpropanolamine (PPA), which is found in antihistamine drugs (causes catastrophic strokes, primarily in young and middle-aged women)
- Hypercoagulable states

Incidence/Prevalence

It is estimated that there are more than 4.7 million stroke survivors in the United States. About 730,000 strokes occur each year, and more than 150,000 deaths result. About 25% of strokes occur in people under 65 years of age. The number of strokes occurring in the younger population is increasing as a result of chronic intravenous (IV) drug abuse. Those using crack cocaine experience an increased incidence of stroke resulting from changes in the clotting mechanism caused by the drugs, spasm of cerebral vessels or hemodynamic stress from the sudden increase in systolic blood pressure.

Between 5% and 15% of all clients who have had strokes have a recurrence within 1 year. By 5 years, about 40% have recurrence, and half of those die from stroke complications (Goldszmidt & Caplan, 2003). Strokes tend to occur more often in the southern United States ("stroke belt"), which is probably related to the geographic distribution of the older population, an increased use of tobacco, obesity, and a diet higher in fats.

HEALTH PROMOTION/ILLNESS PREVENTION

Individuals with predisposing health conditions should be aware that they could have a stroke unless they change their lifestyle. Teach them the importance of seeking professional health care and being compliant with the recommended treatment plan. Also remind them that other risk factors contribute to stroke, some of which can be avoided, such as smoking, a sedentary lifestyle, and high-fat diet (Chart 48-2). Recommend a diet high in fruits and vegetables and low in saturated and trans fats. Light to moderate alcohol consumption may reduce the risk of stroke, but a higher consumption

may increase it. Additional information about diet, weight control, and smoking cessation can be found in the Cardiac Unit and in the discussion on obesity in Chapter 64.

Nurses or other health care providers can assess a client's risk for stroke by completing a Stroke Risk Screening tool (Figure 48-3).

◆COLLABORATIVE MANAGEMENT
◆Assessment

HISTORY

An accurate history is important in the diagnosis of a stroke. The information obtained assists in identifying the area of the brain involved as well as the cause. Obtain a history of the client's activity when the stroke began. Ischemic strokes often occur during sleep, whereas hemorrhagic strokes tend to occur during activity. Next ask the client or a family member how the symptoms progressed. Be sure to elicit a history of the onset of the stroke. Symptoms of an embolic or hemorrhagic stroke tend to occur abruptly, whereas thrombotic strokes generally have a more gradual progression. Determine the severity of the symptoms, such as whether they worsened after the initial onset (hemorrhagic stroke) or began to improve (embolic stroke). It is important to determine whether the symptoms come and go, possibly indicating a transient ischemic attack (TIA) or a reversible ischemic neurologic deficit (RIND).

During the interview, observe the client's level of consciousness (LOC), and assess for indications of intellectual or memory impairments or difficulties with speech or hearing. Question the client or family member about the presence of any sensory or motor changes, visual problems, problems with balance or gait, and changes in reading or writing abilities.

In addition, ask about the client's medical history, with specific attention directed toward a history of head trauma, diabetes, hypertension, heart disease, anemia, obesity, and headache. Obtain a list of current medications, including prescribed, over-the-counter (OTC), and recreational (illicit) drugs. Always ask about herbal supplements. Medications that could contribute to stroke include anticoagulants, aspirin, vasodilators, and illegal drugs as well as OTC products containing ephedra or herbal products that affect blood clotting. To complete the history, obtain data about the client's social history, including education, employment, travel, leisure activities, and personal habits (e.g., smoking, diet, exercise pattern, drug and alcohol use).

PHYSICAL ASSESSMENT/CLINICAL MANIFESTATIONS

NEUROLOGIC ASSESSMENT. Perform a neurologic assessment of the client. Specific neurologic signs and other manifestations depend on the extent and location of the ischemia and the arteries involved (Chart 48-3).

COGNITIVE CHANGES. The client may exhibit a variety of cognitive problems in addition to changes in level of consciousness (LOC). LOC may vary, depending on the extent of increased intracranial pressure (ICP) caused by the stroke and on the location of the stroke. LOC changes may also vary according to concurrent conditions, such as drug or alcohol intoxication as well as hypoxemia or metabolic disturbances. Always assess for indications of the following:

- Denial of the illness
- Spatial and **proprioceptive** (awareness of body position in space) dysfunction

STROKE RISK SCREENING

Site and address of Screening _____ Date:_____/_____/_____

PART I - DEMOGRAPHICS, AGE AND ETHNICITY

Name: (last)_____ (first) _____ (middle initial)_____

Gender: __ Male ___Female   Highest Level of Education: ____ High School or less __ College __ Graduate School

Address: _____ (city)_____ (state)_____ (zip)_____ (county)_____

Phone: Home (___)_____ Work (___)_____ Date of Birth:___/___/_____ Age today_____

Do you have a primary health care provider? .... _____Yes_____No
Have you seen a health care provider in the past year? .... _____Yes_____No
Do you have medical insurance?.. _____Yes_____No

Ethnicity/Race: _____ African American _____Caucasian ____Hispanic White _____Hispanic Non-White

_____ Asian/Pacific Islander _____ American Indian or Alaskan Native _____ Other or Unknown

PART II - HISTORY FOR KNOWN AND ESTABLISHED HIGH RISK FACTORS FOR STROKE

1. Have you ever been told that you have high blood pressure?.. _____Yes_____No

2. Do you take medication for high blood pressure?.. _____Yes_____No

3. Do you have a history of abnormal heart rate or rhythm called atrial fibrillation?.......................... _____Yes_____No

4. Have you ever been checked for or been told that you have narrowing of the arteries to the brain?.......... _____Yes_____No

5. Have you had a heart attack, heart bypass surgery, angioplasty or another disease of the heart?............ _____Yes_____No

6. Have you had a previous stroke, mini-stroke or TIA?.. _____Yes_____No

7. Do you have diabetes mellitus (DM) or are you on insulin or medication for high blood sugar?.............. _____Yes_____No

8. Have you ever smoked cigarettes?... _____Yes_____No

9. Do you currently smoke cigarettes?... _____Yes_____No

PART III - HISTORY FOR SIGNIFICANT BUT SLIGHTLY LOWER RISK FACTORS FOR STROKE

10. Has a family member had a stroke or heart attack when they were less than 45 years of age?................ _____Yes_____No

11. Do you consume more than two ounces of alcohol per day on a daily basis?................................. _____Yes_____No

12. Do you have a cholesterol level greater than 200?... _____Yes_____No

PART IV - HISTORY OF OTHER/UNCOMMON IMPORTANT RISK FACTORS FOR STROKE

13. Do you smoke cigarettes and take birth control pills?... _____Yes_____No

14. Do you have Sickle Cell Anemia?... _____Yes_____No

15. Do you use one or more of the following drugs: Cocaine, Crack, Heroin, Amphetamines?..................... _____Yes_____No

16. Are you overweight or obese? .... _____Yes_____No

17. Do you consider your activity level as generally inactive?.. _____Yes_____No

Figure 48-3 ■ Stroke Risk Screening Tool.

PART V - BLOOD PRESSURE AND PULSE

Blood Pressure (BP) recorded sitting _____(Systolic)_____(Diastolic) _____ Right Arm _____Left Arm

Radial Pulse rate for 60 seconds (beats/minute) _____ Irregular pulse rate?........_____Yes_____No

PART VI - IDENTIFICATION OF RISK FOR STROKE AND RECOMMENDATION

1._____ **Low Risk for Stroke:**

Under the age of 55, responded "**NO**" to questions 1-17 (self-reported risk factors) and was not identified to have an irregular pulse rate or a measured Systolic BP equal to or greater than or equal to 140 or Diastolic equal to or greater than 90.

RECOMMENDATION: Take this completed screening form to your health care provider at your next appointment.

2._____ **Moderate Risk for Stroke:**

Age equal to or greater than 55 with no self-reported risk factors and no risk factors identified on screening

OR - Age up to 64 with one self-reported risk factor, or an irregular pulse rate or a measured Systolic BP equal to or greater than 140 or a Diastolic equal to or greater than 90.

RECOMMENDATION: Notify your health care provider within a week with the results of your screening and request an appointment for an evaluation and care to prevent a stroke.

3._____ **High Risk for Stroke:**

Age equal to or greater than 65 with one self-reported risk factor, or irregular pulse, or a measured Systolic BP equal to or greater than 140 or a Diastolic BP equal to or greater than 90.

OR - Any age with **two or more risk factors**, either self-reported and/or identified on measurement of an irregular pulse or Systolic BP equal to or greater than 140 or a Diastolic equal to or greater than 90.

RECOMMENDATION: Notify your health care provider <u>TODAY</u> with the results of your screening and request an appointment for an evaluation of your risks for stroke and care to prevent a stroke.

4._____ **PRESENTS WITH WARNING SIGNS OF STROKE, OR TIA (MINI-STROKE)**
_____ **RECOMMENDATION: CALL OR HAVE SOMEONE CALL 9-1-1 IMMEDIATELY!**

PART VII - THE EARLY WARNING SIGNS OF STROKE

* SUDDEN WEAKNESS, NUMBNESS, OR PARALYSIS OF THE FACE, ARM OR LEG, ON ONE OR BOTH SIDES OF THE BODY

* SUDDEN BLURRED VISION OR BLINDNESS IN ONE OR BOTH EYES

* SUDDEN DIFFICULTY SPEAKING, SLURRING OF SPEECH OR DIFFICULTY UNDERSTANDING

* SUDDEN SEVERE HEADACHE WITH SUDDEN ONSET THAT OCCURS WITHOUT APPARENT REASON

* SUDDEN LOSS OF BALANCE, DIZZINESS, OR FALLING WITHOUT ANY APPARENT REASON

CALL 9-1-1 IMMEDIATELY IF YOU EXPERIENCE ANY OF THESE SYMPTOMS

I have received a screening for the risk of stroke and agree to follow up with the recommendations. I understand this is only a screening. I agree that this data can be entered into a database for research without identifying me by name.

(Signature of Participant) _____**Signature of Health care provider**_____

The **Stroke Risk Screening** was developed in 1999 jointly by the Division on Research, Delaware Nurses Association and Ellen Barker, MSN, RN, CNRN, Neuroscience Nursing Consultants, Wilmington, Delaware. Marian P. LaMonte, M.D., M.S.N., Assistant Professor of Neurology and Co-Director of the Maryland Brain Attack Center, University of Maryland Medical Center, Baltimore, Maryland, served as Nurse/Neurologist advisor. There is no Copyright and permission is not needed to duplicate this form.

Figure 48-3 ■ *cont'd.*

CHART 48-3

KEY FEATURES of
Stroke Syndromes

Middle Cerebral Artery Strokes
- Contralateral hemiparesis: arm > leg
- Contralateral sensory deficit
- Homonymous hemianopsia
- Unilateral neglect or inattention
- Aphasia, anomia, alexia, agraphia, and acalculia
- Impaired vertical sensation
- Spatial deficit
- Perceptual deficit
- Visual field deficit
- Altered level of consciousness: drowsy to comatose

Posterior Cerebral Artery Strokes
- Perseveration
- Aphasia, amnesia, alexia, agraphia, visual agnosia, and ataxia
- Loss of deep sensation
- Decreased touch sensation
- Possible choreoathetoid movements
- Stupor; coma

Internal Carotid Artery Strokes
- Contralateral hemiparesis
- Sensory deficit
- Hemianopsia, blurred vision, blindness
- Aphasia (dominant side)

Internal Carotid Artery Strokes
- Headache
- Bruit

Anterior Cerebral Artery Strokes
- Contralateral hemiparesis: leg > arm
- Bladder incontinence
- Personality and behavior changes
- Aphasia, gait apraxia, and amnesia
- Positive grasp and sucking reflex
- Perseveration
- Sensory deficit (lower extremity)
- Memory impairment
- Apraxic gait

Vertebrobasilar Artery Strokes
- Headache and vertigo
- Coma
- Memory loss and confusion
- Flaccid paralysis
- Areflexia, ataxia, and vertigo
- Cranial nerve dysfunction
- Dysconjugate gaze
- Visual deficits (uniorbital) and homonymous hemianopsia
- Sensory loss: numbness

CHART 48-4

KEY FEATURES of
Left and Right Hemisphere Strokes

Feature	Left Hemisphere*	Right Hemisphere
Language	Aphasia Agraphia Alexia (word blindness)	Impaired sense of humor
Memory	Possible deficit	Disorientation to time, place, and person Inability to recognize faces
Vision	Inability to discriminate words and letters Reading problems Deficits in the right visual field	Visual spatial deficits Neglect of the left visual field Loss of depth perception
Behavior	Slowness Cautiousness Anxiety when attempting a new task Depression or a catastrophic response to illness Sense of guilt Feeling of worthlessness Worries over future Quick anger and frustration Intellectual impairment	Impulsiveness Lack of awareness of neurologic deficits Confabulation Euphoria Constant smiling Denial of illness Poor judgment Overestimation of abilities (risk for injury)
Hearing	No deficit	Loss of ability to hear tonal variations

*Location for speech in all but 15% to 20% of people.

- Impairment of memory, judgment, or problem-solving and decision-making abilities
- Decreased ability to concentrate and attend to tasks

Dysfunction in one or more of these areas may be more pronounced, depending on the hemisphere involved (Chart 48-4).

The right cerebral hemisphere is more involved with visual and spatial awareness and proprioception. A person who has a stroke involving the right cerebral hemisphere is often unaware of any deficits and may be disoriented to time and place. Personality changes include impulsivity (poor impulse control) and poor judgment. The left cerebral hemisphere, the dominant hemisphere in all but about 15% to 20% of the population, is the center for language, mathematic skills, and analytic thinking. Therefore a left hemisphere stroke results in **aphasia** (inability to use or comprehend language), **alexia** (reading problems), and **agraphia** (difficulty with writing). Persons with left-hemisphere strokes tend to be slow and cautious.

MOTOR CHANGES. The motor examination provides information about which part of the brain is involved. A right **hemiplegia** (paralysis on one side of the body) or **hemiparesis** (weakness on one side of the body) indicates a stroke involving the left cerebral hemisphere because the motor nerve fibers cross in the medulla before entering the spinal cord and periphery. Conversely, a left hemiplegia or hemiparesis indicates a stroke in the right cerebral hemisphere. If the brainstem or cerebellum is affected, the client may experience hemiparesis or quadriparesis and ataxia.

In collaboration with the physical and occupational therapist, gauge the client's muscle tone. The client with **hypotonia,** or **flaccid paralysis,** is unable to overcome the forces of gravity, and the extremities tend to fall to the side. The extremities feel heavy, and muscle tone is inadequate for balance, equilibrium, or protective mechanisms. **Hypertonia (spastic paralysis)** tends to cause fixed positions or contractures of the involved extremities. Range of motion (ROM) of the joints is restricted, and shoulder subluxation may easily occur from either spasticity or flaccidity. Also assess proprioception, head and trunk control, balance, coordination, and gait.

Loss of inhibitory nervous control from the cerebral cortex results in a spastic (upper motor neuron), uninhibited bladder. Bowel function may also be affected.

SENSORY CHANGES. The sensory examination evaluates the client's response to touch and painful stimuli. In addition to diminished motor function, decreased sensation typically occurs on the affected side of the body. The client who has had a stroke may also be unable to write, comprehend reading material, use an object correctly **(agnosia)**, or carry out a purposeful motor activity **(apraxia)**.

Evaluate for indications of **neglect syndrome,** which is particularly evident with strokes in the right cerebral hemisphere. In this syndrome, the client is unaware of the existence of his or her left or paralyzed side. The typical picture is that of the client sitting in a wheelchair, leaning to the left with the arm caught in the wheelchair wheel. When questioned, the client often states that everything is fine and believes that he or she is sitting up straight in the chair. Another typical example of neglect syndrome is the client who washes or dresses only one side of the body.

Another important part of the nursing assessment focuses on visual ability. Infarction or ischemia involving the carotid artery may cause pupillary abnormalities, **ptosis** (eyelid drooping), visual field deficits, or pallor and petechiae of the conjunctiva. **Amaurosis fugax,** a brief episode of blindness in one eye, results from retinal ischemia caused by ophthalmic or carotid artery insufficiency. **Hemianopsia,** or blindness in half of the visual field, results from damage to the optic tract or occipital lobe. Most often this deficit occurs as homonymous hemianopsia, in which there is blindness in the same side of both eyes (Figure 48-4). The client with this condition must turn his or her head to scan the complete range of vision. Otherwise, he or she does not see half of the visual field. For example, the client eats only half of a meal because that is the only portion seen. Clients with brainstem or cerebellar damage may experience abnormal eye movements.

CRANIAL NERVE FUNCTION. Assessment of the client's ability to chew reflects cranial nerve (CN) V. Assessment of the client's ability to swallow reflects CNs IX and X. In addition, note any facial paralysis or paresis (CN VII), absent gag reflex (CN IX), or impaired tongue movement (CN XII). The client who has difficulty chewing or swallowing foods and liquids is at risk for aspiration pneumonia and may become constipated from inadequate fluid intake.

CARDIOVASCULAR ASSESSMENT. Clients with embolic strokes may have a heart murmur, dysrhythmias, or hypertension. It is not unusual for the client to be admitted to the hospital with a blood pressure greater than 180-200/110-120 mm Hg. Although a somewhat higher blood pressure (150/100 mm Hg) is needed to maintain cerebral perfusion after a stroke, pressures above this limit may lead to another stroke.

PSYCHOSOCIAL ASSESSMENT

A typical client with a stroke is older than 60 years of age, is hypertensive, and has varying degrees of motor weakness and level of consciousness. Language and cognitive deficits,

as well as behavior and memory problems, may also occur. It is possible for stroke to occur at much younger ages.

Determine the client's reaction to the illness, especially in relation to changes in body image, self-concept, and ability to perform activities of daily living (ADLs). In collaboration with the client's family and friends, identify any difficulties in coping mechanisms or personality changes.

Determine the client's financial status and occupation because these aspects may be altered by the residual neurologic deficits of the stroke. Clients who do not have disability or health insurance may worry about how their family will cope financially with the disruption in their lives. Early involvement of social services or psychological counseling may enhance coping skills.

Assess for **emotional lability,** especially if the frontal lobe of the brain has been affected. In such cases, the client laughs and then cries unexpectedly for no apparent reason. It is important that the nurse explain these uncontrollable emotions to the family or significant others so they do not feel responsible for these reactions.

LABORATORY ASSESSMENT

Clinical history and presentation are usually sufficient to identify a stroke. No definitive laboratory tests confirm its diagnosis. Elevated hematocrit and hemoglobin levels are often associated with a severe or major stroke as the body attempts to compensate for lack of oxygen to the brain. An elevated white blood cell count may indicate the presence of an infection, possibly subacute bacterial endocarditis or a response to physiologic stress as well as inflammation. The health care provider typically orders a prothrombin time (PT) or International Normalized Ratio (INR) as well as a partial thromboplastin time (PTT) to establish baseline coagulation information in case anticoagulation therapy is initiated. These diagnostic tests may also provide supportive evidence that a hemorrhagic stroke has occurred. If there is no indication of increased intracranial pressure (ICP), a lumbar puncture may be performed to obtain cerebrospinal fluid (CSF) for analysis. Blood in the spinal fluid or a high red blood cell count in the CSF in all samples obtained is indicative of a subarachnoid hemorrhage.

RADIOGRAPHIC ASSESSMENT

Computed tomography (CT) and CT angiography (CTA) assist in the differential diagnosis of a stroke. The primary purpose of the initial scan is to identify the presence of cerebral hemorrhage. Cerebral aneurysms, if large enough, may be identified. For a client with an ischemic or occlusive stroke, the head CT is usually initially negative. After the first 24 hours, CT shows progressive changes of ischemia, infarction, and associated cerebral edema. This test is invaluable in establishing baseline information for future comparison in case the client's condition deteriorates. In addition, the scans enable the physician to identify pathologic changes that may mimic a stroke, such as a brain tumor or cerebral hematoma, both of which may be unrelated to cerebrovascular disease.

OTHER DIAGNOSTIC ASSESSMENTS

Magnetic resonance imaging (MRI) may show the presence of edema, ischemia, and tissue necrosis earlier than a CT scan. Information about the status of the cerebral vessels is

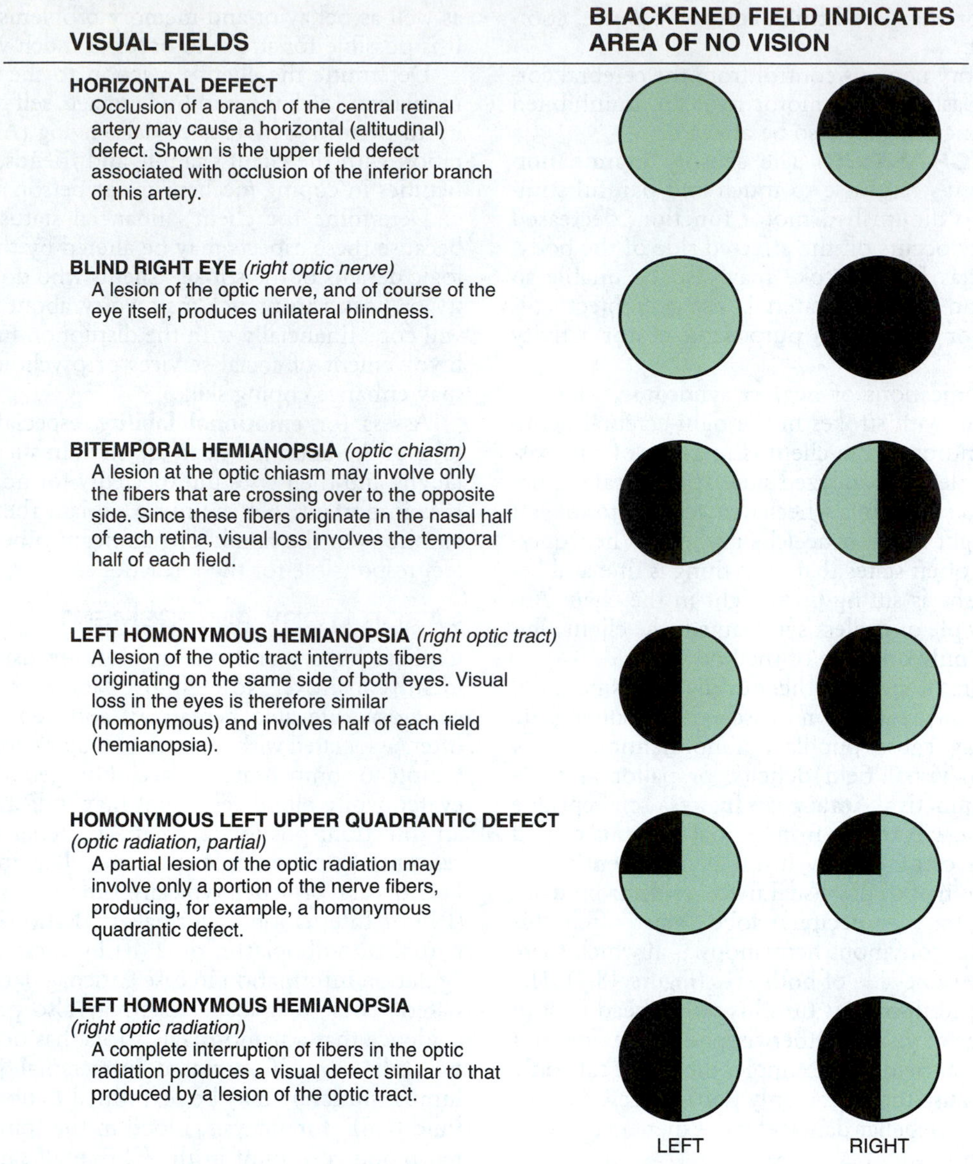

VISUAL FIELDS

**BLACKENED FIELD INDICATES
AREA OF NO VISION**

HORIZONTAL DEFECT
Occlusion of a branch of the central retinal artery may cause a horizontal (altitudinal) defect. Shown is the upper field defect associated with occlusion of the inferior branch of this artery.

BLIND RIGHT EYE *(right optic nerve)*
A lesion of the optic nerve, and of course of the eye itself, produces unilateral blindness.

BITEMPORAL HEMIANOPSIA *(optic chiasm)*
A lesion at the optic chiasm may involve only the fibers that are crossing over to the opposite side. Since these fibers originate in the nasal half of each retina, visual loss involves the temporal half of each field.

LEFT HOMONYMOUS HEMIANOPSIA *(right optic tract)*
A lesion of the optic tract interrupts fibers originating on the same side of both eyes. Visual loss in the eyes is therefore similar (homonymous) and involves half of each field (hemianopsia).

HOMONYMOUS LEFT UPPER QUADRANTIC DEFECT
(optic radiation, partial)
A partial lesion of the optic radiation may involve only a portion of the nerve fibers, producing, for example, a homonymous quadrantic defect.

LEFT HOMONYMOUS HEMIANOPSIA
(right optic radiation)
A complete interruption of fibers in the optic radiation produces a visual defect similar to that produced by a lesion of the optic tract.

LEFT   RIGHT

Figure 48-4 ■ Visual field defects produced by selected lesions in the visual pathways. (Modified from Bates, B. [2000]. Bates' guide to physical examination and history taking [7th ed.]. Philadelphia: J.B. Lippincott.)

obtained by angiography, digital subtraction angiography, diffusion/perfusion-weighted MRI, or magnetic resonance angiography (MRA). These studies reveal abnormal vessel structures (aneurysm location) or identify the area of vessel wall rupture and vasospasm. Following angiography, a narrowed vessel can be treated by catheter injection of papaverine or by using angioplasty techniques. Diffusion/perfusion MRI or MRA helps to locate areas that are underperfused but not yet infarcted. Single-photon emission computed tomography (SPECT) studies can also provide information on regional perfusion of blood flow in the brain.

To assist in the determination of a cardiac cause of a stroke, the health care provider may request an electrocardiogram (ECG), a Holter monitor test, cardiac enzymes evaluation, and an echocardiogram. As with other neurovascular diseases, it is not unusual to find the following changes on the ECG: inverted T wave, ST depression, and prolongation of the Q-T interval in the cardiac cycle.

?⃝ Critical Thinking Challenge
You have been floated from a medical unit to the emergency department (ED) for the night shift. Two clients present with possible stroke—a middle-aged black man and an older white woman. The man's history reveals that he is a construction worker who collapsed on the job. His wife states that he has been noncompliant with his antihypertensive medications and he "drinks too much." The female client has a history of diabetes mellitus type 2 and mild hypertension, but she has been very diligent in following her physician's treatment plan.
1. What other information would you want to obtain from these clients or their families or significant others?
2. What factors do you already know put these clients at risk for stroke?
3. What physical assessment should you perform at this time?
4. What diagnostic testing would you anticipate for these clients?

evolve For suggested answer guidelines, go to http://evolve.elsevier.com/Iggy/.

◆Analysis

COMMON NURSING DIAGNOSES AND COLLABORATIVE PROBLEMS

The following are the most common nursing diagnoses for clients with a stroke:

1. Ineffective Tissue Perfusion (Cerebral) related to interruption of arterial blood flow and a possible increase in ICP
2. Impaired Physical Mobility and Self-Care Deficit related to neuromuscular impairment or cognitive impairment
3. Disturbed Sensory Perception related to altered sensory reception, transmission, and integration
4. Unilateral Neglect related to effects of disturbed perceptual abilities or hemianopsia
5. Impaired Verbal Communication related to decreased circulation in the brain
6. Impaired Swallowing related to neuromuscular impairment
7. Total Urinary Incontinence and Bowel Incontinence related to neurologic dysfunction

ADDITIONAL NURSING DIAGNOSES AND COLLABORATIVE PROBLEMS

In addition to the common nursing diagnoses, clients with stroke may have one or more of the following:

- Risk for Aspiration related to impaired swallowing
- Disturbed Body Image related to biophysical or cognitive disability
- Ineffective Role Performance related to health alterations
- Risk for Falls related to visual difficulties, urgency or incontinence, decreased lower extremity strength, impaired balance, difficulty with gait, or proprioceptive deficits
- Sexual Dysfunction related to altered body function
- Constipation related to lack of adequate fluid intake or insufficient physical activity
- Imbalanced Nutrition: Less Than Body Requirements related to impaired swallowing

Additional collaborative problems include the following:

- Potential for Deep Vein Thrombosis or Pulmonary Embolism
- Potential for Increased Intracranial Pressure
- Potential for Seizures
- Potential for Hypoxemia
- Potential for Atelectasis and Pneumonia
- Potential for Hypercarbia

◆Planning and Implementation

INEFFECTIVE TISSUE PERFUSION (CEREBRAL)

NOC ◼ **PLANNING: EXPECTED OUTCOMES.** The client with a stroke is expected to have an adequate blood flow through the cerebral vasculature to maintain brain function. Indicators include that the following will be noncompromised in this client:

- Neurologic function
- Intracranial pressure
- Systolic blood pressure
- Diastolic blood pressure

CHART 48-5

KEY FEATURES of
Increased Intracranial Pressure

- Decreased level of consciousness (lethargy to coma)
- Behavior changes: restlessness, irritability, and confusion
- Headache
- Nausea and vomiting
- Change in speech pattern
- Aphasia
- Slurred speech
- Change in sensorimotor status
- Pupillary changes: dilated and nonreactive pupils ("blown pupils") or constricted and nonreactive pupils
- Cranial nerve dysfunction
- Ataxia
- Seizures
- Cushing's triad
- Abnormal posturing (see Chapter 44)
  - Decerebrate (extensor)
  - Decorticate (flexion)

INTERVENTIONS. Interventions are determined primarily by the type and extent of the stroke. For selected clients with ischemic strokes, early intervention with systemic thrombolytic therapy to dissolve the clot is indicated to address neurologic deficits if implemented within 3 hours of the onset of stroke.

Unless major medical complications occur, the health care provider manages the client conservatively with drug therapy and aggressive rehabilitation to promote an optimal level of well-being and function. In some cases, as with cerebral hemorrhage causing progressive damage, the physician may need to intervene surgically to prevent further neurologic dysfunction.

NONSURGICAL MANAGEMENT. Nursing interventions are initially aimed at monitoring for neurologic changes or complications associated with stroke. The client is at risk for continued progression of the stroke or increased intracranial pressure (ICP) (Chart 48-5). Perform a neurologic assessment when the client is admitted to the hospital and at intervals as indicated thereafter, including the beginning of each nursing shift. Periodic neurologic checks using the Glasgow Coma Scale (GCS) (see Chapter 44) or other neurologic assessment tools are indicated at least every 2 to 4 hours or more frequently, depending on the client's condition.

NIC **Intracranial Pressure Monitoring.** The client is most at risk for increased ICP resulting from edema during the first 72 hours after onset of the stroke (Chart 48-6). Be alert for symptoms of increased ICP, and report any deterioration in the client's neurologic status to the health care provider *immediately*. *The first sign of increased ICP is a declining level of consciousness (LOC).*

Current nursing practice for the care of clients with ischemic strokes is to elevate the head of the bed (HOB) to 30 degrees. However, evidence to support this practice is lacking. Wojner, El-Mitwalli, and Alexandrov (2002) found that lowering the HOB increases blood flow to the ischemic brain, which decreases further infarction (see the Evidence-Based Practice for Nursing box on p. 1038). The physician or clinical pathway may designate the desired HOB position. Maintain the head in a midline, neutral position to facilitate venous drainage from the brain.

In collaboration with other team members, plan care to avoid activities and procedures that may increase ICP,

NIC **INTERVENTION ACTIVITIES for**
The Client with a Stroke

Intracranial Pressure Monitoring: *Measurement and interpretation of client data to regulate intracranial pressure*

- Assist with ICP monitoring device insertion.
- Provide information to family/significant others.
- Calibrate and level the transducer.
- Set alarms.
- Record ICP pressure readings and analyze waveforms.
- Note client's change in response to stimuli.
- Monitor cerebral perfusion pressure.
- Monitor client's ICP and neurologic response to care activities.
- Monitor intake and output.
- Monitor insertion site for infection.
- Monitor temperature and WBC count.
- Administer pharmacologic agents to maintain ICP within specified range.
- Space nursing care to minimize ICP elevation.
- Notify health care provider of elevated ICP that does not respond to treatment protocols.

NIC intervention activities selected from Dochterman, J.M., & Bulechek, G.M. (Eds.). (2004). *Nursing interventions classification (NIC)* (4th ed.). St. Louis: Mosby. No part of this work is to be altered without prior written permission from the Publisher.
ICP, Intracranial pressure; *WBC,* white blood cell.

particularly if the client has focal neurologic deficits and indications of cerebral edema. Extreme hip and neck flexion should be avoided. Extreme hip flexion may increase intrathoracic pressure, which may make ICP more difficult to control. Extreme neck flexion interferes with venous drainage from the brain, also making ICP more difficult to control.

Additional nursing considerations include avoiding the clustering of nursing procedures (e.g., giving a bath followed immediately by changing the bed linen) within a short time. This is because the effect on ICP elevation is more dramatic when multiple activities are clustered within a narrow time interval. Hyperoxygenating the client before suctioning may also be appropriate to avoid even transient hypoxemia and resultant ICP elevation from dilation of cerebral arteries. Fully assess the need for suctioning because it may increase ICP. A quiet environment is particularly important for the client experiencing a headache, which is common with an aneurysm or increased ICP. The client may have **photophobia** (sensitivity to light); therefore the room lights should be kept low.

Monitor vital signs closely, at least every 4 hours. Notify the health care provider if the blood pressure exceeds acceptable levels. Generally, the health care provider allows the client to be slightly hypertensive (150/100 mm Hg) to facilitate adequate cerebral tissue perfusion. A higher blood pressure could lead to a hemorrhagic stroke or rebleeding of an aneurysm (if present).

Clients admitted to a critical care unit are connected to a cardiac monitor and observed for dysrhythmias. The critical care nurse performs a cardiac assessment, with particular attention directed toward auscultation of heart sounds to identify the presence of cardiac murmurs or atrial fibrillation (AF). Murmurs or AF may place the client at increased risk for emboli. Close physical assessment for indications of hemodynamic stability is indicated. Invasive hemodynamic monitoring may be needed to monitor and evaluate physiologic stability and response to therapy. (See also Chapter 37 for a discussion of AF.)

EVIDENCE-BASED PRACTICE for Nursing

Head elevation: A critical new look at traditional practice

Wojner, A.W., El-Mitwalli, A., & Alexandrov, A.V. Effect of head positioning on intracranial blood flow velocities in acute ischemic stroke: A pilot study. *Critical Care Nurse Quarterly*, 25(4), 57-66.

Evidence has been lacking regarding the current nursing practice of elevating the head of the bed (HOB) to 30 degrees following an acute ischemic stroke. The practice might be taken from studies of clients with traumatic brain injury. This small pilot study of 11 clients examined cerebral artery mean flow velocities (MCA-MFV) when the HOB was placed in various positions. On average, a 9.2% increase in MCA-MFV occurred when the HOB was lowered to 15 degrees from a 30-degree elevation. An additional increase of 3.9% resulted when the bed was lowered from 15 degrees to a flat position. The researchers concluded that the clients in the sample benefited from lowering the HOB because the total increase was 13.1% ($p = 0.054$).

Level of Evidence: 6—The study sample is small and not randomized, but it illustrates the need for further study and has questioned a traditional practice that has not been research based in the past.

Critique. No substantial research has been conducted that examined HOB positioning in clients immediately following an ischemic stroke. This study clearly demonstrated that in this small convenience sample whose average age was 60 years, there was an increase in cerebral blood flow that could possibly reduce additional infarction. The authors did not state the race or ethnic origin of the sample, so it is assumed that the sample population was white. Additional studies using larger numbers, varying ages, and an ethnically diverse group might help to validate these early findings.

Implications for Nursing. This study begins to provide an evidence base for changing practice in the positioning of clients after an acute ischemic stroke. Further study needs to be conducted to ensure that clients have optimal clinical outcomes.

Drug Therapy. The medications prescribed by the health care provider for a stroke depend on the type of stroke and the resulting neurologic dysfunction. In general, the goals of drug therapy are to prevent further thrombotic episodes (anticoagulation), increase blood flow, and protect the neurons (cytoprotection).

Thrombolytic Therapy. Intravenous (systemic) thrombolytic therapy for an acute ischemic stroke (AIS) dissolves the cerebral artery occlusion to re-establish blood flow and prevent cerebral infarction. Recombinant tissue plasminogen activator (rt-PA [Retavase]) was the first definitive drug with Food and Drug Administration (FDA) approval for the treatment of acute ischemic stroke. Thrombolytics activate plasminogen, which degrades the thrombus by breaking down fibrin. Fibrin breakdown results in the release of fibrin degradation products, such as D-dimers and other D-polymers (Goldszmidt & Caplan, 2003).

Clients must meet strict eligibility criteria for rt-PA administration. Contraindications to thrombolytic therapy include, but are not limited to, stroke or serious head injury in the past 3 months, hemorrhagic stroke, recent myocardial infarction (MI), increased partial thromboplastin time (PTT), anticoagulant therapy, or pregnancy. When considering thrombolytic therapy, the client should be quickly evaluated for any concurrent clinical state that might increase bleeding risk. Some health care facilities refer to an admission of a client having a stroke as a **Code Gray**

(Nolan, Naylor, & Burns, 2003). This label alerts the health care team of the importance of treating the client quickly.

For treatment of ischemic or occlusive stroke, the initial head CT should be negative. The presence of changes on head CT indicating progression of ischemia or infarction rules out systemic thrombolytic therapy because the time interval from symptom onset to medical evaluation exceeds 3 hours. The rt-PA should be given within 3 hours of the onset of symptoms. However, when the occlusion affects the basilar artery, thrombolysis may be effective even after 12 to 18 hours of ischemia (Goldszmidt & Caplan, 2003).

Catheter-directed thrombolytic therapy may be attempted if systemic therapy is not effective in improving the client's condition. As an option, catheter-directed therapy into an obstructed vessel may be initiated without attempting the systemic method based on agency protocols. This type of therapy should be prescribed within 6 hours of the ischemic event. Current lytic agents for this purpose include urokinase (Abbokinase), t-PA (alteplase), and rt-PA (Retavase). These agents may also be used with heparin and a platelet inhibitor such as abciximab (ReoPro).

Anticoagulants. The use of **anticoagulants** and **antiplatelet agents** to treat stroke is controversial and depends on the health care provider's preference. The principal drugs used are aspirin, heparin, low–molecular weight heparin (enoxaparin [Lovenox]), and warfarin (Coumadin). If the client received thrombolytic therapy, an IV anticoagulant is usually prescribed as a follow-up treatment.

The provider typically prescribes sodium heparin (Hepalean✽) subcutaneously or via a continuous IV infusion to prevent the progression of transient ischemic attacks (TIAs) or evolving strokes. This drug is also effective in prevention of deep vein thrombosis (DVT), a hazard of immobility. Baseline prothrombin time (PT) and partial thromboplastin time (PTT) values are usually obtained before initiating of heparin therapy, 6 to 8 hours after the start of the infusion, and every morning while the client is receiving heparin therapy. The therapeutic goal is to achieve 1.5 to 2 times the client's normal baseline PT and PTT values. PT is used to monitor oral anticoagulant therapy, whereas PTT is used to monitor heparin therapy. The World Health Organization advocates use of the International Normalized Ratio (INR) to monitor warfarin therapy. The target INR value for most clients with strokes is 2.0 to 3.0; for strokes of cardiac origin, the goal is usually 3.0 to 4.5.

Sodium heparin and other anticoagulants, such as warfarin (Coumadin, Warfilone✽), can cause bleeding. Observe for signs of blood in the urine or stool, epistaxis, bleeding gums, and easy bruising. Anticoagulant therapy is contraindicated in clients who have ulcers, uremia, or hepatic failure.

Enteric-coated or other forms of aspirin (Ecotrin, Ancasal✽) have proved useful primarily in the prevention of recurrent stroke or embolic stroke. These drugs prevent blood clotting by reducing platelet adhesiveness. Other commonly used **antiplatelet medications** include ticlopidine hydrochloride (Ticlid), clopidogrel (Plavix), and dipyridamole (Persantine, Apo-Dipyridamole✽). These agents can cause bruising, hemorrhage, and liver disease. Always teach the client to report any unusual bruising or bleeding to the health care provider. Liver function and coagulation studies are carefully monitored during the course of drug therapy. Clopidogrel should be taken with food to prevent gastric distress.

Other Drugs. To treat seizures, lorazepam (Ativan), a benzodiazepine, is administered with close neurologic and cardiorespiratory monitoring. For long-term anticonvulsant therapy, the health care provider may also prescribe antiepileptic drugs (AEDs), such as phenytoin (Dilantin), gabapentin (Neurontin), or topiramate (Topamax). Calcium channel blockers (e.g., nimodipine [Nimotop]) are used to treat or prevent cerebral vasospasm following a subarachnoid hemorrhage, which usually occurs between 4 and 14 days after the stroke, inhibits blood flow to the area, and worsens ischemia. These drugs work by relaxing the smooth muscles of the vessel wall and reducing the incidence and severity of the spasm. Neurologic functioning is improved and further deterioration from ischemia is prevented. In addition, calcium channel blockers possibly dilate collateral vessels to ischemic areas of the brain. Stool softeners, analgesics for pain, and antianxiety drugs may also be prescribed.

Monitoring for Other Complications. The client with an aneurysm or arteriovenous malformation (AVM) must be monitored for the presence of hydrocephalus and vasospasm. **Hydrocephalus** (increased CSF within the ventricular and subarachnoid spaces) may occur as a consequence of blood in the CSF, which prevents it from being reabsorbed properly by the arachnoid villi. It may also occur resulting from cerebral edema, interfering with flow of CSF out from the ventricular system. Eventually the ventricles become enlarged and, if hydrocephalus is left untreated, increased intracranial pressure (ICP) occurs. Observe for clinical manifestations of hydrocephalus, which mirror those of ICP elevation, including a change in the level of consciousness (LOC). Clinical findings may also include headache, alterations in pupils, seizures, poor coordination, gait disturbances (if ambulatory), and behavior changes.

Vasospasm, or a narrowing of the cerebral vessels in response to stimulus such as bleeding or irritation, leads to cerebral ischemia and infarction. Clinical manifestations may include decreased LOC, motor and reflex changes, and increased neurologic deficits (e.g., CN dysfunction, motor weakness and aphasia). The symptoms may fluctuate with the occurrence and degree of vasospasm present.

Rebleeding or rupture is a common complication for the client with an aneurysm or AVM. It may occur within 24 hours of the initial bleed or rupture and up to 7 to 10 days later. It is manifested by severe headache, nausea and vomiting, a decreased LOC, and additional neurologic deficits. Potential consequences of aneurysm rebleed may be catastrophic.

Carotid Artery Angioplasty. Although angioplasty was introduced in the mid-1980s, it was rarely used on the carotid arteries. However, with the development and refinement of vascular stents, carotid artery angioplasty has become more common. A device called a **distal protection device (DSP)** can make carotid angioplasty safer than endarterectomy. The DSP is placed beyond the stenosis, which catches any debris that breaks off during the angioplasty/stenting procedure. This interventional radiology procedure is done under moderate sedation and may eventually be performed as an outpatient procedure.

Other Nonsurgical Techniques. New early techniques are being tried for clients who are not candidates for thrombolytic therapy. For example, hypothermia treatment started during the first few hours after onset of a stroke may result in preservation of neurologic function in select clients. Techniques for cooling need further evaluation with well-structured research to identify optimal client selection criteria, target temperature, and duration of therapy. Cytoprotective drugs such as sodium channel blockers, opioid antagonists, free radical scavengers, magnesium, estrogens, gamma-aminobutyric acid (GABA) antagonists, glutamate receptor antagonists, calcium channel blockers, and membrane stabilizers are being tested as a therapy for stroke. A clot-dissolving substance in vampire bat saliva is also being tested and may be used to develop a new drug to treat occlusive strokes. No conclusive results have been demonstrated, and research is ongoing. Cell and tissue transplants are also being investigated for their potential benefit in replacing dead or damaged neurons and restoring otherwise lost brain function.

SURGICAL MANAGEMENT. Some clients are candidates for surgery to prevent or treat strokes. The surgical procedure depends on the cause of the stroke.

Endarterectomy. Carotid endarterectomy is the most widely used surgical procedure to prevent progressing stroke in symptomatic clients with recurrent TIAs or carotid stenosis. The purpose of a **carotid endarterectomy** is to remove atherosclerotic plaque from the inner lining of the carotid artery. The goal is to open the artery enough to re-establish blood flow and decrease stroke risk.

Extracranial-Intracranial Bypass. In an **extracranial-intracranial bypass**, the surgeon performs a craniotomy and bypasses the blocked artery by making a graft or a bypass from the first artery to the second artery. This procedure establishes blood flow around the blocked artery and re-establishes blood flow to the involved areas. The two most common techniques are the superficial middle temporal artery-to-middle cerebral artery (STA-MCA) graft and the occipital-to-posterior inferior cerebellar artery (PICA) bypass. Clinical trials have shown little or no differences in the effectiveness and benefit of this procedure in preventing stroke. Despite this finding, this procedure continues to be performed.

Management of Arteriovenous Malformations. The usual treatment of an arteriovenous malformation (AVM) is interventional therapy to occlude abnormal arteries or veins and prevent bleeding from the vascular lesion. The same procedure may be performed to occlude the vessels surrounding an aneurysm. Under fluoroscopic guidance, the physician inserts a microcatheter into the carotid artery, typically using a femoral artery approach, and threads it to the vessel to be embolized. The physician then injects an embolic agent, such as platinum coils, detachable silicone balloons, liquid acrylic, or polyvinyl alcohol, to embolize the involved arteries (Figure 48-5). If the AVM is large, the physician may elect to occlude the artery gradually to allow a gradual change in the blood supply to the surrounding brain. In this case, the embolization procedure is carried out over 1 to 2 weeks. Whenever possible, the involved vessels are totally removed surgically. The surgeon ligates the vessels and removes the defect. Gamma radiation delivered through the Gamma Knife produces fibrous thickening of the endothelial lining of the vessels to prevent further vessel enlargement and ultimately eliminated the lesion from the cerebral circulation. Improved microsurgical techniques have significantly reduced morbidity and mortality rates, and these procedures are becoming the treatment of choice in many medical centers.

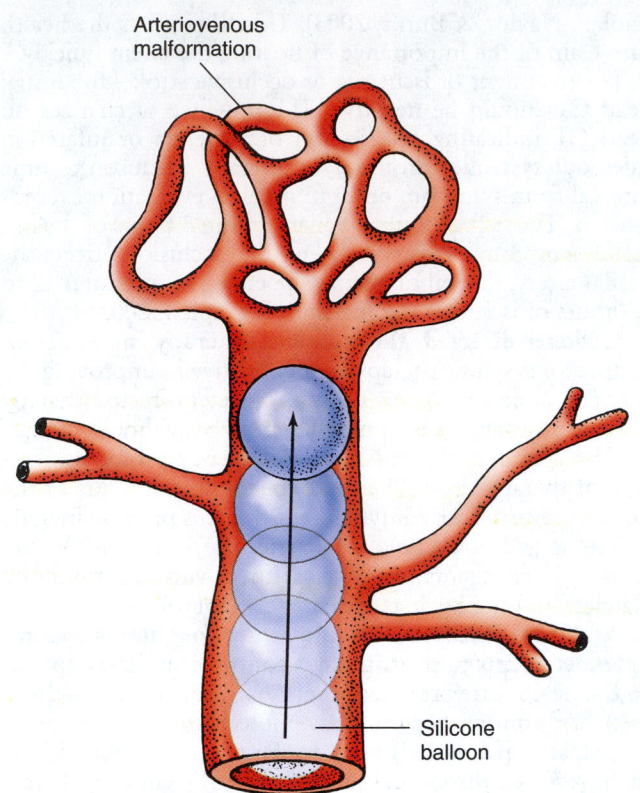

Figure 48-5 ■ Embolization procedure to treat an arteriovenous malformation. The embolic agent travels to the area to cause vessel thrombosis.

Management of Cerebral Aneurysms. Cerebral aneurysms may be repaired via a craniotomy as soon as the client's condition is stabilized. Surgery may be postponed for clients with ruptured aneurysms that caused stupor or coma because their condition makes them high-risk surgical candidates. During surgery, the aneurysm is clipped or a clamp is placed at the base, or neck, of the aneurysm to prevent blood from entering the area. If the aneurysm does not have a neck, it may be wrapped with muscle, muslin, or a plastic coating to reinforce the wall and prevent rebleeding. Timing of the surgery and specific interventions are usually determined by individual physician preferences. Visitors may be limited, and measures to decrease the client's stress and increase comfort are usually initiated.

A less invasive method for treating cerebral aneurysms is interventional radiology. An interventional neuroradiologist directs a small catheter into the femoral artery and advances the catheter into the aneurysm. Specially designed, detachable platinum wire coils are advanced into the aneurysm, which helps to seal the area with a clot. It is predicted that this method will soon treat most intracranial aneurysms, thus avoiding craniotomies and their complications.

Management of Intracranial Bleeding. For some clients who have hemorrhagic strokes, blood clots may be removed via a craniotomy to relieve intracranial pressure (ICP). Particular indications for clot removal would be a progressively worsening neurologic examination and extension of the intracranial lesion with significant ICP elevation. Craniotomies are discussed on p. 1053.

Critical Thinking Challenge

The two clients who presented in the ED with possible strokes have been diagnosed through history, physical examination, and diagnostic testing. The middle-aged man has a small intracerebral bleed and a current blood pressure of 210/120. The woman has a resolving transient ischemic attack (TIA) and a current blood pressure of 160/92. Both clients are being admitted to the hospital as soon as beds are available.

1. What do you suspect is the cause of the male client's intracerebral bleed?
2. The ED techs can take vital signs as part of their responsibility. Would you delegate that activity to a tech when caring for these clients? Why or why not?
3. Which client will be your priority for nursing care? Why?
4. The female client is placed on clopidogrel (Plavix) and is given her first dose while in the ED. Why did the physician prescribe this medication for her?

evolve For suggested answer guidelines, go to http://evolve.elsevier.com/Iggy/.

IMPAIRED PHYSICAL MOBILITY; SELF-CARE DEFICIT

NOC **PLANNING: EXPECTED OUTCOMES.** The client with a stroke is expected to be able to move purposefully in his or her own environment independently, with or without assistive device. Indicators include that the following will be noncompromised in this client:

- Balance and coordination
- Gait
- Transfer performance

The client is also expected to perform basic personal care activities and household tasks. Indicators include that the client will not be compromised in the following:

- Bathing self
- Dressing self
- Feeding self
- Maintaining personal cleanliness
- Toileting
- Performing household tasks

INTERVENTIONS. Clients who have experienced a stroke may exhibit flaccid or spastic paralysis. It is not unusual for the client to have a spastic arm and flaccid leg on the affected side. The affected leg often regains function more quickly than the arm. The nurse or family member performs passive range-of-motion (ROM) exercises at least every 2 to 3 hours for the involved extremities. The client is taught how to do active ROM exercises for the unaffected side. When able, he or she may perform passive exercises on the affected side. Physical therapy consultation should be initiated on admission, and intervention should continue through discharge.

Careful positioning is necessary to maintain proper body alignment and decrease spasticity or increase muscle tone in flaccid extremities. The affected hand or lower leg may need splinting to prevent contractures. Collaborate with the physical and occupational therapists (PT/OT) to determine the most appropriate splinting technique and client positions when lying, sitting, and transferring from the bed to a chair.

A major complication of impaired physical mobility is the development of deep vein thrombosis (DVT). Provide care to prevent this complication by applying sequential compression stockings or pneumatic compression boots, changing the client's position frequently, and mobilizing the client. Always report any indications of DVT to the health care provider, and document your assessment in the client's chart.

The rehabilitation therapists also evaluate the client in the ability to perform basic activities of daily living (ADLs) and household tasks that will be performed on discharge to home. After a thorough evaluation, the PT and OT develop a treatment plan to promote client independence, with or without assistive or adaptive devices. Therapy begins in the hospital setting and continues after discharge in most cases.

DISTURBED SENSORY PERCEPTION

PLANNING: EXPECTED OUTCOMES. The major concern of clients with sensory or perceptual changes is adapting to the deficits. Therefore the client with stroke is expected to adapt to sensory or perceptual changes in vision, proprioception (position sense), and sensation and to be free from injury.

INTERVENTIONS. Clients with right hemisphere brain damage typically have difficulty with visual-perceptual or spatial-perceptual tasks. They have problems with depth and distance perception and with discrimination of right from left or up from down. Because of these problems, they have difficulty performing routine activities of daily living (ADLs). Caregivers help the client adapt to these disabilities by using frequent verbal and tactile cues and by breaking down tasks into discrete steps. Always approach the client from the unaffected side, which should face the door of the room.

The client who has experienced a stroke may have difficulties with ambulating, lack depth perception, and proprioception. Objects should be placed within the client's field of vision; a mirror may help in visualizing more of the environment. If the client has diplopia (double vision), a patch may be placed over the affected eye. Ensure a safe environment by removing clutter from the room.

The client with a left hemisphere lesion generally experiences memory deficits and may show significant changes in the ability to carry out simple tasks. To assist with memory problems, reorient the client to the month, year, day of the week, and circumstances surrounding hospital admission. Establish a routine or schedule that is as structured, repetitious, and consistent as possible. Information is presented in a simple, concise manner. A step-by-step approach is often most effective because the client can master one step before moving to the next. When possible, the family or significant other should bring in pictures and other familiar objects.

The client may be unable to plan and execute tasks in an organized manner. Apraxia, or the inability to perform previously learned motor skills or commands, may be present. Typically, the client with apraxia exhibits a slow, cautious, and hesitant behavior style. Physical therapy involvement will assist the client in compensating for loss of position sense.

UNILATERAL NEGLECT

PLANNING: EXPECTED OUTCOMES. The client with stroke is expected to adjust and use techniques to compensate for one-sided neglect.

INTERVENTIONS. Unilateral neglect, or neglect syndrome, occurs most commonly in clients who have had a right cerebral stroke. However, it can occur in any client who experiences hemianopsia, in which the vision of one or both eyes is affected. This problem places the client at additional risk for injury because of an inability to recognize his or her physical impairment or because of a lack of proprioception.

Teach the client to touch and use both sides of the body. For example, encourage the client to wash both the affected and unaffected sides of the body. When dressing, remind the client to dress the affected side first. If hemianopsia is present, teach the client to turn his or her head from side to side to expand the visual field. This scanning technique is also useful when the client is eating or ambulating.

IMPAIRED VERBAL COMMUNICATION

NOC **PLANNING: EXPECTED OUTCOMES.** Ideally, the client with a stroke is expected to receive, interpret, and express spoken, written, and nonverbal messages. However, some clients may need to develop strategies for alternative methods of communication, such as pictures or nonverbal language.

INTERVENTIONS. Language or speech problems are usually the result of a stroke involving the dominant hemisphere. The left cerebral hemisphere is the speech center in all but 15% to 20% of the population. Speech and language problems may be the result of aphasia or dysarthria. Although aphasia is caused by cerebral hemisphere damage, **dysarthria** is due to a loss of motor function to the tongue or to the muscles of speech, causing slurred speech. Involvement of the speech-language pathologist as early as possible in the hospitalization will maximize the client's chances for optimal recovery.

Aphasia can be classified in a number of ways. Most commonly, aphasia is classified as expressive, receptive, or global (mixed) (Table 48-2). **Expressive (Broca's, or motor) aphasia** is the result of damage in Broca's area of the frontal lobe. It is a motor speech problem in which the client generally understands what is said but is unable to communicate verbally. He or she also has difficulty writing. Rote speech and automatic speech, such as responses to a greeting, are often intact. The client is aware of the deficit and may become frustrated and angry.

Receptive (Wernicke's, or sensory) aphasia is due to injury involving Wernicke's area in the temporoparietal area. The client is unable to understand the spoken and often the written word. Although he or she may be able to talk, the language is often meaningless. Neologisms (made-up words) are common parts of speech.

More often, the client exhibits dysfunction in both the areas of expression and reception; this is known as a global, or mixed, aphasia. Reading and writing ability are equally affected. Few clients exhibit either expressive *or* receptive aphasia. In most cases, one type is dominant but two or more types are present.

Collaborate with the speech-language pathologist (SLP) in working with the client who has aphasia or dysarthria. The aphasic client requires repetitive directions to understand or complete a task. Each task should be broken down into component parts and given one step at a time. Face the client and speak slowly and clearly. The client should be given sufficient time to understand and process the information and to respond. Encourage the client to communicate and reinforce this behavior positively.

Family members or significant others and staff repeat the names of objects used on a routine basis. For example, state,

---

TABLE 48-2   Types of Aphasia

Expressive
- Referred to as Broca's, or motor, aphasia
- Difficulty speaking
- Difficulty writing

Receptive
- Referred to as Wernicke's, or sensory, aphasia
- Difficulty understanding spoken words
- Difficulty understanding written words
- Speech often meaningless
- Neologisms

Global (Mixed)
- Combination of difficulty understanding words and speech
- Difficulty with reading and writing

"This is the toothbrush" when assisting the client to brush his or her teeth. If necessary, a picture board or communication board should be developed by the SLP for the client with Broca's aphasia. This board consists of a picture of an activity (e.g., someone eating) and the printed description below. The client can point to the activity or object desired.

It is difficult to understand a client with dysarthria. The same techniques used for the client with aphasia can be used for dysarthria. Facial muscle exercises may be performed to strengthen the muscles used for speech. Many clients who are dysarthric are also aphasic.

IMPAIRED SWALLOWING

NOC **PLANNING: EXPECTED OUTCOMES.** The client with a stroke is expected to have safe passage of fluids and solids from the mouth to the stomach. Indicators include that the client will have noncompromised ability to do the following:
- Maintain food in the mouth
- Handle oral secretions
- Chew
- Deliver bolus to hypopharynx in time with swallow reflex
- Clear oral cavity

INTERVENTIONS. Before feeding, assess the client's ability to swallow. Observe for facial drooping, drooling, and a weak, hoarse voice. To assess the swallowing reflex, place the thumb and the index finger on either side of the client's Adam's apple, or laryngeal protuberance, and ask him or her to swallow. You should be able to feel the larynx elevate. Next check the gag and cough reflex. Collaborate with the SLP, who specializes in swallowing evaluation, to determine the extent of the swallowing problem. In some cases, the health care provider may order a barium swallow to detect the specific cause of the swallowing problem.

Positioning the client to facilitate the swallowing process is extremely important. He or she should eat all meals sitting in a chair or sitting straight up in bed. The head and neck are positioned slightly forward and flexed. In general, clients with swallowing problems are able to tolerate or swallow soft or semisoft foods and fluids (mechanically soft or dental diet, junior baby foods, custards, scrambled eggs) better than thin liquids (water, juice, or milk) or a regular meal. Powdered thickener (Thick-It) may be added to thicken foods to a more manageable consistency.

Collaborate with the dietitian to find an appropriate diet for the client with dysphagia. Monitor the client's weight at least twice a week to ensure that he or she is receiving adequate nutrition. Supplements such as milkshakes and Ensure may be needed to meet caloric and protein requirements. Calorie counts may be necessary to evaluate nutritional intake fully.

Foods that stimulate saliva production and thus facilitate swallowing include beef broth and sweet, sour, or salty foods. Instruct the client to place food in the back of the mouth on the unaffected side to prevent trapping food in the affected cheek.

Some clients are able to swallow without difficulty but are at risk for aspiration because they are easily distracted and impulsive. These clients require a distraction-free environment with minimal disruption from television, visitors, or environmental noise. Observe for indications of fatigue because this can significantly interfere with the desire and ability to eat.

TOTAL URINARY INCONTINENCE; BOWEL INCONTINENCE

NOC **PLANNING: EXPECTED OUTCOMES.** The client with a stroke is expected to control elimination of urine and stool. Indicators include that the client will consistently demonstrate the ability to do the following:
- Recognize the urge to void and defecate
- Maintain predictable pattern of urinary and bowel elimination
- Respond to urge in timely manner
- Get to toilet between urge and passage of urine or stool
- Empty bladder and bowel completely

INTERVENTIONS. The client may be incontinent of urine and stool because of an altered level of consciousness, impaired innervation, or an inability to communicate the need to urinate or defecate. Before beginning an education program to correct these problems, the cause must first be established. Typically, the client who has had a stroke can relearn both bowel and bladder control. To begin a bladder training program, place the client on the bedpan or the commode or offer the urinal every 2 hours. Encourage a total fluid intake of at least 2000 mL daily unless contraindicated. Catheterizations to check for residual urine after voiding (postvoiding residuals) may be done in the early part of the bladder retraining program to ensure that the client is emptying the bladder. A bedside ultrasound can also be used for this purpose and is less invasive. Retained urine can lead to a urinary tract infection.

Before establishing a bowel training program, determine the client's normal time for bowel elimination and any routine that helps to ensure an acceptable evacuation. This routine is followed, if possible, and the client is placed on the bedpan or commode at the same time as the previous schedule at home. Collaborate with the dietitian to provide a diet high in bulk and fiber. Encourage the client to drink apple or prune juice to help promote bowel elimination. A stool softener (Colace) may be prescribed. Suppositories or digital stimulation may also assist in re-establishing a bowel routine. Chapter 10 provides a complete discussion of bowel and bladder training programs.

Community-Based Care

The client with a stroke without complications may be discharged within 2 to 3 days to home, a rehabilitation center, or a long-term care facility, depending on the extent of the disability and the availability of family or caregiver support. Some clients experience no significant neurologic dysfunc-

tion and are able to return home and live independently or with minimal support. Other clients are able to return home but require ongoing assistance with activities of daily living as well as supervision to prevent accidents or injury. Speech, physical, or occupational therapy may continue in the home or on an ambulatory care basis. Clients admitted to a rehabilitation or long-term care facility require continued or more complex nursing care as well as extensive physical, occupational, recreational, speech-language, or cognitive therapy, which is coordinated by a case manager. The goal of rehabilitation is to maximize the client's abilities in all aspects of life.

HOME CARE MANAGEMENT

Collaboration with the case manager is needed if the client is discharged to the home setting. Needs for assistive or adaptive and safety equipment must be identified. The extent of this assessment depends on the disabilities experienced by the client. The home of the client with hemiparesis should be free from scatter rugs or other obstacles in the walking pathways. The bathtub and toilet should be equipped with grab bars. Anti-skid patches or strips should be placed in the bathtub to prevent slipping. The PT or OT works with the client and the family or significant others to obtain all needed assistive devices *before* the client is discharged from the hospital, rehabilitation setting, or long-term care facility. Appointments for outpatient speech, physical, and occupational therapy must also be arranged before discharge. Involvement of the case manager and utilization of critical pathways have been shown to be very effective in facilitating optimal timing of diagnostic testing, consultations with SLT and physical therapy, as well as facilitating discharge to home or rehabilitation.

HEALTH TEACHING

The teaching plan for the client with a stroke includes the medication schedule, ambulation/transfer skills, communication skills, safety precautions, dietary management, activity levels, and self-care skills. Health teaching should focus on tasks that must be performed by the client and the family after hospital discharge. Provide both written and verbal instruction in all these areas. Return demonstrations assist in evaluating the family members' competency in tasks required for the client's care.

The client must take the prescribed medication to prevent another stroke and to keep hypertension under control. Teach the client and the family the name of the drug, the dosage, the timing of administration and how to take it, and possible side effects. In collaboration with the PT and OT, teach the client how to climb stairs safely, if he or she is able; transfer from the bed to a chair; get into and out of a car; and use any aids for mobility. The client and family members are also taught how to use any equipment needed to increase independence in self-care skills. The most important information provided is what to do in an emergency and whom to call for nonemergency questions.

It is not unusual for clients, particularly older white men, to become depressed within 6 months after discharge. In general, this depression is self-limiting, but the client may require antidepressants for a short time. Emotional lability is also common. The family is advised to avoid being overprotective and is assisted in establishing realistic and achievable goals.

Families may feel overwhelmed by the continuing demands placed on them. Depending on the location of the lesion, the client may be anxious, slow, cautious, hesitant, and lack initiative (left hemisphere lesions), or he or she may be impulsive and seemingly unaware of any deficit. Family members and other caregivers need to spend time away from the client on a routine basis to continue to provide full-time care without sacrificing their own physical and emotional health. Refer the family to social services for further support and counseling.

HEALTH CARE RESOURCES

Available resources include a variety of publications from the American Heart Association, including *Stroke: A Guide for Families* and *Stroke: Why Do They Behave That Way?* The National Stroke Association also provides publications and videotapes for caregivers and clients. *Recovering After a Stroke: A Patient and Family Guide* is available from the Agency for Healthcare Research and Quality (http://www.ahrq.gov), formerly the Agency for Health Care Policy and Research. Refer the client and family members or significant others to local stroke support groups.

◆ Evaluation: Outcomes

Evaluate the care of the client with stroke on the basis of the identified nursing diagnoses and collaborative problems. The expected outcomes are that the client:

- Has an adequate blood flow through the cerebral vasculature to maintain brain function
- Moves purposefully in his or her own environment with or without assistive devices
- Learns to adapt to sensory and perceptual changes
- Adjusts and uses techniques to compensate for one-sided neglect
- Receives, interprets, and expresses messages or develops strategies for alternative communication methods
- Has safe passage of fluids and solids from the mouth to the stomach
- Controls elimination of urine and stool

Specific indicators for these outcomes are listed for each nursing diagnosis under the Planning and Implementation section (see earlier).

TRAUMATIC BRAIN INJURY

Traumatic brain injury (TBI) occurs as a result of an external force applied to the head and brain causing disruption of physiologic stability locally, at the point of injury, as well as globally with elevations in ICP and potentially dramatic changes in blood flow within and to the brain. These changes may produce a diminished or altered state of consciousness. TBI may result in the impairment of cognitive abilities or physical functioning as well as a disturbance of behavior or emotional functioning. These impairments may be either temporary or permanent and may cause partial or total functional disability or psychosocial maladjustment. In the United States, TBI has taken more lives of people 18 to 34 years of age than all other causes combined for that age group. The annual cost of care for TBI survivors in the United States is higher than that for stroke survivors.

PATHOPHYSIOLOGY

Various terms are used to describe the brain injuries that occur when a mechanical force is applied either directly or indirectly to the brain. A force produced by a blow to the head is a direct injury, whereas a force applied to another body part with a rebound effect to the brain is an indirect injury. The brain responds to these forces by movement within the rigid cranial vault. The brain may also rebound or rotate on the brainstem, causing diffuse axonal injury (shearing injuries). The moving brain may be contused or lacerated as it moves over the inner surfaces of the cranium, which is irregularly shaped and sharp. Damage most commonly occurs to the frontal and temporal lobes of the brain, especially the raised surfaces of the gyri. Movement or distortion of the brain within the cranial cavity is possible due to multiple factors. The first factor is how the brain is supported. The brain is supported by cerebrospinal fluid (CSF) within the cranial cavity. As such, when external force is applied to the head, the brain can be injured by the internal surfaces of the skull and meninges. The second factor is the consistency of brain tissue. It is exceedingly fragile and prone to injury.

Primary Brain Injury

Primary brain damage results from the physical stress (force) within the brain tissue caused by open or closed trauma. An **open head injury** occurs when there is a skull fracture or when the skull is pierced by a penetrating object. The integrity of the brain and the dura is violated, and there is exposure to outside, or environmental, contaminants. Damage may occur to the underlying vessels, dural sinus, brain, and cranial nerves. A **closed head injury** is the result of blunt trauma; the integrity of the skull is not violated. It is the more serious of the two types of injury, and the damage to brain tissue depends on the degree and mechanisms of injury.

Brain injury may also be described as mild, moderate, or severe. A Glasgow Coma Scale (GCS) score of 13 to 15 and a loss of consciousness for 0 to 15 minutes characterize a mild TBI (MTBI). A moderate TBI often includes a period of loss of consciousness (LOC) up to 6 hours and may be accompanied by other systemic injury and a GCS score of 9 to 12. A short critical care stay maybe needed for close monitoring. After injury, these clients may have difficulty with work, learning, and role function. Severe head injury (GCS score of 3 to 8 and LOC greater than 6 hours) is more serious and requires management in critical care with ongoing monitoring of multiple physiologic parameters, including hemodynamic stability and intracranial pressure (ICP).

OPEN HEAD INJURY

The types of fractures associated with an open head injury are linear, depressed, open, and comminuted. A **linear fracture** is a simple, clean break in which the impacted area of bone bends inward and the area around it bends outward; linear fractures account for about 80% of all skull fractures. In a **depressed fracture,** the bone is pressed inward into the brain tissue to at least the thickness of the skull. In an **open fracture,** the scalp is lacerated, creating a direct opening to the brain tissue. A **comminuted fracture** involves fragmentation of the bone with depression of bone into the brain tissue.

A unique fracture is a basilar skull fracture. It occurs at the base of the skull, usually extending into the anterior, middle, or posterior fossa and results in cerebrospinal fluid (CSF) leakage from the nose or ears. Of significance with this fracture is the potential development of hemorrhage caused by damage to the internal carotid artery; damage to cranial nerves (CN) I, II, VII, and VIII; and infection.

Most penetrating injuries to the skull are caused by gunshot wounds (GSWs) and knife injuries. The degree of injury to brain tissue depends on the velocity, mass, shape, and direction of impact. High-velocity injuries produce the greatest damage to brain tissue. As with any open head injury, the client with a penetrating injury is at high risk for infection from the object that pierced the skull and from other environmental contaminants.

CLOSED HEAD INJURY

Closed head injuries are caused by blunt trauma and lead to concussions, contusions, and lacerations of the brain. The damage to the brain may be mild, as occurs in a concussive injury, or it may be more severe, causing diffuse axonal injury or widespread injury to the white matter of the brain.

A **mild concussion** is characterized by a brief LOC. Possibly as many as 30% of these clients experience "post-concussion" syndrome (PCS). The mechanism of injury is typically acceleration/deceleration with shearing stress on the reticular formation. PCS symptoms may include headache, irritability, memory deficits, fatigue and sleep disturbances, and depression (Mateo, 2003). Severity of concussion is measured by duration of unconsciousness.

Diffuse axonal injury (DAI) is usually related to high-speed acceleration/deceleration as with automobile accidents. In DAI significant damage occurs to axons in the white matter. Lesions may also be found in the corpus callosum, midbrain, cerebellum, and upper brainstem. Depending on severity, small areas of hemorrhage may be found on computed tomography (CT) scanning followed by possible enlargement of the lateral ventricles. Severe DAI may present with immediate coma, and most survivors require long-term care.

A **contusion** is a bruising of the brain tissue and is most commonly found at the site of impact (coup injury) or in a line opposite the site of impact (**contrecoup injury**) (Figure 48-6). The base of the frontal and temporal lobes is most often involved.

A **laceration** causes actual tearing of the cortical surface vessels, which may lead to secondary hemorrhage and significant cerebral edema and inflammation. This condition is more serious than a contusion.

Types of Force

Other factors that must be considered in the dynamics of head injury are the type of force and the mechanisms of injury involved (Figure 48-7). An **acceleration injury** is caused by an external force contacting the head, suddenly placing the head in motion. A **deceleration injury** occurs when the moving head is suddenly stopped or hits a stationary object. These forces may be sufficient to cause the cerebrum to rotate about the brainstem, resulting in shearing, straining, and distortion of the brain tissue, particularly of the axons in the brainstem and cerebellum. Small areas of hemorrhage may develop around the blood vessels that sustain the impact of these forces (stress), with destruction of adjacent brain tissue. Particularly affected are the basal nuclei and the hypothalamus.

Secondary Responses and Insults

Secondary responses to brain injury include any neurologic damage that occurs after the initial injury. Secondary injuries or responses increase the morbidity and mortality af-

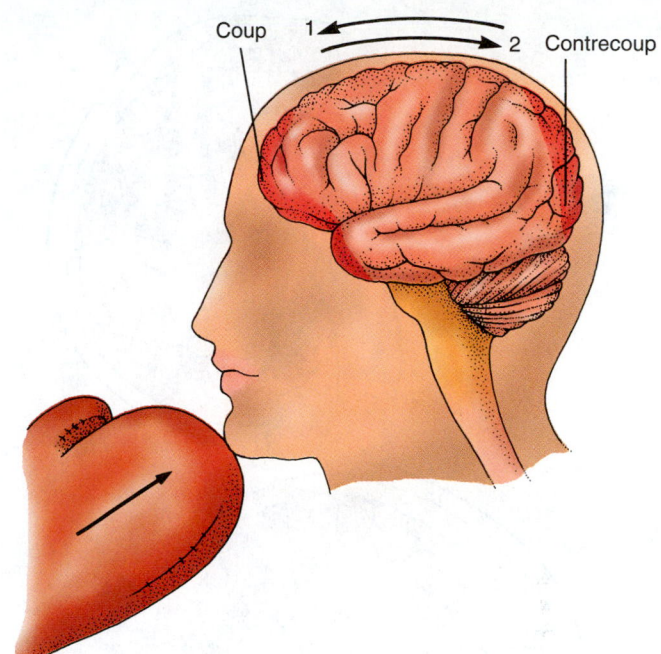

Figure 48-6 ■ Coup (site of impact) injury to frontal area of brain, and contrecoup injury to frontal and temporal areas of the brain.

ter head trauma. The most common response is the development of increased intracranial pressure (ICP) attributable to edema, hemorrhage, hematoma development, impaired cerebral autoregulation, or hydrocephalus. Hypoxemia, hypercapnia (increased carbon dioxide), or systemic hypotension may precipitate increased ICP. Damage to the brain tissue occurs primarily because the delivery of oxygen and glucose to the brain is interrupted.

INCREASED INTRACRANIAL PRESSURE

The cranial contents include brain tissue, blood, and cerebrospinal fluid (CSF). These components are encased in the relatively rigid skull. Within this space, there is little room for any of the components to expand or increase in volume. Through the processes of accommodation and compliance, ICP is maintained at its normal level of 10 to 15 mm Hg despite transient increases in pressure that occur with straining during defecation, coughing, or sneezing. According to the Monro-Kellie hypothesis, any increase in the volume of one component must be compensated for by a decrease in the volume of one of the other components.

As a first response to an increase in the volume of any of these components, the CSF is shunted or displaced from the cranial compartment to the spinal subarachnoid space or the rate of CSF absorption is increased. An additional response, if needed, is a decrease in cerebral blood volume by displacement of cerebral venous blood into the sinuses. As long as the brain is able to compensate for the increase in volume and remain compliant, increases in ICP are minimal.

Increased ICP is the leading cause of death from head trauma in clients who reach the hospital alive. It occurs when compliance no longer takes place and the brain cannot accommodate further volume changes. As ICP increases, cerebral perfusion decreases, leading to tissue hypoxia, a decrease in serum pH level, and an increase in the level of carbon dioxide. This process causes cerebral vasodilation, edema, and a

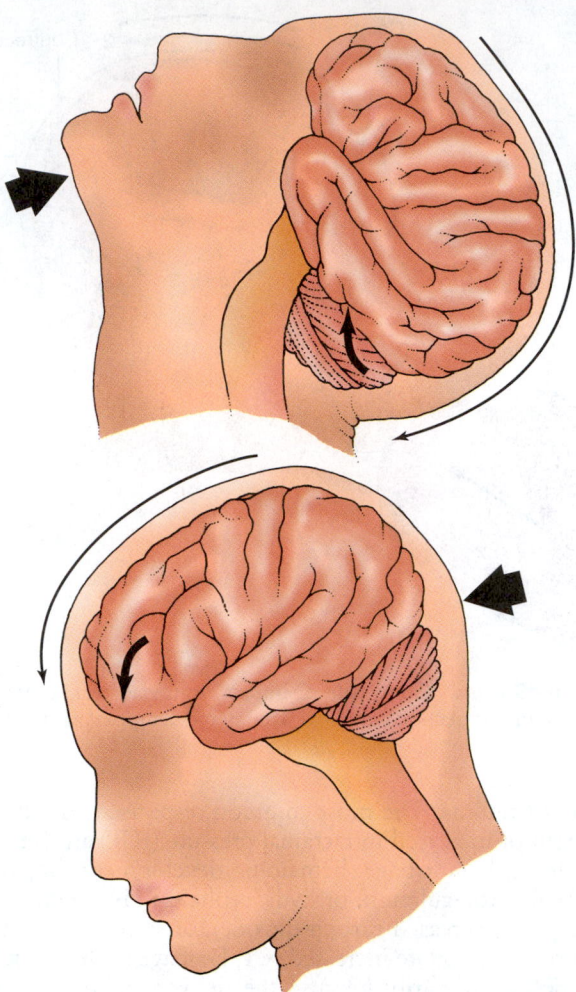

Figure 48-7 ■ Head movement during acceleration-deceleration injury, which is typically seen in motor vehicle accidents.

further increase in ICP, and the cycle continues. If the condition remains untreated, the brain may herniate downward toward the brainstem or laterally from a unilateral lesion within one cerebral hemisphere, causing irreversible brain damage and possibly death (**brain herniation syndromes**).

Two types of edema may cause increased ICP: vasogenic edema and cytotoxic edema. A third type (interstitial edema) occurs in the presence of acute brain swelling. Vasogenic edema is seen most often as a cause of increased ICP in the adult. It is characterized by an increase in the volume of brain tissue. This increase is caused by an abnormal permeability of the walls of the cerebral vessels, which allows protein-rich plasma infiltrate to leak into the extracellular space of the brain. The fluid collects primarily in the white matter.

Cytotoxic, or cellular, edema may occur as a result of a hypoxic insult, which causes a disturbance in cellular metabolism, the sodium pump, and active ion transport. The brain is quickly depleted of available oxygen, glucose, and glycogen and converts to anaerobic metabolism. The sodium pump fails, and sodium enters the cells and pulls water from the extracellular space. A concomitant decrease occurs in the serum sodium level to less than 120 mEq/L. As a result, an abnormal accumulation of fluid in the brain cells and a decrease in the extracellular fluid space occur. Cytotoxic edema may lead to vasogenic edema and a further increase in ICP.

Interstitial edema occurs in the presence of acute brain swelling and is associated with elevated blood pressure or increased CSF pressure. Edema develops rapidly in the perivascular and periventricular white space and can be controlled through measures to reduce blood pressure, decrease CSF pressures, or increase the **cerebral perfusion pressure (CPP)**. The CPP is the pressure gradient over which the brain is perfused. It is influenced by oxygenation, cerebral blood volume, blood pressure, cerebral edema, and ICP and is determined by subtracting the mean ICP from the mean arterial pressure. Maintenance of a CPP above 70 mm Hg is generally accepted as an appropriate goal of therapy.

HEMORRHAGE

Hemorrhages, which cause brain hematoma or clot formation, may occur as part of the primary injury and begin at the moment of impact. They may also be a secondary event arising from vessel damage and occur somewhat later or worsen later in the client's clinical course. Classically they are caused by vascular damage from the shearing force of the trauma or direct physical damage from skull fractures or penetrating injury. All hematomas are potentially life threatening because they act as space-occupying lesions and are surrounded by edema. Three types of hemorrhages include **epidural, subdural, and intracerebral hemorrhage**. Subarachnoid hemorrhage may also occur following head trauma. The pathophysiology of subarachnoid hemorrhage is discussed under Stroke earlier in this chapter.

EPIDURAL HEMATOMA. An **epidural hematoma** results from arterial bleeding into the space between the dura and the inner table of the skull (Figure 48-8). It is often caused by a fracture of the temporal bone, which houses the middle meningeal artery. Epidural hematomas may be characterized by the presence of a "lucid interval" that lasts for minutes, during which time the client is awake and talking. This follows a momentary unconsciousness that occurred within minutes of the injury. Following the initial lucid interval, symptoms progress very quickly with potentially catastrophic ICP elevation and structural changes. The client becomes increasingly symptomatic, loses consciousness, and may become increasingly unstable. An epidural hematoma is a neurosurgical emergency.

SUBDURAL HEMATOMA. A **subdural hematoma (SDH)** results typically from venous bleeding into the space beneath the dura and above the arachnoid (see Figure 48-8). It results most often from a tearing of the bridging veins within the cerebral hemispheres or from a laceration of brain tissue. Bleeding from this injury occurs more slowly than from an epidural hematoma and mirrors the slower development of symptoms. SDHs are subdivided into acute, subacute, and chronic. An acute SDH presents within 48 hours after impact; the subacute SDH, between 48 hours and 2 weeks; and the chronic SDH, from 2 weeks to several months following injury. SDHs have the highest mortality rate.

INTRACEREBRAL HEMORRHAGE. An intracerebral hemorrhage (ICH) is the accumulation of blood within the brain tissue caused by the tearing of small arteries and veins in the subcortical white matter (see Figure 48-8). ICH may act as a space-occupying lesion and may be potentially devastating, depending on its location. ICH may also produce significant brain edema and ICP elevations. A brainstem hemorrhage occurs as a result of direct trauma, fractures, or torsion injuries to the brainstem.

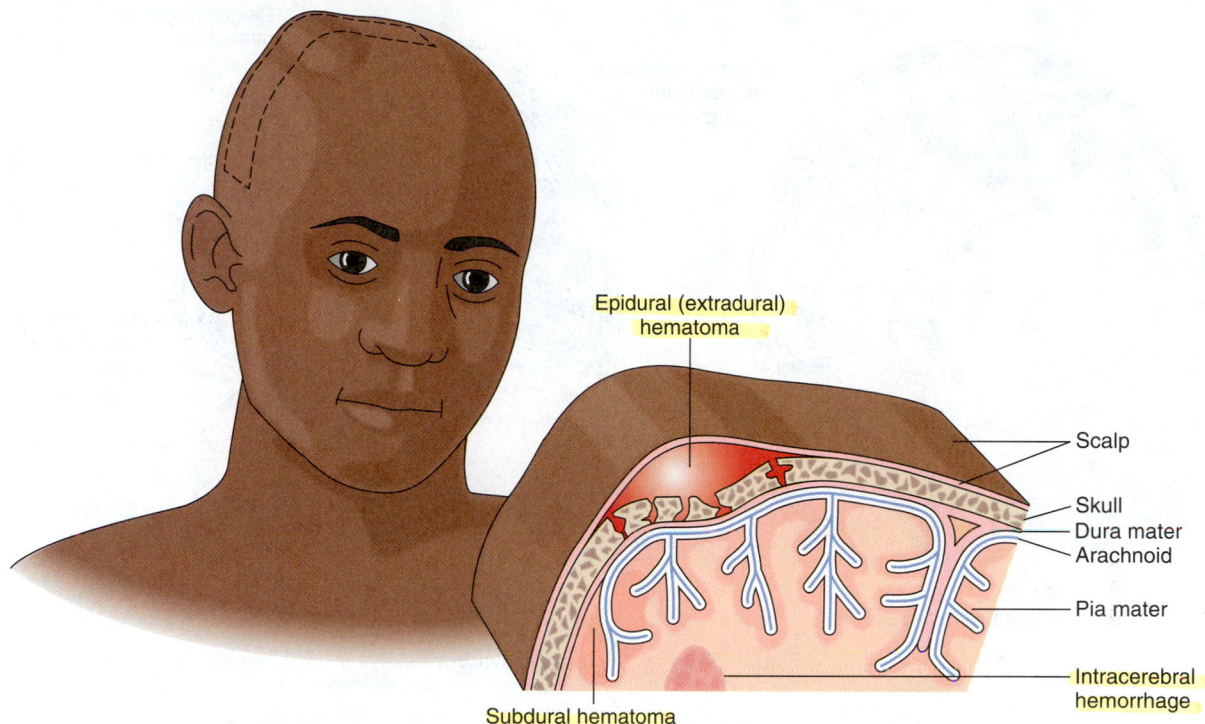

Figure 48-8 ■ Epidural hematoma (outside the dura mater of the brain), subdural hematoma (under the dura mater), and intracerebral hemorrhage (within the brain tissue).

LOSS OF AUTOREGULATION

Through the process of cerebral autoregulation, blood flow to the brain remains relatively constant despite variations in systemic blood pressure. A loss of autoregulation causes the cerebral blood flow to fluctuate passively with the systemic blood pressure. Systemic hypertension may cause an increase in ICP (from an increase in cerebral blood flow) and the potential for vasogenic edema. Hypoxemia and hypercapnia cause marked cerebral vasodilation and therefore an increase in cerebral blood flow, which contributes to increased ICP.

HYDROCEPHALUS

Hydrocephalus is an abnormal increase in CSF volume. It may caused by impaired reabsorption of CSF at the arachnoid villi (from subarachnoid hemorrhage or meningitis). This is called a communicating hydrocephalus. It may also be caused by interference or blockage with CSF outflow from the ventricular system (from cerebral edema, tumor or debris). The ventricles may dilate from the relative increase in CSF volume. Ultimately, if not treated, this increase in CSF volume may lead to increased ICP.

BRAIN HERNIATION

In the presence of increased ICP, the brain tissue may shift and herniate downward. Of the several types of herniation syndromes (Figure 48-9), uncal (transtentorial) herniation is one of the most clinically significant because it is life threatening. It is caused by a shift of one or both areas of the temporal lobe, known as the uncus. This shift creates pressure on the third cranial nerve. Late findings include dilated and nonreactive pupils, ptosis, and a rapidly deteriorating level of consciousness. Central herniation is caused by a downward shift of the brainstem and the diencephalon from a supratentorial lesion. It is clinically manifested by Cheyne-Stokes respirations, pinpoint and nonreactive pupils, and potential hemodynamic instability.

A shift of the cingulate gyrus below the falx cerebri is known as cingulate herniation. Cingulate herniation is diagnosed most frequently on head computed tomography (CT). It is a sign of brain decompensation and poor intracranial compliance. A type of infratentorial herniation, cerebellar tonsillar herniation, occurs when the cerebellar tonsils shift and compress the medulla. This may lead to respiratory and cardiovascular compromise or arrest. All herniation syndromes are potentially life threatening, and the physician must be notified immediately when they are suspected.

Etiology

The most common causes of traumatic brain injury (TBI) in the United States are accidents involving motor vehicles, including both automobiles and motorcycles. All too often, alcohol and drugs are contributing factors to the accident. Falls, acts of violence, and sports-related injuries are the next most common causes.

Incidence/Prevalence

Each year seven million people in the United States sustain some type of TBI. Of these, 500,000 require hospitalization and 100,000 are permanently disabled, with 2000 remaining in a persistent vegetative state (Hickey, 2003). Summer and spring months, evenings, nights, and weekends are associated with the greatest number of injuries.

HEALTH PROMOTION/ILLNESS PREVENTION

Head injuries occur three times more often in males than in females. Males tend to play more sports, take more risks when

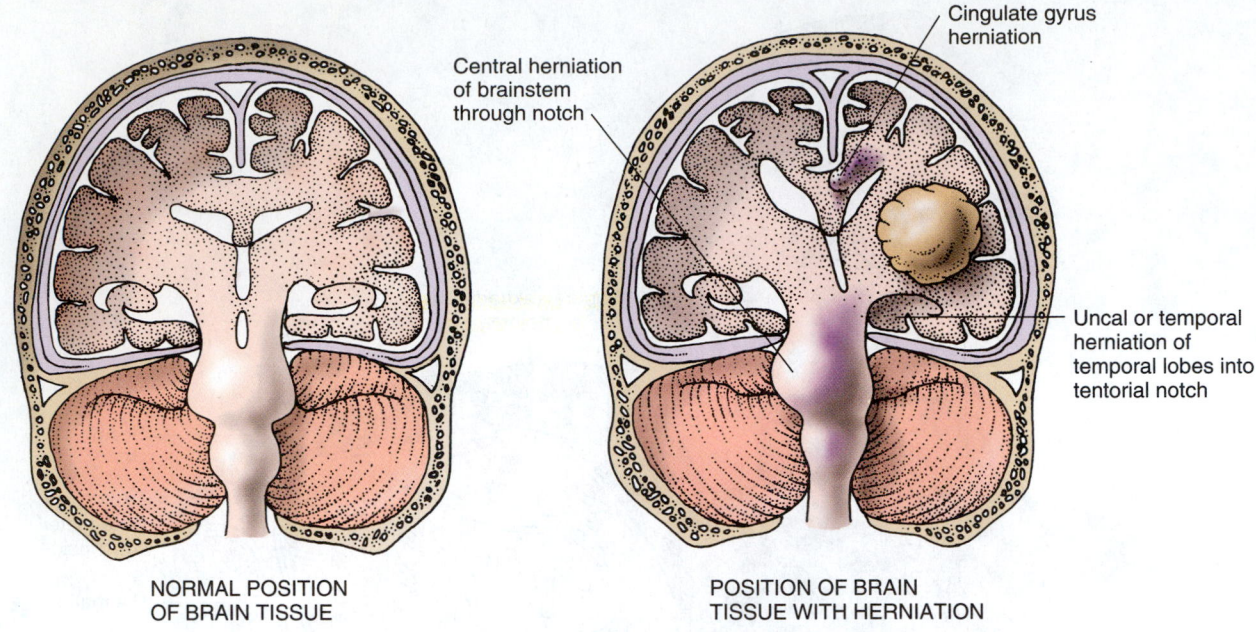

Central herniation
of brainstem
through notch

Cingulate gyrus
herniation

Uncal or temporal
herniation of
temporal lobes into
tentorial notch

NORMAL POSITION
OF BRAIN TISSUE

POSITION OF BRAIN
TISSUE WITH HERNIATION

Figure 48-9 ■ Herniation syndromes.

driving, and consume large amounts of alcohol. More than 70% of these injuries occur in people between 10 and 39 years of age. Therefore, teach adolescents and young adults to do the following:

- Avoid driving when drinking.
- Follow the game rules for sports.
- Be cautious when engaging in sports (e.g., do not try to "show off" on ski slopes).
- Avoid vehicular speeding.
- Wear helmet and other protective gear when engaging in contact sports or driving motorcycles/all-terrain vehicles (ATVs).
- Avoid dangerous risk-taking activities unless trained to participate in them.

◆COLLABORATIVE MANAGEMENT
◆Assessment

HISTORY

Obtaining an accurate history from a client who has sustained craniocerebral trauma may be difficult because of either the seriousness of the injury or the presence of amnesia. It is not unusual for the client to experience **amnesia** (loss of memory) for the events before or after the injury. The client with a serious head injury is often admitted to the hospital unconscious or in a confused and combative state. If the client is unable to provide information, the history can be obtained from rescue workers or witnesses to the injury. Always ask when, where, and how the injury occurred. Did the client lose consciousness? If so, for how long? Has there been a change in the level of consciousness (LOC)? If trauma is related to drug or alcohol intoxication, it may be difficult to differentiate neurologic changes from head trauma from those produced by intoxication.

Obtain as much information about the events as possible immediately after the injury. Clients with a severe injury may have several different presentations. The client may be completely unresponsive after the injury; alternatively, the client may initially be responsive and deteriorate rapidly within a few minutes to several hours. In another typical presentation, the client is initially unconscious for a few minutes as a result of the primary brain injury, returns to a normal level of consciousness, and then rapidly deteriorates as a consequence of secondary insult to the brain.

Determine whether the client experienced any seizure activity before or after the injury and whether there is a history of a seizure disorder. It is important to obtain precise information about the circumstances of falls, particularly in the older client (Chart 48-7). Other pertinent information includes hand dominance, any diseases of or injuries to the eyes, and any allergies to medications or food, particularly seafood. People allergic to seafood are often allergic to the intravenous (IV) contrast media used in diagnostic tests. Inquire about a history of alcohol or drug use and abuse because drugs or alcohol may mask the symptoms of increased ICP.

PHYSICAL ASSESSMENT/CLINICAL MANIFESTATIONS

No two injuries are alike. The client with a TBI may have a variety of manifestations depending on the severity of injury and the resulting increase in intracranial pressure (ICP) (see Chart 48-5). The goals of the nursing assessment are the establishment of baseline data and the early detection of and prevention of increased ICP, systemic hypotension, hypoxia, or hypercapnia (increased blood levels of carbon dioxide). The early detection of subtle changes in the client's neurologic status enables the health care team to prevent or treat potentially life-threatening complications.

Because it is estimated that 5% to 20% of clients with TBI have associated cervical spinal cord injuries, all clients with head trauma are treated as though they have spinal cord injury until radiographic studies prove otherwise. Assess for indicators of spinal cord injury, such as loss of motor and sensory function, tenderness along the spine, and abnormal head tilt. The client may experience respiratory problems and diaphragmatic breathing, and his or her re-

CHART 48-7

NURSING FOCUS on the OLDER ADULT
Head Injury

- Head injury is the fifth leading cause of death in older adults.
- The 65- to 75-year age-group has second highest incidence of head injury of all age-groups.
- Falls and motor vehicle accidents are the most common cause of head injury.
- The following factors contribute to high mortality:

  Falls causing subdural hematomas (closed head injuries), especially chronic subdural hematomas

  Poorly tolerated systemic stress, which is increased by admission to a high-stimuli environment

  Medical complications, such as hypotension, hypertension, and cardiac problems

  Decreased protective mechanisms, which make clients susceptible to infections (especially pneumonia)

  Decreased immunologic competence, which is further diminished by head injury

flexes may be diminished or absent. The client may also experience severe hemodynamic instability from an existing spinal cord injury.

AIRWAY AND BREATHING PATTERN ASSESSMENT. The *first priority* is the assessment of the client's airway and breathing pattern. Hypoxia and hypercapnia are best detected through arterial blood gas analysis, but the nursing assessment is vital to identify the client at risk for respiratory-related complications. Direct observation of chest wall movement and lung auscultation are paramount. Any suspicion of respiratory inadequacy should be reported immediately to the physician. The client's lung ventilation should be supported as appropriate, and they may need controlled ventilation through an endotracheal tube. Injuries to the brainstem may cause a change in the client's breathing pattern, such as Cheyne-Stokes respirations, central neurogenic hyperventilation, and/or apnea.

VITAL SIGNS ASSESSMENT. The mechanisms of autoregulation are often impaired as the result of craniocerebral trauma. The more serious the injury, the more severe the impact on autoregulation. Depending on the severity of the injury, the nurse or assistive nursing personnel monitors the client's blood pressure and pulse to detect possible changes in cerebral blood flow caused by impaired autoregulation as a result of hypotension or hypertension. The **Cushing reflex,** a classic yet late sign of increased ICP, is manifested by severe hypertension with a widened pulse pressure and bradycardia. As ICP increases, the pulse becomes thready, irregular, and rapid. Cerebral blood flow increases in response to hypertension, and vasogenic edema may occur, further increasing ICP. In contrast, hypotension and tachycardia are symptomatic of hypovolemic shock. This decrease in blood volume may lead to decreased cerebral perfusion pressure and eventually to ischemia and infarct of the brain tissue.

Hypovolemic shock is usually due to intra-abdominal bleeding or bleeding into the soft tissue around major fractures—not to intracranial bleeding. Cardiac dysrhythmias may result from chest trauma, bruising of the heart, or interference with the autonomic nervous system. Cardiac dysrhythmias may also result from severe ICP elevations and brainstem pressure.

NEUROLOGIC ASSESSMENT. Many hospitals use the Glasgow Coma Scale to assess neurologic status (see Chapter 44). The *most important* variable to assess is level of con-

sciousness. A decrease or change in level of consciousness is typically the *first sign* of deterioration in neurologic status. Changes in consciousness or orientation are due to injury to the cerebral cortex and may also involve damage to the reticular formation. A decrease in arousal or increased sleepiness and coma are caused by pressure on the reticular activating system within the brainstem. Early indicators of a change in level of consciousness include behavior changes (e.g., restlessness or irritability), which are often subtle in nature.

EYE ASSESSMENT. Elicit a history of previous eye injury or medications that affect pupillary dilation and constriction, such as anticholinergics and adrenergics. Check pupils for size and reaction to light. Any changes in pupil size, shape, and reactivity must be reported to the health care provider immediately because such changes indicate an increase in ICP. Pupillary changes or eye signs differ depending on which areas of the brain are damaged. Pinpoint and nonresponsive pupils are indicative of brainstem dysfunction at the level of the pons. Of particular importance is the **ovoid pupil,** which is regarded as the midstage between a normal-sized pupil and a dilated pupil. This finding indicates the development of increased ICP. Pupils that are fixed (nonreactive) and dilated are a poor prognostic sign, resulting from a marked increase in ICP. Clients with this problem are sometimes referred to as having "blown" pupils.

Check gross vision if the client's condition permits. Have the client read any printed material (e.g., the nurse's name tag) or count the number of fingers that you hold within the client's visual field. Loss of vision is usually caused by injury to the occipital lobe, which produces temporary cortical blindness.

If the client is able to cooperate, the health care provider or neurosurgical nurse tests CN III, IV, and VI. Extraocular movements may be diminished because of the presence of increased ICP and hydrocephalus. Damage to the optic chiasm, optic tract, or optic radii may cause visual-field deficits or diplopia. In the unconscious client, additional oculocephalic and oculovestibular tests are performed to test the integrity of the brainstem and of CN III, VI, and VII.

MOTOR ASSESSMENT. Assess for bilateral motor responses to avoid missing lateralizing signs. The client's motor loss or dysfunction usually appears contralateral to the site of the lesion. For example, a left-sided hemiparesis is indicative of an injury to the right cerebral hemisphere. A deterioration in motor function or the development of abnormal posturing (**decerebrate** or **decorticate posturing**) or flaccidity is another indicator of increased ICP. These changes are attributable to dysfunction within the pyramidal system or cerebral peduncles. Brainstem or cerebellar injury may cause ataxia, decreased or increased muscle tone, and weakness.

ADDITIONAL NEUROLOGIC ASSESSMENT. If the client is able to cooperate, a full neurologic assessment is completed as outlined in Chapter 44. Particular attention is given to cranial nerves I, V, VII, IX, and X. The first cranial nerve is often damaged where the frontal lobe passes over the irregularly shaped bones of the anterior and middle fossa; this results in the loss of smell (anosmia). CN V, VII, IX, and X are important for chewing and swallowing abilities and phonation. The client's ability to speak must be assessed, with particular attention directed toward differentiating aphasias (caused by injury to the cerebral cortex) from communication impairments (caused by damage to the cranial nerves and cerebellum). Damage to the cranial nerves occurs from disruption of the nerve trunk, either intracranially or along its extracranial course in the skull or face. Cranial nerve damage may result from direct trauma or compression associated with pressure or hemorrhage.

Assess for additional signs of increased ICP (see Chart 48-5). These include severe headache, nausea, vomiting, seizures, and papilledema (seen by ophthalmoscopic examination). **Papilledema,** also known as a **choked disc,** is edema and hyperemia of the optic disc. It is always a sign of increased ICP. Headache and seizures are a response to the injury and may or may not be associated with increased ICP. Findings on the neurologic examination should be interpreted over time, in response to interventions, and may also indicate progression of injury. Always remember that the client with a head injury is at risk for potentially devastating ICP elevations.

Carefully observe the client's ears and nose for any signs of cerebrospinal fluid (CSF) leaks that result from a basilar skull fracture. CSF placed on a white absorbent background can be distinguished from other fluids by the "halo" sign, a yellowish stain surrounded by bloody drainage. CSF tests positively for glucose when a strip testing method (Dipstix) is used, but this method of determining a CSF leak is not always reliable. If there is a CSF leak, the client should be assessed for any signs of **nuchal rigidity** (stiff neck), which may indicate infection or blood in the CSF. Nuchal rigidity is not checked until a spinal cord injury has been ruled out.

The client's head is palpated carefully to detect the presence of fractures or hematomas. The nurse looks for areas of ecchymosis (bruising), tender areas of the scalp, and lacerations.

Clients with a *minor* head injury should be assessed for manifestations of post-concussion syndrome. Symptoms include a wide array of physical and cognitive problems that range from persistent headache, weakness, and dizziness to personality and behavior changes, loss of memory, and problems with perception, reasoning abilities, and concept formation. The symptoms may persist for a few days or weeks to several months after the injury. For some clients, severe physical and cognitive problems remain despite a relatively benign initial clinical presentation and normal diagnostic test findings.

PSYCHOSOCIAL ASSESSMENT

The person who has had a moderate or severe head injury is never the same as before the injury. Most often, the client with a major head injury has personality changes manifested by temper outbursts, depression, risk-taking behavior, and denial of disability. The client may become talkative and develop a very outgoing personality. Memory, especially recent or short-term memory, is affected and should not be confused with problems of aphasia. The ability to learn new information and concentration may be affected. Finally, the client may exhibit problems with insight and planning. All these problems may lead to difficulties within the family structure and with social and work-related interactions. Coping strategies that have been used in the past must be assessed to determine the client's ability to adapt to the changes in physical and cognitive abilities. Although they have no focal signs, clients with a mild head injury may still have symptoms of disability 1 year after injury.

Assess family dynamics, particularly if the client is discharged to the family's care directly from the acute care hospital. The family or significant others must also cope with changes in the client's physical appearance and cognitive abilities. Many families are angry with the client for being injured, especially when his or her behavior or their own behavior resulted in an injury that could have been prevented. They may feel guilty that they did not or were not able to prevent the injury. The family or significant others may feel overwhelmed by the complexity of care required and the long recovery period. Both the family and the client need to develop coping strategies to deal with the potential role reversals and role changes caused by the injury. Consultation with social services or utilization of available counseling services may assist the family in developing appropriate coping strategies.

> ### Critical Thinking Challenge
>
> A female college student who had been treated for clinical depression attempted suicide by jumping from her fourth-floor dormitory room. Although she has multiple orthopedic injuries, she sustained only a mild traumatic brain injury (MTBI). You are assigned to care for her in the step-down surgical unit. When you enter her room, you find that her family is visiting and she is crying.
>
> 1. What should you do at this time? Give a rationale for your answer.
> 2. What are some reasons she is so upset? (Think of all the possibilities.)
> 3. The neurologist explained to the client's mother that she could have long-lasting neurologic problems as a result of the MTBI. What problems might she have, and how might they compound her existing health problems?

evolve For suggested answer guidelines, go to http://evolve.elsevier.com/Iggy/.

LABORATORY ASSESSMENT

There are no laboratory tests to diagnose a primary brain injury; however, several laboratory tests are used to diagnose or indicate measures to prevent secondary brain insult. Arterial blood gases (ABGs) are analyzed, with particular attention given to oxygen and carbon dioxide levels. The health care provider also orders a complete blood count (CBC) and determination of serum glucose and electrolyte levels and osmolarity. These tests are performed to monitor hemodynamic status or to identify electrolyte imbalance or the presence of infection. Severe electrolyte imbalances can also contribute to secondary injury as well as increase the risk of seizures.

RADIOGRAPHIC ASSESSMENT

The health care provider immediately orders computed tomography (CT) scanning to identify the extent and scope of injury to the brain. This diagnostic test can identify the presence of a lesion that requires surgical intervention, such as epidural or subdural hematoma. Radiography and CT scanning of the cervical spine and the skull are done to rule out fractures and dislocations. A chest x-ray is done to identify fractured ribs or other chest injuries. A flat plate of the abdomen, abdominal ultrasound, or abdominal CT may be obtained to assist in the diagnosis of abdominal bleeding or bowel laceration.

OTHER DIAGNOSTIC ASSESSMENTS

Magnetic resonance imaging (MRI) is particularly useful in the diagnosis of diffuse axonal injury, but it is not recommended for clients with ICP monitoring devices or other invasive monitoring devices. As the client's condition stabilizes, the physician may order other diagnostic tests to identify the extent of injury to the brain. For example, the integrity of the cerebral vessels is measured through the use of Doppler flow studies or an arteriogram; cerebral perfusion is measured by cerebral blood flow studies. Evoked potentials provide information on the functioning sensory pathways and may be useful in predicting outcome.

◆ Interventions

The client with a *severe* head injury is admitted to the critical care unit or a trauma center. Clients with moderate head injuries are admitted to either the general nursing unit or the critical care unit, where they are closely observed for at least 24 hours. Clients with mild TBI may possibly be sent home from the emergency department with instructions (Chart 48-8).

NONSURGICAL MANAGEMENT. Nursing interventions for all clients with a head injury are directed toward preventing or detecting increased ICP, promoting fluid and electrolyte balance, and monitoring the effects of treatments and medications.

Assessment of Vital Signs. Take and record the client's vital signs at least every 1 to 2 hours and as indicated based on client acuity. The health care provider may prescribe medications to prevent severe hypertension or hypotension. The client in the critical care unit is connected to a cardiac monitor to detect any cardiac dysrhythmias. Nonspecific ST-segment or T-wave changes may occur, possibly in response to stimulation of the autonomic nervous system or an increase in the level of circulating catecholamines. Documents and report cardiac irregularities to the health care provider.

The client with a head injury is often admitted with a fever—a defense mechanism in the presence of trauma or an indication of inflammatory response. Fever as a consequence of infection may develop later in the course of the disease. A third cause of fever is a central fever caused by hypothalamic damage. It is manifested by an absence of sweating and no diurnal (daily) variation; this type of fever is high and lasts several days to weeks. In addition, this type of fever responds better to cooling (hypothermia blanket, sponge bath) than to the administration of antipyretic drugs such as acetaminophen (Tylenol, Ace-Tabs ✱).

Positioning. Position the client to avoid extreme flexion or extension of the neck and to maintain the head in the midline, neutral position. Log roll the client during turning to avoid extreme hip flexion, and keep the head of the bed elevated at least 30 degrees or as recommended by the health care provider. Head positioning should be based on both intracranial pressure (ICP) and systemic blood pressure. If increasing head elevation lowers ICP but also significantly lowers systemic blood pressure, the client does not benefit and may actually be harmed. Base head elevation on cerebral perfusion pressure when possible. All these measures enhance venous drainage, which helps prevent increased ICP.

Pulmonary Ventilation and Management. Prophylactic hyperventilation during the first 20 hours after injury is usually avoided because it may produce ischemia by causing cerebral vasoconstriction with a resulting decrease in cerebral blood volume and ICP. In acute neurologic deterioration, however, hyperventilation may be used for brief periods of central ICP elevations pending use of other therapies.

The client who requires mechanical ventilation is ventilated to maintain a partial pressure of arterial carbon dioxide ($PaCO_2$) of about 35 mm Hg. One major goal is to prevent hypercarbia. Carbon dioxide is a very potent vasodilator that can contribute to increases in ICP. The $PaCO_2$ must not be allowed to fall significantly, which may result in tissue hypoxia caused by *severe* vasoconstriction. Arterial oxygen levels (PaO_2) are maintained between 80 and 100 mm Hg to prevent cerebral vasodilation resulting from hypoxemia. Arterial blood gas values are monitored at least twice daily and after each change in the ventilator setting.

Pulmonary secretions tend to pool as the result of a decreased level of consciousness, an ineffective cough, or an altered breathing pattern. The secretions may be thick because of the diuretics or fluid intake restriction that may be used to prevent cerebral edema. Chest physiotherapy and frequent turning may be needed as indicated by the results of the respiratory assessment, with close attention given to the ICP response.

The client with increased ICP should be carefully observed when suctioned. If the client is intubated, he or she should be manually hyperventilated carefully with 100% oxygen before each pass of the catheter. Overly aggressive hyperventilation with endotracheal suctioning may be dangerous because of the cerebral vasoconstriction caused by even transient hypocapnia (low arterial carbon dioxide levels). This may increase the risk of cerebral ischemia as a secondary event. The

---

CHART 48-8

CLIENT EDUCATION GUIDE
Minor Head Injury

- If the person is sleeping, wake him or her every 3 to 4 hours for the first 2 days, asking his or her name, where he or she is, and the name of the caregiver.
- Expect the person to complain of headache, nausea, or dizziness for at least 24 hours. If these symptoms are severe or do not improve, contact the physician immediately or take the person back to the emergency department.
- For a headache, give acetaminophen (Tylenol) every 4 hours as needed.
- Avoid giving the person sedatives, sleeping pills, or alcoholic beverages for at least 24 hours unless the physician instructs otherwise.
- Do not allow the person to engage in strenuous activity for at least 48 hours.
- Do not allow nose blowing or ear cleaning for 48 hours.
- If any of the following symptoms occur, take the person back to the emergency department immediately:
    Blurred vision
    Drainage from the ear or nose
    Weakness
    Slurred speech
    Progressive sleepiness
    Vomiting
    Worsening headache
    Unequal pupil size
- Keep follow-up appointments with the health care provider.

client should be allowed a rest period of a few minutes after suctioning to prevent increased ICP. Lidocaine given IV or endotracheally may be used to suppress the cough reflex, which would increase ICP.

Drug Therapy. Glucocorticoids (dexamethasone [Decadron, Dexasone]) and methylprednisolone sodium succinate [Solu-Medrol, Medrol]) have no demonstrated benefit in the management of increased ICP as a result of head injury or cerebral infarction. Mannitol (Osmitrol), an **osmotic diuretic,** is used to treat cerebral edema by pulling water out of the extracellular space of the edematous brain tissue, but it does not cross the blood-brain barrier. It is most effective when given in boluses rather than as a continuous infusion. Furosemide (Lasix), a loop diuretic, is often used as adjunctive therapy to reduce the incidence of rebound from mannitol and also enhances its therapeutic action. Furosemide also reduces edema and blood volume, decreases sodium uptake by the brain, and decreases the production of CSF at the choroid plexus.

Administer mannitol through a filter in the IV tubing or, if given by IV push, draw it up through a filtered needle to eliminate microscopic crystals. Monitor the client receiving either osmotic or loop diuretics for intake and output and severe dehydration as well as for indications of acute renal failure, weakness, edema, and changes in urine output. Serum electrolyte and osmolarity levels are measured every 6 hours. Mannitol is used to obtain a serum osmolarity of 310 to 320 mOsm/L, depending on physician preference and the goals of therapy. A Foley catheter must be inserted to maintain strict measurement of output. The client's serum and urine osmolarity are checked daily.

Opioids, such as morphine sulfate or fentanyl citrate, may be used with ventilated clients to decrease agitation and control restlessness if the agitation is caused by pain. Fentanyl has fewer hemodynamic consequences than morphine and may therefore be a safer agent to manage pain. These agents may be reversed with naloxone (Narcan), but opioid reversal should be avoided if at all possible to reduce risk of withdrawal and rebound pain and agitation. Sedatives such as lorazepam (Ativan) and midazolam (Versed) may be used for anxiety to promote comfort and treat agitation. Sedatives and opioids may mask the neurologic assessment and potentially lower blood pressure. As such, they should be administered in small incremental doses to a predetermined endpoint with close assessment of hemodynamic stability and neurologic status.

Neuromuscular blocking agents (NMBAs), such as vecuronium bromide or cisatracurium (Nimbex), may be used for the client following head trauma if the client is experiencing dangerous agitation or if the increased activity is causing ICP elevations (Arbour, 2000). NMBAs have no analgesic and sedative effects and *must never be used without aggressive sedation/analgesia.* NMBAs are associated with an increased risk of pneumonia and other complications. Therefore they are not used routinely.

Antiepileptic drugs, such as phenytoin (Dilantin), to prevent seizures that occur initially more than 7 days **(late-onset seizures)** following injury are not recommended. However, they may be recommended as an option to prevent seizure activity that may occur within 7 days following injury **(early-onset seizures).** Acetaminophen (Tylenol, Ace-Tabs✱) and aspirin (acetylsalicylic acid [ASA], Ancasal✱)

are given to clients who are febrile (temperature greater than 101° F [39° C]) to reduce fever.

Induction of Barbiturate Coma. Clinical trials in the use of **barbiturate coma** have been disappointing yet remain an option for clients whose ICP cannot be controlled by other means. Pentobarbital sodium (Nembutal, Novopentobarb✱) or sodium thiopental are the drugs of choice (Censullo & Sebastian, 2003). These drugs decrease the metabolic demands of the brain and cerebral blood flow, stabilize cell membranes, decrease the formation of vasogenic edema, and produce a more uniform blood supply. The provider adjusts the dosage to maintain complete unresponsiveness. Barbiturate coma is optimally managed using hemodynamic assessment, ICP monitoring, and electroencephalographic (EEG) monitoring to document endpoints. As a consequence, it is difficult to recognize subtle or unsubtle neurologic changes. The client requires mechanical ventilation, sophisticated hemodynamic monitoring, and ICP monitoring. Complications of barbiturate coma include decreased gastrointestinal motility, cardiac dysrhythmias, hypotension, and fluctuations in body temperature. **Therapeutic hypothermia** is being widely researched as a better option for lowering elevated ICP (Bayir, Clark, & Kochanek, 2003).

Fluid and Electrolyte Management. The client with craniocerebral trauma is at risk for diabetes insipidus (DI) and the syndrome of inappropriate antidiuretic hormone (SIADH) because the pituitary gland may be injured or compressed from cerebral edema (see Chapter 14). Fluid overload can occur and cerebral edema can be worsened in the client with multiple trauma from the rapid administration of IV fluids, plasma expanders, or corticosteroids. Fluids management may be titrated to optimize volume resuscitation but minimize brain swelling and ICP elevation. Fluid management is also influenced by the response to diuretic therapy and an evaluation of laboratory values. Serum osmolarity should be maintained below 310 to 320 mOsm as ordered by the physician. Check urine specific gravity every 1 to 4 hours. Monitor serum and urine osmolarity and electrolytes frequently.

Strategies for Sensory/Perceptual Alterations. The client with a *major* head injury following the acute phase of management may exhibit changes in the following areas: sense of smell; ability to taste, swallow, or feel the presence of food within the oral cavity; and vision, pain, and temperature sensation. As a result, the client is at risk for nutritional deficits, which may interfere with the healing process. The client may be injured from falling over objects outside the field of vision, or burn injuries could occur because of the inability to perceive variations in water temperatures.

Ensure that mealtime and the surrounding environment are a pleasant experience, and position the client to maximize swallowing ability. The speech-language pathologist identifies strategies to prevent food from accumulating in the cheek of the affected side. In general, clients who have swallowing problems are able to tolerate or swallow soft or semisoft foods and liquids (mechanical soft or dental diet, junior baby foods, custards, scrambled eggs) better than thin liquids (water, juice, or milk). Powdered thickener (Thick-It) may be added to thicken foods to a more manageable consistency. Collaborate with the dietitian to find a diet appropriate for the client with dysphagia.

If a large lesion of the parietal lobe is present, the client may experience a loss of sensation for pain, temperature, touch, and proprioception, which prevents the client from responding appropriately to environmental stimuli. A hazard-free environment is necessary to prevent injury (e.g., from burns if the client's coffee is too hot or from falls if the siderails on the bed are not kept up). A sensory stimulation program should be integrated into the comatose or stuporous client's routine care activities. Sensory stimulation is done to facilitate a meaningful response to the environment. Present visual, auditory, or tactile stimuli one at a time and explain the purpose and the type of stimulus presented. For example, show a picture of the client's mother and say, "This is a picture of your mother." The picture is shown several times, and the same words are used to describe the picture. If auditory tapes are used, they should not be longer than 10 to 15 minutes. If the stimulus is presented for a longer period, it simply becomes "white" noise, or meaningless background noise.

The client may be disoriented and experience a short-term memory loss. Always introduce yourself to the client before any interaction. Explanations of procedures and activities should be short and simple and given immediately before and throughout the procedure. A sleep-wake cycle must be maintained, with scheduled rest periods. Orient the client to time (day, month, and year), and place and explain the reason for the hospitalization. Reassure the client that he or she is safe and that family members know where he or she is. Ask the family to bring in familiar objects, such as pictures. Orientation cues within the environment, such as a large clock with numbers or a single-date calendar, should be provided.

Behavioral Management. The client is at risk for seizure activity, and actions are taken as outlined in the discussion of epilepsy (see Chapter 45). Keep the bed in low position with the side rails up. Hand mittens may be applied if the client attempts to pull out the IV line or nasogastric tube. Restraining any extremity increases agitation and fear. The client's behavior is observed and documented at least every hour. Alternatives to restraints should be attempted according to hospital policy. For example, covering the client's IV site with the I.V. House or other device may prevent dislodgment. Keeping the client's hands busy with activity pillows or puzzles accomplishes the same goal.

Orient the client to the surroundings as needed, and provide a quiet environment. Closely monitor the client's response to television programs or the radio. Often he or she is unable to differentiate these situations or programs from what is happening within his or her own environment.

Strategies for Preventing Complications of Immobility. Chapter 10 discusses mobility and activities of daily living (ADLs) skills in detail as well as ways to prevent complications of immobility.

Nutrition Management. The client who is moderately to severely injured usually has a decreased level of consciousness, at least temporarily. As a result, the client is unable to chew or swallow and must receive nutrition and fluids by an alternative method. The client initially receives IV fluids until he or she has stabilized. If there is no improvement in level of consciousness, long-term nutritional support via enteral feeding is usually instituted. A small-lumen nasogastric or nasoduodenal tube or a percutaneous endoscopic gastrostomy (PEG) tube is used for continuous or intermittent feeding. Small-bore tubes decrease the risk for aspiration in a client who is at high risk. Care of the client receiving enteral feeding is described in Chapter 64.

With the use of either type of tube, the client should be weighed daily. Collaborate with the dietitian to determine whether caloric needs are being met, and monitor serum albumin and prealbumin levels to assess adequacy of protein intake. Assess the client daily for signs of dehydration, such as dry mucous membranes and poor skin turgor. Supplements such as milkshakes and Ensure may be needed to meet the client's caloric and protein requirements if he or she is not receiving total enteral nutrition.

SURGICAL MANAGEMENT. The physician may elect to insert an intracranial pressure (ICP) monitoring device to evaluate the client's ICP more closely. All devices are inserted through a burr hole that is placed in the skull using a twist drill. Each device is connected to an electronic transducer that converts ICP to electronic impulses and provides information that can be viewed real-time using a monitor at the client's bedside. The monitor is able to record the pressure waves and provide a digital readout of the pressure.

Intracranial Pressure Monitoring. Various types of devices for monitoring ICP are used. An **intraventricular catheter (IVC)** is a small tube that is inserted into the anterior horn of the lateral ventricle of the nondominant cerebral hemisphere. The advantage of this system is that cerebrospinal fluid (CSF) can be drained to decrease ICP, and specimens can be obtained for laboratory analysis. The **subarachnoid screw or bolt** is a hollow device placed into the subarachnoid space for direct pressure measurement. A disadvantage of the system is that CSF cannot be drained to treat increased ICP; however, it is less invasive, which lowers the risk of infection (Table 48-3).

An **epidural catheter** or sensor is a transducer that is placed between the skull and the dura, leaving the dura intact. A similar device is the **subdural catheter**, which is placed under the dura mater. Its major advantage is the decreased risk of infection from an open dural space. The **fiberoptic transducer-tipped pressure sensor** is a commonly used device for ICP monitoring. It is easily transported and can be placed in the subdural or subarachnoid space, in the ventricle, or directly into brain tissue. The critical care nurse follows the agency's protocols for the management of these devices.

Craniotomy. In extreme cases in which the client's ICP cannot be controlled, the physician may elect to perform a craniotomy to remove ischemic tissue or the tips of the temporal lobes. The removal of nonvital brain tissue allows expansion of brain tissue without further compromise of ICP. A craniotomy may also be performed to remove epidural or subdural hematomas. Care of the client with a craniotomy is discussed under Postoperative Care (Brain Tumor), p. 1058.

Community-Based Care

The client with a *major* head injury requires case management and ongoing rehabilitation following the acute phase of hospitalization. Information on the selection of a head injury rehabilitation facility can be obtained from the National Head Injury Foundation (NHIF). Other preparation includes the development of a detailed client care plan to be

TABLE 48-3 Advantages and Disadvantages of Intracranial Pressure Monitoring Devices

Monitoring Device	Advantages	Disadvantages
Intraventricular catheter (IVC)	Allows accurate measurement of intracranial pressure (ICP) Allows drainage or sampling of cerebrospinal fluid (CSF) Allows instillation of contrast media Provides reliable evaluation of cerebral compliance	Provides additional site for potential infection Most invasive method for monitoring ICP Must be balanced and recalibrated frequently Catheter can become occluded by blood or tissue Insertion can be difficult with small or collapsed ventricles CSF leakage can occur around insertion site Associated with increased infection rate
Subarachnoid bolt or screw	Lower infection rates than with IVC Quickly and easily placed Can be used with small or collapsed ventricles Does not penetrate brain parenchyma	Tendency for dampened waveform Less accurate at high ICP May become occluded by blood or tissue Must be balanced and recalibrated frequently (i.e., every 4 hr and whenever client is repositioned) Baseline drift and tendency for dampened waveform Does not provide for CSF sampling
Subdural/epidural catheter or sensor	Least invasive Decreased risk for infection Easily and quickly placed	Increasing baseline drift over time; therefore accuracy and reliability are questionable Does not provide for CSF sampling or drainage
Fiberoptic transducer tipped catheter	Can be placed in subdural or subarachnoid space, in ventricle, or into brain tissue Easily transported Requires zeroing only once (during insertion) Baseline drift to 1 mm Hg/day Decreased risk of infection Less waveform artifact No need to adjust transducer to client's position Easy to insert	Does not provide for CSF sampling or drainage Cannot be recalibrated after placement Probe needs periodic replacement Fragile fiberoptic cable easily damaged and broken

given to the rehabilitation facility. This enables the provision of consistent care and decreases the initial anxiety related to the changes the client may experience. The discharge summary states medications, including dosage, possible reactions, and special preparation; the current client care plan; techniques used to motivate or calm the client; and strategies to assist the family to adapt to the situation.

The goal of rehabilitation after head injury is to maximize the client's ability to return to his or her highest level of functioning. Rehabilitation activities such as occupational therapy (OT), physical therapy (PT), and speech therapy may continue in the home after discharge from the rehabilitation facility. Adaptation of the home environment to accommodate the client safely may be needed. The family may require assistance in obtaining adaptive devices needed for ADLs and ambulation.

HOME CARE MANAGEMENT

Little home care preparation is needed for the client with a concussion unless he or she is experiencing post-traumatic symptoms. The client's home should be assessed for potential hazards before discharge from the hospital. Functioning smoke and fire alarms must be present because the client with a head injury often loses the sense of smell. This information can be obtained from the admission data or by a home visit. Home adaptations and referrals to outside agencies should be completed before discharge. Case management and use of critical pathways can facilitate optimal timing of diagnostic testing, clinical consults, and involvement of other health care providers, such as physical/occupational therapy.

HEALTH TEACHING

The staff nurse or case manager provides the client and family with both written and verbal instructions. The teaching

plan for the client with craniocerebral trauma includes a review of seizure precautions and strategies to adapt to sensory dysfunction and to cope with the personality or behavior problems that may arise. Explain the purpose, dosage, schedule, and route of administration of any medications. The client is encouraged to participate in activities as tolerated. Demonstrations and return demonstrations of care activities may facilitate the competence of family members in skill performance. Stress the importance of regular follow-up visits with therapists and health care providers.

With the family and the client, reinforce the same strategies used in the hospital to treat sensory or perceptual changes. In addition, the family or significant others are taught about the importance of not moving furniture or other objects in the home to a different place because this can lead to an injury in the client with visual problems or might confuse the client with cognitive impairments.

Clients with personality and behavior problems respond best to a structured and consistent environment. Instruct the family to develop a home routine that provides structure, repetition, and consistency. The family must also be reminded about the importance of reinforcing positive behaviors and not reinforcing negative behaviors.

Teach the client who has sustained a *minor* head injury (e.g., a concussion) that post-concussion syndrome may occur. As stated earlier, this syndrome is a group of clinical manifestations including, but not limited to, the following:

- Personality changes
- Irritability
- Headaches
- Dizziness
- Restlessness
- Nervousness
- Insomnia

- Memory loss
- Depression

Many clients with head injuries experience some of these manifestations during recovery. However, some clients have these problems for weeks, months, or even years to the extent that they interfere with daily activities such as employment. The prolonged pattern is classified as post-trauma syndrome. The exact cause of the phenomenon is not known, but physiologic and psychological theories have been espoused. Support groups and professional counseling are the most effective interventions.

Most clients with moderate to severe craniocerebral trauma are discharged with physical and cognitive disabilities. Changes in personality and behavior are not unusual. The family must learn to cope with the client's increased fatigue, irritability, temper outbursts, depression, and memory problems. These clients often require constant supervision at home, and eventually the families feel socially isolated. Instruct the family to plan for regular respite care, either in a structured day-care respite program or through relief provided by a friend or neighbor. Family members, particularly the primary caretaker, may become depressed and experience feelings of loneliness. They may also experience isolation, increased responsibilities, and role reversals. In addition, the family may feel angry with the client because of the additional responsibilities (financial or emotional) that his or her care has placed on them. To help the family cope with these problems, suggest that they join and actively participate in a local head injury support group.

The client needs assistance in identifying realistic expectations for discharge. Because of cognitive deficits, it may not be possible for the client to return to his or her previous employment or educational pursuits. The client may experience a sense of isolation and loneliness because personality and behavior changes make it difficult to resume or maintain the social contacts he or she had before the injury.

HEALTH CARE RESOURCES

The nurse or case manager refers families and significant others and clients to the National Head Injury Foundation (NHIF) as well as to the local or state group for information and support. The NHIF and its state chapters maintain lists of rehabilitation facilities for clients with head injuries. The NHIF will send family members and other interested persons guidelines for selecting a rehabilitation facility. Families should inquire about the facility's experience in caring for the person with a head injury, how many admissions the facility has had in the previous 2 to 3 years, and the results or outcome statistics on those clients (e.g., how many went home and at what functional recovery level—poor, fair, or good). Other helpful groups include the National Easter Seal Society and the National Institute of Handicapped Research.

BRAIN TUMORS

Brain tumors can arise anywhere within the brain structures and are named according to the cell or tissue from which they originate. *Primary* tumors originate within the central nervous system (CNS) and rarely metastasize outside this area. *Secondary* brain tumors result from metastasis from other areas of the body, such as the lungs, breast, kidney, and gastrointestinal tract.

PATHOPHYSIOLOGY

Regardless of origin, the tumor expands and invades, infiltrates, compresses, and displaces normal brain tissue. This leads to the following problems:

- Cerebral edema/brain tissue inflammation
- Increased intracranial pressure (ICP)
- Focal neurologic deficits
- Obstruction of the flow of cerebrospinal fluid (CSF)
- Pituitary dysfunction

Complications of Cerebral Tumors

Cerebral edema, or more specifically vasogenic edema, results from changes in capillary endothelial tissue permeability, which allows plasma to seep into the extracellular spaces. This leads to increased ICP and, depending on the location of the primary lesion, brain herniation syndromes may occur. A variety of focal neurologic deficits result from edema, infiltration, distortion, and compression of surrounding brain tissue. The cerebral blood vessels may become compressed because of edema and increased ICP. This compression leads to ischemia of the area supplied by the vessel. In addition, the tumor may infiltrate the walls of the vessel, causing it to rupture and hemorrhage into the tumor bed or adjacent brain tissue. About 33% of clients who have brain tumors experience seizure activity attributable to interference with the brain's normal electrical activity.

Increased ICP may also result from hydrocephalus related to obstruction of the flow of CSF or displacement of the lateral ventricles by the expanding lesion. Typically, a tumor obstructs the aqueduct of Sylvius or one of the ventricles or encroaches on the subarachnoid space. Posterior fossa tumors may obstruct the flow of CSF from the fourth ventricle to the foramen of Luschka or Magendie. With any brain tumor, the obstruction of normal CSF flow causes hydrocephalus and eventually leads to increased ICP.

Pituitary dysfunction may occur as the tumor compresses the pituitary gland and causes the syndrome of inappropriate antidiuretic hormone (SIADH) or diabetes insipidus (DI). These disorders result in severe fluid and electrolyte imbalances and can be life threatening (see Chapter 66 for a complete description).

Classification of Tumors

Brain tumors are usually classified as either malignant or benign (Table 48-4). Benign tumors are generally associated with a favorable outcome, which is often not the case with malignant tumors. However, benign tumors may be malignant by virtue of their location. If the tumor cannot be completely removed or treated, it continues to grow. As it invades other brain tissue, cerebral edema, focal neurologic deficits, and increased ICP occur. Herniation of brain tissue may eventually lead to death. Benign tumors also may undergo histologic changes and become malignant.

A second classification system is based on location. **Supratentorial** tumors, which occur most often in adults, are located in the area above the tentorium cerebelli, the tentlike fold of dura that surrounds the cerebellar hemisphere and supports the occipital lobe. In other words, supratentorial tumors are located within the cerebral hemispheres. Located beneath the tentorium is the **infratentorial** area, the area of the brainstem structures and cerebellum.

TABLE 48-4 Classification of Brain Tumors

Benign	Malignant
▪ Acoustic neuroma	▪ Astrocytoma
▪ Meningioma	Grade 2
▪ Pituitary adenoma	Grade 3
▪ Astrocytoma	Grade 4 (also known as
Grade 1 (may undergo	glioblastoma multiforme)
changes and become	▪ Oligodendroglioma
malignant)	▪ Ependymoma
▪ Chondroma	▪ Medulloblastoma
▪ Craniopharyngioma	▪ Chondrosarcoma
▪ Hemangioblastoma	▪ Glioma
	▪ Lymphoma

A third classification system depends on the cellular, histologic, or anatomic origins of the tumor. The nervous system is composed of two types of cells: (1) neurons, which are responsible for nerve impulse conduction; and (2) neuroglial cells, which provide support, nourishment, and protection for neurons. Four specific types of cells are neuroglial cells: astrocytes, oligodendroglia, ependymal cells, and microglia. When classifying tumors according to this system, tumors are named by their cell type. For example, an astrocytoma is a tumor of astrocytes.

GLIOMAS

Gliomas are malignant tumors. They account for 60% of all brain tumors in adults and arise from the neuroglial cells of the brain and brainstem. Malignant gliomas have a peak incidence in people 40 to 60 years of age. They infiltrate and invade surrounding brain tissue. The most common type of glioma is the astrocytoma, which may be found anywhere within the cerebral hemispheres. It is usually treated by surgery to remove as much tumor bulk as possible, followed by radiation and chemotherapy. Oligodendrogliomas, another type of glioma, are generally located within the frontal lobes of the brain. These tumors are slow-growing and are usually calcified. Surgical removal is possible, and the long-term prognosis is good. A glioblastoma is a highly malignant, grade 3 or higher, rapidly growing, invasive astrocytoma. Although improved surgical techniques and advanced treatment have improved the outlook and quality of life for a client with this type of tumor, fewer than 15% of affected clients survive 18 months after diagnosis.

Ependymomas arise from the lining of the ventricles and are difficult to treat surgically because of their location. The treatment of choice involves radiation and shunting procedures to control the hydrocephalus caused by the blocking of normal CSF flow by the tumor. Chemotherapy may also be used to treat these tumors.

Gliomas are graded according to their cellular differentiation or how closely the tumor cells resemble normal cells. Grade 1 tumors are well differentiated, grade 2 tumors are moderately differentiated, and grade 3 tumors are poorly differentiated. Grade 3 tumors can rapidly change to grade 4 tumors, which are also very poorly differentiated. A grade 3 or 4 astrocytoma is referred to as glioblastoma multiforme and is associated with a poor outcome. Grade 1 and 2 tumors may undergo cellular changes and become grade 3 or 4 tumors.

MENINGIOMAS

Meningiomas arise from the coverings of the brain (the meninges). They are the most common benign tumor, with a peak incidence at age 50 years. Females are affected more than males by a 2:1 ratio. This tumor is encapsulated, globular, and well demarcated and causes compression and displacement of adjacent brain tissue. Although complete removal of the tumor is possible, it tends to recur. It tends to occur in areas where the meninges predominate.

PITUITARY TUMORS

Pituitary tumors that occur in the anterior lobe account for 10% to 25% of brain tumors and may cause endocrine dysfunction. The most common type of pituitary tumor is the adenoma, which is subdivided into chromophobe, secretory, and nonsecretory adenomas. These tumors are benign and often occur in young and middle-aged adults. The presenting symptoms are often visual disturbances. These tumors also produce hypopituitary signs, such as loss of body hair, diabetes DI, sterility, visual field defects, and headaches.

ACOUSTIC NEUROMAS

Acoustic neuromas arise from the sheath of Schwann cells in the peripheral portion of cranial nerve VIII. They are also referred to as cerebellar pontine angle (CPA) tumors to describe their anatomic location. Acoustic neuromas compress brain tissue and tend to surround adjacent cranial nerves (VII, V, IX, X), making surgical removal difficult without causing permanent cranial nerve dysfunction. Females are twice as likely as males to have acoustic neuromas. Common symptoms include hearing loss, **tinnitus** (ringing in the ears), and dizziness or vertigo.

METASTATIC TUMORS

Metastatic, or secondary, tumors account for nearly 30% of brain tumors. Metastatic cells from the lungs, breast, colon, pancreas, and kidney can travel to the brain via the blood and the lymphatic system. Multiple metastatic lesions are not uncommon.

Etiology

The exact cause of brain tumors is unknown. Several areas under investigation include genetic changes, heredity, errors in fetal development, ionizing radiation, electromagnetic fields, environmental hazards, diet, viruses, and injury. Recently, the use of cellular phones has been investigated in the development of brain tumors, but findings are inconclusive.

Incidence/Prevalence

Brain tumors account for less than 2% of all cancer deaths. About 18,000 people per year are diagnosed with a primary brain tumor in the United States. Another 150,000 have metastatic brain tumors. Brain tumors in the adult population are seen primarily in clients 40 to 60 years of age, and the survival rate is low compared with other cancers.

◆ COLLABORATIVE MANAGEMENT
◆ Assessment

The clinical manifestations of brain tumors vary with the site of the tumor (Chart 48-9). In general, symptoms of a brain tumor include the following:

- Headaches that are usually more severe on awakening in the morning
- Nausea and vomiting
- Visual symptoms
- Seizures

CHART 48-9
KEY FEATURES of
Common Brain Tumors

Cerebral Tumors
- Headache (most common feature)
- Vomiting unrelated to food intake
- Changes in visual acuity and visual fields; diplopia (visual changes caused by papilledema)
- Hemiparesis or hemiplegia
- Hypokinesia
- Hyperesthesia, paresthesia, decreased tactile discrimination
- Seizures
- Aphasia
- Changes in personality or behavior

Brainstem Tumors
- Hearing loss (acoustic neuroma)
- Facial pain and weakness
- Dysphagia, decreased gag reflex
- Nystagmus
- Hoarseness
- Ataxia and dysarthria (cerebellar tumors)

- Changes in mentation or personality
- **Papilledema** (swelling of the optic disc)

Neurologic deficits result from the destruction, distortion, or compression of brain tissue. *Supratentorial* tumors usually result in paralysis, seizures, memory loss, cognitive impairment, language impairment, or vision problems. *Infratentorial* tumors produce ataxia, autonomic nervous system dysfunction, vomiting, drooling, hearing loss, and vision impairment. As the tumor grows, ICP increases, and the symptoms become progressively more severe.

Diagnosis is based on the history, neurologic assessment, clinical examination, and results of neurodiagnostic testing. Noninvasive diagnostic studies such as computed tomography (CT), magnetic resonance imaging (MRI), and skull films are conducted first. The CT and MRI identify the size, location, and extent of the tumor. The MRI may be used for initial diagnostic evaluation and is a more sensitive diagnostic study, whereas the CT is often used for follow-up during the hospital course.

Cerebral angiography is usually not indicated to diagnose a brain tumor but may be used to provide additional information about vascular supply to the tumor. Electroencephalography (EEG), lumbar puncture (LP), myelography, brain scan, and positron emission tomography (PET) may be indicated to provide further information about the size, location, and characteristics of the tumor. LP should not be performed if the client is exhibiting signs of ICP elevation to prevent brain herniation. Laboratory tests may also be ordered to evaluate endocrine function, renal status, and electrolyte balance.

◆Interventions

When possible, obtain a history from both the client and the family, including current signs and symptoms. A complete neurologic assessment is needed to establish baseline data and to determine the nature and extent of neurologic deficits.

NONSURGICAL MANAGEMENT. The goal of treatment of brain tumors is to decrease tumor size, improve quality of life, and improve survival time. The type of treatment selected depends on the tumor size and location, client symptoms and general condition, and whether the tumor is recurrent. The treatment of brain tumors may include radiation, chemotherapy, and surgery. A number of experimental treatment modalities are being investigated, including blood-brain barrier disruption, recombinant deoxyribonucleic acid (DNA), monoclonal antibodies, new antineoplastic drugs, immunotherapy, and hyperthermia.

Radiation Therapy. Radiation therapy may be used alone, after surgery, or in combination with chemotherapy and surgery. Chapter 28 discusses radiation treatment for cancer in detail. An anti-tenascin radioactive monoclonal antibody treatment (81C6) that is directly injected into the cavity where the tumor was removed is being investigated. The antibodies deliver radiation directly into the brain but are less potent than traditional radiation (Wood, 2004).

Drug Therapy. The health care provider may prescribe a variety of medications to treat the tumor as well as manage the client's symptoms and prevent complications.

Chemotherapy. Chemotherapy may be given alone, in combination with radiation and surgery, and with tumor progression. Although these drugs may control tumor growth or decrease tumor burden, the benefit usually is very short-lived. Chemotherapy usually involves more than one agent and may be given IV, intra-arterially, or intrathecally through an Ommaya reservoir placed in a cranial ventricle.

The most commonly used drugs are alkylating agents, especially nitrosoureas such as carmustine (BCNU) and lomustine (CCNU). A combination of procarbazine, lomustine, and vincristine (PCV) may be given for selected clients. Tamoxifen may also be used for selected types of tumors. A newer drug, temozolomide (Temodar), crosses the blood-brain barrier and is widely used today. It is administered orally, unlike most other agents. Side effects of these drugs are similar to those of any chemotherapeutic medication. Chapter 28 describes nursing implications for care of a client receiving chemotherapy.

Most chemotherapeutic agents have difficulty crossing the blood-brain barrier. Therefore direct drug delivery to the tumor is an emerging practice. Disk-shaped drug wafers called Gliadel wafers may be placed directly into the cavity created during surgical tumor removal. The major drug in the wafer is carmustine. This therapy is usually used for newly diagnosed high-grade malignant gliomas, but recurrent tumors may also be treated with this method. Other drugs that are awaiting approval from the Food and Drug Administration (FDA or have been recently approved include erlotinib (Tarceva) for malignant glioma, gefitinib (Iressa), and tipifarnib (Zarnestra) (Wood, 2004). New drugs are continuously emerging for all types of cancers.

Other Drugs. Analgesics, such as codeine and acetaminophen (Tylenol, Ace-Tabs✶), are given for headache. Dexamethasone (Decadron) is usually given to control cerebral edema. Research supports the efficacy of administering glucocorticoids for the treatment of edema resulting from brain tumors. Phenytoin (Dilantin) may be used to prevent or treat seizure activity. Histamine blockers such as ranitidine hydrochloride (Zantac, Apo-Ranitidine✶) or proton pump inhibitors such as pantoprazole (Protonix) are given to decrease gastric acid secretion and prevent the development of stress ulcers. Metoclopramide (Reglan) and other antiemetics are used to treat nausea and vomiting.

Radiosurgery. Radiosurgical procedures are an alternative to surgery. These techniques include the modified linear accelerator using accelerated x-rays (LINAC), a particle accelerator using beams of protons (cyclotron), and isotope seeds implanted in the tumor (brachytherapy). The Gamma Knife and CyberKnife are newer treatments.

Gamma Knife. The Gamma Knife is a type of stereotactic radiosurgical procedure that uses a single high dose of ionized radiation to focus 201 beams of gamma radiation produced by the radioisotope cobalt 60 to destroy intracranial lesions selectively without damaging surrounding healthy tissue (Figure 48-10). Combining neurodiagnostic imaging tools—including magnetic resonance imaging (MRI), computed tomography (CT), magnetic resonance angiography (MRA), and angiography—with the Gamma Knife allows for precise localization of deep-seated or anatomically difficult lesions. Treatment usually takes less than an hour, and clients require only overnight hospitalization. Advantages of this technique include its noninvasive nature; a lower risk than the traditional craniotomy; surgical precision; and decreased cost, morbidity, length of hospital stay, and recovery time.

The Gamma Knife is used primarily for brain tumors or arteriovenous malformations (AVMs) that are in an inaccessible location and therefore unresectable by craniotomy. Tumors typically treated in this manner are acoustic neuromas, meningiomas, and metastatic tumors. The procedure may also be used with clients who refuse conventional surgery, for clients whose age and physical condition preclude general anesthesia, as an adjunct to radiation therapy, and for recurrent or residual AVM or tumors after embolization or craniotomy. Additional potential applications of Gamma Knife radiosurgery are being evaluated.

Other Radiosurgical Procedures. The LINAC has an advantage over the Gamma Knife in that the Gamma Knife uses a rigid head frame that is difficult to position. The LINAC employs a skull-conforming mask. In another system called the CyberKnife, no frame is needed.

SURGICAL MANAGEMENT. The most important modality in the treatment of brain tumors is a biopsy to determine the specific pathology. A craniotomy is the most common surgical treatment and may be done to improve symptoms related to the lesion or to decrease pressure effects. The challenge for the surgeon is to remove the tumor as completely as possible without damaging normal tissue. Complete removal is possible with some benign tumors,

which results in a "surgical cure." Postoperatively, the client is usually admitted to the critical care unit.

Postoperative Care. The Plan of Care on pp. 1059 to 1063 highlights the major aspects of postoperative nursing care following a craniotomy. The focus of postoperative care is to monitor the client to detect changes in status and to prevent or minimize complications, especially increased intracranial pressure (ICP). Assess neurologic and vital signs every 30 minutes for the first 4 to 6 hours after surgery and then every hour. If the client is stable for 24 hours, the frequency of these checks may be decreased to every 2 to 4 hours, depending on the agency's policy. Potential neurologic deficits include a decreased level of consciousness, motor weakness or paralysis, aphasia, visual changes, and personality changes. Periorbital edema and ecchymosis of one or both eyes is not unusual and is treated with cold compresses to decrease swelling. Irrigate the affected eye with warm saline solution or artificial tears to improve client comfort. If the client is still recovering from anesthesia, has a decreased level of consciousness, or may not be able to protect the airway, he or she may remain intubated and receive controlled ventilation.

The client in the critical care unit is routinely connected to the cardiac monitor. Dysrhythmias may occur after posterior fossa surgery, or they may result from fluid and electrolyte imbalance. Other nursing interventions include strict recording of the client's intake and output and possibly fluid restriction to 1500 mL daily as clinically indicated. Range-of-motion exercises to all extremities are performed at least every 2 to 3 hours. Assist the client to turn, cough, and breathe deeply every 2 hours. To prevent the development of deep vein thrombosis, sequential compression stockings or pneumatic compression boots are kept in place until the client is ambulating.

Positioning. Clients who have undergone supratentorial surgery should have the head of the bed elevated 30 degrees or as tolerated to promote venous drainage from the head. Position the client to avoid extreme hip or neck flexion and maintain the head in a midline, neutral position. The client may be turned side-to-side or remain supine. If a large tumor has been removed, it is recommended that the client be placed on the nonoperative side to prevent displacement of the cranial contents by gravity. The client with an infratentorial craniotomy should be kept flat and positioned on either side for 24 to 48 hours. This prevents pressure on the neck-area incision site. It also prevents pressure on the internal tumor excision site from higher cerebral structures. The client should receive nothing by mouth (NPO status) for 24 hours because edema around the medulla and lower cranial nerves may place the client at risk for vomiting and aspiration.

Monitoring the Dressing. Check the head dressing every 1 to 2 hours for signs of drainage. Mark the area of drainage once during each shift for baseline comparison. A small or moderate amount of drainage is expected. Some clients may have a Hemovac, Jackson-Pratt, or other surgical drain in place for 24 hours after surgery. Measure the drainage every 8 hours and record the amount and color; a typical amount of drainage is 30 to 50 mL per shift (8 hours). Follow the manufacturer's and surgeon's instructions to maintain suction within the drain. Excessive amounts of drainage (a saturated head dressing or drainage greater than 50 mL/8 hr should be reported immediately to the physician.

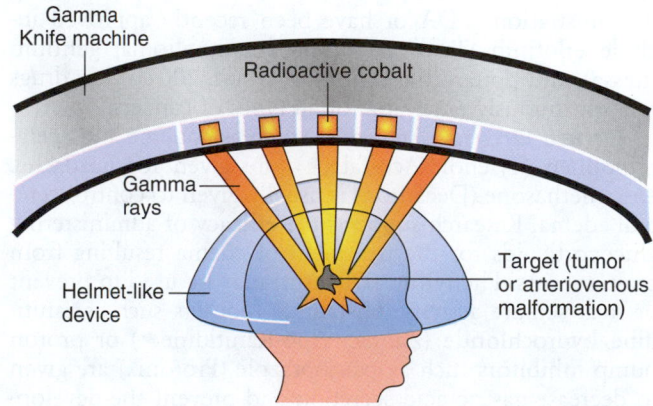

Figure 46-10 ■ A Gamma Knife treatment. The treatment beams are widely dispersed over the surface of the head to prevent damage to healthy brain tissue. The beams are intense only at the point of target.

Text continued on p. 1064.

■ PLAN of CARE   MEDICAL DIAGNOSIS: CRANIOTOMY

NURSING DIAGNOSIS NO. 1 ■ Decreased Intracranial Adaptive Capacity

	Expected Outcomes	Nursing Interventions	Rationales
RELATED FACTORS Decreased cerebral perfusion <60-70 mm Hg Sustained increase in intracranial pressure (ICP) = >15-20 mm Hg Systemic hypotension with intracranial hypertension Brain injuries **DEFINING CHARACTERISTICS** Baseline ICP ≥10-15 mm Hg Disproportionate increase in ICP following a single environmental or nursing maneuver stimulus	Baseline ICP remains ≤15-20 mm Hg Has an ICP that remains stable following nursing activities or environmental stimuli Remains oriented to time, place, person, and situation Has a level of consciousness (LOC) that remains stable	**NIC** **Cerebral Perfusion Promotion** Monitor neurologic status. Calculate and monitor cerebral perfusion pressure (CPP). Monitor client's ICP and neurologic response to care activities. Monitor central venous pressure (CVP) if central venous access is present. Also perform regular physical examinations to assess fluid balance (edema, rales/crackles on lung auscultation), as well as jugular venous distension. Monitor pulmonary artery wedge pressure (PAWP) and pulmonary artery pressure (PAP). Monitor respiratory status (e.g., rate, rhythm, and depth of respirations; Po_2, Pco_2, pH, and bicarbonate levels). Maintain Pco_2 level at 35 mm Hg to avoid hypercarbia. Monitor $Paco_2$, Sao_2, and hemoglobin levels and cardiac output, if available. Administer colloid, blood products, and crystalloid, as appropriate. Administer and titrate vasoactive drugs, as ordered. Maintain serum glucose level within normal range. Consult with physician to determine optimal head of bed (HOB) placement (e.g., 0, 15, or 30 degrees), and monitor the client's responses to head positioning. Avoid neck flexion or extreme hip/knee flexion.	A decrease or change in LOC is typically the first sign of a deterioration in neurologic status. A CPP ≥60-70 mm Hg is needed to provide adequate oxygenation and nutrition to brain tissue. ICP may elevate in response to stimulation from care activities. An elevation in ICP decreases CPP. CVP measures fluid status. ICP elevates with fluid overload. Elevated PAWP and PAP indicates ineffective pumping force of the heart and increased fluid pressure in the lungs, upper extremities, head, and neck. Adequate gas exchange is required for tissue oxygenation. CO_2 is a powerful vasodilator, which causes cerebral vasodilation and increases ICP. $Paco_2$, Sao_2, and hemoglobin levels and cardiac output are determinants of tissue oxygen delivery. Volume expanders maintain hemodynamic parameters. Vasoactive drugs maintain hemodynamic parameters. The brain does not store glucose and needs a constant supply for cellular energy. Hypoglycemia can cause brain damage. Hyperglycemia is associated with increased morbidity and mortality. The client's head should be positioned to best facilitate drainage of blood and cerebrospinal fluid. Absence of neck or hip flexion enhances venous drainage, which prevents increased ICP.

Continued

PLAN of CARE   MEDICAL DIAGNOSIS: CRANIOTOMY—cont'd

NURSING DIAGNOSIS NO. 1 ■ Decreased Intracranial Adaptive Capacity—cont'd

Expected Outcomes	Nursing Interventions	Rationales
	Administer and monitor the effects of osmotic and loop-active diuretics and corticosteroids.	Osmotic diuretics are used to treat cerebral edema by pulling fluid out of edematous brain tissue. A loop-active diuretic may be used to counteract rebound from the osmotic diuretic.
	Administer pain medication, as appropriate.	Pain may increase ICP and other stress-related complications.
	Test stool and nasogastric (NG) drainage for blood.	Clients receiving anticoagulant medication should be observed for signs of bleeding.
	NIC Intracranial Pressure Monitoring	
	Check client for nuchal rigidity or other meningeal signs.	Nuchal rigidity indicates irritation of the meninges and may indicate inflammation or infection, such as meningitis.
	Administer antibiotics.	Antibiotics will treat an infectious process and lower the risk of systemic or intracranial infection.
	Record ICP pressure readings and analyze waveforms.	ICP pressure readings and the characteristics of the waveforms provide indicators of changes in CPP, ICP, and intracranial compliance.
	Other Interventions	
	Give simple, clear explanations.	Increased ICP may affect cognition and make information processing difficult.
	Keep surroundings as quiet and calm as possible.	Stimulation may cause ICP to increase.
	Continuing Care Considerations	
	Provide the client and family with written explanations and instructions.	Brain injury and/or anxiety may affect cognition.
	Refer the family to the National Head Injury Foundation (NHIF), as appropriate.	The foundation provides information and support for clients and their families who are dealing with head injury.

NURSING DIAGNOSIS NO. 2 ■ Impaired Memory

	Expected Outcomes	Nursing Interventions	Rationales
RELATED FACTORS Neurologic impairment Hypoxia, acute **DEFINING CHARACTERISTICS** Inability to recall factual information Inability to recall recent events Inability to learn or retain new skills or information Observed or reported experience of forgetting	Able to recall factual information Able to recall recent or past events Able to learn or retain new skills or information No verbal report or observation of forgetting Able to perform previously learned skill (specify) Has cognitive functions that remain stable No verbal report or observation of impaired memory No verbal report or observation of diminished ability to learn	**NIC Memory Training** Discuss with the client and family any practical memory problems experienced. Reminisce about past experiences with the client, as appropriate. Implement visual imagery, mnemonic devices, memory games, memory cues, association techniques, list making, computers, name tags, or rehearsing of information.	Determine the extent of memory problems and the client's and family's response to those difficulties. Reminiscing about past experiences may assist the client to remember problem-solving skills and techniques previously used. Appropriate memory techniques can assist the client with storage and retrieval of information.

NURSING DIAGNOSIS NO. 2 ■ Impaired Memory—cont'd		
Expected Outcomes	**Nursing Interventions**	**Rationales**
	D Assist in associated learning tasks, as appropriate.	Practice in learning and recalling verbal and pictorial information as presented helps the client to exercise memory and information retrieval.
	Provide for orientation training, as appropriate.	The client can rehearse personal information and dates to improve retention of key information.
	D Have the client engage in games such as matching pairs of cards, as appropriate.	Matching games provide an opportunity for concentration.
	Question the client about a recent outing or other recent notable event.	Questioning the client about a recent event provides an opportunity to use memory for recent events.
	Provide for picture recognition memory, as appropriate.	Pictures trigger memories from storage areas of the brain that are different from those used for speech.
	Structure the teaching methods according to the client's organization of information.	The client's organization of information will determine the logical sequence of learning for the individual.
	Encourage the client to participate in group memory training programs, as appropriate.	Group support and understanding of memory difficulties makes memory problems less threatening.
	Monitor the client's behavior during therapy.	The client may get agitated and frustrated during therapy, which signals the need to stop the session.
	Other Interventions	
	D Encourage the client to use previously learned skills.	Distant memory may remain intact and provide a sense of control to the client.
	Assist the family to understand that assaultive behavior may be the result of poor memory.	Aggressive or combative behavior by the client may signal a threat to self-esteem from memory loss.
	Continuing Care Considerations	
	Collaborate with the client and family to manage tasks that may be difficult for the client (e.g., paying bills).	The client may need to have financial or other protection.

NURSING DIAGNOSIS NO. 3 ■ Impaired Physical Mobility			
	Expected Outcomes	**Nursing Interventions**	**Rationales**
RELATED FACTORS Discomfort Sensoriperceptual impairments Musculoskeletal impairment Neuromuscular impairment Intolerance to activity	Has full or improved range of motion in all joints Has smooth, coordinated movements Able to turn without assistance	**NIC** **Exercise Therapy: Joint Mobility** Collaborate with physical therapy in developing and executing an exercise program.	The physical therapist is the primary health care professional responsible for developing and executing an exercise program.
DEFINING CHARACTERISTICS Limited ability to perform gross motor skills Limited ability to perform fine motor skills Uncoordinated or jerky movement Limited range of motion Difficulty turning	Has stable posture during performance of activities of daily living Has no movement-induced tremor Has skin that remains intact with no bruising or rashes Able to perform fine motor skills Able to perform gross motor skills	Initiate pain control measures before beginning joint exercise. **D** Dress the client in nonrestrictive clothing.	Initiating pain control measures before joint exercise increases the likelihood of client comfort and willingness to engage in the exercise. Nonrestrictive clothing permits full range of joint motion.

Continued

D Indicates tasks that can be delegated to unlicensed assistive nursing personnel at the discretion of the nurse.

≣PLAN of CARE   MEDICAL DIAGNOSIS: CRANIOTOMY—*cont'd*

NURSING DIAGNOSIS NO. 3 ■ Impaired Physical Mobility—*cont'd*

Expected Outcomes	Nursing Interventions	Rationales
	D Encourage active range-of-motion exercises according to regular, planned schedule.	Regular periods of active range-of-motion exercise maximize the exercise benefit to joints.
	Assist the client to develop a schedule for active range-of-motion exercises.	Regular exercise maximizes the benefit of the exercise.
	D Encourage ambulation, if appropriate.	Ambulation is a form of active joint exercise and also improves cardiovascular tone.
	NIC **Positioning**	
	Premedicate the client before turning, as appropriate.	Premedicating the client before turning will increase client comfort and decrease resistance to repositioning from fear of pain.
	D Place the client in the designated therapeutic position.	The designated therapeutic position should cause no undue stress on muscles or joints.
	D Position the client in proper body alignment.	Proper body alignment preserves the functionality of muscles and bony skeleton.
	D Minimize friction and shearing forces when positioning and turning the client.	Friction and shearing forces will cause damage to the skin and underlying tissues.
	D Turn using the log roll technique.	The log roll technique keeps the spinal column in alignment during the turn, which prevents injury to the spinal nerves.
	Apply a foot board to the bed.	A foot board will prevent foot drop.
	D Elevate the head of the bed, as appropriate.	The head of the bed may be elevated to provide countertraction or for comfort if permitted.
	D Turn the client as indicated by skin condition.	Clients should be turned at least every 2 hours and have small position shifts more frequently to prevent pressure injury.
	D Place frequently used objects within reach.	Placing frequently used objects within reach permits the client safe and convenient access.
	Other Interventions	
	Instruct the client in the use of assistive devices.	The client will need instruction to properly use canes, crutches, walkers, splints, or other assistive devices.
	Continuing Care Considerations	
	Refer the client to rehabilitative services, as appropriate.	Ongoing support from physical therapists, occupational therapists, and others may be needed to help the client resume activities of daily living.
	Refer the client to a vocational counselor, as appropriate.	Long-term physical impairment may require the client to change employment.
	Collaborate with community organizations to inform the public about injury prevention.	Injury prevention saves the individual and society as a whole an enormous economic burden.

D Indicates tasks that can be delegated to unlicensed assistive nursing personnel at the discretion of the nurse.

PLAN of CARE   MEDICAL DIAGNOSIS: CRANIOTOMY—cont'd

NURSING DIAGNOSIS NO. 4 ■ Risk for Infection

	Expected Outcomes	Nursing Interventions	Rationales
RELATED FACTORS Invasive procedures Insufficient knowledge to avoid exposure to pathogens Trauma or injury Tissue destruction and increased environmental exposure Increased environmental exposure to pathogens Immunosuppression (steroids)	Denies fatigue Denies weakness Denies nausea Has a blood pressure that remains ±10 mm Hg of baseline Has no observable alterations in personality No verbal report or observation of urgency Has skin with warm undertones Has a heart rate that remains regular, strong, and between 60 and 100 beats/min No verbal report or observation of altered eating habits No verbal report or observation of vomiting Denies headache No verbal report or observation of diarrhea Has a body temperature that remains between 97° and 99.6° F (36.1° and 37.5° C)	**NIC Infection Protection** Monitor for systemic and localized signs and symptoms of infection. Monitor absolute granulocyte count, white blood cell (WBC) count, and differential results. Obtain cultures, as needed. Inspect the condition of any surgical incision/wound. Maintain asepsis for the client at risk. **D** Encourage deep breathing and coughing, as appropriate. **D** Promote sufficient nutritional intake. **D** Encourage fluid intake, as appropriate. **D** Encourage rest. **NIC Infection Control** Administer antibiotic therapy, as appropriate. **Continuing Care Considerations** Teach the client and family about the signs and symptoms of infection and when to report them to the health care provider.	Elevated temperature, pulse, respirations, and fever indicate systemic infection. Redness, heat, swelling, and pain indicate local infection. Elevations in these laboratory tests demonstrate the body's response to infection. Purulent wound drainage indicates infection. A culture will identify the causative agent and indicate the appropriate antibiotic therapy. A surgical incision may be slightly reddened and swollen from tissue damage but remain free of the purulent drainage, excess swelling, or excess local pain that indicates infection. Asepsis will minimize client exposure to pathogenic agents and thus minimize the incidence of infection. Coughing and deep breathing clears the lungs of secretions that may encourage the growth of pathogenic microbes. Adequate nutrition is essential for immune system cell formation and for the repair of damaged body tissues to provide protection against external pathogens. Adequate fluid intake provides for renal clearance of toxins produced by pathogens. Mending tissues requires energy. A fatigued client is stressed and requires greater expenditure of energy to accomplish tasks. Antibiotic therapy should assist the body to destroy pathogens. Early intervention to treat infection prevents untoward complications from the infection and its therapy.

Monitoring Laboratory Values. The laboratory studies monitored postoperatively include complete blood count (CBC), serum electrolyte levels and osmolarity, coagulation studies, and arterial blood gas (ABG) measurements.

The client's hematocrit and hemoglobin concentration may be abnormally low from blood loss during surgery or elevated if the blood was replaced. Hyponatremia (low serum sodium) may occur as a result of fluid volume overload, syndrome of inappropriate antidiuretic hormone (SIADH), or steroid administration. Hypokalemia (low serum potassium) may cause cardiac irritability. Weakness, a change in level of consciousness, and confusion are symptoms of hyponatremia and hypokalemia. Hypernatremia may be caused by meningitis, dehydration, or diabetes insipidus (DI). It is manifested by muscle weakness, restlessness, extreme thirst, and dry mouth. Additional signs of dehydration such as poor skin turgor, thickened lung secretions, and hypotension may be present. Untreated hypernatremia may lead to seizure activity. ABG values are monitored to ensure adequate cerebral oxygenation. DI should be considered if the client voids large amounts of very dilute urine with an increasing serum osmolarity and electrolyte concentration.

Ventilating the Client. Often the client is electively mechanically ventilated and hyperventilated for the first 24 to 48 hours after surgery to prevent increased intracranial pressure (ICP). The goal of controlled ventilation is to keep the partial pressure of arterial carbon dioxide ($PaCO_2$) at about 35 mm Hg, with normal arterial oxygen levels. This is designed to avoid cerebral vasodilation from hypercarbia (increased carbon dioxide) with the resulting rise in ICP. If the client is awake or attempting to breathe at a rate other than that set on the ventilator, medications such as fentanyl citrate or midazolam (Versed) are given to treat pain and anxiety as well as to promote rest and comfort. The client who is intubated is suctioned if indicated by the findings of frequent respiratory assessments. Remember to hyperoxygenate the client carefully before suctioning.

Drug Therapy. Medications routinely given postoperatively include antiepileptic drugs, histamine blockers, proton pump inhibitors, and corticosteroids, such as dexamethasone (Decadron). Analgesics such as codeine are given for pain, and acetaminophen is given for fever or mild pain. Some physicians may elect to administer prophylactic antibiotics to prevent infection.

Preventing Postoperative Complications. Postoperative complications are listed in Table 48-5.

Increased Intracranial Pressure. The major postoperative complication of supratentorial surgery is increased ICP from cerebral edema, hemorrhage, or obstruction of the normal flow of cerebrospinal fluid (CSF). Symptoms of increased ICP include severe headache, deteriorating level of consciousness, restlessness, irritability, and dilated or pinpoint pupils that are slow to react or nonreactive to light. Treatment of increased ICP is the same as that described in the Interventions section of Traumatic Brain Injury on p. 1051.

Hematomas. Subdural and epidural hematomas and intracranial hemorrhage are manifested by severe headache, a change in level of consciousness, progressive neurologic deficits, and herniation syndromes. Bleeding into the posterior fossa may lead to sudden cardiovascular and respiratory arrest. Treatment of a hematoma necessitates surgical re-

---

TABLE 48-5 Postoperative Complications of Craniotomy

Increased intracranial pressure (ICP)
Hematomas
- Subdural hematoma
- Epidural hematoma
- Subarachnoid hemorrhage

Hypovolemic shock
Hydrocephalus
Respiratory complications
- Atelectasis
- Hypoxia
- Pneumonia
- Neurogenic pulmonary edema

Wound infection
Meningitis
Fluid and electrolyte imbalances
- Dehydration
- Hyponatremia
- Hypernatremia

Seizures
Cerebrospinal fluid (CSF) leak
Cerebral edema

---

moval, whereas an intracranial hemorrhage is treated with aggressive medical management (e.g., osmotic diuretics and ICP monitoring).

Hydrocephalus. Hydrocephalus is caused by obstruction of the normal CSF pathway from edema, an expanding lesion such as a hematoma, or blood in the subarachnoid space. Rapidly progressive hydrocephalus produces the classic symptoms of increased ICP. Slowly progressive hydrocephalus is manifested by headache, decreased level of consciousness, irritability, blurred vision, and urinary incontinence. Emergently, an intraventricular catheter (**ventriculostomy**) may be placed to drain CSF for rapidly deteriorating neurologic function. If long-term treatment is required for chronic hydrocephalus, a surgical shunt is inserted to drain CSF to another area of the body. A ventriculoperitoneal or, less often, a ventriculoatrial or lumbar peritoneal shunt procedure is usually performed. A major complication of the shunting procedure is a subdural hematoma from the tearing of bridging veins. An external lumbar drain may also be used temporarily. Additional information about shunts may be found in neuroscience nursing textbooks.

Respiratory Problems. Respiratory complications include atelectasis, pneumonia, and neurogenic pulmonary edema. Atelectasis and pneumonia can be prevented by providing appropriate pulmonary hygiene, turning the client frequently, and encouraging the client to take frequent deep breaths to expand the lungs each hour. The provision of humidified air and incentive spirometry are useful techniques to prevent these complications. Other treatment modalities include endotracheal or oral tracheal suctioning and chest physiotherapy. These measures may cause an increase in ICP. However, close monitoring of the client's status and ICP waveforms allows him or her to receive the benefits of aggressive pulmonary hygiene despite the potential risk.

Neurogenic pulmonary edema is an infrequent but life-threatening complication of neurologic insult such as traumatic brain injury (TBI), brain tumors, or surgery. Its symptoms are the same as those of acute pulmonary edema, but there are no associated cardiac problems. In spite of aggressive treatment, most clients with neurogenic pulmonary edema do not survive the insult.

Wound Infection. Wound infections occur more often in older and debilitated clients and in clients with a history of diabetes, long-term steroid use, obesity, and previous infections. The client may contribute to the problem by rubbing or scratching the wound. If infection is present, the wound appears reddened and puffy. It may begin to separate, is sensitive to touch, and feels warm. The client may or may not be febrile. Treatment is based on the degree and extent of the infection. The nurse may treat a localized infection by simply cleaning it with alcohol or by applying local antibiotics. For more severe infections, systemic antibiotic administration may be required. If the underlying bone is involved, it may need to be removed.

Meningitis. Meningitis is an inflammation of the meninges and may occur as a result of surgery or wound infection, a cerebrospinal fluid (CSF) leak, or contamination during surgery. (See the discussion of meningitis in Chapter 45 for a more complete explanation of this complication.)

Fluid and Electrolyte Imbalances. Complications related to fluid and electrolyte imbalance include DI, syndrome of inappropriate antidiuretic hormone (SIADH), and cerebral salt wasting (CSW). DI is seen most often after supratentorial surgery, especially procedures involving the pituitary gland or hypothalamus. Failure of the posterior pituitary gland to secrete antidiuretic hormone (ADH) leads to failure of the renal tubules to reabsorb water. The client's urine output increases dramatically (it may be up to 10 L/day), and the urine specific gravity drops to below 1.005. Urine osmolarity decreases, whereas serum osmolarity increases. The client may become dehydrated, and hypovolemic shock may develop if this condition is left untreated. Fluid replacement to replace urinary losses and prevent dehydration may be accomplished by having the client increase oral intake or use IV fluids if he or she can do so. Hormonal replacement may also be necessary, especially if fluid loss is greater than 6 L/24 hr. Aqueous vasopressin is short-acting, lasting only 6 to 8 hours. Desmopressin acetate (DDAVP) may be administered for long-term replacement therapy.

Syndrome of inappropriate antidiuretic hormone (SIADH) occurs when the posterior pituitary gland secretes too much ADH, causing water retention. The urine output decreases dramatically, with a urine output of less than 20 mL/hr. Sodium concentration in the urine is normal or elevated, whereas the serum sodium level falls. Other indications of SIADH are loss of thirst, irritability, muscle weakness, and decreased level of consciousness. SIADH is treated by fluid restriction, which is usually sufficient to correct the hyponatremia. Slow, controlled IV infusion of 3% hypertonic sodium may be needed for severe hyponatremia (<118 mEq/L).

Cerebral salt-wasting (CSW) is thought to result from the extrarenal influence of atrial natriuretic factor (ANF). ANF cells are located in the hypothalamus and the right atrium and regulate fluid volume. CSW is believed to be the primary cause of hyponatremia in the neurosurgical population. It is characterized by hyponatremia, decreased serum osmolarity, and decreased blood volume. Serum vasopressin and ANF levels can differentiate CSW and SIADH. CSW is treated with the replacement of sodium and isotonic fluid volume.

Clients with complications related to fluid and electrolyte imbalance undergo strict measurement of their intake and output. An accurate daily weight measurement is an essential aspect of nursing care. The nurse assesses carefully for indications of fluid overload or dehydration during treatment. Serum electrolyte levels and osmolarity are measured daily (or more often if clinically indicated). Chapters 15 and 16 provide additional information on fluid and electrolyte imbalances, and Chapter 66 provides further discussion of SIADH and DI.

❓ *Critical Thinking Challenge*

A young woman was employed as an accountant for a well-known firm. She was planning to be married in 6 months but began to have frequent headaches with occasional nausea and vomiting. After a thorough medical evaluation, she was diagnosed as having a grade 3 astrocytoma. She is scheduled for a craniotomy before radiation via a Gamma Knife and chemotherapy with PCV.

1. What preoperative teaching would you provide for this client?
2. What postoperative complications should you look for? How will you know if she develops any of these problems, and what should you do if she does?
3. What can you tell her to expect during the Gamma Knife procedure?
4. What health teaching does she need regarding her PCV treatments? (Hint: You might need to refer to Chapter 28 to help answer this question.)
5. How can you help her meet her psychosocial needs while her tumor is being treated?

evolve For suggested answer guidelines, go to http://evolve.elsevier.com/Iggy/.

Community-Based Care

The client with a brain tumor is managed at home if possible. The nurse or case manager mobilizes health resources to support the client and family at home. Maintaining a reasonable quality of life is an important goal for recovery and rehabilitation.

HOME CARE MANAGEMENT

Unless the client has a significant degree of disability, no special preparation for home care is needed. Clients with hemiparesis need assistance to ensure that their home is accessible according to their method of mobility (e.g., cane, walker, wheelchair). The environment should be made safe to prevent falls. For example, scatter rugs should be removed and grab bars placed in the bathroom.

Information about the selection of rehabilitation or chronic care facility, if needed, can be obtained from the social worker or discharge planner. The selected facility should have experience in providing care for neurologically impaired clients. A psychologist should be available to provide input in the evaluation of the cognitive disabilities often exhibited by the client.

HEALTH TEACHING

It is important that the client and family fully understand the importance of any recommended follow-up health care appointments. The discharge summary should state the name of the person who has given the follow-up information.

Information given to the client and the family or significant others includes the name of the medications, the dosage, the timing of administration, the number of days to take the medication, and any side effects. Explain what to do or whom to call if any adverse reactions occur. Remind the client to refrain from taking any over-the-counter medications unless authorized by the health care provider.

Instruct the client to maintain a program of regular physical exercise within the limits of any disabilities. Referral to the dietitian may be necessary to ensure adequate caloric intake for the client receiving radiation or chemotherapy.

Seizures are a potential complication that can occur at any time for as long as 1 year or more postoperatively. Provide the client and the family with information about seizure precautions and what to do if a seizure occurs.

If long-term changes or disability is expected, the client needs to be prepared for major lifestyle changes. Chapter 10 discusses coping with disability in more detail.

HEALTH CARE RESOURCES

Refer the client and the family or significant others to the American Brain Tumor Association or the National Brain Tumor Foundation. The American Cancer Society is also an appropriate community resource for clients with malignant tumors. Home care agencies are available to provide both the physical and rehabilitative care that the client may need at home. Hospice services and palliative care may be needed for the terminally ill client. Brain tumor support groups may also be a valuable asset to the client and family.

BRAIN ABSCESS

A **brain abscess** is a purulent infection of the brain in which pus forms in the extradural, subdural, or intracerebral area of the brain. The causative organisms are most often bacteria, which invade the brain directly or indirectly. Cerebral abscesses may be a complication of meningitis infection.

PATHOPHYSIOLOGY

In general, organisms from the ear, sinus, or mastoid area enter the brain by traveling along the wall of the cerebral veins, and therefore they may spread to any area of the brain. At times, the organisms (especially those from the ear) erode the bone, form a tract, and enter the brain directly. Septic emboli from the heart, the lungs, or a dental or peritonsillar abscess may break off and enter the systemic circulation. These organisms may become lodged in a cerebral vessel and produce a localized infection. Penetrating trauma, open head injuries, and neurosurgical procedures provide a potential means for the direct entry of an organism into the brain. In the past 15 years, the number of clients with a brain abscess as a consequence of immunosuppression, organ transplantation, and acquired immunodeficiency syndrome (AIDS) has increased rapidly.

The organisms cause a local infection, and acute inflammation surrounds the involved area. Within a few days, necrosis of the tissue takes place, and pus formation and liquefaction of the tissue occur. This is followed by the development of cerebral edema resulting from localized vascular congestion and tissue swelling in response to inflammation. During the subsequent 2 weeks, the area becomes encapsulated, first by fibrous granulation tissue and later by collagenous connective tissue. The abscess usually occurs deep within the cerebral hemisphere and involves the white matter of the brain. Occasionally the abscess does not become encapsulated but instead spreads through the brain tissue to the subarachnoid space and ventricular system.

The organism varies with the source of the abscess. *Streptococci* are the most common organisms and are often found with other anaerobes such as *Bacteroides*. *Enterobacteriaceae* such as *Escherichia coli* and *Proteus* organisms may also be combined with *Streptococcus*. Yeast and fungi are now implicated in 9% to 17% of cases of cerebral abscess formation, particularly in clients who are immunosuppressed. *Toxoplasma gondii* is the most commonly seen central nervous system (CNS) opportunistic infection in the AIDS population.

Most brain abscesses occur in the frontal and temporal lobes. It is estimated that 5% to 20% of affected clients have more than one abscess. Mortality rates vary from 30% to 60%; abscesses that occur in immunosuppressed clients are associated with a higher mortality rate.

◆COLLABORATIVE MANAGEMENT
◆Assessment

PHYSICAL ASSESSMENT/CLINICAL MANIFESTATIONS

The clinical manifestations of a brain abscess are insidious and are similar to some of the manifestations of meningitis. The client may present with headache, fever, and focal neurologic deficits or nonspecific signs and symptoms. Perform a complete neurologic assessment. The client may be mildly lethargic or somewhat confused. The pupillary response to light is normal in the early stages. As increased intracranial pressure (ICP) progresses, the pupils may become sluggish, unequal, dilated, and nonresponsive to light. The client's level of consciousness declines to a state in which he or she loses the ability to interact with the environment. Airway and respiratory function may also be altered.

Examination of the client's visual fields often reveals a **temporal field blindness** (decrease in peripheral vision laterally). If the abscess affects the cerebral hemispheres, nystagmus and a dysconjugate gaze may be noted. Motor examination reveals a generalized weakness. More significant motor problems, such as hemiplegia, may be apparent in the presence of a frontal lobe abscess. An ataxic gait is seen with a cerebellar abscess. Sensory impairment varies, although the client often exhibits no sensory deficits. The client may have varying degrees of aphasia in the presence of a frontal or temporal lobe abscess. Seizure activity may occur because of irritation of the cortical tissue. Late in the disease process, more severe symptoms of increased ICP occur and include severe headache, coma, a widened pulse pressure, bradycardia, and irregular respirations. The client with AIDS often presents with systemic infection, CNS involvement, and lymphoma.

Some clients may have atypical presentations. Clients with atypical presentations include age extremes, such as older adults (age-related compromise in immune function) and pediatric populations (immature immune system), those receiving steroid therapy, immune-modulating drugs, and clients with later stages of human immunodeficiency virus (HIV) infection (immune system compromise). Particularly in the earlier stages, the inflammatory response (arising from immune system function) is responsible for much of the clinical presentation, particularly if cerebral abscess formation is a consequence of meningitis infection. Any clinical state that affects immune system function or the inflammatory response can lead to an atypical clinical presentation. The risk is that the client may progress to severe abscess formation before the onset of "classic" manifestations.

DIAGNOSTIC TESTS

A complete blood count (CBC) and erythrocyte sedimentation rate (ESR) are typically performed. The white blood cell count (WBC) and ESR are usually elevated, indicating the presence of infection. If the abscess is encapsulated, the WBC may be normal. Obtain specimens for aerobic and, when possible, and anaerobic cultures of the blood, ear, nose, and throat to determine the primary source of infection.

The health care provider orders a computed tomography (CT) scan to determine the presence of cerebritis, hydrocephalus, or a midline shift. Magnetic resonance imaging (MRI) is also useful in detecting the presence of an abscess early in the course of the disease. An EEG can localize the lesion in most cases and shows high-voltage, slow-wave activity; electra-cerebral silence may be noted in the area of the abscess. Radiography of the sinuses and the mastoid is often indicated. A lumbar puncture may be performed if meningitis is also suspected and the client does not exhibit indications of ICP elevation.

◆Interventions

Medications are prescribed by the physician to treat the abscess. Typically used antibiotics include penicillin G benzathine (Bicillin) and nafcillin sodium (Nafcil, Unipen). Metronidazole (Flagyl, Novonidazol✦) or vancomycin may be used if an anaerobic organism is the causative agent. Antibiotic dosing may be adjusted upward to ensure adequate CNS penetration. These agents are particularly useful in the early stages (cerebritis) of abscess formation. A combination of antibiotics is used, particularly if the abscess resulted from septic emboli. Antiepileptic drugs, such as phenytoin (Dilantin), may be used prophylactically to prevent seizures. The medication schedule is strictly followed to maintain therapeutic blood levels. Analgesics may be prescribed to treat headache.

The physician may surgically drain an encapsulated abscess via a burr hole to reduce the mass effect of the lesion. In certain cases a craniotomy may be performed to remove the abscess. The decision to perform surgery is based on the client's general condition, the stage of abscess development, and the site of the abscess. Provide routine preoperative and postoperative care for the client undergoing a craniotomy, as discussed earlier under Postoperative Care (Brain Tumor), p. 1058.

The client with a brain abscess is discharged to home if few or no neurologic deficits are present. Clients with severe dysfunction are usually transferred to long-term care or a rehabilitation facility. Thirty percent of surviving clients have neurologic deficits.

GET READY for the NCLEX Examination!

KEY POINTS

Safe Effective Care Environment

- When caring for a client experiencing a stroke ("brain attack"), assess airway, breathing, and circulation status first.

- Monitor clients with stroke, brain tumor, traumatic brain injury (TBI), and brain abscess for signs and symptoms of increased intracranial pressure (ICP).
- Be aware that the *first* sign of increasing ICP is a decreased level of consciousness (LOC); notify the health care provider immediately if this occurs.
- Monitor for other signs and symptoms of increased ICP as described in Chart 48-5.
- Keep the head of the bed at 30 degrees or as otherwise ordered and the head in a neutral position to prevent increasing ICP and promote venous drainage.
- Collaborate with the case manager to plan care for clients being discharged from the hospital with stroke, brain tumor, TBI, or brain abscess.
- Collaborate with other members of the health care team, especially physical and occupational therapists, and speech-language pathology (SLP), following the acute phase of a stroke.
- Be aware that clients having strokes and traumatic brain injuries are at risk for falls.
- For clients receiving thrombolytics and anticoagulants, monitor carefully for bleeding.

Health Promotion and Maintenance

- Teach clients with risk factors for strokes to avoid or manage them to prevent the chance of having a stroke; risk factors are listed in Chart 48-2.
- Teach the client with hemianopsia to turn his or her head to scan from side to side.
- Remind clients, their families, and significant others to employ home safety measures for clients who have had a stroke.
- Teach young adults, especially men, to avoid risk-taking behaviors, such as driving a motorcycle without a helmet.
- Teach clients with critically ill neurologic problems about their medications, including adverse effects (e.g., antiplatelet drugs for clients who had a stroke).

Psychosocial Integrity

- Recognize that clients with strokes, especially men, may become depressed; monitor for signs of depression, and teach families about what to observe and report to the health care provider.
- Teach the family and significant others of clients with TBI that mood disorders, including depression, are very common, even in mild injury.
- Refer clients with brain tumors and their families to health care resources, such as the American Brain Tumor Association and American Cancer Society, and suggest a brain tumor support group.
- Refer clients who have had a stroke to a local stroke support group.

Physiological Integrity

- Recall that the two major classifications of strokes are ischemic and hemorrhagic; thrombotic and embolic strokes are common types of ischemic strokes.
- Remember that hemorrhagic strokes result most often from severe hypertension, ruptured aneurysms, and arteriovenous malformations (AVMs).
- Assess common clinical manifestations of stroke as listed in Charts 48-3 and 48-4.

- Determine the specific speech and language problems manifested by stroke clients; expressive and receptive aphasia are common.
- In collaboration with the speech-language pathologist (SLP), determine whether the client experiencing a stroke has impaired swallowing; if so, modify the diet and implement swallowing precautions.
- Be aware that traumatic brain injury TBI can be either open head injury or closed head injury and can range in severity from mild to severe.
- Recognize that the priority concern for a client with TBI is prevention and management of increased ICP; interventions are described in Chart 48-6.
- Recall that brain tumors may be benign or malignant, as listed in Table 48-4.
- Note that a brain abscess is an infection within the brain that produces localized inflammation and pus; assess for signs and symptoms similar to those for meningitis (e.g., fever and headache).
- Observe for postoperative complications of craniotomy as listed in Table 48-5.

ADDITIONAL STUDY RESOURCES

Go to your Student CD-ROM for Review Questions for the NCLEX Examination.

Go to http://evolve.elsevier.com/Iggy/ for Integrated Management of Care Questions for the NCLEX Examination.

SELECTED BIBLIOGRAPHY

Asterisk indicates a classic or definitive work on this subject.

*American Brain Tumor Association. (1996). *A primer of brain tumors*. Des Plaines, IL: American Brain Tumor Association.

Arbour, R. (2000). "Mastering neuromuscular blockade". *Dimensions of Critical Care Nursing, 19*(5), 4-18.

Arbour, R. (2004). Intracranial hypertension: Monitoring and nursing assessment. *Critical Care Nurse, 24*(5), 19-34.

Armstrong, T., & Gilbert, M.R. (2000). Metastatic brain tumors: Diagnosis, treatment and nursing interventions. *Clinical Journal of Oncology Nursing, 4*(5), 217-225.

Bader, M.K., & Palmer, S. (2000). Keeping the brain in the zone: Applying the severe head trauma guidelines to practice. *Critical Care Nursing Clinics of North America, 12*(4), 413-427.

Bayir, H., Clark, R.S.B., & Kochanek, P.M.. (2003). Promising strategies to minimize secondary brain injury after head trauma. *Critical Care Medicine, 31*(1 suppl), S-112- S-117.

Becskee, T., & Jallo, G. (2002). Subarachnoid hemorrhage. eMedicine Journal. Accessed February 7, 2002, from http://www.emedicine.com.

*Blank-Reid, C. (1996). How to have a stroke at an early age: The effects of crack, cocaine, and other illicit drugs. *Journal of Neuroscience Nursing, 28*(1), 19-27.

*Bohan, E.M., & Weingart, J. (1998). Neurosurgical management of primary brain tumors: Diagnosis, treatment and future trends. *Journal of Neuroscience Nursing, 30*(6), 361-362.

Bonnono, C., et al. (2000). Emergi-paths and stroke teams: An emergency department approach to acute ischemic stroke. *Journal of Neuroscience Nursing, 32*(6), 298-305.

Brown, D.M., & and Levine, S.R. (2003). Highlights from the 28th international stroke conference. Accessed April 20, 2003, from http://www.medscape.com/viewarticle/451138_print.

Censullo, J.L., & Sebastian, S. (2003). Pentobarbital sodium coma for refractory intracranial hypertension. *Journal of Neuroscience Nursing, 35*(5), 252-262.

Davis, A. (2000). Mechanisms of traumatic brain injury: Biomechanical, structural and cellular considerations. *Critical Care Nurse Quarterly, 23*(3), 1-13.

Del Castillo, M.A. (2001). Monitoring neurologic patients in intensive care. *Curr Opin in Crit Care, 7*, 49-60.

Felberg, R.A., and Naidech, A.M. (2003). The 5 Ps of acute ischemic stroke treatment: Parenchyma, pipes, penumbra and prevention of complications. *Southern Medical Journal, 96*(4), 336-342.

Fernandes H.M., et al. (2000) Continuous monitoring of ICP and CPP following ICH and its relationship to clinical, radiological and surgical parameters. *Acta Neurochir (Suppl), 76*, 463-466.

Georgiadis, D., et al. (2001). Influence of positive end-expiratory pressure in intracranial pressure and cerebral perfusion pressure in patients with acute stroke. *Stroke 32*, 2088-2092.

Goldszmidt, A.J., & Caplan, L.R. (2003). *Stroke essentials*. Royal Oak, MI: Physicians' Press.

Guidelines for cerebral perfusion pressure. (2000). *Journal of Neurotrauma, 17*(6/7), 507-512.

Harvey, J. (2004). Countering "brain attacks." *Nursing Management, 35*(8), 27-32.

Hickey, J.V. (2003). *The clinical practice of neurological and neurosurgical nursing* (5th ed.). Philadelphia: J.B. Lippincott.

Hilton, G. (2000) Cerebral oxygenation in the traumatically brain-injured patient: Are ICP and CPP enough? *Journal of Neuroscience Nursing, 32*, 278-282.

Hinkle, J.L., & Bowman, L. (2003). Pharmacology update: Neuroprotection for ischemic stroke. *Journal of Neuroscience Nursing, 35*(2), 114-118.

Hlatky, R., et al. (2003). Intracranial hypertension and cerebral ischemia after severe traumatic brain injury. Retrieved May 14, 2003, from http://www.medscape.com/viewarticle/452766_print.

Hung, O.R., et al. (2000). Head elevation reduces head-rotation associated increased ICP in patients with intracranial tumors. *Canadian Journal of Anesthesia, 47*(5), 415-420.

*Indications for intracranial pressure monitoring. (2000). *Journal of Neurotrauma, 17*, 479-491.

Intracranial pressure treatment threshold. (2000). *Journal of Neurotrauma, 17*(6/7), 493-495.

Jacobi, J., et al. (2002). Clinical practice guidelines for the sustained use of sedatives and analgesics in the critically ill adult. *Critical Care Medicine, 30*(1), 119-141.

*Jauch, E.C., & Elias, B. (1999). Intracerebral hemorrhage: Pathophysiology and management. *Air Medical Journal, 18*(2), 62-67.

Kelley, R.E., & Minagar, A. (2003). Cardioembolic stroke: An update. *Southern Medical Journal, 96*(4), 343-349.

Kondziolka, D., et al. (2002). The role of cell therapy in stroke. Accessed January 26, 2003, from http://www.medscape.com/viewarticle/446194_print.

Libby, P. (2002). Atherosclerosis: The new view. *Scientific American, May*, 47-55.

Littlejohns, L.R., & Bader, M.K. (2001). Guidelines for the management of severe head injury: Clinical application and changes in practice. *Critical Care Nurse, 21*(6), 48-65.

Liu, J.K., et al. (2003). Conduits for cerebrovascular bypass and lessons learned from the cardiovascular experience. Accessed April 24, 2003, from http://www.medscape.com/viewarticle/451256_print.

Lutz, B.J. (2004). Determinants of discharge destination for stroke patients. *Rehabilitation Nursing, 29*(5), 154-163.

March, K. (2000a). Intracranial pressure monitoring and assessing intracranial compliance in brain injury. *Critical Care Nursing Clinics of North America, 12*, 429-436.

March, K. (2000b). Application of technology in the treatment of traumatic brain injury. *Critical Care Nursing Quarterly, 23*(3), 26-37.

Mateo, M.A. (2003). Evaluation of patients with mild traumatic brain injury. *Lippincott's Case Management, 8*(5), 203-207.

NIH Consensus Development Panel on rehabilitation of Persons with Traumatic Brain Injury. (2000). Rehabilitation of persons with traumatic brain injury. *Journal of the American Medical Association, 282*(10), 974-986.

Nolan, S., Naylor, G., & Burns, M. (2003). Code Gray—An organized approach to inpatient stroke. *Critical Care Nurse Quarterly, 26*(4), 296-302.

Recommendations for intracranial pressure monitoring technology. (2000). *Journal of Neurotrauma,* 17 (6/7), 497-506.

Resuscitation of blood pressure and oxygenation. (2000). *Journal of Neurotrauma, 17*(6/7), 471-478.

Rhoney, D.H., & Parker, D. (2001). Use of sedative and analgesic agents in neurotrauma patients: Effects on cerebral physiology. *Neurological Research, 23,* 237-259.

Robertson, C.S. (2001) Management of cerebral perfusion pressure after traumatic brain injury. Anesthesiology, *95,* 1513-1517.

Roth, P., & Farls, K. (2000). Pathophysiology of traumatic brain injury. *Critical Care Nursing Quarterly, 23*(3), 14-25.

Shepard, S. (2001). Head trauma. Accessed February 7, 2002, from http://www.medscape.com.

Smillova, A., & Walker, E. (2000). Meningococcemia: A critical care emergency. *Critical Care Nurse, 20*(5), 28-38.

Stubgen, J.-P., & Caronna, J.J. (2002). Coma. In J. E. Parillo & R.P. Dellinger (Eds.), *Critical care medicine: Principles of diagnosis and management in the adult.* St. Louis: Mosby.

Thompson, H.J. (2000). Managing patients with lumbar drainage devices. *Critical Care Nurse, 20*(5), 59-68.

Tolias, C., & Sgouros, S. (2001). Initial evaluation and management of CNS injury. *eMedicine Journal, 2*(10). Accessed November 29, 2001 from http://www.emedicine.com/med/topic3216.htm.

Torbey, M.T., & Bhardwaj, A. (2001). How to manage blood pressure in critically ill neurologic patients. *The Journal of Critical Illness, 16*(4), 179-192.

Tummala, R.P., et al. (2003). Extracranial-intracranial bypass for symptomatic occlusive cerebrovascular disease not amenable to carotid endarterectomy. Accessed April 24, 2003, from http://www.medscape.com/viewarticle/451261_print.

Vinas, F.C. (2001). Bedside invasive monitoring techniques in severe brain-injured patients. *Neurological. Research, 23,* 157-166.

Winkleman, C. (2000). Effect of backrest position on intracranial and cerebral perfusion pressures in traumatically brain-injured adults. *American Journal of Critical Care, 9,* 373-382.

Wojner, A.W., El-Mitwalli, A., & Alexandrov, A.V. (2002). Effect of head positioning on intracranial blood flow velocities in acute ischemic stroke: A pilot study. *Critical Care Nurse Quarterly, 25*(4), 57-66.

Wong, F.W.H. (2000). Prevention of secondary brain injury. *Critical Care Nurse, 20*(5), 18-27.

Wood, D. (2004). Into the brain: Unlocking new brain cancer treatments. *Cure: Cancer Updates, Research, and Education, 3*(1), 22-30.

Xavier, A.R., et al. (2003). Neuroimaging of stroke: A review. *Southern Medical Journal, 96*(4), 367-379.

Zuccarelli, L.A. (2000). Altered cellular anatomy and physiology of acute brain injury and spinal cord injury. *Critical Care Nursing Clinics of North America, 12*(4), 403-412.

Zweifler, R.M. (2003). Management of acute stroke. *Southern Medical Journal, 96*(4), 380-385.

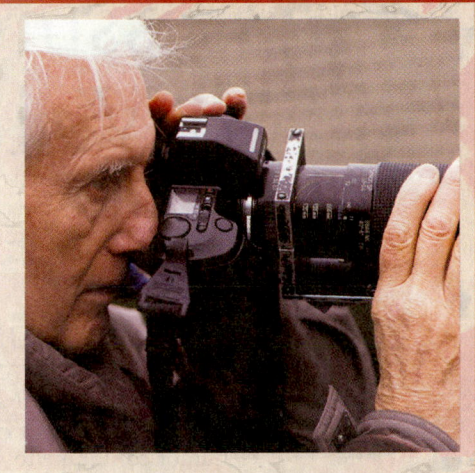

PROBLEMS of SENSATION

Management of Clients with Problems of the Sensory System

Assessment of the Eye and Vision

M. LINDA WORKMAN

 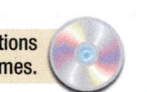
Vision is considered by many people to be their most important sense. Vision begins with the eye and is fully perceived in the brain. Many conditions can affect the eye and change vision temporarily or permanently. Changes in the eye and vision can provide information about the client's general health status and problems that might occur in self-care.

ANATOMY AND PHYSIOLOGY REVIEW

Structure

The eyeball, a round, ball-shaped organ about 2.5 cm long and 2.3 cm in diameter, is located in the front part of the eye orbit. The **orbit** is the bony socket of the skull that surrounds and protects the eye along with the attached muscles, nerves, vessels, and tear-producing glands.

LAYERS OF THE EYEBALL

The eye has three layers, or coats (Figure 49-1). The external layer is the **sclera** (the opaque tissue making up the "whites" of the eye) and the transparent cornea on the front of the eye.

The middle layer, or **uvea,** is heavily pigmented. This layer consists of the choroid, the ciliary body, and the iris. The choroid, a dark brown membrane between the sclera and the retina, lines most of the sclera. The choroid has many blood vessels that supply nutrients to the retina.

The ciliary body connects the choroid with the iris and secretes aqueous humor. The **iris** is the colored portion of the external eye; its center opening is the **pupil.** The muscles of the iris contract and relax to control pupil size and the amount of light entering the eye.

The innermost layer is the **retina,** a thin, delicate structure made up of sensory receptors that transmit impulses to the optic nerve. The retina contains blood vessels and two types of photoreceptors called rods and cones. The rods work at low light levels and provide peripheral vision. The cones are active at bright light levels and provide color and central vision.

The **optic fundus** is the area at the inside back of the eye that can be seen with an ophthalmoscope. This area contains the **optic disc,** a creamy pink to white depressed area in the retina (Figure 49-2). The optic nerve enters the eyeball at this point. The optic disc is sometimes called the "blind spot" because it contains only nerve fibers and no photoreceptor cells. To one side of the optic disc is a small, yellow-

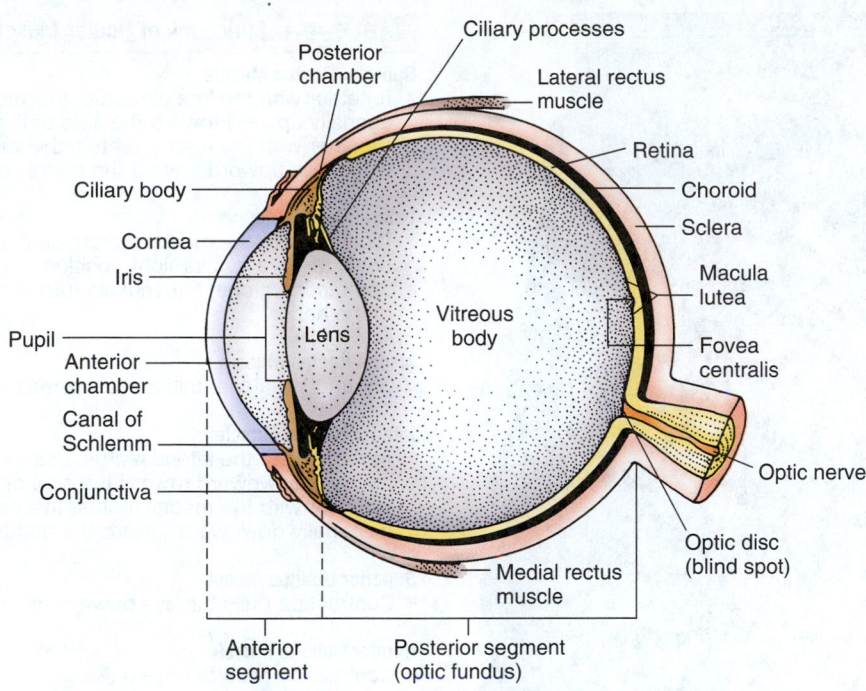

Figure 49-1 ■ Anatomic features of the eye.

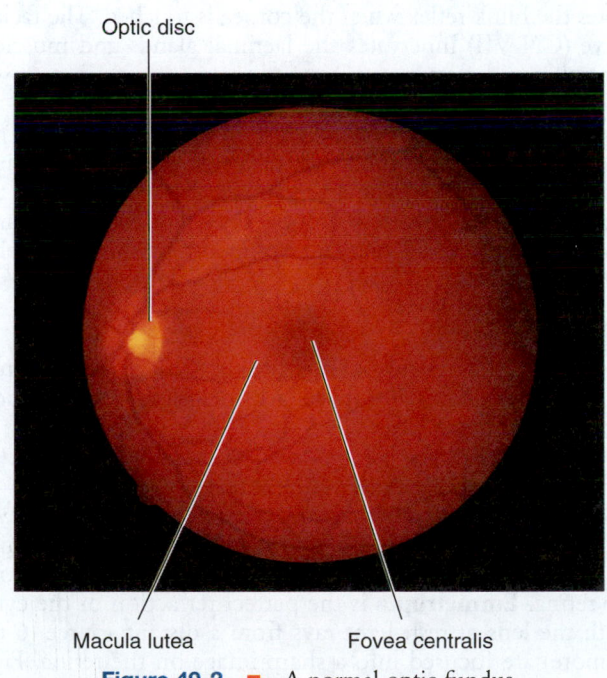

Figure 49-2 ■ A normal optic fundus.

ish pink area called the macula lutea. The center of the macula is the *fovea centralis*, where vision is the most acute.

REFRACTIVE STRUCTURES AND MEDIA

Light waves pass through the following structures on the way to the retina: cornea, aqueous humor, lens, and vitreous humor. Each of these structures has a different density, which causes the light waves to bend **(refract)** to some degree and focus images on the retina. These structures are the eye's refracting media.

The **cornea** is the clear layer that forms the external coat on the front of the eye (see Figure 49-1). The **aqueous humor** is a clear, watery fluid that fills the anterior and posterior chambers of the eye. Aqueous humor is continually produced by the ciliary processes and passes from the posterior chamber, through the pupil, and into the anterior chamber. This fluid drains through the canal of Schlemm into the blood to maintain a balanced intraocular pressure (IOP), the pressure within the eye.

The **lens** is a circular, convex structure that lies behind the iris and in front of the vitreous body. It is normally transparent. The lens bends the rays of light entering through the pupil so that they focus properly on the retina. The curve of the lens changes to focus on near or distant objects.

The **vitreous body** is a clear, thick gel that fills the vitreous chamber (the space between the lens and the retina). This gel transmits light and shapes the eye.

EXTERNAL STRUCTURES

The eyelids are thin, movable folds of skin that protect the eyes, shut out light during sleep, and keep the cornea moist. The upper eyelid is larger than the lower one. The **canthus** is the place where the two eyelids meet at the corner of the eye.

The **conjunctivae** are the mucous membranes of the eye. The palpebral conjunctiva is a thick membrane with many blood vessels that lines the under surface of each eyelid. Located over the sclera is the thin, transparent bulbar conjunctiva.

Tears are produced by a small **lacrimal gland,** which is located in the upper outer part of each orbit (Figure 49-3). Tears flow across the front of the eye, toward the nose, and into the inner canthus. They drain through the **punctum** (an opening at the nasal side of the lid edges), into the lacrimal duct and sac, and then into the nose through the nasolacrimal duct.

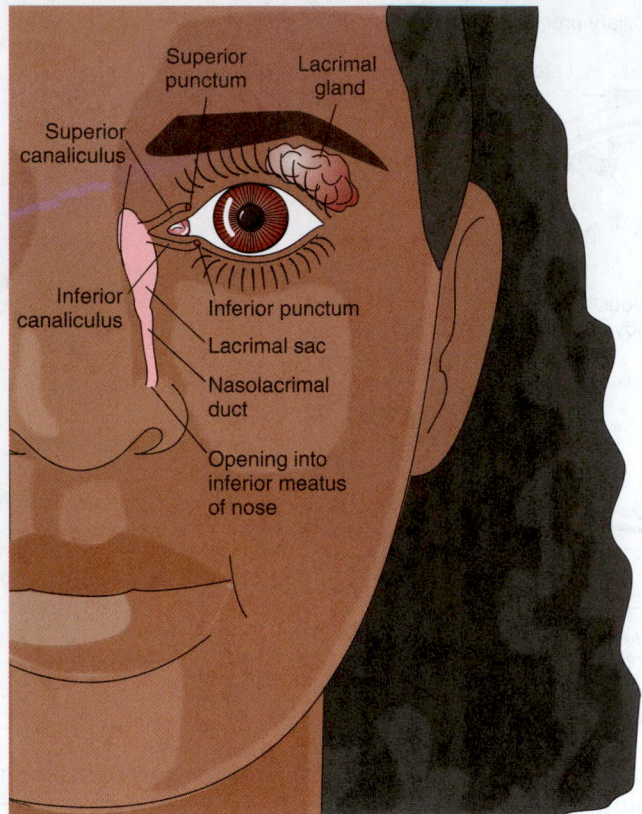

Figure 49-3 ■ Anterior view of the eye and adjacent structures.

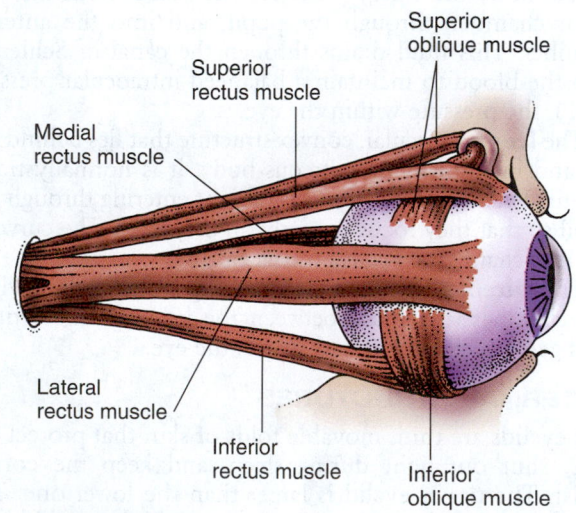

Figure 49-4 ■ The extraocular muscles.

MUSCLES

Six voluntary muscles rotate the eye and coordinate eye movements (Figure 49-4). Table 49-1 lists the functions of these muscles. Coordinated eye movements ensure that the retina of each eye receives an image at the same time so only a single image is seen.

NERVES

The muscles around the eye are innervated by cranial nerves (CN) III (oculomotor), IV (trochlear), and VI (abducens). The **optic nerve** (CN II) is the nerve of sight, connecting the op-

---

TABLE 49-1 Functions of Ocular Muscles

Superior Rectus Muscle
- Together with the lateral rectus, this muscle moves the eye diagonally upward toward the side of the head.
- Together with the medial rectus, this muscle moves the eye diagonally upward toward the middle of the head.

Lateral Rectus Muscle
- Together with the medial rectus, contraction of this muscle holds the eye in a straight position.
- Contracting alone, this muscle turns the eye toward the side of the head.

Medial Rectus Muscle
- Contracting alone, this muscle turns the eye toward the nose.

Inferior Rectus Muscle
- Together with the lateral rectus, this muscle moves the eye diagonally downward toward the side of the head.
- Together with the medial rectus, this muscle moves the eye diagonally downward toward the middle of the head.

Superior Oblique Muscle
- Contraction pulls the eye downward.

Inferior Oblique Muscle
- Contraction pulls the eye upward.

---

tic disc to the brain. Part of the trigeminal nerve (CN V) stimulates the blink reflex when the cornea is touched. The facial nerve (CN VII) innervates the lacrimal glands and muscles controlling lid closure.

BLOOD VESSELS

The ophthalmic artery brings oxygenated blood to the eye and structures in the orbit. This artery branches to supply blood to the retina. The ciliary arteries supply the sclera, choroid, ciliary body, and iris. Venous drainage occurs through the two ophthalmic veins.

Function

The four eye functions that provide clear images of near and far objects are refraction, pupillary constriction, accommodation, and convergence.

REFRACTION

The different curved surfaces and refractive media of the eye allow light to pass through to the retina. Each surface and media bends (refracts) light differently to focus an image on the retina. **Emmetropia** is the perfect refraction of the eye: With the lens at rest, light rays from a distant source (6 m or more) are focused into a sharp image on the retina. Figure 49-5 shows the normal refraction of light within the eye. Images fall on the retina inverted and reversed left to right. For example, an object in the lower nasal visual field strikes the upper outer area of the retina.

Errors of refraction are common. **Hyperopia** (also called hypermetropia or farsightedness) occurs when the eye does not refract light enough. As a result, images actually fall (converge) behind the retina (see Figure 49-5). Vision beyond 20 feet is normal, but near vision is poor. Hyperopia is corrected with a convex lens in eyeglasses or contact lenses.

Myopia (nearsightedness) occurs when the eye overrefracts or overbends the light. As a result, images are focused in front of the retina (see Figure 49-5). Near vision is normal, but dis-

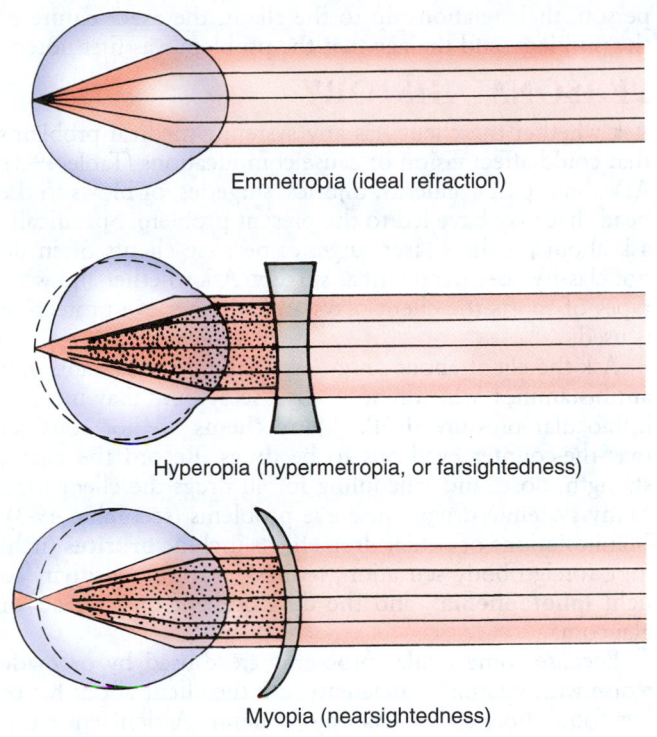

Emmetropia (ideal refraction)

Hyperopia (hypermetropia, or farsightedness)

Myopia (nearsightedness)

Figure 49-5 ■ Refraction and correction in emmetropia, hyperopia, and myopia.

CHART 49-1

NURSING FOCUS on the OLDER ADULT
Changes in the Eye Related to Aging

Structure/Function	Change
Appearance	Eyes appear to be sunken. Arcus senilis forms. Sclera yellows or appears blue.
Cornea	Cornea flattens, which causes blurring of vision.
Ocular muscles	Muscle strength is reduced, which results in a diminished capacity to maintain an upward gaze and to maintain a single image.
Lens	Elasticity is lost, which increases the near point of vision. Lens hardens and becomes compact. Cataracts form.
Iris	Decrease in ability to dilate results in small pupil size and poor adaptation to darkness.
Pupil	Pupil size is smaller. Aperture size takes longer to change, which reduces the ability to see in dim light.
Color vision	Discrimination among colors of short wavelength (green, blue, violet) decreases.
Tears	Diminished tear production results in dry eyes, increasing discomfort and risk for infection.

---

tance vision is poor. Myopia is corrected with a biconcave lens in eyeglasses or contact lenses.

Astigmatism is a refractive error caused by unevenly curved surfaces on or in the eye, especially of the cornea. These uneven surfaces distort vision.

PUPILLARY CONSTRICTION

The pupil controls the amount of light that enters the eye. If the level of light to one or both eyes is increased, both pupils constrict (become smaller). The amount of constriction depends on how much light is available and how well the retina can adapt to light changes. Pupillary constriction is called **miosis,** and pupillary dilation is called **mydriasis.** Drugs can alter pupillary constriction.

ACCOMMODATION

The healthy eye can focus images sharply on the retina whether the image is close to the eye or distant. The process of maintaining a clear visual image when the gaze is shifted from a distant to a near object is known as **accommodation.** The eye is able to adjust its focus by changing the curve of the lens.

Eye Changes Associated with Aging

Changes inside the eye cause visual acuity to decrease with age. Age-related changes of the nervous system and in the eye support structures also reduce visual function (Chart 49-1).

Age-Related Structural Changes

In the older adult, decreased eye muscle tone reduces the ability to keep gaze focused on a single object. The lower eyelid may relax and fall away from the eye (ectropion), exposing more of the eye and leading to dry-eye symptoms.

Arcus senilis, an opaque, bluish white ring within the outer edge of the cornea, is caused by fat deposits (Figure 49-6). Although it is very common, not all older people have arcus senilis. Its presence does not affect vision.

The clarity and shape of the cornea change with age. After age 65, the cornea flattens and the curve of its surface becomes irregular. This change causes or worsens astigmatism and distorts or blurs vision.

Fatty deposits cause the sclera to develop a yellowish tinge. A bluish color may be seen as the sclera thins. With increasing age, the iris has less ability to dilate, which leads to difficulty in adapting to dark environments. Older adults may need additional light for reading.

Age-Related Functional Changes

The lens yellows with aging, reducing the ability of the eye to transmit and focus light. The aging lens hardens, shrinks, and loses elasticity. As the lens loses elasticity, the ability of the eye to accommodate is gradually lost. The **near point of vision** (the closest distance at which the eye can see an object clearly) increases. Near objects (especially reading material) must be placed farther from the eye to be seen clearly. This age-related change is called **presbyopia.** In addition, the **far point** (farthest point at which an object can be distinguished) decreases. Thus the older person has a narrower visual field.

As a person ages, general color perception decreases, especially among the colors of green, blue, and violet. More light is needed to stimulate the visual receptors. Intraocular pressure (IOP) is slightly higher in older adults.

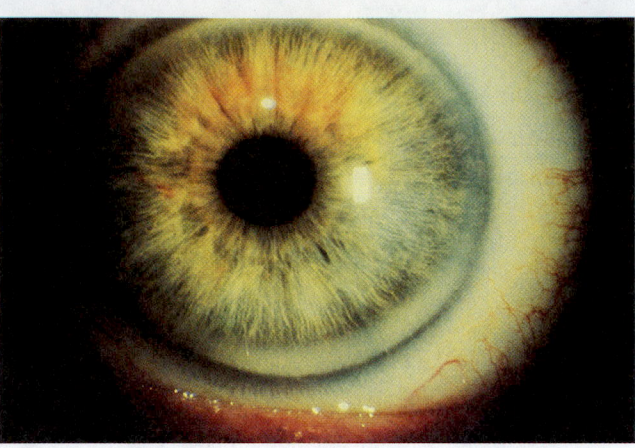

Figure 49-6 ■ Arcus senilis of the iris.

CHART 49-2

Eye and Vision Assessment
USING GORDON'S FUNCTIONAL HEALTH PATTERNS

Cognition Perceptual Pattern
- Do you have any difficulty seeing objects at a distance?
- Do you have any difficulty reading fine print or doing close work?
- Do you wear eyeglasses or contact lenses?
- What type of light do you use for reading?
- Do you wear sunglasses or a hat when outdoors?
- Do you have frequent headaches?
- Have you noticed any change in your ability to see things at night?
- When did you last have your eyes examined?
- Do you go to an ophthalmologist or an optometrist?
- When were you last tested for glaucoma?

Based on Gordon, M. (2002). *Manual of nursing diagnosis* (10th ed.). St. Louis: Mosby.

ASSESSMENT TECHNIQUES

History

Collect subjective information from the client to determine whether problems with the eye or vision have an impact on daily functioning. Chart 49-2 lists some questions to ask when assessing eye and vision history.

DEMOGRAPHIC DATA

Age is an important factor to consider when assessing the visual processes and eye structure. The incidence of glaucoma and cataract formation increases with aging. Presbyopia commonly begins in the 40s.

Gender also may be important. For example, retinal detachments are more common in men, and dry-eye symptoms are more common in women.

FAMILY HISTORY AND GENETIC RISK

Ask the client about a family history of eye problems. Some conditions, such as a refractive error, show a familial tendency. In addition, some genetic problems lead to visual impairment in adulthood. Table 49-2 lists some eye and vision problems that may have a genetic basis. When a client tells you that other relatives, especially first-degree relatives, have eye problems, be sure to record the gender of the affected

person, their relationship to the client, the exact nature of the problem, and the age that the problem was first noted.

PERSONAL HISTORY

Ask whether the client has any systemic medical problems that could affect vision or cause complications (Table 49-3). Ask about past accidents, injuries, surgeries, or blows to the head that may have led to the present problem. Specifically ask about previous laser surgeries because clients often do not classify laser treatment as surgery. Ask whether and what types of sports the client plays and whether eye protection is used.

Ask the client about drugs, especially decongestants and antihistamines, which tend to dry the eye and may increase intraocular pressure (IOP). Many clients do not consider over-the-counter eyedrops to be drugs. Record the name, strength, dose, and scheduling for all drugs the client uses. Many systemic drugs cause eye problems (see Table 49-3). Manifestations of ocular drug effects include **pruritus** (itching), foreign body sensation, redness, tearing, sensitivity to light **(photophobia),** and the development of cataracts or glaucoma.

Because some ocular problems are caused by or made worse with vitamin deficiencies, ask the client about his or her food choices. For example, vitamin A deficiency can cause eye dryness, keratomalacia, and blindness.

Ask the client about his or her work and specifically how the eyes are used. In some occupations, such as computer programming, constant exposure to monitor screens may lead to eyestrain and the need for eyeglasses. Machine operators are at risk for eye injury because of the high speeds at which particles can be thrown at the eye. Ask the client who works in industrial settings about the use of protective eyewear, such as goggles. Chronic exposure to infrared or ultraviolet light may cause photophobia and cataract formation.

CURRENT HEALTH PROBLEMS

Ask the client about the onset of visual changes. Did the change occur rapidly or slowly? *A client with a sudden or persistent loss of vision within the past 48 hours should be seen immediately by an ophthalmologist, as should the client experiencing trauma, a foreign body in the eye, sudden ocular pain, or sudden redness.* Determine whether the same symptoms are present to the same degree in both eyes.

Ask the following questions if ocular injury or eye trauma is involved:

- How long ago did the injury occur?
- What was the client doing when it happened?
- If a foreign body was involved, what was its source?
- Was any first aid administered at the scene? If so, what actions were taken?

Physical Assessment
INSPECTION

Look for head tilting, squinting, or other noticeable actions that offer clues to compensatory stances for attaining clear vision. For example, clients with double vision may cock the head to the side in an attempt to focus the two images into one, or they may close one eye to see more clearly.

TABLE 49-2 Genetic Disorders Affecting the Eye and Vision in Adults

Disorder	Eye and Vision Problems	Related Health Problems	Inheritance Pattern
Retinitis pigmentosa	Increased pigmentation leading to night blindness and reduced visual fields, eventually progressing to total blindness	None consistently present	AR (85%-90% AD (10%) XL (<1%)
Cone-rod retinal dystrophy	Colorblindness, night blindness, reduced peripheral vision, eventually progressing to total blindness	None consistently present	AR
Bothnia retinal dystrophy	Atrophy of rods, night blindness, eventually progressing to total blindness	None consistently present	AD
Ocular albinism	Decreased visual acuity, myopia, colorblindness	None consistently present	XL
Pericentral pigmentary retinopathy	Progressive retinal degeneration and atrophy in young adults, progressing to total blindness by 6th and 7th decades of life	None consistently present	AD
Alström syndrome	Retinal atrophy and progressive blindness	Diabetes mellitus, obesity	AR
Usher syndrome	Progressive retinal pigmentation and total blindness	Progressive hearing loss	AR
Amyloidosis	Corneal dystrophy, reduced acuity	Cutaneous amyloidosis	XL
Choroidal sclerosis	Progressive degeneration of choroidal capillaries and retinal epithelial atrophy, blindness	None consistently present	XL
Rieger syndrome	Early onset glaucoma	None consistently present	AD

AD, Autosomal dominant; *AR,* autosomal recessive; *XL,* X-linked.

TABLE 49-3 Extraocular Conditions Affecting the Eye and Vision

Systemic Disorders	Drugs
■ Diabetes mellitus	■ Antihistamines
■ Hypertension	■ Decongestants
■ Lupus erythematosus	■ Antibiotics
■ Sarcoidosis	■ Opioids
■ Thyroid dysfunction	■ Anticholinergics
■ Acquired immunodeficiency syndrome	■ Cholinergic agonists
■ Cardiac disease	■ Sympathomimetics
■ Multiple sclerosis	■ Oral contraceptives
■ Pregnancy	■ Antineoplastic agents
	■ Corticosteroids
	■ Carbonic anhydrase inhibitors
	■ Beta blockers

Assess for symmetry in the appearance of the eyes. Check the eyes to determine whether they are equal distance from the nose, the same size, and of the same degree of prominence. Assess the eyes for their placement in the orbits and for symmetry of movement. **Exophthalmos** (proptosis) is protrusion of the eye. **Enophthalmos** is the sunken appearance of the eye.

Assess the eyebrows and eyelashes for hair distribution, and determine the direction of the eyelashes. Eyelashes normally point outward and away from the eyelid. Assess the eyelids for **ptosis** (drooping), redness, lesions, or swelling. The lids normally close completely, with the upper and lower lid edges touching. When the eyes are open, the upper lid covers a small portion of the iris. The edge of the lower lid lies below the line between the cornea and sclera. No sclera should be visible between the eyelid and the iris.

Scleral and Corneal Assessment

Examine the sclera for color; it is usually white. A yellow color may indicate jaundice or systemic problems. In dark-skinned people the normal sclera may appear yellow, and small, pigmented dots may be visible (Jarvis, 2004).

The cornea is best observed by directing a light at it from the side using several angles. The cornea should be transparent, smooth, shiny, and bright. Any cloudy areas or specks may be the result of accidents or injuries.

Assess the blink reflex by bringing a fist quickly toward the client's face; clients with vision will blink. This reflex can also be assessed by expelling a syringe full of air toward the eyes. The client blinks if the reflex is intact.

Pupillary Assessment

The pupils are usually round and of equal size. About 5% of people normally have a noticeable difference in the size of their pupils **(anisocoria).** Pupil size varies in people exposed to the same amount of light. Pupils are smaller in older adults. People with myopia have larger pupils; people with hyperopia have smaller pupils. The normal pupil diameter is between 3 and 5 mm.

Observe the pupils for their response to light. Increasing light causes constriction, whereas decreasing light causes dilation. Constriction of both pupils is the normal response to direct light and to accommodation. Assess pupillary reaction to light by asking the client to look straight ahead while quickly bringing the beam of a penlight in from the side and directing it at the right pupil. Constriction of the right pupil is a direct response to shining the penlight into that eye. Constriction of the left pupil when light is shined at the right pupil is known as a **consensual response.** Assess the direct and consensual responses for each eye.

Evaluate each pupil for speed of reaction. The pupil should immediately constrict when a light is directed at it. This rapid response is termed **brisk.** If the pupil takes more than 1 second to constrict, the response is termed **sluggish.** Pupils that fail to react are termed **nonreactive** or **fixed.** Compare the reactivity speed of right and left pupils and document any difference.

In assessing for accommodation, hold the index finger about 18 cm from the client's nose and move it toward the

Video Clip: External Eye ▶

Video Clip: Pupil Responses ◀

nose. The client's eyes normally converge during this movement, and the pupils constrict equally. When accommodation stops, the pupils begin to enlarge and return to their normal size.

MEASUREMENT OF VISION

Vision is measured by various tests. First test each eye separately, and then test both eyes together. Clients who wear corrective lenses are tested both without and with their lenses.

Acuity

Visual acuity tests measure both distance and near vision. The Snellen chart, or "eye chart," is a simple tool to measure distance vision. This chart has letters, numbers, pictures, or a single letter presented in various positions (Figure 49-7). Have the client stand 20 feet from the chart, cover one eye, and use the other eye to read the line that appears most clear. If the client can do this accurately, ask him or her to read the next lower line. Repeat this sequence to the last line on which the client can correctly identify most characters. Repeat the procedure with the other eye. Record findings as a comparison between

what the client can read at 20 feet and the distance at which a person with normal vision can read the same line. For example, 20/50 means that the client is able to see at 20 feet from the chart what a "healthy eye" can see at 50 feet.

For clients who are in a confined space that does not permit a 20-foot distance to the eye chart or who cannot see the 20/400 character, visual acuity is assessed by holding fingers in front of their eyes and asking them to count (Figure 49-8). This procedure is repeated five times. Acuity is recorded as "count fingers vision at 5 feet," or the farthest distance at which the client can count the fingers correctly.

Clients who cannot count fingers are tested for hand motion (HM) acuity. Stand about 2 to 3 feet in front of the client. Ask the client to cover the eye not being tested. Direct a light onto your hand from behind the client. Demonstrate the three possible directions in which the hand can move during the test (stationary, left-right, or up-down). Move your hand slowly (1 second per motion) and ask the client, "What is my hand doing now?" Repeat this procedure at least five times. Visual acuity is recorded as HM at the farthest distance at which the client correctly identifies most of the hand motions.

If the client cannot detect hand movement, test acuity by measuring light perception (LP). Ask the client first to cover the left eye. In a darkened room, direct the beam of a penlight at the client's right eye from a distance of 2 to 3 feet for 1 to 2 seconds. Instruct the client to say "on" when the beam of light is perceived and "off" when it is no longer detected. Repeat this procedure five times. If the client identifies the presence or absence of light three times correctly, acuity is recorded as LP.

Near-Vision Testing

Near vision is tested for clients who have difficulty reading and in clients over 40 years of age. Use a small, handheld Snellen chart called a Rosenbaum Pocket Vision Screener (Figure 49-9) or a Jaeger card. Ask the client to hold the card 14 inches away from his or her eyes and read the characters. Test each eye separately and then together. Record the value of the lowest line on which the client can identify more than half the characters.

Assessment of Visual Fields

A **confrontation test** is used to examine the client's visual fields, or peripheral vision. During the test, sit facing the client and ask him or her to look directly into your eyes while you look into the client's eyes. Cover your right eye, and have the client cover his or her left eye so that you both have the same

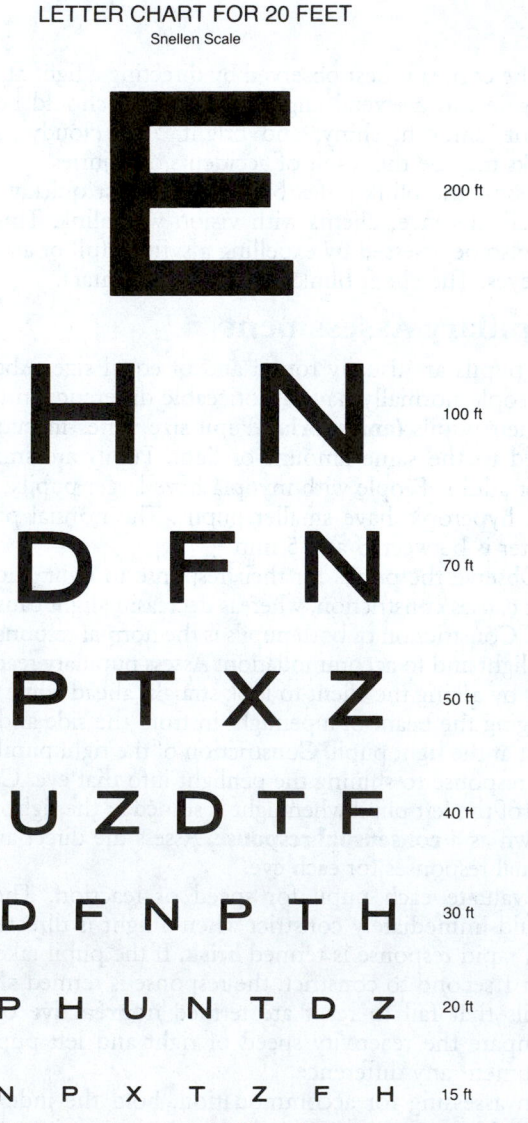

Figure 49-7 ■ A typical Snellen chart. (Courtesy of the National Society to Prevent Blindness, Schaumburg, IL.)

LETTER CHART FOR 20 FEET
Snellen Scale

E — 200 ft

H N — 100 ft

D F N — 70 ft

P T X Z — 50 ft

U Z D T F — 40 ft

D F N P T H — 30 ft

P H U N T D Z — 20 ft

N P X T Z F H — 15 ft

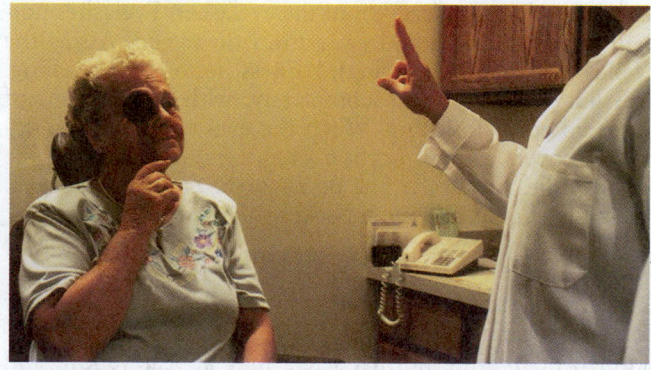

Figure 49-8 ■ Client counting fingers during determination of visual acuity.

visual field. Then move a finger or an object from a nonvisible area into the client's line of vision. The client with normal peripheral vision should notice the object at about the same time you do. Repeat this examination by covering your left eye and the client covering his or her right eye.

This test provides only a crude estimate of the client's visual fields but can reveal large-field defects such as **hemianopia** (blindness in one half the field of vision), **quadrantanopia** (blindness in one fourth of the field of vision), or large **scotomas** (blind spots in the visual field).

Assessment of Extraocular Muscle Function

Assessment of extraocular muscle function uses three tests: the corneal light reflex, the six cardinal positions of gaze, and the cover-uncover test. Also observe for parallelism of the eyes and smoothness of ocular movements.

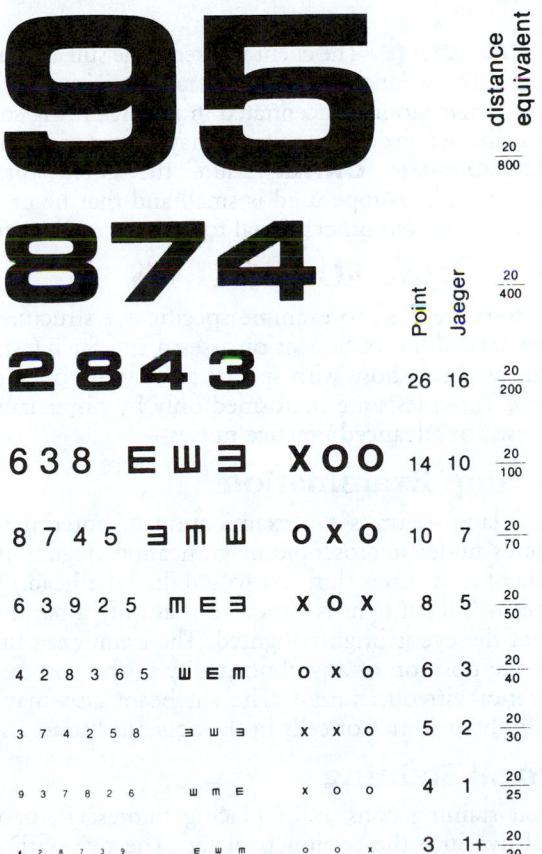

ROSENBAUM POCKET VISION SCREENER

Card is held in good light 14 inches from eye. Record vision for each eye separately with and without glasses. Presbyopic patients should read thru bifocal segment. Check myopes with glasses only.

DESIGN COURTESY J. G. ROSENBAUM, M.D., CLEVELAND, OHIO

PUPIL GAUGE (mm.)

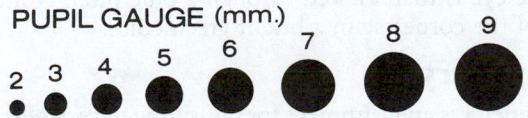

Figure 49-9 ■ A Rosenbaum Pocket Vision Screener. (Courtesy J.G. Rosenbaum, M.D., Cleveland, OH).

The corneal light reflex determines alignment of the eyes. After asking the client to stare straight ahead, shine a penlight at both corneas from a distance of 12 to 15 inches. The bright dot of light reflected from the shiny surface of the cornea should be in a symmetric position (e.g., at the 1 o'-clock position in the right eye and at the 11 o'clock position in the left eye). An asymmetric reflex indicates a deviating eye and possible muscle imbalance.

Use the six cardinal positions of gaze to assess muscle function (Figure 49-10). The eye will not turn to a particular position if the muscle is weak or if the controlling nerve is affected. Ask the client to hold his or her head still and to move the eyes to follow a small object such as a pen. Move the object to the client's right (lateral), upward and right (temporal), down and right, left (lateral), upward and left (temporal), and down and left (see Figure 49-10). While the client moves the eyes to these positions, observe for parallel eye movements and any deviation of movement. **Nystagmus,** an involuntary and rapid twitching of the eyeball, is a normal finding for the far lateral gaze. It may also be caused by abnormal nerve function or prolonged reduced vision.

Another method of assessing muscle function is the cover-uncover test. Ask the client to use both eyes to look at a specific fixed point, such as your nose. Then place a card over one of the client's eyes, and observe the uncovered eye to see if it moves to fix on the object. If muscle function is normal, the eye does not move. If the eye moves, it was not focused on the fixed point before the other eye was covered. Then remove the cover and observe for any movement in the eye just uncovered. Record the presence and direction of any eye movement deviation.

Assessment of Color Vision

Several methods are used to test color vision. The most commonly used tool is the **Ishihara chart,** which shows numbers composed of dots of one color within a circle of dots of a different color (Figure 49-11). Test each eye separately by asking the client what numbers he or she sees on the chart. Reading the numbers correctly indicates normal color vision.

Psychosocial Assessment

A client with changes in visual perception may be anxious or fearful about a possible loss of vision. Clients with severe visual defects may be unable to perform normal activities of daily living and may need to change their leisure activities. The sense of dependency resulting from reduced vision can affect self-esteem. Ask the client how he or she feels about the vision changes and assess the effectiveness of coping techniques. Discuss his or her concerns with family members to determine whether support is available. Also assess the client's knowledge and use of services for the visually impaired.

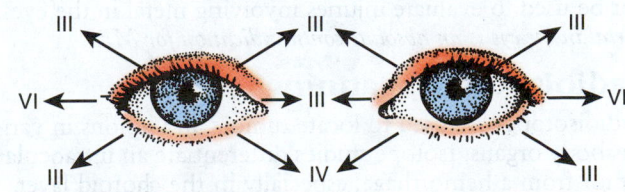

Figure 49-10 ■ Checking extraocular movements in the six cardinal positions indicates the functioning of cranial nerves III, IV, and VI.

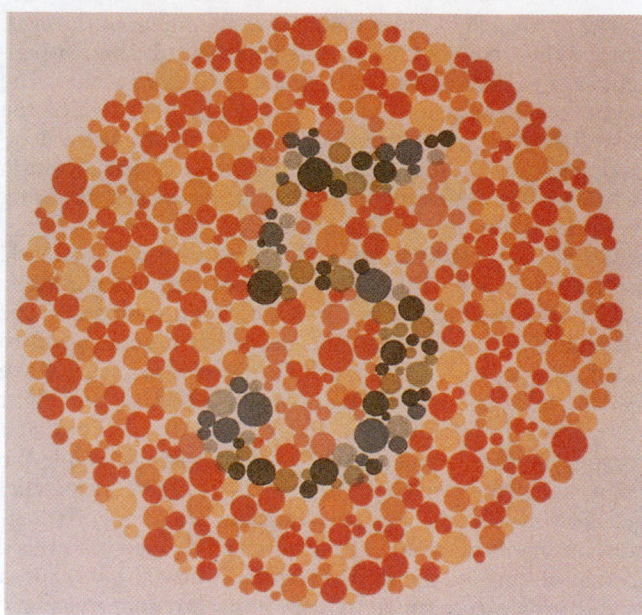

Figure 49-11 ■ An Ishihara chart for testing color vision.

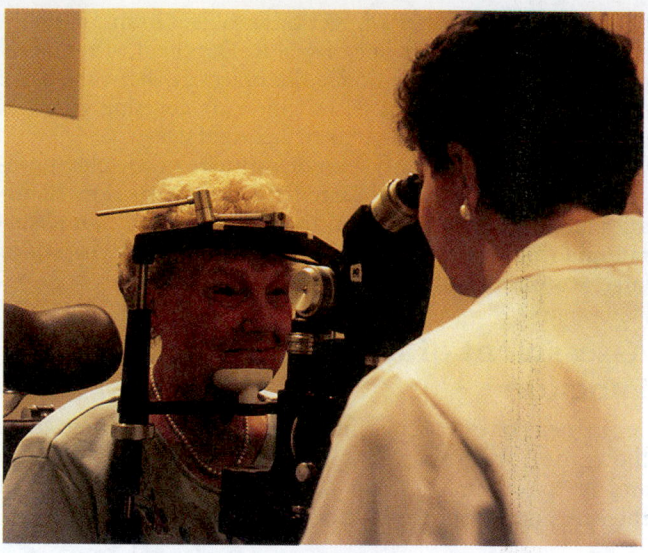

Figure 49-12 ■ Slit-lamp ocular examination.

Diagnostic Assessment

LABORATORY TESTS

Cultures and smears of corneal or conjunctival swabs and scrapings help to diagnose infections. Obtain a sample of the exudate for culture before antibiotics or topical anesthetics are instilled. Take swabs from the conjunctivae and any ulcerated or inflamed areas.

RADIOGRAPHIC EXAMINATIONS

Computed Tomography

Computed tomography (CT) is a useful diagnostic tool for looking at the eyes, bony structures around the eye, and the extraocular muscles. CT is also used for detecting tumors in the orbital space. The use of contrast dye is common unless trauma is suspected. Usually two sets of CT scans are performed, one set taken in the supine position (called axial images) and one set taken with the head tipped back as far as possible (called coronal images). The coronal images provide the "front view" needed to determine the extent of many eye problems. Inform the client that this test is not painful but does require that he or she be positioned in a confined space and keep the head still during the procedure.

Magnetic Resonance Imaging

Magnetic resonance imaging (MRI) has replaced CT in many settings for looking at the orbits and the optic nerves. MRI is also useful for evaluating ocular tumors. MRI cannot be used to evaluate injuries involving metal in the eyes. *Metal in the eye is an absolute contraindication for MRI.*

Radioisotopic Scanning

Radioisotopes are used to locate tumors and lesions in various body organs. Isotope studies differentiate an intraocular tumor from a hemorrhage, especially in the choroid layer.

CLIENT PREPARATION. After the informed consent process, the client receives a tracer dose of the radioactive isotope, either orally or by injection.

PROCEDURE. The client is asked to lie still and breathe normally. The scanner measures the radioactivity emitted by the radioactive atoms concentrated in the area being studied. Clients who are anxious or agitated may require sedation.

FOLLOW-UP CARE. Assure the client that the amount of radioisotope used is small and that he or she is not radioactive. No other special follow-up care is required.

OTHER DIAGNOSTIC TESTS

Many tests are used to examine specific eye structures but are not needed for routine vision assessment. Such tests may be indicated for those with special risks, symptoms, or exposures. These tests are performed only by physicians, optometrists, or advanced practice nurses.

Slit-Lamp Examination

The slit lamp permits the examination of anterior ocular structures under microscopic magnification (Figure 49-12). The client leans on a chin rest to stabilize the head. A narrow beam (slit) of light is aimed so that only a narrow segment of the eye is brightly lighted. The examiner can then locate the position of any abnormality in the cornea, lens, or anterior vitreous humor. The slit beam also may help identify the presence of cells in the aqueous humor.

Corneal Staining

Corneal staining consists of placing fluorescein or other topical dye into the conjunctival sac. The dye outlines irregularities of the corneal surface that are not easily visible. Corneal staining is used for corneal trauma, problems caused by a contact lens, or the presence of foreign bodies, abrasions, ulcers, or other corneal disorders.

This procedure is noninvasive and is performed under aseptic conditions. The dye is applied topically to the eye, and the eye is then viewed through a blue filter. Nonintact areas of the cornea stain a bright green color.

Tonometry

A **tonometer** is an instrument for measuring **intraocular pressure (IOP)**. Normal IOP readings are 10 to 21 mm Hg. About 5% of clients with healthy eyes have a slightly higher pressure.

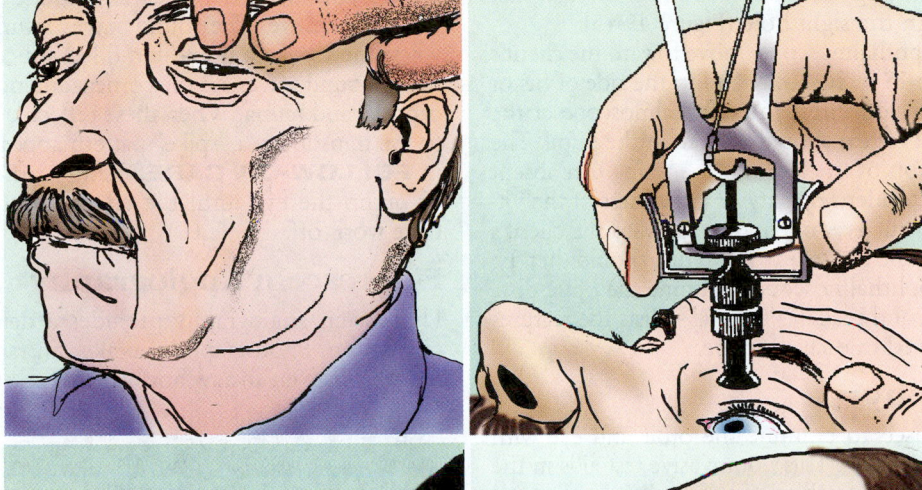

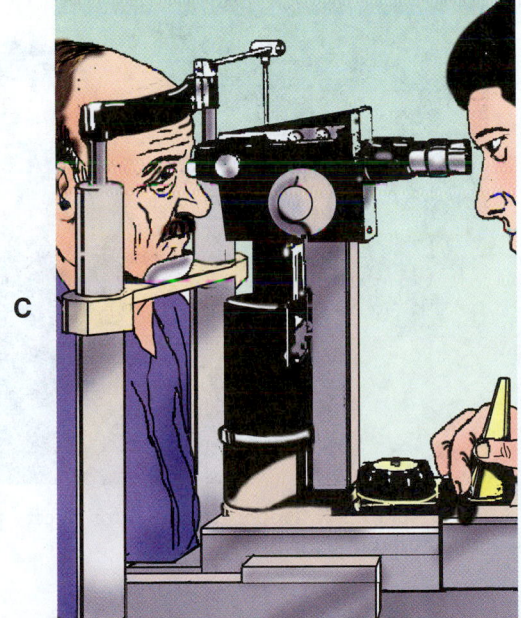

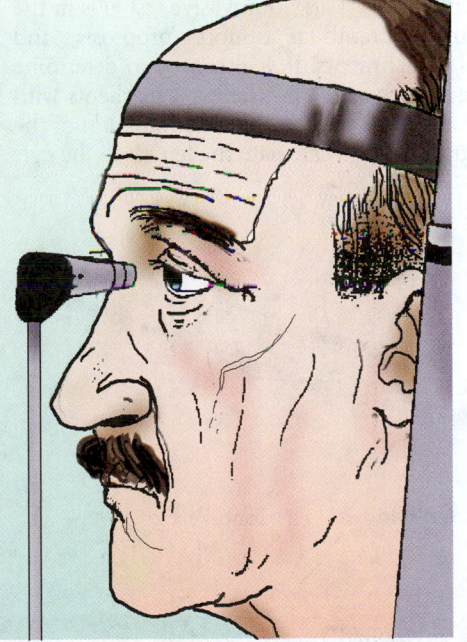

Figure 49-13 ■ Methods of intraocular pressure estimation. **A,** Finger palpation is useful only when a large difference exists between the intraocular pressure of the two eyes, as in unilateral angle-closure glaucoma. **B,** Schiötz tonometry can be learned readily. Because the tonometer is relatively inexpensive, it can be used in every physician's office to screen for chronic simple glaucoma. **C,** The air-puff tonometer can be used for screening large numbers of clients but is far more expensive than Schiötz's tonometer. **D,** Goldman's applanation tonometer, used with a slit-lamp, is the standard instrument for glaucoma diagnosis and management for most ophthalmologists. It is expensive and requires considerable skill.

Tonometer readings are indicated for all clients older than 40 years of age. Adults with a family history of glaucoma should have their IOP measured once or twice a year.

Intraocular pressure varies throughout the day. It is often higher in the morning but may peak at any time of the day. Therefore always document the time of IOP measurement.

Several methods and instruments are available to measure IOP (Figures 49-13 and 49-14). Some involve direct contact with the eye, whereas others use a noncontact technique. Table 49-4 compares the advantages and disadvantages of each method.

Ophthalmoscopy

The ophthalmoscope allows viewing of the eye's external and interior structures. It is easiest to examine the fundus when the room is dark because the pupil will dilate. When performing ophthalmoscopy, hold the instrument with your right hand when examining the right eye and with your left hand when examining the left eye. Stand on the same side as the eye being examined. Tell the client to look straight ahead at an object on the wall behind you. Placing your thumb on the client's eyebrow can help you know the distance from the ophthalmoscope to the client. Hold the ophthalmoscope firmly against your face and align it so that your eye sees through the sight hole (Figure 49-15).

When using the ophthalmoscope, move toward the client's eye from about 12 to 15 inches away and to the side of his or her line of vision. As you direct the ophthalmoscope at the pupil, a red glare **(red reflex)** should be seen in the pupil. The red reflex is a reflection of the light on the retina. An absent red reflex may indicate a lens opacity or cloudiness of the vitreous. With both of your eyes open, move toward the client's pupil while following the red reflex. The retina should then be visible through the ophthalmoscope. Examine the optic disc, optic vessels, fundus, and macula. Table 49-5 lists the features that should be observed in each structure.

Ultrasonography

Ultrasonography is used to examine the orbit and eye with high-frequency sound waves. This noninvasive test aids in the diagnosis of trauma, intraorbital tumors, proptosis, and choroidal or retinal detachments. It is also used to determine gross outline changes in the eye and the orbit in clients with cloudy corneas or lenses that reduce direct examination of the fundus. Ultrasonography helps calculate the length of the eye,

one of the measurements used to determine the strength of the intraocular lens implant needed after cataract removal.

CLIENT PREPARATION. Explain the test to the client and instill anesthetic drops into the lower lid. Caution the client to avoid rubbing the eye. Seat the client upright with his or her chin in the chin rest.

PROCEDURE. The probe is touched against the client's anesthetized cornea and sound waves are bounced through the eye. The sound waves return to the transducer when they strike a non–fluid-filled structure. Structures that reflect sound waves are the cornea, anterior and posterior lens capsule, and retina. When these reflected sound waves return to the transducer, a "spike" pattern appears on the screen.

FOLLOW-UP CARE. Remind the client not to rub or bump the eye until the effects of the anesthetic drops have worn off.

Fluorescein Angiography

Fluorescein angiography provides a detailed image of eye circulation. Photographs are taken in rapid succession after the dye is given intravenously. This test is useful for assess-

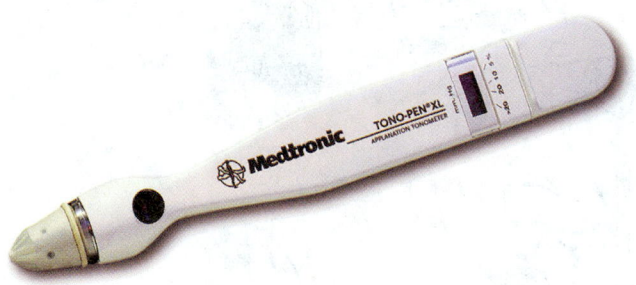

Figure 49-14 ■ The Tono-Pen.

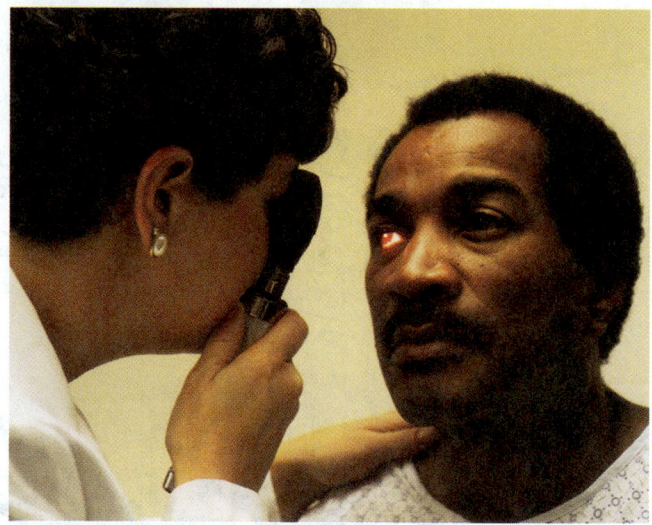

Figure 49-15 ■ Proper technique for direct ophthalmoscopic visualization of the retina.

TABLE 49-4 Types of Tonometry		
Type of Tonometry	**Advantages**	**Disadvantages**
Noncontact (air-puff) tonometer A puff of air indents the cornea	No direct contact with the client's cornea No anesthesia needed Very rapid	Less accurate than direct contact methods The puff of air is unpleasant and may startle the client
Schiötz tonometer A small pressure gauge is placed on the cornea, and a weighted plunger is depressed	Reliable readings Portable Low cost	Touches the client's cornea Requires topical anesthetic May abrade or infect the cornea
Goldman's applanation tonometer The machine exerts a force against the cornea	Highly accurate Rapid	Touches the client's cornea Requires topical anesthetic Danger of infection Machine is expensive
Tono-Pen XL A penlight-sized appliance is placed against the cornea and exerts a force against the cornea	Rapid Portable Accurate Uses a sleeve to prevent infection	Touches the client's cornea Requires topical anesthetic

ing problems of retinal circulation (e.g., diabetic retinopathy, retinal hemorrhage, and macular degeneration) or for the diagnosis of intraocular tumors.

CLIENT PREPARATION. Explain the procedure to the client, and instill mydriatic eyedrops (cause pupil dilation) 1 hour before the test. Chart 49-3 lists the best practice for correct eyedrop instillation. Check that the informed consent has been signed by the client or responsible person. Warn that the dye may cause the skin to appear yellow for several hours after the test. The stain is eliminated through the urine, which also changes color.

PROCEDURE. Intravenous access must be obtained. After the needle is in the vein, 5 mL of a 10% solution of fluorescein is injected. A digital camera is set up with equipment to photograph retinal and choroidal blood vessels as the dye passes through them. The results can be viewed immediately on a computer screen. The procedure takes only minutes because the vessels fill quickly.

FOLLOW-UP CARE. After the test, encourage clients to drink fluids to help eliminate the dye. Emphasize that any yellow or green staining of the skin will disappear in a few hours. After the test, the urine will be bright green until the dye is excreted. Instruct the client to avoid direct sunlight until pupil dilation returns to normal.

TABLE 49-5 Structures to Assess by Direct Ophthalmoscopy

Red Reflex
- Presence or absence

Optic Disc
- Color
- Margins (sharp or blurred)
- Cup size
- Presence of rings or crescents

Optic Blood Vessels
- Size
- Color
- Kinks or tangles
- Light reflection
- Narrowing
- Nicking at arteriovenous crossings

Fundus
- Color
- Tears or holes
- Lesions
- Bleeding

Macula
- Presence of blood vessels
- Color
- Lesions
- Bleeding

CHART 49-3

BEST PRACTICE for
Instillation of Ophthalmic Drops

- Wash your hands.
- Don gloves if secretions are present.
- Explain the procedure to the client.
- Check the name, strength, and expiration date of the solution.
- Stand behind the client.
- Instruct the client to tilt the head backward, open the eyes, and look up.
- Have the client's head rest against your body.
- Pull the lower lid downward against the cheekbone.
- Hold the medication bottle like a pencil, with the tip down.
- Rest the wrist holding the bottle on the client's cheek.
- Without touching the tip of the bottle to the client's conjunctiva, squeeze the bottle gently and release the correct number of drops into the conjunctival pocket.
- Gently release the lower eyelid.
- Instruct the client to close the eyes gently, without squeezing the lids together.

Electroretinography

Electroretinography is the process of graphing the retina's response to light stimulation. This test is helpful in detecting and evaluating blood vessel changes from disease or drugs. The graph is obtained by placing a contact lens electrode on an anesthetized cornea. Lights at varying speeds and intensities are flashed, and the neural response is graphed. The measurement from the cornea is identical to the response that would be obtained if electrodes were placed directly on the retina.

Preparation includes instilling an anesthetic into the eye. Afterward, remind the client to avoid rubbing the eye until the effects of the anesthetic have disappeared.

Critical Thinking Challenge

The client is a 90-year-old woman who has experienced many vision changes within the last year. She has bilateral cataracts, macular degeneration, and has had retinal bleeding. Her other health problems include hypertension and chronic heart failure. She is being evaluated today with fluorescein angiography to determine whether surgical intervention is needed. She lives alone, no longer drives, and is accompanied today by her 60-year-old son. She is extremely anxious and repeats over and over again, "I want you to fix my eyes so I can do everything that I used to do."

1. How would you address this client's expectations of having her eyes "fixed?"
2. What could you do to reduce her anxiety over the angiography?
3. Should you include her son during any explanations or procedures? Why or why not?

evolve For suggested answer guidelines, go to http://evolve.elsevier.com/Iggy/.

GET READY for the NCLEX Examination!

KEY POINTS

Safe Effective Care Environment

- Wash your hands before moving a client's eyelids.
- If a client has discharge from one eye, examine the eye without the discharge first.
- Use contact precautions with any client who has drainage from the eyes.
- Avoid performing an examination using an ophthalmoscope on a confused or uncooperative client.

Health Promotion and Maintenance

- Teach clients not to rub their eyes.
- Teach clients who have discharge from one eye to use a tissue to wipe the drainage and discard the tissue. Use a clean tissue on the second eye.
- Identify clients at risk for eye injury as a result of work environment or leisure activities.
- Encourage all clients to wear eye protection when performing yard work, working in a woodshop or metal shop, using chemicals, or are in any environment where drops or particulate matter are airborne.

Psychosocial Integrity

- Pace your interview to match the learning needs and style of the individual client.
- Allow the client the opportunity to express fear or anxiety regarding a possible change in vision status.
- Refer clients newly diagnosed with permanent vision impairment to local resources and support groups.
- Explain all diagnostic procedures, restrictions, and follow-up care to the client scheduled for tests.
- Offer large print or auditory educational materials for the client with decreased visual acuity.

Physiological Integrity

- Ask the client about vision problems in any other members of the family because some vision problems have a genetic component.
- Test the visual acuity of both eyes immediately of any person who experiences an eye injury.

ADDITIONAL STUDY RESOURCES

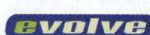 Go to your Student CD-ROM for Review Questions for the NCLEX Examination.

Go to http://evolve.elsevier.com/Iggy/ for Integrated Management of Care Questions for the NCLEX Examination.

SELECTED BIBLIOGRAPHY

Berne, R., et al. (2004). *Physiology* (5th ed.). St. Louis: Mosby.

Bron, A. (2001). The architecture of the corneal stroma. *British Journal of Ophthalmology, 85*(4), 379-381.

Bron, A. (2002). Danger: Ultraviolet light! *Insight (American Society of Ophthalmic Registered Nurses), 27*(3), 80-81.

Ebersole, P., Hess, P., & Luggen, A. (2004). *Toward healthy aging: Human needs and nursing response* (6th ed.). St. Louis: Mosby.

Garber, N. (2000a). A guide to performing basic manifest refractometry. *Journal of Ophthalmic Nursing and Technology, 19*(2), 84-95.

Garber, N. (2000b). Performing direct ophthalmoscopy. *Journal of Ophthalmic Nursing and Technology, 19*(3), 120-133.

Gordon, M. (2002). *Manual of nursing diagnosis* (10th ed.). St. Louis: Mosby.

Jarvis, C. (2004). *Physical examination and health assessment* (4th ed.). Philadelphia: W. B. Saunders.

Nussbaum, R., McInnes, R., & Willard, H. (2001). *Thompson & Thompson: Genetics in medicine* (6th ed.). Philadelphia: W.B. Saunders.

Pagana, K., & Pagana, T. (2002). *Mosby's manual of diagnostic and laboratory tests* (2nd ed.). St. Louis: Mosby.

Sackett, C., & Schenning, S. (2002). The age-related eye disease study: The results of the clinical trial. *Insight (American Society of Ophthalmic Registered Nurses), 27*(1), 5-7.

Sackett, C., & Schenning, S. (2003). Eye safety in the workplace. *Insight (American Society of Ophthalmic Registered Nurses), 27*(4), 101-102.

Segal, W., et al. (2001). Disinfection of Goldman tonometers after contamination with hepatitis C virus. *American Journal of Ophthalmology, 131*(2), 184-187.

Smith, S. (2003). Reducing ophthalmic drug-related injuries in older patients. *Insight (American Society of Ophthalmic Registered Nurses), 28*(2), 33-34.

Vaughan, D., Asbury, T., & Riordan-Eva, P. (Eds.). (2004). *General ophthalmology* (16th ed.). New York: McGraw-Hill.

Interventions for Clients with Eye and Vision Problems

M. LINDA WORKMAN

LEARNING OUTCOMES

After studying this chapter, you should be able to:

1. Describe how to correctly instill ophthalmic drops and ointment into the eye.
2. Explain the consequences of increased intraocular pressure (IOP).
3. Identify common actions, conditions, and positions that increase IOP.
4. Prioritize educational needs for the client after cataract surgery with and without lens replacement.
5. Compare myopia with hyperopia for pathophysiology and the correction needed for each.
6. Describe the pathologic bases, manifestations, and nursing care priorities for primary open-angle glaucoma and acute angle-closure glaucoma.
7. Describe the mechanism of action, side effects, and nursing implications of drug therapy for glaucoma.
8. Identify the nursing care priorities for the donor when corneal donation is planned.
9. Explain how diabetes mellitus and hypertension affect vision.
10. Develop a community-based teaching plan for the client after corneal transplantation.
11. Describe the common visual deficits for the client with dry macular degeneration.
12. Identify nursing interventions to promote home safety for the client with reduced vision.

Go to your Student CD-ROM for Review Questions for the NCLEX Examination keyed to these Learning Outcomes.

Many conditions affect vision. Some conditions occur gradually, such as cataracts, and others can result from an acute insult or illness. Even when reduced vision is temporary, the client must make some changes in function or lifestyle.

EYELID DISORDERS

The eyelid is composed of thin skin attached to small muscles. It protects the eye surface and spreads tears. Eyelid problems can be related to changes in the structure, function, or position of the eyelid. Lid structure may also be altered by age (Figures 50-1 and 50-2).

Blepharitis

PATHOPHYSIOLOGY

Blepharitis, an inflammation of the eyelid edges, occurs most often in the older adult and those with dry-eye syndrome (see Keratoconjunctivitis Sicca, p. 1090). Reduced

tear production often leads to bacterial infection of the eye structures, because tears inhibit bacterial growth.

◆COLLABORATIVE MANAGEMENT

Clients usually have itchy, red, and burning eyes. **Seborrhea** (greasy, itchy scaling) of the eyebrows and eyelids is often present. On close inspection, greasy scales and mattering may be seen where the eyelashes exit the eyelid.

Blepharitis is controlled with eyelid care using warm, moist compresses followed by gentle scrubbing with dilute baby shampoo. Instruct the client to avoid rubbing the eyes, because this action can spread the infection to other eye structures.

Entropion

PATHOPHYSIOLOGY

An **entropion** is the turning inward of the eyelid causing the lashes to rub against the eye. Entropion can be caused by eyelid muscle spasms or by scarring and deformity of the

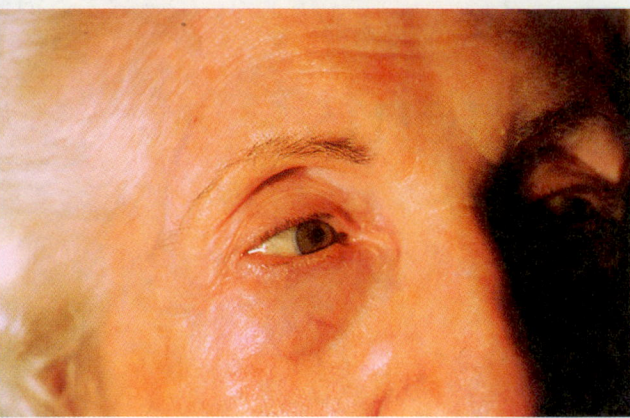

Figure 50-1 ■ Eyelid eversion (ectropion).

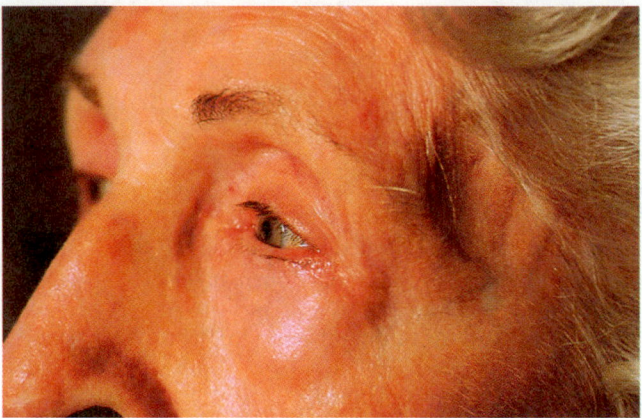

Figure 50-2 ■ "Bags" under the eyes.

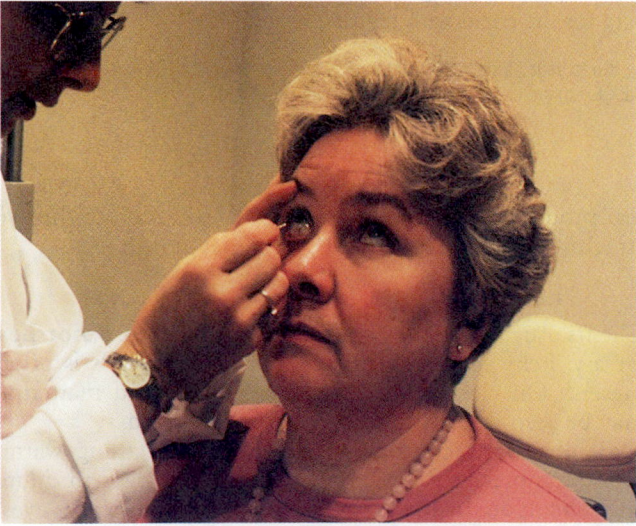

Figure 50-3 ■ Application of ophthalmic ointment.

eyelid as a result of trauma. Entropion occurs often among older adults because of age-related loss of tissue support.

◆COLLABORATIVE MANAGEMENT

The client usually reports "feeling something in my eye." Pain and tears may also be present. The eyelid is turned inward, and the conjunctiva is red. Corneal abrasion may result from constant irritation.

Surgery corrects eyelid position by either tightening the orbicular muscles and moving the eyelid to a normal position or by preventing inward rotation of the eyelid. After surgery, the eye is covered with a patch, and the client is discharged a few hours later.

Demonstrate instillation of eyedrops and evaluate the client's ability to instill the drops. Instruct the client to leave the patch in place until he or she is seen by the ophthalmologist and to report any pain or drainage under the patch. Teach the client or family member how to clean the suture line with a cotton swab and the prescribed solution. A small amount of antibiotic ointment may be applied (Figure 50-3). Chart 50-1 describes how to apply ophthalmic ointment; Chart 50-2 lists important information on ophthalmic drugs.

Ectropion
PATHOPHYSIOLOGY

An **ectropion** is the turning outward and sagging of the eyelid (see Figure 50-1), which often occurs with aging. It is caused by relaxation of the orbicular muscle. This lid position reduces the washing action of tears, leading to corneal drying and ulceration.

◆COLLABORATIVE MANAGEMENT

Clients often have constant tears and a sagging lower eyelid. Surgery can restore proper lid alignment. After surgery, the eye is covered with a patch and the client is discharged. Nursing care is the same as for an entropion.

Hordeolum
PATHOPHYSIOLOGY

A hordeolum, or stye, can be external or internal. An external hordeolum is an infection of the sweat glands in the eyelid at the place where the eyelashes exit from the eyelid. A red, swollen, tender area is found on the skin surface side of

CHART 50-2

DRUG THERAPY for Eye Problems

Drug	Nursing Interventions*,†	Rationales
Topical Anesthetics Proparacaine HCl, or proxymeta-caine (AK-Taine, Alcaine, Ocu-Caine, Ophthetic) Tetracaine HCl, cocaine HCl (Pontocaine)	Remind the client not to rub or touch the eye while it is anesthetized. Patch the eye if the client leaves the facility before the anesthetic wears off. Do not use discolored solution. Store the bottle tightly closed.	Touching may injure the eye. The use of a patch prevents injury, such as corneal abrasion. Discoloration is a sign of altered drug composition. Air may cause drug contamination and oxidation.
Topical Steroids Prednisolone acetate (Ocu-Pred, Ophtho-Tate ✱) Prednisolone phosphate (Inflamase) Dexamethasone (Dexair, Dexotic, Maxidex) Betamethasone (Betnesol) Fluorometholone (Fluor-Op, Liquifilm)	Shake vigorously before use. Monitor the client for signs of corneal ulceration. Advise the client not to share eyedrops with others.	Medication is a suspension; shaking is required to distribute the medication evenly in the solution. Steroid use predisposes the client to local infection. Disease transmission is possible when sharing eyedrops.
Anti-Infective Agents Gentamicin (Alcomicin ✱, Garamycin, Genoptic) Tobramycin (Tobrex) Ciprofloxacin (Ciloxan) Erythromycin (Ilotycin) Chlortetracycline (Aureomycin) Sulfisoxazole (Gantrisin) Ofloxacin (Ocuflox)	Be sure to obtain a specimen for culture before use. Clean exudate from the eyes before administering drops. Reinforce the importance of completing the prescribed medication regimen.	Use of an antibiotic before a culture specimen is obtained may alter culture results. Cleansing decreases the risk of contaminating the medication and increases contact of the conjunctiva with the medication. Compliance is critical to maintain a therapeutic level of medication.
Antibiotic-Steroid Combinations Tobramycin with dexamethasone (TobraDex) Neomycin sulfate with polymyxin B sulfate and dexamethasone (Maxitrol)	This is the same as for each component alone.	This is the same as for each component alone.
Topical Antiviral Agents Idoxuridine (Herplex, Stoxil) Trifluridine (Viroptic) Vidarabine (Vira-A)	Refrigerate and protect from light. Monitor the client for itching lids and burning eyes.	Cool temperatures and absence of light ensures medication stability. Sensitivity to this drug is common.
Nonsteroidal Anti-Inflammatory Agents Flurbiprofen (Ocufen) Diclofenac (Voltaren) Ketorolac (Acular)	Monitor the client for bleeding in the eye. Instruct the client not to wear soft contact lenses during therapy with these drugs.	These drugs disrupt platelet aggregation. These drugs interact with contact lens materials and increase the risk for infection.
Agents for Glaucoma **Alpha-2 Adrenergic Agonist** Brimonidine tartrate (Alphagan)	Do not give to clients who take an MAOI (monoamine oxidase inhibitor). Teach clients not to insert soft contact lenses for at least 15 minutes after instilling the drug.	Drug can precipitate hypertensive crisis. Soft contact lenses absorb the preservative.
Sympathomimetics Epinephrine (Epifrin, Glaucon) Dipivefrin HCl (Propine) Apraclonidine (Iopidine)	Do not use with soft contact lenses. Clients taking epinephrine eyedrops for glaucoma need to discontinue epinephrine therapy before starting dipivefrin. Do not give this drug to clients who have a hypersensitivity to the drug clonidine.	Drug discolors soft contact lenses. Taking the two drugs together increases the side effects and can cause an acute angle-closure glaucoma. This drug contains the same active ingredient as clonidine.

⚠️ **Med Error Alert!** All of these drugs are administered by the eye instillation route, not the oral route. Oral administration of these agents can cause systemic side effects in addition to not having the correct effect on the eyes.

*When instilling eyedrops, teach clients to use nasal punctal occlusion to reduce the risk for systemic absorption and side effects.
†When more than one topical ophthalmic drug is prescribed, teach clients to separate the instillation of each drug by at least 5 minutes.

Continued

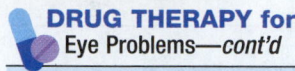

CHART 50-2

DRUG THERAPY for Eye Problems—cont'd

Drug	Nursing Interventions*,†	Rationales
Agents for Glaucoma—cont'd		
Beta-Adrenergic Blockers Levobunolol HCl (Betagan Liquifilm) Betaxolol HCl (Betoptic) Metipranolol HCl (Metipranolol, OptiPranolol) Carteolol HCl (Ocupress) Timolol (Betimol, Timoptic) Levobetaxolol (Betaxon)	Use of any beta-adrenergic blocker is contraindicated in clients with severe asthma or chronic obstructive pulmonary disease. Caution diabetic clients using beta-adrenergic blockers to check blood glucose levels frequently. Teach clients who are taking these drugs along with systemic beta-adrenergic blockers to take their pulse at least twice per day.	These drugs, if absorbed systemically, constrict bronchiolar smooth muscle and narrow the airways. These drugs mask the hypoglycemic symptoms. These drugs can potentiate the effects of systemic beta-adrenergic drugs on heart rate and blood pressure.
Mitotics, Direct-Acting Acetylcholine chloride Carbachol (Carboptic, Carbastat, Isopto Carbachol, Miostat) Pilocarpine (Isopto Carpine, Pilocar, Akarpine, Pilopine)	Do not use this class of drugs in clients with corneal abrasion. Caution clients to not exceed the dose or scheduling of this drug class.	Drug increases penetration of drug and the risk for side effects. Drug excess can lead to systemic side effects.
Mitotics, Cholinesterase Inhibitors Demecarium bromide (Humorsol) Echothiophate iodide (Phospholine Iodide)	Tell clients that pupil changes may not be present for the first 24 hours. Teach clients to have their intraocular pressure measured more frequently when using this drug.	Drug has a slow onset of action and a long duration of action. Tolerance develops quickly with this drug; a rest period of several days restores response.
Carbonic Anhydrase Inhibitors Dorzolamide (TruSopt) Brinzolamide (Azopt)	Do not give this class of drugs to clients who have a known hypersensitivity to sulfonamides. Teach clients to not wear contact lenses during or within 15 minutes of instilling these drugs.	Drug contains similar proteins, and allergic reactions are possible. Contact lenses absorb the drug and may cloud or discolor.
Prostaglandin Agonist Latanoprost (Xalatan)	Inform clients that a change in the color of the iris does not interfere with vision.	Many clients have increased iris pigmentation that may be permanent.
Travoprost (Travatan)	Drug should not be used in pregnant clients or those who may become pregnant.	Drug has been associated with increased pregnancy loss.
Bimatoprost (Lumigan)	Pigment changes are the same as for latanoprost.	
Unoprostone isopropyl (Rescula)	Same pigment changes as with latanoprost.	

*When instilling eyedrops, teach clients to use nasal punctal occlusion to reduce the risk for systemic absorption and side effects.
†When more than one topical ophthalmic drug is prescribed, teach clients to separate the instillation of each drug by at least 5 minutes.

the eyelid. An internal hordeolum is caused by an infection of the eyelid sebaceous glands. The most common causative organisms are *Staphylococcus aureus, Staphylococcus epidermidis,* and *Streptococcus.* The hordeolum usually affects only one eyelid at a time. Vision is not affected.

◆ COLLABORATIVE MANAGEMENT

Small, beady, swollen areas may be seen on the skin side of the eyelid or on the conjunctival side of the eyelid. As the hordeolum forms, it fills with purulent material, causing pain.

Treatment includes the use of warm compresses four times a day and an antibacterial ointment. When the lesion opens, the purulent material drains and the pain subsides.

Nursing interventions include applying compresses and instructing the client in this application. Chart 50-3 lists the proper technique for application of an eye compress.

After compresses have been applied, instill antibiotic ointment. Advise the client that ointments may cause blurred vision, and tell him or her to remove the ointment from the eyes before driving or operating machinery. To remove the ointment, tell the client to close the eye and then gently wipe the closed eyelid from the nasal side of the eye outward.

Chalazion

PATHOPHYSIOLOGY

A **chalazion** is an inflammation of a sebaceous gland in the eyelid. It begins with redness and tenderness (similar to the hordeolum), followed by a gradual painless swelling at the gland. In its fully developed state, no inflammatory signs are present.

CHART 50-3

CLIENT EDUCATION GUIDE
Application of an Ocular Compress

1. Wash your hands.
2. Fold a clean washcloth into fourths.
3. Soak the washcloth with running tap water that is warm to your inner wrist. (If cool compresses are needed, follow the same steps using cold running tap water.)
4. Place the cloth over your closed eye.
5. Keep the cloth in place with minimal pressure until the cloth cools.
6. Refold the washcloth so that a different "fourth" will be held against the eye.
7. Resoak the cloth with running tap water.
8. Repeat applications three times for as many times each day as prescribed by your physician.

◆COLLABORATIVE MANAGEMENT

Most chalazia protrude on the inside of the eyelid. The client has eye fatigue, light sensitivity, and excessive tears.

Treatment includes the use of warm compresses for 15 minutes four times a day, followed by instillation of ophthalmic ointment. If the chalazion is large enough to affect vision, is cosmetically displeasing to the client, or recurs frequently, it may be removed surgically.

After surgery, antibiotic ointment is instilled and the eye is covered with a patch. Best practices for application of a nonpressure eye patch are listed in Chart 50-4.

Instruct the client to leave the eye patch in place for about 6 hours, then remove the patch and apply warm, wet compresses. Instill antibiotic eyedrops after use of the compresses.

CHART 50-4

BEST PRACTICE for
Application of an Eye Patch

Nonpressure Eye Patch
1. Assemble the equipment:
   - Eye patch
   - Skin preparation
   - Nonallergenic paper tape
2. Explain the procedure to the client.
3. Wash your hands.
4. Apply a skin preparation to the client's forehead and cheek.
5. Instruct the client to close both eyes gently.
6. Place a patch over the closed eyelid.

8. Cover the patch with overlapping pieces of tape.

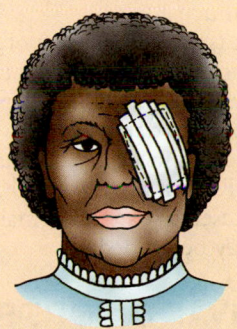

Pressure Eye Patch
1. Assemble the equipment:
   - Two eye patches for each eye requiring treatment
   - Skin preparation pad
   - Nonallergenic paper tape
2-5. Follow corresponding steps under Nonpressure Eye Patch.
6. Fold one eye patch in half, place it over the closed eyelid, and apply a second eye patch (unfolded) over the folded one.

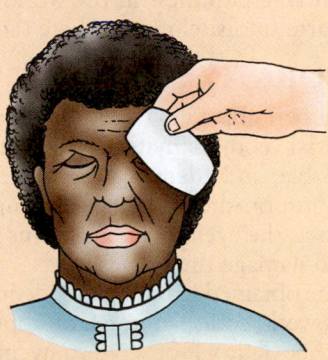

7. Apply tape from the cheek to the middle of the forehead in a diagonal line.

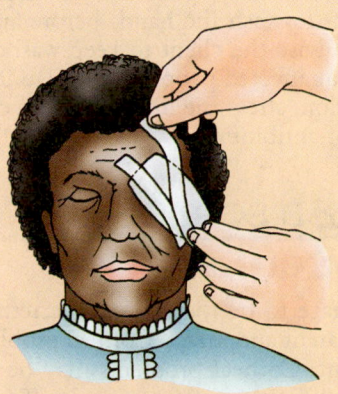

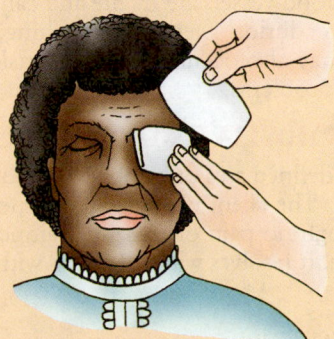

7, 8. Follow corresponding steps under Nonpressure Eye Patch.

Tell the client to immediately report increasing redness, purulent drainage, or reduced vision to the ophthalmologist.

KERATOCONJUNCTIVITIS SICCA

PATHOPHYSIOLOGY

The lacrimal system moistens the eye surface with tears and removes tears from the eye. Problems arise from reduced tear production, infection, or inflammation in the lacrimal system.

Keratoconjunctivitis sicca, or dry-eye syndrome, results from changes in tear composition, lacrimal gland malfunction, or altered tear distribution. Decreased tear production can also occur with the use of some drugs, such as antihistamines, beta-adrenergic blocking agents, or anticholinergic drugs. Diseases associated with decreased tear production include rheumatoid arthritis, leukemia, sarcoidosis, and multiple sclerosis. Radiation or chemical burns to the eye also decrease tear production. Injury to the facial nerve (cranial nerve VII) inhibits tears. Eye dryness may follow vision-enhancing surgery.

◆ COLLABORATIVE MANAGEMENT

The client may feel as if a foreign body is in the eye, burning and itching eyes, and photophobia (sensitivity to light). The corneal light reflex is dulled or distorted. Tears may contain strands of mucus.

Treatment depends on the severity of the manifestations. Restasis, a cyclosporine ophthalmic emulsion, may be prescribed to increase tear production. Artificial tears (HypoTears, Refresh) are prescribed for daytime use to reduce dryness and can be used as often as necessary. A lubricating ointment (Lacri-Lube S.O.P., Refresh P.M.) is used at night. If the dry-eye syndrome is caused by an abnormal eyelid position or function, surgery may be needed.

CONJUNCTIVAL DISORDERS

The conjunctiva is a thin mucous membrane that covers and protects the eye. Because of its location, the conjunctiva is subject to trauma and infection.

Hemorrhage

PATHOPHYSIOLOGY

Conjunctival blood vessels are fragile and can break with increased pressure during sneezing, coughing, or vomiting. Hemorrhages may also occur with hypertension, trauma, or blood clotting problems.

◆ COLLABORATIVE MANAGEMENT

The small, well-defined area of hemorrhage is bright red under the conjunctiva. The client is usually concerned about its appearance although no pain or visual impairment occurs with the hemorrhage. It resolves within 14 days without treatment.

Conjunctivitis

PATHOPHYSIOLOGY

Conjunctivitis is an inflammation or infection of the conjunctiva. Inflammation occurs from exposure to allergens or irritants and is not contagious. Infectious conjunctivitis occurs with bacterial or viral infection and is readily transmitted from person to person.

◆ COLLABORATIVE MANAGEMENT

Manifestations of allergic conjunctivitis include edema, a sensation of burning, engorgement of blood vessels ("bloodshot" appearance), excessive tears, and itching.

Treatment includes the instillation of vasoconstrictors and corticosteroid eyedrops. Instruct the client to avoid using makeup until all symptoms have subsided.

Bacterial conjunctivitis, or "pink eye," is usually caused by *Staphylococcus aureus, Haemophilus influenzae,* or *Pseudomonas aeruginosa.* Manifestations include blood vessel dilation, mild conjunctival edema, tears, and discharge. The discharge is watery at first and then becomes thicker, with shreds of mucus.

Cultures of the drainage are obtained to identify the organism. Treatment is aimed at controlling the infection. Appropriate topical antibiotics are given.

Nursing interventions focus on preventing the spread of the disease to the other eye or to other people. Document the amount, color, and type of drainage. Review hygiene with the client, including handwashing after touching the eye and before instilling eyedrops. Warn the client not to touch the unaffected eye without first washing the hands and to avoid sharing washcloths and towels with others.

Trachoma

PATHOPHYSIOLOGY

Trachoma is a chronic, bilateral scarring form of conjunctivitis caused by *Chlamydia trachomatis.* Trachoma is the chief cause of preventable blindness in the world. The incidence is highest in warm, moist climates where sanitation is poor.

◆ COLLABORATIVE MANAGEMENT

The incubation period is 5 to 14 days. At first, trachoma resembles bacterial conjunctivitis. Manifestations include tears, photophobia, and edema of the eyelids and conjunctiva. Follicles form on the upper eyelid conjunctiva. As the disease progresses, the eyelid scars and turns inward, causing the eyelashes to damage the cornea.

Specimens are obtained for culture to identify the causative organism. A 4-week course of oral or topical tetracycline (Achromycin, Apo-Tetra✹) or erythromycin (Apo-Erythro-EC✹, E-Mycin, E.E.S.) is given. Azithromycin (Zithromax) can be used once per week for 1 to 3 weeks.

Nursing interventions focus on infection control. Instruct the client to wash the hands before and after touching the eyes. Advise the client to keep washcloths separate from those of unaffected people and to launder them separately. In addition, stress the importance of completing the entire course of antibiotics.

CORNEAL DISORDERS

PATHOPHYSIOLOGY

For a sharp image to be focused on the retina, the cornea must be transparent and intact. Corneal problems lead to visual impairment. Corneal problems may be caused by degeneration of the cornea (keratoconus) (Figure 50-4); deposits in the cornea, reducing the refracting power (dystrophies); irritation or infection (keratitis); or ulceration of the corneal surface. Table 50-1 lists common causes of corneal disorders.

◆COLLABORATIVE MANAGEMENT
◆Assessment

The client with a corneal disorder usually has pain, reduced vision, photophobia, and eye secretions. Cloudy or purulent (pus-filled) fluid may be present on the eyelids or eyelashes. Wear gloves during the examination when drainage is present.

The cornea may look hazy or cloudy. An altered corneal light reflex may occur. The cornea may no longer be intact, and patchy areas may be visible on examination. When fluorescein stain is used, these areas appear green.

No definitive tests confirm corneal disease, although microbial culture and corneal scrapings can help determine which organism is causing a corneal ulcer. For culture, obtain swabs from the ulcer and its edges. For corneal scrapings, the cornea is anesthetized with a topical agent, and a sterile spatula is used to remove samples from the center and edge of the ulcer.

◆Interventions

NONSURGICAL MANAGEMENT. Treatment for a corneal disorder is aimed at reducing symptoms, restoring corneal clarity, and enhancing the client's ability to use the remaining vision.

TABLE 50-1   Common Causes of Corneal Disorders

Keratoconus
- Autosomal recessive trait
- Down syndrome
- Aniridia
- Marfan syndrome
- Atopic allergy
- Retinitis pigmentosa

Keratitis (Exposure)
- Ectropion/entropion
- Exophthalmos
- Neurologic deficits

Keratitis (Acanthamoeba)
- Protozoal infection

Corneal Ulcers
- Mechanical injury
- Chemical injury
- Drying
- Infection

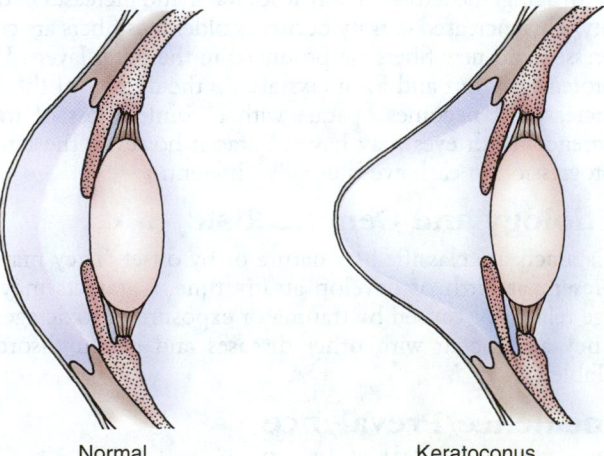

Figure 50-4 ■ Profiles of a normal eyeball and one with keratoconus.

Normal   Keratoconus

Drug Therapy. Antibiotics, antifungals, and antivirals are prescribed to reduce or eliminate microorganisms. Usually, a broad-spectrum antibiotic is prescribed first and may be changed when culture results are known. Steroids may be used with antibiotics to reduce the inflammatory response in the eye. Drugs can be given topically as eyedrops, injected subconjunctivally, or injected intravenously (IV). Chart 50-5 lists best practices for instilling eyedrops.

Vision Enhancement. Assist clients in using their functional vision, suggesting sunglasses and indirect lighting if glare creates difficulties. Inform clients about magnifiers and special light fixtures.

SURGICAL MANAGEMENT. Keratoplasty (corneal transplant) is the surgical removal of diseased corneal tissue and replacement with tissue from a human donor cornea. This process restores vision by removing corneal deformities and replacing them with healthy corneal tissue.

Preoperative Care. Corneal transplantation is performed when the donor tissue becomes available. Usually the client is quite anxious. Use a calm approach to assess the client's knowledge of the surgery and of expected care before and after surgery.

Examine the client's eyes for signs of infection and report any redness, drainage, or edema to the ophthalmologist. Instill antibiotic drops into the eye to reduce the risk for infection. IV access is placed before surgery.

Operative Procedures. Usually regional anesthesia is used. The nerves around and behind the eye are numbed so that the client cannot move or see out of the eye. The surgeon removes the center 7 to 8 mm of the diseased cornea (Figure 50-5) with a **trephine,** an instrument that works like a cookie cutter. The same trephine is used to cut the tissue graft from the donor cornea. The donor corneal graft is sutured into place on the eye. Figure 50-6 shows the eye after transplantation.

Postoperative Care. After the procedure is completed, a subconjunctival antibiotic injection is given and an antibiotic ointment instilled. The eye is covered with a pressure patch and a protective shield. This dressing is left in place until the next day. Usually, the surgeon removes this dressing.

Notify the ophthalmologist of changes in vital signs or of drainage on the dressing. Instruct the client to lie on the nonoperative side to reduce intraocular pressure (IOP).

CHART 50-5

BEST PRACTICE for
Eyedrop Administration

- Administer drugs at frequent, precise intervals. *The timing of administration is critical.* Clients with eye problems are often given several broad-spectrum antibiotics. If each drug is administered every hour, create separate dosage schedules. For example, give antibiotic A at 7:00, 8:00, 9:00, and 10:00. Then give antibiotic B at 7:30, 8:30, 9:30, and 10:30.
- If two medications must be administered *at the same time, separate the instillation by 5 minutes.* For example, a client with glaucoma and a bacterial ulcer receives timolol (Apo-Timop✱, Timoptic) at 7:00 and tobramycin (Tobrex) at 7:05.
- If the same medication is required for both eyes and one eye is infected, use *separate* bottles of medication.
- Clearly label each bottle with "left" or "right" for the appropriate eye.
- Wear gloves when ocular drainage is present.
- Wash your hands before and after administering eyedrops.

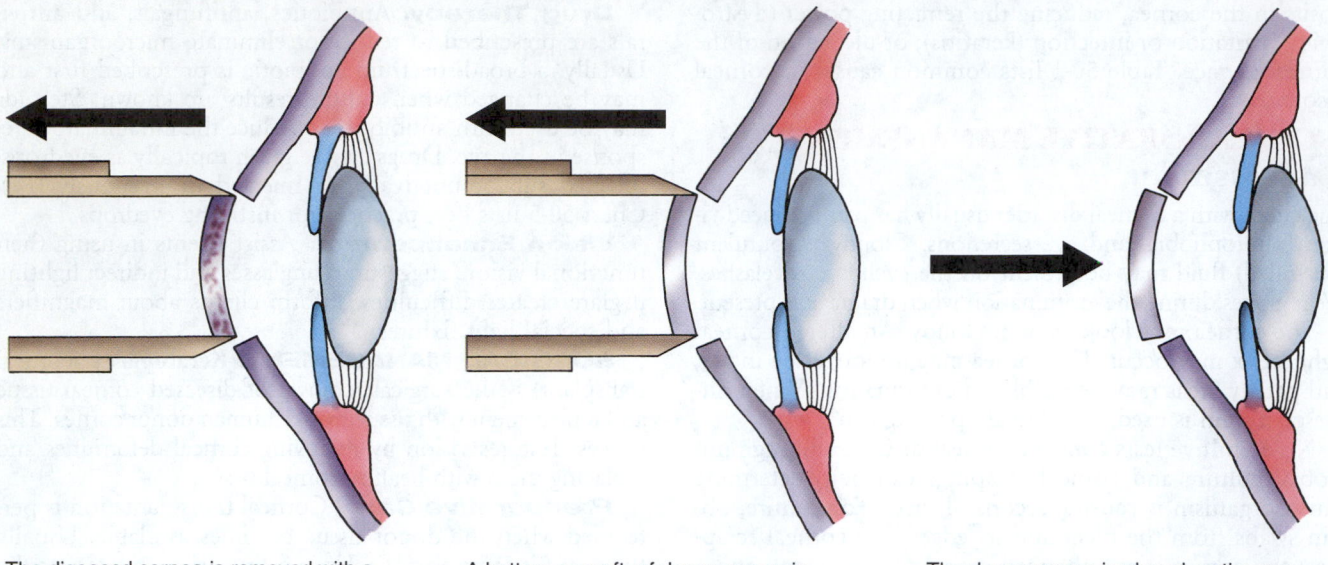

The diseased cornea is removed with a trephine.

A button, or graft, of donor cornea is removed with the same trephine so the cuts are identical.

The donor cornea is placed on the eye and stitched into place with suture material that is finer than a human hair.

Figure 50-5 ■ The steps involved in corneal transplantation (penetrating keratoplasty).

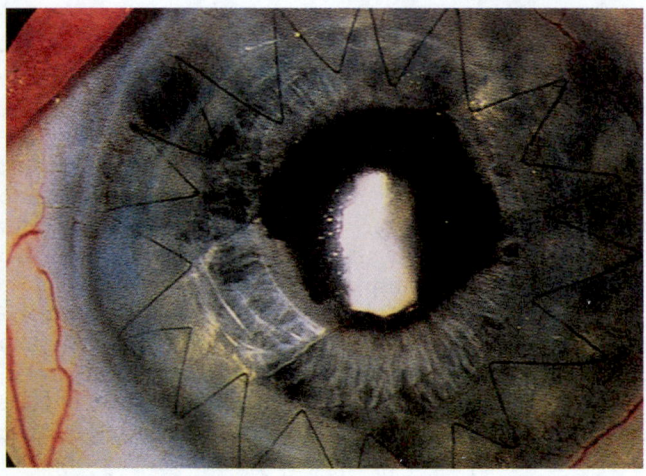

Figure 50-6 ■ The appearance of the eye with sutures in place after corneal transplantation. (Courtesy of John A. Costin, MD.)

During the early period after surgery, the client cannot see out of the affected eye because of the eye patch and shield.

If the patches are to remain in place after discharge, show the client how to apply a patch and obtain a return demonstration. Instruct the client to wear the shield at night for the first month after surgery and whenever he or she is around small children or pets. Complications after surgery include bleeding, wound leakage, infection, and graft rejection.

Although the cornea has no blood supply, graft rejection is possible. Inflammation starts in the donor cornea near the graft edge and moves toward the center. Vision is reduced and the cornea becomes cloudy. Frequent applications of topical corticosteroids are used. If rejection continues, the graft becomes opaque and blood vessels branch into the opaque tissue.

Eye Donation. Corneal tissue is obtained from a local eye or tissue bank. An eye bank obtains its supply of corneal tissue from volunteer donors. These donors must be free of infectious disease or cancer at the time of death. If a deceased client is a potential eye donor, follow the steps listed below:

- Raise the head of the bed 30 degrees.
- Instill antibiotic eyedrops, such as Neosporin or tobramycin.
- Close the eyes and apply a *small* ice pack to the closed eyes.
- Contact the family and physician to discuss eye donation.

CATARACT

PATHOPHYSIOLOGY

The lens is a biconvex, transparent, refractive elastic structure suspended behind the iris. A cataract is an opacity of the lens that distorts the image projected onto the retina (Figure 50-7). With aging, the lens gradually loses water and increases in density. This increased density occurs as older lens fibers are compressed and new fibers are produced in the outer layers. Lens proteins dry out and form crystals. As the density of the lens increases, it becomes opaque with a painless loss of transparency. Both eyes may have cataracts; however, the rate of progression in each eye is usually different.

Etiology and Genetic Risk

Cataracts are classified by nature or by onset. They may be present at birth or develop at any time. Cataracts may be age related or caused by trauma or exposure to toxic agents. They also occur with other diseases and ocular disorders (Table 50-2).

Incidence/Prevalence

Cataracts develop in 5 to 10 million people worldwide every year. The age-related cataract is the most common type. Some

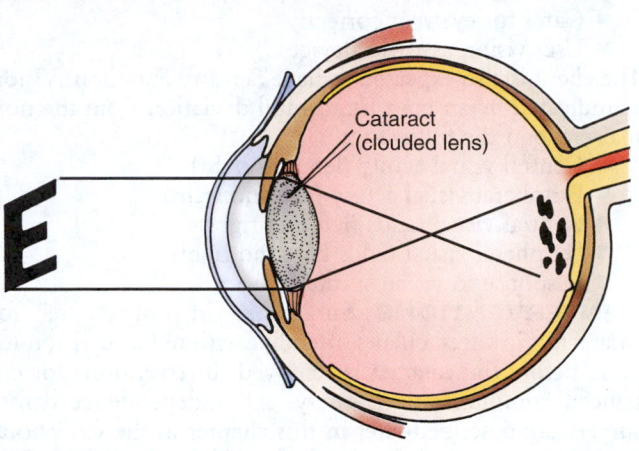

Figure 50-7 ■ The visual impairment produced by the presence of a cataract.

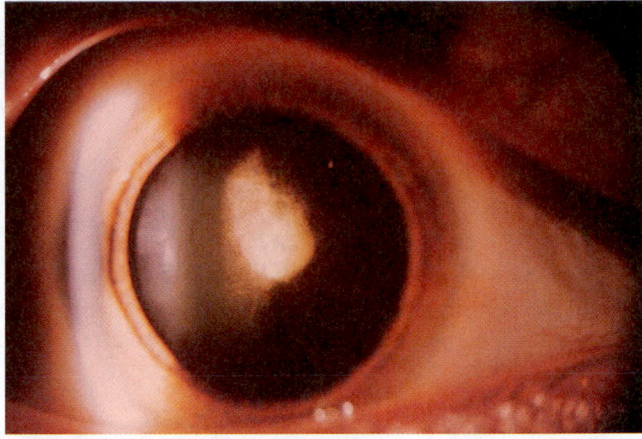

Figure 50-8 ■ The appearance of an eye with a mature cataract. (Courtesy of John A. Costin, MD.)

TABLE 50-2 Common Causes of Cataracts	
Age-Related Cataracts ■ Lens water loss and fiber compaction	**Associated Cataract** ■ Diabetes mellitus ■ Hypoparathyroidism ■ Down syndrome ■ Chronic sunlight exposure
Traumatic Cataracts ■ Blunt injury to eye or head ■ Penetrating eye injury ■ Intraocular foreign bodies ■ Radiation exposure, therapy	**Complicated Cataracts** ■ Retinitis pigmentosa ■ Glaucoma ■ Retinal detachment
Toxic Cataracts ■ Corticosteroids ■ Phenothiazine derivatives ■ Miotic agents	

CHART 50-6

KEY FEATURES of
Cataracts

Early
■ Blurred vision
■ Decreased color perception

Late
■ Diplopia
■ Reduced visual acuity progressing to blindness
■ Absence of red reflex
■ Presence of white pupil

degree of cataract formation is expected in all people older than 70 years of age (Vaughan, Asbury, & Riordan-Eva, 2004).

HEALTH PROMOTION/ILLNESS PREVENTION

Although most cases of cataracts in North America are age related, the onset of cataract formation occurs earlier with heavy sun exposure or exposure to other sources of ultraviolet light. Wearing sun glasses that limit penetration of ultraviolet light is a major way to reduce cataract formation. Additionally, cataracts are caused by direct eye injury. Urging all people to wear eye and head protection during sports, such as baseball, or any activity that increases the risk for the eye being hit by objects in motion, can help reduce the incidence of cataracts.

◆ COLLABORATIVE MANAGEMENT
◆ Assessment
HISTORY

Age is important because cataracts are most prevalent in the older adult. Ask about the following predisposing factors:
■ Recent or past trauma to the eye
■ Exposure to radioactive materials or x-rays
■ Systemic disease (such as diabetes mellitus, hypoparathyroidism, Down syndrome, or atopic dermatitis)

■ Use of corticosteroids, chlorpromazine, or miotic drugs
■ Intraocular disease (such as recurrent uveitis)

Ask the client to describe his or her vision. For example, you might say, "Tell me what you can see well and what you have difficulty seeing." This technique helps determine the impact of visual deficits on the client.

PHYSICAL ASSESSMENT/CLINICAL MANIFESTATIONS

Early manifestations of cataracts include slightly blurred vision and decreased color perception (Chart 50-6). As lens cloudiness continues, the client may have vision reduced to such an extent that daily activities are adversely affected. Blurred and double vision may occur. Without surgical intervention, visual impairment can progress to blindness. *No pain or eye redness is associated with age-related cataract formation.*

Visual acuity is very reduced. Vision is tested using a Snellen chart and brightness acuity testing (see Chapter 49). Evaluate the client's acuity under various lighting conditions, which can help determine the degree of visual disability.

Examine the lens with the direct ophthalmoscope and describe any observed densities by size, shape, and location. As the cataract matures, the opacity makes it difficult to see the retina and the red reflex may be absent. When this occurs, the pupil is white (Figure 50-8).

PSYCHOSOCIAL ASSESSMENT

Loss of vision is gradual, and the client may not be aware of the change until reading or driving is affected. Fear of losing one's eyesight can be overwhelming, and the client may have great anxiety during an eye evaluation.

◆Analysis

COMMON NURSING DIAGNOSES AND COLLABORATIVE PROBLEMS

The most common nursing diagnosis for clients with cataracts is Disturbed Sensory Perception: Visual related to altered sensory reception.

ADDITIONAL NURSING DIAGNOSES AND COLLABORATIVE PROBLEMS

In addition to the most common nursing diagnosis, clients with cataracts may have one or more of the following:

- Fear related to sensory impairment, loss of eyesight, scheduled surgery, or inability to regain eyesight
- Risk for Injury related to decreased vision
- Social Isolation related to reduced visual acuity, fear of injury, or fear of embarrassment
- Self-Care Deficit (dressing/grooming) related to perceptual impairment
- Deficient Knowledge (Cataract Pathophysiology and Treatment) related to lack of information or misconceptions
- Impaired Home Maintenance related to age, limited vision, or activity restrictions imposed by surgery

Critical Thinking Challenge

The client is a 62-year-old woman who works as a stockbroker. She has recently been diagnosed with bilateral cataracts. She lives in the Denver area and her hobbies include long-distance biking and downhill skiing. She has a glass or two of wine with dinner every night. She smoked when she was in college but has not smoked for more than 30 years. She is surprised by her diagnosis because she is a vegetarian and keeps herself physically fit. She also tells you that neither her parents nor any of her four brothers and sisters have cataracts.

1. How should you explain the influence of genetics on the development of cataracts?
2. What factors may have influenced the development of her cataracts?
3. What additional personal and family information should you obtain from this client?

evolve For suggested answer guidelines, go to http://evolve.elsevier.com/Iggy/.

◆Planning and Implementation

DISTURBED SENSORY PERCEPTION: VISUAL

PLANNING: EXPECTED OUTCOMES. The client with cataracts is expected to have Vision Compensation Behavior as indicated by consistent demonstration of the following behaviors:

- Monitors symptoms of vision deterioration
- Positions self to advantage vision
- Uses adequate lighting for activity being performed
- Wears eyeglasses or contact lenses correctly

- Cares for eyewear correctly
- Uses vision assistive devices

The client is also expected to have Sensory Function: Vision as indicated by an increase to mild deviation from the normal range in the following:

- Central visual acuity (left and right)
- Peripheral visual acuity (left and right)
- Central visual fields (left and right)
- Peripheral visual fields (left and right)
- Response to visual stimuli

INTERVENTIONS. Surgery is the only "cure" for cataracts. However, clients often live with reduced vision for years before the cataract is removed. Interventions for enhanced communication, safety, and independence before surgery are described later in this chapter in the Collaborative Management section for Reduced Vision (see p. 1108).

Preoperative Care. The health care provider gives the client accurate information so that he or she can make informed decisions about treatment. Teach about the nature of cataracts, their progression, and their treatment.

Because cataract surgery is usually an outpatient procedure and most clients are older, adequate preoperative teaching is problematic. Assess how the client's vision affects the activities of daily living, especially dressing, eating, and ambulating.

Stress to the client that care after surgery requires the instillation of different types of eyedrops several times a day for 2 to 4 weeks. Careful assessment of eye appearance is also needed. If the client is unable to perform these tasks, help him or her make arrangements for this care.

An IV infusion may be started in the operating room. A sedative is given before surgery, and oral acetazolamide (Acetazolam✱, Diamox) may be given on the morning of surgery to reduce intraocular pressure (IOP). A series of ophthalmic drugs are instilled just before surgery to dilate the pupils and cause vasoconstriction. Other eyedrops are instilled to induce paralysis to prevent lens movement. When the client is in the surgical area, a local anesthetic is injected into the muscle cone behind the eye for anesthesia and eye paralysis.

Operative Procedures. Extraction of the lens can be intracapsular or, more commonly, extracapsular (Figure 50-9). The front portion of the capsule is opened and removed. Usually the surgeon then uses sound waves to break the cataractous lens into small pieces, a process known as **phacoemulsion.** The small pieces are then sucked out. The posterior lens capsule is left inside the eye to anchor the replacement lens.

In intracapsular surgery, the surgeon removes the lens and capsule completely. A disadvantage of this approach is that the protective posterior capsule is removed, placing the eye at greater risk for retinal detachment and resulting in the loss of a supportive structure for the intraocular lens (IOL) implant.

After the lens with the cataract is removed, the eye has no accommodative power and has lost most of its refractive ability **(aphakia).** A replacement lens is needed to focus light rays in the retina. Most often, a small, clear, plastic lens is implanted at the time of cataract removal. Replacement lenses can be selected to allow correction of a specific refractive error. Some clients have distant vision restored to 20/20 and may need glasses only for reading or close work. Some replacement lenses have multiple focal planes and may correct all vision for a client to the extent that glasses or contact lenses are not needed at all or are only minimally needed.

EXTRACAPSULAR
CATARACT EXTRACTION

INTRACAPSULAR
CATARACT EXTRACTION

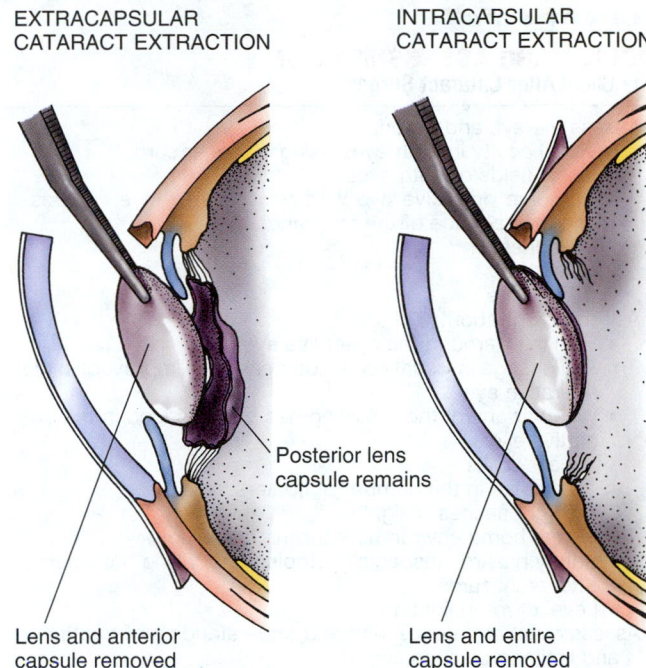

Posterior lens
capsule remains

Lens and anterior
capsule removed

Lens and entire
capsule removed

Figure 50-9 ■ Surgical approaches to lens removal for cataracts.

Postoperative Care. Immediately after surgery, antibiotics are given subconjunctivally. Usually an antibiotic plus steroid ointment also is instilled. The eye is usually left unpatched and often the client is discharged within an hour after surgery. Instruct the client to wear dark glasses outdoors or in brightly lit environments until the pupil responds to light.

The ophthalmologist examines the eye with a slit-lamp microscope the next day. Antibiotic-steroid eyedrops, such as tobramycin combined with dexamethasone (TobraDex), are instilled.

Mild itching is normal, as is a "bloodshot appearance." The eyelid may be slightly swollen; however, significant swelling or bruising is abnormal. Cool compresses may be beneficial. Discomfort at the site is controlled by a mild analgesic such as acetaminophen (Abenol✳, Tylenol) or acetaminophen with oxycodone (Endocet✳, Percocet, Tylox). Instruct the client to avoid aspirin because of its effects on blood clotting.

Pain early after surgery may indicate a complication, such as increased IOP or hemorrhage. Instruct the client to contact the ophthalmologist if pain occurs with nausea or vomiting.

To reduce increases in IOP (the major complication after surgery), teach the client and family about activity restrictions. Activities that can cause a sudden rise in IOP are listed in Table 50-3.

Another major complication is infection. Instruct the client to observe for increasing redness of the eye, a change in visual acuity, tears, and photophobia. Creamy white, dry, crusty drainage on the eyelids and lashes is normal. Yellow or green drainage indicates infection and must be reported.

Bleeding into the anterior chamber of the eye also may occur, usually several days after surgery. Blood may come from the incision, iris, or ciliary body. Instruct the client to report any change in vision immediately to the ophthalmologist.

TABLE 50-3 Activities That Increase Intraocular Pressure

- Bending from the waist
- Sneezing, coughing
- Blowing the nose
- Straining to have a bowel movement
- Vomiting
- Sexual intercourse
- Keeping the head in a dependent position
- Wearing tight shirt collars

Most clients experience a dramatic improvement in vision as early as the day of surgery. Caution the client that final best vision will not be present until 4 to 6 weeks after surgery.

Critical Thinking Challenge

Your 62-year-old client with bilateral cataracts is scheduled to have an extracapsular cataract removal with immediate intraocular lens implantation for her left eye (the one with the worse vision). She asks why both eyes can't be done at the same time so that she will not have to go "through all of this rigmarole twice." She also is concerned about her facial appearance after surgery and whether any bruising will be present.

1. Should both eyes be done at the same time? Why or why not?
2. How will her appearance be changed during the first week after surgery?

evolve For suggested answer guidelines, go to http://evolve.elsevier.com/Iggy/.

Community-Based Care

The client is usually discharged within 2 hours after cataract surgery. Nursing interventions focus on helping the client and family with plans for return to the home, assisted living, or extended care setting.

HOME CARE MANAGEMENT

If the client has difficulty instilling eyedrops, a supportive neighbor, friend, or family member can be taught the procedure. Adaptive equipment that positions the bottle of eyedrops directly over the eye can also be purchased.

HEALTH TEACHING

Review the following indications of complications after cataract surgery with the client and family before discharge:

- Sharp, sudden pain in the eye
- Bleeding or increased discharge
- Lid swelling
- Decreased vision
- Flashes of light or floating shapes

Tell the client to avoid activities that might increase IOP (see Table 50-3). The client may wash his or her hair a day or two after surgery, but only with the head tilted back, such as in a beauty salon or barber shop, to avoid getting water in the eye. For the first week after surgery, advise the client to stand in the shower with the face held away from the showerhead.

Cooking and light housekeeping are permitted, but vacuuming should be avoided for several weeks because of the forward flexion involved and the rapid, jerky movements required. Advise the client to refrain from driving, operating machinery, and participating in certain sports, such as golf, until given specific permission from the ophthalmologist.

CHART 50-7

NIC INTERVENTION ACTIVITIES for
The Client Requiring Topical Eye Medication

Medication Administration: *Eye: Preparing and instilling ophthalmic medications*
- Follow the five rights of medication administration.
- Note client's medical history and history of allergies.
- Determine client's knowledge of medication and understanding of method of administration.
- Position client supine or sitting in a chair with neck slightly hyperextended; ask client to look at ceiling.
- Instill medication onto the conjunctival sac using aseptic technique.
- Apply gentle pressure to nasolacrimal duct if medication has systemic effects.
- Instruct client to close eye gently to help distribute medication.
- Monitor for local, systemic, and adverse effects of medication.

NIC intervention activities selected from Dochterman, J.M., & Bulechek, G.M. (Eds.). (2004). *Nursing interventions classification (NIC)* (4th ed.). St. Louis: Mosby. No part of this work is to be altered without prior written permission from the Publisher.

Review the procedure for instilling eyedrops with the client or caretaker. If the client is concerned that the drops may not be correctly instilled, advise him or her to refrigerate the eyedrops. Then, when the eyedrop falls into the conjunctival sac, the client will notice a cool feeling. Eyedrops are often prescribed for 4 to 6 weeks after cataract surgery (Chart 50-7). Chart 50-8 lists items to cover in the focused assessment of a client in the home environment after cataract surgery.

HEALTH CARE RESOURCES

If the client lives alone and has no family or significant others, arrange for a home care nurse to assess the client and the home situation. If the client is unable to instill eyedrops independently, a friend, neighbor, or family member can be taught this technique.

Critical Thinking Challenge

Your 62-year-old client had the cataract removed from her left eye and a multifocal lens implanted on Friday afternoon. She plans to go back to work on Monday and does not want her co-workers to know about the surgery. (She worries that people will think she is "old" and not on the cutting edge of her profession.)
1. Should she go back to work on Monday? Why or why not?
2. What accommodations will she have to make at her work place?
3. What specific activities will you tell her to avoid?

evolve For suggested answer guidelines, go to http://evolve.elsevier.com/Iggy/.

◆Evaluation: Outcomes

Evaluate the care of the client with cataracts on the basis of the identified nursing diagnoses. The expected outcomes include that the client having cataracts will:
- Demonstrate Vision Compensation Behavior
- Remain free from injury

The client having cataract surgery will:
- Have improved Sensory Function: Vision
- Recognize manifestations of complications

CHART 50-8

HOME CARE ASSESSMENT of
The Client After Cataract Surgery

Assess the eye and vision:
- Visual acuity in both eyes using a Jaeger card
- Visual fields of both eyes
- Compare operative eye with nonoperative eye for presence or absence of the following:
    Redness
    Tearing
    Drainage

Ask the client about:
- Pain in or around the operative eye
- Any change in visual acuity (decreased or improved) in the operative eye
- Whether any of the following has been noticed in the operative eye:
    Dark spots
    Increase in the number of floaters
    Bright flashes of light

Assess the home environment for the following:
- Safety hazards (especially tripping and falling hazards)
- Kitchen hazards
- Level of room lighting

Assess client adherence with and understanding of treatment and limitations, such as:
- Signs and symptoms to report
- Medication regimen
- Activity restrictions

Assess functional ability:
- Activities of daily living
- Compliance with medication regimen

Specific indicators for these outcomes are listed for each nursing diagnosis under the Planning and Implementation section (see earlier).

GLAUCOMA

PATHOPHYSIOLOGY

Glaucoma is a group of ocular diseases resulting in increased IOP. Intraocular pressure (IOP) is the fluid (aqueous humor) pressure within the eye. A normal IOP of 10 to 21 mm Hg is maintained when there is a balance between production and outflow of aqueous humor. IOP can be raised by decreasing the outflow of aqueous fluid or by overproducing aqueous humor. In people with glaucoma, aqueous humor builds up inside the eye, and the increased pressure reduces blood flow to the optic nerve and retina. The sensitive nerve tissue becomes ischemic and dies. Tissue damage usually starts in the periphery and moves inward toward the fovea centralis. Left untreated, glaucoma can result in blindness. Glaucoma is commonly painless and the client may be unaware of a gradual reduction in vision.

Etiology

There are several causes and types of glaucoma (Table 50-4). Glaucoma is classified as primary, secondary, or associated. In primary glaucoma, the most common form, the structures involved in circulation and reabsorption of the aqueous humor undergo direct pathologic change.

Primary open-angle glaucoma (POAG), the most common form of primary glaucoma, is usually bilateral and asymptomatic in the early stages. There is reduced outflow

TABLE 50-4   Common Causes of Glaucoma

Primary Glaucoma
- Aging
- Heredity
- Central retinal vein occlusion

Associated Glaucoma
- Diabetes mellitus
- Hypertension
- Severe myopia
- Retinal detachment

Secondary Glaucoma
- Uveitis
- Iritis
- Neovascular disorders
- Trauma
- Ocular tumors
- Degenerative disease
- Eye surgery

CHART 50-9

KEY FEATURES of
Glaucoma

Early
- Increased intraocular pressure
- Diminished accommodation

Late
- Diminished visual fields (loss of peripheral vision)
- Decreased visual acuity not correctable with glasses
- Halos around lights
- Headache or eye pain (acute closed-angle glaucoma)
- Increased cup-disc ratio
- Pale optic disc

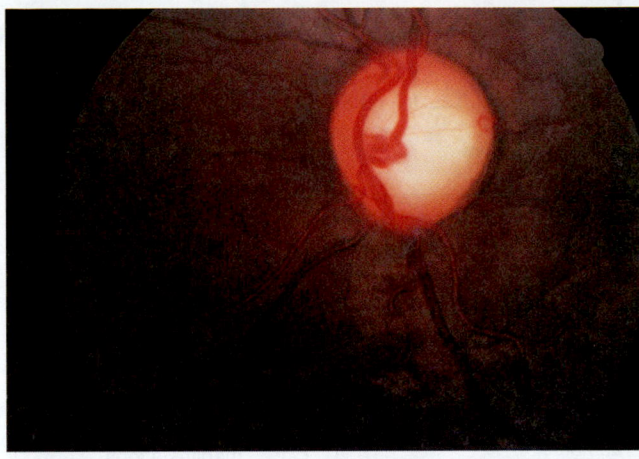

Figure 50-10 ■ The optic fundus of a client with glaucoma.

of aqueous humor through the chamber angle. Because the fluid cannot leave the eye at the same rate it is produced, IOP gradually increases.

Angle-closure glaucoma (also called closed-angle glaucoma, narrow-angle glaucoma, or acute glaucoma) is less common, has a sudden onset, and is an emergency. The basic problems are a narrowed angle and forward displacement of the iris. Movement of the iris against the cornea narrows or closes the chamber angle, obstructing the outflow of aqueous humor. This can happen suddenly and without warning.

Secondary glaucoma results from ocular diseases that cause a narrowed angle or an increased volume of fluid within the eye. This can happen suddenly and without warning.

Incidence/Prevalence

Glaucoma is a common cause of blindness in affluent countries. It is age related, occurring in about 10% of people older than 80 years of age (McCance & Huether, 2002).

◆COLLABORATIVE MANAGEMENT

Primary open-angle glaucoma develops slowly, usually without symptoms. The gradual loss of visual fields may go unnoticed because central vision is unaffected. At times, the client may have foggy vision, reduced accommodation, mild aching in the eyes, or headaches and may require frequent changes in eyeglass prescriptions. Late manifestations occur after irreversible damage to optic nerve function and include visual field losses along with decreased visual acuity not correctable with eyeglasses. Chart 50-9 lists other manifestations of glaucoma. The Concept Map on p. 1098 addresses assessment and nursing care issues for clients who have glaucoma.

◆Assessment

PHYSICAL ASSESSMENT/CLINICAL MANIFESTATIONS

Ophthalmoscopic examination of the client with glaucoma shows cupping and atrophy of the optic disc. The disc becomes wider and deeper and turns white or gray (Figure 50-10).

To determine the extent of peripheral field losses, visual fields are measured. In chronic open-angle glaucoma, the visual fields first show a small crescent-shaped defect that gradually progresses to a larger field defect. In acute angle-closure glaucoma, the visual fields can quickly decrease.

The manifestations of acute angle-closure glaucoma differ from those of open-angle glaucoma. The onset of symptoms is acute, and the client has sudden, severe pain around the eyes that radiates over the face. Headache or brow pain, nausea, and vomiting also may occur. Other manifestations include seeing colored halos around lights and sudden blurred vision with decreased light perception.

On examination, the sclera may appear reddened and the cornea foggy. Ophthalmoscopic examination reveals a shallow anterior chamber, cloudy aqueous humor, and a moderately dilated, nonreactive pupil.

OTHER DIAGNOSTIC ASSESSMENTS

TONOMETRY. Intraocular pressure (IOP), as measured by tonometry, is elevated in glaucoma. If an elevated reading is found during routine screening examination, take several readings over a period of time at various times of the day to determine a pattern, because IOP varies during the day. In open-angle glaucoma, the tonometry reading is between 22 and 32 mm Hg (normal is 10 to 21 mm Hg). In angle-closure glaucoma, the tonometry reading may be 30 mm Hg or higher.

TONOGRAPHY. Tonography combines the use of an electronic indentation tonometer with a recording device. The outflow of aqueous humor from the eye is measured while a weight rests on the globe. The slope of the graph indicates IOP changes. A steep downhill tracing (normal) indicates adequate drainage. A flat tracing indicates reduced outflow, as in glaucoma.

GONIOSCOPY. A special lens that eliminates the corneal curve helps view the drainage angle in the anterior chamber. The entire 360-degree circumference of the angle

CONCEPT MAP Glaucoma

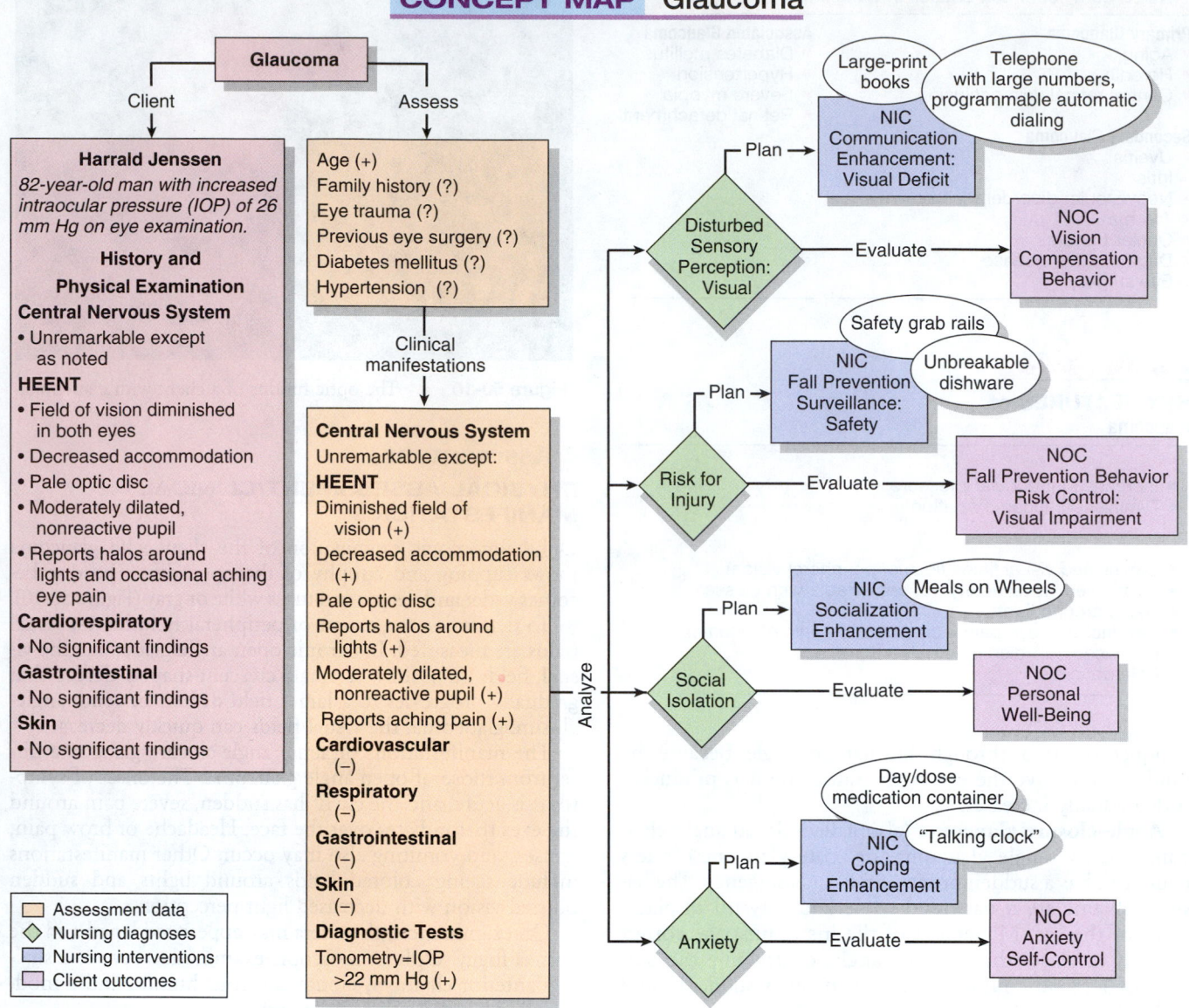

Concept Map by Elaine Bishop Kennedy, EdD, RN

between the iris and the cornea is examined. Adhesions, abnormal blood vessels, sites of trauma, and other changes as possible causes of secondary glaucoma can be seen.

◆Interventions

NONSURGICAL MANAGEMENT. Blindness from glaucoma can be prevented by early detection, lifelong treatment, and a regimen of close monitoring and follow-up care. Some degree of vision loss occurs, although use of topical agents that reduce ocular hypertension have been found to delay or prevent damage from glaucoma. (See the Evidence-Based Practice for Nursing box on p. 1099.) Chart 50-10 lists ways to assist the older client with impaired vision to remain as independent as possible.

Drug Therapy. Drug therapy for glaucoma focuses on reducing IOP through the following mechanisms:

- Constricting the pupil so that the ciliary muscle is contracted, allowing better circulation of the aqueous humor to the site of absorption
- Reducing the production of aqueous humor

Pupillary Constriction. Drugs that constrict the pupil and contract the ciliary muscle **(miotics),** such as pilocarpine hydrochloride (Isopto Carpine, Pilocar, Spersacarpine✱), are commonly used to treat glaucoma. In acute angle-closure glaucoma, pupil constriction is helpful because it enhances aqueous outflow. Carbachol (Isopto Carbachol, Miostat) may be used with or in place of pilocarpine. Echothiophate iodide (Phospholine Iodide) produces miosis and increases outflow. Remind the client that miotics may cause blurred vision for 1 to 2 hours after use and that vision in low light environments is difficult because of the pupillary constriction. Another group of drugs that improve outflow of aqueous humor are the prostaglandin agonists. Drugs from this class include latanoprost (Xalatan), travoprost (Travatan), bimatoprost (Lumigan), and unoprostone (Rescula). Nursing interventions for these drugs are listed in Chart 50-2.

Inhibition of Aqueous Humor. Beta blockers such as timolol (Apo-Timop✱, Timoptic) and levobunolol (Betagan) are used to decrease IOP. When used as eyedrops,

EVIDENCE-BASED PRACTICE for Nursing

Encourage clients to adhere to their ocular hypotensive drug therapy

Kass, M., et al. (2002). The ocular hypertension treatment study: Medication delays or prevents the onset of primary open-angle glaucoma. *Archives of Ophthalmology, 120*(6), 701-713.

The purpose of this multicenter, randomized, controlled clinical trial was to determine whether topical ocular hypotensive agents could delay or prevent the onset of primary open-angle glaucoma (POAG). The study subjects were 1500 individuals between 40 and 80 years of age who were identified as having mild to moderate elevations of intraocular pressure (IOP of 24 to 32 mm Hg) in at least one eye and who had no evidence of damage from glaucoma (as determined by visual field examination). The subjects were randomized to one of two groups, an observation-only control group or a treatment group receiving daily ocular hypotensive drugs with a goal of lowering IOP by at least 20%. Subjects in both groups were followed at 6-month intervals for 5 years. Purposive sampling of 400 African-American subjects was performed to ensure adequate representation of this population who are at high risk for glaucoma. The two groups were statistically homogeneous for baseline measures, ages, education, socioeconomic factors, gender, and study completion.

Measures performed at follow-up visits included IOP, slit-lamp examination, direct ophthalmoscopy, optic disc photographs, refraction, visual acuity, and full threshold visual field tests performed by clinicians who were masked to the participant category and to the previous examination findings for each subject.

At the conclusion of the study, subjects receiving the ocular hypotensive drugs had an average reduction in IOP of 22.5% and those in the observational group had an average reduction in IOP of 4.0%. A total of 36 subjects in the treatment group developed glaucoma compared to 89 subjects in the observation group. The researchers concluded that intervention with ocular hypotensive agents could delay or prevent glaucoma in clients with an elevated IOP.

Level of Evidence: 1—Well-designed, randomized, controlled clinical trial at multiple sites of adequate quality.

Critique. The study was well designed and well controlled to answer the questions posed. The multicentered nature of the study contributes to its validity but has the potential to reduce the reliability. The researchers used appropriate methods to ensure reliability. The large sample size also increases the generalizability of the findings.

Implications for Nursing. Many clients are not aware that they have ocular hypertension until glaucoma is present and vision is affected. In addition, many people are poorly adherent to drug regimens involving eyedrops. The results of this study can be used as an inducement for nurses to strongly encourage all clients to have yearly eye examinations that include measurement of intraocular pressure. Explaining the findings of this study to clients under treatment for ocular hypertension could improve client adherence to the treatment regimen and delay vision loss.

beta blockers reduce aqueous humor production without causing pupillary constriction.

Carbonic anhydrase inhibitors, such as acetazolamide (Acetazolam✳, Diamox) and methazolamide (Neptazane), reduce aqueous humor production to help maintain a lowered IOP. Epinephrine 0.5% to 2% and dipivefrin hydrochloride (Propine) also reduce aqueous humor production. *Epinephrine-containing agents are not used in angle-closure glaucoma because they dilate the pupil.*

Osmotic drugs may be given angle-closure glaucoma as part of emergency treatment to rapidly reduce IOP. Such agents include oral glycerin (Osmoglyn) and IV mannitol (Osmitrol).

SURGICAL MANAGEMENT

Laser Surgery. When drugs for the client with open-angle glaucoma are not effective at controlling IOP, laser surgery is indicated.

Preoperative Care. Nursing interventions include informing the client about laser technology, expected sights and sounds often heard during this procedure, and expected outcomes.

Operative Procedures. A laser trabeculoplasty burns the trabecular meshwork, scarring it and causing the meshwork fibers to tighten. Fiber tightening increases the size of the spaces between the fibers, improving outflow of aqueous humor and a reduction in IOP. Topical or local anesthesia is used. Clients may have a temporary increase in IOP immediately after this procedure.

Laser surgery is also indicated for clients with angle-closure glaucoma. The laser makes a hole near the edge of the iris, allowing aqueous humor to flow from the posterior chamber to the anterior chamber and then into the drainage meshwork.

Postoperative Care. Instruct the client to arrange for transportation home because driving is prohibited right after the surgery. Because laser procedures can sometimes increase IOP, the pressure should be re-evaluated 1 hour after surgery and before discharge. An ocular steroid, such as prednisolone acetate (Ocu-Pred, Ophtho-Tate✳), may be prescribed.

Standard Surgical Therapy. For open-angle glaucoma that fails to respond to drug and laser therapy and for some cases of angle-closure glaucoma, surgery is needed. This surgery either creates a new drainage channel for aqueous humor or destroys the structures that produce it.

Glaucoma surgery is performed either in a hospital or on an outpatient basis. The usual length of stay is several hours to several days.

After surgery, the ophthalmologist injects an antibiotic under the conjunctiva. The eye is then covered with a patch and a protective shield is applied over it. Instruct the client to avoid taking aspirin, to avoid lying on the operative side, and to report any brow pain, severe eye pain, or nausea.

The most serious complication after glaucoma surgery is choroidal hemorrhage. If IOP is too low, fluid may enter the suprachoroid space and cause a choroidal detachment. Extra fluid in this space may break blood vessels located there. Manifestations of choroidal hemorrhage include the following:

- Acute pain deep in the eye
- Decreased vision
- Vital sign changes

VITREOUS HEMORRHAGE

PATHOPHYSIOLOGY

The vitreous is the gel that fills the posterior two thirds of the eye and maintains the eye's shape. Vitreous hemorrhage (bleeding into the vitreous cavity) may result from aging, systemic diseases, or trauma, or it may occur spontaneously. With aging, the vitreous may spontaneously detach from the retina. Torn blood vessels allow bleeding into the vitreous. Diseases that disrupt the retinal blood vessels, such as

NURSING FOCUS on the OLDER ADULT
Promote Independent Living in Clients with Impaired Vision

Medications

- Having a neighbor, relative, friend, or visiting nurse visit once a week to measure the proper medications for each day may be helpful.

  If the client is to take medications more than once each day, it is helpful to use a container of a different shape (with a lid) each time. For example, if the client is to take medications at 9 AM, 1 PM, and 9 PM, the 9 AM medications would be placed in a round container, the 1 PM medications in a square container, and the 9 PM medications in a triangular container.

  It is helpful to place each day's medication containers in a separate box with raised letters on the side of the box spelling out the day.
- "Talking clocks" are available for the client with low vision.

Communication

- Telephones with large, raised block numbers may be helpful. The best models are those with black numbers on a white phone or white numbers on a black phone.
- Telephones that have a programmable, automatic dialing feature are very helpful. Programmed numbers should include those for the fire department, police, relatives, friends, neighbors, and 911.

Safety

- It is best to leave furniture the way the client wants it and not move it.
- Throw rugs are best eliminated.
- Appliance cords should be short and kept out of walkways.
- Lounge-style chairs with built-in footrests are preferable to footstools.
- Nonbreakable dishes, cups, and glasses are preferable to breakable ones.
- Cleansers and other toxic agents should be labeled with large, raised letters.
- Hook-and-loop (Velcro) strips at hand level may help to mark the locations of switches and electrical outlets.

Food Preparation

- Meals on Wheels is a service that many older adults find helpful. This service brings meals at mealtime, cooked and ready to eat. The cost of this service varies, depending on the client's ability to pay.
- Many grocery stores offer a "shop by telephone" service. The client can either complete a computer booklet indicating types, amounts, and brands of items desired, or the store will complete this booklet over the telephone by asking the client specific information. The store then delivers groceries to the client's door (many stores also offer a "put away" service) and charges the client's bank card.
- A microwave oven is a safer means of cooking than a standard stove, although many older clients are afraid of microwave ovens. If the client has and will use a microwave oven, others can prepare meals ahead of time, label them, and freeze them for later use. Also, many complete, microwavable frozen dinners that comply with a variety of dietary restrictions are available.
- Friends or relatives may be able to help with food preparation. Often relatives do not know what to give an older person for birthdays or other gift-giving occasions. One suggestion is a homemade prepackaged frozen dinner that the client enjoys.

Personal Care

- Handgrips should be installed in bathrooms.
- The tub floor should have a nonskid surface.
- Male clients should use an electric shaver rather than a razor.
- Choosing a hairstyle that is becoming but easy to care for (avoiding parts) helps in independent living.
- Home hair care services may be available.

Diversional Activity

- Some clients are able to use large-print books, newspapers, and magazines (available through local libraries and vision services).
- Books, magazines, and some newspapers are available on audiotape.
- Clients experienced in knitting or crocheting may be able to create items fashioned from straight pieces, such as afghans.
- Card games, dominoes, and some board games that are available in large, high-contrast print may be helpful for clients with low vision.

---

hypertension and diabetes mellitus, also cause blood leakage into the vitreous.

◆COLLABORATIVE MANAGEMENT

The main manifestation of vitreous hemorrhage is reduced visual acuity. The degree of reduced vision varies with the severity of the hemorrhage. A mild hemorrhage may cause the client to see a red haze or "floaters." A moderate hemorrhage may cause the client to see "black streaks" or "tiny black dots." Severe hemorrhage may reduce visual acuity to hand motion. Eye examination shows a reduced red reflex because light rays are blocked from reaching the retina. Ultrasonography is used to determine the location and extent of the hemorrhage.

A vitreous hemorrhage may absorb slowly with no treatment. Leaking blood vessels can be sealed with laser therapy. If the hemorrhage is still present several weeks to months later, a **vitrectomy** (surgical removal of the vitreous) is indicated.

UVEITIS

PATHOPHYSIOLOGY

The uveal tract has three related parts: the iris, the ciliary body, and the choroid. A common problem within these structures is inflammation, or **uveitis.** Uveitis may occur in the anterior or posterior portion of the eye.

Anterior uveitis is inflammation of the iris, inflammation of the ciliary body, or both. The cause of anterior uveitis is unknown, but often follows exposure to allergens, infectious agents, trauma, or systemic disease (rheumatoid arthritis, herpes simplex, herpes zoster). It can follow any local or systemic bacterial infection. Manifestations include aching around the eye; tearing; blurred vision; photophobia; a small, irregular, nonreactive pupil; and a "bloodshot" appearance of the sclera.

Posterior uveitis is the common term for **retinitis** (inflammation of the retina) and **chorioretinitis** (inflammation of both the choroid and the retina). Posterior uveitis occurs with tuberculosis, syphilis, and toxoplasmosis.

The onset of symptoms is slow and painless. Visual impairment in the affected eye results from fluid, fibrin, and cells leaking into the vitreous cavity. The pupil is small, nonreactive, and irregularly shaped. Black dots are visible against the red background of the fundus. Lesions appear as grayish yellow patches on the retinal surface.

◆COLLABORATIVE MANAGEMENT

Treatment of uveitis includes resting the ciliary body with a cycloplegic agent. The pupil is dilated to prevent adhesions between the iris and the lens. Steroid drops are given hourly to reduce the inflammation and to prevent adhesion of the iris to the cornea and lens. Ocular injections of steroids are used in posterior uveitis or when topical steroids have been ineffective. Analgesics that contain neither aspirin nor opioids are prescribed for pain. Systemic antibiotic therapy may be started for posterior uveitis or when infection is present with anterior uveitis.

Cool or warm compresses are applied for ocular pain. Darkening the room and wearing sunglasses reduce the discomfort of photophobia. Because of blurred vision from the cycloplegic drops, instruct the client not to drive or operate machinery. Review the manifestations of bacterial and fungal ulcers and those of increased intraocular pressure (IOP).

RETINAL DISORDERS

Hypertensive Retinopathy
PATHOPHYSIOLOGY

Many Americans have hypertension. Hypertension causes blood vessel changes in the eyes that damage the retina and reduce vision. Hypertensive retinopathy is classified by grades. With each increasing grade, progressive changes occur in the retina.

◆COLLABORATIVE MANAGEMENT

As blood pressure increases, retinal arterioles narrow and take on a classic "copper wire" appearance (Figure 50-11). Nicking, or narrowing, of the vessel at arteriovenous crossings is present. If blood pressure remains elevated, areas of ischemia, known as soft exudates or "cotton wool" spots, develop from blood vessel occlusion. Small hemorrhages may be seen. The client may also have headaches and vertigo. Left untreated, hypertensive retinopathy can cause retinal detachment.

Treatment focuses primarily on management of the systemic hypertension (see Chapter 39) and controlling IOP.

Diabetic Retinopathy
PATHOPHYSIOLOGY

Diabetic retinopathy is a retinal blood vessel complication. The longer the person has diabetes, the greater the incidence and severity of retinopathy (McCance & Huether, 2002). Poor glucose control worsens the retinopathy. Good control lessens the disease severity. The two types of diabetic retinopathy are background retinopathy and proliferative retinopathy.

In **background diabetic retinopathy,** the cells of the retinal vessels die and fluid leaks into the eye. As this fluid is

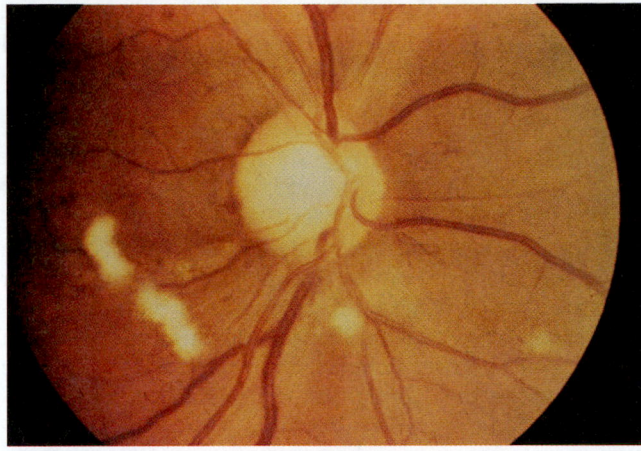

Figure 50-11 ■ The optic fundus of a client with hypertension.

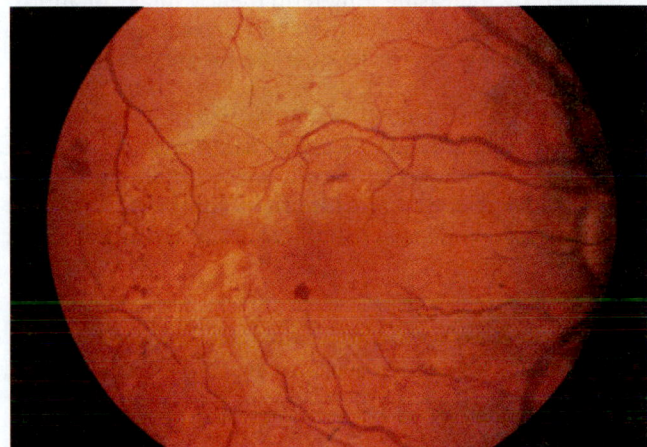

Figure 50-12 ■ The optic fundus of a client with diabetes.

absorbed, thick yellow-white hard exudates, are formed. The capillaries lose their ability to transport needed oxygen and nutrients. Small outpouches **(microaneurysms)** form in the walls of capillaries. These fragile capillaries bleed easily and cause hemorrhages in the nerve layer of the retina (Figure 50-12). Visual acuity is reduced by retinal ischemia or by macular edema.

In clients with **proliferative diabetic retinopathy,** a network of fragile new blood vessels develops, leaking blood and protein into the surrounding tissue. These new blood vessels are stimulated by retinal hypoxia that results from poor capillary perfusion of retinal tissues. New blood vessels grow in the retina, onto the iris, and into the back of the vitreous. The vitreous contracts and pulls away from the retina, causing blood vessels to break and bleed into the vitreous.

◆COLLABORATIVE MANAGEMENT

Treatment of diabetic retinopathy depends on the severity of retinal damage. Laser therapy can seal microaneurysms and decrease bleeding. Scattering of laser burns across the retina can decrease the retina's need for oxygen and control the growth of new blood vessels.

A vitrectomy is performed if frequent bleeding into the vitreous occurs and fibrin bands threaten to detach the retina. Fibrin bands within the vitreous are severed and removed. A laser may be used in the eye during surgery to seal leaking or bleeding blood vessels.

Macular Degeneration

PATHOPHYSIOLOGY

Macular degeneration (deterioration of the macula, the area of central vision) can be atrophic (age related, or *dry*) or exudative *(wet)*. Age-related degeneration is caused by gradual blockage of retinal capillaries, allowing retinal cells in the macula to become ischemic and necrotic. Rod and cone photoreceptors die. Central vision declines, and clients describe "mild blurring and distortion." This type of degeneration is more common and progresses at a faster rate among smokers than among nonsmokers. Current research findings suggest that the risk for atrophic macular degeneration can be reduced by increasing long-term dietary intake of antioxidants and the carotenoids lutein and zeaxanthin. The same dietary treatments appear to slow the progression of macular degeneration.

Clients with exudative ("wet") degeneration have a sudden decrease in vision after a serous detachment of pigment epithelium in the macula. Newly formed blood vessels invade this injured area and cause fluid and blood to collect under the macula (like a blister), resulting in scar formation and visual distortion.

> ### Critical Thinking Challenge
>
> The client is a 75-year-old man who was diagnosed with age-related "dry" macular degeneration after he was involved in a car accident in which he failed to stop at an intersection and hit another car at a low rate of speed. No injuries resulted from the car accident although the client received a citation for a moving violation. The client is very upset with the diagnosis. His wife has never driven nor has she managed the household accounts. He is concerned about "going blind" and wants to know if the LASIK procedure would restore his vision.
> 1. Can the client continue to drive? Why or why not?
> 2. Will a LASIK procedure be helpful for this problem? Why or why not?
> 3. How will you address the issue of "going blind?"
>
> 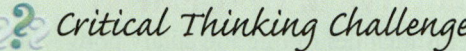 For suggested answer guidelines, go to http://evolve.elsevier.com/Iggy/.

◆COLLABORATIVE MANAGEMENT

Treatment of age-related macular degeneration aims to help the client maximize remaining vision. The loss of central vision reduces the ability to read, write, recognize safety hazards, and drive. Suggest alternative strategies (such as large-print books and public transportation) and referrals to community organizations that provide a wide range of adaptive equipment.

Management of clients with exudative or "wet" macular degeneration is geared toward slowing the process and identifying further changes in visual perception. Fluid and blood may resorb in some clients with exudative degeneration. Laser therapy to seal the leaking blood vessels in or near the macula can limit the extent of the damage. Another method used with some success at sealing or destroying the leaking retinal blood vessels is photodynamic therapy (Gottlieb, 2002; Rechtman et al., 2002). In this treatment, the client is given an IV agent to increase photosensitivity (Verteporfin). After the agent is absorbed, a special nonheating light is applied in the specific area to activate the agent. Activation causes local formation of oxygen radicals that occlude the leaking vessels and prevent excessive formation of new vessels.

> ### Critical Thinking Challenge
>
> Your client with macular degeneration (dry) wants to know if continuing to use his limited vision will increase the progression of the macular degeneration. He also worries that he will "lose his mind" if he has to give up all his usual activities.
> 1. How will you address his concerns?
> 2. How will you proceed to assist the client and his wife in maintaining independence and quality of life?
>
> 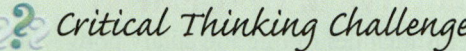 For suggested answer guidelines, go to http://evolve.elsevier.com/Iggy/.

Retinal Holes, Tears, and Detachments

PATHOPHYSIOLOGY

A retinal hole is a break in the retina. Retinal holes can be caused by trauma or can occur with aging. A retinal tear is a more jagged and irregularly shaped break in the retina. It can result from traction on the retina. A retinal detachment is the separation of the retina from the epithelium. Detachments are classified by the nature of their development.

Rhegmatogenous detachments occur following a hole or tear in the retina caused by mechanical force, creating an opening for the vitreous to move under the retina. When sufficient fluid collects in this space, the retina detaches. *Traction* detachments occur when the retina is pulled away from the support tissue by bands of fibrous tissue in the vitreous. *Exudative* detachments are caused by fluid collecting under the retina. These often occur with a systemic disease or with ocular tumors. No retinal break occurs.

◆COLLABORATIVE MANAGEMENT

The onset of a retinal detachment is usually sudden and painless because no pain fibers are located in the retina. Clients may suddenly see bright flashes of light **(photopsia)** or floating dark spots in the affected eye. During the initial phase of the detachment or if the detachment is partial, the client may describe the sensation of a curtain being pulled over part of the visual field. The visual field loss corresponds to the area of detachment.

◆Assessment

On ophthalmoscopic examination, detachments are seen as gray bulges or folds in the retina that quiver. Depending on the cause of the detachment, a hole or tear also may be seen at the edge of the detachment.

◆Interventions

If a retinal hole or tear is discovered before it causes a detachment, the defect may be closed or sealed. Closure prevents fluid from collecting under the retina and reduces the risk for a detachment. Treatment involves creating an inflammatory response that will bind the retina and choroid together around the break. The inflammatory response can be created with the application of **cryotherapy** (a freezing probe), **photocoagulation** (laser), or **diathermy** (high-frequency current).

Spontaneous reattachment of the retina is rare. Surgical repair is usually needed to place the retina in contact with the underlying structures. A common repair procedure is scleral buckling.

Preoperative Care. The client is usually anxious and fearful about a possible permanent loss of vision. Provide information and reassurance to allay fears.

Activity is often restricted before surgery to prevent further tearing or detachment and to promote drainage of any fluid under the retina. An eye patch is placed over the client's affected eye to reduce eye movement. Topical drugs are given before surgery to inhibit pupil constriction and accommodation.

Operative Procedures. The surgery is performed with the client under general anesthesia. In scleral buckling, the ophthalmologist repairs wrinkles or folds in the retina so that the retina can assume its normal smooth position. To promote reattachment, a small piece of silicone is placed against the sclera and held in place by an encircling band (Figure 50-13). This device keeps the retina in contact with the choroid and sclera to promote attachment. Any fluid under the retina is drained.

A gas or silicone oil placed inside the eye can be used to promote retinal reattachment. These agents float up against the retina to hold it in place until healing occurs.

Postoperative Care. After surgery, an eye patch and shield are applied. Monitor the client's vital signs and check the eye patch and shield for any drainage.

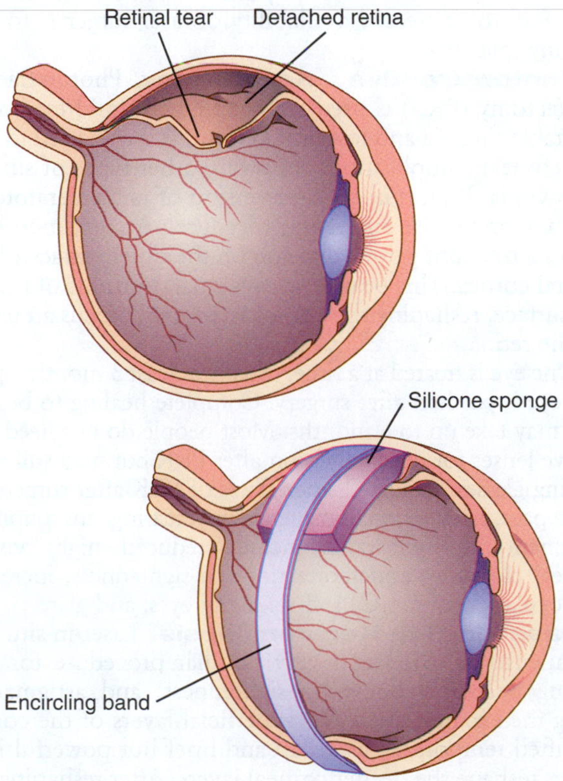

Activity after surgery varies. If gas or oil has been used, position the client on his or her abdomen to allow the gas to float against the retina. Instruct the client to lie with the head turned so that the affected eye is facing up, for several days or until the gas has been absorbed. As an alternative, he or she can sit on the side of the bed and place the head on an over-the-bed table. Bathroom privileges are allowed once the client is fully awake.

The client may have nausea and pain after surgery. Give analgesics and antiemetics as prescribed. Report any sudden increase in pain or pain occurring with nausea to the surgeon because these symptoms may indicate the development of complications. Instruct the client to avoid activities that increase intraocular pressure (IOP) (see Table 50-3).

In the first week after retinal detachment surgery, the client must avoid reading, writing, and close work, such as sewing, because these activities cause rapid eye movements and promote detachment. Teach the client the manifestations of infection and detachment. Instruct the client to notify the nurse or physician if any signs or symptoms occur.

Retinitis Pigmentosa

PATHOPHYSIOLOGY

Several types of retinal disorders can cause progressive degeneration of the retina and lead to blindness. Retinitis pigmentosa (RP) is a condition in which retinal nerve cells degenerate and the pigmented cells of the retina grow and move into the sensory areas of the retina, causing further degeneration.

Genetic Considerations

Different forms of this disorder can be inherited as an autosomal dominant trait, an autosomal recessive trait, or an X-linked recessive trait (Nussbaum, McInnes, & Willard, 2001). Mutations in several genes have been identified as being responsible for retinitis pigmentosa and screening of people who are at high risk is available in some medical centers (Majewski, et al., 2003).

◆COLLABORATIVE MANAGEMENT

The most common early manifestation of retinitis pigmentosa is night blindness, often occurring in childhood. Over time, decreased visual acuity progresses to total blindness. Examination of the retina shows heavy pigmentation in a lacy pattern. Cataracts may accompany this disorder.

No current therapy has proved effective in preventing or slowing the degenerative process. Because some retinal destruction resembles that seen with vitamin A deficiency, a regimen of vitamin A, along with decreased exposure of the retina to bright light, is being tried. An experimental treatment of a retinal microchip implant (artificial retina) is under investigation (Smith, 2002).

REFRACTIVE ERRORS

PATHOPHYSIOLOGY

The ability of the eye to focus images on the retina depends on the length of the eye from front to back and the refractive power of the lens system. **Refraction** is the bending of

Figure 50-13 ■ The scleral buckling procedure for repair of retinal detachment.

light rays. Problems in either eye length or refraction can result in refractive errors.

Myopia

In **myopia** (nearsightedness), the refractive ability of the eye is too strong for the eye length. Images are bent and fall in front of, not on, the retina.

Hyperopia

In **hyperopia,** or **hypermetropia** (farsightedness), the refractive ability of the eye is too weak, causing images to be focused behind the retina. A short eye length may contribute to the development of hyperopia.

Presbyopia

As people age, the lens loses its elasticity and is less able to alter its shape to focus the eye for close work **(presbyopia).** As a result, images fall behind the retina. Presbyopia usually occurs in people in their 30s and 40s.

Astigmatism

Astigmatism occurs when the curve of the cornea is uneven. Because light rays are not refracted equally in all directions, the image does not focus on the retina.

◆COLLABORATIVE MANAGEMENT
◆Assessment

Refractive errors are diagnosed through a process known as **refraction.** The client is asked to view an eye chart while lenses of different strengths are systematically placed in front of the eye. With each lens strength, the client is asked whether the lenses sharpen or worsen vision. The strength of the lens needed to focus the image on the retina is expressed in measurements called diopters.

◆Interventions

NONSURGICAL MANAGEMENT. Errors of refraction can be corrected with a lens that focuses light rays on the retina (see Figure 49-5). Hyperopic vision is corrected to bring the image forward onto the retina with a concave lens. Myopic vision is corrected with a convex lens to move the focused image back to the retina.

Eyeglasses. Eyeglasses are used to correct refractive errors. Advantages of eyeglasses are ease of use, durability, availability, and low cost. Disadvantages include a change in appearance, the weight of the frame on the nose, and reduced peripheral vision (vision is corrected only when the client looks through the center of the lens).

Contact Lenses. Contact lenses also correct refractive errors. Round plastic disks rest against the cornea and fit under the eyelid.

Hard Lenses. Hard contact lenses correct errors in two ways, by changing the shape of the cornea and by providing direct refraction. Changing corneal shape increases its refracting ability. Direct refraction from the contact lens places the specific refractive power and shape needed in front of the eye so that light rays are correctly focused onto the retina.

Complications of hard contact lens wear include corneal edema, which occurs when the lenses are worn for an extended period. Corneal abrasions can result from overwear, which dries the cornea and causes minute breaks, or from the irritation of the contact lens against the cornea.

Soft Lenses. Soft contact lenses are larger but better tolerated than hard contact lenses. They resemble the thickness of plastic wrap and can be worn for longer periods because this type of lens allows greater corneal access to moisture and oxygen. Most problems with wearing soft lenses are related to lens deterioration, deposits in the lens, and failure to follow correct lens care practices.

There are two types of soft contact lenses: daily-wear lenses (worn during waking hours) and extended-wear lenses. Extended-wear contact lenses can be worn continuously for several days to several weeks, depending on the client's environment, activities, and tolerance of the lenses.

SURGICAL MANAGEMENT. Surgery is a popular alternative for the treatment of refractive errors. Vision-enhancing surgeries include radial keratotomy, photorefractive keratectomy, laser in-situ keratomileusis (LASIK), and placement of Intacs corneal ring segments. All surgical procedures are much more expensive than eyeglasses or any type of contact lens. These procedures, performed as outpatient surgery, are rarely covered by insurance.

Radial Keratotomy. Radial keratotomy (RK) is an outpatient surgical procedure for the treatment of mild to moderate myopia. Eight to 16 diagonal incisions are made through 90% of the peripheral cornea. Because the central cornea is not incised, vision is not reduced. These incisions flatten the cornea, which allows the image to be focused closer to the retina.

Most clients have several days of moderate discomfort after surgery. Slight overcorrection or undercorrection of the refractive error is possible, in which case the client still must wear some form of visual correction after the surgery. Other complications include corneal scarring and chronic dry eyes. This procedure is less popular now in North America as a result of increased availability of laser surgeries to correct myopia.

Photorefractive Keratotomy. Photorefractive keratectomy (PRK) is used for people with mild to moderate stable myopia and low astigmatism. It is also used to correct corneal complications following other types of surgery for myopia. PRK is not a laser version of radial keratotomy but a completely different procedure. An excimer laser pulses a brief but powerful beam on the outer surface of the central cornea. This beam removes small portions of the tissue surface, reshaping the cornea to properly focus an image on the retina.

One eye is treated at a time, usually at least 3 months apart. The eye is patched after surgery. Complete healing to best vision may take up to 6 months. Most people do not need corrective lenses for distance vision after PRK but may still need reading glasses. Expected side effects of PRK after surgery include pain, hazy vision, light sensitivity, tearing, and pupil enlargement. Complications include reduced night vision, corneal clouding, undercorrection, far-sightedness, increased intraocular pressure (IOP), chronic dry eyes, and glare.

Laser In-Situ Keratomileusis. Laser-in-situ keratomileusis (LASIK) is a very popular procedure for correcting near-sightedness, far-sightedness, and astigmatism using the excimer laser. The superficial layers of the cornea are lifted temporarily as a flap and brief but powerful laser pulses reshape the deeper corneal layers. After reshaping the deeper layers, the corneal flap is placed back into its original position.

Usually both eyes are treated at the same time. Most clients have improved vision within an hour after surgery; complete healing to best vision may take up to 4 weeks.

This procedure is thought to be superior to PRK because the outer corneal layer is not damaged. Pain is less than for PRK, and the time to best vision is reduced. A wider variety of refractive errors can be treated with LASIK than with PRK.

After LASIK correction of refractive errors, many clients no longer require eyeglasses or contact lenses. Overcorrection or undercorrection is possible, however, and some clients may need a mild prescription for a continued refractive error.

The risk for complications is reported to be less than for other types of vision-enhancing surgery, although clients must be informed that serious complications are possible. Complications include corneal clouding, chronic dry eyes, and refractive errors. Some clients have developed blurred vision and other refractive errors months to years after this surgery as a result of keratectasia (Kymionis et al, 2003; Rojas & Manche, 2002). This problem is related to the formation of the corneal flap during surgery and laser-thinning of the cornea. The cornea then becomes unstable and does not refract appropriately.

Intacs Corneal Ring. Intacs corneal ring placement enhances vision for near-sightedness. This surgery does not involve the use of a laser and has the advantage of being reversible. With this procedure, the shape of the cornea is changed by placing a flexible ring in the outer edges of the cornea (outside of the optical zone).

Intacs ring placement is performed on both eyes during one surgery under local anesthesia. Healing to best vision is immediate. Overcorrection or undercorrection of refraction is possible; however, removal, replacement, or adjustment of ring tightness can enhance satisfaction. In addition, replacements can be made if the client's vision changes further as a result of aging. Because the ring is applied to the cornea outside of the optical zone, the risk for corneal clouding or scarring is lower than with other surgical procedures.

TRAUMA

Trauma to the eye or orbital area can result from almost any activity. Care varies depending on the area of the eye affected and whether the globe of the eye has been penetrated.

Hyphema
PATHOPHYSIOLOGY

A **hyphema** is a hemorrhage in the anterior chamber. It occurs when a force is applied to the eye and breaks the blood vessels.

◆COLLABORATIVE MANAGEMENT

If the hyphema is large, it may block the pupil and reduce vision, possibly causing pain and photophobia. Hemolysis of the blood occurs, and the blood is filtered out of the eye through the trabecular meshwork. If the blood particles obstruct the meshwork, increased intraocular pressure (IOP) results.

The client with a hyphema is treated by bedrest in semi-Fowler's position to use gravity as an aid in keeping the hyphema away from the optical center of the cornea. Minimal or no sudden eye movements are permitted for 3 to 5 days to decrease the risk for rebleeding. Cycloplegic eyedrops may be prescribed to place the eye at rest, and the eye is protected by a patch and shield. Television and reading are restricted. A hyphema usually resolves in 5 to 7 days.

Contusion
PATHOPHYSIOLOGY

A contusion of the eyeball and surrounding tissue is caused by traumatic contact with a blunt object. The force of the blow pushes the eye back in the socket. The globe is compressed, and stretching of the ocular soft tissues occurs, which can produce damage and possibly rupture the globe.

Results of the injury may not be seen immediately. These results include edema of the eyelids, subconjunctival hemorrhage, corneal edema, and hyphema.

◆COLLABORATIVE MANAGEMENT

Periorbital ecchymosis, or "black eye," a common contusion injury, is usually caused by blunt trauma. Bleeding into the soft tissue occurs, creating the bruise. The color fades gradually and disappears in 10 to 14 days. Visual acuity is usually not affected, although orbital pain, photophobia, eyelid edema, and diplopia may be present.

Treatment begins at the time of injury. Ice is applied immediately. The client should have a thorough eye examination to rule out any other eye injuries.

Foreign Bodies
PATHOPHYSIOLOGY

Eyelashes, dust, fingernails, dirt, and airborne particles can come in contact with the conjunctiva or cornea and irritate or abrade the surface. If nothing is seen on the cornea or conjunctiva, the eyelids are everted to examine the conjunctivae.

◆COLLABORATIVE MANAGEMENT

The client usually has a feeling of something being in the eye and may have blurry vision. Pain occurs if the corneal surface is injured. Tearing and photophobia may be present.

Evaluation of vision is done before treatment. The eye of any client with a suspected corneal abrasion is examined with fluorescein, followed by irrigation with normal saline (0.9%) to gently remove the particles. Best practices for ocular irrigation are listed in Chart 50-11.

After the foreign body is removed and if an eye patch is applied, tell the client how long the patch must be left in place (patching over corneal abrasions is controversial). Follow-up with the ophthalmologist is needed.

Lacerations
PATHOPHYSIOLOGY

Lacerations are wounds caused by sharp objects and projectiles. Lacerations can occur to any part of the eye, but the most commonly injured areas are the eyelids and the cornea.

◆COLLABORATIVE MANAGEMENT

Initially, close the eye and apply a small ice pack to decrease bleeding. The client should receive medical attention as soon as possible.

BEST PRACTICE for
Ocular Irrigation

1. Assemble equipment:
   - Normal saline IV (1000-mL bag)
   - Macrodrip IV tubing
   - IV pole
   - Eyelid speculum
   - Topical anesthetic (proparacaine hydrochloride)
   - Gloves
   - Collection receptacle (emesis basin works well)
   - Towels
   - pH paper
2. Quickly obtain a history from the client while flushing the tubing with normal saline:
   - Nature and time of the injury
   - Type of irritant or chemical (if known)
   - Type of first aid administered at the scene
   - Any allergies to the "caine" family of medications
3. Evaluate the client's visual acuity *before* treatment:
   - Ask the client to read your name tag with the affected eye while covering the good eye.
   - Ask the client to "count fingers" with the affected eye while covering the good eye.
4. Put on gloves.
5. Place a strip of pH paper in the cul-de-sac of the client's affected eye.
6. Instill proparacaine hydrochloride eyedrops as prescribed.
7. Place the client in a supine position with the head turned slightly toward the affected eye.
8. Have the client hold the affected eye open, or position an eyelid speculum.
9. Direct the flow of normal saline across the affected eye from the nasal corner of the eye toward the outer corner of the eye.
10. Assess the client's comfort during the procedure.
11. If both eyes are affected, irrigate them simultaneously using separate personnel and equipment.

If the client can open the eye, check visual acuity and clean the eyelids. Minor lacerations of the eyelid can be sutured in an emergency department, an urgent care center, or an ophthalmologist's office. A microscope is needed in the operating room if the client has a laceration that involves the eyelid margin, affects the lacrimal system, involves a large area, or has jagged edges.

Corneal lacerations are an emergency because eye contents may prolapse through the laceration. Manifestations include severe eye pain, photophobia, tearing, decreased visual acuity, and inability to open the eyelid. If the laceration is the result of a penetrating injury, an object may be seen protruding from the eye. *The object is removed only by the ophthalmologist, because it may be holding eye structures in place.*

Antibiotics are given to reduce the risk for infection. Depending on the depth of the laceration, scarring may develop. If the scar alters vision, a corneal transplant may be needed later. If the eye contents have prolapsed through the laceration or if the injury is severe, enucleation (surgical eye removal) may be indicated.

Penetrating Injuries

PATHOPHYSIOLOGY

Clients with penetrating eye injuries have the poorest chance of retaining vision in the injured eye. Glass, high-speed metal or wood particles, BB pellets, and bullets are common causes of penetrating injuries. The particles can enter the eye and lodge in or behind the eyeball.

◆COLLABORATIVE MANAGEMENT

The client usually has some eye pain and says he or she "suddenly felt something hit my eye." An entrance wound may be visible. Depending on the location of the entrance and the resting place of the projectile, vision may be affected.

X-rays and computed tomography (CT) scans of the orbit are usually performed. Computer-generated reconstructions of the CT images are created to study this complex area to ensure the orbit is intact and to look for fractures that might entrap orbital muscles. *Magnetic resonance imaging (MRI) is contraindicated because the procedure may move any metal-containing projectile and cause more injury.*

Surgery is usually needed to remove the foreign object. In some cases, foreign bodies need to be removed by a vitrectomy. IV antibiotics are started before surgery to reduce the risk for infection. A tetanus booster is given if necessary.

Assess and document visual acuity. If the client cannot see print, determine whether he or she can count fingers or see hand motions. If the client cannot see movement, assess his or her ability to see light.

OCULAR MELANOMA

PATHOPHYSIOLOGY

Melanoma is the most common malignant eye tumor in adults. This tumor occurs most often in the uveal tract among people in their 30s and 40s.

Because of its rich blood supply, a melanoma can spread easily. Spread occurs by extension through the sclera or invasion of other eye structures into nearby tissue and the brain.

◆COLLABORATIVE MANAGEMENT
◆Assessment

Manifestations of melanoma may not be readily apparent; the tumor may be discovered during a routine examination. Blurring of vision may occur if the macular area is invaded. Visual acuity is reduced if the tumor grows inward toward the center of the eye from the choroid and alters the visual pathway. Increased intraocular pressure (IOP) can result if the tumor invades the canal of Schlemm and obstructs flow of aqueous humor. A change in iris color may occur if the tumor infiltrates the iris. Sudden loss of a portion of the visual field may result from tumor invasion of the space under the retina, producing retinal detachment.

Diagnostic tests for a melanoma depend on the size and tumor growth rate. Ultrasonography is performed to determine the tumor's location and size.

◆Interventions

Treatment also depends on the tumor's size and growth rate, as well as the condition of the other eye. Small lesions of the iris not affecting the iris root are monitored until growth is observed. Tumors of the choroid are treated by surgical enucleation or by radiation therapy with a radioactive plaque.

SURGERY. **Enucleation** (surgical removal of the entire eyeball) is performed under general anesthesia. After the eye is removed, a ball implant is inserted to provide a base for the socket prosthesis and to ensure the best cosmetic result.

CHART 50-12

BEST PRACTICE for
Insertion and Removal of an Ocular Prosthesis

Insertion

1. Assemble equipment:
   - Prosthesis
   - Gloves
   - Towel
2. Explain the procedure to the client.
3. Wash your hands.
4. Cover the work area with a cloth or towel.
5. Don gloves.
6. Remove the prosthesis from its container and rinse it with tepid water.
7. Lift the client's upper lid using your nondominant hand.

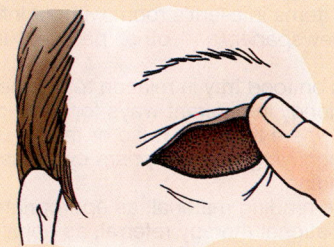

8. Place the prosthesis between the thumb and forefinger of your dominant hand. The notched end of the prosthesis should be closest to the client's nose.

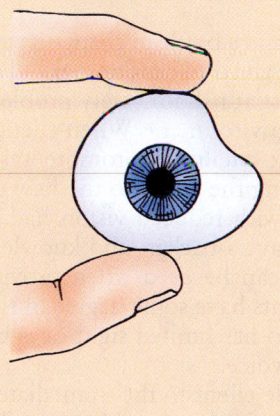

9. Insert the prosthesis with the top edge slipping under the upper lid. Continue until most of the iris is covered by the upper lid.

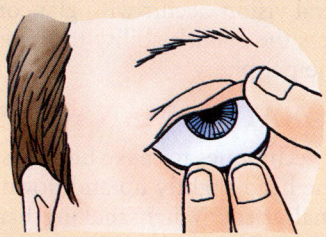

10. Gently release the upper eyelid.
11. Retract the lower lid slightly until the bottom edge of the prosthesis slips behind it.

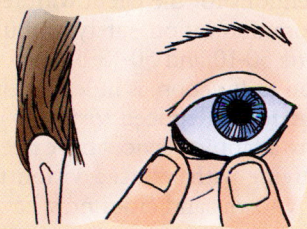

12. Release your hands slowly.

Removal

1. Assemble equipment:
   - Normal saline-filled labeled container
   - Gloves
2. Explain the procedure to the client.
3. Wash your hands.
4. Don gloves.
5. Instruct the client to sit up and tilt the head slightly downward.
6. Place your hand against the client's cheek, palm side up.
7. Pull the lower lid slightly down and laterally.
8. Allow the prosthesis to slide out onto your hand, or pull gently if necessary.
9. Place the prosthesis in a container filled with normal saline labeled with the client's name. Cover the container.

The implant is covered with surrounding tissue, muscles, and conjunctiva. A plastic conformer is placed over the conjunctiva to maintain the shape of the eyelids until a prosthesis can be fitted. After the dressing is removed, a pressure patch is placed over the eye for 24 hours.

Until the prosthesis is fitted (about 1 month after surgery), an antibiotic-steroid ointment is inserted into the cul-de-sac once a day. Best practices for the insertion and removal of the prosthesis are listed in Chart 50-12.

RADIATION. Radiation therapy can reduce the size and thickness of melanomas. The radioactive plaque, a round, flat disk about the size of a dime and containing a radioactive material, is sutured to the sclera overlying the tumor site. The length of time the plaque remains sutured to the sclera depends on the size of the tumor and the dose of radiation to be delivered.

Complications of radiation therapy include vascular changes, retinopathy, glaucoma, necrosis of the sclera, and cataract formation. Vitreous hemorrhage may develop as the tumor becomes smaller and pulls or breaks blood vessels.

While the plaque is in place, the eye may or may not be covered with a patch. Cycloplegic eyedrops and an antibiotic-steroid combination are given. Teach the client how to instill eyedrops.

REDUCED VISION

PATHOPHYSIOLOGY

Different forms of reduced vision may affect any or all aspects of vision, including color, light, image, movement, and acuity. Some periods of reduced vision may be temporary, such as when cataracts obscure vision but surgery has not yet been planned or performed. Clients are legally blind if their best visual acuity with corrective lenses is 20/200 or less in the better eye or if the widest diameter of the visual field in that eye is no greater than 20 degrees.

Blindness can occur in one or both eyes. When one eye is affected, the field of vision is narrowed and depth perception is impaired.

Central vision can be impaired by diseases involving the macula, such as macular edema or macular degeneration. Loss of peripheral vision occurs with glaucoma. The loss of side vision affects the client's ability to drive and awareness of hazards in the periphery.

◆COLLABORATIVE MANAGEMENT

Teach the client techniques to make better use of existing vision. Moving the head slightly up and down can enhance a three-dimensional effect. When shaking hands or pouring water, the client can line up the object and move toward it. He or she should choose a position that favors the good eye; for example, people with vision in the right eye should position people and items on their right.

Nursing interventions for the client with reduced sight fall into the areas of communication, safety, ambulation, self-care, and support. Charts 50-10 and 50-13 list ways to help clients with reduced vision to function as independently as possible.

Communication. Reduced vision is a common occurrence and many adaptive devices have been developed to help the person living with reduced vision to maintain independence. Many towns and cities now have auditory traffic signals so that persons with reduced vision can know when it is safe to cross a street. Curbs in these areas may have high contrast color paint to let the person know when to step up or down. Libraries have large-print books and books on tape. "Talking" clocks, watches, and timers are available. Playing cards, games, restaurant menus, calendars, and instruction booklets are available in large print sizes. Computer keyboards with high contrast and larger letters in the keys are available as are large screens. Direct the client with reduced vision to the local resources to obtain adaptive items and to learn how best to use them.

Safety. For clients at home with reduced vision, the home is the place where the client feels most safe. He or she is familiar with room and item location. For example, they may have counted the number of footsteps needed to move from one area to another within the home. It is important to stress to family and friends that changes in item location should not be made without input from the person with reduced vision.

Even people who have experienced gradually reduced vision over time and who use Vision Compensation Behaviors in the home may benefit from having a person with vision assist in making adaptations in the home. Such adaptations may include the following:

- Using tape and a heavy black marker, mark
  the 350-degree temperature setting on the oven
  the 70-degree temperature setting on the heating or cooling thermostat
- Paint or mark light switches in a deep color that contrasts with the surrounding wall.
- Label canned goods with large, bold, black letters on white tape.
- Teach the client to feel for the crease in paper milk cartons that indicates the place to open the spout.
- Help the client differentiate different drugs by altering the shape or contours of a bottle. Rubber bands can be

CHART 50-13

NIC **INTERVENTION ACTIVITIES for**
The Client with Reduced Vision

Communication Enhancement: Visual Deficit: *Assistance in accepting and learning alternate methods for living with diminished vision*
- Identify yourself when you enter the client's space.
- Note client's reaction to diminished vision (e.g., depression, withdrawal, or denial).
- Accept client's reaction to diminished vision.
- Assist client in setting new goals to learn how to "see" with other senses.
- Build on client's remaining vision, as appropriate.
- Walk one or two steps ahead of the client, with client's hand on your elbow.
- Describe environment to client.
- Do not move items in client's room without informing client.
- Read mail, newspaper, and other pertinent information to client.
- Identify items on food tray in relation to numbers on a clock.
- Fold paper money in different ways for easy identification.
- Inform client where to locate radio or talking books.
- Provide a magnifying glass or prism eyeglasses, as appropriate, for reading.
- Provide braille reading material, as appropriate.
- Initiate occupational therapy referral, as appropriate.
- Refer client with visual problems to appropriate agency.

NIC intervention activities selected from Dochterman, J.M., & Bulechek, G.M. (Eds.). (2004). *Nursing interventions classification (NIC)* (4th ed.). St. Louis: Mosby. No part of this work is to be altered without prior written permission from the Publisher.

wound around a bottle to change its texture. Raised symbols can be glued to caps to make identification easier. The client is most at risk for safety problems in an unfamiliar or changing environment. When clients with reduced vision must be hospitalized, promote safety and independence by orienting the client to the new environment.

Most clients with reduced vision had full sight at some time and thus have a background knowledge regarding size and shape that can be used when providing information. Many blind clients have some degree of sight. When talking with a client who has limited sight or is blind, always use a normal tone of voice.

First orient the client to the immediate environment, including the size of the room. Use one object in the room, such as a chair or hospital bed, as the focal point during your description. Guide the client to the focal point and orient him or her to the environment from that point. For example, you might say, "To the left of the bed is a chair." Then describe all other objects in relation to the focal point. Go with the client to other important areas, such as the bathroom, so that the client can learn their locations. Highlight the location of the toilet, sink, and toilet paper holder. *Never leave the client with reduced vision in the center of an unfamiliar room.*

Clients with reduced vision prefer to establish the location of important objects, such as the call bell, water pitcher, and clock. Once their location has been fixed, do not move these items without the client's consent. Do not move the location of chairs, stools, and wastebaskets without consulting the client.

At mealtime, set up food on the tray using clock placement. For example, "There is sliced ham at 6 o'clock; peas are located at 3 o'clock; to the right of the plate is coffee; salt and pepper are next to the coffee."

Ambulation. When helping a client with reduced vision to ambulate, allow him or her to grasp your arm at the elbow. Keep the arm close to your body so that the client can detect your direction of movement. Alert the client when obstacles are in the path ahead.

Clients may use a cane to detect obstacles, such as furniture, walls, or curbs. The cane is held in the dominant hand several inches off the floor and sweeps the ground where the client's foot will be placed next. The laser cane sends out signals to help detect obstacles.

Self-Care. The ability to control the environment is important to the client with reduced vision. Knock on the door before entering the hospital room or any other environment of a client with reduced vision. State your name and the reason for visiting when entering the room.

Support. Clients' reaction to the loss of sight is similar to the reaction to loss of a body part. Newly blind clients may need a period of grieving for the "dead" (nonseeing) eye. Clients often feel hopeless and angry. With time, anger usually gives way to acceptance. The ability to cope may begin within days, but some clients mourn for months or years.

Clients benefit from the honest support that you can provide. They need to hear that it is normal to mourn, to cry, and to feel the loss. Help clients move toward acceptance by encouraging the mastery of one task at a time and by providing positive reinforcement for each success.

GET READY for the NCLEX Examination!

KEY POINTS

Safe Effective Care Environment

- Use contact precautions with any client who has drainage from the eye or lacrimal apparatus.
- Avoid performing an ophthalmoscopic examination on a confused or uncooperative client.
- Orient the client with reduced vision to his or her immediate surroundings, including how to call for help and where the bathroom is located.
- Identify the room of a client with reduced vision.

Health Promotion and Maintenance

- Identify clients at risk for visual impairment as a result of work environment or leisure activities.
- Encourage all clients to wear eye protection when performing yard work, working in a woodshop or metal shop, using chemicals, or are in any environment where drops or particulate matter are airborne.
- Encourage all adult clients older than 40 years of age to have an eye examination with measurement of intraocular pressure every year.
- Encourage all clients to use polarizing sunglasses whenever outdoors in bright sunlight.
- Teach all clients to wash their hands before and after touching the eyes.

Psychosocial Integrity

- Use a normal tone of voice to talk with a client who has a vision problem and normal hearing.

- Pace your interview to match the learning needs and style of the individual client.
- Knock on the door before entering the room of a client with reduced vision and introduce yourself.
- Allow the client the opportunity to express fear or anxiety regarding a change in vision.
- Refer clients newly diagnosed with visual impairment to appropriate local resources and support groups.
- Explain all diagnostic procedures, restrictions, and follow-up care to the client scheduled for tests.

Physiological Integrity

- Ask the client about vision problems in any other members of the family, because many vision problems have a genetic component.
- Teach clients the proper technique to use for self instillation of eyedrops and eye ointment.
- Stress the importance of completing an antibiotic regimen when an infection is present in the eye.
- Teach clients who are at risk for increased intraocular pressure what activities to avoid (see Table 50-3).
- Teach clients with an infection of the eye or eyelid not to rub the eye (to avoid infecting the other eye).
- Never attempt to remove any object protruding from the eye.

ADDITIONAL STUDY RESOURCES

Go to your Student CD-ROM for Review Questions for the NCLEX Examination.

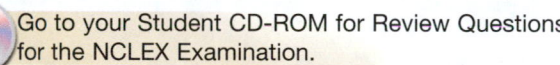
Go to http://evolve.elsevier.com/Iggy/ for Integrated Management of Care Questions for the NCLEX Examination.

SELECTED BIBLIOGRAPHY

Ackley, B., & Ladwig, G. (2002). *Nursing diagnosis handbook: A guide to planning care* (5th ed.). St. Louis: Mosby.

American Cancer Society. (2005). *Cancer facts and figures 2005*. Report No. 00-300M-No. 5008.05. Atlanta: Author.

Barnie, D. (2002). Restoring vision in older patients. *RN, 65*(1), 30-36.

Bickerton, R. (2000). Identifying and treating ocular emergencies. *Journal of Ophthalmic Nursing and Technology, 19*(5), 224-229.

Collins, M., et al. (2001). Effect of laser in situ keratomileusis (LASIK) on the corneal endothelium three years postoperatively. *American Journal of Ophthalmology, 131*(1), 1-6.

Craffey, A. (2000). Look on the bright side: A case study of uveitis. *Insight (American Society of Ophthalmic Registered Nurses), 25*(4), 119-124.

Dochterman, J., & Bulechek, G. (Eds.). (2004). *Nursing interventions classification (NIC)* (4th ed.). St. Louis: Mosby.

Ebersole, P., Hess, P., & Luggen, A. (2004). *Toward healthy aging: Human needs and nursing response* (6th ed.). St. Louis: Mosby.

Facts and Comparisons. (2004). *Drug facts and comparisons* (58th ed.). St. Louis: Author.

Gordon, M., et al. (2002). The ocular hypertension treatment study: Baseline factors that predict the onset of primary open-angle glaucoma. *Archives of Ophthalmology, 120*(6), 714-720.

Jarvis, C. (2004). *Physical examination and health assessment* (4th ed.). Philadelphia: W. B. Saunders.

Kass, M., et al. (2002). The Ocular Hypertension Treatment Study: Medication delays or prevents the onset of primary open-angle glaucoma. *Archives of Ophthalmology, 120*(6), 701-713.

Kushner, B., & Kowal, L. (2003). Diplopia after refractive surgery: Occurrence and prevention. *Archives of Ophthalmology, 121*(3), 315-321.

Kymionis, G., et al. (2003). Management of post-LASIK corneal ectasia with Intacs inserts: One-year results. *Archives of Ophthalmology, 121*(3), 322-326.

Majewski, J., et al. (2003). Age-related macular degeneration—A genome scan in extended families. *American Journal of Human Genetics, 73*(3), 540-550.

McCance, K., & Huether, S. (2002). *Pathophysiology: The biologic basis for disease in adults and children* (4th ed.). St. Louis: Mosby.

Milder, L., & Smith, S. (2002). Refractive surgery: An overview. *Insight (American Society of Ophthalmic Registered Nurses), 27*(2), 46-49.

Moore, L. (2000). Severe visual impairment in older women. *Western Journal of Nursing Research, 22*(5), 571-595.

Moore, L., & Miller, M. (2003). Older men's experiences of living with severe visual impairment. *Journal of Advanced Nursing, 43*(1), 10-18.

Moorhead, S., Johnson, M., & Maas, M. (Eds.). (2004). *Nursing outcomes classification (NOC)* (3rd ed.). St. Louis: Mosby.

Nicholls, P. (2004). Consult stat: Traumatic glaucoma can arise years after an injury. *RN, 67*(10), 65.

Nussbaum, R., McInnes, R., & Willard, H. (2001). *Thompson & Thompson: Genetics in medicine* (6th ed.). Philadelphia: W. B. Saunders.

Pagana, K., & Pagana, T. (2002). *Mosby's manual of diagnostic and laboratory tests* (2nd ed.). St. Louis: Mosby.

Ramponi, D. (2000). Go with the flow during an eye emergency. *Nursing2000, 30*(8), 54-56.

Rapaport, M. (2000). Eyelid dermatitis. *Dermatology Nursing, 12*(5), 352-354.

Rechtman, E., et al. (2002). An update on photodynamic therapy in age-related macular degeneration. *Expert Opinion on Pharmacotherapy, 3*(7), 931-938.

Rojas, M., & Manche, E. (2002). Phototherapeutic keratectomy for anterior basement membrane dystrophy after laser in situ keratomileusis. *Archives of Ophthalmology, 120*(6), 722-727.

Sackett, C., & Schenning, S. (2002). The age-related eye disease study: The results of the clinical trial. *Insight (American Society of Ophthalmic Registered Nurses), 27*(1), 5-7.

Shelswell, N. (2002). Perioperative patient education for retinal surgery. *AORN Journal, 75*(4), 801-807.

Smith, S. (2002). Eye on research: Retinal microchip implants. *Journal of the American Society of Ophthalmic Registered Nurses, 27*(3), 88.

Smith, S. (2003). Reducing ophthalmic drug-related injuries in older patients. *Insight (American Society of Ophthalmic Registered Nurses), 28*(2), 33-34.

Vaughan, D., Asbury, T., & Riordan-Eva, P. (Eds.) (2004). *General ophthalmology* (16th ed.). New York: McGraw-Hill.

Assessment of the Ear and Hearing

JUDY MALKIEWICZ

LEARNING OUTCOMES

After studying this chapter, you should be able to:

1. Describe the key elements to inspect when performing assessment of the external ear.
2. Describe age-related changes in the structure of the ear and hearing.
3. Identify 10 common drugs that affect hearing.
4. Demonstrate the correct use of an otoscope.
5. Describe the landmarks of the tympanic membrane (eardrum).
6. Compare air conduction of sound with bone conduction of sound.
7. Demonstrate the correct use of a tuning fork in performing the Weber and Rinne tests for hearing.
8. Prioritize educational needs for the client about to undergo pure-tone audiometry and electronystagmography.

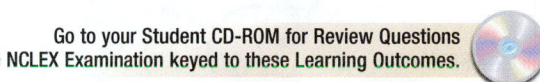

Go to your Student CD-ROM for Review Questions
for the NCLEX Examination keyed to these Learning Outcomes.

Ear and hearing problems are common among adults of all ages. Assessment of the ear and hearing is an important skill for nurses in any care environment. Many problems with the ear and hearing develop over a long period, and hearing may also be affected by many drugs. An understanding of the anatomy and physiology of the ear is essential. Table 51-1 defines terms commonly used in assessing the ear and hearing.

ANATOMY AND PHYSIOLOGY REVIEW

Structure

The ear has three divisions or parts: the external ear, the middle ear, and the inner ear. Each part is important to the hearing process.

EXTERNAL EAR

The external ear develops in the embryo at the same time as the kidneys and urinary tract. Any person with a defect of the external ear should also be examined for possible problems or defects of the renal and urinary systems.

The external ear **(pinna),** which is composed of cartilage covered by skin, is embedded in the temporal bone on both sides of the head at the level of the eyes. The ear is attached to the head by skin and cartilage at about a 10-degree angle. The external ear extends from the pinna through the external

canal to the **tympanic membrane** (eardrum) (Figure 51-1). The external ear canal is slightly S-shaped and lined with **cerumen** (wax)-producing glands (which help protect and lubricate the ear canal), sebaceous glands, and hair follicles. The hair follicles and cerumen protect the eardrum and the middle ear. In the adult, the distance from the opening of the external canal to the eardrum is about 1 to 1½ inches (2.5 to 3.75 cm). The external ear includes the **mastoid process,** the bony ridge located over the temporal bone behind the pinna.

MIDDLE EAR

The middle ear begins at the medial side of the eardrum. It consists of the **epitympanum,** a compartment containing the three bony **ossicles** (Figure 51-2): the malleus, the incus, and the stapes. The beginning of the eustachian tube also opens in the middle ear.

The eardrum **(tympanic membrane)** is a thick, transparent sheet of tissue providing a barrier between the external ear and the middle ear. The landmarks on the eardrum include the annulus, the pars flaccida, and the pars tensa. The eardrum is attached to the first bony ossicle, the **malleus** (hammer), at the **umbo** (Figure 51-3). The bony ossicles behind the eardrum are joined loosely, moving with vibrations from the eardrum.

The pars flaccida and pars tensa are parts of the eardrum. The pars flaccida is that portion of the eardrum above the short process of the malleus; the pars tensa is that portion surrounding the long process of the malleus. The eardrum is usually transparent, opaque, or pearly gray, and it moves

1111

when air is injected into the external canal. The umbo is seen through the eardrum membrane as a white dot at the end of the long process of the malleus. The short process of the malleus, the long process of the malleus, and the umbo are structures that can be seen through the transparent eardrum.

The middle ear is separated from the inner ear by the round window and the oval window. The eustachian tube begins at the floor of the middle ear at the proximal end and opens at the distal end in the throat. The distal opening in the throat is surrounded by adenoid lymphatic tissue (Figure 51-4). The eustachian tube allows the pressure on both sides of the eardrum to equalize. Secretions from the middle ear drain through it.

INNER EAR

The inner ear, which lies on the other side of the oval window, contains the semicircular canals, the cochlea, the vestibule, and the distal end of the eighth cranial nerve (see Figure 51-2). The **semicircular canals** are tubes made of car-

tilage that contain fluid and hair cells. These canals are connected to the sensory nerve fibers of the vestibular portion of the eighth cranial nerve. The fluid and hair cells within the canals help to maintain the sense of balance.

The **cochlea,** the spiral organ of hearing, is divided into the scala tympani and the scala vestibuli. Reissner's membrane stretches across the scala vestibuli and forms the duct of the cochlea, or the scala media. The scala media is filled with **endolymph,** a fluid similar to intracellular fluid. The scala tympani and scala vestibuli are filled with **perilymph.** Endolymph and perilymph protect the cochlea and the semicircular canals by allowing these structures to "float" in the fluids and be cushioned against abrupt head movements.

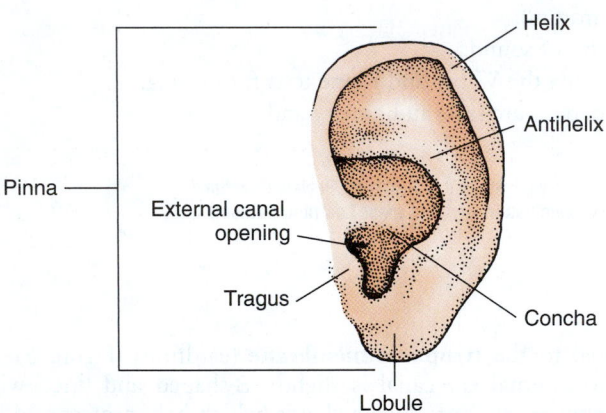

Figure 51-1 ■ Anatomic features of the external ear.

TABLE 51-1	Terminology Commonly Used in Ear and Hearing Assessment

cerumen Waxlike secretion of the external ear canal
conductive hearing loss Hearing loss resulting from a physical disruption in the transmission of sound waves
decibel A unit of sound for expressing loudness
masking The process of hiding a specific sound from one ear while the other ear is tested for its ability to hear that sound
Ménière's disease An intermittent but progressive deterioration of hearing and balance
otitis media Inflammation/infection of the middle ear
otosclerosis Formation of spongy bone around structures of the middle and inner ear, leading to low-tone hearing impairment
ototoxic Damaging to the structures important for hearing
presbycusis Age-related degenerative changes in the ear, leading to decreased hearing acuity
sensorineural Hearing loss resulting from neural defects
spondee Words of two syllables on which equal stress is placed during pronunciation
tympanic membrane The eardrum; a thin membrane that separates the middle ear from the external ear canal. This membrane vibrates when sound waves strike it
vestibular Relating to the functions of the ear for the sense of balance and position

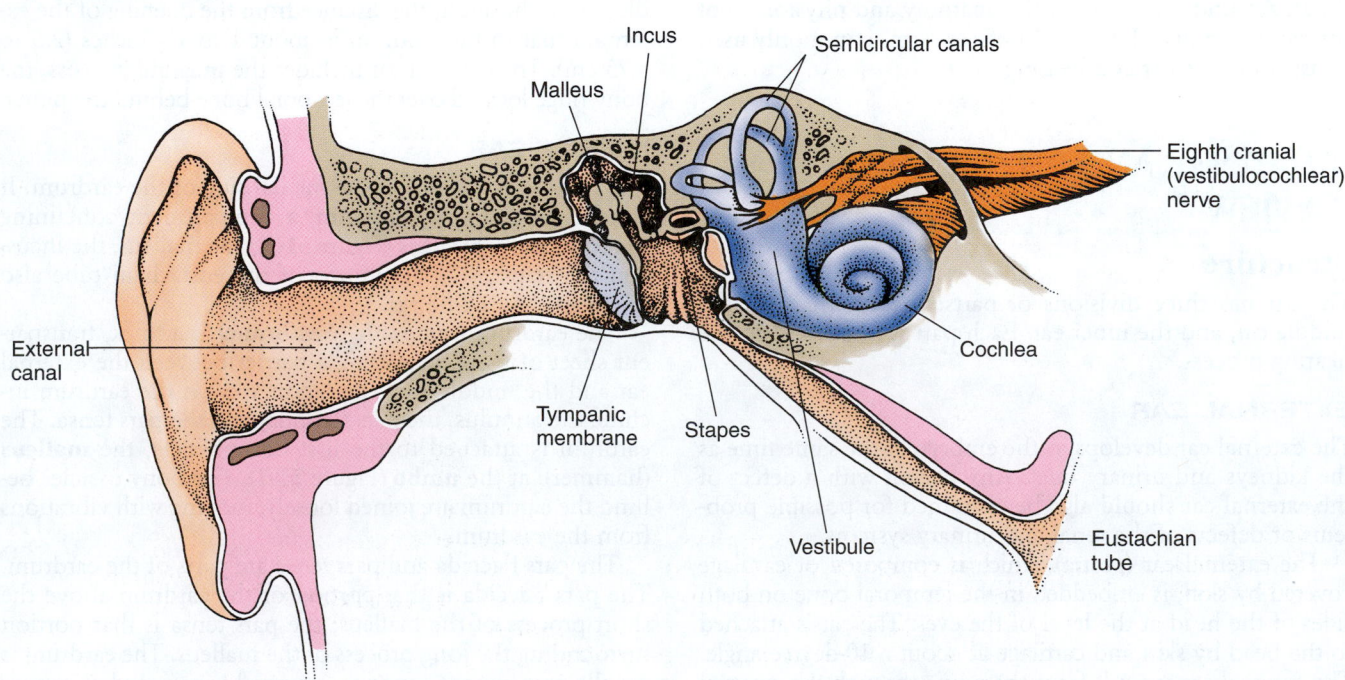

Figure 51-2 ■ Anatomic features of the internal ear.

The **organ of Corti** is the receptor end-organ of hearing located on the basilar membrane of the cochlea. The cochlea contains hair cells that detect vibration from sound and stimulate the eighth cranial nerve.

Function

The ear's main function is hearing, which occurs when sound is delivered through the air to the external ear canal and the temporal bone covering the mastoid air cells. The sound waves strike the mastoid and the movable eardrum, which is connected to the first bony ossicle. The sound wave vibrations are transferred from the eardrum to the malleus, the incus, and the stapes. From the stapes the vibrations are transmitted to the cochlea. Receptors there **transduce** (change) the vibrations into action potentials, conducted to the brain as nerve impulses by the cochlear portion of the eighth cranial (or auditory) nerve. Sound is processed and interpreted by the brain.

Ear and Hearing Changes Associated with Aging

Ear and hearing changes related to aging are listed in Chart 51-1. Some of these changes are harmless; others pose serious threats to the hearing ability of older clients and call for nursing interventions.

All older adults should be screened for hearing acuity. Many scales or tools can be used to obtain the client's perception of hearing loss. These scales may not be any more helpful than just asking, "Do you have a hearing problem now?" (see the Evidence-Based Practice for Nursing box on p. 1114).

ASSESSMENT TECHNIQUES

History

First obtain a thorough history from the client. Informal hearing assessment begins as you observe the client listening to and answering questions. The client's posture and appropriateness of responses provide additional information about his or her hearing acuity.

During the interview, sit in adequate light, facing the client, which allows him or her to see you speaking. Be careful to use ordinary language. Also assess demographic data, personal and family history, socioeconomic status, current health problems, and the use of any remedies for

RIGHT TYMPANIC MEMBRANE

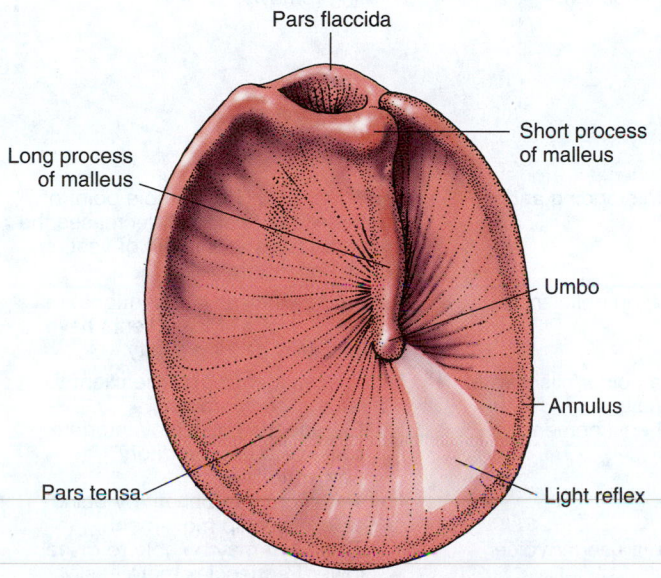

Figure 51-3 ■ Landmarks on the tympanic membrane.

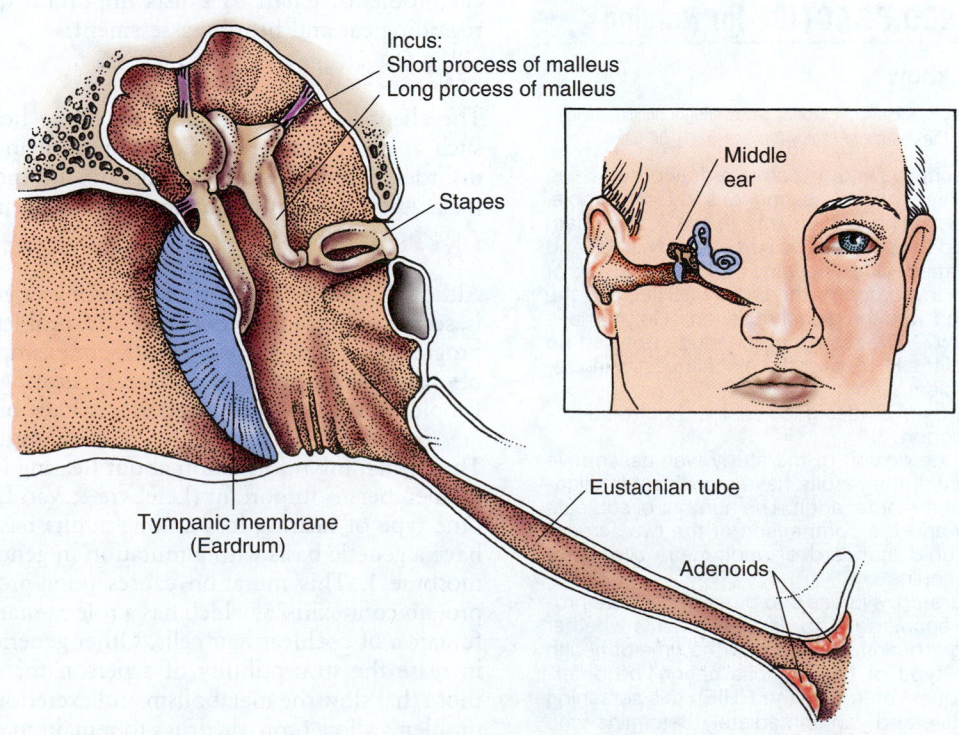

Figure 51-4 ■ Anatomic features and attached structures of the middle ear.

CHART 51-1

NURSING FOCUS on the OLDER ADULT
The Ear and Hearing

Physiologic Change	Nursing Interventions	Rationales
The pinna becomes elongated because of normal loss of subcutaneous tissue and decreased tissue elasticity.	When asked, explain that larger-appearing ears are associated with the normal aging process.	Explanation allays anxiety about the change in ear size.
Hair becomes coarser and longer, especially in men.		
Cerumen-producing glands decrease in number and function.	Irrigate ear canal weekly.	Irrigation removes excess cerumen, preventing impaction and enhancing transmission of sound waves.
Cerumen tends to be drier in older clients; it becomes impacted, which causes hearing loss.	Place 1 or 2 drops of oil into ear canal 8 hr before irrigation.	Oil softens impacted cerumen, facilitating removal.
The tympanic membrane loses elasticity; it may normally appear dull and retracted.		
Bony ossicles have decreased movement.		
The cochlea undergoes degenerative changes.		
Disturbed vestibular function results in occasional dizziness, vertigo, and sensations of unsteadiness in 50%-60% of older adults.	Assist the client with standing and initial ambulation.	The nurse provides a stable point of reference. Assistance decreases the risk of falling as a result of vestibular disorientation.
Hearing acuity diminishes with advancing age.	Establish that a hearing deficiency exists.	Determine whether interventions are needed. Not all older clients have diminished hearing acuity.
The ability to hear high-frequency sounds is nearly gone by age 60 years, which affects speech reception and increases auditory reaction time greatly. Clients have particular difficulty with the *f, s, sh,* and *pa* sounds. Some older clients hear a persistent noise (tinnitus). Presbycusis (a sensorineural type of hearing loss) is common in older adults.	When speaking to an older client with a hearing deficiency: ■ Provide a quiet environment. ■ Face the client. ■ Speak slowly in a deeper voice.	This makes it easier for the client to hear and communicate. ■ Extraneous noise may interfere with the client's auditory perception. ■ The client can benefit by being able to see lip movement. ■ The client may be able to discern lower frequencies more easily.

EVIDENCE-BASED PRACTICE for Nursing

Sometimes clients know best

Gates, G., Murphy, M., Rees, T., & Fraher, A. (2003). Screening for handicapping hearing loss in the elderly. *The Journal of Family Practice,* 52(1), 56-62.

This prospective descriptive study compared two screening methods to identify unrecognized hearing loss in older people. The 546 subjects, continuing participants in the Framingham Heart Study, consented to using the two screening methods and had audiometry performed. One screening method consisted of the Hearing Handicap Inventory for the Elderly (HHIE), and the other screening method was the global question, "Do you have a hearing problem now?" The results of the study revealed no improved specificity of the HHIE over the global questioning related to a hearing problem.

Level of Evidence: 3—Well-designed trial without randomization, with a large cohort.

Critique. Although the design of the study was descriptive rather than experimental, the results have significant implications for health care of the older adult. The number of subjects involved in the study and the comparison of the two screening methods to the gold standard of audiometry allows for generalization of the findings.

Implications for Nursing. Nurses and other health care professionals should be encouraged to ask their clients whether they are experiencing a hearing problem at the time of health history. Although the type of hearing loss cannot be determined by the global question (or by the HHIE), this screening method is cost-effective and can immediately determine who should undergo audiometry.

ear problems. Chart 51-2 lists important questions to ask regarding ear and hearing assessment.

DEMOGRAPHIC DATA

The client's gender is important. Some hearing disorders, such as otosclerosis, are more common in women. Other disorders, such as Ménière's disease, are more common in men. Age is also an important factor in hearing loss.

FAMILY HISTORY AND GENETIC RISK

Although most hearing loss as a result of a genetic mutation is seen in childhood, some genetic problems can lead to progressive hearing loss in adults. For example, 70% of people with Down syndrome develop hearing loss as adults. People with osteogenesis imperfecta have bilateral and progressive hearing loss in the second or third decade of life. Thus obtaining information about hearing loss among family members is important (Lefebvre & Van De Water, 2000). One type of hearing loss among adults has been found to have a genetic basis with a mutation in gene *GJB2* on chromosome 1. This mutation causes poor production of the protein connexin-26, which has a role in maintaining proper function of cochlear hair cells. Other genetic problems that increase the susceptibility of a person for hearing loss are those that slow the metabolism and excretion of drugs. Such problems allow ototoxic drugs to remain in a client's system longer and do more damage to the hearing system.

Ear and Hearing Assessment
USING GORDON'S FUNCTIONAL HEALTH PATTERNS

Cognitive-Perceptual Pattern
- Do you have any hearing difficulty?
- Do you use any type of hearing aid?
- Do you notice that you have the volume of the television or radio set at an increased level?
- Are you sitting closer to the television or radio in order to hear more clearly?
- Do you have difficulty in your ability to hear or follow conversations in a noisy environment, such as a restaurant?
- Do you have difficulty hearing high-pitched sounds like the doorbell?

Health Perception/Health Management Pattern
- Have you had your hearing checked?
- If you are or were exposed to environmental noise, have you consistently used appropriate hearing protection?
- Do you avoid cleaning your ear canals with foreign objects such as toothpicks or paper clips?
- Have you discussed with your health care provider the side effects of any drugs you may be taking that might affect your ear and hearing?

Based on Gordon, M. (2002). *Manual of nursing diagnosis* (10th ed.). St. Louis: Mosby.

Specific questions to ask the client include the following:
- Who in your family has hearing problems?
- In those who have hearing problems, are the problems present in men and women equally, or are they present more in one gender?
- At what age was hearing loss diagnosed in your relative(s)?
- Are both ears affected?

PERSONAL HISTORY

Personal history includes information on past or current manifestations of ear pain, ear discharge, vertigo, tinnitus, decreased hearing, and difficulty understanding people when they talk or difficulty hearing environmental noises. Ask the client about the following:
- Ear trauma
- Ear surgery
- Past infections
- Excessive cerumen
- Ear itch
- Any invasive instruments routinely used to clean the ear
- Type and pattern of ear hygiene
- Exposure to loud noise or music
- Air travel (especially in unpressurized aircraft)
- Swimming habits and the use ear protection when swimming
- History of hereditary factors and health problems causing changes in the blood supply to the ear (heart disease, hypertension, diabetes)
- History of vitiligo (a pigment disorder in which there may be a loss of melanin-containing cells [and their protective function] in the inner ear, resulting in hearing loss)
- History of smoking (nicotine increases the carboxyhemoglobin in the blood, reducing the oxygen supply to the cochlea, and possibly increasing sensory cell damage)
- History of vitamin B_{12} and folate deficiency (associated with age-related hearing loss)

TABLE 51-2 Ototoxic Drugs

Drug Type	Drug
Antibiotics	Amikacin Capreomycin Chloramphenicol Dihydrostreptomycin Erythromycin Gentamicin (Garamycin, Cidomycin) Kanamycin Metronidazole (vestibulotoxicity rarely) Neomycin Netilmicin Streptomycin Tobramycin
Diuretics	Acetazolamide (Apo-Acetazolamide, Diamox) Ethacrynic acid (Edecrin) Bumetanide Furosemide (Apo-Furosemide✲, Lasix, Furoside✲)
Nonsteroidal anti-inflammatory agents	Ibuprofen (Advil, Nuprin, Motrin) Indomethacin (Indocin) Naproxen (Aleve, Naprosyn, Anaprox) Feldene, Dolobid, Lodine, Relafen, Toradol, Voltaren Salicylates (aspirin, Disalcid, Bufferin, Ecotrin, Trilisate, Ascriptin, Empirin, Excedrin, Fiorinal)
Chemotherapy agents	Actinomycin Bleomycin Cisplatin (Abiplatin, Platinol) Carboplatin Nitrogen mustard (Mustargen) Vincristine
Miscellaneous	Carbamazepine Hydroxychloroquine (Plaquenil) Quinine (Legatrin, NovoQuinine✲, Quinamm) Quinidine (Apo-Quinidine✲, Cardioquin, Quinidex)

If the client uses a hearing aid, determine how well it works, the date of the last hearing test, the type of test given, and the results. Ask the client about other problems that may impair hearing, such as allergies; upper respiratory infections; hypothyroidism; arteriosclerosis; head trauma; and recent head, facial, or dental surgery. A thorough drug history is crucial because many drugs are ototoxic (Table 51-2).

Ask the client about his or her occupation and any hobbies that involve exposure to loud environmental noise or music. Also determine whether the client uses protective ear devices or any devices inserted into the ear, such as a telephone headset or a stethoscope.

SOCIOECONOMIC STATUS

Assess the client's socioeconomic status to determine the availability of health care. Clients of lower socioeconomic status often do not seek health care for ear-related problems until hearing damage is extensive. Clients at any socioeconomic level, however, might hesitate to have their hearing loss diagnosed because of the fear of needing to wear a hearing aid.

CURRENT HEALTH PROBLEMS

Assess current ear-related health problems by asking whether the client has noticed any "trouble with" his or her ears, ear pain, or discharge, including any earwax. Ask about any change in hearing, such as intolerance for sound levels that do not bother other people (hyperacusis), or other problems, such as ringing in the ears. If a change in hearing is reported, ask whether one or both ears are involved and whether the change was sudden or gradual. Also ask the client about any problems with dizziness, sensations of being "off balance" or **vertigo** (sense of spinning movement).

Physical Assessment

Inspection and palpation are the only examination techniques used to assess the ear. Begin the examination by placing the client in either a sitting or a supine position. Do not attempt to examine an uncooperative or confused client. Remove any hearing aids during the examination. After the otoscopic examination, inspect the hearing aid for cracks, debris, and a proper fit. Ear examination is divided into external ear and mastoid assessment, otoscopic assessment, and auditory assessment.

EXTERNAL EAR AND MASTOID ASSESSMENT

Inspect the mastoid process for redness and swelling, which indicate inflammation. To assess for tenderness, gently tap with one finger over the mastoid process, compress the tragus with one finger, and gently manipulate the pinna forward and backward. Any tenderness suggests an inflammatory process in either the external ear or the mastoid.

Inspect the entire external ear for shape, location of attachment to the head, and condition of the visible external canal. The normal pinna is uniformly shaped without skin tags or deformity. The pinna should be attached vertically to the side of the head at a posterior angle of no greater than 10 degrees. It should fall within or touch the eye-occiput line, an imaginary line drawn from the greatest protuberance on the occiput to the lateral canthus of the eye. Record any variation from the normal ear shape and attachment.

Abnormalities of the pinna include swelling, nodules, and lesions. In chronic gout, collection of uric acid crystals results in hard, irregular, painless nodules called **tophi** on the helix and antihelix portions of the pinna. Other painless nodules on the pinna might be due to basal cell carcinoma or rheumatoid arthritis. Small, crusted, ulcerated, or indurated lesions on the pinna that fail to heal could be squamous cell carcinoma.

The normal external canal is free from lesions, dry, clean, and not reddened. Assess for the following problems:

- Furuncles
- Large amounts of cerumen
- Scaliness
- Redness
- Swelling of or drainage from the ear associated with a foreign object (insects or other substances), trauma, or infection

Also record any other drainage (blood, cerebrospinal fluid, pus, or serous fluid) and its character.

OTOSCOPIC ASSESSMENT

An instrument called an otoscope is used to examine the ear. Many types are available. An **otoscope** (Figure 51-5) consists of a light, a handle, a magnifying lens, and a pneu-

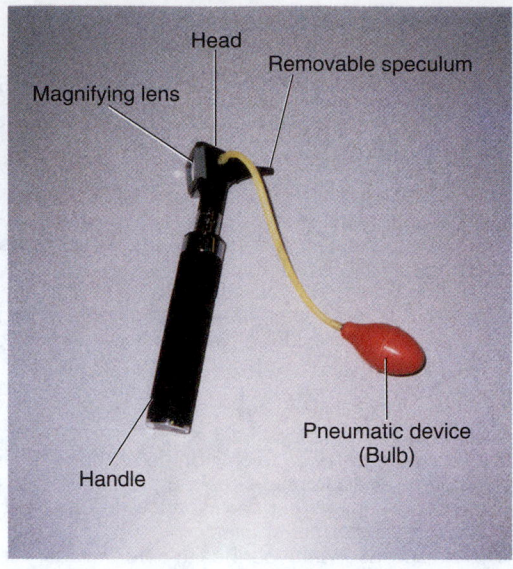

Figure 51-5 ■ Functional components of an otoscope.

matic bulb for injecting air into the external canal to test mobility of the eardrum.

Specula of various diameters attach to the head of the otoscope. Select the largest that most comfortably fits the client's external canal. *Never blindly insert the speculum into the external canal because of the risk of perforating the eardrum.*

If the client has any pain during external ear examination, cautiously attempt an otoscopic examination. (The speculum will cause extreme pain if it comes in contact with inflamed tissue in the external canal.) Become familiar with and memorize all the structures of the eardrum and middle ear before attempting to visualize them with an otoscope.

When performing an otoscopic examination, tilt the client's head slightly away and hold the otoscope upside down, like a large pen (Figure 51-6). This position permits your hand to lie against the client's head for support. If the client moves, both your hand and the otoscope also move, preventing damage to the external canal or eardrum. Hold the otoscope in the dominant hand and gently pull the pinna up and back with the nondominant hand. Visualize the external canal while you slowly insert the speculum. Use caution and avoid jamming the speculum into the walls of the external canal, which causes pain.

After the pinna is correctly displaced and the otoscope is comfortably introduced in the external canal, observe the eardrum for color, intactness, and shape. Assess for lesions and the amount and consistency of cerumen and hair. The normal external canal is skin colored, intact, and without lesions. It contains various amounts of soft cerumen and has small, fine hairs.

Next assess the eardrums for intactness; normal structures seen through the eardrum (the long and short processes of the malleus and the umbo); portions of the eardrum itself (light reflex, pars flaccida, and pars tensa); and the color, shape, and mobility of the membrane as well as any lesions. Figure 51-7 shows an otoscopic view of a normal eardrum. *The normal eardrum is always intact.* The long process of the malleus is seen through the eardrum as a whitish streak extending from the short process of the malleus to the umbo.

Video Clip: External Ear

Video Clip: Ear Canal

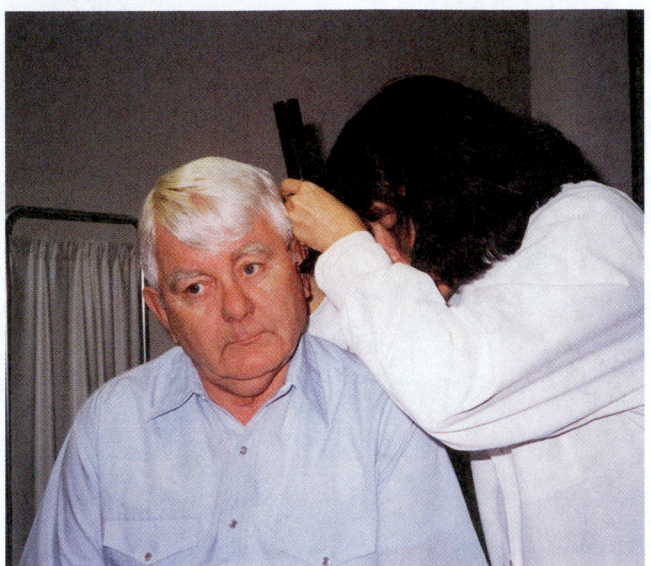

Figure 51-6 ■ Proper technique for an otoscopic examination.

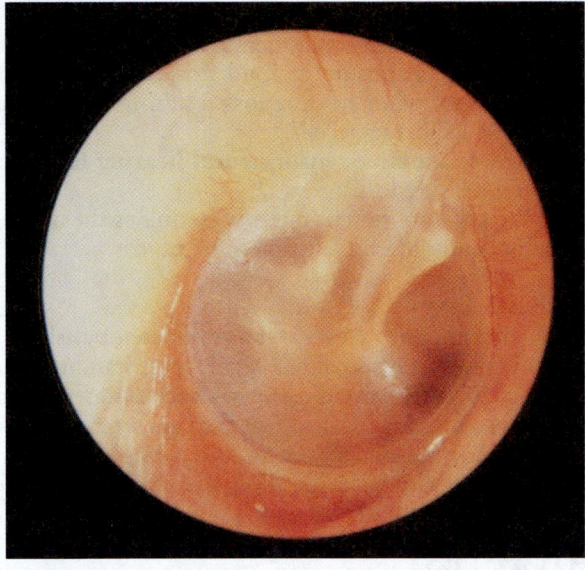

Figure 51-7 ■ Otoscopic view of a normal tympanic membrane.

In some people with allergies, visible blood vessels may be present on the long process, although this finding also occurs as an early indication of otitis media.

The short process of the malleus is seen through the eardrum as a white structure that seems more three-dimensional (projecting out toward the otoscope) than the other structures on the eardrum. The umbo appears as a round, white dot.

The long and short processes of the malleus, in addition to the umbo, are always easily identified in the normal ear. Abnormal variations are caused by serous otitis and otitis media, among other disorders.

Reflection of the otoscope's light off of the eardrum is the **light reflex,** a clearly demarcated triangle of light in the normal ear. The base of the triangle is on the annulus, and the point of the triangle is on the umbo. When the light reflex is spotty or multiple because of a changed eardrum shape from either retraction or bulging, the light reflex is termed **diffuse.**

The eardrum is normally shiny, transparent, and opaque or pearly gray. Abnormal variations include redness (as seen in otitis media) and dullness or retraction (as seen in serous otitis).

The normal eardrum is slightly concave, allowing the pars tensa portion to move gently on testing with a puff of air from the pneumatic bulb on the otoscope.

The normal eardrum is free of lesions. The most common lesion is scarring caused by previous ear infection and perforation. A scar thickens the eardrum, which makes it difficult or impossible to see through the membrane at the point of the scar and reduces the mobility of the eardrum.

Test the mobility of the eardrum by gently injecting a small puff of air through the pneumatic bulb into the external canal and watching the pars tensa portion for movement. The normal eardrum moves gently. Decreased or absent mobility results from scarring, retraction, bulging, the presence of fluid in the middle ear, and decreased mobility of the ossicles associated with aging.

CULTURAL CONSIDERATIONS

Cerumen is generally moist and tan or brown in black clients and white clients. It is dry and light brown to gray in Asians and Native Americans/American Indians. The color of the lining of the external ear canal varies with the client's skin tone. Clients with more moist earwax may form cerumen impactions more easily than do clients with drier, flaky earwax.

Critical Thinking Challenge

The client is an older woman who lives with her son's family. The family immigrated from Mexico 3 years ago. She speaks limited English and is fluent in Spanish. She arrives at the clinic with her 15-year-old granddaughter, who is bilingual in English and Spanish. They tell you that Abuela's (Grandmother's) left ear has been painful for some time. She seems reluctant to tell you how she has tried to treat her ear at home. You are about to perform an external and otoscopic examination on her.

1. How will you explain these procedures to the client?
2. Describe variations in home treatments for ear pain.
3. Describe the otoscopic examination results you would expect if her eardrum is infected.

evolve For suggested answer guidelines, go to http://evolve.elsevier.com/Iggy/.

Auditory Assessment

After completing bilateral external ear and otoscopic examinations, assess the client's hearing acuity. Sound is transmitted by air conduction and bone conduction. Air conduction of sound is normally more sensitive than bone conduction. If hearing acuity is decreased, the hearing loss is categorized as follows:

■ **Conductive hearing loss,** which results from any physical obstruction of sound wave transmission (such as a foreign body in the external canal, a retracted or bulging tympanic membrane, or fused bony ossicles)

- **Sensorineural hearing loss,** which results from a defect in the cochlea, the eighth cranial nerve, or the brain itself. Exposure to loud noises and music may cause this type of hearing loss resulting from damage of the cochlear hair cells.
- **Mixed conductive-sensorineural hearing loss,** a profound hearing loss.

Each of the auditory function tests determines the degree of hearing loss and differentiates the type of loss.

VOICE TEST

A simple hearing acuity test can be conducted by asking the client to block one external ear canal while standing 1 to 2 feet (30 to 60 cm) away. Quietly whisper a statement and then ask the client to repeat it. Test each ear separately. If the client does not respond correctly, use a louder whisper. If you suspect the client is lip-reading, use your hand to block the view of your mouth.

WATCH TEST

A ticking watch is used to test hearing acuity for high-frequency sounds. Hold a ticking watch about 5 inches (12.7 cm) from each of the ears and ask whether the ticking is heard. The client with normal hearing should be able to hear it.

AUDIOSCOPY

The lightweight audioscope allows you to visualize the external ear and eardrum. Hearing can be measured at a 40-decibel (dB) intensity at frequencies of 510, 1000, 2000, and 4000 cycles per second (cps), or hertz (Hz). The audioscope is larger than a standard otoscope, and you can easily use it to assess hearing.

TUNING FORK TESTS

Hearing acuity can be tested by the Weber and Rinne tuning fork tests. Tuning fork tests are useful, although limited, in distinguishing between conductive and sensorineural hearing losses. The frequency range of the tuning fork used for these tests corresponds to that of normal speech: 512 or 1024 Hz. To perform this assessment, stand in front of the sitting client.

Animation: Weber Test ▶

Weber Tuning Fork Test

To perform the Weber tuning fork test, strike the tuning fork to make it vibrate. Place the vibrating tuning fork on the middle of the client's head, at the midline of the forehead, or above the upper lip over the teeth. Many clients object to the vibration over the upper lip; so the preferred site is the midline of the skull (Figure 51-8). Take care to hold the vibrating tuning fork by the stem only, not by the vibrating fork. Ask the client in which ear the sound is louder. The normal test result is sound heard equally in both ears. If the client hears the sound louder in one ear, the term *lateralization* describes the side on which the sound is the loudest.

Rinne Tuning Fork Test

The Rinne tuning fork test compares hearing by air conduction with hearing by bone conduction. Sound is normally heard two to three times longer by air conduction than by bone conduction. Perform the Rinne tuning fork test by placing the vibrating tuning fork stem on the client's mastoid process. When the client indicates that he or she no longer hears the sound, quickly bring the tuning fork in front of the

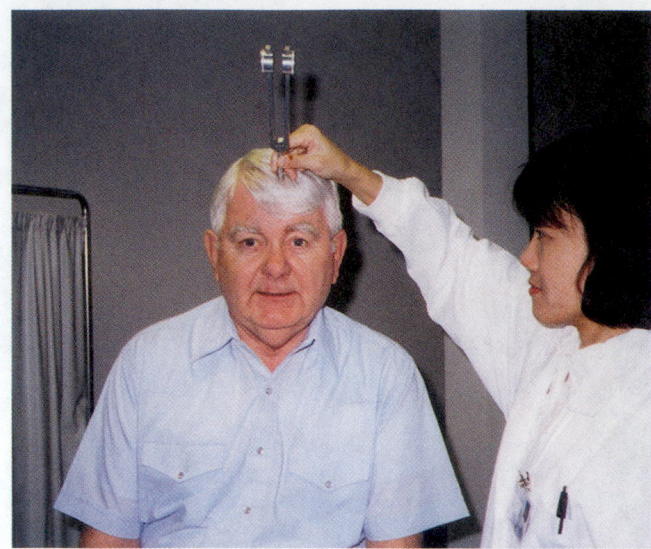

Figure 51-8 ■ Correct placement of the tuning fork for the Weber test.

pinna without touching the client, and ask whether he or she still hears the sound (Figure 51-9). Record the duration of both phases, bone conduction followed by air conduction, and compare the times. The client normally continues to hear the sound two times longer in front of the pinna after not hearing it with the tuning fork touching the mastoid process.

Psychosocial Assessment

The client may become irritable, frustrated, and depressed by an inability to hear and respond appropriately. The inability to hear often isolates the client from the world. Depression may result from the sensory isolation of hearing loss. You must be sensitive to the client and conduct the interview at a pace appropriate for that person.

Ask about social and work relationships to determine whether the client is isolated because of hearing problems. In addition, encourage the client to express feelings related to hearing loss and discuss changes in daily living activities for coping. Also obtain information from family members, especially if the client does not acknowledge having a hearing problem. Throughout the assessment, remain patient and empathetic.

Diagnostic Assessment
LABORATORY TESTS

Laboratory tests generally are not of value in determining hearing acuity. For an external ear infection, microbial culture and antibiotic sensitivity tests can determine the causative organism and the most appropriate antibiotic.

RADIOGRAPHIC EXAMINATIONS
Computed Tomography

Computed tomography (CT), with or without contrast enhancement, reveals the structures of the ear in great detail by multiple x-ray scans of the head. These scans are then av-

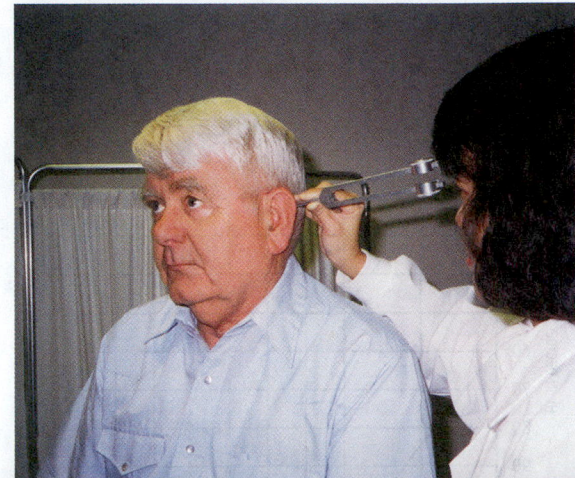

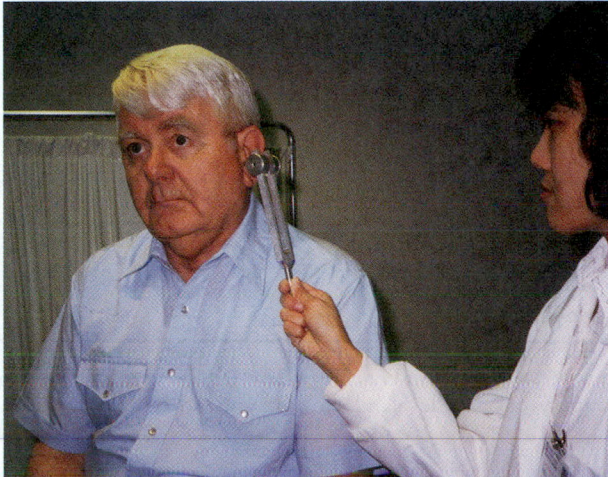

Figure 51-9 ■ Correct placement of the tuning fork for the Rinne test.

eraged by a computer. CT is especially helpful in diagnosing acoustic tumors.

OTHER DIAGNOSTIC ASSESSMENTS

Magnetic Resonance Imaging

Magnetic resonance imaging (MRI) is a noninvasive, nonradioactive diagnostic tool that uses a computer to generate images. Because of its superior contrast resolution, no bony artifacts can obscure tissue. Therefore MRI has great sensitivity to soft-tissue changes. Clients with internal metal vascular clips cannot have MRI.

Auditory Brainstem-Evoked Response

Auditory brainstem-evoked response (ABR) assesses hearing in clients who are unable to indicate or unreliable in indicating their recognition of sound stimuli during hearing testing. This test helps to diagnose both conductive and sensorineural hearing losses. Electrodes are placed on the scalp during the test. After the test, the client's hair should be cleansed to remove the electrode gel.

To prepare the client for ABR testing, you must do the following:
- Tell the client that no fasting or sedation is needed
- Carefully explain the procedure and its purpose

- Inform the client that the procedure usually takes about 30 minutes

Electronystagmography

Electronystagmography (ENG) is a cost-effective test that is sensitive in detecting both central and peripheral disease of the vestibular system in the ear. The ENG detects **nystagmus** (involuntary eye movements) that can be recorded. (The eyes and ears depend on each other for good balance.) Electrodes are taped to the skin near the eyes, and one or more procedures (caloric testing, changing gaze position, or changing head position) are performed to stimulate nystagmus. Failure of nystagmus to occur with cerebral stimulation suggests an abnormality in the vestibulocochlear apparatus, the cerebral cortex, the auditory nerve, or the brainstem. To prepare the client for ENG, you must do the following:
- Carefully explain the procedure and its purpose. The examiners will be asking the client to name names or do simple math problems during the test to ensure the client stays alert.
- Tell the client to fast for several hours before the test and to avoid caffeine-containing beverages for 24 to 48 hours before the test.
- Tell clients with pacemakers that they should not have the test.
- Carefully introduce fluids after the test to prevent nausea and vomiting.

Caloric Testing

Caloric testing is performed to evaluate the vestibular (inner-ear) portion of the auditory nerve. Water warmer or cooler than body temperature is infused into the ear. A normal response is the onset of **vertigo** (spinning sensation) and nystagmus (involuntary eye movements) within 20 to 30 seconds. To prepare the client for caloric testing, you must do the following:
Carefully explain the procedure and its purpose.
- Tell the client to fast for several hours before the test.
- Tell the client that the affected side will be tested first.
- Explain that the client will be maintained on bedrest after the procedure with careful introduction of fluids to prevent nausea and vomiting.

Dix-Hallpike Test for Vertigo

The Dix-Hallpike test for vertigo is performed by assisting the client to a sitting position on an examination table. Stand to the side of the client, and quickly reposition him or her from sitting to supine with the head extending beyond the end of the table. This change of position is done first to one side and then to the other side. A client with benign positional vertigo will have a burst of nystagmus after a delay of 5 to 10 seconds.

To prepare the client for the Dix-Hallpike test, you must do the following:
- Carefully explain the procedure and its purpose.
- Tell the client that he or she should keep the eyes open and try not to blink.
- Explain that double vision may occur during the test.

Audiometry

Audiometry is the measurement of hearing acuity. **Frequency** is the highness or lowness of tones (expressed in

TABLE 51-3 Decibel Intensity and Safe Exposure Time for Common Sounds

Sound	Decibel Intensity (dB)	Safe Exposure Time*
Threshold of hearing	0	
Whispering	20	
Average residence or office	40	
Conversational speech	60	
Car traffic	70	>8 hr
Motorcycle	90	8 hr
Chain saw	100	2 hr
Rock concert, front row	120	3 min
Jet engine	140	Immediate danger
Rocket launching pad	180	Immediate danger

*For every 5-dB increase in intensity, the safe exposure time is cut in half.

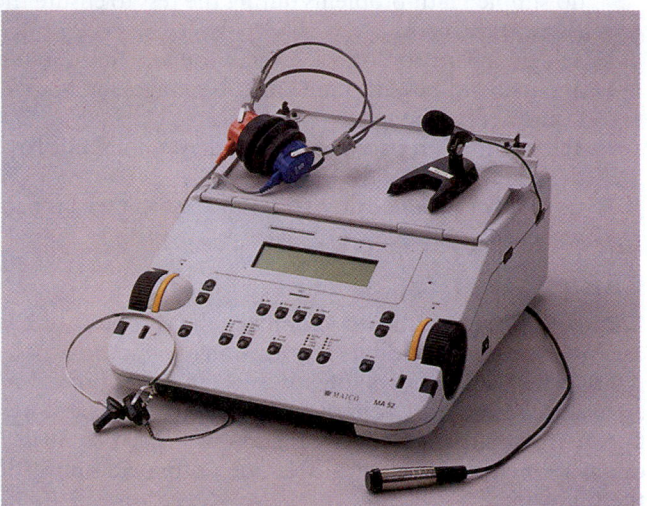

Figure 51-10 ■ A pure-tone audiometer. (Courtesy of Maico, Inc., Minneapolis, MN.)

hertz). The greater the number of vibrations per second, the higher the frequency (pitch) of the sound; the fewer the number of vibrations per second, the lower the pitch.

Intensity of sound is expressed in decibels. The lowest intensity at which a young, normal ear can detect sound (about 51% of the time) is 0 dB. Sound at 110 dB is so intense (loud) that it is painful for most people with normal hearing. Conversational speech is around 60 dB, and a soft whisper is around 20 dB (Table 51-3). A hearing loss of 45 to 51 dB renders the person unable to hear speech without a hearing aid. A person with a hearing loss of 90 dB may not be able to hear speech even with a hearing aid.

Threshold is the lowest level of intensity at which pure tones and speech are heard by a client (about 50% of the time).

Pure tones are generated by an **audiometer** (Figure 51-10) to determine hearing acuity. The two types of audiometry are pure-tone audiometry and speech audiometry.

Pure-Tone Audiometry

Tones generated by an audiometer are presented to the client at frequencies for hearing speech, music, and other common sounds. Pure-tone audiometry is performed by air-

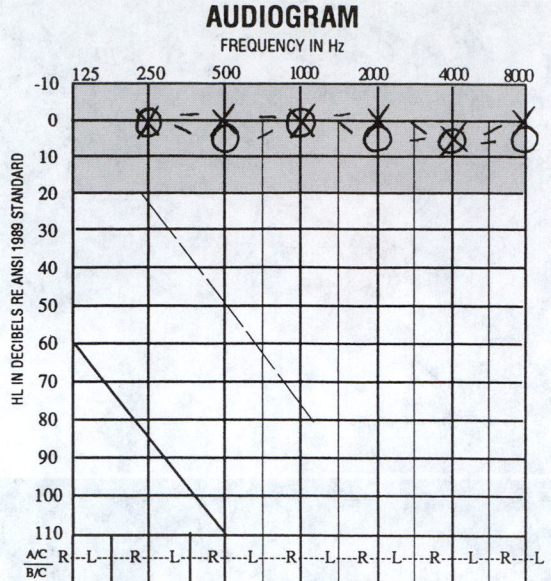

Audiogram Key	Left	Right		Left	Right
AC Unmasked	x	o	AC Masked	□	Δ
BC Unmasked	>	<	BC Masked	]	[
No Response	↓	↙	SF		S

Figure 51-11 ■ Audiogram pattern depicting normal hearing. (Courtesy of the Cleveland Hearing and Speech Center, Cleveland, OH.)

conduction testing or bone-conduction testing. The results of pure-tone audiometry are plotted on an **audiogram** (Figure 51-11). For some clients, the hearing of one ear is "masked" while the hearing of the other ear is tested.

AIR-CONDUCTION TEST

Pure-tone air-conduction testing determines whether a client hears normally or has a hearing loss. It is designed to test air-conduction hearing sensitivity (through earphones) at frequencies of 125, 251, 510, 751, 1000, 1510, 2000, 3000, 4000, 6000, and 8000 Hz, but thresholds are usually confined to the frequencies of 251, 510, 1000, 2000, 4000, and 8000 Hz. The intensities for the pure tones generally range from 10 to 110 dB.

CLIENT PREPARATION. Place the client in a sound-isolated room in which background noise does not exceed American National Standards Institute noise standards. Sit facing the client because his or her facial expressions are often helpful in evaluating responses. Hearing-impaired clients may benefit from lip-reading your instructions. Instruct the client as follows:

"I am going to test your hearing. The object of the test is to find the point at which you can just barely hear the tones. The tones will sound like soft bells or tuning forks. Every time you hear one, no matter how soft, signal by raising your hand (or pushing the button) on the side you hear the tone." (If the client cannot raise a hand or push a button because of physical or motor disabilities, a yes-no verbal response can be used.)

"When you no longer hear the tone, lower your hand (or release the button). This lets me know when you hear the tone and when it goes away."

PROCEDURE. Test the ear with the better hearing first. Before beginning the test, adjust the audiometric equipment by doing the following:

1. Setting the frequency control at 1000 Hz and the hearing level control at 40 dB.
2. Putting on the earphones and listening to the tone while switching from one ear to the other.
3. In each earphone, listening to the tone while gradually turning the hearing level control toward 0 dB.
4. Testing the signal cord and light to make sure they are working.

Best practices for conduction audiometry to obtain a profile of the client's hearing for pure tones from low to high frequencies are listed in Chart 51-3. No special follow-up care is needed.

BONE-CONDUCTION TEST

Pure-tone bone-conduction testing determines whether the hearing loss detected by air-conduction testing is due to conductive or sensorineural factors or to a combination of the two. It is used only when the results of air-conduction testing are abnormal. There are restrictions on both the frequency and the intensity of the sound produced by the device. The frequencies are usually restricted to those between 251 and 4000 Hz. Because a bone-conduction oscillator requires great power to vibrate the skull, maximal outputs for bone conduction are also lower.

CLIENT PREPARATION. Explain that hearing sensitivity for bone conduction is going to be checked. The sounds and how the client should respond are the same as those for the air-conduction test.

PROCEDURE. The ear with greater acuity is tested first. If neither ear is "better," it makes no difference which is tested first.

The bone-conduction vibrator is placed behind the pinna, firmly on the mastoid process. Then follow steps 4 through 9 of Chart 51-3. Remember that restrictions are placed on both the intensity and the frequency used in bone-conduction testing. Restrictions are usually described on the face of the audiometer. No special follow-up care is needed.

INTERPRETATION OF RESULTS

Audiometric evaluation determines whether the client's hearing is within normal limits or, with a hearing impairment, whether the hearing loss is conductive, sensorineural, or mixed. The type of loss can be determined by the shape of the audiogram after completion of pure-tone air- and bone-conduction audiometry.

For an experienced clinician, the audiometer is a useful tool for evaluating the extent and type of hearing loss. For interpreting the results of a hearing test, the expertise of the person who performed the test and the reliability of the client's responses must be considered. In reality the audiogram is the diagnostician's best estimate of hearing, based on observations of the client's hearing behavior in the testing situation.

Figure 51-11 is an audiogram showing normal results of air- and bone-conduction tests. Hearing is considered normal when the pure-tone thresholds are at 10 dB or better. The line

CHART 51-3

BEST PRACTICE for
Pure-Tone Air-Conduction Audiometry

1. After explaining the procedure to the client, place the earphones on the client. Make sure that the side marked *left* is on the left ear and the side marked *right* is on the right ear. The earphones must cover the ears.
2. If the client reports a hearing difference between the two ears, test the ear with better hearing first.
3. Begin the testing at 1000 Hz. This frequency is near the middle of the ear's sensitivity spectrum, and it has been demonstrated to have good test-retest reliability.
4. Adjust the audiometer so that the tone is inaudible unless the interrupter switch is depressed. Start with the hearing level control at its lowest setting, either 0 or −10 dB. Depress the interrupter switch, and gradually increase the intensity of the tone until the client signals that the tone is heard. Increase the intensity of the tone beyond this point by about 20 dB to give the client an opportunity to hear it well.
5. Now reduce the intensity of the tone in 5-dB steps until the client indicates that the tone is no longer heard. Note the last intensity level, in 5-dB decrement steps, at which the client signaled. The last point at which the client indicated that the tone was still heard should be his or her threshold for hearing for that frequency. The threshold can be tested for reliability by increasing the tone by 20 dB once again and then descending in 5-dB steps until once again the lowest point in intensity is reached.
6. If you have succeeded in obtaining a consistent threshold at 1000 Hz, change the frequency control to 500 Hz and start again. The preferred method is to test the lower frequencies first (500 and 250 Hz) and then move higher, usually to 2000, 4000, and 8000 Hz. At each frequency, the procedure is the same as for 1000 Hz.
7. After you have completed the threshold measurements on the first ear, switch the output selector to the opposite earphone. Proceed in the same manner to obtain thresholds for the other ear, also beginning at 1000 Hz.
8. If the thresholds of the second ear seem to differ by 40 dB or more from those of the first ear, masking of the better-hearing ear is indicated to rule out its participation in the test.
9. In operating the interrupter switch, make sure that you do not fall into rhythmic patterns that the client can follow. The pattern of tonal presentations should be irregular so that the client cannot predict when the tone will be presented.

at 0 dB on the audiogram represents the hearing thresholds of a young person with normal hearing. Figure 51-12 shows audiogram graphs of various types of hearing loss.

Speech Audiometry

In speech audiometry, the client's ability to hear spoken words is measured through a microphone connected to an audiometer. The two components of speech audiometry are the speech reception threshold and speech discrimination.

SPEECH RECEPTION THRESHOLD

The **speech reception threshold** is the minimum loudness at which a client can repeat simple words. In testing this threshold, try to determine how intense (or loud) a simple speech stimulus must be before the client can hear it well enough to repeat it correctly. In one common test, lists of two-syllable words called **spondee** are used (i.e., words in which there is generally equal stress on each syllable, such as *airplane*, *railroad*, and *cowboy*).

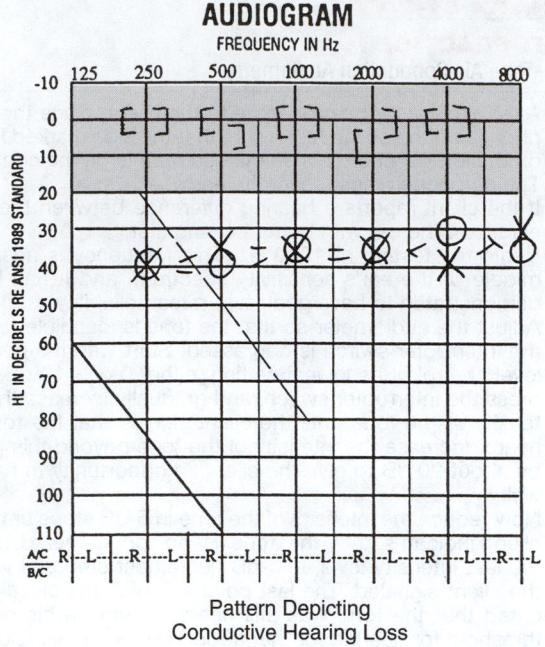

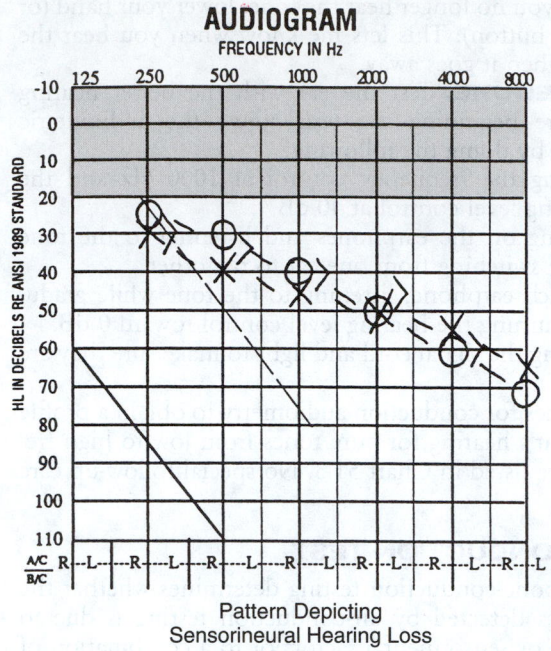

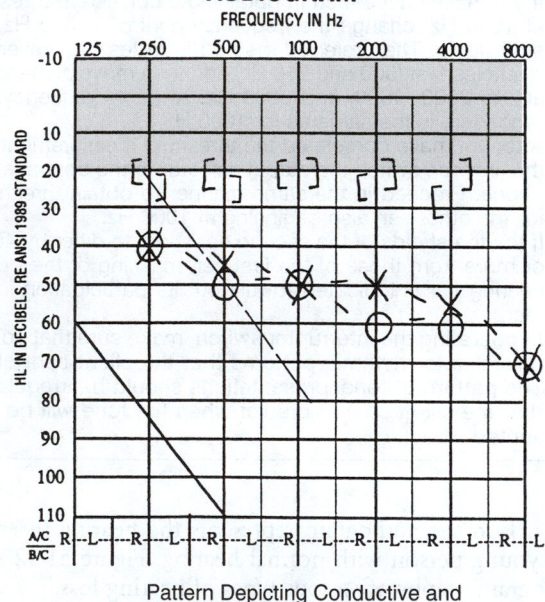

Audiogram Key	Left	Right		Left	Right
AC Unmasked	x	o	AC Masked	□	Δ
BC Unmasked	>	<	BC Masked	]	[
No Response	↓	↙	SF		S

Figure 51-12 ■ Audiogram patterns depicting various types of hearing loss. (Courtesy of the Cleveland Hearing and Speech Center, Cleveland, OH.)

The speech reception threshold measured by the audiometer is the hearing level at which the client can repeat simple words correctly 50% of the time. The test is conducted in a manner similar to the pure-tone tests, but the microphone is activated through the audiometer. The intensity dial on the audiometer regulates word level intensity.

SPEECH DISCRIMINATION

Speech discrimination testing determines the client's ability to discriminate among similar sounds or among words that contain similar sounds. The ability to understand speech is the most important measurable aspect of human hearing. Speech discrimination testing assesses understanding of speech. A hearing loss may decrease sensitivity to sound and impair understanding of what is being said.

A standard format contains lists of 25 to 50 **monosyllabic** (one-syllable) words, such as *carve, day, toe,* and *ran,* phonemically balanced (designed to include the phonemes of American English in the proper proportion) and with equal word difficulty between lists. The lists are presented to the client through earphones at a selected loudness level, generally about 30 to 40 dB above the speech reception threshold, or at the client's most comfortable listening level. A percentage score is derived from the number of words repeated correctly.

Tympanometry

Tympanometry assesses mobility of the eardrum and structures of the middle ear by systematically varying air pressure in the external auditory canal. The progression or resolution of serous otitis and otitis media can be accurately monitored with this procedure.

Tympanometry is helpful in distinguishing middle-ear pathologic conditions, such as otosclerosis, ossicular disarticulation, otitis media, and perforation of the eardrum. It is also useful for assessing patency of the eustachian tube and for check recovery of middle-ear function after surgery.

Critical Thinking Challenge

Your client is a 24-year-old man who arrives at the clinic on his motorcycle from his construction job. He is wearing a headset with a compact disc (CD) player hooked to his belt. You are to perform a hearing assessment on him.

1. What should you tell him regarding the preparation and actual audiometry procedures?
2. What recommendations would you make to him regarding the protection of his hearing in the future?

evolve For suggested answer guidelines, go to http://evolve.elsevier.com/Iggy/.

GET READY for the NCLEX Examination!

KEY POINTS

Safe Effective Care Environment

- Use a separate speculum cover for each ear when conducting an otoscopic examination.
- Slowly and gently introduce the otoscopic speculum into the external ear canal during assessment.
- Use contact precautions with any client who has drainage from the ear canal.
- Do not perform an otoscopic examination on a confused or uncooperative client.
- Use the suggestions presented under the History section to enhance communication with a client who has a hearing impairment.

Health Promotion and Maintenance

- Teach clients the proper way to clean the pinna and external ear canal.
- Identify clients at risk for hearing impairment as a result of work environment or leisure activities.
- Encourage all clients, even if they already have a hearing impairment, to use ear protection in loud environment.
- Inform all clients who smoke that smoking increases the risk for development of hearing problems.
- Assist clients interested in smoking cessation to find an appropriate smoking cessation program.

Psychosocial Integrity

- Pace your interview to match the learning needs and style of the individual client.

- Allow the client the opportunity to express fear or anxiety regarding a change in hearing status.
- Refer clients newly diagnosed with hearing impairment to local resources and support groups.
- Explain all diagnostic procedures, restrictions, and follow-up care to the client scheduled for tests.

Physiological Integrity

- Ask the client about hearing problems in any other members of the family because many hearing problems have a genetic component, such as osteogenesis imperfecta, retinitis pigmentosa, Usher's syndrome, Waardenburg's syndrome, Alport's syndrome, and Treacher Collins syndrome.
- Ask the client whether any ototoxic drugs have ever been used (Table 51-2).

ADDITIONAL STUDY RESOURCES

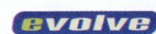 Go to your Student CD-ROM for Review Questions for the NCLEX Examination.

evolve Go to http://evolve.elsevier.com/Iggy/ for Integrated Management of Care Questions for the NCLEX Examination.

SELECTED BIBLIOGRAPHY

Asterisk indicates a classic or definitive work on this subject.

Baker, C. (2002). Caring for patients with hearing impairments. *Dermatology Nursing, 14*(1), 49, 52.

Benjamin, B., et al. (1994). *A color atlas of otorhinolarynogology.* Philadelphia: Lippincott-Raven.

Bess, F.H., & Humes, L.E. (2003). *Audiology: The fundamentals* (3rd ed.). Baltimore: Williams & Wilkins.

Borg-Stein, J., Rauch, S., & Krabak, B. (2001). Evaluation and management of cervicogenic dizziness. *Critical Reviews in Physical and Rehabilitation Medicine, 13*(4), 255-264.

Boys Town National Research Hospital. Retrieved April 2003 from http://www.boystownhospital.org/services/AudioVest/basic.asp#Basic.

Dean, W.A., & Davidson, M. (2002). Hearing loss in adults: Physical limitation, psychosocial barrier. *Clinician Reviews, 12*(6), 62-67.

Demers, K. (2002). Try this: Hearing screening. *Home Health Care Nurse, 20*(2), 132-133.

Diagnostic tests (February 22, 2003). Retrieved April 2003 from http://www.vestibular.org/tests.html.

Dowden, C. (2002). What is the best treatment for impacted cerumen? *The Journal of Family Practice, 51*(2), 117-119.

Ebersole, P., Hess, P., & Luggen, A. (2004). *Toward healthy aging: Human needs and nursing response* (6th ed.). St. Louis: Mosby.

Fields, R. Borderlands: An El Paso Community College local history project: Food, spices double as folk cures. Retrieved June 2003 from http://www.epcc.edu/ftp/Homes/monicaw/borderlands/09_food.htm.

Finesilver, C. (2002). A new age for childhood diseases: Down syndrome. *RN, 64*(11), 43-49.

Gates, G., et al. (2003). Screening for handicapping hearing loss in the elderly. *The Journal of Family Practice, 52*(1), 56-62.

Gill-Body, K. (2001). Current concepts in the management of patients with vestibular dysfunction. *PT: Magazine of Physical Therapy, 9*(12), 40-58.

Gordon, M. (2002). *Manual of nursing diagnosis* (10th ed.). St. Louis: Mosby.

Hain, T. Ototoxic mezdication. Retrieved April 2003 from http://www.tchain.com/otoneurology/disorders/bilat/ototoxins.html.

Jarvis, C. (2004). *Physical examination and health assessment* (4th ed.). Philadelphia: W.B. Saunders.

Kuurila, K., et al. (2002). Hearing loss in Finnish adults with osteogenesis inperfecti: A nationwide study. *Annals of Otology, Rhinology & Laryngology, 111*(10), 939-946.

Lefebvre, P., & Van De Water, T. (2000). Connexins, hearing and deafness: Clinical aspects of mutations in the connexin 26 gene. *Brain Research Reviews, 32,* 159-162.

Lucas, L., & Matthews-Flint, L. (2001). Sound advice about hearing aids. *Nursing 2001, 31*(2), 59-61.

Lucas, L., & Matthews-Flint, L. (2003). Heed the word about hearing impairment. *Nursing 2003, 33*(10), 32hn1-32hn3.

*Lusk, S.L. (1997). Noise exposures: Effects of hearing and prevention of noise induced hearing loss. *AAORN Journal, 45*(8), 397-405, 409-410.

Martin, F.N. (2000). *Introduction to audiology* (7th ed.). Boston: Allyn & Bacon.

McCance, K., & Huether, S. (2002). *Pathophysiology: The biologic basis for disease in adults and children* (4th ed.). St. Louis: Mosby.

McConnell, E. (2002). How to converse with a hearing-impaired patient. *Nursing 2002, 32*(8), 20.

National Council on Aging. (2000). The consequences of untreated hearing loss in older persons. *ORL-Head and Neck Nursing, 18*(1), 12-16.

Nussbaum, R., McInnes, R., & Willard, H. (2001). *Thompson & Thompson: Genetics in medicine* (6th ed.). Philadelphia: W.B. Saunders.

Pagana, K., & Pagana, T. (2002). *Mosby's manual of diagnostic and laboratory tests* (2nd ed.). St. Louis: Mosby.

Phillips, M. (2003). Genetics of hearing loss. *MEDSURG Nursing, 12*(6), 386-390, 411.

Sheehan, J. (2000). Caring for the deaf: Do you do enough? *RN, 63*(3), 69-72.

Sommer, S., & Sommer, N. (2002). When your patient is hearing impaired. *RN, 65*(12), 28-32.

*Ventry, I., & Selsnick, S. (1983). Identification of elderly people with hearing problems. *American Speech-Language Hearing Association, July,* 37-42.

Zadeh, M., & Selesnick, S. (2001). Evaluation of hearing impairment. *Comprehensive Therapy, 27*(4), 302-310.

Interventions for Clients with Ear and Hearing Problems

JANICE HOOT MARTIN

LEARNING OUTCOMES

After studying this chapter, you should be able to:

1. Compare the clinical manifestations and interventions for external otitis with those of otitis media.
1. Describe how to correctly instill medications into the ear.
3. Describe the mechanisms of action, side effects, and nursing interventions of drug therapy for ear infections.
4. Explain the procedures to safely remove impacted cerumen from the ear canal of an older client.
5. Prioritize educational needs for the client with Ménière's disease.
6. Describe the mechanisms of action, side effects, and nursing implications of drug therapy for Ménière's disease.
7. Compare the causes and interventions for conductive hearing loss with those for sensorineural hearing loss.
8. Prioritize nursing care needs for the client after tympanoplasty.
9. Prioritize educational needs for the client after stapedectomy.
10. Identify an appropriate method for communicating with a client who has recently become hearing impaired.
11. Develop a community-based teaching plan for a client who is learning to use a hearing aid.

Go to your Student CD-ROM for Review Questions
for the NCLEX Examination keyed to these Learning Outcomes.

The ears play an important role in daily functioning. Ear disorders can cause many problems ranging from hearing difficulty to problems of balance and functional ability. Hearing problems can lead to confusion, mistrust, social isolation, and the inability to give and receive accurate information. Disorders of the ear and of hearing are often easily treated with proper diagnosis; however, early recognition and intervention are necessary to prevent additional damage and to promote a maximal level of wellness.

CONDITIONS AFFECTING THE EXTERNAL EAR

The external ear is the outermost part of the ear structures and is subject to outside factors that can cause problems. Disorders of the external ear include congenital malformation (birth defects), trauma, and infectious or noninfectious lesions of the pinna, auricle, or auditory canal. Ear structures (external, middle, and inner ear) develop at different times during fetal life; thus the presence of birth defects in one area does not necessarily mean that other areas also will be affected. Abnormalities of the external ear range from crumpling or falling forward of the pinna to complete absence (**atresia**) of the auditory canal. In addition, trauma can damage or destroy the auricle and external canal. Surgical reconstruction can re-form the pinna with skin grafts and plastic prostheses. Trauma to the auricle resulting in a hematoma requires the removal of blood via needle aspiration to prevent calcification and hardening, which is often referred to as a **cauliflower** or **boxer's ear.**

Benign cysts or polyps of the auricle or external canal are surgically removed if they block the canal and affect hearing. Cancer cells, most often basal cell carcinoma, can also be found on the pinna. In general, treatment consists of simple excision. As the lesion becomes larger, its location near the skull and facial nerve makes treatment more difficult.

TABLE 52-1 Comparison of Features Between External Otitis and Otitis Media

Etiology	Clinical Manifestations	Treatment
External Otitis		
Allergic reactions	Pain	Topical antibiotics
Bacterial or fungal infection	Itching	Corticosteroids
Swimming	Hearing loss	Oral analgesics
Local trauma	Plugged feeling in ear	Local heat
	Redness and edema	
Otitis Media		
Bacterial or viral infection	Exudate	Systemic antibiotics
Fluid accumulation	Pain	Analgesics
	Pressure in ear	Local heat
	Hearing loss	Antipyretics
	Tinnitus	Antihistamines
	Fever	Decongestants
	Malaise	Myringotomy
	Nausea or vomiting	
	Bulging tympanic membrane	
	Fluid behind tympanic membrane	

CHART 52-1

BEST PRACTICE for
Instillation of Eardrops

1. Gather the solutions to be administered.
2. Check the labels to ensure correct dosage and time.
3. Remove and discard any ear packing.
4. Irrigate the ear if the eardrum is intact.
5. Place the bottle of eardrops (with the top on tightly) in a bowl of warm water for 5 minutes.
6. Tilt the client's head in the opposite direction of the affected ear and place the drops in the ear.
7. With the head tilted, gently move the head back and forth five times.
8. Insert a cotton ball into the opening of the ear canal to act as packing.

External Otitis

PATHOPHYSIOLOGY

External otitis is a painful condition caused when irritating or infective agents come into contact with the skin of the external ear. The result to the external ear canal or the auricle is either an allergic response or inflammation with or without infection. Affected skin becomes red, swollen, and tender to touch or movement. Swelling of the ear canal can lead to hearing loss due to canal obstruction. Allergic external otitis is commonly caused by contact with cosmetics, hair sprays, earphones, earrings, or hearing aids. The most common infectious organisms, usually bacterial or fungal, are *Pseudomonas aeruginosa, Streptococcus, Staphylococcus,* and *Aspergillus.* Table 52-1 compares external otitis and otitis media.

External otitis occurs more often in hot, humid environments, especially in the summer, and is commonly referred to as **swimmer's ear** because of the high incidence in people involved in water sports. In addition, clients who have traumatized their external ear canal with sharp or small objects (such as hairpins or cotton-tipped applicators) or through headphones are more susceptible to external otitis.

Necrotizing or *malignant otitis* is the most virulent form of external otitis. Organisms spread beyond the external ear canal into the ear and skull. The high mortality rate seen with malignant external otitis results from complications such as meningitis, brain abscess, and destruction of cranial nerve VII.

COLLABORATIVE MANAGEMENT
Assessment

Manifestations of external otitis include many problems, ranging from mild itching to pain with movement of the pinna or tragus. Clients have pain with movement of the pinna and tragus or when upward pressure is applied to the external canal. They report feeling as if the ear is plugged and hearing is reduced.

Use caution during otoscopic examination to avoid pressing on the walls of the external canal, which causes pain. Drainage from the ear is often greenish white. To prevent cross-contamination, dispose of the otoscope tip and wash your hands before examining the opposite ear. Hearing loss in the affected ear can be severe when inflammation obstructs the ear canal and prevents sounds from reaching the eardrum (**tympanic membrane).**

Interventions

Treatment focuses on reducing inflammation, edema, and pain. Heat is applied locally for 20 minutes three times a day, using towels warmed with water and then wrapped in a plastic bag, or heating pads placed on a low setting. Bedrest limits head movements, thereby reducing pain.

Topical antibiotic and steroid therapies are most effective in decreasing inflammation and pain. Review best practices for instilling eardrops with the client, as shown in Chart 52-1. Observe the client to make sure that he or she uses proper technique. If edema obstructs the external canal, an earwick is inserted past the blockage, with medicated drops applied to the outside end (Figure 52-1). A long piece of gauze dressing serves as an earwick, which the health care provider inserts using forceps to push carefully through the blocked external auditory canal to the eardrum. The earwick may be removed when medication can flow freely into the canal. Thorough handwashing is strictly enforced. Systemic oral or intravenous antibiotics are used in severe cases, especially when cellulitis is present or the auricular lymph nodes are enlarged.

Analgesics, including opioids, may be needed for pain relief during the initial days of therapy. Acetylsalicylic acid (aspirin, Entrophen✶), ibuprofen (Advil), or acetaminophen (Tylenol, Abenol✶) may relieve less severe pain.

After the inflammation has subsided, diluted alcohol may be dropped into the ear to keep it clean and dry and to prevent recurrence. Teach the client not to use cotton-tipped applicators to dry the ears, because this use could damage the canal and increase the risk for infection or inflammation. Recommend that clients with recurrent episodes of external otitis use ear plugs when engaging in water sports.

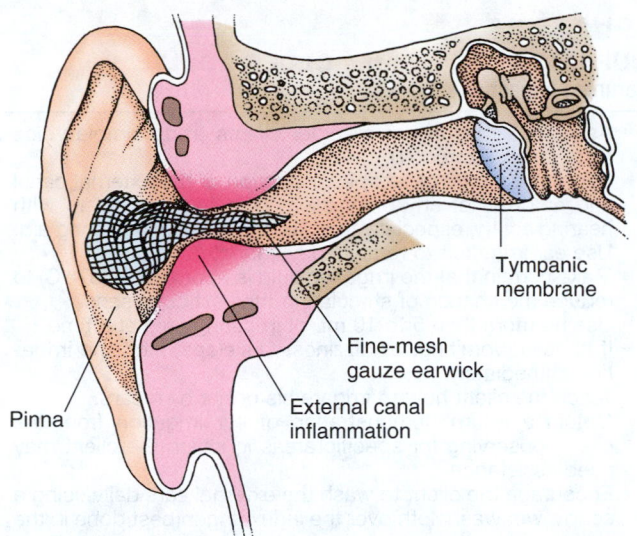

Figure 52-1 ■ Earwick for instillation of antibiotics into the external canal. When edema occludes the external auditory canal, it is difficult for antibiotic solutions to enter the canal adequately. An earwick is placed through the meatus. Solutions placed on the external portion of the earwick are absorbed through the canal.

Furuncle

PATHOPHYSIOLOGY

A **furuncle** is a localized external otitis caused by bacterial infection, usually *Staphylococcus*, of a hair follicle. Most furuncles occur on the outer half of the external canal.

◆COLLABORATIVE MANAGEMENT

The manifestations of a furuncle include intense local pain to light touch. The area is swollen and red, with tight skin covering the area, possibly with a purulent head. No drainage is seen unless the furuncle has ruptured. Hearing is impaired if the lesion blocks the canal.

Treatment consists of local and systemic antibiotics and local heat application. An earwick may be used with one-half strength Burow's solution to relieve pain. The furuncle may need to be incised and drained if it does not resolve with the use of antibiotics.

Cerumen or Foreign Bodies

PATHOPHYSIOLOGY

Many objects can enter or be placed in the external ear canal. **Cerumen** (wax) is the most common cause of an impacted canal. Vegetables, beads, pencil erasers, and insects are other common items that may also enter the ear, with or without the client's help. Although uncomfortable, cerumen or foreign bodies are rarely true emergencies, and can be carefully removed by a health care professional. Remember, cerumen impaction in the older adult is common and research has shown that removal of cerumen from residents of a long-term care facility not only improves hearing but also improves mental status (see the Evidence-Based Practice for Nursing box above).

EVIDENCE-BASED PRACTICE for Nursing

Effect of cerumen impaction on cognition in older adults

Moore, A., et al. (2002). Cerumen, hearing, and cognition in the elderly. *Journal of the American Medical Directors Association, 3*(3), 136-139.

The purpose of this study was to confirm the high incidence of cerumen impaction among older adult residents admitted to skilled nursing facilities and to evaluate the impact of hearing loss caused by cerumen impaction on cognition in these residents. The design was a prospective pretest-posttest design conducted in a 160-bed long-term care facility. Subjects included 29 newly admitted residents who were older than 65 years of age. All residents were tested using the Folstein Mini-Mental Status Exam (MMSE) [mental status measure] and electronic audiometry [hearing measure]. The residents were divided into two groups, those without 50% cerumen occlusion and those with 50% cerumen occlusion. The intervention included removal of cerumen in those residents with 50% or more occlusion. Residents were tested for mental status and hearing both before and after cerumen removal. Residents with less than 50% cerumen occlusion were used as a control.

As suspected, a large percentage of the residents (65.5%) had cerumen occlusions of more than 50%. A statistically significant hearing improvement was found for 80% of the residents who had cerumen removed. Additionally, mental status was significantly improved for residents after removal of cerumen.

Level of Evidence: 3—Well-designed trial without randomization; single pretest and post-test.

Critique. This was a well-designed study with reliable and valid measurement tools. Statistical significance was found even though there was small variability in the measurement score for the hearing (improvement, no change, loss of frequency). The sample size was ample although it may not be representative of other long-term care facilities. Further study is needed to determine whether the mental status changes again as cerumen impaction develops again or whether these findings are similar for clients hospitalized with acute illnesses.

Implications for Nursing. Nurses are responsible for assessing the mental status of clients and making judgments based on these findings. This study suggests that hearing loss has a direct effect on mental status and that the simple task of cerumen removal to improve hearing will also improve mental status in a significant number of clients. Nursing care aimed at improving sensory hearing that leads to improved mental status might also lead to improved client outcomes and adherence to health care needs.

◆COLLABORATIVE MANAGEMENT
◆Assessment

Clients have a sensation of fullness in the ear, with or without hearing loss, and may have ear pain, itching, or bleeding from the ear. The object may be visible with direct inspection.

◆Interventions

When the occluding material is cerumen, irrigate the canal with a mixture of water and hydrogen peroxide at body temperature (Figure 52-2), following best practices for proper irrigation (Chart 52-2). Wax removal by irrigation is a slow process and may take more than one sitting. When cerumen obstruction is the cause of hearing loss, its removal improves hearing. Between 50 and 70 mL of solution is the maximum amount that the client can tolerate at one sitting. *Do not irrigate an ear that has an eardrum perforation or otitis media.*

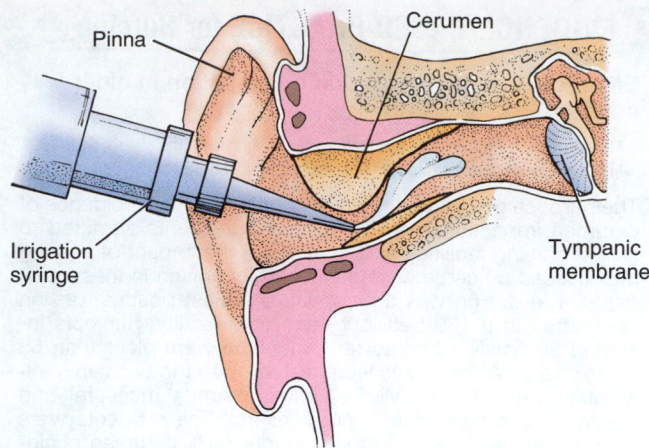

Figure 52-2 ■ Irrigation of the external canal. Cerumen and debris can be removed from the ear by irrigation with warm water. The stream of water is aimed above or below the impaction to allow back pressure to push it out rather than further down the canal.

CHART 52-2

BEST PRACTICE for
Ear Irrigation

1. Gather the proper equipment: basin, syringe, otoscope, towel.
2. Warm tap water to body temperature.
3. Fill a syringe with warm water.
4. Place a towel around the client's neck.
5. Place a basin under the ear to be irrigated.
6. Use an otoscope to check the location of the impacted cerumen; ascertain that the eardrum is intact and that the client does not have otitis media.
7. Place the tip of the syringe at an angle so that the fluid pushes on one side and not directly on the impaction (this helps to loosen the impaction instead of forcing it further into the canal).
8. Watch the fluid return for signs of cerumen plug removal.
9. Continue to irrigate the ear with about 70 mL of fluid.
10. If the cerumen does not drain out, wait 10 minutes and repeat the irrigation procedure.
11. Monitor the client for signs of nausea.
12. If the client becomes nauseated, stop the procedure.
13. If the cerumen cannot be removed by irrigation, the client may place mineral oil into the ear three times a day for 2 days to soften dry, impacted cerumen, after which irrigation may be repeated.

If the cerumen is thick and dry or cannot be removed easily, the health care provider may prescribe a ceruminolytic product such as Cerumenex to soften the wax before trying to remove it. Another way to soften cerumen is to add 3 drops of glycerin or mineral oil to the ear at bedtime and 3 drops of hydrogen peroxide twice a day. After several days of this treatment, the cerumen is more easily removed by irrigation. In some cases, a small curette or cerumen spoon may be used to scoop out the wax. Only trained health care providers should use this method, because damage to the canal or the eardrum is likely with improper technique. Refer to Chart 52-3 for nursing care considerations of older adult clients with cerumen impaction.

Irrigation is *not* used when the foreign object is vegetable matter, because this material expands when wet, making the

---

CHART 52-3

NURSING FOCUS on the OLDER ADULT
Cerumen Impaction

- Assess the hearing of all older clients using simple voice tests (see Chapter 51).
- Perform a gentle otoscopic inspection of the external canal and eardrum of any older client who has a problem with hearing acuity, especially the client who wears a hearing aid.
- Use ear irrigation to remove any impacted cerumen.
- Make certain that the irrigating fluid is about 98° F (37° C) to reduce the chance of stimulating the vestibular sense.
- Use no more than 5 to 10 mL of irrigating fluid at a time.
- If nausea, vomiting, or dizziness develops, stop the irrigation immediately.
- Teach the client how to irrigate his or her own ears.
- Obtain a return demonstration of ear irrigation from the client, observing for specific areas in which the client may need assistance.
- Encourage the client to wash the external ears daily using a soapy, wet washcloth over the index finger (best done in the shower or while washing the hair).

---

impaction worse. The object needs to be physically removed by an experienced health care provider.

Insects are killed before removal unless they can be coaxed out by a flashlight or a humming noise. Mineral oil or diluted alcohol is instilled into the ear to suffocate the insect, which is then removed with ear forceps.

If the client has local irritation, an antibiotic or steroid ointment may be applied to prevent infection and reduce local irritation. Hearing acuity is tested if hearing loss is not resolved by removal of the object.

In rare cases, surgical removal of the foreign object is required. The object is removed through the transcanal route using a wire bent at a 90-degree angle. The wire is looped around the object, and the object is pulled out. Because this procedure is painful, general anesthesia is necessary.

CONDITIONS AFFECTING THE MIDDLE EAR

Otitis Media

PATHOPHYSIOLOGY

The three most common forms of otitis media are acute otitis media, chronic otitis media, and serous otitis media. Each type affects the middle ear but has slightly different causes, incidences, and pathologic changes. If otitis progresses or remains untreated, permanent conductive hearing loss may occur. Otitis media is less common in adults than in children.

Acute otitis media and chronic otitis media, also known as suppurant or purulent otitis media, are similar. An infecting agent introduced into the middle ear causes inflammation of the mucosa, leading to swelling and irritation of the ossicles within the middle ear. A purulent inflammatory exudate follows. Acute disease has a sudden onset and a duration of 3 weeks or less. Chronic otitis media often follows repeated acute episodes, has a longer duration, and causes greater middle-ear injury.

The eustachian tube and mastoid, connected to the middle ear by a sheet of cells, are also affected by the infection. If the eardrum membrane perforates and infective materials

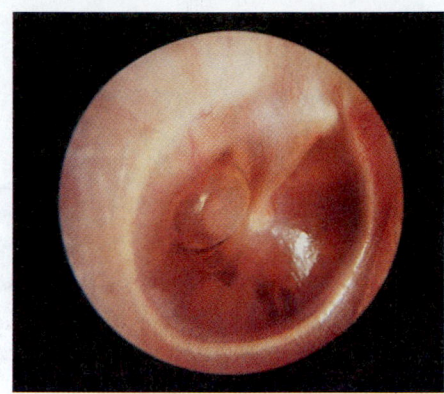

Figure 52-3 ■ Otoscopic view of otitis media.

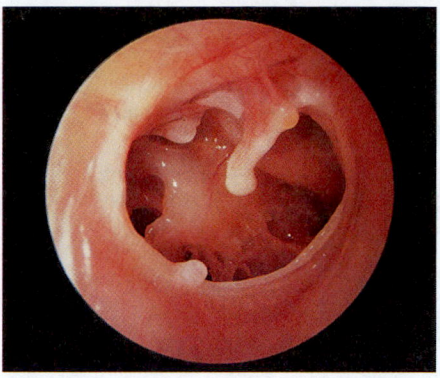

Figure 52-4 ■ Otoscopic view of a perforated tympanic membrane.

spill into the external ear, external otitis also develops, which thickens and scars the middle ear if left untreated. Necrosis of the ossicles destroys middle-ear structures.

◆ COLLABORATIVE MANAGEMENT

◆ Assessment

The chief complaint of the client with acute or chronic otitis media is ear pain with or without movement of the external ear. Pain with chronic otitis media is much less severe than that occurring with acute otitis media. As the pressure in the middle ear increases, there is a sensation of fullness in the ear. Hearing is reduced and distorted. The client may notice a sticking or cracking sound in the ear on yawning or swallowing or may have tinnitus in the form of a low hum or a low-pitched sound. Conductive hearing loss may occur as sound wave transmission is obstructed. Headaches are common, and systemic symptoms such as malaise, fever, nausea, and vomiting can occur. As the pressure on the middle ear pushes against the inner ear, the client may have dizziness or vertigo.

Otoscopic examination findings vary, depending on the stage of the disease. The eardrum is initially retracted, which allows landmarks of the ear to be seen clearly. At this early stage, the client has only vague ear discomfort. As the disease progresses, the eardrum's blood vessels dilate and appear red (Figure 52-3). In the third stage, the eardrum becomes red, thickened, and bulging, with loss of landmarks. Decreased eardrum mobility is evident on inspection with a pneumatic otoscope. Pus may be seen behind the membrane.

If the disease progresses, the eardrum spontaneously **perforates** (breaks open) and pus or blood drains from the ear (Figure 52-4). This discharge may be pulsating when viewed through the otoscope. When the membrane ruptures, the client notices a marked decrease in pain as the pressure on middle-ear structures is relieved (Figure 52-5). Tympanic perforations from any cause may heal if the underlying problem is controlled. The membrane covering initially appears thinner over the healed perforation. A simple central perforation does not interfere with hearing unless the ossicles of the middle ear are damaged or the perforation is large. However, repeated perforations with extensive scarring can cause hearing loss.

Cultures of drainage after a perforation from uncontrolled otitis media may reveal the infecting agent. Cultures are taken only when previous treatment has been ineffective. When the eardrum is not perforated, a needle aspiration or myringotomy draws fluid for culture.

◆ Interventions

NONSURGICAL MANAGEMENT. Treatment can be as simple as putting the client in a quiet environment. Bedrest limits head movements that intensify the pain. Heat may be applied by using a heating pad adjusted to a low setting. Application of cold may occasionally relieve pain.

Systemic antibiotic therapy decreases pain by reducing inflammation. Topical antibiotics are not used to treat otitis media. Analgesics such as aspirin and acetaminophen (Tylenol, Abenol✦) or nonsteroidal anti-inflammatory drugs (NSAIDs) such as ibuprofen (Advil) relieve pain and reduce fever. When the client has severe pain, opioid analgesics such as codeine and meperidine hydrochloride (Demerol) also may be used.

Antihistamines and decongestants are prescribed to decrease mucus production and to decrease fluid in the middle ear. The body can then reabsorb the fluid, reducing pressure and pain.

SURGICAL MANAGEMENT. If the pain persists after antibiotic therapy and the eardrum continues to bulge, a **myringotomy** (surgical opening of the pars tensa of the eardrum) is performed. A myringotomy drains middle-ear fluids and immediately relieves pain.

Preoperative Care. Reassure the client that the myringotomy will relieve pain and is usually performed without anesthesia. Many people are concerned about a perforation and its effect on hearing. To relieve some of this anxiety, discuss the reasons for the procedure and encourage the client to use techniques such as deep breathing before and during the procedure. Systemic antibiotic therapy continues before and after this procedure. Clean the external canal with a bacteriostatic solution such as povidone-iodine (Betadine) before the myringotomy.

Operative Procedures. The small surgical incision is performed in an office or clinic setting and heals rapidly. Another approach is the removal of fluid from the middle ear with a needle. For relief of pressure caused by serous otitis media, a small **grommet** (polyethylene tube) may be surgically placed through the tympanic membrane to allow continuous drainage of middle-ear fluids (Figure 52-6).

Postoperative Care. Take care to keep the external ear and canal free of other substances while the incision is healing. Instruct the client to keep his or her head dry by not washing the hair or showering for several days. Other instructions after surgery are listed in Chart 52-4.

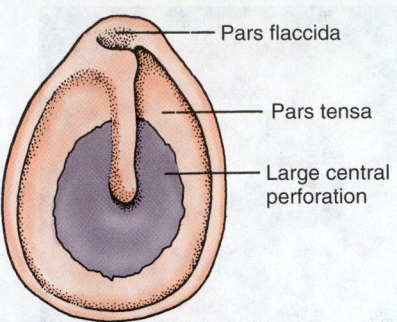

With a **large central perforation,**
clients complain of significant hearing loss.

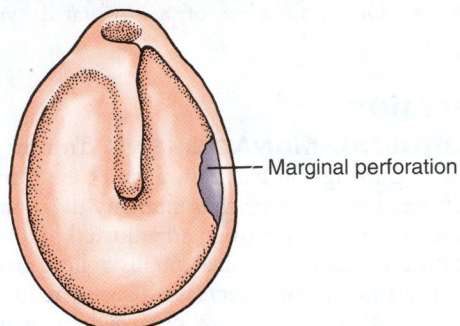

With a **marginal perforation,**
clients might complain of significant hearing loss.

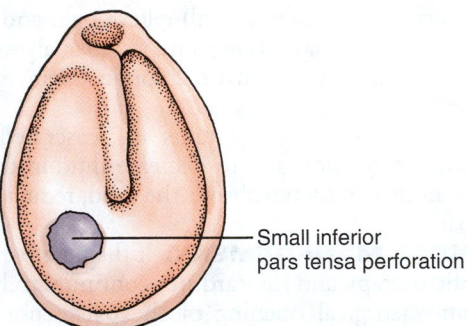

With a **small inferior pars tensa perforation,**
clients do not complain of much interference with hearing.

Figure 52-5 ■ Perforations of the tympanic membrane. Central perforations heal more quickly than marginal perforations. Marginal perforations that do not heal allow cholesteatoma formation.

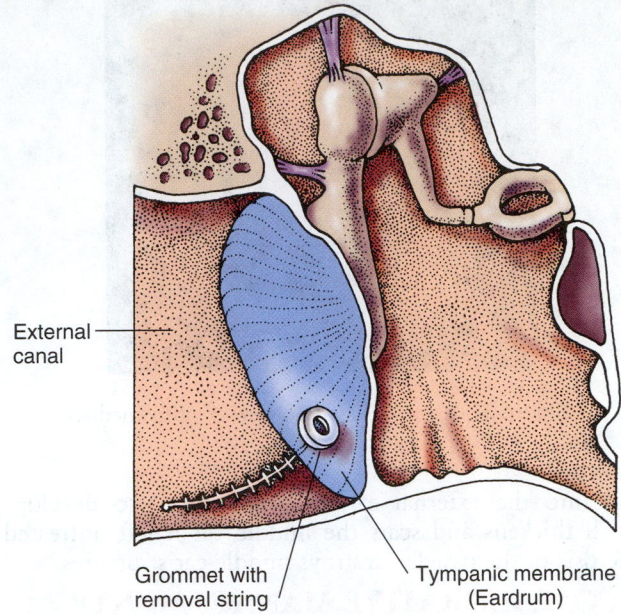

Figure 52-6 ■ Grommet through the tympanic membrane. A small grommet is placed through the tympanic membrane away from the margins, which allows prolonged drainage of fluids from the middle ear. The grommet can be removed later and the tympanic membrane allowed to heal naturally or patched with a small piece of homogenous tissue.

CHART 52-4

CLIENT EDUCATION GUIDE
Recovery from Ear Surgery

- Avoid straining when you have a bowel movement.
- Do not drink through a straw for 2 to 3 weeks.
- Avoid air travel for 2 to 3 weeks.
- Avoid excessive coughing for 2 to 3 weeks.
- Stay away from people with colds.
- If you need to blow your nose, blow gently, one side at a time, with your mouth open.
- Avoid getting your head wet, washing your hair, and showering for 1 week.
- Keep your ear dry for 6 weeks by placing a ball of cotton coated with petroleum jelly (such as Vaseline) in your ear. Change the cotton ball daily.
- Avoid rapidly moving the head, bouncing, and bending over for 3 weeks.
- Change your ear dressing every 24 hours as directed.
- Report excessive drainage immediately to your physician.

Mastoiditis

PATHOPHYSIOLOGY

The lining of the middle ear is continuous with the lining of the mastoid air cells, which are embedded in the temporal bone. **Mastoiditis** is an infection of the mastoid air cells caused by untreated or inadequately treated otitis media. This infection can be acute or chronic. Antibiotic therapy is aimed at treating the middle-ear infection before it progresses to mastoiditis.

◆COLLABORATIVE MANAGEMENT
◆Assessment

The manifestations of mastoiditis include swelling behind the ear and pain with minimal movement of the tragus, the pinna, or the head. Pain is not relieved by myringotomy. **Cellulitis** (infection spreading laterally through the tissues of the skin) develops on the skin or external scalp over the mastoid process. Otoscopic examination shows a red, dull, thick, immobile eardrum with or without perforation. Lymph nodes behind the ear are tender and enlarged. Clients may have low-grade fever, malaise, ear drainage, and anorexia.

◆Interventions

NONSURGICAL MANAGEMENT. Intravenous antibiotics are prescribed to prevent the spread of infection. These drugs have limited use in actual mastoiditis treatment because they do not easily penetrate the infected bony structure of the mastoid. Cultures of the ear drainage determine which antibiotics should be most effective.

SURGICAL MANAGEMENT. Surgical removal of the infected tissue is needed if the infection does not respond to antibiotic therapy within a few days. A simple or modified radical mastoidectomy with tympanoplasty is the most common treatment. All infected tissue must be removed so that the infection does not spread to other structures. A tympanoplasty is then performed to reconstruct the ossicles and the eardrum to restore hearing. Client preparation, the operative procedure, and follow-up care for tympanoplasty are discussed on pp. 1137 and 1138.

Complications occur when infective material is not removed completely or when other structures are contaminated. Such complications include damage to cranial nerves VI and VII, decreasing the client's ability to look laterally (cranial nerve VI) and causing a drooping of the mouth on the affected side (cranial nerve VII). Other complications include vertigo, meningitis, brain abscess, chronic purulent otitis media, and wound infection.

Trauma
PATHOPHYSIOLOGY

Trauma and damage may occur to the eardrum and ossicles by infection, by direct damage, or through rapid changes in the middle-ear cavity pressure. Foreign objects placed in the external canal exert pressure on the eardrum and cause perforation. If the objects continue through the canal, the bones of the stapes, incus, and malleus may be damaged. Blunt injury to the skull and ears can also damage middle-ear structures through fractures extending to the middle ear. Slapping of the external ear increases the pressure in the ear canal, tearing the eardrum when the pressure is great enough. The eardrum has a limited stretching ability and gives way under high pressure. Excessive nose blowing and rapid changes of pressure that occur with nonpressurized air flight (**barotrauma**) can cause an increase in pressure within the middle ear. High pressure damages the ossicles and can perforate the eardrum.

◆COLLABORATIVE MANAGEMENT

Most eardrum perforations heal within 1 or 2 weeks. Repeated perforations, especially from chronic otitis media, heal more slowly, with scarring. Depending on the amount of damage to the ossicles, hearing may or may not return. Hearing aids can improve hearing in this type of hearing loss. Surgical reconstruction of the ossicles and eardrum through a tympanoplasty or a myringoplasty may also improve hearing (see later discussion of nursing care under Tympanoplasty, pp. 1137 and 1138).

Preventive measures should be taken to avoid trauma. Instruct clients to avoid inserting objects into the external canal. Ear protectors should be used when blunt trauma is likely, especially in sports such as boxing.

Neoplasms
PATHOPHYSIOLOGY

Tumors of the middle ear are rare. The most common type of tumor is the *glomus jugulare*, a highly vascular benign lesion arising from the jugular vein. Malignant ear tumors include adenocarcinoma, adenoid cystic carcinoma, and mucoepidermoid carcinoma. The growth of any lesion within the middle-ear fossa disrupts conductive hearing, erodes the ossicles, and may spread to the inner ear and adjacent cranial nerves.

◆COLLABORATIVE MANAGEMENT

Clients have progressive hearing loss and tinnitus. Infection and pain rarely occur with *glomus jugulare* tumors. Otoscopic examination reveals bulging of the eardrum or a mass extending to the external ear canal. The many blood vessels of the *glomus jugulare* tumor give it a reddish color and a visible pulsation when seen through the eardrum.

Diagnosis is made by physical examination, tomography, and angiography. Tumors are removed by surgery, which often destroys hearing in the affected ear. If all of the edges of the tumor can be seen clearly through the eardrum, a transcanal approach is used to remove the lesion. When the tumor edges extend past the eardrum, more testing is needed to determine the extent of involvement. Radiation therapy is used to decrease the vascularity of the *glomus jugulare* tumor but is not the preferred method of treatment.

Benign lesions are removed because, with continued growth of the neoplasm, other structures can be affected, further damaging the facial or trigeminal nerve. When possible, reconstruction of the middle-ear structures is performed later to restore conductive hearing.

CONDITIONS AFFECTING THE INNER EAR

Tinnitus
PATHOPHYSIOLOGY

Tinnitus (continuous ringing or noise perception in the ear) is a common ear or hearing disorder. Diagnostic testing cannot confirm tinnitus. However, some tests are performed to assess for hearing loss and to rule out other ear problems. Tinnitus can have disturbing emotional consequences for the person afflicted with this disorder.

◆COLLABORATIVE MANAGEMENT

Symptoms of tinnitus range from mild ringing, which can go unnoticed during the day, to a loud roaring in the ear, which can interfere with thinking and attention span. When clients report tinnitus, you must be alert to the many factors that cause tinnitus: presbycusis, **otosclerosis** (irregular bone growth around ossicles), Ménière's disease, certain drugs, exposure to loud noise, and other inner-ear problems.

The exact pathophysiology and treatment of tinnitus vary with the underlying cause. When no cause can be found or the disorder is untreatable, therapy focuses on ways to mask the tinnitus with background sound, noisemakers, and music during sleeping hours. Ear mold hearing aids can amplify sounds to drown out the tinnitus during the day. The American Tinnitus Association assists clients in coping with tinnitus when other therapy is unsuccessful.

Vertigo and Dizziness
PATHOPHYSIOLOGY

Vertigo and dizziness are common manifestations of many ear disorders. Dizziness is a disturbed sense of a person's proper relationship to space. Clients vary greatly in defining dizziness. Vertigo is often used interchangeably with dizziness, but the definition, as well as the cause, is somewhat different. True **vertigo** is a real sense of whirling or turning in space.

The visual system, the vestibular system (cochlea, semicircular canals), and the proprioceptive system (muscles and nerve endings) combine to give input to the brain about balance. Problems in any of these areas leads to a disturbed sense of balance or motion. Factors affecting the ear that cause vertigo include Ménière's disease, labyrinthitis, acoustic neuromas, motion sickness, and drug or alcohol ingestion.

◆ COLLABORATIVE MANAGEMENT

Manifestations of vertigo include nausea, vomiting, falling, nystagmus, hearing loss, and tinnitus. Until the cause of the vertigo can be treated, each manifestation is treated. Advise clients to:

- Restrict head motions and move more slowly.
- Maintain adequate hydration, especially after vomiting.
- Take drugs with antivertiginous effects, such as dimenhydrinate (Dramamine, Gravol✱), diazepam (Valium, Apo-Diazepam✱), and scopolamine (Transderm Scop, Transderm-V✱).

Many clients are dissatisfied with treatment because side effects of the drugs, especially drowsiness, can be worse than the vertigo. Caution clients to maintain a safe, uncluttered environment to prevent accidents during periods of vertigo and to use a cane or walker to maintain balance. Also instruct them not to drive or operate machinery when taking these drugs.

Labyrinthitis

PATHOPHYSIOLOGY

Labyrinthitis is an infection of the labyrinth, which may occur as a complication of acute or chronic otitis media. Infection results from an erosion of the bony capsule, allowing organisms to invade the inner ear. Labyrinthitis often results from the growth of a **cholesteatoma** (benign overgrowth of squamous cell epithelium) from the middle ear into the semicircular canal. Labyrinthitis may follow middle-ear or inner-ear surgery when infection is present. Labyrinthitis may be part of a systemic viral infection such as an upper respiratory infection or infectious mononucleosis.

◆ COLLABORATIVE MANAGEMENT

Manifestations include hearing loss, tinnitus, spontaneous nystagmus to the affected side, and vertigo with nausea and vomiting. **Meningitis** (infection of the brain covering) is a common complication of labyrinthitis.

Treatment of labyrinthitis includes the use of systemic antibiotics such as ampicillin (Omnipen, Apo-Ampi✱). Advise clients to stay in bed in a darkened room until manifestations are reduced. Antiemetics, such as chlorpromazine hydrochloride (Thorazine, Novo-Chlorpromazine✱), and antivertiginous medications, such as dimenhydrinate (Dramamine, Gravol✱), relieve symptoms.

The client also needs psychosocial support. Hearing loss on the affected side may be permanent, although vertigo subsides as the inflammation resolves. Persistent balance problems may improve with gait training and physical therapy.

Ménière's Disease

PATHOPHYSIOLOGY

Ménière's disease has three features: tinnitus, one-sided sensorineural hearing loss, and vertigo, occurring in attacks that can last for several days. Clients are almost totally incapacitated during an attack, and several days are needed for full recovery. The pathology of Ménière's disease is either overproduction or decreased reabsorption of endolymphatic fluid, causing a distortion of the entire inner-canal system. This distortion decreases hearing from dilation of the cochlear duct, vertigo because of damage to the vestibular system, and tinnitus from unknown cause. The initial hearing loss is reversible, but repeated damage to the cochlea from increased fluid pressure, leads to permanent hearing loss.

The cause of Ménière's disease is unknown but it often occurs with infections, allergic reactions, and fluid imbalances. Long-term stress may have a role in Ménière's disease.

◆ COLLABORATIVE MANAGEMENT
◆ Assessment

Ménière's disease usually first occurs in people between the ages of 20 and 50 years. The prevalence is greater in men and in white individuals. Times of severe, debilitating attacks alternate with symptom-free periods. Clients often have certain manifestations before an attack of vertigo, such as headaches, increasing tinnitus, and a feeling of fullness in the affected ear. Manifestations are usually unilateral.

Clients describe the tinnitus as a continuous, low-pitched roar or a humming sound, which worsens just before and during a severe attack. Hearing loss is initially of the low-frequency tones but worsens to include all levels after repeated episodes. In the early stages of Ménière's disease, periods of remission are marked by normal or nearly normal hearing, but permanent hearing loss develops as the attacks increase.

Clients describe the vertigo as periods of whirling, which might even cause them to fall. The vertigo is so intense that even while lying down, clients hold the bed or ground to prevent the whirling sensation. Severe vertigo usually lasts 3 to 4 hours, but clients may feel dizzy long after the attack. Nausea and vomiting are common. Other manifestations include rapid eye movements **(nystagmus)** and severe headaches.

◆ Common Nursing Diagnoses and Collaborative Problems

Nursing diagnoses that may apply to clients with Ménière's disease include the following:

- Anxiety related to loss of control
- Risk for Injury related to loss of balance
- Powerlessness related to loss of control
- Activity Intolerance related to perception of dizziness
- Risk for Deficient Fluid Volume related to nausea and vomiting
- Fear related to potential of hearing loss

◆ Interventions

NONSURGICAL MANAGEMENT. Instruct clients to make slow head movements to prevent worsening of the vertigo. Dietary and lifestyle changes, such as salt and fluid restrictions that reduce the amount of endolymphatic fluid, are helpful. Advise clients to stop smoking because of the blood vessel constricting effects.

Drug therapy aims to control the vertigo and vomiting and restore normal balance. Mild diuretics are prescribed to decrease endolymph volume. Nicotinic acid has been found to be useful because of its vasodilatory effect. Antihistamines such as diphenhydramine hydrochloride (Benadryl, Allerdryl✦) and dimenhydrinate (Dramamine, Gravol✦) help reduce the severity of or stop an acute attack. Antiemetics such as chlorpromazine hydrochloride (Thorazine, Novo-Chlorpromazine✦), droperidol (Inapsine), and trimethobenzamide hydrochloride (Arrestin, Tigan) help control the nausea and vomiting. Diazepam (Valium, Apo-Diazepam✦) calms the client; controls vertigo, nausea, and vomiting; and allows the client to rest quietly during an attack.

SURGICAL MANAGEMENT. Surgical treatment of Ménière's disease is a last resort because the hearing in the affected ear is often sacrificed. When medical therapy is ineffective and the client's hearing level has decreased significantly, surgery is performed. The most radical procedure involves resection of the vestibular nerve or total removal of the labyrinth **(labyrinthectomy),** performed via the transcanal route. The footplate of the stapes is moved aside, and the labyrinth is removed through the oval window.

Another procedure performed early in the course of the disease is endolymphatic decompression with drainage and a shunt. The endolymphatic sac is drained, and a small tube is inserted to improve fluid drainage. Some clients report relief of vertigo with retention of their hearing.

If endolymphatic decompression has been performed, movement of the vestibular structures of the inner ear causes postoperative vertigo. Reassure the client that the vertigo is temporary as a result of the surgical procedure, not the disease.

❓ Critical Thinking Challenge

The client is a 52-year-old man who is the conductor of a symphony in a large city. He is admitted to the emergency department with severe dizziness and vomiting. He tells you he was eating dinner in a restaurant when his symptoms began suddenly. He has had such episodes in the past and has been diagnosed with Ménière's disease. He tells you he would rather die than lose his hearing because music is his life.

1. What vital signs should you take first for this client? Why?
2. What nursing diagnoses are appropriate at this time for this client?
3. What interventions can you initiate for the symptoms he has before he is seen by a physician?
4. What lifestyle changes can you suggest for his chronic problem?

evolve For suggested answer guidelines, go to http://evolve.elsevier.com/Iggy/.

Acoustic Neuroma
PATHOPHYSIOLOGY

An **acoustic neuroma** is a benign tumor of cranial nerve VIII. The tumor is destructive as it grows, often damaging structures in the cerebellum. Depending on the size and exact location of the tumor, damage to hearing, facial movements, and sensation can occur. The presence of an acoustic neuroma can cause many neurologic manifestations as the tumor enlarges in the brain.

◆COLLABORATIVE MANAGEMENT

Manifestations begin with tinnitus and progress to gradual sensorineural hearing loss in most clients. Later, clients have constant mild vertigo. As the tumor enlarges, nearby cranial nerves are damaged.

Acoustic neuromas are diagnosed with computed tomography (CT) scanning and magnetic resonance imaging (MRI). Audiograms detect sensorineural hearing loss. Cerebrospinal fluid assays show increased pressure and the presence of protein.

Surgical removal via a craniotomy is performed, and the remaining hearing is sacrificed. Extreme care is taken to preserve the function of the facial nerve (cranial nerve VII). Routine postcraniotomy care is discussed in Chapter 48. Acoustic neuromas rarely recur after surgical removal.

HEARING LOSS
PATHOPHYSIOLOGY

Hearing loss is one of the most common physical handicaps in North America. Hearing loss may be conductive, sensorineural, or a combination of the two (Figure 52-7). Conductive hearing loss occurs when sound waves are blocked from contact with inner-ear nerve fibers because of external-ear or middle-ear disorders. If the inner-ear nerve, or sensory, fibers that lead to the cerebral cortex are damaged, the hearing loss is termed sensorineural. Combined hearing loss is known as mixed conductive-sensorineural.

The differences in conductive and sensorineural hearing loss are listed in Table 52-2. Disorders that cause conductive hearing loss are often corrected with no or minimal permanent damage. Sensorineural hearing loss is often permanent, and measures must be taken to prevent further damage or to amplify sounds as a means to improve hearing.

Etiology and Genetic Risk
COMMON CAUSES OF CONDUCTIVE HEARING LOSS

Any inflammatory process or obstruction of the external or middle ear by cerumen or foreign objects leads to conductive hearing loss. Changes in the eardrum such as bulging, retraction, and perforations may indicate damage to middle-ear structures, which leads to conductive hearing loss. Tumors, scar tissue buildup, and overgrowth of soft bony tissue **(otosclerosis)** on the ossicles from previous middle-ear surgery also lead to conductive hearing loss.

COMMON CAUSES OF SENSORINEURAL HEARING LOSS

When the inner ear or auditory nerve (cranial nerve VIII) is damaged, sensorineural hearing loss develops. Prolonged exposure to loud noise can damage the hair cells of the cochlea. Many drugs are toxic **(ototoxic)** to the inner-ear structures, and their effects on hearing can be transient or permanent, dose related or non–dose related, and affect one or both ears. When ototoxic drugs (such as those listed in Table 51-2) are given to clients with reduced renal function, increased ototoxicity can result because drug elimination is slower. Older clients are especially at risk for ototoxicity because of reduced kidney function.

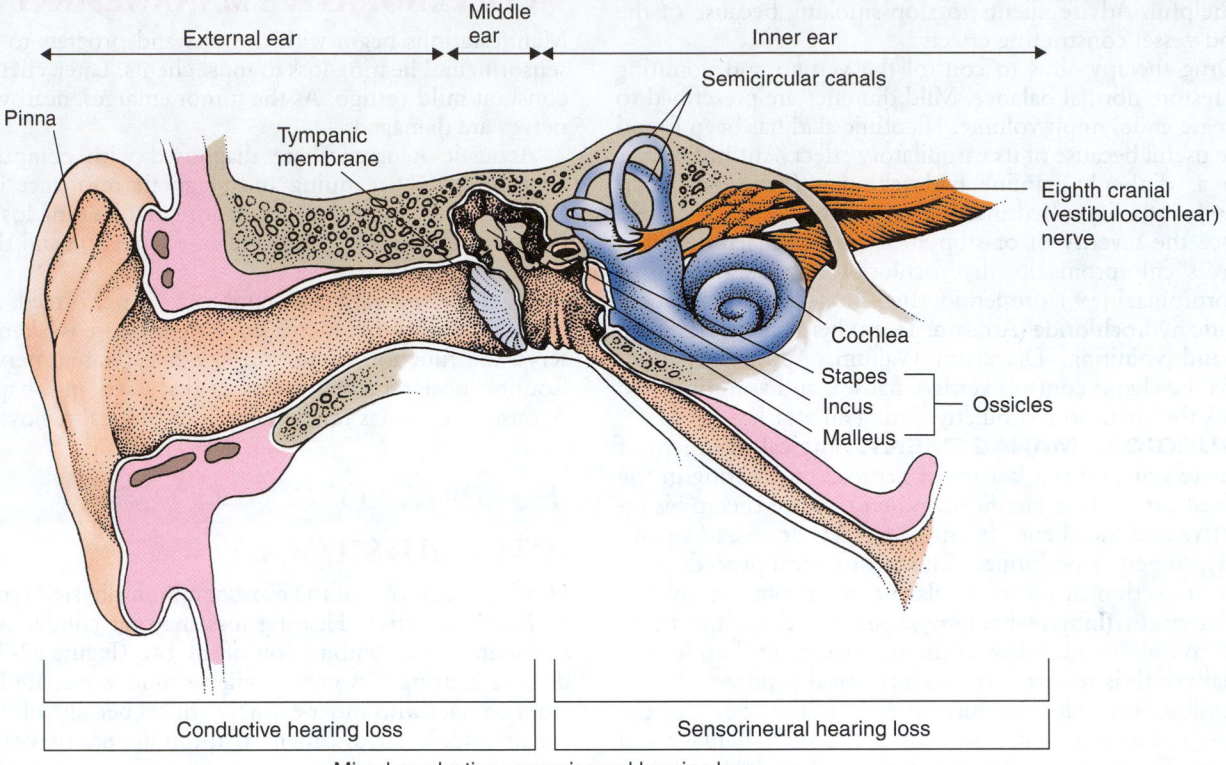

Figure 52-7 ■ Anatomy of hearing loss. Hearing loss can be divided into three types: (1) conductive (difficulty in the external or the middle ear), (2) sensorineural (difficulty in the inner ear or the acoustic nerve), and (3) mixed conductive-sensorineural (a combination of the two).

TABLE 52-2 Differential Features of Conductive and Sensorineural Hearing Loss

Conductive Hearing Loss	Sensorineural Hearing Loss
Causes	
Cerumen	Prolonged exposure to noise
Foreign body	Presbycusis
Perforation of the tympanic membrane	Ototoxic substances
Edema	Ménière's disease
Infection of the external ear or middle ear	Acoustic neuroma
Tumors	Diabetes mellitus
Otosclerosis	Labyrinthitis
	Infection
	Myxedema
Assessment Findings	
Evidence of obstruction with otoscope	Normal appearance of external canal and tympanic membrane
Abnormality in tympanic membrane	Tinnitus common
Speaking softly	Occasional dizziness
Hearing best in a noisy environment	Speaking loudly
Rinne test: air conduction greater than bone conduction	Hearing poorly in loud environment
Weber test: lateralization to affected ear	Rinne test: air conduction less than bone conduction
	Weber test: lateralization to unaffected ear

Presbycusis is a sensorineural hearing loss that occurs as a result of aging. This hearing loss is caused by degeneration or atrophy of the ganglion cells in the cochlea, loss of elasticity of the basilar membrane, or a decreased blood supply to the inner ear. Research findings suggest that deficiencies of vitamin B_{12} and folic acid may play a role in presbycusis. Other causes include atherosclerosis, hypertension, infections, prolonged fever, Ménière's disease, diabetes mellitus, and ear surgery. Each disorder appears to accelerate degenerative changes of the cochlea. Trauma to the ear or the head also contributes to sensorineural hearing loss.

Genetic Considerations

In some cases, hearing loss in adults can have a genetic origin. Some syndromes in which a single gene mutation results in many abnormal manifestations also increase the risk for progressive hearing loss in adults. Two such syndromes are Usher's syndrome and Alport's syndrome. Usher's syndrome, in addition to hearing loss, occurs with blindness as a result of retinitis pigmentosa. This syndrome has an autosomal recessive pattern of inheritance. Alport's syndrome, which causes abnormal renal function in addition to progressive hearing loss, has many forms and patterns of inheritance, including autosomal dominant, autosomal recessive, and X-linked recessive (Online Mendelian Inheritance in Man, 2000). One type of adult-onset progressive hearing loss that does not have any other physical problems is associated with a mutation in the GJB2 gene on chromosome 1. This problem has an autosomal dominant pattern of inheritance.

Incidence/Prevalence

Because hearing loss may be gradual and affect only some aspects of hearing, many adults are unaware that their hearing is impaired. The actual incidence of hearing loss is not known, although about 30% to 35% of people ages 65 to 75

CHART 52-5

NIC INTERVENTION ACTIVITIES for
Care of the Ears

Ear Care: *Prevention or minimization of threats to ear or hearing*
- Monitor for drainage from ears, as appropriate.
- Irrigate the ear, as appropriate.
- Avoid placing sharp objects in the ear.
- Administer eardrops, as appropriate.
- Explain the relationship between balance and the inner ear, as appropriate.
- Monitor for episodes of dizziness associated with ear problems, as appropriate.
- Determine if cerumen in the ear canal is causing pain or hearing loss.
- Instill mineral oil in the ear to soften impacted cerumen before irrigation.
- Irrigate the ear canal with a WaterPik (or similar device) on a low setting using warm water (80° to 90°F), as appropriate.
- Demonstrate proper technique for ear irrigation to caregiver, as appropriate.
- Monitor frequency of ear infections.
- Instruct clients how to administer eardrops, as appropriate.
- Instruct how to monitor and regulate high-volume noise exposure.
- Instruct client to wear hearing protection for exposure to high-intensity noise.
- Instruct client with pierced ears how to avoid infection at the insertion site.
- Encourage use of ear plugs for swimming, if client is susceptible to ear infections.

NIC intervention activities selected from Dochterman, J.M., & Bulechek, G.M. (Eds.). (2004). *Nursing interventions classification (NIC)* (4th ed.). St. Louis: Mosby. No part of this work is to be altered without prior written permission from the Publisher.

years have a hearing loss. As many as half of the people older than 85 years of age have some degree of hearing loss (National Institute on Deafness and Other Communications Disorders, 1999).

HEALTH PROMOTION/ILLNESS PREVENTION

For most people, hearing is as an important factor in social interactions and to gain knowledge. With special care to the ears, hearing can be preserved at maximal levels (Chart 52-5).

◆COLLABORATIVE MANAGEMENT
◆Assessment

HISTORY

Ask clients how long they have noticed a difference in their hearing and whether the changes occurred suddenly or gradually. Age is an important factor, because some ear and hearing changes occur with advanced age. Chronic otitis media occurs more often in the older adult. Ask about occupational exposure to loud or continuous noises, as well as current or previous use of ototoxic drugs. Also ask about any history of external-ear or middle-ear infection and whether eardrum perforation occurred with the infection. Ask clients about any direct trauma to the ears. Because some types of hearing loss have a genetic predisposition, ask whether any family members are hearing impaired.

When pain occurs with acute-onset hearing loss, ask about recent upper respiratory infection and allergies affecting the nose and sinuses.

CHART 52-6

FOCUSED ASSESSMENT of
The Client with Suspected Hearing Loss

Assess whether the client has any of the following ear complaints:
- Pain
- Feeling of fullness or congestion
- Dizziness or vertigo
- Tinnitus
- Difficulty understanding conversations, especially in a noisy room
- Difficulty hearing sounds
- The need to strain to hear
- The need to turn the head to favor one ear or the need to lean forward to hear

Assess visible ear structures, particularly the external canal and tympanic membrane:
- Position and size of the pinna
- Patency of the external canal; presence of cerumen or foreign bodies, edema, or inflammation
- Condition of the tympanic membrane: intact, edema, fluid, inflammation

Assess functional ability, including:
- Frequency of asking people to repeat statements
- Withdrawal from social interactions or large groups
- Shouting in conversation
- Failing to respond when not looking in the direction of the sound
- Answering questions incorrectly

PHYSICAL ASSESSMENT/CLINICAL MANIFESTATIONS

Chart 52-6 lists focused assessment techniques for clients with suspected hearing loss. Hearing loss may be sudden or gradual and often affects both ears. The ability to hear high-frequency soft, consonants, especially *s, sh, f, th,* and *ch* sounds, is lost first. Clients often state that they have no problem with hearing but cannot understand specific words. They might think that the speaker is mumbling. They often experience high-pitched, continuous bilateral tinnitus. Vertigo may be present, depending on the extent of inner-ear involvement.

TUNING FORK TESTS. Tuning fork tests help diagnose hearing loss (see Chapter 51). With the Weber test, the client can usually hear sounds well in the ear with a conductive hearing loss because of bone conduction. With the Rinne test, the client reports that sound transmitted by bone conduction is louder and more sustained than that transmitted by air conduction.

OTOSCOPIC EXAMINATION. An otoscopic examination is performed to assess the external ear canal, the eardrum, and structures of the middle ear visible through the eardrum (see Chapter 51). Findings from examination vary, depending on the cause of the hearing loss.

Obstruction of the external ear canal can result in hearing loss. Inspect the canal, looking for the following:
- Whether the canal is open
- The amount and character of cerumen present
- The integrity of the skin lining the canal
- The presence of redness, exudates, lesions, or foreign objects

Middle-ear infections can also reduce hearing. In infection or inflammation, the eardrum appears red, thickened, and bulging, with a loss of landmarks. Loss of eardrum mobility is seen with inspection through a pneumatic otoscope. Document the presence of any scars or perforations on the eardrum. With close observation, you may be able to see exudate behind the membrane.

PSYCHOSOCIAL ASSESSMENT

For persons with a hearing loss, communication can become a struggle, and they may isolate themselves because of the difficulty in talking and listening. Social isolation can lead to depression, fear, and despair. You must be sensitive to emotional changes that may be related to reduced hearing and a decline in conversational skills.

LABORATORY ASSESSMENT

No laboratory test diagnoses hearing loss. However, some laboratory findings can indicate problems that affect hearing.

White blood cell counts are elevated in the client with acute or chronic otitis media. Microbial culture and antibiotic sensitivity tests can determine the causative organism and the most appropriate drug therapy when infection causes hearing loss.

The client with hearing loss from peripheral neuropathy may have other systemic diseases, including poorly controlled diabetes mellitus. The blood glucose level may be elevated, and the blood may be positive for serum acetone.

RADIOGRAPHIC ASSESSMENT

Radiographic assessment can determine nonauditory problems affecting hearing ability. Some hearing problems can be diagnosed using radiographic techniques. Skull x-rays are used to determine bony involvement in otitis media and the location of otosclerotic lesions, and computed tomography (CT) and magnetic resonance imaging (MRI) are used to determine soft-tissue involvement and the presence and location of tumors.

OTHER DIAGNOSTIC ASSESSMENTS

Audiometry can help to determine the extent and type of hearing loss. An audiogram shows whether hearing loss is only conductive or whether it has a sensorineural component. This is important in determining possible causes of the hearing loss and in planning interventions.

Critical Thinking Challenge

You are the home care nurse for a 74-year-old woman with diabetes, stasis ulcers, and rheumatoid arthritis who lives alone at home. She has had a conductive hearing loss for 10 years and has been using a hearing aid successfully for that time. She has had a kidney infection for the past 2 weeks and was seen by her internist for this problem. At first she was taking Septra orally (prescribed by her internist) for the infection but when her symptoms didn't subside, she went to an urgent care center and was started on streptomycin 8 days ago. The other drugs she takes routinely are insulin, bumetanide, and ibuprofen. She says her hearing has decreased during the last 4 days.

1. What questions should you ask this client?
2. Exactly how will you test her hearing in this setting?
3. What interventions could you perform immediately for her change in hearing?
4. Can you determine whether she has any sensorineural hearing loss? Why or why not?
5. What drugs or health factors could be contributing to her difficulty hearing?

evolve For suggested answer guidelines, go to http://evolve.elsevier.com/Iggy/.

◆ Analysis

COMMON NURSING DIAGNOSES AND COLLABORATIVE PROBLEMS

The following are priority nursing diagnoses for clients with any degree of hearing impairment:

1. **Disturbed Sensory Perception (Auditory)** related to obstruction, infection, damage to the middle ear, or damage to the auditory nerve
2. **Impaired Verbal Communication** related to reduced sensory perception (auditory)

ADDITIONAL NURSING DIAGNOSES AND COLLABORATIVE PROBLEMS

In addition to the common nursing diagnoses, clients with hearing loss or impairment may have one or more of the following:

- **Deficient Knowledge** related to treatment and prevention
- **Activity Intolerance** related to pain
- **Social Isolation** related to pain and decreased hearing
- **Risk for Injury** related to altered auditory perception and infection
- **Acute Pain** related to an inflammatory process and fluid in the middle ear
- **Impaired Physical Mobility** related to vertigo

◆ Planning and Implementation

DISTURBED SENSORY PERCEPTION (AUDITORY)

NOC **PLANNING: EXPECTED OUTCOMES.** The client with hearing loss or impairment is expected to either experience an increase in auditory sensory perception to a functional level or maintain existing levels of hearing. Indicators include the following:

- Mild to no loss of high pitch tones
- Mild to no loss of ability to distinguish conversation from background environmental noise
- Turning to sound
- Maintaining auditory discrimination of discrete sounds

INTERVENTIONS. Interventions aim at identifying the problem, halting the pathologic processes, and improving auditory sensory perception.

NONSURGICAL MANAGEMENT. Interventions include early detection of hearing impairment, use of drug therapy and comfort measures, and use of assistive devices to amplify or augment the client's auditory perception.

Early Detection. Early detection helps correct the problem causing the hearing loss. When hearing loss is gradual, the client can compensate. Assess for indications of hearing loss, as listed in Chart 52-6.

Drug Therapy. Drug therapy is aimed at either correcting the underlying pathologic change or reducing the side effects of disorders occurring with hearing loss. Local (topical) antibiotics are given to clients with external otitis. Systemic antibiotics are needed when clients have other auditory infections. By treating the infection, antibiotics reduce local edema and improve hearing. When pain occurs with hearing disorders, analgesics are used, depending on the location and type of pain. Many ear disorders disturb equilibrium, causing vertigo and dizziness with nausea and vomiting. Antiemetic, antihistamine, antivertiginous, and benzodiazepine drugs can help correct nausea, vertigo, and dizziness.

Assistive Devices. Many devices are useful for clients with permanent, progressive hearing loss. Telephone amplifiers increase telephone volume, allowing the caller to speak in a normal voice. Flashing lights activated by the ringing telephone or a doorbell alert clients visually. In some cases, clients may have a specially trained dog to help them be aware of sounds (ringing telephones or doorbells, cries of other people, and potential dangers), in much the same way that a seeing eye dog assists a blind person.

Small, portable audio amplifiers can assist you in communicating with clients with hearing loss but who have chosen not to use a hearing aid. The use of audio amplifiers or allowing clients to use a stethoscope helps you to communicate with anyone who requires additional volume to hear speech.

Hearing Aids. A hearing aid is a miniature electronic amplifier that is usually used for clients with conductive hearing loss. Hearing aids are less effective for sensorineural hearing loss and may make hearing worse by amplifying background noise. The amplifier can be worn in one or both ears. Local agencies offer special classes for the hearing impaired that help the user benefit from this device.

Offer some special tips to help the client adjust to the hearing aid. Hearing with a hearing aid can be different from natural hearing. Encourage the client to start using the hearing aid slowly, at first wearing it only at home and only during part of the day. Listening to television and the radio and reading aloud can help the client get used to new sounds. The tone or volume of the hearing aid can be adjusted. The most important and difficult aspect of a hearing aid is the amplification of background noise, as well as voices. The client must learn to concentrate and filter out background noises.

The client must also learn to care for the hearing aid (Chart 52-7). Hearing aids are delicate devices that should be handled only by people who know how to care for them properly. The cost of the aids varies greatly but is a significant investment.

Cochlear Implants. Cochlear implantation may help clients with sensorineural hearing loss. A small computer converts sound waves into electronic impulses. Electrodes are placed by the internal ear, with the computer at-tached to the external ear. The electronic impulses then directly stimulate nerve fibers. Some clients have a 50% return of their hearing with this method.

SURGICAL MANAGEMENT. Many surgical interventions are available for clients with specific disorders leading to hearing loss.

Tympanoplasty. Tympanoplasty reconstructs the middle ear to improve hearing caused by conductive hearing loss. The procedures vary from simple reconstruction of the eardrum **(myringoplasty)** to replacement of the ossicles within the middle ear. A type I tympanoplasty is used for a myringoplasty; a type II tympanoplasty is used in cases of greater damage and to provide more extensive reconstruction (Figure 52-8).

CHART 52-7

CLIENT EDUCATION GUIDE
Hearing Aid Care

- Keep the hearing aid dry.
- Clean the ear mold with mild soap and water while avoiding excessive wetting.
- Clean debris from the hole in the middle of the part that goes into your ear with a toothpick or a pipe cleaner.
- Turn off the hearing aid and remove the battery when not in use.
- Check and replace the battery frequently.
- Keep extra batteries on hand.
- Keep the hearing aid in a safe place.
- Avoid dropping the hearing aid or exposing it to temperature extremes.
- Adjust the volume to the lowest setting that allows you to hear, to prevent feedback squeaking.
- Avoid using hair spray, cosmetics, oils, or other hair and face products that might come into contact with the receiver.
- If the hearing aid does not work:
  Change the battery.
  Check the connection between the ear mold and the receiver.
  Check the on/off switch.
  Clean the sound hole.
  Adjust the volume.
  Take the hearing aid to an authorized service center for repair.

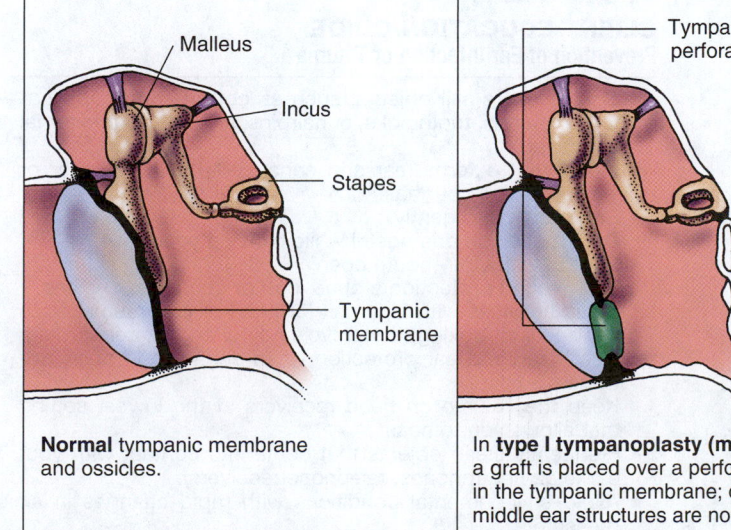
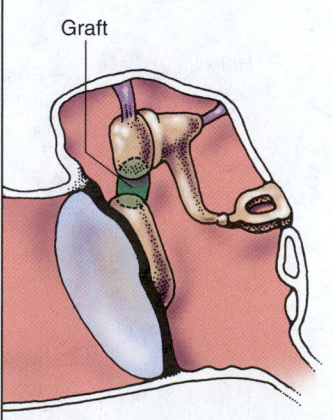

Normal tympanic membrane and ossicles.

In **type I tympanoplasty (myringoplasty)**, a graft is placed over a perforation in the tympanic membrane; other middle ear structures are normal.

In **type II tympanoplasty (ossiculoplasty)**, the malleus, which has become disconnected from the tympanic membrane, is grafted to reconnect the structures.

Figure 52-8 ■ A normal tympanic membrane and two types of tympanoplasties.

Preoperative Care. The client requires specific instructions before surgery. Systemic antibiotics reduce the risk for infection. Before surgery, irrigate the ear with a solution of equal parts of vinegar and sterile water to restore normal ear pH. Teach the client to follow other measures to decrease the risks for infection, such as avoiding people with upper respiratory infections, getting adequate rest, eating a balanced diet, and maintaining an adequate fluid intake.

Assure the client that hearing loss immediately after surgery is normal because of canal packing, and that hearing will improve on packing removal. Explain the importance of deep breathing and coughing after surgery but emphasize that forceful coughing increases middle-ear pressure and must be avoided.

Operative Procedures. Surgery is performed only when the middle ear is free of infection and if the condition of the eustachian tube does not promote continued infection. If an infection is present, the graft is more likely to become infected and not heal properly. Surgery of the eardrum and ossicles requires the use of a microscope and is a delicate procedure. Local anesthesia can be used, although general anesthesia is often used to prevent the client from moving.

The surgeon can repair the eardrum with many materials, including muscle fascia, a skin graft, and venous tissue. If the ossicles are damaged, more extensive surgery is needed for repair or replacement. The ossicles are reached via a transcanal approach, an endaural incision, or the postauricular route with a mastoidectomy (Figure 52-9).

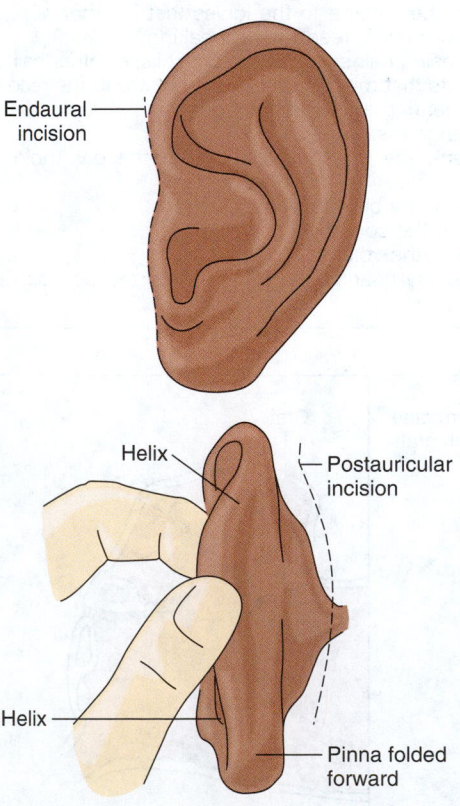

Figure 52-9 ■ Surgical approaches for the ear. The endaural approach is used when the external canal is too small to use for a transcanal approach (not shown because no external incision is used). The postauricular approach is used for more extensive repair of the middle-ear and inner-ear structures.

The surgeon removes diseased tissue and cleans the middle-ear cavity. The ossicles are assessed for damage and the extent of needed repair or replacement. The surgeon uses the client's cartilage or bone, cadaver ossicles, stainless steel wire, or special polymers (Teflon) to repair or replace the ossicles.

Postoperative Care. An antiseptic-soaked gauze, such as iodoform gauze (Nu Gauze), is packed in the ear canal. If a postauricular or endaural incision is used, a dressing is placed over the incision. Keep the dressing clean and dry, using sterile technique for changes. Keep the client flat, with the head turned to the side and the operative ear facing up for at least 12 hours after surgery. Give prescribed antibiotics to prevent infection.

Clients often report hearing improvement after removal of the canal packing. Until that time, communicate as with a hearing-impaired client, directing conversation to the unaffected ear. Instruct the client in care and activity restrictions (see Chart 52-4).

Stapedectomy. A partial or complete stapedectomy with a prosthesis corrects hearing loss. This procedure is most effective for clients with hearing loss related to otosclerosis.

Preoperative Care. To prevent infection, the client must be free from external otitis at surgery. Instruct the client to follow measures that prevent middle-ear or external-ear infections (Chart 52-8).

Review with the client the expected outcomes and possible complications of the surgery. Hearing is initially worse after a stapedectomy. The success rate of this procedure is high; however, there is always a risk of failure that might lead to total deafness on the affected side. Possible complications include prolonged vertigo, infection, and facial nerve damage. A decision to proceed with surgery should be made with the client's full knowledge and understanding of these complications.

Operative Procedures. A stapedectomy is usually performed through the external ear canal with the client under local anesthesia. The head and neck of the stapes and, less often, the footplate are removed. After removal of the bone, a small hole is drilled in the footplate and a prosthesis in the shape of a piston is connected between the incus

---

CHART 52-8

CLIENT EDUCATION GUIDE
Prevention of Ear Infection or Trauma

- Do not use small objects, such as cotton-tipped applicators, matches, toothpicks, or hairpins, to clean your external ear canal.
- Wash your external ear and canal daily in the shower or while washing your hair.
- Blow your nose gently.
- Do not occlude one nostril while blowing your nose.
- Sneeze with your mouth open.
- Wear sound protection around loud or continuous noises.
- Avoid activities with high risk for head or ear trauma, such as wrestling, boxing, motorcycle riding, and skateboarding; wear head and ear protection when engaging in these activities.
- Keep the volume on head receivers at the lowest setting that allows you to hear.
- Frequently clean objects that come into contact with your ear (e.g., headphones, telephone receivers).
- Avoid environmental conditions with rapid changes in air pressure.

and the footplate (Figure 52-10). Sounds cause the prosthesis to vibrate as the stapes did. After stapedectomy, up to 90% of clients have restoration of practical hearing.

Postoperative Care. Inform the client that improvement in hearing may not occur until 6 weeks after surgery. Initially, the ear packing interferes with hearing. Swelling in the ear after surgery reduces hearing until the edema has resolved. Drugs for pain help reduce discomfort, and antibiotics are given to reduce the risk for infection. Instruct the client to follow the procedures in Chart 52-4.

The surgical procedure is performed in an area where cranial nerves VII, VIII, and X can be damaged by trauma or by swelling after surgery. Assess for facial nerve damage or muscle weakness and changes in tactile sensation or taste. Vertigo, nausea, and vomiting are common after surgery because of the nearness to inner-ear structures.

Antivertiginous drugs, such as meclizine hydrochloride (Antivert, Bonamine✱), and antiemetic drugs, such as droperidol (Inapsine), are given. Take care to prevent injury, especially during times of increased vertigo. Assist the client with ambulating during the first 1 to 2 days after surgery. Keep bed siderails up and remind the client to move his or her head slowly when changing position to avoid vertigo.

IMPAIRED VERBAL COMMUNICATION

NOC PLANNING: EXPECTED OUTCOMES. The client with hearing loss or impairment is expected to become proficient in hearing compensation behaviors to maintain or improve expressive and receptive communication. Indicators include that the client consistently demonstrates the following behaviors:

- Uses hearing assistive devices
- Cares for external hearing assistive devices
- Uses sign language, lip reading, or closed captioning (for television viewing)
- Accurately interprets messages received
- Uses nonverbal language
- Exchanges messages accurately with others

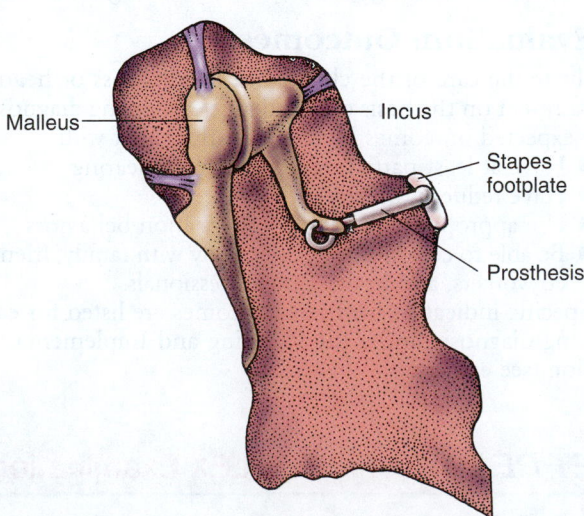

Figure 52-10 ■ Prosthesis used with stapedectomy. The stapes is removed, leaving the footplate. After a hole is drilled in the footplate, a metal or plastic prosthesis is connected to the incus and inserted through the hole to act as a vibration device, much as the stapes worked before the development of otosclerosis.

INTERVENTIONS. Interventions focus on facilitating communication and reducing anxiety.

Use best practices for communicating with a hearing-impaired client that are listed in Chart 52-9. Shouting to the client is of little benefit, because the sound may be projected at a higher frequency, making him or her less able to understand. The most obvious means of communicating with such a client is by the written word (if he or she is able to see, read, and write) or with pictures of familiar phrases and objects. Many television programs are now closed captioned (subtitled).

Assistive Devices. Assistive devices, described on p. 1137, can greatly increase communication for the client with a hearing impairment.

Lip-Reading. Lip-reading and sign language can also enhance communication. In lip-reading classes, clients are taught the special cues to look for when lip-reading and how to understand body language. However, the best lip-reader still misses more than 50% of what is being said. Because hearing is assisted by even minimal lip-reading, urge clients to wear their eyeglasses when talking with someone to see lip movement.

Sign Language. For clients with more severe hearing loss, special languages have been developed, including American Sign Language (ASL). Such languages combine speech with hand movements that signify letters, words, and phrases. These languages take time and effort to learn, and many people are unable to learn them, just as many people cannot learn foreign languages. However, as the hearing-impaired person becomes less able to function, motivation to learn may increase.

Managing Anxiety. A major source of anxiety is the possibility of permanent hearing loss. Provide honest and accurate information about the likelihood of hearing returning. When the hearing impairment is likely to be permanent or become more profound, reassure clients that communication and social interaction can be maintained.

To reduce anxiety and prevent social isolation, clients use remaining resources to make social contact satisfying. The most obvious way to decrease social isolation is by improving communication (as previously described). Ask about past or present diversional activities to identify the

CHART 52-9

BEST PRACTICE for
Communicating with a Hearing-Impaired Client

- Position yourself directly in front of the client.
- Make sure that the room is well lighted.
- Get the client's attention before you begin to speak.
- Move closer to the better-hearing ear.
- Speak clearly and slowly.
- Do not shout (shouting raises the frequency of the sound and often makes understanding more difficult).
- Keep hands and other objects away from your mouth when talking to the client.
- Attempt to have conversations in a quiet room with minimal distractions.
- Have the client repeat your statements rather than just indicating assent.
- Rephrase sentences and repeat information to aid in understanding.
- Use appropriate hand motions.
- Write messages on paper if the client is able to read.

client's most satisfying activities and social interactions and determine the amount of effort necessary to continue them. Activities can be altered to maximize client satisfaction. Someone accustomed to large gatherings might choose smaller groups instead. A quiet evening meal at home with friends might substitute for dinner in a noisy restaurant.

Community-Based Care

Lengthy hospitalization is rare for most clients with ear and hearing disorders. If surgical repair is necessary and the procedure is completed without complications, the procedure may be completed as an outpatient, or the hospital stay is usually only 1 day.

HOME CARE MANAGEMENT

Clients who have persistent vertigo, either with the disorder or as a side effect of surgery, remain in danger of falling. Assess the home for potential hazards and to determine whether family members or significant others are available to assist with meal preparation and other activities of daily living. A nurse case manager can, in collaboration with the home care nurse, assist clients and their families in determining the best ways to maintain adequate self-care abilities, maintain a safe environment, decide about assistance needs, and provide needed care.

HEALTH TEACHING

Give clients written instructions about how to take drugs and when to return for follow-up care. If the client cannot read, give these instructions to a family member who may assist with care. Teach clients how to instill eardrops (see Chart 52-1) and irrigate the ears (see Chart 52-2), and ask for a return demonstration.

To promote health and prevent infections after surgery, clients are instructed to follow the suggestions in Chart 52-8. For clients who use a hearing aid, teach them how to use it effectively.

HEALTH CARE RESOURCES

If clients do not have family or friends to help during the time before surgery, a referral to a home care agency is needed. Help with meal preparation, cleaning, and personal hygiene can be arranged by the hospital discharge planners.

Follow-up hearing tests are scheduled for clients when the lesions are well healed, in about 6 to 8 weeks. Audiograms done before and after treatment are compared, and evaluation for further intervention to improve hearing begins. A complication of an unsuccessful surgery is continued disability or complete loss of hearing in the affected ear. Surgery is performed on the ear with the greatest hearing loss. If the surgery does not improve hearing, clients must decide to either attempt surgical correction of the other ear or continue to use an amplification device. When the underlying disorder causing the hearing impairment is progressive, this decision is difficult. Support clients by listening to their concerns and giving additional information when needed.

Costs to the person with a hearing impairment can be extensive. Information and support can come from several organizations that publish informative articles to help clients reduce hearing loss (Table 52-3). Many public and private

---

TABLE 52-3   Agencies Offering Services for Ear and Hearing Disorders

House Ear Institute
2100 West Third Street, Fifth Floor
Los Angeles, CA 90057
Voice: (800) 352-8888
TTY: (213) 484-2642
Internet: http://www.hei.org

National Information Center on Deafness
Gallaudet University
800 Florida Avenue NE
Washington, DC 20002
Voice: (202) 651-5051
TTY: (202) 651-5000
E-mail: nidc@gallux.gallaudet.edu
Internet: http://www.gallaudet.edu

American Academy of Otolaryngology/Head and Neck Surgery
One Prince Street
Alexandria, VA 22314
Voice: (703) 519-1589
TTY: (703) 836-4444
Internet: http://www.entnet.org

American Speech-Language-Hearing Association
10801 Rockville Pike
Rockville, MD 20852
Voice/TTY: (301) 897-5700
Voice: (800) 638-8255
Internet: http://www.asha.org

Self-Help for Hard of Hearing People, Inc. (SHHH)
7910 Woodmont Avenue, Suite 1200
Bethesda, MD 20814
Voice: (301) 657-2248
TTY: (301) 657-2249
Fax: (301) 913-9413
E-mail: info@hearingloss.org
Internet: http://www.hearingloss.org

---

agencies offer hearing evaluations as well as supply information and counseling for clients with hearing disorders.

◆ Evaluation: Outcomes

Evaluate the care of the client with hearing loss or hearing impairment on the basis of the identified nursing diagnoses. The expected outcomes include that the client will:
- Have at least partial improvement of hearing
- Have reduced anxiety
- Use appropriate hearing compensation behaviors
- Be able to communicate effectively with family, friends, co-workers, and health care professionals

Specific indicators for these outcomes are listed for each nursing diagnosis under the Planning and Implementation section (see earlier).

GET READY for the NCLEX Examination!

KEY POINTS

Safe Effective Care Environment

- Use a separate speculum cover for each ear when conducting an otoscopic examination.

- Slowly and gently introduce the otoscopic speculum into the external ear canal during assessment.
- Use contact precautions with any client who has drainage from the ear canal.
- Avoid performing an otoscopic examination on a confused or uncooperative client.
- Use the suggestions presented under "History" to enhance communication with a client who has a hearing impairment.
- Initiate fall precautions with clients with vertigo or dizziness and assist with ambulation.

Health Promotion and Maintenance

- Teach clients the proper way to clean the pinna and external ear canal.
- Identify clients at risk for hearing impairment as a result of work environment or leisure activities.
- Encourage all clients, even if they already have a hearing impairment, to use ear protection in loud environment.
- Teach clients how to properly care for their hearing aids.
- Instruct clients to avoid closing off one nares when blowing the nose.
- Tell clients who engage in water sports and who are at risk for external otitis either to wear earplugs when in the water or to rinse the ear canal with drops of dilute alcohol after any immersion of the head in water.
- Teach proper ear hygiene for cleaning cerumen from external canal.
- Urge everyone to avoid exposure to loud noises for extended periods of time without proper OSHA-approved ear protection.

Psychosocial Integrity

- Pace your interview to match the learning needs and style of the individual client.
- Allow the client the opportunity to express fear or anxiety regarding a change in hearing status.
- Refer clients newly diagnosed with hearing impairment or any chronic ear problem to appropriate local resources and support groups.
- Explain all diagnostic procedures, restrictions, and follow-up care to the client scheduled for tests.
- Teach family members ways to communicate with a hearing impaired client with and without a hearing aid.

Physiological Integrity

- Ask the client about hearing problems in any other members of the family, because many hearing problems have a genetic component.
- Check the hearing of any client receiving an ototoxic medication (Table 51-2) for more than 5 days.
- Teach clients the proper technique to use for self-instillation of eardrops and ear irrigation.
- Stress the importance of completing an antibiotic regimen when an infection is present in the ear.
- Follow the guidelines in Chart 52-2 when irrigating the ear canal.
- Avoid ear canal irrigation if the eardrum is perforated or if the canal contains vegetative matter.

ADDITIONAL STUDY RESOURCES

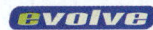 Go to your Student CD-ROM for Review Questions for the NCLEX Examination.

evolve Go to http://evolve.elsevier.com/Iggy/ for Integrated Management of Care Questions for the NCLEX Examination.

SELECTED BIBLIOGRAPHY

Asterisk indicates a classic or definitive work on this subject.

Ackley, B., & Ladwig, G. (2002). *Nursing diagnosis handbook: A guide to planning care* (5th ed.). St. Louis: Mosby.

Alper, C., Myers, E., & Eibling, D. (2001). Decision making in ear, nose, and throat disorders, Philadelphia: W. B. Saunders.

Baker, C. (2002). Caring for patients with hearing impairments. *Dermatology Nursing, 14*(1), 49, 52.

Ball, A. (2002). Caring for older people who have a hearing disability. *Nursing Older People, 14*(4), 39.

Battaglia, S., Sabri, A., & Jackson, C. (2002). Management of chronic otitis media in the only hearing ear. *Laryngoscope, 112*(4), 681-685.

Berry, J., et al. (2002). Patient-based outcomes in patients with primary tinnitus undergoing tinnitus retraining therapy. *Archives of Otolaryngology: Head and Neck Surgery, 128*(10), 1153-1157.

Burton, M. (2000). Hall and Colman's diseases of the ear, nose, and throat *(15th ed.). New York: Churchill Livingstone.*

Canalis, R., & Lambert, P. (2000). *The ear comprehensive otology.* Philadelphia: Lippincott Williams & Wilkins.

Carmen, R., & Uram, S. (2002). Hearing loss and anxiety in adults. *Hearing Journal, 55*(4), 48, 50, 52-54.

Cattel, C., Manna, R., & Carbonin, P. (2003). Case report: a swollen and red ear. *Journal of the American Geriatrics Society, 51*(1),138-139.

Chasin, M. (2000). Middle ear implants: what are surgically-implanted hearing aids and who are they for? *Hearing Loss, 21*(3), 13-15.

Dean, W. A., & Davidson, M. (2002). Hearing loss in adults: Physical limitation, psychosocial barrier. *Clinician Reviews, 12*(6), 62-67.

Demers, K. (2001). Try this: best practices in nursing care to older adults. Hearing screening. *Journal of Gerontological Nursing, 27*(11), 8-9.

Devaiah, A. (2000). Clinical indicators useful in predicting response to the medical management of Meniere's disease. *Laryngoscope, 110*(11), 1884-1889.

*Dhillon, R., & East, C. (1999). *Ear, nose, and throat, and head and neck surgery: An illustrated colour text.* New York: Churchill Livingstone.

Dochterman, J., & Bulechek, G. (Eds.). (2004). *Nursing interventions classification (NIC)* (4th ed.). St. Louis: Mosby.

Dowden, C. (2002). What is the best treatment for impacted cerumen? *The Journal of Family Practice, 51*(2), 117-119.

Ebersole, P., Hess, P., & Luggen, A. (2004). *Toward healthy aging: Human needs and nursing response* (6th ed.). St. Louis: Mosby.

Erber, S., & Garstecki, D. (2002). Hearing loss and hearing aid related stigma: Perceptions of women with age-normal hearing. *American Journal of Audiology, 11*(2), 83-91.

Facts and Comparisons. (2004). *Drug facts and comparisons* (58th ed.). St. Louis: Author.

Garber, S., et al. (2002). Payment under public and private insurance and access to cochlear implants. *Archives of Otolaryngology B Head & Neck Surgery, 128*(10), 1145-1152.

Gates, G., et al. (2003). Screening for handicapping hearing loss in the elderly. *The Journal of Family Practice, 52*(1), 56-62.

Green, C., & Pope, C. (2001). Effects of hearing impairment on use of health services among the elderly, *Journal of Aging & Health, 13*(3), 315-328.

Grossan, M. (2000). Safe, effective techniques for cerumen removal. *Geriatrics, 55*(1), 80-86.

Humes, L., et al. (2002). Longitudinal changes in hearing aid satisfaction and usage in the elderly over a period of one or two years after hearing aid delivery. *Ear & Hearing, 23*(5), 428-438.

Jafek, B., & Murrow, B. (2001). *ENT secrets.* Philadelphia: Hanley & Belfus

Larrabee, T. (2002). Prescribing practices that promote antibiotic resistance: Strategies for change. *Journal of Pediatric Nursing, 17*(2), 126-132.

Lucas, L., & Matthews-Flint, L. (2001). Sound advice about hearing aids. *Nursing2001, 31*(2), 59-61.

Lucas, L., & Matthews-Flint, L. (2003). Heed the word about hearing impairment. *Nursing 2003, 33*(10), 32hn1-32hn3.

McCance, K., & Huether, S. (2002). *Pathophysiology: The biologic basis for disease in adults and children* (4th ed.). St. Louis: Mosby.

McConnell, E. (2002). How to converse with a hearing-impaired patient. *Nursing 2002, 32*(8), 20.

Meyer, S., & Megerian, C. (2000). Patients' perceived outcomes after stapedectomy for otosclerosis. *ENT-Ear, Nose & Throat Journal, 79*(11), 846-856.

Moore, A., et al. (2002). Cerumen, hearing, and cognition in the elderly. *Journal of the American Medical Directors Association, 3*(3), 136-139.

Moorhead, S., Johnson, M., & Maas, M. (Eds.). (2004). *Nursing outcomes classification (NOC)* (3rd ed.). St. Louis: Mosby.

National Council on the Aging. (2000). The consequences of untreated hearing loss in older persons. *ORL-Head and Neck Nursing, 18*(1), 12-16.

*National Institute on Deafness and Other Communication Disorders. (1999). What is presbycusis? NIH Publication No. 97-4233. Available at http://www. nidcd.nih.gov/.

Ng, M., & Nipako, J. (2000). Otosclerosis: Causes, surgical and medical treatment. *Hearing Loss, 21*(2), 26-28.

*Nusbaum, N. (1999). Aging and sensory senescence. *Southern Medical Journal, 92*(3), 267-275. Also available at http://www.medscape.com/SMA/SMJ/1999/v92.n03/smj9203.02.nusb/smj9203.02.nusb-01.html.

Nussbaum, R., McInnes, R., & Willard, H. (2001). *Thompson & Thompson: Genetics in medicine* (6th ed.). Philadelphia: W. B. Saunders.

Online Mendelian Inheritance in Man, OMIM (TM). McKusick-Nathans Institute for Genetic Medicine, Johns Hopkins University (Baltimore, MD) and National Center for Biotechnology Information, National Library of Medicine (Bethesda, MD), 2000. Available at http://www.ncbi.nlm.nih.gov/omim/.

Pagana, K., & Pagana, T. (2002). *Mosby's manual of diagnostic and laboratory tests* (2nd ed.). St. Louis: Mosby.

Phillips, M. (2003). Genetics of hearing loss. *MEDSURG* Nursing, 12(6), 386-390, 411.

Pichichero, M. (2000). Acute otitis media: Part I. Improving diagnostic accuracy, *American Family Physician,* 61 (7), 2052-2056.

Ruholl, L. (2003). Tips for teaching the elderly. *RN,* 66(5), 48-52.

*Sanna, M. (1999). *Color atlas of otoscopy: From diagnosis to surgery.* New York: Thieme.

Sheehan, J. (2000). Caring for the deaf: Do you do enough? *RN,* 63(3), 69-72.

Sommer. S., & Sommer, N. (2002). When your patient is hearing impaired. *RN,* 65(12), 28-32.

Summerfield, A.Q., Marshall, D., Barton, G., & Bloor, K. (2002). A cost-utility scenario analysis of bilateral cochlear implantation. *Archives of Otolaryngology-Head and Neck Surgery, 128*(11), 1255-1262.

Wilson, S., & Lopez, R. (2002). What is the best treatment for impacted cerumen? *The Journal of Family Practice,* 51(2), 117.

Woodson, G. (2001). Ear, nose, and throat disorders in primary care. Philadelphia: W. B. Saunders.

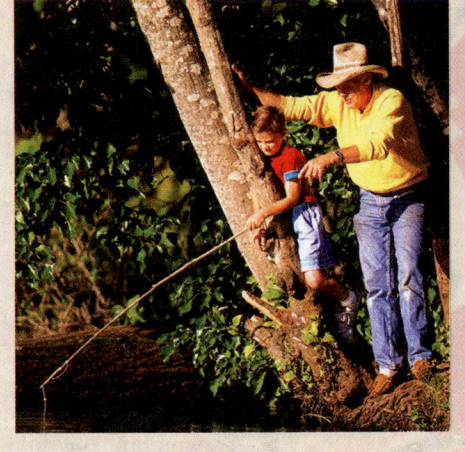

PROBLEMS of MOBILITY

Management of Clients with Problems of the Musculoskeletal System

Assessment of the Musculoskeletal System

CATHY A. MURRAY

LEARNING OUTCOMES

After studying this chapter, you should be able to:

1. Recall the anatomy and physiology of the musculoskeletal system.
2. Explain how physiologic aging changes of the musculoskeletal system affect care of older adults.
3. Conduct a musculoskeletal history using Gordon's Functional Health Patterns.
4. Evaluate important assessment findings in a client with a musculoskeletal health problem.
5. Explain the use of laboratory testing for a client with a musculoskeletal health problem.
6. Identify the use of radiography in diagnosing musculoskeletal health problems.
7. Plan follow-up care for clients undergoing musculoskeletal diagnostic testing.
8. Develop a teaching plan for clients undergoing arthroscopic procedures.

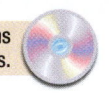

Go to your Student CD-ROM for Review Questions for the NCLEX Examination keyed to these Learning Outcomes.

The musculoskeletal system is the second largest body system; it includes the bones, joints, and skeletal muscles, as well as their supporting structures. Disease, surgery, and trauma often affect one or more parts of this system, yet nurses often overlook assessment of this system. This chapter does not include diagnostic testing related to arthritis or specific tests for osteoporosis. Descriptions of those tests are found in Chapters 24 and 54 under discussions of those diseases.

ANATOMY AND PHYSIOLOGY REVIEW

Skeletal System

The skeletal system consists of 206 bones and multiple joints. The growth and development of these structures occur during childhood and adolescence and are not discussed in this text.

BONES
Types

Bone can be classified in two ways, by shape and by structure. In regard to shape, *long bones,* such as the femur, are cylindrical with rounded ends and often bear weight. *Short bones,* such as the phalanges, are small and bear little or no weight. *Flat bones,* such as the scapula, protect vital organs and often contain blood-forming cells. Bones that have unique shapes are known as *irregular bones.* The carpal bones in the wrist and the small bones in the inner ear are examples of irregular bones. The *sesamoid bone* is the least common type and develops within a tendon; the patella is a typical example.

Structure

The second way bone is classified is by structure or composition. As shown in Figure 53-1, the outer layer of bone, or **cortex,** is composed of dense, compact bone tissue. The inner layer, in the medulla, contains spongy, cancellous tissue. Almost every bone has both tissue types but in varying quantities. The long bone typically has a shaft, or **diaphysis,** and two knoblike ends, or **epiphyses.**

The structural unit of the cortical, compact bone is the haversian system, which is detailed in Figure 53-1. The haversian system is a complex canal network containing microscopic blood vessels, which supply nutrients and oxygen to bone, and lacunae, which are small cavities that house osteocytes (bone cells). The canals run longitudinally within the hard, cortical bone tissue.

The softer, **cancellous** tissue contains large spaces, or trabeculae, which are filled with red and yellow marrow. **Hematopoiesis** (production of blood cells) occurs in the red marrow. The yellow marrow contains fat cells, which can be dislodged and enter the bloodstream to cause fat embolism

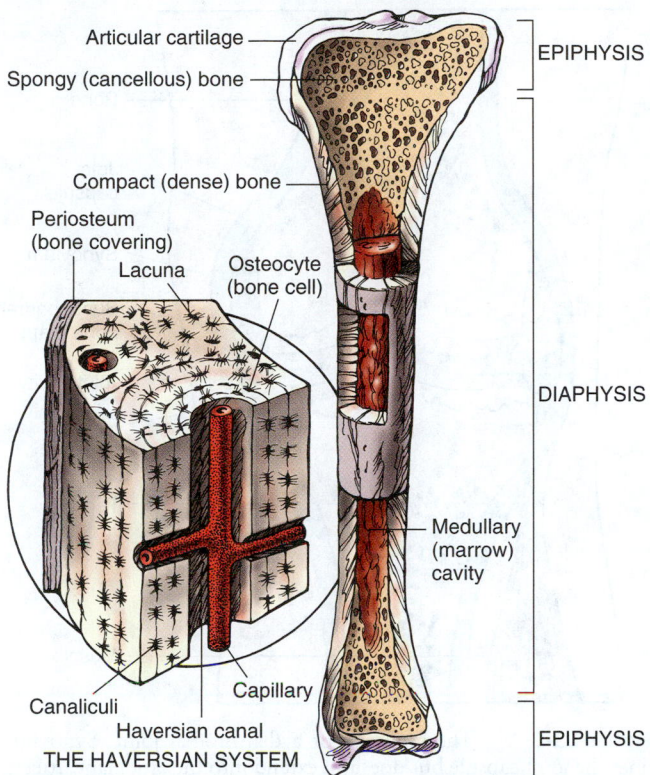

Figure 53-1 ■ The structure of a typical long bone. The cortex, or outer layer, is composed of dense, compact tissue. The microscopic structure of this compact cortical tissue is the haversian system.

syndrome (FES), a life-threatening complication. Volkmann's canals connect bone marrow vessels with the haversian system and periosteum, the outermost covering of the bone. Osteogenic cells, which later differentiate into **osteoblasts** (bone-forming cells) and **osteoclasts** (bone-destroying cells), are found in the deepest layer of the periosteum.

Bone also contains a **matrix** (also called *osteoid*) consisting chiefly of collagen, mucopolysaccharides, and lipids. Deposits of inorganic calcium salts (carbonate and phosphate) in the matrix provide the hardness of bone.

Bone is a very vascular tissue; its estimated total blood flow is between 200 and 400 mL/min. Each bone has a principal nutrient artery, which enters near the middle of the shaft and branches into ascending and descending vessels. These vessels supply the cortex, the marrow, and the haversian system. Sympathetic and afferent (sensory) fibers constitute the sparse nerve supply to bone. Sympathetic nerve fibers control dilation of blood vessels. Afferent nerve fibers transmit pain signals experienced by clients who have primary lesions of the bone.

Function

The skeletal system:
- Provides a framework for the body and allows the body to be weight bearing, or upright
- Supports the surrounding tissues (e.g., muscle and tendons)
- Assists in movement through muscle attachment and joint formation

- Protects vital organs, such as the heart and lungs
- Manufactures blood cells in red bone marrow
- Provides storage for mineral salts (e.g., calcium and phosphorus)

Growth and Metabolism

After puberty, bone reaches its maturity and maximal growth. Bone is a dynamic tissue, however, that undergoes a continuous process of formation and resorption, or destruction, at equal rates until the age of 35 years. In later years, bone resorption accelerates, decreasing bone mass and predisposing clients to injury. (See Chapter 54 for a discussion of the effects of aging on bone metabolism.)

Numerous minerals and hormones, including the following, affect bone growth and metabolism:
- Calcium
- Phosphorus
- Calcitonin
- Vitamin D
- Parathyroid hormone (PTH)
- Growth hormone
- Glucocorticoids
- Estrogens and androgens
- Thyroxine
- Insulin

CALCIUM AND PHOSPHORUS

Bone accounts for about 99% of the calcium in the body and 90% of the phosphorus. The serum concentrations of calcium and phosphorus maintain an inverse relationship; for example, as calcium levels rise, phosphorus levels decrease. When serum levels of calcium and phosphorus are altered, calcitonin and PTH work to maintain equilibrium. If the calcium level of the blood is decreased, the bone, which stores calcium, releases calcium into the vascular system in response to PTH stimulation.

CALCITONIN

Calcitonin is produced by the thyroid gland and *decreases* the serum calcium concentration if it is increased above its normal level. Calcitonin inhibits bone resorption and increases renal excretion of calcium and phosphorus as needed to maintain equilibrium.

VITAMIN D

Vitamin D and its metabolites are produced in the body and transported in the blood to promote the absorption of calcium and phosphorus from the small intestine. They also seem to enhance PTH activity in the release of calcium from the bone. A decrease in the body's vitamin D level can result in osteomalacia in the adult. An external source of vitamin D may be given to clients at risk for or diagnosed with osteomalacia. Vitamin D metabolism and osteomalacia are detailed in Chapter 54.

PARATHYROID HORMONE

When serum calcium levels are lowered, parathyroid hormone (PTH, or parathormone) secretion increases and stimulates bone to promote osteoclastic activity and *release* calcium to the blood. PTH reduces the renal excretion of calcium and facilitates its absorption from the intestine. Conversely, when serum calcium levels increase, PTH secretion diminishes to preserve the bone calcium supply; this is an example of the feedback loop system of the endocrine system.

GROWTH HORMONE

Growth hormone secreted by the anterior lobe of the pituitary gland is responsible for increasing bone length and determining the amount of bone matrix formed before puberty. During childhood, an increased secretion results in gigantism, and a decreased secretion results in dwarfism. In the adult, an increase causes acromegaly, which is characterized by bone and soft-tissue deformities (see Chapter 66).

GLUCOCORTICOIDS

Adrenal glucocorticoids regulate protein metabolism, either increasing or decreasing catabolism to reduce or intensify the organic matrix of bone. They also aid in regulating intestinal calcium and phosphorus absorption.

ESTROGENS AND ANDROGENS

Estrogens stimulate osteoblastic activity and inhibit PTH. When estrogen levels decline at menopause, women are susceptible to low serum calcium levels with subsequent bone loss (osteoporosis). Androgens, such as testosterone, promote anabolism and increase bone mass. External sources of estrogen and testosterone may be prescribed for clients at risk for or diagnosed with osteoporosis.

THYROXINE AND INSULIN

Thyroxine is one of the principal hormones secreted by the thyroid gland. Its primary function is to increase the rate of protein synthesis in all types of tissue, including bone. Insulin works together with growth hormone to build and maintain healthy bone tissue.

JOINTS

A **joint** is a space in which two or more bones come together. This is also referred to as *articulation* of the joint. The primary function of a joint is to provide movement and flexibility in the body.

Types

There are three types of joints in the body:

- Synarthrodial, or completely immovable, joints (e.g., in the cranium)
- Amphiarthrodial, or slightly movable, joints (e.g., in the pelvis)
- Diarthrodial (synovial), or freely movable, joints (e.g., the elbow and knee)

Although any of these joints can be affected by disease or injury, the diarthrodial joints are most commonly involved.

Structure and Function

The **diarthrodial,** or **synovial, joint** is the most common type of joint in the body. Synovial joints are so named because they are the only type lined with synovium, a membrane that secretes synovial fluid for lubrication and shock absorption. As illustrated in Figure 53-2, the synovium lines the internal portion of the joint capsule but does not normally extend onto the surface of the cartilage at the spongy bone ends. Articular cartilage consists of a collagen fiber matrix impregnated with a complex ground substance. Clients with inflammatory types of arthritis often have syn-

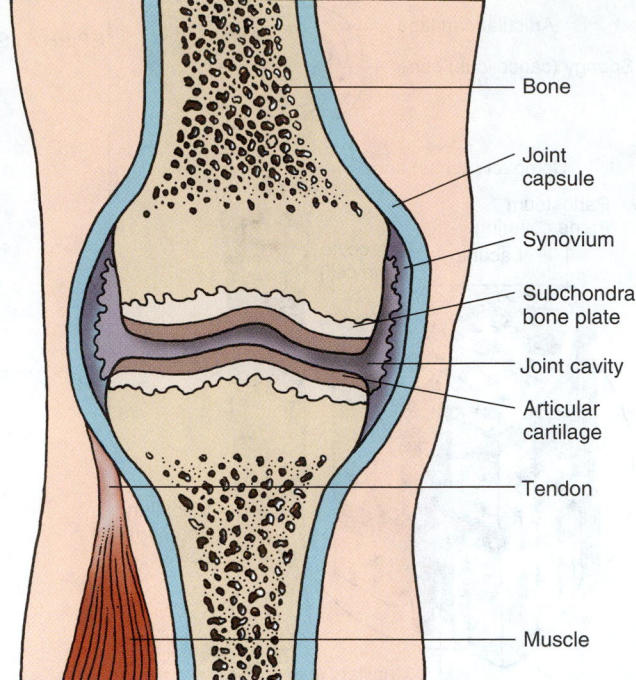

Figure 53-2 ■ The structure of a diarthrodial joint. Synovium lines the joint capsule but does not extend into the articular cartilage.

ovitis (synovial inflammation) and breakdown of the cartilage. **Bursae,** small sacs lined with synovial membrane, are located at joints and bony prominences to prevent friction between bone and structures adjacent to bone. These structures can also become inflamed, causing bursitis.

Synovial joints are subtyped by their anatomic structures. *Ball-and-socket* joints (shoulder, hip) permit movement in any direction. *Hinge* joints (elbow) allow motion in one plane, flexion, and extension. The knee is often classified as a hinge joint, but it rotates slightly, as well as flexes and extends. It is best described as a *condylar* type of synovial joint. The gliding movement of the wrist is characteristic of the *biaxial* joint. *Pivot* joints permit rotation only, as in the radioulnar area.

Muscular System

There are three types of muscle in the body: smooth muscle, cardiac muscle, and skeletal muscle. Smooth, or nonstriated, involuntary muscle is responsible for contractions of organs and blood vessels and is controlled by the autonomic nervous system. Cardiac muscle, or striated, involuntary muscle is also controlled by the autonomic nervous system. The smooth and cardiac muscles are discussed with the body systems to which they belong in the assessment chapters.

Structure

In contrast to smooth and cardiac muscle, skeletal muscle is **striated,** voluntary muscle controlled by the central and peripheral nervous systems. The junction of a peripheral motor nerve and the muscle cells that it supplies is sometimes referred to as a motor end plate. Muscle fibers are held in place by connective tissue in bundles, or fasciculi. The entire mus-

CHART 53-1

NURSING FOCUS on the OLDER ADULT
Changes in the Musculoskeletal System Related to Aging

Physiologic Change	Nursing Interventions	Rationales
Decreased bone density	Teach safety tips to prevent falls. Reinforce need to exercise, especially weight-bearing exercise.	Porous bones are more likely to fracture. Exercise slows bone loss.
Increased bone prominence	Prevent pressure on bone prominences.	There is less soft tissue to prevent skin breakdown.
Kyphotic posture: widened gait, shift in the center of gravity	Teach proper body mechanics; instruct the client to sit in supportive chairs with arms.	Correction of posture problems prevents further deformity; the client should have support for bony structures.
Cartilage degeneration	Provide moist heat, such as a shower or warm, moist compresses.	Moist heat increases blood flow to the area.
Decreased ROM	Assess the client's ability to perform ADLs and mobility.	The client may need assistance with self-care skills.
Muscle atrophy, decreased strength	Teach isometric exercises.	Exercises increase muscle strength.
Slowed movement	Do not rush the client; be patient.	The client may become frustrated if hurried.

ROM, Range of motion; *ADLs*, activities of daily living.

cle is surrounded by dense, fibrous tissue, or fascia, which contains the muscle's blood, lymph, and nerve supply.

Function

The primary function of skeletal muscle is movement of the body and its parts. When bones, joints, and supporting structures are adversely affected by injury or disease, the adjacent muscle tissue is often involved, limiting mobility. During the aging process, muscle fibers decrease in size and number, even in well-conditioned people. Atrophy results when muscles are not regularly exercised, and they deteriorate from disuse.

Supporting Structures

In addition to the articular cartilage of joints, several types of cartilage occur in other areas. *Costal* cartilage connects the sternum to the rib cage. *Hyaline* cartilage is in the septum of the nose, larynx, and trachea. The external ear and epiglottis contain *yellow* cartilage. In all areas, the tissue is flexible and elastic and can withstand enormous tension.

Other important supporting structures that are susceptible to injury include **tendons** (bands of tough, fibrous tissue that attach muscles to bones) and **ligaments,** which attach bones to other bones at joints.

Musculoskeletal Changes Associated with Aging

As one ages, bone density often decreases, causing postural changes and predisposing a person to fractures (osteoporosis). Synovial joint cartilage can become less elastic and compressible as a person ages. As a result of these cartilage changes and continued use of joints, trauma to the joint cartilage can occur. The result is sometimes described as osteoarthritis (OA); however, genetic defects in cartilage may contribute to joint disease. The most common joints affected are the weight-bearing joints of the hip, knee, and cervical and lumbar spine, but joints in the shoulder and upper extremity, feet and hands can be affected. Refer to Chapter 24 for a complete discussion of OA. Muscle tissue

atrophy occurs, but increased activity and exercise can slow the progression of atrophy and restore muscle strength. Collectively, these changes cause decreased coordination, muscle strength loss, gait changes, and predisposition to falls with injury. Chart 53-1 lists the major anatomic and physiologic changes and suggested nursing interventions.

CULTURAL CONSIDERATIONS

The body proportions of African Americans differ from those of white individuals, Asian Americans, and Native Americans/ American Indians. African-American men typically have denser bones than African American women. White women have the least amount of bone density of any group, which makes them more likely to have osteoporosis and fractures (Jarvis, 2004).

Many African Americans and some white individuals have a **lactose intolerance** (inability to convert lactose to glucose and galactose). Milk and dairy products are high in lactose, but are also rich in calcium, a bone-building mineral. Therefore, lactose-intolerant individuals need to obtain their calcium from other food sources, such as dark, green leafy vegetables.

ASSESSMENT TECHNIQUES

History

In the assessment of a client with an actual or potential musculoskeletal problem, a detailed history aids the nurse in identifying diagnoses and subsequent interventions (Chart 53-2).

DEMOGRAPHIC DATA

Young men are at the greatest risk for trauma related to motor vehicle crashes. Older adults are at the greatest risk for falls that result in fractures and soft-tissue injury (see Chapter 5).

FAMILY HISTORY AND GENETIC RISK

Certain disorders have a familial or genetic tendency. Osteoporosis (age-related bone loss), for instance, often occurs in several generations of a family, and bone cancer tends to

Musculoskeletal Assessment
USING GORDON'S FUNCTIONAL HEALTH PATTERNS

Activity-Exercise Pattern
- Do you have sufficient energy for desired/required activities?
- What is your exercise pattern? Type of exercise? Regularity?
- What spare time (leisure) activities do you engage in?
- What is your perceived ability for (code for level according to key below):

Feeding?	Level 0: Full self-care
Bathing?	Level I: Requires use of equipment or
Toileting?	device
Bed mobility?	Level II: Requires assistance or supervi-
Dressing?	sion of another person
Grooming?	Level III: Requires assistance or
General mobility?	supervision of another person and
Cooking?	equipment or device
Home maintenance?	Level IV: Is dependent and does not
Shopping?	participate

Cognitive-Perceptual Pattern
- Do you experience any discomfort?
- Do you have pain? If so, how do you manage it?
- What is the easiest way for you to learn things?
- Do you have any difficulty learning?

Based on Gordon, M. (2002). *Manual of nursing diagnosis* (10th ed.). St. Louis: Mosby.

be genetically linked. The risk for osteoarthritis may also be strongly linked to genetic factors. Chapters 24 and 54 provide a more complete description of musculoskeletal disease processes that have strong genetic links.

PERSONAL HISTORY

Accidents, illnesses, lifestyle and medications may relate to a client's current problem. When taking a personal health history, question the client about current level of physical activity, all traumatic injuries, participation in sports and sports injuries, regardless of the date of occurrence. An injury to the lumbar spine 30 years previously may contribute to a client's current complaint of low back pain. A motor vehicle accident or sports injury can be the cause of osteoarthritis years after the event.

Previous or concurrent diseases may affect musculoskeletal status. For example, a client with diabetes who is treated for a foot ulcer is at high risk for acute or chronic osteomyelitis (bone infection). In addition, diabetes slows the healing process. It is also important to determine a history of previous hospitalizations and illnesses or complications.

Ask about previous and current use of medications. Some drugs, such as steroids, can affect calcium metabolism and promote bone loss. Other drugs may be taken to relieve musculoskeletal pain. Inquire about herbal, vitamin and mineral supplements, or biologic compounds that may be used for arthritis and other musculoskeletal problems, such as glucosamine and chondroitin. Complementary and alternative therapies are commonly employed by clients with various types of arthritis and arthralgias (joint aching) (see Chapter 24).

DIET HISTORY

An evaluation of the client's diet history will help determine any risks of inadequate nutrition. For example, most people, especially women, do not consume adequate amounts of calcium. Asking a client for a recall of a typical day of food intake helps identify deficiencies and excesses in the diet. Lactose intolerance is a common problem and can affect ad-

equate calcium intake. People who cannot afford to buy food are especially at risk for undernutrition.

Inadequate protein or insufficient vitamin C or D in the diet inhibits healing of bone and tissue. Obesity places excess stress and strain on bones and joints, with resultant fractures and trauma to joint cartilage. In addition, obesity inhibits mobility in clients with musculoskeletal problems, which predisposes them to complications such as respiratory and circulatory problems.

SOCIOECONOMIC STATUS

When assessing a client with a possible musculoskeletal alteration, inquire about lifestyle. A person's occupation can cause or contribute to an injury. For instance, fractures are not uncommon in clients whose jobs require manual labor, such as housekeepers and mechanics. Certain occupations, such as computer-related jobs, may predispose a person to carpal tunnel syndrome (entrapment of the median nerve in the wrist). Construction workers and health care workers may experience back injury from prolonged standing and excessive lifting. Amateur and professional athletes often experience acute musculoskeletal injuries, such as joint dislocations and fractures, or chronic disorders, such as joint cartilage trauma, which can lead to osteoarthritis.

Socioeconomic status may be related to the client's occupation and therefore affect the likelihood of musculoskeletal problems. For example, an executive working in an office is less likely to sustain a musculoskeletal injury than is a painter or roofer engaged in manual labor and activities such as climbing ladders.

CURRENT HEALTH PROBLEMS

Collect data pertinent to the client's presenting complaint as follows:
- Date and time of onset
- Factors that cause or exacerbate (worsen) the problem
- Course of the problem (e.g., intermittent or continuous)
- Clinical manifestations (as expressed by the client) and the pattern of their occurrence
- Measures that improve clinical manifestations (e.g., heat)

The most common complaint of people with musculoskeletal problems is pain. The pain may be acute or chronic, depending on its onset and duration. Use the PQRST model or other tool to elicit a complete assessment of the client's pain:

P Provoking incident? (Was there a certain incident or event that precipitated the pain or caused an exacerbation of the pain?)

Q Quality of pain? (What does the pain feel like in descriptive terms? For example, is it burning, throbbing, stabbing?)

R Region, radiation, and relief? (Exactly where is the pain located? Does the pain travel or radiate? Does anything help relieve the pain?)

S Severity of the pain? (How severe is the pain? The client may use a pain scale [see Chapter 7] or describe how the pain has interfered with his or her ability to function.)

T Time? (How long does the pain last? When does it occur? Is it worse at night or during the day? If the pain awakens a person at night, the source of the pain is most likely inflammatory, not degenerative.)

With any pain assessment, it is always best if the client describes the pain in his or her own words and points to its location, if possible.

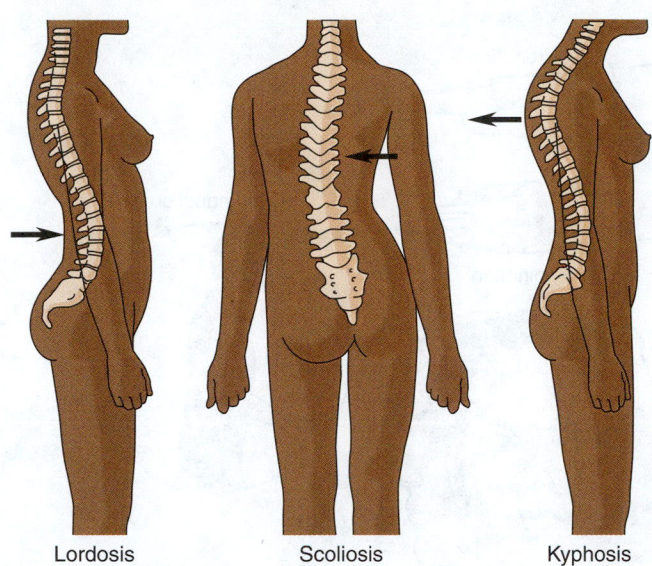

Lordosis   Scoliosis   Kyphosis

Figure 53-3 ■ Common spinal deformities.

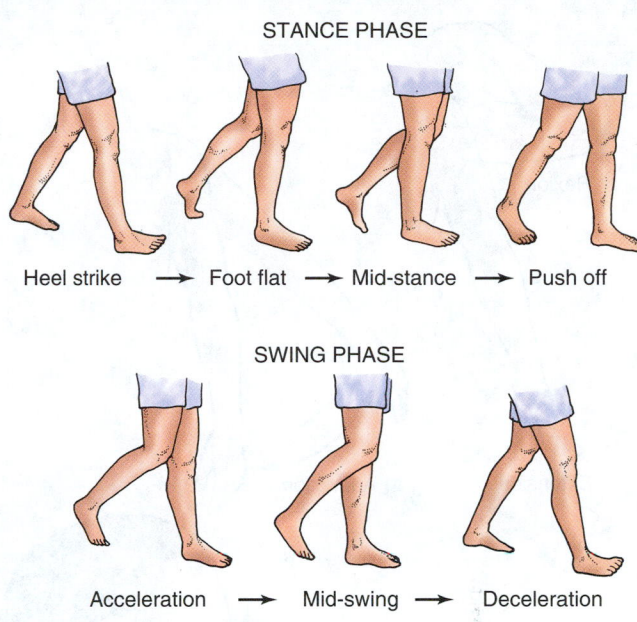

STANCE PHASE

Heel strike → Foot flat → Mid-stance → Push off

SWING PHASE

Acceleration → Mid-swing → Deceleration

Figure 53-4 ■ The phases of gait.

Physical Assessment

Although bones, joints, and muscles are usually assessed simultaneously in a head-to-toe approach, each subsystem is described separately for emphasis and understanding. For physical assessment of the musculoskeletal system, the nurse incorporates inspection, palpation, range of motion (ROM), which may be active (AROM) or passive (PROM), and special techniques for specific problems. A general assessment is described in this chapter. More specific assessment techniques are discussed in the interventions chapters that follow for each musculoskeletal problem.

ASSESSMENT OF THE SKELETAL SYSTEM
General Inspection

Observe the client's posture, gait, and general mobility for gross deformities and impairment. Note unusual findings and collaborate with the physical or occupational therapist for an in-depth physical assessment.

POSTURE

Posture includes the person's body build and alignment when standing and walking. Assess the curvature of the spine and the length, shape, and symmetry of extremities. Figure 53-3 illustrates some common spinal deformities. Muscle mass is also inspected for size and symmetry.

GAIT

Most clients with musculoskeletal problems eventually have a problem with gait. The two phases of normal, automatic gait are the stance phase and the swing phase (Figure 53-4).

The nurse or therapist evaluates the client's balance, steadiness, and ease and length of stride; any limp or other asymmetric leg movement or deformity is noted. An abnormality in the stance phase of gait is called an **antalgic** gait. When part of one leg is painful, the person shortens the stance phase on the affected side. An abnormality in the swing phase is called a **lurch**. This abnormal gait occurs

Video Clip: Gait

when the muscles in the buttocks and/or legs are too weak to allow the person to change weight from one foot to the other. In this case, the shoulders are moved either side-to-side or front-to-back for help in shifting the weight from one leg to the other. Some clients, such as those with chronic hip pain and muscle atrophy from arthritic disorders, have a combination of an antalgic gait and lurch.

MOBILITY

In collaboration with the physical or occupational therapist, monitor the client's need for or use of ambulatory devices, such as canes and walkers, during transfer from bed to chair and while walking and climbing stairs. Assess mobility by asking the client to perform activities of daily living (ADLs) such as dressing and bathing. Pain and deformity may limit physical mobility and function. A complete discussion of functional assessment is found in Chapter 10.

After performing a functional assessment, assess major bones, joints, and muscles by inspection, palpation, and determination of ROM. Pay special attention to areas that are affected or may be affected, according to the client's history or current complaint.

A **goniometer** is a tool that may be used by physical therapists or nurses to provide an exact measurement of ROM. Active range of motion (AROM) can be evaluated by asking the client to move each joint through the ROM himself or herself. If a client is unable to actively move a joint through range of motion, ask the client to relax the muscles in the extremity. Hold the part with one hand above and one hand below the joint to be evaluated and allow passive range of motion to evaluate joint mobility. Movements shown in Figure 53-5 may be used to evaluate active and passive ROM. Circumduction is a movement that can also be evaluated in the shoulder by having the client move the arm in circles from the shoulder joint. As long as the client can function to meet personal needs, a limitation in ROM may not be significant. For each anatomic location, the skin is observed for color, elasticity, and lesions that may relate to musculoskeletal dysfunction. This also includes inspection of skin over bony prominences.

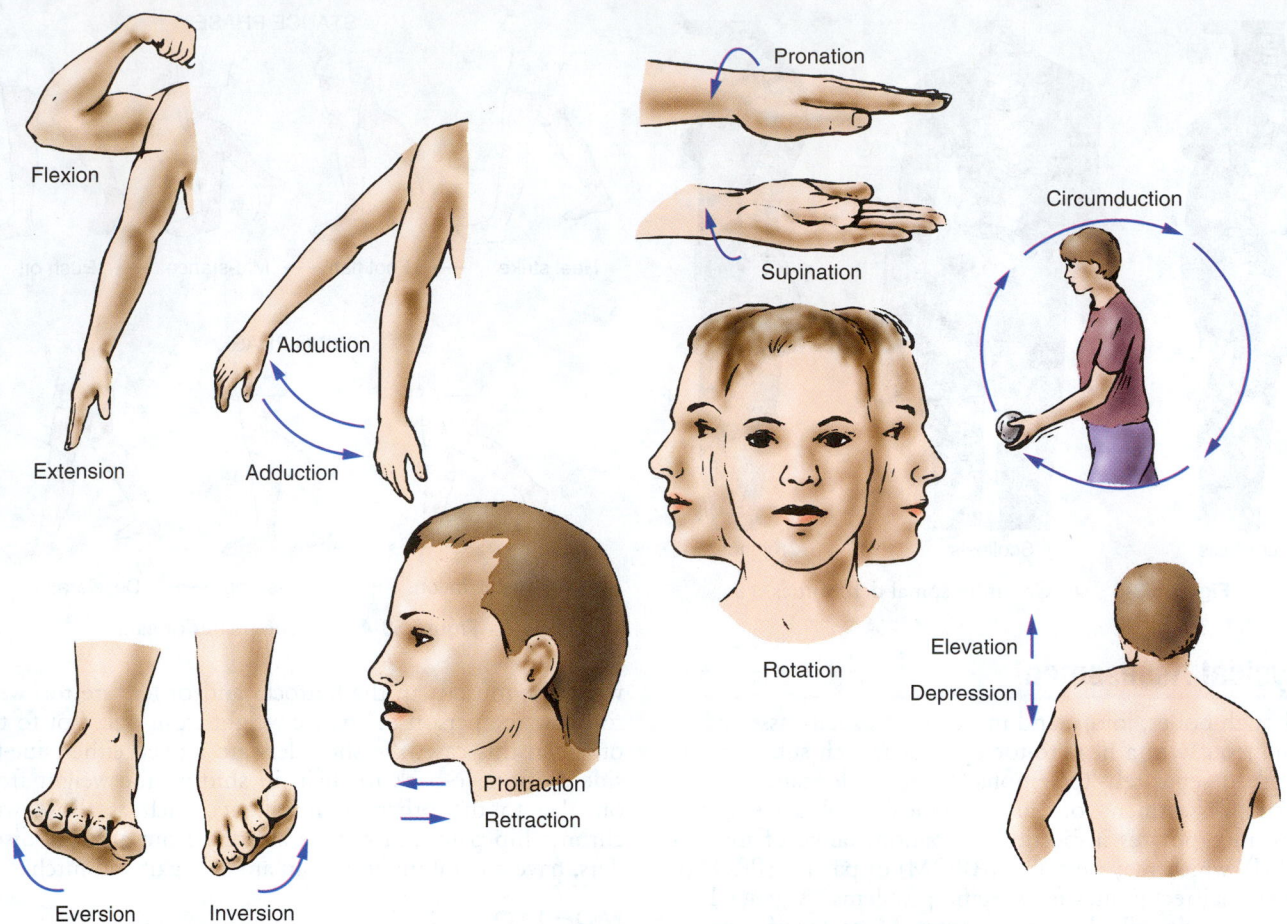

Figure 53-5 ■ Movements of the skeletal muscles. (Modified from Jarvis, C. [2000]. *Physical examination and health assessment* [3rd ed.]. Philadelphia: W. B. Saunders.)

Assessment of the Head and Neck

Inspect and palpate the skull for shape, symmetry, tenderness, and masses. The temporomandibular joints (TMJs) are best evaluated by palpation. Ask the client to open his or her mouth while palpating the TMJs. Common abnormal findings are tenderness or pain, **crepitus** (a grating sound), and a spongy swelling caused by excess synovium and fluid.

Then inspect and palpate each vertebra of the spine in the neck. Clinical findings may include malalignment; tenderness; or inability to flex, extend, and rotate the neck as expected.

Assessment of the Spine

The thoracic spine, lumbar spine, and sacral spine are evaluated in the same manner as the neck. Spinal alignment problems are common (see Figure 53-3). Place both hands over the lumbosacral area and apply pressure with the thumbs along the spine to elicit tenderness. Many clients do not complain of discomfort until the area is palpated. **Lordosis** is a common finding in pregnancy and in abdominal obesity. During screening for **scoliosis**, ask the client to flex forward from the hips and inspect for a lateral curve in the spine.

Assessment of the Upper Extremities

Assess both extremities at the same time. For example, both shoulders are inspected and palpated for size, swelling, deformity, malalignment, tenderness or pain, and mobility. A shoulder injury may prevent the client from combing his or her hair with the affected arm, but severe arthritis may inhibit movement in both arms. Assess the elbows and wrists in a similar way.

Because the hand has multiple joints in a single digit, assessment of hand function is perhaps the most critical part of the examination. Inspect and palpate the metacarpophalangeal (MCP), proximal interphalangeal (PIP), and distal interphalangeal (DIP) joints. The same digits are compared on the right and left hands (Figure 53-6). Determine the range of motion (ROM) for each joint by observing active movement. If movement is not possible, evaluate passive motion. For a quick and easy assessment of ROM, the client is asked to make a fist and then appose each finger to the thumb. If he or she can perform these maneuvers, ROM of the hand is not seriously restricted.

Assessment of the Lower Extremities

Evaluation of the hip joint relies primarily on determination of its degree of mobility, because the joint is deep and difficult to inspect or palpate. The client with hip pain usually experiences pain in the *groin* area, or the pain may radiate to the knee. The knee is readily accessible for nursing assessment, particularly when the client is sitting and the knee is flexed. Fluid accumulation, or **effusion**, is easily detected in the knee joint; limitations in movement with accompanying pain are common findings. The knees may be malaligned, as

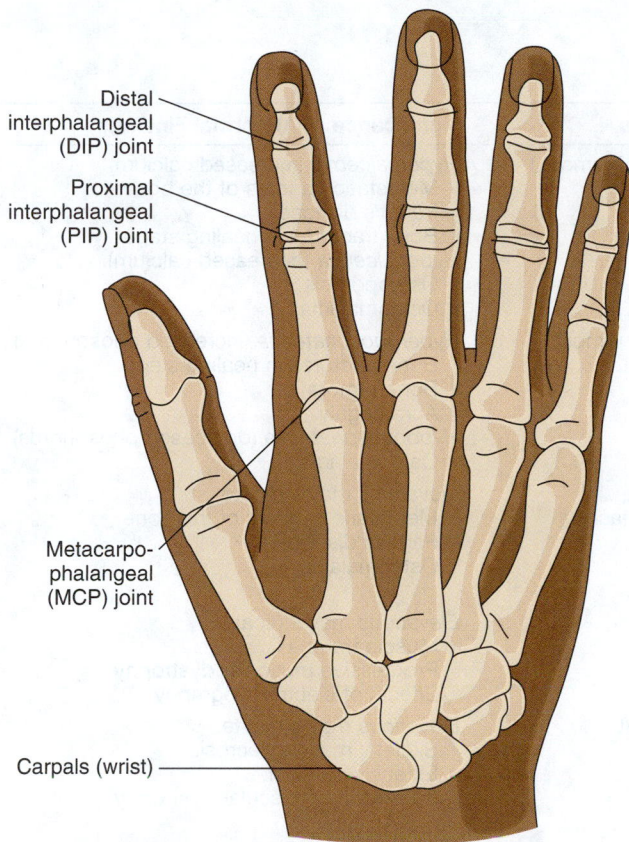

Figure 53-6 ■ The small joints of the hand.

- Distal interphalangeal (DIP) joint
- Proximal interphalangeal (PIP) joint
- Metacarpo-phalangeal (MCP) joint
- Carpals (wrist)

TABLE 53-1	Lovett's Scale for Grading Muscle Strength
Rating	**Description**
5	Normal: ROM unimpaired against gravity with full resistance
4	Good: can complete ROM against gravity with some resistance
3	Fair: can complete ROM against gravity
2	Poor: can complete ROM with gravity eliminated
1	Trace: no joint motion and slight evidence of music contractility
0	Zero: no evidence of muscle contractility

ROM, Range of motion.

squeeze a sphygmomanometer (blood pressure cuff) bulb to record the level of pressure achieved. This method provides a precise measurement that can be used to observe improvement or deterioration of muscle ability. In another method, apply resistance by holding the extremity and asking the client to move against resistance. For example, place your hands on the client's upper arms and ask the client to try to raise the arms. Although movement against resistance is not easily quantified, several scales are available for grading the client's strength. A commonly used scale is delineated in Table 53-1.

Psychosocial Assessment

The data from the history and physical examination provide clues for the nurse in anticipating psychosocial problems. For instance, the client with multiple fractures who requires extensive immobilization and therapy is at high risk for sensory deprivation. Prolonged absence from employment or permanent disability may cause the client to lose his or her job or occupation. Further stress may be experienced if chronic pain ensues and he or she cannot cope with numerous stressors simultaneously. Deformities resulting from musculoskeletal disease or injury can affect a person's body image and self-concept. Assessment of a client's support systems and coping mechanisms from previous stressful situations will assist in planning for possible stressors that may occur with a current injury or illness.

Diagnostic Assessment

LABORATORY TESTS

Chart 53-3 lists the common laboratory tests used in assessing clients with musculoskeletal disorders. There is no special client preparation or follow-up care for any of these tests. Teach the client the purpose of the test and the procedure that can be expected. Additional tests performed for clients with connective tissue diseases, such as rheumatoid arthritis, are described in Chapter 24.

Serum Calcium and Phosphorus

The concentrations of calcium and phosphorus, or phosphate (inorganic phosphorus), have an inverse relationship. In a healthy state, when the calcium level decreases, the phosphorus level increases, and vice versa. Disorders of bone and the parathyroid gland are often reflected in an alteration of the serum calcium or phosphorus level.

in **genu valgum** ("knock-knee") or **genu varum** ("bow-legged") deformities.

The ankles and feet are often neglected in the physical examination; however, they contain multiple bones and joints that can be affected by disease and injury. Observe and palpate each joint and test for ROM.

Neurovascular Assessment

While completing a physical assessment of the musculoskeletal system, it is important to include assessment of peripheral vascular and peripheral nerve integrity. As with other physical assessment, always compare one extremity to the other, beginning with the injured side. Neurovascular assessment includes inspection of skin color, temperature, and capillary refill distal to an injury or cast. Palpation of pulses in the extremities below level of injury and assessment of sensation, movement, and pain in the injured part give a complete neurovascular assessment. If pulses are not palpable, a Doppler should be used to evaluate pulses in the extremities. See Chart 55-3 for more detail of neurovascular assessment.

ASSESSMENT OF THE MUSCULAR SYSTEM

During the skeletal assessment, evaluate the size, shape, tone, and strength of major skeletal muscles. The circumference of each muscle may be measured and compared symmetrically for an estimation of muscle mass.

In addition to inspecting and palpating the skeletal muscles, ask the client to demonstrate muscle strength. For instance, to determine grip strength, ask the client to

▶ **Video Clips: Muscular Development and Strength**

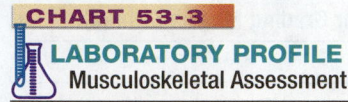

CHART 53-3

LABORATORY PROFILE
Musculoskeletal Assessment

Test	Normal Range for Adults	Significance of Abnormal Findings
Serum calcium	9.0-10.5 mg/dL (2.25-2.75 mmol/L) *Older adults:* decreased	*Hypercalcemia* (increased calcium) ■ Metastatic cancers of the bone ■ Paget's disease ■ Bone fractures in healing stage *Hypocalcemia* (decreased calcium) ■ Osteoporosis ■ Osteomalacia
Serum phosphorus	3.0-4.5 mg/dL (0.97-1.45 mmol/L) *Older adults:* decreased	*Hyperphosphatemia* (increased phosphorus) ■ Bone fractures in healing stage ■ Bone tumors ■ Acromegaly *Hypophosphatemia* (decreased phosphorus) ■ Osteomalacia
Alkaline phosphatase (ALP)	30-120 units/L *Older adults:* slightly increased	*Elevations* may indicate: ■ Metastatic cancers of the bone ■ Paget's disease ■ Osteomalacia
Serum muscle enzymes Creatine kinase (CK)	Total CK: *Men:* 55-170 units/L *Women:* 30-135 units/L	*Elevations* may indicate: ■ Muscle trauma ■ Progressive muscular dystrophy ■ Effects of electromyography
Lactate dehydrogenase (LDH)	Total LDH: 100-190 units/L LDH_1: 17%-27% LDH_2: 27%-37% LDH_3: 18%-25% LDH_4: 3%-8% LDH_5: 0% to 5%	*Elevations* may indicate: ■ Skeletal muscle necrosis ■ Extensive cancer ■ Progressive muscular dystrophy
Aspartate aminotransferase (AST)	0-35 units/L *Older adults:* increased	*Elevations* may indicate: ■ Skeletal muscle trauma ■ Progressive muscular dystrophy
Aldolase (ALD)	3.0-8.2 units/dL	*Elevations* may indicate: ■ Polymyositis and dermatomyositis ■ Muscular dystrophy

Alkaline Phosphatase

Alkaline phosphatase (ALP) is an enzyme normally present in blood. The concentration of ALP increases with bone or liver damage. In metabolic bone disease and bone cancer, the enzyme concentration rises in proportion to the osteoblastic activity, which indicates bone formation. The level of ALP is normally slightly increased in older adults.

Serum Muscle Enzymes

The major muscle enzymes affected in skeletal muscle disease or injuries are as follows:

- Creatine kinase (CK-MM)
- Aspartate aminotransferase (AST)
- Aldolase (ALD)
- Lactic dehydrogenase (LDH)

As a result of damage, the muscle tissue releases additional amounts of these enzymes, which increases serum levels.

The serum CK level begins to rise 2 to 4 hours after muscle injury and is elevated early in muscle disease, such as muscular dystrophy. The CK molecule has two subunits: M (muscle) and B (brain). Three isoenzymes have been identified. Skeletal muscle CK (CK-MM, or CK_3) is the only isoenzyme that rises in concentration with damage to skeletal muscle.

AST is moderately elevated (three to five times normal) in certain muscle diseases, such as muscular dystrophy and der-matomyositis. The levels of the isoenzymes aldolase A (ALD-A) and LDH_5 also increase in clients with these disorders.

RADIOGRAPHIC EXAMINATIONS
Standard Radiography

The skeleton is readily visible on standard x-rays. Anteroposterior and lateral projections are the initial screening views. Other approaches, such as oblique or stress views, depend on the part of the skeleton to be evaluated and the necessity of the x-ray.

Observations of bone density, alignment, swelling, and intactness are made. The conditions of joints can be determined, including the size of the joint space, the smoothness of articular cartilage, and synovial swelling. Soft-tissue involvement may be evident but not clearly differentiated.

Inform the client that the x-ray table is hard and cold and instruct him or her to remain still during the filming process.

Tomography and Xeroradiography

Whereas standard x-rays superimpose one structure on another, **tomography** produces planes, or slices, for focus and blurs the images of other structures. This procedure is helpful in detailing the musculoskeletal system, because the many close structures make visualization difficult.

Xeroradiography highlights the contrast between structures. Margins and edges can be clearly seen (edge enhancement). Disadvantages of xeroradiography are the higher radiation dose to the client and inability of xeroradiography to determine tissue densities.

Myelography

Myelography involves the injection of contrast medium, or dye, into the subarachnoid space of the spine, usually by spinal puncture. The vertebral column, intervertebral disks, spinal nerve roots, and blood vessels can be visualized. Although this test is still performed, it is far less popular; computed tomography (CT) and magnetic resonance imaging (MRI) have often replaced such invasive, and potentially painful, diagnostic techniques. The post-test care is similar to that for lumbar puncture, except that the client is usually placed in a sitting position to prevent the contrast medium from getting into the brain. (See Chapter 44.)

Arthrography

An **arthrogram** is an x-ray study of a joint after contrast medium (air or solution) has been injected to enhance its visualization. Double-contrast arthrography, which uses both air and contrast, may be performed when a traumatic injury is suspected. The physician can often determine bone chips, torn ligaments, or other loose bodies within the joint.

The most common joints studied are the knee and the shoulder. The client is questioned about allergy to contrast media. Most joints are now studies by magnetic resonance imaging.

Computed Tomography

Computed tomography (CT) has gained wide acceptance for the detection of musculoskeletal problems, particularly those of the vertebral column. The scanned images can be used to create additional images from other angles or to create three-dimensional images, and therefore view complex structures from any position. CT scans may be requested with intravenous (IV) contrast if tumor or postsurgical changes are suspected. The nurse or radiology technologist should ask the client about iodine-based contrast allergies. The current class of CT scans takes less than 20 minutes per body part. Because scanners are faster, claustrophobia (fear of small spaces) is rarely an issue.

❓ Critical Thinking Challenge

An older adult comes to the oncology clinic for follow-up of her treatment for breast cancer. She has been experiencing severe lower back pain for the past 2 weeks. The physician suspects metastatic cancer to her bone.

1. What assessment should you perform at this time? Consider a complete assessment, including interview, physical assessment, and psychosocial assessment.
2. For the following laboratory values, what changes might you expect in this client and why?
   Alkaline phosphatase
   Calcium
   Phosphorus
3. What other diagnostic assessment would you anticipate the physician to request?

evolve For suggested answer guidelines, go to http://evolve.elsevier.com/Iggy/.

OTHER DIAGNOSTIC TESTS

Bone and Muscle Biopsy

In a **bone biopsy**, the physician extracts a specimen of bone for microscopic examination. This invasive test may confirm the presence of infection or neoplasm, but it is not commonly done today. One of two techniques may be used to retrieve the specimen: needle (closed) biopsy or incisional (open) biopsy.

Muscle biopsy is done for the diagnosis of atrophy (as in muscular dystrophy) and inflammation (as in polymyositis). The procedure and care for clients undergoing muscle biopsy are the same as those for clients undergoing bone biopsy.

Electromyography

Electromyography (EMG) is usually accompanied by nerve conduction studies for determining the electrical potential generated in an individual muscle. EMG helps in the diagnosis of neuromuscular, lower motor neuron, and peripheral nerve disorders.

CLIENT PREPARATION. Inform the client that EMG may cause temporary discomfort, especially when the client is subjected to episodes of electrical current. For selected clients, mild sedation is prescribed. The physician may also prescribe a temporary discontinuation of skeletal muscle relaxants several days before the procedure to prevent medication from having effects on the test results.

PROCEDURE. The test may be performed at the bedside or in an EMG laboratory. When both EMG and nerve conduction studies are done, nerve conduction is usually tested first. Flat electrodes are placed along the nerve to be evaluated, and low electrical currents are passed through the electrodes to the nerve and muscle innervated. If nerve conduction is accomplished, the muscle contracts.

For testing muscle potential, multiple needle electrodes varying from $\frac{1}{2}$ to 3 inches (1.3 to 7.5 cm) are inserted. The client may be asked to perform activities for measurement of muscle potential during minimal and maximal contraction. The degree of nerve and muscle activity is recorded on an oscilloscope, which provides a graphic readout for later interpretation.

FOLLOW-UP CARE. A few medical complications are associated with EMG. The nurse provides comfort measures and inspects the needle sites for hematoma formation. The application of ice can prevent this complication. The client may also complain of increased pain and anxiety after the test.

Arthroscopy

The **arthroscopy** may be used as a diagnostic test or a surgical procedure. An arthroscope is a fiberoptic tube inserted into a joint for direct visualization; the knee and shoulder are most commonly evaluated. In addition, synovial biopsy and surgical procedures to repair traumatic injury can be accomplished through the arthroscope.

CLIENT PREPARATION. Because the knee is most commonly "scoped," the care described for the client undergoing arthroscopy relates to that joint. Arthroscopy is performed on an ambulatory basis or as same-day surgery. Clients who cannot flex their knees at least 40 degrees or who have infected knees are not candidates for the procedure. The client must be able to flex the knee. Joint infection may worsen from the mechanical trauma of arthroscope insertion.

If the procedure is surgical, the client may have a physical therapy consultation before arthroscopy to learn the leg exercises that are necessary after the test. Straight-leg raises (SLRs) and quadriceps setting exercises (isometrics with the leg extended) are practiced in sets of 10 each. Range-of-motion (ROM) exercises are also taught but may not be allowed immediately after arthroscopic surgery. The nurse in the surgeon's office or at the surgical center can teach these exercises or reinforce the information provided by the physical therapist. The nurse also explains the procedure and post-test care.

PROCEDURE. The client is usually given local, light general, or epidural anesthesia, depending on the purpose of the procedure. In some settings, a large pneumatic tourniquet is used around the thigh to minimize bleeding during the procedure. Medications promoting vasoconstriction for control of bleeding may be used alone or in conjunction with the tourniquet.

The knee is flexed to at least 40 degrees, and the knee is irrigated. As shown in Figure 53-7, the arthroscope is inserted through a small incision less than $\frac{1}{4}$ inch (0.6 cm) long. Multiple incisions may be required to allow inspection at a variety of angles. After the procedure, a dressing may be applied, depending on the amount of manipulation during the test or surgery.

FOLLOW-UP CARE. Evaluate the neurovascular status of the client's affected limb frequently, in accordance with the nursing standard of care. Monitor distal pulses, warmth, color, capillary refill, pain, movement, and sensation of the affected extremity.

Encourage the client to perform exercises as taught before the examination, if appropriate. For the mild discomfort experienced after the diagnostic arthroscopy, the physician prescribes a mild analgesic, such as acetaminophen (Tylenol, Ace-Tabs❋). If postoperative, the client has short-term activity restrictions, depending on the musculoskeletal problem. Ice is often used for 24 hours, and the extremity should be elevated for 24 to 48 hours. When arthroscopic surgery is performed, the health care provider usually prescribes an opioid-analgesic combination, such as oxycodone and acetaminophen (Percocet, Tylox).

Although complications are not common, monitor and teach the client to observe for the following:

- Swelling
- Hypothermia (decreased body temperature) resulting from the use of the tourniquet during the procedure
- Increased joint pain attributable to mechanical injury
- Thrombophlebitis
- Infection

Severe joint or limb pain after discharge may indicate a possible complication and warrants that the client contacts the physician immediately. The health care provider may see the client about 1 week after the test to check for complications.

Bone Scan

The **bone scan** is a radionuclide test in which radioactive material is injected for visualization of the entire skeleton. It is used primarily to detect tumors, arthritis, osteomyelitis, osteoporosis, vertebral compression fractures, and unexplained bone pain. Bone scans are used less commonly today as magnetic resonance imaging (MRI) becomes more available. However, it is very useful for detecting hairline fractures in clients with unexplained bone pain and diffuse metastatic bone disease.

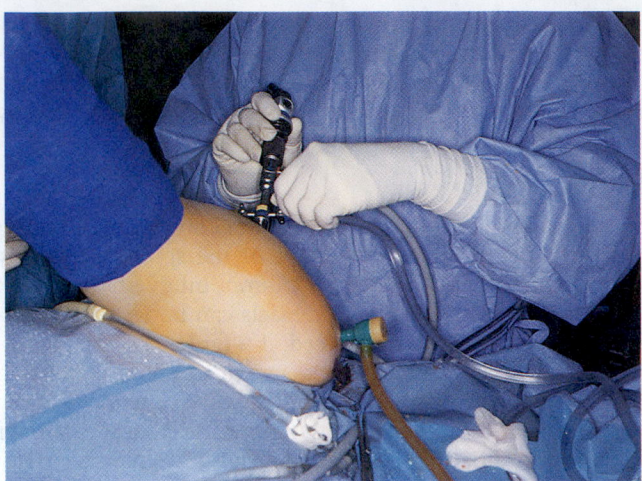

Figure 53-7 ■ An arthroscope is used in the diagnosis of pathologic changes in the joints. This client is undergoing arthroscopy of the shoulder.

Gallium/Thallium Scans

The **gallium** or **thallium scan** is similar to the bone scan but is more specific and sensitive in detecting bone problems. Gallium citrate (^{67}Ga) is the radioisotope most commonly used. This substance also migrates to brain, liver, and breast tissue and therefore is used in examination of these structures when disease is suspected.

For clients with osteosarcoma, thallium (^{201}Tl) is better than gallium or technetium for diagnosing the extent of the disease. Thallium has traditionally been used for the diagnosis of myocardial infarctions, but can be used for additional evaluation of cancers of the bone.

CLIENT PREPARATION. Because bone takes up gallium slowly, the nuclear medicine physician or technician administers the isotope 1 to 2 days before scanning. Other tests that require contrast media or other isotopes cannot be given during this time.

Instruct the client that the radioactive material poses no threat because it readily deteriorates in the body. Because gallium is excreted through the intestinal tract, it tends to collect in feces before the scanning procedure.

PROCEDURE. Depending on the tissue to be examined, the client is taken to the nuclear medicine department 1 to 2 days after injection. The procedure takes 30 to 60 minutes, during which time the client must lie still for accurate test results to be achieved. Mild sedation may be necessary to facilitate relaxation and cooperation during the procedure for confused older clients or those in severe pain.

FOLLOW-UP CARE. No special care is required after the test. The radioisotope is excreted in stool and urine, but no precautions are taken in handling the excreta. Encourage the client to push fluids to facilitate urinary excretion.

Magnetic Resonance Imaging

Magnetic resonance imaging (MRI), with or without the use of contrast media, can be used to diagnose musculoskeletal disorders. It is more accurate than computed tomography (CT) and myelography for many spinal and knee problems. MRI is most appropriate for joints, soft tissue, and bony tumors that involve soft tissue. CT is still the test of choice for injuries or pathology that involve only bone.

CHART 53-4

BEST PRACTICE for
The Client Preparing for Magnetic Resonance Imaging

- Is the client pregnant?
- Does the client have ferromagnetic fragments or implants, such as an older style aneurysm clip?
- Does the client have a pacemaker or electronic implant?
- Can the client lie still in the supine position for 45 to 60 minutes (may require sedation)?
- Does the client need life support equipment available?
- Can the client communicate clearly and understand verbal communication?

The image is produced through the interaction of magnetic fields, radio waves, and atomic nuclei showing hydrogen density. Simply put, the radio waves "bounce" off the body tissues being examined. Because each tissue has its own density, the computer image clearly distinguishes normal and abnormal tissues. For some tissues, the cross-sectional image is better than that produced by radiography or CT. The lack of hydrogen ions in cortical bone makes it easily distinguishable from soft tissues. The test is particularly useful in identifying problems with muscles, tendons, and ligaments.

Ensure that the client removes all metal objects and checks for clothing zippers and metal fasteners. Although joint implants made of titanium or stainless steel are safe, pacemakers and surgical clips are not. Chart 53-4 lists questions that the nurse or technician should consider in preparing the client for MRI. Open MRIs prevent the claustrophobia that occurs with the older, encased machines.

Gadolinium-DTPA (diethylenetriamine-pentaacetic acid) is the contrast agent approved for MRI. It is most commonly used to diagnose degenerative vertebral disease and recurrent disk herniation—sometimes referred to as the failed back surgery syndrome (Patel & Lauerman, 1997).

Ultrasonography

Sound waves produce an image of the tissue in ultrasonography. An ultrasound procedure may be used to visualize the following:

- Soft-tissue disorders, such as masses and fluid accumulation
- Traumatic joint injuries
- Osteomyelitis
- Surgical hardware placement

A jelly-like substance applied to the skin over the site to be examined promotes the movement of a metal probe. No special preparation or post-test care is necessary. A quantitative ultrasound (QUS) may be done for determining fractures or bone density.

Critical Thinking Challenge

A young male client complains of severe left knee pain following a ski trip last weekend. The orthopedic surgeon suspects damage to the meniscus and schedules the client for an arthroscopy.

1. As his office nurse, what health teaching will you need to provide to prepare the client for this procedure?
2. What immediate post-test care will the client require?
3. What discharge instructions will the postanesthesia care unit (PACU) nurse need to review?

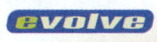 For suggested answer guidelines, go to http://evolve.elsevier.com/Iggy/.

GET READY for the NCLEX Examination!

KEY POINTS

Safe Effective Care Environment

- Be aware that older adults are at high risk for falls due to decreased bone density.
- Ask the client about allergy to iodine-based contrast media prior to diagnostic testing, such as computerized tomography (CT).
- Monitor the client for bleeding following an open bone biopsy.
- Assess the client to ensure that he or she is an appropriate candidate for magnetic resonance imaging; use the guidelines in Chart 53-4.

Health Promotion and Maintenance

- Teach clients to eat a diet sufficient in vitamin D, calcium, and protein to promote bone healing.
- Teach the client that mild discomfort can be expected during electromyography, a test to assess the electrical potential of muscles and their innervation.
- Instruct the client to report swelling, infection, and increased pain following an arthroscopy.

Psychosocial Integrity

- Assess the client's support systems and coping mechanisms when musculoskeletal trauma or disease affects his or her body image.
- Ask about the client's occupation because heavy, manual labor may cause back injury and other musculoskeletal trauma.

Physiological Integrity

- Assess the client's pain using the P-Q-R-S-T model.
- Assess the client's mobility, including gait, posture, and muscle strength.
- Interpret the client's laboratory values that are related to musculoskeletal disease (see Chart 53-3).
- Evaluate the neurovascular status of the client's affected extremity after an arthroscopic procedure.
- Encourage clients to drink additional fluids after tests that require contrast media or radioisotopes to help eliminate these substances.

ADDITIONAL STUDY RESOURCES

Go to your Student CD-ROM for Review Questions for the NCLEX Examination.

Go to http://evolve.elsevier.com/Iggy/ for Integrated Management of Care Questions for the NCLEX Examination.

SELECTED BIBLIOGRAPHY

Asterisk indicates a classic or definitive work on this subject.

Gordon, M. (2002). *Manual of nursing diagnosis* (10th ed.). St. Louis: Mosby.

Jarvis, C. (2004). *Physical examination and health assessment* (3rd ed.). Philadelphia: W. B. Saunders.

Maher, A. B. (2002). Assessment of the musculoskeletal system. In A.B. Maher, S.W. Salmond, & T.A. Pellino (Eds.). *Orthopaedic nursing* (3rd ed.) Philadelphia: W. B. Saunders.

*Mangini, M. (1998). Physical assessment of the musculoskeletal system. *Nursing Clinics of North America, 33*(4), 643-652.

*Martsolf, D.S. (1999). Cultural aspects of orthopaedic nursing. *Orthopaedic Nursing, 18*(2), 65-71.

*Neal, L. (1997). Basic musculoskeletal assessment: Tips for the home health nurse. *Home Healthcare Nurse, 15*(4), 227-235.

*O'Hanlon-Nichols, T. (1998). Basic assessment series: A review of the adult musculoskeletal system. *American Journal of Nursing, 98*(6), 48-52.

Pagana, K.D., & Pagana, T.J. (2002). *Mosby's diagnostic and laboratory test reference* (2nd ed.). St. Louis: Mosby.

*Patel, P.R., & Lauerman, W.C. (1997). The use of magnetic resonance imaging in the diagnosis of lumbar disc disease. *Orthopaedic Nursing, 16*(1), 59-65.

Interventions for Clients with Musculoskeletal Problems

CATHY A. MURRAY

Musculoskeletal disorders include metabolic bone diseases, such as osteoporosis and Paget's disease, bone tumors and lesions, and a variety of deformities and syndromes. Whereas the older adult is at the greatest risk for the development of most of these health problems, young persons and adults can experience these musculoskeletal disorders. The incidence of bone cancer is increasing in both the younger and the older population. As technologic advances occur and clients survive longer with primary cancers, metastatic lesions become more prevalent. This chapter focuses on selected disorders not covered in Chapter 24 on arthritis and other connective tissue diseases.

METABOLIC BONE DISEASES

Osteoporosis

PATHOPHYSIOLOGY

Osteoporosis is a metabolic disease in which bone demineralization results in decreased density and subsequent fractures. Osteoporosis is often referred to as a "silent disease" because the first indication of osteoporosis in most persons follows some kind of a fracture. The wrist, hip, and vertebral column are most often affected (National Osteoporosis Foundation, 2003a).

TABLE 54-1 Causes of Secondary Osteoporosis

Diseases/Conditions
- Diabetes mellitus
- Hyperthyroidism
- Hyperparathyroidism
- Cushing's syndrome
- Growth hormone deficiency
- Metabolic acidosis
- Female hypogonadism
- Paget's disease
- Osteogenesis imperfecta
- Rheumatoid arthritis
- Prolonged immobilization
- Marfan syndrome
- Bone cancer
- Cirrhosis
- Chronic airway limitation

Drugs (Chronic Use)
- Corticosteroids
- Heparin
- Anticonvulsants
- Ethanol (alcohol)
- Drugs that induce hypogonadism (decreased levels of sex hormones)
- High levels of exogenous (external) thyroid hormone

CHART 54-1

BEST PRACTICE for
Assessing Risk Factors for Primary Osteoporosis

Assess for the following:
- Client's age older than 60 years of age
- Family history of osteoporosis
- White or Asian race
- Thin, lean body build
- Low lifetime calcium intake
- Estrogen deficiency
- Androgen deficiency
- Smoking history
- High alcohol intake
- Lack of physical exercise or prolonged immobility

Bone is a dynamic tissue that is constantly undergoing changes in a process referred to as bone remodeling. Osteoporosis and **osteopenia** (low bone mass) occur when there is a disruption in the bone remodeling process. This disruption can be described when **osteoclastic** (bone resorption) activity is greater than **osteoblastic** (bone building) activity. The result is a decreased **bone mineral density (BMD).** BMD determines bone strength and peaks between 30 and 35 years of age. Before and during the peak years, osteoclastic activity is followed by osteoblastic activity at a constant rate. After the peak years, bone resorption activity exceeds bone-building activity, and bone density decreases. BMD decreases rapidly in postmenopausal women as serum estrogen levels diminish. About 40% to 45% of a woman's bone mass is lost during her life span. **Trabecular**, or **cancellous** (spongy), bone is lost first, followed by loss of **cortical** (compact) bone. This results in thin, fragile bone tissue that is susceptible to fracture.

The World Health Organization (WHO) has developed a standard for osteoporosis diagnosis based on BMD values using T-scores. A T-score is obtained during dual-energy x-ray absorptiometry. A T-score is the number of standard deviations above or below the average BMD for young, healthy white women. **Osteopenia** is present when the T-score is between 1 and 2.5. **Osteoporosis** in postmenopausal women is defined as a BMD T-score more than 2.5 standard deviations below normal (or −2.5 or below) (National Institutes of Health, 2000).

The exact pathophysiology of osteoporosis is unclear, but two theories of disease development have been advocated. First, osteoporosis may result from decreased osteoblastic activity. The osteoblasts, or bone-forming cells, may have a shortened life span or may be less efficient in the client with osteoporosis. The second and more popular theory suggests an increase in osteoclastic (bone resorption) activity. The latter theory has gained increased recognition over the past decade and has resulted in treatment directed toward measures to prevent rapid bone resorption.

Classification of Osteoporosis

Osteoporosis can be classified as generalized or regional. **Generalized osteoporosis** involves many structures in the skeleton and is further divided into two categories, primary and secondary. *Primary* osteoporosis is more common and occurs in postmenopausal women and in men in their sixth or seventh decade of life. Estrogen presumably prevents or decreases the rate of bone resorption in women and is unavailable in sufficient quantities after menopause. Even though men do not experience the rapid bone loss that women experience after menopause, they do experience decreasing levels of testosterone and altered ability to absorb calcium. This results in a slower loss of bone mass in men, especially those over 75 years of age. *Secondary* osteoporosis results from an associated medical condition, such as hyperparathyroidism; long-term drug therapy, such as with corticosteroids; or prolonged immobility, such as that seen with spinal cord injury (Table 54-1). Treatment of the secondary type is directed toward the cause of the osteoporosis when possible.

Regional osteoporosis occurs when a limb is immobilized related to a fracture, injury, paralysis, or joint inflammation. Immobilization for periods of time greater than 8 to 12 weeks can result in this type of osteoporosis. Bone loss also occurs when persons spend prolonged time in a gravity-free or weightless environment.

Etiology and Genetic Risk

The exact cause of primary osteoporosis is unknown; however, numerous risk factors have been identified (Chart 54-1). About 98% of peak bone mass is achieved by around 20 years of age in most women. The rate of bone loss accelerates after menopause. These two factors together determine bone density. Building strong bone as a young person may be the best defense against osteoporosis in later adulthood (National Osteoporosis Foundation, 2003a). Young women need to be aware of appropriate health and lifestyle practices that can prevent this potentially disabling disease (see the Meeting Healthy People 2010 Objectives box on p. 1159). A nursing study by Berarducci et al. (2000) found that most health care providers focus on the risk of osteoporosis in women older than 50 years of age and do not assess risk as often in women 49 years of age and younger (see the Evidence-Based Practice for Nursing box on p. 1159).

Primary osteoporosis most often occurs in women after menopause as a result of decreased estrogen levels. Women

Meeting HEALTHY PEOPLE 2010 Objectives

OSTEOPOROSIS

Objective 2.10: Reduce the proportion of adults who are hospitalized for vertebral fractures associated with osteoporosis.

- Teach women of all ages about osteoporosis as a disease and cause of potentially life-threatening fractures.
- Teach young and middle-aged women the need to practice a lifestyle that reduces the risk factors for osteoporosis (e.g., no smoking, increased exercise, increased calcium intake).
- Teach middle-aged and older adults to have bone mineral density screening tests to determine their bone loss percentage (often available at no or minimal cost at local health fairs or pharmacies).
- Remind clients to use proper body mechanics, such as using large leg muscles rather than back muscles for lifting.
- If clients are at high risk for osteoporosis, tell them to avoid jarring activities such as jogging or horseback riding.
- If clients are at high risk for osteoporosis, tell them to consult with a health care provider and comply with preventive treatment.

EVIDENCE-BASED PRACTICE for Nursing

Do health care providers assess knowledge of osteoporosis in young women?

Berarducci, A., et al. (2000). Health-promoting educational practices related to osteoporosis. *Applied Nursing Research, 13*(4), 173-180.

This descriptive study was designed to determine whether health care providers educate women of all ages about osteoporosis, including assessing risk factors for the disease. The researchers surveyed 90 health care providers in southwest Florida. Forty-nine surveys were returned, and 47 were usable. The responses of the providers showed significant differences between women 49 years of age and younger and women older than 50 years of age. Health care providers routinely assessed risk factors in older women and educated these women, but they did not identify risk factors or provide education for younger women.

Level of Evidence: 6—Study sample is small and not randomized.

Critique. Although the sample size was small and the subjects constituted a convenience sample, this research is one of the few studies that address the issue of health promotion to prevent osteoporosis in young women. The study cannot be generalized and needs to be repeated using a larger sample in a larger geographic area.

Implications for Nursing. Nurses and other health care professionals in any setting have a responsibility to educate all women, regardless of age, about the risk factors for osteoporosis and how to reduce them. Other studies have supported the belief that lifestyle changes in young adulthood can prevent or minimize the risk for osteoporosis as women age.

lose about 2% of their bone mass every year in the first 5 years after menopause. For women of any age who cannot take estrogen replacement, such as breast cancer survivors, the risk of osteoporosis increases.

In addition, body build seems to predict the occurrence of the disease. Osteoporosis occurs more often in thin, lean-built white and Asian women, particularly those who do not exercise regularly. Obese women can store estrogen in their tissues for use as necessary to maintain a normal level of serum calcium. Exercise decreases bone resorption and stimulates bone formation. Immobilization, such as prolonged bedrest, produces rapid bone loss.

The relationship of osteoporosis to dietary factors is becoming more well-established. A diet deficient in calcium and vitamin D stimulates the parathyroid gland to produce parathyroid hormone (PTH). PTH triggers the release of calcium from the bony matrix. Malabsorption, caused by disease or drugs, also contributes to low serum calcium levels. Institutionalized or homebound people who are not exposed to sunlight may be at a higher risk because they do not receive adequate vitamin D for the metabolism of calcium.

Protein deficiency may contribute to the incidence of bone demineralization, although this theory is controversial. Because 50% of serum calcium is protein bound, protein is needed for calcium utilization; however, excessive protein intake may increase calcium loss in the urine. Protein is needed for bone healing when a fracture occurs.

Alcohol consumption and cigarette smoking are other possible risk factors. Although the exact mechanisms are not known, these substances may promote acidosis, which in turn increases bone loss. Alcohol also has a direct toxic effect on bone tissue, resulting in decreased bone formation and increased bone resorption (Leslie, 2000). Excessive caffeine intake can increase calcium loss in the urine.

Osteoporosis is also reported in persons who participate in excessive exercise or experience eating disorders, such as anorexia nervosa or bulimia. Excessive exercise and eating disorders can result in a low body mass index with resulting amenorrhea and estrogen deficiency in adolescents and young women.

Genetic factors may play a role for both men and women, but this hypothesis has not been confirmed (Orwell, 2000). Several of the suspected risk factors, such as body build, are determined in part by heredity. History of fracture in a first-degree relative may be a risk factor; however, heredity or a genetic influence alone probably is not predictive for osteoporosis.

Incidence/Prevalence

Osteoporosis is a major health problem in the United States and many countries. A World Congress on Osteoporosis was convened in 2000 to explore how to best prevent and treat this costly health problem. The estimated cost for osteoporosis-related health care in the United States alone was more than $17 billion in 2001 with continual cost increases each year (National Osteoporosis Foundation, 2003a).

Osteoporosis is a potential health problem for more than 44 million Americans. About 10 million persons have the disease and about 34 million persons 50 years of age and older experience osteopenia and are at risk for development of osteoporosis. Women remain the largest group affected by osteoporosis at about 80%, and 20% of men experience osteoporosis. Persons of all ethnic backgrounds are at risk (National Osteoporosis Foundation, 2003a).

Osteoporosis results in more than 1.5 million fractures each year, 300,000 of which are hip fractures. In people older than 90 years of age, one third of women and one fifth of men experience at least one hip fracture. The mortality rate for older clients with hip fractures is very high, especially within the first 6 months, and the debilitating effects can be devastating (McClung, 2000).

HEALTH PROMOTION/ILLNESS PREVENTION

The focus of osteoporosis prevention is to minimize risk factors, as described earlier under the Assessment section (see Chart 54-1). For example, for clients who ingest inadequate amounts of calcium, teach them which foods should be included. Clients who have sedentary lifestyles should be taught about the importance of exercise and what types of exercise they should do. Weight-bearing exercises are preferred; activities that cause jarring, such as horseback riding, should be avoided to prevent further damage.

Rather than wait until adulthood, osteoporosis education should begin in childhood to prevent possible pain and disability later in life. Lypaczewski, Lappe, and Stubby (2002) published the short-term results of an educational intervention on bone health for 50 prepubertal Girl Scouts and their mothers. The program stressed the importance of exercise and increased dietary calcium intake for both children and women to prevent osteoporosis. The authors suggested that nurses must take opportunities to teach bone health to school-age children as one way to improve health of future adults.

◆COLLABORATIVE MANAGEMENT
◆Assessment

A complete health history with assessment of risk factors is important in the prevention, early detection, and treatment of osteoporosis. Clients who have risk factors for osteoporosis are at increased risk for fractures when falls occur. A fall risk assessment may be included in the health history. Assess for fall risk factors, including the following:

- Delirium
- Dementia
- Immobility
- Muscular weakness
- History of falls
- Visual or hearing deficits
- Current medications

Chapter 5 discusses falls in older adults in more detail.

PHYSICAL ASSESSMENT/CLINICAL MANIFESTATIONS

When performing a musculoskeletal assessment, inspect and palpate the vertebral column. The classic "dowager's hump," or kyphosis of the dorsal spine, is usually present (Figure 54-1). The client often states that height has been shortened, perhaps as much as 2 to 3 inches (5 to 7 cm) within the previous 20 years. Height and weight should be measured and compared with previous measurements if they are available.

Accompanying the spinal deformity is the complaint of back pain, which often occurs after lifting, bending, or stooping. The pain may be sharp and acute in onset. Pain is worse with activity and is relieved by rest. Palpation of the vertebrae, particularly the lower thoracic and lumbar vertebrae, usually increases the client's discomfort. Therefore palpation should be gentle.

Back pain accompanied by tenderness and voluntary restriction of spinal movement suggests one or more compression vertebral fractures, the most common type of osteoporotic fracture. Movement restriction and spinal de-

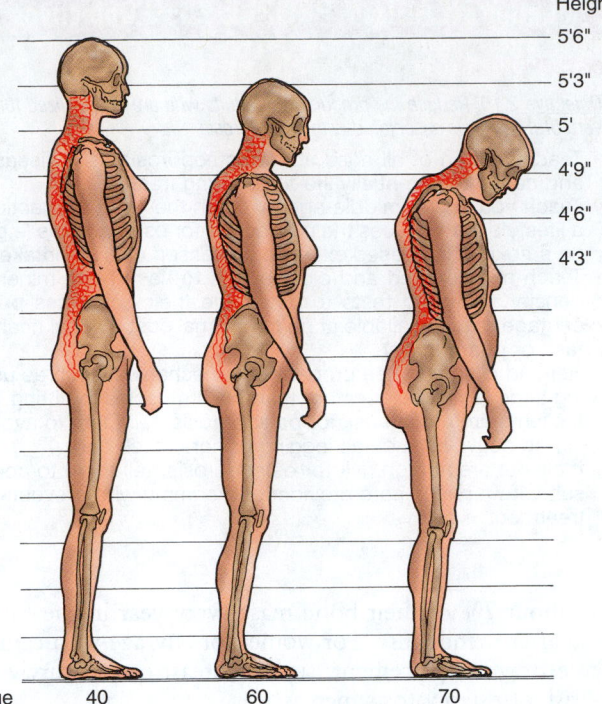

Figure 54-1 ■ A normal spine at age 40 years of age and osteoporotic changes at ages 60 and 70 years of age. These changes can cause a loss of as much as 6 inches in height and can result in the so-called dowager's hump (far right) in the upper thoracic vertebrae.

formity may result in constipation, abdominal distention, reflux esophagitis, and respiratory compromise in severe cases. The most likely area for fracture occurrence is between T8 and L3.

Fractures are also common in the distal end of the radius and the upper third of the femur (hip). The nurse directs special attention to these areas as part of the physical assessment.

PSYCHOSOCIAL ASSESSMENT

Women often associate osteoporosis with menopause, getting older, and becoming less independent. The disease can result in suffering, deformity, and disability that can affect the client's well-being and life satisfaction. The quality of life may be further impacted by pain, insomnia, depression, and **fallophobia** (fear of falling).

Assess the client's concept of body image, especially if the client is severely kyphotic. For example, the client may have difficulty finding clothes that fit properly. Social interactions may be curtailed because of a change in appearance or the physical limitations of being unable to sit in chairs in restaurants, movie theaters, and other places. Alterations in sexuality may occur as a result of poor self-esteem or the discomfort imposed by positioning during intercourse.

Because osteoporosis readily predisposes a client to fractures, the client must be extremely cautious about activities. As a result, the threat of fracture can create anxiety and fear and result in further limitation of social or physical activities. Assessment for the presence of these feelings assists in individualization of treatment and client teaching. For example, the client may not exercise as prescribed for fear that a fracture will occur.

LABORATORY ASSESSMENT

There are no definitive laboratory tests that confirm a diagnosis of primary osteoporosis, although a number of biochemical markers can provide information about bone modeling. A battery of tests can be performed to rule out secondary osteoporosis or other metabolic bone diseases, such as osteomalacia and Paget's disease. These include determination of serum calcium, vitamin D, phosphorus, and alkaline phosphatase levels.

Urinary calcium levels may also be assessed. Serum protein measurements and thyroid function tests are performed to exclude hyperthyroidism.

A simple, specific, and sensitive test to evaluate bone resorption is being used with clients with spinal cord injury and others at risk. The uPYR Crosslinks assay measures urinary concentrations of pyridinium, a collagen substance found in bone and cartilage. An increase in urinary levels indicates increased bone resorption (loss). The advantage of this test is its ability to detect bone loss early. In addition, no special client preparation is required. The disadvantage of the test is its cost, which is high because the test is relatively new. However, pyridinium and other biochemical markers of bone modeling may be used in the future as a routine screening test.

RADIOGRAPHIC ASSESSMENT

X-rays of the spine and long bones show loss of bone density and the presence of fractures. However, radiographic findings of bone density changes are evident only after a 25% to 40% bone loss has occurred.

In the past decade, technologic advances have enabled the detection of early changes in bone density. A popular screening and diagnostic tool is **dual-energy x-ray absorptiometry (DEXA).** Many physicians recommend that women in their 40s have a baseline DEXA scan so that later bone changes can be detected and compared. DEXA is a painless scan that measures bone mineral density (BMD) in the hip, wrist, or vertebral column. It is the best tool currently available for diagnosis and follow-up evaluation of treatment of osteoporosis. No special client preparation or follow-up care is required.

Qualitative ultrasound (QUS) of the heel or calcaneus is an effective and low-cost screening tool that can detect osteoporosis and predict risk for hip fracture. The test requires no special preparation, is quick, and has no radiation exposure or specific follow-up care.

◆ Common Nursing Diagnoses and Collaborative Problems

The most common nursing diagnoses and collaborative problems that apply to clients with diagnosed osteoporosis include the following:
- Risk for Falls related to being female 65 years of age or older and environmental hazards
- Impaired Physical Mobility related to decreased muscle strength, pain, and musculoskeletal impairment
- Acute Pain and/or Chronic Pain related to effects of acute physical illness (fracture) or chronic disability

The primary collaborative problem for clients with the disease is Potential for Fractures. (See the Plan of Care box below and on pp. 1162 to 1165.)

◆ Interventions

Because the client is predisposed to fractures, medications, nutritional therapy, and exercise are used to retard bone resorption and form new bony tissue. Client education can help prevent osteoporosis or slow the progress. These measures help reduce the chance of fracture and subsequent

Text continued on p. 1165.

▰ PLAN of CARE   MEDICAL DIAGNOSIS: OSTEOPOROSIS

NURSING DIAGNOSIS NO. 1   ■   Imbalanced Nutrition: Less Than Body Requirements

	Expected Outcomes	Nursing Interventions	Rationales
RELATED FACTORS Inability to ingest or digest food or absorb nutrients due to biologic, psychological, or economic factors	Has muscle tone ≥4+ Has skin with warm undertones No verbal report or observation of altered eating habits	**NIC** **Nutrition Management** Determine, in collaboration with the dietitian as appropriate, the number of calories and type of nutrients needed to meet nutrition requirements.	Individual client needs for nutrients and calories should be the basis of a sound dietary plan.
DEFINING CHARACTERISTICS Reported or evidence of lack of food Misconceptions Lack of information or misinformation		Provide appropriate information about nutritional needs and how to meet them.	Clients need accurate and timely information to make informed decisions about nutritional needs and how to meet them.
		Other Interventions Teach the client and family about nutritional supplements, as appropriate.	Additional vitamins and minerals, calories, dietary fiber, or other nutritional components may need to be added to the diet of a client who is unable to eat a nutritionally adequate diet.
		Teach the client and family about the prevention of constipation.	Clients on diets low in fiber may need additional fluids and supplemental fiber to maintain bowel regularity.

Continued

≡ PLAN of CARE   MEDICAL DIAGNOSIS: OSTEOPOROSIS—cont'd

NURSING DIAGNOSIS NO. 1 ■ Imbalanced Nutrition: Less Than Body Requirements—cont'd

Expected Outcomes	Nursing Interventions	Rationales
	Continuing Care Considerations Refer the client to appropriate community nutritional programs, as needed.	Resources such as Weight Watchers, Overeaters Anonymous, and Take Off Pounds Sensibly provide support for the client attempting to maintain appropriate body weight.
	Refer the client to community support groups and encourage attendance, as appropriate.	Clients may need support to maintain healthy eating patterns. In addition, support groups can offer advice on how to overcome common problems.
	Encourage the client and family to use the home nutritional therapy team.	The home nutritional therapy team is able to monitor and adjust the nutritional plan of care to maximize client nutritional status.

NURSING DIAGNOSIS NO. 2 ■ Impaired Physical Mobility

	Expected Outcomes	Nursing Interventions	Rationales
RELATED FACTORS Discomfort Pain Lack of knowledge regarding value of physical activity Musculoskeletal impairment Intolerance to activity Decreased strength and endurance **DEFINING CHARACTERISTICS** Postural instability during performance of routine activities of daily living Gait changes Reaction time: Decreased	Has full or improved range of motion in all joints Has smooth, coordinated movements Has stable posture during performance of activities of daily living Has no movement-induced tremor Has skin that remains intact with no bruising or rashes Able to perform fine motor skills Able to perform gross motor skills	**NIC** **Exercise Therapy: Joint Mobility** Collaborate with physical therapy in developing and executing an exercise program. Initiate pain control measures before beginning joint exercise. **D** Dress the client in nonrestrictive clothing. **D** Protect the client from trauma during exercise. **D** Encourage ambulation, if appropriate. **Continuing Care Considerations** Refer the client to a vocational counselor, as appropriate.	Physical therapists are the primary health care professionals responsible for developing and executing an exercise program. Initiating pain control measures before joint exercise increases the likelihood of client comfort and willingness to engage in the exercise. Nonrestrictive clothing permits full range of joint motion. Stretching exercises may cause the client to be off balance. Ambulation is a form of active joint exercise and also improves cardiovascular tone. Long-term physical impairment may require the client to change his or her employment.

NURSING DIAGNOSIS NO. 3 ■ Ineffective Health Maintenance

	Expected Outcomes	Nursing Interventions	Rationales
RELATED FACTORS Lack of material resources Ineffective individual coping **DEFINING CHARACTERISTICS** Demonstrated lack of knowledge regarding basic health practices	Able to accurately perform needed health care tasks No verbal report or observation of lack of equipment, financial, and/or other resources	**NIC** **Health System Guidance** Identify and facilitate communication among health care providers, client, or family, as appropriate.	Faulty communication may increase the time delays for service or foster distrust among the health care providers, client, and family.

D Indicates tasks that can be delegated to unlicensed assistive nursing personnel at the discretion of the nurse.

NURSING DIAGNOSIS NO. 3 ■ Ineffective Health Maintenance—*cont'd*

	Expected Outcomes	Nursing Interventions	Rationales
Expressed interest in improving health behaviors Reported or observed lack of equipment, financial, and/or other resources	Able to ask for or seek out assistance Practices basic health maintenance activities	Give written instructions for the purpose and location of posthospitalization and outpatient activities, as appropriate.	Written instructions provide clear information that can be referred to for memory assistance.
		Identify and facilitate transportation needs for obtaining health care services.	Ensuring that the client/family has suitable, timely transportation increases the likelihood that appointments will be kept as scheduled.
		NIC Support System Enhancement Determine the adequacy of existing social networks.	The client's/family's perception of the adequacy of social networks provides the basis of planning.
		Identify degree of family support.	Family support is not guaranteed, even with proximity.
		Determine barriers to using support systems.	The client/family needs to plan ways to overcome barriers as needed, because they may impair health maintenance.
		Encourage the client to participate in social and community activities.	Participation in social and community activities provides the client with the opportunity to form friendships that may provide emotional support.
		Assess community resource adequacy to identify strengths and weaknesses.	Understanding the strengths and weaknesses of available community resources permits realistic expectations of assistance from those sources.
		Refer to a community-based promotion, prevention, treatment, and/or rehabilitation program, as appropriate.	A community-based promotion, prevention, treatment, and/or rehabilitation program may provide the client/family with essential services and emotional support.
		Other Interventions Teach the client and family about the care necessary to manage their health state.	Lack of knowledge will render efforts at health maintenance less effective.
		Continuing Care Refer the family to appropriate counseling services.	Families in distress may be unable to provide essential support to a family member with a health maintenance problem.

NURSING DIAGNOSIS NO. 4 ■ Risk for Falls

	Expected Outcomes	Nursing Interventions	Rationales
RELATED FACTORS Age 65 or older History of falls Use of assistive devices (e.g., walker, cane) Impaired physical mobility Impaired balance Difficulty with gait Cluttered environment Throw or scatter rugs	No falls No injuries	**NIC Fall Prevention** Identify characteristics of the environment that may increase potential for falls (e.g., slippery floors and open stairways).	Removal or modification of the environment to prevent falls decreases the risk for injury.
		Monitor gait, balance, and fatigue level with ambulation.	Tired, unsteady clients are more likely to fall and suffer injury.

Continued

NURSING DIAGNOSIS NO. 4 ■ Risk for Falls—cont'd

Expected Outcomes	Nursing Interventions	Rationales
	D Assist the unsteady client with ambulation and provide assistive devices (e.g., cane and walker).	Assistance with mobility and assistive devices serves to steady gait and diminish fall risk.
	D Provide adequate lighting.	Increased visibility assists the client to locate hazards and avoid them.
	D Place a mechanical bed in the lowest position or provide a sleeping surface close to the floor, as needed.	For clients who are at high risk for falling out of bed, placing the bed in a low position or providing a sleeping surface close to the floor diminishes the distance that the client may fall, thereby lowering the force of the fall.
	D Assist with toileting at frequent, scheduled intervals.	Frequent toileting assists the client to remain continent and decreases the necessity for unassisted attempts to toilet himself or herself.
	D Ensure that the client wears shoes that fit properly, fasten securely, and have nonskid soles, and ensure that the client wears prescription glasses, as appropriate, when out of bed.	Nonskid, properly fitting shoes and corrected vision increase the client's ability to remain stable and to see hazards.
	D Instruct the client to call for assistance with movement, as appropriate.	Giving assistance to unsteady clients prevents falls.
	Other Interventions	
	Collaborate with other health care team members to minimize the side effects of medications that contribute to falling (e.g., orthostatic hypotension and unsteady gait).	Clients should be evaluated carefully for adverse effects that create an injury hazard. Medications should be reviewed and dosages altered to minimize the adverse effects whenever possible.
	Provide safety equipment (e.g., nonslip, nontrip floor surfaces, grab bars in the bathroom, nonslip surfaces in tubs, and nonglare lighting).	Environmental safety equipment permits the unsteady client to ambulate safely.
	Continuing Care Considerations	
	Encourage the client to develop a routine physical exercise program that includes walking.	Exercise helps strengthen muscles and improves coordination.
	Have the client's doors, thresholds, and steps clearly marked.	Having clearly identified geographic markers will help the client maneuver over and through uneven spots with fewer bumps or falls.
	Instruct the client to remain indoors during inclement weather to avoid ice and other slippery outdoor surfaces.	Outdoor surfaces made slippery with water or ice increase the risk of falls.

D Indicates tasks that can be delegated to unlicensed assistive nursing personnel at the discretion of the nurse.

PLAN of CARE   MEDICAL DIAGNOSIS: OSTEOPOROSIS—*cont'd*

NURSING DIAGNOSIS NO. 5   ■   Disturbed Body Image

	Expected Outcomes	Nursing Interventions	Rationales
RELATED FACTORS Biophysical Developmental changes Trauma or injury **DEFINING CHARACTERISTICS** Verbal report of feelings that reflect an altered view of one's body in appearance, structure, or function Actual change in structure and/or function	Acknowledges changes in body that reflect a realistic appraisal of altered appearance or function	**NIC** **Body Image Enhancement** Use anticipatory guidance. Assist the client to discuss changes caused by aging, as appropriate. Assist the client to discuss stressors affecting body image. Identify the significance of the client's culture, religion, race, gender, and age on body image. Determine the client's and family's perceptions of the alteration in body image versus reality. Assist the client to identify actions that will enhance appearance. **Other Interventions** **D** Provide an atmosphere of caring and acceptance.	Anticipatory guidance prepares the client for predictable changes in body image. The client may be unaware of the normal body changes caused by aging and may associate negative feelings about those changes. Stressors affecting body image may be due to congenital condition, injury, disease, or surgery. Culture, religion, race, gender, and age influence the client's perception of a positive or negative body image. The client's and family's perceptions of the alteration in body image may vary significantly from the reality of the change. Assisting the client to enhance his or her appearance will improve his or her self-concept. A client with traumatic changes in body parts or functioning may be especially sensitive to cues that indicate an aversive reaction.

complications. The role of drug therapy has increased over the past decade and helps to prevent fractures related to osteoporosis.

Drug Therapy. The health care provider may prescribe hormone replacements, calcium supplements, vitamin D, bisphosphonates (BPs), selective estrogen receptor modulators (SERMs), calcitonin, or a combination of several drugs to treat, as well as prevent, osteoporosis (Chart 54-2). Other agents have been given, but with limited success. Estrogen and combination hormone therapy are the least expensive of the drugs used for osteoporosis, but they do increase other health risks for women.

Hormone Replacement Therapy. Hormone replacement therapy (HRT) has been used as a primary *prevention* strategy for reducing bone loss in the postmenopausal woman. However, recent studies by the Women's Health Initiative demonstrated that long-term effects of HRT may increase a woman's risk of breast cancer, cardiovascular disease, and stroke. Warnings for drugs such as conjugated estrogens/medroxyprogesterone (Prempro, Premphase) state that the use of these drugs for prevention of osteoporosis must be carefully evaluated by the health care provider and the client. If taken, the benefit of the medication should outweigh the risks to the client (U.S. Food and Drug Administration, 2003).

Parathyroid Hormone. The use of parathyroid hormone is approved for *treatment* of osteoporosis in men and women. Clients must be instructed to self-administer teriparatide (Forteo) as a daily subcutaneous injection. Teriparatide stimulates new bone formation, thus increasing BMD. Reduced risk of fracture in hip, spine, and wrist is reported in women and reduced risk of hip fracture is reported in men (National Osteoporosis Foundation, 2003b). For clients taking this medication, teach them the signs and symptoms of hypercalcemia, including the following:

■ Fatigue
■ Anorexia
■ Nausea/vomiting
■ Constipation
■ Polyuria

Calcium. Intake of calcium alone is not a treatment for osteoporosis, but calcium is an important part of a prevention program to promote bone health. Most persons cannot ingest sufficient quantities of calcium in the diet, and therefore calcium supplements may be used. Calcium carbonate, found in over-the-counter (OTC) drugs such as Tums or Os-Cal, is one of the most cost-effective supplement formulas. Calcium citrate, available OTC as Citracal, is often recommended for those persons who experience gastric upset when

CHART 54-2

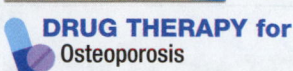

DRUG THERAPY for Osteoporosis

Drug	Usual Dosage	Nursing Interventions	Rationales
Calcium (e.g., Os-Cal, Tums, Caltrate-600, Citracal)	1-1.5 g in divided doses PO	Give a third of daily dose at bedtime. Push fluids.	Calcium is most readily utilized by the body when the client is fasting and immobile. Increased fluid intake aids in preventing the formation of calcium-based urinary stones.
		Assess for a history of urinary stones.	Calcium supplements are not given to clients who are susceptible to urinary stone formation.
		Monitor serum calcium level.	Hypercalcemia, or calcium excess, is a side effect of calcium supplementation.
		Monitor urinary calcium level (no more than 4 mg/kg in 24 hr).	The kidneys attempt to excrete excess calcium.
		Observe for signs of hypercalcemia.	Hypercalcemia can result in urinary stones, cardiac dysrhythmias, and an increase or decrease in skeletal muscle tone.
Estrogen or estrogen/progesterone (e.g., Premarin, Prempro)	0.425-1.25 mg PO for 25 days/mo 0.625 mg conjugated estrogens/2.5 mg medroxyprogesterone acetate (Prempro) (dose may be lower)	Assess for history of tumors, hypertension, thromboembolic disease, or liver or gallbladder disease.	Estrogen therapy is withheld from clients with susceptibility to an exacerbation of one or more of these problems.
		Teach the importance of gynecologic examinations every 6 months.	Endometrial and breast cancer can result from estrogen therapy.
		Teach breast self-examination.	Clients can detect potentially malignant lesions early so that treatment can begin immediately.
		Observe for vaginal bleeding.	Vaginal bleeding is a side effect of estrogen therapy and a sign of possible endometrial cancer.
		Monitor blood pressure.	Hypertension and other cardiovascular complications may result from combined estrogen-progesterone therapy.
		Observe for thrombus formation.	Deep vein thrombosis is a complication of combined estrogen-progesterone therapy.
		Monitor serum liver enzyme and cholesterol levels.	An elevation of liver enzyme levels may be indicative of liver involvement resulting from estrogen. An elevated cholesterol level can result in hypertension and thrombus formation.
Alendronate (Fosamax)	5 mg PO daily	Take early in AM with 8 oz water; do not lie down until after breakfast.	Although not common, esophagitis or esophageal ulcers may result from alendronate therapy.
Risedronate (Actonel)	5 mg daily	Give ≥30 min before a meal (preferably breakfast); follow interventions for alendronate	Same as for alendronate.
		Observe for CNS side/adverse effects, such as drowsiness, anxiety, agitation	Drug can cause CNS effects that may not be tolerated.
Ibandronate (Boniva)	2.5 mg daily	Same as for alendronate.	Same as for alendronate.
Raloxifene (Evista)	60 mg daily	Teach client to monitor weight and BP frequently.	Drug causes increased water and sodium retention.
		Monitor liver function tests (LFTs) in collaboration with health care provider.	Raloxifene can cause increased LFTs or worsen hepatic disease (should not be given to client who has liver disease).
Calcitonin (e.g., Calcimar [salmon], Cibacalcin [human], Miacalcin [salmon; nasal spray])	100 International Units SC or IM daily 200 International Units intranasally daily, alternating nostrils	Rotate injection sites for parenteral administration.	Injection sites become irritated and reddened.
		Monitor for flushing, headache, nausea, and vomiting.	These are common side effects of calcitonin.
		Monitor renal function, calcium, and vitamin D levels.	Toxicity from calcitonin can cause renal problems.

Med Error Alert! *Do not confuse Fosamax with Flomax, a selective alpha-adrenergic blocker used for benign prostatic hyperplasia (BPH).*

SC, Subcutaneous.

taking a calcium supplement. Teach clients to take calcium supplements with food and 6 to 8 ounces of water. It is best to divide the daily dose, with one third of the daily dose being taken in the evening. Supplements should be started in high-risk persons in young adulthood to assist in building peak bone mass (Sedlak & Doheny, 2002).

Clients should take calcium supplements under the supervision of a health care provider. **Hypercalcemia** (excess serum calcium) can cause serious damage to the urinary system. The amount of calcium prescribed is affected by the addition of HRT and the presence of risk factors for osteoporosis. Chart 16-13 lists the clinical manifestations associated with hypercalcemia.

In the United States the typical daily intake of dietary calcium is between 450 and 550 mg. The recommended daily allowance (RDA) of calcium is 1200 mg. Many clinicians and researchers believe that the RDA is insufficient to meet the calcium requirements of postmenopausal women, who may require as much as 1500 mg or more daily to prevent osteoporosis. An increased calcium intake may prevent bone loss in men as well. The nurse teaches the client to consume foods rich in calcium, such as milk and dairy products and dark green, leafy vegetables (see Chapter 14 for a list of foods high in calcium).

Vitamin D. Vitamin D supplementation may be necessary for the institutionalized or homebound client or for those who do not meet daily requirements. An adequate level of vitamin D is needed for optimal calcium absorption in the intestines. The prescribed dosage is usually 400 to 800 International Units/day. Higher doses can produce toxic effects, such as hypercalcemia and hyperphosphatemia.

Bisphosphonates. Bisphosphonates (BPs) inhibit bone resorption by binding with crystal elements in bone, especially spongy, trabecular bone tissue. Three BPs, alendronate (Fosamax), ibandronate (Boniva), and risedronate (Actonel), are commonly used for the *prevention and management* of osteoporosis and hypercalcemia associated with cancer. They are also approved for use in the prevention and treatment of osteoporosis in men and postmenopausal women. New bisphosphonates are being approved every year.

Although side effects are not common, when they do occur, they tend to be serious. **Esophagitis** (inflammation of the esophagus) and esophageal ulcers have been reported with the use of BPs, especially when the tablet is not completely swallowed. Teach clients taking this drug to take it early in the morning with 8 ounces of water and wait 30 minutes before eating. They should remain upright during the 30 minutes before eating. If chest pain occurs, a symptom of esophageal irritation, instruct them to discontinue the drug and contact their health care provider. Clients with poor renal function, hypocalcemia, or gastrointestinal reflux disease (GERD) should not take BPs.

Selective Estrogen Receptor Modulators. Selective estrogen receptor modulators (SERMs), a newer class of drugs, are designed to mimic estrogen in some parts of the body while blocking its effect elsewhere. Raloxifene (Evista) is used for *prevention and management* of osteoporosis in postmenopausal women. It increases BMD, reduces bone resorption, and lowers serum cholesterol. The drug should not be given to women who have a history of venous thromboembolism (VTE) (Leslie, 2000). Research continues to evaluate the effect of raloxifene as a cardiovascular protective agent.

Calcitonin. Calcitonin is a thyroid hormone that inhibits osteoclastic activity, thus decreasing bone loss. It is used for the *treatment* of osteoporosis, Paget's disease, and hypercalcemia associated with cancer. The drug also has an analgesic effect after vertebral fracture, thereby promoting early recovery.

Calcitonin (salmon) can be given intramuscularly, subcutaneously, or intranasally (Miacalcin). Nasal administration is preferred because it improves compliance, minimizes side effects, and is convenient. However, the effect of salmon calcitonin may decrease after use for two or more years. Clients may require a holiday from this treatment to maintain effectiveness. The nurse teaches the client to alternate nostrils to prevent nasal mucosal irritation, a common side effect. Salmon calcitonin must be refrigerated.

Other Agents. Androgens, such as testosterone propionate (Testex, Malogen✦), have been successful in decreasing bone resorption and increasing bone growth. Androgens may decrease bone resorption in men, particularly in older men. When given to postmenopausal women, however, androgens cause masculine traits and may lead to liver disease.

Diet Therapy. The dietary considerations for the treatment of a client with a diagnosis of osteoporosis are the same as those for preventing the disease. Adequate amounts of protein, magnesium, vitamin K, and trace minerals are needed for bone formation. Calcium and vitamin D intake needs to be increased, and alcohol and caffeine consumption should be discouraged. For the client who has sustained a fracture, intake of protein, vitamin C, and iron is increased to promote bone healing. Education for persons of all ages must focus on the importance of adequate intake of calcium to build strong bones (Lypaczewski, Lappe, Stubby, 2002).

Fall Prevention. The client must be careful to prevent falls and other activities that can cause a fracture. A hazard-free environment is necessary to meet this goal, and the nurse must teach the client about its importance.

Many hospitals and long-term care facilities have risk management programs in which clients are assessed for their risk for falls. For those at high risk, programs such as the Falling Star protocol have reduced falls by making the staff aware of the client's high risk. In this program, a star is placed at the head of the bed to designate a person at high risk. Chapter 5 discusses fall prevention in health care agencies and at home in more detail.

Hip protectors are inexpensive devices that can prevent hip fracture if the client experiences a fall. A **hip protector** is a pad that is worn while ambulating. If the client falls onto his or her trochanter, the probability of hip fracture is lessened.

Exercise. Exercise is important in the prevention and management of osteoporosis. It also plays a vital role in pain management, cardiovascular function, and an improved sense of well-being.

In collaboration with the health care provider, the physical therapist prescribes exercises for strengthening the abdominal and back muscles. These exercises improve posture and provide an improved support for the spine. Abdominal isometrics, deep breathing, and pectoral stretching are stressed in order to increase pulmonary capacity. Exercises for the extremity muscles include isometric, resistive, and range-of-motion (ROM) exercises. The nurse encourages active ROM exercises, which improve joint mobility and increase muscle tone.

In addition to exercises for muscle strengthening, a general weight-bearing exercise program is implemented. Walking for 30 minutes three times a week, swimming, or bicycling are recommended activities. Teach the client that certain high-impact recreational activities, such as bowling and horseback riding, may cause vertebral compression and should be avoided.

Pain Management. The pain management program depends on the intensity and duration of the pain. With treatment, pain from spinal fractures often resolves 6 to 8 weeks after injury; treatment usually includes drug therapy and orthotic devices. The health care provider prescribes analgesics (opioid and non-opioid) during the acute phase of the pain (i.e., from the time of injury to as long as several weeks afterward). Muscle relaxants, which ease the discomfort associated with muscle spasms, are often used for spinal fractures. Nonsteroidal anti-inflammatory drugs (NSAIDs) are beneficial for pain relief and for decreasing spinal nerve root inflammation from crushed vertebrae. However, monitor for problems associated with NSAIDs, such as gastrointestinal bleeding and heart failure, particularly in older adults.

Orthotic Devices. Known as dorsolumbar orthoses, orthotic devices immobilize the spine during the acute pain phase and provide spinal column support (Figure 54-2). The physical therapist or orthotist custom fits the client for this lightweight device. Teach the client to inspect the skin for irritation and report tolerance to the device.

Community-Based Care

Clients with osteoporosis are usually managed at home. However, some experience fractures that may require hospitalization. In any setting, assess for risk factors of osteoporosis and provide health teaching as appropriate, and described under the Interventions section above.

The client with osteoporosis who has one or more fractures can be discharged to the home setting. In some instances, the client is discharged to a long-term care facility for rehabilitation or permanent residence when support systems are not available. Case managers, social workers, and discharge planners assist in preparing clients and their families for placement in long-term care facilities. Chapter 55 discusses continuing care for clients who experience fractures.

The National Osteoporosis Foundation provides information to clients and health care professionals regarding the disease and its treatment. Large metropolitan hospitals often have osteoporosis specialty clinics and support groups for clients with osteoporosis.

Osteomalacia

PATHOPHYSIOLOGY

Osteomalacia is described as softening of the bone tissue and is characterized by inadequate mineralization of osteoid. Mineralized osteoid results in mature compact and cancellous (spongy) bone. In osteomalacia, normal remodeling of the bone is disrupted and mineralization or calcification does not occur. Osteomalacia is the adult equivalent of rickets, or vitamin D deficiency, in children.

Vitamin D deficiency is the most important factor in development of osteomalacia. In its natural form, vitamin D is obtained from the ultraviolet radiation of the sun, from certain foods, and as a nutritional supplement. In combination with calcium and phosphorus, the vitamin is necessary for bone formation.

Osteomalacia is frequently confused with osteoporosis because of similar characteristics shared by the two disease processes. Table 54-2 shows a comparison and contrast of osteoporosis and osteomalacia.

> **CONSIDERATIONS FOR OLDER ADULTS**
>
> Osteomalacia is not thought to be common, but researchers and clinicians are exploring its incidence in older adults. Although there are no accurate statistical data to indicate the incidence of osteomalacia in the United States, health care professionals are continuing to study its occurrence in nursing homes and other residences for older adults.

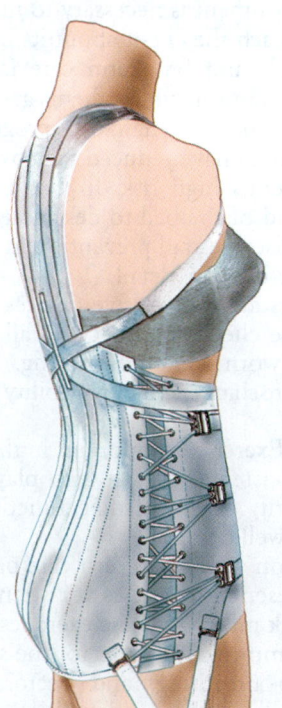

Figure 54-2 ■ A dorsolumbar orthosis. (Courtesy Truform Orthotics and Prosthetics, Cincinnati, OH.)

TABLE 54-2 Differential Features of Osteoporosis and Osteomalacia

Characteristic	Osteoporosis	Osteomalacia
Definition	Decreased bone mass	Demineralized bone
Pathophysiology	Lack of calcium	Lack of vitamin D
Radiographic findings	Osteopenia, fractures	Pseudofractures, Looser's zones, fractures
Calcium level	Normal	Low or normal
Phosphate level	Normal	Low or normal
Parathyroid hormone	Normal	High or normal
Alkaline phosphatase	Normal	High

Etiology and Genetic Risk

In addition to primary vitamin D deficiency related to lack of sunlight exposure or dietary intake, vitamin D deficiency attributable to various pathologic conditions may result in osteomalacia (Table 54-3). Malabsorption of the vitamin from the small bowel is a common postsurgical complication of partial or total gastrectomy and bypass or resection surgery of the small intestine. Disease of the small bowel, such as Crohn's disease, may cause decreased vitamin absorption.

Liver and pancreatic disorders interrupt vitamin D metabolism and decrease the production of usable substance. Chronic renal insufficiency interferes with the synthesis of calcitriol, the most active vitamin metabolite. Osteomalacia can also be caused by malignant bone tumors (**oncogenic** or **tumor-induced osteomalacia**).

Conditions that contribute to phosphate depletion (hypophosphatemia) lead to osteomalacia. Osteomalacia is also a complication of the intake of certain drugs, particularly anticonvulsants, barbiturates, and fluoride. The exact mechanism for the drug effects is not known. Genetic deviations in vitamin D or phosphate metabolism may commonly cause bone changes seen in osteomalacia.

Incidence/Prevalence

Osteomalacia is rarely seen in the United States and Western Europe, however, it is more common in nonindustrialized nations or in countries where famine is common. In the United States, older adults are most at risk. This group may have inadequate exposure to sunlight or intake of vitamin D–fortified foods. Persons who adhere to very restrictive vegetarian diets without adequate supplement of vitamin D can also be at risk. The risk for osteomalacia should be assessed in any person who has poor nutritional intake related to homelessness or severe drug or alcohol abuse or who is very poor.

HEALTH PROMOTION/ILLNESS PREVENTION

Because the nursing diagnoses for osteomalacia are the same as those for osteoporosis, client outcomes are also similar. An increase in vitamin D through dietary intake, sun exposure, and drug supplementation is promoted. Teach the at-risk client about foods high in vitamin D and the importance of frequent sun exposure for the manufacture of the vitamin.

Some persons are lactose intolerant or choose not to use dairy products related to strict vegetarian diets. Many products

are available for persons who need to make dietary choices other than dairy products. Soy and rice milk, tofu, and other soy products are readily available. Instruct clients to choose those products that are fortified with vitamin D. Other foods rich in vitamin D are eggs, swordfish, chicken, liver, as well as cereals and bread products enriched with vitamin D.

◆ COLLABORATIVE MANAGEMENT
◆ Assessment

Important data to collect for a client with osteomalacia or suspected osteomalacia include age, exposure to sunlight, and skin pigmentation. The older adult who has been homebound or chronically institutionalized is at the greatest risk. People who have dark skin and consume minimal protein are more at risk than light-skinned people with the same dietary habits. Take a thorough diet history to determine the intake of foods containing vitamin D and calcium.

Assessment will also include any history of chronic disease processes of the gastrointestinal tract including inflammatory bowel disease, gastric or intestinal bypass surgery, or any syndrome that interferes with absorption from the gastrointestinal tract. A history of renal or liver dysfunction may lead to ineffective metabolism of vitamin D. Drugs such as phenytoin (Dilantin) or fluoride preparations may interfere with metabolism of vitamin D.

PHYSICAL ASSESSMENT/CLINICAL MANIFESTATIONS

Osteomalacia is easily confused with osteoporosis. Many of the clinical manifestations are similar, and both disorders may occur at the same time.

In the early stages of osteomalacia, the manifestations are nonspecific. Muscle weakness and bone pain are often misdiagnosed as arthritis or other connective tissue disorder. In some cases, proximal muscle weakness in the shoulder and pelvic girdle areas is the only complaint.

Muscle weakness in the lower extremities may cause a waddling and unsteady gait, which contributes to falls and subsequent fractures. Hypophosphatemia leads to an inadequate production of muscle cell adenosine triphosphate, thus resulting in a decrease in muscle cell energy. If hypocalcemia is present, muscle cramping may accompany the weakness.

Assessment of muscle strength and observation of the client's gait will be made. Document complaints of muscle cramps and bone pain. Skeletal discomfort is often vague and generalized. The spine, ribs, pelvis, and lower extremities are most often affected. The client usually describes the pain as aggravated by activity and worse at night.

In addition to the client's subjective complaint of pain, palpate the affected bones for tenderness. Bone tenderness can be elicited by pressure on the tibia or rib cage. Observation of skeletal malalignment as in long-bone bowing or spinal deformity may be similar to that seen in osteoporosis. In extreme cases, the pelvis narrows, so that vaginal childbirth is difficult.

If osteomalacia is untreated, vertebral, rib, and long-bone fractures may occur. The client may be misdiagnosed as having bone cancer or osteoporosis.

DIAGNOSTIC ASSESSMENT

Table 54-2 shows the changes in laboratory values that help support the diagnosis of osteomalacia. X-rays of bone tissue with osteomalacia reveal a decrease in the trabeculae of

TABLE 54-3 Causes of Osteomalacia

Vitamin D Disturbance	Kidney Disease
Inadequate production	Chronic renal failure
Lack of sunlight exposure	Renal tubular disorders
Dietary deficiency	■ Acidosis
Abnormal metabolism	■ Hypophosphatemia
Drug therapy	
■ Phenytoin (Dilantin)	**Familial Metabolic Error**
■ Fluoride	Hypophosphatemia
■ Barbiturates	
Liver disease	
Renal disease	
Inadequate absorption	
■ Postgastrectomy	
■ Malabsorption syndrome	
Inflammatory bowel disease	

cancellous bone and lack of osteoid sharpness. The classic diagnostic finding specific to the disease, however, is the presence of radiolucent bands (Looser's lines or zones). Looser's zones are pseudofractures; they represent stress fractures that have not mineralized. They often appear symmetrically in the medial area of the femoral neck, ribs, and inferior pubic rami and may progress to complete fractures with minimal trauma. Bone biopsy of these areas may be necessary for complete diagnosis. DEXA scan may assist in diagnosis of osteomalacia.

◆Interventions

The major treatment for osteomalacia is vitamin D. The recommended daily allowance (RDA) of vitamin D is 400 International Units. Because older adults are at risk for bone demineralization from aging, as well as for osteomalacia, a safe and adequate daily requirement may be as high as 600 to 800 International Units. Chart 54-3 lists interventions for helping older clients meet the daily requirement of vitamin D. Other interventions for clients with osteomalacia are discussed under Health Promotion/Illness Prevention.

> ### ❓ Critical Thinking Challenge
>
> An older woman who lives in an assisted-living complex tells you that she had a recent DEXA scan that revealed beginning osteoporosis. She is very upset because she has always had a "normal" scan, and thought she was not a high risk for the disease. Her mother suffered a fractured hip and died of complications in a nursing home. The client is worried that this complication could happen to her and wants to know how she can "slow this disease down."
>
> 1. What further information do you need to complete her history?
> 2. What physical assessment should you perform?
> 3. What health teaching is appropriate at this time?
> 4. What options does she have for treatment?
> 5. Is this client also at risk for osteomalacia? Why or why not?
>
> **evolve** For suggested answer guidelines, go to http://evolve.elsevier.com/Iggy/.

Paget's Disease of the Bone

PATHOPHYSIOLOGY

Paget's disease, or **osteitis deformans**, is a metabolic disorder of bone remodeling, or turnover, in which increased resorption or loss results in bone deposits that are weak, enlarged, and disorganized.

CHART 54-3

NURSING FOCUS on the OLDER ADULT

Meeting the Daily Requirement for Vitamin D

- Advise clients to get sun exposure for at least 5 minutes weekly, even in the summer and winter.
- Recommend that clients eat food high in calcium to promote vitamin D absorption and utilization in the small intestines.
- Suggest that clients eat natural and fortified foods containing vitamin D, including milk and dairy products, such as ice cream (or ice milk), yogurt, and cheese.
- Recommend that clients exercise on a regular basis (at least three times a week for 20 to 30 minutes) to prevent bone loss.

Three pathophysiologic phases of the disorder have been described: active, mixed, and inactive. In the first phase (the active phase), a prolific increase in osteoclasts (cells that break down bone) causes massive bone destruction and deformity. The osteoclasts of pagetic bone are large and multinuclear, unlike the osteoclasts of normal bone tissue.

In the mixed phase, the osteoblasts (bone-forming cells) react to compensate in forming new bone. The result is bone that is vascular, structurally weak, and deformed. Paget's disease occurs in one bone or in multiple sites. The most common areas of involvement are the vertebrae, the femur, the skull, the sternum, and the pelvis.

When the osteoblastic activity exceeds the osteoclastic activity, the inactive phase occurs. The newly formed bone becomes sclerotic and very hard. The number of osteoclasts begins to return toward normal.

Bone biopsy specimens have revealed an antigen from a respiratory virus and measles. Because the disorder is present in monozygotic twins, a familial autosomal dominant pattern has been suggested. The disease has been noted in up to 30% of people with a positive family history for Paget's disease.

Paget's disease is the second most common bone disease, after osteoporosis, in the older population. The exact cause of Paget's disease is unknown but it may be the result of a latent viral infection contracted in young adulthood and manifesting as a disease 20 to 40 years later. The risk for developing Paget's disease increases as a person ages, particularly in those 80 years old and older.

> ### CONSIDERATIONS FOR OLDER ADULTS
>
> About 1 to 3 million people in the United States suffer from Paget's disease. It is primarily a disease of older adults and occurs in a very small percentage of those younger than 40 years of age.

> ### CULTURAL CONSIDERATIONS
>
> Because Paget's disease occurs more often in Europe and less often in Asia, there may be a link between the disease and ethnic origin. This linkage has not been well researched.

◆COLLABORATIVE MANAGEMENT

◆Assessment

Of clients with Paget's disease, 80% are asymptomatic. The disease may be confined to one bone. The disease is often accidentally discovered during a routine laboratory or radiographic examination. In more severe disease, the manifestations are diverse and potentially fatal (Chart 54-4).

Assessment should include history of fracture and a thorough pain assessment. Bone pain causes the client to seek medical attention. The pain is aching, poorly described, deep, and worsened by pressure and weight bearing. It is most noticeable at night or when the client is resting, and the pain is typically mild to moderate. Back pain and headache are common complaints.

The pain associated with the disorder may result from metabolic bone activity, secondary arthritis, impending fracture, or nerve impingement. Arthritis occurs at the joints of the affected bones, but its relationship to Paget's disease is unclear. Nerve impingement is particularly common in the lumbosacral area of the vertebral column, presenting as back pain that radiates along one or both lower extremities.

In addition to these assessments, inquire about any changes in hearing, vision, swallowing, balance, or speech. As bony changes progress in the skull and temporal regions, deficits in these areas may appear.

PHYSICAL ASSESSMENT/CLINICAL MANIFESTATIONS

MUSCULOSKELETAL AND NEUROLOGIC ASSESSMENT.
Posture, stance, and gait are observed to identify gross bony deformities. Because of the enlargement of the vertebrae, loss of normal spinal curvature, and lower extremity malalignment, the client is usually short. Long-bone bowing in the arms and legs with subsequent varus deformity of the elbows and knees may be asymmetric. Flexion contracture in the hip joint is often present.

When performing a musculoskeletal assessment in a client with Paget's disease, pay particular attention to the size and shape of the skull, which is typically soft, thick, and enlarged. Involvement of the temporal bone may lead to deafness and vertigo, whereas basilar complications can compress any of the cranial nerves and result in neurologic compromise. Assess the client for impairments in vision, swallowing, and speech. **Platybasia**, or basilar invagination, causes brainstem manifestations that threaten life. In some cases, the bony enlargement of the skull blocks cerebrospinal fluid (CSF), resulting in hydrocephalus.

Pathologic fractures may be the presenting clinical manifestation of the disorder. Up to 30% of clients with Paget's disease can sustain at least one incomplete or complete fracture. The femur and the tibia are most often affected, and fracture of these bones can result from minimal trauma. The fracture line is usually perpendicular to the long axis of the bone, and healing is unpredictable because of abnormal metabolic activity within the bone.

The most dreaded complication of Paget's disease is neoplasm, most commonly osteogenic sarcoma (see the discussion later under Malignant Bone Tumors, p. 1176). Sarcomas occur in about 1% of clients with pagetic bone. They appear primarily in the pelvis, the femur, and the humerus and carry a grave prognosis because of early metastasis to the lung or extensive local invasion. They are often multifocal, and they occur more often in men. When severe bone pain is present in a client with Paget's disease, neoplasm is suspected.

SKIN ASSESSMENT.
Assess the skin for its color and temperature. In people with Paget's disease, the skin is typically flushed and warm because of increased vascularity. In addition, the nurse assesses the client's energy level. The client usually complains of apathy, lethargy, and fatigue.

OTHER MANIFESTATIONS.
Other, less common manifestations of Paget's disease include hyperparathyroidism and gout. Secondary hyperparathyroidism leads to an increase in serum and urinary calcium levels. In severe cases, calcium excess results from prolonged immobilization. Calcium deposits occur in joint spaces or as stones in the urinary tract. **Hyperuricemia** (serum uric acid excess) and gout occur because the increased metabolic activity of bone creates an increase in nucleic acid catabolism.

In a few cases, increased vascularity causes an increase in cardiac output, resulting in heart failure. Cardiac complications tend to occur only when more than a third of the skeleton is involved.

LABORATORY ASSESSMENT

Increases in serum alkaline phosphatase (ALP) and urinary hydroxyproline levels are the primary laboratory findings indicating the probability of Paget's disease. Overactive osteoblasts cause the alteration in ALP level. Clients who are receiving medications to manage Paget's disease should have an assessment of ALP three or four times a year to assess treatment effectiveness.

The 24-hour urinary hydroxyproline level reflects bone collagen turnover and indicates the degree of disease severity. The higher the hydroxyproline, the more severe the disease.

The calcium levels in blood and urine are normal or elevated. The immobilized client is more likely to have an increase in calcium levels as a result of calcium moving from bone into the blood.

Paget's disease often causes an elevation of uric acid because nucleic acid from overactive bone metabolism increases. This finding may be misinterpreted as primary gout.

RADIOGRAPHIC ASSESSMENT

Radiologic studies are the primary means of diagnosis of Paget's disease. X-rays of pagetic bone reveal radiolucent, or punched-out, areas indicative of increased bone resorption. Depending on the phase of the disease, the overall bone mass is enlarged and the cortices are thickened. Malalignment deformities, fractures, and secondary arthritic changes may be present.

Computed tomography (CT) is useful in the detection of sarcomas, changes in the skull, and spinal cord or nerve compression.

OTHER DIAGNOSTIC ASSESSMENTS

Magnetic resonance imaging (MRI) may also be used for the same purpose as the CT scan. Bone biopsy may also be used to rule out suspicion of malignancy.

CHART 54-4

KEY FEATURES of
Paget's Disease of the Bone

Musculoskeletal Manifestations
- Bone and joint pain (may be in a single bone) that is aching, poorly described, and aggravated by walking
- Low back and sciatic nerve pain
- Bowing of long bones
- Loss of normal spinal curvature
- Enlarged, thick skull
- Pathologic fractures
- Osteogenic sarcoma

Skin Manifestations
- Flushed, warm skin

Other Manifestations
- Apathy, lethargy, fatigue
- Hyperparathyroidism
- Gout
- Urinary or renal stones
- Heart failure from fluid overload

◆ Interventions

Nonsurgical or surgical management may be necessary to reduce pain. Nonsurgical interventions are used initially.

NONSURGICAL MANAGEMENT. Drug therapy is the primary intervention used for treatment and pain relief. Not only can drugs relieve pain, but they also may cause the disease to go into remission for a period of time by reducing pagetic bone resorption. Other pain relief measures are also used.

Drug Therapy. The purpose of drug therapy in Paget's disease is to relieve pain and to decrease bone resorption. Management of mild to moderate pain may include the use of aspirin or nonsteroidal anti-inflammatory drugs (NSAIDs), such as ibuprofen (Motrin, Apo-Ibuprofen✱). When the calcium level is more than twice the normal value and the disease is widespread, the physician usually prescribes more potent drugs, such as calcitonin, selected bisphosphonates, alendronate (Fosamax), or mithramycin.

Calcitonin. Calcitonin is a thyroid hormone and is one of the treatments of choice for Paget's disease. It seems to retard bone resorption and, subsequently, relieve pain. The drug often causes a dramatic decrease in the alkaline phosphatase level in a few weeks. Calcitonin is approved for parenteral administration in treating Paget's disease. Side effects include nausea, flushing, and skin rash. Skin testing should be done before administration of the first dose.

Bisphosphonates. Etidronate (Didronel), an older bisphosphates (BP), may be prescribed orally in a dose of 5 mg/kg/day. Etidronate must be given in a 6-month on and 6-months off schedule. The dosage is kept to a minimum because high dosages may increase the risk of pathologic fracture. The major disadvantage is that the drug is poorly absorbed from the small intestine. Etidronate should be taken on an empty stomach 1 to 2 hours after breakfast or at bedtime with water or juice. Milk or milk products inhibit the drug's absorption. Diarrhea may occur in a few clients, but this problem can be treated with an antidiarrheal medication.

Calcitonin and etidronate are often the first drugs prescribed and are often used in combination. If repeated courses of these drugs are not effective, mithramycin or other BPs may be added to the drug regimen. Alendronate (Fosamax) and tiludronate (Skelid) are BPs that are also approved for treatment of Paget's disease.

Mithramycin. Mithramycin (Mithracin) is a potent antineoplastic and antibiotic with many side effects and is rarely used. It is reserved for clients with marked hypercalcemia or severe disease with neurologic compromise. Observe for signs of toxicity to the liver, gastrointestinal tract, and kidneys. Liver and kidney function studies and intake and output are monitored daily. Because mithramycin also suppresses platelets, daily platelet counts and bleeding precautions are taken. When liver enzyme levels become extremely high, drug therapy is interrupted temporarily.

The nurse and health care provider monitor the client's alanine phosphatase levels periodically to determine drug effectiveness. Periodic x-rays may also be ordered to assess bone changes during and after drug therapy.

Other Interventions. In addition to administering medication, implement physical measures to reduce pain. These measures may include application of heat and gentle massage. An exercise program may be started with the help of a physical therapist. Exercise may be difficult because of pain and danger of fracture. Nonimpact exercise should be used, but the client may benefit from strengthening and weight-bearing exercises. ROM and gentle stretching should be taught to the client. The client may be fitted for an orthotic device to immobilize and provide support for the vertebrae or long bones. Additional interventions for pain relief, such as relaxation techniques, are discussed in Chapter 7.

Measures to promote bone health are also important and include a diet rich in calcium. Diet therapy for bone health is described earlier under the interventions for Osteoporosis.

Provide the client with information to contact the local chapter of the Paget's Disease Foundation and the Arthritis Foundation. These resources provide information and support for the client and family or significant others. Dietary instruction should be similar to information given to the person with osteoporosis.

SURGICAL MANAGEMENT. When a client with Paget's disease has secondary arthritis and pain relief is not achieved, he or she may undergo a tibial osteotomy, or partial or total joint replacement (see Chapter 24). Surgical decompression and stabilization of the spine may be used to retain function, decrease pain, and reduce potential cardiac and respiratory complications.

OSTEOMYELITIS

PATHOPHYSIOLOGY

Invasion by one or more pathogenic microorganisms stimulates the inflammatory response in bone tissue, a condition known as **osteomyelitis.** The inflammation produces an increased vascularity and edema often involving the surrounding soft tissues. Once inflammation is established, the vessels in the area become thrombosed and release exudate into bony tissue. Ischemia of bone tissue follows and necrotic bone results. This area of necrotic bone separates from surrounding bone tissue and **sequestrum** is formed. The presence of sequestrum retards bone healing and causes superimposed infection, often in the form of bone abscess. As shown in Figure 54-3, the cycle repeats itself as the superimposed infection leads to further inflammation, vessel thromboses, and necrosis.

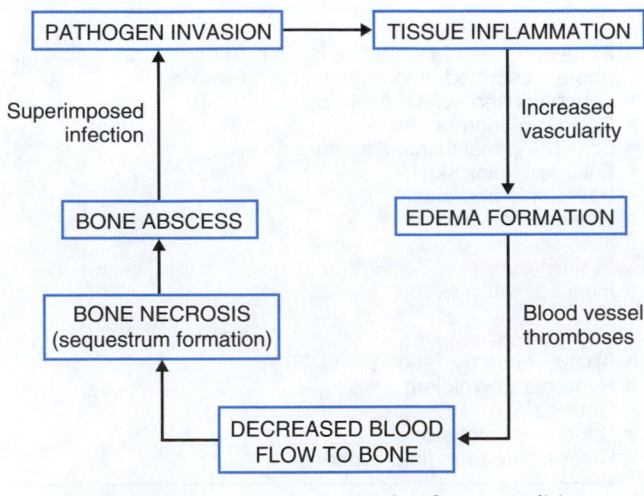

Figure 54-3 ■ Infection cycle of osteomyelitis.

Osteomyelitis is categorized as **exogenous,** in which infectious organisms enter from outside the body as in an open fracture, or **endogenous,** in which organisms are carried by the bloodstream from other areas of infection in the body. Endogenous osteomyelitis may also be referred to as **hematogenous** osteomyelitis. A third category is **contiguous,** in which bone infection results from skin infection of adjacent tissues. Osteomyelitis can be further divided into two major types: acute osteomyelitis and chronic osteomyelitis.

Etiology

Each type of bone infection has its own causative factors. Pathogenic microbes favor bone that has a rich vascular supply and a marrow cavity. **Acute hematogenous** infection results from bacteremia, underlying disease, or nonpenetrating trauma. Urinary tract infections, particularly in older men, tend to spread to the lower vertebrae. Long-term intravenous (IV) catheters, such as Hickman catheters, are primary sources of infection. Clients undergoing long-term hemodialysis and IV drug abusers are also at risk for osteomyelitis. *Salmonella* infections of the gastrointestinal tract may spread to bone. Clients with sickle cell anemia and other hemoglobinopathies often experience multiple episodes of salmonellosis, which can cause bone infection.

Poor dental hygiene and gum infection can be a causative factor in **contiguous** osteomyelitis in facial bones. Minimal trauma of the nonpenetrating type can cause hemorrhages or small-vessel occlusions, leading to bone necrosis. Regardless of the source of infection, many infections are caused by *Staphylococcus aureus.* Treatment of infection may be complicated further by the presence of methicillin-resistant *Staphylococcus aureus,* which is becoming more common in institutionalized persons.

CONSIDERATIONS FOR OLDER ADULTS

Malignant external otitis media involving the base of the skull is sometimes seen in older adults with diabetes. The most common cause of contiguous spread in older adults, however, is found in clients with diabetes or peripheral vascular disease who have slow-healing foot ulcers. Multiple organisms tend to be responsible for the resulting osteomyelitis.

In contrast, penetrating trauma leads to acute osteomyelitis by direct inoculation. A concurrent soft-tissue infection may be present as well. Animal bites, puncture wounds, and bone surgery can result in bone infection. The most common offending organism is *Pseudomonas aeruginosa,* but other gram-negative bacteria may be found.

If bone infection is misdiagnosed or inadequately treated, **subchronic** or **chronic osteomyelitis** occurs. Inadequate treatment results when the treatment period is too short or when the treatment is delayed or inappropriate. About 50% of cases of chronic osteomyelitis are caused by gram-negative bacteria. Remaining infections may be the result of a mixture of gram-negative and gram-positive organisms. Although bacteria are the most common causes of osteomyelitis, fungal organisms and virus also may cause infection.

Incidence/Prevalence

Hematogenous osteomyelitis is the most common type of osteomyelitis. Osteomyelitis occurs more often in children but is becoming increasingly common in adults, particularly older adults. Acute infection is more common in children; subchronic and chronic infection is more common in adults. Men experience osteomyelitis more frequently than women related to a higher incidence of blunt or penetrating trauma. Accompanying conditions such as malnutrition, alcoholism, renal or liver disease, and immunosuppressive disorders increase the risk and complicate effective treatment. Bone tissue in the vertebrae and long bones are common sites of infection. The adult with a compromised vascular supply is at greatest risk for chronic infection. Advanced age and concurrent disease may prolong the course of the infection for as long as a year or more.

◆COLLABORATIVE MANAGEMENT
◆Assessment

Bone pain, with or without other manifestations, is a common complaint of clients with bone infection. The pain is described as a constant, localized, pulsating sensation that intensifies with movement.

The client with *acute* osteomyelitis manifests fever, usually with temperature greater than 101° F (38° C). The area around the infected bone swells and is tender when palpated. Erythema (redness) and heat may also be present. When there is severe vascular compromise, clients may not feel discomfort because of nerve damage from lack of blood supply.

When vascular insufficiency is suspected, assess circulation in the distal extremities. Draining ulcers may be present on the feet or hands, indicating inadequate healing ability as a result of poor circulation.

Fever, swelling, and erythema are less common in those with *chronic* osteomyelitis. Ulceration resulting in sinus tract formation, localized pain, and drainage are more characteristic of chronic infection (Chart 54-5).

The client with osteomyelitis usually has an elevated white blood cell (leukocyte) count, which may be double the normal value. In chronic infection, normal values or slight elevations may be seen.

The erythrocyte sedimentation rate (ESR) may be normal early in the course of the disease but rises as the condition progresses. The rate may remain elevated for as long as 3 months after drug therapy is discontinued.

If bacteremia is present, a potentially life-threatening complication that could lead to septic shock, a blood culture identifies the offending organisms to determine which an-

---

CHART 54-5

KEY FEATURES of
Acute and Chronic Osteomyelitis

Acute Osteomyelitis
- Fever; temperature usually above 101° F (38° C)
- Swelling around the affected area
- Erythema of the affected area
- Tenderness of the affected area
- Bone pain that is constant, localized, and pulsating; intensifies with movement

Chronic Osteomyelitis
- Ulceration of the skin
- Sinus tract formation
- Localized pain
- Drainage from the affected area

tibiotics should be used in treatment. Both aerobic and anaerobic blood cultures should be collected at the initiation of therapy. About 50% of clients with acute hematogenous infection have positive blood cultures.

Although bone changes cannot be detected early with standard x-rays, changes in blood flow can be seen early in the course of the disease by radionuclide scanning. A bone scan, using technetium or gallium, is extremely helpful in the diagnosis of osteomyelitis and identifies most cases. In some cases, magnetic resonance imaging (MRI) may be more sensitive than traditional bone scanning in the diagnosis of osteomyelitis.

The definitive diagnosis of osteomyelitis may be made by bone biopsy. A culture of soft tissue or of the sinus tract may not identify the offending microbes invading the bone. Often the organisms affecting soft tissue and bone are different, and each must be treated.

◆ Common Nursing Diagnoses and Collaborative Problems

Nursing diagnoses and collaborative problems that may apply to clients with osteomyelitis include the following:

- Acute Pain or Chronic Pain related to inflammation
- Hyperthermia related to pathogenic invasion of the bone
- Ineffective Tissue Perfusion (peripheral) related to tissue swelling
- Potential for Sepsis and Septic Shock

◆ Interventions

The specific treatment protocol depends on the type and number of microbes present in the infected tissue. If other measures fail to resolve the infectious process, surgical management may be needed.

NONSURGICAL MANAGEMENT. To reverse osteomyelitis, the health care provider initiates antibiotic therapy as soon as possible. Contact precautions prevent the spread of the offending organism to other clients and health care personnel (see Chapter 29 for a discussion of contact precautions).

Drug Therapy. IV antibiotic therapy is usually prescribed for several weeks for acute osteomyelitis. More than one antibiotic may be needed to combat the presence of multiple types of organisms. The hospital or home care nurse gives the drugs at specifically prescribed times so that therapeutic serum levels are achieved. The nurse must become familiar with the actions, side effects, toxicity, interactions, and precautions for administration of the drugs. Family members in the home setting may be taught how to administer the antibiotics.

The optimal drug regimen for clients with chronic osteomyelitis is not well established. Prolonged therapy for more than 3 months may be needed to eliminate the infection. Because of the cost of lengthy hospital stays, clients are typically discharged to the home setting with long-term vascular access catheters, such as the peripherally inserted central catheter (PICC), for medication administration. After discontinuation of IV drugs, oral antibiotic therapy may be needed for weeks or months. Clients and families must understand the complications of inadequate treatment or failure to follow-up with health care providers. Teach the client and family that antibiotic therapy must be continued over a long period of time to be effective. Even when symptoms of the disease appear to be improved, the full course of IV and oral antibiotics must be completed.

In addition to parenteral or oral drug administration, the wound may be irrigated, either continuously or intermittently, with one or more antibiotic solutions. Use sterile technique at all times. A technique in which beads are impregnated with an antibiotic and packed into the wound can provide direct contact of the antibiotic with the offending organism.

Medications are also needed to control pain. Clients experience acute and chronic pain, and must receive regimen drug therapy for control. Chapter 7 describes pharmacologic and nonpharmacologic interventions for both acute and chronic pain.

Infection Control. If an open wound or ulcer is present in the hospital or long-term care setting, the client's treatment usually includes standard precautions for limited infections in which the wound is covered. This practice may vary according to health care agency policy. Contact precautions are reserved for more severe infections, particularly when the purulent material cannot be adequately contained by a dressing. The open area is covered, and strict aseptic technique is used when dressings are changed to prevent further contamination. Wounds may be managed through the window of a cast, which must remain dry during dressing or irrigation procedures.

Hyperbaric Oxygen Therapy. A treatment to increase tissue perfusion for clients with chronic, unremitting osteomyelitis is the use of a hyperbaric chamber or portable device to administer hyperbaric oxygen (HBO) therapy. These devices are usually available in large teaching hospitals and may not be accessible to all clients who might benefit from them. With HBO therapy, the affected area is exposed to a high concentration of oxygen that diffuses into the tissues to promote healing. In conjunction with high-dose antibiotic therapy and surgical debridement, HBO has proved very useful in treating a number of anaerobic infections.

SURGICAL MANAGEMENT. Antibiotic therapy alone may not be sufficient to meet the goals of treatment. Surgical techniques are used to minimize the disfigurement that heretofore has been a devastating result of severe osteomyelitis. Most often, surgery is reserved for clients with chronic osteomyelitis.

Sequestrectomy. Because bone cannot heal in the presence of necrotic tissue, a sequestrectomy is performed to debride the infected bone and allow revascularization of tissue.

Bone Grafts. The excision of devitalized and infected bone often results in a sizable cavity, or bone defect. The use of cancellous bone grafts to obliterate bone defects began in the 1940s and is still widely used. One of the most popular surgical techniques is the Papineau procedure, or open cancellous bone graft, which is used primarily with large bone and soft-tissue defects.

The surgeon excises necrotic bone, grafts the bone, and covers the skin, if necessary. The donor bone is most often taken from the client's posterior ileum, but can be taken from other sites. If needed, the surgeon performs a skin graft, usually a simple split-thickness graft, often between 8 and 16 weeks after the bone graft.

Bone Segment Transfers. When infected bone is extensively resected, reconstruction with microvascular bone transfers may be useful. In general, a bone transfer is reserved for larger skeletal defects.

The most common donor sites are the client's fibula and iliac crest. The bone graft may have an attached muscle or skin flap, if necessary. The steps of the procedure are similar to those of cancellous grafting in that debridement precedes bone transfer.

Nursing care of the client after surgery is similar to that for any postoperative client (see Chapter 22). However, the important difference is that neurovascular (NV) assessments must be done frequently because the client experiences swelling after the surgical procedure. Elevate the affected extremity to increase venous return, and thus control swelling. Assess the client's NV status, including the following:

- Pain
- Movement
- Sensation
- Warmth
- Temperature
- Distal pulses
- Capillary refill (not as reliable as the above indicators)

Muscle Flaps. If the bony defect is relatively small, a muscle flap may be the only surgery required. Local muscle flaps are used in the treatment of chronic osteomyelitis when soft tissue does not obliterate the dead space, or cavity, resulting from bone debridement. The flap provides wound coverage and enhances blood flow to promote healing. A split-thickness skin graft is often applied several days after the muscle flap.

Amputation. When the previously described surgical procedures are not appropriate or successful, the affected limb may need to be amputated. The physical and psychological care for a client who has undergone an amputation is discussed in Chapter 55.

For all of the surgical procedures and their recovery phases, long-term antibiotic treatment is necessary. The preoperative and postoperative nursing care is similar to that for repair of musculoskeletal trauma.

Critical Thinking Challenge

An older adult has a history of type II diabetes and peripheral vascular disease. He was recently admitted to your medical unit with a draining foot ulcer. A blood culture reveals septicemia, and an MRI scan shows osteomyelitis. The client is placed on IV antibiotic therapy and analgesics for pain control. Today, his wife tells you that the doctor told her that her husband will be going home on IV antibiotics. She is angry that he has not taken better care of himself, and she doesn't know if she can take care of him at home because she is not well herself.

1. What is your best response to the client's wife at this time?
2. Who should you collaborate with when planning the client's discharge to home?
3. If the wife refuses to care for him at home, what options for care might he have?
4. What health teaching is needed for both the client and his wife after he is discharged?
5. What infection control measures will you use while he is hospitalized, and what measures will be necessary at home?

evolve For suggested answer guidelines, go to http://evolve.elsevier.com/Iggy/.

BONE TUMORS

Benign Bone Tumors

Benign (noncancerous) bone tumors are often asymptomatic and may be discovered on routine x-ray examination or as the cause of pathologic fractures. The cause of benign bone tumors is not known. Tumors may arise from several types of tissue. The major classifications include **chondrogenic** tumors (from cartilage), **osteogenic** tumors (from bone), and **fibrogenic** tumors (from fibrous tissue and found most often in children) (Table 54-4). As with other neoplasms, the cause of bone tumors is unknown. Although many specific benign tumors have been identified, only the common ones are described in the following sections.

CHONDROGENIC TUMORS
Osteochondroma

The most common benign bone tumor is the **osteochondroma**. Although its onset is usually in childhood, the tumor grows until skeletal maturity and may not be diagnosed until adulthood. The tumor may be a single growth or multiple growths and can occur in any bone. The femur and the tibia are most often involved.

On gross appearance, the tumor has a large cartilaginous cap with a bony stalk protruding from the bone. As the cap grows, the tumor ossifies (calcified) and may become malignant (cancerous). About 10% of osteochondromas change into sarcomas. Osteochondromas account for about 40% of all benign bone tumors and typically affect males more often than females.

Chondroma

The **chondroma,** or endochondroma, is closely related to the osteochondroma in histologic (cellular) presentation. Unlike the osteochondroma, however, the chondroma is a lesion of mature hyaline cartilage affecting primarily the hands and the feet. The ribs, the sternum, the spine, and the long bones may also be involved. Chondromas are slow growing and often cause pathologic fractures after minor injury.

Chondromas are found in people of all ages, occur in both males and females, and can affect any bone.

OSTEOGENIC TUMORS
Osteoid Osteoma

The **osteoid osteoma** is distinguished by its pinkish, granular appearance, resulting from the proliferation of osteoblasts. Unlike other tumors, a single lesion is usually less than 0.4

TABLE 54-4   Classification of Primary Bone Tumors

Benign	Malignant
Chondrogenic	***Chondrogenic***
Osteochondroma	Chondrosarcoma
Chondroma	
	Osteogenic
Osteogenic	Osteosarcoma
Osteoid osteoma	
Osteoblastoma	***Fibrogenic***
Giant cell tumor	Fibrosarcoma
	Unknown Origin
	Ewing's sarcoma

inch (1 cm) in diameter. Any bone can be affected, but the femur and the tibia are most often involved. When the osteoid osteoma occurs in the spinal column and sacrum, the clinical manifestations resemble those of the lumbar disk syndrome. The client complains of unremitting bone pain, probably attributable to the increase in prostaglandin levels associated with the tumor.

About 10% of all benign bone tumors are osteoid osteomas. The lesion occurs in children and young adults, with predominance among males.

Osteoblastoma

Often called *giant osteoid osteoma*, the **osteoblastoma** affects the vertebrae and long bones. The tumor is larger than the osteoid osteoma and lies in cancellous bone. Its reddish, granular appearance facilitates diagnosis.

The lesion accounts for less than 1% of primary bone tumors and affects adolescent boys and young adults of both genders.

Giant Cell Tumor

The origin of the **giant cell tumor** remains uncertain. This lesion is aggressive and can be extensive. On gross examination, the lesions are gray to reddish brown and may involve surrounding soft tissue. Although classified as benign, giant cell tumors can metastasize (spread) to the lung.

Unlike most other benign bone tumors, giant cell tumors affect women older than 20 years of age; the peak incidence occurs in clients in their 30s.

◆COLLABORATIVE MANAGEMENT
◆Assessment

PHYSICAL ASSESSMENT/CLINICAL MANIFESTATIONS

If a client experiences clinical manifestations of a benign bone tumor, pain is the most frequent complaint. The pain can range from mild to moderate, as seen with chondromas, to unremitting and intense, as is typical with osteoid osteomas. Pain can be caused by direct tumor invasion into soft tissue, compressing peripheral nerves, or by a resulting pathologic fracture.

In addition to collecting information regarding the nature of the client's pain, observe and palpate the suspected involved area. When the tumor affects the lower extremities or the small bones of the hands and feet, local swelling may be detected as the neoplasm enlarges. In some cases, muscle atrophy or muscle spasm may be present. Palpate the bone and muscle to detect these changes and elicit tenderness.

DIAGNOSTIC ASSESSMENT

Routine radiography and conventional tomography are extremely beneficial in localizing and visualizing neoplasms of the bone. Benign tumors are characterized by sharp margins, intact cortices, and smooth, uniform periosteal bone.

Computed tomography (CT) is less useful, except in complex anatomic areas, such as the spinal column and sacrum. The test is helpful in evaluating the extent of soft-tissue involvement.

When the diagnosis of a benign tumor is uncertain, an open or needle biopsy of the bone is performed. The open surgical method is preferred to obtain a sufficient amount of tissue.

Magnetic resonance imaging (MRI) may be especially helpful in viewing problems of the spinal column.

◆Interventions

The physician uses drug therapy and surgery in combination when possible. Nondrug pain relief measures are also used. Depending on the client's preference and tolerance, measures such as application of heat or cold may be helpful to relieve pain.

In addition to prescribing analgesics to reduce pain, the health care provider usually prescribes one or more nonsteroidal anti-inflammatory drugs (NSAIDs) to inhibit prostaglandin synthesis and thus relieve pain in the client with an osteoid osteoma. Observe for drug actions and side effects, administering the drug after meals or with milk and crackers.

The most common surgical procedure used for clients with benign bone tumors is curettage, or simple excision of the tumor tissue. If the tumor is small, surgery may not be indicated. When the lesion is extremely extensive, as in a giant cell tumor, the neoplasm is removed with care to restore or maintain the function of the adjacent joint, most often the knee. In some cases, the knee is replaced with a prosthetic device, and less often, is fused **(arthrodesis).** Bone grafting may be needed. The nursing care for clients undergoing these surgical procedures is discussed in Chapter 24.

Malignant Bone Tumors

Malignant bone tumors may be **primary** (those that originate in bone; see Table 54-4) or **secondary** (those that originate in other tissues and metastasize to bone). Primary tumors occur most often in people between 10 and 30 years of age and make up a small percentage of bone cancers. As for other forms of cancer, the exact cause of bone cancer is unknown. Metastatic lesions most often occur in the older age-group and account for most bone cancers.

Primary Tumors
OSTEOSARCOMA

Osteosarcoma, or osteogenic sarcoma, is the most common type of primary malignant bone tumor. More than 50% occur in the distal femur, followed in decreasing order of occurrence by the proximal tibia and humerus. Flat-bone and long-bone incidence is about equal in people older than 25 years of age.

The lesion is relatively large, causing pain and swelling of short duration. The involved area is usually warm, because the vascularity to the site increases. The central portion of the mass is sclerotic from increased osteoblastic activity; the periphery is soft, extending through the bone cortex in the classic sunburst appearance associated with the neoplasm. An inward expansion into the medullary canal is also common.

Osteosarcoma may be osteoblastic, chondroblastic, or fibroblastic, depending on the tissue of origin. Regardless of its source, the lesion typically metastasizes to the periphery of the lung within 2 years of treatment; metastasis usually results in death.

Osteosarcoma occurs more often in males than in females (2:1), between ages 10 and 30 years, and in older clients with Paget's disease. Clients who have received radiation for other forms of cancer or who have benign lesions are also at high risk.

EWING'S SARCOMA

Although **Ewing's sarcoma** is not as common as other tumors, it is the most malignant. Like other primary tumors, it causes pain and swelling. In addition, systemic manifestations, particularly low-grade fever, leukocytosis, and anemia, characterize the lesions. The pelvis and the lower extremity are most often affected. Pelvic involvement is a poor prognostic sign.

On a cellular level, the tumor is similar to bone lymphoma. On x-ray examination the characteristic mottled destructive pattern and "onion skin" appearance of the bone surface distinguish the neoplasm as Ewing's sarcoma. Like other malignant tumors, it is not encapsulated and often extends into soft tissue. Death results from metastasis to the lungs and other bones.

Five percent of all malignant bone tumors are Ewing's sarcoma. Although the tumor can be seen in clients of any age, it usually occurs in children and young adults in their 20s. Men are affected more often than women.

CHONDROSARCOMA

In contrast to the client with osteosarcoma, the client with **chondrosarcoma** experiences dull pain and swelling for a long period. The tumor typically affects the pelvis and proximal femur near the diaphysis. Arising from cartilaginous tissue, the lesion destroys bone and often calcifies. The client with chondrosarcoma usually has a better prognosis than the client with osteogenic sarcoma.

Chondrosarcoma occurs in middle-aged and older people, with a slight predominance in men, and accounts for fewer than 10% of all malignant bone tumors.

FIBROSARCOMA

Arising from fibrous tissue, **fibrosarcomas** can be divided into subtypes, of which malignant fibrous histiocytoma (MFH) is the most malignant. Most often, the clinical presentation of MFH is gradual, without specific symptoms. Local tenderness, with or without a palpable mass, occurs in the long bones of the lower extremity. As with other bone cancers, the lesion can metastasize to the lungs.

Although MFH affects people of all ages, it typically occurs in middle-aged men. Fortunately, the lesion is not common.

Metastatic Bone Disease

PATHOPHYSIOLOGY

Primary tumors of the prostate, breast, kidney, thyroid, and lung are called *bone-seeking* cancers; they metastasize to the bone more often than other primary tumors. The vertebrae, pelvis, femur, and ribs are the bone sites commonly affected. Simply stated, primary tumor cells, or seeds, are carried to bone through the bloodstream. Almost all metastatic lesions are of epithelial origin and begin in the bone marrow. **Pathologic fractures** are a major concern in man-

agement. The most commonly affected areas for fracture are the acetabulum and the proximal femur.

Metastatic bone tumors greatly outnumber primary malignant neoplasms. Metastatic bone disease primarily affects people older than 40 years of age. In clients with a history of cancer and local pain, metastasis is suspected. The incidence of bone metastasis ranges from 20% to 70%, depending on the statistical reporting source. It is suspected that the reported incidence of metastasis is grossly understated.

◆COLLABORATIVE MANAGEMENT
◆Assessment

HISTORY

The data collected for the client suspected of having a malignant tumor are similar to the data required for the client with a benign growth. In addition, ask whether the client has had previous radiation therapy for cancer and elicit information about the client's general health.

PHYSICAL ASSESSMENT/CLINICAL MANIFESTATIONS

The clinical manifestations seen in the client with a primary malignant tumor or metastatic disease vary, depending on the specific type of lesion. Most often, the client has a group of nonspecific complaints, including pain, local swelling, and a tender, palpable mass. Marked disability may be present in advanced metastatic bone disease.

In a client with Ewing's sarcoma, a low-grade fever may occur because of the systemic features of the neoplasm. For this reason, Ewing's sarcoma is often confused with osteomyelitis. Fatigue and pallor resulting from anemia are also common.

In performing a musculoskeletal assessment, inspect the involved area and palpate the mass for size characteristics and tenderness. The client's ability to perform mobility tasks and activities of daily living (ADLs) is also determined. If possible, observe the client performing mobility tasks and record the results on a functional assessment tool (see Chapter 10). The degree of disability can then be determined for comparison with later measurements after medical and nursing intervention.

PSYCHOSOCIAL ASSESSMENT

Often, clients with malignant bone tumors are young adults whose socially productive lives are just beginning. They need support systems to help cope with the diagnosis and its treatment. Family, significant others, and health care professionals are major components of the needed support. Determine what systems are available to clients.

Clients often experience a loss of control over their lives when a diagnosis of malignancy is made. As a result, they become anxious and fearful about the outcome of their illness. Coping with the diagnosis becomes a challenge. All clients go through the grieving process; initially, there is denial. Identify the anxiety level and assess the stage or stages of the grieving process. Explore any maladaptive behavior, indicating ineffective coping mechanisms. Chapter 28 further elaborates on the psychosocial assessment for clients with malignancy.

LABORATORY ASSESSMENT

The client with a primary malignant or metastatic bone tumor typically shows elevated serum alkaline phosphatase (ALP) levels, indicating the body's attempt to form new bone by increasing osteoblastic activity. The client with Ewing's sarcoma or metastatic bone lesions often has normocytic anemia. In addition, leukocytosis is common with Ewing's sarcoma. The progression of Ewing's sarcoma may be evaluated by elevated serum lactate dehydrogenase (LDH) levels.

In some clients with bone metastasis from the breast, kidney, or lung, the serum calcium level is elevated. Massive bone destruction stimulates release of the mineral into the bloodstream.

In clients with Ewing's sarcoma and bone metastasis, often the erythrocyte sedimentation rate (ESR) is elevated, which is probably attributable to secondary tissue inflammation.

RADIOGRAPHIC ASSESSMENT

As with benign bone tumors, routine x-rays and computed tomography (CT) allow for adequate visualization of malignant lesions. Although each tumor type has its own characteristic radiographic pattern, certain findings are common to all. Malignant tumors typically show poor margination, bone destruction, irregular periosteal new bone, and cortical breakthrough.

Metastatic lesions may increase or decrease bone density, depending on the amount of osteoblastic and osteoclastic activity. CT is helpful in determining the extent of soft-tissue damage.

OTHER DIAGNOSTIC ASSESSMENTS

The client may have magnetic resonance imaging and a bone scan. In some cases, a bone biopsy may be performed. After biopsy, the cancer is staged according to the grade of the tumor. One popular method is the TNM staging system, which uses determinations of *t*umor size, *n*odal involvement, and evidence of *m*etastasis.

Another surgical staging method is to correlate the tumor grade (high or low), tumor site (intracompartmental or extracompartmental), and presence of metastatic disease (positive or negative). Staging guides the health care team in their decision regarding treatment.

◆Analysis

COMMON NURSING DIAGNOSES AND COLLABORATIVE PROBLEMS

The following are priority nursing diagnoses for clients with malignant bone tumors:

1. Acute Pain and Chronic Pain related to physical injury (direct tumor invasion into soft tissue)
2. Anticipatory Grieving related to a change in body image or impending death
3. Disturbed Body Image related to the effects of illness treatment, including surgery

A primary collaborative problem is Potential for Fractures.

ADDITIONAL NURSING DIAGNOSES AND COLLABORATIVE PROBLEMS

In addition to the common nursing diagnoses and collaborative problems, clients with malignant bone tumors may have one or more of the following:

- Fear and Anxiety related to the medical diagnosis, possible disfiguring surgery, or impending death
- Ineffective Coping related to inadequate level of confidence in ability to cope
- Compromised Family Coping related to prolonged disease
- Dysfunctional Grieving related to actual loss
- Impaired Physical Mobility related to pain and musculoskeletal impairment
- Imbalanced Nutrition: Less Than Body Requirements related to an increased metabolic process
- Disturbed Sleep Pattern related to pain
- Self-Care Deficit (Total) related to impaired physical mobility and weakness
- Ineffective Role Performance related to a temporary or permanent inability to maintain the family or community role
- Spiritual Distress related to fear of death

◆Planning and Implementation

ACUTE PAIN; CHRONIC PAIN

NOC PLANNING: EXPECTED OUTCOMES. The client with a malignant bone tumor is expected to take personal actions to control pain. Indicators include that the client will consistently demonstrate the ability to:

- Recognize pain onset
- Use preventive measures
- Use analgesics appropriately
- Use nonanalgesic relief measures
- Report pain control

INTERVENTIONS. Because the pain is often due to direct tumor invasion, treatment is aimed at reducing the size of or removing the tumor. A combination of nonsurgical and surgical management is often used to promote client comfort and eliminate the complications of bone cancer.

NONSURGICAL MANAGEMENT. In addition to analgesics for local pain relief, chemotherapeutic agents and radiation therapy are often administered to cause tumor regression. In clients with vertebral metastatic disease, bracing and immobilization with cervical traction reduce back pain.

Drug Therapy. The physician may prescribe chemotherapy to be given alone or in combination with radiation or surgery. Certain proliferating tumors, such as Ewing's sarcoma, are sensitive to cytotoxic medications. Others, such as chondrosarcomas, are often totally drug resistant. Chemotherapy seems to work best for small, metastatic lesions and may be administered before or after surgery. For most tumors, the physician prescribes a combination of agents. At present, there is no universally accepted protocol of chemotherapeutic agents. The drugs selected are determined in part by the primary source of the cancer in metastatic disease. For example, when metastasis occurs from breast cancer, estrogens and progesterone may be used.

Observe the client carefully for side and toxic effects and monitors laboratory tests diligently. Chapter 28 discusses the nursing care associated with the administration of cytotoxic agents.

Radiation Therapy. Radiation is used for selected types of malignant tumors. For clients with Ewing's sarcoma and early osteosarcoma, radiation may be the treatment of choice in reducing tumor size and thus pain.

For clients with metastatic disease, radiation is given primarily for palliation. The therapy is directed toward the painful sites to provide a more comfortable life span. One or more treatments are given, depending on the extent of disease. With precise planning, radiation therapy can be used with minimal complications. The nursing care for clients receiving radiation therapy is described in Chapter 28.

SURGICAL MANAGEMENT. The treatment of primary bone tumors is surgery, often combined with radiation or chemotherapy.

Preoperative Care. Preoperatively, thoroughly evaluate the client to assist the physician in the selection of the surgical procedure to be performed. In addition to the nature, progression, and extent of the tumor, the client's age and general health state are taken into consideration. Chemotherapy may be administered preoperatively.

As for any client preparing for cancer surgery, the client with bone cancer needs psychological support from the nurse and other members of the health care team. Assess the level of understanding of the client and the family or significant others. As a client advocate, encourage the expression of concerns and questions and provide information regarding hospital routines and procedures. Spiritual support is important to some clients, who may prefer to contact their own clergy, rabbi, or spiritual leader or talk with the clergy affiliated with the hospital. Assist in arranging for spiritual assistance if needed.

Postoperative needs are anticipated and planned for as much as possible before the client undergoes surgery. Remind the client what to expect postoperatively and how to help ensure adequate recovery.

Operative Procedures. Wide or radical resection procedures are commonly performed for clients with bone sarcomas. Wide excision is removal of the lesion surrounded by an intact cuff of normal tissue and leads to cure of low-grade tumors only. A radical resection includes removal of the lesion, the entire muscle, bone, and other tissues directly involved. It is the only procedure adequate for high-grade tumors.

Bone defects that result from tumor removal include the following:

- Total joint replacements with prosthetic implants, either whole or partial
- Custom metallic implants
- Allografts from the iliac crest, rib, or fibula

As an alternative to total replacement, an allograft may be implanted with internal fixation for those clients who do not have metastases. This is a common procedure for sarcomas of the proximal femur. Allograft procedures for the knee are also performed, particularly in young adults. Preoperative chemotherapy is given to enhance the likelihood of success. **Allografts** with adjacent tendons and ligaments are harvested from cadavers and can be frozen or freeze-dried for a prolonged period. The graft is fixed with a series of bolts, screws, or plates. Observe for signs of hemorrhage, infection, or fracture.

For clients with metastatic disease, intractable pain is surgically treated with percutaneous **cordotomy** (cutting of the spinal nerve roots). **Cryosurgery** (cold application) may reduce pain and tumor size.

Postoperative Care. The surgical incision for a limb salvage procedure is often extensive. A pressure dressing with wound suction is typically maintained for several days.

The client who has undergone a limb salvage procedure has resulting impaired physical mobility and a self-care deficit. The nature and extent of the alterations depend on the location and extent of the surgery.

Promotion of Physical Mobility. Usually, muscle strengthening and range-of-motion (ROM) exercises begin immediately postoperatively and continue for at least a year. After upper extremity surgery, the client can engage in active-assistive exercises by using the opposite hand to help achieve motions such as forward flexion and abduction of the shoulder. Continuous passive motion (CPM) using a CPM machine may be initiated as early as the first postoperative day for either upper extremity or lower extremity procedures.

After lower extremity surgery, the emphasis is on strengthening the quadriceps muscles by using passive and active motion when possible. Maintaining muscle tone is an important prerequisite to weight bearing, which progresses from toe touch or partial weight bearing to full weight bearing by 3 months postoperatively.

The client who has had a bone graft has a plaster cast that remains in place for several months. Weight bearing is prohibited until there is evidence that the graft is incorporated into the adjacent bone tissue.

During the recovery phase, the client also needs assistance with activities of daily living (ADLs), particularly if the surgery involves the upper extremity. Assist if needed, but at the same time try to encourage the client to do as much as possible unaided.

Neurovascular Assessment. Surrounding tissues, including nerves and blood vessels, may be sacrificed during surgery. Vascular grafting is common, but the lost nerve is usually not replaced. Assess the neurovascular status of the affected extremity and its digits thoroughly and frequently. Splinting or casting of the limb may also cause neurovascular compromise and needs to be checked for proper placement.

Pelvic lesions, although not commonly seen, are also excised. Reconstruction generally entails bone fusion with muscle and nerve preservation. A hip spica cast or brace may be necessary until graft incorporation has occurred. The client may need a cane for ambulation.

The major complications peculiar to reconstructive surgery for which you should observe are superficial and deep wound infection, dislocation or loosening of the implants, and rapid neurovascular compromise. Report an increase in pain or temperature, or a rapid deterioration in circulatory status to the physician promptly.

Psychological Support. In addition to needing psychological help in coping with physical disabilities, the client may need help coping with the surgery and its effects postoperatively. Having identified the available support systems preoperatively, you can help mobilize them for use after surgery.

As a result of most of the surgical procedures, the client experiences an alteration in body image. Suggest ways to minimize cosmetic changes. For example, a lowered shoulder can be covered by a custom-made pad worn under clothing. The client can cover lower extremity defects with pants.

ANTICIPATORY GRIEVING

NOC PLANNING: EXPECTED OUTCOMES. The client with a malignant bone tumor is expected to adjust to actual or impending loss. Indicators include that the client will have the ability to:

- Resolve feelings about loss
- Verbalize reality of loss

- Discuss unresolved conflicts
- Seek social support
- Progress through stages of grief

INTERVENTIONS. The nurse's most important role is to be an active listener and to encourage the client and family or significant others to verbalize their feelings. Counselors and members of the clergy or spiritual leaders may provide additional assistance in promoting acceptance of the diagnosis, treatment, or, possibly, impending death. Chapter 9 provides information about death and dying.

Regardless of the prognosis, a diagnosis of bone cancer is a major stressor that causes the client and family or significant others to grieve. Help the client and others to cope with the loss and resolve the grief (Chart 54-6).

The nurse also acts as an advocate for the client and the family and often promotes the physician-client relationship. For instance, the client may not completely understand the medical or surgical treatment plan but may be hesitant to question the physician. The nurse's intervention increases communication, which is essential in successful management of the client with cancer.

DISTURBED BODY IMAGE

NOC **PLANNING: EXPECTED OUTCOMES.** The client with a malignant bone tumor is expected to experience a positive perception of his or her own appearance and body func-

tions. Indicators include that the client will have a consistently positive:
- Internal picture of self
- Satisfaction with body appearance
- Adjustment to changes in health status
- Adjustments to body changes due to surgery

INTERVENTIONS. The client's self-perception of body image is closely associated with his or her ability to accept the illness. Recognize and accept the client's view about the body image alteration. A trusting nurse-client relationship allows the client freedom to verbalize negative feelings. Emphasize the client's strengths and remaining capabilities. Establish realistic mutual goals regarding lifestyle (see Chart 54-6).

POTENTIAL FOR FRACTURES

PLANNING: EXPECTED OUTCOMES. As with other bone diseases in which pathologic fracture is a possible complication (e.g., osteoporosis), the client with a malignant bone tumor is expected to avoid falls and minimize trauma to prevent fractures. In people with metastatic bone disease, fractures occur more readily and are not as preventable because of resulting destructive bone resorption. A more realistic outcome for people with metastatic disease, then, may be that the client's pain will be minimized through treatment of the fracture.

INTERVENTIONS. Radiation or surgery may be required to reinforce or replace the diseased bone to prevent fracture. In recent years, surgical techniques have also been improved for fracture fixation.

NONSURGICAL MANAGEMENT. Newer techniques in radiation therapy have improved the incidence of bone healing for actual and impending pathologic fractures. To improve muscle tone and, consequently, to reduce the risk for fracture, the client performs strengthening exercises. Physical therapy on an ambulatory basis is commonly prescribed.

One of two bisphosphonates, zoledronic acid (Zometa) and pamidronate (Aredia), may be used to inhibit bone resorption and subsequent hypercalcemia. Both medications are given by IV infusion and place clients at risk for flulike symptoms, hypokalemia, hypomagnesemia, and hypophosphatemia. Inform clients that osteonecrosis of the jaw may also occur, especially in those who have dental procedures (Aschenbrenner, 2005).

SURGICAL MANAGEMENT. The principles of surgery for metastatic fractures include the following:
- Replacing as much defective bone as possible
- Being thorough in technique to avoid a second procedure
- Aiming to return the client to a functional state with a minimum of hospitalization and immobilization

Fractures of the proximal femur are very common. Prosthetic replacement reinforced with polymethylmethacrylate ("bone glue") is preferred over open reduction with internal fixation (ORIF) when feasible. The surgeon uses intramedullary rods and compression screws for more distal fractures. Prophylactic fixation may be indicated for microscopic fractures that cause chronic pain. Chapter 55 discusses the nursing management for clients undergoing repair of a fractured hip.

Community-Based Care

After medical treatment for a primary malignant tumor, the client is usually managed at home with follow-up care. The client with metastatic disease may remain in the home or,

---

CHART 54-6

NIC **INTERVENTION ACTIVITIES for**
The Client with Bone Cancer (Psychosocial Care)

Grief Work Facilitation: *Assistance with the resolution of a significant loss*
- Identify the loss.
- Assist the client to identify the nature of the attachment to the lost object or person.
- Assist the client to identify the initial reaction to the loss.
- Encourage expression of feelings about the loss.
- Instruct in phases of the grieving process, as appropriate.
- Support progression through personal grieving stages.
- Include significant others in discussion and decisions, as appropriate.
- Assist client to identify personal coping strategies.
- Communicate acceptance of discussing loss.
- Identify sources of community support.
- Reinforce progress made in the grieving process.
- Assist in identifying modifications needed in lifestyle.

Body Image Enhancement: *Improving a client's conscious and unconscious perceptions and attitudes toward his/her body*
- Assist client to discuss changes caused by illness or surgery, as appropriate.
- Help client determine the extent of actual changes in the body or its level of functioning.
- Assist client to determine the influence of a peer group on the client's perception of present body image.
- Identify the effects of the client's culture, religion, race, sex, and age in terms of body image.
- Monitor whether client can look at the changed body part.
- Determine if a change in body image has contributed to increased social isolation.
- Assist client to identify actions that will enhance appearance.
- Identify support groups available to client.

when home support is not available, may be admitted to a long-term care facility for extended or hospice care. A case manager may assist with management of the client's care.

HOME CARE MANAGEMENT

In collaboration with the occupational therapist, evaluate the client's home environment for structural barriers that may hinder mobility. The client may be discharged with a cast, crutches, or a wheelchair.

Accessibility to eating and toileting facilities is essential to promote independence. Because the client with metastatic disease is susceptible to pathologic fractures, potential hazards that may contribute to falls or injury should be removed.

HEALTH TEACHING

For the client receiving intermittent chemotherapy on an ambulatory basis, emphasize the importance of keeping appointments. Review the expected, side, and toxic effects of the medications with the client. Teach the client how to treat minor side effects and when to alert the health care provider. If the drugs are administered at home via long-term IV catheter, explain the care involved with daily dressing changes and potential catheter complications. Chapter 17 describes the health teaching required for a client receiving infusion therapy at home.

The client receiving radiation therapy is also taught the importance of keeping appointments and recognizing the complications of treatment. Review interventions that can be used at home for minor complications.

If the client has undergone surgery, he or she has a wound and limited mobility. Teach the client, family, and/or significant others how to care for the wound. Help the client learn how to perform activities of daily living (ADLs) and mobility activities independently. Physical and occupational therapists assist in ADL teaching and provide or recommend assistive and adaptive devices if necessary. The physical therapist also teaches the proper use of ambulatory aids, such as crutches, and exercises.

Pain management can be a major problem, particularly in the client with metastatic bone disease. Discuss the various options for pain relief, including relaxation and music therapy. Emphasize the importance of those techniques that worked during hospitalization.

The client with bone cancer typically fears that the malignancy will return. Acknowledge this fear, but reinforces confidence in the health care team and medical treatment chosen.

Realistic goals regarding return to work, recreational activities, and so forth are mutually established. Encourage the client to resume a functional lifestyle, but caution that it should be gradual. Certain activities, such as participating in sports, may be prohibited.

The client with advanced metastatic bone disease needs to prepare for death. The nurse and other support personnel assist the client through the stages of death and dying (see Chapter 9). Identify resources that can help the client write a will, visit with distant family members, or do whatever he or she thinks is needed to die in peace. In the later stages of the disease, hospice care may be an option. Nurses working in this area of care can be most helpful in managing end-of-life care.

HEALTH CARE RESOURCES

In addition to family and significant others, cancer support groups are helpful to the client with bone cancer. Some or-

ganizations, such as I Can Cope, provide information and emotional support; others, such as CanSurmount, are geared more toward client and family education.

The hospital staff nurse, discharge planner, or case manager also ensures that follow-up care, including nursing care and physical or occupational therapy, is available in the home. The client with terminal cancer may choose to become part of a hospice program (see Chapter 9).

◆Evaluation: Outcomes

Evaluate the care of the client with a malignant bone tumor on the basis of the identified nursing diagnoses and collaborative problems. The expected outcomes may include that the client will:

- Demonstrate ability to control pain
- Adjust to actual or impending loss
- Experience positive perception of own appearance and body function

Specific indicators for these outcomes are listed for each nursing diagnosis and collaborative problem under the Planning and Implementation section (see earlier).

DISORDERS OF THE HAND

Carpal Tunnel Syndrome

PATHOPHYSIOLOGY

Carpal tunnel syndrome (CTS) is a common condition in which the median nerve in the wrist becomes compressed, causing pain and numbness. The carpal tunnel is a rigid canal lying between the carpal bones and a fibrous tissue sheet called the flexor retinaculum. As seen in Figure 54-4, a group of nine tendons enveloped by synovium share space with the median nerve in the carpal tunnel. When the synovium becomes swollen or thickened, the nerve is compressed.

The median nerve supplies the motor, sensory, and autonomic function for the first three digits of the hand and the palmar aspect of the fourth digit. Because of the median nerve's proximity to other structures, wrist flexion causes nerve impingement against the flexor retinaculum; extension causes increased pressure in the distal portion of the carpal tunnel.

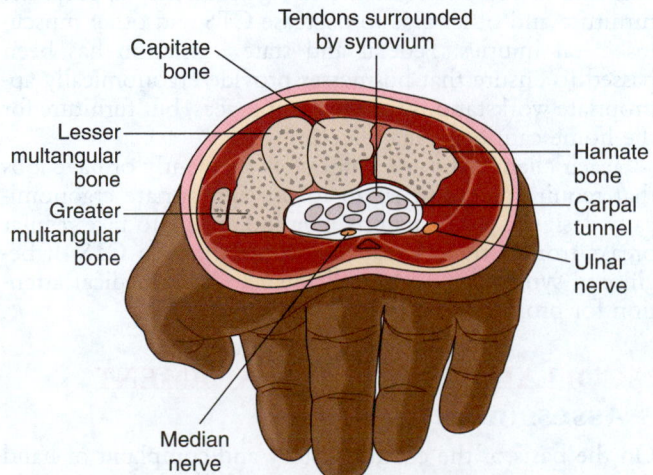

Figure 54-4 ■ Anatomy of the carpal tunnel.

Etiology and Genetic Risk

CTS usually presents as a chronic problem; acute cases are rare. Excessive hand exercise, edema or hemorrhage into the carpal tunnel, or thrombosis of the median artery can lead to acute CTS. Clients with a Colles' fracture of the wrist or hand burns are particularly at risk for rapid CTS development.

In most cases, however, the causative factors may not result in neurologic deficit for years. CTS is a common complication of certain metabolic and connective tissue diseases. For example, **synovitis** (inflammation of the synovium) occurs in clients with rheumatoid arthritis. The hypertrophied synovium compresses the median nerve. In other chronic disorders such as diabetes mellitus, inadequate blood supply can cause median nerve neuropathy, or dysfunction, resulting in CTS.

CTS is the most **common repetitive strain injury (RSI)—** the fastest growing type of occupational injury. People whose jobs require repetitive hand activities involving pinch or grasp during wrist flexion, such as factory workers, computer operators, and jackhammer operators, are predisposed to CTS. CTS can also result from overuse in sports activities such as golf, tennis, or racquetball.

In a few cases, CTS may be a familial or congenital problem, manifesting in adulthood. Space-occupying lesions, such as ganglia, tophi, and lipomas, can also result in nerve compression.

Incidence/Prevalence

CTS occurs in adults of all ages but peaks between ages 30 and 60 years of age. Women are five times more likely to experience the problem than men. Most often, CTS affects the dominant hand, but it can occur in both hands simultaneously. Children and adolescents are also beginning to experience CTS as a result of the increased use of computers in everyday life.

HEALTH PROMOTION/ILLNESS PREVENTION

Many businesses have recognized the hazards of repetitive motion as a primary cause of occupational injury and disability. Both men and women in the labor force are experiencing increasing numbers of repetitive strain injuries (RSIs). Occupational health nurses have played an important role in the development of ergonomically appropriate furniture and other aids to decrease CTS and other musculoskeletal injuries. Federal and state legislation has been passed to ensure that businesses provide ergonomically appropriate workstations for their employees, but furniture for the home cannot be mandated.

Teach clients who use computers frequently or have jobs that require repetitive strain to use appropriate ergonomically designed work stations. Remind clients to take regular breaks from activities that predispose them to CTS. If beginning symptoms occur, tell them to seek medical attention for prompt, early treatment.

◆COLLABORATIVE MANAGEMENT
◆Assessment

On the basis of the client's history and complaint of hand pain and numbness, a medical diagnosis is often made without further assessment. Question clients regarding the na-

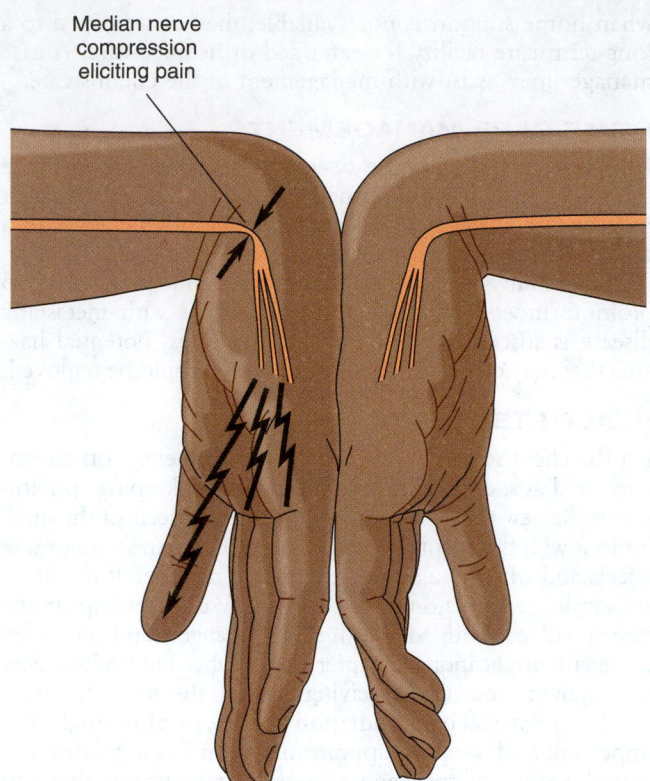

Median nerve compression eliciting pain

Figure 54-5 ■ Phalen's maneuver for detection of carpal tunnel syndrome.

ture, intensity, and location of the pain. Clients often state that the pain is worse at night as a result of flexion or direct pressure during sleep. The pain may radiate to the arm, the shoulder and neck, or the chest.

In addition to the complaint of numbness, clients with carpal tunnel syndrome (CTS) may also experience **paresthesia** (painful tingling). Sensory changes usually precede motor manifestations by weeks or months.

PHYSICAL ASSESSMENT/CLINICAL MANIFESTATIONS

The health care provider performs several tests to elicit abnormal sensory findings. Phalen's wrist test, sometimes called **Phalen's maneuver,** produces paresthesia in the median nerve distribution (palmar side of the thumb, index, and middle finger, and radial half of the ring finger) within 60 seconds. The client is asked to relax the wrist into flexion or place the back of the hands together and flex both wrists simultaneously (Figure 54-5). Most clients with CTS have a positive Phalen's test result.

The same sensation can be elicited by tapping lightly over the area of the median nerve in the wrist **(Tinel's sign).** If the test is unsuccessful, a blood pressure cuff can be placed on the upper arm and inflated to the client's systolic pressure. The result is often pain and tingling.

Motor changes begin with a weak pinch, clumsiness, and difficulty with fine movements and then progress to muscle weakness and wasting. The nurse may test for pinching ability and ask the client to perform a fine-movement task, such as threading a needle. Strenuous hand activity worsens the subjective complaints.

In addition to inspecting for muscle atrophy and task performance, observe the wrist for swelling. Palpate the area and note unusual findings. Autonomic changes may be evidenced by skin discoloration, nail changes (e.g., brittleness), and increased or decreased palmar sweating.

DIAGNOSTIC ASSESSMENT

Routine x-rays are ordered to visualize bone changes, space-occupying lesions, and synovitis. If these causative factors are not suspected, a client with CTS may not have x-rays done.

The health care provider may order electromyography (EMG), magnetic resonance imaging (MRI), or ultrasonography when a definitive diagnosis is uncertain. Problems of the cervical spine and spinal nerves can mimic the clinical manifestations of CTS. EMG testing reveals nerve dysfunction before muscle atrophy is observed. MRI is very useful for helping to diagnose CTS. The most common finding is an enlarged median nerve within the carpal tunnel. The newest technique for diagnosis is the use of ultrasound.

◆Interventions

The health care provider uses conservative measures before surgical intervention. With either type of treatment, however, CTS can recur.

NONSURGICAL MANAGEMENT. Drug therapy and immobilization of the wrist are the major components of nonsurgical management. Teach the client the importance of these modalities in the hope of preventing surgical intervention.

The most commonly prescribed drugs for the relief of pain and inflammation, if present, are nonsteroidal anti-inflammatory drugs (NSAIDs). In addition to or instead of systemic medications, the physician may inject corticosteroids directly into the carpal tunnel. If the client responds to the medication, several additional weekly or monthly injections are given. As with any medication, monitor the effects of drug therapy. NSAIDs are given with or after meals to reduce gastric irritation.

A splint may be used to immobilize the wrist during the day, during the night, or both. Many clients experience temporary relief with splinting. The occupational therapist places the wrist in the neutral position or in slight extension. Even when a splint is not used, instruct the client to minimize hand activities, at least temporarily.

SURGICAL MANAGEMENT. Surgery is necessary in about half of clients with CTS. Surgery can relieve the pressure on the median nerve by providing nerve decompression.

Preoperative Care. The nurse in the physician's office or same-day surgical center reinforces the teaching provided by the surgeon regarding the nature of the surgery. Postoperative care is reviewed so that the client knows what to expect.

Operative Procedures. The two most common surgeries are the open carpal tunnel release (OCTR) and the newer endoscopic carpal tunnel release (ECTR). When CTS is a complication of rheumatoid arthritis, a **synovectomy** (removal of excess synovium) through a small inner-wrist incision may resolve the problem. Removal of a space-occupying lesion, if present, also decompresses the nerve. Whatever the cause of nerve compression, the physician removes it either by cutting or by the newer laser technique. In some cases, CTS recurs months to years after surgery.

An alternative to OCTR is the endoscopic release. The surgeon makes a very small incision (less than $\frac{1}{2}$ inch [1.2 cm]) through which the endoscope is inserted. The surgeon then uses special instruments, which may include a laser, to free the trapped median nerve.

Postoperative Care. Although ECTR is less invasive and costs less than the open procedure, the client may experience pain and numbness for a longer time postoperatively as compared with recovery from OCTR. Major surgical complications are rare following CTS surgery.

After surgery, monitor vital signs and check the dressing carefully for drainage and tightness. If the endoscopic procedure has been performed, the dressing is very small. The surgeon may require that the client's hand and arm be elevated above heart level for several days to reduce swelling from surgery. Check the neurovascular status of the digits every hour during the immediate postoperative period, encouraging the client to move all fingers of the affected hand frequently. Offer pain medication and assure the client that he or she will be given a prescription for analgesics for use at home during recovery.

Hand movements, including lifting heavy objects, may be restricted for 4 to 6 weeks after surgery. The client can expect weakness and discomfort for weeks or perhaps months. Teach the client to report any changes in neurovascular status.

The client must realize that the surgical procedure might not be a cure. For instance, synovitis may recur in the client with rheumatoid arthritis and may recompress the median nerve. Multiple operations and other treatments are not uncommon with CTS.

The client may need assistance with routine daily tasks or even self-care activities during recovery. Ensure the client that assistance in the home should be available; this is usually provided by the family or significant others.

❓ Critical Thinking Challenge

You are a nurse working for a large factory in an urban area. One of the employees comes to you complaining of pain and tingling in his right hand, and he is right-handed. He has been working at the factory for 37 years and has worked every piece of equipment there during that period. He is upset that "this place" doesn't care about its workers and makes them work too long in one station without adequate breaks. He plans to file a complaint for worker's compensation and notify the local Occupational Safety and Health board to report this problem.

1. What history questions should you ask him at this time?
2. What physical assessment findings would you expect and why?
3. What options does he have for management of his health problem?
4. How should you respond to his perception regarding the employer's lack of caring for its employees?

evolve For suggested answer guidelines, go to http://evolve.elsevier.com/Iggy/.

Dupuytren's Contracture

Dupuytren's contracture, or deformity, is a slowly progressive contracture of the palmar fascia, resulting in flexion of the fourth or fifth digit of the hand. The third digit is occasionally affected. Although Dupuytren's contracture is a fairly common problem, the cause is unknown. It usually occurs in older men, tends to occur in families, and can be bilateral.

When function becomes impaired, surgical release is required. A partial or selective fasciectomy (removal of fascia) is performed. After removal of the dressing and drain, a splint may be used. Nursing care is similar to that for the client with carpal tunnel repair.

Ganglion

A **ganglion** is a round, cystlike lesion, often overlying a wrist joint or tendon. The synovium surrounding the tendon degenerates, allowing the tendon sheath tissue to become weak and distended. Ganglia are painless on palpation, but they can cause joint discomfort after prolonged joint use or minor trauma, such as a strain. The lesion can disappear and then recur. Ganglia are most likely to develop in people between 15 and 50 years of age.

Although the fluid within the lesion can be aspirated, total excision is preferred. The postoperative care is the same as that for the client undergoing other hand surgery.

DISORDERS OF THE FOOT

Hallux Valgus

The **hallux valgus** deformity, sometimes referred to as a bunion, is a common foot problem. The great toe deviates laterally at the metatarsophalangeal (MTP) joint (Figure 54-6). Although hallux valgus is often congenital, it can occur as a result of arthritis or poorly fitted shoes. As the deviation worsens, the bony prominence enlarges and causes pain, particu-

larly when shoes are worn. Women are affected more often than men.

The surgical procedure, a simple **bunionectomy,** involves removal of the bony overgrowth and bursa. When other toe deformities accompany the condition or if the bony overgrowth is large, several osteotomies, or bone resections, may be performed. Fusions may also be performed. Screws or wires are often inserted to stabilize the bones during the healing process. If both feet are affected, one foot is usually treated at a time. Most clients are allowed partial weight bearing while wearing an orthopedic boot or shoe.

Hammertoe

Often clients have hammertoes and hallux valgus deformities simultaneously. As shown in Figure 54-7, a **hammertoe** is the dorsiflexion of any MTP joint with plantar flexion of the adjacent proximal interphalangeal (PIP) joint. The second toe is most often affected. As the deformity worsens, corns may develop on the dorsal side of the toe and calluses may appear on the plantar surface. Clients are uncomfortable when wearing shoes and walking.

Hammertoe is often treated by surgical correction of the deformity with **osteotomies** (bone resections) and the insertion of wires or screws for fixation. The postoperative course is similar to that for the client with hallux valgus repair. The client uses crutches until full weight bearing is allowed several weeks postoperatively.

Morton's Neuroma

In the client with **Morton's neuroma,** or plantar digital neuritis, a small tumor grows in a digital nerve of the foot. The client usually describes the pain as an acute, burning sensa-

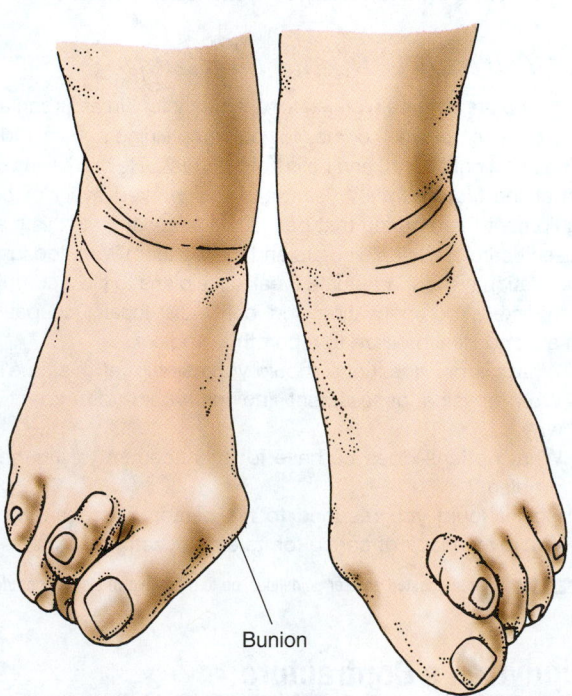

Figure 54-6 ■ Appearance of hallux valgus with a bunion.

Bunion

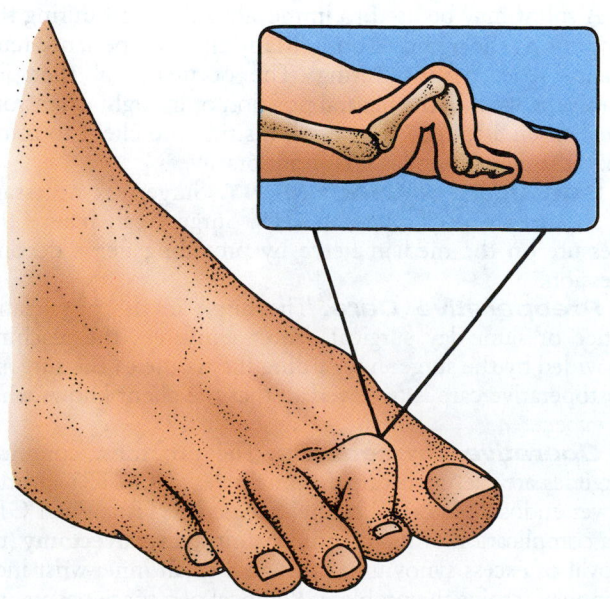

Figure 54-7 ■ Hammertoe of the second metatarsophalangeal joint.

tion in the web space. The pain involves the entire surface of the third and fourth toes.

Treatment involves surgical removal of the neuroma and application of a pressure dressing. Ambulation is usually permitted immediately after surgery.

Tarsal Tunnel Syndrome

Tarsal tunnel syndrome is the ankle version of carpal tunnel syndrome (CTS). The posterior tibial nerve in the ankle becomes compressed, resulting in loss of sensation and pain in a portion of the foot. Typically, the median and lateral plantar branches, which supply the sole of the foot and the distal phalanges, are affected by the nerve compression. Diagnosis and treatment are similar to those for CTS.

Plantar Fasciitis

Plantar fasciitis is an inflammation of the plantar fascia, which is located in the area of the arch of the foot. It is often seen in middle-aged and older adults, as well as in athletes, especially runners. In ambulatory care settings, plantar fasciitis accounts for 10% of running injuries. Obesity is also a contributing factor.

Clients complain of pain in the arch of the foot, especially when getting out of bed. The pain is worsened with weight bearing. Although most clients experience unilateral plantar fasciitis, the problem can affect both feet.

More than 90% of clients respond to conservative management, which includes rest, ice, stretching exercises, strapping of the foot to maintain the arch, shoes with good support, and orthotics. Nonsteroidal anti-inflammatory drugs (NSAIDs) or steroids may be needed to control pain and inflammation. If conservative measures are unsuccessful, endoscopic surgery to remove the inflamed tissue may be required.

Nursing care involves teaching the client about the importance of complying with the treatment plan and coordinating care with the physical therapist for instruction in exercise.

Other Problems of the Foot

Table 54-5 cites other common foot problems. Although clients are usually not hospitalized for these conditions, the nurse may recognize a foot disorder and alert the physician.

OTHER DISORDERS OF THE SKELETON

Scoliosis
PATHOPHYSIOLOGY

In early scoliosis, changes in muscles and ligaments on the concave side of the spinal column occur. These structures shorten and over time progressive deformity of the vertebra result. The vertebra rotate, begin to compress, and the spinal column begins to move into a lateral curve, a condition known as **scoliosis** (see Figure 53-3). As the degree of curvature increases, damage to the vertebral bodies occurs. The degree of the curvature increases during periods of growth, such as in adolescence. Curvature of greater than 50 degrees results in an unstable spine and curvature of greater than 60

degrees in the thoracic spine results in compromise of cardiopulmonary function.

The exact cause of scoliosis is not well understood. The process may result from some deviation in the balance mechanism located in the central nervous system. Females are affected more often than males and onset is often in adolescence. Children are screened for scoliosis during the middle school years. Information about caring for children with scoliosis is presented in most pediatric nursing textbooks.

Three types of scoliosis can be described: congenital, neuromuscular, and idiopathic. Congenital scoliosis occurs during embryonic development. Neuromuscular scoliosis can result from a neuromuscular condition in childhood or adulthood, such as cerebral palsy or spinal cord tumors. Idiopathic scoliosis is the most common form of scoliosis and results from no known cause.

Scoliosis can be further classified as structural or nonstructural. Nonstructural scoliosis results from a cause outside the spine itself, such as a leg length discrepancy. Structural scoliosis follows some deviation of the spinal column.

◆ **COLLABORATIVE MANAGEMENT**
◆ **Assessment**

Complete history of the client with spinal deformity should include onset of problem, in adolescence or adulthood and what treatments may be been used in the past. Clients who experienced surgery for scoliosis during adolescence are returning with progressive, debilitating back pain from degenerative disk disease below the fusion. A loss of lumbar curvature, or **lordosis**, described as "flat back" syndrome, may be present. A thorough pain assessment must be completed for those clients presenting with complaint of back pain.

The client is observed from the front and back, while standing and during forward flexion from the hips. Physical examination reveals asymmetry of hip and shoulder height, prominence of the thoracic ribs and scapula on one side, and visible curve in the spinal column. Observation from the side may reveal kyphosis of the thoracic spine. Leg length discrepancy must be ruled out.

TABLE 54-5 Treatment of Common Foot Problems

Description/Cause	Treatment
Corn Induration and thickening of the skin caused by friction and pressure, painful conical mass	Surgical removal by podiatrist
Callus Flat, poorly defined mass on the sole over a bony prominence caused by pressure	Padding and lanolin creams; overall good skin hygiene
Ingrown Nail Nail sliver penetration of the skin, causing inflammation	Removal of sliver by podiatrist; warm soaks; antibiotic ointment
Hypertrophic Ungual Labium Chronic hypertrophy of nail lip caused by improper nail trimming; results from untreated ingrown nail	Surgical removal of necrotic nail and skin; treatment of secondary infection

◆Interventions

Methods of treating adult scoliosis differ from those used for children. The adult spinal column is less flexible and therefore less likely to respond to exercises, weight reduction, bracing, and casting for correction of the deformity. In the adult, the disorder is progressive and can result in an additional one degree of deviation each year.

Adults with less than 50 degrees of curvature of the spine may be treated conservatively but those with greater than 50 degrees of curvature may require surgical intervention. The procedure consists of surgical fusion and insertion of instrumentation or rods to stabilize the spine. The surgeon performs spinal fusion by packing cancellous bone chips, usually from the iliac crest, between the affected vertebrae for support and stabilization. Both an anterior and a posterior approach may be needed. If so, the surgeon may perform both procedures during the same operative day or may stage them 7 to 10 days apart. The metal instrumentation supports the spine and immobilizes the fused area during healing.

The nursing care of the client undergoing corrective surgery for scoliosis is similar to that for the client undergoing a laminectomy or spinal fusion (see Chapter 46). Some procedures may require several days of immobilization postoperatively while other procedures allow the client to begin mobility the next day after surgery. A thoracolumbosacral orthosis (TLSO) is typically used to support the vertebral column (see Figure 54-2).

The client usually returns to work in about 3 weeks and can resume activities such as swimming and bicycling. Recreational sports, such as tennis, are usually resumed in 6 weeks. Other surgical procedures may prevent the client from performing these activities until 3 to 6 months postoperatively.

Osteogenesis Imperfecta

Osteogenesis imperfecta (OI) is a rare genetic disorder in which the bones are fragile and fracture easily resulting in bone deformity. The pathophysiology of the disease involves errors in synthesis of collagen, a connective tissue. OI is described by the Sillence classification system. The Sillence system describes four types of OI based on inheritance as autosomal dominant or autosomal recessive and clinical findings of each type. Types I and IV are more mild manifestations of the disease and can persist into adulthood. Types II and III are more severe and can result in fractures in utero, during the birth process, or in early childhood. Types II and III are associated with a high mortality rate.

Clinical manifestations include osteoporosis, history of multiple fractures, bony deformity, and poor skeletal development. Blue sclerae; soft, brownish teeth; and hearing loss may also be found upon assessment. Serum alkaline phosphatase will be elevated. In children with milder types of OI, child abuse is often considered until the diagnosis of OI can be made.

The treatment is palliative, and the client's life span is often shortened. The physician prescribes steroids, calcium, vitamin C, and, possibly, sodium fluoride. Physical therapy, casting or bracing, and telescoping intramedullary rods are used to maintain mobility and promote ambulation if possible. Research is ongoing in the use of bisphosphonates for treatment of OI. The nurse refers the client to the Osteogenesis Imperfecta Foundation in the United States or to the Brittle Bones Society in other countries for information and support.

MUSCULAR DISEASES

Progressive Muscular Dystrophies

PATHOPHYSIOLOGY

At least nine types of **muscular dystrophy (MD)** have been clinically identified. They can be broadly categorized as slowly progressive or rapidly progressive. The slowly progressive types are most commonly seen in adults. Most pediatric nursing books describe the care for clients with MD in detail. Five forms of MD are often seen in adults. Each type has its own distinct characteristics and causes, but all are progressive (Table 54-6).

The exact pathophysiologic mechanisms are unknown, but three theories have been advocated. The vascular theory suggests that a lack of blood flow causes the typical degeneration of muscle tissue seen in MD. Microscopic necrotic areas in atrophied muscle tissue support this hypothesis, although this finding does not explain the marked degree of degeneration often seen in the disease.

The neurogenic theory proposes a disturbance in nerve-muscle interaction. Research has failed, however, to locate the nature of the disturbance.

The most popular belief is the membrane theory. This theory suggests that cell membranes are genetically altered, causing a compromise in cell integrity. An increase in the activity of muscle proteolytic enzymes may accompany the membrane alteration, leaving the muscle cell vulnerable to degeneration. Increased enzyme activity has been documented in the client with atrophied muscles.

The cause of MD is unknown, but there may be a genetic influence for most of the major types. Some forms of MD are transmitted as autosomal dominant or recessive traits, whereas others are sex linked.

The most commonly occurring type of MD is the severe X-linked recessive variety initially described by Guillaume Duchenne in 1868. Each year, 20 to 33 cases are reported per 100,000 live male births. In an X-linked recessive disorder, one half of the male children of an unaffected mother, or carrier, manifest the disease. Becker's dystrophy is also inherited in an X-linked recessive manner, but it is less common than Duchenne's dystrophy. The other types of MD seen in adults can occur in either gender.

◆COLLABORATIVE MANAGEMENT

Diagnosis of MD is often difficult because the clinical manifestations are similar to those of other muscular disorders. Muscle biopsy often confirms the diagnosis. Muscle weakness and trophic changes are characteristic of all types of MD. Serum muscle enzyme values may be elevated, and electromyographic (EMG) findings are often abnormal.

Management of the client with MD is supportive and involves the entire health care team. Physical and occupational therapy helps the client maintain as much function and independence as possible. Major organ or body system involvement is medically managed, but the life span is often short-

TABLE 54-6 Differential Features of Common Muscular Dystrophies

Onset	Genetics	Clinical Manifestations	Progression
Duchenne (Severe X-Linked) Dystrophy			
18 mo-4 yr	Sex-linked recessive; expression in males	Symmetric pelvic and shoulder girdle muscle weakness; waddling gait; cardiac involvement common; mental retardation in one third of clients	Severely progressive, leading to inability to walk between 7 and 11 yr of age; death from cardiac or respiratory failure in 20s or 30s
Becker (Benign X-Linked) Dystrophy			
5-25 yr	Sex-linked recessive; expression in males	Wasting of pelvic and shoulder muscles; normal cardiac and mental function	Gradual progression; inability to walk 25 yr after onset; usually normal life span
Limb-Girdle Dystrophy			
Usually 20s or 30s	Usually autosomal dominant; expression in either gender	Upper extremity and neck muscles and lower extremity and hip muscle weakness	Extremely variable; severe disability within 10-20 yr after onset; life span shortened by 10-20 yr
Facioscapulohumeral (Landouzy-Dejerine) Dystrophy			
Usually in 20s	Autosomal dominant; expression in either gender	Facial and shoulder girdle muscle involvement	Usually benign; normal life span
Myotonic (Steinert) Dystrophy			
Birth to 40s	Autosomal dominant; expression in either gender	Muscle atrophy with multiple organ involvement (e.g., heart, lungs, smooth muscle, and endocrine system)	Usually gradual if onset in adulthood

ened from these manifestations of the disease. With the exception of prednisone, no drug has been found to slow the progression of the disorder, although immunosuppressive agents, anabolic steroids, and growth factors have been tried.

An experimental treatment, myoblast transfer therapy (MTT), has been supported by the Food and Drug Administration (FDA). MTT involves injections of healthy muscle cells (myoblasts) taken from a donor and multiplied in a laboratory. The cells are then given to the client with MD, where they theoretically fuse with each other and the recipient's unhealthy muscle cells. Effective gene therapy may also be an option for curing MD in the future.

Nursing interventions focus on making the client as comfortable as possible and reinforcing techniques and exercises taught in the physical therapy program. The nurse's role in caring for a client with cardiac or other organ involvement is the same as for any client with dysfunction of these areas.

Other Muscular Disorders

Most muscular disorders are classified as neuromuscular disorders, such as myasthenia gravis, or as connective tissue diseases, such as polymyositis. Therefore these disorders are discussed in Chapters 47 and 24, respectively.

GET READY for the NCLEX Examination!

KEY POINTS

Safe Effective Care Environment

- Assess clients with osteoporosis for risk for falls; fractures are common in these clients.

- Use strict aseptic technique when caring for clients with an open wound associated with osteomyelitis.
- Differentiate key features of acute and chronic osteomyelitis as listed in Chart 54-5; acute osteomyelitis can lead to bacteremia, a potentially life-threatening complication.
- For clients who have surgery for bone cancer, report postoperative manifestations of infection, dislocation, or neurovascular compromise to the surgeon promptly.

Health Promotion and Maintenance

- Teach clients at risk for osteoporosis to minimize risk factors, such as stopping smoking, decreasing alcohol intake, exercising regularly, and increasing dietary calcium.
- Remind clients at risk for osteoporosis to have screening tests, such as the DEXA scan.
- Remind clients taking bisphosphonates (BPs) to take them early in the morning, at least 30 minutes before breakfast with a full glass of water, and to remain sitting upright during that time to prevent esophagitis, a common complication of BP therapy.
- Instruct older adults to have at least 5 minutes of sun per week and to eat vitamin D–fortified foods to prevent osteomalacia.
- Teach clients who have repetitive hand activities to be alert to clinical manifestations of carpal tunnel syndrome, the fastest growing occupational injury; use techniques to avoid repetitive strain.

Psychosocial Integrity

- Assist clients with osteoporosis to overcome fear of falling, or fallophobia, which prevents them from socializing or going outside their homes; collaborate with the physical therapist to determine whether ambulatory devices such as canes are indicated.

- Help clients with bone cancer cope with their illness as described in Chart 54-6.
- Refer clients with musculoskeletal problems to appropriate community resources, such as the Paget's Disease Foundation and the National Osteoporosis Foundation.

Physiological Integrity

- Most clients are unaware that they have osteoporosis until they experience a fracture, the most common complication of the disease.
- Secondary generalized or regional osteoporosis can be caused by any of the risk factors listed in Table 54-1.
- Osteomalacia, caused by a deficiency in vitamin D, can be caused by the factors listed in Table 54-3.
- Assess for key features of Paget's disease as summarized in Chart 54-4.
- Remember that bone tumors can be benign or malignant, as summarized in Table 54-4.
- Be aware that carpal tunnel syndrome (CTS) can be treated conservatively with medications and splinting; the goal of surgery is to release the pressure from the median nerve in the wrist.
- Assess clients having CTS surgery for changes in neurovascular status.
- Be aware that even minor hand and foot problems can be very painful; common foot problems are described in Table 54-5.
- Recognize that most major types of muscular dystrophy are genetic and manifest usually in childhood; care is supportive.

ADDITIONAL STUDY RESOURCES

Go to your Student CD-ROM for Review Questions for the NCLEX Examination.

Go to http://evolve.elsevier.com/Iggy/ for Integrated Management of Care Questions for the NCLEX Examination.

SELECTED BIBLIOGRAPHY

Asterisk indicates a classic or definitive work on this subject.

Aschenbrenner, D.S. (2005). Drug watch: new warnings and safety concerns: medications and adverse effects. *American Journal of Nursing, 105*(1), 29.

Bayles, C.M., Cochran, K., & Anderson, C. (2000). The psychosocial aspects of osteoporosis in women. *Nursing Clinics of North America, 35*(1), 279-286.

Berarducci, A., et al. (2000). Health-promoting educational practices related to osteoporosis. *Applied Nursing Research, 13*(4), 173-180.

Carroll, K.L. (2002). Alterations in musculoskeletal function in children. In K.L. McCance & S.E. Huether (Eds.), *Pathophysiology: The biologic basis for disease in adults and children* (pp. 1409-1433). St. Louis: Mosby.

Crowther, C.L., & Mourad, L.A. (2002). Alterations in musculoskeletal function. In K.L. McCance & S.E. Huether (Eds.), *Pathophysiology: The biologic basis for disease in adults and children* (pp. 1364-1408). St. Louis: Mosby.

*Dowd, R., & Cavalieri, R.J. (1999). Help your patient live with osteoporosis. *American Journal of Nursing, 99*(4), 55, 57-60.

Geier, K.A. (2001). Osteoporosis in men. *Orthopaedic Nursing, 20*(6), 49-56.

*Hall, J., & Riley, R.E. (1999). Nutritional strategies to reduce the risk of osteoporosis. *MEDSURG Nursing, 8*(5), 281-293.

*Hunt, A.H. (1996). The relationship between height change and bone mineral density. *Orthopaedic Nursing, 15*(3), 57-71.

Lehne, R.A. (2001). *Pharmacology for nursing care.* Philadelphia: W. B. Saunders.

Leslie, M. (2000). Issues in the nursing management of osteoporosis. *Nursing Clinics of North America, 35*(1), 189-197.

*Lewis, T., et al. (1999). Caring for the patient with Paget's disease of the bone. *Nurse Practitioner, 24*(7), 53, 57-58.

Lypaczewski, G., Lappe, J., & Stubby, J. (2002). "Mom & me" and healthy bones: An innovative approach to teaching bone health. *Orthopaedic Nursing, 21*(2), 35-43.

*Mahon, S.M. (1998). Osteoporosis: A concern for cancer survivors. *Oncology Nursing Forum, 25*(5), 843-851.

McClung, B.L. (2000). *Nursing practice guideline: Clinical management of patients at risk for or diagnosed with osteoporosis.* New York: Medical Information Services.

National Institutes of Health. (2000). *Consensus statements: Osteoporosis prevention, diagnosis, and therapy.* Accessed July 27, 2003, from http://www.consensus.nih.gov/cons/111/111_statement.htm.

*National Osteoporosis Foundation. (1995). *Position paper: Current perspective on diagnosis, prevention, and treatment of osteoporosis.* Washington, DC: Author.

National Osteoporosis Foundation. (2003a). *Disease statistics.* Accessed July 26, 2003, from http://www.nof.org/osteoporosis/stats.htm.

National Osteoporosis Foundation. (2003b). *Medications to prevent and treat osteoporosis.* Accessed July 26, 2003, from http://www.nof.org/patientinfo/medications.htm.

Orwell, E. (2000). Men with osteoporosis. Presented at the World Congress on Osteoporosis 2000, June 17, 2000, Chicago.

Peterson, J.A. (2001). Osteoporosis overview. *Geriatric Nursing, 22*(1), 17-23.

*Piasecki, P.A. (1996). Nursing care of the patient with metastatic bone disease. *Orthopaedic Nursing, 15*(4), 25-33.

*Quaschnick, M.S. (1996). The diagnosis and management of plantar fasciitis. *Nurse Practitioner, 21*(4), 50-63.

Rodts, M.F. (2002). Disorders of the spine. In A.B. Maher, S.W. Salmond, & T.A. Pellino (Eds.), *Orthopaedic nursing* (pp. 515-550). Philadelphia: W. B. Saunders.

Sedlak, C.A. & Doheny, M.O. (2002). Metabolic conditions. In A.B. Maher, S.W. Salmond, & T.A. Pellino (Eds.), *Orthopaedic nursing* (pp. 423-467). Philadelphia: W. B. Saunders.

Sedlak, C.A., Doheny, M.O., & Estok, P.J. (2000). Osteoporosis in older men: Knowledge and health beliefs. *Orthopaedic Nursing, 19*(3), 38-46.

Sedlak, C.A., et al. (1998). Osteoporosis prevention in young women. *Orthopaedic Nursing, 17*(3), 53-60.

Taft, L.B., Looker, P.A., & Cella, D. (2000). Osteoporosis: A disease management opportunity. *Orthopaedic Nursing, 19*(2), 67-76.

*Tawil, R. (1999). Outlook for therapy in the muscular dystrophies. *Seminars in Neurology, 19*(1), 81-86.

U.S. Food and Drug Administration. (2003). *FDA approves new labeling and provides new advice to postmenopausal women who use or who are considering using estrogen and estrogen with progestin.* Accessed July 26, 2003, from http://www.fds.gov/bbs/topics/factsheets/2003/fsl.htm.

Interventions for Clients with Musculoskeletal Trauma

MARY R. HERON EVANS

Go to your Student CD-ROM for Review Questions
for the NCLEX Examination keyed to these Learning Outcomes.

Musculoskeletal injury accounts for about 66% of all injuries and is one of the primary causes of disability in the United States. Trauma to the musculoskeletal system ranges from simple muscle strain to multiple bone fractures with severe soft-tissue damage. With advancing age, a person is more likely to develop decreased bone mass (osteoporosis), which causes fractures. Hip, wrist, vertebral, and pelvic fractures are common in late adulthood.

FRACTURES

PATHOPHYSIOLOGY

A **fracture** is a break or disruption in the continuity of a bone. Fractures can occur anywhere in the body and at any age. All fractures have the same basic pathophysiologic mechanism and nursing management, regardless of fracture type or location.

Classification of Fractures

A fracture is classified by the extent of the break as follows:
- *Complete fracture.* The break is across the entire width of the bone in such a way that the bone is divided into two distinct sections.
- *Incomplete fracture.* The fracture does not divide the bone into two portions because the break is through only part of the bone.

A fracture is described by the extent of associated soft-tissue damage as **open** (or **compound**) or **closed** (or **simple**). The skin surface over the broken bone is disrupted in a compound fracture, which causes an external wound. These fractures are often graded to define the extent of tissue damage. Grade I is the least severe injury, and skin damage is minimal. In grade II an open fracture is accompanied by skin and muscle contusions. The most severe injury is grade III, in which there is damage to skin, muscle, nerve tissue, and blood vessels; the wound is more than

2.4 to 3.2 inches (6 to 8 cm) in diameter. A closed (simple) fracture does not extend through the skin and therefore has no visible wound.

Figure 55-1 illustrates common types of fractures. The nurse needs to be familiar with the differences in these types because they often dictate the specific nursing care required for the client. In addition to being identified by type, fractures are characterized by their cause. A **pathologic (spontaneous) fracture** occurs after minimal trauma to a bone that has been weakened by disease. For example, a client with bone cancer or osteoporosis can easily sustain a pathologic fracture. A **fatigue or stress fracture** results from excessive strain and stress on the bone. **Compression fractures** are produced by a loading force applied to the long axis of cancellous bone. They commonly occur in the vertebrae of clients with osteoporosis.

Stages of Bone Healing

When a bone is broken, the body immediately begins the healing process to repair the injury and restore the body's equilibrium. Within 48 to 72 hours after the injury, a hematoma forms at the site of the fracture because bone is extremely vascular. Blood supply to and within the bone usually diminishes because of the injury, which causes an area of bone necrosis. The dead cells prompt the migration of fibroblasts and osteoblasts to the fracture site as part of the inflammatory process. This then prompts the formation of fibrocartilage, providing the foundation for bone healing (within 3 days to 2 weeks).

As a result of vascular and cellular proliferation, the fracture site is surrounded by new vascular tissue known as a callus (within 2 to 6 weeks). **Callus** formation is the beginning of a nonbony union. As healing continues, it is transformed

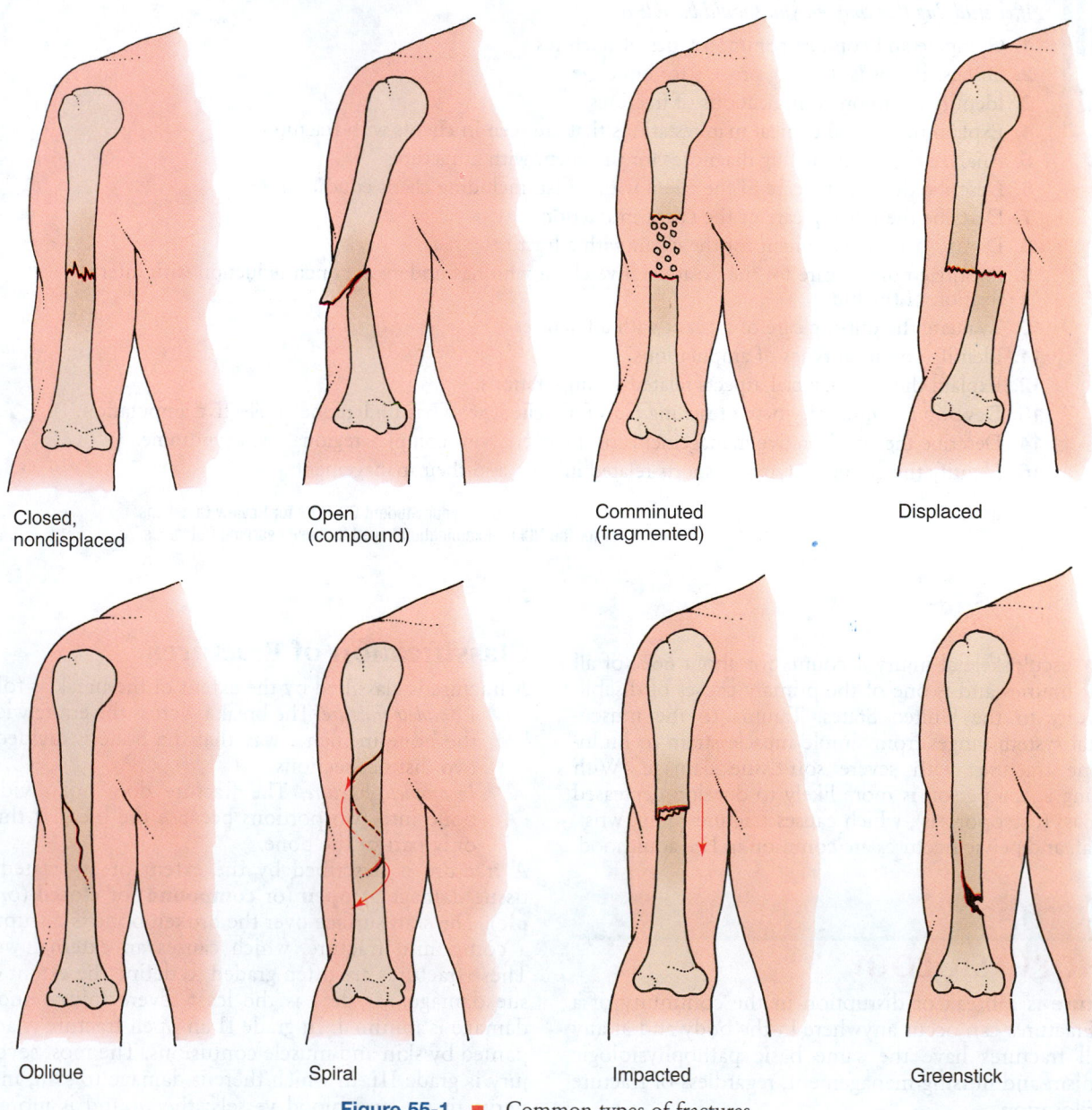

Closed, nondisplaced	Open (compound)	Comminuted (fragmented)	Displaced

Oblique	Spiral	Impacted	Greenstick

Figure 55-1 ■ Common types of fractures.

from a loose, fibrous tissue into bone (within 3 weeks to 6 months). Excess callus is resorbed. During the final phase of healing, consolidation, and remodeling, bone continues to be resorbed and deposited in response to stress, reshaping to meet mechanical demands. This process may start as early as 6 weeks after fracture and can continue for up to 1 year. Figure 55-2 summarizes the stages of bone healing.

In young, healthy adult bone, healing takes about 6 weeks. In the older person who has reduced bone mass, healing time is lengthened; complete healing often takes 3 to 6 months. Other factors that affect healing include the severity of the trauma, the type of bone injured, inadequate immobilization, infections at the fracture site, and ischemic or avascular necrosis (AVN).

CONSIDERATIONS FOR OLDER ADULTS

Healing can be affected by a number of factors in addition to the aging process. Bone formation and strength rely on adequate nutrition. Calcium, phosphorus, vitamin D, and protein are necessary for the production of new bone (see Chapter 54). For women the loss of estrogen after menopause is detrimental to the body's ability to form new bone tissue. Concurrent diseases can also affect the rate at which bone heals. For instance, peripheral vascular diseases, such as arteriosclerosis, reduce arterial circulation to bone; thus the bone receives less oxygen and lesser amounts of nutrients, both of which are needed for repair.

Complications of Fractures

Regardless of the type or location of the fracture, several limb- and life-threatening complications can result from the injury. The nurse must be able to recognize the clinical manifestations of impending complications so that treatment can be started immediately. In some cases, careful monitoring and assessment can prevent these complications.

ACUTE COMPARTMENT SYNDROME

Compartments are sheaths of inelastic fascia that support and partition muscles, blood vessels, and nerves in the body. **Acute compartment syndrome (ACS)** is a serious condition in which increased pressure within one or more compartments causes massive compromise of circulation to the area. The most common sites for ACS in clients experiencing musculoskeletal trauma are the compartments in the lower leg and the dorsal and volar compartments of the forearm.

PREVENTION. The pressure to the compartment can be from an external or internal source. Tight, bulky dressings and casts are examples of external pressure. Blood or fluid accumulation is a common source of internal pressure. ACS is not limited to clients with musculoskeletal problems; clients with severe burns, extensive insect bites, or massive infiltration of intravenous (IV) fluids are also susceptible to compartment syndrome. In these situations, edema increases pressure in one or more compartments.

Identify clients who may be at risk for ACS and monitor them closely. If ACS is suspected, notify the health care provider immediately and, if possible, implement interventions to relieve the pressure. For example, for the client with constricting bulky dressings, loosen the bandage or tape. If the client has a cast, request an order to cut the cast. In some agencies, protocols permit this procedure without a physician's order.

PATHOPHYSIOLOGIC CHANGES. The primary pathophysiologic changes of increased compartment pressure are sometimes referred to as the ischemia-edema cycle. Capillaries within the viable muscle dilate, which raises capillary pressure. Capillaries then become more permeable because of the release of histamine by the ischemic muscle tissue. As a result, plasma proteins leak into the interstitial fluid space, and edema occurs. Edema causes pressure on nerve endings and subsequent pain. Blood flow to the area is reduced, and further ischemia results. Sensory deficits

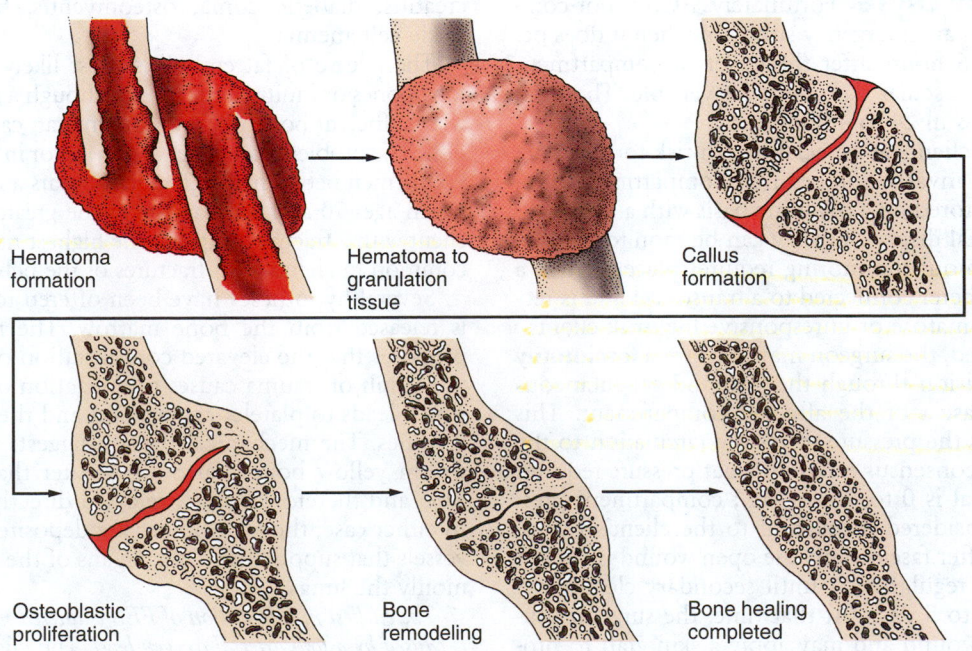

Hematoma formation

Hematoma to granulation tissue

Callus formation

Osteoblastic proliferation

Bone remodeling

Bone healing completed

Figure 55-2 ■ The stages of bone healing.

CHART 55-1

KEY FEATURES of
Compartment Syndrome

Physiologic Change	Clinical Findings
Increased compartment pressure	No change
Increased capillary permeability	Edema
Release of histamine	Increased edema
Increased blood flow to area	Pulses present Pink tissue
Pressure on nerve endings	Pain
Increased tissue pressure	Referred pain to compartment
Decreased tissue perfusion	Increased edema
Decreased oxygen to tissues	Pallor
Increased production of lactic acid	Unequal pulses Flexed posture
Anaerobic metabolism	Cyanosis
Vasodilation	Increased edema
Increased blood flow	Tense muscle swelling
Increased tissue pressure	Tingling Numbness
Increased edema	Paresthesia
Muscle ischemia	Severe pain unrelieved by medication
Tissue necrosis	Paresis/paralysis

(e.g., paresthesia) generally appear before changes in vascular or motor signs. The color of the tissue pales, and pulses begin to weaken but rarely disappear; the affected area is usually palpably tense, and pain can be elicited with passive motion of the extremity. If the condition is not treated, cyanosis, tingling, numbness, paresis, and severe pain occur. Chart 55-1 summarizes the sequence of pathophysiologic events in compartment syndrome and the associated clinical assessment findings.

EMERGENCY CARE. Fortunately, ACS is not common, but it creates an emergency situation when it does occur. Within 4 to 6 hours after the onset of compartment syndrome, neuromuscular damage is irreversible. The limb can become useless in 24 to 48 hours.

In a few cases, clients at especially high risk for ACS are monitored by an invasive procedure. Compartment pressures can be monitored on a one-time basis with a handheld device with a digital display, or they can be monitored continuously. Continuous monitoring requires placement of a wick or slit-tip catheter connected to a transducer and is recommended for comatose or unresponsive high-risk clients.

If ACS is verified, the surgeon may perform a **fasciotomy** by making an incision through the skin and subcutaneous tissues into the fascia of the affected compartment. This procedure relieves the pressure to restore circulation to the affected area. No consensus exists on what pressure requires fasciotomy (normal is 0 to 8 mm Hg); compartment pressures must be considered in relation to the client's hemodynamic status. After fasciotomy, the open wound is packed and dressed on a regular basis until secondary closure occurs, usually in 4 to 5 days. At that time, the surgeon usually debrides the wound and may apply a skin graft to promote healing.

POSSIBLE RESULTS. Although uncommon, specific problems resulting from compartment syndrome include infection, persistent motor weakness in the affected extremity, contracture, and myoglobinuric renal failure. In extreme cases, amputation becomes necessary.

Infection from the necrotic tissue may become severe enough that amputation of the limb is warranted. *Motor weakness* from injured nerves is not reversible, and the client may require braces or other orthotic devices for assistance in movement. Volkmann's *contractures* of the forearm, which can begin within 12 hours of the pressure increase, result from shortening of the ischemic muscle and from nerve involvement.

Myoglobinuric renal failure, from muscle tissue breakdown **(rhabdomyolysis),** is a potentially fatal complication of compartment syndrome. It commonly occurs when large or multiple compartments are involved. Injured muscle tissues release myoglobulin (muscle protein) into the circulation, where it can occlude the distal convoluted tubule and precipitate acute renal failure. Although the exact pathophysiologic mechanisms are unknown, it is suspected that myoglobulin has a direct toxic effect on the kidney. Damaged muscle cells also release potassium, which cannot be excreted because of the renal failure. The resulting hyperkaliemia may cause cardiac dysrhythmias and cardiac arrest.

SHOCK

Bone is quite vascular; therefore there is a risk of bleeding with bone injury. In addition, trauma can sever adjacent arteries and cause hemorrhage; consequently, hypovolemic shock can develop rapidly. (The pathophysiology of hypovolemic shock is described in Chapter 40.)

FAT EMBOLISM SYNDROME

Fat embolism syndrome (FES) is a serious complication, usually resulting from a fracture, in which fat globules are released from the yellow bone marrow into the bloodstream. FES may also occur, although less often, with pancreatitis, diabetic coma, osteomyelitis, blunt trauma, or sickle cell anemia.

The release of fat emboli is most likely with fractures of long bones or multiple fractures, although a break in any bone with sufficient bone marrow content can cause the complication. The problem can occur at any age or in either gender, but young men between ages 20 and 40 years and older adults between ages 70 and 80 years are at the greatest risk. The older client with a fractured hip has the highest risk, but FES is also common in clients with fractures of the pelvis.

Several hypotheses have been offered to explain how fat is released from the bone marrow. The metabolic theory proposes that the elevated concentration of catecholamines as a result of trauma causes mobilization of free fatty acids, which leads to platelet aggregation and the formation of fat globules. The mechanical theory suggests that the pressure within yellow bone marrow is greater than capillary pressure, and therefore fats are released directly from the bone. In either case, the fat globules are deposited in small blood vessels that supply the major organs of the body, most commonly the lungs.

The earliest manifestation of FES is altered mental status, which is caused by a low arterial oxygen level. The client then typically experiences respiratory distress, tachycardia, tachypnea, fever,

CHART 55-2

KEY FEATURES of
Pulmonary Emboli: Fat Embolism Versus Blood Clot Embolism

Fat Embolism	Blood Clot Embolism
Definition	
Obstruction of the pulmonary vascular bed by fat globules	Obstruction of the pulmonary artery by a blood clot or clots
Origin	
95% from fractures of the long bones; occurs usually within 48 hr	85% from deep vein thrombosis in the legs or pelvis; can occur anytime
Assessment Findings	
Altered mental status (earliest sign)	Same as for fat embolism, except no petechiae
Increased respirations, pulse, temperature	
Chest pain	
Dyspnea	
Crackles	
Decreased Sao$_2$	
Petechiae (50%-60%)	
Retinal hemorrhage (not common)	
Mild thrombocytopenia	
Treatment	
Bedrest	Preventive measures (e.g., leg exercises, antiembolism stockings, SCDs)
Gentle handling	
Oxygen	
Hydration (IV fluids)	Bedrest
Possibly steroid therapy	Oxygen
Fracture immobilization	Possibly mechanical ventilation
	Anticoagulants
	Thrombolytics
	Possible surgery: pulmonary embolectomy, vena cava umbrella

Sao$_2$, Arterial oxygen saturation; SCD, sequential compression device.

and **petechiae** (a macular, measles-like rash over the neck, upper arms, or chest and abdomen). Petechiae are characteristic of fat emboli, but the physiologic basis for their development is not known.

Laboratory findings in FES include the following:
- Increased erythrocyte sedimentation rate (ESR)
- Decreased serum calcium levels
- Decreased red blood cell and platelet counts
- Increased serum lipase level

These changes in blood values are poorly understood, but they aid in diagnosis of the condition.

Fat embolism usually occurs within 48 hours of the fracture and can result in respiratory failure or death, often from pulmonary edema. When the lungs are affected, the complication may be misdiagnosed as a pulmonary embolism from a blood clot (Chart 55-2). Care of the client is similar to that for those with pulmonary emboli, with the primary exception that FES is not treated with anticoagulant agents.

VENOUS THROMBOEMBOLISM

Venous thromboembolism (VTE) includes deep vein thrombosis (DVT) and its complication, pulmonary embolism (PE). DVT often develops in people who are immobile because of trauma, surgery, or disability. It is the *most common* complication of lower extremity surgery or trauma and the most often fatal complication of musculoskeletal surgery. A person who smokes, is obese, has heart disease, is taking oral contraceptives or hormones, or has a history of thromboembolitic complications is at increased risk for DVT. The incidence of life-threatening embolic conditions is highest in older adults, particularly during the first 2 to 3 days after musculoskeletal surgery, usually hip repair.

Certain fracture sites are more often associated with life-threatening thrombi. For example, DVT that leads to PE is more likely to develop in clients with fractures of the lower extremities and pelvis. Local venous stasis secondary to trauma or surgical procedures (e.g., use of tourniquets in lower extremity injuries) increases the chance of VTE in clients with musculoskeletal trauma. A further discussion of VTE is found in Chapter 39.

INFECTION

Anytime there is trauma to tissues, the body's defense system is disrupted. Wound infections are the most common type of infection resulting from orthopedic trauma; they range from superficial skin infections to deep wound abscesses. Infection can also be caused by implanted hardware used to repair a fracture surgically, such as pins, plates, or rods. Clostridial infections can result in gas gangrene or tetanus and can prevent the bone from healing properly.

Bone infection, or **osteomyelitis,** is most common with open fractures in which skin integrity is lost and after surgical repair of a fracture (see Chapter 54). For clients experiencing this type of trauma, the risk of hospital-acquired **(nosocomial)** infections is increased.

ISCHEMIC NECROSIS

Ischemic necrosis is sometimes referred to as aseptic or avascular necrosis or **osteonecrosis.** Blood supply to the bone is disrupted, which results in the death of bone tissue. This problem is most often a complication of hip fractures or any fracture in which there is displacement of bone. Surgical repair of fractures also can lead to necrosis because the hardware can interfere with circulation.

FRACTURE BLISTERS

Fracture blisters are associated most commonly with high-energy fractures and twisting injuries in the lower extremities. Extensive tissue edema allows fluid to move into the weakened space between the epidermis and the dermis. The increased colloidal osmotic pressure then pulls more fluid into the space. Fracture blisters can lead to wound infection and delayed fracture treatment, which may then contribute to potential nonunion. Nursing measures that can assist in preventing or minimizing fracture blisters include maintaining proper immobilization before definitive treatment and elevation to limit edema.

DELAYED UNION, NONUNION, AND MALUNION

Delayed union describes a fracture that has not healed within 6 months of injury. Some fractures never achieve union; that is, they never completely heal (nonunion); others heal incorrectly (malunion). These problems are most common in clients with tibial fractures, fractures for which a number of different treatment techniques have been used (e.g., cast, traction), and pathologic fractures. Union may also be delayed or not achieved in the older client. If bone does not heal, the client typically experiences pain and immobility from deformity.

Etiology and Genetic Risk

The primary cause of a fracture is trauma from a motor vehicle accident or fall and is spread over all socioeconomic groups. The trauma experienced may be a direct blow to the bone or an indirect force from muscle contractions or pulling forces on the bone. Sports, vigorous exercise, and malnutrition are contributing factors. Bone diseases, such as osteoporosis, increase the risk of a fracture in older adults. Genetic factors that increase risk of fracture will be discussed with the specific problems throughout the text.

Incidence/Prevalence

The incidence of fractures depends on the location of the injury. Rib fractures are the most common type in the adult population. Femoral shaft fractures occur most often in young and middle-aged adults. The incidence of proximal femur (hip) fractures is highest in older adults. Humeral fractures are common in adults; the older the person, usually the more proximal the fracture. Wrist (Colles') fractures are typically seen in middle and late adulthood.

> ### ☀ WOMEN'S HEALTH CONSIDERATIONS
>
> It is estimated that more than 1.5 million fractures occur annually in the United States as a result of osteoporosis, and most occur in middle-aged and older women. By age 80, one in five women has suffered a hip fracture.

HEALTH PROMOTION/ILLNESS PREVENTION

The introduction of airbags and seatbelts has decreased the number of severe injuries and deaths, but it has increased the number of lower extremity and ankle fractures, especially in older adults. Nurses need to encourage the use of seatbelts and support legislation for improved vehicle design and reevaluation of the federal standards for motor vehicle safety. Health promotion and illness prevention activities should focus on decreasing falls and motor vehicle crashes. Such activities might include programs regarding the following:

- Osteoporosis screening and education
- Fall prevention
- Home assessment and modification
- Drinking and driving
- Medication safety
- Older adults and driving

◆COLLABORATIVE MANAGEMENT

◆Assessment

HISTORY

Collect data to determine the cause of the fracture, which helps in developing an individualized plan of care for the client.

PRECEDING EVENTS. Ask the client to recall the specific events up to the time of the injury. Some type of

force, such as incisional, crush, acceleration or deceleration, shearing, or friction, leads to most musculoskeletal injuries. As a result, several body systems are often affected.

Incisional (as from a knife wound) and crush injuries cause hemorrhage and disrupt blood flow to major organs. Acceleration or deceleration injuries cause direct trauma to the spleen, brain, and kidneys when these organs are moved from their fixed locations in the body. Shearing and friction damage the skin and cause a high level of wound contamination.

By asking about the events leading to the injury, you can determine which forces have been experienced and therefore which body systems or parts of the body to assess. For example, a forward fall often results in Colles' fracture of the wrist because the person tries to catch himself or herself with an outstretched hand. Knowing the mechanism of injury also helps the nurse to determine whether other types of injury, such as head and spinal cord injury, might be present.

OTHER HISTORY. A medication history, including substance abuse (recreational drug use), is important regardless of the client's age. For example, a young adult may have had an excessive amount of alcohol, which contributed to a motor vehicle accident or to a fall at the work site. Many older adults also consume alcohol and an assortment of prescribed and over-the-counter drugs, which can cause dizziness and loss of balance.

A medical history elicits possible causes of the fracture and gives clues as to how long it will take for the bone to heal. Certain diseases, such as bone cancer and Paget's disease, cause pathologic fractures that often do not achieve union.

Ask about the client's occupation and recreational activities. Some occupations are more hazardous than others; for instance, construction work is potentially more physically dangerous than office work. Certain hobbies and recreational activities are also extremely hazardous (e.g., skiing, in-line skating). Contact sports, such as football and ice hockey, often result in musculoskeletal injuries, including fractures. Other activities do not have such an obvious potential for injury but can cause fractures nonetheless. For instance, daily jogging and frequent marching in a band can lead to fatigue fractures.

Because inadequate nutrition contributes to fractures and can inhibit bone healing, take a complete diet history. Health-promotion counseling is a major focus for comprehensive health care today.

PHYSICAL ASSESSMENT/CLINICAL MANIFESTATIONS

BODY SYSTEM ASSESSMENT. The client with a fracture often sustains trauma to other body systems. Consequently, assess all major body systems *first* for life-threatening complications, including head, thoracic, and abdominal injuries. The assessment of these areas is described elsewhere in this text.

MUSCULOSKELETAL ASSESSMENT. When inspecting the site of a possible fracture, look for a change in bone alignment. The bone may appear deformed, or a limb may be internally or externally rotated. Accompanying these deviations may be an alteration in the length of the extremity (usually a shortening) or a change in bone shape. Ask the client to move the involved body part, but if pain is elicited, stop the movement immediately. Range of motion (ROM) is

CHART 55-3

BEST PRACTICE for
Assessment of Neurovascular Status in Clients with Musculoskeletal Injury

Assessment Technique	Normal Findings
Skin Color Inspect the area distal to the injury.	No change in pigmentation compared with other parts of the body.
Skin Temperature Palpate the area distal to the injury (the dorsum of the hands is most sensitive to temperature).	The skin is warm.
Movement Ask the client to move the affected area or the area distal to the injury (active motion).	The client can move without discomfort.
Move the area distal to the injury (passive motion).	No difference in comfort compared with active movement.
Sensation Ask the client if numbness or tingling is present (paresthesia).	No numbness or tingling.
Palpate with a paper clip (especially the web space between the first and second toes or the web space between the thumb and forefinger).	No difference in sensation in the affected and unaffected extremities. (Loss of sensation in these areas indicates perineal nerve or median nerve damage.)
Pulses Palpate the pulses distal to the injury.	Pulses are strong and easily palpated; no difference in the affected and unaffected extremities.
Capillary Refill (least reliable) Press the nail beds distal to the injury until blanching occurs (or the skin near the nail if nails are thick and brittle).	Blood returns (return to usual color) within 3 sec (5 sec for older clients).
Pain Ask the client about the location, nature, and frequency of the pain.	Pain is usually localized and is often described as stabbing or throbbing. (Pain out of proportion to the injury and unrelieved by analgesics might indicate compartment syndrome.)

typically decreased. When the affected part is moved, the nurse may hear **crepitation,** a grating sound created by bone fragments.

Observe the skin for integrity. If the skin is intact (closed fracture), the area over the fracture may be **ecchymotic** (bruised) from bleeding into the underlying soft tissues. **Subcutaneous emphysema,** the appearance of bubbles under the skin because of air trapping, is not uncommon but is seen later.

Swelling at the fracture site is rapid and can result in marked neurovascular compromise. Perform a thorough neurovascular assessment and compare the injured area with its symmetric counterpart. Skin color and temperature, sensation, mobility, pain, and pulses are assessed distal to the fracture site. If the fracture involves an extremity, check the nails for capillary refill by applying pressure to the nail and observing for the speed of blood return. If nails are brittle or thick, the skin adjacent to the nail is assessed. *Checking for capillary refill is not as reliable as other indicators of perfusion.* Chart 55-3 describes the procedure for a neurovascular assessment, which evaluates circulation, movement, and sensation.

For an open fracture, determine the degree of soft-tissue damage and the amount of overt bleeding. The area may be lightly palpated for tenderness, but a sterile glove is worn if the skin is disrupted.

Clients often complain of moderate to severe pain at the site of the fracture or in an adjacent or distal area. For example, clients with a fractured hip may have groin pain or pain referred to the back of the knee. Pain is usually due to muscle spasm and edema, which result from the fracture. In clients with one or more fractured ribs, severe pain occurs when deep breaths are taken. Assess respiratory status, which may be severely compromised from pain or pneumothorax (air in the pleural cavity).

SPECIAL ASSESSMENT CONSIDERATIONS. For fractures of the shoulder and upper arm, the physical assessment is best done with the client in a sitting or standing position, if possible, so that shoulder drooping or other abnormal positioning can be seen. Support the affected arm and flex the elbow to promote comfort during the assessment. For more distal areas of the arm, the assessment is done with the client in a supine position so that the extremity can be elevated to reduce swelling.

Place the client in a supine position for assessment of the lower extremities and pelvis. A client with an impacted hip fracture may be able to walk for a short time after injury, although this is not recommended. The client with any type of hip fracture has pain in addition to decreased ROM in the hip.

Some fractures can cause internal organ damage, resulting in hemorrhage. When a pelvic fracture is suspected, assess vital signs, skin color, and the level of consciousness for indications of possible hypovolemic shock. The urine is checked for blood, which indicates damage to the urinary system, often the bladder. If the client is unable to void, the nurse suspects damage to the urethra.

PSYCHOSOCIAL ASSESSMENT

The psychosocial status of a client with a fracture depends on the extent of the injury and other complications. Hospitalization is usually not required for a single, uncomplicated fracture, and the client may return to usual daily activities within a few days. Healing is usually complete in a young adult in 4 to 6 weeks.

In contrast, a client suffering multiple trauma can be hospitalized for weeks and may undergo many surgical procedures, treatments, and prolonged rehabilitation. For these clients, disruptions in lifestyle can create a high level of stress.

The stresses that result from a chronic condition affect relationships between the client and family members or significant others. Assess the client's feelings about himself or herself as a person, and ask about how he or she coped with previously experienced stressful events. Body image and sexuality may be altered by deformity, treatment modalities for fracture repair, or long-term immobilization.

Critical Thinking Challenge

A 30-year-old man arrives at the emergency department via ambulance. He was the driver of a motorcycle involved in a collision with an SUV. Paramedics report that the client was hit from the side; the bike fell on him, and he was trapped underneath the SUV. Initial reports from the ambulance en route describe an individual in shock with a mangled left leg below the knee and a left wrist fracture. The client was wearing a helmet at the time of the crash.

1. What information given above is helpful in predicting other injuries this client may have sustained?
2. What are the priority assessments you should perform when he arrives at the hospital?
3. What assessments of the leg injury will determine the type and grade of the fracture?
4. What initial assessments of the injured leg should you perform?

evolve For suggested answer guidelines, go to http://evolve.elsevier.com/Iggy/.

LABORATORY ASSESSMENT

No special laboratory tests are available for assessment of fractures. The client's hemoglobin and hematocrit levels are often low because of bleeding caused by the injury. If extensive soft-tissue damage accompanies the fracture, the erythrocyte sedimentation rate (ESR) may be elevated, which indicates the expected inflammatory response. If the ESR increases during fracture healing, the client may have a bone infection. During the healing stages, serum calcium and phosphorus levels are often increased as the bone releases these elements into the blood.

RADIOGRAPHIC ASSESSMENT

The health care provider orders standard x-rays and tomograms to confirm a diagnosis of fracture. These reveal the bone disruption, malalignment, or deformity. If the x-ray film does not show a fracture but the client is symptomatic, the x-ray is usually repeated with additional views.

The computed tomography (CT) scan is useful in detecting fractures of complex structures, such as the hip and pelvis. It also identifies compression fractures of the spine.

OTHER DIAGNOSTIC ASSESSMENTS

Although not commonly used, the health care provider may order a bone scan (with technetium or gallium) for help in detecting certain types of fractures, particularly pathologic fractures. It is impossible for fractures of small bones or occult fractures to be visualized by conventional x-rays as early as by a bone scan. In addition, the bone scan can better determine fracture complications, such as delayed bone healing, nonunion, infection, and ischemic necrosis.

Magnetic resonance imaging (MRI) is useful in determining the amount of soft-tissue damage that may have occurred with the fracture. It is also very helpful in visualizing vertebral and skull fractures.

◆Analysis

COMMON NURSING DIAGNOSES AND COLLABORATIVE PROBLEMS

The following are priority nursing diagnoses for clients with fractures:

1. Risk for Peripheral Neurovascular Dysfunction related to fractures (bone and soft-tissue trauma)
2. Acute Pain related to biologic injury (bone disruption, soft-tissue damage, muscle spasm, and edema)
3. Risk for Infection related to trauma
4. Impaired Physical Mobility related to pain
5. Imbalanced Nutrition: Less Than Body Requirements related to additional metabolic need for healing of bone and soft tissues

ADDITIONAL NURSING DIAGNOSES AND COLLABORATIVE PROBLEMS

In addition to the common nursing diagnoses, clients with fractures may have one or more of the following:

- Activity Intolerance related to pain and impaired mobility
- Constipation related to opioids and prolonged immobility (particularly in older adults)
- Ineffective Coping related to prolonged immobility, hospitalization, or lifestyle changes
- Compromised Family Coping related to prolonged hospitalization or lifestyle changes
- Self-Care Deficit related to pain and immobility
- Disturbed Body Image related to deformity and/or treatment modality
- Sexual Dysfunction related to pain and immobility
- Disturbed Sleep Pattern related to chronic pain or prolonged hospitalization
- Fear related to possible nursing home placement or death (particularly in older adults)
- Impaired Skin Integrity and Impaired Tissue Integrity related to bone injury and immobility

The following collaborative problems may be appropriate for clients with *severe* fractures:

- Potential for Acute Compartment Syndrome
- Potential for Hypovolemic Shock
- Potential for Fat Embolism Syndrome
- Potential for Venous Thromboembolism
- Potential for Ischemic Necrosis
- Potential for Delayed Healing, Malunion, or Nonunion

◆Planning and Implementation

RISK FOR PERIPHERAL NEUROVASCULAR DYSFUNCTION

NOC **PLANNING: EXPECTED OUTCOMES.** The client with a fracture is expected to have adequate blood flow through the small vessels of the extremities to maintain tissue function. Indicators include that the client will have noncompromised:

- Capillary refill
- Sensation
- Skin color
- Muscle function
- Extremity skin color
- Pedal pulses

CHART 67-4

BEST PRACTICE for
Emergency Care of the Client with an Extremity Fracture

EMERGENCY CARE

1. Remove the client's clothing (cut if necessary) to inspect the affected area while supporting the injured area above and below the injury. Do not remove shoes because this can cause increased trauma.
2. Apply direct pressure on the area if there is bleeding and pressure over the proximal artery nearest the fracture.
3. Keep the client warm and in a supine position.
4. Check the neurovascular status of the area distal to the extremity: temperature, color, sensation, movement, and capillary refill. Compare affected and unaffected limbs.
5. Immobilize the extremity by splinting; include joints above and below the fracture site. Recheck circulation after splinting.
6. Cover the affected area with a dressing (preferably sterile).

INTERVENTIONS. A fracture can happen anywhere, and it may be accompanied by multiple injuries to vital organs. In some cases, one or more fractures occur in the community setting, often as a result of an accident (e.g., fall, vehicle).

EMERGENCY CARE: FRACTURE. For any client who experiences trauma, first assess for respiratory distress, bleeding, and head injury. If any of these is present, provide lifesaving care before being concerned about the fracture. In the community setting, provide emergency interventions until medical treatment in a hospital is available, or call 911 for the emergency team.

The fracture injury is then assessed (Chart 55-4). If the person is clothed, the emergency team member (first responder) cuts away clothing from the fracture site for best visualization. Bleeding is controlled by direct pressure on the area and digital pressure over the proximal artery nearest the fracture. At the same time, to prevent shock, check vital signs, place the client in a supine position, and keep him or her warm.

The emergency team also does the following:

- Inspects the fracture site for intactness of skin, swelling, and deformity (e.g., shortening and rotation)
- Palpates the area *lightly* to determine temperature (coolness), decreased sensation, and blanching
- Assesses distal pulses by comparing affected and unaffected extremities, if applicable
- Assesses for motor function by asking the client to move an area distal to the fracture (e.g., if a femoral fracture is suspected, he or she is asked to move the ankle and foot on the affected side; the upper portion of the leg remains immobilized)

To prevent further damage, reduce pain, and increase circulation, the emergency team immobilizes the area of the fracture by splinting. Any object or device that extends to the joints above and below the fracture can be used as a splint. At the scene of an accident, the emergency team may need to improvise by using available materials, such as a board. If the skin is broken, loosely apply a clean (preferably sterile) cloth to prevent further contamination of the wound. Neurovascular assessment is rechecked after splinting.

In the emergency department, physician's office, or clinic, fracture management begins with reduction and immobilization of the fracture:

- Reduction, or realignment of the bone ends for proper healing, is accomplished by a closed method (e.g., traction) or an open (surgical) procedure.

CHART 55-5

NIC INTERVENTION ACTIVITIES for
The Client at Risk for Peripheral Neurovascular Dysfunction

Circulatory Care (Arterial Insufficiency/Venous Insufficiency): *Promotion of arterial and venous circulation*

- Perform a comprehensive appraisal of peripheral circulations (e.g., check peripheral pulses, edema, capillary refill, color, and temperature).
- Monitor degree of discomfort or pain.
- Protect the extremity from injury.
- Place extremity in a dependent position, as appropriate.

Peripheral Sensation Management: *Prevention or minimization of injury or discomfort in the client with altered sensation*

- Monitor for paresthesia: numbness, tingling, hyperesthesia, and hypoesthesia.
- Monitor fit of bracing devices, prostheses, shoes, and clothing.
- Administer analgesics, as necessary.
- Discuss or identify causes of abnormal sensations or sensation changes.

NIC intervention activities selected from Dochterman, J.M., & Bulechek, G.M. (Eds.) (2004). *Nursing interventions classification (NIC)* (4th ed.). St. Louis: Mosby. No part of this work is to be altered without prior written permission from the Publisher.

- Immobilization is achieved by the use of bandages, casts, traction, internal fixation, or external fixation. The health care provider selects the treatment method on the basis of the type, location, and extent of the fracture. These interventions prevent further injury and reduce discomfort.

NONSURGICAL MANAGEMENT. Nonsurgical management typically involves closed reduction and immobilization with a bandage, splint, cast, or traction. For each modality, the nurse's *primary* concern is assessment and prevention of neurovascular dysfunction or compromise (Chart 55-5). Assess the neurovascular status of the client who has sustained a fracture every hour for the first 24 hours and every 4 to 8 hours thereafter (see Chart 55-3). Elevate the fractured extremity higher than the heart, and apply ice for the first 24 to 48 hours, as appropriate, to reduce edema. Assess dressings, splints, casts, and traction for neurovascular compromise. The client will usually complain of discomfort that is unrelieved by analgesics if the bandage, splint, or cast is too tight.

Pay particular attention to *early* signs and symptoms of acute compartment syndrome (ACS) by doing a thorough pain assessment. The client with early ACS typically complains of severe, diffuse pain that is not relieved by analgesics; pain during passive motion is greater than pain during active motion. If the client presents with this complaint, notify the health care provider *immediately*. Additional preventive measures and interventions for ACS are described earlier in this chapter under Complications of Fractures.

Closed Reduction. Closed reduction is the most common nonsurgical method for managing a simple fracture. While applying a manual pull, or traction, on the bone, the health care provider manipulates the bone ends so that they realign. Anesthesia or analgesia is typically used during this procedure to minimize pain. An x-ray verifies that the bone ends are approximated before the bone is immobilized.

Bandages and Splints. For certain areas of the body, such as the scapula and clavicle, an elastic bandage or commercial mobilizer may be used to immobilize the bone during healing. Because upper extremity bones do not bear

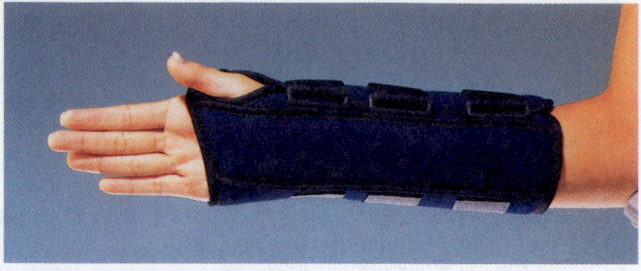

Figure 55-3 ■ A universal wrist and forearm splint used for immobilization. (Courtesy Smith & Nephew, Inc., Orthopaedics Divisions, Memphis, TN.)

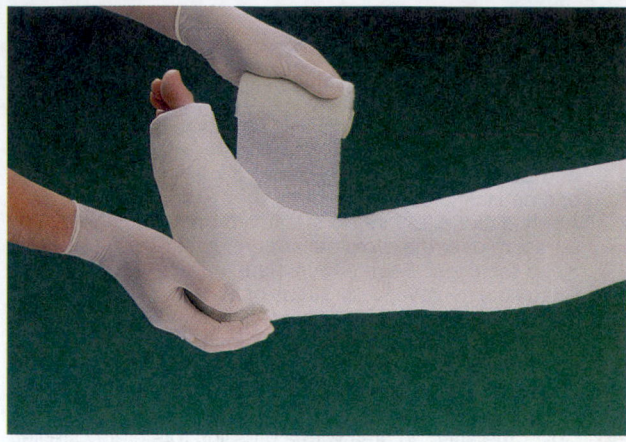

Figure 55-4 ■ Application of fiberglass synthetic cast. (Courtesy Smith & Nephew, Inc., Orthopaedics Divisions, Memphis, TN.)

weight, splints may be sufficient to keep bone fragments in place. Figure 55-3 illustrates the use of a wrist splint for fracture immobilization. Thermoplast, a durable, flexible material for splinting, allows custom fitting to the client's body part.

The nurse's primary responsibility is to assess the area distal to the bandage or splint for neurovascular compromise. The client usually complains of increased discomfort that is not relieved by analgesics if the splint or bandage is too tight. Reinforce the need for elevation as appropriate and teach how to assess for circulatory changes. The client is reminded to keep the device as dry and clean as possible to prevent skin breakdown and infection.

Casts. For more complex fractures or fractures of the lower extremity, the physician or orthopedic technician applies a cast to hold bone fragments in place after reduction. A **cast** is a rigid device that immobilizes the affected body part while allowing other body parts to move. It also allows early mobility and reduces pain. Although its most common use is for fractures, a cast may be applied for correction of deformities (such as clubfoot) or for prevention of deformities (such as those seen in some clients with rheumatoid arthritis).

Cast Materials. Several types of materials are used to make casts. The traditional plaster-of-Paris (anhydrous calcium sulfate) cast requires application of a well-fitted stockinette under the material. If the stockinette is too tight, it may impair circulation; if it is too loose, wrinkles can lead to the development of pressure ulcers and subsequent skin breakdown. Padding is applied over the stockinette, followed by wet plaster rolls wrapped around the extremity or other body part. The cast feels hot because an immediate chemical reaction occurs, but it soon becomes damp and cool. This type of cast takes 24 to 72 hours to dry, depending on the size and location of the cast. A wet cast feels cold, smells musty, and is grayish. The cast is dry when it feels hard and firm, is odorless, and has a shiny white appearance.

On occasion, the plaster cast may have rough edges, which can crumble and cause skin irritation. Petaling the cast will resolve this problem, if the underlying stockinette does not cover the edges of the cast. Small strips of tape are placed over the rough edges to protect the skin. If the skin under the cast was disrupted, the health care provider, orthopedic technician, or specially trained nurse cuts a window into the cast so that the wound can be observed and cared for. A window is also an access for taking pulses, removing wound drains, or relieving abdominal distention when the client is in a body or spica cast.

If the cast is too tight, it may be cut with a cast cutter to relieve pressure or allow tissue swelling. The health care

provider may choose to bivalve the cast (i.e., cut it lengthwise into two equal pieces) if bone healing is almost complete. Either half of the cast can be removed for inspection or for provision of care. The two halves are then reunited by an elastic bandage wrap.

Synthetic materials for casts include fiberglass and polyester-cotton knit (Figure 55-4). These materials are lighter than plaster and require minimal drying time. Fiberglass casts are dry in 10 to 15 minutes and can bear weight 30 minutes after application. Polyester-cotton knit casts take 7 minutes to dry and can withstand weight bearing in about 20 minutes. Some health care providers use synthetic casts for upper extremities and plaster-of-Paris casts for lower extremities because plaster casts can bear more weight for a longer time. However, synthetic casts are used much more commonly overall.

Types of Casts. Casts can be generally divided into four main groups: arm casts, leg casts, cast braces, and body or spica casts. Table 55-1 describes specific casts that are used for various parts of the body.

When a client is in bed with an *arm cast,* the arm is elevated above the heart to reduce swelling. The hand should be higher than the elbow. Ice may be prescribed for the first 24 to 48 hours. When the client is out of bed, the arm is supported with a sling placed around the neck to alleviate fatigue caused by the weight of the cast. The sling should distribute the weight over a large area of the shoulders and trunk, not just the neck. Some health care providers prefer that after the first few days in an arm cast, particularly a short-arm cast, the client not use a sling; this encourages normal movement of the mobile joints and enhance bone healing.

A *leg cast* permits mobility and requires the client to use ambulatory aids, such as crutches. A cast shoe, sandal, or boot that attaches to the foot or a rubber walking pad attached to the sole of the cast assists in ambulation (if weight bearing is allowed) and helps prevent damage to the cast. The affected leg is elevated on several pillows to reduce swelling, and ice is applied for the first 24 hours or as prescribed.

A *cast brace* enables the client to bend unaffected joints while the fracture is healing. The fracture must show signs of healing and minimal tissue edema before application of

TABLE 55-1 Types of Casts Used for Musculoskeletal Trauma

Type and Characteristics of Cast	Use
Upper Extremity Casts	
Short-arm cast (SAC) (extends from below the elbow to and including part of the hand)	Stable fractures of the wrist (metacarpals, carpals, or distal radius)
Long-arm cast (LAC) (includes the upper arm to and including part of the hand)	Unstable fractures of the wrist, distal humerus, radius, or ulna
Hanging-arm cast (same as LAC but heavier, with added loop at the mid-forearm)	Fractures of the humerus that cannot be aligned by LAC (light traction is possible while the client is in bed or by an attached strap that extends around the neck).
Thumb spica (gauntlet) cast (similar to SAC with the thumb casted in abduction)	Fractures of the thumb
Shoulder spica cast (the shoulder is casted in abduction with the elbow flexed)	Unstable fractures of the shoulder girdle or humerus; dislocations of the shoulder
Lower Extremity Casts	
Short-leg cast (SLC) (from below the knee to the base of the toes)	Fractures of the ankle, metatarsals, or foot
Long-leg cast (LLC) (from the mid-upper thigh to the base of the toes)	Unstable fractures of the tibia, fibula, or ankle
Walking cast (a walking device on the bottom of SLC or LLC)	Same as for SLC or LLC
Leg cylinder (similar to SLC, but the ankle and foot are not casted)	Stable fractures of the tibia, fibula, or knee
Long-leg cylinder (similar to LLC, but the ankle and foot are not casted)	Stable fractures of the distal femur, proximal tibia, or knee
Cast Braces (or Brace Casts)	
Patellar weight-bearing cast (similar to SLC or leg cylinder)	Midshaft or distal shaft fractures of the femur
External polycentric knee hinge cast (a hinge connects the lower and upper leg and allows 90 degrees of knee flexion)	Same as for the patellar weight-bearing cast
Body Casts	
Hip spica (extends from below the nipple line down the affected leg [single], down the leg and half of the unaffected leg [1½], or down both legs [double])	Dislocation of the hip; pelvic or hip injuries
Risser's cast (the body jacket extends from the shoulders to beyond the iliac crests and hips, with a large opening over the anterior chest)	Scoliosis; thoracic spinal fractures
Halo cast (the body jacket contains a halo brace)	Fractures of the cervical spine

this cast. Two cylindrical casts are made and connected by a hinge to allow joint movement. As healing occurs, the casts may be removed and replaced with a soft brace. Commercial immobilizers, which serve the same function as a cast brace, are available and may be used in some cases.

A *body cast* encircles the trunk of the body; a **spica cast** encases a portion of the trunk and one or two extremities. A client with either of these casts presents a special challenge for nursing care. Potential complications related to severe impairment in mobility include the following:

- Skin breakdown
- Respiratory dysfunction, such as pneumonia and atelectasis
- Constipation
- Joint contractures

Cast syndrome (superior mesenteric artery syndrome), an uncommon but serious complication, is most often seen in orthopedic clients who have been placed in a hip spica or body cast. Partial or complete upper intestinal obstruction results in classic symptoms: abdominal distention, epigastric pain, nausea, and vomiting. The vomiting often occurs after meals, and clients may have normal bowel sounds. Partial obstruction occurs initially from compression of the third portion of the duodenum between the superior mesenteric artery and the

aorta. This progresses to complete obstruction from duodenal edema caused by continued vomiting and distention. Placing a window in the abdominal portion of the cast or bivalving the cast may be sufficient to relieve pressure on the duodenum. Management of intestinal obstruction is the same as for any client with this complication.

Cast Care. Before the cast is applied, explain the purpose of the cast and the procedure for its application. With a plaster cast, it is particularly important to warn the client about the heat that will be felt immediately after the wet cast is applied. The new cast is not covered; this facilitates air-drying.

When a client with a wet plaster cast is moved and turned, the cast is handled with the palms of the hands to prevent indentations and resultant areas of pressure on the skin. The client is turned every 1 to 2 hours to allow air to circulate and dry all parts of the cast. If the client is hospitalized, a sign is placed at the head of the bed as a reminder that the cast is wet and requires special handling. If the health care provider requests that the cast be elevated to reduce swelling, a cloth-covered pillow is used instead of one encased in plastic, which could cause the cast to retain heat and prevent drying. Elevation of the casted extremity reduces edema but may impair arterial circulation to the affected limb. Uniform support is needed while the cast is drying to prevent development of pressure points.

For preventing contamination by urine or feces, the perineal area of a dry long leg or body cast is encased in a plastic protective covering. Fracture pans are preferred over traditional bedpans because they are smaller and more comfortable for the client. Care is taken to prevent spillage onto the cast.

Check to ensure that the cast is not too tight and frequently monitor the client's neurovascular status, usually every hour for the first 24 hours after application. You should be able to insert a finger between the cast and the skin. Ice may be applied for the first 24 to 36 hours to reduce swelling and inflammation.

Once the plaster cast is dry, it is inspected at least once every 8 hours for drainage, cracking, crumbling, alignment, and fit. Plaster casts act like sponges and absorb drainage, whereas synthetic casts act like a wick, pulling drainage away from the drainage site. Padding can also absorb wound drainage. Drainage on any cast should always be measured and documented in the client record; however, sources disagree on whether drainage should be circled on the cast because it may increase anxiety. Immediately report to the health care provider any sudden increases in the amount of drainage or change in the integrity of the cast. After swelling decreases, it is not uncommon for the cast to become too loose and need replacement. If the client is not admitted to the hospital, he or she is given instructions regarding cast care, as discussed later under Community-Based Care, p. 1205.

Cast Complications. During hospitalization, assess for other complications resulting from casting that can be serious and life threatening, such as infection, circulation impairment, and peripheral nerve damage. If the client returns home after cast application, the client and family are taught how to monitor for these complications and when to notify the health care provider.

Infection most often results from the breakdown of skin under the cast (pressure necrosis). If pressure necrosis occurs, the client typically complains of a very painful "hot spot" under the cast, and the cast may feel warmer in the affected area. Smell the area for mustiness or an unpleasant odor that would indicate infected material. If the infection progresses, a fever may develop.

Circulation impairment and peripheral nerve damage can result from constriction of the cast. Perform frequent neurovascular assessments as described in Chart 55-3. A client with a new cast may require hourly assessments. A client with a cast that is 3 or 4 days old usually requires assessments every 4 to 8 hours.

The client with a cast may be immobilized for a prolonged period, depending on the extent of the fracture and the type of cast. Assess for complications of immobility, such as skin breakdown, pneumonia, atelectasis, thromboembolism, and constipation. Before the cast is removed, inform the client that the cast cutter will not injure the skin but that heat may be felt during the procedure.

Because of prolonged immobilization, a joint may become contracted, usually in a fixed state of flexion, or degenerative arthritis may develop from lack of weight bearing, which is necessary for cartilage viability. Muscle can also atrophy from lack of exercise during prolonged immobilization of the affected body part, usually an extremity.

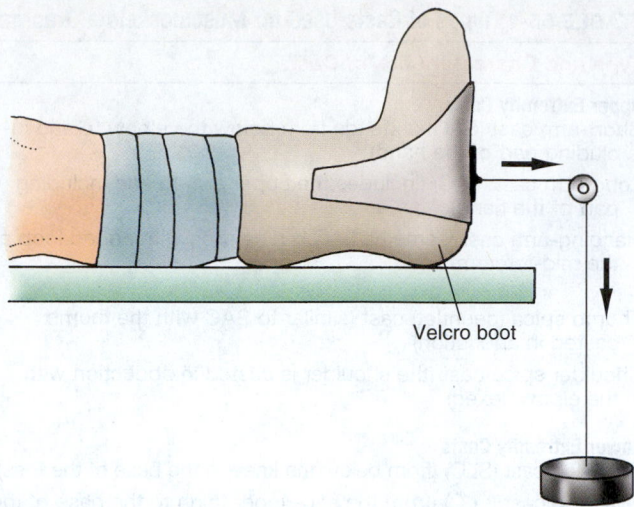

Figure 55-5 ■ Buck's traction with a hook-and-loop fastener (Velcro) boot, commonly used for hip fractures.

Velcro boot

Traction. **Traction** is the application of a pulling force to a part of the body to provide reduction, alignment, and rest. Traction can also decrease muscle spasm (thus relieving pain) and prevent or correct deformity and tissue damage. A client in traction is usually hospitalized longer, but in some cases home care is possible even for skeletal traction.

Mechanical traction can be either of the following:

- Continuous, as in fracture treatment
- Intermittent, for relief of muscle spasm in other types of musculoskeletal/neurologic trauma, such as cervical nerve root compression

Traction may also be classified as running traction or balanced suspension. In running traction, the pulling force is in one direction and the client's body acts as countertraction. Moving the body or bed position can alter the countertraction force. Balanced suspension provides the countertraction so that the pulling force of the traction is not altered when the bed or client is moved. This allows for increased client movement and facilitates care.

Types of Traction. Traction is typically one of five types: skin traction, skeletal traction, plaster traction, brace traction, or circumferential traction. Skin traction involves the use of a Velcro boot (Buck's traction) (Figure 55-5), belt, or halter, which is secured around a body part. The primary purpose of skin traction is to decrease painful muscle spasms that accompany fractures. The weight is used as a pulling force is limited (5 to 10 pounds [2.3 to 4.5 kg]) to prevent injury to the skin.

In skeletal traction, pins, wires, tongs (e.g., Crutchfield), or screws are surgically inserted directly into bone. These allow the use of longer traction time and heavier weights (usually 15 to 30 pounds [6.8 to 13.6 kg]). Skeletal traction aids in bone realignment.

Plaster traction combines skeletal traction and a plaster cast. A brace traction device exerts a pull for correction of alignment deformities. Circumferential traction uses a belt around the body, such as pelvic traction for low back problems. Table 55-2 describes commonly used types of traction for various parts of the body.

Traction Care. The nurse may set up or assist in the setup of traction. In larger or specialty hospitals or units, or-

TABLE 55-2 Types of Traction Used for Musculoskeletal Trauma

Type and Characteristics of Traction	Use
Upper Extremity Traction	
Sidearm skin or skeletal traction (the forearm is flexed and extended 90 degrees from the upper part of the body)	Fractures of the humerus with or without involvement of the shoulder and clavicle
Overhead or 90-90 traction, skin or skeletal (the elbow is flexed and the arm is at a right angle to the body over the upper chest)	Same as above (depends on the physician's preference)
Plaster traction (pins inserted through the bone are fixed in the cast)	Fractures of the wrist
Lower Extremity Traction	
Buck's extension traction (skin) (the affected leg is in extension)	Fractures of the hip or femur preoperatively Prevention of hip flexion contractures Hip dislocation
Russell's traction (similar to Buck's traction, but a sling under the knee suspends the leg)	Fractures of the hip or end of the femur
Balanced skin or skeletal traction (the limb is usually elevated in a Thomas splint with Pearson's attachment, or a Böhler-Braun splint is used)	Fractures of the femur or pelvis (acetabulum)
Spinal Column and Pelvic Traction	
Cervical halter (a strap under the chin)	Cervical muscle spasms, strain/sprain, or arthritis
Cervical skeletal (e.g., halo brace, Crutchfield tongs)	Cervical fractures of the spine Muscle spasms
Pelvic belt (a strap around the hips at the iliac crests is attached to weights at the foot of the bed)	Pain, strain, sprain, or muscle spasms, in the lower back
Pelvic sling (a wide strap around the hips is attached to an overhead bar to keep the pelvis off the bed)	Pelvic fractures; other pelvic injuries

thopedic technicians may set up traction. Once traction is applied, maintain the correct balance between traction pull and countertraction force. Weights are not usually removed without an order; they are not usually lifted manually or allowed to set on the floor. Weights should be freely hanging at all times. Teach this important point to staff members on the unit and to other personnel, such as those in the radiology department.

Inspect the skin at least every 8 hours for signs of irritation or inflammation. When possible, remove the belt or boot that is used for skin traction every 8 hours to inspect under the device.

When skeletal traction is used, pay particular attention to the points of entry of pins, wires, or screws for signs of inflammation or infection. A small amount of clear fluid drainage ("weeping") is expected. Most health care providers prefer that pin care is preformed every day. No standardized method or protocol for pin care has been established throughout the United States. Some health care providers and nurse specialists believe that cleaning the pins disrupts the skin's natural barrier to infection and advise against this practice. In any case, observe pin sites at least every 8 hours for drainage, color, odor, and severe redness, which indicate inflammation and possible infection. Infection of the pin tract may result in osteomyelitis.

The nurse is responsible for checking traction equipment to ensure its proper functioning. All ropes, knots, and pulleys are inspected at least every 8 hours for loosening, fraying, and positioning. Check the weight for consistency with the health care provider's order. At times the health care provider or qualified technician changes the weight without notifying the nurse or modifying the written order; contact the person responsible to confirm the change. Sometimes one of the weights is accidentally displaced by a staff member or visitor who bumps into it. Replace the weights if they are not correct, and notify the health care provider or orthopedic technician.

If the client complains of severe pain from muscle spasm, the weights may be too heavy or the client may need realignment. Report the pain to the health care provider if body realignment fails to reduce the discomfort. Also assess the neurovascular status of the affected body part to detect circulatory compromise and subsequent tissue damage. The circulation is usually monitored every hour for the first 24 hours after traction is applied and every 4 hours thereafter.

SURGICAL MANAGEMENT. For some types of fractures, casts and traction are not appropriate or sufficient treatment techniques. Surgical intervention may be needed to realign the bone for the healing process.

Preoperative Care. For stabilizing the fracture, the client may be placed in traction before surgery. This procedure is typical for managing a fractured hip when Buck's traction may be used preoperatively (see Figure 55-5). Teach the client and family or significant others what to expect during and after the surgery. The preoperative care for a client undergoing musculoskeletal surgery is similar to that for any client preparing for surgery with general or epidural anesthesia. (See Chapter 20 for a thorough discussion of preoperative nursing care.)

Operative Procedures. Open reduction with internal fixation (ORIF) is a common method of reducing and immobilizing a fracture. When this method is not feasible, external fixation with closed reduction is used. Although nurses do not decide which surgical technique is used, understanding the procedures enhances client teaching and care.

Open Reduction with Internal Fixation. Because ORIF permits early mobilization, it is often the preferred surgical method for an older adult who is susceptible to the complications of immobility.

Open reduction allows the surgeon direct visualization of the fracture site. **Internal fixation** uses metal pins, screws, rods, plates, or prostheses to immobilize the fracture during healing. The surgeon makes an incision to gain access to the broken bone and implants one or more devices. A newer bioabsorbable plate was recently introduced for internal fixation. This device is strong enough to fix the fracture but is reabsorbed by the body in about 3 months.

After the bone achieves union, the metal hardware may be removed, depending on the location and type of fracture (e.g., fractured ankle). Specific types of internal fixation devices are discussed later under Fractures of Specific Sites, p. 1206.

External Fixation. An alternative modality for the initial management of fractures is the external fixation apparatus, as shown in Figure 55-6. After fracture reduction, the physician makes small percutaneous incisions so that pins may be implanted into the bone. All pins are self-drilling. The pins are held in place by an external metal frame to prevent bone movement.

ADVANTAGES AND DISADVANTAGES. External fixation has several advantages over other immobilization techniques:

- There is minimal blood loss in comparison with internal fixation.
- The device allows early ambulation and exercise of the affected body part while relieving pain.
- The device maintains alignment in closed fractures that will not maintain position in a cast and stabilizes comminuted fractures that require bone grafting.
- In open fractures, in which skin and tissue trauma accompanies the fracture, the device permits easy access to the wound and promotes healing. This method is often preferred over the use of a window in a cast for wound care.

A disadvantage of external fixation is pin-tract infection. Pin-tract infections can lead to osteomyelitis, which is serious and difficult to treat (see Chapter 54). For prevention of these infections, some agencies have a pin-care procedure that is performed several times a day. The procedure is similar to that described earlier for skeletal traction pins (see Traction Care, pp. 1200 and 1201). As with skeletal traction, the need for special cleaning of the pins and the area around the pins is controversial. Regardless of whether pin care is done, inspect the pin sites at least daily for severe redness, swelling, and purulent drainage.

CARE OF THE CLIENT WITH AN EXTERNAL FIXATOR. As with any fracture treatment, assess the neurovascular status of the extremity distal to the fracture. External fixators may be used for an extremity or for fractures of the pelvis. External fixation is not definitive treatment for fractures. After a fixator is removed, the client may be placed in a cast until healing is complete.

The client with an external fixator may experience a disturbed body image. The frame may be large and bulky, and the affected area may have massive tissue damage with dressings. Be sensitive to this possibility in planning care.

CIRCULAR EXTERNAL FIXATION. The Ilizarov technique of circular external fixation is sometimes used to treat new fractures (closed, comminuted fractures and open fractures

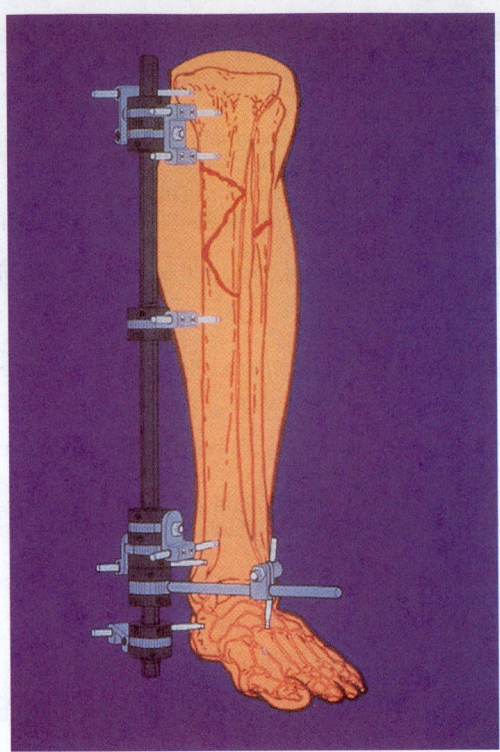

Figure 55-6 ■ The Hex-Fix external fixations system for tibial fractures. (Courtesy of Smith & Nephew, Inc., Orthopaedics Divisions, Memphis, TN.)

with bone loss) as well as malunion or nonunion of fractures. It may also be used to treat congenital bone deformities, especially in children. This procedure originated in Russia about 50 years ago and was introduced in the United States in 1986.

A circular external fixation device stimulates bone growth. Unlike the traditional fixator, the Ilizarov external fixator promotes rotation, angulation, shortening, lengthening, or widening of bone while allowing healing of the soft-tissue defect. The nursing care of the client with this device is similar to the care of the client with other external fixation systems except in one major exception: if the device is being used for filling bone gaps, using bone transport or distraction, the client must be taught how to manually turn the four-sided nuts (clickers), usually four times a day, unless he or she has an automated device. Daily distraction rates vary among clients, but 1 mm daily is common. Screening and teaching are particularly important because the client adjusts and cares for the apparatus for a prolonged time.

Postoperative Care. The postoperative care for a client undergoing ORIF or external fixation is similar to that provided for any client undergoing surgery (see Chapter 22). Because bone is a vascular, dynamic body tissue, the client is at risk for certain complications specific to fractures and musculoskeletal surgery. These problems (e.g., fat embolism and venous thromboembolism) were discussed earlier under Complications of Fractures, p. 1191.

Procedures for Nonunion. Some surgical repairs are not successful because the bone does not heal. Several additional options are available to the surgeon to promote bone union, such as electrical bone stimulation, bone grafting, and the newest therapy, ultrasound fracture treatment.

For selected clients, **electrical bone stimulation** may be successful. This procedure is based on research showing that bone has inherent electrical properties that are used in healing. The exact mechanism of action is unknown. Several types of devices have been developed. A noninvasive system uses magnetic coils applied on the skin or over a cast to deliver a pulsed magnetic field. There are no known risks with this system, although clients with pacemakers cannot use this device on an upper extremity. Implanted direct-current stimulators are placed directly in the fracture site and have no external apparatus. Both systems require about 6 months of treatment, and weight bearing is at the discretion of the health care provider.

Another method of treating nonunion is **bone grafting**. A bone graft may also replace diseased bone or increase bone tissue for joint replacement. In most cases, chips of bone are taken from the client's iliac crest or other site and are packed or wired between the bone ends to facilitate union. Allografts from cadavers may also be used. These grafts are frozen or freeze-dried and stored under sterile conditions in a bone bank.

Bone banking from living donors is becoming increasingly popular. If qualified, clients undergoing total hip replacement may donate their femoral heads to the bank for later use as bone grafts for other clients. Careful screening ensures that the bone is healthy and that the donor has no communicable disease. The bone cannot be donated without the client's written consent.

One of the newest modalities for fracture healing is **low-intensity pulsed ultrasound** (Exogen therapy). Used for slow-healing fractures or for new fractures as an alternative to surgery, ultrasound treatment has yielded excellent results. The client applies the treatment for about 20 minutes each day. It has no contraindications or adverse effects.

ACUTE PAIN

NOC **PLANNING: EXPECTED OUTCOMES.** The client with a fracture is expected to take personal actions to control pain. Indicators include that the client will consistently demonstrate the ability to:
- Use preventive measures
- Use nonanalgesic relief measures
- Use analgesic relief measures appropriately
- Report changes in pain symptoms or sites to health care professional
- Report uncontrollable pain symptoms to health care professional
- Report that pain is controlled

INTERVENTIONS. The nonsurgical or surgical management of fractures through reduction and immobilization helps reduce pain and prevents neurovascular injury. However, the client often requires drug therapy and other pain relief measures.

Drug Therapy. Musculoskeletal pain related to soft-tissue damage, bone disruption, and muscle spasm is one of the most severe types of pain that can be experienced. The client often has the pain for a prolonged time, which makes pain management difficult. The health care provider commonly prescribes opioid analgesics, anti-inflammatory drugs, and muscle relaxants.

For clients with chronic, severe pain, opioid and nonopioid drugs are alternated or given together to manage pain both centrally and peripherally. The nurse and client mutually decide on the best times for the strong pain relievers to be administered (e.g., before a complex dressing change, physical therapy, and at bedtime). Observe the client carefully for the effectiveness of the medication and its side effects. An early sign of acute compartment syndrome (ACS) is often the sudden inability of pain medication to relieve pain. Chapter 7 discusses the various methods of pain management, including epidural analgesia and patient-controlled analgesia.

Complementary and Alternative Therapies. With chronic, severe pain, the client cannot depend solely on drugs for relief. The client uses temporary pain relief measures, such as ice or heat, depending on the cause of the pain. If swelling causes pressure on the affected area, ice and elevation of the affected body part may be appropriate. Muscle spasms are best relieved by application of heat and massage. Other physical measures include a warm, soothing bath, a back rub, and the use of therapeutic touch.

If these measures are not effective in reducing pain, distraction, imagery, or music therapy may be used as alternatives. Teach the client relaxation techniques, such as deep breathing, for use during periods of severe pain. Chapters 4 and 7 discuss these techniques in detail.

RISK FOR INFECTION

NOC **PLANNING: EXPECTED OUTCOMES.** The client with a fracture is expected to be free of a wound or bone infection. Indicators include that the client will have none of the following:
- Foul-smelling discharge
- Purulent drainage
- Fever
- Lethargy
- Wound-site culture colonization (if wound present)
- White blood cell (WBC) elevation

INTERVENTIONS. When caring for a client with a fracture, particularly an open fracture, use strict aseptic technique for dressing changes and wound irrigations. Manifestations of local inflammation with purulent drainage are reported immediately to the health care provider. Other infections, such as pneumonia and urinary tract infection, may occur days after the fracture. The client's vital signs are monitored every 4 to 8 hours because increases in temperature and pulse often indicate systemic infection.

For most clients with an open fracture, the health care provider prescribes one or more broad-spectrum antibiotics prophylactically. This treatment is especially important for fractures requiring surgical repair.

IMPAIRED PHYSICAL MOBILITY

NOC **PLANNING: EXPECTED OUTCOMES.** The client with a fracture is expected to be free of physiologic consequences of impaired mobility. Indicators include that the client will have none of the following:
- Pressure ulcers
- Constipation
- Urinary retention
- Contracted joints
- Pneumonia
- Venous thrombosis

The client is also expected to move purposefully in his or her own environment independently with or without an assistive device. Indicators include that the following will not be compromised for the client:

- Balance
- Coordination
- Muscle movement
- Transfer performance
- Ambulation

INTERVENTIONS. The interventions necessary for this diagnosis can be grouped into two types: those that help to prevent complications of impaired mobility and those that help to increase mobility.

Prevention of Complications. The nurse plays a vital role in preventing and assessing for complications in immobilized clients with fractures. Additional information about nursing care for preventing problems associated with immobility is found in Chapter 10 and earlier in this chapter in the discussion of specific complications under Complications of Fractures, p. 1191.

Promotion of Mobility. The use of crutches or a walker increases mobility and assists in ambulation. The client may progress to use of a cane.

Crutches. Crutches are the most commonly used ambulatory aid for many types of musculoskeletal trauma (e.g., fractures, sprains, amputations). In most agencies, the physical therapist fits the client for crutches and teaches him or her how to ambulate with them on flat surfaces and stairs. The nurse's role may be to reinforce the instructions and evaluate whether the client is using the crutches correctly. However, in emergency department and ambulatory settings, nurses routinely teach clients how to use crutches.

Walking with crutches requires strong upper extremities, balance, and coordination. For this reason, crutches are not used as often for older adults. The therapist pads the tips and axillary bars of the crutches; padding prevents the tips

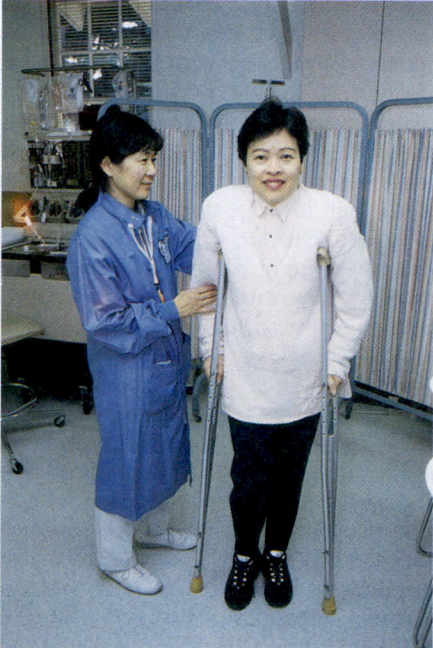

Figure 55-7 ■ Assisting the client with crutch walking. Note how the therapist guards the client and how the client's elbows are at no more than 30 degrees of flexion.

from slipping and the bars from damaging the axillae. To prevent pressure on the axillary nerve, there should be two to three finger breadths between the axilla and the top of the crutch when the crutch tip is at least 6 inches (15 cm) diagonally in front of the foot. The crutch is adjusted so that the elbow is flexed no more than 30 degrees when the palm is on the handle (Figure 55-7).

There are several types of gaits for walking with crutches. The most common one for musculoskeletal injury is the three-point gait, which allows minimal weight bearing on the affected leg.

Walkers and Canes. A walker is most often used by the older client who needs additional support for balance. The physical therapist assesses the strength of the upper extremities and the unaffected leg. Strength is improved with exercise as needed.

A cane is sometimes used if the client needs only minimal support for an affected leg. The straight cane offers the least support. A hemi-cane or quad-cane provides a broader base for the cane and therefore more support. The cane is placed on the *unaffected* side and should create no more than 30 degrees of flexion of the elbow. The top of the cane should be parallel to the greater trochanter of the femur.

IMBALANCED NUTRITION: LESS THAN BODY REQUIREMENTS

NOC **PLANNING: EXPECTED OUTCOMES.** The client with a fracture is expected to maintain an adequate dietary intake to meet metabolic needs. Indicators include that the client will have no deviation from normal range in the following:

- Nutrient intake
- Food intake
- Fluid intake
- Hematocrit

INTERVENTIONS. Nursing interventions focus on meeting the client's nutritional needs. The dietitian assesses the client's food likes and dislikes and collaborates with him or her to plan meals that are both appealing and nutritional. For promotion of bone and tissue healing, the client needs a high-protein, high-calorie diet. Supplements of vitamins B and C are also required for tissue nutrition. Clients with fractures may be immobilized for extended periods; thus they are predisposed to hypocalcemia, which results in loss of calcium from bone and in subsequent bone fragility. Teach the client to increase the intake of foods high in calcium, particularly milk and milk products if the client can tolerate them.

A negative nitrogen balance can develop 7 to 10 days after injury in an immobilized client because of an increase in catabolism without compensatory protein intake. Suggest frequent small feedings and supplements of high-protein liquids, such as Boost or Carnation Instant Breakfast preparations. Milk shakes are an excellent protein and calorie supplement as well as a source of calcium.

Because of less weight bearing on long bones, the immobilized client with a fracture often becomes anemic. Blood loss from the injury or reparative surgery contributes to the anemic state. Encourage intake of foods high in iron content. The health care provider may prescribe a daily multivitamin with iron supplement.

Critical Thinking Challenge

Following initial assessment in the emergency department, your client, who was injured in a motorcycle accident, has a closed reduction of the wrist fracture and application of a long-arm cast. He is alert and oriented when he arrives on the orthopedic unit.

1. What assessments should you perform to evaluate the client's injured arm?
2. What is a potential cause of compartment syndrome in this client's fractured arm?
3. What symptoms would raise suspicion of compartment syndrome?

evolve For suggested answer guidelines, go to http://evolve.elsevier.com/Iggy/.

Community-Based Care

The client with an uncomplicated fracture is usually discharged to home from the emergency department. Older adults with hip or other fractures or clients with multiple trauma are hospitalized and then transferred to home, a rehabilitation setting, or a long-term care facility for rehabilitation. To ensure continuity of care, the case manager or the discharge planner in the hospital communicates the plan of care to the health care agency receiving the client (see the Evidence-Based Practice for Nursing box below).

HOME CARE MANAGEMENT

If the client is discharged to home, the nurse, therapist, or case manager assesses the home environment for structural barriers to mobility, such as stairs. Most clients are taught how to use stairs, but older adults may not be able to perform this difficult task.

HEALTH TEACHING

The client with a fracture may be discharged from the hospital, emergency department, office, or clinic with a bandage, splint, cast, or external fixator. Provide verbal and written instructions on the care of these devices. Chart 55-6 describes care of the affected extremity after removal of the cast.

The client may also need to continue wound care at home. Instruct the client and caregiver about how to assess and dress the wound to promote healing and prevent infection. Teach the client also how to recognize complications (see Complications of Fractures, p. 1191) and when and where to seek professional health care if complications occur.

Additional educational needs depend on the type of fracture and fracture repair. Care of external fixators and casts is discussed earlier in this chapter under Cast Care (p. 1199) and External Fixation (p. 1202).

HEALTH CARE RESOURCES

Identify potential or actual problems in the hospital and arrange for follow-up care at home. For example, professional counseling for depression may need to continue after discharge from the hospital. A social worker may need to help the client apply for funds to pay medical bills. If there is severe bone and tissue damage, be realistic and help the client understand the long-term nature of the recovery period, particularly if he or she experiences a major complication, such as infection, while in the hospital. Multiple treatment techniques and surgical procedures required for complications can be mentally and emotionally draining for the client and family. A vocational counselor may be needed to help the client seek a different type of job, depending on the nature of the fracture.

The client with a severe injury and multiple treatment modalities may need follow-up care in the home by a home care nurse. An older or incapacitated client may need assistance with activities of daily living (ADLs), which is provided by home care aides. The nurse in the hospital anticipates the client's needs and arranges for these services, usually with the assistance of the case worker or discharge planner.

It is extremely important for the hospital nurse to communicate the client's needs to the nurse or aide who will care for the client at home. A physical therapist may come to the home, or the client may go to a clinic, hospital, or private office for follow-up physical therapy after discharge

---

EVIDENCE-BASED PRACTICE for Nursing

Improving client outcomes through trauma case management

Curtis, K., et al. (2002). The impact of trauma case management on patient outcomes. *The Journal of Trauma Injury, Infection, and Critical Care, 53*(3), 477-482.

This study examined the use of nurse case managers for trauma clients with injury severity scores (ISS) of 8-15, length of stay, length of stay for age over and under age 50, missed injury detection, complication rated overall, over/under age 50, and utilization and days/client of allied health intervention (physical, occupational, or other therapies).

Results demonstrated a trend toward reduced length of stay overall, more so in the older and more severely injured. The trauma case management greatly improved the missed injury detection rates and coordinated allied health use more efficiently. Staff surveys exhibited dramatic improvement in the effectiveness of client care. There was an overall reduction in complication rates, especially in the older group of clients; however, it was not statistically significant.

Level of Evidence: 6—This study serves as a pilot study for future research regarding the utilization of nurse case managers, a growing trend.

Critique. The sample sizes of both the control (327) and study (149) groups were relatively small, which makes generalization more difficult. Also, the use of age 50 to divide the older and younger populations is an unusual age and makes interpretation of data more difficult to relate to other studies.

Implications for Nursing. Nurses play an important role in improving client care and follow-up. Nurses should (1) coordinate care between various health care providers, (2) listen to all the client's complaints and concerns, and (3) be alert for early signs and symptoms of complications.

CHART 55-6

CLIENT EDUCATION GUIDE
Care of the Extremity After Cast Removal

- Remove scaly, dead skin carefully by soaking; do not scrub.
- Move the extremity carefully. Expect discomfort, weakness, and decreased range of motion.
- Support the extremity with pillows or your orthotic device until strength and movement return.
- Exercise slowly as instructed by your physical therapist.
- Wear support stockings or elastic bandages to prevent swelling (for lower extremity).

from the hospital. An occupational therapist assists with retraining in the home environment for ADLs; adaptations in the home enable the client to be independent.

The cost to individuals and society at large is enormous (see the Resource Management box at right). The cost for direct medical care, rehabilitation, lost wages, and lost productivity is more than $224 billion each year (http://www.cdc.gov). Each year about 90,000 people sustain injuries serious enough to cause long-term disability. Injury is a definable, correctable event with specific identifiable risks. It is imperative that nurses be active in educating the public on prevention of injury through programs that highlight the major risk factors, including alcohol, illicit drugs, and firearms among the young and falls in older adults.

◆Evaluation: Outcomes

Evaluate the care of the client with a fracture on the basis of the identified nursing diagnoses and collaborative problems. The expected outcomes include that the client:

- Has adequate blood flow through the small vessels to maintain tissue perfusion
- Takes personal actions to control pain
- Is free of infection
- Is free of physiologic consequences of impaired mobility
- Moves purposefully independently in his or her own environment with or without an assistive device
- Meets metabolic needs

Specific indicators for these outcomes are listed for each nursing diagnosis under the Planning and Implementation (see earlier).

FRACTURES OF SPECIFIC SITES

Upper Extremity Fractures

Fractures of the Clavicle

Fractures of the clavicle typically result from a fall on an outstretched hand, a fall on the shoulder, or a direct injury. Most clavicular fractures are self-healing; a splint or bandage is used for immobilization. Complicated fractures, although uncommon, may require open reduction with internal fixation (ORIF) by pins, wires, or screws.

Fractures of the Scapula

Scapular fractures are not common and are usually caused by direct impact to the area. Serious internal trauma, including pneumothorax, pulmonary contusion, and fractured ribs, can accompany these fractures.

The shoulder is immobilized with a sling and swathe or a shoulder immobilizer until the fracture heals, usually in 2 to 4 weeks. Intra-articular neck and glenoid fractures may require surgical intervention with plate and screw fixation.

Fractures of the Humerus

Fractures of the proximal humerus, particularly impacted or displaced fractures, are common in the older adult. An impacted injury is usually treated conservatively with a sling for immobilization. A displaced fracture often requires ORIF with pins or a prosthetic device.

Humeral shaft fractures are generally corrected by closed reduction and application of a hanging-arm cast or splint. If necessary, the fracture is repaired surgically (with an intramedullary rod or metal plate and screws) or with external fixation. Nonunion of the bone and radial nerve palsy are frequent complications of this fracture. Bone grafting facilitates union; prolonged splinting is necessary while the radial nerve regenerates.

A direct blow to the condyles of the distal humerus can cause either or both condyles to fracture, usually in a T- or Y-shaped configuration. The most serious complication is damage to the brachial or median nerve. Condylar fracture is usually treated by ORIF with a series of screws, although skeletal traction and casting can be used.

Fractures of the Olecranon

Fractures of the olecranon are relatively common in adults and typically result from a fall on the elbow. Many are successfully treated by closed reduction and application of a cast. The healing process usually takes more than 2 months, and several additional months may be needed before full use of the elbow is achieved. ORIF is performed for displaced fractures, and a splint is worn during the healing phase.

Fractures of the Radius and Ulna

Forearm fractures of the ulna without accompanying injury to the radius are rare. As with other fractures of long bones, closed reduction with casting may be the appropriate treatment. If the fracture is displaced, ORIF with intramedullary rods or plates and screws is required.

Fractures of the Wrist and Hand

One or more of the bones in the wrist and hand can break, but the most common fracture is of the carpal scaphoid bone in young adult men. This is also one of the most misdiagnosed fractures because it is poorly visualized on an x-

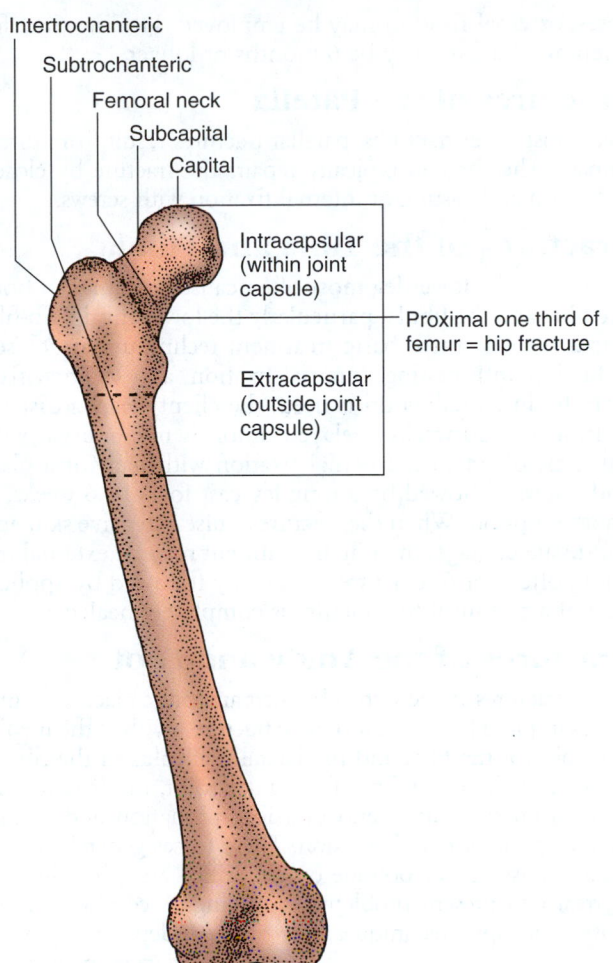

Intertrochanteric
Subtrochanteric
Femoral neck
Subcapital
Capital

Intracapsular
(within joint
capsule)

Proximal one third of
femur = hip fracture

Extracapsular
(outside joint
capsule)

Figure 55-8 ■ Types of hip fractures.

ray film. Closed reduction and casting for 6 to 12 weeks is the treatment of choice. If the bone does not heal, open reduction and bone grafting are performed.

Fractures of the metacarpals and phalanges are usually not displaced, which makes their treatment less difficult than that of other fractures. Metacarpal fractures are immobilized for 3 to 4 weeks. Phalangeal fractures are immobilized in finger splints for 10 to 14 days.

Lower Extremity Fractures

Fractures of the Hip

Hip fractures include those involving the upper third of the femur and are classified as **intracapsular** (within the joint capsule) or **extracapsular** (outside the joint capsule). These types are further divided according to fracture location (Figure 55-8).

Falls cause most hip fractures; impaction or displacement, especially of the femoral neck, often results. If the degree of osteoporosis is so severe that it prevents surgical intervention, the client may be incapacitated for the remainder of his or her life. The cost of hip fractures is increasing as baby boomers age and increased Medicare funds are needed (see the Evidence-Based Practice for Nursing box above).

EVIDENCE-BASED PRACTICE for Nursing

Evaluating costs for older adults with musculoskeletal injury

Bishop, C.E., et al. (2002). Medicare spending for injured elders: Are there opportunities for savings? *Health Affairs, 21*(6), 215-223.

This study examined Medicare spending for injuries in 1999 on all paid claims from a randomly selected 5% sample. The study found that fractures were the most common and costly injury (67% / $5.5 billion), followed by open wounds (11% / $873 million), then internal injuries (6% / $503 million). Sprains and strains accounted for 4% of the injuries and resulted in an additional $323 million expenditure. More than 70% of these unintentional injuries are musculoskeletal.

Level of Evidence: 2—The study used a large sample and randomized the sample.

Critique. The 5% randomly selected sample and calculation of costs for the HMO portion of Medicare may or may not be accurate. Because the study reviewed paid claims, it did identify expenses that would be missed by more traditional studies, which review only hospitalization or emergency department records. The findings related to cost for fractures generally confirm other studies related to the cost of fractures and incidence of fractures in this age group.

Implications for Nursing. Results of this study and prior research can be used to develop guidelines reduce the incidence and related cost of musculoskeletal injuries in older adults. Nurses should (1) continue osteoporosis screening and education to increase bone mineral density for both women and men; (2) provide fall prevention education; (3) support special programs for older drivers to reduce injuries to pedestrians, passengers, and drivers; (4) teach about medication safety; and (5) encourage exercise programs to increase gait, strength, and coordination.

CONSIDERATIONS FOR OLDER ADULTS

Hip fractures occur most often in older persons, particularly women who have osteoporosis. Repair of hip fracture is rapidly becoming the most common surgical procedure for people older than 85 years of age. As many as one third of older clients who sustain a hip fracture die within 1 year of injury from medical complications caused by the fracture or by the immobility that occurs after the fracture. About 50% cannot return home or live independently after the fracture (Schmitt, 2000). Because of the poor prognosis of clients experiencing hip fractures, public education on osteoporosis and fracture prevention is crucial. Studies suggest that older, thin, white women are at the greatest risk for hip fracture.

The treatment of choice is surgical repair, when possible, to allow the older client to get out of bed. Buck's traction may be applied before surgery, which should be scheduled within 24 hours of injury if at all possible. Depending on the exact location of the fracture, open reduction with internal fixation (ORIF) may include an intramedullary rod, pins, a prosthesis, or a fixed sliding plate (such as a compression screw). The client with a compression screw can usually ambulate a few days after surgery and has a decreased chance of infection and nonunion in comparison with clients for whom other procedures are used. If the femoral neck or head is fractured, a prosthetic device is implanted. Depending on the age of the client and prior mobility status, the surgeon replaces the femoral head only or performs a total hip replacement. Figures 55-9 and 55-10 illustrate examples of these devices used for ORIF of the hip. Nonsurgical options are Buck's traction and skeletal traction, followed by use of a cast brace (Taggart, 1999).

CONSIDERATIONS FOR OLDER ADULTS

Older clients often have peripheral vascular disease, connective tissue disease, or diabetes. Therefore they are at high risk for problems caused by skin or skeletal traction because of inadequate circulation and sensation. Traction of any type is not the ideal treatment for the older client because it necessitates a prolonged period of immobilization; serious complications can result, such as pneumonia and pulmonary emboli. Abrasions, ulcers, and other skin problems should be reported to the health care provider. Care must be taken to avoid pressure on the bony prominences and superficial nerves. Pressure on the peroneal nerve at the point where it passes around the neck of the fibula must also be avoided, or footdrop could occur.

Hip fractures are very common. Nurses in all health care settings need to know how to care for the special needs of the older adult with a hip fracture (see the Plan of Care on pp. 1209 to 1217). Some of the postoperative care is similar to that needed by older clients undergoing total hip replacement (see Chapter 22).

Fractures of the Femur

Fractures of the lower two thirds of the femur usually result from trauma (often from a motor vehicle accident). A femoral fracture is seldom immobilized by casting because the powerful muscles of the thigh become spastic, which causes displacement of bone ends. Extensive hemorrhage is associated with femoral fracture.

Skeletal traction, followed by a cast brace or hip spica cast, is the typical nonsurgical treatment. Surgical treatment is ORIF with nails, rods, or a compression screw. In a few cases, external fixation may be employed. Healing time for a femoral fracture may be 6 months or longer.

Fractures of the Patella

Like most other fractures, patellar fractures result from direct impact. The surgeon typically repairs the fracture by closed reduction and casting or internal fixation with screws.

Fractures of the Tibia and Fibula

Trauma to the lower leg most often causes fractures of both the tibia and the fibula, particularly the lower third ("tib-fib" fractures). The three basic treatment techniques are closed reduction with casting, internal fixation, and external fixation. If closed reduction is used, the client wears a cast for at least 8 to 10 weeks. Delayed union is not unusual with this type of fracture. Internal fixation with nails or a plate and screws, followed by a long leg cast for 4 to 6 weeks, is another option. When the fractures cause extensive skin and soft-tissue damage, the initial treatment may be external fixation, often for 6 to 10 weeks, usually followed by application of a cast until the fracture is completely healed.

Fractures of the Ankle and Foot

Ankle fractures are described by their anatomic place of injury. For example, a bimalleolar (Pott's) fracture involves the medial malleolus of the tibia and the lateral malleolus of the fibula. Because of the instability of the ankle joint, the fracture can result from supination and eversion, pronation and abduction, or pronation and eversion. These forces generally create spiral, transverse, or oblique breaks, which are often difficult to treat and present problems in healing. A combination of closed and open techniques may be used, depending on the

Text continued on p. 1217.

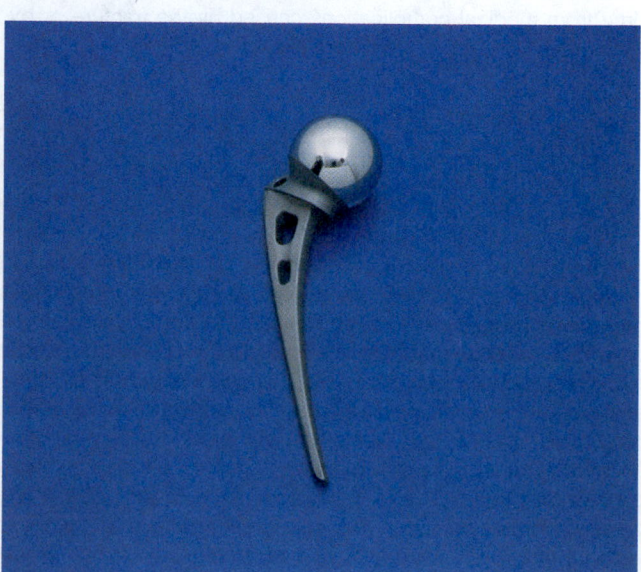

Figure 55-9 ■ The Moore prosthesis, which is used for hip fractures. (Courtesy of Smith & Nephew, Inc., Orthopaedics Divisions, Memphis, TN.)

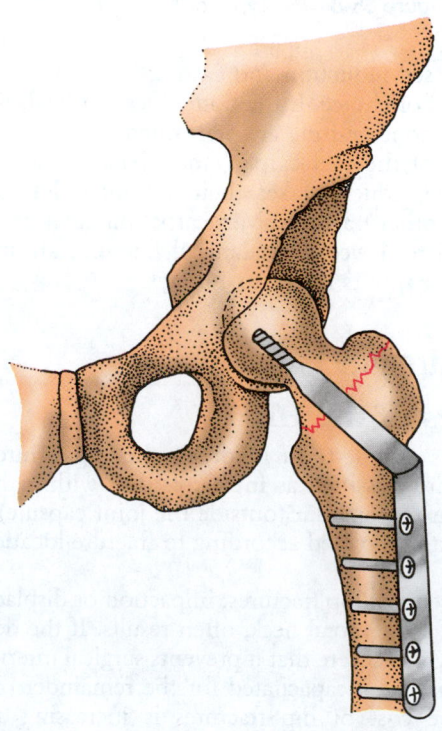

Figure 55-10 ■ A compression hip screw used for open reduction with internal fixation (ORIF) of the hip.

PLAN of CARE   MEDICAL DIAGNOSIS: FRACTURES

NURSING DIAGNOSIS NO. 1   ■   Risk for Peripheral Neurovascular Dysfunction

	Expected Outcomes	Nursing Interventions	Rationales
RELATED FACTORS Trauma or injury Vascular obstruction Orthopedic surgery Fracture Mechanical compression (e.g., tourniquet, cane, cast, brace, dressing, restraint)	No verbal report or observation of altered interpretation or response to stimuli No verbal report or observation of guarding or protective gestures Has skin with warm undertones Has a pulse that remains strong and equal at all pulse points No verbal report or observation of delayed healing Denies paresthesias or numbness	**NIC Peripheral Sensation Management** Monitor for paresthesia: numbness, tingling, hyperesthesia, and hypoesthesia. Monitor for thrombophlebitis and deep vein thrombosis. Instruct the client or family to examine the skin daily for alterations in skin integrity. **Other Interventions** Assist the client to develop a plan to manage the stress in his or her life. Administer hemorheologic and antiplatelet agents as prescribed. Prepare the client for surgical intervention as ordered by the physician. **D** Instruct the client to avoid crossing his or her legs. **D** Instruct the client to completely abstain from tobacco products. **D** Instruct the client to abstain from caffeine. **Continuing Care Considerations** Teach the client and family how to assess tissue perfusion to the affected extremity. Instruct the client about the therapeutic regimen. **D** Remove safety hazards in the home.	Changes in sensation are clinical indicators of changes in circulation or nerve functioning. Pooling of blood from impaired circulation or impaired mobility may facilitate the formation of thrombophlebitis and deep vein thrombosis. Frequent skin inspection may prevent breaks in skin integrity. Emotional stress may cause vasoconstriction. Hemorheologic agents increase the flexibility of red blood cells, and antiplatelet agents inhibit the platelet aggregation that could impede blood flow in the extremities. Procedures such as percutaneous transluminal angioplasty, laser-assisted angioplasty, atherectomy, or arterial revascularization may be needed to restore peripheral tissue perfusion. Crossing the legs will interfere with blood flow. Nicotine causes vasoconstriction. Caffeine causes vasoconstriction. Pain, pallor, paresthesias, pulselessness, paralysis, and poikilothermia are indicators of poor tissue perfusion. The client needs to follow foot care instructions, cease smoking, and avoid exposure of the affected extremity to heat/cold to prevent further injury to the extremity. Fall prevention and prevention of injury to the lower extremities is essential if the client has circulatory or nervous system impairments.

D Indicates tasks that can be delegated to unlicensed assistive nursing personnel at the discretion of the nurse.

Continued

▤ PLAN of CARE   MEDICAL DIAGNOSIS: FRACTURES—*cont'd*

NURSING DIAGNOSIS NO. 2 ■ Acute Pain

	Expected Outcomes	Nursing Interventions	Rationales
RELATED FACTORS Injury agents: Biologic, chemical, physical, psychological **DEFINING CHARACTERISTICS** Verbal or coded report of pain Observed evidence of pain Protective gestures Facial mask Self-focus	Denies experiencing pain greater than 5 on a 0 to 10 pain scale No verbal report or observation of guarding or protective gestures No verbal report or observation of self-focusing behavior No verbal report or observation of facial mask of pain	**NIC Pain Management** Perform a comprehensive pain assessment that includes location, characteristics, onset/duration, frequency, quality, intensity or severity of pain, and precipitating factors. **D** Observe for nonverbal cues of discomfort, especially in those who are unable to communicate effectively. Consider cultural influences on the pain response. Determine the needed frequency of making an assessment of client comfort, and implement a monitoring plan. **D** Reduce or eliminate factors that precipitate or increase the pain experience. Encourage the client to monitor his or her own pain and to intervene appropriately. Use pain control measures before pain becomes severe. Provide information about the pain, such as causes, how long it will last, and anticipated discomforts from procedures. Teach the use of non-pharmacologic techniques before, after and, if possible, during painful activities; before pain occurs or increases; and along with other pain relief measures. **NIC Analgesic Administration** **D** Monitor vital signs before and after administering opioid analgesics with a first-time dose or if unusual signs are noted. Choose the IV rather than the IM route for frequent pain medication injections, when possible. Administer analgesics around-the-clock. Set positive expectations regarding the effectiveness of analgesics.	A plan for pain management must be based on the client's unique responses to pain. Nonverbal cues provide support for the existence of pain. Cultural stereotypes may lead to an inaccurate assessment of pain. Initial pain management strategies may require frequent evaluation to adjust dosing to maintain adequate comfort. Preventing a pain experience is preferred to trying to control or eliminate pain. The client is the best person to manage his or her own pain. Medicating the client in a timely manner prevents pain from reaching acutely unpleasant levels. The client is better able to monitor his or her own discomfort and to intervene appropriately when informed. Nonpharmacologic techniques help the client to establish a sense of control over his or her pain experience. Opioid analgesics may depress respirations or cause other adverse effects. The IV route avoids tissue trauma and the unpredictable absorption of medication. Administration around-the-clock prevents the peaks and troughs of analgesia, especially with severe pain. Positive expectations will optimize the client's response to the analgesics.

D Indicates tasks that can be delegated to unlicensed assistive nursing personnel at the discretion of the nurse.

PLAN of CARE   MEDICAL DIAGNOSIS: FRACTURES—cont'd

NURSING DIAGNOSIS NO. 2 ■ Acute Pain—cont'd

Expected Outcomes	Nursing Interventions	Rationales
	Institute safety precautions for a client who is receiving opioid analgesics, as appropriate.	Opioid analgesics may impair the client's judgment and/or coordination.
	After each administration of the analgesic, evaluate the effectiveness at regular and frequent intervals, especially after the initial dose; in addition, observe for any signs or symptoms of untoward effects.	Frequent evaluation of analgesic effectiveness permits the nurse to adjust the dose and timing interval to the client's need and provides an early warning of adverse responses.
	Instruct the client to request a PRN pain medication before the pain becomes severe.	Pain may be managed with lower doses of analgesics and fewer untoward effects if PRN pain medications are used before pain becomes severe.
	Inform the client that drowsiness sometimes occurs during the first 2 to 3 days of opioid administration and then subsides.	Drowsiness poses a hazard to the client, making accidents more likely to occur.
	Correct any misconceptions or myths that the client or family members may hold regarding analgesics, particularly opioids.	A client's misconceptions may prevent him or her from using opioid analgesics.
	Teach about the use of analgesics, strategies to decrease side effects, and expectations for involvement in decisions about pain relief.	Information about analgesics and the expectations for client involvement increase the client's sense of control over his or her pain.
	NIC **Environmental Management: Comfort**	
	Determine sources of discomfort, such as damp dressings, tubing position, constrictive dressings, wrinkled bed linens, and environmental irritants.	Control of environmental discomforts may decrease the need for pharmacologic intervention.
	Monitor skin, especially over bony prominences, for signs of pressure or irritation.	Skin irritation or tissue damage add a source of discomfort.
	D Prevent unnecessary interruptions and allow for rest periods.	Rest may improve the client's pain tolerance.
	D Provide a clean, comfortable bed.	Clean bed linens decrease exposure to infectious agents and increase the client's sense of well-being.
	D Facilitate hygiene measures to keep the client comfortable.	Hygiene measures may improve the client's overall sense of well-being.
	D Position the client to facilitate comfort.	The nurse may decrease sources of discomfort by using principles of body alignment, supporting with pillows, supporting joints during movement, splinting over incisions, and immobilizing painful body parts.

Continued

PLAN of CARE   MEDICAL DIAGNOSIS: FRACTURES—*cont'd*

NURSING DIAGNOSIS NO. 2 ■ Acute Pain—*cont'd*

Expected Outcomes	Nursing Interventions	Rationales
	Other Interventions Refer the client to the Pain Advisory Committee.	The Pain Advisory Committee is a multidisciplinary committee with wide expertise in pain relief interventions.
	Consider the use of alternative therapies such as yoga, meditation, spirituality, and/or religion.	The experience of meditation and prayer and the reflection on meaning may help the client to relax, thereby easing the muscle tension that contributes to pain sensation.
	Consider the use of alternative therapies such as imagery, aromatherapy, music, touch, and laughter/humor.	Cognitive and behavioral strategies may be used as adjuncts to or in place of pharmacologic or surgical interventions for chronic pain. Each therapy has a different mode of action, which may or may not benefit the client.
	Consider using other cutaneous skin stimulation techniques such as massage and/or vibration to complement pain management strategies.	Massage may cause muscle relaxation, which decreases pain signals; vibration interrupts pain signal transmission to decrease pain perception.
	Continuing Care Considerations Refer the client to an advanced practice nurse pain specialist, social worker, home care nurse, and/or psychologist, as appropriate.	The health care team members are able to provide continuing support for the client facing chronic pain.

NURSING DIAGNOSIS NO. 3 ■ Risk for Infection

	Expected Outcomes	Nursing Interventions	Rationales
RELATED FACTORS Invasive procedures Trauma or injury Inadequate secondary defenses (decreased hemoglobin, leukopenia, suppressed inflammatory response) Inadequate primary defenses (broken skin, traumatized tissue, decrease in ciliary action, stasis of body fluids, changes in pH secretions, altered peristalsis)	Denies fatigue Denies weakness Denies nausea Has no observable alterations in personality Has skin with warm undertones Has a heart rate that remains regular, strong, and between 60 and 100 beats/min Has a body temperature that remains between 97° and 99.6° F (36.1° and 37.5° C)	**NIC** **Infection Protection** Monitor for systemic and localized signs and symptoms of infection. Monitor absolute granulocyte count, white blood cell (WBC) count, and differential results. Inspect the condition of any surgical incision/wound. **D** Provide appropriate skin care to edematous areas. **D** Maintain asepsis for the client at risk.	An elevated temperature, pulse, and respirations indicate systemic infection; redness, heat, swelling, and pain indicate local infection. Elevations in these laboratory tests demonstrate the body's response to infection. A surgical incision may be slightly reddened and swollen from tissue damage but remain free of the purulent drainage, excess swelling, or excess local pain that indicate infection. Edematous skin is particularly susceptible to injury, and edematous tissue may encourage the growth of pathogenic agents. Asepsis will minimize the client's exposure to pathogenic agents and thus minimize the incidence of infection.

D Indicates tasks that can be delegated to unlicensed assistive nursing personnel at the discretion of the nurse.

PLAN of CARE   MEDICAL DIAGNOSIS: FRACTURES—*cont'd*

NURSING DIAGNOSIS NO. 3 ■ Risk for Infection—*cont'd*

Expected Outcomes	Nursing Interventions	Rationales
	D Encourage coughing and deep breathing, as appropriate.	Coughing and deep breathing clears the lungs of secretions that may encourage the growth of pathogenic microbes.
	D Promote sufficient nutritional intake.	Adequate nutrition is essential for the formation of immune system cells and for the repair of damaged body tissues to provide protection against external pathogens.
	D Encourage fluid intake, as appropriate.	Adequate fluid intake provides for renal clearance of the toxins produced by pathogens.
	Report positive cultures to infection control personnel.	Early intervention to treat infection improves the client's response to therapy.
	NIC **Infection Control** Administer antibiotic therapy, as appropriate.	Antibiotic therapy should assist the body to destroy pathogens.
	Continuing Care Considerations Numerous visitors should be limited, and visits from individuals with known infections should be discouraged.	Visitors may provide a needed diversion for the client, but too many visitors may cause fatigue and bring unwanted exposure to pathogens.
	Teach the client and family about the signs and symptoms of infection and when to report them to the health care provider.	Early intervention to treat infection prevents untoward complications from the infection and its therapy.

NURSING DIAGNOSIS NO. 4 ■ Impaired Physical Mobility

Expected Outcomes	Nursing Interventions	Rationales
RELATED FACTORS Medications Prescribed movement restrictions Pain Musculoskeletal impairment **DEFINING CHARACTERISTICS** Limited ability to perform gross motor skills Limited range of motion Difficulty turning	**Has full or improved range of motion in all joints** Has smooth, coordinated movements Able to turn without assistance Has skin that remains intact with no bruising or rashes Able to perform gross motor skills	NIC **Exercise Therapy: Joint Mobility** Collaborate with physical therapy in developing and executing an exercise program.	Physical therapists are the primary health care professionals responsible for developing and executing an exercise program.
		Explain to the client and family the purpose of and plan for joint exercises.	An informed client and family is more likely to comply with a joint exercise regimen.
		Initiate pain control measures before beginning joint exercise.	Initiating pain control measures before joint exercise increases the likelihood of client comfort and his or her willingness to engage in the exercise.
		D Dress the client in nonrestrictive clothing.	Nonrestrictive clothing permits full range of joint motion.
		D Protect the client from trauma during exercise.	Stretching exercises may cause the client to be off balance.
		D Assist the client to an optimal body position for passive/active joint movement.	Neutral alignment is the optimal positioning for joint movement.

Continued

PLAN of CARE **MEDICAL DIAGNOSIS: FRACTURES—cont'd**

NURSING DIAGNOSIS NO. 4 ■ Impaired Physical Mobility—cont'd

Expected Outcomes	Nursing Interventions	Rationales
	D Encourage active range-of-motion exercises, according to a regular, planned schedule.	Periods of regular active range-of-motion exercise maximize the exercise benefit to the joints.
	D Perform passive range-of-motion (PROM) or assisted range-of-motion (AROM) exercises, as indicated.	The use of PROM or AROM exercises depends on the client's ability to initiate muscle and joint movement, the restrictions imposed by medical therapies, and the client's endurance.
	Assist the client to develop a schedule for active range-of-motion exercises.	Regular exercise maximizes the benefit of the exercise.
	D Encourage the client to sit in bed, on the side of the bed ("dangle"), or in a chair, as tolerated.	Sitting in bed, on the edge of the bed, or in a chair exercises the joints by the shift in position.
	D Encourage ambulation, if appropriate.	Ambulation is a form of active joint exercise and also improves cardiovascular tone.
	NIC **Positioning**	
	D Provide a firm mattress.	A firm mattress offers support.
	D Encourage the client to get involved in positioning changes, as appropriate.	Involving the client in positioning changes actively exercises the muscles and joints and permits the client a measure of control in the positioning process.
	Premedicate the client before turning, as appropriate.	Premedicating the client before turning will increase comfort and decrease resistance to repositioning from fear of pain.
	D Position in proper body alignment.	Proper body alignment preserves the functionality of the muscles and bony skeleton.
	D Immobilize or support the affected body part, as appropriate.	Immobilization or support of the affected body part permits healing and decreases further injury.
	D Provide support to edematous areas (e.g., pillow under the arms, scrotal support), as appropriate.	Support to edematous areas is necessary because edematous tissue is more susceptible to pressure injury.
	D Provide appropriate support for the neck.	The neck should be kept in neutral alignment, neither hyperflexed nor hyperextended.
	D Avoid placing the client in a position that increases pain.	Repositioning should provide the client with a measure of comfort. Pain may indicate improper body positioning.
	D Minimize friction and shearing forces when positioning and turning the client.	Friction and shearing forces will cause damage to the skin and underlying tissues.
	D Turn the client using the log roll technique.	The log roll technique keeps the spinal column in alignment during the turn, thereby preventing injury to the spinal nerves.

D Indicates tasks that can be delegated to unlicensed assistive nursing personnel at the discretion of the nurse.

PLAN of CARE   MEDICAL DIAGNOSIS: FRACTURES—cont'd

NURSING DIAGNOSIS NO. 4 ■ Impaired Physical Mobility—cont'd

Expected Outcomes	Nursing Interventions	Rationales
	▶ Position the client to avoid placing tension on the wound, as appropriate.	Tension on a wound will cause pain and impede healing.
	Apply a foot board to the bed.	A foot board will prevent foot drop.
	▶ Elevate the affected limb 20 degrees or more, above the level of the heart.	Elevating the affected limb 20 degrees or more, above the level of the heart, improves venous return.
	Monitor traction devices.	Traction devices need to be monitored for proper setup.
	Maintain the position and integrity of the traction.	The traction must be intact and in the prescribed position to provide the desired therapeutic effect.
	▶ Elevate the head of the bed, as appropriate.	The head of the bed may be elevated to provide countertraction or comfort if permitted.
	Develop a written schedule for repositioning, as appropriate.	A written schedule for repositioning permits all health care workers to participate in repositioning.
	▶ Use a hand roll or trochanter roll, as appropriate.	Hand rolls and trochanter rolls support the limbs.
	▶ Place frequently used objects within reach.	Placing frequently used objects within reach permits the client safe and convenient access.
	▶ Place the bed-positioning switch within easy reach.	Placing the bed-positioning switch within easy reach permits the client to change positions safely and conveniently.
	Place the call light within reach.	Placing the call light within reach allows the client to summon assistance conveniently.
	Other Interventions Instruct the client in the use of assistive devices.	The client will need instruction to properly use canes, crutches, walkers, splints, or other assistive devices.
	Continuing Care Considerations Refer the client to rehabilitative services, as appropriate.	Ongoing support from physical therapists, occupational therapists, and others may be needed to help the client resume his or her activities of daily living.
	Refer the client to a vocational counselor, as appropriate.	Long-term physical impairment may require a change in employment.
	Collaborate with community organizations to inform the public about injury prevention.	Injury prevention saves the individual—and society as a whole—an enormous economic burden.

Continued

PLAN of CARE MEDICAL DIAGNOSIS: FRACTURES—cont'd

NURSING DIAGNOSIS NO. 5 ■ Imbalanced Nutrition: Less Than Body Requirements

	Expected Outcomes	Nursing Interventions	Rationales
RELATED FACTORS Inability to ingest or digest food or absorb nutrients due to biologic, psychological, or economic factors **DEFINING CHARACTERISTICS** Poor muscle tone Lack of interest in food Capillary fragility Information: Lack of or misinformation	Has muscle tone ≥4+ Denies changes in taste sensation Has bowel sounds that remain at 3 to 5 per quadrant per minute Has skin with warm undertones No verbal report or observation of altered eating habits No verbal report or observation of alteration in appetite Weight remains within ±5 pounds of desired weight	**NIC Nutrition Management** Determine, in collaboration with a dietitian as appropriate, the number of calories and type of nutrients needed to meet nutrition requirements. Provide appropriate information about nutritional needs and how to meet them. **NIC Weight Gain Assistance** Monitor the daily calories consumed. Monitor levels of serum albumin, lymphocytes, and electrolytes. Provide oral care before meals, as needed. Ensure that the client is in a sitting position before eating or feeding. Assist clients with eating or feed them, as appropriate. Administer medications to reduce nausea and pain before eating, as appropriate. Encourage increased calorie intake. Provide the client with a variety of high-calorie and nutritious foods from which to select. Consider the client's food preferences as governed by personal choices and cultural and religious preferences. **Other Interventions** Teach the client and family about high-calorie, high-protein meal planning, as appropriate. Teach the client and family about nutritional supplements, as appropriate. Teach the client and family about preventing constipation.	Individual client needs for nutrients and calories should be the basis for a sound dietary plan. Clients need accurate and timely information to make informed decisions about nutritional needs and how to meet them. Calorie consumption that is inadequate for individual need causes weight loss. Serum albumin and lymphocyte production and electrolyte levels reflect nutritional intake. A clean mouth improves taste sensation. The sitting position minimizes the risk of aspiration and prevents an increasingly full stomach from pressing on the diaphragm. Clients who are unable to feed themselves should be fed to maintain adequate nutrition. Medicating for nausea and pain before a meal improves the client's willingness to expend the energy to eat. Clients with a diminished appetite need reminders and encouragement to consume adequate nutrition. Monotony in food choices may lead to disinterest in the foods offered. Selecting appropriate foods according to personal, cultural, and religious preferences increases the likelihood that the client will eat the food. Meal planning that considers the client's and family's budget and other resources increases the likelihood that appropriate meals will be prepared. Additional vitamins and minerals, calories, dietary fiber, or other nutritional components may need to be added to the diet of a client who is unable to eat a nutritionally adequate diet. Clients on low-fiber diets may need additional fluids and supplemental fiber to maintain bowel regularity.

PLAN of CARE   MEDICAL DIAGNOSIS: FRACTURES—cont'd

NURSING DIAGNOSIS NO. 5 ■ Imbalanced Nutrition: Less Than Body Requirements—cont'd

Expected Outcomes	Nursing Interventions	Rationales
	Continuing Care Considerations	
	Refer the client to appropriate community nutritional programs, as needed.	Resources such as Weight Watchers, Overeaters Anonymous, and Take Off Pounds Sensibly provide support to the client who is attempting to maintain appropriate body weight.
	Refer the client to community support groups and encourage attendance, as appropriate.	Clients may need support to maintain healthy eating patterns. In addition, support groups can offer advice on how to overcome common problems.
	Encourage the client and family to use the home nutritional therapy team.	The home nutritional therapy team is able to monitor and adjust the nutritional plan of care to maximize the client's nutritional status.

severity and extent of the fracture. An arthrodesis (fusion) may be needed if the bone does not heal.

Treatment of fractures of the foot or phalanges is similar to that of other fractures, with either closed or open reduction. Phalangeal fractures are more painful than, but not as serious as, most other types of fractures.

Fractures of the Ribs and Sternum

Chest trauma may cause fractures of the ribs or sternum; the most commonly fractured ribs are numbers 4 through 8. The major concern with rib and sternal fractures is the potential for puncture of the lungs, heart, or arteries by bone fragments or ends. Fractures of the lower ribs may damage underlying organs, such as the liver, spleen, or kidneys. These fractures tend to heal spontaneously without surgical intervention. The client is often uncomfortable during the healing process and requires analgesia.

Fractures of the Pelvis

Because the pelvis is very vascular and is close to major organs and blood vessels, associated internal damage is the chief concern in fracture management. After head injuries, pelvic fractures are the second most common cause of death from trauma. In young adults, pelvic fractures typically result from motor vehicle accidents or falls from buildings; falls are the most common cause in older adults. The major concern related to pelvic injury is venous oozing or arterial bleeding. Loss of blood volume leads to hypovolemic shock.

Internal abdominal trauma is assessed by checking for the presence of blood in the urine and stool and by watching the abdomen for the development of rigidity or swelling. The trauma team may use peritoneal lavage, computed tomography (CT) scanning, or ultrasound (the newest diagnostic modality) for assessment of hemorrhage. Ultrasound is noninvasive, rapid, reliable, and cost effective, and it can be done at the bedside.

There are many classification systems for pelvic fractures. A system that is particularly useful divides fractures of the pelvis into two broad categories: non–weight-bearing fractures and weight-bearing fractures.

When a non–weight-bearing part of the pelvis is fractured, such as one of the pubic rami or the iliac crest, treatment can be as minimal as bedrest on a firm mattress or bed board. This type of fracture can be quite painful, and the client may need stool softeners to facilitate defecation because of hesitancy to move. Well-stabilized fractures usually heal in 2 months.

A weight-bearing fracture, such as multiple fractures of the pelvic ring creating instability or a fractured acetabulum, necessitate external fixation or open reduction with internal fixation (ORIF) or both. Progression to weight bearing depends on the stability of the fracture after fixation. Some clients can fully bear weight within days of surgery, whereas others managed with traction may not be able to bear weight for as long as 12 weeks.

Compression Fractures of the Spine

Most vertebral fractures are associated with osteoporosis rather than acute spinal injury. Multiple hairline fractures, called **compression fractures,** result when bone mass diminishes. The client experiences pain, deformity, and occasional neurologic compromise. As discussed in the Osteoporosis section of Chapter 54, the client's quality of life is reduced by the negative emotional impact of this problem.

Nonsurgical management with bedrest, analgesics, and physical therapy has been the traditional treatment. However, two new procedures have been successful in managing vertebral fractures in clients with osteoporosis. **Vertebroplasty** and **kyphoplasty** are both minimally invasive surgeries in which bone cement is injected directly into the fracture site to provide immediate pain relief. Kyphoplasty includes the additional step of using an inflated balloon to restore height to the vertebra. For most clients, these procedures are very successful in controlling pain (http://www.spine-health.com).

Fractures at Other Sites

Because the skull and vertebral column protect the brain and spinal cord, these acute fractures are described in Chapters 46 and 48. The nurse must be aware of the special care required for these clients because of possible neurologic damage resulting from these fractures. Fractures of the mandible or nose and other facial trauma are discussed elsewhere in the text.

AMPUTATIONS

PATHOPHYSIOLOGY

An **amputation** is the removal of a part of the body. The nurse recognizes that the psychosocial ramifications of the procedure are often more devastating than the physical impairment that results. The loss experienced is complete and permanent and causes a change in body image and often in self-esteem. As with other types of loss, the client can be expected to progress through phases of the grieving process.

Surgical Amputation

Amputations range from removal of part of a digit to removal of nearly half the entire body. The surgeon performs an amputation by one of two methods: open (guillotine) method or closed (flap) method. Surgical amputations are often referred to as "elective" surgeries.

The open method is used for clients who have, or are likely to develop, an infection. The wound remains open, and drains allow exudate to escape from the site until the infection clears. The surgeon may suture the skin flaps over the wound at a later time. In the closed technique, the surgeon pulls the skin flaps over the bone end and sutures them in place as part of the amputation procedure. One or more drains are typically inserted.

In either the closed or open method, the surgeon attempts to preserve as much of the part as possible and to keep major joints intact for maximal postoperative mobility.

Traumatic Amputation

Not all amputations are surgically planned. Some, classified as traumatic amputations, occur when a body part is severed unexpectedly (e.g., by a chain saw). Because the amputated part in these clients is usually healthy, attempts to replant it may be made.

One of the most likely replantations involves one or more digits. The current recommendation for prehospital care is that the severed digit be wrapped in a cool, dry cloth and moistened with normal saline, if possible, or bottled water. The digit should then be placed in a sealed plastic bag. The bag is placed in ice water, never directly on ice. Contact between the digit and the water is avoided to prevent tissue damage. Any semidetached parts of the digit should not be removed.

Levels of Amputation

LOWER EXTREMITY

Lower extremity amputations are performed much more frequently than upper extremity amputations. Five types of lower extremity amputations may be performed (Figure 55-11).

The loss of any or all of the small toes presents a minor disability. Loss of the great toe is significant because it af-

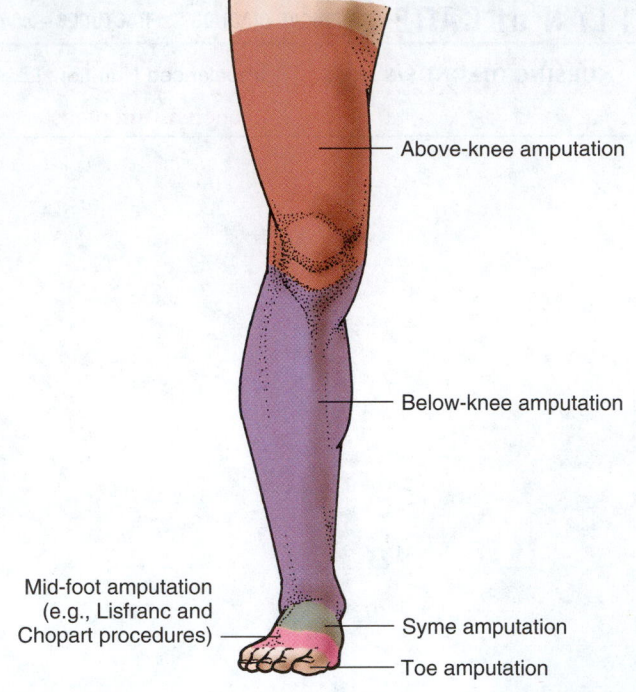

Figure 55-11 ■ Common levels of lower extremity amputation.

Above-knee amputation

Below-knee amputation

Mid-foot amputation (e.g., Lisfranc and Chopart procedures)

Syme amputation

Toe amputation

fects balance, gait, and "push off" ability during walking. Midfoot amputations (e.g., the Lisfranc amputation and the Chopart amputation) and the Syme amputation are common procedures for peripheral vascular disease. In the Syme amputation, most of the foot is removed but the ankle remains. The advantage of this surgery over traditional amputations below the knee is that weight bearing can be accomplished without use of a prosthesis and without pain.

An intense effort is made to preserve knee joints with below-knee amputation (BKA) rather than above-knee amputation (AKA). When the cause for the amputation extends beyond the knee, however, above-knee or higher amputations are performed. Hip disarticulation, or removal of the hip joint, and hemipelvectomy procedures are more common in younger clients than in older clients, who cannot easily handle the cumbersome prostheses required for ambulation. The higher the level of amputation, the more energy is required for ambulation. These higher-level procedures are typically done for cancer of the bone, osteomyelitis, or trauma.

UPPER EXTREMITY

Fewer than 10% of all amputations are upper extremity amputations. An amputation of any part of the upper extremity is generally more incapacitating than one of the leg. The arms and hands are necessary for activities of daily living (ADLs), such as feeding, bathing, dressing, and driving a car. As much length as possible is saved to maintain function. Early replacement with a prosthetic device is vital for the client with this type of amputation.

Complications of Amputations

The following are common complications of elective or traumatic amputations:

- Hemorrhage
- Infection
- Phantom limb pain

- Problems associated with immobility
- Neuroma
- Flexion contractures

HEMORRHAGE

When a person loses part or all of an extremity either by surgery or by trauma, major blood vessels are severed, which causes bleeding. If the bleeding is uncontrolled, the client is at risk for hypovolemic shock and possibly death.

INFECTION

As with any surgical procedure or trauma, infection can occur in the wound or the bone (osteomyelitis). The older adult who is debilitated and confused is at the greatest risk because excreta may soil the wound, or the client may remove the dressing and pick at the incision.

PHANTOM LIMB PAIN

Phantom limb pain (PLP) is a frequent complication of amputation. Most clients experience phantom limb sensation in the early postoperative period, most often after an AKA. Sensation is perceived in the phantom foot or hand and diminishes over time. When phantom limb sensation persists and is unpleasant or painful, it is referred to as PLP. PLP is more common in clients who have experienced chronic limb pain before surgery and rare in those who experience traumatic amputations.

No one theory explains or predicts PLP. Three theories continue to be researched:

- Peripheral nervous system theory
- Central nervous system theory
- Psychological theory

The peripheral nervous system theory implies that sensations remain as a result of severing peripheral nerves during the amputation. The central nervous system theory states that PLP results from a loss of inhibitory signals that are usually generated through afferent impulses from the amputated limb. When many sensory fibers are destroyed by amputation, the loss of inhibitory influences allows repetitive neural activity, which results in pain. Neither of these physiologic theories completely explains PLP. Most likely, a psychological component helps to predict and explain this phenomenon. Stress, anxiety, and depression often worsen or trigger an episode of PLP but are not likely to be the causative factors.

When experiencing PLP, the client complains of pain in the removed body part, most often shortly after surgery. The pain is often described either as an intense burning or crushing sensation or as cramping. Some clients say they feel as if the removed part is in a distorted, uncomfortable position; they experience numbness and tingling (sometimes called phantom limb sensation) as well as pain.

Some clients report that the most distal area of the removed part feels as if it is retracted into the residual limb end. For most clients, the pain is triggered by touching the residual limb, by temperature or barometric pressure changes, by concurrent illness, by fatigue, or by emotional stress. Routine activities, such as urination, can trigger the pain in other clients. If pain is long-standing, especially if it existed before the amputation, any stimulus can cause it, including touching any part of the body.

Pain does interfere with the amputee's activities of daily living. Some clients report that residual limb pain (RLP) ac-counted for more pain-related impairment than PLP or back pain (Marshall et al., 2002).

PROBLEMS ASSOCIATED WITH IMMOBILITY

Because the client experiences reduced mobility as a result of surgery, the complications of immobility can readily occur. These problems are discussed earlier under Complications of Fractures, p. 1191.

NEUROMA

Neuroma—a sensitive tumor consisting of nerve cells found at severed nerve endings—forms most often in amputations of the upper extremity but can occur anywhere.

FLEXION CONTRACTURES

Flexion contractures of the hip or knee are seen in clients with amputations of the lower extremity. This complication must be avoided so that the client can ambulate with a prosthesis.

Etiology

Most knowledge about amputations was obtained during World War II, when trauma often necessitated a loss of one or more body parts. Today, with highly sophisticated microsurgery for revascularization of tissues, amputations related to trauma are less likely to be needed. Limb salvage procedures, such as those described in Chapter 54 (under Surgical Management in the section on malignant bone tumors), have reduced the need for amputation.

Traumatic amputations most often result from accidents. A person may be cleaning lawn mower blades or a snow blower without disconnecting the machine. A motor vehicle or industrial machine accident may also cause an amputation. Individuals with a family history of peripheral vascular disease and diabetes have a higher risk for amputation.

Incidence/Prevalence

Surgical amputations are not as common as they were in the past because the success rates of revascularization and limb salvage techniques have improved over the last 30 years. However, more than 100,000 amputations are performed yearly in the United States, about half of these in clients with coexisting diabetes.

CONSIDERATIONS FOR OLDER ADULTS

The primary indication for surgical amputation is *ischemia* from peripheral vascular disease in the older client. The rate of lower extremity amputation, for example, is much greater among clients with diabetes than among other clients because of peripheral neuropathy and peripheral vascular disease (Collins et al., 2002). In addition, these older diabetic clients have visual, cardiac, and kidney problems. A client with an amputation of one leg because of poor circulation will often have an amputation of the other leg within 5 years. Older adults of advanced age may not be candidates for prostheses because of the energy required for ambulation. The more proximal (higher) the amputation in the lower extremity, the more energy required for ambulation.

CULTURAL CONSIDERATIONS

The incidence of lower extremity amputations is greater in the black and Hispanic populations because the incidence of

Continued

major diseases leading to amputation, such as diabetes and arteriosclerosis, is greater in this population. Limited access to health care for these minority groups may also play a major role in limb loss (Collins et al., 2002).

HEALTH PROMOTION/ILLNESS PREVENTION

The typical client undergoing the procedure is a middle-aged or older man with diabetes and a lengthy history of smoking. The client most likely has failed to care for his feet properly, which has resulted in a nonhealing, infected foot ulcer and possibly gangrene. Therefore compliance with the disease management plan may help prevent the need for later amputation.

The second largest group with amputations consists of young men who experience motorcycle or other vehicular accidents or who are injured at work by industrial equipment. These men may either experience a traumatic amputation or undergo a surgical amputation because of a severe crushing injury and massive soft-tissue damage. Teach young male adults the importance of taking safety precautions to prevent injury at work and to avoid speeding or driving while drinking alcohol.

◆COLLABORATIVE MANAGEMENT
◆Assessment

PHYSICAL ASSESSMENT/CLINICAL MANIFESTATIONS

When the client has peripheral vascular disease, the nurse's primary concern preoperatively is to assess circulation in other parts of the body. Assess skin color, temperature, sensation, and pulses in both affected and unaffected extremities. Capillary refill is evaluated by applying pressure to the nail bed and waiting for the brisk return of normal color. In the older adult, however, this test may be difficult to do because the nails may be thick and opaque. In this situation, the skin near the nail bed can be assessed (see Chart 55-3). Capillary refill may not be as reliable as other indicators.

PSYCHOSOCIAL ASSESSMENT

People react differently to the loss of a body part. Be aware that an amputation of a portion of one finger can be traumatic to the client; therefore the loss must not be underestimated. The client undergoing an amputation faces a complete, permanent loss. Evaluate the client's psychological preparation for a planned amputation, and expect him or her to experience the grieving process. Adjustment to a traumatic, unexpected amputation is often more difficult than accepting a planned one. The young client may be bitter, hostile, and uncooperative. In addition to loss of a body part, the client may lose a job, the ability to participate in favorite recreational activities, or a social relationship if the other person cannot accept the body change.

The client is faced with an altered self-concept. The physical alteration that results from an amputation affects body image and self-esteem. For example, a client may think that an intimate relationship with a mate is no longer possible. An older adult may feel a loss of independence. Assess the client's feelings about himself or herself to identify areas in which he or she needs emotional support.

Attempt to determine the client's willingness and motivation to withstand prolonged rehabilitation after the amputation. Asking questions about how the client has dealt with previous life crises can provide clues. The client's willingness to change careers or other activities is also determined. Adjustment to the amputation and rehabilitation is less difficult if the client is willing to make necessary changes.

In addition to assessing the client's psychosocial status, assess the family's or significant others' reaction to the surgery. The family's response usually correlates directly with the client's progress during recovery and rehabilitation. The family can be expected to grieve for the loss and must be allowed to adjust to the change in the client.

Also assess the client's coping abilities, and help him or her to identify personal strengths and weaknesses. Ascertain that the client's religious or spiritual beliefs have been determined because certain groups require that the amputated body part be stored for later burial with the rest of the body or be buried immediately.

DIAGNOSTIC ASSESSMENT

Routine preoperative x-rays, such as a chest x-ray, are done as appropriate for any client undergoing surgery. The surgeon determines which tests are performed to assess for viability of the limb. A large number of noninvasive techniques are available to assist the physician in this evaluation. For complete accuracy, the health care provider does not rely on any single test.

One procedure is measurement of segmental limb blood pressures, which can also be used by the nurse at the bedside. In this test, an ankle-brachial index (ABI) is calculated by dividing ankle systolic pressure by brachial systolic pressure. A normal ABI is greater than or equal to 1.

Blood flow in an extremity can also be assessed by many other noninvasive tests, including Doppler ultrasonography, laser Doppler flowmetry, and transcutaneous oxygen pressure ($TcPO_2$). The ultrasonography measures the velocity of blood flow in the limb. The $TcPO_2$ measures oxygen pressure to indicate blood flow in the limb. Angiography is the most commonly used invasive method; however, it is not helpful in predicting healing of amputations. Transcutaneous oxygen pressure has proved reliable for predicting healing.

◆Interventions

Clients undergoing amputation today are not confined to a wheelchair. Advancements in the design of prosthetics have enabled clients to become independent in ambulation. Therefore complications from extended bedrest are not common, even for older adults.

Assessment of Tissue Perfusion. *The nurse's primary focus is to monitor for signs indicating that there is sufficient tissue perfusion but no hemorrhage.* The skin flap at the end of the residual limb should be pink in a light-skinned person and not discolored (lighter or darker than other skin pigmentation) in a dark-skinned client. The area should be warm but not hot. Assess the closest proximal pulse for strength and compare it with that in the other extremity. If the client has bilateral vascular disease, however, comparison of limbs is not an accurate way of measuring blood flow.

Management of Pain. Phantom limb pain (PLP) must be distinguished from stump pain because they are managed differently. Pain management related to stump pain is not unlike that for any client in pain (see Chapter 7). If the client complains of PLP, recognize that the pain is real. It is not therapeutic to remind the client that the limb cannot be hurting because it is missing. To prevent increased pain, handle the residual limb carefully when assessing the site or changing the dressing.

Drug Therapy. Some studies have shown that opioids are not as effective for PLP as they are for residual limb pain. For unknown reasons, IV infusions of calcitonin (Miacalcin, Calcimar) during the week after amputation can reduce phantom limb pain. The health care provider prescribes other medications on the basis of the type of PLP the client experiences. For instance, beta-blocking agents such as propranolol (Inderal, Apo-Propranolol✱, Detensol✱) are used for constant, dull burning. Anticonvulsants, such as carbamazepine (Tegretol) and gabapentin (Neurontin), may be used for knifelike pain; antispasmodics such as baclofen may be prescribed for muscle spasms or cramping.

Complementary and Alternative Therapies. More than 50 treatments for PLP have been used worldwide. Transcutaneous electrical nerve stimulation (TENS) has had the most consistent pain relief rates. Other treatment measures include the following:

- Ultrasound therapy
- Massage
- Exercises
- Biofeedback
- Distraction therapy
- Hypnosis
- Psychotherapy

These modalities are described in Chapters 4 and 7.

Prevention of Infection. The surgeon typically prescribes broad-spectrum prophylactic antibiotics for several days postoperatively. The initial pressure dressing and drains are usually removed by the surgeon 48 to 72 hours after surgery. The nurse does the following:

- Inspects the wound site for signs of inflammation (e.g., redness and swelling)
- Monitors the healing process
- Records the characteristics of drainage, if present
- Changes the soft dressing every day until the sutures are removed

The below-the-knee limb may be casted in the operating room for protection, prevention of edema, and prevention of knee contractures. On the third postoperative day, a window is opened in the distal end of the cast to inspect the suture line.

Promotion of Ambulation. The nurse or health care provider consults with a physical therapist to initiate exercises as soon as possible after surgery. If the amputation is a planned one, the therapist often works with the client before surgery to start muscle-strengthening exercises and to evaluate the need for aids, such as crutches. If the client can be instructed preoperatively in the use of these devices, learning how to ambulate after surgery is facilitated.

Exercise. For clients with above-knee amputations (AKAs) or below-knee amputations (BKAs), teach range-of-motion (ROM) exercises for prevention of flexion contractures, particularly of the hip and knee. A trapeze and an overhead frame, as shown in Figure 55-12, aid in strengthening the upper extremities and allow the client to move independently in bed.

A firm mattress is essential for preventing contractures with a lower extremity amputation. Assist the client into a

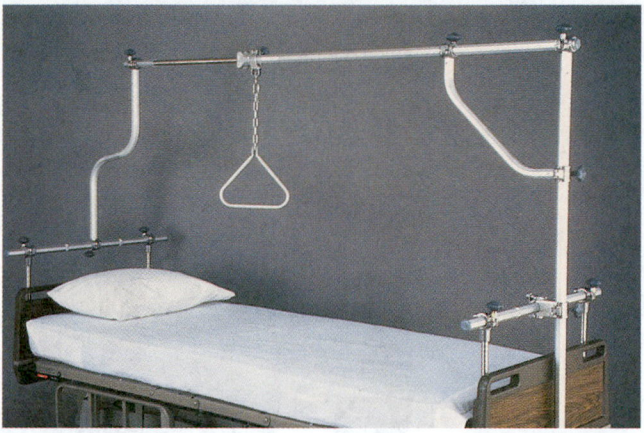

Figure 55-12 ■ The placement of an overhead frame and trapeze on a bed.

prone position every 3 to 4 hours for 20- to 30-minute periods. This position may be uncomfortable initially, but it is necessary to prevent hip flexion contractures. Instruct the prone client to pull the residual limb close to the other leg and contract the gluteal muscles of the buttocks. For BKAs, also teach the client to push the residual limb down toward the bed while supporting it on a pillow. After the sutures are removed, the physical therapist may begin resistive exercises with a "sling-and-spring" apparatus, which can also be used at home.

Elevation of a lower-leg residual limb on a pillow while the client is in a supine position is controversial. Some practitioners advocate avoiding this procedure at all times because it promotes hip or knee flexion contracture. Others allow elevation for the first 24 hours to reduce swelling and subsequent discomfort. Inspect the residual limb daily to ensure that it lies completely flat on the bed.

Prostheses. Following an amputation, arrange for the client to see a certified prosthetist-orthotist (CPO) so that planning can begin for the client's postoperative needs. Arrangements for replacing an upper extremity are especially important so that the client can provide self-care. Some clients are fitted with a temporary prosthesis at the time of surgery. Other clients, particularly older clients with vascular disease, are fitted after the residual limb has healed.

The client being fitted with a lower extremity prosthesis should bring a sturdy pair of shoes to the fitting. The prosthesis will be adjusted to that heel height.

Several devices help to shape and shrink the residual limb in preparation for the prosthesis. Rigid, removable dressings are preferred because they decrease edema, protect and shape the limb, and allow easy access to the wound for inspection. The Jobst air splint, a plastic inflatable device, is sometimes used for this purpose. This device is usually inflated to 20 mm Hg for 22 of every 24 hours. One of its disadvantages is air leakage.

Wrapping with elastic bandages can be effective in reducing edema, shrinking the limb, and holding the wound dressing in place. Most surgeons prefer elastic bandages over a shrinker sock, although it is easier for the client to apply a sock than to wrap elastic bandages.

For wrapping to be effective, reapply the bandages every 4 to 6 hours or more often if they become loose. Figure-eight wrapping prevents restriction of blood flow. Decrease

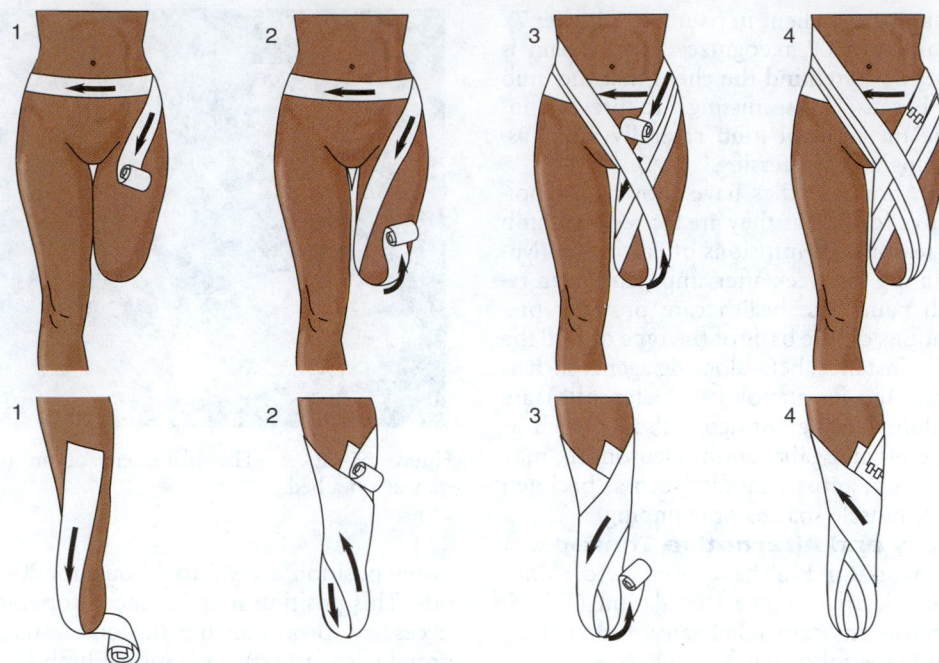

Figure 55-13 ■ A common method of wrapping an amputation stump. *Top,* Wrapping for above-knee amputation. *Bottom,* Wrapping for below-knee amputation.

the tightness of the bandages while wrapping in a distal-to-proximal direction. After wrapping, anchor the bandages to the most proximal joint, such as above the knee for BKAs (Figure 55-13).

The design of and materials for prostheses have improved dramatically over the years. Computer-assisted design and manufacturing (CAD-CAM) is now available for a custom fit. One of the most important developments in lower extremity prosthetics is the ankle-foot prosthesis. The Flex-Foot is used by more active amputees.

Promotion of Body Image. The client often experiences feelings of inadequacy as a result of losing a body part, especially the older adult who was in poor health before surgery. If possible, arrange for the client to meet with a rehabilitated amputee. If the client is older, an older amputee is the ideal person with whom the client should interact.

Use of the word *stump* for referring to the remaining portion of the limb (residual limb) is controversial. Clients have reported feeling as if they were part of a tree when the term was used. However, some rehabilitation specialists who routinely work with amputees believe the term is appropriate because it forces the client to realize what has happened and enhances adjustment to the amputation.

Assess the client's verbal and nonverbal references to the affected area. Some clients behave euphorically and seem to have accepted the loss. Do not jump to the conclusion that acceptance has occurred. Ask the client to describe his or her feelings about changes in body image and self-esteem. The client may verbalize acceptance but refuse to look at the area during a dressing change. This inconsistent behavior is not unusual and should be noted.

Promotion of Lifestyle Adaptations. The client may believe that it will be impossible to return to a previous lifestyle, including intimate relationships, his or her job, and recreational activities. With advancements in prostheses, many

clients can return to their jobs and other activities. Professional athletes who use prostheses are quite successful in sports. Clients with amputations ski, hike, bowl, and participate in other physically demanding activities. More than 20,000 amputees in the United States currently participate actively in sports; about a fourth of these individuals are engaged in organized competition.

If a job or career change is necessary, consult with a social worker for evaluation of the client's other skills that could be used in another capacity. A supportive family or significant other is important for the client's adjustment to this change. The client may also think that an intimate relationship is no longer possible because of physical changes. Work with the sexual partner to help in the client's adjustment to the amputation. Professional assistance from a sex counselor or psychologist may be needed.

Help the client to set realistic goals and to take one day at a time. Help him or her to recognize personal strengths, which are emphasized and taken into account in setting goals. If the goals are not realistic, frustration and disappointment may dampen the client's motivation during rehabilitation. Basic principles of rehabilitation are discussed in Chapter 10.

Community-Based Care

The client is discharged directly to home or to a rehabilitation facility, depending on the extent of the amputation. In the few cases in which rehabilitation is not feasible (e.g., for a debilitated, confused older client), he or she may be discharged to a long-term care facility. The case manager or discharge planner coordinates this transfer.

HOME CARE MANAGEMENT

The client with a lower extremity amputation needs to have enough room at home to maneuver a wheelchair if the leg prosthesis is not yet available. He or she must be able to use

CHART 55-7

HOME CARE ASSESSMENT of
The Client with a Lower Extremity Amputation in the Home

Assess the residual limb for the following:
- Adequate circulation
- Infection
- Healing
- Flexion contracture
- Dressing/elastic wrap

Assess the client's ability to perform activities of daily living (ADLs) in the home.

Evaluate the client's ability to use ambulatory aids and care for the prosthetic device (if available).

Assess the client's nutritional status.

Assess the client's ability to cope with body image change.

toileting facilities and have access to areas necessary for self-care, such as the kitchen. Structural changes may be required before the client goes home.

HEALTH TEACHING

After the sutures are removed (several weeks after surgery), the client begins residual limb care. The home care nurse teaches the client how to care for the residual limb and how to care for the prosthesis if it is available. The limb should be rewrapped three times a day with an elastic bandage applied in a figure-eight manner (see Figure 55-13) by the client or family member. After the residual limb is healed, it is cleaned each day with the rest of the body during bathing with soap and water, and it is inspected for signs of inflammation or skin breakdown.

Prostheses require special care for ensuring their reliability and proper function, and the prosthetist plays an important role in the rehabilitation team effort. Prostheses are custom made, taking into account the client's level of amputation, lifestyle, and occupation. Proper teaching regarding correct cleansing of the socket and inserts, wearing the correct liners, assessing shoe wear, and a schedule of follow-up care is essential before discharge.

A client who seems to adjust to the amputation during hospitalization may realize that it is difficult to cope with the loss after discharge from the hospital. The nurse in the hospital setting should tell the client that this can happen. During the hospital stay, help the client to identify strong support systems on which he or she can rely after discharge. The home care or rehabilitation nurse reinforces this supporting information.

HEALTH CARE RESOURCES

For the older adult or for the client with an extensive amputation, such as a hemipelvectomy, the case manager or discharge planner arranges for follow-up care in the home by a home care nurse (Chart 55-7). Physical therapy may continue in the home or on an ambulatory care basis.

The client with an upper extremity amputation may need occupational therapy to relearn activities of daily living (ADLs). The nurse or case manager also makes arrangements for vocational or family counseling as needed. Some clients are discharged to a rehabilitation facility for 2 to 3 weeks for these services. Chapter 10 describes the rehabilitation phase of health care in detail. Teach the client to explore support groups for amputees that may be available in the client's community.

Critical Thinking Challenge

Four days ago, an adolescent client had closed reduction and external fixation for a severely comminuted left tibia and fibula. Today he becomes febrile, has an elevated white blood cell count, and a decreased hematocrit level. He returns to the operating suite for debridement and exploration, where his surgeon finds extensive tissue loss and damage. After this surgery, he recommends a BKA for the client.

1. What teaching will the client and family require in preparation for surgery?
2. What psychosocial assessment and interventions will this client need?
3. What can you tell him about changes in his lifestyle after the BKA?

evolve For suggested answer guidelines, go to http://evolve.elsevier.com/Iggy/.

CRUSH SYNDROME

When multiple compartments in the leg or arm are injured, crush syndrome (CS) can occur. CS is a potentially life-threatening, systemic complication after a severe crush injury. Its pathophysiologic mechanism is similar to that of acute compartment syndrome (see p. 1191).

Specific causes of CS include the following:
- Wringer-type injuries
- Natural disasters, such as earthquakes
- Work-related injuries, such as being trapped under heavy equipment or material
- Drug or alcohol overdose, when one or more limbs may be compressed by body weight for a prolonged time

Regardless of the cause, CS is characterized by the following:
- Acute compartment syndrome
- Hypovolemia
- Hyperkalemia
- **Rhabdomyolysis** (myoglobulin release from skeletal muscle into the bloodstream)
- Acute tubular necrosis (ATN) resulting from hypovolemia and rhabdomyolysis

Nursing assessments include signs and symptoms of hypovolemia, hyperkalemia, and compartment syndrome. Treatments focus on preventing acute tubular necrosis secondary to myoglobin release and cardiac dysrhythmias related to hyperkalemia. Adequate IV fluids, diuretics, and low-dose dopamine to enhance renal perfusion may be prescribed. An output of 100 to 200 mL/hr is the goal. Sodium bicarbonate is given to treat acidosis. Kayexalate may reduce serum potassium adequately, but hemodialysis may be required if potassium levels remain high or renal failure occurs.

COMPLEX REGIONAL PAIN SYNDROME

PATHOPHYSIOLOGY

Complex regional pain syndrome (CRPS), formerly called **reflex sympathetic dystrophy (RSD),** is a poorly understood complex disorder that includes debilitating pain, atrophy, autonomic dysfunction (excessive sweating, vascular changes), and motor impairment (most notably muscle paresis). It is probably caused by an abnormally hyperactive sympathetic nervous system. CRPS most often results from traumatic injury and commonly occurs in the feet and hands. In some cases, specific nerve injuries are present, but in others no definable injury can be identified.

The syndrome tends to progress through three classic stages. In stage 1, which lasts 1 to 3 months, the client complains of locally severe, burning pain; edema; vasospasm; and muscle spasm. Over the next 3 months, clients in stage 2 have more severe, diffuse pain and edema, muscle atrophy, and spotty osteoporosis, as shown on x-ray examination. In stage 3, the final stage, the client presents with marked muscle atrophy, intractable (unrelenting) pain, severely limited mobility of the affected area, contractures, and marked, diffuse osteoporosis. Timing of diagnosis is important because the syndrome is more difficult to treat when diagnosed in the later stages.

◆COLLABORATIVE MANAGEMENT

The first priority of management is pain relief. Nurses play an important role in pain management, which includes drug therapy and an array of nonpharmacologic modalities. Chapter 7 discusses pain management in detail.

In collaboration with the physical and occupational therapist, the nurse also assists in maintaining adequate range of motion (ROM). The skin of a client with CRPS tends to alternate between warm, swollen, and red to cool, clammy, and bluish. Skin care needs to be gentle, with minimal stimulation.

A new procedure to control hyperhidrosis (excessive sweating), the **endoscopic thoracic sympathectomy (ETS),** has also been successful for some clients with CRPS. Only one extremely small incision is made in the axilla, through which an endoscope is inserted. The surgeon identifies and cuts the sympathetic nerve branches involved. Topical skin adhesive is used to close the microincision. The client is discharged to home a few hours later with a follow-up examination the next day. Usual activities can resume a few days later.

Assist the client in coping with CRPS, realizing that psychotherapy may be indicated. The Reflex Sympathetic Dystrophy Syndrome Association (RSDSA) is available to help clients organize or locate support groups and other resources for clients with this syndrome.

SPORTS-RELATED INJURIES

In addition to the bone and muscle problems already discussed, trauma can cause cartilage, ligament, and tendon injury. Many musculoskeletal injuries are the result of participation in sports (professional and amateur) or other strenuous physical activities. The popularity of all-terrain vehicles (ATVs) and skateboarding has increased injuries in younger clients. Sports injuries have become so common that large metropolitan hospitals have sports medicine clinics and physicians who specialize in this field.

Although the specific types of injury are numerous, this chapter includes only the most common ones seen in a hospital or ambulatory care setting. The principles of injury to one part of the body are analogous to those of similar injuries in other parts. For example, a tendon rupture in a knee is cared for in the same manner as a tendon rupture in the wrist. Chart 55-8 lists general emergency measures for sports-related injuries.

CHART 55-8

BEST PRACTICE for
Emergency Care of Sports-Related Injuries

EMERGENCY CARE

- Do not move the victim until spinal cord injury is ascertained (see Chapter 46 for assessment of spinal cord injury).
- Immobilize the injured part, and immobilize the joint above and below the injury by applying a splint.
- Apply ice intermittently for the first 24 to 48 hours (heat may be used thereafter).
- Elevate the affected limb to decrease swelling.
- Always assume the area is fractured until x-ray studies are done.
- Assess neurovascular status in the area distal to the injury.

Because the knee is most often injured, it is discussed as a typical example of other areas of the body. Trauma to the knee results in **internal derangement,** a broad term for disturbances of an injured knee joint. When surgery is required to resolve the problem, most surgeons prefer to perform the procedure through an arthroscope when possible. A general description of arthroscopy is presented in Chapter 53.

Knee Injuries: Meniscus
PATHOPHYSIOLOGY

There are two semilunar cartilaginous structures, or menisci, in the knee joint: the medial meniscus and the lateral meniscus. These pads act as shock absorbers, but they can tear. Tearing is usually a result of twisting the leg when the knee is flexed and the foot is placed firmly on the ground. The medial meniscus is much more likely to tear than the lateral meniscus because it is less mobile. Internal rotation causes a tear in the medial meniscus; external rotation causes a tear in the lateral meniscus.

Tears can be anterior or posterior, longitudinal or transverse. In the medial meniscus, a longitudinal tear, or "bucket handle" injury, often causes the knee to lock; that is, the torn cartilage jams between the femur and the tibia and prevents extension of the knee. Surgery is often required for this type of injury. In transverse tears, the knee does not lock, and surgery may not be required.

◆COLLABORATIVE MANAGEMENT

The client with a torn meniscus typically has pain, swelling, and tenderness in the knee. A clicking or snapping sound can often be heard when the knee is moved.

A common diagnostic technique is the **McMurray test.** The examiner flexes and rotates the knee and then presses on the medial aspect while slowly extending the leg. The test result is positive if clicking is palpated or heard. A negative finding, however, does not rule out a tear.

For a locked knee, the treatment may be manipulation followed by casting for 3 to 6 weeks. If the problem recurs, a partial or total **meniscectomy** is performed. An open meniscectomy requires a surgical incision for removal of all or part of the meniscus and is rarely performed. Most surgeons prefer to remove only the affected portion, during a closed meniscectomy, which can be accomplished through an arthroscope as a same-day surgical procedure. As described in Chapter 53, an arthroscope is a metal tubular instrument used for examination or surgery of joints. One or more small incisions (less than ¼ inch [0.6 cm] long) are made in the knee for insertion of the arthroscope. The surgeon threads a cutting device through the arthroscope for removal of the torn cartilage while the knee is irrigated. The surgeon may use a laser during the procedure, depending on the type and severity of the injury. A bulky pressure dressing is applied after the procedure, and the affected leg is wrapped in elastic bandages.

As for any postoperative client, check the surgical dressing for bleeding and monitor vital signs after the client is readmitted to the unit. Perform circulation checks, as outlined in Chart 55-3, usually every hour for the first few hours and then every 4 hours.

The client begins leg exercises immediately after surgery to strengthen the leg, prevent thrombophlebitis, and reduce swelling. Quadriceps setting, in which the client straightens the leg while pushing the knee against the bed, is done in sets of 10 or more. Straight-leg raises are also performed as soon as the client awakens from anesthesia. Range-of-motion (ROM) exercises are usually not started for several days.

To prevent the client from bending the affected knee, the physician may order a knee immobilizer, such as the one shown in Figure 55-14. Elevate the leg on one or two pillows according to the physician's preference, and apply ice to reduce postoperative swelling. Full weight bearing is restricted for several weeks, depending on the amount of cartilage removed. The client is usually discharged from the hospital with crutches in less than 23 hours.

Knee Injuries: Ligaments

PATHOPHYSIOLOGY

The cruciate and collateral ligaments in the knee are predisposed to injury, often from sports or vehicular accidents. The anterior cruciate ligament (ACL) is the most commonly torn ligament in the knee. Athletes often experience ACL injuries during skiing or gymnastics.

When the ACL is torn, the person feels a snap; the knee gives way because of ACL laxity. Within hours, the knee is swollen, stiff, and painful.

◆COLLABORATIVE MANAGEMENT

Physical examination by the health care provider shows positive ligamentous laxity. The diagnosis of ACL deficiency is confirmed by x-rays, magnetic resonance imaging (MRI), or assessment with an arthrometer (an instrument for measuring the amount of tibial displacement).

Treatment may be nonsurgical or surgical, depending on the severity of the injury and the anticipated activity of the client. Exercises, bracing, and limits on activities while the ligament heals may be sufficient. If medical management is not effective, surgery may be needed.

The surgeon repairs the tear by reattaching the torn portions of the ligament, and the leg is placed in a cast. If the ligament cannot be repaired, reconstructive surgery may be performed with the use of autologous grafts. Since the early 1980s, the Food and Drug Administration (FDA) has approved several artificial knee ligaments. The Gore-Tex ligament is a permanent implant. A ligament augmentation device is used temporarily while the autograft heals. Both of these materials can be implanted through an arthroscope.

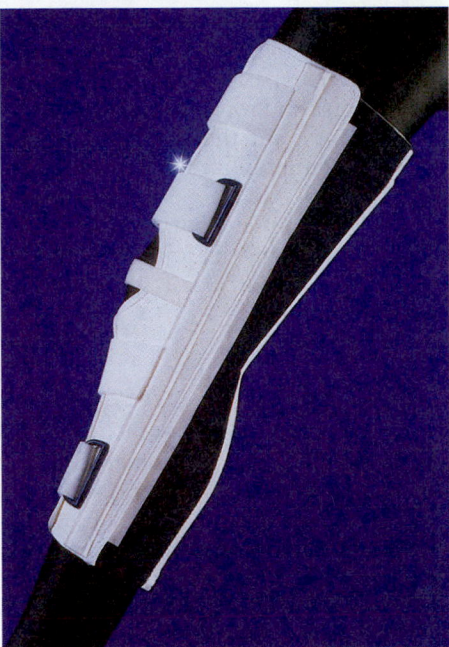

Figure 55-14 ■ A knee immobilizer. (Courtesy Zimmer, Inc., Warsaw, IN.)

Complete healing of knee ligaments after surgery can take 6 to 9 months or longer. Nursing management is similar to the care of any client in a cast, which is described earlier in this chapter under Cast Care, p. 1199. These clients may have postoperative orders for a continuous passive motion machine (CPM). CPM use is discussed with the postoperative care of the total knee client in Chapter 24.

Tendon Ruptures

Rupture of the Achilles tendon is common in adults who participate in strenuous sports. In the older adult, quadriceps tendon rupture may occur from a fall down several steps. For severe damage, the tendon is surgically repaired and the leg is immobilized in a cast for 6 to 8 weeks. If the tendon is beyond repair, a **tendon transplant** (also known as tendon reconstruction) is performed. A tendon is removed from one part of the body and transplanted to the affected area. The nursing care for these clients is similar to that discussed earlier for a client with a cast (see Cast Care, p. 1199).

Dislocations and Subluxations

Dislocation of a joint occurs when the articulating surfaces are no longer in proximity. If the dislocation is not complete, the joint is partially dislocated, or subluxed. Dislocation can occur in any diarthrodial (synovial) joint but is common in the shoulder, hip, knee, and fingers. This injury is most often the result of trauma but can be congenital or pathologic (resulting from joint disease, such as arthritis).

The following are the typical manifestations of dislocation:
- Pain
- Immobility
- Alteration in contour of the joint

■ Deviation in length of the extremity
■ Rotation of the extremity

The health care provider performs a closed manipulation, or reduction, of the joint and forces it back into its original position while the client is anesthetized or under conscious sedation. The joint is immobilized by a cast or immobilizer until healing occurs.

Recurrent dislocations are common in the knee and shoulder. For this problem, the joint is fixed with wires to prevent further displacement; a cast, splint, or traction is applied for 3 to 6 weeks.

Strains

A strain is excessive stretching of a muscle or tendon when it is weak or unstable. Strains are sometimes referred to as muscle pulls. Falls, lifting of heavy items, and exercise often cause this injury.

Strains are classified according to their severity:

■ A first-degree (mild) strain causes mild inflammation but little bleeding. Swelling, ecchymosis, and tenderness are usually present.

■ A second-degree (moderate) strain involves tearing of the muscle or tendon fibers without complete disruption. Muscle function may be impaired.

■ A third-degree (severe) strain involves a ruptured muscle or tendon with separation of muscle from muscle, tendon from muscle, or tendon from bone. Severe pain and disability result from severe strains.

Management usually involves cold and heat applications, exercise, and activity limitations. The health care provider may prescribe anti-inflammatory drugs to decrease inflammation and pain. Muscle relaxants may also be used. In third-degree strains, surgical repair of the ruptured muscle or tendon may be necessary.

Sprains

A sprain is excessive stretching of a ligament. Twisting motions from a fall or sports activity typically precipitate the injury. Sprains are classified according to severity:

■ A first-degree (mild) sprain involves tearing of a few fibers of a ligament. Function of the joint is not impaired.

■ In a second-degree (moderate) sprain, more fibers are torn, but stability of the joint remains intact.

■ A third-degree (severe) sprain causes marked instability of the joint.

■ Pain and swelling characterize ligament injuries. The treatment for mild (first-degree) sprains is minimal:

■ Rest

■ Use of ice for the first 24 to 48 hours

■ Application of a compression bandage for a few days to reduce swelling and provide joint support

■ Elevation

Second-degree sprains require immobilization (elastic bandage and Air Stirrup ankle brace, splint, or cast) and partial weight bearing while the tear heals. For severe ligament damage (third-degree sprain), immobilization for 4 to 6 weeks is necessary. Surgery may be recommended, particularly for chronic instability, as discussed earlier under Knee Injuries: Ligaments, p. 1225.

For more specific client education, refer to the Clinical Pathway on the Evolve website.

Rotator Cuff Injuries

The musculotendinous, or rotator, cuff of the shoulder functions to stabilize the head of the humerus in the glenoid cavity during shoulder abduction. The rotator cuff typically undergoes degenerative changes as one ages. Young adults usually sustain a tear of the cuff by substantial trauma, such as may occur during a fall, while throwing a ball, or with heavy lifting. Older adults tend to have small tears related to aging, repetitive motions, or falls.

Clients with a torn rotator cuff have shoulder pain and cannot initiate or maintain abduction of the arm at the shoulder. When the arm is abducted, the client usually drops the arm because abduction cannot be maintained (drop arm test).

The health care provider usually treats the client conservatively with nonsteroidal anti-inflammatory drugs (NSAIDs), physical therapy, sling support, and ice/heat applications while the tear heals.

For clients who do not respond to conservative treatment or for those who have a complete tear, the surgeon repairs the cuff. After surgery, the affected arm is usually immobilized in a sling for several weeks. Pendulum exercises are started on the third or fourth postoperative day and progress to active exercises in about 2 weeks. If the surgery is extensive, the client's arm may be immobilized for a longer time before exercises begin.

GET READY for the NCLEX Examination!

KEY POINTS

Safe Effective Care Environment

■ Identify the client at risk for acute compartment syndrome; loosen bandages or request that the client's cast be cut if neurovascular compromise.

■ As a priority, assess neurovascular status frequently in clients with musculoskeletal injury, traction, or cast as described in Chart 55-3.

■ Identify clients at risk for venous thromboembolism (VTE), and monitor for early signs of this potentially fatal complication.

■ Implement interventions to prevent complications of immobility in clients having musculoskeletal injury or surgery.

■ Observe for hemorrhage in the client having an amputation.

Health Promotion and Maintenance

■ Encourage the use of seat belts in motor vehicles and helmets for skateboarding to help prevent serious injury.

■ Educate individuals in the community about the importance of osteoporosis screening, medication safety, fall prevention, and programs for older drivers.

■ Teach clients and their family members and significant others how to care for casts or traction at home.

■ Reinforce teaching for ambulating with crutches, walkers, or canes.

■ Teach exercises to clients with leg amputation to prevent hip flexion contractures.

- Provide health care resource information for clients with musculoskeletal trauma, such as RSDS Association for clients with complex regional pain syndrome.
- Teach clients to take precautions when operating machinery to avoid traumatic amputations or other severe injury.

Psychosocial Integrity

- Be aware that clients with severe musculoskeletal trauma may have a prolonged hospitalization and recovery period.
- For clients with severe trauma or amputation, assess the client's coping skills and encourage verbalization.
- Recognize that the client having an amputation may need to adjust to an altered lifestyle; however, new custom prosthetics improve mobility.
- Help the client with an amputation or other musculoskeletal trauma to set realistic goals and take one day at a time.
- Be aware that clients with complex regional pain syndrome may require psychotherapy.

Physiological Integrity

- Be aware that open fractures cause a higher risk for infection than do closed fractures.
- Assess clients with fractures for complications, such as VTE, infection, and acute compartment syndrome.
- Differentiate fat embolism syndrome from pulmonary (blood clot) embolism as outlined in Chart 55-2.
- Provide emergency care of the client experiencing a fracture as described in Chart 55-4.
- Provide appropriate cast care, depending on the type of cast (plaster or synthetic); check for pressure necrosis under the cast by feeling for heat, assessing the client's pain level, and smelling the cast for an unpleasant odor.
- Provide pin care for clients with skeletal traction or external fixator; assess for manifestations of infection at the pin sites.
- Provide postoperative care for the client having a hip repair as described in the Client Care Plan.
- Postoperatively, assess for and manage phantom limb pain in the client who has an amputation.
- Provide emergency care for clients experiencing a sports-related injury as outlined in Chart 55-8.

ADDITIONAL STUDY RESOURCES

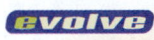 Go to your Student CD-ROM for Review Questions for the NCLEX Examination.

Go to http://evolve.elsevier.com/Iggy/ for Integrated Management of Care Questions for the NCLEX Examination.

SELECTED BIBLIOGRAPHY

Asterisk indicates a classic or definitive work on this subject.

Altizer, L. (2002). Fractures. *Orthopaedic Nursing, 21*(6), 51-58.

Altizer, L. (2003). Hand and wrist fractures. *Orthopaedic Nursing, 22*(2), 131-138.

Bartley, M.K., & Telford, G. (2004). The latest in trauma care. *Critical Care Choices 2004*, 26-29.

Bishop, C.E., et al. (2002). Medicare spending for injured elders: Are there opportunities for savings? *Health Affairs, 21*(6), 215-223.

Collins, T.C., et al. (2002). Lower extremity nontraumatic amputation among veterans with peripheral arterial disease: Is race an independent factor? *Medical Care, 40*(1), Suppl I106-I116.

Curtis, K., et al. (2002). The impact of trauma cast management on patient outcomes. *The Journal of TRAUMA Injury, Infection, and Critical Care, 53*(3), 477-482.

Fletcher, D.D., et al. (2002). Trends in rehabilitation after amputation for geriatric patients with vascular disease: Implications for future health resource allocation. *Archives of Physical Medicine and Rehabilitation, 83*(10), 1389-1393.

Geier, K. (2001). Osteoporosis in men. *Orthopaedic Nursing, 20*(6), 49-56.

Harvey, C. (2001). Compartment syndrome: When it is least expected. *Orthopaedic Nursing, 20*(3), 15-25.

Injury fact book 2001-2002. Available at http://www.cdc.gov.

Jacobs, D.J., et al. (2003). Practice management guideline for geriatric trauma: The EAST practice management guidelines work group. *The Journal of TRAUMA Injury, Infection, and Critical Care, 54*(2), 391-416.

Kyphoplasty—A new treatment for osteoporotic fractures. Available at http://www.spine-health.com.

Maher, A.B. (2001). Trauma. In D.C. Schoen (Ed.), *Core curriculum for orthopaedic nursing* (4th ed.) Pitman, NJ: National Association of Orthopaedic Nurses.

Maher, A.B., Salmond, S.W., & Pellino, T.A. (Eds.). (2002). *Orthopaedic nursing* (3rd ed.) Philadelphia: W.B. Saunders.

Marshall, H.M., et al. (2002). Pain site and impairment in individuals with amputation pain. *Archives of Physical Medicine & Rehabilitation, 83*(8), 1116-1119.

Michaels, A., et al. (2001). Traditional injury scoring underestimates the relative consequences of orthopedic injury. *The Journal of TRAUMA Injury, Infection, and Critical Care, 50*(3), 389-396.

Miller, R.L.S. (2003). Reflex sympathetic dystrophy. *Orthopaedic Nursing, 22*(2), 91-101.

Moran, S.G., et al. (2003). Relationship between age and lower extremity fractures in frontal motor vehicle collisions. *The Journal of TRAUMA Injury, Infection, and Critical Care, 54*(2), 261-265.

National Osteoporosis Foundation. (2003). *Physician's guide to prevention and treatment of osteoporosis*. Washington D.C.: National Osteoporosis Foundation.

Pudelek, B. (2002). Geriatric trauma: Special needs for a special population. *AACN Clinical Issues, 13*(1), 61-72.

*Roberts, D. (1999). Introduction to bone: Structure and function, fractures, and osteoporosis. In C.M. Ceccio, J.A. Deuschle, & D.R. Eckhouse-Ekeberg (Eds.), *An introduction to orthopaedic nursing* (2nd ed., pp. 3-16). Pitman, NJ: National Association of Orthopaedic Nurses.

Rudman, N., & McIlmail, D. (2000). Emergency department evaluation and treatment of hip and thigh injuries. *Emergency Medicine Clinics of North America, 18*(1), 29-66.

Schmitt, M. (2000) Osteoporosis: Focus on fractures. *Patient Care for the Nurse Practitioner, 3*(2), 61-71.

Swiontkowski, M.F., et al. (2002). Factors influencing the decision to amputate or reconstruct after high-energy lower extremity trauma. *The Journal of TRUAMA Injury, Infection, and Critical Care, 52*(4), 641-649.

*Taggart, H. (1999). Caring for the elderly hip fracture patient. In C.M. Ceccio, J.A. Deuschle, & D.R. Eckhouse-Ekeberg (Eds.), *An introduction to orthopaedic nursing* (2nd ed., pp. 113-122). Pitman, NJ: National Association of Orthopaedic Nurses.

PROBLEMS of DIGESTION, NUTRITION, and ELIMINATION

Management of Clients with Problems of the Gastrointestinal System

Assessment of the Gastrointestinal System

KARRIE K. DIETZEN

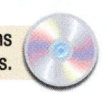
The gastrointestinal (GI) system includes the GI tract (alimentary canal), consisting of the mouth, esophagus, stomach, small and large intestines, and rectum. The salivary glands, liver, gallbladder, and pancreas secrete substances into the GI tract by connecting ducts (Figure 56-1). The adult GI tract is about 25 feet long (mouth to anus). The main function of the GI tract, with the aid of organs such as the pancreas and the liver, is the digestion of food and the elimination of waste. The GI tract is susceptible to many pathologic conditions, including structural problems, impaired motility, infection, and cancer.

ANATOMY AND PHYSIOLOGY REVIEW

Overview of the Gastrointestinal System

Structure

The GI tract consists of a hollow muscular tube surrounded by four tissue layers. The **lumen**, inner wall, of the GI tract consists of four layers: mucosa, submucosa, muscularis, and serosa. The **mucosa**, the innermost layer, includes a thin layer of smooth muscle and specialized exocrine gland cells.

The mucosa is surrounded by the submucosa, which is made up of connective tissue. Submucosa layer is surrounded by the muscularis. The muscularis is composed of both circular and longitudinal smooth muscles, which work to keep contents moving through the tract. The outermost layer, serosa, is composed of connective tissue. Although the GI tract is continuous from the mouth to the anus, it is divided into specialized regions. The mouth, pharynx, esophagus, stomach, and small and large intestines each perform a specific function. In addition, the secretions of the salivary, gastric, and intestinal glands; liver; and pancreas empty into the GI tract to aid digestion.

Function

The functions of the GI tract include secretion, digestion, absorption, motility, and elimination. Food and fluids are ingested, swallowed, and propelled along the lumen of the GI tract to the anus for elimination. The smooth muscles contract to move food from the mouth to the anus. Before food can be absorbed, it must be broken down to a liquid, called **chyme.** Digestion is the mechanical and chemical process whereby complex foodstuffs are broken down into simpler forms that can be used by the body. During digestion, the stomach secretes hydrochloric acid, the liver se-

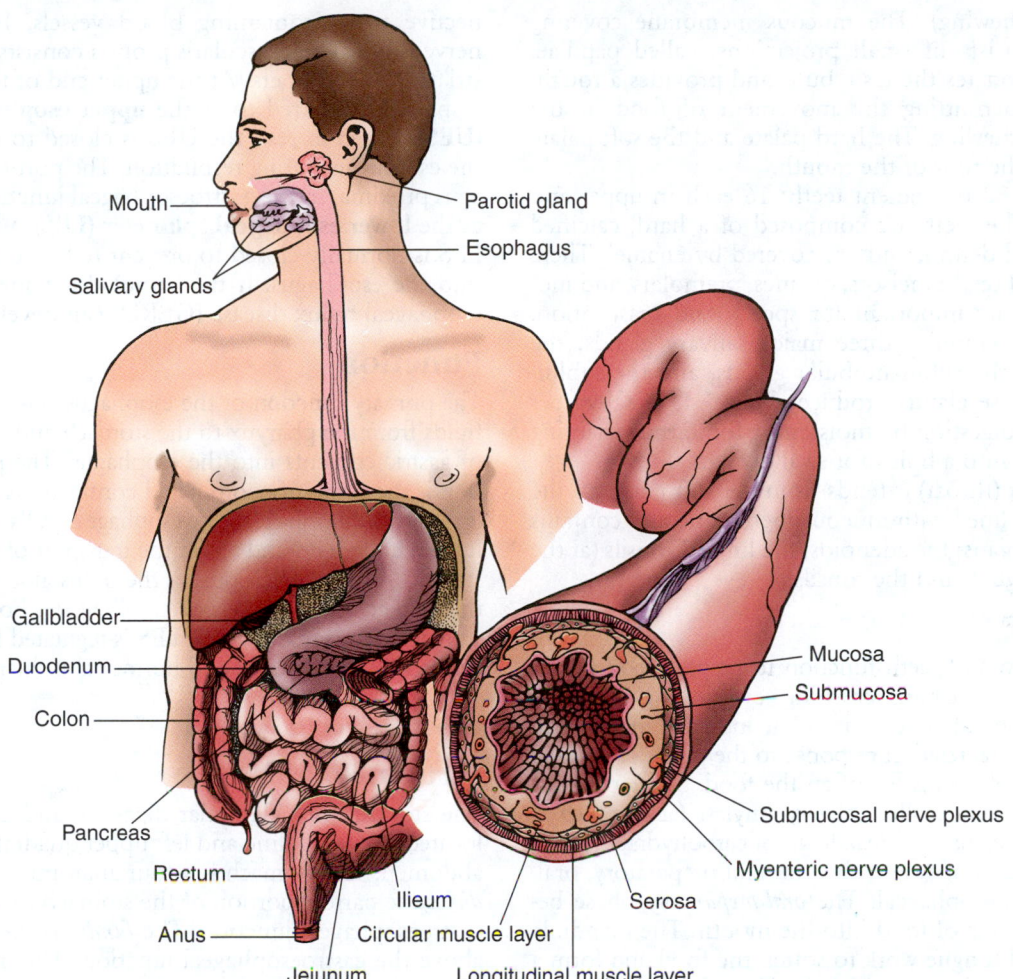

Figure 56-1 ■ The gastrointestinal system (GI tract) can be thought of as a tube (with necessary structures) extending from the mouth to the anus for a 25-foot length. The structure of this tube (shown enlarged) is basically the same throughout its length.

cretes bile, and digestive enzymes are released from accessory organs, aiding in food breakdown. After the digestive process is complete, absorption takes place. **Absorption** is carried out as the nutrients produced by digestion move from the lumen of the GI tract into the body's circulatory system for uptake by individual cells.

Nerve Supply

Innervation of the GI tract occurs in two ways. First, intrinsic contractile stimulation is provided by two internal nerve plexuses: the *myenteric* plexus (an outer plexus found in the longitudinal and circular smooth muscle) and the *submucosal* plexus (an inner nerve plexus in the submucosa). These nerve plexuses connect with each other along the entire length of the GI tract to maintain the tone of the smooth muscle and to stimulate movements.

The second type of innervation is provided by the autonomic nervous system, which connects with nerve fibers from the intrinsic nerve plexuses. Parasympathetic stimulation is provided primarily by the vagus nerve (cranial nerve X). The vagus nerve innervates the esophagus, the stomach, and to a lesser extent, the small intestine, the gallbladder, and part of the large intestine. This stimulation causes increased motor

and secretory activity and relaxation of sphincters. Sympathetic stimulation via the thoracic and lumbar splanchnic nerves is provided to all parts of the GI tract. It slows movement, inhibits secretions, and contracts sphincters.

Blood Supply

The blood supply to the GI tract originates from the aorta and branches to the many arteries throughout the length of the tract. The venous system that carries absorbed nutrients away from the lumen of the GI tract consists of the gastric vein, the splenic vein, and other veins that drain into the portal vein of the liver. This blood circulates through the liver to the hepatic vein and returns to the heart via the inferior vena cava.

ORAL CAVITY

Structure

The oral cavity (mouth) includes the buccal mucosa, lips, tongue, hard palate, soft palate, teeth, and salivary glands. The buccal mucosa is the mucous membrane lining the inside of the mouth. The lips are external to the mouth and are pink-red. The tongue is involved in speech, taste, and mastication (chewing). The mucous membrane covering the tongue consists of small projections, called papillae, which accommodates the taste buds and provides a roughened surface, permitting the movement of food in the mouth during chewing. The hard palate and the soft palate together form the roof of the mouth.

Adults have 32 permanent teeth: 16 each in upper and lower arches. The teeth are composed of a hard, calcified substance called dentin, and are covered by enamel. There are four types of teeth: incisors, canines, premolars, and molars. The teeth are important for speech and mastication. The oral cavity contains three major salivary glands: the parotid glands, the submandibular glands, and the sublingual glands. These glands produce about 1 L of saliva per day to assist in digestion by moistening food, thus enabling it to be formed into a bolus for swallowing.

The **pharynx** (throat) extends from the soft palate to the esophagus. It is lined with mucous membrane and contains three pairs of organs: the adenoids, the lingual tonsils (at the base of the tongue), and the tonsils.

Function

The different types of teeth function to prepare food for digestion by cutting, tearing, crushing, or grinding the food. Swallowing begins after food is taken into the mouth and chewed. Saliva is secreted in response to the presence of food in the mouth and begins to soften the food. Saliva contains mucin and an enzyme called salivary amylase (also known as ptyalin), which begins the breakdown of carbohydrates.

The four phases of swallowing are oral preparatory, oral, pharyngeal, and esophageal. The *oral preparatory* phase begins with the intake of food into the mouth. The mandible (jaw), teeth, and tongue work to soften the food and form a bolus. The tongue acts to move the bolus toward the back of the mouth. The *oral* phase begins with the movement of the bolus toward the back of the mouth. The tongue presses the bolus against the hard palate, toward the glossopalatine arch, elevating the larynx, which forces the food bolus to pass into the pharynx, triggering the swallowing reflex. The oral phase is under voluntary control of the individual.

The *pharyngeal* phase begins as the swallowing reflex is triggered. As the bolus is forced into the pharynx, the soft palate elevates, which seals the nasal cavity. At this time, the swallowing reflex also inhibits respiration and allows the opening of the esophagus so that the food can enter. The oral and pharyngeal phases are extremely rapid, usually taking less than 1 second. The pharyngeal phase is under both voluntary and involuntary control of the individual.

The *esophageal* phase begins when the bolus enters the esophagus at the cricopharyngeal juncture. A peristaltic wave passes the food to the stomach, which takes about 9 seconds. The esophageal phase is completely under involuntary control.

ESOPHAGUS
Structure

The esophagus is a muscular canal about 10 inches (24 cm) long; it extends from the pharynx to the stomach and passes through the hiatus in the center of the diaphragm. The wall of the esophagus consists of mucosa, submucosa, and muscularis propria. The mucosal layer is composed of squamous epithelial cells. The submucosa is composed of loose connective tissue containing blood vessels, lymphatics, and nerve fibers. The muscularis propria consists of smooth and striated muscle fibers. At the upper end of the esophagus is a sphincter referred to as the **upper esophageal sphincter (UES).** When at rest, the UES is closed to prevent air into the esophagus during respiration. The portion of the esophagus proximal to the gastroesophageal junction is referred to as the **lower esophageal sphincter (LES).** When at rest, the LES is normally closed to prevent reflux of gastric contents into the esophagus. If this is not done adequately, gastroesophageal reflux disease (GERD) can develop.

Function

The primary function of the esophagus is to propel food and fluids from the pharynx to the stomach and to prevent reflux of gastric contents into the esophagus. The propulsive function is the result of coordinated contractions of the muscular layers of the esophagus. The esophageal walls secrete mucus to lubricate the food and aid in the transport of the bolus to the stomach. As peristalsis pushes the bolus along the esophagus, the cardiac sphincter relaxes to allow the bolus to enter the stomach. The activity of the LES is regulated by smooth muscle, as well as by neural and hormonal influences.

STOMACH
Structure

The stomach is a glandular digestive and endocrine organ located in the midline and left upper quadrant (LUQ) of the abdomen. The stomach has four anatomic regions. The *cardia* is the narrow portion of the stomach that is distal to the gastroesophageal junction. The *fundus* is the area to the left above the gastroesophageal junction. The main area of the stomach is referred to as the *body* or *corpus*. The *antrum* (pylorus) is the distal portion of the stomach and is separated from the duodenum by the pyloric sphincter. Both ends of the stomach are guarded by sphincters (cardiac and pyloric), which aid in the transport of food through the gastrointestinal (GI) tract and prevent backflow (Figure 56-2).

The surface of the stomach is covered with *rugae*, or folds of mucosa and submucosa that extend longitudinally.

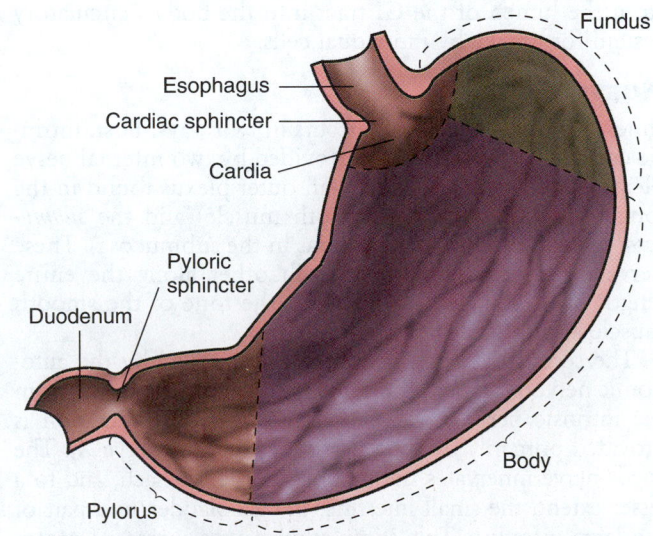

Figure 56-2 ■ The anatomy of the stomach.

Smooth muscle cells that line the stomach are responsible for gastric motility. The stomach is also richly innervated with intrinsic and extrinsic nerves. Parietal cells lining the wall of the stomach secrete hydrochloric acid, whereas chief cells secrete pepsinogen (a precursor to pepsin, a digestive enzyme). Parietal cells also produce intrinsic factor, which works to facilitate the absorption of vitamin B_{12}. Absence of the intrinsic factor causes pernicious anemia.

Function

The stomach performs several functions. Following ingestion of food, the stomach functions as a food reservoir. The primary function of the stomach is to begin the digestive process by using both mechanical movements and chemical secretions. Gastric secretion can be divided into three phases: cephalic, gastric, and intestinal.

The *cephalic phase* begins with the sight, smell, and taste of food and is regulated by the vagus nerve. Sympathetic nerve fibers activate neurons in the GI nerve plexus, which then initiate secretory and contractile activity. The *gastric phase* begins with the presence of food in the stomach. The G-cells in the antrum secrete the hormone gastrin, which promotes the secretion of hydrochloric acid and pepsinogen. Hydrochloric acid transforms inactive pepsinogen into active pepsins, which aid in the digestion of proteins. The secretion of mucus and bicarbonate protect the stomach from mechanical and chemical damage. The fluids secreted into the stomach are collectively referred to as gastric juice (Table 56-1).

The stomach also mixes or churns the food, breaking apart the large food molecules and mixing them with gastric secretions to form chyme, which then empties into the duodenum. The *intestinal phase* begins as the chyme passes from the stomach into the duodenum, causing distention. The intestinal phase is mediated by secretin, a hormone that inhibits further acid production and decreases gastric motility.

PANCREAS
Structure

The pancreas is a fish shaped gland that lies retroperitoneally in the upper abdominal cavity behind the stomach and extends horizontally from the duodenal C-loop to the spleen. The pancreas is divided into portions known as the head, the body, and the tail (Figure 56-3).

Function

Two major cellular bodies within the pancreas have separate functions: exocrine and endocrine. The *exocrine* part of the pancreas constitutes about 80% of the organ and consists of acinar cells, which secrete the enzymes that are necessary for the digestion of carbohydrates, fats, and proteins (trypsin, chymotrypsin, amylase, and lipase) (Table 56-2). The *endocrine* part of the pancreas is made up of the islets of Langerhans, with alpha cells producing glucagon and beta cells producing insulin. Although the islet cells account for less than 2% of the volume of the pancreas, the hormones produced

TABLE 56-1	Gastrointestinal Hormones	
Hormone	**Source**	**Effect**
Gastrin	Secreted by the gastric mucosa in the presence of peptides	Stimulates gastric motility and secretion of hydrochloric acid
Secretin	Secreted by the duodenum in the presence of hydrochloric acid	Stimulates the secretion of pancreatic juice and bile from the liver
Pancreozymin	Secreted by the duodenum in the presence of hydrochloric acid and peptides	Stimulates the secretion of pancreatic juice
Cholecystokinin	Secreted by the duodenum in the presence of amino acids and fatty acids	Stimulates the secretion of pancreatic enzymes and bile from the gallbladder

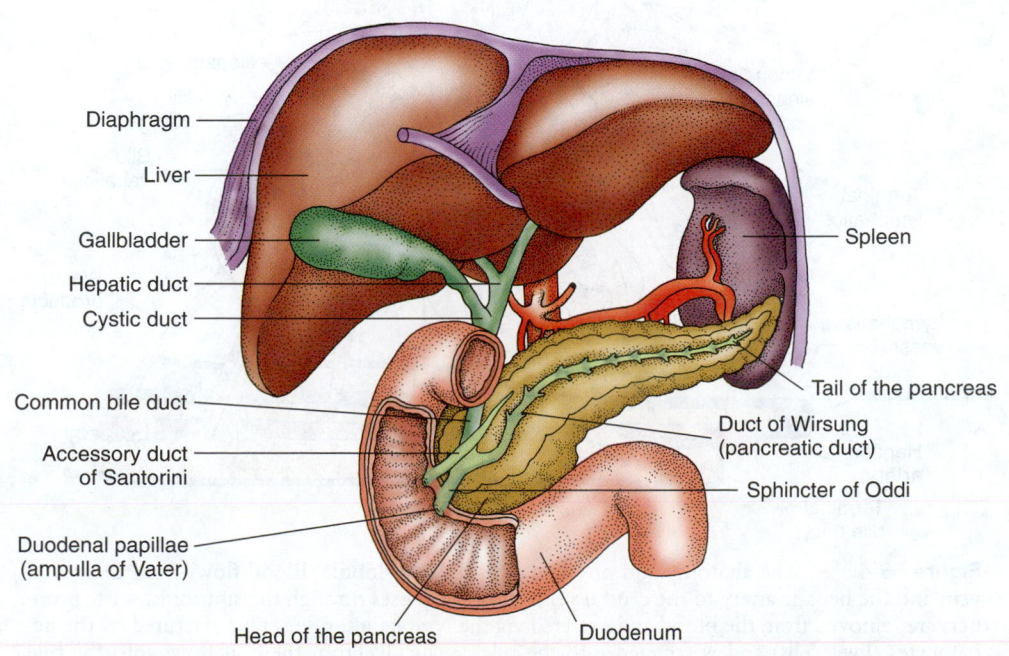

Diaphragm
Liver
Gallbladder
Hepatic duct
Cystic duct
Common bile duct
Accessory duct of Santorini
Duodenal papillae (ampulla of Vater)
Head of the pancreas
Duodenum
Spleen
Tail of the pancreas
Duct of Wirsung (pancreatic duct)
Sphincter of Oddi

Figure 56-3 ■ The anatomy of the pancreas, the liver, and the gallbladder.

are essential in the regulation of metabolism. Chapter 65 describes the endocrine function of the pancreas.

LIVER AND GALLBLADDER
Structure

The liver is the largest organ in the body and is mainly located in the right upper quadrant (RUQ) of the abdomen. The liver is divided into two major regions: a larger right lobe and a smaller left lobe. It is made up of functioning units called lobules (Figure 56-4). The right and left hepatic ducts transport bile from the liver. The liver receives its blood supply from the hepatic artery and the hepatic portal vein. About 1500 mL of blood flows through the liver every minute.

The gallbladder is a pear-shaped bulbous sac that is located in a depression on the inferior surface of the liver. The gallbladder has three portions: the neck, which is continu-

TABLE 56-2 Major Digestive Enzymes and Bile

Substance	Source	Substrate	End Product
Salivary amylase (ptyalin)	Salivary glands	Starch	Dextrins, maltose
Gastric pepsin (protease)	Stomach	Proteins	Polypeptides
Gastric lipase	Stomach	Emulsified fats	Fatty acids* and glycerol*
Bile (contains no enzymes)	Liver; stored and released from the gallbladder	Unemulsified fats	Emulsified fats
Trypsin	Pancreas	Proteins and polypeptides	Polypeptides and amino acids*
Chymotrypsin	Pancreas	Proteins and polypeptides	Polypeptides and amino acids*
Carboxypeptidase	Pancreas	Polypeptides	Smaller polypeptides
Amylase	Pancreas	Starch	Maltose, lactose, and sucrose
Lipase	Pancreas	Bile and emulsified fats	Glycerol* and fatty acids*
Enterokinase	Duodenal mucosa	Trypsinogen	Trypsin
Peptidases	Intestine	Peptides	Amino acids*
Lactase	Intestine	Lactose (milk sugar)	Glucose* and galactose*
Maltase	Intestine	Maltose (malt sugar)	Glucose*
Sucrase	Intestine	Sucrose (cane sugar)	Glucose* and fructose*

*End product ready for digestion.

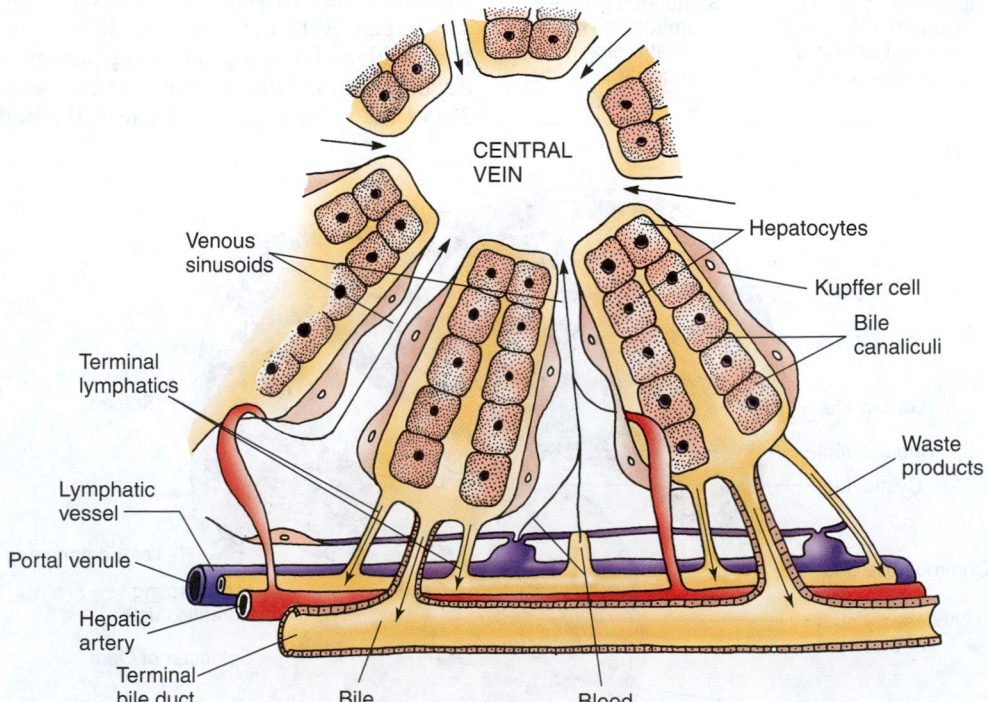

Figure 56-4 ■ The anatomy and physiology of the liver lobule. Blood flows from the portal vein and the hepatic artery to the central vein. As blood passes through the sinusoids, waste products are removed from the blood and excreted via the lymphatics. Bile is manufactured by the hepatocytes (liver cells) and is secreted into the bile canaliculi. From there, it flows into the bile ducts and then to the gallbladder.

ous with the cystic duct; the body, or main portion; and the fundus, the lower bulbous section. The gallbladder is drained by the cystic duct, which joins with the hepatic duct from the liver to form the common bile duct.

Function

The liver performs more than 400 functions in three major categories: storage, protection, and metabolism. The liver stores several minerals and vitamins, such as the following:

- Copper
- Iron
- Magnesium
- Vitamin B_2
- Vitamin B_{12}
- Folic acid
- Vitamin B_6
- Fat-soluble vitamins A, D, E, and K

The protective function of the liver involves phagocytic **Kupffer cells**, which are part of the body's reticuloendothelial system. They engulf harmful bacteria and anemic red blood cells. The liver also detoxifies potentially harmful compounds (such as drugs, chemicals, and alcohol) that are ingested.

The liver functions in the metabolism of proteins considered vital for human survival. It breaks down amino acids to remove ammonia, which is then converted to urea and is excreted via the kidneys. In addition, the liver synthesizes several plasma proteins, including albumin, prothrombin, and fibrinogen. The liver's role in carbohydrate metabolism involves storing and releasing glycogen as the body's energy requirements change. The liver synthesizes, breaks down, and temporarily stores fatty acids and triglycerides.

The liver forms and continually secretes bile. **Bile** is essential for the emulsification of fat. The secretion of bile increases in response to gastrin, secretin, and cholecystokinin. Bile is secreted into small ducts that empty into the common bile duct and into the duodenum at the sphincter of Oddi. However, if the sphincter is closed, the bile goes to the gallbladder for storage.

The gallbladder collects, concentrates, and stores the bile that has come from the liver. It releases the bile into the duodenum via the common bile duct when fat is present.

SMALL INTESTINE
Structure

The small intestine is the longest and most convoluted portion of the digestive tract, measuring 16 to 19 feet (5 to 6 m) in length in an adult. It is composed of three different regions: duodenum, jejunum, and ileum. The *duodenum* is the first 12 inches (30 cm) of the small intestine and is attached to the distal end of the pylorus. It is C-shaped, curving left around the head of the pancreas and bending behind the transverse portion of the large intestine. The common bile duct and pancreatic duct join to form the ampulla of Vater, emptying into the duodenum at the duodenal papilla. This papillary opening is surrounded by muscle known as the **sphincter of Oddi**. The 8-foot (2.5 m) portion of the small intestine that follows the sphincter of Oddi is the *jejunum*. The last 8 to 12 feet (2.5 to 4 m) of the small intestine is called the *ileum*. The ileocecal valve separates the entrance of the ileum from the cecum of the large intestine.

The inner surface of the small intestine has a velvety appearance because of numerous mucous membrane finger-like projections. These projections are called intestinal villi. In addition to the intestinal villi, the small intestine has circular folds of mucosa and submucosa, which increase the surface area for digestion and absorption.

Function

The small intestine has three main functions: movement (mixing and peristalsis), digestion, and absorption. Because the intestinal villi increase the surface area of the small intestine, the small intestine is the major organ of absorption of the digestive system. The small intestine mixes and transports the chyme by movements called segmental contractions. The contents are moved back and forth over short distances, thereby allowing the chyme to mix with many digestive enzymes. The ileocecal valve opens only to allow the passage of chyme. It takes an average of 3 to 10 hours for the contents to be propelled by peristalsis through the small intestine. The intestinal glands secrete intestinal juice containing epithelial cells that are used to replace surface epithelial cells of the villi as they are lost. The intestinal cells also produce cells that contain enzymes aiding in the digestion of proteins, carbohydrates, and lipids (see Tables 56-1 and 56-2).

LARGE INTESTINE
Structure

The large intestine extends about 5 to 6 feet in length from the ileocecal valve to the anus and is lined with columnar epithelium that has absorptive and mucous cells. It begins with the *cecum*, a dilated pouchlike structure that is inferior to the ileocecal opening. At the base of the cecum is the vermiform appendix, which has no known digestive function. The large intestine then extends upward from the cecum as the colon. The colon consists of four divisions: ascending colon, transverse colon, descending colon, and sigmoid colon. The sigmoid colon empties into the rectum.

Following the sigmoid colon, the large intestine bends downward to form the rectum. The last 6 to 8 inches (3 to 4 cm) of the large intestine is called the anal canal, which opens to the exterior of the body through the anus. The anal canal is surrounded by sphincter muscles.

Function

The large intestine's functions are movement, absorption, and elimination. Movement in the large intestine consists mainly of segmental contractions, like those in the small intestine, to allow enough time for the absorption of water and electrolytes. In addition, three or four strong peristaltic contractions per day are triggered by colonic distention in the proximal large intestine to propel the contents toward the rectum, where the material is stored until the urge to defecate occurs.

Absorption of water and some electrolytes occurs in the large intestine to reduce the fluid volume of the chyme, which creates a more solid material, the feces, for elimination.

Gastrointestinal Changes Associated with Aging

Like other systems, physiologic changes occur as individuals age, especially when they become 65 years of age or older. Changes in digestion, nutrition, and elimination are common, and affect nursing care as outlined in Chart 56-1.

CHART 56-1

NURSING FOCUS on the OLDER ADULT
Changes in the Gastrointestinal System Related to Aging

Physiologic Change	Disorders Related to Change	Nursing Interventions	Rationales
Stomach Atrophy of the gastric mucosa is characterized by a decrease in the ratio of gastrin-secreting cells to somatostatin-secreting cells. This change leads to decreased hydrochloric acid levels (hypochlorhydria).	Decreased hydrochloric acid levels lead to decreased absorption of iron and vitamin B_{12} and to proliferation of bacteria. Atrophic gastritis occurs as a consequence of bacterial overgrowth.	Encourage bland foods high in vitamins and iron. Assess for epigastric pain.	Bland foods help prevent gastritis. Assessment helps detect gastritis.
Large Intestine Peristalsis decreases, and nerve impulses are dulled.	Decreased sensation to defecate can result in postponement of bowel movements, which leads to constipation and impaction.	Encourage a high-fiber diet and 1500 mL of fluid intake daily (if not contraindicated). Encourage as much activity as tolerated.	These interventions increase the sensation of needing to defecate.
Pancreas Distention and dilation of pancreatic ducts change. Calcification of pancreatic vessels occurs with a decrease in lipase production.	Decreased lipase level results in decreased fat absorption and digestion. Steatorrhea, or excess fat in the feces, occurs because of decreased fat digestion.	Encourage small, frequent feedings. Assess for diarrhea.	Small, frequent feedings help prevent steatorrhea. Diarrhea may be steatorrhea.
Liver A decrease in the number and size of hepatic cells leads to decreased liver weight and mass. This change and an increase in fibrous tissue lead to decreased protein synthesis and changes in liver enzymes. Enzyme activity and cholesterol synthesis are diminished.	Decreased enzyme activity depresses drug metabolism, which leads to accumulation of drugs—possibly to toxic levels.	Assess all clients for adverse effects of all drugs, even those administered in normal doses.	Assessment detects drug toxicity.

ASSESSMENT TECHNIQUES

History

One method of assessing gastrointestinal (GI) functioning is to use the nutritional-metabolic and elimination patterns found in Gordon's Functional Health Patterns (Chart 56-2). The goal of the health history is to determine the events related to the current health problem.

DEMOGRAPHIC DATA

Collect demographic data about the client, such as age, gender, culture, and occupation. This information can provide information regarding predispositions to particular GI system disorders.

FAMILY HISTORY AND GENETIC RISK

Inquire about a family history of gastrointestinal (GI) disorders. Some GI health problems have a genetic predisposition. For example, familial adenomatous polyposis (FAP) is an inherited autosomal dominant disorder that predisposes the client to colon cancer.

PERSONAL HISTORY

A thorough review of the client's overall health status is an important part of every nursing history. Question the client regarding previous GI disorders or abdominal surgeries. Ask about prescription medications being taken, including how much, when the drugs are administered, and why they have been prescribed. It is also important to explore whether the client takes over-the-counter medications, which he or she may use independently. In particular, you should ask whether aspirin, nonsteroidal anti-inflammatory drugs (NSAIDs) (such as ibuprofen), laxatives, herbal preparations, or enemas are routinely taken. Large amounts of aspirin or NSAIDs can predispose the client to peptic ulcer disease and GI bleeding. Long-term use of laxatives or enemas can cause dependence on such stimulation and result in constipation. Some herbal preparations can affect absorption and elimination, or enhance the action of certain medications.

Finally, investigate the client's travel history. Ask the client whether he or she has traveled outside of the country recently. This information may provide clues as to the origin of symptoms such as diarrhea.

CHART 56-2

Gastrointestinal Assessment
USING GORDON'S FUNCTIONAL HEALTH PATTERNS

Nutritional-Metabolic Pattern
- What is your typical daily food intake? Describe a day's meals, snacks, and vitamins.
- How much salt do you typically add to your food? Do you use salt substitutes?
- How is your appetite? Any recent change?
- Do you have any difficulty chewing or swallowing?
- Do you wear dentures? How well do they fit?
- Do you ever experience indigestion or "heartburn"? How often? What seems to cause it? What helps it?
- Do you have pain, diarrhea, gas, or any other problems? Do any specific foods cause this for you?
- What is your typical daily fluid intake? What types of fluids (water, juices, soft drinks, coffee, tea)? How much?
- Have you had any recent change in your weight? Weight gain? Weight loss? How much?
- Have you noticed a change in the tightness of your rings or shoes? Tighter? Looser?
- Have you noticed any difference in the size of your abdomen?

Elimination Pattern
- What is your usual bowel elimination pattern? Frequency? Character? Discomfort? Laxatives?
- Do you have any pain or bleeding associated with bowel movements?
- Have you experienced any changes in your usual bowel pattern?
- When was your last rectal examination?
- Have you ever had an endoscopy or a colonoscopy?
- What is your usual urinary elimination pattern? Frequency? Amount? Color? Odor? Control?
- Have you noticed a change in the amount of urine?

Based on Gordon, M. (2002). *Manual of nursing diagnosis* (10th ed.). St. Louis: Mosby.

DIET HISTORY

A diet history is important when assessing GI system function. Many conditions manifest themselves as a result of alterations in dietary intake and absorption of nutrients. The goal of a nutritional assessment is to gather information about how well the client's nutritional needs are being met. You should inquire about any special diet and whether there are any known food allergies. Ask the client to describe the usual foods that are eaten daily and the times that meals are taken.

Illness changes dietary intake, so explore with the client any changes that have occurred in eating habits as a result of illness. **Anorexia** (loss of appetite for food) can occur with GI disease. Assess changes in taste and any difficulty or pain with swallowing (dysphagia) that could be associated with esophageal disorders. Also ascertain whether abdominal pain or discomfort accompanies eating, and whether the client has experienced any nausea, vomiting, or **dyspepsia** (indigestion or heartburn). Unknown food allergies often cause these symptoms. Inquire about any unintentional weight loss, because some cancers of the GI tract may present in this manner. It is also important to assess alcohol and caffeine consumption, because both substances are associated with many GI disorders, such as gastritis and peptic ulcer disease.

CULTURAL CONSIDERATIONS

Cultural and religious patterns are important in obtaining a complete diet history. The nurse determines whether cultur-ally based foods pose a problem for the client. For example, the spices or hot pepper used in cooking in many cultures can aggravate or precipitate GI tract complaints, such as indigestion. Note religious patterns such as fasting or abstinence.

About 80% to 90% of black individuals are lactose intolerant. A much smaller percentage of white individuals also have this problem. Lactose intolerance causes bloating, cramping, and diarrhea as a result of lack of the enzyme lactase. Lactase is needed to convert lactose in milk and other dairy products to glucose and galactose.

SOCIOECONOMIC STATUS

The client's socioeconomic status may have a profound impact on his or her nutritional status. Knowledge of the client's socioeconomic status can provide valuable clues for determining his or her ability to obtain food, medications, and medical care. People who have limited budgets, such as some older adults or the unemployed, may not be able to purchase foods required for a balanced diet. In addition, they may substitute less expensive, and perhaps less effective, over-the-counter medications for prescription medications. Necessary medical care may be delayed, and clients may not seek health care until conditions are well advanced. Clients who are financially restricted may benefit from suggestions for managing nutrition while on a budget.

CURRENT HEALTH PROBLEMS

Because GI clinical manifestations are often vague and difficult for the client to describe, it is important to obtain a chronologic account of the current problem, symptoms, and any treatments taken. Furthermore, explore the characteristics associated with each symptom, including the location, quality, quantity, timing (onset, duration), and factors that may aggravate or alleviate the symptom (see Chart 56-2).

For example, a change in bowel habits is a significant complaint. Obtain the following information from the client:
- Pattern of bowel movements
- Color and consistency of the feces
- Occurrence of diarrhea or constipation
- Effective action taken to relieve diarrhea or constipation
- Presence of frank blood or tarry stools
- Presence of abdominal distention or gas

An unintentional weight gain or loss is another symptom that warrants further investigation. Assess the following:
- Normal weight
- Weight gain or loss
- Period of time for weight change
- Changes in appetite or oral intake

Smoking predisposes the client to several types of cancer, especially oral cancer, because nicotine and other chemicals found in tobacco are GI irritants. Obtain the client's smoking history, including the number of packs of cigarettes smoked per day times the number of years smoked. For example, if the client smoked two packs of cigarettes per day for 20 years, then he or she would have a 40-year cigarette smoking history. Also ask about any history or current use of cigars, pipe tobacco, or chewing tobacco.

Pain is a common complaint in clients with GI tract disorders. The mnemonic **PQRST** may be helpful in assisting you to organize the current problem assessment (Jarvis, 2004):

P: Precipitating or palliative. What brings it on? What makes it better? Worse? When did you first notice it?

Q: Quality or quantity. How does it look, feel, or sound? How intense/severe is it?

R: Region or radiation. Where is it? Does it spread anywhere?

S: Severity scale. How bad is it (on a scale of 1 to 10)? Is it getting better, worse, or staying the same?

T: Timing. Onset—Exactly when did it first occur? Duration—How long did it last? Frequency—How often does it occur?

Abdominal pain is often vague and difficult to evaluate. Asking the client to apply descriptors to the type of pain, such as burning, gnawing, or stabbing, is often helpful. The location of the pain can be determined by asking the client to point to the involved site. Ask about the relationship of food intake to the onset or worsening of pain. For example, a high-fat meal often triggers gallbladder pain.

Changes in the skin can result from several GI tract disorders, such as liver and biliary system obstruction. Ask the client about whether these clinical manifestations have occurred, or assess whether they are present:

- Skin discolorations or rashes
- Itching
- Jaundice
- Increased susceptibility to bruising
- Increased tendency to bleed

Physical Assessment

Physical assessment of the gastrointestinal (GI) system involves a comprehensive examination of the client's nutritional status, the mouth and pharynx, the abdomen, and the extremities. Nutritional assessment is discussed in detail in Chapter 64.

MOUTH AND PHARYNX

Assessment of the mouth involves inspection and palpation. To begin the examination of the mouth, put on gloves, face the client, and inspect the lips for color, moisture, cracking, or lesions. You will need a penlight and a tongue depressor to continue inspecting the inner surfaces of the lips and the oral mucosa, starting on the client's left side and moving in a clockwise fashion. Carefully palpate the U-shaped area under the tongue for nodules, because oral malignancies are most likely to develop in this area. The tongue is inspected for color, coating, ulcers, and variations in size and shape.

It is important to examine the teeth for evidence of dental caries and note the absence of teeth. Tooth discoloration may be the result of excessive tobacco use. Refer the client to a dentist if you detect abnormalities or decay.

The gums should be pink, moist, and smooth. Dark-skinned clients may have a dark line on the margins of the gingiva. If the client wears dentures, they are removed to facilitate a thorough examination of the mouth. Throughout this examination, be alert to any significant mouth odors that suggest disease. For instance, a fruity smell may indicate uncontrolled diabetes mellitus.

Oral lesions or nodules are noted. For example, lesions from Kaposi's sarcoma may be seen in clients with acquired immunodeficiency syndrome (AIDS).

ABDOMEN

In preparation for examination of the abdomen, the client is instructed to empty his or her bladder and then to lie in a supine position with knees bent, keeping the arms at the sides to prevent inadvertent tensing of the abdominal muscles.

The abdominal examination usually begins at the client's right side and proceeds in a systematic fashion (Figure 56-5):

- Right upper quadrant (RUQ)
- Left upper quadrant (LUQ)
- Left lower quadrant (LLQ)
- Right lower quadrant (RLQ)

Table 56-3 lists the organs that lie in each of these areas.

If areas of pain or discomfort are noted from the history, this area is examined last in the examination sequence. This sequence should prevent the client from tensing abdominal muscles because of the pain, which would make the examination difficult. Examine any area of tenderness cautiously and instruct the client to state whether it is too painful. Observe the client's face for signs of distress or pain.

Assess the abdomen by using the four techniques of examination, but in a sequence different from that used for other body systems: inspection, auscultation, percussion, and then palpation. This sequence is preferred so that palpation and percussion do not increase intestinal activity and hence increase bowel sounds. Palpation is not performed if appendicitis or an abdominal aneurysm is suspected.

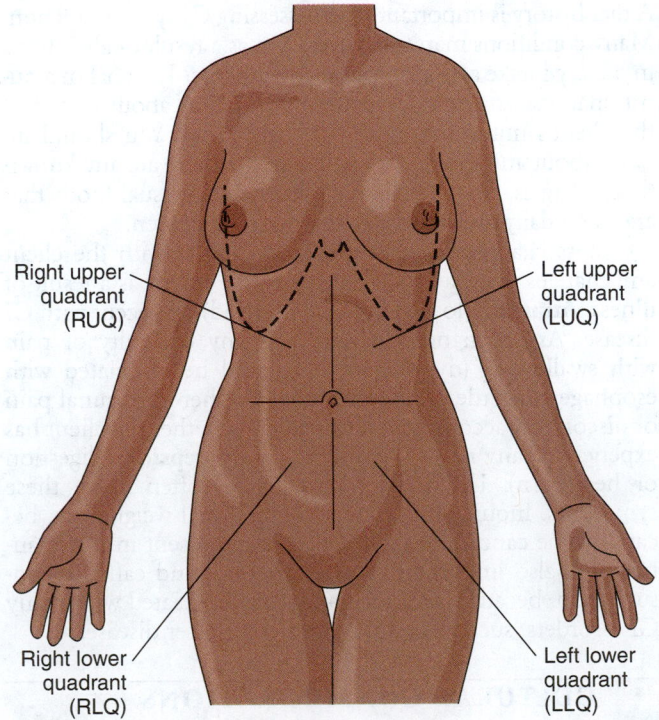

Right upper quadrant (RUQ)

Left upper quadrant (LUQ)

Right lower quadrant (RLQ)

Left lower quadrant (LLQ)

Figure 56-5 ■ A topographic division of the abdomen into quadrants.

Inspection

Inspect the skin and note the following:

- Overall symmetry of the abdomen
- Presence of discolorations (rashes, lesions, striae, petechiae, scars, distended superficial veins, jaundice, and any other pigmentation changes)
- Abdominal distention
- Bulging flanks
- Taut, glistening skin

Assess the shape of the abdomen by observing its contour and symmetry. The contour of the abdomen can be rounded, flat, concave, or distended. It is best determined when standing at the side of the bed or treatment table and looking down on the abdomen. View the abdomen at eye level from the side. Note whether the contour is symmetric or asymmetric. Asymmetry of the abdomen can indicate problems affecting the underlying body structures (see Table 56-3). Note the shape and position of the umbilicus for any deviations. The presence of ecchymosis around the umbilicus **(Cullen's sign)** is an indication of intra-abdominal bleeding.

Finally, observe the client's abdominal movements, including the normal rising and falling with inspiration and expiration, and note any distress during movement. Occasionally, pulsations may be visible, particularly in the area of the abdominal aorta. Peristaltic movements are rarely seen on inspection unless the client is thin and has markedly increased peristalsis. If these movements are observed, note the quadrant of origin and the direction of peristaltic flow. This finding is reported to the health care provider, because it may indicate an intestinal obstruction.

Auscultation

Video Clip: Abdomen, Bowel Sounds

Auscultation of the abdomen is performed with the diaphragm of the stethoscope because bowel sounds are usually high pitched. The stethoscope is placed lightly on the abdominal wall while listening for bowel sounds in all four quadrants, beginning in the RLQ at the ileocecal valve area.

Bowel sounds are created as air and fluid move through the GI tract. They are normally heard as relatively high-pitched gurgles every 5 to 15 seconds, with a normal frequency range of 5 to 30 per minute. Bowel sounds are characterized as normal, hypoactive, or hyperactive. Listen for the character and frequency of the sounds. Bowel sounds may be irregular, so you must listen for *at least* 1 full minute in each quadrant to confirm the absence of bowel sounds. Bowel sounds are diminished or absent after abdominal surgery or in the client with peritonitis or paralytic ileus. Increased bowel sounds, especially loud gurgling sounds, result from hypermotility of the bowel **(borborygmus).** These sounds are usually heard in the client with diarrhea or gastroenteritis or above a complete intestinal obstruction.

Video Clip: Percussion, Abdomen

When auscultating the abdomen, also listen for vascular sounds or **bruits** ("swooshing" sounds) over the abdominal aorta, the renal arteries, and the iliac arteries. A bruit heard over the aorta usually indicates the presence of an aneurysm. *If this sound is heard, do not percuss or palpate the abdomen. Notify the health care provider of your findings!*

TABLE 56-3 Location of Body Structures in Each Abdominal Quadrant

Right Upper Quadrant (RUQ)	Left Upper Quadrant (LUQ)	Left Lower Quadrant (LLQ)	Right Lower Quadrant (RLQ)	Midline
Most of the liver	Left lobe of the liver	Part of the descending colon	Cecum	Abdominal aorta
Gallbladder	Stomach	Sigmoid colon	Appendix	Uterus (if enlarged)
Duodenum	Spleen	Left ureter	Right ureter	Bladder (if distended)
Head of the pancreas	Body and tail of the pancreas	Left ovary and fallopian tube	Right ovary and fallopian tube	
Hepatic flexure of the colon	Splenic flexure of the colon	Left spermatic cord	Right spermatic cord	
Part of the ascending and transverse colon	Part of the transverse and descending colon			

Percussion

Video Clip: Percussion, Liver

Percussion may be used during the abdominal assessment to determine the size of solid organs; to detect the presence of masses, fluid, and air; and to estimate the size of the liver and spleen. This part of the physical assessment is usually performed by a physician or advanced practice nurse (APN). The examiner elicits percussion notes by placing the middle finger of the nondominant hand over the abdominal area to be percussed, striking his or her finger lightly with the tip of the middle finger of the dominant hand several times. Each quadrant is systematically assessed by comparing sounds over different areas. The **percussion notes** normally heard in the abdomen are termed **tympanic** (the high-pitched, loud, musical sound of an air-filled intestine) or **dull** (the medium-pitched, softer, thudlike sound over a solid organ, such as the liver).

Video Clip: Percussion, Spleen

To percuss the size of the liver span, the physician or APN begins from below the right nipple in the midclavicular line and is careful to percuss between ribs. The percussion note should change from resonance of the lung tissue to dullness of the liver when the upper liver border is reached. The examiner marks the area where percussion tones change, then percusses up from the iliac crest in the midclavicular line until the percussion note changes from tympany of the bowel to dullness of the liver at the lower border. Again, this area is marked. The distance between the two marks is the approximate liver span, which is normally 2.4 to 5 inches (6 to 12 cm). An enlarged liver span indicates **hepatomegaly** (liver enlargement).

The examiner may also use percussion techniques to determine the size and position of the spleen at the tenth intercostal space in the left midaxillary line. Dullness heard forward of the midaxillary line or in the left anterior axillary line indicates enlargement of the spleen **(splenomegaly).** Mild to moderate splenomegaly can be detected before the spleen becomes palpable. Percussion can also be used to detect a distended bladder. Dullness is heard over a distended bladder.

Palpation

The purpose of palpation is to determine the size and location of abdominal organs and to assess for the presence of masses or tenderness. Palpation of the abdomen consists of two types: light palpation and deep palpation. Only physi-

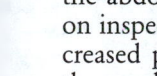

cians and APNs, such as clinical nurse specialists and nurse practitioners, should perform deep palpation. Deep palpation is used to further determine the size and shape of abdominal organs and masses.

The technique of *light palpation* is used to detect large masses and areas of tenderness and to help the client achieve muscular relaxation. Place the first four fingers of the palpating hand close together and then place them lightly on the abdomen and proceed smoothly and systematically from quadrant to quadrant. The abdomen is depressed to a depth of 0.5 to 1 inch (1.25 to 2.5 cm), and the assessment proceeds with a rotational movement of the palpating hand. Any areas of tenderness or guarding are noted, because these areas are examined last and cautiously during deep palpation. While performing light palpation, be alert to signs of rigidity which, unlike voluntary guarding, is a sign of peritoneal inflammation. Areas of pain should be evaluated for rebound tenderness **(Blumberg's sign).** With fingers placed at a 90-degree angle in relation to the abdomen, the examiner pushes slowly and deeply, releasing quickly. Pain felt on release is a positive sign for rebound tenderness and should be reported to the health care provider.

Psychosocial Assessment

Psychosocial assessment focuses on how the current complaint affects the client's lifestyle. Remember that clients are often reluctant to discuss elimination problems, which are very personal. The interview focus is whether there has been any interruption of, or disturbance to, usual activities, including employment. Question the client about recent stressful events. Emotional stress has been associated with the development or exacerbation of irritable bowel syndrome (IBS) and other GI disorders.

Critical Thinking Challenge

A middle-aged female client is seen in the emergency department where you work complaining of RUQ abdominal pain and cramping for the last 2 days. Because she travels extensively for her job, her usual dietary pattern consists of eating at restaurants several times weekly. The symptoms began 1 to 2 hours after eating a dinner of fried or spicy foods.

1. About which specific areas of the history should you seek further information or clarification?
2. What physical assessment findings would you be most likely to find during the abdominal examination?

evolve For suggested answer guidelines, go to http://evolve.elsevier.com/Iggy/.

Diagnostic Assessment

LABORATORY TESTS

To make an accurate assessment of the many possible causes of gastrointestinal (GI) system abnormalities, laboratory testing of blood, urine, and stool specimens may be performed.

Blood Tests

A *complete blood count (CBC)* aids in the diagnosis of anemia and infection; it also detects changes in the blood's formed elements. In adults, GI bleeding is the most frequent cause of anemia.

Because the liver is the main site of all proteins involved in coagulation, the prothrombin time is useful in evaluating the levels of these clotting factors. *Prothrombin time (PT)* measures the rate at which prothrombin is converted to thrombin, a process that is dependent on most of the vitamin K–associated clotting factors. Severe acute or chronic liver damage leads to a prolonged PT secondary to impaired synthesis of clotting proteins.

Many *electrolytes* are altered in GI tract dysfunction. For example, calcium is absorbed in the GI tract and may be measured to detect malabsorption. Excessive vomiting or diarrhea causes electrolyte depletion, thus requiring replacement.

Assays of serum enzymes are important in the evaluation of liver damage. **Aspartate aminotransferase (AST)** and **alanine aminotransferase (ALT)** are two enzymes found in the liver and other organs. These enzymes are elevated in most liver disorders, but they are highest in conditions that cause necrosis, such as severe viral hepatitis.

Elevations in serum **amylase** and **lipase** are indicative of acute pancreatitis. In acute pancreatitis, serum amylase levels begin to elevate within 24 hours of onset and remain elevated for up to 5 days. Serum amylase and lipase are not elevated when extensive pancreatic necrosis is present because there are few pancreatic cells manufacturing the enzymes. Serum amylase and lipase measurements are the best indicators of the presence of acute pancreatitis, with elevations in 80% to 85% of pancreatitis cases (Avunduk, 2002).

Bilirubin is the primary pigment in bile, which is normally conjugated and excreted by the liver and biliary system. It is measured as total serum bilirubin, conjugated (direct) bilirubin, and unconjugated (indirect) bilirubin. These measurements are important in the evaluation of jaundice and in the evaluation of liver and biliary tract functioning. Elevations in direct and indirect bilirubin levels can indicate impaired secretion or conjugation.

The serum level of ammonia is also measured to evaluate hepatic function. Ammonia is normally used to rebuild amino acids or is converted to urea for excretion. Elevated ammonia levels are seen in conditions that cause severe hepatocellular injury, such as cirrhosis of the liver or fulminant hepatitis (Pagana & Pagana, 2002).

Two primary **oncofetal antigens**—CA19-9 and CEA—are evaluated to diagnose, monitor the success of cancer therapy, and assess for the recurrence of cancer in the GI tract. These antigens may also be increased in benign GI conditions. Chart 56-3 lists blood tests commonly used by the health care provider in the diagnosis of GI disorders.

Urine Tests

The presence of amylase can be detected in the urine. In acute pancreatitis, there is increased renal clearance of amylase. Amylase levels in the urine remain high even after serum levels return to normal. This becomes an important finding in clients who are symptomatic for 3 days or longer (Pagana & Pagana, 2002).

Urine urobilinogen is a form of bilirubin that is converted by the intestinal flora and excreted in the urine. Its measurement is useful in the evaluation of hepatic and biliary obstruction, because the presence of bilirubin in the urine often precedes the development of jaundice (Chart 56-4).

CHART 56-3

LABORATORY PROFILE
Gastrointestinal Assessment

Test	Normal Range for Adults	Significance of Abnormal Findings
Calcium (total)	9.0-10.5 mg/dL (Values decrease in older adults)	*Decreased* values indicate possible: Malabsorption Renal failure Acute pancreatitis
Potassium	3.5-5.0 mEq/L or 3.5-5.0 mmol/L	*Decreased* values indicate possible: Vomiting Gastric suctioning Diarrhea Drainage from intestinal fistulas
Albumin	3.5-5.0 g/dL	*Decreased* values indicate possible: Hepatic disease
Alanine aminotransferase (ALT)	3-35 International Units/L or 8-20 units/L (SI units)	*Increased* values indicate possible: Liver disease Hepatitis Cirrhosis
Aspartate aminotransferase (AST)	5-40 units/L	*Increased* values indicate possible: Liver disease Hepatitis Cirrhosis
Lactate dehydrogenase (LDH)	115-225 International Units/L	*Increased* values indicate possible: Damaged liver caused by hepatitis and other hepatocellular disorders
Alkaline phosphatase	30-85 International Units/L or 42-128 units/L (SI units)	*Increased* values indicate possible: Hepatic disease Biliary obstruction
Bilirubin Total serum	0.1-1.0 mg/dL	*Increased* values indicate possible: Hemolysis Biliary obstruction Hepatic damage
Conjugated (direct)	0.1-0.3 mg/dL	*Increased* values indicate possible: Biliary obstruction
Unconjugated (indirect)	0.2-0.8 mg/dL	*Increased* values indicate possible: Hemolysis Hepatic damage
Ammonia	15-110 mg/dL	*Increased* values indicate possible: Hepatic disease such as cirrhosis
Xylose absorption	*5-g* dose *in 2 hr:* >20 mg/dL or >1.3 mmol/L *25-g dose in 2 hr:* >25 mg/dL or >1.7 mmol/L	*Decreased* values in blood and urine indicate possible: Malabsorption in the small intestine
Serum amylase	56-90 International Units/L or 25-125 units/L (SI units)	*Increased* values indicate possible: Acute pancreatitis
Serum lipase	0-110 units/L	*Increased* values indicate possible: Acute pancreatitis
Cholesterol	<200 mg/dL	*Increased* values indicate possible: Pancreatitis Biliary obstruction *Decreased* values indicate possible: Liver cell damage
Carbohydrate antigen 19-9 (CA19-9)	<37 units/mL	*Increased* values indicate possible: Cancer of the pancreas, stomach, colon Acute pancreatitis Inflammatory bowel disease
Carcinoembryonic antigen (CEA)	*Nonsmoker:* <2.5 ng/mL *Smoker:* up to 5 ng/mL	*Increased* values indicate possible: Colorectal, stomach, pancreatic cancer Ulcerative colitis Crohn's disease Hepatitis Cirrhosis

LABORATORY PROFILE
Common Urine and Stool Tests Used in Gastrointestinal Assessment

Test	Normal Range for Adults	Significance of Abnormal Findings
Urine bilirubin	Negative	*Increased* values indicate possible: Biliary obstruction Cirrhosis Hepatitis
Urobilinogen	Urine 0.1-1.0 Ehrlich unit/mL	*Increased* values indicate possible: Hepatitis Cirrhosis *Absence* indicates possible obstructive jaundice
Urine amylase	Various levels, depending on unit of measure	*Increased* values indicate possible: Acute pancreatitis Pancreatic obstruction
Stool for occult blood (FOBT)	Negative	*Presence* indicates possible: Carcinoma Peptic ulcer Ulcerative colitis
Ova and parasites	Negative	*Presence* is diagnostic of infection.
Fecal fat	<5 g/24 hr with normal diet	*Increased* values indicate possible: Crohn's disease Malabsorption syndrome Pancreatic disease

Stool Tests

Several stool examinations are used in the evaluation of GI tract dysfunction (see Chart 56-4). Stool studies are conducted to evaluate the function and integrity of the GI tract. Stool testing for occult blood is called the **fecal occult blood test (FOBT)**. The FOBT measures the presence of blood in the stool from GI bleeding, a common finding associated with colorectal cancer.

Stool samples are collected to test for ova and parasites to aid in the diagnosis of parasitic infection. Stool samples tested for fecal fats are evaluated for steatorrhea and malabsorption. Fat is normally absorbed in the small intestine in the presence of biliary and pancreatic secretions. In malabsorption, fat is abnormally excreted in the stool.

Another common stool examination is for the presence of a bacterial infection called *Clostridium difficile*. This test is indicated on clients who have been on antibiotic therapy. The antibiotic therapy depresses the natural intestinal flora causing an overgrowth of *C. difficile*. The bacterium releases a toxin, which causes colonic epithelium necrosis resulting in severe diarrhea (Pagana & Pagana, 2002).

WOMEN'S HEALTH CONSIDERATIONS

Compared with women of lower socioeconomic status, women of higher socioeconomic status are more likely to have regular physical examinations that include an annual FOBT and a proctosigmoidoscopy every 3 to 5 years after the age of 50. An annual FOBT may reduce mortality from colorectal cancer in women. Most physicians include an FOBT as part of the gynecologic examination.

RADIOGRAPHIC EXAMINATIONS

Radiographic examinations and similar diagnostic procedures are useful in detecting structural and functional disorders of the gastrointestinal (GI) system. Your role is to prop-erly prepare the client for the examination, to provide an explanation of the procedure, and to provide the necessary postprocedure care. As with most invasive procedures, many of the diagnostic tests outlined here require a witnessed and signed informed consent.

Plain Films of the Abdomen

A plain film of the abdomen is generally the first x-ray study that the health care provider requests when diagnosing a GI problem. This film, taken in the supine position, has the ability to reveal abnormalities such as masses, tumors, and strictures or obstructions to normal movement. Patterns of bowel gas appear light on the abdominal film and can be useful in detecting an obstruction (ileus). There is no required client preparation except to wear a hospital gown and remove any jewelry or belts, which may interfere with the film.

When abdominal pain is severe or when there is a suspicion of bowel perforation, a set of films called an *acute abdomen series* is requested. This procedure consists of a chest x-ray, supine abdomen film, and an upright abdomen film. The chest x-ray may reveal a hiatal hernia and an upright abdomen film may show air in the peritoneum for a bowel perforation.

Upper Gastrointestinal Series and Small Bowel Series

An **upper GI radiographic series** is an x-ray visualization from the oral part of the pharynx to the duodenojejunal junction. The upper GI series is used to detect disorders of structure or function of the esophagus (barium swallow), stomach, or duodenum. An extension of the upper GI series, the small bowel follow-through (SBFT), continues tracing the barium through the small intestine—up to and including the ileocecal junction—to detect disorders of the jejunum or ileum.

CLIENT PREPARATION. Remind the client to withhold foods or liquids for 8 hours before the test. If possible, opioid analgesics and anticholinergic medications are withheld for 24 hours before the test, because they decrease intestinal tract motility.

Instruct the client about the barium preparation and the need to drink about 16 ounces of the barium. The radiology nurse or technician explains that a rotating examination table will be used to assist the client in assuming the vertical, supine, prone, and lateral positions required for this test.

PROCEDURE. The procedure takes about 30 minutes for the radiologist to perform. Fluoroscopy is used to trace the barium through the esophagus and stomach. The client stands against the x-ray table for this part of the test. The table then moves the client to a lying position for more views of the stomach and duodenum. Lying in a prone position, the client drinks more barium as quickly as possible while x-rays are taken. To attempt to make the client as comfortable as possible, a pillow for the head and a sheet to prevent chilling are supplied whenever possible. The position changes help to coat the mucosa and identify gastroesophageal reflux and hiatal hernia.

If a small bowel radiographic series is included, the client drinks additional barium, and more x-rays are taken at specific intervals. This series can take several hours, depending on how long it takes the barium to reach the cecum.

FOLLOW-UP CARE. After either of these series, teach the client to drink plenty of fluids to help eliminate the barium. The client may be given a mild laxative or stool softener to assist in its elimination. The radiology nurse or technician instructs the client that stools may be chalky white for 24 to 72 hours as barium is excreted. The client is informed that when all barium is passed, brown stools return. If the client is at home, he or she is instructed to report abdominal fullness, pain, or a delay in return to brown stools.

Barium Enema

A **barium enema** examination, also known as a **lower GI series**, is a radiographic visualization of the large intestine. This test is usually ordered for a client with a complaint of blood or mucus in the stool or a change in bowel pattern, such as diarrhea or constipation. A barium enema can also detect bowel obstruction from the twisting of the colon upon itself **(volvulus)**. This test is usually contraindicated in clients when colon perforation or fistula is suspected because there is the potential for barium to enter the venous circulation, causing cardiac arrest.

CLIENT PREPARATION. Adequate client preparation for a barium enema study is very important. The client consumes only clear liquids 12 to 24 hours before the examination to reduce the amount of fecal matter in the bowel. The client is allowed nothing by mouth (NPO) after midnight on the night before the test. In addition, the health care provider prescribes a potent laxative. Oral liquid preparations, such as magnesium citrate or GoLYTELY, are used for cleaning the bowel the evening before the examination. In some cases, a cleansing enema is needed or required according to the agency's procedure.

PROCEDURE. To begin the barium enema examination, a rectal catheter with an inflatable balloon is inserted. About 500 to 1500 mL of barium is instilled slowly by gravity, and the client is instructed to hold the barium.

Films are taken with the client in supine, prone, and lateral positions. He or she may experience abdominal cramps and the urge to defecate as the barium enema is given. This procedure can be extremely uncomfortable, especially for older adults. The client is instructed to take slow, deep breaths and to hold the anal sphincter as tightly closed as possible. The test takes about 45 minutes to 1 hour. In some cases, a double-contrast study (ACBE) is requested. In this study, air is instilled to enhance the contrast and outline small lesions.

FOLLOW-UP CARE. After the study is completed, the client is allowed to expel the barium. The radiology nurse or technician teaches the client to drink plenty of fluids to assist in eliminating the barium. A laxative is given to help remove the barium from the intestinal tract. The client is informed that the stools will be chalky white for about 24 to 72 hours, until all barium is expelled.

Percutaneous Transhepatic Cholangiography

Percutaneous transhepatic cholangiography (PTC) is an x-ray study of the biliary duct system using an iodinated dye instilled via a percutaneous needle inserted through the liver into the intrahepatic ducts. This procedure may be performed when a client has jaundice or persistent upper abdominal pain, even after cholecystectomy, but is rarely done as a diagnostic procedure any more. Information about dilated biliary ducts can be obtained using ultrasound and ERCP (discussed later).

CLIENT PREPARATION. A laxative is usually given to the client the evening before the procedure. The client is NPO for 12 hours before the test. It is important to ask about allergies to iodine or seafood. Steroids are administered if the client has one of these allergies. Coagulation tests are monitored, because impaired clotting is a contraindication to this procedure. Before the procedure begins, an intravenous (IV) infusion is started for the administration of sedatives.

PROCEDURE. The client is placed in a supine position on the fluoroscopy table. The site is prepared and draped, and a local anesthetic is injected into the skin. During the test, the client is instructed to hold his or her breath on expiration while a needle is inserted into the liver under x-ray visualization. The dye is injected slowly until the biliary tree is filled. X-ray images are taken as the dye reaches the biliary duct system. A tilt table may be used to place the client in various positions to visualize the entire biliary tree. At the end of the test, the biliary ducts are aspirated of the contrast medium. The procedure usually takes 30 minutes to 1 hour.

FOLLOW-UP CARE. After a PTC, the client is confined to bed for several hours. The client's vital signs are checked frequently, because there is a risk of hemorrhage and sepsis. The client is placed on the right side with a firm pillow or sandbag placed against the lower ribs and abdomen. Observe the lower right rib cage area for signs of bleeding, hematoma, ecchymosis (bruising), or bile leakage with each postprocedure vital sign assessment.

Computed Tomography of the Gastrointestinal System

Computed tomography (CT), also referred to as a CT scan, is a noninvasive cross-sectional x-ray visualization that can detect tissue densities and abnormalities in the abdomen, liver, pancreas, spleen, and biliary tract. CT may be performed with or without contrast media.

The client is instructed that he or she will need to lie still in a rather enclosed space of the machine. The client is instructed to remove jewelry or metal. If the use of a contrast medium is scheduled, ask about allergies to seafood and iodine. The client is NPO for at least 4 hours before the test if a contrast medium is to be used. IV access will be required for injection of the contrast medium. The client is advised that a warm, flushing feeling may be felt on injection. The client who is mildly claustrophobic may require a mild sedative to tolerate the study.

The radiologic technician instructs the client to lie still and to hold his or her breath when asked. The client is placed on the examining table, and a series of x-ray images are taken. The contrast medium may be given by IV injection for a second set of images. The test takes about 1 to 2 hours to complete.

No particular follow-up care is needed after a CT scan unless sedatives were administered. If the client was sedated, monitor vital signs until the client is alert and fully awake.

OTHER DIAGNOSTIC TESTS

Endoscopy

Endoscopy is direct visualization of the gastrointestinal (GI) tract by means of a flexible fiberoptic endoscope. Endoscopes of various sizes are used for different areas of the GI tract. Visualization of the esophagus, stomach, biliary system, and bowel is possible. Endoscopy is usually ordered to evaluate bleeding, ulceration, inflammation, masses, tumors, and cancerous lesions. Obtaining specimens for biopsy and cytologic studies is also possible through the endoscope. There are several types of endoscopic examinations.

Esophagogastroduodenoscopy

Esophagogastroduodenoscopy (EGD), a visual examination of the esophagus, stomach, and duodenum, is accomplished using a fiberoptic endoscope. The distal end of the endoscope is flexible, allowing visualization of the entire area. This procedure has significantly reduced the number of upper GI series that are done.

The client preparing for an upper GI endoscopic examination is usually placed on NPO status 6 to 8 hours before the procedure. Instruct the client that a flexible tube will be passed down the esophagus while he or she is under conscious sedation. Midazolam hydrochloride (Versed), meperidine (Demerol), and fentanyl (Fentanyl, Sublimaze) are commonly used medications to sedate the client. Atropine may be administered to dry secretions. In addition, a local anesthetic is sprayed to inactivate the gag reflex and facilitate passage of the tube. Explain that this anesthetic will depress the gag reflex and that swallowing will be difficult. If the client has dentures, they are removed. Evaluate the strength of the gag reflex before giving the anesthetic spray, so that you can adequately assess the return of the client's gag reflex following the procedure.

After the medications are administered, the client is usually placed in the left lateral decubitus (Sims', or side-lying) position with a towel or basin at the mouth for secretions. A bite block is inserted to prevent the client from biting

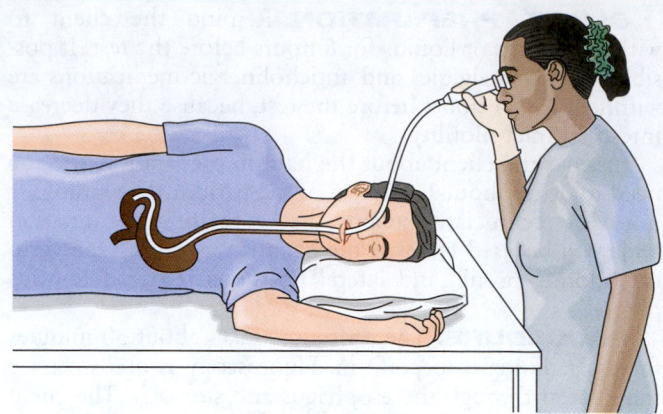

Figure 56-6 ■ Esophagogastroduodenoscopy allows visualization of the esophagus, the stomach, and the duodenum. If the esophagus is the focus of the examination, the procedure is called esophagoscopy. If the stomach is the focus, the procedure is called gastroscopy.

down on the endoscope and to protect the client's teeth. The physician passes the tube through the mouth and into the esophagus (Figure 56-6). The procedure takes about 20 to 30 minutes.

After the test, vital signs are checked frequently (usually every 30 minutes) until the sedation wears off. The siderails of the bed are raised during this time. The client remains NPO until the gag reflex returns (usually in 1 to 2 hours). *Do not offer fluids or food by mouth until the gag reflex is intact to prevent aspiration!* Monitor for signs of perforation, such as pain, bleeding, or fever. The client is instructed not to drive for 12 hours following the procedure. He or she is informed that a hoarse voice or sore throat may persist for several days following the test. Throat lozenges can be used to relieve throat discomfort.

Endoscopic Retrograde Cholangiopancreatography

Endoscopic retrograde cholangiopancreatography (ERCP) includes visual and radiographic examination of the liver, gallbladder, bile ducts, and pancreas to identify the cause and location of obstruction. After the cannula is inserted into the common bile duct, a radiopaque dye is inserted, followed by several x-ray images. The physician may perform a **papillotomy**, a small incision in the sphincter around the ampulla of Vater, to remove gallstones.

The client is prepared in the same manner as for an EGD, including being NPO for 6 to 8 hours before the test. The client will require IV access for the administration of sedation. Ask about prior exposure to x-ray dye and any sensitivities or allergies. If the client has dentures, they are removed. It is important to evaluate the strength of the gag reflex before giving the anesthetic spray, so that you can adequately assess the return of the client's gag reflex following the procedure.

The endoscopic portion of an ERCP is similar to that of an EGD, except that the endoscope is advanced farther, to the duodenum and into the biliary tract. Once the cannula is in the common duct, contrast medium is injected, and x-rays are taken to evaluate the biliary tract. A tilt table assists in distributing the contrast medium to all branches of the biliary tree. The client is placed in a left lateral position for the cannulization of the common bile duct; once the cannula is placed, the client is placed in a prone position. Following examination of the biliary tree, the cannula is directed into the pancreatic duct for examination. The ERCP lasts from 30 minutes to 2 hours.

After the test, assess vital signs frequently, usually every 15 minutes, until the client is stable. Check to ensure that the gag reflex has returned before offering fluids or food. Monitor the client for several postprocedure complications, including cholangitis, perforation, sepsis, and pancreatitis. The client will complain of pain if any of these complications occur. These problems do not occur immediately after the procedure but may take several hours to 2 days to develop. Colicky abdominal pain can occur secondary to the air instilled during the procedure. The client is instructed to report abdominal pain, fever, nausea, or vomiting that fails to resolve. He or she remains on NPO status until the gag reflex returns.

Small Bowel Capsule Enteroscopy

Enteroscopy is the visualization of the small intestine. Capsule endoscopy (M2A) is a small bowel enteroscopy that visualizes the entire small bowel, including the distal ileum. It is used to evaluate and locate the source of GI bleeding. Before the development of the M2A Capsule Endoscope, visualization of the small intestine was inadequate, and physicians relied primarily on barium x-rays for diagnosing disorders of the small intestine (Yu, 2002).

Prepare the client by explaining the procedure, the purpose, and what to expect during the testing. The client must fast (water only) for 8 to 10 hours before the test and be NPO for the first 2 hours of the testing.

At the time of the procedure the client's abdomen is marked for the location of the sensors, and the eight-lead sensors (Sensor Array) are applied. The client wears an abdominal belt that houses a recorder (DataRecorder) to capture the transmitted images. After the capsule is taken with a glass of water, the client may return to normal activity for the remainder of the study. The client can resume a normal diet 4 hours after capsule ingestion. At the conclusion of the procedure, the client returns to the facility with the capsule equipment for downloading to a central computer. The procedure lasts about 8 hours (Yu, 2002).

Because the M2A Capsule Endoscope is a single-use device that is propelled through the GI tract by peristalsis and excreted naturally, explain to the client the capsule will be excreted in the stool. No other follow-up is necessary.

Colonoscopy

Colonoscopy is an endoscopic examination of the entire large bowel. The physician may also obtain tissue biopsy specimens or remove polyps through the colonoscope. A colonoscopy is also used to evaluate the cause of chronic diarrhea or locate the source of GI bleeding. An alternative to this invasive procedure is the **virtual colonoscopy**, which is not invasive and uses a scanner to view the colon.

CLIENT PREPARATION. The client should have a liquid diet for 12 to 24 hours before a colonoscopy and is usually NPO 6 to 8 hours before the procedure.

An oral liquid preparation for cleaning the bowel (e.g., polyethylene glycol electrolyte solution [GoLYTELY] or

---

CHART 56-5

BEST PRACTICE for
Care of the Client After a Colonoscopy

- Do not allow the client to take anything by mouth until sedation wears off and the client is alert.
- Take vital signs every 15 to 30 minutes until the client is alert.
- Keep the siderails up until the client is alert.
- Assess for rectal bleeding or blood clots.
- Remind the client that fullness and mild abdominal cramping are expected for several hours.
- Assess for manifestations of bowel perforation, including *severe* abdominal pain and guarding. Fever may occur later.
- Assess for manifestations of hypovolemic shock, including dizziness, light-headedness, decreased blood pressure, tachycardia, pallor, and altered mental status (may be the first sign).
- If the procedure is performed in an ambulatory care setting, arrange for another person to drive the client home.

---

sodium phosphate [Phospho-Soda]) is given to the client the evening before the examination and may be repeated the morning of the study. The solutions should be chilled to make them more palatable. Instruct the client to drink the preparation quickly. These solutions produce a watery diarrhea that begins in about 1 hour. The bowel clears in 4 to 5 hours. In some cases, the client may require laxatives, suppositories (e.g., bisacodyl [Dulcolax]), or one or more cleansing enemas. IV access is necessary for the administration of conscious sedation. A bowel preparation is needed for both the endoscopic procedure and the virtual colonoscopy.

PROCEDURE. The physician prescribes medication to aid in relaxation, usually midazolam hydrochloride (Versed) and/or an opiate. Initially, the client is placed on the left side with the knees drawn up while the endoscope is passed into the rectum to the cecum. Air may be instilled for better visualization. The entire procedure lasts about 30 to 60 minutes. Atropine sulfate is kept available in case of bradycardia resulting from vasovagal response.

FOLLOW-UP CARE. Check vital signs every 15 minutes until the client is stable. Siderails are kept up until the client is fully alert. Observe for signs of perforation (causes severe pain) and hemorrhage. Instruct the client that a feeling of fullness, cramping, and passage of flatus are expected for several hours after the test. If a polypectomy or tissue biopsy was performed, there may be a small amount of blood in the first stool after the colonoscopy. However, excessive bleeding should be reported immediately to the health care provider (Chart 56-5). If the procedure was performed in an ambulatory care setting, the client will need another person to provide transportation home. The client should avoid driving for 8 to 12 hours after the procedure because of the effects of sedation.

If a polyp is detected during a virtual colonoscopy, the client must have an endoscopic procedure at a later time to have it removed. Therefore the advantage of the invasive method is that both diagnostic testing and minor surgical procedures can be done at the same time.

Proctosigmoidoscopy

Proctosigmoidoscopy is an endoscopic examination of the rectum and sigmoid colon using a flexible or rigid scope. The purpose of this test is to screen for colon cancer, investigate the source of GI bleeding, or diagnose or monitor inflammatory bowel disease. If proctosigmoidoscopy is used as an alternative to colonoscopy for colorectal cancer screening, it is recommended that screening begin at 50 years of age.

The client should have a liquid diet for at least 24 hours before a sigmoidoscopy; a cleansing enema or sodium biphosphate (Fleet's) enema is usually given the morning of the procedure. A laxative may also be prescribed the evening before the test.

For a proctosigmoidoscopy, the client is placed on the left side in the knee-chest position or on a special table in the proctoscopic position. No sedation is required. The endoscope is lubricated and inserted into the anus to the required depth for visualization. Tissue biopsy may be performed during this procedure. The examination usually lasts about 30 minutes.

The client is informed that mild gas pain and flatulence may be experienced from air instilled into the rectum during the examination. If a biopsy was obtained, a small amount of bleeding may be observed. Instruct the client that excessive bleeding should be reported immediately to the health care provider.

? Critical Thinking Challenge

In the endoscopy clinic today, you are assigned to a middle-aged man who is having his first colonoscopy. He tells you that his aunt died of colon cancer 5 years ago and he is very worried about the procedure. The client also mentions that he's not sure his wife will be able to leave work to pick him up after the test.

1. How should you respond to his comments about his worries and his aunt's death?
2. What would you tell him about what he can expect during the procedure?
3. What discharge instructions will he need after the procedure is finished? When can you discharge him? Will he be able to drive home alone? Why or why not?

evolve For suggested answer guidelines, go to http://evolve.elsevier.com/Iggy/.

Gastric Analysis

Gastric analysis measures the hydrochloric acid and pepsin content for evaluation of aggressive gastric and duodenal disorders (e.g., Zollinger-Ellison syndrome). There are two tests in gastric analysis: basal gastric secretion and gastric acid stimulation. Basal gastric secretion measures the secretion of hydrochloric acid between meals. If only small amounts of secretion are collected, a follow-up gastric stimulation test is given.

The client is NPO for at least 12 hours before the test. Alcohol, tobacco, and medications that may affect gastric secretion are avoided for 24 hours before the study. A nasogastric (NG) tube is inserted and gastric residual contents are aspirated and discarded.

The NG tube is attached to suctioning equipment for collecting the contents at 15-minute intervals for 1 hour. Samples are collected and labeled with basal acid output (BAO), time, and volume of each specimen.

For the gastric acid stimulation test, the NG tube is left in place, and a drug that stimulates gastric acid secretion (e.g., pentagastrin or betazole dihydrochloride [Histalog]) is

given subcutaneously. Fifteen minutes after injection of the drug, specimens are again collected at 15-minute intervals for 1 hour. Samples are collected and labeled with maximal acid output (MAO), time, and volume of each specimen.

Depressed levels of gastric secretion suggest the presence of gastric carcinoma. Increased levels of gastric secretion indicate Zollinger-Ellison syndrome and duodenal ulcers (see Chapter 59).

After the test is completed, the NG tube is removed and the client can resume normal eating patterns. No other follow-up is necessary.

Ultrasonography

Ultrasonography is a technique in which high-frequency, inaudible vibratory sound waves are passed through the body via a transducer; the echoes of the sound waves created are then recorded. The echoes are converted into images and photographed for analysis. Ultrasound testing is commonly used to image soft tissues, such as the liver, the spleen, the pancreas, the gallbladder, and the biliary system. The advantages of ultrasonography are that it is painless, noninvasive, and requires no radiation.

The client may be fasting depending on the abdominal organs to be examined. Inform the client that it will be necessary to lie still during the study. He or she is instructed to drink 1 to 2 L of fluid just before the test, because a full bladder is necessary for accurate visualization.

The client is placed in a prone or supine position. The technician applies insulating gel to the end of the transducer and on the area of the abdomen under study. This gel allows airtight contact of the transducer with the skin. The technician moves the transducer back and forth over the skin until the desired images are obtained. The study takes about 15 to 30 minutes. No follow-up care is necessary after ultrasonography.

Endoscopic Ultrasonography

Endoscopic ultrasonography (EUS) provides images of the gastrointestinal (GI) wall and high-resolution images of the digestive organs. The ultrasonography is performed through the endoscope. This procedure is useful in diagnosing the presence of lymph node tumors, mucosal tumors, and tumors of the pancreas, stomach, and rectum. The client preparation and follow-up care are similar to the preparation and follow-up care for both endoscopy and ultrasonography.

Liver-Spleen Scan

A liver-spleen scan uses IV injection of a radioactive material that is taken up primarily by the liver and secondarily by the spleen. The scan evaluates the liver and the spleen for tumors or abscesses, organ size and location, and vascularity. This scan is useful in evaluating hepatocellular disease.

Instruct the client about the need to lie still during the scanning. The client is assured that the colloid injection has only small amounts of radioactivity and is not dangerous. Ask female clients of childbearing age if they may be pregnant or are currently breastfeeding. The radionuclide can be found in breast milk, and radiation from x-rays should be avoided in pregnancy.

The technician or the physician gives the radioactive injection through an IV line, and a wait of about 15 minutes is necessary for uptake. The client is placed in many different positions while the scanning takes place. No follow-up care is necessary after a liver scan.

The client should be instructed that the radionuclide is eliminated from the body through the urine in 24 hours. Careful handwashing following toileting will decrease the exposure to any radiation present in the urine.

GET READY for the NCLEX Examination!

KEY POINTS

Safe Effective Care Environment

- Check for the return of the gag reflex after an upper endoscopic procedure before offering fluids or food; aspiration may occur if the gag reflex is not intact.
- Monitor vital signs carefully for the client having any endoscopic procedure and conscious sedation.
- Monitor clients having a percutaneous transhepatic cholangiogram (PTC) for bleeding, the most common and life-threatening complication.

Health Promotion and Maintenance

- Teach clients to limit caffeine and alcohol in their diets to reduce risk of gastrointestinal health problems.
- If the client is having an endoscopic procedure on an ambulatory basis, remind him or her to have someone available to drive him or her home due to the effects of conscious sedation.
- Teach clients having invasive colon diagnostic procedures to follow instructions carefully for the bowel preparation before testing; the bowel must be clear to allow visualization of the colon.
- Instruct the client to drink plenty of fluids and take a laxative as prescribed to eliminate barium if used during diagnostic testing.
- Teach clients having a PTC to report pain following the procedure, which could indicate bleeding.

Psychosocial Integrity

- Because most clients do not openly express their elimination patterns and complaints, provide support and education.
- Remember that problems of digestion, nutrition, and elimination can markedly affect lifestyle.

Physiological Integrity

- Assess and report any complications of GI testing to the health care provider.
- Review laboratory results, report abnormal findings to the health care provider.

ADDITIONAL STUDY RESOURCES

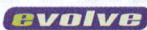 Go to your Student CD-ROM for Review Questions for the NCLEX Examination.

Go to http://evolve.elsevier.com/Iggy/ for **evolve** Integrated Management of Care Questions for the NCLEX Examination.

SELECTED BIBLIOGRAPHY

Avunduk, C. (2002). *Manual of gastroenterology: Diagnosis and therapy* (3rd ed.). Philadelphia: Lippincott Williams & Wilkins.

Carpenito, L.J. (2001). *Nursing diagnosis: Application to clinical practice* (9th ed.). Philadelphia: Lippincott Williams & Wilkins.

Donley, K.M. (2003). Surfing an acidic wave: pH monitoring technologies swim in sea of innovation. *EndoNurse, 3*(1), 22-24.

Dykes, C.M. (2001). Virtual colonoscopy: A new approach for colorectal cancer screening. *Gastroenterology Nursing, 24*(1), 5-11.

Given Imaging. (2002). M2A Capsule Endoscopy: Given diagnostic system. (Available from Given Imaging, Inc., Oakbrook Technology Center, 5555 Oakbrook Parkway, # 355, Norcross, GA 30093.

Gordon, M. (2002). *Manual of nursing diagnosis* (10th ed.). St. Louis: Mosby.

Huether, S.E. (2002). Structure and function of the digestive system. In K.L. McCance & S.E. Huether (Eds.), *Pathophysiology: The biologic basis for disease in adults & children* (4th ed., pp. 1231-1260). St. Louis: Mosby.

Jarvis, C. (2004). *Physical examination and health assessment* (4th ed.). Philadelphia: W. B. Saunders.

National Institutes of Health. (2000). National digestive disease information clearinghouse publications. Available at http://www.nih.gov.

Pagana, K.D. & Pagana, T.J. (2002). *Mosby's manual of diagnostic and laboratory tests* (2nd ed.). St. Louis: Mosby.

Price, A.S. (2003). Primary and secondary prevention of colorectal cancer. *Gastroenterology Nursing, 26*(2), 73-81.

Shier, D., Butler, J., & Lewis, R. (2003). Digestive system. In *Hole's human anatomy and physiology* (10th ed., pp. 655-702). Boston: McGraw-Hill.

Skidmore-Roth, L. (2004). *Mosby's nursing drug reference*. St. Louis: Mosby.

Society of Gastroenterology Nurses and Associates. (2004). *Gastroenterology nursing: A core curriculum* (3rd ed.). St. Louis: Mosby.

Whitney, E.N., et al. (2000). Nutrition assessment: History, drug history, and physical examination. In *Nutrition for health and health care* (2nd ed., pp. 299-319). St. Paul, MN: West.

Yu, M. (2002). M2A Capsule Endoscopy: A breakthrough diagnostic toll for small intestine imaging. *Gastroenterology Nursing, 25*(1), 24-27.

Interventions for Clients with Oral Cavity Problems

KARRIE K. DIETZEN

Oral cavity disorders can severely impact speech, nutrition, body image, and overall quality of life. Although there are numerous oral health problems, this chapter discusses the most common disorders. Nurses play an important role in maintaining and restoring oral cavity health in their clients through nursing interventions and client education. Chart 57-1 lists ways for clients to maintain a healthy oral cavity.

STOMATITIS

PATHOPHYSIOLOGY

Stomatitis is characterized by painful single or multiple ulcerations of the oral mucosa that appear as inflammation and denudation of the oral mucosa, impairing the protective lining of the mouth. These ulcerations are commonly referred to as canker sores. The ulceration causes pain, and open areas predispose the individual to bleeding and infection. Mild erythema (redness) may respond to topical treatments, whereas extensive stomatitis may require treatment with opioid analgesics. Stomatitis is classified according to the cause of the inflammation. *Primary stomatitis* includes aphthous (noninfectious) stomatitis, herpes simplex stoma-

titis, and traumatic ulcers. *Secondary stomatitis* generally results from infection by opportunistic viruses, fungi, or bacteria in clients who are immunocompromised.

A common type of secondary stomatitis is caused by *Candida albicans.* **Candidiasis,** also called moniliasis, is a fungal infection resulting from an overgrowth of normal flora. In most cases, antibiotic therapy destroys the normal flora that usually prevents fungal infections; thus candidiasis can occur in clients receiving long-term antibiotic therapy. Candidiasis of the oral cavity is also common in clients undergoing immunosuppressive therapy (chemotherapy, radiation, steroid therapy, or antirejection medication). In addition, the mouth is susceptible to the effects of human immunodeficiency virus (HIV) disease; therefore HIV-positive individuals commonly present with candidiasis.

CONSIDERATIONS FOR OLDER ADULTS

Older adults are especially at high risk for candidiasis because aging causes a decrease in immune function. The risk increases for clients who are diabetic, malnourished, or under emotional stress. Older adults who wear dentures may use soft denture liners that provide comfort but can also be colonized by *C. albicans,* contributing to denture stomatitis.

CHART 57-1

CLIENT EDUCATION GUIDE
Maintaining a Healthy Oral Cavity

- Perform a self-examination of your mouth every month; report any unusual finding.
- Be sure to eat a balanced diet.
- Brush and floss your teeth every day. Set a routine and keep to it.
- Manage your stress as much as possible; learn how to maintain your emotional health.
- Avoid contact with agents that may cause inflammation of the mouth, such as mouthwashes that contain alcohol.
- If possible, avoid medications that may cause inflammation of the mouth or reduce the flow of saliva.
- Be aware of any changes in the occlusion of your teeth, mouth pain, or swelling; seek medical attention promptly.
- See your dentist regularly: have problems attended to promptly.
- If you wear dentures, make sure they are in good repair and fit properly.

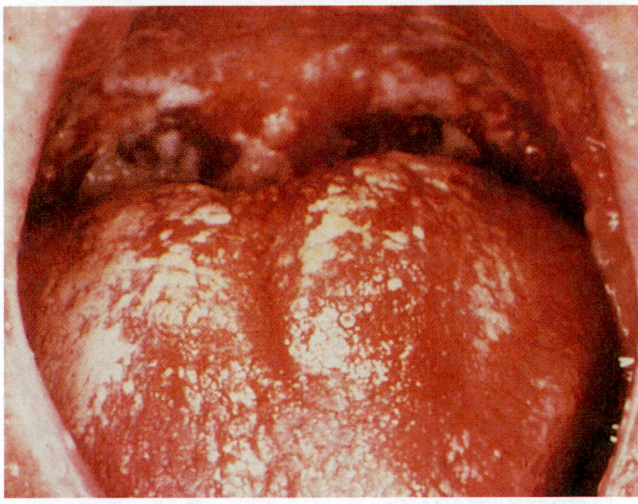

Figure 57-1 ■ Oral candidiasis. (From Radford, J., & Thatcher, N. [1988]. The toxicity of cancer chemotherapy in adults. Cancer Care, 5, 4-7.)

Etiology and Genetic Risk

Stomatitis can result from infection, allergy, vitamin deficiency, systemic disease, irritants (e.g., tobacco and alcohol), chemotherapy, or radiation. Infectious agents, such as bacteria and viruses, may have a role in the development of recurrent stomatitis. Although viruses have not been successfully cultured from aphthous lesions, recurrent lesions have been associated with latent zoster or cytomegalovirus (CMV).

Certain foods may trigger allergic responses that result in the formation of aphthous ulcers, although this remains controversial. Foods such as coffee, potatoes, cheese, nuts, citrus fruits, and gluten may be precipitating factors. In some cases, strict elimination diets have resulted in the improvement of ulcers. Deficiencies in complex B vitamins, folate, zinc, and iron associated with malnutrition can contribute to the formation of recurrent stomatitis. Recurrent aphthous ulcers (RAU) are reported to run in families, but may be environmental rather than genetic (Rini & Bloom, 2002).

Systemic diseases such as HIV infection, chronic renal failure, and inflammatory bowel disease can also predispose a person to stomatitis. Treatment of cancer with antineoplastic agents or radiation can predispose an individual to the development of painful stomatitis or mucositis. The severity of stomatitis is related to the type and dose of therapy as well as to client-related factors, such as pretreatment oral health. (See Chapter 28 for nursing care of the client undergoing radiation and chemotherapy.)

Incidence/Prevalence

Aphthous stomatitis is the most common oral lesion. Recurrent aphthous lesions have been found to affect at least 30% of the population (Scully & Shotts, 2001). Data for other types of stomatitis are not readily available.

WOMEN'S HEALTH CONSIDERATIONS

A hormonal influence has been suggested in relation to women and aphthous stomatitis. Women generally have a higher prevalence of the disorder, with an increased incidence of oral ulceration during the luteal phase of the menstrual cycle. A moderation or absence of lesions during pregnancy has been attributed to increased steroid levels.

◆ COLLABORATIVE MANAGEMENT
◆ Assessment

HISTORY

When performing an oral assessment, collect information concerning possible etiologic factors, such as recent infections, a history of stomatitis, nutritional compromise, oral hygiene habits, oral trauma, stress, or immunocompromise. A medication history should also be collected, including over-the-counter (OTC) agents and herbals. Document the course of the current outbreak, and ascertain whether episodes of stomatitis are recurrent. Ask the client if the lesions interfere with swallowing or eating.

PHYSICAL ASSESSMENT/CLINICAL MANIFESTATIONS

The symptoms of stomatitis range in severity from a dry, painful mouth to open ulcerations, predisposing the client to infection. Mouth ulcerations can alter nutritional status as a result of difficulty with food ingestion or swallowing. When they are severe, stomatitis and the accompanying edema have the potential to compromise the airway.

Stomatitis lesions appear most commonly on the buccal mucosa, soft palate, oropharyngeal mucosa, and lateral and ventral areas of the tongue. The painful lesions appear as shallow ulcerations covered by a whitish gray pseudomembrane and outer erythematous ring (Jarvis, 2004).

In oral candidiasis, a type of yeast infection, white plaque-like lesions appear on the tongue, palate, pharynx, and buccal mucosa (Figure 57-1). When these patches are wiped away, the underlying surface appears red and sore (Walton, Miller, & Tordecilla, 2001). Clients rarely complain of actual pain but describe the lesions as dry or hot.

While examining the oral cavity, wear nonsterile gloves for protection against infection. Adequate lighting, including a flashlight or penlight, and a tongue blade facilitate the examination. Assess the oral cavity for lesions, coating, cracking, and fissures. Characteristics of the lesions are described in terms of location, size, shape, color, and drainage. Any odors are noted and described.

If lesions are noted along the pharynx, and the client reports dysphagia or pain on swallowing, you should suspect that the lesions might extend down the esophagus. Additional diagnostic testing may be required.

The physical examination should also include examination of the cervical and submandibular lymph nodes for swelling. Any elevation in temperature is noted.

LABORATORY ASSESSMENT

Laboratory tests are usually not needed. However, serum albumin, vitamin B$_{12}$, folate, and iron levels may be obtained if nutritional status appears to be compromised. A complete blood count may reveal the presence of infection, neutropenia, or anemia. Cytologic; routine, viral, or bacterial cultures; and Gram stain testing can assist in distinguishing organisms causing the stomatitis ulcerations.

◆ Interventions

Interventions for stomatitis are aimed toward the promotion of oral health through meticulous oral hygiene and careful food selection.

Oral Hygiene. When providing oral care for your client, use a soft-bristled toothbrush or disposable foam swabs to stimulate gums and clean the oral cavity. Encourage frequent rinsing of the mouth with any of the following: sodium bicarbonate solution, warm saline, or hydrogen peroxide solution. The client should avoid commercial mouthwashes because they have high alcohol content, causing a burning sensation in irritated or ulcerated oral mucosa.

Instruct the client or provide mouth care every 2 hours and twice at night if the stomatitis is not controlled. Frequent gentle mouth care enhances debridement of ulcerated lesions and can prevent superinfections. Frequent oral care also promotes a general feeling of well-being. Chart 57-2 lists measures for special oral care.

Drug Therapy. Medications used include antimicrobials, immune modulators, symptomatic topicals, and complementary and alternative therapies.

Antimicrobial Agents. Antimicrobials, including antibiotics and antifungals, may be necessary for control of infection in the client with stomatitis. Tetracycline syrup (swish/swallow) 250 mg/10 mL four times daily for 10 days may be prescribed, especially for RAU. The client rinses for 2 minutes and swallows the syrup, thus obtaining both topical and systemic therapy. Minocycline swish/swallow and chlorhexidine mouthwashes may also be used.

A regimen of intravenous (IV) acyclovir (Zovirax) is typically prescribed for immunocompromised clients who contract herpes simplex stomatitis. Acyclovir is typically administered to clients with normal renal function at a dose of 5 mg/kg, infused at a constant rate over a 1-hour period, every 8 hours for 7 days. Clients with competent immune systems may be given acyclovir in oral or topical form.

For fungal infections, nystatin (Mycostatin) oral suspension 600,000 units four times daily for 7 to 10 days is the agent most often used. The client swishes and swallows the topical preparation. Ice pop troches (lozenges) of the antifungal preparation allow the medication to slowly dissolve, and the cold provides an analgesic effect.

Anti-Inflammatory Agents and Immune Modulators. Topical triamcinolone in benzocaine (Kenalog in Orabase) and oral dexamethasone elixir used as a swish/

---

expectorate preparation are commonly used for stomatitis, especially recurrent aphthous ulcers (RAU).

Immune modulating agents that may be prescribed include the following:

- Oral levamisole
- Topical amlexanox (Aphthasol)
- Topical granulocyte-macrophage colony-stimulating factor (GM-CSF)
- Thalidomide

The exact mechanism for how these drugs work is not clear. However, they may inhibit release of mediators that contribute to the inflammation seen in clients with RAU (Rini & Bloom, 2002).

Symptomatic Topical Agents. Other agents can be used to minimize pain, such as over-the-counter (OTC) benzocaine anesthetics (e.g., Orabase, Anbesol) and camphor phenol (Campho-Phenique).

Fifteen mL of 2% viscous lidocaine every 3 hours (maximum of 8 doses per day) can be used as a gargle or mouthwash.

Critical Thinking Challenge

You are a nurse on a busy medical-surgical nursing unit where you are caring for an older adult with cellulitis and type 2 diabetes mellitus. She was on oral antibiotics at home before admission yesterday and is now receiving IV antibiotics. The client's daughter states that her mother is not eating well and complains that her mouth is burning and sore. When you check her oral cavity, you note white patches that can be partially scraped away.

1. What problem do you think this client has and why?
2. What risk factors does she have for her oral cavity problem?
3. What treatment will she most likely receive as a result of her problem?
4. How will you describe the special oral care this client needs to your nursing assistant?

evolve For suggested answer guidelines, go to http://evolve.elsevier.com/Iggy/.

ORAL TUMORS

Oral cavity tumors can be benign, premalignant, or malignant. Whether benign or malignant, tumors of the oral cavity impact many daily functions. Activities such as swallowing, chewing, and speaking can be affected. Pain accompanying the tumor can also impose limitations on daily activities and self-care. Oral cavity tumors affect body image, especially if treatment involves removal of the tongue or part of the mandible, or requires a tracheostomy.

Premalignant Lesions

Leukoplakia

PATHOPHYSIOLOGY

Leukoplakia presents as slowly developing changes in the oral mucous membranes that are characterized by thickened, white, firmly attached patches. These patches appear slightly raised and sharply circumscribed. Ninety percent of leukoplakial lesions are benign; however, about 7% of lesions become malignant after a mean of 8 years (Palkhivala, 2003). Although leukoplakia can be found anywhere on the oral mucosa, lesions on the lips or tongue are more likely to progress to malignancy.

Etiology

Leukoplakia results from mechanical factors that cause long-term oral mucous membrane irritation, such as poorly fitting dentures, chronic cheek nibbling, or broken or poorly repaired teeth. In addition, oral hairy leukoplakia can be found in clients with HIV infection. The use of tobacco products has also been implicated in the development of leukoplakia, which is sometimes referred to as "smoker's patch." Oral leukoplakia can be confused with oral candidal infection. However, unlike candidal infection, leukoplakia cannot be removed by scraping.

Incidence/Prevalence

Leukoplakia is the most common oral lesion among adults. Oral hairy leukoplakia is an early manifestation of HIV infection and is highly correlated with progression from HIV infection to acquired immunodeficiency syndrome (AIDS). Leukoplakia not associated with HIV infection is more often seen in people over 40 years of age. Men have twice the incidence of leukoplakia that women have, but this ratio is changing because increasing numbers of women are smoking.

Erythroplakia

Erythroplakia presents as a red, velvety mucosal lesion on the surface of the oral mucosa. There is a higher degree of malignant transformation in erythroplakia than in leukoplakia. As such, these lesions should be regarded with suspicion and analyzed by biopsy. Erythroplakia is most commonly found on the floor of the mouth, tongue, palate, and mandibular mucosa, and it can be difficult to distinguish from inflammatory or immune reactions.

Malignant Tumors

Squamous Cell Carcinoma

PATHOPHYSIOLOGY

More than 90% of oral cancers are squamous cell carcinomas that begin on the surface of the epithelium. Over a period of many years, premalignant (or dysplastic) changes begin. Cells begin to vary in size and shape; alterations in the thickness of the lining of the epithelium develop, resulting in atrophy. These tumors usually grow slowly, and the lesions may be large before the onset of symptoms unless ulceration is present. Mucosal erythroplasia is the earliest sign of oral carcinoma. Oral lesions that appear as red, raised, eroded areas are suspicious for carcinoma.

The American Joint Committee on Cancer has devised the TNM (tumor, node, metastasis) classification system for tumors of the lip and oral cavity. Each lesion is defined by the following:

T—the size of the tumor or degree of penetration
N—the presence, size, number, and location of cervical lymph nodes involved
M—the presence of distant metastasis (spread)

Etiology

Squamous cell carcinoma is the most common oral malignancy. It can be found on the lips, tongue, buccal mucosa, and oropharynx. The major risk factors in the development of oral cancers are increasing age, tobacco use, and alcohol ingestion. Ninety-five percent of all oral cancers occur in people over 40 years of age. Tobacco use in any form (e.g., smoking or chewing tobacco) can increase the risk of cancer. Alcohol ingestion can potentiate the carcinogenic effects of tobacco products.

An increased rate of oral carcinoma is found in individuals with certain occupations, such as textile workers, plumbers, and coal and metal workers. Additional factors, such as sun exposure, poor dietary habits, poor oral hygiene, and infection with the human papillomavirus (HPV) may also contribute to oral cancer (Neville & Day, 2002).

Incidence/Prevalence

Carcinomas of the oral cavity account for about 3% of all cancers in men and 2% of all cancers in women in the United States. Nearly 30,000 new cases are diagnosed each year, with almost 8000 deaths, or 2% of all cancer deaths (American Cancer Society, 2004; Weinberg & Estefan, 2002). Most cancers occur in middle-aged and older individuals, although in recent years more younger adults have been affected, most likely as a result of sun exposure. Oral and oropharyngeal cancers are more common in black individuals than in white individuals, but the reason for this disparity is not known.

Basal Cell Carcinoma

Basal cell carcinoma of the oral cavity occurs primarily on the lips. The lesion is asymptomatic and resembles a raised scab. With time, the lesion evolves into a characteristic ulcer with a raised pearly border. Basal cell carcinomas do not metastasize but can aggressively involve the skin of the face. The major etiologic factor in basal cell carcinoma is exposure to sunlight.

Basal cell carcinoma occurs as a result of the failure of basal cells to mature into keratinocytes. It is the second most common type of oral cancer, but it is much less common than squamous cell carcinoma.

Kaposi's Sarcoma

Kaposi's sarcoma is a malignant lesion that arises in blood vessels. Kaposi's sarcoma is usually painless and appears as a raised purple nodule or plaque. In the mouth the hard palate is the most common site of Kaposi's sarcoma, but it can also be found on the gums, tongue, or tonsils. It is most often associated with AIDS. (See Chapter 25 for a complete discussion of Kaposi's sarcoma.)

Health Promotion/Illness Prevention

In the past decade, dentists and other physicians have begun systematically screening their clients for oral cancer. Oral examination has become a part of the routine dental examination. Individuals should visit a dentist at least once per year for professional dental hygiene and oral examination.

In addition to medical screening, prevention strategies for oral cancer include minimizing sun exposure, including tanning beds, tobacco cessation, and decreasing alcohol intake. Teach clients to follow the guidelines in Chart 57-1 to maintain oral health.

◆ COLLABORATIVE MANAGEMENT
◆ Assessment

HISTORY

A priority for nurses in the prevention and detection of oral cancers is the identification of high-risk groups. Individuals at high risk for developing oral cancer tend to use large amounts of alcohol and tobacco and are over 40 years of age. It is important to conduct a functional assessment. Ask about occupation and exposure to known oral carcinogens or irritants, such as sunlight or other source of ultraviolet radiation. A family history of cancer and a history of previous oral cancer alert health care providers to be especially observant for signs of cancer.

Begin by assessing the client's routine oral hygiene regimen and use of dentures or oral appliances, which might add to discomfort or mechanically irritate the mucosa. Ask the client about oral bleeding, which might indicate an ulcerative lesion. Determine the status of the client's past and current appetite and nutritional state, including difficulty with chewing or swallowing. A continuing trend of weight loss may be related to metastasis, heavy alcohol intake, difficulty in eating or chewing, or an underlying disorder.

PHYSICAL ASSESSMENT/CLINICAL MANIFESTATIONS

Common signs and symptoms of oral carcinoma include unusual lumps or thickening of the buccal mucosa or red or white patches appearing on the gums, tongue, or oral mucous membranes. Cancers of the lip are strongly associated with chronic exposure to the sun and often present as a sore that fails to heal. Soreness, pain, or a burning sensation may also be present. In later stages, the client may experience difficulty chewing or swallowing. Advanced cancers of the tongue can cause pain that radiates to the ear. Cervical lymph nodes may become enlarged, hardened, and fixed secondary to metastatic invasion.

An examination of the oral cavity requires adequate lighting for proper visualization. Thoroughly inspect the oral cavity for any lesions, evidence of pain, or restriction of movement. Using a tongue blade, visually examine all areas of the oral cavity. Carefully note any alteration in speech attributable to tongue restriction. Following inspection, the advanced practice nurse uses bimanual palpation of any vis-

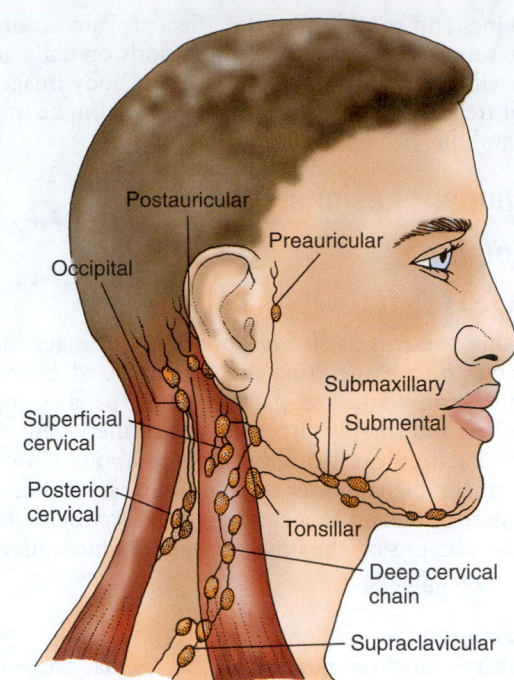

Figure 57-2 ■ The lymph nodes of the cervical region.

ible nodules to determine size and fixation. The cervical lymph nodes should also be palpated (Figure 57-2).

PSYCHOSOCIAL ASSESSMENT

The functioning and appearance of the oral cavity are strongly linked with body image and quality of life. Therefore, it is important to assess the impact of oral lesions on the client's self-concept. In addition, assess the client for any educational or cultural needs regarding instruction or therapy. Evaluate the client's support system and past mechanisms of coping.

RADIOGRAPHIC ASSESSMENT

The purpose of radiologic diagnostic tests for cancer of the oral cavity is to assess the extent and spread of the tumor. Computed tomography (CT) scans are helpful in determining the extent of the tumor and lymphatic or bone involvement.

OTHER DIAGNOSTIC ASSESSMENTS

Biopsy is the definitive method for diagnosis of oral cancer. Therefore the physician obtains a needle biopsy specimen of the oral tissue to assess for malignant or premalignant changes. Incisional biopsies may also be performed. An intraoral biopsy can be done with the client under local anesthesia. In very small lesions, an excisional biopsy can permit complete tumor removal. Magnetic resonance imaging (MRI) is useful in detecting perineural involvement and in evaluating thickness in cancers of the tongue. Both CT and MRI can be used to determine metastatic spread to the liver or lungs if further staging of the disease is warranted.

An aqueous solution of toluidine blue 1% can be applied to oral lesions to determine if they are malignant. This preparation stains malignant lesions, leaving normal tissue unaffected. However, a lesion that is the result of an inflammatory process may also pick up the stain, leading to a false-positive result. Although a biopsy is still needed to confirm a cancer diagnosis, toluidine blue may be useful for screening high-risk individuals.

◆Analysis

COMMON NURSING DIAGNOSES AND COLLABORATIVE PROBLEMS

The following are priority nursing diagnoses for clients with malignant tumors of the oral cavity:

1. Risk for Ineffective Airway Clearance related to obstructed airway by the tumor, edema, or secretions
2. Impaired Oral Mucous Membrane related to pathologic conditions from the tumor

ADDITIONAL NURSING DIAGNOSES AND COLLABORATIVE PROBLEMS

In addition to the common nursing diagnoses, clients with tumors of the oral cavity may have one or more of the following:

- Impaired Verbal Communication related to physical barrier or anatomic defect
- Disturbed Body Image related to surgery
- Acute Pain related to physical injury
- Risk for Infection related to invasive procedures
- Impaired Swallowing related to oral cavity or oropharyngeal abnormalities
- Imbalanced Nutrition: Less Than Body Requirements related to inability to ingest food
- Potential for Metastasis

◆Planning and Implementation

RISK FOR INEFFECTIVE AIRWAY CLEARANCE

NOC **PLANNING: EXPECTED OUTCOMES.** The client with a malignant tumor of the oral cavity is expected to have open, clear tracheobronchial passages for air exchange. Indicators include that the client will have noncompromised:

- Ease of breathing
- Respiratory rate
- Respiratory rhythm
- Ability to move sputum out of airway

INTERVENTIONS. Extensive tumor involvement and tenacious secretions can inhibit airway patency. Nursing measures for maintaining airway patency is a primary focus. Assessment should be centered on the client's dyspnea, inability to cough effectively, or inability to swallow.

NONSURGICAL MANAGEMENT. Assess for difficulty breathing and decreased air exchange and dysphagia. Institute measures to increase air exchange, remove secretions, and prevent aspiration (Chart 57-3).

NIC **Airway Management.** Assess for dyspnea resulting from the obstructive presence of the tumor or from excessive secretions. Assess the quality, rate, and depth of respirations, and auscultate the lungs for decreased or absent ventilation or for the presence of adventitious sounds. If oral secretions are excessive or thick, aid the client in expectorating secretions. To increase air exchange, place the client in a semi-Fowler's or high Fowler's position to maximize ventilation potential. Secretions can be mobilized by encouraging fluids to help liquefy secretions, by chest physiotherapy, and by measures to encourage effective coughing.

CHART 57-3

NIC **INTERVENTION ACTIVITIES for**
The Client with Oral Cancer

Airway Management: *Facilitation of patency of air passages*
- Position client to maximize ventilation potential.
- Remove secretions by encouraging coughing or by suctioning.
- Instruct how to cough effectively.
- Auscultate breath sounds, noting areas of decreased or absent ventilation and presence of adventitious sounds.
- Administer humidified air or oxygen, as appropriate.
- Position to alleviate dyspnea.
- Monitor respiratory and oxygenation status, as appropriate.

Cough Enhancement: *Promotion of deep inhalation by the client with subsequent generation of high intrathoracic pressures and compression of underlying lung parenchyma for the forceful expulsion of air*
- Assist client to a sitting position with the head slightly flexed, shoulders relaxed, and knees flexed.
- Encourage client to take several deep breaths.
- Encourage client to take a deep breath, hold it for 2 seconds, and cough two or three times in succession.
- Instruct client to inhale deeply, bend forward slightly, and perform three or four huffs (against an open glottis).
- Instruct client to inhale deeply several times, to exhale slowly, and to cough at the end of exhalation.
- Instruct client to follow coughing with several maximal inhalation breaths.
- Promote systemic fluid hydration, as appropriate.

Aspiration Precautions: *Prevention or minimization of risk factors in the client at risk for aspiration*
- Monitor level of consciousness, cough reflex, gag reflex, and swallowing ability.
- Monitor pulmonary status.
- Maintain an airway.
- Position upright 90 degrees or as far as possible.
- Feed in small amounts.
- Avoid liquids or use thickening agent.
- Offer foods or liquids that can be formed into a bolus before swallowing.
- Cut food into small pieces.
- Request medication in elixir form.
- Break or crush pills before administration.
- Keep head of bed elevated 30 to 45 minutes after eating.

NIC intervention activities selected from Dochterman, J.M., & Bulechek, G.M. (Eds.) (2004). *Nursing interventions classification (NIC)* (4th ed.). St. Louis: Mosby. No part of this work is to be altered without prior written permission from the Publisher.

If oral secretions remain problematic, oral suction equipment with a dental tip or a tonsil tip (Yankauer catheter) can be used.

If edema is associated with oral cavity lesions, the client may receive steroids for reducing inflammation. Antibiotics may be prescribed if infection is present because infection can increase inflammation and edema. A cool mist supplied by a face tent may assist with oxygen transport and control of edema.

NIC **Cough Enhancement.** Measures that promote deep inhalation generate high intrathoracic pressure, which assists the client in producing an effective cough to mobilize secretions. Assist the client to a sitting position with the head slightly flexed and the knees flexed. Then instruct the client to take several deep breaths, hold the breath for 2 seconds, and then cough two to three times in succession. He or she is instructed to follow coughing with several maximal inhalation breaths. The client can also be instructed to enhance coughing by inhaling deeply several times and coughing at the end of exhalation.

NIC Aspiration Precautions. Aspiration precautions prevent or minimize the risk factors associated with aspiration. The client's level of consciousness, gag reflex, and ability to swallow are assessed. To prevent aspiration, place the client sitting upright at 90 degrees (high Fowler's position). As a precaution, suction equipment should be kept nearby. Clients at risk of aspiration should be fed in small amounts. Thickened liquids can be used as an aid to prevent aspiration.

SURGICAL MANAGEMENT. The client with an oral lesion may require a tracheostomy. This may be due to the extent of surgical excision required to remove the tumor, or it may be due to excessive edema. A tracheostomy re-establishes a patent airway and can be performed by the physician with the client under local or general anesthesia. The tracheostomy tube is usually left in place until edema resolves and the airway is patent. If the tumor is the major cause of the oral airway blockage, however, the tracheostomy may be maintained through the perioperative period until oral healing begins. In some cases, it may be permanent. After postoperative edema resolves, the client is **decannulated** (i.e., the tracheostomy tube is removed). (Refer to Chapter 31 for nursing care of the client with a tracheostomy.)

IMPAIRED ORAL MUCOUS MEMBRANE

NOC PLANNING: EXPECTED OUTCOMES. The client with a malignant tumor of the oral cavity is expected to maintain or re-establish structural intactness and normal physiologic function of mucous membranes. Indicators include that the client will not have the following:

- Mucous membrane lesions
- Induration
- Erythema

INTERVENTIONS. Both the presence of tumors of the oral cavity and the effects of treatment of oral tumors pose threats to the integrity of the oral mucosa. Oral cavity lesions can be treated by surgical excision, by nonsurgical treatments such as radiation or chemotherapy, or by a combination of treatments (referred to as multimodal therapy). Multimodal therapy is the treatment option that incurs the most cost. Nursing interventions focus primarily on the restoration and maintenance oral health.

NONSURGICAL MANAGEMENT. The purpose of nonsurgical management is to promote tissue healing and to maintain and promote oral hygiene for the client with oral lesions.

Oral Care. It is important to work with the client to establish an oral hygiene routine. Ideally, oral hygiene is performed every 2 hours for ulcerated lesions, infection, or in the immediate postoperative period. Modifications might be needed because of oral discomfort, bleeding, or edema. Oral care with a soft-bristled toothbrush is preferred. In the event of a fall in the platelet count below 40,000/mm³, the client should be switched to an ultrasoft "chemobrush." The use of "toothettes" or a disposable foam brush is discouraged because these products may not adequately control bacteremia-promoting plaque. Lubricant can be applied to moisten the lips and oral mucosa as needed.

Clients with ulcerative or bleeding lesions should avoid using commercial mouthwashes and lemon-glycerin swabs. Commercial mouthwashes contain alcohol, and lemon-

glycerin swabs are acidic. These substances can cause a burning sensation and contribute to drying of the oral mucous membranes. Encourage frequent rinsing of the mouth with sodium bicarbonate solution, warm saline, or hydrogen peroxide solution (see also Chart 57-2).

Radiation Therapy. Radiation therapy has been used alone as well as in conjunction with surgery and chemotherapy in the treatment of cancer of the oral cavity. The goal of radiation therapy is tumor eradication while preserving function and appearance. There are several ways to apply radiotherapy. In collaboration with the client, the physician chooses the best mode on the basis of the tumor site and staging.

Radiation therapy for oral cancers can be given by external beam or interstitial implantation. External-beam radiation passes through the skin or mucous membrane to the tumor site. Typically, treatments are given as five daily treatments per week over a 6- to 9-week period. Special precautions are taken to minimize the dose of radiation to the brain or spinal cord. Another option is the implantation of radioactive substances (interstitial radiation therapy) either to boost the dosage or to deliver a radiation dose close to the tumor bed. This form of implant therapy can be curative in early stage lesions in the floor of the mouth or anterior tongue or to add an additional boost of radiation to a tumor that received external-beam radiation.

Interstitial radiation is used for smaller lesions that do not infiltrate surrounding tissues. The following can be radioactive materials:

- Seeds, which are permanently implanted into the tissue (usually for tumors unable to be completely excised or in neck nodes)
- Needles or wires, which are removed at the end of therapy
- Radiation catheters or holders, which are loaded with radioactive materials
- A "mold" of radioactive material placed directly over the lesion for a specific time

With the exception of radioactive seeds, which have a low level of activity, clients receiving interstitial radiation are usually hospitalized for the duration of treatment. Radiation isolation precautions must be instituted while the materials are active or in place. A tracheostomy may be required with interstitial implants because of edema and increased oral secretions. (See Chapter 28 for nursing care of clients undergoing radiation therapy.)

Chemotherapy. The client may receive one or more chemotherapeutic agents. The advantages of chemotherapy instead of, or as an adjunct to, surgery or radiation for cancer of the oral cavity continue to be evaluated.

It is important to instruct the client undergoing chemotherapy about the anticipated side effects of the medication, which vary with each antineoplastic agent. Administer antiemetic medications as prescribed and provide other comfort measures as needed (see Chapter 28 for care of clients receiving chemotherapy).

SURGICAL MANAGEMENT. The physician can often excise small, noninvasive lesions of the oral cavity in an ambulatory setting with local anesthesia. The surgical defect is usually small enough to be closed by sutures. These smaller lesions are also responsive to carbon dioxide laser therapy or *cryotherapy* (extreme cold application), which can be performed as an ambulatory care procedure in a surgical center (but may require general anesthesia).

Small oral cancers are equally responsive to radiation therapy and to surgery. More invasive lesions (stage III and IV) require more extensive surgical excision and result in a greater loss of function and disfigurement. Not all lesions can be excised by the peroral approach (through the mouth). The goal of surgical resection is removal of the tumor with a surgical margin that is free of tumor involvement.

Preoperative Care. Before excision of a lesion in the oral cavity, it is important to assess and document the client's level of understanding of the disease process, the rationale for the surgery, and the planned intervention. Problems associated with cancer therapy can be minimized or optimally managed with client preparation and instruction (Robins-Sadler et al., 2003). Information is reinforced as needed. Family members or other caregivers are included in the health teaching.

For small, local excisions, postoperative restrictions include a liquid diet for a day and then advancing as tolerated. There are no activity limitations, and postoperative analgesics are prescribed.

Instructions for the client undergoing large surgical resections may include, but are not limited to, the following postoperative expectations:

- Placement of a temporary tracheostomy and the concomitant nursing care (oxygen therapy and suctioning)
- Temporary loss of speech due to the tracheostomy
- Frequent monitoring of postoperative vital signs
- Nothing by mouth (remain on NPO status) until intraoral suture lines are healed
- Need to have IV lines in place for medication delivery and hydration
- Postoperative medications and activity (out of bed on the first postoperative day)
- Possibility of surgical drains

Because communication is interrupted, you need to assess the client's ability to read and write. In collaboration with the client, select the method of communication to use postoperatively with staff and family members (e.g., Magic Slate, computer, picture board, or pad and pencil).

Operative Procedures. Three factors influence the extent of surgery performed for oral cancers: the size and location of the tumor, tumor invasion into the bone, and the presence of metastasis to neck lymph nodes. Small, noninvasive tumors located near the mouth opening can be excised periorally (inside the mouth). Otherwise, an external approach may be used. The most extensive oral operations are composite resections, which combine partial or total **glossectomy** (tongue removal) and partial mandibulectomy. In the *commando* (co-mandible) *procedure,* the surgeon excises a segment of the mandible with the oral lesion, usually in conjunction with a radical neck dissection (see Chapter 32).

Metastasis to cervical lymph nodes usually indicates a poor prognosis for clients with cancer of the oral cavity. In clients with cervical node metastasis, a neck dissection may also be performed. A radical neck dissection involves the removal of submental; submandibular; upper, mid, and lower jugular; and posterior triangular levels of the cervical lymph nodes, along with cranial nerve XI, the internal jugular vein, and the sternocleidomastoid muscle. Modified and selective neck dissections may be done in individuals with minimal lymph node involvement.

CHART 57-4

FOCUSED ASSESSMENT of
The Postoperative Older Adult with Oral Cancer

- Assess the mouth and surrounding tissues for candidiasis, mucositis, pain, and loss of appetite and taste.
- Monitor the client's weight.
- Monitor nutritional and fluid intake.
- Assess for difficulty in eating or speech.
- Assess pain status and measures used to control pain.
- Monitor the client's response to medications.
- Identify psychosocial problems, such as depression, anxiety, and fear.

Postoperative Care. Airway management is a priority postoperatively for the client with cancer of the oral cavity. The client will have a temporary or permanent tracheostomy, requiring intensive nursing care to promote airway clearance. In addition, care must be taken to protect the surgical incision site from mechanical damage and infection. Nursing interventions to relieve pain or discomfort and promote nutrition are also important. Older adults are a special risk for surgery and need to be monitored very carefully (Chart 57-4).

Maintaining Airway Patency. After extensive excision or resection, the most important nursing intervention is maintaining airway patency. The client may not recall on awakening from anesthesia that a tracheostomy tube is in place and may initially panic because of the inability to speak. Remind the client why he or she cannot speak, and provide reassurance that the vocal cords are intact (unless a total laryngectomy has been performed, then the loss of voice is permanent). Ensure that the predetermined method of communication is available for the client, family members, and staff.

Nursing interventions are aimed at keeping the temporary tracheostomy patent. Frequent suctioning, using sterile technique, may be required for excessive secretions. Humidified oxygen may be prescribed to help liquefy secretions in the early postoperative phase. After the immediate postoperative phase, the client may be able to cough effectively enough to decrease the need for suctioning. After oral edema has decreased and the tracheostomy tube has been changed to a noncuffed type, the client can speak by plugging the stoma with the fingertip. Collaboration between the nurse and physician determine the appropriateness of instructing the client in this technique. (See Chapter 31 for care of the client with a tracheostomy.)

When the client has been determined to have an adequate airway through the aerodigestive tract and can effectively clear secretions by coughing, the tracheostomy tube may be removed. When the tracheostomy tube is removed, an airtight dressing is placed over the site, and the tracheostomy incision heals without the need for sutures.

Clients who have undergone extensive resection may have slurred speech or difficulty in speaking. A consultation with a speech-language pathologist may be indicated.

Protecting the Operative Area. The surgical incision site requires careful attention to avoid infection. It is important to provide gentle mouth care for cleaning away thick secretions and stimulating the flow of saliva. The delivery of oral care depends on the nature and extent of the surgical procedure. Oral care should be provided every 4 hours in the early postoperative phase. The presence of unusual odors from the mouth can indicate infection. In the early postoperative phase, care must be taken to avoid disruption of the suture line during oral hygiene.

Elevate the head of the bed to at least 30 degrees to assist in decreasing edema by gravity. If skin grafting was done, the nurse inspects the donor site (generally on the anterior thigh) during every nursing shift for bleeding or signs of infection. (See Chapter 32 for specific nursing care of the client with a radical neck dissection.)

Relieving Pain. To provide optimal pain relief in the postoperative period, rely on subjective and objective data to assess the need for analgesics and the effectiveness of the medications given. The goal of pain medication during this period is relief of pain while allowing the client to function at an optimal level. Clients who have undergone surgery for oral carcinomas describe their pain as throbbing or pounding. IV morphine is usually the initial postoperative pain medication given. Tylox or Percocet (Percodan plus acetaminophen) may be used for systemic relief of moderate pain.

Promoting Nutrition. Clients who have undergone extensive resections of the oral cavity remain on NPO status for several days. This allows healing in the oral cavity before food contacts the incision. Nasogastric feeding or total parenteral nutrition may be needed during this time (see Chapter 64).

When oral fluid intake is begun, it is important to assess for and document difficulty in swallowing, aspiration, or leakage of saliva or fluids from the suture line. Nursing care should also include the monitoring of weight and hydration. Nutritional supplementation may be used to improve the client's quality of life (see the Legal/Ethical Issues box above). Clients who experience weight loss or who are having difficulty maintaining hydration may be candidates for the surgical placement of a gastrostomy tube.

Encourage the client to perform swallowing exercises. A speech-language pathologist is often consulted to assist with swallowing techniques. A swallowing impairment may be temporary or permanent.

Community-Based Care

Continuing care for the client with an oral tumor depends on the severity of the tumor, the treatment for the tumor, and available support systems. Most clients are maintained at home during follow-up care. Ongoing nutritional management remains a vital part of the treatment plan. In addition, the client and family may benefit from a community-based support group for cancer victims.

HOME CARE MANAGEMENT

If radiation therapy is part of the client's treatment plan, home care considerations include preparatory information and management strategies. Complications due to radiation to the head or neck can be acute or delayed. Acute effects include treatment-related mucositis, stomatitis, and alterations in taste. Long-term effects such as xerostomia (excessive mouth dryness) and dental decay require ongoing oral care, the use of saliva substitutes, and follow-up dental visits. Although ongoing dental care is important, the possible adverse effects that radiation has on the cellular elements of the bone make elective oral surgical procedures, such as tooth extraction, impossible in the area of the radiation. Fatigue is a common side effect of radiation and chemotherapy.

≡ LEGAL/ETHICAL ISSUES

NUTRITIONAL SUPPLEMENTATION IN CLIENTS UNDERGOING RADIATION TREATMENTS

Maintaining optimal nutritional status for individuals with oral carcinoma is a difficult task, considering the many aspects of digestion impacted by the disease and treatment. Radiation therapy can pose additional challenges to nutrition because of the decreased saliva flow and alterations in taste that can result. Not only does increasing evidence point to nutritional status as a predictor of overall survival, but the ability to eat and enjoy food is an important component of quality of life.

The purpose of the study by McCarthy and Weihofen (1999) was to describe the effect of nutritional supplements on the food intake of clients undergoing radiotherapy. Forty clients beginning external-beam radiation therapy were given weekly dietary counseling. The daily food intake was recorded 3 days per week for 4 weeks. One half of the subjects were assigned to ingest a nutritional supplement between meals and at bedtime. Findings suggested that those who ingested the nutritional supplements significantly increased their total caloric and protein intake while not reducing their food-derived caloric and protein intake. Based on this study, the addition of nutritional supplements to the normal food intake for clients undergoing radiotherapy for the treatment of oral cancer may be a viable option in helping to maintain adequate nutrition.

From McCarthy, D., & Weihofen, D. (1999). The effect of nutritional supplements on food intake in patients undergoing radiotherapy. *Oncology Nursing Forum, 26*(5), 897-900.

The client whose tracheostomy has been removed is often taking a soft diet by mouth before discharge. Occasionally, however, clients are discharged from the hospital while still requiring tracheostomy suction, oral suction, and nasogastric feedings. Suction equipment, nutritional supplies, and nursing care can be provided by home care companies. (See Chapter 64 for home care preparation for the client receiving home parenteral nutrition and Chapter 31 for home care preparation for the client with a tracheostomy.)

HEALTH TEACHING

It is vitally important to instruct the client and family about medications, diet or feedings, any treatments (such as tracheostomy care, suture line care, and dressing changes), and early symptoms of infection before hospital discharge.

Alterations in taste and dysphagia make maintaining adequate nutrition a challenge for the oral cancer client. Alterations in taste occur when the taste buds are included in the radiation treatment field. Taste sensation begins to return several weeks after the completion of treatment.

Changes in taste include aversions for meat, such as beef or pork, and metallic tastes in the mouth. Teach clients to add seasonings to foods, to use gravies or sauces to make foods more palatable, and to use high-protein foods such as cheeses, milk, eggs, puddings, and legumes in place of meat. Instruct clients with dysphagia in swallowing exercises. Recommend thickened liquids because thin liquids, such as water, are difficult to control during swallowing. In collaboration with the dietitian, instruct the client and family on how to assess the nutritional intake of the client who is just beginning to eat. Liquid dietary supplements are usually recommended at this time. If bleeding or stomatitis is present, a diet of soft foods is recommended so as to not cause further injury to the mucous membranes.

Instruct the client or family members to inspect the oral cavity daily for areas of redness, indicating the onset of stomatitis. Meticulous oral hygiene should be continued in the post-operative phase, especially with adjuvant chemotherapy or radiation. When instructing the client, reinforce the oral hygiene routine, emphasizing the need for frequent rinsing of the oral cavity to reduce the number of microorganisms and to maintain adequate hydration. The client should use a chemobrush, rinse the chemobrush with hydrogen peroxide and water after each use, and change chemobrushes weekly.

Saliva production is greatly reduced as a consequence of radiation. The resulting xerostomia results in the inability to eat dry foods. Instruct the client regarding the use of saliva substitutes.

Skin reactions are also a common side effect of radiation. Instruct the client to avoid sun exposure, to avoid perfumed lotions or powders, and to cleanse the face or neck area with a gentle nondeodorant soap.

Assess and document the client and family's understanding of health teaching. The client and family should provide a return demonstration of learned skills. This activity increases retention of the health information provided.

HEALTH CARE RESOURCES

Clients who have undergone composite resection often require community services because they have both physical and psychosocial needs. Depression related to a change in body image is common. Excision of a portion of the mandible can leave a facial defect that may be difficult to hide. A social worker or other health care professional may be needed for client and family counseling. Clients who have undergone a total glossectomy may be able to speak with special training and the use of an intraoral prosthesis fashioned by a maxillofacial prosthodontist. The prosthesis is similar to dentures, with augmentation to approximate the oral articulating surfaces.

A social worker or case manager provides assistance in obtaining special equipment or nutritional resources required by the client at home. The case manager assesses the financial needs of the client and makes referrals to government, community, and religious organizations as needed. Refer the client to the American Cancer Society for local support groups.

? Critical Thinking Challenge

A middle-aged man with a long history of smoking is admitted to your surgical unit for surgery for oral cancer. His cancer involves the epiglottis and tongue on the left side. The surgeon performs a commando procedure in which part of his mandible and tongue are removed as well as lymph nodes and muscle tissue from his neck (radical neck dissection). Postoperatively he has a tracheostomy and is receiving oxygen via a tracheostomy mask.

1. What is your priority for care for this client? Why?
2. How will you meet his communication needs?
3. How will you meet his nutritional needs at this time?
4. What health teaching will he and his wife need before discharge to home?

evolve For suggested answer guidelines, go to http://evolve.elsevier.com/Iggy/.

◆ Evaluation: Outcomes

Evaluate the care of the client with a malignant tumor of the oral cavity on the basis of the identified nursing diagnoses and collaborative problems. The expected outcomes include that the client will:

- Maintain open, clear tracheobronchial passages for air exchange
- Maintain the structural intactness and physiologic integrity of the oral mucous membrane

Specific indicators for each of these outcomes are listed for each nursing diagnosis under the Planning and Implementation section (see earlier).

DISORDERS OF THE SALIVARY GLANDS

Acute Sialadenitis

PATHOPHYSIOLOGY

Acute sialadenitis, the inflammation of a salivary gland, can be caused by infectious agents, irradiation, or immunologic disorders. Salivary gland inflammation can have a bacterial or viral etiology. Acute sialadenitis can be caused by infection with cytomegalovirus (CMV). The most common bacterial organisms are *Staphylococcus aureus, Staphylococcus pyogenes, Streptococcus pneumoniae,* and *Escherichia coli.* This disorder most commonly affects the parotid or submandibular gland in adults.

A decrease in the production of saliva (as in dehydrated or debilitated clients or in those who are on NPO status postoperatively for an extended time) usually precipitates acute sialadenitis. The bacteria or viruses enter the gland through the ductal opening in the oral cavity. Systemic medications, such as phenothiazines and the tetracyclines, can also precipitate an episode of acute sialadenitis. Untreated infections of the salivary glands can evolve into abscesses, which can rupture and spread infection into the tissues of the neck and the mediastinum.

Clients who receive radiation for the treatment of cancers of the head and neck or thyroid may develop decreased salivary flow, predisposing them to acute or persistent sialadenitis. The effect of radiation on the salivary glands is rapid and dose related. Immunologic disorders such as HIV infection can cause enlargement of the parotid gland that result from secondary infection. Sjögren's syndrome, an autoimmune disorder, is characterized by chronic salivary gland enlargement and inflammation (see Chapter 24).

◆COLLABORATIVE MANAGEMENT
◆Assessment

During the initial interview, assess for any predisposing factors for sialadenitis, such as ionizing radiation to the head or neck area. Collect a thorough medication history and ask about systemic illnesses, such as HIV infection.

The presence of dehydration can be noted by assessing the oral cavity and the skin for turgor. Other assessment findings include pain and swelling of the face over the affected gland. Cranial nerve function is tested because the branches of the facial nerve lie close to the salivary glands. Fever and general malaise also occur, and purulent drainage can often be massaged from the affected duct in the oral cavity (Chart 57-5).

CHART 57-5

KEY FEATURES of
Sialadenitis

- Swelling on the sides of the face or under the tongue, which increases when the client eats
- Alteration in the quantity or appearance of saliva
- Pain, especially during eating
- Purulent drainage from the affected duct

◆ Interventions

Collaborative management includes the administration of IV fluids and measures such as the following to treat the underlying cause and increase the flow of saliva:

- Hydration
- Application of warm compresses
- Massage of the gland
- Use of a saliva substitute
- Use of **sialogogues** (substances that stimulate the flow of saliva)

Sialagogues include lemon slices and fruit- or citrus-flavored candy. Massage is accomplished by milking the edematous gland with the fingertips toward the ductal opening. Elevation of the head of the bed promotes gravity drainage of the edematous gland.

Acute sialadenitis is best prevented by adherence to routine oral hygiene. This practice prohibits infections from ascending to the salivary glands from the oral cavity.

Postirradiation Sialadenitis

The salivary glands are sensitive to ionizing radiation, such as from radiation therapy or radioactive iodine treatment of thyroid cancers. Exposure of the glands to radiation produces **xerostomia** (very dry mouth caused by a severe reduction in the flow of saliva) within 24 hours. Radiation to the salivary glands can also produce pain and edema, which generally abate after several days.

Xerostomia may be temporary or permanent, depending on the dose of radiation and the percentage of total salivary gland tissue irradiated. Little can be done to relieve the client's dry mouth during the course of radiation therapy. Frequent sips of water and frequent mouth care, especially before meals, are the most effective interventions. After the course of radiation therapy has been completed, saliva substitutes may provide moisture for 2 to 4 hours at a time. Over-the-counter solutions are available, or solutions may be mixed with methylcellulose (Cologel), glycerin, and saline.

Salivary Gland Tumors

PATHOPHYSIOLOGY

Of all oral tumors, those of the salivary glands are relatively rare. Initially, malignant tumors present as slow-growing, painless masses. Involvement of the facial nerve, more common with malignant tumors, results in facial weakness or paralysis (partial or total) on the affected side. Needle aspiration biopsy and open biopsy are useful procedures in establishing a diagnosis.

◆ COLLABORATIVE MANAGEMENT
◆ Assessment

It is important to collect information about any prior radiation exposure because radiation to the head and neck areas is associated with the occurrence of salivary gland tumors. Salivary gland malignancies present as localized, firm masses. In advanced stages of salivary gland tumors, you may note a large preauricular mass accompanied by facial nerve paralysis. Submandibular and minor salivary gland tumors may be tender or painful. Tumor invasion of the hypoglossal nerve causes impaired movement of the tongue, and a loss of sensation can follow. Pay particular attention to assessment of the facial nerve because of its close proximity to the salivary glands. Assess the client's ability to do the following:

- Wrinkle the brow
- Raise the eyebrows
- Squeeze the eyes shut
- Wrinkle the nose
- Pucker the lips
- Puff out the cheeks
- Grimace or smile

◆ Interventions

The treatment of choice for both benign and malignant tumors of the salivary glands is surgical excision. However, radiation therapy is often used for salivary gland cancers that are large, have recurred, show evidence of residual disease after excision, or are highly malignant.

Clients who have undergone **parotidectomy** (surgical removal of the parotid glands) or submandibular gland surgery are at risk for weakness or loss of function of the facial nerve because the nerve courses directly through the gland. Facial nerve repair with autogenous nerve grafting can be done at the time of surgery. A combination of surgery with postoperative radiation is common for advanced disease. Care for clients following parotidectomy is similar to that required for clients having oral cancer surgery, described on pp. 1254 and 1255.

GET READY for the NCLEX Examination!

KEY POINTS

Safe Effective Care Environment

- Be aware that airway management is the priority for care for clients having surgery for oral cancer.
- Place clients having oral cancer surgery in a high-Fowler's, sitting position to facilitate breathing and prevent aspiration.
- Be sure to assess for swallowing ability before offering liquids or food to the client who has had oral cancer surgery to prevent aspiration.

Health Promotion and Maintenance

- Teach clients to seek medical attention for oral lesions that do not heal; these lesions could be oral carcinomas.
- Remind clients to visit their dentist regularly for dental hygiene and oral examination.
- Instruct clients to avoid harsh commercial mouthwashes if they have oral lesions.

- Teach clients to avoid tobacco, alcohol, and sun exposure to decrease their chance of having oral cancer.
- Instruct clients with acute sialadenitis to use sialagogues to stimulate saliva, such as citrus foods or candies.

Psychosocial Integrity

- Recognize that clients with stomatitis are often unable to eat or swallow without discomfort.
- Be aware that those who have had surgery for oral cancer may have difficulty coping with the disease.
- Remember that clients having oral cancer may have an impaired body image because of their reconstructive surgery.
- Refer clients with oral cancer to support groups, such as those available through the American Cancer Society.

Physiological Integrity

- Remember that stomatitis usually manifests as painful single or multiple ulcerations within the mouth.
- Recognize that stomatitis can be caused by a variety of organisms; candida infections are very common in clients who receive antibiotic therapy and in those who are immunocompromised.
- Provide gentle oral care for clients with oral lesions, including the need for chemobrushes and warm saline, hydrogen peroxide, or sodium bicarbonate.
- Be aware that clients with stomatitis receive antimicrobials, anti-inflammatory agents, immune modulators, and topical agents for relief of symptoms, including pain.
- Differentiate leukoplakia and erythroplakia: leukoplakia presents as thin, white patches, and erythroplakia presents as red, velvety lesions.
- Provide care for clients having cancer surgery as summarized in Chart 54-3.
- Be aware that sialadenitis can occur as result of radiation therapy.
- For clients with salivary gland tumors, assess for facial nerve involvement.
- Remember that a parotidectomy involves the removal of the salivary glands; postoperative are is similar to that for clients who have oral cancer surgery.

ADDITIONAL STUDY RESOURCES

Go to your Student CD-ROM for Review Questions for the NCLEX Examination.

Go to http://evolve.elsevier.com/Iggy/ for Integrated Management of Care Questions for the NCLEX Examination.

SELECTED BIBLIOGRAPHY

Asterisk indicates a classic or definitive work on this subject.

Anonymous. (2001). Oral care update. *Nursing Management, 34*(5), S1.

Capenito-Moyet, L.J. (2003). *Nursing care plans & documentation: Nursing diagnosis and collaborative problems* (10th ed.). Philadelphia: Lippincott, Williams, & Wilkins.

Chia-Hui Chen, C. (2003). The Geriatric Oral Health Assessment Index (GOHAI). *Try This: Best Practices in Nursing for Older Adults, 14*(6), 5-6.

Fitzpatrick, J. (2000). Oral health needs of dependent older people: Responsibilities of nurses and care staff. *Journal of Advanced Nursing, 32*, 1325-1332.

Freer, S.K. (2000). Use of an oral assessment tool to improve practice. *Professional Nurse, 15*(10), 635-639.

Greenlee, R., et al. (2000). Cancer statistics, 2000. *Ca: A Cancer Journal for Clinicians, 50*(1), 7-33.

Jarvis, C. (2004). *Physical examination and health assessment* (4th ed.). Philadelphia: W.B. Saunders.

*Mandel, S., & Mandel, R. (1999). Persistent sialadenitis after radioactive iodine therapy: Report of two cases. *Journal of Oral Maxillofacial Surgery, 57*(7), 738-741.

McCance, K.L., & Huether, S.E. (2002). *Pathophysiology: The biologic basis for disease in adults & children* (4th ed.). St. Louis: Mosby.

*McCarthy, D., & Weihofen, D. (1999). The effect of nutritional supplements on food intake in patients undergoing radiotherapy. *Oncology Nursing Forum, 26*(5), 897-900.

Miller, M., & Kearney, N. (2001). Oral care for patients with cancer: A review of the literature. *Cancer Nursing, 24*(4), 241-254.

Neville, B.W., & Day, T.A. (2002). Oral cancer and precancerous lesions. *CA: A Cancer Journal for Clinicians, 52*(4), 195-215.

Palkhivala, A. (2003). Leukoplakia. *Dermatology Times, 24*(5), 36-39.

*Pearson, L. (1996). A comparison of the ability of foam swabs and toothbrushes to remove dental plaque: Implications for nursing practice. *Journal of Advanced Nursing, 23*, 62-69.

*Peterson, M.J., & Baughman, R. (1996). Recurrent aphthous stomatitis: Primary care management. *Nurse Practitioner, 21*(5), 36-47.

*Ransier, A., et al. (1995). A combined analysis of a toothbrush, foam brush, and a chlorhexidine-soaked foam brush in maintaining oral hygiene. *Cancer Nursing, 18*(5), 393-396.

Rini, A., & Bloom, K.C. (2002). Down in the mouth: Update on treatment of oral aphthous ulcers. *The Clinical Advisor, February,* 67-72.

Robins-Sadler, G., et al. (2003). Managing the oral sequelae of cancer therapy. *MedSurg Nursing, 12*(1), 28+.

Scully, C., & Shotts, R. (2001). Mouth ulcers and other causes of orofacial soreness and pain. *Western Journal of Medicine, 174*(6), 421+.

Walton, J.C., Miller, J., & Tordecilla, L. (2001). Elder oral assessment and care. *MEDSURG Nursing, 10*(1), 37-44.

Weinberg, M.A., & Estefan, D.J. (2002). Assessing oral malignancies. *American Family Physician, 65*(7), 1379-1384.

58

Interventions for Clients with Esophageal Problems

CONSTANCE VISOVSKY

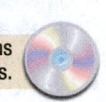
The esophagus is a hollow tube located behind the trachea, passing through the diaphragm at the esophageal hiatus and extending to the gastroesophageal junction. The function of the esophagus is to allow the passage of food from the mouth to the stomach. Disorders of the esophagus can be of inflammatory, structural, motor, and neoplastic origin. Collaborative management involves dietary and lifestyle modifications in conjunction with medical and surgical therapies. Gastroesophageal reflux and related esophageal disorders affect as much as 20% of the population in the United States (Hubbard, 2002). Approximately two million ambulatory care visits yearly can be attributed to GERD. Impaired gastroesophageal motility resulting from achalasia or diverticula is responsible for 400,000 visits to health care providers annually.

GASTROESOPHAGEAL REFLUX DISEASE

Gastroesophageal reflux disease (GERD) is the most common upper gastrointestinal disorder in the United States. It occurs as a result of the backward flow **(reflux)** of gastrointestinal contents into the esophagus. Reflux produces symptoms by exposing the esophageal mucosa to the irritating effects of gastric or duodenal contents, resulting in inflammatory changes of the esophageal mucosa. A person with acute symptoms of inflammation is often described as having **reflux esophagitis,** a hallmark of GERD. Reflux esophagitis is graded according the extent and severity of the lesions.

PATHOPHYSIOLOGY

Several physiologic factors are implicated in the development of GERD (Hubbard, 2002):

- Inappropriate relaxation of the lower esophageal sphincter
- Irritation from the refluxed material
- Delayed gastric emptying
- Abnormal esophageal clearance

The reflux of gastric contents into the esophagus is normally prevented by the presence of two high-pressure areas that remain relatively contracted in the resting phase. A 3-cm (1.2-inch) segment at the proximal end of the esophagus is called the upper esophageal sphincter (UES). Another 2- to 4-cm (0.8- to 1.6-inch) portion just proximal to the gastroesophageal junction is called the **lower esophageal sphincter (LES).** The function of the LES is supported by its anatomic placement in the abdomen, where the surrounding pressure is significantly higher than in the low-pressure thorax. Sphincter function is also supported by the acute angle (angle of His) that is formed as the esophagus enters the stomach. Esophageal reflux can occur when the following occur:

- Gastric volume or intra-abdominal pressure is elevated
- The sphincter tone of the LES is decreased
- The LES undergoes inappropriate relaxation

An individual experiencing reflux may be asymptomatic and relatively unaware that reflux is occurring. However, the esophagus has only limited resistance to the damaging effects of the acidic gastrointestinal (GI) contents. The pH of acid secreted by the stomach ranges from 1.5 to 2.0, whereas the pH of the distal esophagus is normally neutral (6.0 to 7.0). Repeated exposure of the esophageal mucosa to highly acid gastric secretions is associated with the development of erosive esophagitis.

Refluxed material is returned to the stomach by a combination of gravity, saliva, and peristalsis. The effectiveness of the clearance mechanism is very important. An inflamed esophagus cannot eliminate the refluxed material as quickly or efficiently as a healthy one, and therefore the duration of exposure increases with each reflux episode. Hyperemia (increased blood flow) and erosion occur in the esophagus in response to the chronic inflammation. Gastric acid and pepsin are responsible for the tissue injury. Minor capillary bleeding often accompanies the erosion, but frank hemorrhage is rare.

During the process of healing, the body may substitute a columnar epithelium (**Barrett's epithelium**) for the normal squamous cell epithelium of the lower esophagus. Although this new tissue is more resistant to acid and therefore supports esophageal healing, it is considered premalignant and is associated with an increased risk of cancer in clients with prolonged GERD (Field, 2003). The fibrosis and scarring that accompany the healing process can produce esophageal stricture, resulting in a narrowing of the esophageal lumen. The stricture leads to progressive difficulty in swallowing. Uncontrolled esophageal reflux also creates a risk for other serious complications, such as esophageal ulceration, hemorrhage, and aspiration pneumonia. GERD has been implicated as one of the causes of adult-onset asthma, laryngitis, and dental deterioration.

Etiology

The most common cause of GERD is inappropriate relaxation of the LES, which allows the reflux of gastric contents into the esophagus and exposure of the esophageal mucosa to gastric contents from impaired esophageal clearance. Nighttime reflux tends to result in prolonged exposure of the esophagus to acid because recumbency tends to impair peristalsis and gravity clearance mechanisms.

Gastric distention caused by the ingestion of large meals or by conditions associated with delayed gastric emptying predispose the client to reflux. A number of individual factors, including certain foods and medications, have been identified as influencing the tone and contractility of the LES (Table 58-1). Clients who have a nasogastric tube often experience compromised esophageal sphincter function. The tube keeps the cardiac sphincter open and allows acidic contents from the stomach to enter the esophagus. Other factors that increase intra-abdominal and intragastric pressure (e.g., pregnancy, wearing tight belts, obesity, bending

TABLE 58-1 Factors Contributing to Decreased Lower Esophageal Sphincter Pressure	
■ Fatty foods ■ Caffeinated beverages, such as coffee, tea, and cola ■ Chocolate ■ Citrus fruits ■ Tomatoes and tomato products ■ Nicotine in cigarette smoke	■ Calcium channel blockers ■ Nitrates ■ Peppermint, spearmint ■ Alcohol ■ Anticholinergic drugs ■ High levels of estrogen and progesterone ■ Nasogastric tube placement

over, and ascites) overcome the gastroesophageal pressure gradient maintained by the LES and allow reflux to occur.

Incidence/Prevalence

Gastroesophageal reflux disease (GERD) affects about 5% to 7% of the world population and 20% of the U.S. population (Hubbard, 2002). Forty percent of the population reports experiencing symptoms of heartburn once monthly, and 20% report experiencing symptoms weekly (Fennerty et al., 2002). GERD can occur at any age, but it is more common in people over 45 years of age. The incidence of GERD may be underestimated because many people with mild disease relate the symptoms to episodes of stress or dietary indiscretion.

◆ COLLABORATIVE MANAGEMENT
◆ Assessment

HISTORY

Ask the client about a history of heartburn or atypical chest pain associated with the reflux of gastrointestinal contents. Assess the client for dysphagia (difficulty swallowing) or odynophagia (painful swallowing), either of which can indicate the development of a stricture. Ask the client whether he or she has been newly diagnosed asthma or has experienced morning hoarseness or pneumonia. These symptoms are suggestive of severe reflux reaching the pharynx or mouth or pulmonary aspiration.

PHYSICAL ASSESSMENT/CLINICAL MANIFESTATIONS

The clinical manifestations of reflux may vary substantially in severity (Chart 58-1).

DYSPEPSIA. Heartburn, also known as **dyspepsia,** is the characteristic symptom of GERD. Clients often describe this pain as a substernal or retrosternal burning sensation that tends to move up and down the chest in a wavelike fashion. Because heartburn might not be viewed as a serious concern, clients may delay seeking treatment for GERD. If the heartburn is severe, the pain may radiate to the neck or jaw or may be referred to the back. The pain typically worsens when the client bends over, strains, or is in a recumbent position.

With severe GERD, the pain occurs after each meal and persists for 20 minutes to 2 hours. Clients usually experience prompt relief by ingesting fluids or antacids or by maintaining an upright posture.

REGURGITATION. **Regurgitation** of food particles or fluids is common. The client reports the occurrence of warm fluid traveling up the throat, unaccompanied by nausea. If the fluid reaches the level of the pharynx, he or she notes a

KEY FEATURES of
Gastroesophageal Reflux Disease

- Dyspepsia (heartburn)
- Regurgitation (may lead to aspiration or bronchitis)
- Coughing, hoarseness, or wheezing at night
- Water brash (hypersalivation)
- Dysphagia
- Odynophagia (painful swallowing)
- Epigastric pain
- Belching
- Flatulence
- Nausea
- Pyrosis (retrosternal burning)
- Globus (feeling of something in back of throat)
- Pharyngitis
- Dental caries (severe cases)

sour or bitter taste in the mouth. This effortless regurgitation can even occur when the client is in an upright position. The danger of aspiration is increased if regurgitation occurs when the client is in a recumbent (lying down) position.

The client experiencing regurgitation should be carefully monitored for crackles in the lung, which is an indication of associated aspiration. Assess the client for coughing, hoarseness, or wheezing at night, which may be related to recumbent regurgitation. Assessment for bronchitis may be necessary in clients experiencing long-term regurgitation.

HYPERSALIVATION. A reflex salivary hypersecretion known as **water brash** occurs in response to reflux. Water brash must be carefully distinguished from regurgitation. The client reports a sensation of fluid in the throat, but unlike with regurgitation, there is no bitter or sour taste.

DYSPHAGIA AND ODYNOPHAGIA. Chronic GERD can involve **dysphagia** (difficulty swallowing). Dysphagia usually indicates a narrowing of the esophagus because of stricture or inflammation. Careful assessment is required if a client reports progressive or persistent dysphagia because it usually indicates the development of a stricture or cancer. Assessment of the client should include the following:

- The degree of dysphagia
- Whether dysphagia occurs with the ingestion of solids, liquids, or both
- Whether dysphagia is intermittent or occurs with each swallowing effort

Odynophagia (painful swallowing) is a possible symptom of GERD, but it is relatively rare in people with uncomplicated reflux disease. Severe and long-lasting chest pain may be present if spasms occurring in the esophagus cause the muscle to contract with excess force. The resulting pain can be agonizing and may last for hours.

OTHER MANIFESTATIONS. Other symptoms include chronic cough that occurs mostly at night or when the client is in a recumbent position, asthma, and atypical chest pain. Cough and symptoms of asthma occur when refluxed acid is spilled over into the tracheobronchial tree (Field, 2003). *Atypical chest pain* is thought to be caused by stimulation of pain receptors in the esophageal wall and by esophageal spasm. This type of chest pain can mimic angina and needs to be carefully differentiated from cardiac disease.

Eructation (belching), flatulence (gas), or bloating after eating are other common complaints. Nausea and vomiting occur infrequently, and unplanned weight loss is rare.

DIAGNOSTIC ASSESSMENT

The most accurate method of diagnosing gastroesophageal reflux disease (GERD) is **24-hour ambulatory pH monitoring** (McCormick, 2004). This test involves placing a small catheter through the nose into the distal esophagus. The client is asked to keep a diary of activities and symptoms, and the pH is continuously monitored and recorded. Ambulatory pH monitoring is very useful in establishing a diagnosis in clients with atypical symptoms.

Endoscopy, in particular esophagogastroduodenoscopy (EGD), is useful in diagnosing or evaluating reflux esophagitis or in monitoring complications such as Barrett's esophagus. Endoscopy requires the use of conscious sedation during the procedure and the clients must have someone accompany them home after recovery. During the procedure, tissue samples can be obtained for biopsy, and strictures can be dilated (see Chapter 56).

Esophageal manometry, or motility testing, can be performed when the diagnosis is uncertain. Water-filled catheters are inserted via the client's nose or mouth and slowly withdrawn while measurements of LES pressure and peristalsis are recorded. When used alone, manometry is not sensitive or specific enough to establish a diagnosis of GERD.

◆ Common Nursing Diagnoses and Collaborative Problems

Nursing diagnoses that may apply to clients with GERD include the following:

- Acute Pain and Chronic Pain related to physical (esophageal irritation) injury
- Risk for Aspiration related to incompetent LES
- Impaired Swallowing related to stricture or inflammation

◆ Interventions

Inform the client that GERD is a chronic disorder that requires ongoing management. Clients will need to make lifestyle modifications and adhere to medication regimens for the successful treatment of GERD.

NONSURGICAL MANAGEMENT. The goals of treatment for GERD are the relief of symptoms, treatment of esophagitis, and prevention of complications such as strictures or Barrett's esophagus. Although GERD can be controlled by diet therapy, education, lifestyle changes, and drug therapy, it is important to note that, even after esophagitis is healed, 40% to 80% of clients relapse in 6 months after their medication is discontinued.

Diet Therapy. Diet therapy is used to relieve symptoms in clients with relatively mild GERD. In collaboration with the dietitian, explore the client's basic meal patterns and food preferences. Collaborate with the dietitian, client, and family to plan modifications that may decrease reflux symptoms. For adherence at home to be successful, it is essential that family members who do the shopping and cooking be included in this discussion.

Advise the client to limit or eliminate foods that decrease LES pressure, such as chocolate, fat, and mints. The client should also restrict spicy and acidic foods (e.g., orange juice, tomatoes) until esophageal healing can occur because these foods irritate the inflamed tissue and cause heartburn.

Large meals increase the volume of and pressure in the stomach and delay gastric emptying. Therefore, teach the client to eat four to six small meals each day rather than three large ones. Carbonated beverages should also be avoided because they increase pressure in the stomach. Encourage clients to avoid evening snacks and to eat no food for at least 3 hours before going to bed. Reflux episodes are most damaging at night. Clients may have the most difficulty adhering to the restriction of evening snacks. Advise the client to eat slowly and chew thoroughly to facilitate digestion and prevent eructation (belching).

Client Education. Teach the client about the risk factors for the development of reflux, including contributing lifestyle factors. Lifestyle factors that can exacerbate the disease need to be reviewed, and the client should be given instructions on ways to avoid recurrence. Educate the client regarding the need for ongoing monitoring, particularly if the client has developed strictures, ulcerations, or Barrett's esophagus.

Lifestyle Changes. The control of GERD involves lifestyle adjustments to promote health and control reflux (Chart 58-2). Instruct the client to elevate the head of the bed by 6 inches for sleep to prevent nighttime reflux. This can be done by placing blocks under the head of the bed or by using a large, wedge-style pillow instead of a standard pillow (Hubbard, 2002). Emphasize the importance of this intervention, and investigate all possible approaches for achieving compliance.

Instruct the client to sleep in the left lateral decubitus (side-lying) position to minimize the effects of nighttime episodes of reflux. Nighttime reflux is extremely common, and infrequent swallowing in combination with a recumbent position significantly impairs esophageal clearance. Smoking and alcohol cause decreased LES pressure. Explore the possibility and means of smoking cessation, and make appropriate referrals for the client. Ask the client about the normal pattern and amount of alcoholic beverages. If appropriate, assist the client in finding appropriate alcohol cessation programs.

For the obese client, collaborate with the dietitian to examine approaches to weight reduction. Decreasing intra-abdominal pressure often reduces reflux symptoms. Wearing constrictive clothing, lifting heavy objects or straining, and working in a bent-over or stooped position should be avoided. Emphasize that these general adaptations are an essential and effective component of disease management and can produce prompt results in uncomplicated cases.

Drug Therapy. Some medications lower LES pressure and cause reflux, such as oral contraceptives, anticholinergic agents, sedatives, tranquilizers, beta-adrenergic agonists, nitrates, and calcium channel blockers (Hubbard, 2002). The possibility of eliminating those medications in reflux should be explored with the health care provider.

Three principles guide drug therapy for gastroesophageal reflux:

- Inhibit gastric acid secretion
- Accelerate gastric emptying
- Protect the gastric mucosa (Chart 58-3)

Antacids. In uncomplicated cases of GERD, antacids may be effective for occasional episodes of heartburn. Antacids act by elevating the pH level of the gastric contents, thereby deactivating pepsin. They are inadequate for the control of frequent symptoms because their duration of action is too short and their nighttime effectiveness is minimal.

Antacids containing aluminum hydroxide or magnesium hydroxide may be used. Maalox and Mylanta consist of a

---

CHART 58-2

CLIENT EDUCATION GUIDE
Health Promotion Modifications to Control Reflux

- Eat four to six small meals a day.
- Limit or eliminate fatty foods, coffee, tea, cola, and chocolate.
- Reduce or eliminate from your diet any food or spice that increases gastric acid and causes pain.
- Limit or eliminate alcohol and tobacco.
- Do not snack in the evening, and take no food for 2 to 3 hours before you go to bed.
- Eat slowly, and chew your food thoroughly to reduce belching.
- Remain upright for 1 to 2 hours after meals, if possible.
- Elevate the head of your bed 8 to 12 inches using wooden blocks or a foam wedge. Never sleep flat in bed.
- If you are overweight, lose weight.
- Do not wear constrictive clothing.
- Avoid heavy lifting, straining, and working in a bent-over position.
- Chew "chewable" antacids thoroughly and follow with a glass of water.

---

combination of these two agents. Clients often tolerate them better because they produce fewer side effects, such as constipation and diarrhea. Instruct the client to take the antacid 1 hour before and 2 to 3 hours after each meal. Some antacids are prepared as double-strength (DS) suspensions or tablets. The advantage of DS preparations is that the client can take a smaller amount of the drug. For example, 30 mL of regular Mylanta equals 15 mL of Mylanta-II (DS preparation).

Gaviscon, a combination of aluminum hydroxide and magnesium carbonate, is a commonly used and very effective medication for GERD. It forms a viscous foam that floats on top of the gastric contents and theoretically decreases the incidence of reflux. If reflux occurs, the foam enters the esophagus first and buffers the acid in the refluxed material. Remind the client to take this drug when food is in the stomach.

Histamine Receptor Antagonists. Histamine blockers, such as famotidine (Pepcid), ranitidine (Zantac), cimetidine (Tagamet), and nizatidine (Axid) decrease acid. With histamine receptor antagonists available over the counter (OTC) and widely advertised for heartburn, many clients self-medicate before seeking professional assistance from their health care provider. When clients who have self-medicated with OTC preparations experience uncontrolled symptoms, the health care provider usually prescribes a *higher* dose of a histamine receptor antagonist.

Cimetidine (Tagamet) is not used as often as the longer-acting preparations. It has an inhibitory effect on the elimination of certain other medications, and therefore significant drug interactions can occur in clients taking warfarin (Coumadin), theophylline (Theo-Dur), phenytoin (Dilantin), nifedipine (Procardia), or propranolol (Inderal). Ranitidine and the other preparations are longer acting, and less frequent dosing is necessary. They also appear to produce fewer side effects and are safe for long-term administration. Although these drugs do not affect the occurrence of reflux directly, they do reduce gastric acid secretion, improve symptoms, and promote healing of inflamed esophageal tissue.

Proton Pump Inhibitors. The proton pump inhibitors (PPIs), such as omeprazole (Prilosec), lansoprazole (Prevacid), rabeprazole (Aciphex), pantoprazole (Protonix), and esomeprazole (Nexium), are the *main* treatment for

CHART 58-3

DRUG THERAPY for
Gastroesophageal Reflux Disease (GERD)

Drug	Usual Dosage	Nursing Interventions	Rationales
Antacids			
Aluminum or magnesium salts (Mylanta, Maalox)	30 mL PO between meals and as needed (PRN) throughout the day and at bedtime	Give 1 hr before meals, 2-3 hr after meals and at bedtime. Give PRN as instructed by physician. Observe the client for constipation or diarrhea. Suggest the use of combination mixtures or alternating use of aluminum and magnesium products.	Aluminum products produce constipation, and magnesium products induce diarrhea. Balancing their effects is important for client adherence.
Gaviscon, antacid plus alginic acid	1 tablet or 10-20 mL PO throughout the day and at bedtime	Give after meals and at bedtime.	Alginic acid forms a viscous foam that floats on top of the gastric contents, impeding reflux or buffering its effects when it occurs.
Histamine receptor antagonists			
Cimetidine (Tagamet) (Peptol)	300 mg PO four times daily or 900-1200 mg PO at bedtime	Observe the client for side effects; fatigue, headache, and diarrhea are common. Instruct client about potential toxicity with some medications.	Tagamet causes interactions with common medications and is not used as often.
Ranitidine (Zantac)	150 mg PO twice daily	Administer with meals and at bedtime.	Ranitidine and famotidine are more potent, longer-acting drugs but produce fewer side effects.
Famotidine (Pepcid)	40 mg PO daily or 20 mg PO twice daily		
Nizatidine (Axid)	150 mg PO twice daily	Use cautiously and in reduced dosages in clients with renal disease. Observe for dysrhythmias. Do not mix with tomato-based, mixed-vegetable juices; apple juice is the preferred choice.	Clients need an adequate creatinine clearance to prevent drug toxicity. Dysrhythmias are common adverse effects of the drug. Nizatidine may be less potent when mixed with tomato-based, mixed-vegetable juices.
Metoclopramide (Reglan)	10 mg PO three or four times daily	Instruct the client to take the drug before meals. Teach the client to report any neurologic or psychotropic side effects, such as restlessness, anxiety, ataxia, or hallucinations.	This drug increases the rate of gastric emptying. Long-term drug use produces adverse effects in up to one third of clients.
Proton Pump Inhibitors			
Omeprazole (Prilosec, Losec ✻)	20-30 mg PO daily	Instruct the client to take the drug before meals. Observe the client for typical side effects: abdominal cramping, diarrhea, headache.	Gastric acid suppression is greater than 90%. Action is prolonged, but gastrointestinal effects are severe in some clients.
Lansoprazole (Prevacid)	15 mg PO daily for gastroesophageal reflux disease (GERD) Up to 60 mg PO for gastrointestinal ulcers or Zollinger-Ellison syndrome	Instruct the client to take the drug before meals. For the client who has difficulty swallowing or has a nasogastric tube, open the capsule and mix granules in apple juice (or applesauce if not tube fed).	Same as omeprazole. The drug is safe to administer by opening (not crushing) the capsule.
Rabeprazole (Aciphex)	60 mg PO daily (may increase to 120 mg in two divided doses)	Do not crush, break, or chew delayed release tablets. Teach client to wear sunscreen.	This form of the drug is released into the body slowly throughout the day The drug predisposes the client to burns.
Pantoprazole (Protonix, Protonix IV)	40 mg daily or 40 mg IV daily for 7-10 days	Do not crush, break, or chew delayed release tablets.	This form of the drug is released slowly into the body throughout the day.
Esomeprazole (Nexium)	20-40 mg PO daily	Do not administer with digoxin, rabeprazole, or iron salts.	This drug may alter the effect and absorption of these agents.

GERD. These agents provide effective, long-acting inhibition of gastric acid secretion through inhibition of the proton pump of the gastric parietal cell. PPIs reduce gastric acid secretion by about 90% over a 24-hour period and can be given in a single daily dose. If once-a-day dosing fails to control symptoms, twice-daily dosing is appropriate. PPIs promote rapid tissue healing, but recurrence is common when the drug is stopped.

Other Drugs. Prokinetic drugs may used to increase gastric emptying and improve lower esophageal sphincter (LES) pressure and esophageal peristalsis. Metoclopramide (Reglan) is a prokinetic agent that acts to increase the rate of gastric emptying. It does not affect gastric acid secretion or directly heal esophageal tissue. Its use is also associated with a high incidence of neurologic and psychotropic side effects such as fatigue, anxiety, ataxia, and hallucinations. Long-term use is not recommended.

Endoscopic Therapies. In the past decade, several noninvasive endoscopic procedures have been approved for GERD. Three of these newer techniques are the Stretta procedure, the Enteryx procedure, and the Bard EndoCinch Suturing System (BESS). Although not as common as other treatment measures, these methods are becoming more popular.

In the Stretta procedure, the physician applies radiofrequency (RF) energy through needles placed near the gastroesophageal junction. The RF energy inhibits the activity of the vagus nerve, thus reducing discomfort for the client (McCormick, 2004).

The Enteryx procedure also requires an endoscopy and needles. The physician injects a soft, spongy permanent implant made of liquid polymeric material into the LES muscle. This technique tightens the LES and prevents reflux. Similarly, the BESS procedure tightens the LES, but the physician sutures near the sphincter. Chart 58-4 outlines discharge instructions for endoscopic therapies.

The advantage of these therapies compared with surgery include the following:

- Moderate sedation (rather than general anesthesia)
- Ambulatory procedure (rather than an inpatient stay)
- Shorter procedure (45 minutes versus several hours)

CHART 58-4

CLIENT EDUCATION GUIDE
Postoperative Instructions for Clients Having Endoscopic Therapies for Gastroesophageal Reflux Disease (e.g., Stretta Procedure)

- Remain on clear liquids for 24 hours after the procedure.
- After the first day, consume a soft diet, such as custard, pureed vegetables, mashed potatoes, and applesauce.
- Avoid nonsteroidal anti-inflammatory drugs and aspirin for 10 days.
- Continue medications as prescribed, usually proton pump inhibitors.
- Ingest liquid medications whenever possible.
- Do not allow nasogastric tubes for at least 1 month because esophageal perforation could occur.
- Contact the health care provider if the following problems occur:
    Chest or abdominal pain
    Bleeding
    Dysphagia
    Shortness of breath
    Nausea or vomiting

- 1 to 2 days absence from work (rather than 2 to 3 weeks)
- No antibiotics and lower complication rate

❓ Critical Thinking Challenge

You are a nurse in an internist's office and take the history of a middle-aged man with complaint of heartburn. He tells you that he especially has problems when he eats tomatoes, onions, and citrus fruits or juice. For the past month he has been taking over-the-counter Tagamet or Prilosec, and finds that Prilosec is best.

1. What other data should you collect from this client and why?
2. What diagnostic testing might he have to confirm a diagnosis of GERD?
3. Why does he get more relief from the Prilosec compared with Tagamet?
4. If the client is diagnosed with GERD, what health teaching does this client need?

evolve For suggested answer guidelines, go to http://evolve.elsevier.com/Iggy/.

SURGICAL MANAGEMENT. A very small percentage of clients with GERD require antireflux surgery. It is usually indicated for otherwise healthy clients who have failed to respond to medical treatment or have developed complications related to GERD. Various surgical procedures may be used through conventional open techniques or laparoscope.

Laparoscopic Nissen fundoplication (LNF) is the gold standard for surgical management. A discussion of this procedure can be found in the next section under Surgical Management (Hiatal Hernia). Clients who have surgery are encouraged to continue following the basic antireflux regimen of antacids and diet therapy because the rate of recurrence is significant.

Placement of the synthetic Angelchik esophageal antireflux prosthesis may be used for clients with severe reflux. The surgeon performs a laparotomy (abdominal approach) and ties a C-shaped silicone prosthesis filled with gel around the distal esophagus. The prosthesis anchors the LES in the abdomen and reinforces sphincter pressure. This device is not used as often as in previous years because of complications, such as long-term dysphagia and migration of the prosthesis. About 25% of clients with Angelchik devices have them removed.

HIATAL HERNIA

Hiatal hernias, also called diaphragmatic hernias, involve the protrusion of the stomach through the esophageal hiatus of the diaphragm into the thorax. The esophageal hiatus is the opening in the diaphragm through which the esophagus passes from the thorax to the abdomen. Clients with hiatal hernias may be completely asymptomatic or may experience daily symptoms similar to those of clients with GERD.

PATHOPHYSIOLOGY

The two major types of hiatal hernias are sliding hernias and paraesophageal (rolling) hernias.

Sliding Hernia

Sliding hernias are the most common type of hernia and account for 90% of the total number of hiatal hernias. The esophagogastric junction and a portion of the fundus of the

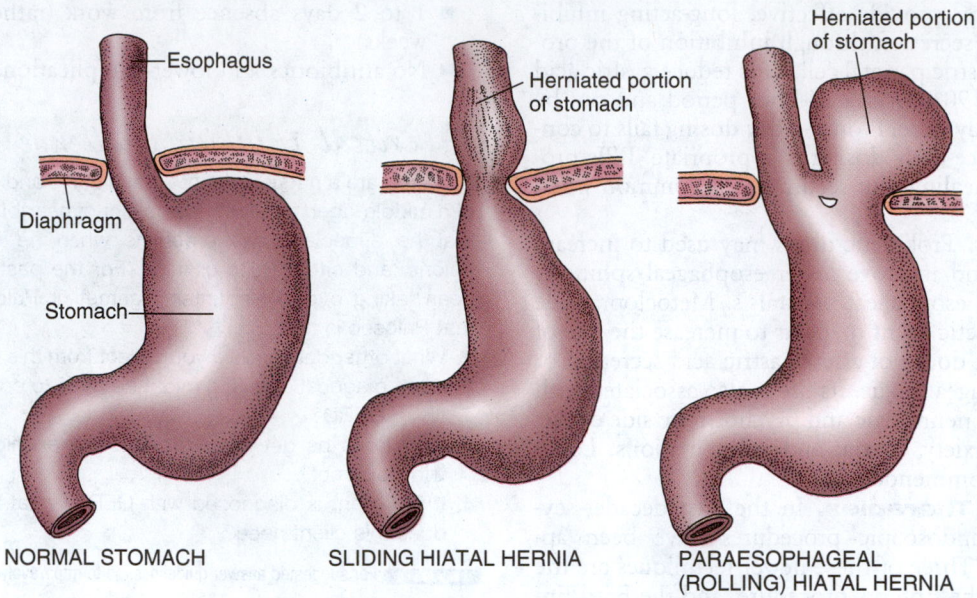

Figure 58-1 ■ A comparison of the normal stomach and sliding and paresophageal (rolling) hiatal hernias.

stomach slide upward through the esophageal hiatus into the thorax (Figure 58-1). The hernia generally moves freely and slides into and out of the thorax during changes in position or intra-abdominal pressure. Although **volvulus** (bowel twisting) and obstruction do occur rarely, the major concern in a client with a sliding hernia is the development of esophageal reflux and its complications. The development of reflux appears to be related to chronic exposure of the lower esophageal sphincter (LES) to the low pressure of the thorax, which significantly reduces the effectiveness of the LES. Symptoms associated with LES pressure are worsened by positions that favor reflux, such as bending or lying supine.

Rolling Hernia

With paraesophageal hernias, the gastroesophageal junction remains in its normal intra-abdominal location, but the fundus (and possibly portions of the stomach's greater curvature) rolls through the esophageal hiatus and into the thorax beside the esophagus (see Figure 58-1). The herniated portion of the stomach may be small or quite large; in rare cases, the stomach completely inverts into the thorax. Reflux is rarely a concern because the LES remains anchored below the diaphragm, but the risks of volvulus, obstruction, and strangulation are high. The development of iron deficiency anemia is common because slow bleeding secondary to venous obstruction causes the gastric mucosa to become engorged and ooze. Significant bleeding or hemorrhage is rare.

Etiology

Sliding hiatal hernias develop from muscle weakening in the esophageal hiatus, which loosens the esophageal supports and permits the lower portion of the esophagus to rise into the thorax. Congenital weaknesses, trauma, obesity, or surgery may also play a significant role. The development of the hernia is the result of the combined effects of weakened

support structures and prolonged increases in abdominal pressure.

Paraesophageal hernias are thought to develop from an anatomic defect occurring when the stomach is not properly anchored below the diaphragm rather than from muscle weakness. Paraesophageal hernias can also be caused by previous esophageal surgeries, including sliding hernia repair.

Incidence/Prevalence

Hiatal hernia is one of the most common disorders affecting the upper gastrointestinal tract, and it affects women more often than men. Hiatal hernias have been reported in up to 20% of adults.

◆COLLABORATIVE MANAGEMENT
◆Assessment

Assess the client for heartburn, regurgitation, pain, dysphagia, and belching. An assessment of general physical appearance and nutritional status is also included. Note the location, onset, duration, quality, and aggravating and alleviating factors associated with the presence of pain. The primary symptoms of sliding hiatal hernias are associated with reflux. Auscultate the thorax and lungs because pulmonary symptoms similar to asthma may be triggered by episodes of aspiration, particularly at night. A detailed history is crucial in attempting to differentiate angina from noncardiac chest pain caused by gastroesophageal reflux. Symptoms resulting from hiatal hernia typically worsen after a meal or when the client is in a recumbent position (Chart 58-5).

In clients with paraesophageal (rolling) hernias, assess for symptoms related to the stretching or displacement of thoracic contents by the hernia. Clients may report a feeling of fullness after eating and may even experience breathlessness or a feeling of suffocation if the hernia interferes with

CHART 58-5
KEY FEATURES of
Hernias

Sliding Hiatal Hernias	Paraesophageal Hernias
■ Heartburn	■ Feeling of fullness after eating
■ Regurgitation	■ Breathlessness after eating
■ Chest pain	■ Feeling of suffocation
■ Dysphagia	■ Chest pain that mimics angina
■ Belching	■ Worsening of manifestations in a recumbent position

breathing. Some clients experience chest pain associated with reflux that mimics angina.

The barium swallow study with fluoroscopy is the most specific diagnostic test for identifying hiatal hernia. Paraesophageal hernias are usually clearly visible, and sliding hernias can often be observed as the client is moved through a series of positions that increase intra-abdominal pressure.

Clients with sliding hernias usually experience symptoms of reflux. Therefore any or all of the diagnostic tests used for gastroesophageal reflux disease (GERD) may be used to evaluate the extent of reflux and the degree of esophageal damage (see Diagnostic Assessment [GERD], p. 1262).

◆ Interventions

Clients with hiatal hernias may be managed either medically or surgically. The health care provider's choice of management is based on the severity of the client's symptoms and the risk of serious complications. Sliding hiatal hernias are most commonly treated medically. Large paraesophageal hernias can become strangulated or obstructed; therefore early surgical repair is encouraged.

NONSURGICAL MANAGEMENT. The interventions for clients with hiatal hernia closely follow those outlined for clients with GERD and include drug therapy, diet therapy, lifestyle modifications, and client education. The health care provider typically prescribes antacids and histamine receptor antagonists, such as ranitidine (Zantac), in an attempt to control reflux and its symptoms.

Diet therapy is also an integral part of the conservative management of hiatal hernia and follows the guidelines discussed earlier for GERD, p. 1262.

Encourage the client to avoid eating in the late evening and to avoid foods associated with reflux. In collaboration with the dietitian, teach the client to modify the diet to reduce body weight (if appropriate). Obesity increases intra-abdominal pressure and worsens both the hernia and the symptoms of reflux. Explain the underlying condition to increase the client's understanding of the disorder and increase adherence to the treatment regimen. Teaching about positioning, as described earlier for GERD (p. 1263) is also extremely important. It is essential that clients do the following:

- Sleep at night with the head of the bed elevated 6 inches.
- Remain upright for several hours after eating.
- Avoid straining or excessive vigorous exercise.
- Refrain from wearing clothing that is tight or constrictive around the abdomen.

SURGICAL MANAGEMENT. Surgery may be required when the risk of complications is high or when damage from chronic reflux becomes severe.

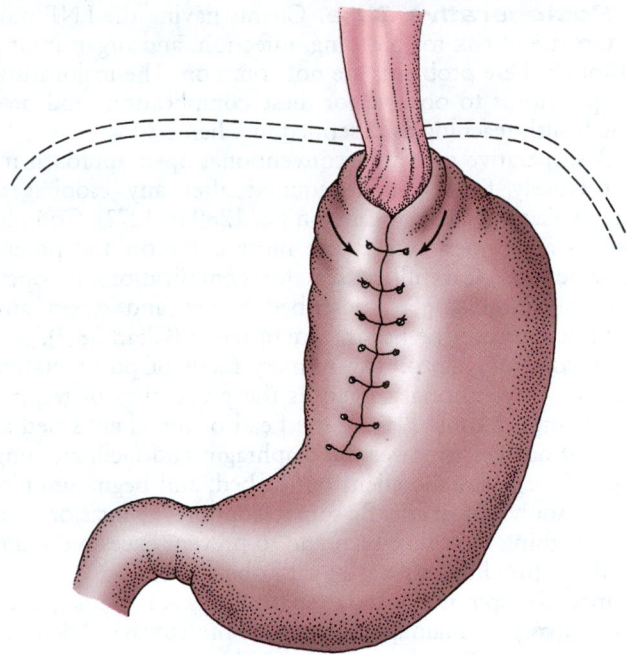

Figure 58-2 ■ Open surgical approach for Nissen fundoplication for gastroesophageal reflux disease or hiatal hernia repair.

Preoperative Care. If the surgery is not urgent, the surgeon encourages clients who are overweight to lose weight before surgery. They are advised to quit or significantly reduce smoking. As part of preoperative teaching, you should reinforce the surgeon's instructions and prepare the client for the postoperative course.

You must know which surgical approach is chosen to develop an appropriate teaching plan. For example, for the trans-thoracic surgical approach, teach the client about chest tubes. Inform the client that a nasogastric tube will be inserted during surgery and will remain in place for several days. Oral intake is started gradually with clear liquids after peristalsis is re-established or to stimulate peristalsis. Instruct the client about techniques for effective deep breathing and use of the incentive spirometer. These measures are essential to prevent postoperative respiratory complications. The high incision makes deep breathing extremely painful for the client. Educate the client concerning the aspects of postoperative pain, and assure the client that adequate postoperative analgesia will be administered.

Operative Procedures. Although several hiatal hernia repair procedures are in use, each involves reinforcement of the lower esophageal sphincter (LES) through some degree of fundoplication. The surgeon wraps a portion of the stomach fundus around the distal esophagus to anchor it and reinforce the LES. The eventual recurrence for either type of hernia following surgical repair is 10% to 15% over 5 years.

Laparoscopic Nissen fundoplication (LNF) is the most common surgical technique for hiatal hernia repair. However, a small percentage of clients are not candidates for laparoscopic procedures and require a conventional open fundoplication (Figure 58-2). In laparoscopic surgery, the repair is performed through several (usually five) 1/2-inch incisions in the abdomen.

Postoperative Care. Clients having the LNF procedure are at risk for bleeding, infection, and organ injury, although these problems are not common. The major nursing priority is to observe for these complications and provide health teaching as described in Chart 58-6.

Postoperative care after conventional open approach repair closely follows that required after any esophageal surgery (see the Plan of Care on pp. 1269 to 1272). Complications after open surgery are more common and potentially serious. Carefully assess for complications of open fundoplication surgery, described below, and report any complications to the health care provider (Chart 58-7).

Respiratory Care. The primary focus of postoperative care for conventional surgery is the prevention of respiratory complications. Elevate the head of the client's bed at least 30 degrees to lower the diaphragm and facilitate lung expansion. Assist the client out of bed, and begin ambulation as soon as possible. Be sure to support the incision during coughing to reduce pain and to prevent excessive strain on the suture line, especially with obese clients.

Incentive spirometry and deep breathing are routinely used after surgery to maintain patency of the airways. Adequate pain control with analgesics is essential for postoperative deep breathing and coughing, and it should be administered as needed. Clients with a smoking history or chronic airway lim-

itation (e.g., chronic obstructive pulmonary disease, asthma) require more aggressive respiratory management by the respiratory therapist to prevent atelectasis and pneumonia. Clients with large hiatal hernias are at high risk for developing respiratory complications.

Nasogastric Tube Management. Postoperative management for open surgery also involves the care of the nasogastric (NG) tube. Inserting a large-diameter NG tube during surgery prevents the fundoplication wrap from becoming too tight around the esophagus. The NG drainage is initially dark brown with old blood but should become normal yellowish green within the first 8 hours after surgery. Check the NG tube every 4 to 8 hours for proper placement in the stomach. The NG tube should be properly anchored so it cannot be displaced because it cannot be safely reinserted without risking perforation of the incision. Follow the surgeon's requests for care of the client with an NG tube.

Frequent assessment of the patency of the tube is essential to keep the stomach decompressed; this prevents retching or vomiting, which can strain or rupture the stomach sutures. The NG tube is irritating; therefore provide frequent oral hygiene to increase comfort. Assess the client's hydration status regularly, including accurate measures of intake and output. Adequate fluid replacement helps to thin respiratory secretions.

Nutritional Care. The client may begin oral intake with clear fluids after peristalsis is re-established or in an effort to stimulate peristalsis. Some surgeons create a temporary gastrostomy for feeding to allow for undisturbed healing of the repair. The client gradually progresses to a near-normal diet during the first 6 weeks. A few foods, such as caffeinated or carbonated beverages and alcohol, are either restricted or eliminated. The food storage area of the stomach is reduced by the surgery, and meals need to be both smaller and more frequent.

The first oral feedings should be carefully supervised because temporary dysphagia is common. Persistent dysphagia usually indicates that the fundoplication is too tight, and dilation may be required.

Another common complication of fundoplication surgery is the **gas bloat syndrome,** in which clients are unable to voluntarily eructate (belch). The syndrome is usually temporary but may persist, even in clients who have the lap-aroscopic approach. Teach the client to avoid drinking carbonated beverages and to avoid eating gas-producing foods (especially high-fat foods), chewing gum, and drinking with a straw.

Many clients acquire the habit of **aerophagia** (air swallowing) from attempting to reverse or clear acid reflux. Teach these clients to relax consciously before and after meals, to eat and drink slowly, and to chew all food thoroughly. Air in the stomach that cannot be removed by belching can be extremely uncomfortable. Frequent position changes and ambulation are often effective interventions for eliminating air from the gastrointestinal tract. If gas pain is still present, clients are encouraged to take simethicone, 80 mg four times daily as needed. Be sure to remind the client to crush and dissolve the medication in water before taking.

Community-Based Care

Clients undergoing one of the open surgical repairs require activity restrictions during the 3- to 6-week postoperative recovery period. For laparoscopic surgery, activity is typically restricted for a shorter time, and the client can return to his or her usual lifestyle more quickly, usually in a few days to

Text continued on p. 1272.

CHART 58-6

CLIENT EDUCATION GUIDE
Postoperative Instructions for Clients Having Laparoscopic Nissen Fundoplication (LNF)

- Stay on a soft diet for about a week, including mashed potatoes, puddings, custard, and milkshakes; avoid carbonated beverages, tough foods, and raw vegetables that are difficult to swallow.
- Remain on antireflux medications as prescribed for at least a month.
- Do not drive for a week after surgery; do not drive if taking opioid pain medication.
- Walk every day, but do not do any heavy lifting.
- Remove gauze dressings 2 days after surgery and shower; do not remove Steri-strips until 10 days after surgery.
- Wash incisions with soap and water, rinse well, and pat dry; report any redness or drainage from the incisions to your surgeon.
- Report fever above 101° F, nausea, vomiting, or uncontrollable bloating or pain.
- Schedule an appointment for follow-up with your surgeon in 3 to 4 weeks.

CHART 58-7

BEST PRACTICE for
Assessment of Postoperative Complications Related to Fundoplication Procedures

Complication	Assessment Findings
Temporary dysphagia	The client has difficulty swallowing when oral feeding begins.
Gas bloat syndrome	The client has difficulty belching to relieve distention.
Atelectasis, pneumonia	The client experiences dyspnea, chest pain, or fever.
Obstructed nasogastric tube	The client experiences nausea, vomiting, or abdominal distention. The nasogastric tube does not drain.

PLAN of CARE   MEDICAL DIAGNOSIS: ESOPHAGEAL SURGERY

NURSING DIAGNOSIS NO. 1 ■ Ineffective Breathing Pattern

	Expected Outcomes	Nursing Interventions	Rationales
RELATED FACTORS Pain Musculoskeletal impairment **DEFINING CHARACTERISTICS** Altered chest excursion	No verbal report or observation of dyspnea Respiratory rate remains between 11 and 22 breaths/min Has respirations that remain regular and deep	**NIC Airway Management** Place the client in semi-Fowler's position, if possible. Encourage the client to cough frequently, or suction the client as necessary. **D** Encourage the client to take slow, deep breaths; to turn; and to cough. **D** Assist the client with an incentive spirometer, as appropriate. **D** Regulate fluid intake to optimize fluid balance. **NIC Respiratory Monitoring** **D** Monitor the rate, rhythm, depth, and effort of respirations. Note chest movement, watching for symmetry, the use of accessory muscles, and supraclavicular and intercostal muscle retractions. Auscultate breath sounds, noting areas of decreased/absent ventilation and the presence of adventitious sounds. Note changes in SaO_2, SvO_2, end tidal CO_2, and arterial blood gas (ABG) values, as appropriate. **D** Monitor the client's respiratory secretions. **Other Interventions** Provide pain relief. **Continuing Care Considerations** Teach the client relaxation techniques. **D** Encourage the client to engage in regular physical exercise. Encourage the client to enroll in a smoking cessation program, as indicated.	Semi-Fowler's position ensures that abdominal contents do not press against the diaphragm and restrict chest expansion. Coughing or suction will rid the airway of secretions. Effective aeration and coughing will help rid the body of secretions. Frequent position changes will prevent secretions from pooling in one area. Incentive spirometry encourages the client to deep breathe. Fluids will help keep lung secretions thin and easier to cough out of the airways. Changes in respiratory rate, rhythm, depth, or effort may signal a descent into respiratory failure. The use of accessory muscles indicates an increased respiratory effort. Absent breath sounds or adventitious breath sounds indicate poor gas exchange or poor movement of air through the airways. These tests indicate the effectiveness of gas exchange or gas transport. Changes in the color, consistency, or odor of the secretions may indicate infection. Deep breathing and coughing causes diaphragmatic movement and may increase pain. Stress management and relaxation techniques help to control the anxiety resulting from hypoxia. Cardiopulmonary efficiency and endurance improve with exercise. Smoking damages the airways and alveoli.

D Indicates tasks that can be delegated to unlicensed assistive personnel at the discretion of the nurse.

Continued

▤ PLAN of CARE   MEDICAL DIAGNOSIS: ESOPHAGEAL SURGERY—cont'd

NURSING DIAGNOSIS NO. 2 ■ Imbalanced Nutrition: Less Than Body Requirements

	Expected Outcomes	Nursing Interventions	Rationales
RELATED FACTORS Inability to ingest or digest food or absorb nutrients due to biologic factors: Surgery **DEFINING CHARACTERISTICS** Pain: Abdominal with or without pathology Perceived inability to ingest food	Has bowel sounds that remain at 3 to 5 per quadrant per minute Denies abdominal pain No verbal report or observation of diarrhea Weight remains within ±5 pounds of desired weight	Determine, in collaboration with a dietitian as appropriate, the number of calories and type of nutrients needed to meet nutrition requirements. **D** Provide foods appropriate for the client—blenderized or commercial formula via nasogastric or gastrostomy tube, or total parental nutrition—as ordered by physician. **D** Create a pleasant and relaxing environment at mealtime. **Other Interventions** Teach the client and family about high-calorie, high-protein meal planning, as appropriate. Administer medication such as simethicone (crushed and dissolved in water) as ordered. Teach the client to consciously relax before and after meals. Teach the client and family about nutritional supplements, as appropriate. Teach the client and family about preventing constipation. **Continuing Care Consideration** Encourage the client and family to use the home nutritional therapy team.	Individual client needs for nutrients and calories should be the basis for a sound dietary plan. Diet therapy and type of surgery dictate the type and form of foods that may be offered to the client. A pleasant and relaxing environment at mealtime improves digestion. Meal planning that considers the client's and family's budget and other resources increases the likelihood that appropriate meals will be prepared. Simethicone may alleviate or eliminate painful gastrointestinal gas. Clients may have the habit of aerophagia to clear acid reflux. The excess air may be extremely uncomfortable. Additional vitamins and minerals, calories, dietary fiber, or other nutritional components may need to be added to the diet of clients who are unable to eat a nutritionally adequate diet. Clients on low-fiber diets may need additional fluids and supplemental fiber to maintain bowel regularity. The home nutritional therapy team is able to monitor and adjust the nutritional plan of care to maximize the client's nutritional status.

NURSING DIAGNOSIS NO. 3 ■ Acute Pain

	Expected Outcomes	Nursing Interventions	Rationales
RELATED FACTORS Injury agents (biologic, chemical, physical, psychological): Surgery **DEFINING CHARACTERISTICS** Verbal or coded report of pain Observed evidence of pain	Denies experiencing pain greater than a 5 on a 0 to 10 pain scale No verbal report or observation of guarding or protective gestures No verbal report or observation of an alteration in sleep patterns No verbal report or observation of self-focusing behavior	**NIC** **Pain Management** Perform a comprehensive pain assessment that includes location, characteristics, onset/duration, frequency, quality, intensity or severity of pain, and precipitating factors. Consider the cultural influences on the pain response.	A plan for pain management must be based on the client's unique responses to pain. Cultural stereotypes may lead to an inaccurate assessment of pain.

D Indicates tasks that can be delegated to unlicensed assistive personnel at the discretion of the nurse.

▤ PLAN of CARE   MEDICAL DIAGNOSIS: ESOPHAGEAL SURGERY—cont'd

NURSING DIAGNOSIS NO. 3 ■ Acute Pain—*cont'd*

Expected Outcomes	Nursing Interventions	Rationales
No verbal report or observation of facial mask of pain No verbal report or observation of an alteration in activity level	Select and implement a variety of measures to facilitate pain relief, as appropriate.	Pharmacologic, nonpharmacologic, and interpersonal strategies may provide pain relief depending on the client's unique responses to the therapeutic interventions.
	Use pain control measures before pain becomes severe.	Medicating the client in a timely manner prevents pain from reaching acutely unpleasant levels.
	Teach the use of nonpharmacologic techniques before, after and, if possible, during painful activities; before pain occurs or increases; and along with other pain relief measures.	Nonpharmacologic techniques help the client establish a sense of control over his or her pain experience.
	NIC Analgesic Administration	
	Choose the IV rather than the IM route for frequent pain medication injections, when possible.	The IV route avoids tissue trauma and the unpredictable absorption of medication.
	D Institute safety precautions for clients who are receiving opioid analgesics, as appropriate.	Opioid analgesics may impair the client's judgment and/or coordination.
	Document the client's response to the analgesic and any untoward effects.	Documentation provides the health care team with the information needed to accurately evaluate the client's response to the analgesic regimen.
	Implement actions to decrease the untoward effects of analgesics.	Actions taken to prevent the predictable but unwanted effects of narcotic analgesics (e.g., constipation) increase client comfort.
	Instruct the client to request PRN pain medication before the pain is severe.	Pain may be managed with lower doses of analgesics and fewer untoward effects if PRN drugs are used before pain becomes severe.
	NIC Patient-Controlled Analgesia (PCA) Administration	
	Consult with the client, family members, and physician to adjust lockout interval, basal rate, and demand dosage.	The client's response to the analgesic will determine the PCA settings.
	Teach the client and family to monitor pain intensity, quality, and duration.	This information will help the client and family determine when to administer a bolus dose of analgesic, if appropriate, or when to request an increase in basal rate of the analgesic.
	Teach the client and family members to monitor respiratory rate and blood pressure.	This information will help the health care team to adjust the analgesic doses to the client's responses and decrease the untoward effects.

Continued

▤ PLAN of CARE   MEDICAL DIAGNOSIS: ESOPHAGEAL SURGERY—cont'd

NURSING DIAGNOSIS NO. 3 ■ Acute Pain—cont'd

Expected Outcomes	Nursing Interventions	Rationales
	Teach the client and family how to use the PCA device.	The PCA device will not be used if the client and/or family do not know how to use or are afraid of the device.
	NIC Environmental Management: Comfort	
	D Facilitate hygiene measures to keep the client comfortable.	Hygiene measures may improve the client's overall sense of well-being.
	D Position the client to facilitate comfort.	The nurse may decrease sources of discomfort by using principles of body alignment, supporting with pillows, supporting joints during movement, splinting over incisions, and immobilizing painful body parts.
	Other Interventions	
	Refer the client to the Pain Advisory Committee.	The Pain Advisory Committee is a multidisciplinary committee with wide expertise in pain relief interventions.
	Consider the use of alternative therapies such as yoga, meditation, spirituality, and/or religion.	The experience of meditation and prayer and the reflection on meaning may help the client to relax, thereby easing the muscle tension that contributes to pain sensation.
	Consider the use of alternative therapies such as imagery, aromatherapy, music, touch, and laughter/humor.	Cognitive and behavioral strategies may be used as adjuncts to or in place of pharmacologic or surgical interventions for chronic pain. Each therapy has a different mode of action that may or may not benefit the client.
	Consider using other cutaneous skin stimulation techniques such as massage and/or vibration to complement pain management strategies.	Massage may cause muscle relaxation, which decreases pain signals; vibration interrupts pain signal transmission to decrease pain perception.
	Continuing Care Considerations	
	Refer the client to an advanced practice nurse pain specialist, social worker, home care nurse, and/or psychologist, as appropriate.	Health care team members are able to provide continuing support to the client who is facing chronic pain.

D Indicates tasks that can be delegated to unlicensed assistive personnel at the discretion of the nurse.

a week. For long-term management, teach the client and family about appropriate diet modifications. The use of stool softeners or bulk laxatives is recommended for the first postoperative weeks until healing is complete. Instruct the client to avoid straining and to prevent constipation. Teach the client to inspect the healing incision daily and to notify the health care provider if swelling, redness, tenderness, discharge, or fever occurs. Advise the client to avoid contact with people with respiratory infections and to contact the health care provider if symptoms of a cold or influenza develop. Persistent coughing can cause the incision or the fundoplication to dehisce. The client is also advised to avoid smoking.

Consult with the dietician to educate the family and significant others about dietary changes. Full support is essential for the client to modify the size and timing of meals successfully. Relatively few ongoing diet restrictions are needed, but overeating or eating the wrong types of foods can produce discomfort if the client cannot belch. Instruct the client to report the recurrence of reflux symptoms to the health care provider.

Although severe surgical complications are relatively rare, conditions such as gas bloat syndrome and dysphagia are common and may persist. Prepare the client for these problems and for the potential that reflux may not be completely controlled or may occur again. Although surgery controls the condition, a cure is rare, and lifestyle modifications need to be ongoing.

ACHALASIA

PATHOPHYSIOLOGY

Achalasia is an esophageal motility disorder believed to result from esophageal **denervation** (loss of nerve impulse passage). Its exact cause is unknown. A genetic basis to the disorder has been proposed as suggested by occasional familial clustering and phenotype (observable characteristics) association. As a result, the lower esophageal sphincter (LES) fails to relax properly with swallowing and in which the normal peristalsis of the esophagus is replaced with abnormal contractions. Achalasia is characterized by chronic and progressive dysphagia. Over time, peristaltic failure plus spasm can produce a massively dilated esophagus, which further slows food passage (Strader, 2001). Epigastric pain, a sensation of food sticking in the lower esophagus, and regurgitation of ingested food may also occur (Goroll & Mulley, 2000). Nighttime regurgitation of food occurs in 33% of people and can be the cause of cough, aspiration, or pneumonia (Strader, 2001). If left untreated, progressive dysphagia can result in weight loss.

Achalasia is an uncommon disorder that usually occurs between 20 and 40 years of age. Both genders appear to be equally affected. About 5% to 10% of individuals with this disorder develop esophageal squamous cell carcinoma. Complications of achalasia also include esophageal candidiasis, lower esophageal diverticula, airway obstruction, and aspiration pneumonia.

◆ COLLABORATIVE MANAGEMENT
◆ Assessment

Assess for the primary symptoms of achalasia, such as dysphagia and regurgitation of solids, liquids, or both. Ask the client about the presence of chest pain associated with these symptoms. Inquire about factors that aggravate the symptoms (e.g., body position or diet changes) as well as medications or home treatments that relieve the symptoms. Ask the client about a history of previous esophageal surgery or trauma, which can compound the progressive dysphagia. A respiratory history and current respiratory-associated symptoms are particularly important with regard to their direct relationship to reflux, regurgitation, and aspiration.

Take a nutritional history to determine the effect of the esophageal symptoms. Collect information about dietary habits, food tolerances, and weight loss. Note the presence of **halitosis** (foul mouth odor), which can be caused by the regurgitation of previously ingested food. Auscultate the

lungs for adventitious sounds secondary to pulmonary aspiration of retained saliva and food. The client's current and usual weight should be noted and compared for weight loss resulting from dysphagia.

A barium swallow is the most sensitive test for visualizing the esophagus and is likely to show esophageal dilation with a persistent beaklike narrowing at the terminal esophagus, the hallmark of a nonrelaxing LES. A chest x-ray can show a distorted and dilated tubular esophagus, the absence of a gastric air bubble, and occasionally a tubular mediastinal mass next to the aorta. Esophageal manometry typically reveals an increased LES pressure and incomplete sphincter relaxation when the client swallows. Endoscopy is used to evaluate the appearance of the esophageal mucosa, especially for changes associated with cancer or the presence of candida.

◆ Interventions

The symptoms associated with achalasia can be treated with a variety of approaches. A combination of dietary measures, pharmacologic agents, esophageal dilation, and surgery is used.

Drug and Diet Therapy. Mild cases of achalasia can be managed with calcium channel blockers (nifedipine [Procardia]) or nitrates (sublingual nitroglycerin) to reduce LES pressure. Drug therapy is given for symptom relief and is not recommended as an alternative to more definitive therapy. Achalasia can also be treated with the direct injection of botulinum toxin (Botox) into the LES muscle via endoscopy. Botulinum toxin acts to denervate cholinergic nerves in the distal esophagus by suppression of acetylcholine release. Ninety percent of clients have improvement after this procedure; however, repeated regular dosing is required, and the long-term effects are unknown.

Advise the client to experiment with changes in diet because they can often ease the pressure and reflux associated with achalasia. Discuss any food habits he or she has noted that aggravate or relieve the symptoms. Semisoft foods are often better tolerated, as are warm foods and liquids. Eating four to six smaller meals rather than three large meals during the day facilitates the passage of food. Collaborate with the dietitian for additional suggestions about diet changes and nutritional balance. Nocturnal reflux of foods and liquids from the dilated esophagus into the hypopharynx and oral cavity often can be prevented if the client sleeps with the head of the bed elevated or in a semi-sitting position. Advise the client to experiment with various changes in position while eating because such changes can reduce pressure sensations during meals. Some clients benefit from arching the back while swallowing. Caution the client to avoid wearing restrictive clothing, which can increase esophageal pressure and regurgitation.

Esophageal Dilation. More severe cases of achalasia require dilation of the LES. The traditional treatment involves the passage of progressively larger sizes of esophageal bougies (dilators) using polyurethane balloons on a catheter. The procedure is performed on an ambulatory care basis. Large-diameter metal **stents** may be used to keep the esophagus open for longer durations.

After the procedure, monitor the client for complications of bleeding and signs of perforation, such as chest and shoulder pain, elevated temperature, **subcutaneous emphysema** (air under the skin), or **hemoptysis** (coughing up blood). Teach the client to expectorate rather than swallow any secretions that are be produced. Instruct the client to take nothing by mouth (NPO) for 1 hour and to limit dietary intake to liquids for 24 hours. The procedure may be repeated in 2 to 3 months if needed. Most clients report improvement in swallowing.

Esophagomyotomy. Surgical procedures for the client with achalasia are aimed at facilitating the passage of food. **Esophagomyotomy,** in which the LES is incised, has been used successfully for decades. Open thoracic and abdominal approaches can be used, but laparoscopic surgery has become more common. An antireflux wrap (**fundoplication**) may or may not be part of the procedure.

Conventional esophagomyotomy is a more complex surgical treatment for achalasia. Using an open approach, general anesthesia is required, and the client is hospitalized for several days. A thoracotomy approach permits exposure of the esophagus. The surgeon cuts muscle fibers around the LES to open the sphincter and thereby provide less obstruction to food passage.

For long-term refractory achalasia, the surgeon may attempt excision of the affected portion of the esophagus, with or without replacement by a segment of colon or jejunum (partial esophagectomy).

Postoperative care for clients undergoing trans-thoracic esophagomyotomy includes managing chest tubes and drains, assessing healing of the thoracotomy or abdominal incision, pain control, and managing NG feedings. (See Chapter 22 for general postoperative care and Chapter 33 for care of the client with a thoracotomy.)

Laparoscopic surgery permits a shorter length of stay and fewer complications compared with either open surgical approach. Clients receive conscious sedation rather than general anesthesia. Teach clients having laparoscopic surgery to report complications, such as bleeding and fever. Instruct the client as described in Chart 58-6.

ESOPHAGEAL TUMORS

PATHOPHYSIOLOGY

Esophageal tumors can be benign or malignant. However, benign esophageal tumors, known as leiomyomas, are extremely uncommon. These tumors are removed if they cause discomfort but otherwise require no specific treatment. Most malignant esophageal tumors arise from the epithelium. Squamous cell carcinomas of the esophagus are located in the upper two thirds of the esophagus. Adenocarcinomas are more commonly found in the distal third and at the gastroesophageal junction, and these tumors account for 50% of all esophageal cancers (Brooks-Brunn, 2000). The local and regional lymphatic spread of the disease differs according to the site of the original tumor. Esophageal tumors exhibit rapid local growth because there is no serosal layer to limit their extension. Because the esophageal mucosa is richly supplied with lymphatics, there is early spread of tumors to lymph nodes. Esophageal tumors can protrude into the esophageal lumen and can cause thickening of the lumen or invade deeply into surrounding tissue. In rare cases the lesion may be confined to the epithelial layer (in situ). In the most cases, the tumor is relatively large and well established on diagnosis. More than 50% of esophageal cancers **metastasize** (spread throughout the body).

Etiology and Genetic Risk

In Western societies, the two primary risk factors associated with the development of squamous cell carcinoma of the esophagus are tobacco use and heavy alcohol intake. The compounds in tobacco smoke may be responsible for the genetic mutations seen in one half of esophageal tumors. A smoker has two to six times the risk of eventually developing esophageal cancer than does a nonsmoker. Some alcoholic beverages contain potent carcinogens that may be responsible for the development of esophageal tumors. Smoking and alcohol ingestion act together in the development of esophageal cancer.

Long-term, untreated gastroesophageal reflux disease (GERD) can play a role in esophageal cancer development. For individuals with Barrett's esophagus, the risk of developing esophageal cancer is increased 30 to 150 times as compared with the general population. Exposure to acid and pepsin leads to the replacement of normal distal squamous mucosa with columnar epithelium as a response to tissue injury, known as **Barrett's esophagus.** This tissue undergoes dysplasia and, ultimately, malignant transformation. In other parts of the world where esophageal cancer is common, the incidence of squamous cell carcinoma appears to be linked to high levels of nitrosamines (which are found in pickled and fermented foods) and foods high in nitrate. Diets that are chronically deficient in fresh fruits and vegetables have also been implicated in the development of squamous cell carcinoma.

Certain genetic factors may have a role in the development of esophageal cancer. It has been proposed that esophageal cancers result from mutations in suppressor genes and proto-oncogenes (see Chapter 11 for a more complete discussion). Overexpression and mutations of the $p53$ tumor suppressor gene have been found in persons with esophageal cancer. In addition, the presence of the $p53$ gene may be an indication of advanced disease. Tumor cells with a mutated $p53$ gene have demonstrated resistance to chemotherapy.

Incidence/Prevalence

Esophageal cancer, the second most common cancer of the thoracic cavity, accounts for 6% of all cancers of the GI tract, and mortality from the disease remains very high (American Cancer Society, 2003). In 2003 about 14,000 new cases of esophageal cancer were diagnosed and as many related deaths in the United States (American Cancer Society, 2003). The incidence of squamous cell carcinoma of the esophagus has remained stable, but the rate of adenocarcinoma has continued to rise 4% to 5% per year. This increased rate seems to be directly related to the increase in cases of GERD.

CULTURAL CONSIDERATIONS

Squamous cell carcinoma is more commonly found in African-American men, whereas adenocarcinoma is more prevalent in white men. Squamous cell carcinoma of the esophagus is the seventh leading cause of cancer deaths in African Americans. By contrast, white men have a higher prevalence of adenocarcinoma of the esophagus (Brooks-Brunn, 2000).

◆ COLLABORATIVE MANAGEMENT
◆ Assessment

HISTORY

Assess for risk factors related to the development or symptoms of esophageal cancer, such as the client's racial and cultural background, age, gender, history of alcohol consumption, tobacco use, dietary habits, and other esophageal problems (e.g., dysphagia, stricture, reflux). Ask the client about the ingestion of pickled foods, changes in appetite, changes in taste, or a decline in weight. Cancer of the esophagus is a silent tumor in its early stages, with few signs to identify on assessment. By the time the tumor causes symptoms, it usually has spread rather extensively.

PHYSICAL ASSESSMENT/CLINICAL MANIFESTATIONS

Dysphagia (difficulty swallowing) is the most common symptom of esophageal cancer, but it may not be present until the lumen of the esophagus is significantly narrowed. Dysphagia is both persistent and progressive. It is initially associated with swallowing solids, particularly meat, and then progresses rapidly over a period of weeks or months to difficulty in swallowing soft foods and liquids. Late in the disease, even saliva can induce choking. Clients usually report a sensation that food is sticking in the throat or in the substernal area. Careful assessment of the dysphagia is an important part of the diagnosis because dysphagia associated with other esophageal disorders is not usually continuous. Weight loss often accompanies dysphagia and can exceed 20 pounds.

Odynophagia (painful swallowing) is present in most clients and is reported as a steady, dull, substernal pain that may radiate. The presence of severe or persistent pain often indicates tumor invasion of the mediastinal structures. Assess for the occurrence of regurgitation, vomiting, foul breath, and chronic hiccups, which often accompany advanced disease. In most clients, pulmonary complications develop at some point. Assess for the presence of chronic cough, increased secretions, and a history of recent infections. Tumors in the upper esophagus may involve the larynx and thus cause hoarseness. Chart 58-8 summarizes the clinical manifestations of esophageal tumors.

PSYCHOSOCIAL ASSESSMENT

The diagnosis of esophageal cancer is a great source of anxiety to the client. The disease is accompanied by distressing symptoms and is often terminal. The fear of choking can place unusual stress on normal mealtimes. Assess the client's response to the diagnosis and prognosis, and explore his or her coping strengths and resources. The impact of the disease on the usual pattern of activities is also assessed. Determine the availability of support systems and the potential financial impact of the disease and its treatment. Refer the client and family members to psychological counseling, pastoral care, and the social worker as needed.

RADIOGRAPHIC ASSESSMENT

A barium swallow study with fluoroscopy is usually the first diagnostic test ordered to evaluate dysphagia. In a barium swallow, the margins of a tumor may be seen. However, to

---

CHART 58-8

KEY FEATURES of
Esophageal Tumors

- Persistent and progressive dysphagia (most common feature)
- Feeling of food sticking in the throat
- Odynophagia (painful swallowing)
- Severe, persistent chest or abdominal pain or discomfort
- Regurgitation
- Chronic cough with increasing secretions
- Hoarseness
- Anorexia
- Nausea and vomiting
- Weight loss (often more than 20 pounds)
- Changes in bowel habits (diarrhea, constipation, bleeding)

---

make a definitive diagnosis of cancer, a tissue biopsy via endoscopy is needed.

OTHER DIAGNOSTIC ASSESSMENTS

The definitive diagnosis of esophageal cancer is made by esophagogastroduodenoscopy (EGD) with biopsies of the esophagus and tumor. During an EGD, the esophagus is inspected and tissue specimens are obtained for cytologic studies and disease staging. Multiple tissue samples may be required when the suspected tumor is in the distal esophagus, because clear tissue samples are difficult to obtain. A complete staging workup is performed to determine the extent of the disease.

A computed tomography (CT) scan assists in identifying metastatic disease, which might be present in the chest or abdomen. Positron emission tomography (PET) is a newer technology that may identify metastatic disease with more accuracy than a CT scan. An endoscopic ultrasound (EUS) is a staging technique that can help determine the size and depth of tumor invasion. (These tests are described elsewhere in Chapter 56.)

Critical Thinking Challenge

You are caring for an older adult recently diagnosed with esophageal cancer. He states he smoked two packs of cigarettes per day for 30 years but quit 5 years ago. He also states that he drinks alcohol occasionally but tends to eat late at night and as a result often has heartburn. He also complains of food "sticking" in his throat.

1. What lifestyle factors in this client's history would predispose him to esophageal cancer?
2. What questions would you ask him regarding symptoms he might be experiencing as a result of his diagnosis?
3. What complications will he experience if his dysphagia worsens?

evolve For suggested answer guidelines, go to http://evolve.elsevier.com/Iggy/.

◆ Analysis

COMMON NURSING DIAGNOSES AND COLLABORATIVE PROBLEMS

The following is a priority nursing diagnosis for adult clients with esophageal cancer:

- **Imbalanced Nutrition: Less Than Body Requirements** related to impaired swallowing

ADDITIONAL NURSING DIAGNOSES AND COLLABORATIVE PROBLEMS

In addition to the common nursing diagnosis, the client with esophageal cancer may develop any of the following resulting from the impact of the disease and its treatment:

- Risk for Aspiration related to impaired swallowing secondary to esophageal strictures
- Impaired Swallowing related to obstruction by the tumor or the effects of radiotherapy
- Acute Pain or Chronic Pain related to the physical injury (pressure of the tumor mass in the esophagus or mediastinum)
- Ineffective Coping and Compromised Family Coping related to the effects of the disease and to the terminal prognosis
- Anticipatory Grieving related to declining physical status and terminal prognosis
- Spiritual Distress related to impending death

The additional collaborative problem is Potential for Metastasis resulting from the close proximity of the esophagus to other body structures.

◆ Planning and Implementation

IMBALANCED NUTRITION: LESS THAN BODY REQUIREMENTS

NOC PLANNING: EXPECTED OUTCOMES. The major concern for a client with esophageal cancer is weight loss secondary to dysphagia. Therefore the client is expected to maintain adequacy of his or her usual pattern of nutrient intake. Indicators include that the client will have totally adequate:

- Caloric intake
- Protein and fat intake
- Carbohydrate intake
- Vitamin and mineral intake

INTERVENTIONS. Interventions to maintain or improve the nutritional status of the client must focus on treatments that remove or shrink the obstructive tumor. Methods to reduce the effects of treatment that can impact nutritional status are also a priority.

NONSURGICAL MANAGEMENT. Treatment options for cancer of the esophagus that can assist in both disease and nutrition management include the following:

- Nutrition therapy
- Swallowing therapy
- Chemotherapy
- Radiation therapy
- Photodynamic therapy
- Esophageal dilation
- Endoscopic therapies
- Surgical removal of the tumor

The treatment of esophageal cancer often involves a combination of the above therapies (**multimodal therapies**). Clients with cancer of the esophagus can experience many problems, and relieving symptoms becomes an essential consideration.

NIC Nutrition Therapy. The purpose of nutrition therapy is the administration of food and fluids to support the client who is malnourished or at high risk of becoming malnourished. A thorough nutritional assessment provides members of the health care team with baseline information concerning the client's nutritional status. The dietitian determines the caloric needs of the client to meet nutritional requirements. Weigh the client daily. Careful positioning is essential for a client who is experiencing frequent regurgitation or who has prosthetic tubes to keep the esophagus patent. Teach the client to remain upright for several hours after meals and to avoid lying completely flat. The head of the bed should remain elevated to a 30-degree angle or more to prevent reflux.

Semisoft foods and thickened liquids are preferred because they are easier to swallow. The total number of calories taken in daily and the amount of fluids ingested are monitored daily to monitor progress toward nutritional goals. Liquid nutritional supplements (e.g., Boost, Ensure) are used between feedings to increase caloric intake. Ongoing efforts are made to preserve the ability to swallow, but feeding tubes may be needed temporarily when dysphagia is severe. In clients with complete obstruction or life-threatening fistula formation, it may be necessary to create a gastrostomy or jejunostomy. Laboratory and clinical indicators of nutritional status are also monitored on a regular basis. The client and family are encouraged to meet with the dietician for diet teaching and planning.

NIC Swallowing Therapy. Consult with the speech-language pathologist to assist the client with oral exercises to improve swallowing. A lollipop given to the client to suck on can enhance tongue strength. The client is instructed to reach for food particles on the lips or chin using the tongue. In preparation for swallowing, you should assist the client to position the head in forward flexion (chin tuck). The client is then instructed to place food at the back of the mouth. Monitor the client for the sealing of lips and for tongue movements while eating and also check for pocketing of food after swallowing. It is important to monitor for signs of aspiration. Family members and caregivers are taught how to feed the client, monitor for aspiration, and institute appropriate measures if choking occurs. Chart 58-9 provides a summary of NIC interventions.

Chemotherapy. The use of chemotherapy in the treatment of esophageal cancer has been only moderately effective. It can be given as a primary treatment if the client is not a candidate for surgery. However, chemotherapy is most often given in combination with radiation therapy. This treatment is thought to provide the client with the best chance of cure. The rationale behind this approach is to shrink the tumor and eliminate any tumor that may be in the local lymph nodes, improving the odds for a complete surgical resection. The two most commonly used chemotherapeutic agents are 5-fluorouracil (5-FU) and cisplatin. Cisplatin and 5-FU make the tumor cells more sensitive to the effects of radiation.

Radiation Therapy. Radiation therapy to manage esophageal cancer is only moderately effective and can be used alone or in combination with other modalities. Radiation given alone can provide palliation of symptoms by shrinking the tumor. It is contraindicated for clients with tracheoesophageal fistula, mediastinitis, mediastinal hemorrhage, or infiltration of the cancer to the trachea or bronchus. Normal esophageal tissue is very sensitive to the effects of radiation, and although higher doses of radiation demonstrate better results, esophageal stricture or stenosis can result in 30% to 50% of clients requiring esophageal dilation.

Radiation therapy is typically administered in 20 episodes over 4 weeks. In the first weeks of treatment, it produces edema and epithelial desquamation, which often create

CHART 58-9

NIC   **INTERVENTION ACTIVITIES for**
The Client with Esophageal Problems

Nutrition Therapy: *Administration of food and fluids to support metabolic processes of a client who is malnourished or at high risk for becoming malnourished*
- Determine—in collaboration with the dietitian, as appropriate—the number of calories and type of nutrients needed to meet nutrition requirements.
- Assist client to a sitting position before eating or feeding.
- Encourage client to select semisoft food, if lack of saliva hinders swallowing.
- Monitor food/fluid ingested and calculate daily caloric intake, as appropriate.
- Determine need for enteral tube feedings.

Swallowing Therapy: *Facilitating swallowing and preventing complications of impaired swallowing*
- Collaborate with speech therapist to instruct client/family about swallowing exercise regimen.
- Explain rationale of the swallowing regimen to client/family.
- Provide a lollipop for client to suck on to enhance tongue strength, if appropriate.
- Assist client to position head in forward flexion in preparation for swallowing ("chin tuck").
- Assist client to place food at back of mouth and on unaffected side.
- Monitor for signs and symptoms of aspiration.
- Instruct family/caregiver how to position, feed, and monitor client.
- Instruct client/caregiver on emergency measures for choking.

NIC intervention activities selected from Dochterman, J.M., & Bulechek, G.M. (Eds.). (2004). *Nursing interventions classification (NIC)* (4th ed.). St. Louis: Mosby. No part of this work is to be altered without prior written permission from the Publisher.

acute esophagitis and odynophagia (painful swallowing). Profound anorexia, nausea, and vomiting may also result. Symptoms persist until treatment is completed. Assess the client frequently to determine the incidence and severity of symptoms. Systemic analgesics are often required to control discomfort, and topical lidocaine (Viscous Xylocaine) can be administered before each attempt at oral feeding.

Assist the client to modify the diet to meet nutritional needs and maintain comfort. Small, frequent, soft or semiliquid meals are offered. Sweet, light foods are often tolerated best, and protein powder may be used to supplement the nutritional content of the diet. An accurate record of calorie counts, intake and output, and daily weights should be maintained. Assess skin turgor and mucous membranes regularly. In collaboration with the health care provider and dietitian, assess the need for enteral nutrition if oral intake is insufficient. Frequent, gentle mouth care is important for clients receiving radiation therapy because clients are at risk for monilial esophagitis. Chapter 28 describes additional nursing interventions for the client undergoing radiation therapy.

Photodynamic Therapy. Photodynamic therapy (PDT) was originally used for the treatment of skin cancer. In 1995 it was approved for use as a palliative treatment for individuals with advanced esophageal cancer, who are not candidates for surgery. The client is injected with porfimer sodium (Photofrin), a light-sensitive drug that acts to amass cancer cells. Two days after the injection, a fiberoptic probe with a light at the tip is threaded into the esophagus. The light activates the Photofrin, destroying only cancer cells.

PDT is far less invasive than surgery and is performed on an ambulatory care basis under conscious sedation.

The side effects of Photofrin are rare but include nausea, fever, and constipation. After the procedure, the client is given written guidelines concerning photosensitivity measures. Instruct the client to avoid exposure to sunlight for 1 month. Sunglasses and protective clothing that covers all exposed body areas are essential. The client may experience chest pain secondary to tissue damage and will require pain relief with opioid analgesics for a short time. Remind the client to follow a clear liquid diet for 3 to 5 days after the procedure and advance to full liquids as tolerated.

Esophageal Dilation. Esophageal dilation may be performed as necessary throughout the course of the disease to achieve temporary but immediate relief of dysphagia. Esophageal dilation can be performed on an ambulatory care basis. Dilators are used to tear soft tissue, thereby widening the esophageal lumen. In most cases, malignant tumors can be dilated safely, but perforation remains a significant risk. Large metal stents may be used to keep the esophagus open for longer durations. A stent covered with graft material can be used to seal a perforation. Bacteremia can also occur. To reduce the risk of endocarditis, the American Heart Association recommends prophylaxis with antibiotics. The treatment is repeated as often as needed to preserve the client's ability to swallow.

Endoscopic Therapies. When clients are not candidates for surgery or the tumor is too large to remove surgically, laser therapy or electrocoagulation may be performed as a palliative measure. Both of these methods destroy cancer cells to improve swallowing.

SURGICAL MANAGEMENT. The goals of surgical resection vary from palliation to cure. **Esophagectomy** is the removal of all or part of the esophagus. An **esophagogastrostomy** involves the removal of part of the esophagus and proximal stomach. The remaining stomach may be "pulled up" to take the place of the esophagus, or the jejunum or colon may be used as a conduit. Conventional open surgical techniques can take 6 to 8 hours and are associated with significant morbidity and mortality. Mortality as a result of open surgery ranges from 10% to 20%. Complications (e.g., fistula formation, abscess, respiratory complications) occur in 20% to 50% of individuals.

For clients with early stage cancer, a **minimally invasive esophagectomy (MIE)** via laparoscopy may be performed. However, most clients require the conventional open surgery because of tumor size and metastasis.

Preoperative Care. Preoperative preparation for clients undergoing esophagectomy or esophagogastrostomy can be quite extensive, especially before conventional techniques. Clients are advised to stop smoking 2 to 4 weeks before surgery to enhance their pulmonary functioning. Client preparation may include 5 days to 2 to 3 weeks of nutritional support in an effort to improve nutritional status and decrease postoperative morbidity. Ideally this supplementation is given orally, but many clients require tube feeding or parenteral nutrition. The role of parenteral nutritional support in these clients remains controversial. Monitor the client's weight, intake and output, and fluid and electrolyte balance. A preoperative dental evaluation may be required to remove pre-existing dental caries. Provide meticulous oral care four times daily to decrease the risk of postoperative infection.

Preoperative nursing care also focuses on teaching and on psychological support regarding the surgical procedure and preoperative and postoperative instructions. Educate the client about the following:

- The number and sites of all incisions and drains
- The placement of a jejunostomy tube for initial enteral feedings
- The need for chest tubes if the pleural space is entered
- The purpose of the nasogastric tube
- The need for intravenous (IV) infusion

Instruct the client about routines for turning, coughing, deep breathing, and chest physiotherapy. Emphasize the crucial nature of postoperative respiratory care. If colon interposition (resecting a piece of colon and creating an esophagus) is planned, the client also undergoes a complete bowel preparation with laxatives and enemas before surgery.

The client facing a serious illness and extensive surgery can be expected to display feelings of grief and anxiety. Encourage the client to talk about personal feelings and fears, and involve the family or significant others in all preoperative teaching and discussions. A primary nurse or case manager can be extremely helpful in providing continuity of care and support to the entire family.

Operative Procedures. In the MIE procedure, the surgeon makes four or five small incisions in the chest and abdomen. The lower esophagus and gastric fundus are removed. The remaining portion of the esophagus is then anastomosed (reconnected) to the stomach.

For most clients, an open subtotal or total esophagectomy is required because tumors are often quite large and involve distant lymph nodes. The diseased portion of the esophagus is removed, and the cervical portion is anastomosed (connected) to the stomach. The cervical portion of the stomach is then brought up into the thorax through the esophageal hiatus (Figure 58-3). A **pyloromyotomy** is created to prevent gastric motility disturbances. Finally, a jejunostomy tube may be placed for postoperative enteral feeding.

For clients with early stage tumors of the lower third of the esophagus, a transhiatal esophagectomy is the preferred surgical approach. The surgery is performed through an upper midline cervical incision. With this approach there is no entry into the pleural space, reducing respiratory complications. For clients with tumors in the upper esophagus, a radical neck dissection and laryngectomy may also be needed if the disease has spread to the larynx. The surgeon may perform a **colon interposition** when the tumor involves the stomach or the stomach is otherwise unsuitable for anastomosis. A section of right or left colon is removed and brought up into the thorax to substitute for the esophagus (see Figure 58-3).

Postoperative Care. These surgical procedures pose cardiovascular risks for the client. Intraoperative hypotension can result from pressure on the posterior heart. Pulmonary edema can occur when mediastinal lymph nodes and lymphatics are resected due to decreased pulmonary clearance and lymphatic congestion. The stress placed on the heart by extensive surgery can increase the risk of myocardial ischemia and dysrhythmias, especially if the client has underlying coronary disease.

The client with compromised nutritional status or prior radiation or chemotherapy is predisposed to an increased risk of infection. For clients who undergo more radical surgical procedures, there is a serious risk of leakage at the anastomosis site. This situation is especially true with colon interpositions because several anastomosis sites are vulnerable to the effects of tension, poor blood supply, and delayed healing. Mediastinitis resulting from an anastomotic leak can lead to fatal sepsis.

The client requires meticulous postoperative care and is at risk for multiple serious complications. The Plan of Care on pp. 1269 to 1272 outlines client interventions for esophageal surgery.

Respiratory Care. *Respiratory care is the highest postoperative priority.* For the client having traditional surgery, intubation with mechanical ventilation is needed for at least the

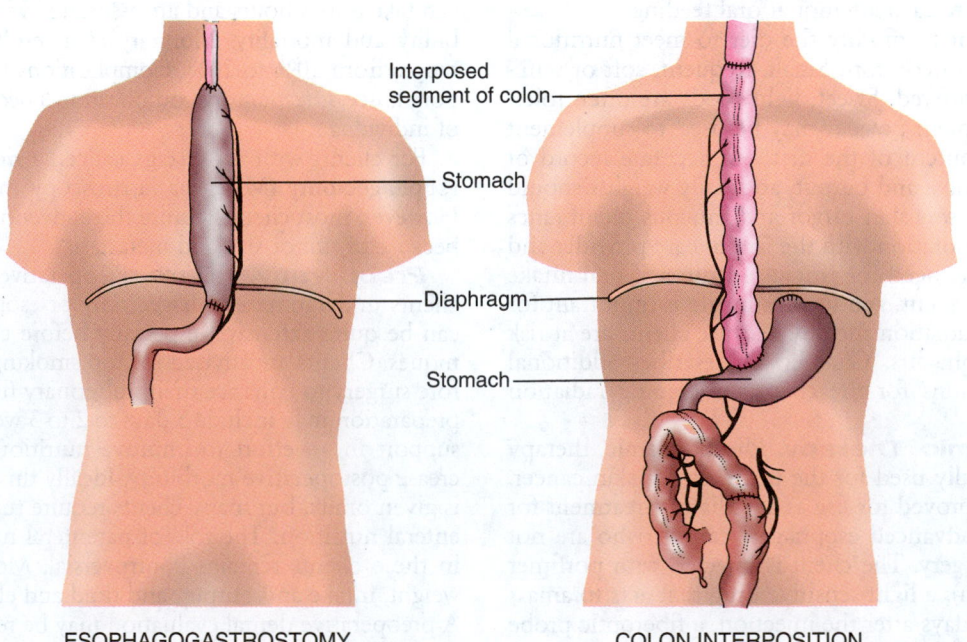

ESOPHAGOGASTROSTOMY   COLON INTERPOSITION

Interposed segment of colon

Stomach

Diaphragm

Stomach

Figure 58-3 ■ Open surgical approaches to the treatment of esophageal cancer.

first 24 hours. Postoperative pulmonary complications include atelectasis and pneumonia. The risk of postoperative pulmonary complications is increased in the client who has received preoperative radiation. Once the client is extubated, deep breathing, turning, and coughing routines should begin. Chest physiotherapy is initiated as ordered, usually every 2 to 4 hours. Assess the client for decreased breath sounds and shortness of breath every 1 to 2 hours. Incisional support and adequate analgesia are essential for effective coughing and should be administered regularly if the client's vital signs remain stable. Keep the client in a semi-Fowler's or high Fowler's position to support ventilation and prevent reflux. The health care provider prescribes prophylactic antibiotics and supplemental oxygen; blood gases are ordered regularly. Ensure the patency of the chest tube drainage system, and monitor for changes in the volume or color of the drainage.

Cardiovascular Care. Cardiovascular complications, particularly hypotension, can occur secondary to pressure placed on the posterior heart, and usually respond well to IV fluid administration. Monitor for manifestations of fluid volume overload, particularly in older clients and in those who have undergone lymph node dissection. Assess for edema, crackles in the lungs, and increased jugular venous pressure. In the immediate postoperative phase, the client may be admitted to the intensive care unit. Critical care nurses assess hemodynamic parameters such as cardiac output, cardiac index, and systemic vascular resistance every 2 hours to monitor for myocardial ischemia. Atrial fibrillation is a dysrhythmia that results from irritation of the vagus nerve during surgery and must be managed.

Wound Management. Wound management is another significant postoperative concern for conventional surgery because the client typically has multiple incisions and drains. Provide incisional support during turning and coughing to prevent dehiscence. Wound infection usually occurs 4 to 5 days after surgery. Postoperative leakage from the site of anastomosis is a dreaded complication that can appear 2 to 10 days after surgery. If an anastomotic leak occurs, all oral intake is discontinued and is not resumed until the leak has healed. Nutrition may be given through the jejunostomy tube during the healing process. Carefully assess for fever, fluid accumulation, general signs of inflammation, and symptoms of early shock (e.g., tachycardia, tachypnea), and report these findings to the health care provider immediately.

Nasogastric Tube Management. A nasogastric (NG) tube is placed intraoperatively to decompress the suture line. Monitor the NG tube for patency and carefully secure the tube to prevent dislodgment, which can disrupt the sutures at the anastomosis. *Do not independently irrigate or reposition the NG tube in clients who have undergone esophageal surgery!* The initial nasogastric drainage is bloody but should change to a greenish yellow color by the end of the first postoperative day. The continued presence of blood may indicate bleeding at the suture line. Oral hygiene should be provided to the client every 2 to 4 hours while the tube is in place (Chart 58-10).

Nutritional Care. The nutritional management of the client who has undergone an esophageal surgery is an early postoperative concern. After conventional surgery, on the second postoperative day, initial feedings begin through the jejunostomy tube. The feedings are slowly increased over the next several days. Feeding by this method can be discontinued once the client is taking adequate oral nutrition. However, some clients may require jejunostomy feedings for about 1 month if small amounts of aspiration are detected.

Before beginning oral feedings, a cine-esophagram study is performed to detect the presence of anastomotic leaks, strictures, or signs of aspiration. If no leaks are detected, an esophageal diet is begun, starting with liquids. If liquids are well tolerated, the client's diet is advanced to include semi-solid foods and then solid foods. The client should be placed in an upright position and supervised during all initial swallowing efforts. The food storage area of the stomach has been radically decreased, and gravity is the client's only real defense against reflux. The client is instructed to consume six to eight meals per day and to ingest fluids between, rather than with, meals to prevent diarrhea. Diarrhea can occur 20 minutes to 2 hours after eating and can be symptomatically managed with loperamide (Imodium) before meals. The diarrhea is thought to be the result of **vagotomy syndrome,** which develops as a result of the interruption of vagal fibers to the abdominal viscera during surgery. This syndrome is diminished by pyloroplasty. Assessment for signs of anastomotic leakage should be continued throughout hospitalization.

> ### ? Critical Thinking Challenge
>
> Your client has been told he is not a candidate for curative surgery for his esophageal cancer and will be receiving combination chemoradiation as a palliative treatment.
> 1. What should you teach the client about these treatments?
> 2. What other types of services should you anticipate this client will require?
> 3. What psychological issues is this client facing?
>
> **evolve** For suggested answer guidelines, go to http://evolve.elsevier.com/Iggy/.

Community-Based Care

Clients with esophageal cancer have many challenges to face once they are discharged home. The combination treatment regimens cause long-lasting side effects, such as fatigue and

---

CHART 58-10

BEST PRACTICE for
Managing the Client with a Nasogastric Tube After Esophageal Surgery

- Check for tube placement every 4 to 8 hours.
- Ensure that the tube is patent (open) and draining; drainage should turn from bloody to yellowish green by the end of the first postoperative day.
- Secure the tube well to prevent dislodgment.
- Do not irrigate or reposition the tube without a physician's order.
- Provide meticulous oral and nasal hygiene every 2 to 4 hours.
- Keep the head of the bed elevated to at least 30 degrees.
- When the client is permitted to have a small amount of water, place the client in an upright position and observe for dysphagia (difficulty swallowing).
- Observe for leakage from the anastomosis site, as indicated by fever, fluid accumulation, and manifestations of early shock (tachycardia, tachypnea, altered mental status).

weakness. These complex treatments also require the client to be knowledgeable about symptom management and to know when to report issues of concern to the health care provider. (See Chapter 28 for care of the client undergoing radiation therapy and chemotherapy.)

HOME CARE MANAGEMENT

The client having minimally invasive surgery has a shorter hospital stay and fewer complications compared with conventional surgical clients. Clients with MIE usually stay several days in the hospital and return to usual activities sooner than those having traditional surgical procedures. Many clients have chemotherapy and radiation after surgery.

Once the client is discharged home, ongoing respiratory care is a priority. Give the client and family members instructions about ambulation and incentive spirometer use. Encourage the client to be as active as possible and to avoid excessive bedrest because this can lead to complications. Teach the family to protect the client from infection and to contact the health care provider immediately if signs of respiratory infection develop.

HEALTH TEACHING

Teach the client and family to inspect the incisions daily for redness, tenderness, swelling, odor, and discharge because proper wound healing is still a concern at the time of discharge. Instruct the client and family to report a temperature greater than 101° F (38.3° C). Prepare written instructions about the signs of anastomosis leakage and the importance of reporting them to the health care provider immediately. Instruct the client and family members to report the presence of fever and a swollen, painful neck incision, which indicate a cervical anastomotic leak.

Nutritional support also remains a concern. Encourage the client to continue increasing oral feedings as tolerated. Instruct the client to eat small, frequent meals containing high-calorie, high-protein foods that are soft and easily swallowed. Instruct the client to use supplemental eggnogs and milkshakes between meals, and instruct the client to eat slowly. Individuals who have undergone esophageal resection can lose up to 10% of their body weight. Teach the client to monitor his or her weight at home and to report a weight loss of 5 pounds or more. If sufficient oral intake is not possible, the family may need instruction about tube feedings or parenteral nutrition at home.

Emphasize the importance of remaining upright after meals. Dysphagia or odynophagia may recur because of stricture, reflux, or cancer recurrence. These symptoms should be promptly reported to the health care provider. Despite radical surgery, the client with cancer of the esophagus still has a terminal illness and a relatively short life expectancy. Emphasis is placed on maximizing quality of life. (See Evidence-Based Practice for Nursing box above). Realistic planning is important as the client's condition eventually worsens, and the client and family are assisted to plan for the future together. Assist family members in exploring formal and informal sources of support. Help the family or significant others arrange for hospice care when it is needed.

HEALTH CARE RESOURCES

Referrals to community or home care organizations should be initiated to assist the family in providing care in the home. The client may need transportation to the radiation treatment center five times per week for up to 6 weeks. Oncology nursing care may be needed to monitor and evaluate the client who is receiving chemotherapy at home through venous access devices or portable infusion pumps. Inform the client and family about the services available through the American Cancer Society. Familiarize the family with area hospice services for future planning.

◆ Evaluation: Outcomes

Evaluate the care of the client with esophageal cancer on the basis of the identified nursing diagnoses. The major expected outcome is that the client will be able to consume adequate nutrition and maintain a stable weight. Other outcomes for postoperative esophageal surgical clients are outlined in the Plan of Care on pp. 1269 to 1272. Specific indicators for this outcome are listed for the nursing diagnosis under the Planning and Implementation section (see earlier).

DIVERTICULA

PATHOPHYSIOLOGY

Diverticula are sacs resulting from the herniation of esophageal mucosa and submucosa into surrounding tissue. Diverticula may develop anywhere along the length of the esophagus. No environmental risk factors are known to be involved in the development of esophageal diverticula. The incomplete or late opening of the cricopharyngeal muscle during swallowing leads to high pressures in the hypopharynx and leads to *Zenker's diverticulum*, the most common

---

EVIDENCE-BASED PRACTICE for Nursing

What is the quality of life for a client who has undergone esophagectomy for cancer?

Sweed, M.R., et al. (2002). Quality of life after esophagectomy for cancer. *Oncology Nursing Forum, 29*(7), 1127-1131.

The purpose of this longitudinal, descriptive pilot study was to evaluate the quality of life (QOL) in 23 clients who had undergone esophagectomy for esophageal cancer. The European Organization for Research and Treatment of Cancer (EORTC) questionnaire was used to measure QOL at four time points. This tool contains five subscales that measure function, three symptom subscales, a global health status, a QOL scale, and six single items scored from 0 to 100, with higher scores equaling a higher response level. Measures were taken at baseline (before chemoradiation), 2 weeks following esophagectomy, 3 months after surgery and 6 months after surgery.

The study supported previous findings of weight loss, diarrhea, and acid reflux occurring post-esophagectomy. Increased hoarseness was also found, but it could not be attributed to the surgery itself. The study concluded that overall QOL remains stable after esophagectomy, but severity of symptoms can affect QOL.

Level of Evidence: 6—This research was a descriptive pilot that serves as a basis for future study.

Critique. Although the study is limited by the small sample size and some findings that were not statistically significant, it provides important beginning data on symptoms that affect QOL after curative esophagectomy for esophageal cancer. This study should be replicated with a larger sample to confirm findings to assist in helping nurses to develop interventions to improve QOL in this population.

Implications for Nursing. Nurses need to be supportive and yet realistic when caring for clients with esophageal cancer and surgery. Expected changes in QOL tend to occur when symptoms become more severe.

form. Zenker's diverticulum occurs most often in older adults. Clients complain of dysphagia, regurgitation, nocturnal cough, and halitosis (bad breath). Clients with esophageal diverticula can be at risk for esophageal perforation because the mucosa is without the protection of the normal esophageal muscle layer.

COLLABORATIVE MANAGEMENT

Esophageal diverticula are diagnosed by barium swallow and esophagogastroduodenoscopy (EGD). If endoscopy is done, it must be performed with strict care because of the risk of perforation. Diet therapy and positioning are the major interventions for controlling symptoms related to diverticula. The dietitian assists the client in exploring variations in the size and frequency of meals and in food texture and consistency. Semisoft foods and smaller meals are often best tolerated and may reduce or relieve the symptoms of pressure and reflux. Nocturnal reflux associated with diverticula is managed by instructing the client to sleep with the head of the bed elevated and to avoid the recumbent position for at least 2 hours after eating. Counsel the client to avoid vigorous exercise after meals. Advise the client to avoid restrictive clothing and frequent stooping or bending.

Surgical management is aimed at excising the diverticula and reapproximating the mucosa. Postoperatively the client takes nothing by mouth for several days to promote healing. During that period, the client receives IV fluids for hydration, tube feedings, and then oral fluid and food. Provide pain relief measures, and monitor for complications such as bleeding or perforation. A nasogastric (NG) tube is placed during surgery for decompression and is *not* irrigated or repositioned unless specifically ordered by the surgeon.

Community-based care includes teaching the client and family about the following:
- Tube feeding and resuming an oral diet
- Positioning guidelines to prevent reflux
- Warning signs of complications

Community resources are usually not needed for uncomplicated cases.

ESOPHAGEAL TRAUMA

PATHOPHYSIOLOGY

Trauma to the esophagus can result from blunt injuries, chemical burns, surgery or endoscopy, or the stress of protracted severe vomiting (Table 58-2). Trauma may affect the esophagus directly, impairing swallowing and nutrition, or it may create problems and complications in related structures such as the lungs or mediastinum. The incidence of most forms of esophageal trauma is low in adults. When excessive

TABLE 58-2   Common Causes of Esophageal Perforation
- Straining
- Seizures
- Trauma
- Foreign objects
- Instrument or tubes
- Chemical injury
- Complications of esophageal surgery
- Ulcers

force is exerted on the esophageal mucosa, it may perforate or rupture, allowing the caustic acid secretions to enter the mediastinal cavity. These tears are associated with a high mortality rate related to shock, respiratory impairment, or sepsis.

Chemical injury is usually a result of the accidental or intentional ingestion of caustic substances. The oral cavity is also usually damaged, and the damage is rapid and severe. Acid burns tend to affect the superficial layers of the esophagus, whereas alkaline substances cause deeper penetrating injuries. Strong alkalis can cause full perforation of the esophagus within 1 minute. Additional problems may include aspiration pneumonia and hemorrhage. Strictures may develop as scar tissue forms.

COLLABORATIVE MANAGEMENT

Clients with esophageal trauma are initially evaluated and treated in the emergency department. Assessment focuses on the nature of the injury and the circumstances surrounding it. Assess for the presence of an airway, chest pain, dysphagia, vomiting, or bleeding. If the risk of extending the damage is not excessive, an x-ray or endoscopic study may be ordered to evaluate tears or perforation. A computed tomography (CT) scan of the chest can be done to assess for the presence of mediastinal air.

After the injury, keep the client NPO (nothing by mouth) to prevent further leakage of esophageal secretions. Esophageal and gastric suction can be used for drainage and to rest the esophagus. Esophageal rest is maintained for at least 10 days after injury to allow for initial healing of the mucosa. Total parenteral nutrition (TPN) is prescribed to provide calories and protein for wound healing while the client is not eating.

To prevent sepsis, broad-spectrum antibiotics are prescribed. High-dose corticosteroids may be administered to suppress inflammation and prevent strictures. In addition, opioid and nonopioid analgesics are prescribed for pain management. When caustic burns involve the oral cavity, topical agents, such as 50/50 diphenhydramine hydrochloride (Benadryl) and kaolin with pectin (Kapectolin) or topical lidocaine (Viscous Xylocaine), may be used for topical analgesia and local anti-inflammatory action.

If nonsurgical management is not effective in healing traumatized esophageal tissue, the client may need surgery to remove the damaged tissue. The client with severe injuries may require resection of part of the esophagus with a gastric pull-through and repositioning or replacement by a bowel segment. (See Surgical Management [Esophageal Tumors], p. 1277.)

GET READY for the NCLEX Examination!

KEY POINTS

Safe Effective Care Environment

- Teach client and family to recognize the symptoms of dysphagia.
- Remain with the dysphasic client during meals to prevent or assist with choking episodes.
- Teach the client oral exercises aimed at improving swallowing.

Health Promotion and Maintenance

- Consult with dietitian, client, and family regarding dietary restrictions for clients with GERD.
- Stress the importance of recognizing and controlling reflux through dietary and medications to avoid further esophageal damage that could lead to Barrett's esophagus.
- Teach the client to elevate the head of the bed by 6 inches for sleep to prevent nighttime reflux.
- Instruct the client to sleep in the left lateral decubitus position to minimize the effects of nighttime episodes of reflux.
- Teach the client with esophageal cancer to monitor his or her body weight and to notify the health care provider for a loss of 5 pounds or greater.
- Teach the client to avoid alcoholic beverages, smoking, and other substances as listed in Chart 58-2 because they lead to increased gastroesophageal reflux.
- Teach the client to prevent gas bloat syndrome by avoiding drinking carbonated beverages, eating gas-producing foods, chewing gum, and drinking with a straw.
- Review post-procedure instructions for clients having endoscopic therapies for GERD as outlined in Chart 58-4.

Psychosocial Integrity

- Allow the client the opportunity to express fear or anxiety regarding the diagnosis of esophageal cancer and related treatment regimen of surgery, chemotherapy, and radiation.
- Explain all procedures, restrictions, medications, and follow-up care to the client and family.
- Refer the client or family members to psychological counseling, hospice, pastoral care, and the social worker as needed.

Physiological Integrity

- For clients with GERD, teach the importance of strict adherence to antireflux agents in preventing esophageal damage (see Chart 58-3).
- Be aware that laparoscopic Nissen fundoplication (LNF) is the most common surgical procedure for clients with GERD and hiatal hernia; LNF may also be performed for clients with achalasia.
- Recall that achalasia is an esophageal motility disorder caused by esophageal denervation, which can lead to severe complications, such as carcinoma and aspiration pneumonia.
- Assess for complications and provide postoperative care for clients having the LNF procedure as described in Charts 58-6 and 58-7.
- Teach the client having open esophageal surgery about incisions, drains, and jejunostomy tube placement before he or she undergoes surgery for esophageal cancer.
- For the client with a nasogastric (NG) tube, check the NG tube every 4 to 8 hours for proper placement and anchorage; follow guidelines as outlines in Chart 58-10.
- Assess the postoperative esophageal surgical client for pulmonary and cardiac complications of surgery, and report changes to the health care provider.
- Assess clients for key features of esophageal tumors as listed in Chart 58-8.
- Provide care for clients with esophageal surgery as discussed in the Plan of Care.

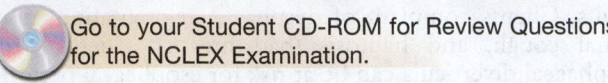

ADDITIONAL STUDY RESOURCES

Go to your Student CD-ROM for Review Questions for the NCLEX Examination.

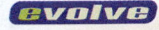

Go to http://evolve.elsevier.com/Iggy/ for Integrated Management of Care Questions for the NCLEX Examination.

SELECTED BIBLIOGRAPHY

American Cancer Society. (2003). *Cancer facts and figures 2003*. Report No. 01-300M-No. 5008.03. Atlanta: Author.

Arbogast, D. (2002). Enteral feedings with comfort and safety. *Clinical Journal of Oncology Nursing, 6*(5), 275-282.

Brooks-Brunn, J.A. (2000). Esophageal cancer: An overview. *MEDSURG Nursing, 9*(5), 248-254.

Bruce, S. (2001). Photodynamic therapy: Another option in cancer treatment. *Clinical Journal of Oncology Nursing, 5*(3), 95-100.

Daly, B. (2000). The special challenges of withholding artificial nutrition and hydration. *Journal of Gerontological Nursing, 26*(9), 25-31.

Fackler, W.K., & Richter, J.E., (2000). Refractory GERD: What next? *Consultant*, May, pp. 973-983.

Fennerty, B., et al. (2002). New paradigms for the treatment of acid-related reflux disorders. *Patient Care for the Nurse Practitioner, Special Edition*, Fall, 3-12.

Field, S. (2003). Detecting patients with hidden GERD. *Clinical Advisor*, 23-34.

Goroll, A., & Mulley, A. (2000). Evaluation of dysphagia and suspected esophageal chest pain. *Primary Care Medicine* (4th ed., pp. 389-394). Philadelphia: Lippincott Williams & Wilkins.

Hemminger, L.L., & Wolfsen, H.C. (2002). Photodynamic therapy for Barrett's esophagus and high-grade dysplasia: results of a patient satisfaction survey. *Gastrointestinal Nursing, 25*(4), 139-141.

Hubbard, P.M. (2002). Update on gastroesophageal reflux disease. *The American Journal for Nurse Practitioners, 2*, 9-18.

Maguire, M. (2000). Nutritional care of surgical oncology patients. *Seminars in Oncology Nursing, 16*(2), 128-134.

McCormick, D.G. (2004). Stretta procedure for the treatment of gastroesophageal reflux disease. *Gastroenterology Nursing, 27*(1), 22-28.

Nilsson, G., et al. (2002). Patient's experience of illness, operation and outcome with reference to gastroesophageal reflux disease. *Journal of Advanced Nursing, 40*(3), 307-315.

Parkman, H., MacMillan Rooney, W., & Rogers, H. (2000). Empiric therapy for nonulcer dyspepsia. *Patient Care for the Nurse Practitioner, 3*(1), 23-34.

Rayhorn, N., Argel, N., & Demchak, K. (2003). Understanding gastroesophageal reflux disease. *Nursing 2003, 33*(10), 36-41.

Rockney, A.D. (2002). What you need to know about Barrett's esophagus. *Gastroenterology Nursing, 25*(6), 237-240.

Strader, S.L. (2001). Esophageal motor disorders: Achalasia and esophageal spasm. *Journal of the American Academy of Nurse Practitioners, 13*(11), 502-507.

Sweed, M., et al. (2002). Quality of life after esophagectomy for cancer. *Oncology Nursing Forum, 29*(7), 1127-1131.

Terrado, M., Russell, C., & Bowman, J. (2001). Dysphagia: An overview. *MEDSURG Nursing, 10*(5), 233-248.

Interventions for Clients with Stomach Disorders

JACQUELYN R. GIBBS

Although only a few diseases affect the stomach, they can be very serious and in some cases life threatening. The most common disorders include gastritis, peptic ulcer disease, Zollinger-Ellison syndrome, and gastric carcinoma (cancer).

GASTRITIS

Gastritis is defined as inflammation of the gastric mucosa (stomach lining). It can be scattered or localized and can be classified according to cause, cellular changes, or distribution of the lesions. Gastritis can be designated as erosive (acute gastritis, stress ulcers) or nonerosive (chronic gastritis). Although the mucosal changes accompanying acute gastritis typically resolve after several months, this is not true for chronic gastritis.

PATHOPHYSIOLOGY

Prostaglandins provide a protective mucosal barrier that prevents the stomach from digesting itself by a process called acid **autodigestion.** If there is a break in the protective barrier, mucosal injury occurs. The resulting injury is compounded by histamine release and vagal nerve stimulation. Hydrochloric acid can then diffuse back into the mucosa and injure small vessels. This back-diffusion results in edema, hemorrhage, and erosion of the stomach's lining. The pathologic changes of gastritis include vascular congestion, edema, acute inflammatory cell infiltration, and degenerative changes in the superficial epithelium of the stomach lining.

The early pathologic manifestation of gastritis is a thickened, reddened mucous membrane with prominent **rugae**, or folds. As the disease progresses, the walls and lining of the stomach thin and atrophy. With progressive gastric atrophy from chronic mucosal injury, the function of the parietal (acid-secreting) cells decreases and the source of intrinsic factor is lost. The intrinsic factor is critical for absorption of vitamin B_{12}. When body stores of vitamin B_{12} are eventually depleted, **pernicious anemia** results. The amount and concentration of acid in stomach secretions gradually decrease until the secretions consist of only mucus and water.

Chronic gastritis is associated with an increased risk of gastric cancer as the persistent inflammation extends deep into the mucosa, causing destruction of the gastric glands and cellular changes. Hemorrhage may occur after an episode of acute gastritis or with ulceration caused by chronic gastritis.

Acute Gastritis

Inflammation of the gastric mucosa or submucosa after exposure to local irritants can result in **acute gastritis**. Various degrees of mucosal necrosis and inflammatory reaction occur in acute disease. The diagnosis cannot be based solely on clinical symptoms. Complete regeneration and healing usually occur within a few days. If the stomach muscle is not involved, complete recovery usually occurs with no residual evidence of gastric inflammatory reaction.

Chronic Gastritis

Chronic gastritis appears as a patchy, diffuse (spread out) inflammation of the mucosal lining of the stomach. Chronic gastritis usually heals without scarring, but it can progress to hemorrhage and the formation of an ulcer.

Chronic gastritis may be categorized as type A, type B, or atrophic. Type A (nonerosive) chronic gastritis refers to an inflammation of the glands, as well as the fundus and body of the stomach. Type B chronic gastritis usually affects the glands of the antrum but may involve the entire stomach. In atrophic chronic gastritis, diffuse inflammation and destruction of deeply located glands accompany the condition. Chronic atrophic gastritis affects all layers of the stomach, thus decreasing the number of cells. The muscle becomes thickened, and inflammation is present. Chronic atrophic gastritis is characterized by total loss of fundal glands, minimal inflammation, thinning of the gastric mucosa, and intestinal metaplasia (abnormal tissue development).

Etiology and Genetic Risk

ACUTE GASTRITIS

The onset of infection with *Helicobacter pylori* can result in acute gastritis. *H. pylori* is a gram-negative, spiral-shaped bacterium that penetrates the mucosal gel layer of the gastric epithelium. Although it is uncommon, other forms of bacterial gastritis from organisms such as staphylococci, streptococci, *Escherichia coli*, or salmonella can cause life-threatening consequences such as sepsis and extensive tissue necrosis (death). Other infectious causes of acute gastritis can be found in clients with immunosuppressive disorders. In clients with acquired immunodeficiency syndrome (AIDS), for example, gastric erosions can be found with herpes simplex viral infection and disseminated cytomegalovirus (CMV) infection.

Nonsteroidal anti-inflammatory drug (NSAID) use poses a risk for the development of acute gastritis. Gastritis occurs in 5% to 25% of NSAID users, but the exact mechanism of the role of NSAIDs in the development of gastritis is not well understood. Other drugs, including alcohol, cytotoxic agents, caffeine, and corticosteroids, have also been implicated; however, scientific evidence is lacking. Acute gastritis is also caused by local irritation from radiation therapy and accidental or intentional ingestion of corrosive substances, including acids or alkalis (e.g., lye and drain cleaners). In the client who is allowed nothing by mouth (NPO), gastritis may result from lack of stimulation of normal secretions. Acute stress-induced gastritis, characterized by multiple shallow erosions of the proximal stomach, may be present in 80% to 100% of critically ill clients.

CHRONIC GASTRITIS

Type A gastritis has been associated with the presence of antibodies to parietal cells and intrinsic factor; therefore an autoimmune pathogenesis for this type of gastritis has been proposed. Parietal cell antibodies have been found in 90% of clients with pernicious anemia and in more than one half of individuals with type A gastritis. A genetic link to this disease, with an autosomal dominant pattern of inheritance, has been noted in the relatives of clients with pernicious anemia.

The most common form of the disease is **type B gastritis**, caused by *H. pylori* infection. There is a direct correlation between the number of organisms and the degree of cellular abnormality present. Although serum antibodies have been isolated in some clients, it is believed that these antibodies are not representative of an autoimmune process but are the result of prolonged inflammation. Fifty percent of clients who have gastric ulcers have associated chronic gastritis.

Chronic local irritation and toxic effects caused by alcohol ingestion, radiation therapy, and smoking have been implicated in the development of chronic gastritis. Surgical procedures that involve the pyloric sphincter, such as the Billroth II procedure, can lead to gastritis by causing reflux of alkaline secretions into the stomach. Other systemic disorders such as Crohn's disease, graft-versus-host disease, and uremia can also precipitate the development of chronic gastritis.

Atrophic gastritis is a type of chronic gastritis that is seen most often in older adults. It can occur after exposure to toxic substances in the workplace (e.g., benzene, lead, and nickel) or *H. pylori* infection, or it can be related to autoimmune factors.

Although atrophic gastritis is often present in people with gastric cancer, it is not always considered a precancerous lesion. Gastric carcinoma develops in fewer than 10% of clients who have atrophic gastritis. Chart 59-1 lists guidelines for preventing gastritis.

Incidence/Prevalence

About 2.7 million people in the United States have gastritis. The incidence of gastritis is higher in men than in women; although it has been suggested that more women have chronic

---

CHART 59-1

CLIENT EDUCATION GUIDE
Gastritis Prevention

- Avoid drinking excessive amounts of alcoholic beverages.
- Use caution in taking large doses of aspirin, nonsteroidal anti-inflammatory drugs (e.g., ibuprofen), and corticosteroids. Prolonged use of small doses of corticosteroids may also cause gastritis.
- Avoid excessive intake of caffeine-containing beverages.
- Avoid eating contaminated foods or drinking contaminated water.
- Stop smoking.
- Protect yourself against exposure to toxic substances in the workplace, such as lead and nickel.
- Seek medical treatment if you are experiencing symptoms of esophageal reflux (see Chapter 58).

atrophic gastritis. Acute and chronic forms of the disease are more prevalent in heavy smokers and persons who abuse alcohol. The incidence of chronic gastritis increases with age.

HEALTH PROMOTION/ILLNESS PREVENTION

Balanced diet, regular exercise, and stress reduction techniques help prevent gastritis. A balanced diet includes following the recommendations of the U.S. Department of Agriculture (USDA) food pyramid and limiting intake of foods and spices that can cause gastric distress such as tea, coffee, cola, chocolate, mustard, paprika, cloves, pepper, and hot spices. Alcohol and tobacco consumption should be avoided. Regular exercise maintains peristalsis, which helps prevent gastric contents from irritating the gastric mucosa. Stress reduction techniques can include cardiovascular exercise, meditation, reading, and/or yoga depending on individual preferences. Psychotherapy may also be considered.

Excessive use of aspirin and other NSAIDs should also be avoided. Clients with problems such as back pain that find themselves needing to take NSAIDs frequently need to see their health care provider promptly so the pain can be managed under medical supervision. If a family member or significant other has *H. pylori* infection or has had it in the past, then testing should be considered. This test could diagnose, treat, and eradicate the bacteria before it causes gastritis.

◆COLLABORATIVE MANAGEMENT
◆Assessment

PHYSICAL ASSESSMENT/CLINICAL MANIFESTATIONS

Physical assessment findings may include abdominal tenderness and bloating, **hematemesis** (vomiting blood), or **melena** (traces of blood in the stool). In stress-induced gastritis, symptoms of intravascular volume depletion and shock may be present.

ACUTE GASTRITIS. Symptoms of acute gastritis can range from mild to severe. Epigastric discomfort, anorexia, cramping, nausea, and vomiting may be present. In some cases, gastric hemorrhage is the presenting symptom (Chart 59-2). The symptoms last only a few hours or days and vary with the cause. Aspirin-related gastritis may result in dyspepsia

---

CHART 59-2

KEY FEATURES of
Gastritis

Acute Gastritis
- Rapid onset of epigastric pain or discomfort
- Nausea and vomiting
- Hematemesis (vomiting blood)
- Gastric hemorrhage
- Dyspepsia (heartburn)
- Anorexia

Chronic Gastritis
- Vague complaint of epigastric pain that is relieved by food
- Anorexia
- Nausea or vomiting
- Intolerance of fatty and spicy foods
- Pernicious anemia

(heartburn). Gastritis from alcohol abuse may cause vomiting and hematemesis. Gastritis or food poisoning caused by endotoxins, such as staphylococcal endotoxin, has an abrupt onset; severe nausea and vomiting often occur within 5 hours of ingestion of the contaminated food.

CHRONIC GASTRITIS. Chronic gastritis causes few symptoms. Clients may complain of nausea, vomiting, or upper abdominal discomfort. Periodic epigastric pain may simulate ulcer-like distress, which is relieved on ingestion of food. Some clients may have anorexia, and pain may be exacerbated by eating fatty or spicy foods (see Chart 59-2).

DIAGNOSTIC ASSESSMENT

Esophagogastroduodenoscopy (EGD) via an endoscope with biopsy is the gold standard for diagnosing gastritis, as well as detecting the presence of *H. pylori*. The health care provider uses biopsy to establish a definitive diagnosis of the type of gastritis. If lesions are patchy and diffuse, biopsy of several suspicious areas may be necessary to avoid misdiagnosis. A cytologic examination of the biopsy specimen is performed to confirm or rule out gastric cancer.

◆Common Nursing Diagnoses and Collaborative Problems

Nursing diagnoses and collaborative problems that may apply to clients with gastritis include the following:
1. Acute Pain or Chronic Pain related to physical injury (inflammation)
2. Nausea related to gastric irritation
3. Deficient Knowledge related to unfamiliarity with information resources
4. Potential for Hemorrhage

◆Interventions

Clients with gastritis are not often seen in the acute care setting unless they have an exacerbation ("flare up") of acute or chronic gastritis that results in fluid and electrolyte imbalance or bleeding. Management is directed toward supportive care for relieving the symptoms and removing the cause of discomfort.

Acute gastritis is treated symptomatically and supportively because the healing process is spontaneous, usually occurring within a few days. When the cause is removed, pain and discomfort usually subside. If hemorrhage is severe, a blood transfusion may be necessary. Fluid replacement is indicated in clients with severe fluid loss. Surgery, such as partial gastrectomy, pyloroplasty, and/or vagotomy, may be indicated for clients with major bleeding or ulceration. Treatment of chronic gastritis varies with the cause. General treatment goals include the elimination of causative agents, treatment of any underlying disease (e.g., uremia, Crohn's disease), and avoidance of toxic substances (e.g., alcohol, tobacco, nonsteroidal anti-inflammatory drugs [NSAIDs]).

NONSURGICAL MANAGEMENT. The identification and elimination of the causative factors, such as *H. pylori* infection, is the primary treatment modality. Drugs and diet therapy are also used in the treatment of gastritis.

Drug Therapy. In the acute phase, the health care team directs actions toward relief of pain and discomfort. The health care provider may prescribe medications that block and buffer gastric acid secretions to relieve pain.

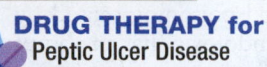

CHART 59-3

DRUG THERAPY for
Peptic Ulcer Disease

Drug	Usual Dosage	Nursing Interventions	Rationales
Antacids			
Magnesium hydroxide with aluminum hydroxide (Maalox, Mylanta)	50-80 mEq 1 hr and 3 hr after meals and at bedtime	Give 2 hr after meals and at bedtime.	Hydrogen ion load is high after ingestion of foods.
		Use liquid rather than tablets.	Suspensions are more effective than chewable tablets.
		Do not give other drugs within 1-2 hr of antacids.	Antacids interfere with absorption of other drugs.
		Assess the client for a history of renal disease.	Hypermagnesemia may result. These antacids have a high sodium content.
			These antacids contain magnesium, which cannot be excreted by poorly functioning kidneys, thus causing toxicity.
		Assess the client for a history of heart failure.	Inadequate renal perfusion from heart failure decreases the ability of the kidneys to excrete magnesium, thus causing toxicity.
		Observe the client for the side effect of diarrhea.	Magnesium often causes diarrhea.
Aluminum hydroxide (Amphojel)	50-80 mEq 1 hr and 3 hr after meals and at bedtime	Give 1 hr after meals and at bedtime.	Hydrogen ion load is high after ingestion of food.
		Use liquid rather than tablets if palatable.	Suspensions are more effective than chewable tablets.
		Do not give other drugs within 1-2 hr of antacids.	Antacids interfere with absorption of other drugs.
		Observe the client for the side effect of constipation. If constipation occurs, consider alternating with magnesium antacid.	Aluminum causes constipation, and magnesium has a laxative effect. Aluminum binds with phosphates in the gastrointestinal (GI) tract.
		Use for clients with renal failure.	This antacid does not contain magnesium.
H₂ Antagonists			
Ranitidine (Zantac)	150 mg PO twice daily or 300 mg PO at bedtime; 50 mg IV q6h or 8 mg/hr IV (continuous)	Give single dose at bedtime for treatment of GI ulcers. **NOTE:** IV ranitidine may also be given to prevent surgical stress ulcers.	Bedtime administration suppresses nocturnal acid production.
Famotidine (Pepcid)	40 mg PO once daily or in two divided doses; 20 mg IV q12h	Give single dose at bedtime.	Bedtime administration suppresses nocturnal acid production. Compliance may improve with less frequent administration.
Nizatidine (Axid)	150 mg PO twice daily or 300 mg at bedtime	Give single dose at bedtime.	Bedtime administration suppresses nocturnal acid production. Compliance may improve with less frequent administration.

H₂-receptor antagonists are typically used to block gastric secretions. The most common agents include ranitidine (Zantac), famotidine (Pepcid), and nizatidine (Axid). Sucralfate (Carafate, Sulcrate✲), a mucosal barrier fortifier, may also be prescribed. Antacids used as buffering agents include aluminum hydroxide combined with magnesium hydroxide (Maalox) and aluminum hydroxide combined with simethicone and magnesium hydroxide (Mylanta). Antisecretory agents (proton-pump inhibitors) such as omeprazole (Prilosec) or esomeprazole magnesium (Nexium) may also be used to suppress gastric acid secretion (Chart 59-3). Monitor for symptom relief and side effects of these medications and notify the health care provider of any untoward effects or worsening of gastric distress.

Clients with chronic gastritis may require vitamin B₁₂ for prevention or treatment of pernicious anemia. If *H. pylori* is found in biopsy specimens, the health care provider may treat the infection and reverse or prevent impairment of mucosal defenses. A common drug regimen for *H. pylori* infection includes triple therapy, which may include bismuth subsalicylates (Pepto-Bismol) or a proton-pump inhibitor such as omeprazole (Prilosec), and a combination of two antibiotics such as metronidazole (Flagyl, Novonidazol✲) and tetracycline or clarithromycin and amoxicillin.

The nurse, health care provider, or pharmacist instructs clients about the medications associated with gastric irritation. These medications include chemotherapeutic agents, corticosteroids, erythromycin (E-Mycin, Erythromid✲), and

CHART 59-3

DRUG THERAPY for
Peptic Ulcer Disease—cont'd

Drug	Usual Dosage	Nursing Interventions	Rationales
Mucosal Barrier Fortifiers			
Sucralfate (Carafate, Sulcrate ✱)	1 g PO four times daily or 2 g twice daily	Give 1 hr before and 2 hr after meals, and at bedtime. Do not give within 30 min of giving antacids or other drugs.	Food may interfere with drug's adherence to mucosa. Antacids may interfere with effect.
Antisecretory Agents			
Omeprazole (Prilosec, Losec ✱)	20 mg PO twice daily or 40 mg at bedtime	Have the client take capsule whole; do not crush. Give single dose at bedtime for ulcer disease.	Delayed-release capsules allow absorption after granules leave the stomach. Bedtime administration suppresses nocturnal acid production.
Lansoprazole (Prevacid)	15 or 30 mg PO at bedtime	Give single dose at bedtime for ulcer disease; do not crush.	Bedtime administration suppresses nocturnal acid production.
Rabeprazole (AcipHex)	20 mg PO once daily	Take following the morning meal. Do not crush capsule.	Drug promotes healing and symptom relief of duodenal ulcers. Drug is a sustained-release capsule.
Pantoprazole (Protonix)	40 mg PO or IV daily	Do not crush. IV form must be given with filter and in a separate line.	Drug is enteric-coated. Given IV, drug precipitates easily.
Esomeprazole (Nexium)	20 or 40 mg PO daily	Give 1 hr before meals. Assess for hepatic impairment.	Food decreases absorption. Clients with severe hepatic problems need a low dose.
Prostaglandin Analogues			
Misoprostol (Cytotec)	200 mcg PO four times daily	Take with food. Avoid magnesium-containing antacids.	Drug protects against nonsteroidal anti-inflammatory drug (NSAID)–induced ulcers. Both misoprostol and magnesium-containing antacids can cause diarrhea.
Antimicrobials			
Clarithromycin (Biaxin)	500 mg PO three times daily	Antimicrobials should be given as part of therapy to eradicate Helicobacter pylori infection. The selection of the specific drug depends on its effectiveness, side effects, and drug interactions.	*H. pylori* is a gram-negative bacterium implicated in the development of peptic ulcer disease (PUD).
Amoxicillin (Amoxil)	1 g PO twice daily		
Tetracycline	500 mg PO four times daily		
Metronidazole (Flagyl)	250 mg PO three times daily and at bedtime		

NSAIDs, such as aspirin, naproxen (Naprosyn), and ibuprofen (Motrin, Advil, Amersol ✱, Novo-Profen ✱).

The health care provider may change the dose, frequency, or type of medication if symptoms of gastric irritation appear or persist. Instruct clients to avoid stomach-irritating over-the-counter (OTC) medications, such as aspirin and ibuprofen.

Diet Therapy. Instruct the client with gastric disease to limit intake of any foods and spices that cause distress. Tea, coffee, cola, chocolate, mustard, paprika, cloves, pepper, and hot spices may increase discomfort. Alcohol and tobacco should also be avoided.

After the client has an acute episode of gastritis, help him or her identify foods that cause discomfort. New foods should be introduced one at a time. Avoidance of substances that cause symptoms is important. Most clients seem to progress better with a soft, bland diet and smaller, more frequent meals.

Stress Reduction. Assist the client with various techniques that reduce stress and discomfort, such as progressive relaxation, cutaneous stimulation, guided imagery, and distraction. (See Chapter 4 for a discussion of these therapies.)

SURGICAL MANAGEMENT. Partial gastrectomy, pyloroplasty, vagotomy, or even total gastrectomy may be indicated for clients who have major bleeding caused by severe erosive gastritis. Such surgery is necessary only if more conservative measures have not controlled the bleeding. Surgical interventions are discussed under Surgical Management (Peptic Ulcer Disease), p. 1296.

PEPTIC ULCER DISEASE

A **peptic ulcer** is a mucosal lesion of the stomach or duodenum. The term *peptic ulcer* is used to describe both gastric and duodenal ulcers. **Peptic ulcer disease (PUD)** results when gastric mucosal defenses become impaired and no longer protect the epithelium from the effects of acid and pepsin (Figure 59-1).

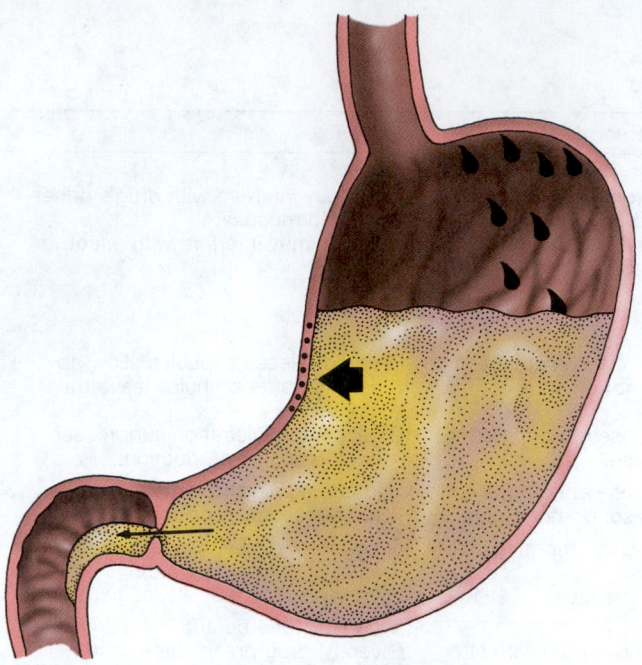

Conditions favoring the development of **gastric ulcers** are normal gastric acid secretion and delayed stomach emptying with *increased diffusion of gastric acid back into the stomach tissues.*

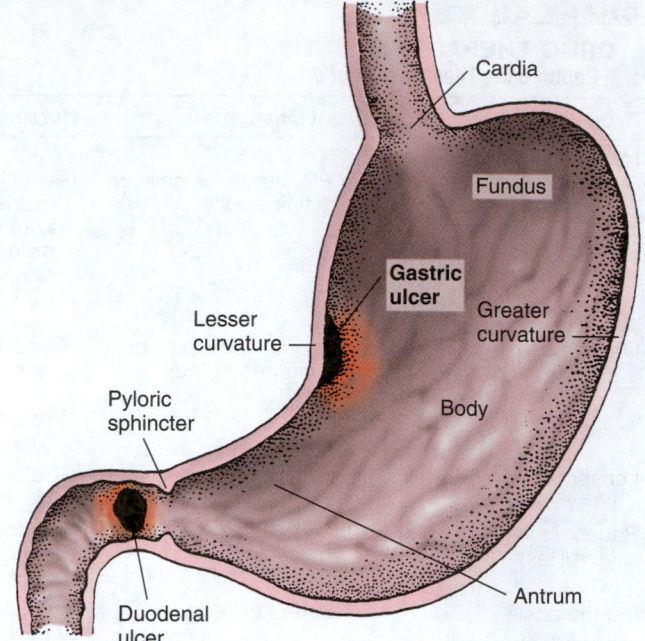

Figure 59-2 ■ The most common sites for peptic ulcers.

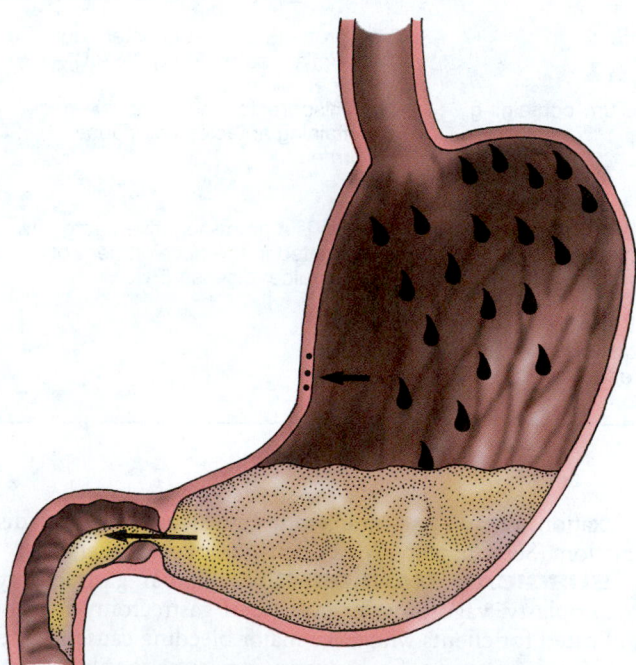

Conditions favoring the development of **duodenal ulcers** are normal diffusion of acid back into stomach tissues with *increased secretion of gastric acid* and *increased stomach emptying.*

Figure 59-1 ■ The pathophysiology of peptic ulcer.

PATHOPHYSIOLOGY

Gastric Ulcers

Acid, pepsin, and *H. pylori* infection play an important role in the development of gastric ulcers. The gastric mucosal barrier overlies the epithelium. The secretion of mucus and bicarbonate provides a first line of defense in maintaining a near-normal pH on the gastric epithelium and protects the mucosal barrier against acid. Gastromucosal prostaglandins increase the barrier's resistance to ulceration. The integrity of the barrier is enhanced by the rich blood supply of the mucosa of the stomach and duodenum.

When a break in the mucosal barrier occurs, hydrochloric acid injures the epithelium. Gastric ulcers may then result from back-diffusion of acid or dysfunction of the pyloric sphincter (see Figure 59-1). Without normal functioning of the pyloric sphincter, bile refluxes (backs up) into the stomach. This reflux of bile acids may break the integrity of the mucosal barrier and produce hydrogen ion back-diffusion, which leads to mucosal inflammation. Toxic agents and bile then destroy the lipid plasma membrane of the gastric mucosa.

Gastric emptying is often delayed in clients with gastric ulceration. This causes regurgitation of duodenal contents, which compounds the gastric mucosal injury. A decreased blood flow to the gastric mucosa may also alter the defense barrier and thereby allow ulceration to occur. Characteristically, gastric ulcers are deep and penetrating, and they usually occur on the lesser curvature of the stomach, near the pylorus (Figure 59-2).

Duodenal Ulcers

Most duodenal ulcers occur in the first portion of the duodenum. Duodenal ulcers present as deep, sharply demarcated lesions that penetrate through the mucosa and submucosa into the muscularis propria (muscle layer). The floor of the ulcer consists of a necrotic area residing on granulation tissue and surrounded by areas of fibrosis.

The characteristic feature of a duodenal ulcer is high gastric acid secretion, although a wide range of secretory levels is found. In clients with duodenal ulcers, pH levels are low in the duodenum for long periods. Protein-rich meals, calcium, and vagal excitation stimulate acid secretion. Combined with hypersecretion, a rapid emptying of food from the stomach reduces the buffering effect of food and delivers a large acid bolus to the duodenum (see Figure 59-1). Inhibitory secretory mechanisms and pancreatic secretion may be insufficient to control the acid load.

Many clients with duodenal ulcer disease have confirmed *H. pylori* infection. *H. pylori* produces substances that damage the gastric mucosa. Urease produced by *H. pylori* catalyzes the hydrolysis of urea to ammonia. Hydrogen ions are then released in response to the presence of ammonia and contribute further to gastric mucosal damage.

Stress Ulcers

Stress ulcers are acute gastric mucosal lesions occurring after an acute medical crisis or trauma. Stress ulcers have been associated with head injury, major surgery, burns, respiratory failure, shock, and sepsis. Bleeding caused by gastric erosion is the principal manifestation of acute stress ulcers. Multifocal lesions associated with stress ulcers occur in the proximal portion of the stomach and duodenum. These lesions begin as focal areas of ischemia and evolve into erosions and ulcerations that may progress to massive hemorrhage. Little is known of the exact etiology of stress ulcers; however, in the presence of elevated levels of hydrochloric acid, ischemic areas can progress to erosive gastritis and subsequent ulcerations. Stress ulcers are associated with lengthened hospital stay by as much as 11 days and mortality rates greater than 50% (Rotello, 2003).

Complications of Ulcers

The most common complications of PUD are hemorrhage, perforation, pyloric obstruction, and intractable disease.

HEMORRHAGE

Hemorrhage occurs in about 15% to 25% of clients with PUD and is the most serious complication (Figure 59-3). It tends to occur more often in clients with gastric ulcers and in older adults. Of those with an initial bleed, 40% experience a recurrence of bleeding if underlying infection with *H. pylori* remains untreated or if therapy does not include an H_2 antagonist. With massive bleeding, the client vomits bright red or coffee-ground blood (**hematemesis**). Hematemesis usually indicates bleeding at or above the duodenojejunal junction (**upper gastrointestinal [GI] bleeding**).

Minimal bleeding from ulcers is manifested by occult blood in a tarry stool (melena). Melena may occur in clients with gastric ulcers but is more common in those with duodenal ulcers. Gastric acid digestion of blood typically results in a granular dark vomitus (coffee-ground appearance); the digestion of blood within the duodenum and small intestine may result in a black stool.

PERFORATION

Gastric and duodenal ulcers can perforate or bleed. Perforation occurs when the ulcer becomes so deep that the entire thickness of the stomach or duodenum is worn away. The stomach or duodenal contents can then leak into the surrounding abdomen. In clients with perforation, the gastroduodenal contents (acid peptic juice, bile, and pancreatic juice) empty through the anterior wall of the stomach or duodenum into the peritoneal cavity. Sudden, sharp pain begins in the midepigastric region and spreads over the entire abdomen. The amount of pain correlates with the amount and type of GI contents spilled. The characteristic pain causes the

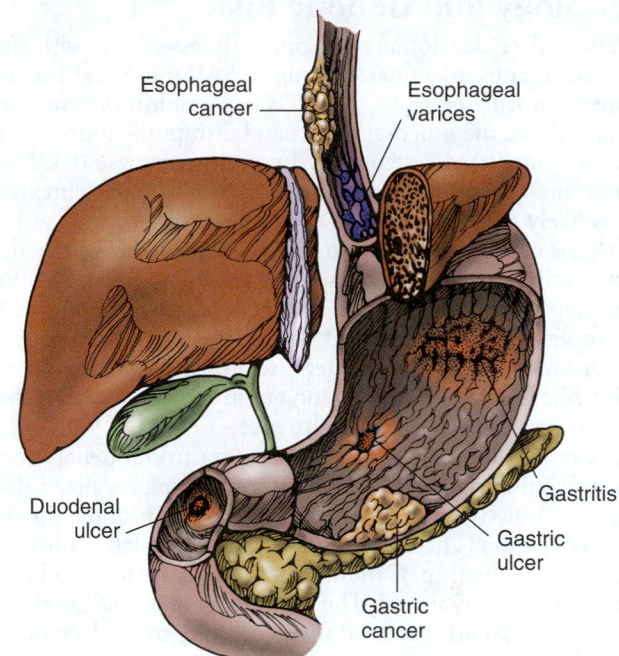

Figure 59-3 ■ Common causes of upper gastrointestinal bleeding.

client to be apprehensive. The abdomen is tender, rigid, and boardlike. The client assumes the knee-chest ("fetal") position to decrease the tension on the abdominal muscles. The client may become desperately ill within hours. Chemical peritonitis soon occurs; bacterial septicemia and hypovolemic shock follow. Peristalsis diminishes, and paralytic ileus develops. Peptic ulcer perforation is considered a surgical emergency and can be life threatening.

PYLORIC OBSTRUCTION

Pyloric obstruction (blockage) occurs in a small percentage of clients and is manifested by vomiting caused by stasis and gastric dilation. Obstruction occurs at the pylorus (the gastric outlet) and is caused by scarring, edema, inflammation, or a combination of these factors.

Symptoms of gastric outlet obstruction include abdominal bloating, nausea, and vomiting. When vomiting persists, the client may experience hypochloremic (metabolic) alkalosis from loss of large quantities of acid gastric juice (hydrogen and chloride ions) in the vomitus. Hypokalemia may also result from the vomiting or metabolic alkalosis. The health care provider typically hospitalizes the client so he or she may receive intravenous (IV) fluid and electrolyte replacement.

INTRACTABLE DISEASE

One third of all clients with ulcers have a single episode with no recurrence. However, intractability may develop from complications of ulcers, excessive stressors in the client's life, or an inability to adhere to long-term therapy. The client no longer responds to conservative management, or recurrences of symptoms interfere with activities of daily living (ADLs). In general, the client continues to have recurrent pain and discomfort despite treatment. Clients who fail to respond to traditional treatments or who have a relapse following discontinuation of therapy should be referred to a gastroenterologist.

Etiology and Genetic Risk

Peptic ulcer development is primarily associated with non-steroidal anti-inflammatory drug (NSAID) use and bacterial infection with *H. pylori*. NSAIDs (e.g., aspirin or ibuprofen) break down the mucosal barrier and disrupt the mucosal protection mediated systemically by cyclooxygenase (COX) inhibition. COX-2 inhibitors, such as celecoxib (Celebrex), are less likely to cause mucosal damage but place clients at high risk for cardiovascular events, such as myocardial infarction. In addition, NSAIDs cause the depletion of endogenous prostaglandins, resulting in local gastric mucosal injury. GI complications from NSAID use can occur at any time, even after long-term uncomplicated use. NSAID-related ulcers are difficult to treat, even with long-term therapy, because these ulcers have a high rate of recurrence.

Certain drugs may contribute to gastroduodenal ulceration by altering gastric secretion, producing localized damage to mucosa and interfering with the healing process. Theophylline (Theo-Dur) and caffeine stimulate hydrochloric acid production. Caffeine may contribute to vascular stasis and mucosal anoxia. The use of corticosteroids is also associated with an increased incidence of peptic ulceration.

H. pylori infection is transmitted from person to person, but the exact mode of transmission remains uncertain. Studies have suggested that it is spread either fecally–orally or by mouth-to-mouth contact, such as by kissing or perhaps by ingesting contaminated food or water (Perry, 2002).

Genetic factors may be important. Some studies found that 50% of children with PUD have a first- or second-degree relative with PUD. First-degree relatives of clients with duodenal ulcers have a threefold increase in the prevalence of duodenal (but not gastric) ulcers, and relatives of clients with gastric ulcers have a threefold increase in the prevalence of gastric (but not duodenal) ulcers (Soll, 2002).

Incidence/Prevalence

In the United States, PUD affects about 4.5 million people annually. One in 10 Americans develops an ulcer at some time in his or her life (see the Resource Management box above). Physician office visits and hospitalizations for PUD have decreased in the last few decades. The mortality rate has also decreased in the last few decades and is about 1 death per 100,000 cases. The hospitalization rate is about 30 clients per 100,000 cases. Duodenal ulcers are increasing in older women, which may be the result of increased NSAID use for arthritic pain (Fantry, 2003).

HEALTH PROMOTION/ILLNESS PREVENTION

Health promotion and illness prevention practices are the same as for gastritis. For critically ill clients, health care providers may consider prophylactic therapy to prevent stress ulcers from occurring. This includes focusing on optimal oxygenation and circulation, which may involve finding and treating the underlying cause of bleeding aggressively. In addition health care providers may consider starting a client on enteral nutrition. Enteral nutrition is suggested to have a beneficial effect on the stomach mucosa because the artificial enteral products are alkaline. Finally, health care providers may consider drug therapy with H_2 antagonists, antacids, sucralfate, or antisecretory agents to prevent stress ulcers from occurring (McCarthy, 2003).

◆COLLABORATIVE MANAGEMENT
◆Assessment

HISTORY

Collect data related to the causes and risk factors for peptic ulcer disease (PUD). Question the client about dietary factors that can influence the development of PUD, such as alcohol intake and tobacco use. Note if certain foods, such as tomatoes, or caffeinated beverages precipitate or worsen symptoms. Information regarding actual or perceived daily stressors is also elicited.

A history of current or past medical conditions focuses on gastrointestinal (GI) tract problems, particularly any history of diagnosis or treatment for *H. pylori* infection. A complete evaluation of all prescription and OTC medications is obtained. Specifically inquire whether the client is taking corticosteroids, aspirin, or other nonsteroidal anti-inflammatory drugs (NSAIDs). Also ask whether the client has ever undergone radiation treatments.

A history of GI upset, pain and its relationship to eating and sleep patterns, and actions taken to relieve pain is also important. Inquire about any changes in the character of the pain, because this may signal the development of complications. For example, if pain that was once intermittent and relieved by food and antacids becomes constant and radiates to the back or upper quadrant, this may indicate impending ulcer perforation. It is important to note that many individuals with active duodenal or gastric ulcers report having no ulcer symptoms.

TABLE 59-1   Differential Features of Gastric and Duodenal Ulcers

Feature	Gastric Ulcer	Duodenal Ulcer
Age	Usually 50 yr or older	Usually 50 yr or older
Gender	Male/female ratio of 1.1:1	Male/female ratio of 1:1
Blood group	No differentiation	Most often type O
General nourishment	May be malnourished	Usually well nourished
Stomach acid production	Normal secretion or hyposecretion	Hypersecretion
Occurrence	Mucosa exposed to acid-pepsin secretion	Mucosa exposed to acid-pepsin secretion
Clinical course	Healing and recurrence	Healing and recurrence
Pain	Occurs 30-60 min after a meal; at night: rarely	Occurs $1\frac{1}{2}$-3 hr after a meal; at night: often awakens client between 1 and 2 AM
	Accentuated by ingestion of food	Relieved by ingestion of food
Response to treatment	Healing with appropriate therapy	Healing with appropriate therapy
Hemorrhage	Hematemesis more common than melena	Melena more common than hematemesis
Malignant change	Perhaps in less than 10%	Rare
Recurrence	Tends to heal and recurs often in the same location	60% recur within 1 yr; 90% recur within 2 yr
Surrounding mucosa	Atrophic gastritis	No gastritis

PHYSICAL ASSESSMENT/CLINICAL MANIFESTATIONS

Physical assessment findings may reveal epigastric tenderness, usually located at the midline between the umbilicus and the xiphoid process. If perforation into the peritoneal cavity is present, the client exhibits a rigid, boardlike abdomen accompanied by rebound tenderness. Initially, auscultation of the abdomen may reveal hyperactive bowel sounds, but these may diminish with progression of the disorder.

Dyspepsia (indigestion), which is defined as discomfort centered around the epigastrium or upper abdomen, is the most commonly reported symptom associated with PUD. It is typically described as sharp, burning, or gnawing. Some clients may perceive discomfort as a sensation of abdominal pressure or of fullness or hunger.

> ### CONSIDERATIONS FOR OLDER ADULTS
> Both duodenal and gastric ulcers occur more often following the sixth decade of life. Pain is less often the initial complaint in the older client. In this age group, **melena** (occult blood) is often the presenting sign. Acute confusion and dizziness may also occur as a result of the lack of oxygen to the brain.

Gastric ulcer pain often occurs in the upper epigastrium with localization to the left of the midline and may be relieved by food. *Duodenal* ulcer pain is usually located to the right of the epigastrium (Table 59-1). The pain associated with a duodenal ulcer occurs 90 minutes to 3 hours after eating and often awakens the client at night. Pain may also be exacerbated by certain foods (e.g., tomatoes, hot spices, fried foods, onions, alcohol, or caffeine drinks) and certain medications (e.g., aspirin, NSAIDs, or corticosteroids).

Vomiting may be a symptom accompanying ulcer disease, most commonly with pyloric sphincter dysfunction. It results from gastric stasis associated with pyloric obstruction. Appetite is generally maintained in clients with a peptic ulcer unless pyloric obstruction is present.

To assess for fluid volume deficit, which can occur secondary to bleeding, take orthostatic vital signs of all clients suspected of having PUD. Orthostatic changes are characterized by a decrease of more than 20 mm Hg in systolic blood pressure, a decrease of 10 mm Hg in diastolic blood pressure, and/or an increase in pulse when the client rises from a lying to an erect (sitting or, if possible, standing) position. Also assess for dizziness, especially when the client is upright, because this is another symptom of fluid volume deficit.

PSYCHOSOCIAL ASSESSMENT

Assess the impact of ulcer disease on the client's lifestyle, occupation, family, and social and leisure activities. Questions about lifestyle, occupation, and leisure can yield important information. Evaluate the impact that lifestyle changes will have on the client. This assessment determines the client's ability to comply with the prescribed treatment regimen and to obtain the needed social support to alter his or her lifestyle.

LABORATORY ASSESSMENT

Hemoglobin and hematocrit values may be low, indicating bleeding. The stool specimen may be positive for occult (not apparent on visual inspection) blood if bleeding is present.

RADIOGRAPHIC ASSESSMENT

A barium examination of the GI tract can be used to establish a duodenal ulcer. A duodenal ulcer appears as a discrete crater in the duodenal bulb. This is often the initial test for a client who does not have severe symptoms. If perforation is suspected, the health care provider usually requests an upright abdomen series to demonstrate free air in the peritoneum. In any instance where free air is a possibility, barium should not be used.

OTHER DIAGNOSTIC ASSESSMENTS

The major diagnostic test for PUD is esophagogastroduodenoscopy (EGD), which is the most accurate means of establishing a diagnosis. Visualization of the ulcer crater by EGD allows the health care provider to take specimens for *H. pylori* testing and for biopsy and cytologic studies for ruling out gastric cancer (see the Legal/Ethical Issues box on p. 1292). EGD may be repeated at 4- to 6-week intervals while the health care provider evaluates the progress of healing in response to therapy.

≡LEGAL/ETHICAL ISSUES

QUALITY OF CARE FOR MEDICARE CLIENTS WITH PEPTIC ULCER DISEASE

Economic constraints on the health care system have resulted in efforts to provide cost-effective, high-quality care. To improve the quality of care delivered to Medicare beneficiaries with peptic ulcer disease (PUD), a chart review of 2644 Medicare beneficiaries was conducted to measure compliance with National Institutes of Health (NIH) guidelines for the detection and treatment of *Helicobacter pylori* in PUD.

In this particular study, only 57% of hospitalized Medicare recipients with PUD were tested for *H. pylori*. In addition, only 74% of clients with known *H. pylori* infection were treated with appropriate antimicrobial therapy. Medical record review also noted that 74% of clients were screened for nonsteroidal anti-inflammatory drug (NSAID) use. Only 24% had documented counseling regarding the risks associated with NSAID use, and only 2% had documented education of the ulcer-associated risks of NSAID use.

Although limited documented education may be in part to blame for the poor quality of care regarding *H. pylori*–related ulcers, NIH clinical practice guidelines for the diagnosis and treatment of peptic ulcer disease are clearly underutilized. Quality improvement initiatives are needed to improve the care delivered to Medicare beneficiaries with PUD. *H. pylori* screening and treatment guidelines need to be enforced to ensure that appropriate treatment is received, especially by older adults.

Data from Offman, J., et al. (2000). The quality of care for Medicare patients with peptic ulcer disease. *American Journal of Gastroenterology 95*(1), 106-113.

A common noninvasive test for *H. pylori* involves IgG serologic testing. Infection with *H. pylori* causes immunoglobulin antibodies to form. Although antibody assays have a high sensitivity and specificity (>95%) for detecting *H. pylori*, antibody assays cannot be used to document elimination of the organism, because antibody levels can remain elevated despite successful treatment.

Urea breath testing has been employed to detect *H. pylori* when endoscopy is not clinically indicated. To perform this test, the client must be on NPO status after midnight on the night before the test. The client drinks a carbon-enriched urea solution. The presence of *H. pylori* causes the bacteria to break down the solution and release carbon dioxide, which the client exhales in a collection container for analysis. The carbon dioxide excreted in the breath is then measured and compared with a baseline measurement to determine the presence of *H. pylori*. In addition to its noninvasive nature, this test assesses the entire stomach and may prove especially helpful in determining whether treatment was successful. The breath test is 96% to 98% accurate.

Stool tests may also be used to detect *H. pylori*. The test detects *H. pylori* antigen in the stool (National Digestive Diseases Information Clearinghouse, 2002).

A complete medication history needs to be obtained before diagnostic testing is done for *H. pylori*. False-negative results could be obtained if the client has received antibiotic treatment, used a bismuth preparation (Pepto-Bismol), or used a proton-pump inhibitor within the 4-week period before testing for *H. pylori*. Other medications, such as misoprostol, sucralfate, or an H_2-blocker administered within the week before the test may also yield a false-negative result. Use of over-the-counter medications (OTC), such as Pepcid AC, Tagamet, and Zantac, can also affect test results.

◆Analysis

COMMON NURSING DIAGNOSES AND COLLABORATIVE PROBLEMS

The priority nursing diagnosis for clients with peptic ulcer disease (PUD) is Acute Pain or Chronic Pain related to physical (gastric and/or duodenal mucosal) injury.

The collaborative problem that is of most concern is Potential for Gastrointestinal (GI) Bleeding.

ADDITIONAL NURSING DIAGNOSES AND COLLABORATIVE PROBLEMS

In addition to the common nursing diagnosis and collaborative problem, clients with PUD may have one or more of the following:

- Deficient Knowledge related to management of PUD
- Imbalanced Nutrition: Less Than Body Requirements related to anorexia, nausea, or diet constraints
- Disturbed Sleep Pattern related to discomfort
- Risk for Falls related to orthostatic hypotension
- Fatigue related to loss of blood and chronic illness
- Nausea related to gastrointestinal irritation
- Ineffective Health Maintenance related to lack of knowledge regarding health practices to prevent ulcer formation
- Fear related threat to well-being or potential death

Possible collaborative problems include the following:

- Potential for Shock
- Potential for Metabolic Alkalosis

◆Planning and Implementation

ACUTE PAIN; CHRONIC PAIN

NOC **PLANNING: EXPECTED OUTCOMES.** PUD causes significant discomfort that impacts many aspects of daily living. The client with PUD is expected to take personal actions to control pain. Indicators include that the client will:

- Report that pain is controlled.
- Use available resources.
- Use previous measures.
- Report uncontrolled symptoms to health care professionals.

INTERVENTIONS. Interventions to manage pain related to PUD are accomplished with specific ulcer therapy and dietary modifications. One of the primary purposes for employing drug therapy in the management of PUD is to reduce or eliminate pain. Analgesics are not the mainstay of pain relief for PUD. Instead, the ulcer drug regimen itself promotes relief of pain by eradicating *H. pylori* infection and promoting healing of gastric mucosa.

CONSIDERATIONS FOR OLDER ADULTS

Older adults tend to use over-the-counter (OTC) remedies, often delaying appropriate treatment for symptoms of PUD. In addition, they often suffer from one or more chronic illnesses that require the use of medications that can precipitate or worsen PUD. Older adults may also be at increased risk for complications and death following acute peptic ulcer bleeding.

Perform a comprehensive pain assessment that includes the following aspects of pain:

- Location
- Characteristics
- Onset/duration
- Frequency
- Quality
- Severity
- Precipitating and alleviating factors

Any changes in the characteristics or location of peptic ulcer pain are carefully assessed, because such changes often accompany the development of complications. Teach the client to eliminate irritants (e.g., spicy foods) that can precipitate or increase pain from ulcer disease.

Measures to promote adequate rest and sleep may be necessary, because ulcer pain can cause the client to awaken. Assist the client in achieving compliance with the medication regimen, because adherence to the drug regimen promotes relief of pain and discomfort. Monitor the client's satisfaction with the level of pain relief.

Drug Therapy. The primary goals of drug therapy in the treatment of PUD are (1) to provide pain relief, (2) to eradicate *H. pylori* infection, (3) to heal ulcerations, and (4) to prevent recurrence (see Chart 59-3). Several different regimens can be used to achieve these goals. In selecting a therapeutic drug regimen, the health care provider must consider the efficacy of the treatment, the anticipated side effects, the ability of the client to comply with the regimen, and the cost of the treatment.

Although numerous drugs have been evaluated for the treatment of *H. pylori* infection, no single agent has been used successfully against the organism. Current practice involves using a combination of agents to achieve treatment goals. The most successful regimen used is a triple therapy consisting of a bismuth compound or a proton-pump inhibitor such as omeprazole (Prilosec), and a combination of two antibiotics such as metronidazole (Flagyl, Novonidazol✱) and tetracycline or clarithromycin and amoxicillin. Although this regimen is the most effective and least expensive, adherence to the regimen is difficult for most clients. A client must consume medications four times daily for up to 14 days, and adverse effects occur in 20% to 30% of individuals, especially in older adults. Some strains of *H. pylori* have begun to demonstrate metronidazole resistance, raising concerns about long-term treatment with this regimen.

Hyposecretory Drugs. Hyposecretory drugs produce a reduction in gastric acid secretions. These drugs include antisecretory agents, H_2-receptor antagonists, and prostaglandin analogues (see Chart 59-3).

Antisecretory Agents. These medications are also called proton pump inhibitors and have emerged as the drug class of choice for treating clients with acid-related disorders (Horn, 2000). Omeprazole (Prilosec), lansoprazole (Prevacid), rabeprazole (Aciphex), pantoprazole (Protonix), and esomeprazole magnesium (Nexium) suppress the H, K-ATPase enzyme system of gastric acid production. Omeprazole, lansoprazole, and esomeprazole magnesium are each available as delayed-release capsules designed to release their contents outside of the stomach. Omeprazole and lansoprazole may be dissolved in a solution of sodium bicarbonate and given through any feeding tube. Bicarbonate protects the dissolved omeprazole and lansoprazole granules

in gastric acid. Therefore the drugs are still absorbed correctly. These capsules can also be opened. The enteric-coated capsules can be put in apple juice or orange juice and given through a large-bore feeding tube (McCarthy, 2003). Rabeprazole (Aciphex) and pantoprazole (Protonix) are enteric-coated tablets that quickly dissolve after the tablet has moved through the stomach and cannot be crushed before administration. Pantoprazole (Protonix) is also available in an IV form, which may be helpful for clients who are NPO.

H_2-Receptor Antagonists. Drugs that block histamine-stimulated gastric secretions are effective in the management of ulcer disease. These medications may be used for indigestion and heartburn. Lower-dose forms are available in over-the-counter (OTC) products. H_2-receptor antagonists block the action of the H_2 receptors of the parietal cells, thus inhibiting gastric acid secretion. The most common drugs are ranitidine (Zantac), famotidine (Pepcid), and nizatidine (Axid). These drugs are typically administered in a single dose at bedtime and are used for 4 to 6 weeks in combination with other therapy.

Prostaglandin Analogues. Prostaglandins are naturally abundant in the gastrointestinal (GI) tract. Prostaglandin analogues have been shown to be effective in clinical trials in the treatment of duodenal ulcers. They reduce gastric acid secretion and enhance gastric mucosal resistance to tissue injury. Misoprostol (Cytotec), the most commonly used drug in this category, *helps prevent* NSAID-induced ulcers. Some NSAIDs are being manufactured in combination with misoprostol. A significant adverse effect of this drug is uterine contraction; therefore its use is contraindicated in pregnant women.

Antacids. Antacids buffer gastric acid and prevent the formation of pepsin. Antacids have demonstrated effectiveness in accelerating the healing of duodenal ulcers. Liquid suspensions are the most therapeutic form, but tablets may be more convenient and enhance compliance. The most widely used preparations are mixtures of aluminum hydroxide and magnesium hydroxide. This combination overcomes the unpleasant GI side effects of either of these preparations when used alone. Mylanta and Maalox are examples of this type of combination antacid formulation. The aluminum and magnesium hydroxide combination products neutralize well at small doses. These products must be administered cautiously to those with renal impairment. These substances cannot be eliminated adequately by the kidneys and are consequently retained in excessive amounts in the body.

Instruct the client that to achieve a therapeutic effect, sufficient antacid must be ingested to neutralize the hourly production of acid. For optimal effect, teach the client to take antacids about 2 hours after meals to reduce the hydrogen ion load in the duodenum. Antacids may be effective from 30 minutes to 3 hours after ingestion. Antacids taken with an empty stomach are quickly evacuated; thus the neutralizing effect is reduced. Calcium carbonate (Tums) is a potent antacid, but it triggers gastrin release, causing a rebound acid secretion. Therefore its use in acid inhibition is not recommended.

Antacids can interact with certain drugs, such as phenytoin (Dilantin), tetracycline, and ketoconazole, and interfere with their effectiveness. Determine what other drugs the client is using before a specific antacid is prescribed. Medications are administered 1 to 2 hours before or after the antacid. Inform the client that flavored antacids, especially wintergreen, should be avoided. The flavoring increases the emptying time of the stomach; thus the desired effect of the antacid is negated.

Teach the client with past or present heart failure to avoid antacids containing a high sodium content, such as aluminum hydroxide, magnesium hydroxide, sodium bicarbonate, and simethicone combination products (Gelusil and Mylanta). Magaldrate (Riopan) has the lowest sodium concentration.

Mucosal Barrier Fortifiers. Sucralfate (Carafate) is sulfonated disaccharide that forms complexes with proteins at the base of a peptic ulcer. This protective coat prevents further digestive action of both acid and pepsin.

Sucralfate does not inhibit acid secretion. Rather, it binds bile acids and pepsins, reducing injury from these substances. Sucralfate may be used in conjunction with H_2-receptor antagonists and antacids but should not be administered within 1 hour of the antacid. Sucralfate is given on an empty stomach 1 hour before each meal and at bedtime. The main side effect of this drug is constipation.

Diet Therapy. The value of diet in the management of ulcer disease is highly controversial. There is no evidence that dietary restriction reduces gastric acid secretion or promotes tissue healing, although a bland diet may assist in relieving symptoms. Food itself acts as an antacid by neutralizing gastric acid for 30 to 60 minutes. An increased rate of gastric acid secretion, called rebound, may follow. If diet therapy is used, it may be directed toward neutralizing acid and reducing hypermotility, which may alleviate symptoms.

Instruct the client to avoid substances that increase gastric acid secretion. This includes caffeine-containing beverages (coffee, tea, and cola). Both caffeinated and decaffeinated coffees should be avoided, because coffee contains peptides that stimulate gastrin release.

In collaboration with the dietitian, teach the client to exclude any foods that cause discomfort. A bland, nonirritating diet is recommended during the acute symptomatic phase. Bedtime snacks are avoided because they may stimulate gastric acid secretion. Eating six smaller daily meals may help, but this regimen is no longer a regular part of therapy. There is no evidence to support the theory that eating six daily meals promotes healing of the ulcer. This practice actually stimulates gastric acid secretion. Clients should avoid alcohol and tobacco because of their stimulatory effects on gastric acid secretion.

Complementary and Alternative Therapies. The use of Kundalini yoga meditation techniques is currently being studied to see how they can help manage gastrointestinal disorders such as peptic ulcer disease. Kundalini yoga techniques have been demonstrated to have a dramatically beneficial effect on obsessive-compulsive disorders and anxiety disorders. Many have suggested that GI disorders result from the dysfunction of both the GI tract itself and the brain. This means that stress is thought to make GI disorders such as peptic ulcer disease worse. Yoga is thought to alter the activities of the central and autonomic nervous system (Shannahoff-Khalsa, 2002).

Other modalities include herbs, such as powders of slippery elm and marshmallow root, quercetin, and licorice.

These herbs are thought to heal inflamed tissue and increase blood flow to the gastric mucosa. Other substances include zinc, vitamin C, essential fatty acids, acidophilus, vitamins E and A, and glutamine. All of these substances enhance healing.

POTENTIAL FOR GASTROINTESTINAL BLEEDING

PLANNING: EXPECTED OUTCOMES. Fluid volume loss secondary to the development of complications is a risk associated with PUD. Blood loss due to hemorrhage can carry significant morbidity and mortality. Fluid volume loss secondary to vomiting can lead to dehydration and electrolyte imbalances. The client with peptic ulcer disease (PUD) is expected to maintain vascular, cellular, and intracellular perfusion. Indicators include that the client will:

- Have intact mental status
- Have stable blood pressure
- Have warm, dry skin
- Excrete at least 30 mL/hr of urine

INTERVENTIONS. Monitoring and early recognition of complications are critical to the successful management of PUD. Interventions aimed at managing complications associated with PUD include prevention and/or management of bleeding, perforation, and gastric outlet obstruction. In some cases, surgical treatment of complications becomes necessary.

NIC HYPOVOLEMIA MANAGEMENT. The purpose of managing hypovolemia is to expand intravascular fluid in a client who is volume depleted. Monitor vital signs and observe for fluid loss from bleeding and vomiting. Carefully monitor the client's fluid status, including intake and output. Fluid replacement in older adults should be closely monitored to prevent fluid overload. An infusion pump is used to ensure accurate delivery of the desired volume. Serum electrolytes are also monitored, because depletions from vomiting or nasogastric suctioning must be replaced. Ensure that two large-bore peripheral IV catheters are inserted so that both fluids and blood lost to vomiting and/or hemorrhage can be replaced. Volume replacement with isotonic crystalloid solutions (0.9 normal saline solution, or lactated Ringer's solution) should be started immediately, because adequate fluid volume replacement is essential. The health care provider may order blood products, such as packed red blood cells, to expand volume and correct abnormalities in the complete blood count (CBC). For clients with active bleeding, fresh frozen plasma may be given if the prothrombin time is 1.5 times higher than the midrange control value. To prevent injury from falls secondary to orthostatic hypotension, the client is assisted with ambulation. Orthostatic hypotension is common in clients with decreased fluid volume.

NIC BLEEDING REDUCTION: GASTROINTESTINAL. The purpose of activities to reduce bleeding is to limit the amount of blood loss from the upper and lower gastrointestinal (GI) tract resulting from complications related to PUD. Monitor the client for manifestations indicating GI bleeding. All excretions are observed for the presence of frank (obvious) or occult (not apparent on visual inspection) bleeding. With GI bleeding, the presence of frank blood or coffee-ground vomitus may be observed. Stools can contain frank blood or appear black and tarry.

CHART 59-4

KEY FEATURES of
Gastrointestinal Bleeding

- Coffee-ground vomitus
- Tarry stools or frank (obvious) blood in stools
- Melena (occult blood)
- Decreased blood pressure
- Increased weak and thready pulse
- Decreased hemoglobin and hematocrit
- Vertigo
- Acute confusion (in older adults)
- Dizziness
- Syncope

Occult blood loss may be detected by stool examination and may be accompanied by progressive iron deficiency anemia (Chart 59-4).

Monitor the client's hematocrit, hemoglobin, and coagulation studies for changes from the baseline measurements. Monitor vital signs frequently. With mild bleeding (less than 500 mL), slight feelings of weakness and mild perspiration may be present. When blood loss exceeds 1 L/24 hr, manifestations of shock may be manifested, such as hypotension, chills, palpitations, diaphoresis, and a weak, thready pulse. (See Chapter 40 for the treatment of shock.)

Immediately notify the health care provider of major bleeding. Transfusion therapy may be required to replace blood loss. (See Chapter 43 for nursing interventions for clients undergoing blood transfusion.) The health care provider may prescribe H_2 blockers to avoid extremes in gastric pH levels. If appropriate and as prescribed, insert a nasogastric (NG) tube, monitor secretions, and perform nasogastric lavage to decompress the stomach and alleviate bleeding. In addition, instruct the client and family to avoid the use of anti-inflammatory medications that can precipitate or worsen GI bleeding. NIC interventions and activities are summarized in Chart 59-5.

NONSURGICAL MANAGEMENT. Because prevention or early detection of complications is critical in obtaining a satisfactory outcome, monitor the client carefully and immediately report changes to the health care provider. The type of nonsurgical intervention selected will depend on the type and severity of the complication.

The goals of therapeutic interventions for bleeding secondary to PUD are as follows:

- Stop the acute bleeding episode
- Prevent rebleeding

A combination of several different therapeutic interventions, including endoscopic therapy, acid suppression, NG tube placement, and saline lavage, can be used to control acute bleeding and prevent rebleeding. Therapeutic trials have been conducted to determine the optimal treatment for bleeding due to peptic ulcers. Endoscopic therapy and suppression of gastric acid are the primary therapies used to control active bleeding caused by PUD. H_2-receptor antagonists, proton pump inhibitors, and antacids are the primary medications used to treat this bleeding.

Endoscopic Therapy. Endoscopic therapy via an esophagogastroduodenoscopy (EGD) can assist in achieving homeostasis during an acute bleeding episode. The primary methods of endoscopic therapy are (1) thermal contact using a heater probe or multielectrocoagulation, (2) injection

CHART 59-5

NIC INTERVENTION ACTIVITIES for
The Client with Peptic Ulcer Disease

Hypovolemia Management: *Expansion of intravascular fluid volume in a client who is volume depleted*
- Monitor vital signs, as appropriate.
- Monitor fluid status, including intake and output, as appropriate.
- Monitor for fluid loss (e.g., bleeding, vomiting, diarrhea, perspiration, and tachypnea).
- Arrange availability of blood products for transfusion, if necessary.
- Administer blood products (e.g., platelets and fresh frozen plasma), as appropriate.
- Monitor for blood reaction, if appropriate.

Bleeding Reduction: *Gastrointestinal: Limitation of the amount of blood loss from the upper and lower gastrointestinal tract and related complications*
- Monitor for signs and symptoms of persistent bleeding (e.g., check all secretions for frank or occult blood).
- Hematest all excretions and observe for blood loss in emesis, sputum, feces, urine, NG tube drainage, and wound drainage, as appropriate.
- Document color, amount, and character of stools.
- Monitor coagulation studies and complete blood count (CBC) with WBC differential.
- Insert nasogastric tube to suction and monitor secretions, if appropriate.
- Perform nasogastric lavage, as appropriate.
- Avoid extremes in gastric pH level by administration of appropriate medication (e.g., antacids or histamine-blocking agent).
- Instruct the client and/or family on the need for blood replacement, as appropriate.
- Instruct the client and/or family to avoid the use of antiinflammatory medications (e.g., aspirin and ibuprofen).

NIC intervention activities selected from Dochterman, J.M., & Bulechek, G.M. (Eds.). (2004). *Nursing interventions classification (NIC)* (4th ed.). St. Louis: Mosby. No part of this work is to be altered without prior written permission from the Publisher. *WBC,* White blood cell.

of the bleeding site with diluted epinephrine, (3) laser therapy, and (4) clipping the bleeding vessel with a mechanical clip. All methods are effective in achieving blood clot formation. Thermal contact and injection with epinephrine are most commonly used. Laser therapy is costly and therefore is used less often. Clipping is used mostly when a bleeding vessel is visible. Generally, endoscopic therapy is beneficial for clients with active bleeding; however, ulcers that continue to bleed or continue to rebleed despite endoscopic therapy may require surgical repair. Sometimes endoscopists (physicians) may scope a client daily during an acute bleed of a peptic ulcer to assess and possibly re-treat the ulcer if it continues to bleed or begins bleeding again. Sometimes this regimen will prevent the client from having to have surgery.

Pre-EGD nursing care involves inserting a large-bore IV catheter. A large catheter allows the client to receive IV conscious sedation (e.g., midazolam [Versed] and meperidine [Demerol]) to remain comfortable during the procedure. In addition, ensure that the client remains NPO six hours before the procedure. This prevents the risk of aspiration and allows the endoscopist (physician) to visualize and treat the ulcer. A client must sign a consent before the EGD after the physician informs the client about the procedure. During the EGD, a trained endoscopy nurse and technician assist the physician with the procedure. Post-EGD care involves checking the vital signs, heart rhythm, and oxygen saturation frequently until they return to baseline. In addition, assess the client's ability to swallow saliva frequently. The client's gag reflex may initially be absent after an EGD due to the anesthetizing (numbing) the throat with a spray before the procedure. The client will not be able to resume a pre-procedure diet until the gag reflex is intact.

Acid Suppression. Aggressive acid suppression is used to prevent rebleeding. When acute bleeding is stopped and clot formation has taken place within the ulcer crater, the clot remains in contact with gastric contents. Acid-suppressive agents are used to stabilize the clot by raising the pH level of gastric contents. Several drugs are used to achieve acid suppression in clients with a bleeding episode. H_2-receptor antagonists prevent acid from being produced by parietal cells. Proton pump inhibitors prevent the transport of acid across the parietal cell membrane, whereas antacids buffer acid produced in the stomach.

Somatostatin analogue may also be used and has shown excellent hemostatic results. Somatostatin analogue is actually a synthetic gastrointestinal (GI) hormone that suppresses gastric acid secretion by a direct action on parietal and chief cells. Somatostatin analogue vasoconstricts splanchnic arteries, which reduces hemorrhage (Yabuki et al., 2002).

Nasogastric Tube Placement. Upper GI bleeding may require the health care provider or nurse to insert a nasogastric (NG) tube to:
- Ascertain the presence or absence of blood in the stomach
- Assess the rate of bleeding
- Prevent gastric dilation
- Administer saline lavage

Nasogastric aspiration is an important part of diagnostic and prognostic evaluation of the client. The presence of red blood in emesis, nasogastric aspirate, or stools is correlated with a poor outcome.

Once the NG tube is placed, confirmation of proper positioning of the tube is determined by x-ray examination. Irrigate the NG tube to maintain its patency and prevent obstruction with clotted blood.

Saline Lavage. Saline lavage requires the insertion of a large-bore NG tube with instillation of saline in volumes of 50 to 200 mL. The saline and blood are repeatedly withdrawn until returns are clear or light pink and without clots. For protection against exposure to blood, practitioners may use the following procedure with a closed system for irrigation and suction. A Y-connector is attached to the NG tube, and an IV bag of normal saline is attached to tubing at one end of the Y-connector. The opposite connector is attached to tubing connected to wall suction. After the stomach is initially drained by suctioning, the tubing attached to the wall suction is clamped, and up to 200 mL of normal saline is allowed to drain into the client through the NG tube. After the saline is instilled, the tube connecting the saline to the NG tube is clamped, and the clamp to suction is released. Instruct the client to lie on the left side during this procedure to limit the flow of saline out of the stomach and prevent aspiration.

NONSURGICAL MANAGEMENT OF PERFORATION. To prevent peritonitis from GI contents that have entered the peritoneum, perforation is managed by immediately replacing fluid, blood, and electrolytes, administering antibiotics, and keeping the client NPO. Maintain nasogastric suction to drain gastric secretions and thus prevent further peritoneal spillage. Carefully monitor intake and output and check vital signs at least hourly and monitor the client for clinical manifestations of septic shock, such as fever, pain, tachycardia, lethargy, or anxiety.

NONSURGICAL MANAGEMENT OF PYLORIC OBSTRUCTION. Pyloric obstruction is caused by edema, spasm, or scar tissue. Symptoms of obstruction related to difficulty in emptying the stomach include feelings of fullness, distention, or nausea after eating, as well as vomiting of copious amounts of undigested food.

Treatment of obstruction is directed toward restoration of fluid and electrolyte balance and decompression of the dilated stomach. Obstruction related to edema and spasm generally responds to medical therapy. First, the stomach must be decompressed with nasogastric suction; next, interventions are directed at correcting metabolic alkalosis and dehydration. The NG tube is clamped after about 72 hours, and the client is checked for retention of gastric contents. If the amount retained is not more than 350 mL in 30 minutes, the health care provider may allow oral fluids. In some cases, surgical intervention may be required.

SURGICAL MANAGEMENT. New guidelines for the treatment of PUD that include *H. pylori* eradication and the development of nonsurgical means of controlling bleeding have led to a decline in the need for surgical intervention. In PUD, surgical intervention is used to:
- Reduce the acid-secreting ability of the stomach
- Treat clients who do not respond to medical therapy
- Treat a surgical emergency that develops as a complication of PUD

Two general surgical approaches are available for PUD—minimally invasive partial gastrectomy and conventional open surgery.

Minimally invasive gastrectomy (MIG) via laparoscopy (a type of endoscope) may be performed to remove a chronic gastric ulcer or treat hemorrhage from perforation. Several small incisions allow access to the stomach and duodenum. The client may have partial gastric removal and/or a vagotomy (vagus nerve cutting) to control acid secretion. The advantages of laparoscopic surgery over traditional procedures include a shorter hospital stay, less postoperative complications, less pain, and better, quicker recovery.

Preoperative Care. Before conventional open-approach surgery, an NG tube is inserted and connected to suction to remove secretions and empty the stomach. This allows surgery to take place without contamination of the peritoneal cavity by gastric secretions. Chart 59-6 describes the procedure for inserting the NG tube and nursing care associated with NG tube maintenance. The NG tube remains in place postoperatively to prevent the accumulation of secretions, which may lead to vomiting or gastrointestinal (GI) distention and pressure on the suture line.

Other preoperative nursing measures for the client undergoing open gastric surgery are the same as those for any client undergoing abdominal surgery and general anesthesia (see Chapter 20).

Operative Procedures. There is no definitive single procedure for PUD. The most commonly performed conventional surgical procedures are gastroenterostomy, vagotomy, and pyloroplasty.

CHART 59-6

BEST PRACTICE for
Nasogastric Tubes

1. Inform the client about the procedure and its potential discomfort.
2. Seat the client with pillows behind the shoulders.
3. Lubricate the tube with a water-soluble lubricant.
4. Measure the length of the tube to be passed.
   a. Measure from the bridge of the nose to the earlobe to the xiphoid process.
   b. Indicate this length with a piece of tape on the tube.

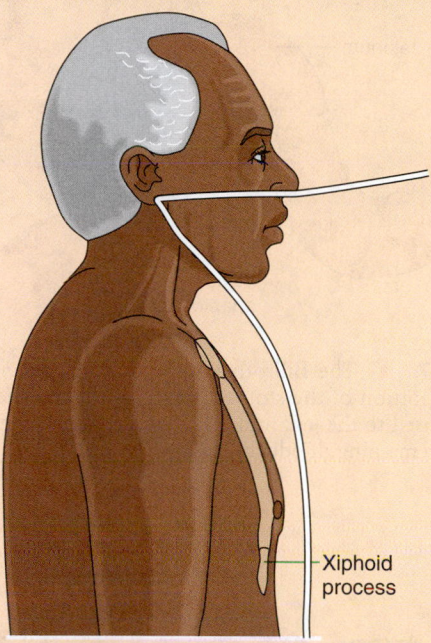

Xiphoid process

5. Determine which nostril is more patent.
6. Encourage the client to swallow or drink water if the level of consciousness and treatment plan permit.

7. Insert the tube.
   a. Pass the tube gently into the nasopharynx. Ask the client to swallow repeatedly while the tube is advanced.
   b. If resistance is met, rotate the tube slowly, aiming downward and toward the closer ear.
   c. In the intubated or semiconscious client, flex the client's head toward the chest while passing the tube.
8. Withdraw the tube immediately if any change is noted in the client's respiratory status.
9. Test for tube placement by using the following techniques:
   a. Obtain a sample of the gastric contents by aspirating with a 50-mL catheter-tipped syringe.
   b. Test the pH of the gastric contents (should be between 1 and 3.5).
   c. Obtain an order for an x-ray study to confirm placement.
10. Connect the tube to suction at low pressure.
    a. The Levin tube is connected to intermittent low suction.
    b. The Salem sump or Anderson tube is connected to continuous low suction.
11. Secure the tube to the client's nose with tape and to the client's gown.
    a. Tie a slipknot around the tube with a rubber band.
    b. Pin a rubber band to the client's gown.
12. Check the client's intake and output every 4 hr or more often, as indicated.
13. Observe the client for nausea, vomiting, abdominal fullness, or distention.
14. If irrigation is indicated, use only a normal saline solution.
15. Observe the client for alterations in fluid and electrolyte balance.
16. If indicated, instruct the client about movement that will not dislodge the tube and cause nasal irritation.
17. Remove the tape securing the tube to the nose daily and PRN to clean skin; reapply tape.

Gastroenterostomy. A simple **gastroenterostomy** permits neutralization of gastric acid by regurgitation of alkaline duodenal contents into the stomach. The surgeon creates a passage between the body of the stomach and the small bowel, often the jejunum (Figure 59-4). The benefit may be offset by interference with acid inhibition of gastrin release, which results in a net increase in acid secretion.

If the gastroenterostomy drains the stomach, it reduces motor activity in the pyloroduodenal area. Drainage of the gastric contents diverts acid from the ulcerated area and facilitates healing. However, the secretory capacity of the parietal cell mass of the stomach has not been reduced, and the gastrin mechanism continues to function. For this reason, a vagotomy is usually combined with gastroenterostomy for reduction of the vagal influences.

Vagotomy. Three types of **vagotomy** have been used in the treatment of duodenal ulcers: truncal vagotomy, selective vagotomy, and proximal gastric vagotomy (Figure 59-5). Vagotomy eliminates the acid-secreting stimulus to gastric cells and decreases the responsiveness of parietal cells. In a truncal vagotomy, the vagal trunks are transected and the antrum is removed. The remaining stomach is anastomosed to the proximal duodenum (Billroth I) or to a loop of jejunum (Billroth II) (Figures 59-6 and 59-7).

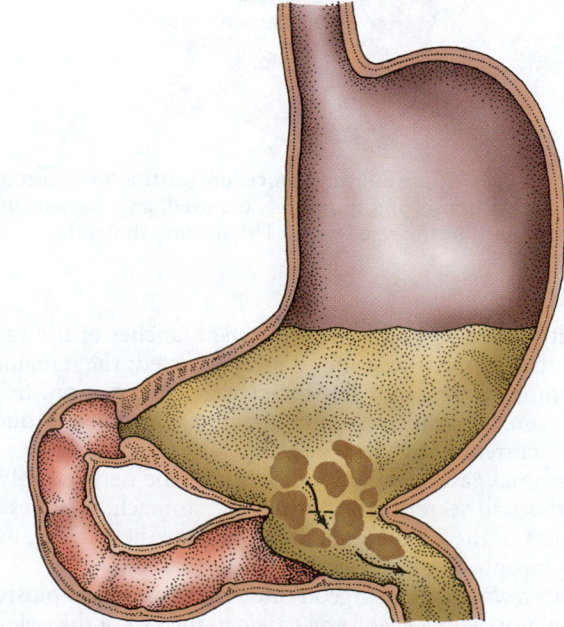

Figure 59-4 ■ Gastroenterostomy (the creation of a passage between the body of the stomach and the jejunum).

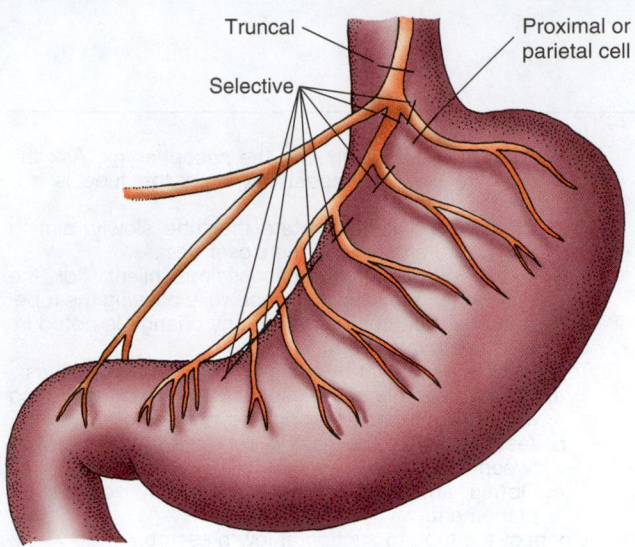

Figure 59-5 ■ Various types of vagotomies.

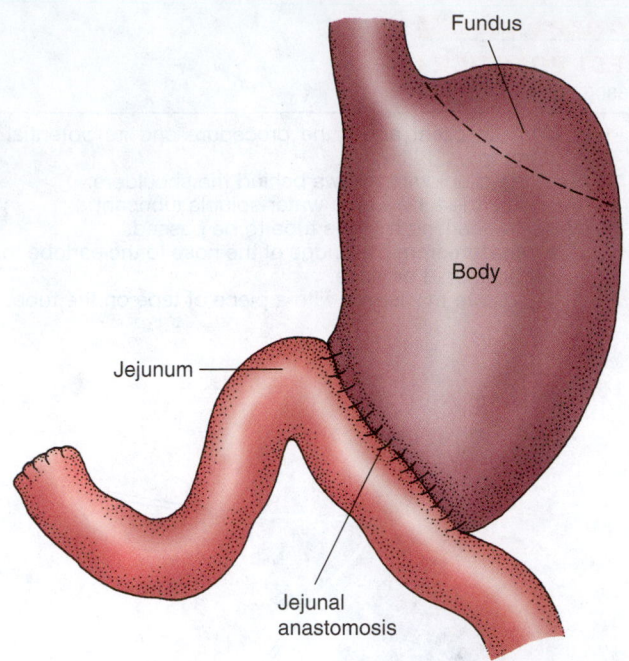

Figure 59-7 ■ The Billroth II procedure (gastrojejunostomy). The lower portion of the stomach is removed, and the remainder is anastomosed to the jejunum. The shading shows the portion removed. A remaining duodenal stump is closed.

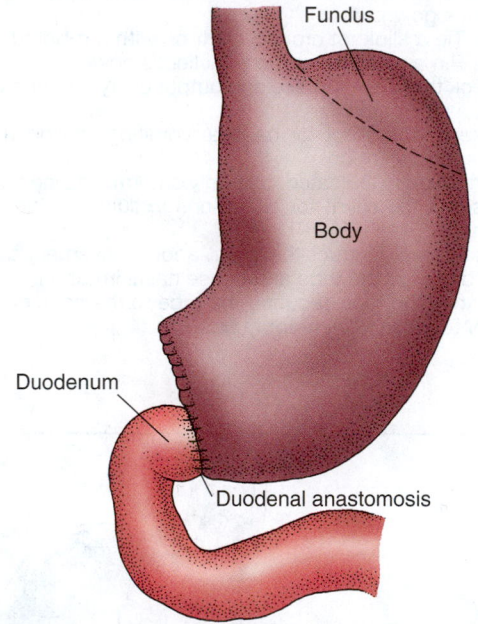

Figure 59-6 ■ The Billroth I procedure (gastroduodenostomy). The distal portion of the stomach is removed, and the remainder is anastomosed to the duodenum. The shading shows the portion removed.

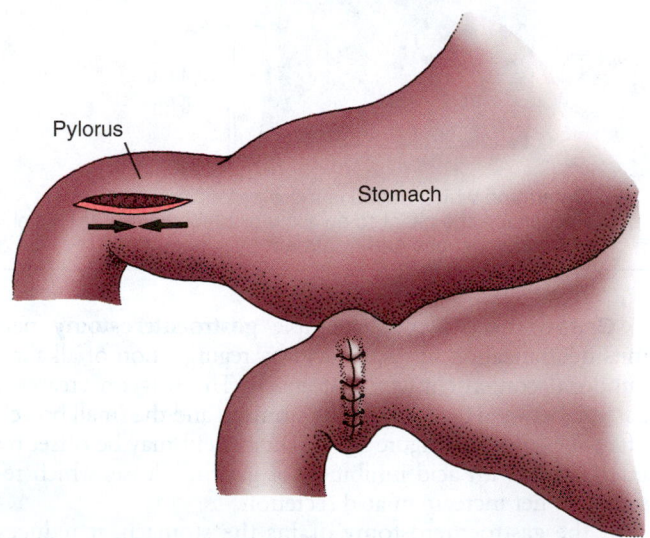

Figure 59-8 ■ The Heineke-Mikulicz pyloroplasty.

With selective vagotomy, only the branches of the vagus nerve that supply the stomach are transected; the remaining abdominal viscera still has intact vagal innervation. Selective vagotomy results in a more complete response, reduced ulcer recurrence, and fewer postoperative complications.

Proximal gastric vagotomy interrupts the nerve supply to only the acid-secreting portion of the stomach; it spares the branches of the vagus nerve that innervate the antrum, making pyloroplasty unnecessary.

Pyloroplasty. The surgeon often performs **pyloroplasty** in conjunction with a vagotomy to widen the exit of the pylorus. This facilitates emptying of stomach contents. The most common procedure is the Heineke-Mikulicz pyloroplasty

(Figure 59-8). In this procedure the surgeon enlarges the pyloric stricture by incising the pylorus longitudinally and sutures the incision transversely.

Postoperative Care. The postoperative care is similar for all of the surgical procedures (see the Plan of Care on pp. 1299 to 1302). Provide the usual postoperative care for clients who have had general anesthesia (see Chapter 22). In addition, monitor the client for the development of postoperative complications.

Nasogastric Tube Management. Monitor the nasogastric (NG) tube for patency and carefully secure the tube to prevent dislodgment; this is critical for preventing the retention of gastric secretions. Monitor the client to make sure that no

▪PLAN of CARE   MEDICAL DIAGNOSIS: GASTRECTOMY

NURSING DIAGNOSIS NO. 1 ▪ Acute Pain

	Expected Outcomes	Nursing Interventions	Rationales
RELATED FACTORS Injury agents: Surgery **DEFINING CHARACTERISTICS** Verbal or coded report of pain Observed evidence of pain	Denies experiencing pain greater than 5 on a 0 to 10 pain scale No verbal report or observation of guarding or protective gestures No verbal report or observation of an alteration in sleep patterns No verbal report or observation of self-focusing behavior No verbal report or observation of facial mask of pain No verbal report or observation of an alteration in activity level	**NIC** **Pain Management** Perform a comprehensive pain assessment that includes location, characteristics, onset/duration, frequency, quality, intensity or severity of pain, and precipitating factors. **D** Reduce or eliminate factors that precipitate or increase the pain experience. Provide information about the pain, such as causes, how long it will last, and anticipated discomforts from procedures. **NIC** **Analgesic Administration** Choose the IV rather than the IM route for frequent pain medication injections, when possible. Administer analgesics around-the-clock. **D** Institute safety precautions for a client who is receiving opioid analgesics, as appropriate. Document the client's response to the analgesic and any untoward effects. Implement actions to decrease the untoward effects of analgesics. Teach about the use of analgesics, strategies to decrease side effects, and expectations for involvement in decisions about pain relief. **NIC** **Patient-Controlled Analgesia (PCA) Administration** Validate that the client can use a PCA device. Document the client's pain, amount and frequency of drug dosing, and response to pain treatment on a pain flow sheet. Teach the client and family how to use the PCA device.	A plan for pain management must be based on the client's unique responses to pain. Preventing a pain experience is preferred to trying to control or eliminate pain. The client is better able to monitor his or her own discomfort and to intervene appropriately when informed. The IV route avoids tissue trauma and the unpredictable absorption of medication. Administration around-the-clock prevents the peaks and troughs of analgesia, especially with severe pain. Opioid analgesics may impair the client's judgment and/or coordination. Documentation provides the health care team with the information needed to accurately evaluate the client's response to the analgesic regimen. Actions taken to prevent the predictable but unwanted effects of opioid analgesics (e.g., constipation) increase client comfort. Information about analgesics and the expectation for involvement increase the client's sense of control over his or her pain. To use a PCA, the client must be able to communicate, comprehend explanations, and follow directions. Information on the pain flow sheet assists the health care team to adjust the analgesic regimen to the client's needs. The device will not be used if the client and/or family do not know how to use or are afraid of the device.

D Indicates tasks that can be delegated to unlicensed assistive nursing personnel at the discretion of the nurse.

Continued

PLAN of CARE MEDICAL DIAGNOSIS: GASTRECTOMY—*cont'd*

NURSING DIAGNOSIS NO. 1 ▪ Acute Pain—*cont'd*

	Expected Outcomes	Nursing Interventions	Rationales
		NIC Environmental Management: Comfort **D** Position the client to facilitate comfort. **Other Interventions** Consider the use of alternative therapies such as imagery, aromatherapy, music, touch, and laughter/humor.	The nurse may decrease sources of discomfort by using principles of body alignment, supporting with pillows, supporting joints during movement, splinting over incisions, and immobilizing painful body parts. Cognitive and behavioral strategies may be used as adjuncts to or in place of pharmacologic or surgical interventions for chronic pain. Each therapy has a different mode of action, which may or may not benefit the client.

NURSING DIAGNOSIS NO. 2 ▪ Ineffective Breathing Pattern

	Expected Outcomes	Nursing Interventions	Rationales
RELATED FACTORS Pain **DEFINING CHARACTERISTICS** Altered chest excursion Depth of breathing: Adult tidal volume 500 mL at rest	No verbal report or observation of dyspnea Respiratory rate remains between 11 and 22 breaths/min Has respirations that remain regular and deep	**NIC Airway Management** **D** Place the client in semi-Fowler's position, if possible. **D** Encourage the client to take slow, deep breaths; to turn; and to cough. **D** Assist the client with an incentive spirometer, as appropriate. **NIC Respiratory Monitoring** **D** Monitor the rate, rhythm, depth, and effort of respirations. Note chest movement, watching for symmetry, the use of accessory muscles, and supraclavicular and intercostal muscle retractions. Auscultate breath sounds, noting areas of decreased/absent ventilation and the presence of adventitious sounds. **Continuing Care Considerations** **D** Encourage the client to engage in regular physical exercise. **D** Encourage the client to enroll in a smoking cessation program, as indicated.	Semi-Fowler's position ensures that the abdominal contents do not press against the diaphragm and restrict chest expansion. Effective aeration and coughing will help rid the body of secretions. Frequent position changes will prevent secretions from pooling in one area. Incentive spirometry encourages the client to deep breathe. Changes in respiratory rate, rhythm, depth, or effort may signal a descent into respiratory failure. The use of accessory muscles indicates increased respiratory effort. Absent or adventitious breath sounds indicate poor gas exchange or poor movement of air through the airways. Cardiopulmonary efficiency and endurance improve with exercise. Smoking damages the airways and alveoli.

D Indicates tasks that can be delegated to unlicensed assistive nursing personnel at the discretion of the nurse.

PLAN of CARE   MEDICAL DIAGNOSIS: GASTRECTOMY—*cont'd*

NURSING DIAGNOSIS NO. 3 ■ Imbalanced Nutrition: Less Than Body Requirements

	Expected Outcomes	Nursing Interventions	Rationales
RELATED FACTORS Inability to ingest or digest food or absorb nutrients due to biologic, psychological, or economic factors **DEFINING CHARACTERISTICS** Satiety immediately after ingesting food Perceived inability to ingest food Abdomen: Cramping Pain: Abdominal with or without pathology Diarrhea	Has bowel sounds that remain at 3 to 5 per quadrant per minute Denies abdominal pain No verbal report or observation of diarrhea Weight remains within ±5 pounds of desired weight	**NIC** **Nutrition Management** Determine, in collaboration with a dietitian as appropriate, the number of calories and type of nutrients needed to meet nutrition requirements. Adjust the diet to the client's lifestyle, as appropriate. **D** Provide foods appropriate for the client—general diet; mechanical soft, blenderized or commercial formula via a nasogastric or gastrostomy tube; or total parental nutrition—as ordered by the health care provider. **D** Create a pleasant, relaxing environment at mealtime. **Other Interventions** Teach the client and family about high-calorie, high-protein meal planning as appropriate, as well as refraining from drinking liquids with meals. Monitor for early signs and symptoms of dumping syndrome—vertigo, tachycardia, syncope, sweating, pallor, palpitations, and the desire to lie down. Teach the client and family about nutritional supplements, as appropriate. **Continuing Care Considerations** Refer the client to appropriate community nutritional programs, as needed.	Individual client needs for nutrients and calories should be the basis for a sound dietary plan. The dietary division of nutrients, calories, and meals should be adjusted to the client's lifestyle to increase compliance. Diet therapy dictates the types and form of foods that may be offered to the client. A pleasant, relaxing environment at mealtime improves digestion. Meals must be nutritionally adequate to promote healing and to avoid events such as reflux and dumping syndrome. Dumping syndrome poses a threat to client safety. Additional vitamins and minerals, calories, dietary fiber, or other nutritional components may need to be added to the diet of a client who is unable to eat a nutritionally adequate diet. Resources such as Weight Watchers, Overeaters Anonymous, and Take Off Pounds Sensibly provide support to the client who is attempting to maintain appropriate body weight.

Continued

≡PLAN of CARE   MEDICAL DIAGNOSIS: GASTRECTOMY—cont'd

NURSING DIAGNOSIS NO. 4 ■ Risk for Infection

	Expected Outcomes	Nursing Interventions	Rationales
RELATED FACTORS Invasive procedures Malnutrition Increased environmental exposure to pathogens Inadequate primary defenses (broken skin, traumatized tissue, decrease in ciliary action, stasis of body fluids, changes in pH secretions, altered peristalsis)	Denies fatigue Denies weakness Denies nausea Has a blood pressure that remains ±10 mm Hg of baseline Has a heart rate that remains regular, strong, and between 60 and 100 beats/min No verbal report or observation of vomiting Has a body temperature that remains between 97° and 99.6° F (36.1° and 37.5° C)	**NIC Infection Protection** Monitor for systemic and localized signs and symptoms of infection. Monitor absolute granulocyte count, white blood cell (WBC) count, and differential results. Inspect the condition of any surgical incision/wound. D Maintain asepsis for the client at risk. D Encourage coughing and deep breathing, as appropriate. D Promote sufficient nutritional intake. D Encourage fluid intake, as appropriate. D Encourage rest. **NIC Infection Control** Administer antibiotic therapy, as appropriate. **Continuing Care Considerations** Numerous visitors should be limited, and visits from individuals with known infections should be discouraged. Teach the client and family about the signs and symptoms of infection and when to report them to the health care provider.	An elevated temperature, pulse, and respirations indicate systemic infection; redness, heat, swelling, and pain indicate local infection. Elevations in these laboratory tests demonstrate the body's response to infection. A surgical incision may be slightly reddened and swollen from tissue damage but remain free of the purulent drainage, excess swelling, or excess local pain that indicate infection. Asepsis will minimize the client's exposure to pathogenic agents and thus minimize the incidence of infection. Coughing and deep breathing clears the lungs of secretions that may encourage the growth of pathogenic microbes. Adequate nutrition is essential for the formation of immune system cells and for the repair of damaged body tissues to provide protection against external pathogens. Adequate fluid intake provides for renal clearance of the toxins produced by pathogens. Mending tissues require energy. A fatigued client is stressed and requires greater expenditure of energy to accomplish tasks. Antibiotic therapy should assist the body to destroy pathogens. Visitors may provide a needed diversion for the client, but too many visitors may cause fatigue and bring unwanted exposure to pathogens. Early intervention to treat infection prevents untoward complications from the infection and its therapy.

D Indicates tasks that can be delegated to unlicensed assistive nursing personnel at the discretion of the nurse.

TABLE 59-2 Diet for Dumping Syndrome

Food Group	Foods Allowed or Encouraged	Foods to Use with Caution	Foods That Must Be Excluded
Soups		Fluids 1 hr before and after meals	Spicy soups
Meat and meat substitutes	8 oz or more per day: fish, poultry, beef, pork, veal, lamb, eggs, cheese, and peanut butter		Spicy meats or meat substitutes
Potato and substitutes	Potato, rice, pasta, starchy vegetables (small amount)		Highly spiced potatoes or substitutes
Bread and cereal	White bread, rolls, muffins, crackers, and cereals (small amount)	Whole-grain bread, rolls, crackers, and cereals	Breads with frosting or jelly, sweet rolls, and coffee cake
Vegetables	Two or more cooked vegetables	Gas-producing vegetables, such as cabbage, onions, broccoli, or raw vegetables	
Fruits	Limit three per day: unsweetened cooked or canned fruits	Unsweetened juice or fruit drinks 30-45 min after meals; fresh fruit	Sweetened fruit or juice
Beverages	Dietetic drinks	Limit to 1 hr after meals; caffeine-containing beverages, such as coffee, tea, and cola; if tolerated, diet carbonated beverages	Milk shakes, malts, and other sweet drinks; regular carbonated beverages and alcohol
Fats	Margarine, oils, shortening, butter, bacon, and salad dressings	Mayonnaise	Any fats with milk products
Desserts	Fruit (see Fruits)	Sugar-free gelatin, pudding, and custard	All sweets, cakes, pies, cookies, candy, ice cream, and sherbet
Seasonings and miscellaneous	Diet jelly, diet syrups, sugar substitutes	Excessive amounts of salt	Excessive amounts of spices, sugar, jelly, honey, syrup, or molasses

General Principles
- Several small meals daily
- Relatively high fat and protein content
- Low roughage
- Relatively low carbohydrate content
- No milk, sweets, or sugars
- Liquid between meals *only*

more than a scant amount of blood drains from the tube and that abdominal distention does not develop. If these problems occur, report them immediately to the surgeon. Irrigation or repositioning of the NG tube is not done after gastric surgery unless specifically prescribed by the surgeon.

Monitoring for Postoperative Complications. Observe the client carefully for possible complications and report them immediately to the health care provider. In the immediate postoperative period, many complications may occur.

A disruption in the patency of the NG tube can result in *acute gastric dilation* postoperatively; this is manifested by epigastric pain and a feeling of fullness, hiccups, tachycardia, and hypotension. Irrigation or replacement of the NG tube by order of the surgeon can relieve these symptoms.

Dumping syndrome is a term that refers to a constellation of vasomotor symptoms after eating, especially following a Billroth II procedure. This syndrome is believed to occur as a result of the rapid emptying of gastric contents into the small intestine, which shifts fluid into the gut, causing abdominal distention. Observe for *early* manifestations of this syndrome, which typically occurs within 30 minutes of eating. Symptoms include vertigo, tachycardia, syncope, sweating, pallor, palpitations, and the desire to lie down.

Late dumping syndrome, which occurs 90 minutes to 3 hours after eating, is caused by a release of an excessive amount of insulin. The insulin release follows a rapid rise in the blood glucose level that results from the rapid entry of high-carbohydrate food into the jejunum. Observe for intestinal manifestations, including dizziness, light-headedness, palpitations, diaphoresis, and confusion.

Dumping syndrome is managed by dietary measures that include decreasing the amount of food taken at one time and eliminating liquids ingested with meals. In collaboration with the dietitian, instruct the client to consume a high-protein, high-fat, low- to moderate-carbohydrate diet (Table 59-2). Pectin administered in the form of a dry powder may *prevent* the syndrome. A somatostatin analogue, octreotide (Sandostatin), 50 to 150 mcg subcutaneously daily, may be prescribed in severe cases. Octreotide is a synthetic form of the hormone, somatostatin, which is found in the gastrointestinal tract. It is thought to inhibit the gastric and pancreatic hormones that probably cause the signs and symptoms of dumping syndrome.

Alkaline **reflux gastropathy,** also known as *bile reflux gastropathy,* is a complication of gastric surgery in which the pylorus is bypassed or removed (e.g., pyloroplasty, gastric resection with gastroduodenostomy [Billroth I procedure], and gastrojejunostomy [Billroth II procedure]). Endoscopic examination reveals regurgitated bile in the stomach and mucosal hyperemia. Symptoms include early satiety, abdominal discomfort, and vomiting.

Delayed gastric emptying is often present after gastric surgery and usually resolves within 1 week. Edema at the anastomosis or adhesions obstructing the distal loop may have mechanical causes. Metabolic causes (e.g., hypokalemia, hypoproteinemia, or hyponatremia) should be considered. The edema is resolved with nasogastric suction, maintenance of fluid and electrolyte balance, and proper nutrition.

Afferent loop syndrome may occur when the duodenal loop is partially obstructed after a Billroth II resection. Pancreatic and biliary secretions fill the intestinal loop, which becomes distended. Painful contractions attempt to propel these secretions from the loop. Monitor for clients reporting abdominal bloating and pain 20 to 60 minutes after eating, often followed by nausea and vomiting. Treatment consists of surgical correction of the incomplete loop obstruction.

Recurrent ulceration occurs in about 5% of clients who have undergone gastric surgery for PUD. Recurrent ulcers can be due to incomplete vagotomy or persistent *H. pylori* infection. Recurrence is most common following vagotomy with antrectomy, and ulcerations tend to occur at the site of anastomosis (stomal or marginal ulcer) or immediately distal in the small intestine. Abdominal pain, usually located in the epigastrium, is the most commonly reported symptom of recurrent peptic ulcer. The health care provider may prescribe H_2-receptor antagonists and proton pump inhibitors to assist with the healing process. The eradication of *H. pylori* in the case of recurrent ulcerations is controversial.

NUTRITIONAL MANAGEMENT. Several problems related to nutrition develop as a result of partial removal of the stomach, including deficiencies of vitamin B_{12}, folic acid, and iron; impaired calcium metabolism; and reduced absorption of calcium and vitamin D. These problems are caused by a shortage of intrinsic factor. The shortage results from the resection and from inadequate absorption because of rapid entry of food into the bowel. In the absence of intrinsic factor, clinical manifestations of pernicious anemia occur. Assess for the development of atrophic glossitis secondary to vitamin B_{12} deficiency. In atrophic glossitis, the tongue takes on a shiny and "beefy" appearance. The client may also have signs of anemia secondary to folic acid and iron deficiency. Monitor the complete blood count (CBC) for signs of megaloblastic anemia and leukopenia. These manifestations are corrected by the administration of vitamin B_{12}. The health care provider may also prescribe folic acid or iron preparations.

⁇ *Critical Thinking Challenge*

A 40-year-old Hispanic client has been experiencing stomach pain for many years "off and on." Recently, the pain has been getting worse and she is fatigued, short of breath, and dizzy with exertion. She notices that the pain hurts most in her right upper quadrant 2 to 3 hours after she eats. The primary health care provider admits the client to the hospital because she is pale and has a blood pressure of 90/50 (normal for her is 130/82) and a pulse of 120 (normal for her is 86).

1. As the nurse admitting this client, what other data should you gather?
2. What are some explanations for why this client did not seek medical attention for this problem sooner?
3. What do you anticipate her complete blood count (CBC) to be?
4. What diagnostic and therapeutic procedures do you anticipate for this client?
5. Would you delegate taking her vital signs to an unlicensed person? Why or why not?
6. What is the priority for her care at this time?

evolve For suggested answer guidelines, go to http://evolve.elsevier.com/Iggy/.

Community-Based Care

Clients may be discharged from the hospital as long as there is no evidence of ongoing bleeding, orthostatic changes, or cardiopulmonary distress or compromise. Clients discharged following treatment for peptic ulcer disease (PUD) and/or complications secondary to the disease must face several challenges in order to manage the disease successfully. Long-term adherence to medication regimens requires the client to take several oral medications on a daily basis. Permanent lifestyle alterations in dietary habits must also be made. Clients must be knowledgeable about complications related to PUD and know when to report symptoms to the health care provider.

HOME CARE MANAGEMENT

Clients are discharged to the home, subacute unit, or skilled nursing facility to continue recuperation. Clients who have undergone surgery or have had complications, such as hemorrhage, may require visits from a home care nurse to assess clinical progress (Chart 59-7).

CHART 59-7

HOME CARE ASSESSMENT of
The Client with Ulcer Disease

Assess gastrointestinal and cardiovascular status, including:
- Vital signs, including orthostatic vital signs
- Skin color
- Presence of abdominal pain (location, severity, character, duration, precipitating factors, and relief measures)
- Character, color, and consistency of stools
- Changes in bowel elimination pattern
- Hemoglobin and hematocrit
- Bowel sounds; palpate for areas of tenderness

Assess nutritional status, including:
- Dietary patterns and habits
- Intake of caffeine and alcohol
- Relationship of food to symptoms

Assess medication history.
- Use of steroids
- Use of nonsteroidal anti-inflammatory drugs (NSAIDs)
- Use of over-the-counter medications

Assess client's coping style.
- Recent stressors
- Past coping style

Assess client's understanding of illness and ability to comply with therapeutic regimen.
- Symptoms to report to health care provider
- Expected and side effects of medications
- Food and drug interactions
- Need for smoking cessation

HEALTH TEACHING

The primary focus of home care preparation is client teaching regarding risk factors for the recurrence of PUD; clients are also taught to recognize and report the development of complications related to the disease process or surgical intervention.

Instruct the client and family or significant others about factors related to the development of an ulcer. A risk assessment assists in identifying gastric irritants and lifestyle stressors that may be contributory to ulcer formation. Strategies for lifestyle changes are developed together with the client. Teach about symptoms that should be brought to the attention of the health care provider after discharge from the hospital, such as abdominal pain; nausea and vomiting; black, tarry stools; and weakness or dizziness. To demonstrate understanding, have the client describe the symptoms.

Also teach the client about diets to be used for avoiding postprandial distention or dumping syndrome. For postsurgical clients, especially those who have undergone partial stomach removal, a smaller meal may be required. In collaboration with the dietitian, instruct the client to:

- Eat small, frequent meals
- Avoid drinking liquids with meals
- Abstain from foods that contribute to discomfort
- Eliminate caffeine and alcohol consumption
- Begin a smoking cessation program
- Receive B_{12} injections, as appropriate
- Lie flat after eating for a short time

The client is also taught to avoid any over-the-counter (OTC) product containing aspirin or other NSAID. Emphasize the importance of adhering to the treatment regimen. Long-term medication compliance is critical for eradicating *H. pylori* infection and achieving healing of the ulcer. The importance of keeping all follow-up appointments is also emphasized, because early detection of recurrence or the development of complications is desirable.

Help the client identify situations that cause stress, describe feelings during stressful situations, and develop a plan for coping with stressors. Encourage the client to learn and use relaxation techniques, such as exercise, biofeedback, humor, and imagery (see Chapter 4). Psychotherapy may be indicated to help some clients cope with excessive anxiety or stress. Ulcer disease is difficult to eradicate, so it is essential for the client and family to understand how modifying living, working, and eating habits minimizes the risk of ulcer recurrence.

HEALTH CARE RESOURCES

Following discharge, home care nursing visits may be indicated if clients and family members or significant others require instruction or assistance with follow-up care, such as dressing changes, monitoring of potential complications, and continued nutritional problems.

◆Evaluation: Outcomes

Evaluate the care of the client with peptic ulcer disease (PUD) on the basis of the identified nursing diagnoses and collaborative problems. The expected outcomes are that the client:

- Maintains hemodynamic stability, free of disease or surgical complications
- Takes personal actions to control pain

Specific indicators for these outcomes are listed for each nursing diagnosis and collaborative problem under the Planning and Implementation section (see earlier).

ZOLLINGER-ELLISON SYNDROME

Zollinger-Ellison syndrome (ZES) is manifested by upper gastrointestinal (GI) tract ulceration, increased gastric acid secretion, and the presence of a non–beta cell islet tumor of the pancreas, called a **gastrinoma**. Affected individuals may have more than one gastrinoma. About two thirds of gastrinomas are malignant. Although most gastrinomas grow slowly, a small portion of them develop rapidly and metastasize widely. Metastasis occurs mainly in the liver and regional lymph nodes. Gastrinoma remains a relatively uncommon disease, with an incidence of one to three new cases per year per million people.

PATHOPHYSIOLOGY

ZES is caused by a non–beta islet cell, gastrin-secreting tumor of the pancreas that stimulates the acid-secreting cells of the stomach to maximal activity. This large quantity of acid causes gastrointestinal ulceration.

In the early course of the disease, symptoms are similar to those of peptic ulcer disease (PUD). However, these symptoms tend to progress, and they respond poorly to traditional ulcer therapy. Diarrhea may be a manifestation of this disorder, occurring in almost half of clients. The diarrhea may be associated with large amounts of hydrochloric acid secreted into the proximal duodenum. **Steatorrhea** (an excessive amount of fat in the feces) results from the inactivation of pancreatic lipase secondary to the large concentrations of acid and decreased amounts of bile acids.

Etiology and Genetic Risk

In 20% to 60% of clients with ZES, the gastrinoma results from an autosomal dominant disorder called multiple endocrine neoplasia type 1 (MEN-1) syndrome. Gastrinomas contain multiple hormones, but adrenocorticotropic hormone (ACTH) is most commonly found. As a result, Cushing's syndrome with increased ACTH levels is reported in about 8% of clients with ZES (Praveen, 2002).

Incidence/Prevalence

ZES occurs in about 1% of clients with duodenal ulcers. Currently, the morbidity and mortality of ZES is low because of better medical and surgical management of the disease. Fewer than 5% of clients develop a complication, such as abdominal perforation or gastric outlet obstruction. All races can be affected (Praveen, 2002).

HEALTH PROMOTION/ILLNESS PREVENTION

Again, health promotion and illness prevention practices are the same as for gastritis and peptic ulcer disease (PUD). In addition, clients with a known family history of Zollinger-Ellison syndrome (ZES) may consider genetic counseling and possible surgery to prevent the syndrome from developing.

◆COLLABORATIVE MANAGEMENT
◆Assessment

Clients may complain of PUD symptoms and may have diarrhea and/or steatorrhea. Inquire whether any relatives have had ZES. Radiographic and endoscopic findings for

ZES are similar to those for PUD. However, infection with *H. pylori* is usually absent. The diagnosis is usually made by radioimmunoassay studies that reveal increased serum gastrin levels in conjunction with the clinical features of the disease.

◆ Interventions

The aim of therapy is to suppress acid secretion in order to control the client's symptoms. The H,K-ATPase inhibitors, such as lansoprazole (Prevacid) and omeprazole (Prilosec, Losec✱) (given as 60 mg daily in a single dose) are the drugs of choice to reduce gastric acid secretion and heal ulcers in clients with ZES. High doses of H₂-receptor antagonists, such as ranitidine (Zantac), are also effective in reducing gastric acid and providing symptom relief.

If medical therapy fails, the health care provider may choose to perform a vagotomy and pyloroplasty to supplement pharmacologic means of controlling hypersecretion. A total gastrectomy is the surgical approach of choice for this disorder when vagotomy, pyloroplasty, and medical therapy are inadequate. Laparoscopic or open gastrectomy may be performed. (See the earlier discussion of these surgeries under Surgical Management [Peptic Ulcer Disease], p. 1296.)

The consequences of the malignant properties of the tumor are now being more widely recognized, and complete surgical resection of the tumor appears to be the optimal treatment. Clients with aggressive disease can also be treated with chemotherapeutic agents such as 5-fluorouracil and doxorubicin to reduce the tumor and control symptoms.

GASTRIC CARCINOMA

Gastric carcinoma refers to malignant neoplasms in the stomach. Most cancers of the stomach are adenocarcinomas. This is a type of cancer that develops in the mucosal cells that form the innermost lining of any portion or all of the stomach. Other types of cancers include lymphomas and sarcomas (Antigenics, 2003). The remaining cases of gastric carcinoma involve the entire stomach. Often there are no symptoms in the early stages and the disease is often advanced when detected.

PATHOPHYSIOLOGY

Gastric adenocarcinoma can be characterized as *intestinal* or *diffuse* (scattered). Intestinal adenocarcinomas result from atrophic gastritis or intestinal metaplasia, both of which are considered precancerous conditions. The diffuse form of the disease is found primarily in areas where gastric cancer is endemic. Early, superficial gastric cancers produce no notable symptoms. On microscopic examination, the cells resemble intestinal metaplasia (abnormal tissue development).

Gastric cancers spread by direct extension through the gastric wall and into regional lymphatics. The intramural lymphatics readily allow horizontal spread within the gastric wall. Extramural lymphatics carry tumor deposits to lymph nodes in more than 50% of operable cases. Direct invasion of and adherence to adjacent organs (e.g., the liver, pancreas, and transverse colon) may also result. Hematogenous spread via the portal vein to the liver and via the systemic circulation to the lungs and bones is the most common mode of metastasis. Peritoneal seeding of cancer cells from the involved gastric serosa to the omentum, peritoneum, ovary, and pelvic cul-de-sac can also occur.

In people with advanced gastric cancer, there is invasion of the muscularis (stomach muscle) or beyond. These lesions are not amenable to curative resection. The overall 5-year survival rate of people with stomach cancer in the United States is about 21%. The 5-year survival rate for early stage cancers of the upper part of the stomach is about 10% to 15%. For early stage cancer of the lower portion of the stomach, the 5-year survival rate is 50% (Antigenics, 2003).

Etiology and Genetic Risk

Recent evidence has provided a strong link between infection with *H. pylori* and the subsequent development of gastric cancer. Metabolic products produced by the organism transform the gastric mucosa while producing a state of chronic inflammation. Such chronic inflammatory states can induce cancer by increasing cell proliferation and free radical formation.

Clients with pernicious anemia, gastric polyps, chronic atrophic gastritis, and **achlorhydria** (absence of secretion of hydrochloric acid) are two to three times more likely to develop gastric cancer.

Gastric cancer seems to be positively correlated with the ingestion of pickled foods, salted fish, salted meat, and nitrates from processed foods, as well as a high consumption of salt. The ingestion of these foods over a long period of time can lead to atrophic gastritis, a precancerous condition.

The role of cigarette smoking and alcohol consumption in the development of gastric carcinoma is controversial, although some studies support the conclusion that smokers are more likely to develop gastric cancer than are nonsmokers.

Genetic factors play a role in the development of gastric cancer. Familial diffuse gastric cancer is a disease with autosomal dominant inheritance in which gastric cancer develops at a young age. Mutations in the E-cadherin gene (CDH1) have been found in many families with hereditary diffuse gastric cancer (Huntsman et al., 2001). Gastric cancer can also be related to mutations in repair genes MLH1 and MSH2. These genes are generally related to an increased risk of colorectal cancer, specifically hereditary nonpolyposis colon cancer (HNPCC), but they also have been related to an increased risk for gastric, ovarian, biliary tract, urinary, and endometrial cancers. This is also inherited in an autosomal dominant fashion.

Gastric surgery, especially a Billroth II procedure, seems to increase the risk for gastric cancer because of the eventual development of atrophic gastritis, which results in changes to the mucosa. Clients with Barrett's esophagus have an increased risk of adenocarcinoma of the gastric cardia (where the stomach connects to the esophagus).

Incidence/Prevalence

Gastric cancer is the second leading cause of cancer death in the world and 5-year survival rates are low (National Cancer Institute, 2000). The American Cancer Society estimated that in 2003, about 22,400 new cases would be diagnosed in the United States and 12,100 people would die of the disease. Men appear to have a slightly greater risk for developing stomach cancer than women. Most people with diagnosed stomach cancer are in their 60s and 70s.

CULTURAL CONSIDERATIONS

In the United States, *H. pylori* is more common in Hispanics (62%) and black individuals (53%) than among non-Hispanic whites (26%). *H. pylori* infection increases the risk of stomach cancer. In the United States, the incidence of stomach cancer is about twice as high among black individuals as it is among non-Hispanic whites. Native Americans/American Indians and Hispanic Americans are also at an increased risk for stomach cancer. The U.S. National Institute of Diabetes and Digestive and Kidney Diseases (NIDDK) is currently focusing research efforts on *H. pylori* and minority populations. The goal of this research is to determine how *H. pylori* is transmitted in these populations so strategies can be developed to decrease *H. pylori* infection in these populations (NIDDK, 2003).

HEALTH PROMOTION/ILLNESS PREVENTION

Clients with gastritis and/or *H. pylori* infection must follow the recommended guidelines from their health care providers to ensure that the gastritis heals correctly and *H. pylori* is eradicated. This helps prevent gastric cancer. In addition, eating a well-balanced diet following the recommendations of the USDA food pyramid and limiting intake of foods that have been attributed to possibly causing gastric cancer such as pickled foods, salted foods, and processed foods can help prevent gastric cancer. Alcohol and tobacco consumption should be avoided. Clients with a family history of gastric cancer or colon, endometrial, biliary tract, ovarian, or urinary tract cancers should consider genetic counseling to determine whether they are more at risk genetically. Proper genetic counseling can help determine whether a client has a high risk for developing cancer and may prevent cancer if prophylactic treatment such as surgery is performed.

COLLABORATIVE MANAGEMENT

Assessment

HISTORY

Question the client regarding the known risk factors for the development of gastric cancer. Elicit information regarding preferred foods, especially pickled, salted, or smoked foods. Information regarding tobacco use and alcohol ingestion is also gathered. Inquire whether the client has ever been diagnosed with or treated for *H. pylori* infection, gastritis, or pernicious anemia. Note whether the client has a history of gastric surgery or polyps. Also inquire whether any of the client's immediate relatives have gastric cancer.

PHYSICAL ASSESSMENT/CLINICAL MANIFESTATIONS

Although clients with *early* gastric cancer may be asymptomatic, indigestion (heartburn) and abdominal discomfort are the *most* common symptoms (Chart 59-8). These symptoms are often ignored, however, or a change in diet or use of antacids relieves them. As the tumor grows, these symptoms become more severe and do not respond to diet changes or antacids. Epigastric or back pain is also an early symptom that may go unrecognized.

CHART 59-8

KEY FEATURES of
Early Versus Advanced Gastric Cancer

Early Gastric Cancer
- Indigestion
- Abdominal discomfort initially relieved with antacids
- Feeling of fullness
- Epigastric, back, or retrosternal pain

(NOTE: Many clients with early gastric cancer have no clinical manifestations.)

Advanced Gastric Cancer
- Nausea and vomiting
- Obstructive symptoms
- Iron deficiency anemia
- Palpable epigastric mass
- Enlarged lymph nodes
- Weakness and fatigue
- Progressive weight loss
- Signs of distant metastasis
  - Virchow's nodes
  - Blumer's shelf
  - "Sister Mary Joseph nodes"
  - Krukenberg's tumor

In *advanced* gastric carcinoma, progressive weight loss, nausea, and vomiting can occur. Vomiting represents pronounced dilation, thickening of the stomach wall, or pyloric obstruction. Obstructive symptoms appear earlier with tumors located near the pylorus than with fundic lesions. Clients with advanced disease may have weakness, fatigue, and anemia.

Physical assessment findings in advanced disease may be absent, or a palpable epigastric mass may suggest hepatomegaly (liver enlargement) from metastatic disease. Hard, enlarged lymph nodes in the left supraclavicular chain, left axilla, or umbilicus may be the result of metastasis from gastric cancer. Masses on the right suggest metastasis in the perigastric lymph nodes or liver. Signs of distant metastasis include the following:

- Virchow's (sentinel or signal) nodes (enlarged supraclavicular lymph nodes, especially on the left)
- Blumer's shelf, resulting from peritoneal seeding that produces a firm mass palpable on rectal or vaginal examination
- "Sister Mary Joseph nodes" (subcutaneous periumbilical deposits)
- Krukenberg's tumor (metastatic ovarian nodules)

LABORATORY ASSESSMENT

In clients with advanced disease, anemia is evidenced by low hematocrit and hemoglobin values. Clients may have macrocytic or microcytic anemia associated with decreased iron or vitamin B_{12} absorption. The stool may be positive for occult blood.

Hypoalbuminemia and abnormal results of liver tests (e.g., bilirubin and alkaline phosphatase) occur with advanced disease and with hepatic metastasis. The level of carcinoembryonic antigen (CEA) is elevated in *advanced* cancer of the stomach.

RADIOGRAPHIC ASSESSMENT

A double-contrast upper gastrointestinal (GI) series is usually the first diagnostic test. The use of a double-contrast medium assists in the detection of small lesions. A polypoid mass, ulcer crater, or thickened fibrotic gastric wall may suggest gastric cancer.

A computed tomography (CT) scan is used to evaluate gastric malignancies. CT scans of the chest, abdomen, and pelvis are used in determining the extent of the disease.

OTHER DIAGNOSTIC ASSESSMENTS

The health care provider uses esophagogastroduodenoscopy (EGD) for definitive diagnosis of gastric cancer. The lesion can be visualized directly, and biopsies of all visible lesions can be obtained to determine the presence of cancer cells. During the endoscopy, an endoscopic ultrasound (EUS) of the gastric mucosa can also be performed. This technology allows the health care provider to evaluate the depth of the tumor and the presence of lymph node involvement that permits more accurate staging of the disease.

◆Interventions

Management of gastric cancer includes drug therapy, radiation, and/or surgery.

NONSURGICAL MANAGEMENT. The treatment of gastric cancer is highly dependent on the stage of the disease. Surgical resection of the tumor is usually combined with chemotherapy and/or radiation. Radiation and chemotherapy commonly prolong survival of clients with advanced gastric disease.

Drug Therapy. The role of chemotherapy in gastric cancer remains uncertain. No specific chemotherapeutic protocol has had a positive effect on survival. Chemotherapy with single agents such as fluorouracil (5-FU), doxorubicin, mitomycin-C, cisplatin, and etoposide have been used, but the use of a combination of agents appears to have superior results. Bone marrow suppression, nausea, and vomiting are common side effects. Chapter 28 discusses chemotherapy in detail.

Radiation Therapy. Although gastric cancers are somewhat sensitive to the effects of radiation, the use of this treatment is limited, because the disease is often widely disseminated to other abdominal organs on diagnosis. Organs such as the liver and kidneys, as well as the spinal cord, have limits as to the amount of radiation they can endure. Postoperative radiation has not significantly increased survival. Intraoperative radiotherapy (IORT) is available at only a few institutions in the United States, because special operative suites, equipment, and personnel are required.

The most common side effects experienced by clients undergoing radiation include impaired skin integrity, fatigue, and anorexia. Nausea, vomiting, and diarrhea may occur about 1 week after treatment is initiated and diminish a month or more after treatment ends. (See Chapter 28 for more information on radiation therapy.) The most common potential problems of IORT are hemorrhage and fistula development.

SURGICAL MANAGEMENT. Surgical resection is the preferred method for treating gastric cancer. The primary surgical procedures for the treatment of gastric cancer are total gastrectomy and subtotal gastrectomy. In early stages, laparoscopic surgery plus adjuvant chemotherapy or radiation may be curative. Clients having laparoscopic surgery have less pain, shorter hospital stays, rare postoperative complications, and quicker recovery.

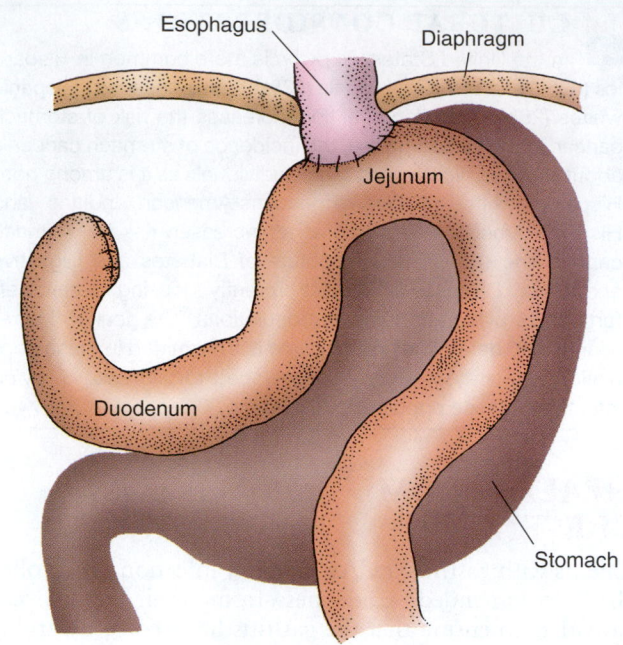

Figure 59-9 ■ Total gastrectomy, with anastomosis of the esophagus to the jejunum (esophagojejunostomy), is the principal medical intervention for extensive gastric cancer.

Most clients with advanced disease are candidates for palliative surgical treatment. Metastasis in the supraclavicular lymph nodes (Virchow's nodes), inguinal lymph nodes, liver, umbilicus, or perirectal wall indicates that the opportunity for cure by resection has been lost. Palliative resection may significantly improve the quality of life for a client suffering from obstruction, hemorrhage, or pain.

Preoperative Care. The health care provider gives the client and family an explanation of the disease and the available treatment options (potentially curative or palliative). Reinforce and clarify the information given. Preoperative care is similar to that provided for the client undergoing general anesthesia and abdominal surgery (see Chapter 20).

Operative Procedures. When the tumor is located in the mid or distal (lower) portions of the stomach, a subtotal gastrectomy is typically performed. The surgeon may use a Billroth I or Billroth II procedure (discussed earlier under Operative Procedures [Peptic Ulcer Disease], pp. 1296 to 1298). The omentum, spleen, and relevant nodes are also removed.

For the client with a resectable growth in the proximal (upper) third of the stomach, a total gastrectomy is performed (Figure 59-9). In this procedure the surgeon removes the entire stomach along with en bloc removal of the lymph nodes and omentum. The surgeon sutures the esophagus to the duodenum or jejunum to reestablish continuity of the GI tract. More radical surgery involving removal of the spleen and distal pancreas is controversial. The overall mortality rate for clients undergoing total gastrectomy surgery is 10% to 15%. For clients with advanced disease, total gastrectomy is performed only when gastric bleeding or obstruction is present.

Clients with tumors at the gastric outlet who are not candidates for subtotal or total gastrectomy may undergo gastroenterostomy for palliation. The surgeon creates a passage between the body of the stomach and the small bowel, often the duodenum (see Figure 59-4).

Postoperative Care. Clients require the standard postoperative care that is given to those who have had general anesthesia (see Chapter 22). Complications after *conventional* gastric surgery may include the following:

- Pneumonia
- Anastomotic leak
- Hemorrhage
- Reflux aspiration
- Sepsis
- Reflux (acute) gastritis (discussed earlier under Acute Gastritis, p. 1284)
- Paralytic ileus
- Bowel obstruction
- Wound infection
- Dumping syndrome (discussed earlier under Monitoring for Postoperative Complications [Peptic Ulcer Disease], p. 1303).

Monitor the client for the development of postoperative complications. Auscultate the lungs for adventitious sounds and monitor for the return of bowel sounds. Monitor vital signs as appropriate to detect signs of infection or bleeding. Aggressive pulmonary exercises and early ambulation can help prevent respiratory complications and deep vein thrombosis. Also inspect the operative site every 8 hours for the presence of redness, swelling, or drainage, which indicates wound infection. Also ensure proper positioning of the client to prevent aspiration from reflux.

Because weight loss is problematic for clients with gastric cancer, nutrition therapy is a vital aspect of preoperative and postoperative management. Preoperatively, compression by the tumor can impede adequate nutritional intake. To correct malnutrition before surgery, the health care provider may prescribe supplements to the diet and/or total parenteral nutrition (TPN). Vitamin, mineral, iron, and protein supplements are essential for correction of nutritional deficits.

Postoperatively, the client's inability to ingest normal-size meals, along with poor nutrient absorption due to decreased stomach size, can prevent the client from taking in adequate nutrition. Therefore the surgeon may place an enteral feeding tube during surgery for continued nutritional support. When feasible, oral intake should begin with fluids and progress to solids as tolerated. For clients who have undergone gastric surgery, regurgitation may result from overeating or from eating too quickly. Experiences with food and fluid are often unsatisfactory for many clients (see the Evidence-Based Practice for Nursing box above).

After oral feedings are restarted, observe the client for signs and symptoms of dumping syndrome and teach the manifestations and management of this syndrome. Advise the client to eat six small meals per day and to consume a diet high in protein and fat but low in carbohydrate-rich foods (see Table 59-2). Liquids should not be taken with meals. Milk and dairy products are usually eliminated because many clients are lactose-intolerant and have symptoms after the ingestion of milk-containing products.

In collaboration with the dietitian, guide the client and family in providing the most nutrients and calories. Counseling about methods of preparation and types of foods that

---

EVIDENCE-BASED PRACTICE for Nursing

What are clients' experiences with food and fluid intake following gastrectomy due to tumor?

Olsson, V., Bergbom, I., & Bosaeus, I. (2002). Patients' experiences of their intake of food and fluid following gastrectomy due to tumor. *Gastroenterology Nursing, 25*(4), 146-153.

The purpose of this qualitative study was to describe clients' experiences of their appetite, hunger, changes in weight, and intake of food and fluid 3 months after gastrointestinal surgery due to tumor. This study was conducted due to the lack of knowledge regarding clients' experiences of intake of food and fluid following gastrointestinal surgery.

Fifteen clients were interviewed regarding their experiences following gastrointestinal surgery. The interviews were tape recorded and transcribed. The interviews were then read several times and repeated phrases and words were identified. Finally, content analysis was performed to identify themes, which included the struggle to eat and drink, bodily estrangement, and nutritional treatment regimens. These three themes consisted of subthemes, such as having no appetite, having difficulty drinking and eating, feeling nauseous, and stress and adaptation.

Some clients felt unhappy because they did not feel hunger, a sensation that made them want to eat and eating was joyful. Eating made many of the clients feel full quickly, which then caused them to dread eating. The full feeling also made them feel nauseous. Many clients felt they were being forced to eat by family members and that food was a medical treatment and not enjoyable. Clients also felt isolated because their eating regimen had to be altered to adhere to medical guidelines.

Level of Evidence: 6—This qualitative research is very small, but serves as a pilot study.

Critique. Although the convenience sample was small, it does give nurses some insight on how to help clients manage nutritional intake after gastrectomy. Qualitative research is an appropriate method for studying this topic. Additional larger studies with diverse subjects are needed to generalize findings.

Implications for Nursing. Nurses need to encourage clients and families to enjoy food after a gastrectomy. They should not view oral nutrition as a medical treatment but as a source of enjoyment. Clients need to be encouraged to eat what they feel like as much as possible. If new eating and drinking habits must be adopted, they should be integrated into the family's existing mealtimes and patterns.

---

increase caloric and protein intake is essential. Maintain intake, output, and calorie counts on a daily basis and record weights at least weekly. Anemia, as well as vitamin B_{12} and folate deficiency, can result following gastrectomy. Oral folate and iron replacement and vitamin B_{12} injections can help correct these deficiencies.

Community-Based Care

Clients who have undergone total gastrectomy and those who are debilitated with advanced gastric cancer are discharged to home with maximal assistance or to a subacute unit or skilled nursing facility. Clients who have undergone subtotal gastrectomy and are not debilitated may be discharged to home with partial assistance for activities of daily living (ADLs). Recurrence of cancer is common, and clients need regular follow-up examinations and radiographic assessments. A case manager may be assigned to ensure continuity of care and thorough follow-up with diagnostic testing.

HOME CARE MANAGEMENT

Gastric cancer is considered a life-threatening illness; therefore the client and family members require physical and emotional care from the health care team. The side effects of gastric cancer treatment can be debilitating, and clients need to learn symptom management strategies. Hospice programs can help both the client and the family cope with these physical and emotional needs.

Clients may fear returning home because of their inability to care for themselves adequately. Enlisting family and health care resources for the client may ease some of this anxiety. The family needs adequate information and support systems to make the transition to home care easier for the client. If the prognosis is poor, the client and family need continued professional support from case managers, social workers and/or nurses to cope with death and dying. (See Chapter 9 for a discussion of end-of-life care.)

HEALTH TEACHING

Instruct the client and family members about any continuing postoperative needs, adjuvant (assistive) treatment, and nutrition therapy. If clients are discharged to home with surgical dressings, teach the client and family to perform dressing changes. Identify the manifestations of incisional infection (e.g., fever, redness, and drainage) that are to be reported.

Clients who will be receiving radiation therapy or chemotherapy require instructions related to the side effects of these treatments. Nausea and vomiting are common side effects of chemotherapy, and instruction in the use of prescribed antiemetics may be needed. (See Chapter 28 for education for clients receiving chemotherapy or radiation therapy.)

In collaboration with the dietitian, educate the client and family concerning the type and quantity of foods that will provide optimal nutritional value. Interventions to minimize dumping syndrome are also emphasized (see Table 59-2).

HEALTH CARE RESOURCES

A home care referral provides ongoing assessment, assistance, and encouragement to the client and family or significant others at home. A home care nurse can help with physical care procedures and can also provide valuable psychological support. Additional referrals to a dietitian, professional counselor, or clergy may be necessary. Referral to a hospice agency can be of great assistance. Hospice care may be delivered in the home or in an institutional setting. Appropriate support groups (e.g., I Can Cope, provided by the American Cancer Society) can be a major resource.

> ### 🎼 Critical Thinking Challenge
>
> One of your clients has just been diagnosed with gastric cancer. The client lives alone and is scheduled for surgery tomorrow. He has just completed a prescribed 2-week series of antibiotics but does not know what it was for. The client lives alone.
>
> 1. Why might the client have taken antibiotics?
> 2. What are some possible postoperative complications that you should anticipate?
> 3. What teaching should you provide to this client if these complications arise?
> 4. What resources might you consider for the client upon discharge?

evolve For suggested answer guidelines, go to http://evolve.elsevier.com/Iggy/.

GET READY for the NCLEX Examination!

KEY POINTS

Safe Effective Care Environment

- For clients with gastric cancer, initiate a consultation or referral to a social worker, grief counselor, and/or community support group.
- For clients undergoing surgical procedures such as esophagogastroduodenoscopy (EGD), make sure that the client has been informed by the physician regarding what the procedure entails, including the benefits and risks and that the client signs a consent form.
- For clients with terminal gastric cancer, encourage them to talk with an attorney or family members regarding their advanced directives.
- Teach clients the importance to of complying with *H. pylori* treatment regimens to eradicate the bacteria, thus preventing its spread.

Health Promotion and Maintenance

- Identify clients at risk for PUD, especially older clients who take large amounts of NSAIDs and clients with *H. pylori*.
- Teach clients behaviors to prevent PUD, such as avoiding large consumption of caffeine, alcohol, coffee, ASA (acetylsalicylic acid), and NSAIDs. Also teach them to avoid contaminated foods and water and smoking.
- Teach clients the importance of complying with *H. pylori* treatment to prevent the risk of gastric cancer.
- Encourage families that have a high incidence of gastric cancer to see a genetic counselor to determine whether specific family members have a high risk for cancer. This action may possibly prevent cancer if prophylactic measures such as surgery are taken.

Psychosocial Integrity

- Allow clients with *H. pylori* to express feelings of anxiety.
- Allow clients with gastric carcinoma to express feelings of grief, fear, and anxiety.
- Address the reactions of family and significant others to the diagnosis of cancer; provide support and education.
- For clients with advanced metastatic gastric cancer, provide end-of-life care, including referral to hospice care.

Physiological Integrity

- For clients who have undergone a gastrectomy, collaborate with the dietitian and instruct the client regarding diet changes to avoid abdominal distention and dumping syndrome.
- Teach clients with abnormal symptoms, such as abdominal tenderness, abdominal pain that is relieved by food or pain or that becomes worse 3 hours after eating, dyspepsia, melena, and/or distention to consult with their physician immediately for a prompt diagnosis and treatment.
- Teach clients that hematemesis is a medical emergency and that they should go to the emergency department for prompt treatment.
- Teach the proper administration of antacids (one to two after meals). Tell clients that antacids can interfere with the effectiveness of certain drugs, such as phenytoin (Dilantin), so other medications must be taken 1 to 2 hours before or after the antacid.

- Teach the client with past or present heart failure to avoid antacids containing a high sodium content. Magaldrate (Riopan) has the lowest sodium concentration.
- Teach the proper administration of H_2 antagonists. Explain that ranitidine, famotidine, and nizatidine are all given at bedtime and sucralfate must be given on an empty stomach.
- Teach the proper administration of antisecretory agents, noting that most cannot be crushed because they are sustained-release or enteric-coated tablets.
- Monitor clients with ulcers for any of the signs and symptoms of GI bleeding that are listed in Chart 59-4. Report any of these symptoms if noted to a physician immediately.
- Post-EGD, monitor the client's vitals signs, heart rhythm, and oxygen saturation frequently until they return to baseline. Assess the gag reflex and ensure that it is intact before giving the client food to prevent aspiration.
- Observe the client for signs and symptoms of dumping syndrome after vagotomy; teach the manifestations and management of this syndrome. Advise the client to eat six small meals per day and to consume a diet high in protein and fat but low in carbohydrate-rich foods. Liquids should not be taken with meals.

ADDITIONAL STUDY RESOURCES

Go to your Student CD-ROM for Review Questions for the NCLEX Examination.

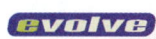 Go to http://evolve.elsevier.com/Iggy/ for Integrated Management of Care Questions for the NCLEX Examination.

SELECTED BIBLIOGRAPHY

Ackley, B.J., & Ladwig, G. B. (2002). *Nursing diagnosis handbook.* St. Louis: Mosby.

Antigenics. (2003). *Gastric cancer.* Retrieved June 19, 2003, from http://www.antigenics.com/diseases/gastriccancer.html.

Barham Solutions. (2003). *Endoscopy Clinic web page.* Retrieved July 9, 2003, from http://www.endo-world.com/peptic.html.

Braunwald, E., et al. (Eds.). *Harrison's manual of medicine* (15th ed., pp. 691). New York: McGraw-Hill.

Carroll, M. (2002). Peptic ulcer disease. *Emedicine.* Retrieved June 16, 2003, from http://www.emedicine.com/PED/topic2341.htm.

Deglin, J.L., & Vallerand, A.J. (2002). *Davis's drug guide for nurses* (8th ed.). Philadelphia: F. A. Davis.

Fantry, G. (2003). Peptic ulcer disease. *Emedicine.* Retrieved June 16, 2003, from http://www.emedicine.com/MED/topic1776.htm.

Giuli, R. (2002). Breast and gastric cancer. *Journal of Surgical Oncology, 2*(8), 1. Retrieved June 19, 2003, from http://www.geocities.com/surgoncnet/roukos.htm.

Horn, J. (2000). The proton-pump inhibitors: Similarities and differences. *Clinical Therapeutics, 22*(3), 266-280.

Huntsman, D.G., et al. (2001). Early gastric cancer in young, asymptomatic carriers of germ-line E-cadherin mutations. *The New England Journal of Medicine, 344*(25), 1904-1909.

Kuremu, R.T. (2002). Surgical management of peptic ulcer disease. *East African Medical Journal, 79*(9), 454-456.

Marshall, J., Collins, S., & Gafni, A. (2000). Prediction of resource utilization and case cost for acute nonvariceal upper gastrointestinal hemorrhage at a Canadian community hospital. *American Journal of Gastroenterology, 94*(7), 1841-1846.

Matheson, A.J. & Jarvis, B. (2001). Lansoprazole: An update of its place in the management of acid-related disorders. *Drugs, 61*(12), 1801-1833.

McCarthy, M.S. (2003). Changing perspectives of stress ulcer prophylaxis. *CME-Today 1*(1), 15-22.

Medical Letter. (2002). Pantoprazole IV (Protonix IV). *Medical Letter on Drugs and Therapeutics, 44*(1129), 41.

National Cancer Institute. (2000). Vitamins, anti-bacterials may prevent stomach cancer. *Stomach Cancer Home Page.* Retrieved June 16, 2003, from http://www.cancer.gov/clinicaltrials/results/vitamins-and-antibacterials1200.

National Cancer Institute. (2001). Radiation and chemotherapy after surgery improves survival in stomach cancer. *Stomach Cancer Home Page.* Retrieved June 16, 2003, from http://www.cancer.gov/clinicaltrials/results/survival-in-stomach-cancer0901.

National Digestive Disease Information Clearinghouse. (2002). *H. pylori* and peptic ulcer. *National Institute of Diabetes and Digestive and Kidney Diseases Home Page.* Retrieved June 27, 2003, from http://www.niddk.nih.gov./health/digest/pubs/hpylori/hypylori.htm.

National Institute of Diabetes and Digestive and Kidney Diseases. (2003). Area of focus #7. Peptic ulcer disease and *Helicobacter pylori.* Retrieved June 27, 2003, from http://www.niddk.nih.gov/federal/planning/Area7.pdf.

Offman, J., et al. (2000). The quality of care for Medicare patients with peptic ulcer disease. *American Journal of Gastroenterology 95*(1), 106-113.

Parkman, H., MacMillan Rodney, W., & Rogers, H. (2001). Empiric therapy for nonulcer dyspepsia. *Patient Care for the Nurse Practitioner, 3*(1), 23-24.

Perry, M. (2002). Peptic ulceration. *Practice Nurse, 24*(8), 39-41.

Praveen, R. (2002). Zollinger-Ellison syndrome. *Emedicine.* Retrieved June 19, 2003, from http://www.emedicine.com/med/byname/zollinger-ellison-syndrome.htm.

Rotello, L.C. (2003). Managing critically ill patients at risk for stress ulcers. *CME-Today, 1*(1), 27-30.

Shannahoff-Khalsa, D. (2002). Stress management for gastrointestinal disorders: The use of Kundalini yoga meditation techniques. *Gastroenterology Nursing, 25*(3), 126-129.

Soll, A.H. (2002). Epidemiology of and risk factors for peptic ulcer disease. *University of California Los Angeles Center for Health Sciences.* Retrieved June 16, 2003, from http://www.uptodate.com/patient_info/topicpages/topics/AcidPep/6089.asp?usd=987106559&r=/patie.

Sukhdeep, P. (2002). Dumping syndrome. *Emedicine.* Retrieved June 30, 2003, from http://www.emedicine.com/medhopic589.htm.

Yabuki, K., et al. (2002). Extensive hemorrhagic erosive gastritis associated with acute pancreatitis successfully treated with a somatostatin analog. *Journal of Gastroenterology, 37*(9), 737-741.

Interventions for Clients with Noninflammatory Intestinal Disorders

MARCIA M. BOEHMKE

LEARNING OUTCOMES

After studying this chapter, you should be able to:

1. Develop a teaching-learning plan for clients with irritable bowel syndrome (IBS).
2. Differentiate the most common types of hernias.
3. Develop a plan of care for a client undergoing a minimally invasive inguinal hernia repair.
4. Interpret assessment findings for clients with colorectal cancer (CRC).
5. Identify health promotion practices to prevent CRC.
6. Discuss the psychosocial aspects associated with CRC and related surgeries.
7. Explain the role of the nurse in managing the client with CRC.
8. Develop a perioperative plan of care for a client undergoing a colon resection and colostomy.
9. Construct a community-based teaching-learning plan for clients requiring colostomy care.
10. Identify community-based resources for clients with CRC.
11. Analyze the differences between small-bowel and large-bowel obstructions.
12. Explain the role of the nurse when caring for clients with nasogastric tubes.
13. Develop a plan of care for a client experiencing intestinal obstruction.
14. Prioritize nursing care for the client with abdominal trauma.
15. Develop a teaching-learning plan for clients having hemorrhoid surgical procedures.
16. Explain the pathophysiology of malabsorption syndrome.

Go to your Student CD-ROM for Review Questions
for the NCLEX Examination keyed to these *Learning Outcomes.*

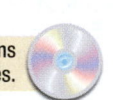

Intestinal disorders commonly present with symptoms of rectal bleeding, changing bowel patterns and abdominal pain. Thorough investigation is imperative to differentiate those caused by a serious condition from those caused by benign processes. Figure 60-1 depicts locations and common causes of gastrointestinal bleeding.

IRRITABLE BOWEL SYNDROME

PATHOPHYSIOLOGY

Irritable bowel syndrome (IBS) is a chronic gastrointestinal (GI) disorder, characterized by the presence of chronic or recurrent diarrhea, constipation, and/or abdominal pain and bloating. It is sometimes referred to as spastic colon, mucous colon, or nervous colon. The disease exacerbates whenever the client is exposed to causative agents.

IBS is believed to be due to impairment in the motor or sensory function of the GI tract. Motility changes, often associated with meals, result in changes in the normal bowel elimination pattern to a pattern of diarrhea, constipation, or alternating diarrhea and constipation. Even with these symptoms, the mucosal lining of the bowel remains essentially unchanged. Symptoms of IBS typically begin to appear in young adulthood. The disease is characterized by remissions and exacerbations ("flare-ups").

Etiology

No structural or infectious etiology has been identified, so the exact cause is unknown. Physical factors, such as diverticular disease, ingestion of coffee or other gastric stimulants, or lactose intolerance may contribute to IBS. There is also considerable evidence to implicate the roles of stress and mental or behavioral illness. Clients who seek medical

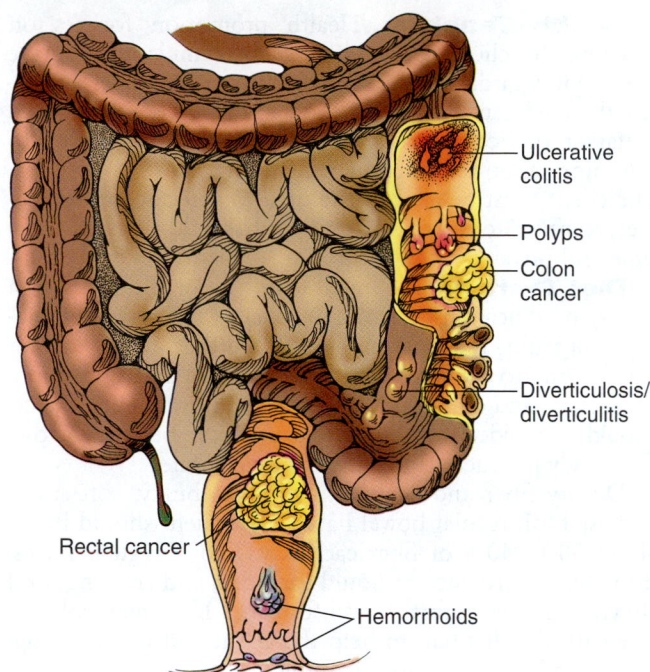

Figure 60-1 ■ Common causes of lower gastrointestinal bleeding.

Labels: Ulcerative colitis; Polyps; Colon cancer; Diverticulosis/diverticulitis; Rectal cancer; Hemorrhoids

EVIDENCE-BASED PRACTICE for Nursing

What are the possible risk factors for irritable bowel syndrome?

Locke, G.R., et al. (2000). Risk factors for irritable bowel syndrome: Role of analgesics and food sensitivities. *American Journal of Gastroenterology, 95*(1), 157-164.

The purpose of this study was to identify additional risk factors for the development of irritable bowel syndrome (IBS), because previous evaluations of traditional risk factors have not led to insight into the pathogenesis of this disorder. Questionnaires were mailed to a sample of 892 individuals residing in Olmsted County, Minnesota, who were stratified by age (30 to 64 years) and gender. Six hundred forty-three individuals returned the surveys. A self-report questionnaire listed gastrointestinal symptoms required for a diagnosis of IBS, measures of potential risk factors, and psychosomatic symptoms. Logistic regression was used in the analysis. The survey controlled for age, gender, and psychosomatic symptoms.

Results showed that 12% of respondents reported IBS symptoms. IBS was significantly associated with the use of analgesics, particularly aspirin. IBS was also correlated with reports of food allergies and ratings of somatic symptoms. The incidence of IBS was higher among subjects taking analgesics and among those reporting multiple food sensitivities.

Level of Evidence: 5—Case control study with adequate sample size.

Critique. Although this study provides early insight into possible risk factors not before associated with IBS, the results must be interpreted with caution. Although the sample size is adequate, the self-selection, cross-sectional design, and limited geographic area lend bias and an inability to generalize the results to the study. Moreover, the self-report method and the fact that the subjects were not necessarily medically evaluated for their symptoms limits the interpretation of the findings.

Implications for Nursing. Although the study results cannot be generalized to the population, nurses collecting history information can include questions concerning analgesic use and food allergies in individuals suspected of having IBS. Individuals who identify themselves as having food sensitivities may also have symptoms of IBS that require investigation. Although analgesics in themselves may not be causative, it is possible that clients with IBS present with other forms of pain induced by the disorder. Careful questioning during the intake history can provide more information into the pathogenesis of IBS.

care for IBS have a higher incidence of panic disorder, anxiety disorder, and major depression than control populations (Lehrer & Lichtenstein, 2004). A familial predisposition has also been noted for some clients.

Incidence/Prevalence

IBS is the most common digestive disorder seen in clinical practice and is estimated to occur in 10% to 22% of the U.S. population. Women are two to three times more likely to have the disease than men. IBS causes 34,000 hospitalizations in the United States each year, and more than 2 million prescriptions are issued for treatment (Lehrer & Lichtenstein, 2004).

◆COLLABORATIVE MANAGEMENT
◆Assessment

HISTORY

Ask the client about a history of abdominal pain, changes in the bowel pattern or consistency of stools, and the passage of mucus. Collect information on all medications the client is taking, because many medications cause GI symptoms similar to those of IBS. A careful dietary history, including the use of caffeinated beverages or beverages sweetened with sorbitol or fructose, which can cause bloating or diarrhea, should be elicited.

The course of the illness is generally specific to the client, and most clients can identify factors that precipitate exacerbations, such as diet, stress, or anxiety. There are no changes in the bowel mucosa and therefore no serious health consequences. Food intolerance may be associated with IBS. Dairy products and grains can contribute to bloating, flatulence, and distention. In one study, individuals who reported intolerances to multiple foods were more likely to report IBS (Locke et al., 2000). Finally, IBS symptoms have

also been associated with analgesic use (see the Evidence-Based Practice for Nursing box above).

PHYSICAL ASSESSMENT/CLINICAL MANIFESTATIONS

There are no specific biomarkers for IBS, but the following characteristic symptoms known collectively as the **Manning criteria** are typically present:

■ Abdominal pain relieved by defecation or associated with changes in stool frequency or consistency
■ Abdominal distention
■ The sensation of incomplete evacuation of stool
■ The presence of mucus with stool passage

Bowel function changes progressively and eventually forms the characteristic pattern.

A flare-up consisting of worsening cramps, abdominal pain, and diarrhea or constipation usually brings the client to the health care provider. The most common symptom of IBS is pain in the left lower quadrant of the abdomen. The client typically reports increased pain after eating and relief after a bowel movement. Nausea may be associated with

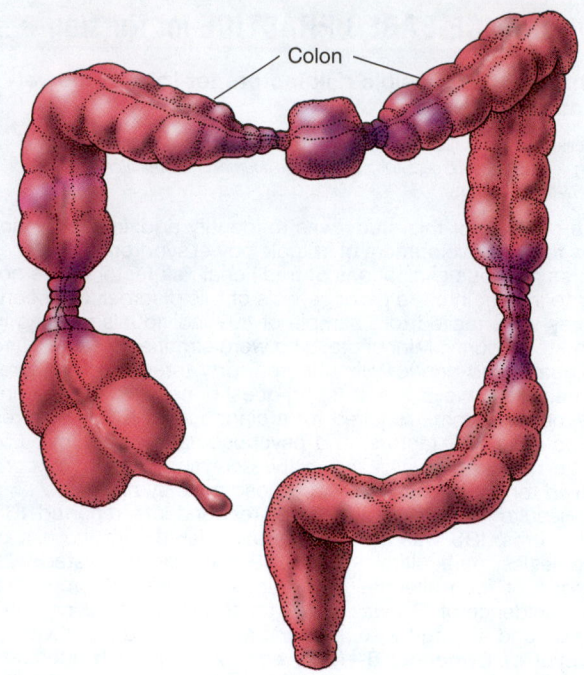

Colon

Figure 60-2 ■ Spastic contractions of the colon as they occur with irritable bowel syndrome.

mealtime and defecation. The crampy abdominal patterns are accompanied by constipation or diarrhea. The constipated stools are small and hard and are generally followed by several softer stools. The diarrheal stools are soft and watery, and mucus is often present in the stools. Clients with IBS often complain of belching, gas, anorexia, and bloating.

The client generally appears well, with a stable weight, and nutritional and fluid levels are within normal ranges. Inspect and auscultate the abdomen. Bowel sounds are generally within normal range and may be somewhat quiet with constipation. On percussion of the abdomen, tympanic sounds may be heard over loops of filled bowel. On palpation, there may be diffuse (widespread) tenderness, which is generally worse if the sigmoid colon is palpable.

DIAGNOSTIC ASSESSMENT

Routine laboratory work (including a complete blood count [CBC], serologic tests, serum albumin, erythrocyte sedimentation rate, and stools for occult blood) is normal in IBS. The health care provider typically orders a barium enema examination for clients suspected of having IBS. Colonic spasm is often noted during the procedure; however, this finding is not diagnostic. In the absence of other diagnostic findings, colonic spasm supports the diagnosis (Figure 60-2).

The evaluation of IBS is not complete without flexible sigmoidoscopy in adults younger than 40 years of age or colonoscopy in adults older than 40 years of age. A colonoscopy often demonstrates intense spastic contractions, which often stimulate painful sensations. Otherwise, the bowel mucosa appears continuous, smooth, and pink.

◆Interventions

The client with IBS is most often cared for on an ambulatory basis. Interventions are directed at education, dietary modification, drug therapy, and stress management. Some clients use complementary and alternative therapies as well.

Health Teaching. Health promotion focuses on teaching the client to avoid problem stimulants. Educate the client regarding the chronic nature of the disorder. Assist the client in identifying food intolerances and needed dietary modifications. Information regarding what constitutes normal bowel function and laxative abuse is provided. The client must be alert to the urge to defecate and evacuate promptly to avoid straining and should plan to allow time and privacy in the bathroom.

Diet Therapy. The initial treatment of IBS focuses on dietary modifications. Instruct the client to eliminate offending or upsetting foods. They should be further advised to limit caffeine and to avoid alcohol, beverages that contain sorbitol or fructose, and other gastric irritants. Milk and milk products should be avoided if lactose intolerance is suspected. Lactose-free or soy products can be used as a substitute.

Dietary fiber and bulk help produce bulky, soft stools and establish regular bowel habits. The client should ingest about 30 to 40 g of fiber each day. Eating regular meals, drinking 8 to 10 cups of liquid each day, and chewing food slowly promote normal bowel function. If needed, collaborate with the dietitian to help the client and family or significant others with meal planning.

Drug Therapy. Drug therapy is directed at the major symptom. The health care provider may prescribe bulk-forming laxatives, antidiarrheal agents, anticholinergic agents, tricyclic antidepressants, and 5-HT$_4$ agonists.

For the treatment of constipation-predominant IBS, bulk-forming laxatives, such as psyllium hydrophilic mucilloid (Metamucil) or calcium polycarbophil (Mitrolan), are generally taken at mealtimes with a glass of water. The hydrophilic properties of these medications help prevent dry, hard, or liquid stools.

Diarrhea-predominant IBS is typically treated with antidiarrheal agents, such as diphenoxylate hydrochloride with atropine sulfate (Lomotil) or loperamide (Imodium) (Chart 60-1). A newer group of drugs called muscarinic (M3)-receptor antagonists also inhibit intestinal motility. Examples of medications in this group currently undergoing clinical trials are darifenacin and zamifenacin.

For IBS in which pain is the predominant symptom, anticholinergics or antispasmodics, such as dicyclomine hydrochloride (Bentyl), help relieve abdominal cramping and intestinal spasm. Tricyclic antidepressants, such as amitriptyline (Elavil), have also been successfully used in this form of IBS. It is unclear whether their effectiveness is due to the antidepressant or anticholinergic effects of the drugs. If clients experience postprandial discomfort (discomfort after eating), they should take these medications 30 to 45 minutes before mealtime.

Recently approved 5-HT$_4$ medications, such as the selective partial agonist tegaserod (Zelnorm) and more potent prucalopride, possess GI prokinetic activity. These drugs are given only to women who have constipation as their primary symptom. Zelnorm imitates the action of serotonin to stimulate peristalsis in the GI tract. The usual dosage is 6 mg twice daily before meals for 4 to 6 weeks. The course may be repeated if needed. Teach clients that the medication should be taken at least 30 minutes before meals because food decreases the drug's absorption. Zelnorm decreases the effects of oral contraceptives, and therefore an additional form of birth control should be used to prevent pregnancy. Prucalopride appears to be a very promising

CHART 60-1

DRUG THERAPY for
Treatment of Irritable Bowel Syndrome (IBS)

Drug	Usual Dosage	Nursing Interventions	Rationales
For Diarrhea-Predominant IBS			
Diphenoxylate hydrochloride and atropine sulfate (Lomotil)	1 tablet 6 times daily; no more than 6 tablets in 24 hr	Teach client to report abdominal distention, pain, and fever.	These symptoms may indicate a bacterial organism in the gastrointestinal (GI) tract. Diarrhea should not be suppressed in the presence of GI infection.
		Teach client to report sedation, dry mouth, urinary retention, and rash.	These are common side effects.
Loperamide (Imodium)	2 mg after each loose stool; maximum of 16 mg daily	Teach client to report abdominal distention, pain, and fever.	These symptoms may indicate a bacterial organism in the GI tract. Diarrhea should not be suppressed if GI infection is present.
For Constipation-Predominant IBS			
Tegaserod (Zelnorm)	6 mg PO twice daily 30 min before meals for 4 to 6 wk (women; dose for men not established)	Teach client to take extra birth control precautions, if appropriate.	The drug decreases effect of oral contraceptives.
		Teach client to report dizziness, irregular pulse, angina.	The drug can cause cardiovascular side effects/adverse effects.
Psyllium (Metamucil, Karacil ✱)	1-2 tsp. in 8 oz. H$_2$O two to three times daily	Teach client to report excessive cramping, rectal bleeding, nausea, or vomiting.	The drug should be discontinued if these problems occur.

drug that is being tested as another choice for clients with IBS who have chronic constipation.

Stress Management. Stress management is based on the client's current and ongoing stressors and available resources. After completing a detailed psychosocial assessment, set expected outcomes and plan appropriate interventions with the client. Relaxation techniques can help the client learn skills for managing the illness. Understanding the illness empowers the client to take certain actions (e.g., diet modification and exercise) that can significantly affect the course of the illness.

If the client is in a stressful work or family situation, personal counseling may be helpful. Make appropriate referrals or assist in making appointments, if necessary. The opportunity to discuss problems and attempt creative problem solving is often helpful. Instruct the client that regular exercise is important for managing stress and promoting regular bowel elimination.

Complementary and Alternative Therapies. Some clients use other modalities as supplements to their medical treatment regimen. The following are examples of therapies that are used to reduce symptoms and reduce discomfort:

- Peppermint and caraway oil combination
- Evening primrose oil
- Chamomile
- Yoga and other relaxation techniques
- Hypnosis
- Acupuncture

Critical Thinking Challenge

A 45-year-old woman is admitted to your hospital unit with acute IBS, severe dehydration, and hyponatremia. On history you find that she is a middle-school teacher who is currently under psychiatric care for acute depression and anxiety disorder. She states that she has a poor memory and has problems with concentration. She is married with no children and states that she is very religious. The client did not want to be admitted because she misses her husband, her primary support system.

1. Why do you think she is dehydrated and has hyponatremia? What other historical data do you need right now?
2. What risk factors does this client have for IBS?
3. What are her primary nursing diagnoses and expected outcomes?
4. What actions should you take at this time?

evolve For suggested answer guidelines, go to http://evolve.elsevier.com/Iggy/.

HERNIATION

PATHOPHYSIOLOGY

A **hernia** is a weakness in the abdominal muscle wall through which a segment of the bowel or other abdominal structure protrudes. Hernias can also penetrate through any other defect in the abdominal wall, through the diaphragm, or through other structures in the abdominal cavity.

The most common types of abdominal hernias (Figure 60-3) are indirect, direct, femoral, umbilical, and incisional.

- An **indirect inguinal hernia** is a sac formed from the peritoneum that contains a portion of the intestine or omentum. The hernia pushes downward at an angle into the inguinal canal. In males, indirect inguinal hernias can become large and often descend into the scrotum.
- **Direct inguinal hernias**, in contrast, pass through a weak point in the abdominal wall.
- **Femoral hernias** protrude through the femoral ring. A plug of fat in the femoral canal enlarges and eventually

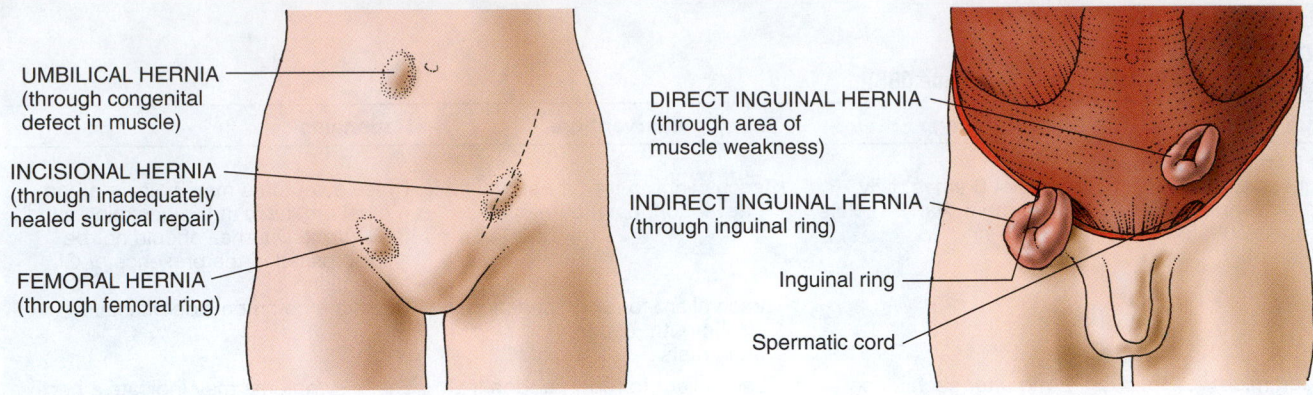

Figure 60-3 ■ Types of abdominal hernia.

pulls the peritoneum and often the urinary bladder into the sac.

- **Umbilical hernias** are congenital or acquired. Congenital umbilical hernias appear in infancy. Acquired umbilical hernias directly result from increased intra-abdominal pressure. They are most commonly seen in obese individuals.
- **Incisional, or ventral, hernias** occur at the site of a previous surgical incision. These hernias result from inadequate healing of the incision, which is most often caused by postoperative wound infections, inadequate nutrition, and obesity.

Hernias may also be classified as **reducible,** irreducible (incarcerated), or strangulated. A hernia is reducible when the contents of the hernial sac can be placed back into the abdominal cavity by gentle pressure. An **irreducible** (incarcerated) hernia cannot be reduced or placed back into the abdominal cavity. Any hernia that is not reducible requires immediate surgical evaluation.

A hernia is **strangulated** when the blood supply to the herniated segment of the bowel is cut off by pressure from the hernial ring (the band of muscle around the hernia). If a hernia is strangulated, there is ischemia and obstruction of the bowel loop. This can lead to necrosis of the bowel and possibly bowel perforation. Signs of strangulation are abdominal distention, nausea, vomiting, pain, fever, and tachycardia.

The most important elements in the development of a hernia are congenital or acquired muscle weakness and increased intra-abdominal pressure. The most significant factors contributing to increased intra-abdominal pressure are obesity, pregnancy, and lifting of heavy objects.

Indirect inguinal hernias, the most common type, are most frequent in men because they follow the tract that develops when the testes descend into the scrotum before birth. Direct hernias occur more often in older adults. Femoral and adult umbilical hernias are most common in obese or pregnant women. Incisional hernias can occur in people who have undergone abdominal surgery.

Defects in the muscle wall result from weakened collagen or widened spaces at the inguinal ligament. These muscle weaknesses can be inherited or acquired as part of the aging process. Increases in intra-abdominal pressure as a result of pregnancy, obesity, abdominal distention, ascites, heavy lifting, or coughing can contribute to their occurrence.

HEALTH PROMOTION/ILLNESS PREVENTION

Even though the muscle weakness cannot be prevented, exercises can be performed to strengthen muscles. Obesity is considered a contributing factor because it causes increased intra-abdominal pressure. Weight control helps to decrease the likelihood of hernias by decreasing pressure on the abdominal muscles. Heavy lifting and straining also increases intra-abdominal pressure and should be avoided.

◆COLLABORATIVE MANAGEMENT
◆Assessment

The client with a hernia typically comes to the health care provider's office or the emergency department with a complaint of a "lump" or protrusion felt at the involved site. The development of the hernia may be associated with straining or lifting.

Perform an abdominal assessment inspecting the abdomen when the client is lying and again when he or she is standing. If the hernia is reducible, it may disappear when the client is lying flat. The advanced practice nurse or other health care provider asks the client to strain or perform the Valsalva maneuver and observes for bulging. The abdomen is auscultated for active bowel sounds. Absent bowel sounds may indicate obstruction and strangulation.

To palpate an inguinal hernia, the health care provider gently examines the ring and its contents by inserting a finger in the ring and noting any changes when the client coughs. The hernia is never forcibly reduced; that maneuver could cause strangulated intestine to rupture.

If a male client suspects a hernia in his groin, the health care provider has him stand for the examination. Using the right hand for the client's right side and the left hand for the client's left side, the examiner invaginates the loose scrotal skin with the index finger, following the spermatic cord upward to the external inguinal cord. At this point, the client is asked to cough, and any palpable herniation is noted.

◆Interventions

The type of treatment selected depends on client factors, as well as the type of hernia.

NONSURGICAL MANAGEMENT. If the client is not a surgical candidate, often an older adult with multiple health problems, the health care provider may prescribe a truss for an inguinal hernia. A **truss** is a pad made with firm material; it is held in place over the hernia with a belt to help keep the abdominal contents from protruding into the hernial sac. If a truss is used, it is applied only after the physician has reduced the hernia if incarcerated. The client usually applies the truss before arising. Teach the client to assess the skin under the truss daily and to protect it with a light layer of powder.

SURGICAL MANAGEMENT. Most hernias are inguinal. Surgical repair of a hernia is the treatment of choice. Surgery is usually performed on an ambulatory care basis for adult clients who have no pre-existing health conditions that would complicate the operative course. In same-day surgery centers, anesthesia may be local, regional, or general, and the surgery is typically laparoscopic. More extensive surgery, such as a bowel resection or temporary colostomy, may be necessary if strangulation results in a gangrenous section of bowel. Clients undergoing extensive surgery are hospitalized for a longer period of time.

A **minimally invasive inguinal hernia repair (MIIHR)** through a laparoscope, also called **herniorrhaphy,** is the surgery of choice. An open, conventional herniorrhaphy may be performed when laparoscopy is not appropriate.

Preoperative Care. In addition to client education about the procedure, the most important preoperative preparation is to teach the client to remain NPO (given nothing by mouth) from midnight the day of surgery. If same day surgery is planned, assist the client in making appropriate arrangements for travel to home and for home care. For clients having an open surgical approach, provide preoperative care as described in Chapter 20.

Operative Procedures. During an MIIHR, the surgeon makes several small incisions, identifies the defect, and covers the weakened area with a mesh patch on the *inside* of the abdominal wall. During a traditional herniorrhaphy, the surgeon makes an abdominal incision and places the contents of the hernial sac back into the abdominal cavity before closing the opening. When a **hernioplasty** is also performed, the surgeon reinforces the weakened *outside* muscle wall with a mesh patch. MIIHR procedures tend to be more successful because the surgeon can reinforce the weakened area inside the abdominal wall and the client has a shorter recovery time. Therefore recurring hernias are not common after laparoscopic herniorrhaphy.

Postoperative Care. The client who has had MIIHR is discharged from the surgical center in 3 to 5 hours. Teach the client to rest for several days before returning to work and a normal routine. Remind the client to observe the small incisions for redness, induration, heat, drainage, and increased pain, and promptly report their occurrence to the surgeon. The client should complain of soreness and discomfort rather than severe, acute pain following laparoscopy.

Postoperative care of the client having an open surgical approach is the same as that described in Chapter 22, except that clients who have undergone surgery for hernias are told to avoid coughing. To promote lung expansion, encourage deep breathing and ambulation. With repair of an indirect inguinal hernia, the physician may suggest a scrotal support and ice bags to be applied to the scrotum to prevent swelling, which often contributes to pain. Elevation of the scrotum with a soft pillow helps prevent and control swelling.

In the immediate postoperative period, the client may experience difficulty voiding. Encourage male clients to stand to allow a more natural position for gravity to facilitate voiding and bladder emptying. Techniques to stimulate voiding, such as allowing water to run, may also be used. A fluid intake of at least 1500 to 2500 mL daily prevents dehydration and maintains urinary function. A "straight" catheterization is required if the client cannot void. Clients usually remain the hospital less than 24 hours.

Most clients have uneventful recoveries after an open hernia repair. Surgeons generally allow clients to return to their usual activities after surgery, with avoidance of straining and lifting for 1 to 2 weeks. Depending on the site and the extent of repair, as well as the client's general physical condition, this period may be extended to 4 to 6 weeks.

Provide oral instructions and a written list of symptoms to be reported, including fever, chills, wound drainage, redness or separation of the incision, and increasing incisional pain. Instruct the client to keep the wound dry and clean with antibacterial soap and water. Showering is usually permitted in a few days.

COLORECTAL CANCER

PATHOPHYSIOLOGY

"Colorectal" refers to the colon and rectum, which together make up the large intestine, also known as the large bowel. Colorectal cancer (CRC) is cancer of the colon or rectum, and is a major health problem worldwide. In the United States, it is one of the most prevalent malignancies, utilizing a significant proportion of health care dollars.

Ninety-five percent of CRCs are adenocarcinomas. **Adenocarcinomas** are tumors that arise from the glandular epithelial tissue of the colon. CRC develops as a multistep process, resulting in a number of molecular changes, such as loss of key tumor suppressor genes and activation of certain oncogenes that alter colonic mucosa cell division. The increased proliferation of the colonic mucosa forms polyps that can be transformed into malignant tumors. Most CRCs are believed to arise from adenomatous polyps that present as a visible protrusion from the mucosal surface of the bowel.

Tumors occur in different areas of the colon, with about two thirds occurring within the rectosigmoidal region. The percentages in Figure 60-4 indicate an increased incidence of cancer in the proximal sections of the large intestine over the past 25 years.

Colorectal cancer (CRC) can metastasize by means of direct extension or by spreading through the blood or lymph. The tumor may spread locally into the four layers of the bowel wall and into neighboring organs. It may enlarge into the lumen of the bowel or spread through the lymphatics or the circulatory system. The circulatory system is entered directly from the primary tumor through blood vessels in the bowel or via the lymphatics. The liver is the most frequent site of metastasis from circulatory spread. Of clients with colorectal cancer, metastasis to the liver develops in 15% to 30% even with surgical resection of the tumor. Metastasis to the lungs, brain, bones, and adrenal glands may also occur. Colon tumors can also spread by peritoneal seeding during surgical resection of the tumor. Seeding occurs when a tumor

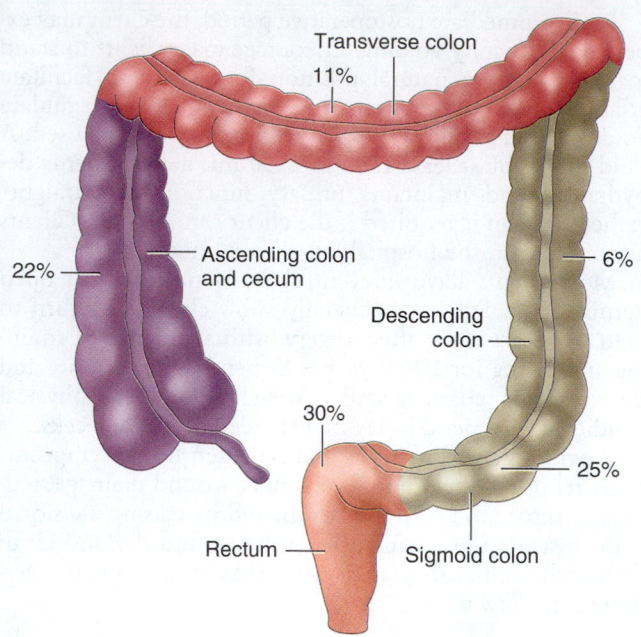

Figure 60-4 ■ The incidence of cancer in relation to colorectal anatomy.

TABLE 60-1	Foods That Affect a Person's Risk for Colorectal Cancer

Foods To Avoid
- Red meat
- Animal fat
- Fatty foods
- Fried meats and fish
- Refined carbohydrates (e.g., concentrated sweets)

Foods To Consume
- Fruits and vegetables, especially cruciferous vegetables from the cabbage family (e.g., broccoli, cabbage, cauliflower, brussels sprouts)
- Whole-grain products
- Adequate fluids, especially water
- Baked or poached fish and poultry

is excised and cancer cells break off from the tumor into the peritoneal cavity.

Complications related to the increasing growth of the tumor locally or through metastatic spread include bowel obstruction or perforation with resultant peritonitis, abscess formation, and fistula formation to the urinary bladder or the vagina. The tumor may invade neighboring blood vessels and cause frank bleeding. A tumor growing into the bowel lumen can gradually obstruct the intestine and eventually block it completely. Tumor extending beyond the bowel wall may place pressure on neighboring organs (uterus, urinary bladder, and ureters) and cause symptoms that mask those of the cancer. Chapter 27 discusses cancer pathophysiology in more detail.

Etiology

Risk factors for the development of colorectal cancer (CRC) include genetic predisposition, personal and dietary factors, and inflammatory bowel disease.

GENETIC CONSIDERATIONS

Individuals with a first-degree relative (sister, sibling, or child) diagnosed with colorectal cancer (CRC) have a threefold to fourfold risk of developing the disease. An autosomal dominant inherited genetic disorder known as **familial adenomatous polyposis (FAP)** accounts for 1% of CRCs. FAP is the result of one or more mutations in the adenomatous polyposis coli gene (APC) (Zangwill, 2004). In these clients, thousands of adenomatous polyps develop over the course of 10 to 15 years and have nearly a 100% chance of becoming malignant. By 20 years of age, most individuals require surgical intervention, usually a colectomy with colostomy, to prevent cancer. New treatment approaches, such as COX-2 drug therapy, are being researched as an alternative to invasive surgical procedures for these clients (Zangwill, 2004). However, COX-2 inhibitors have recently been associated with cardiovascular events, such as myocardial infarction and stroke.

Hereditary nonpolyposis colorectal cancer (HNPCC) is another autosomal dominant disorder and accounts for 10% of all colorectal cancers (CRCs). HNPCC is also caused by gene mutations. Individuals with these mutations have an 80% chance of developing CRC at an average of 45 years of age. They also tend to have a higher incidence of endometrial, ovarian, stomach, and ureteral cancers. Genetic testing is available for these familial CRC syndromes (Zangwill, 2004).

PERSONAL FACTORS

About 75% of all colorectal cancers (CRCs) have no known predisposing cause. Age is considered a risk factor in the development of colorectal cancer, in that 95% of cases are diagnosed in persons over 50 years of age. Clients who have been diagnosed with and treated for CRC have an increased risk of developing a second primary CRC, often at the site of the surgical anastomosis. Those with adenomatous polyps are at an increased risk of developing colorectal cancer. Such individuals need regular follow-up with colonoscopy to visualize and remove polyps.

DIETARY FACTORS

Decreased bowel transit time and certain foods containing chemical mutagens may place individuals at risk for colorectal cancer (Table 60-1). These foods also aid in decreasing bowel transit time, which would increase the time that the bowel is exposed to **carcinogens** (cancer-causing substances). A high-fat diet, particularly animal fat from red meats, increases bile acid secretion and anaerobic bacteria, which are thought to be carcinogenic within the bowel. Fried and broiled meats and fish are also thought to contain chemical mutagens that are carcinogenic. Diets with large amounts of refined carbohydrates that lack fiber decrease bowel transit time as well.

INFLAMMATORY BOWEL DISEASE

Inflammatory bowel diseases (IBDs), such as ulcerative colitis and Crohn's disease, pose an increased risk of colorectal cancer, especially if the disease has had a long, severe course.

Incidence/Prevalence

Colorectal cancer (CRC) is the third most common malignancy (after prostate and lung cancer in men and after breast and lung cancer in women), with an estimated 150,000 new cases each year (Jemal et al., 2002). Americans have a 6% lifetime risk for development of CRC. It is rare before 30 years of age, but incidence increases with age. The median age at diagnosis is 67 years (Ellenhorn, Coia, & Hoff, 2002). The overall incidence is equivalent in men and women, with cancer of the rectum being more common in men. Anal cancers account for about 4% of colorectal cancers.

CULTURAL CONSIDERATIONS

Both black men and black women have an increased frequency of colorectal cancer (CRC) in advanced stages at the time of diagnosis compared with both white men and women; consequently, they also have a greater death rate from CRC. The cause for this difference is not known.

HEALTH PROMOTION/ILLNESS PREVENTION

Individuals at risk can take action to decrease their chance of having CRC. For example, clients whose family members have had hereditary CRC should be genetically tested for FAP and HNPCC. If gene mutations are present, the individual can collaborate with the health care team to decide what treatment plan to implement.

All people, regardless of risk, should modify their diets to decrease fat, refined carbohydrates, and low-fiber foods. Encourage broiled or baked foods, especially those high in fiber and low in animal fat.

Nonsteroidal anti-inflammatory drugs (NSAIDs), including aspirin, decrease the incidence of colon cancer (McCance & Huether, 2002). Regular exercise, daily multivitamins, and female hormonal therapy (e.g., oral contraceptives) also contribute to cancer prevention.

Regular CRC screening, including fecal occult blood testing (FOBT), should be a part of health promotion practices for men and women older than 50 years of age. Individuals who have a personal or family history of the disease should begin screening earlier and more frequently. Teach individuals to follow the American Cancer Society Recommendations for CRC screening listed in Chart 60-2.

◆ COLLABORATIVE MANAGEMENT
◆ Assessment

HISTORY

In taking a history from a client with colorectal cancer, obtain the client's diet history and ask about major risk factors, such as a personal history of breast, ovarian, or endometrial cancer; ulcerative colitis; Crohn's disease; familial polyposis or adenomas; or a family history of colorectal cancer (CRC). Also assess the client's participation in age-specific screening guidelines for CRC (see Chart 60-2).

Ask whether the client has had changes in bowel habits, such as diarrhea or constipation, with or without blood in the stool. The client may also report fatigue (related to anemias), abdominal fullness, pain, or weight loss, which are signs of advanced disease.

PHYSICAL ASSESSMENT/CLINICAL MANIFESTATIONS

The signs of CRC depend on the location of the tumor. However, the most common signs are rectal bleeding, anemia, and a change in the stool. Stools may contain microscopic amounts of blood that are not noticeably visible, or

---

CHART 60-2

BEST PRACTICE for
Screening Recommendations for Men and Women Age 50 and Older at Average Risk for Colorectal Cancer

Procedure: Choice of One of the Following	Interval after Screening Initiated at Age 50 Years	Comments
Fecal occult blood test (FOBT) **OR**	Every year	Procedure: two samples from three consecutive bowel movements obtained at home; tested by physician or nurse
Flexible sigmoidoscopy **OR**	Every 5 yr	
FOBT plus flexible sigmoidoscopy **OR**	FOBT every year; flexible sigmoidoscopy every 5 yr	Procedure for FOBT as above. This combination is preferred over either test alone
Double-contrast barium enema **OR**	Every 5 yr	
Colonoscopy	Every 10 yr	

Data from American Cancer Society. (2003). Colorectal cancer. *CA: A Cancer Journal for Clinicians, 53*(1), 44-51.

---

the client may have mahogany-colored or bright red stools. Gross blood is not usually detected with tumors of the right side of the colon, but is common (but not massive) with tumors of the left side of the colon and the rectum.

Tumors arising in the transverse and descending colon result in symptoms of obstruction as growth of the tumor impedes the passage of stool. The client may complain of "gas pains," cramping, or incomplete evacuation. Tumors arising in the rectosigmoid colon are associated with **hematochezia** (the passage of red blood via the rectum), straining to pass stools, and narrowing of stools. Clients may complain of dull pain. Right-sided tumors can grow quite large without disrupting bowel patterns or appearance, because the stool consistency is more liquid in this part of the colon. These tumors ulcerate and bleed intermittently, so stools can contain dark or mahogany-colored blood. A mass may be palpated in the lower right quadrant, and the client often has anemia secondary to blood loss.

Examination of the abdomen begins with assessment for obvious distention or masses. Visible peristaltic waves accompanied by high-pitched or "tingling" bowel sounds may indicate a partial bowel obstruction from the tumor. Total absence of bowel sounds after listening for 5 full minutes indicates a complete bowel obstruction. Palpation and percussion are performed by the advanced practice nurse or other health care provider to determine whether there is liver or spleen enlargement, or whether there are masses along the colon. The examiner may also perform a digital rectal examination to palpate the rectum and lower sigmoid colon for masses.

PSYCHOSOCIAL ASSESSMENT

The psychological consequences associated with a diagnosis of colorectal cancer (CRC) are many. Clients must cope with a diagnosis that inspires fear and anxiety about treatment, pain, possible disfigurement, and death. In addition, if the cancer is believed to have a genetic origin, there is anxiety concerning implications for the client's immediate family members. Possible loss of health insurance and excessive costs of genetic testing are also sources of fear and anxiety.

LABORATORY ASSESSMENT

Hemoglobin and hematocrit values are usually decreased as a result of the intermittent bleeding associated with the tumor. Colorectal cancer (CRC) that has metastasized to the liver causes liver function tests to be elevated.

A positive test result for occult blood in the stool **(fecal occult blood test [FOBT])** indicates bleeding in the gastrointestinal (GI) tract. These tests can yield false-positive results if certain foods, vitamins, or drugs are ingested before taking the test (Levin et al., 2003). The client should avoid foods such as meat, peroxidase-containing foods (horseradish and beets), and medications, such as aspirin and vitamin C, for 48 hours before giving a stool specimen. Also assess whether the client is taking anti-inflammatory drugs (e.g., ibuprofen, corticosteroids, or salicylates). These medications may be discontinued in consultation with the primary care provider for a designated period before the test. Two separate stool samples should be tested on 3 consecutive days. Negative results do not completely rule out the possibility of CRC.

Carcinoembryonic antigen (CEA), an oncofetal antigen, may be elevated in 70% of people with CRC. There is no relationship between the CEA level and the cancer stage. This antigen is not specifically associated with the colorectal cancer, and it may be elevated in the presence of other benign or malignant diseases and in smokers. CEA is often used to monitor the effectiveness of treatment and identify disease recurrence.

RADIOGRAPHIC ASSESSMENT

A double-contrast barium enema (air and barium are instilled into the colon) provides better visualization of polyps and small lesions than a barium enema alone. This test may demonstrate an occlusion in the bowel, where the tumor is decreasing the size of the lumen.

Computed tomography (CT) of the abdomen, pelvis, lungs, or liver helps confirm the existence of a mass and the extent of disease.

A chest x-ray and liver scan may locate distant sites of metastasis.

OTHER DIAGNOSTIC ASSESSMENTS

A sigmoidoscopy provides visualization of the lower colon using a fiberoptic scope. Polyps can be visualized, and samples can be taken for biopsy. A colonoscopy provides visualization of the entire large bowel from the rectum to the ileocecal valve. As with sigmoidoscopy, polyps can be visualized and removed, and tissue samples can be taken for biopsy. Colonoscopy is the definitive test for the diagnosis of colorectal cancer. A liver scan may locate distant sites of metastasis.

◆Analysis

COMMON NURSING DIAGNOSES AND COLLABORATIVE PROBLEMS

The priority nursing diagnosis for clients with colorectal cancer (CRC) is Anticipatory Grieving related to the diagnosis of a potentially terminal illness, a disturbance in body image, and the possible loss of fecal continence. The priority collaborative problem is Potential for Metastasis.

ADDITIONAL NURSING DIAGNOSES AND COLLABORATIVE PROBLEMS

In addition to the common nursing diagnoses and collaborative problems, clients with colorectal cancer may develop one or more of the following:

- Acute Pain or Chronic Pain related to physical injury agents (e.g., tumor obstruction of the intestine with possible pressure on other organs or chronic physical disability)
- Fatigue related to disease state, anemia, and stress
- Disturbed Body Image related to biophysical factors, illness treatment, and/or surgery
- Ineffective Coping related to uncertainty and high degree of threat
- Imbalanced Nutrition: Less Than Body Requirements related to inability to digest or absorb food due to biologic factors
- Powerlessness related to illness-related regimen

◆Planning and Implementation

ANTICIPATORY GRIEVING

NOC **PLANNING: EXPECTED OUTCOMES.** A client faced with a diagnosis of colorectal cancer is expected to adjust to actual or impending loss. Indicators include that the client will consistently demonstrate the ability to:

- Resolve feelings about loss
- Express spiritual beliefs about death
- Verbalize acceptance of loss
- Report decreased preoccupation with loss
- Report absence of sleep disturbance
- Seek social support
- Progress through stages of grief

INTERVENTIONS. The client and family are faced with a possible loss of or alteration in body functions. Medical and surgical interventions for the treatment of colorectal cancer may result in cure, disease control, or palliation. Interventions are designed to assist the client in formulating effective strategies for expressing feelings of grief and developing coping skills.

Observe and identify the following:

- The client and family's current methods of coping
- Effective sources of support used in past crises
- The client's and family's present perceptions of the health problem
- Signs of anticipatory grief, such as crying, anger, and withdrawal from usual relationships

Encourage the client to verbalize feelings about the diagnosis, treatment, and anticipated alteration in body functions if a colostomy is planned (see later discussion of the operative procedure under Surgical Management, p. 1322). Sadness, anger, feelings of loss, and depression are normal responses to this change in body functions.

If a colostomy is planned, instruct the client what to expect about the appearance and care of the colostomy. Postoperatively, encourage the client to look at and touch the stoma. When the client is physically able, ask him or her to participate in colostomy care. Participation helps to restore the client's sense of control over his or her lifestyle and thus facilitates improved self-esteem.

NIC **Grief Work Facilitation.** The purpose of grief work is to assist the client with the resolution of a significant loss. Assist in identifying the nature of and reaction to the loss. Encourage the client to verbalize feelings and identify fears to help move him or her through the appropriate phases of the grief process. Establish a trusting, ongoing relationship with the client and provide support through the personal grieving stages.

In collaboration with the psychologist or psychiatric clinical nurse specialist and when appropriate, assist the client in identifying personal coping strategies. Encourage the client to implement cultural, religious, and social customs associated with the loss, and identify sources of community support available to the client and family. Modifications in lifestyle can be anticipated in clients with a diagnosis of CRC. Help the client and family to identify the necessary modifications in lifestyle. The chaplain, social worker, or family assists in discussions and decisions concerning treatment, the prognosis, and end-of-life decisions, as appropriate.

NIC **Genetic Counseling.** Genetic counseling entails the use of an interactive helping process focusing on the prevention of a genetic disorder or on the ability to cope with a family member who has a genetically based disorder. Referral to a genetics center for clients with familial CRCs may be needed. Specially trained nurses can discuss the purposes and goals of genetic testing. Privacy and confidentiality need to be ensured. A review of the family history may provide important information concerning the pattern of colorectal cancer inheritance. To make an informed decision, the client and family need information about the advantages, risks, and costs of appropriate genetic tests. Monitor the client's response regarding genetic risk factors. NIC interventions are summarized in Chart 60-3.

CHART 60-3

NIC **INTERVENTION ACTIVITIES for**
The Client with Noninflammatory Intestinal Disorders

Grief Work Facilitation: *Assistance with the resolution of a significant loss*
- Assist the client to identify the nature of the attachment to the lost object or person.
- Assist the client to identify the initial reaction to the loss.
- Encourage expression of feelings about the loss.
- Instruct in phases of the grieving process, as appropriate.
- Support progression through personal grieving stages.
- Include significant others in discussions and decisions, as appropriate.
- Assist client to identify personal coping strategies.
- Encourage client to implement cultural, religious, and social customs associated with the loss.
- Identify sources to community support.
- Assist in identifying modifications needed in lifestyle.

Genetic Counseling: *Use of an interactive helping process focusing on assisting an individual, family, or group, manifesting or at risk for developing or transmitting a birth defect or genetic condition, to cope*
- Provide privacy and ensure confidentiality.
- Determine the client's purpose, goals, and agenda for the genetic counseling session.
- Monitor response when client learns about own genetic risk factors.
- Provide referral to genetic health care specialists, as necessary.

NIC intervention activities selected from Dochterman, J.M., & Bulechek, G.M. (Eds.) (2004). *Nursing interventions classifications (NIC)* (4th ed.). St. Louis: Mosby. No part of this work is to be altered without prior written permission from the Publisher.

POTENTIAL FOR METASTASIS

PLANNING: EXPECTED OUTCOMES. The client with colorectal cancer (CRC) is expected to not have the cancer spread to vital organs; thus the client's life expectancy will be increased and the quality of life will be improved.

INTERVENTIONS. Although surgical resection is the primary means used to control the disease, several adjuvant therapies are employed as well. Adjuvant therapies are administered before or after surgery to affect a cure and to prevent recurrence.

NONSURGICAL MANAGEMENT. The type of therapy used is based on the pathologic staging of the disease. **Dukes' staging classification** may be used to classify colorectal tumors by designating them as A, B, C, or D, according to the depth of invasion into the mucosa and distant spread.

- Dukes' stage A indicates that the tumor has penetrated into, but not through, the bowel wall.
- Stage B indicates that the tumor has penetrated through the bowel wall.
- Stage C indicates that the tumor has penetrated through the bowel wall and that there is lymph node involvement.
- Stage D indicates that the tumor has metastasized to any of a number of distant sites.

Radiation Therapy. The administration of preoperative radiation therapy has not improved overall survival rates for colon cancer but it has been effective in providing local or regional control of the disease. Postoperative radiation has not demonstrated any consistent improvement in survival or recurrence. As a palliative measure, radiation therapy may be used to control pain, hemorrhage, bowel obstruction, or metastasis to the lung in advanced disease. For rectal cancer, unlike the for colon cancer, radiation therapy is almost always a part of the treatment plan. Reinforce information about the radiation therapy procedure to the client and family and monitor for possible side effects (e.g., diarrhea and fatigue). (See Chapter 28 for care of clients undergoing radiation therapy.)

Drug Therapy. Adjuvant *chemotherapy* after primary surgery is recommended for clients with stage II (Dukes' stage B_2) or stage III (Dukes' stage C) disease to interrupt the DNA production of cells and improve survival. The drug of choice is intravenous (IV) 5-fluorouracil (5-FU) with or without leucovorin (folinic acid). These medications cannot discriminate between cancer and healthy cells. Therefore the side effects are diarrhea, mucositis, leucopenia, mouth ulcers, and skin effects.

Oxaliplatin (Eloxatin) is a relatively new platinum analogue chemotherapeutic agent used in combination with 5-FU and leucovorin for clients with treatment-resistant CRC (FOLFOX regimen). The dose-limiting toxicity for this agent is peripheral sensory neuropathy. It may also be used for the initial treatment of advanced colorectal cancer (CRC).

In 1997, irinotecan (Camptosar) was approved as second-line treatment for *metastatic (stage IV or Dukes' D)* disease if it has recurred or progressed after treatment with 5-FU. With this drug, **myelosuppression** (bone marrow suppression, causing **pancytopenia** [decreased blood cells]) and diarrhea are the most frequent dose-limiting toxicities. Camptosar is now given commonly with 5-FU (Saltz regimen). More recently, Camptosar is administered with 48-hour infusions of 5-FU/leucovorin.

In 2004, two new drugs were approved for CRC. Bevacizumab (Avastin) is the first antiangiogenesis medication to be approved for advanced CRC. This type of drug reduces blood flow to the growing tumor cells, thereby depriving them of necessary nutrients needed to grow. Avastin is usually given in combination with other chemotherapeutic agents. Cetuximab (Erbitux), a monoclonal antibody, was also approved for advanced disease. This drug works by binding to a protein (epidural growth factor receptor) to slow cell growth. Erbitux is usually given in combination with another drug.

Current clinical trials using other monoclonal antibodies and a colorectal tumor vaccine are in progress. In addition, new oral agents consisting of a fluorinated pyrimidine and leucovorin are being tested. Additional antiangiogenesis drugs are also being tested. Intrahepatic arterial chemotherapy, often with 5-FU, may be administered to clients with liver metastasis.

Clients with advanced CRC and metastasis also receive drugs for relief of symptoms, such as analgesics and antiemetics. These medications are discussed in Chapter 9.

SURGICAL MANAGEMENT. Surgical removal of the tumor with margins free of disease is the best method of ensuring removal of CRC. The size of the tumor, its location, the extent of metastasis, the integrity of the bowel, and the condition of the client determine which surgical procedure is performed for colorectal cancer (Table 60-2). The most common surgeries performed are **colon resection** (removal of the tumor and regional lymph nodes) with reanastomosis, **colectomy** (colon removal) with *colostomy (temporary or permanent),* and **abdominoperineal (AP) resection**. A **colostomy** is the surgical creation of an opening of the colon onto the surface of the abdomen. An AP resection is performed when rectal tumors are present. The surgeon removes the sigmoid colon, rectum, and anus through combined abdominal and perineal incisions. Most surgeries are done using an open approach, requiring 6 to 7 inch incisions. An alternative is laparoscopic surgery.

Small tumors indicate an early stage of cancer and are well differentiated without evidence of vascular or lymphatic invasion. They can be removed with clean margins and may be treated with local excision and close follow-up. A **transanal approach** without an abdominal incision is the technique most commonly used; this approach decreases the risk for postoperative complications and shortens the hospital stay. Only 5% of clients with colorectal cancer (CRC), however, meet the criteria of early-stage cancer.

Preoperative Care. Reinforce the physician's explanation of the planned surgical procedure. The client is told as accurately as possible what anatomic and physiologic changes will occur with surgery. The location and number of incision sites and drains are also discussed.

Before evaluating the tumor and colon during surgery, the surgeon may not be able to determine whether a colostomy will be necessary. In this case, the client is informed that a colostomy is a possibility. If a colostomy is inevitable, consult an enterostomal therapist (ET) to advise on optimal placement of the ostomy and instruct the client about the rationale and general principles of ostomy care. An ET is a registered nurse who has completed specialized training and is certified in ostomy nursing care. Some are also certified in wound and incontinence care.

The client who requires low rectal surgery (AP resection) is faced with the risk of postoperative sexual dysfunction and urinary incontinence as a result of nerve damage during surgery. The surgeon discusses the risk for these problems with the client before surgery and allows him or her to verbalize concerns and questions related to this risk. Reinforce teaching about abdominal surgery performed with the client under general anesthesia and review the routines for turning and deep breathing (see Chapter 20).

If the bowel is not obstructed or perforated, elective surgery is planned. The client is instructed to thoroughly clean the bowel, or "bowel prep," to minimize bacterial growth and prevent complications. In preparation for the bowel prep, the client is usually instructed to restrict the diet to clear liquids for 1 to 2 days before surgery. Mechanical cleaning is accomplished with laxatives and enemas or with "whole-gut lavage." For whole-gut lavage, the client usually ingests large quantities of a sodium sulfate and polyethylene glycol solution (e.g., GoLYTELY). This solution overwhelms the absorptive capacity of the small bowel and clears feces from the colon.

To reduce the risk of infection, the surgeon may prescribe oral or IV antibiotics to be given the day before surgery. A nasogastric (NG) tube may be placed for decompression of the stomach following surgery. A peripheral IV line is also placed for fluid and electrolyte replacement while the client is taking nothing by mouth (NPO) postoperatively.

The client with colorectal cancer faces a serious illness with long-term consequences of the disease and treatment. A case manager can be very helpful in identifying client and family needs, as well as continuity of care and support.

Operative Procedures. For the conventional open surgical approach, the surgeon makes an incision in the abdomen and explores the abdominal cavity to determine whether the tumor can be removed. For a colon resection, the portion of the colon with the tumor is excised, and the two open ends of the bowel are irrigated before **anastomosis** (reattachment) of the colon. If an anastomosis is not feasible because of the location of the tumor or the bowel is inflamed, a colostomy is created.

TABLE 60-2 Surgical Procedures for Colorectal Cancers in Various Locations

Right-Sided Colon Tumors
- Right hemicolectomy for smaller lesions
- Right ascending colostomy or ileostomy for large, widespread lesions
- Cecostomy (opening into the cecum with intubation to decompress the bowel)

Left-Sided Colon Tumors
- Left hemicolectomy for smaller lesions
- Left descending colostomy for larger lesions

Sigmoid Colon Tumors
- Sigmoid colectomy for smaller lesions
- Sigmoid colostomy for larger lesions
- Abdominoperineal resection for large, low sigmoid tumors (near the anus) with colostomy (the rectum and the anus are completely removed, leaving a perineal wound)

Rectal Tumors
- Resection with anastomosis or pull-through procedure (preserves anal sphincter and normal elimination pattern)
- Colon resection with permanent colostomy
- Abdominoperineal resection with colostomy

A colostomy may be created in the ascending, transverse, descending, or sigmoid colon (Figure 60-5). One of several techniques is used to construct a colostomy. A loop **stoma** (surgical opening) is made by bringing a loop of colon to the skin surface, severing and everting the anterior wall, and suturing it to the abdominal wall. Loop colostomies are usually performed in the transverse colon and are usually temporary. An external rod may be used to support the loop until the intestinal tissue adheres to the abdominal wall. Care must be taken to avoid displacing the rod, especially during appliance changes.

An end stoma is often constructed, most often in the descending or sigmoid colon, when a colostomy is intended to be permanent. It may also be done when the surgeon oversews the distal stump of the colon and places it in the abdominal cavity, preserving it for future reattachment. An end stoma is constructed by severing the end of the proximal portion of the bowel and bringing it out through the abdominal wall.

The least common colostomy is the **double-barrel stoma,** which is created by dividing the bowel and bringing both the proximal and distal portions to the abdominal surface to create two stomas. The proximal stoma (closest to the client's head) is the functioning stoma and eliminates stool; the distal stoma (farthest from the head) is considered nonfunctioning, although it may secrete some mucus. The distal stoma is sometimes referred to as a mucous fistula.

Some surgeons use minimally invasive techniques for colon resection via laparoscopy. Laparoscopic colon resection or total colectomy allows complete tumor removal with an adequate surgical margin and removal of associated lymph nodes. This technique is as safe and effective as the conventional surgical method, but it requires more surgical time.

Postoperative Care. Clients who have undergone an open colon resection without a colostomy receive care similar to that of clients undergoing any abdominal surgery (see Chapter 22). In addition, clients require colostomy and wound management. The client typically has a nasogastric (NG) tube after surgery and receives PCA for the first 24 to 36 hours. After NG tube removal, the diet is slowly progressed from liquids to solid foods as the client can tolerate. The care of clients with an NG tube is discussed under Interventions (Intestinal Obstruction) on p. 1329.

By contrast, clients who have laparoscopic surgery do not have an NG tube and can progress from liquids to solids more quickly. They usually have less pain and are able to ambulate earlier than those who have the conventional approach. The hospital stay is usually shorter for the client with minimally invasive surgery—usually 4 to 5 days.

Colostomy Management. The client who has a colostomy created may return from surgery with an ostomy pouch system in place. If there is no pouch system in place, a petrolatum gauze dressing is usually placed over the

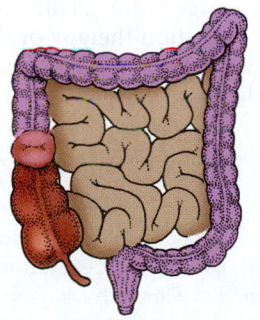

The **ascending colostomy** is done for right-sided tumors.

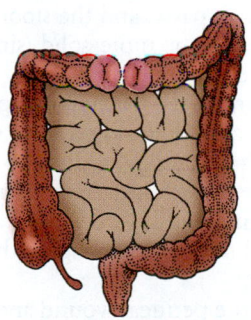

The **transverse (double-barreled) colostomy** is often used in such emergencies as intestinal obstruction or perforation because it can be created quickly. There are two stomas. The proximal one, closest to the small intestine, drains feces. The distal stoma drains mucus.

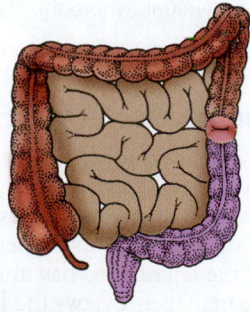

The **descending colostomy** is done for left-sided tumors.

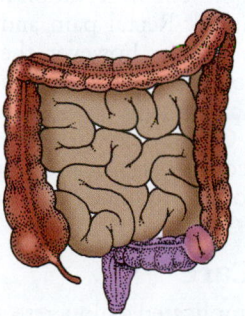

The **sigmoid colostomy** is done for rectal tumors.

Figure 60-5 ■ Different locations of colostomies in the colon.

stoma to keep it moist, and this is covered with a dry, sterile dressing. In collaboration with the enterostomal therapist (ET), place a pouch system as soon as possible. The colostomy pouch system, also called an appliance, allows more convenient and acceptable collection of stool than a dressing does.

Assess the color and integrity of the stoma. A healthy stoma should be reddish pink and moist and will protrude about ¾ inch (2 cm) from the abdominal wall. A small amount of bleeding at the stoma is common.

Report any of the following problems related to the colostomy to the surgeon:

- Signs of ischemia and necrosis (dark red, purplish, or black color; dry, firm, or flaccid)
- Unusual bleeding
- Mucocutaneous separation (breakdown of the suture line securing the stoma to the abdominal wall)

Also assess the condition of the peristomal skin (skin around the stoma) and frequently check the pouch system for proper fit and signs of leakage. The peristomal skin should be intact, smooth, and without redness or excoriation.

The colostomy should start functioning 2 to 4 days postoperatively. When the colostomy begins to function, the pouch may need to be emptied frequently because of excess gas collection. It should be emptied when it is one-third to one-half full of stool. Stool is liquid immediately postoperatively but becomes more solid, depending on where in the colon the stoma was placed. For example, the stool from a colostomy in the ascending colon is liquid, the stool from a colostomy in the transverse colon is pasty, and the stool from a colostomy in the descending colon is more solid (similar to usual stool expelled from the rectum).

Wound Management. For an AP resection, the perineal wound is generally surgically closed, and two bulb suction drains, such as Jackson-Pratt drains, are placed in the wound or through stab wounds near the wound. The drains help prevent drainage from collecting within the wound and are usually left in place for several days, depending on the character and amount of drainage.

Monitoring drainage from the perineal wound and cavity is important because of the possibility of infection and abscess formation. Serosanguineous drainage from the perineal wound may be observed for 1 to 2 months after surgery. Complete healing of the perineal wound may take 6 to 8 months. This wound can be a greater source of discomfort than the abdominal incision and ostomy, and more care may be required. The client may experience phantom rectal sensations because sympathetic innervation for rectal control has not been interrupted. Rectal pain and itching may occasionally occur after healing; however, there is no known physiologic explanation for these sensations. Interventions may include use of antipruritic medications, such as benzocaine, and sitz baths. Continually assess for signs of infection, abscess, or other complications and implement methods for promoting wound drainage and comfort (Chart 60-4).

Community-Based Care

Clients undergoing an uncomplicated colon resection are typically hospitalized for 5 to 7 days. Discharge planning with the assistance of a discharge planner or case manager assists clients and their families in coping with the immedi-

---

CHART 60-4

BEST PRACTICE for
Perineal Wound Care

Wound Care
- Place an absorbent dressing (Kerlix or abdominal pad) over the wound.
- Instruct the client that he or she may:
  Use a feminine napkin as a dressing.
  Wear jockey-type shorts rather than boxers.

Comfort Measures
- If prescribed, soak the wound area in a sitz bath for 10 to 20 minutes three or four times per day.
- Administer pain medication as prescribed and assess its effectiveness.
- Instruct the client about permissible activities. The client should:
  Assume a side-lying position in bed; avoid sitting for long periods.
  Use foam pads or a soft pillow to sit on whenever in a sitting position.
  Avoid the use of air rings or rubber doughnut devices.

Prevention of Complications
- Maintain fluid and electrolyte balance by monitoring intake and output and by monitoring output from the perineal wound.
- Observe incision integrity and monitor wound drains; watch for erythema, edema, bleeding, drainage, unusual odor, and excessive or constant pain.

---

ate postoperative phase of recovery. Following hospitalization for surgery, the client with CRC is usually managed at home. Radiation therapy or chemotherapy is typically done on an ambulatory (outpatient) basis. For the client with advanced cancer, hospice care is an option (see Chapter 9).

Critical Thinking Challenge

A 55-year-old client is admitted to the surgical suite for a colon resection secondary to colorectal cancer (CRC). Although his surgeon believes the cancer is contained and can be removed without having a colostomy, the client is afraid that he may need one. He was recently engaged and is looking forward to his wedding that is scheduled in 6 weeks. His father had colon cancer and died before he was 60 years of age.

1. What further assessment data should you obtain at this time?
2. What collaborative interventions would be useful in view of the client's fears?
3. What should you (the OR nurse) communicate to the postoperative unit where the client will be discharged?

evolve For suggested answer guidelines, go to http://evolve.elsevier.com/Iggy/.

HOME CARE MANAGEMENT

Assess all clients for their ability to perform incision care and activities of daily living (ADLs) within limitations. For clients requiring assistance with these activities, home care visits by nurses or assistive nursing personnel can be provided.

For the client who has undergone a colostomy, the nurse or case manager reviews the home situation to aid the client in arranging for care. Ostomy products should be kept in an area (preferably the bathroom) where the temperature is neither hot nor cold (skin barriers may become stiff or melt in extreme temperatures) to ensure proper functioning. The enterostomal therapist (ET) may serve as a consultant after the client is discharged home to ensure continuity of care.

No changes are needed in sleeping accommodations. A rubber covering may initially be placed over the bed mattress if clients feel insecure about the pouch system. The client may consume his or her usual diet on discharge.

HEALTH TEACHING

Before discharge, clients are instructed to avoid lifting heavy objects or straining on defecation to prevent tension on the anastomosis site. If the client had the open surgical approach, driving should be avoided for 4 to 6 weeks while the incision heals. Clients who had laparoscopy can usually return to all usual activities in 1 to 2 weeks.

A stool softener may be prescribed to keep stools at a soft consistency for ease of passage. Clients are instructed to note the frequency, amount, and character of the stools. In addition to this information, teach all clients with colon resections to watch for and report clinical manifestations of intestinal obstruction and perforation (e.g., cramping, abdominal pain, nausea, and vomiting). A normal diet may be resumed; however, the client is advised to avoid gas-producing foods and carbonated beverages. Four to six weeks may be required to establish the effects of certain foods on bowel patterns.

COLOSTOMY CARE. Rehabilitation after ostomy surgery requires that clients and family members learn the principles of colostomy care and the psychomotor skills needed to facilitate this care. Providing information is important, but the nurse must also allow adequate opportunity for clients to learn the psychomotor skills involved in ostomy care before discharge. Sufficient practice time is planned for clients and family or significant others so that they can handle, assemble, and apply all ostomy equipment. Teach clients and families or other caregivers about the following:

- The normal appearance of the stoma
- Signs and symptoms of complications
- Measurement of the stoma
- The choice, use, care, and application of the appropriate appliance to cover the stoma
- Measures to protect the skin adjacent to the stoma
- Dietary measures to control gas and odor
- Resumption of normal activities, including work, travel, and sexual intercourse

The appropriate pouch system must be selected and fitted to the stoma. Clients with flat, firm abdomens may use either flexible (bordered with paper tape) or nonflexible (full skin barrier wafer) pouch systems. A firm abdomen with lateral creases or folds requires a flexible system. Clients with deep creases, flabby abdomens, a retracted stoma, or a stoma that is flush or concave to the abdominal surface benefit from a convex appliance with a stoma belt. This type of system presses into the skin around the stoma, causing the stoma to protrude. This protrusion helps tighten the skin and prevents leaks around the stoma opening onto the peristomal skin.

Measurement of the stoma is necessary to determine the correct size of the stomal opening on the appliance. The opening should be large enough not only to cover the peristomal skin but also to avoid stomal trauma. The stoma will shrink within 6 to 8 weeks of surgery; therefore it needs to be measured at least once weekly during this time and as

needed if the client gains or loses weight. The client and family caregiver should be taught to trace the pattern of the stomal area on the wafer portion of the appliance and to cut an opening about $1/8$- to $1/16$-inch larger than the stomal pattern to ensure that stomal tissue will not be constricted.

Skin preparation may include clipping peristomal hair or shaving the area to achieve a smooth surface, prevent unnecessary discomfort when the wafer is removed, and minimize the risk of infected hair follicles. The client is advised to avoid using moisturizing soaps to clean the area because the lubricants can interfere with adhesion of the appliance. The client and family caregiver are taught to apply a skin sealant and allow it to dry before application of the appliance (colostomy bag) to facilitate less painful removal of the tape or adhesive. If peristomal skin becomes raw, the client or caregiver checks to see whether the sealant contains alcohol and, if so, reconsiders using it to avoid causing a burning sensation to the skin. Stoma powder or paste, or a combination, may also be used for erythematous peristomal skin. The paste is also used to fill in crevices and creases to create a flat surface for the faceplate of the colostomy bag. If the client develops a fungal rash, an antifungal cream or powder is used, as prescribed.

Control of gas and odor from the colostomy is often a significant goal for clients with new ostomies. Although a leaking or inadequately closed pouch is the usual cause of odor, flatus can also contribute to the odor. Remind the client and family caregiver that although there are generally no forbidden foods for ostomates, certain foods and habits can cause flatus or contribute to odor when the pouch is open. Broccoli, brussels sprouts, cabbage, cauliflower, cucumbers, mushrooms, and peas often cause flatus, as does chewing gum, smoking, drinking beer, and skipping meals. Crackers, toast, and yogurt can help prevent gas. Asparagus, broccoli, cabbage, turnips, eggs, fish, and garlic contribute to odor when the pouch is open. Buttermilk, cranberry juice, parsley, and yogurt will help prevent odor; charcoal filters, pouch deodorizers, or placement of a breath mint in the pouch will eliminate odors. The client should be cautioned not to put aspirin tablets in the pouch because they may cause ulceration of the stoma.

The client with a sigmoid colostomy may benefit from colostomy irrigation to regulate elimination. However, most clients with a sigmoid colostomy can become regulated through diet. An irrigation is similar to an enema, but is administered through the stoma rather than the rectum.

In addition to instructing the client about the clinical manifestations of obstruction and perforation, advise the client with a colostomy to report any fever or sudden onset of pain or swelling around the stoma. Other home care assessment is listed in Chart 60-5.

PSYCHOSOCIAL PREPARATION. The diagnosis of cancer can be emotionally immobilizing for the client and family or significant others, but treatment may be welcomed because it may provide hope for control of the disease. Explore the client's reactions to the illness and perceptions of planned interventions.

The client's reaction to ostomy surgery, which may include disfigurement, may involve the following:

- Fear of not being accepted by others
- Feelings of grief related to disturbance in body image
- Concerns about sexuality

HOME CARE ASSESSMENT of
The Client with a Colostomy

Assess gastrointestinal status, including:
- Dietary and fluid intake and habits
- Presence or absence of nausea and vomiting
- Weight gain or loss
- Bowel elimination pattern and characteristics and amount of effluent (stool)
- Bowel sounds

Assess condition of stoma, including:
- Location, size, protrusion, color, and integrity
- Signs of ischemia, such as dull coloring or dark or purplish bruising

Assess peristomal skin for:
- Presence or absence of excoriated skin, leakage underneath drainage system
- Fit of appliance and effectiveness of skin barrier and appliance

Assess client's and family's coping skills, including:
- Self-care abilities in the home
- Acknowledgment of changes in body image and function
- Sense of loss

Allow the client to verbalize his or her feelings. By teaching how to physically manage the ostomy, help the client begin to restore self-esteem and improve body image. Inclusion of family and significant others in the rehabilitation process may help maintain relationships and raise the client's self-esteem. Anticipatory instruction includes information on leakage accidents, odor control measures, and adjustments to resuming sexual relationships.

HEALTH CARE RESOURCES

Several resources are available to complement nursing care, maintain continuity of care in the home environment, and provide for client needs that the nurse is not able to meet. Make referrals to case managers or social workers, who can provide further emotional counseling to the client and family or significant others, aid in managing the financial concerns that the client and family may have, or arrange home care or extended care (e.g., in a nursing home, group home, or hospice) as needed.

If needed, make a referral to the enterostomal therapist (ET) to aid in preoperative stoma teaching, evaluate the stoma site, and provide consultation for problems in care. The enterostomal therapist (ET) may also conduct an ambulatory care clinic for ongoing client needs.

Information about the United Ostomy Association, a self-help group of people who have ostomies, is provided. Literature, such as the organization's publication *(Ostomy Quarterly)*, and information about a local chapter are given to the client. This organization conducts a visitor program that sends specially trained visitors (who have an ostomy) to talk with clients. After obtaining the client's consent, you can also make a referral to the visitor program so that the visitor can see the client both preoperatively and postoperatively. A physician's consent for visitation is generally necessary.

The local division or unit of the American Cancer Society (ACS) can help provide necessary medical equipment and supplies, home care services, travel accommodations, and other resources for the client who is undergoing cancer treatment or ostomy surgery. Inform the client and family of the programs available through the local division or unit.

Because of short hospital stays, clients with new ostomies receive most of their instruction on colostomy care from nurses working for home care agencies. This resource also facilitates provision for physical care needs, medication management, and emotional support for clients with or without colostomies. If the client has advanced colorectal cancer, a referral for hospice services in the home, nursing home, or other long-term care setting may be appropriate. The home care nurse informs the client and family about what ostomy supplies are needed and where they can be purchased. Price and location are considered before recommendations are made.

◆ Evaluation: Outcomes

Evaluate the care of the client with colorectal cancer on the basis of the identified nursing diagnoses and collaborative problems. The expected outcomes are that the client:
- Adjusts to actual or impending loss
- Is free of complications or metastasis associated with CRC

Specific indicators for these outcomes are listed for each nursing diagnosis and collaborative problem under the Planning and Implementation section (see earlier).

INTESTINAL OBSTRUCTION

PATHOPHYSIOLOGY

Intestinal obstructions can be partial or complete and are classified as mechanical or nonmechanical. In **mechanical obstruction,** the bowel is physically obstructed by disorders outside the intestine (e.g., adhesions or hernias) or by blockages in the lumen of the intestine (e.g., tumors, inflammation, strictures, or fecal impactions). **Nonmechanical obstruction** (also known as paralytic ileus or adynamic ileus because it is a result of neuromuscular disturbance) does not involve a physical obstruction in or outside the intestine. Instead, peristalsis is decreased or absent, resulting in a slowing of the movement or a backup of intestinal contents.

Intestinal contents are composed of ingested fluid and saliva; gastric, pancreatic, and biliary secretions; and swallowed air. In both mechanical and nonmechanical obstructions, the intestinal contents accumulate at and above the area of obstruction. Intestinal distention results from the intestine's inability to absorb the contents and mobilize them down the intestinal tract. To compensate for the lag, peristalsis increases in an effort to move the intestinal contents forward. The increase in peristalsis stimulates more secretions, which leads to additional distention. This causes edema of the bowel with increased capillary permeability. Plasma leaking into the peritoneal cavity and fluid trapped in the intestinal lumen markedly decrease the absorption of fluid and electrolytes into the vascular space. Reduced circulatory blood volume and electrolyte imbalances typically occur. Hypovolemia ranges from mild to extreme (hypovolemic shock).

Specific fluid and electrolyte problems result, depending on the part of the intestine that is blocked. An obstruction high in the small intestine causes a loss of gastric hydrochloride, which can lead to *metabolic alkalosis.* Obstruction below the duodenum but above the large bowel results in loss of both acids and bases, so that acid-base imbalance is usually not compromised. Obstruction at the end of the small intestine and lower in the intestinal tract causes loss of alkaline fluids, which can lead to *metabolic acidosis.*

If the resultant hypovolemia is severe, renal insufficiency or even death can occur. Bacterial peritonitis with or without actual perforation can also result. Bacteria in the intestinal contents lie stagnant in the obstructed intestine. This is not a problem unless the blood flow to the intestine is compromised. However, with so-called closed-loop obstruction (blockage in two different areas) or a **strangulated obstruction** (obstruction with compromised blood flow), the risk for peritonitis is greatly increased. Bacteria without blood supply can form an endotoxin, and release of the endotoxin into the peritoneal or systemic circulation results in septic shock. With a strangulated obstruction, major blood loss into the intestine and the peritoneum can result. Current mortality rates for bowel obstruction range from 3.5% to 6% but may be as high as 14% in older adults.

Etiology

Intestinal obstruction is a common and serious disorder caused by a variety of conditions and is associated with significant morbidity. It can occur anywhere in the intestinal tract, although the ileum in the small intestine (the narrowest part of the intestinal tract) is the most common site.

Mechanical obstruction can result from the following:
- Adhesions
- Tumors
- Hernias
- Fecal impactions (especially in older adults)
- Strictures due to Crohn's disease or radiation
- **Intussusception** (telescoping of a segment of the intestine within itself)
- **Volvulus** (twisting of the intestine)
- Fibrosis due to disorders such as endometriosis
- Vascular disorders (e.g., emboli and arteriosclerotic narrowing of mesenteric vessels) (Figure 60-6).

In individuals age 65 or older, diverticulitis and tumors are the most common causes of obstruction.

Regardless of age, adhesions are the most common cause of mechanical obstruction, accounting for 45% to 60% of cases. Adhesions are bands of granulation and scar tissue that develop as a result of an inflammatory response, encircling the intestine and constricting its lumen.

Paralytic, or **adynamic, ileus** is a nonmechanical obstruction caused by physiologic, neurogenic, or chemical imbalances associated with decreased peristalsis from trauma or the effect of a toxin on autonomic intestinal control. Adynamic ileus occurs to some degree following abdominal surgery or trauma. Paralytic ileus can be caused by handling of the intestines during abdominal surgery; intestinal function is lost for a few hours to several days.

Thoracic diseases such as myocardial infarction, rib fracture, and pneumonia can also cause paralytic ileus. Electrolyte disturbances, especially hypokalemia, predispose the client to ileus. Paralytic ileus can be a consequence of peritonitis, because leakage of colonic contents causes severe irritation and triggers an inflammatory response. Vascular insufficiency to the bowel, also referred to as intestinal ischemia, is a potential cause of adynamic ileus. Vascular insufficiency results when arterial or venous thrombosis or an embolus decreases blood flow to the mesenteric blood ves-

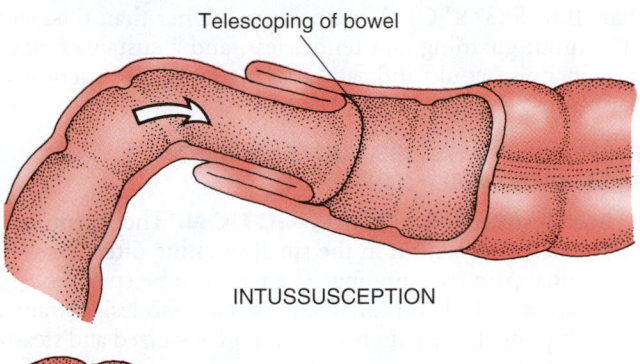

INTUSSUSCEPTION

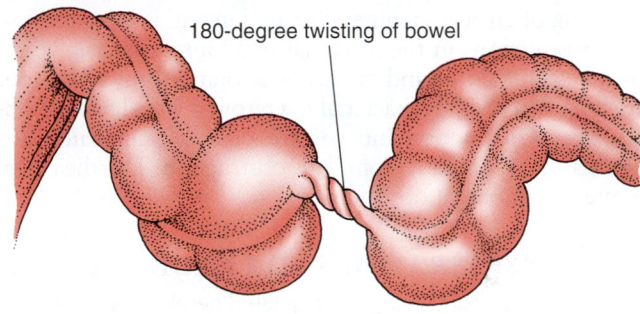

VOLVULUS

Figure 60-6 ■ Two types of mechanical obstruction.

sels surrounding the intestines, as in heart failure or severe shock. Severe insufficiency of blood supply can result in infarction of surrounding organs (e.g., bowel infarction).

Incidence/Prevalence

Obstruction of the intestines occurs in about 20% of all clients who are seen for acute abdominal pain. It is the most common reason for surgery of the small intestine. Because bowel obstruction is a result of other disorders, statistics on the incidence of bowel obstruction are not readily available.

Obstruction of the intestines occurs in all age groups, but the incidence differs with age. In adults, 75% of all obstructions occur in the small intestine and 15% occur in the large intestine.

◆COLLABORATIVE MANAGEMENT
◆Assessment
HISTORY

Collect information concerning the following:
- Past or recent abdominal surgery
- Radiation therapy
- History of inflammatory bowel disease
- Gallstones
- Hernias
- Trauma
- Peritonitis
- Cancer

Question the client about recent nausea or vomiting. Ask about the passage of flatus and the time, character, and consistency of the last bowel movement. Singultus (hiccups) is common with all types of intestinal obstruction.

Assess for a family history of colorectal cancer (CRC) and ask about blood in the stool or a change in bowel pattern. The body temperature with obstruction is rarely higher than 100° F (37.8° C). A temperature higher than this, with or without guarding and tenderness, and a sustained elevation in pulse could indicate a strangulated obstruction or peritonitis.

PHYSICAL ASSESSMENT/CLINICAL MANIFESTATIONS

MECHANICAL OBSTRUCTION. The client with mechanical obstruction in the small intestine often has mid-abdominal pain or cramping. The pain can be sporadic, and the client may feel comfortable between episodes. If strangulation is present, the pain becomes more localized and steady. Vomiting often accompanies obstruction and is more profuse with obstructions in the proximal small intestine. The vomitus may contain bile and mucus or be orange-brown and foul smelling as a result of bacterial overgrowth with low ileal obstruction. **Obstipation** (no passage of stool) and failure to pass flatus accompany complete obstruction. Diarrhea may be present in partial obstruction.

> ### CONSIDERATIONS FOR OLDER ADULTS
> The older adult with a strangulated hernia may not complain of pain but instead may only present with nausea and vomiting. Evaluate the client complaining of any of these symptoms, because they may require immediate medical and eventually surgical intervention.

Mechanical colonic obstruction causes a milder, more intermittent colicky abdominal pain than is seen with small-bowel obstruction. Lower abdominal distention may be present, as well as obstipation, or ribbon-like stools if obstruction is partial. Alterations in bowel patterns and blood in the stools accompany the obstruction if colorectal cancer or diverticulitis is the cause.

On examination of the abdomen, observe for abdominal distention, which is common in all forms of intestinal obstruction. Peristaltic waves may also be visible. Auscultate for proximal high-pitched bowel sounds **(borborygmi)**, which are associated with cramping early in the obstructive process as the intestine tries to push the mechanical obstruction forward. In later stages of mechanical obstruction, bowel sounds are absent, especially distal to the obstruction. Abdominal tenderness and rigidity are usually minimal. The presence of a tense, fluid-filled bowel loop mimicking a palpable abdominal mass may signal a closed-loop, strangulating small-bowel obstruction.

NONMECHANICAL OBSTRUCTION. In most types of nonmechanical obstruction (paralytic, or adynamic, ileus), the pain is described as a constant, diffuse discomfort. Colicky cramping is not characteristic of this type of obstruction. Pain associated with obstruction attributable to vascular insufficiency or infarction is usually severe and constant. On inspection, abdominal distention is typically present. On auscultation of the abdomen, note decreased bowel sounds in early obstruction and absent bowel sounds in later stages. Vomiting of gastric contents and bile is frequent, but the vomitus rarely has a foul odor and is rarely profuse. Obstipation may or may not be present. Chart 60-6 compares small-bowel and large-bowel obstructions.

CHART 60-6

KEY FEATURES of
Small-Bowel and Large-Bowel Obstructions

Small-Bowel Obstructions	Large-Bowel Obstructions
Abdominal discomfort or pain possibly accompanied by visible peristaltic waves in upper and middle abdomen	Intermittent lower abdominal cramping
Upper or epigastric abdominal distention	Lower abdominal distention
Nausea and early, profuse vomiting	Minimal or no vomiting (may contain fecal material)
Obstipation	Obstipation or ribbon-like stools
Severe fluid and electrolyte imbalances	No major fluid and electrolyte imbalances
Metabolic alkalosis	Metabolic acidosis

LABORATORY ASSESSMENT

There is no definitive laboratory test to confirm a diagnosis of mechanical or nonmechanical obstruction. White blood cell (WBC) counts may be normal unless there is a strangulated obstruction, in which case there may be leukocytosis (increased WBCs). Hemoglobin, hematocrit, creatinine, and blood urea nitrogen (BUN) values are often elevated, indicating dehydration. Serum sodium, chloride, and potassium concentrations are reduced because of loss of fluid and electrolytes. Elevations in serum amylase levels may be found with strangulating obstructions, which can damage the pancreas.

High obstruction in the small intestine is likely to show an elevated serum venous carbon dioxide concentration and other values indicative of metabolic alkalosis. Obstruction in the large intestine is likely to show a low serum venous carbon dioxide concentration and other values suggestive of metabolic acidosis.

RADIOGRAPHIC ASSESSMENT

The health care provider obtains flat-plate and upright abdominal x-rays as soon as an obstruction is suspected. Distention of loops of intestine with fluid and gas in the small intestine, in conjunction with the absence of gas in the colon, indicates an obstruction in the small intestine. However, x-ray findings are often normal when a strangulated obstruction actually exists in the small intestine. Therefore obstruction cannot be ruled out on the basis of x-ray findings.

Obstruction of the large intestine often shows gas distention of the colon on abdominal x-rays. A finding of free air under the diaphragm on abdominal x-ray examination indicates a perforated intestine.

OTHER DIAGNOSTIC ASSESSMENTS

The diagnostic examination chosen depends on the suspected location of the obstruction. The physician may perform endoscopy (sigmoidoscopy or colonoscopy) or a barium enema study to determine the cause of the obstruction, except when perforation is suspected. A computed tomography (CT) scan is useful in uncovering the cause and location of the obstruction and may be the diagnostic tool of choice when symptoms are severe.

◆ Interventions

Interventions are aimed at uncovering the cause and relieving the obstruction. Intestinal obstructions can be relieved by nonsurgical or surgical means. If the obstruction is partial and there is no evidence of strangulation, nonsurgical management is the treatment of choice. Decompression of the intestinal tract is initiated along with fluid and electrolyte replacement.

NONSURGICAL MANAGEMENT. Paralytic ileus responds well to nonsurgical methods of relieving obstruction. Nonsurgical approaches are also preferred in the treatment of clients with terminal disease associated with bowel obstruction. In addition to being on NPO status, clients with intestinal obstruction typically have a nasogastric or, more rarely, nasointestinal tube inserted. These tubes provide decompression of the bowel by draining fluid and air and are attached to suction; the type of suction depends on the type of tube inserted.

Nasogastric Tubes. Most clients with an obstruction have at least a **nasogastric (NG) tube** in place unless the obstruction is mild. Salem sump and Anderson tubes are examples of NG tubes that sit distally in the stomach and are attached to *low continuous* suction. Levin tubes are connected to *low intermittent* suction.

At least every 4 hours, assess for proper placement of the tube, tube patency, and output (quality and quantity). The nasal skin is also monitored daily for integrity. Assess for peristalsis by auscultating for bowel sounds with the suction disconnected (suction masks peristaltic sounds).

Question the client regarding the passage of flatus and record the passage, amount, and character of bowel movements daily. Abdominal girth is measured at the same point each day. The client is also assessed for nausea and asked to report this manifestation.

NG tubes must be monitored for proper functioning. Occasionally, NG tubes move out of optimal drainage position or become plugged. In this case, note a decrease in gastric output or stasis of the tube's contents. Assess the client for nausea, vomiting, increased abdominal distention, and placement of the tube. If the NG tube is repositioned or replaced, confirmation of proper placement is obtained by x-ray examination before use. After appropriate placement is established, the contents are aspirated and the tube is irrigated with 30 mL of normal saline every 4 hours or as needed to maintain patency.

Nasointestinal Tubes. The physician *occasionally* inserts nasointestinal (NI) tubes (such as the Miller-Abbott, Cantor, and Harris tubes) for obstruction of the small intestine. These longer tubes extend into the small intestine. Mercury-filled balloons at the end of a lumen act as a bolus of food, stimulating peristalsis and advancing down the intestinal tract. The Cantor and Harris tubes are single-lumen tubes with mercury-filled balloons at the tips and suction ports within the same lumen, proximal to the tip. The Miller-Abbott tube has two separate lumens for mercury and drainage.

Assist with progression of the tube by helping the client change position every 2 hours and, if ordered, by advancing the tube 3 to 4 inches at specified times. These tubes are *never* taped to the nose until they reach a specified position

in the intestine. As the tube is being inserted and advanced, it drains by gravity. Monitor the drainage; if drainage stops, obtain a physician's order to inject 10 mL of air. *Do not irrigate the NI tube with fluid without an order by the health care provider!* If ordered, attach low intermittent suction to the suction lumen when the tube has stopped advancing.

Most health care providers avoid the use of NI tubes because insertion of the mercury-filled lumen is often difficult; the time it takes to insert the tube also delays treatment. Insertion of this tube can be uncomfortable for clients.

Other Nonsurgical Techniques. Most types of nonmechanical obstruction respond to nasogastric decompression in conjunction with medical treatment of the primary disorder. Incomplete mechanical obstruction can sometimes be successfully treated without surgery. Obstruction caused by fecal impaction usually resolves after disimpaction and enema administration. Intussusception may respond to hydrostatic pressure changes during a barium enema.

Fluid and Electrolyte Replacement. IV fluid replacement and maintenance are indicated for all clients with intestinal obstruction, because the client is on NPO status and fluid and electrolyte loss (particularly potassium) through vomiting and nasogastric suction is great. On the basis of serum electrolytes and blood urea nitrogen (BUN) levels, the health care provider orders aggressive fluid replacement with 2 to 4 L of normal saline or lactated Ringer's solution with potassium added. Care must be taken with clients who are susceptible to fluid overload (e.g., the client with a history of heart failure). Monitor lung sounds, weight, and intake and output. Blood replacement may be indicated in strangulated obstruction because of blood loss into the bowel or peritoneal cavity.

Monitor the client's vital signs and other measures of fluid status (e.g., urine output, skin turgor, and mucous membranes). Edema from third spacing is assessed because fluid is lost, mostly from the vascular space, into surrounding spaces (e.g., the peritoneal cavity). In collaboration with the dietitian, the physician may prescribe total parenteral nutrition (TPN) to improve the nutritional status of the client, especially if he or she has had chronic nutritional problems and has been on NPO status for an extended period. Chapter 64 discusses the nursing care of clients receiving TPN.

The client with intestinal obstruction is characteristically thirsty. Provide or delegate frequent mouth care to help maintain moist mucous membranes. A small amount of ice chips may be allowed if the client is not having surgery; however, the health care provider should be consulted first. Ice chips can provide more free water than electrolytes; thus potassium and hydrochloric acid are washed out of the NG tube.

Pain Management. The abdominal distention commonly noted with intestinal obstruction can cause a great deal of discomfort, especially when distention is severe. The colicky, crampy pain that comes and goes with mechanical obstruction and the nausea, vomiting, dry mucous membranes, and thirst contribute to the client's discomfort. Continually assess the character and location of the pain and immediately report any pain that significantly increases or changes from a colicky, intermittent type to a constant discomfort. Such changes can indicate perforation of the intestine or peritonitis.

Opioid analgesics are normally withheld in the diagnostic period so that clinical manifestations of perforation or peritonitis are not masked. Explain to the client and family the rationale for not giving analgesics. In addition, if analgesics such as morphine or meperidine are given, they slow intestinal motility and can cause vomiting. Be alert to this side effect because nausea and vomiting are also signs of NG tube obstruction or worsening bowel obstruction.

Help the client obtain a position of comfort with frequent position changes to promote increased peristalsis. A semi-Fowler's position helps alleviate the pressure of abdominal distention on the chest. Not only is this a good comfort technique, but it also facilitates adequate thoracic excursion and normal breathing patterns.

Discomfort is generally less with nonmechanical obstruction than with mechanical obstruction. With both types of obstruction, discomfort is aggravated by ingestion of food or fluids.

Drug Therapy. If strangulation is thought to be likely, the health care provider prescribes IV broad-spectrum antibiotics. In addition, in cases of partial obstruction or paralytic ileus, medications that enhance gastric motility, such as octreotide acetate (Sandostatin), may be used.

SURGICAL MANAGEMENT. In all cases of complete mechanical obstruction and in many cases of incomplete mechanical obstruction, surgical intervention is necessary to relieve the obstruction. A strangulated obstruction is inevitably complete, and surgical intervention is always required. An **exploratory laparotomy** (a surgical opening of the abdominal cavity to investigate the cause of the obstruction) is initially performed for most clients with obstruction. More specific surgical procedures depend on the cause of the obstruction.

Preoperative Care. Provide preoperative teaching as discussed in Chapter 20. If time permits, all clients who require surgery for obstruction undergo nasogastric intubation and suction before surgery. However, in cases of complete obstruction, surgery should proceed without delay.

Operative Procedures. The surgeon enters the abdominal cavity and explores for obstruction. If adhesions are found to be the cause of the obstruction, the adhesions are lysed (cut and released). Obstruction caused by a tumor or diverticulitis requires a colon resection with primary anastomosis or a temporary or permanent colostomy. If obstruction is caused by intestinal infarction, an embolectomy, thrombectomy, or resection of the gangrenous bowel may be necessary.

Postoperative Care. Postoperative care for the client undergoing an exploratory laparotomy with lysis of adhesions, colon resection, thrombectomy, or embolectomy is similar to that described in Chapter 22. In addition, all clients have an NG tube in place until peristalsis (as characterized by the return of bowel sounds) resumes. The NG tube is removed slowly by first discontinuing suction and then clamping the tube for a scheduled amount of time. Residual drainage is checked at each stage to assess peristalsis without decompression before removing the NG tube entirely.

Critical Thinking Challenge

An older adult from a nursing home is admitted to your medical-surgical unit with severe vomiting and abdominal pain from possible bowel obstruction. She is very "confused" and unable to communicate when you ask her questions. The transfer form from the nursing home states that she is usually alert and oriented but that she began to become confused last night after dinner. She has a long history of diverticulitis and had surgery for colorectal cancer 10 years ago.

1. How will you assess this client's pain level?
2. What fluid, electrolyte, and acid-base imbalances is she likely to have or develop?
3. How will the health care provider determine if she has an obstruction?
4. What do you expect when you listen for bowel sounds?
5. What part of her care would you delegate to the nursing assistant?

evolve For suggested answer guidelines, go to http://evolve.elsevier.com/Iggy/.

Community-Based Care

All clients with intestinal obstruction are hospitalized for monitoring and treatment. The length of stay varies according to the type of obstruction, the treatment, and the presence of complications. Clients who have complicated obstruction, such as strangulation or incarceration, are at greater risk for peritonitis, sepsis, and shock. The hospital stay may be longer than a week, depending on the severity of complications.

Clients with nonmechanical (adynamic) intestinal obstruction are less likely to require a lengthy hospitalization because of the obstruction alone. Adynamic obstruction generally responds to NG intubation and suction within a few days.

HOME CARE MANAGEMENT

For the client who has had an intestinal obstruction, preparation for home care depends on the cause of the obstruction and the treatment required. Clients who have resolution of obstruction without surgical intervention are assessed for their knowledge of strategies to avoid recurrent obstruction. For example, if fecal impaction was the cause of the obstruction, assess the client's ability to carry out a bowel regimen independently. For clients who have undergone surgery, evaluate their ability to function at home with the added tasks of incision care and possibly colostomy care.

HEALTH TEACHING

Instruct the client to report any abdominal pain or distention, nausea, or vomiting, with or without constipation, because these symptoms might indicate recurrent obstruction. The client should be reassured, however, that recurrent paralytic ileus is not usually a problem. The client who has had mechanical obstruction as a result of fecal impaction (often the older adult) needs to have a structured bowel regimen to prevent recurrence (Chart 60-7). Instruct this client to adhere to high-fiber diets, to exercise, and to drink adequate amounts of water daily, unless contraindicated. The physician may also prescribe bulk-forming laxatives to help maintain a consistent elimination pattern.

Instruct the client who has had surgery about incision care, drug therapy, and activity limitations. Drug therapy consists of an oral opioid analgesic, such as oxycodone hydrochloride with acetaminophen (Tylox, Percocet, Endocet✦), to be taken as needed for incisional discomfort. As with any opioid therapy, a stool softener is added to the medication regimen to prevent constipation and possible recurrent obstruction.

CHART 60-7

NURSING FOCUS on the OLDER ADULT
Fecal Impaction

- Teach the client to eat high-fiber foods, including plenty of raw fruits and vegetables and whole-grain products.
- Encourage the client to drink adequate amounts of fluids, especially water.
- Do not routinely administer a laxative; teach the client that laxative abuse decreases abdominal muscle tone and contributes to an atonic colon.
- Encourage the client to exercise regularly, if possible. Walking every day is an excellent exercise for promoting intestinal motility.
- Use natural foods to stimulate peristalsis, such as warm beverages and prune juice.
- Take bulk-forming products, such as Metamucil, to provide fiber.
- Check the client's stool for amount and frequency; oozing of soft or diarrheal stool often indicates a fecal impaction.
- Have the client sit on a toilet or bedside commode, rather than on a bedpan, for elimination.

With resolution of obstruction, educational efforts by the nurse are aimed at prevention of obstruction by examining the cause of the obstruction and how to prevent recurrence. The nurse also reinforces important signs and symptoms to report to the health care provider. The client who had curative treatment of the underlying cause most likely requires less support than the client who underwent treatment of obstruction related to a serious disease that will require further treatment. Encourage the client to express fears and concerns about the future. Assess the client's understanding and needs with regard to treatment plans.

HEALTH CARE RESOURCES

The need for follow-up appointments depends on the cause of the obstruction and the treatment required. If the client is at risk for fecal impaction, arrange for a home care nurse to assess the gastrointestinal (GI) function and dietary habits of the client on an ongoing basis. Arrangements should also be made for the services of a home care nurse if the client needs help with incision or colostomy care. Medicare guidelines or insurance precertification requirements must be met before approval is given for home care visits. The discharge planner or case manager assists in setting up home care follow-up.

ABDOMINAL TRAUMA

PATHOPHYSIOLOGY

Abdominal trauma is defined as injury to the structures located between the diaphragm and the pelvis, which occurs when the abdomen is subjected to blunt or penetrating forces. Organs injured may include the large or small bowel, liver, spleen, duodenum, pancreas, kidneys, and urinary bladder.

At least one half of all blunt abdominal trauma occurs from motor vehicle accidents (MVAs). Other causes of blunt trauma include falls, aggravated assaults, and contact sports. *Penetrating abdominal trauma* is caused by gunshot wounds, stabbing, or impalement with an object. The liver is the most commonly injured organ in blunt and penetrating trauma. The spleen is the most commonly injured organ in blunt abdominal trauma. The small intestine is the third most commonly injured organ in abdominal trauma; 80% of injuries are caused by gunshot wounds (GSWs). Trauma is the leading cause of death in young adults (under 40 years of age) and the fifth leading cause of death in adults in the United States.

Because most abdominal or blunt trauma cases are the result of automobile accidents, encourage health promotion and illness prevention through the wearing of seat belts, which decreases abdominal trauma during accidents.

◆COLLABORATIVE MANAGEMENT
◆Assessment

First, assess any client experiencing trauma for airway, breathing, and circulation (ABC). Once these parameters are stabilized, focus on the risks of hemorrhage, shock, and peritonitis. Mental status, vital signs, and skin perfusion are *priority* nursing assessments, with skin perfusion being the most reliable clinical guide in assessing hypovolemic shock:

- In a person with mild shock, the skin is pale, cool, and moist.
- With moderate shock, diaphoresis is more marked and urine output ceases.
- With severe shock, changes in mental status are manifested by agitation, disorientation, and recent memory loss.

Assess for abdominal trauma by asking the client about the presence, location, and quality of pain. The abdomen, flanks, back, genitalia, and rectum are inspected for contusions, abrasions, lacerations, ecchymosis, penetrating injuries, and symmetry. All of the client's clothes must be removed.

Inspection of the abdomen may reveal distention. To perform an adequate inspection, turn the client while maintaining spinal immobilization. Ecchymosis may signify internal bleeding. Ecchymosis present in the distribution of a lap seat belt should be reported to the health care provider immediately, because investigation for occult injury to the bowel is necessary. Ecchymosis around the umbilicus is known as **Cullen's sign,** and ecchymosis on either flank (known as **Turner's sign**) may indicate retroperitoneal bleeding into the abdominal wall.

Auscultate the abdomen for bowel sounds. Absent or diminished bowel sounds may be caused by the presence of blood, bacteria, or a chemical irritant in the abdominal cavity. Also auscultate for bruits in the abdomen, which could indicate renal artery injury.

During percussion, an abnormal sign associated with abdominal trauma is resonance over the right flank with the client lying on the left side. This is known as **Ballance's sign** and is found with a ruptured spleen. Resonance over the normally dull liver is due to free air, which is pathologic. Palpation for lower rib fractures should increase suspicion of liver or spleen injuries. Injury to the spleen is present in 20% of individuals with left lower rib fractures. Liver injury is present in 10% of individuals with right lower rib fractures. The presence of **Kehr's sign,** left shoulder pain resulting from diaphragmatic irritation, may be present in splenic injury.

Dullness over hollow organs that normally contain gas, such as the stomach and the large and small intestines, may indicate the presence of blood or fluid. Light abdominal palpation identifies areas of tenderness, rebound tenderness, guarding, rigidity, and spasm. If you palpate a mass, it may be blood or a fluid collection.

The client without obvious significant bleeding or definite signs of peritoneal irritation undergoes abdominal radiography, diagnostic peritoneal lavage (DPL), and computed tomography (CT). For peritoneal lavage, the physician inserts a large-bore catheter into the abdomen and allows fluid to enter the abdominal cavity. If the return drainage from the abdomen is pink or grossly bloody, the health care team prepares the client for surgery. Abdominal ultrasound is used to diagnose blunt abdominal trauma and may replace CT and DPL for diagnosis (Levins, 2000). Clients with hemodynamic instability or peritonitis are candidates for immediate laparotomy.

◆Interventions

Nonsurgical and surgical interventions are aimed at preserving or restoring hemodynamic stability, preventing or decreasing blood loss, and preventing complications.

EMERGENCY CARE: ABDOMINAL TRAUMA. Nursing interventions include placement of at least two large-bore IV catheters in the upper extremities. IV catheters are not used in the lower extremities; if the vasculature has been injured, fluid can pool in the abdomen. The health care provider may insert a central venous catheter to assist with rapid fluid volume infusion. IV fluid consists of a balanced saline solution, crystalloids, and possibly blood.

The following physiologic parameters are monitored:

- Arterial blood gases
- Complete blood count (CBC)
- Serum electrolyte, glucose and amylase, and blood urea nitrogen (BUN) determinations
- Liver function tests
- Clotting studies

Measuring arterial blood gases may be of assistance in determining the severity of shock. Hemoglobin and hematocrit values do not initially reflect true blood loss; values can be skewed because of hemoconcentration from volume loss or the dilutional effects of IV fluids. Serial hemoglobin and hematocrit measurements may be more accurate in determining true blood loss. An elevated white blood cell (WBC) count may indicate a ruptured spleen or intestinal injury. Elevated levels of serum transaminases may indicate liver injury. Elevation of serum amylase activity may signal injury to the pancreas or the bowel. All laboratory work is compiled so that values can be compared and subtle changes noted.

Continuous hemodynamic monitoring is begun in the emergency department. Insert an indwelling urinary (Foley) catheter unless there is blood at the urinary meatus. Initially and hourly thereafter, evaluate urine output for bleeding and specific gravity. Laboratory tests indicate the amount of blood and protein in the urine. If there is an open abdominal wound or evisceration, cover it with a sterile dry dressing unless the physician orders otherwise. Unless it is contraindicated, as in the case of a concomitant skull fracture, the physician or nurse inserts a nasogastric (NG) tube, which is kept in place to identify bleeding and to minimize the risk of vomiting and aspiration. Antibiotics are administered as prescribed to reduce the risk of peritonitis.

If the client with known abdominal trauma has no definite clinical manifestations of active bleeding or abdominal injury, he or she is admitted to the hospital for observation. Blunt trauma can cause active, but often not obvious, dam-

age. Assess for abdominal or referred pain and nausea. Every 15 to 30 minutes in the early postinjury period and then hourly, evaluate the following:

- Mental status
- Vital signs
- Clinical findings, such as vomiting, guarding, rigidity, or rebound tenderness
- Skin temperature
- Bowel sounds
- Urine output

Report any change immediately to the health care provider. It is more important to recognize the high risk of an active abdominal injury and assess for general signs of abdominal injury (e.g., hemorrhage and peritonitis) than to identify the exact nature of the abdominal injury. Analgesics for pain are not prescribed at this time so that clinical manifestations are not masked or overlooked. Explain the rationale for withholding analgesics to the client and family or significant others.

SURGICAL MANAGEMENT. For the client with severe abdominal trauma, the surgeon performs an exploratory laparotomy and repairs abdominal injuries immediately if there are definite signs of peritoneal irritation. These signs include rebound tenderness, significant blood loss, evisceration, or a gunshot wound (GSW) with possible peritoneal involvement.

Most stab wounds require exploratory laparotomy, but as many as 25% are superficial and do not involve the peritoneum. Using local anesthesia, the surgeon explores and cleans superficial stab wounds; the client does not require an exploratory laparotomy.

Before discharge from the hospital, the client who has experienced abdominal trauma is taught the signs and symptoms of abdominal bleeding whether or not surgery has been performed. Instruct the client to report abdominal pain, nausea, vomiting, bloody or black stools, fever, weakness, and dizziness.

Hemorrhage can occasionally occur weeks after blunt abdominal trauma, despite medical evaluation. For the client who undergoes surgery or exploration of wounds, provide instructions on wound care before discharge from the hospital.

POLYPS

PATHOPHYSIOLOGY

Polyps in the intestinal tract are small growths covered with mucosa and attached to the surface of the intestine. Although most are benign, polyps are significant in that some have the potential to become malignant.

Polyps are identified by their tissue type. The presence of adenomas always necessitates medical consultation because of their malignant potential. Although only 2% to 5% of adenomas progress to cancer, almost all colorectal cancers develop from an adenoma. Adenomas are further classified as villous or tubular. Of these, villous adenomas pose a greater cancer risk.

Familial adenomatous polyposis (FAP) and hereditary nonpolyposis colorectal cancer (HNPCC) are inherited syndromes characterized by progressive development of colorectal adenomas. Unless these syndromes are treated, colorectal cancer (CRC) inevitably occurs by the fourth to fifth decade of life. These conditions were discussed earlier under Genetic Considerations in the Colorectal Cancer section of this chapter.

Other types of polyps include hyperplastic and hamartomatous polyps. Hyperplastic polyps, which include mucosal and inflammatory varieties, are entirely benign with no malignant potential. Hamartomatous polyps include juvenile and Peutz-Jeghers syndrome polyps. Although both types are generally benign, rare reports of malignant changes have been reported in juvenile polyps.

In addition to being classified by their tissue type, polyps are described according to their appearance (Figure 60-7). Pedunculated polyps are stalklike; a thin stem attaches them to the intestinal wall. They become elongated as peristalsis pulls them into the lumen of the intestine. Polyps attached to the intestinal walls by a broad base are described as sessile. A malignant polyp may be pedunculated or sessile.

◆COLLABORATIVE MANAGEMENT

Polyps are usually asymptomatic and are discovered during routine diagnostic testing, including tests for blood in the stool. However, they can cause gross rectal bleeding, intestinal obstruction, or intussusception (telescoping of the bowel). Diagnostic studies involve a barium enema examination and proctosigmoidoscopy or colonoscopy for ruling out cancer. Biopsy specimens of polyps can be obtained, or the entire polyp can be removed (polypectomy) with the use of an electrocautery snare that fits through the sigmoidoscope or colonoscope. This often eliminates the need for abdominal surgery to remove a suspicious or definitely malignant polyp. The client with FAP often requires a total colectomy (colon removal) to prevent the development of cancer.

Nursing care focuses on client education. Instruct the client about the following:
- The nature of the polyp
- Clinical manifestations to report to the health care provider
- The need for regular, routine monitoring

If the client has undergone a polypectomy, follow-up sigmoidoscopic or colonoscopic examinations are needed, because there is an increased risk of multiple polyps in the client who has had at least one polyp.

Nursing care of the client who has undergone a polypectomy of the colorectal area includes monitoring for abdominal distention and pain, rectal bleeding, mucopurulent rectal drainage, and fever. A small amount of blood might appear in the stool after a polypectomy, but this should be temporary.

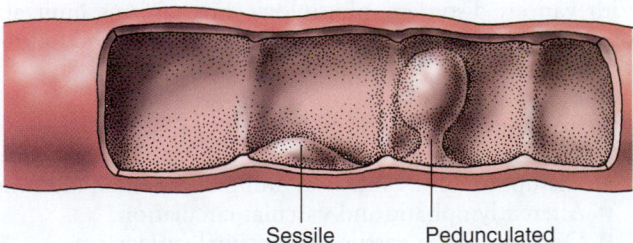

Figure 60-7 ■ Pedunculated and sessile polyps. Pedunculated polyps, such as tubular adenomas, are stalklike. Sessile polyps, such as villous adenomas, are broad based.

HEMORRHOIDS

PATHOPHYSIOLOGY

Hemorrhoids are unnaturally swollen or distended veins in the anorectal region. The veins involved in the development of hemorrhoids are part of the normal structure in the anal region. With limited distention, the veins function as a valve overlying the anal sphincter that assists in continence. Increased intra-abdominal pressure causes elevated systemic and portal venous pressure, which is transmitted to the anorectal veins. Arterioles in the anorectal region shunt blood directly to the distended anorectal veins, which increases the pressure. With repeated elevations in pressure from increased intra-abdominal pressure and engorgement from arteriolar shunting of blood, the distended veins eventually separate from the smooth muscle surrounding them. The result is prolapse of the hemorrhoidal vessels.

Hemorrhoids can be internal or external (Figure 60-8). **Internal hemorrhoids**, which cannot be seen on inspection of the perineal area, lie above the anal sphincter. **External hemorrhoids** lie below the anal sphincter and can be seen on inspection of the anal region. Prolapsed hemorrhoids can become thrombosed or inflamed, or they can bleed.

Etiology

Hemorrhoids are common and not significant unless they cause pain or bleeding. Caused by increased abdominal pressure, the condition exacerbates during pregnancy, constipation with straining, obesity, heart failure, prolonged sitting or standing, and strenuous exercise and weight lifting. Decreased fluid intake can also cause hemorrhoids due to the development of hard stool and subsequent constipation. Straining while evacuating stool causes them to enlarge.

Incidence/Prevalence

One in three individuals, or more than one third of the population of the United States will have hemorrhoids sometime in their lives. For adults over 50 years of age, the numbers

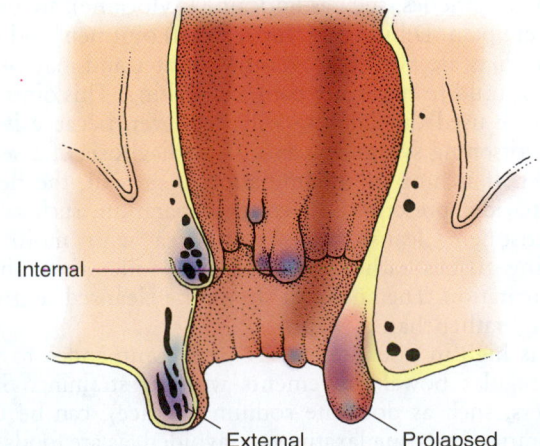

Figure 60-8 ■ Internal, external, and prolapsed hemorrhoids. Internal hemorrhoids lie above the anal sphincter and cannot be seen on inspection of the anal area. External hemorrhoids lie below the anal sphincter and can be seen on inspection of the anal region. Hemorrhoids that enlarge, fall down, and protrude through the anus are called prolapsed hemorrhoids.

increase to 50%, or 1 in every 2. However, only a small percentage of affected individuals actually become symptomatic. Men tend to be affected more often than women. The prevalence of hemorrhoids is highest in affluent countries of the Western World.

HEALTH PROMOTION/ILLNESS PREVENTION

Prevention of constipation is key, and is accomplished by increasing fiber in the diet, such as eating more whole grains, nuts, and raw vegetables and fruits. Encourage individuals to drink plenty of water. Remind the client to avoid straining at stool. Exercise, while encouraged, should be done in moderation with a gradual buildup in intensity. Maintaining a healthy weight also helps prevent hemorrhoids.

◆ COLLABORATIVE MANAGEMENT
◆ Assessment

The most common symptoms of hemorrhoids are bleeding, swelling, and prolapse. Blood is characteristically bright red and is present on toilet tissue or outside the stool. Pain is a common symptom and is often associated with thrombosis, especially if thrombosis occurs suddenly. Other symptoms include itching and a mucous discharge. Diagnosis is made by inspection, digital examination, proctoscopy, or proctoscopic ultrasonography.

◆ Interventions

Interventions are typically conservative and are aimed at reducing symptoms with a minimum of discomfort, cost, and time lost from usual activities.

NONSURGICAL MANAGEMENT. Local treatment and diet therapy are initiated when symptoms begin. Cold packs applied to the anorectal region for a few minutes at a time beginning with the onset of pain and tepid sitz baths three or four times per day are often enough to relieve discomfort, even if the hemorrhoids are thrombosed.

Witch hazel soaks (e.g., Tucks) are also effective for pain. Topical anesthetics, such as lidocaine (Xylocaine), are useful for severe pain. Dibucaine (Nupercainal) ointment and similar products are available over-the-counter and may be applied for mild to moderate pain and itching. This ointment should be used only temporarily, however, because it can mask worsening symptoms and delay diagnosis of a severe disorder. If itching or inflammation is present, the health care provider prescribes a steroid preparation, such as hydrocortisone. Cleansing the anal area with moistened cleansing tissues rather than standard toilet tissue helps avoid irritation. The anal area should be cleansed gently by dabbing, rather than by wiping.

Diets high in fiber and fluids are recommended to promote regular bowel movements without straining. Stool softeners, such as docusate sodium (Colace), can be used temporarily. Irritating laxatives are avoided, as are foods and beverages that can make hemorrhoids worse. Spicy foods, nuts, coffee, and alcohol can be irritating. Remind clients to avoid sitting for long periods of time. The health care provider may prescribe oral analgesics for pain if the hemorrhoids are thrombosed.

Conservative treatment should alleviate symptoms in 3 to 5 days. If symptoms continue or recur frequently, the client may require surgical intervention.

SURGICAL MANAGEMENT. The surgeon can perform several procedures for symptomatic internal hemorrhoids on an ambulatory basis. Ultrasound, sclerotherapy, circular stapling, or simple resection of the hemorrhoids are examples of techniques that can be performed. The type of surgery depends on the degree of prolapse, whether there is thrombosis, and the overall condition of the client.

The harmonic scalpel is an ultrasonically activated instrument that vibrates to coagulate small and medium-size vessels. In sclerotherapy, the surgeon injects a sclerosing agent into the tissues around the hemorrhoids to obliterate the vessels. However, it can be done only for low-grade hemorrhoids. If the hemorrhoid is prolapsed, a circular stapling device is used to excise a band of mucosa above the prolapse and restore the hemorrhoidal tissue back into the anal canal.

Hemorrhoidectomy, or simple resection of the hemorrhoid, tends to cause more pain than the other procedures. Urinary retention can also occur because of rectal spasms and anorectal tenderness. Hemorrhage, which may be internal and not visible or external, is a rare but potential complication.

Teach clients with hemorrhoids about the need to consume high-fiber, high-fluid diets to promote regular bowel patterns before and after surgery. Advise clients to avoid stimulant laxatives, which are habit forming.

For clients who undergo any type of surgical intervention, monitor for bleeding and pain postoperatively and teach clients to report these problems to their health care provider.

Use of moist heat (e.g., sitz baths) three or four times per day can help promote comfort.

The first postoperative bowel movement may be very painful. The physician usually prescribes stool softeners, such as docusate sodium (Colace) to begin preoperatively and continue after surgery. Analgesics and anti-inflammatory medications are administered postoperatively. A mild laxative should be administered if the client has not had a bowel movement by the third postoperative day.

MALABSORPTION SYNDROME
PATHOPHYSIOLOGY

Malabsorption is a syndrome associated with a variety of disorders and intestinal surgical procedures. It interferes with the ability to absorb nutrients and is a result of a generalized flattening of the mucosa of the small intestine. With various disorders, physiologic mechanisms limit absorption of nutrients because of one or more of the following abnormalities:
- Bile salt deficiencies
- Enzyme deficiencies
- Presence of bacteria
- Disruption of the mucosal lining of the small intestine
- Altered lymphatic and vascular circulation
- Decrease in the gastric or intestinal surface area

The nutrient involved in malabsorption depends on the type and location of the abnormality in the intestinal tract.

Deficiencies of bile salts can lead to malabsorption of fats and fat-soluble vitamins. Bile salt deficiencies can result from decreased synthesis of bile in the liver, bile obstruction, or alteration of bile salt absorption in the small intestine.

Enzymes normally found in the intestine split disaccharides (complex sugars) to monosaccharides (simple sugars). Examples of these enzymes are lactase, sucrase, maltase, and isomaltase. Lactase deficiency is the most common disaccharide enzyme deficiency. Without sufficient amounts of this enzyme, the body is not able to break down lactose. Lactase deficiency can be due to genetic transmission, injury to intestinal mucosa from viral hepatitis, bacterial proliferation in the intestine, or sprue. Deficiencies of the other disaccharide enzymes are rare.

Pancreatic enzymes are also necessary for absorption of vitamin B_{12}. With destruction or obstruction of the pancreas or insufficient pancreatic stimulation, these nutrients are malabsorbed. Chronic pancreatitis, pancreatic carcinoma, resection of the pancreas, and cystic fibrosis can cause these malabsorption problems.

Loops of bowel can accumulate intestinal contents, resulting in bacterial overgrowth, when there is a decrease in peristalsis. Bacteria at these sites break down bile salts, and fewer salts are available for fat absorption. These bacteria can also ingest vitamin B_{12}, which contributes to vitamin B_{12} deficiency. This phenomenon can occur after a gastrectomy or with progressive systemic sclerosis and diabetic enteropathy.

Disruption of the mucosal lining of the intestine is responsible for the malabsorption that occurs with celiac (nontropical) sprue, tropical sprue, Crohn's disease, and ulcerative colitis.

In celiac (nontropical) sprue, the absorptive surface area in the small intestine is lost; there is malabsorption of most nutrients. Celiac sprue is thought to be due to a genetic immune hypersensitivity response to gluten or its breakdown products or to result from the accumulation of gluten in the diet with peptidase deficiency.

Tropical sprue is caused by an infectious agent that has not been identified but is thought to be bacterial. Mucosal changes occur in a more widespread manner than in celiac sprue. However, the changes are not as severe as in celiac sprue. Tropical sprue results in malabsorption of fat, folic acid, and vitamin B_{12} in later stages of the disease.

The inflammation in Crohn's disease interferes with the surface of cells absorbing bile salts and therefore leads to fat malabsorption. In ulcerative colitis, protein loss may occur.

Obstruction to lymphatic flow in the intestine can lead to loss of plasma proteins along with loss of minerals (such as iron, copper, and calcium), vitamin B_{12}, folic acid, and lipids. Lymphatic obstruction can be caused by many conditions. Certain cancers, such as lymphoma, inflammatory states, radiation enteritis, Crohn's disease, Whipple's disease, heart failure, and constrictive pericarditis, are causes of lymphatic obstruction.

Interference with blood flow to the intestinal mucosa, which occurs in celiac and superior mesenteric artery disease, results in malabsorption. With intestinal surgery, there is loss of the surface area needed to facilitate absorption. Resection of the ileum results in vitamin B_{12}, bile salt, and other nutrient deficiencies. Gastric surgery is one of the most common causes of malabsorption and maldigestion. Other conditions associated with maldigestion and malabsorption include small-bowel ischemia and radiation enteritis.

◆COLLABORATIVE MANAGEMENT
◆Assessment

Diarrhea is the classic symptom of malabsorption. It occurs secondary to unabsorbed nutrients, which add to the bulk of the stool, and unabsorbed fat. **Steatorrhea** (greater than normal amounts of fat in the feces) is a common sign. Steatorrhea is a result of bile salt deconjugation, nonabsorbed fats, or bacteria in the intestine. Not all clients with malabsorption will have diarrhea; instead, many clients manifest an increased stool mass. Other clinical manifestations include the following:

- Weight loss
- Bloating and flatus (carbohydrate malabsorption)
- Decreased libido
- Easy bruising (purpura)
- Anemia (with iron and folic acid or vitamin B_{12} deficiencies)
- Bone pain (with calcium and vitamin D deficiencies)
- Edema (caused by hypoproteinemia)

Laboratory studies reveal a decrease in mean corpuscular volume (MCV), mean corpuscular hemoglobin (MCH), and mean corpuscular hemoglobin concentration (MCHC). These decreases indicate hypochromic microcytic anemia resulting from iron deficiency. Increased MCV and variable MCH and MCHC values indicate macrocytic anemia resulting from vitamin B_{12} and folic acid deficiencies. Serum iron levels are low in protein malabsorption because of insufficient gastric acid for use of iron. Serum cholesterol levels may be low from decreased absorption and digestion of fat. Low serum calcium levels may indicate malabsorption of vitamin D and amino acids. Low levels of serum vitamin A (retinol) and carotene, its precursor, indicate a bile salt deficiency and malabsorption of fat. Serum albumin and total protein levels are low if protein loss occurs. A quantitative fecal fat analysis is elevated in either malabsorption or maldigestion.

A lactose tolerance test result that shows less than a 20% rise in the blood glucose level over the fasting blood glucose level indicates lactose intolerance. A monosaccharide test validates or rules out lactase deficiency. The xylose absorption test can reveal low urine and serum D-xylose levels if malabsorption in the small intestine is present, a common finding in celiac sprue. An abnormal D-xylose test can indicate bacterial overgrowth in the small intestine.

The Schilling test measures urinary excretion of vitamin B_{12} for diagnosis of pernicious anemia and a variety of other malabsorption syndromes. The bile acid breath test assesses the absorption of bile salt. If the client has bacterial overgrowth, the bile salts will become deconjugated, and the carbon dioxide level in the breath will peak earlier than expected.

Biopsy of the small intestine is performed via an oral endoscopic procedure for diagnosis of tropical sprue or celiac sprue. Ultrasonography is used to diagnose pancreatic tumors and tumors in the small intestine that are causing malabsorption. X-rays of the gastrointestinal (GI) tract reveal pancreatic calcifications, tumors, or other abnormalities that cause malabsorption. Barium enema examination shows mucosal changes representative of celiac sprue or other abnormalities.

◆Interventions

Interventions for most malabsorption syndromes focus on avoidance of dietary substances that aggravate malabsorption and supplementation of nutrients. Surgical or nonsurgical management of the primary disease may be indicated. Drug therapy may also improve or resolve malabsorption.

Dietary management includes a low-fat diet for clients who have gallbladder disease, severe steatorrhea, cystic fibrosis, and progressive systemic sclerosis. A low-fat diet may or may not be indicated for pancreatic insufficiency, because this disorder improves with enzyme replacement. Some clinicians believe that limitation of fat intake is not necessary with enzyme replacement. Dietary intake of fat is actually beneficial to the client because it has a high number of calories. After a total gastrectomy, a high-protein, high-calorie diet and small, frequent meals are recommended. Lactose-free or lactose-restricted diets are available for clients with lactase deficiency, and gluten-free diets are available for clients with celiac sprue.

The physician prescribes nutritional supplements according to the specific deficiency. Common supplements include the following:

- Water-soluble vitamins, such as folic acid and vitamin B complex
- Fat-soluble vitamins, such as vitamin A, vitamin D, and vitamin K
- Minerals, such as calcium, iron, and magnesium
- Pancreatic enzymes, such as pancrelipase (Pancrease, Viokase)

Antibiotics are used to treat tropical sprue, Whipple's disease, and other disorders involving bacterial overgrowth. Tropical sprue is treated with trimethoprim/sulfamethoxazole (Bactrim, Septra). Bacterial overgrowth can be caused by a variety of disorders but is often treated with tetracycline and metronidazole (Flagyl, Novonidazol✱). Steroids are sometimes given in celiac disease to decrease inflammation.

Drug therapy is used to control the clinical manifestations of malabsorption. Antidiarrheal agents, such as diphenoxylate hydrochloride and atropine sulfate (Lomotil), are often used to control diarrhea and steatorrhea (see Chart 60-1). Anticholinergics, such as dicyclomine hydrochloride (Bentyl, Bentylol✱), are often given before meals to inhibit gastric motility. IV fluids may be necessary to replenish fluid losses associated with diarrhea.

CHART 60-8

BEST PRACTICE for
Special Skin Care for Clients with Chronic Diarrhea

- Use medicated wipes or premoistened disposable wipes rather than toilet tissue to clean the perineal area.
- Clean the perineal area well with mild soap and warm water after each stool; rinse soap from the area well.
- If the physician allows, provide a sitz bath several times per day.
- Apply a thin coat of vitamin A & D ointment or other medicated protective barrier, such as aloe products, after each stool.
- Keep the client off the affected buttock area.
- For open areas, cover with thin DuoDerm or Tegaderm occlusive dressing to promote rapid healing.
- Observe for fungal or yeast infections, which appear as dark red rashes. Obtain prescription for medication if this problem occurs.

Provide special measures to protect the skin when diarrhea occurs (Chart 60-8). Conduct an ongoing assessment for clinical manifestations of malabsorption and relate these to activities and dietary intake. For example, clients with steatorrhea are monitored for fluid and electrolyte imbalances and are encouraged to ingest electrolyte-rich liquids liberally. Teach clients the rationale for dietary, drug, and surgical management of nutritional deficiencies and evaluate interventions on the basis of changes in or resolution of clinical manifestations.

▌▌▌ GET READY for the NCLEX Examination!

KEY POINTS

Safe Effective Care Environment

- Be aware that a strangulated hernia can cause ischemia and bowel obstruction, requiring immediate intervention.
- Assess the characteristics of the colostomy stoma, which should be reddish pink and moist; report abnormalities such as ischemia and necrosis (purplish or black) or unusual bleeding to the surgeon.
- Prioritize care for clients experiencing abdominal trauma: First assess airway, breathing, and circulation (ABC), then monitor mental status, vital signs, and skin perfusion to assess for hypovolemic shock.

Health Promotion and Maintenance

- Teach clients with irritable bowel syndrome (IBS) to avoid GI stimulants, such as caffeine, alcohol, and milk and milk products.
- Instruct client on dietary modifications to decrease the occurrence of colorectal cancer (CRC) as listed in Table 60-1.
- Refer clients with familial CRC syndromes for genetic counseling and testing.
- Teach adults over 50 years of age to have routine screening for CRC as listed in Chart 60-2; individuals with genetic predispositions should have earlier and more frequent screening.
- Teach clients and caregivers how to provide colostomy care, including dietary measures, skin care, and ostomy products.
- Refer ostomy clients to the United Ostomy Association and the American Cancer Society for additional information and support groups.
- Teach individuals measures for preventing constipation to minimize hemorrhoid occurrence.
- Teach clients having hemorrhoid surgery to take mild laxatives before and after surgery to decrease discomfort during defecation.

Psychosocial Integrity

- Assess effects of IBS on client lifestyle; recommend stress management techniques.
- Assist the client with CRC with grief work, as listed in Chart 60-3.
- Be aware that having a colostomy is a life-altering event that severely impacts one's body image; issues related to sexuality and fear of acceptance should be discussed.

Physiological Integrity

- Assess clients with IBS for elimination pattern, abdominal pain, and nausea.

- Be aware that minimally invasive inguinal hernia repair is an ambulatory procedure done via laparoscopy; postoperative management requires health teaching regarding rest for a few days and inspection of incisions for signs of infection.
- Monitor clients who have conventional, open herniorrhaphy for ability to void.
- Recognize that surgical procedures for CRC vary depending on tumor location as specified in Table 60-2.
- Consult with the enterostomal therapist (ET) when a client is scheduled for or has a new colostomy.
- Keep the peristomal skin clean and dry; observe for leakage around the pouch seal.
- Provide meticulous perineal wound care for clients having an abdominoperineal (AP) resection, as described in Chart 60-4.
- Recall that bowel sounds are altered in clients with obstruction; absent bowel sounds imply total obstruction.
- Assess the client's nasogastric tube for proper placement, patency, and output at least every 4 hours.
- Monitor clients with bowel obstruction for signs and symptoms of fluid, electrolyte, and acid-base imbalances.
- Be aware that intestinal polyps are usually benign, but can become malignant if not removed.

ADDITIONAL STUDY RESOURCES

Go to your Student CD-ROM for Review Questions for the NCLEX Examination.

Go to http://evolve.elsevier.com/Iggy/ for Integrated Management of Care Questions for the NCLEX Examination.

SELECTED BIBLIOGRAPHY

Asterisk indicates a classic or definitive work on this subject.

*Alderman, J. (1999). Managing irritable bowel syndrome. *ADVANCE for Nurse Practitioners, 7*(1), 40-46.

American Cancer Society. (2003). Colorectal cancer. *CA: A Cancer Journal for Clinicians, 53*(1), 44-51.

American Cancer Society. (2004). *Cancer facts and figures 2004.* Atlanta: Author.

Beackington, E. (2000). Irritable bowel syndrome: An update on treatment options. *Advance for Nurse Practitioners,* October, pp. 32-36.

*Bradley, M., & Pupiales, M. (1997). Essential elements of ostomy care. *American Journal of Nursing, 97*(7), 38-46.

Chung-Park, M. (2002). A look at colorectal cancer screening in women. *Nurse Practitioner, 27*(6), 43-48.

Ellenhorn, J.D.L., Coia, L.R., & Hoff, P.M. (2002). Colorectal and anal cancers. In R. Pazdur, et al. (Eds.). *Cancer management: A multidisciplinary approach* (6th ed., pp. 295-318). Melville, NY: PRR, Inc.

Jacobs, L.A. (2002). Health beliefs of first-degree relatives of individuals with colorectal cancer and participation in health maintenance visits: A population-based survey. *Cancer Nursing, 25*(4), 251-265.

Jarrett, M., Visser, R., Heitkemper, M. (2001). Diet triggers symptoms in women with irritable bowel syndrome: The patient's perspective. *Gastroenterology Nursing, 24*(5), 246-252.

Jemal, A., et al. Cancer statistics, 2002. *A Cancer Journal for Clinicians, 2002, 52*(1), 23-47.

Koloski, N., Talley, N., & Boyce, P. (2000). The impact of functional gastrointestinal disorders on quality of life. *American Journal of Gastroenterology, 95*(1), 67-71.

Lehrer, J.K., & Lichtenstein, G.R. (accessed June 8, 2004). Irritable bowel syndrome. Available at http://www.emedicine.com/med/topic1190.htm.

*Lerman, C., et al. (1999). Genetic testing in families with hereditary nonpolyposis colon cancer. *Journal of the American Medical Association, 281*(17), 1618-1622.

Levin, B., et al. (2003). Emerging technologies in screening for colorectal cancer: CT colonography, immunochemical fecal occult blood tests, and stool screening using molecular markers. *CA: A Cancer Journal for Clinicians, 53*(1), 44-51.

Levins, T.T. (2000). Using ultrasound to assess blunt abdominal trauma. *Nursing2000, 30*(5), 32cc14-32cc15.

Locke, G.R., et al. (2000). Risk factors for irritable bowel syndrome: Role of analgesics and food sensitivities. *American Journal of Gastroenterology, 95*(1), 157-164.

Lustyk, M.K., et al. (2001). Does a physically active lifestyle improve symptoms in women with irritable bowel syndrome? *Gastroenterology Nursing, 24*(3), 129-137.

McCance, K.L., & Huether, S.E. (2002). *Pathophysiology: The biologic basis for disease in adults and children (4th ed.).* St. Louis: Mosby.

Motzer, S.A., et al. (2003). Sense of coherence and quality of life in women with and without irritable bowel syndrome. *Nursing Research, 52*(2), 329-337.

*O'Brien, B. (1999). Coming of age with an ostomy. *American Journal of Nursing, 99*(8), 71-74.

Pontieri-Lewis, V. (2000). Colorectal cancer: Prevention and screening. *MEDSURG Nursing, 9*(1), 9-13.

Schmulson, M., et al. (2000). Correlation of symptom criteria with perception thresholds during rectosigmoid distension in irritable bowel syndrome patients. *American Journal of Gastroenterology, 95*(1), 152-155.

*Shelton, B. (1999). Intestinal obstruction. *AACN Clinical Issues: Advanced Practice in Acute and Critical Care, 10*(4), 478-491.

Shelton, B.K. (2002). Introduction to colorectal cancer. *Seminars in Oncology Nursing, 18*(2), Suppl 2, 2-12.

Toner, B., & Akman, D. (2000). Gender role and irritable bowel syndrome: Literature review and hypothesis. *American Journal of Gastroenterology, 95*(1), 11-16.

Weber, T., et al. (1999). Novel hMLH1 and hMLH2 germline mutations in African-Americans with colorectal cancer. *Journal of the American Medical Association, 281*(24), 2316-2320.

Zangwill, M. (2004). Closing in on colon cancer. *CURE: Cancer updates, research, and education, (3),*1, 46-49.

Interventions for Clients with Inflammatory Intestinal Disorders

MARCIA M. BOEHMKE

LEARNING OUTCOMES

After studying this chapter, you should be able to:

1. Differentiate common types of acute inflammatory bowel disease.
2. Prioritize nursing care for the client who has peritonitis.
3. Discuss the common causes of gastroenteritis.
4. Compare and contrast the pathophysiology and clinical manifestations of ulcerative colitis and Crohn's disease.
5. Analyze priority nursing diagnoses and collaborative problems for clients with chronic inflammatory bowel disease (IBD).
6. Explain the purpose of and nursing implications related to drug therapy for clients with IBD.
7. Formulate a postoperative plan of care for a client undergoing a colon resection/colectomy and colostomy or ileostomy.
8. Identify expected outcomes for clients with chronic IBD.
9. Explain the role of diet therapy in managing the client with diverticular disease.
10. Describe the comfort measures that the nurse can use for the client with an anal abscess, fissure, or fistula.
11. Discuss ways that helminthic infestation, parasitic infection, and food poisoning can be prevented.

Go to your Student CD-ROM for Review Questions for the NCLEX Examination keyed to these Learning Outcomes.

Nonspecific **inflammatory bowel disease (IBD)** is used to describe two conditions of unknown etiology: ulcerative colitis and Crohn's disease. However, IBD is a condition of the small or large intestine or both involving inflammation that can be acute or chronic in duration. Acute conditions are treated and resolved. Chronic forms of IBD are characterized by periods of exacerbation and remission. Inflammatory and infectious intestinal disorders are often difficult to differentiate because many of the characteristics of infectious processes mimic those of more chronic conditions.

ACUTE INFLAMMATORY BOWEL DISORDERS

Appendicitis, peritonitis, and gastroenteritis are the most common acute inflammatory bowel problems. These disorders are potentially life threatening and can have major systemic complications if not treated promptly.

Appendicitis

PATHOPHYSIOLOGY

Appendicitis is acute inflammation of the vermiform appendix—the blind pouch attached to the cecum of the colon that is usually located in the right iliac region, just below the ileocecal valve. The appendix has no known function in adults. Inflammation of the appendix can occur when the lumen (opening) of the appendix is obstructed. Inflammation leads to infection as bacteria invade the wall of the appendix.

When the lumen is blocked, the mucosa continues to secrete fluid until the pressure within the lumen exceeds venous pressure. Blood flow to the appendix is restricted, and infection causes more swelling, which further impedes blood flow. Gangrene from hypoxia or perforation can occur within 24 to 36 hours. If this process occurs slowly, adjacent organs may wall off the area, and a localized abscess develops. If the infectious process occurs rapidly, peritonitis (inflammation of the peritoneum) may result. All complications of peritonitis are serious. Acute appendicitis is the most common cause of acute inflammation in the right lower quadrant. Consequently, it is one of the most common indications for emergency abdominal surgery.

When obstruction is present, calculi composed of fecal material (fecaliths), calcium phosphate–rich mucus, and inorganic salts may be the most common cause of the initial obstruction. Other causes of obstruction include tumors, viral infections, and worms. However, ulceration of the mucosa may be the primary cause of appendicitis. Infection by viral or fungal pathogens has been suggested as the cause of ulceration. Although appendicitis affects a person at any age, the peak incidence is between the ages of 20 and 30 years. Appendicitis affects men and women equally, except before 25 years of age, when males are affected more often than females at a 3:2 ratio.

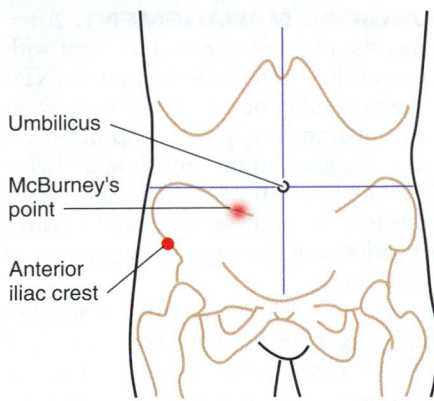

Figure 61-1 ■ McBurney's point is located midway between the anterior iliac crest and the umbilicus in the right lower quadrant. This is the classic area for localized tenderness during the later stages of appendicitis.

> ### CONSIDERATIONS FOR OLDER ADULTS
> Appendicitis is relatively rare at extremes in age; however, perforation is more common in older people, causing a higher mortality rate. The diagnosis of appendicitis is difficult to establish in older adults because symptoms of pain and tenderness are not as pronounced in this age-group. As a result, a significant number of older clients with appendicitis develop perforation due to a delay in diagnosis.

It is thought that chronic infection of the appendix can occur, but this is not usually the cause of abdominal pain that lasts for weeks or months. Recurrent acute appendicitis does sometimes occur, often with complete remission of inflammation between acute attacks. In rare instances, acute appendicitis may be the first manifestation of Crohn's disease.

◆ COLLABORATIVE MANAGEMENT
◆ Assessment
Early history taking and the identification of risk factors such as adolescent males, familial tendency, and intra-abdominal tumors should be obtained from the client. The most common symptom is abdominal pain, which results from contractions of the appendix or distention of its lumen. With *classic* appendicitis, abdominal pain in the epigastric or periumbilical area is the initial symptom. Pain may not be localized, however, and can exist anywhere in the abdomen or flanks. The pain at this time is described as mild or cramping. Nausea and vomiting follow in 50% to 60% of cases. As the inflammation spreads to the peritoneal surface, the pain becomes more steady and severe and the location shifts to the right lower quadrant. Abdominal pain that increases with cough or movement and is relieved by flexion of the right hip or the knees suggests a perforated appendix with peritonitis. Anorexia is a frequent finding associated with acute appendicitis.

Abdominal tenderness on palpation is the most common, important, and reliable symptom. In later stages of inflammation, tenderness becomes more localized and is noted with palpation of the right lower quadrant. This area is referred to as **McBurney's point**; it is located midway between the anterior iliac crest and the umbilicus in the right lower quadrant (Figure 61-1). The nurse may feel tenseness of the muscles (muscle rigidity) over the tender area. Rigidity over the whole abdomen, accompanied by tense positioning and guarding, indicates a perforated appendix with peritonitis.

Perforation (rupture) rarely occurs within 24 hours of the onset of symptoms, but the incidence of peritonitis rises to as high as 80% after 48 hours. **Rebound tenderness** is a term used to describe a sensation of severe pain that occurs after deep pressure is applied and released. This maneuver involves pressing a finger into the abdomen at a point away from the pain and is performed by the physician or advanced-practice nurse.

The client's temperature is usually normal or slightly elevated at 99° to 100.5° F (37.2° to 38° C). A temperature of 101° F (38.2° C) or higher suggests the presence of peritonitis. As the temperature rises, a corresponding rise in pulse rate will be noted.

Because the clinical manifestations associated with many other medical conditions are similar to those of acute appendicitis, arriving at a diagnosis is often difficult. It is important to determine the sequence of symptoms. For example, nausea and vomiting that precede abdominal pain often indicate gastroenteritis.

Clinical manifestations that do not follow the classic pattern can occur as a result of variations in the anatomic location of the appendix. The appendix can be located deep in the pelvis, in the right upper quadrant, or even in the left lower quadrant.

Laboratory findings do not establish the diagnosis, but there is often a moderate elevation of the white blood cell (WBC) count (leukocytosis) to 10,000 to 18,000/mm³ with a "shift to the left" (an increased number of immature WBCs). A WBC elevation greater than 20,000/mm³ may indicate a perforated appendix. An ultrasound study may show the presence of an enlarged appendix. If symptoms are recurrent or prolonged, a barium enema or computed tomography (CT) scan can be diagnostic and may reveal the presence of a fecalith.

◆ Interventions
All clients with suspected or confirmed appendicitis are hospitalized and examined by a surgeon. If the diagnosis is questionable, the health care team observes the client before surgical exploration.

NONSURGICAL MANAGEMENT. After admission to the hospital, the physician keeps the client with suspected or known appendicitis on nothing by mouth (NPO) status to prepare for the possibility of emergency surgery and to avoid aggravating the inflammatory process. Administer intravenous (IV) fluids, as prescribed, to prevent fluid and electrolyte imbalance and to replenish fluid volume. If the semi-Fowler's position can be tolerated, advise the client to maintain this position so that abdominal drainage, if any, can be contained in the lower abdomen.

Once the diagnosis of appendicitis is confirmed, the surgeon schedules surgery. Administer opioid analgesics, as prescribed, while the client is being prepared for surgery. The client with suspected appendicitis should not receive laxatives or enemas, which can cause perforation of the appendix. Heat should never be applied to the abdomen because this may increase circulation to the appendix and result in increased inflammation and perforation.

SURGICAL MANAGEMENT. Surgery is required as soon as possible. If the diagnosis is not definitive but the client is at high risk for complications from suspected appendicitis, the surgeon may perform an exploratory laparoscopy or laparotomy to rule out appendicitis. A **laparoscopy** is a minimally invasive procedure in which the surgeon makes several small incisions near the umbilicus, through which a small endoscope is placed. Various instruments are put through the laparoscope to perform the needed procedure. A **laparotomy** is an open approach in which a large abdominal incision is made.

Preoperative Care. Preoperative teaching is often limited because the client is in pain or may be transferred to the operating suite for emergency surgery. The client is prepared for general anesthesia and surgery (see Chapter 20).

Operative Procedures. An **appendectomy** is the removal of the inflamed appendix. In an open, conventional, and uncomplicated appendectomy, the surgeon removes the appendix through an incision approximately 3 inches (7.5 cm) long in the right lower quadrant. The incision is larger if the appendix is in an atypical position or if peritonitis is present. Most uncomplicated appendectomies today are done via **laparoscopy**.

Postoperative Care. Postoperative care of the client who has undergone an appendectomy includes the care required for any client who has received general anesthesia (see Chapter 22). For clients who have undergone a conventional appendectomy, the incision is located over McBurney's point if the appendix was in the typical location. The incision may be as long as the length of the abdomen, depending on the area explored in surgery and the location of the appendix. Drains may have been inserted during the procedure if an abscess was present or if the appendix perforated.

If peritonitis was present, a nasogastric (NG) tube is placed to decompress the stomach and prevent abdominal distention. IV antibiotics are typically prescribed if peritonitis or abscess is present. Opioid analgesics are administered for pain as needed. The client is typically out of bed on the evening of surgery or the first postoperative day. The client who has had an uncomplicated appendectomy via laparoscopy may stay overnight or may be discharged on the day of surgery. In this case, no NG tubes or drains are needed. The client experiences less pain and recovers much more quickly with this surgical approach. Most clients can return to usual activities in 1 to 2 weeks.

The client who has undergone an open, uncomplicated appendectomy usually recovers rapidly and can resume normal activity in 2 to 4 weeks. If surgery has been complicated by perforation or peritonitis, the client may be hospitalized for as long as 5 to 7 days.

Peritonitis

Peritonitis is an acute inflammation of the visceral/parietal peritoneum and endothelial lining of the abdominal cavity, or peritoneum. Peritonitis can be classified as primary or secondary, localized or generalized. Peritonitis is a life-threatening illness and is associated with several abdominal disorders.

PATHOPHYSIOLOGY

Normally the peritoneal cavity contains approximately 50 mL of sterile fluid (transudate), which serves to prevent friction in the abdominal cavity during peristalsis. When the peritoneal cavity is contaminated by bacteria, the body initially produces an inflammatory reaction that walls off a localized area to fight the infection. This local reaction involves vascular dilation and increased capillary permeability, allowing transport of leukocytes and subsequent phagocytosis of the offending organisms. If this walling off process fails, the inflammation spreads and contamination becomes massive, resulting in diffuse peritonitis.

Complications of Peritonitis

Vascular dilation continues, along with hyperemia (increased blood flow) and a fluid shift. The body responds to the infectious process by shunting extra blood to the area of inflammation. Fluid is shifted from the extracellular fluid (ECF) compartment into the peritoneal cavity, connective tissues, and gastrointestinal (GI) tract ("third spacing"). This shift of fluid out of the vascular space can result in a significant decrease in circulatory volume. The rate of decreasing circulatory volume is proportional to the degree of peritoneal involvement. Severely decreased circulatory volume can result in insufficient perfusion of the kidneys, leading to renal failure with electrolyte imbalance.

Peristalsis slows or stops in response to severe peritoneal infection, and the lumen of the bowel becomes distended with gas and fluid. Fluid that normally flows to the small bowel and the colon for reabsorption accumulates in the intestine in volumes of 7 to 8 L daily. The toxins or bacteria responsible for the peritonitis can also enter the bloodstream from the peritoneal area, leading to bacteremia or **septicemia** (bacterial invasion of the blood).

Respiratory problems can occur as a result of increased abdominal pressure against the diaphragm from intestinal distention and fluid shifts to the peritoneal cavity. Pain can interfere with ventilatory efforts when the client has an increased oxygen demand because of the infectious process.

Types of Peritonitis

Primary peritonitis is an acute bacterial infection that develops as a result of contamination of the peritoneum through the vascular system. Tuberculous peritonitis that arises from a tuberculin infection originating elsewhere in the body is a type of primary peritonitis. Clients with alcoholic cirrhosis and ascites, in the absence of a perforated organ, often manifest peritonitis, which may be due to leakage of bacteria through the wall of the intestine.

Secondary peritonitis is usually caused by bacterial invasion as a result of an acute abdominal disorder. Secondary peritonitis can develop as a result of a gangrenous bowel, perforation of the viscera by blunt or penetrating trauma, or bile leakage.

Etiology

Peritonitis is caused by contamination of the peritoneal cavity by bacteria or chemicals. Bacteria gain entry into the peritoneum by perforation or from an external penetrating wound. The most common causes of bacterial peritonitis are appendicitis and perforations associated with peptic ulcer disease, diverticulitis, a gangrenous gallbladder, or bowel obstruction. Bacterial invasion can also occur from an ascending infection through the reproductive tract, as in salpingitis (fallopian tube inflammation) or a septic abortion. Other causes of peritonitis include perforating tumors, ulcerative colitis, foreign bodies (from trauma), leakage or contamination during a surgical procedure, and infection by skin pathogens in clients undergoing continuous ambulatory peritoneal dialysis (CAPD). Bacteria responsible for peritonitis include *Escherichia coli, Streptococcus, Staphylococcus, Pneumococcus,* and *Gonococcus.* Chemical peritonitis arises from leakage of bile, pancreatic enzymes, and gastric acid.

◆COLLABORATIVE MANAGEMENT
◆Assessment

HISTORY

Question the client regarding a history of abdominal pain and determine whether the pain is localized or generalized. Ask about a history of a low-grade fever or recent spikes in temperature.

PHYSICAL ASSESSMENT/CLINICAL MANIFESTATIONS

Physical findings of peritonitis (Chart 61-1) depend on several factors: the stage of the disease, the ability of the body to localize the process by walling off the infection, and whether the inflammation has progressed to generalized peritonitis. The client typically appears acutely ill, lying still, possibly with the knees flexed. Movement is guarded, and the client may report and show signs of pain (e.g., facial grimacing) with coughing or movement of any type. During inspection, observe for progressive abdominal distention if the inflammation markedly reduces intestinal motility. Aus-

---

CHART 61-1

KEY FEATURES of
Peritonitis

- Rigid, boardlike abdomen (classic)
- Abdominal pain (localized, poorly localized, or referred to the shoulder or thorax)
- Distended abdomen
- Nausea, anorexia, vomiting
- Diminishing bowel sounds
- Inability to pass flatus or feces
- Rebound tenderness in the abdomen
- High fever
- Tachycardia
- Dehydration from high fever (poor skin turgor)
- Decreased urine output
- Hiccups
- Possible compromise in respiratory status

---

cultate for bowel sounds, but these usually disappear with progression of the inflammation.

The cardinal signs of peritonitis are abdominal pain and tenderness. In the client with localized peritonitis, the abdomen is tender on palpation in a well-defined area of the abdomen with rebound tenderness in this area. With generalized peritonitis, tenderness is widespread. *Abdominal wall rigidity is a classic finding, sometimes referred to as a "board-like" abdomen.* The client may have a high fever because of the infectious process, with tachycardia occurring in response to the fever. Assess whether the client has dry mucous membranes and a low urine output. The latter occurs because fluid accumulates in the peritoneal cavity, the GI tract, and connective tissues, resulting in a fluid deficit in the vascular space (dehydration). Nausea and vomiting may also be present. Hiccups may occur as a result of diaphragmatic irritation. Depending on the severity of the peritonitis, the nurse may find that the client has a compromised respiratory status.

DIAGNOSTIC ASSESSMENT

White blood cell (WBC) counts are commonly elevated to 20,000/mm³ with a high neutrophil count. A series of blood culture studies may be done to determine whether septicemia has occurred and to identify the causative organism to enable appropriate therapy. The health care provider orders laboratory tests to assess fluid and electrolyte balance and renal status, including the following:

- Electrolytes
- Blood urea nitrogen (BUN)
- Creatinine
- Hemoglobin
- Hematocrit

Arterial blood gas values are obtained to assess respiratory function and acid-base balance.

Abdominal x-rays may be obtained to assess for free air or fluid in the abdominal cavity, which indicates perforation. The x-rays may also show dilation, edema, and inflammation of the small and large intestines. An abdominal sonogram is also useful in locating the problem.

The physician may perform a diagnostic peritoneal lavage by instilling 1 L of fluid through a peritoneal dialysis catheter. Lavage fluid positive for peritonitis is characterized by the following: more than 500 WBCs/mL of fluid, more than 50,000 red blood cells (RBCs)/mL, or the presence of bacteria on a Gram stain. Bile-stained green fluid may indicate a ruptured gallbladder or perforated intestine, which can lead to chemical peritonitis.

◆Interventions

All clients with peritonitis are hospitalized because of the severe nature of the illness. If complications are extensive, the client may be admitted to a critical care unit. Nursing interventions focus on the early identification of complications.

NONSURGICAL MANAGEMENT. The physician prescribes IV fluids and broad-spectrum antibiotics immediately after establishing the diagnosis of peritonitis. IV fluids are necessary to replace fluids collected in the peritoneum and bowel. Monitor daily weight and intake and output carefully to assess fluid status. A nasogastric (NG) tube is inserted to decompress the stomach and the intestine, and the client is on NPO status. Administer oxygen, as prescribed, according to the client's respiratory status. The health care provider will most likely institute pain management with IV analgesics, such as morphine sulfate administered via a patient-controlled analgesia (PCA) pump. Expect the health care provider to request a surgical consultation in the event that surgery becomes necessary.

SURGICAL MANAGEMENT. Abdominal surgery is the optimal treatment for identifying and repairing the cause of the peritonitis. If the client is so critically ill that surgery would be life threatening, it may be delayed. Surgery focuses on controlling the contamination, removing foreign material from the peritoneal cavity, and draining collected fluid.

The surgeon typically performs an **exploratory laparotomy** to remove or repair the inflamed or perforated organ. The abdominal cavity is opened surgically and explored for inflamed and perforated organs or other abnormalities. For example, an appendectomy is performed for an inflamed appendix; a colon resection, with or without a colostomy, is indicated for a perforated diverticulum or perforated colon secondary to a tumor. Before the abdominal cavity is closed, the surgeon irrigates the peritoneum with antibiotic solutions. Several catheters may also be inserted to drain the cavity and provide a route for irrigation postoperatively.

The preoperative care is similar to that described in Chapter 20 for clients having general anesthesia. Postoperative care is also similar to that for other clients undergoing surgery (see Chapter 22). Clients with peritonitis may have actual or potential multisystem complications. Therefore monitor the level of consciousness, vital signs, respiratory status (respiratory rate and breath sounds), and fluid and electrolyte status (intake and output and laboratory values) at least hourly immediately after surgery.

Positioning. Maintain the client in a semi-Fowler's position to promote drainage of peritoneal contents in the inferior region of the abdominal cavity. This position also facilitates adequate respiratory excursion because the diaphragm and abdominal contents are impinging on respiratory muscles.

Wound Care. The client is likely to have multiple incisions and drains. Because contamination at the time of surgery impedes healing of an incision with edges well approximated (by first intention), incisions are allowed to heal by second or third intention. These incisions necessitate meticulous care involving manual irrigation or packing as ordered by the surgeon. If the surgeon requests peritoneal irrigation through a drain, maintain strict sterile technique during manual irrigation, usually by using a catheter-tipped syringe. Determine that the client is not retaining irrigant by ensuring the absence of abdominal distention or pain and by monitoring irrigant intake and output.

As a result of the loss of fluids from the extracellular space to the peritoneal cavity, IV fluid replacement and maintenance are indicated for all clients with peritonitis. Fluid volume deficit also occurs as a result of NG suctioning and NPO status. Normal saline or a balanced saline solution with potassium is administered IV according to electrolyte, BUN, and serum creatinine values. To assess fluid volume, monitors vital signs, urine output, skin turgor, integrity of mucous membranes, and most importantly weight. Also assess for edema from third spacing.

Community-Based Care

The length of hospitalization depends on the extent and severity of the infectious process. Clients who have a local-ized abscess drained and who respond to antibiotics and IV fluids without multisystem complications are discharged in less than a week. Those who experience complications of peritonitis, along with sepsis or shock, may require mechanical ventilation or hemodialysis, with hospital stays lasting longer. Discharge planning varies with the degree of involvement of all body systems. Some clients may be transferred to a transitional care unit to complete their antibiotic therapy and recovery.

If the client is being discharged to home, assess his or her ability to function at home with the added task of incision care and a diminished activity tolerance. Provide the client and family or significant other with written and oral instructions to report the following:

- Unusual or foul-smelling drainage
- Swelling, redness, or warmth or bleeding from the incision site
- A temperature higher than 101° F (38.2° C)
- The presence of abdominal pain

Also instruct the client in proper handwashing and dressing change techniques, which include directions to dress wounds separately to avoid cross-contamination.

The physician typically prescribes an oral opioid analgesic and possibly an antibiotic. Review information about these medications with the client and caregiver. For clients taking opioid analgesics for any length of time, a stool softener should be prescribed.

Explain diet and activity limitations. Diet depends on the type of surgery performed and the client's specific food tolerances at discharge. All clients are told to refrain from any lifting for *at least* 6 weeks. Other activity limitations are made on an individual basis with the physician's recommendation.

Peritonitis is a life-threatening and consequently frightening illness. Incisional care can be demanding, and activity intolerance can be overwhelming. If complications have resolved, the nurse reassures clients that they can realistically expect to resume their previous lifestyle. Convalescence is often longer than that required for other types of surgery, however, because of the multisystem involvement.

Clients with an incision healing by second or third intention may require dressings, solution, and catheter-tipped syringes to irrigate the wound. A home care nurse may be needed to assess, irrigate, or pack the wound and change the dressing as needed. If a client needs assistance with activities of daily living, a home care aide or temporary placement in a skilled care facility may be indicated. The case manager collaborates with the health care team to determine the most appropriate setting for community-based care.

Gastroenteritis

PATHOPHYSIOLOGY

Acute diarrheal illnesses cause significant morbidity among young children and older adults, especially in less-industrialized nations of the world. **Gastroenteritis** is an increase in the frequency and water content of stools or vomiting as a result of inflammation of the mucous membranes of the stomach and intestinal tract. It primarily affects the small bowel and can be of either viral or bacterial origin. Both forms have similar manifestations and are considered self-limiting in their course unless complications occur. All organisms that are implicated in gastroenteritis cause diarrhea; however, the organisms discussed in this section have distinguishing characteristics.

Authors disagree on classification of the infectious diseases described as gastroenteritis. Some include shigellosis when discussing gastroenteritis; others consider shigellosis separately as a dysentery type of illness. Dysenteries affect the *large* bowel; gastroenteritis affects the *small* bowel. Other authors classify infectious disease of the intestine as bacterial, viral, or parasitic, without using the term *gastroenteritis*.

Food poisoning is sometimes described in conjunction with gastroenteritis, with specific reference to the organism causing the food poisoning. Gastroenteritis, however, differs from food poisoning with regard to transmission in the body, incubation time, and effect on immunity.

The following discussion of gastroenteritis includes the epidemic viral form and the bacterial forms (*Campylobacter, Escherichia coli,* and shigellosis) (Table 61-1). Organisms associated with food poisoning and parasitic infections are discussed under Food Poisoning, p. 1365.

Infection with viral and bacterial organisms can produce gastrointestinal (GI) illnesses in which watery diarrhea is the primary feature. These disorders can be caused by noninflammatory, inflammatory, or penetrating mechanisms. The infecting organism (e.g., enterotoxigenic *E. coli*) can release enterotoxin (a noninflammatory toxic substance specific to the intestinal mucosa), which results in diarrhea. The organism (e.g., *Shigella* or *Campylobacter*) can also attach itself to mucosal epithelium without penetrating it. Cells of the intestinal villi are then destroyed, and malabsorption results. Infections that are mediated by bacterial toxins cause the absorptive capacity of the distal small bowel and proximal colon to be overcome, resulting in diarrhea. Finally, the organism can penetrate the intestine, causing cellular destruction, necrosis, and a potential for ulceration. Diarrhea occurs often with white blood cells (WBCs) or red blood cells (RBCs) present in the stool.

All these situations result in *increased* GI motility, with fluids and electrolytes being secreted into the intestine at rapid rates. Invading organisms have increased capabilities of attaching to the intestinal mucosa if the normal intestinal flora is altered. This can occur in clients who are receiving antibiotics, are malnourished, or are debilitated. Two groups of viruses, the rotaviruses (which affect young children) and Norwalk virus, as well as bacterial pathogens, are primary etiologic agents involved in the development of gastroenteritis.

Types of Gastroenteritis

VIRAL GASTROENTERITIS

Norwalk virus infection can occur year-round and affects adults and children alike. This virus is spread by the oral-fecal route and is responsible for one third of all epidemics of viral gastroenteritis in developed countries. The virus is also a common cause of waterborne epidemics of gastroenteritis.

BACTERIAL GASTROENTERITIS

The following are the three common types of bacterial gastroenteritis:

- *E. coli* diarrhea ("traveler's diarrhea")
- *Campylobacter enteritis* (another "traveler's diarrhea")
- *Shigellosis* (bacillary dysentery)

E. coli is the most common organism implicated in traveler's diarrhea. The reservoirs of *E. coli* are humans, who are often asymptomatic. The organism is transmitted through fecally contaminated food, water, or fomites (any other substance that transmits infection).

The etiologic feature of *Campylobacter* enteritis is the bacterium *Campylobacter jejuni*; reservoirs are domestic or wild animals and birds. *C. jejuni* is transmitted through the fecal-oral route by ingestion of water or food contaminated with feces or by direct contact with infected animals or infants. Incubation ranges from 1 to 10 days. The organism is communicable for several days to weeks throughout the course of the infection (usually 2 to 7 weeks).

Shigellosis is caused by infection with *Shigella* bacteria. Direct or indirect fecal-oral transmission can occur from an infected person or carrier. The incubation period before the illness is 1 to 7 days. The illness can be communicated during the acute phase and for up to 4 weeks after the onset of illness. A person can be a carrier of this illness for months after the acute illness.

Incidence/Prevalence

As a group, acute GI illnesses are the second most common disease worldwide. Acute diarrheal illnesses are the most common cause of morbidity and mortality among children and older adults in Asia, Africa, and Latin America. Gastroenteritis often occurs in epidemic outbreaks.

Campylobacter enteritis occurs worldwide, commonly in epidemic outbreaks. Its incidence is highest during warm

TABLE 61-1	Common Types of Gastroenteritis and Their Characteristics	
Type	**Characteristics**
Viral Gastroenteritis	
Epidemic viral	Caused by many parvovirus-type organisms
	Transmitted by the fecal-oral route in food and water
	Incubation period 10-51 hr
	Communicable during acute illness
Rotarvirus and Norwalk virus	Transmitted by the fecal-oral route and possibly the respiratory route
	Incubation in 48 hr
	Rotavirus is most common in infants and young children
	Norwalk virus affects young children and adults
Bacterial Gastroenteritis	
Campylobacter enteritis	Transmitted by the fecal-oral route or by contact with infected animals or infants
	Incubation period 1-10 days
	Communicable for 2-7 weeks
Escherichia coli diarrhea	Transmitted by fecally contaminated food, water, or fomites
Shigellosis	Transmitted by direct and indirect fecal-oral routes
	Incubation period 1-7 days
	Communicable during the acute illness to 4 wk after the illness
	Humans possibly carriers for months

months. Diarrhea caused by *E. coli* also occurs worldwide, commonly in epidemics. The highest incidence is in areas of poor sanitation during warm months. Shigellosis occurs worldwide in every age-group but most frequently in children under the age of 10 years. Children and older adults are more susceptible to *Shigella* because of their immature or depressed immune systems. Outbreaks of shigellosis are common in areas with crowded living conditions.

◆COLLABORATIVE MANAGEMENT
◆Assessment

The history elicited from the client can provide information related to the potential cause of the illness. Question the client regarding a recent history of travel, especially to tropical regions of Asia, Africa, or Central or South America. Traveler's diarrhea can begin 3 days to 2 weeks after the client's arrival.

The client who has gastroenteritis usually appears ill. Nausea and vomiting can occur with all types of gastroenteritis but are usually limited to the first 1 or 2 days of the illness. All clients with gastroenteritis classically have diarrhea, which varies in consistency and amount with the causative organism.

In clients with epidemic viral gastroenteritis, myalgia (muscle aches), headache, and malaise are often reported. Note any slight abdominal distention, auscultate for hyperactive bowel sounds, and be mindful of any diffuse tenderness on palpation. However, there should be *no* rebound tenderness, which might indicate peritonitis. Depending on the amount of fluids lost through diarrhea and vomiting, the client may have varying degrees of dehydration manifested by the following:

- Poor skin turgor
- Dry mucous membranes
- Orthostatic blood pressure changes
- Hypotension
- Oliguria

In some cases, dehydration may be severe, and shock may occur if diarrhea is prolonged. Dehydration occurs rapidly in older adults and may require hospitalization.

Diarrhea associated with epidemic viral gastroenteritis is typically limited to 24 to 48 hours. Infection with the Norwalk virus is characterized by the rapid onset of nausea, abdominal cramps, vomiting, and diarrhea. The illness is usually mild, lasting 24 to 48 hours. *Campylobacter* enteritis is a more severe disease with foul-smelling stools that contain blood and that can number 20 to 30 per day for up to 7 days. *E. coli* gastroenteritis may or may not involve blood or mucus in the stool; diarrhea can last for up to 10 days. *Shigella* causes stools containing blood and mucus, which can continue for up to 5 days.

As part of the laboratory assessment, Gram stain of stool is usually done before culture. Many white blood cells (WBCs) on Gram stain suggest shigellosis. The presence of WBCs and red blood cells (RBCs) in the stool indicates *Campylobacter* gastroenteritis.

A stool culture that is positive for enterotoxigenic *E. coli* is diagnostic of *E. coli* diarrhea. Culture of stool that is positive for *Shigella* when pus cells or WBCs are present in the stool is diagnostic of shigellosis.

◆Interventions

For clients with most types of gastroenteritis, supportive treatment is instituted. Therapy is focused on fluid replace-

ment, and the amount and route of fluid administration are determined by fluid status.

Fluid Replacement. For mild cases of gastroenteritis, the client is treated on an ambulatory care basis or in the nursing home if he or she is a resident there. If the fluid volume is severely depleted, the client is admitted to the hospital for administration of IV fluids. For older clients at home or in a long-term care setting, oral rehydration therapy (ORT) with commercially prepared rehydration products, such as Resol, may prevent hospitalization.

Obtain a weight, orthostatic blood pressure, and other vital sign measurements at admission. Hypotonic IV fluids, such as half-strength normal saline (0.45% sodium chloride), are infused as prescribed. Monitor the client's vital signs, intake and output, and weight. A rapid gain or loss of 1 kg (2.2 pounds) of body weight is equivalent to the gain or loss of 1 L of fluid. Standard precautions are consistently observed when handling vomitus and stool.

The health care provider may prescribe a potassium supplement to be added to IV fluids if the serum potassium level is low. To help assess renal function and prevent hyperkalemia, verify that the client is voiding before and during potassium replacement. The client is advised to rest in bed, especially during periods of nausea or vomiting.

Depending on the type of gastroenteritis, the local health department may need to be notified. It is mandatory that every case of shigellosis be reported. In some endemic areas, *Campylobacter* enteritis needs to be reported on a case-by-case basis. Other types of gastroenteritis must be reported only if they occur in epidemic proportions.

Diet Therapy. Diet therapy is the same for the client who remains at home as for the client in the hospital. If the client is not actively vomiting, recommend small volumes of clear liquids with electrolytes (e.g., Pedialyte) for 24 hours. The frequency and amount of oral intake can be increased if nausea and vomiting are *not* present. If nausea and vomiting continue, suggest that food and fluids be withheld until these symptoms subside. Advise the client *not* to drink water because it does not contain any electrolytes to replace those lost. After 24 hours, the diet for most clients can be advanced to include saltine crackers, toast, and jelly. When the client can tolerate this diet, bland foods (e.g., nonfat soup, custard, yogurt, cottage cheese, mashed or baked potatoes, cooked vegetables) can be added. Caffeine is avoided because it can increase intestinal motility. The client may progress to a regular diet as tolerated.

Drug Therapy. Drugs that suppress intestinal motility, such as anticholinergics and antiemetics, are *not* routinely given for bacterial or viral gastroenteritis. Use of these drugs can prevent the infecting organisms from being eliminated from the body. If the health care provider determines that antiperistaltic agents are necessary, an initial dose of loperamide (Imodium) 4 mg can be administered orally, followed by 2 mg after each loose stool, up to 16 mg daily. Bismuth subsalicylate (Pepto-Bismol) 30 mL or two tablets every 30 minutes for a maximum of eight doses can be given to reduce the watery volume of the stool.

Treatment with antibiotics may be warranted if the gastroenteritis is due to bacterial infection with fever and severe diarrhea. The health care provider may prescribe norfloxacin (Chibroxin, Noroxin) 400 mg twice daily PO or ciprofloxacin (Cipro) 500 mg twice daily PO for 3 days. If the gastroenteritis is due to shigellosis, anti-infective agents, such as trimethoprim/sulfamethoxazole (Septra DS, Bactrim DS, Roubac✻), are administered.

For relatively short-term diarrhea of 24 to 48 hours' duration, the diagnosis is based primarily on the client's history and clinical manifestations without validation by a stool examination. When diarrhea is severe or persists for long periods, the stool is examined in an effort to determine the causative organism and to begin specific treatment. It should be determined whether the diarrhea is caused by *Salmonella* or by parasites because these organisms respond to specific medications (see Parasitic Infection, p. 1362). Diarrhea that continues longer than 10 days is probably *not* due to gastroenteritis, and a thorough investigation for the cause is warranted.

Skin Care. Frequent stools that are rich in electrolytes and enzymes, as well as frequent wiping and washing of the anal region, can irritate the skin. Teach the client to avoid toilet paper and harsh soaps. Ideally, the client can gently clean the area with warm water or absorbent cotton, followed by thorough drying with absorbent cotton. Cream, oil, or gel can be applied to a damp, warm washcloth to remove excrement adhering to excoriated skin. Hydrocortisone cream or protective barrier cream should be applied to the skin between stools. Witch hazel compresses (e.g., Tucks) and sitz baths for 10 minutes, two to three times daily, can also relieve discomfort.

If leakage of stool is a problem, the client can put absorbent cotton next to the anal orifice and keep it in place with snug underwear. For clients who are incontinent, remind assistive nursing personnel to keep the perineal and buttock areas clean and dry. The use of incontinent pads instead of briefs allows air to circulate to the skin and prevents irritation.

Health Teaching. During the acute phase of the illness, teach the client about the importance of fluid replacement. The client should follow the diet, described earlier under Diet Therapy, p. 1344. Instruction of the client and family about the importance of minimizing the risk of trans-

mission of gastroenteritis is also important. Furthermore, clients are advised to do the following:

- Wash hands meticulously with an antibacterial soap, especially after bowel movements, and maintain good personal hygiene.
- Restrict the use of glasses, dishes, eating utensils, and tubes of toothpaste to themselves only.
- Maintain clean bathroom facilities to avoid exposure to stool.
- Inform the health care provider if symptoms persist beyond 3 days.

Clients adhere to these precautions for up to 7 weeks after the illness or up to several months if *Shigella* was the offending organism. If the client is employed as a food handler, the public health department should be consulted for recommendations about the return to work (Chart 61-2).

CHRONIC INFLAMMATORY BOWEL DISEASE

Chronic inflammatory bowel disease (chronic IBD, also sometimes just called IBD) refers to several inflammatory disorders of the gastrointestinal (GI) tract with no known etiology. Chronic IBDs may be divided into two major groups: ulcerative colitis and Crohn's disease (Table 61-2).

Ulcerative Colitis

PATHOPHYSIOLOGY

Ulcerative colitis (UC) is one of a group of bowel diseases of unknown etiology, characterized by remissions and exacerbations ("flare-ups"). This chronic inflammatory process affects the mucosal lining of the colon or rectum. It can result in loose stools containing blood and mucus, poor absorption of vital nutrients, and thickening of the colon wall. Over time, the client experiences episodes of abdominal discomfort and extraintestinal (other than intestinal) manifestations of the disease that cause disruption of lifestyle. The affected client may have only minor periodic health problems, necessitating only ambulatory care, or the client may have serious problems, such as malnutrition and physical debilitation, requiring multiple hospitalizations.

Ulcerative colitis is characterized by diffuse inflammation of the intestinal mucosa; the result is a loss of surface epithelium with ulceration and possibly abscess formation. Generally the disease begins in the rectum and proceeds in a uni-

---

CHART 61-2

CLIENT EDUCATION GUIDE
Measures to Prevent the Transmission of Gastroenteritis

- Wash your hands meticulously with an antibacterial soap, especially after having a bowel movement.
- Do not share your dishes, glasses, or toothpaste.
- Keep the commode clean to prevent exposure to your stool.
- Do not prepare or handle food that will be consumed by others.

TABLE 61-2 Differential Features of Ulcerative Colitis and Crohn's Disease

Feature	Ulcerative Colitis	Crohn's Disease
Location	Begins in the rectum and proceeds in a continuous manner toward the cecum	Most often in the terminal ileum, with patchy involvement through all layers of the bowel
Etiology	Unknown	Unknown
Peak incidence at age	15-25 yr and 55-65 yr	15-40 yr
Stools	10-20 liquid, bloody stools per day	5-6 soft, loose stools per day, rarely bloody
Common complications	Hemorrhage Perforation Fistulas Nutritional deficiencies	Fistulas Nutritional deficiencies

TABLE 61-3 Complications of Ulcerative Colitis and Crohn's Disease

Complication	Description
Hemorrhage/perforation	Lower gastrointestinal bleeding results from erosion of the bowel wall.
Abscess formation	Localized pockets of infection develop in the ulcerated bowel lining.
Toxic megacolon	Paralysis of the colon causes dilation and subsequent bowel obstruction.
Malabsorption	Essential nutrients cannot be absorbed through the diseased intestinal wall, causing anemia and malnutrition (most common in Crohn's disease).
Bowel obstruction	Obstruction results from toxic megacolon or cancer.
Fistulas	Fistulas can occur anywhere but usually track between the bowel and bladder. Pyuria and fecaluria result.
Colorectal cancer	Clients with ulcerative colitis for 7-10 yr or longer have a high risk for colorectal cancer. This complication accounts for about one third of all deaths related to ulcerative colitis.
Extraintestinal complications	Complications include arthritis, hepatic and biliary disease (especially cholelithiasis), oral and skin lesions, and ocular disorders, such as iritis. The cause is unknown.

form, continuous manner proximally toward the cecum. The process progresses to epithelial cell damage and loss, leaving areas of ulceration, redness, and bleeding in the *acute* stage.

As the disease course progresses, *chronic* changes in the colon occur. Fibrosis and retraction of the bowel result in muscle hypertrophy, deposition of fat and fibrous tissue, and a narrower and shorter colon. With long-term disease, dysplastic changes to the surface epithelium occur. These changes are associated with an increased risk of colon cancer. Complications of UC include the following:

- Intestinal perforation with resultant peritonitis and fistula formation
- Toxic megacolon
- Hemorrhage
- Increased risk of colon cancer
- Abscess formation
- Malabsorption
- Bowel obstruction
- Extraintestinal clinical manifestations, such as arthritis

Table 61-3 describes these common complications.

Etiology and Genetic Risk

The exact cause of UC is unknown. A genetic basis of the disease has been proposed because of the increased incidence seen in families, certain ethnic groups, and twins. Immunologic hypotheses, including autoimmune dysfunction, have been explored because of the extraintestinal manifestations of the disease. One hypothesis suggests that IBD re-

sults from an abnormal response to normal flora present in the intestines; another possibility is that there may be a defect in intestinal permeability that permits antigens to leak through the mucosa, stimulating an inflammatory response. Psychological factors have also been implicated because stress often results in a flare-up of the disease. However, little evidence has been found to relate psychological factors to the cause of the disease.

Incidence/Prevalence

There is a higher geographic distribution of the disease in northern Europe and North America. The annual incidence of ulcerative colitis is about 2 to 10 new cases per 100,000 persons. The prevalence is 40 to 100 cases per 100,000 people in the United States. There is a 10-fold risk of the disease if an individual has a first-degree relative with the disease.

CULTURAL CONSIDERATIONS

Ulcerative colitis is four to five times more common among people of Jewish origin and commonly affects white individuals in developed Western society. It is seen more often in individuals of Jewish European or Ashkenazi origin but not in those of Sephardic origin. Although the disease is more common in white individuals, the incidence in black individuals is increasing.

Peak incidence is between the ages of 15 and 25 years, with another peak occurring between ages of 55 and 65 years. Females are more often affected than men.

◆COLLABORATIVE MANAGEMENT
◆Assessment

HISTORY

Collect data on any family history of inflammatory bowel disease (IBD) and previous and current therapy for the illness, as well as dates and types of surgery. Obtaining a diet history is essential. It should include the client's usual dietary patterns and the relationship of elimination patterns to intolerance of milk and milk products and greasy, fried, spicy, or hot foods. A history of weight loss may be seen in clients with severe disease.

Ask about the symptoms of acute ulcerative colitis, which often include abdominal pain, cramping, urgency, and diarrhea with up to 10 to 20 liquid, bloody stools per day, as well as anorexia and fatigue. Furthermore, question the client regarding his or her usual bowel elimination pattern; the color, consistency, and character of stools; and the presence or absence of blood in all stools. Note any relationship between the occurrence of diarrhea and the timing of meals, pain, emotional distress, and activity. Question the client regarding extraintestinal symptoms such as arthritis, mouth sores, vision problems, and skin disorders.

PHYSICAL ASSESSMENT/CLINICAL MANIFESTATIONS

The client with ulcerative colitis may have symptoms that vary with the acuteness of onset and with complications of the disease process. They may complain of abdominal pain, bloody diarrhea, and **tenesmus** (uncontrollable straining).

Vital signs are usually within normal limits in mild disease. In more severe cases, the client may have a low-grade fever (99° to 100° F [37.2° to 37.8° C]). The physical assessment findings are typically nonspecific, and in milder cases the physical examination may be normal.

Note any mild abdominal distention along the colon. Palpation may reveal areas of increased or localized tenderness. Rebound tenderness may suggest peritonitis. You should further note any localized areas of abdominal pain or cramping over areas of diseased bowel. The client may be febrile and tachycardic, indicating possible complications, such as peritonitis, dehydration, and bowel perforation.

PSYCHOSOCIAL ASSESSMENT

The intestinal and extraintestinal symptoms associated with ulcerative colitis can be taxing. Evaluate the client's understanding of the illness and its impact on his or her lifestyle. Encourage and support the client while simultaneously exploring the following:

- The relationship of life events to disease exacerbations
- Stress factors that produce symptoms
- Family and social support systems
- Concerns regarding the possible genetic basis and associated cancer risks of the disease

Many clients are very apprehensive regarding the frequency of stools and the presence of blood. The uncontrollability of the disease symptoms, particularly diarrhea, can be disruptive and stress producing. More severe illness may limit the client's activities outside the home. As a result of the excessive diarrhea, the client may become dependent on the proximity of a bathroom. Eating may be associated with pain and cramping as well as an increased frequency of stools. Mealtimes may become unpleasant experiences. Frequent visits to health care providers and vigilant monitoring of the colonic mucosa for dysplastic (irregular) changes can be anxiety provoking.

LABORATORY ASSESSMENT

As a result of chronic blood loss, hematocrit and hemoglobin levels may be low, reflecting anemia and a chronic disease state. An increased white blood cell (WBC) count and elevated erythrocyte sedimentation rate (ESR) are consistent with inflammatory disease. Sodium, potassium, and chloride concentrations may be depleted secondary to frequent diarrheal stools and malabsorption resulting from the diseased bowel. Hypoalbuminemia (decreased serum albumin) is found in clients with extensive disease.

Viral and bacterial dysenteries can cause symptoms similar to those of ulcerative colitis. Before an invasive diagnostic workup, the stools are examined for occult blood, ova (eggs), and parasites, and specimens for culture are obtained. Other problems must be ruled out before a definitive diagnosis of ulcerative colitis is made.

RADIOGRAPHIC ASSESSMENT

Barium enemas with air contrast demonstrate differences between Crohn's disease and ulcerative colitis and identify complications, mucosal patterns, and the distribution and depth of disease involvement. In early disease, the barium enema will show incomplete filling as a result of inflammation and fine ulcerations along the bowel contour. These ulcerations appear deeper in more advanced disease.

Critical Thinking Challenge

A 42-year-old client visits the physician's office where you work. She complains of abdominal pain and numerous diarrheal stools each day. She also states that she has abdominal cramping and often feels "bloated." Her activity level has decreased because of her fatigue and the need to stay near a bathroom most of the day.

1. What questions should you ask her to elicit a thorough history?
2. What physical assessment findings would you expect and why?
3. What psychosocial assessment questions would be appropriate?

evolve For suggested answer guidelines, go to http://evolve.elsevier.com/Iggy/.

◆ Analysis

COMMON NURSING DIAGNOSES AND COLLABORATIVE PROBLEMS

The following are priority nursing diagnoses for clients with ulcerative colitis:

1. **Diarrhea** related to inflammation of the bowel mucosa
2. **Acute and Chronic Pain** related to inflammation and ulceration of the bowel mucosa and accompanying skin irritation

The primary collaborative problem is Potential for Gastrointestinal Bleeding.

ADDITIONAL NURSING DIAGNOSES AND COLLABORATIVE PROBLEMS

In addition to the common nursing diagnoses and collaborative problems, clients with ulcerative colitis may have one or more of the following:

- **Imbalanced Nutrition: Less Than Body Requirements** related to inability to absorb food due to biologic factors
- **Disturbed Body Image** related to biophysical factors and possible surgery
- **Activity Intolerance** related to generalized weakness
- **Ineffective Coping** related to high degree of threat and uncertainty
- **Risk for Deficient Fluid Volume** related to diarrhea

◆ Planning and Implementation

DIARRHEA

NOC **PLANNING: EXPECTED OUTCOMES.** A major concern for a client with ulcerative colitis is the occurrence of frequent, bloody diarrhea. Therefore the client is expected to have formed stools. Indicators include that the client will have noncompromised:

- Elimination pattern
- Control of bowel movements
- Stool color
- Stool amount for diet

INTERVENTIONS. Many measures are used to relieve symptoms and to reduce intestinal motility, decrease inflammation, and promote intestinal healing. Medical management is the preferred and initial treatment option.

The purpose of diarrhea management (Chart 61-3) is the prevention and alleviation of diarrhea. It is important to instruct the client with exacerbations of diarrhea to record the

CHART 61-3

NIC INTERVENTION ACTIVITIES for
The Client with Inflammatory Bowel Disease

Diarrhea Management: *Management and alleviation of diarrhea*
- Instruct client/family members to record color, volume, frequency, and consistency of stools.
- Identify factors (e.g., medications, bacteria, tube feedings) that may cause or contribute to diarrhea.
- Teach the client to eliminate gas-forming and spicy foods from diet.
- Suggest trial elimination of foods containing lactose.
- Instruct in low-fiber, high-protein, high-calorie diet, as appropriate.
- Teach client appropriate use of antidiarrheal medications.
- Monitor skin in perianal area for irritation and ulceration.
- Weigh client regularly.
- Perform actions to rest the bowel (NPO, liquid diet).

Pain Management: *Alleviation of pain or a reduction in pain to a level of comfort that is acceptable to the client*
- Perform a comprehensive assessment of pain to include location, characteristics, onset/duration, frequency, quality, intensity or severity of pain, and precipitating factors.
- Evaluate, with the client and the health care team, the effectiveness of past pain control measures that have been used.
- Reduce or eliminate factors that can precipitate or increase the pain experience (e.g., fear, fatigue, monotony, and lack of knowledge).
- Teach the use of nonpharmacologic techniques (e.g., biofeedback, TENS, hypnosis, relaxation, guided imagery, music therapy, distraction, activity therapy, acupressure, hot/cold application, and massage) before, after and, if possible, during painful activities; before pain occurs or increases; and along with other pain relief measures.

NIC intervention activities selected from Dochterman, J.M., & Bulechek, G.M. (Eds.) (2004). *Nursing interventions classification (NIC)* (4th ed.). St. Louis: Mosby. No part of this work is to be altered without prior written permission from the Publisher.
TENS, Transcutaneous electrical nerve stimulation.

color, volume, frequency, and consistency of stools to determine the severity of the problem. In collaboration with the dietitian, assist in identifying factors that may cause or contribute to diarrhea.

Monitor the skin in the perianal area for irritation and ulceration resulting from loose, frequent stools. Stool cultures may be sent for analysis if diarrhea continues. Instruct the client and family members about the appropriate use of antidiarrheal medications. If the client is hospitalized, have the assistive nursing personnel weigh the client daily. Clients at home should weigh themselves one to two times each week.

NONSURGICAL MANAGEMENT. Nonsurgical management includes drug and diet therapy. The provision of physical and emotional rest is also important considerations.

Drug Therapy. The health care provider prescribes a combination of drugs, including salicylate compounds, corticosteroids, immunosuppressants, and antidiarrheals.

Salicylate Compounds. Sulfasalazine (Azulfidine, PMS-Sulfasalazine❖) is one of the primary treatments for ulcerative colitis. It is thought to act by inhibiting prostaglandin synthesis to reduce inflammation. Sulfasalazine is used to prevent recurrences of the disease as well as to treat acute exacerbations of mild to moderate severity. The usual dose of sulfasalazine is 2 to 4 g daily. Remind the client to take the drug with a full glass of water and to increase fluids throughout the

day. The drug should be taken after meals to prevent GI discomfort. Because severe hypersensitivity reactions, blood dyscrasias such as leukopenia and anemia may occur, newer drugs that are less likely to cause these adverse effects are often given as alternatives.

Other 5-aminosalicylic acid agents, such as mesalamine (Asacol, Pentasa, Salofalk❖), olsalazine (Dipentum), and balsalazide (Colazal), are also used for their anti-inflammatory effect. The recommended dose of Asacol is 800 mg three times daily or Pentasa 4 g daily in divided doses for acute illness. Tablets should not be crushed, broken, or chewed. Clients with mild to moderate colitis of the distal bowel may be treated with mesalamine suppositories given two or three times daily or with retention enemas (Rowasa enema) given once daily at bedtime.

Dipentum 1 g daily in divided doses may be used for maintenance therapy. Colazal is used for acute illness at the usual dose of 2.25 g three times daily for 8 to 12 weeks.

Corticosteroids. Oral or IV corticosteroid therapy may be prescribed during exacerbations of the disease. Prednisone (Deltasone, Winpred) 40 to 65 mg daily is usually given orally. For a severely ill client, prednisolone (Delta-Cortef) 45 to 60 mg daily may be given IV. Once clinical improvement has been established, the corticosteroids are tapered over a 2- to 3-month period after discharge because of the long-term adverse effects that commonly occur with steroid therapy. Examples include hyperglycemia (increased blood glucose), osteoporosis, peptic ulcer disease, and increased risk for infection. For clients with rectal symptoms, topical steroids in the form of small-retention enemas may be prescribed. Hydrocortisone rectal foam (Cortifoam) is prescribed as one to two times daily for 2 to 3 weeks and then every other day. Hydrocortisone enemas (Cortenema) are given at bedtime for 21 days, tapered, and discontinued.

Immunosuppressive Drugs. As single agents, immunosuppressive drugs (also known as immunomodulators) are not effective in the treatment of ulcerative colitis. However, when given in combination with steroids, they may help to reduce the amount of steroids necessary to obtain a response. For example, cyclosporine (Gengraf) given at 4 mg/kg/day can be beneficial in severely ill clients who might otherwise require a colectomy. Oral 6-mercaptopurine (Purinethol) may be given at a dose of 1.5 to 2.5 mg/kg/day. Observe for side effects of this medication, which include thrombocytopenia (decreased platelets), leukopenia (decreased white blood cells [WBCs]), anemia, renal failure, infection, headache, GI ulceration, stomatitis (oral cavity inflammation), and hepatotoxicity. Therefore it is important to monitor blood counts and note signs of infection. Other drugs in the same class, such as tacrolimus (Prograf), are being used experimentally for ulcerative colitis when other medications are not effective.

Antidiarrheal Drugs. To provide symptomatic management of diarrhea, antidiarrheal drugs may be prescribed. These drugs are given very cautiously, however, because they can precipitate colonic dilation and toxic megacolon. Common antidiarrheal drugs include diphenoxylate hydrochloride and atropine sulfate (Lomotil) and loperamide (Imodium).

Other Drugs. Although not approved as a first-line medication for ulcerative colitis, infliximab (Remicade) may be used for **refractory disease** (disease that does not respond to any other type of therapy) or for severe complications,

TABLE 61-4 Guidelines for a Low-Fiber Diet

Foods Allowed	Foods Not Allowed
Beverages	
Only 2 glasses of milk, if allowed, boiled or evaporated; strained fruit juices, coffee, tea, and carbonated beverages	Alcohol
Eggs	
Prepared in any manner, except fried	Fried
Cheese	
Cottage, cream, milk, American, and Tillamook (use in small amounts)	Highly flavored
Meats or Poultry	
Roasted, baked, or broiled tender beef, lamb, liver, veal, fish, chicken, or turkey	Tough meats, pork; fried or highly spiced meats
Soups	
Bouillon, broth, and strained cream soups from foods allowed	Any others
Fats	
Butter, margarine, oils, 30 mL (1 oz) of cream daily	None
Vegetables	
Canned or cooked vegetables, such as asparagus, beets, carrots, peas, potatoes, pumpkin, squash, spinach, and young string beans; tomato juice	Raw or whole cooked vegetables (e.g., potato with skin)
Fruits	
Strained fruit juices; cooked or canned apples, apricots, Royal Ann cherries, peaches, pears, dried fruit purée, and ripe banana and avocado; all of the above without skins or seeds	All other raw or cooked fruits
Bread and Crackers	
Refined bread, toast, rolls, and crackers	Pancakes, waffles, and whole-grain bread or rolls
Cereals	
Cooked cereal, such as Cream of Wheat, Malt-O Meal, strained oatmeal, cornmeal, cornflakes, puffed rice, Rice Krispies, and puffed wheat	Whole-grain cereals; other prepared cereals
Potatoes/Rice/Pasta	
White rice, macaroni, noodles, and spaghetti	Fried potato, potato chips, and brown rice
Desserts	
Gelatin desserts, tapioca, angel food or sponge cake, plain custards, water ice or ice cream without fruit or nuts, and rennet or simple puddings	Rich pastries, pies, and anything with nuts or dried fruit
Sweets	
Sugar, jelly, honey, syrups, gumdrops, hard candy, plain creams, milk chocolate	Other candy; jam, marmalade
Miscellaneous Foods	
Cream sauce and plain gravy	Nuts, olives, popcorn, rich gravies, pepper, spices and vinegar

Modified from Williams, S.R. (2001). *Basic nutrition and diet therapy* (11th ed.). St. Louis: Mosby.

such as toxic megacolon. This drug is an immunoglobulin G (IgG) monoclonal antibody that neutralizes the activity of tumor necrosis factor (TNF) to decrease inflammation. It is used more commonly for managing Crohn's disease.

Diet Therapy. The severity of the client's ulcerative colitis determines the type of diet required. Clients may begin with one form of diet therapy and progress to a more advanced diet as symptoms diminish, with the goal of preventing hyperactive bowel activity.

Clients with severe symptoms are kept on NPO status to ensure bowel rest. The physician often prescribes total parenteral nutrition (TPN) for these clients (see Chapter 64).

Clients with slightly less severe symptoms may be given elemental formulas, such as Vivonex, which are absorbed in the upper bowel, thus minimizing bowel stimulation. Clients with significant but less severe symptoms may be restricted to a low-fiber (low-residue) diet. Clients following a low-fiber diet should avoid foods such as whole-wheat grains, nuts, and fresh fruits or fresh vegetables (Table 61-4). Whether fiber needs to be restricted during the chronic phase of the illness remains controversial. If fiber intake does not induce symptoms, the intake of fiber need not be limited. However, because the role of diet in inflammatory bowel disease (IBD) is not well defined, and because individual tolerance to foods vary, clients with controlled symptoms may only need to limit or omit those foods that cause them discomfort or diarrhea.

Typically, lactose-containing foods are poorly tolerated and should be reduced or eliminated. All clients should be cautioned that caffeinated beverages, pepper, alcohol, and smoking are common GI stimulants that could cause discomfort.

Rest. At the onset of treatment, activity is generally restricted because rest can reduce intestinal activity, provide comfort, and promote healing. Ensure that the client has easy access to a bedpan, commode, or bathroom in case of urgency or tenesmus.

Complementary and Alternative Therapies. In addition to dietary changes, complementary and alternative therapies have become very popular to supplement traditional management of ulcerative colitis. Examples include the following:

- Herbs, such as flaxseed
- Selenium
- Vitamin C
- Biofeedback
- Hypnosis
- Yoga
- Acupuncture
- Ayurveda (a combination of diet, yoga, herbs, breathing exercises)

SURGICAL MANAGEMENT. About a fourth of individuals with ulcerative colitis will require a colectomy. Indications for surgery include bowel perforation, toxic megacolon, hemorrhage, colon cancer, and failure of conventional treatment. The surgeon may choose one of several surgical procedures to alleviate these problems.

Total Proctocolectomy with a Permanent Ileostomy. Total proctocolectomy (or colectomy) with a permanent ileostomy has traditionally been the standard surgical procedure for clients undergoing a colectomy.

Preoperative Care. When an ileostomy is indicated, provide an extensive explanation to the client and family or significant other. Preoperative teaching includes aspects that relate to abdominal surgery (see Chapter 20) and those that relate to ileostomy. The surgeon consults with the enterostomal therapist (ET) preoperatively for recommendations on the location of the ostomy (stoma). (An ET is a nurse specializing and certified in skin and ostomy care.) A visit from an **ostomate** (a client with an ostomy) may be appropriate before surgery if the client agrees to this. The surgeon prescribes oral or parenteral antibiotics, such as neomycin sulfate (Mycifradin), as a bowel antiseptic. Mechanical cleansing of the bowel with enemas or laxatives may also be required.

Operative Procedures. During a total proctocolectomy with a traditional permanent **ileostomy,** the colon, rectum, and anus are removed, followed by closure of the anus. The surgeon brings the end of the terminal ileum out through the abdominal wall and forms a stoma, or ostomy. The stoma is usually placed in the right lower quadrant of the abdomen, below the belt line (Figure 61-2). The surgeon makes a perineal incision to remove the rectum and supporting tissues.

Postoperative Care. Initially after surgery the output from the ileostomy is a loose, dark green liquid that may contain some blood. Over time, a process called ileostomy adaptation occurs. The small intestine begins to absorb in-

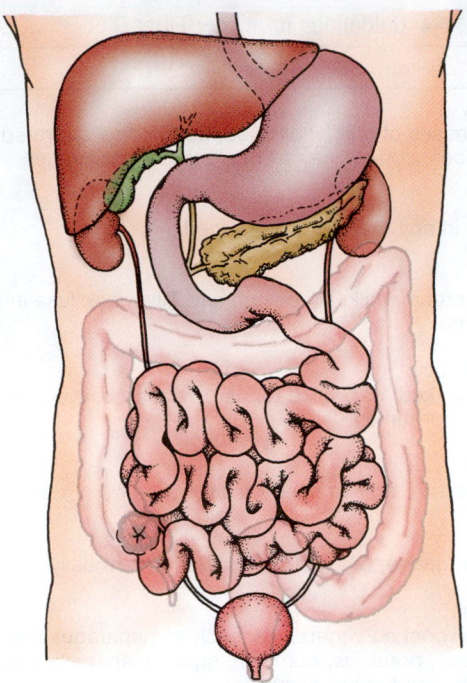

Figure 61-2 ■ Total proctocolectomy with a permanent ileostomy. This involved removal of the colon, the rectum, and the anus with closure of the anus. Note the missing colon, rectum, and anus with the resultant stoma in the right lower quadrant.

creased amounts of sodium and water (a former function of the large intestine, which was removed by surgery). Stool volume decreases, becomes thicker (pastelike), and turns yellow-green or yellow-brown. The effluent (fluid material) usually has little odor or a sweet odor. Any foul or unpleasant odor may be a symptom of some underlying problem (e.g., blockage or infection).

Depending on the frequency and irritation of stool drainage, the client must wear a pouch system at all times. Prevention of skin problems (irritation, excoriation, ulceration) is *a priority* for the client with an ileostomy. The output from the small intestine is rich in proteolytic enzymes and bile salts, which can quickly irritate and injure the skin. A pouch system that has some type of skin barrier (gelatin or pectin) provides sufficient protection for most clients. Other products are also available.

Most clients undergoing surgical intervention for ulcerative colitis have lived with chronic illness for some time. They may view surgery positively as a relief from the multiple problems caused by the disease. Initially, however, they may not perceive life with an ileostomy as a positive alternative.

Total proctocolectomy with a permanent ileostomy results in an alteration in appearance and body function. The goals for a client undergoing this procedure are to become proficient in self-care, to adapt his or her lifestyle to include care of an ostomy, and to resume presurgery activities successfully.

Total Colectomy with a Continent Ileostomy. As an alternative to the traditional ileostomy with an external pouch, the surgeon may create an internal system: a Kock's ileostomy or ileal reservoir. This procedure is sometimes referred to as a continent ileostomy. The surgeon constructs an intra-abdominal pouch or reservoir from the ter-

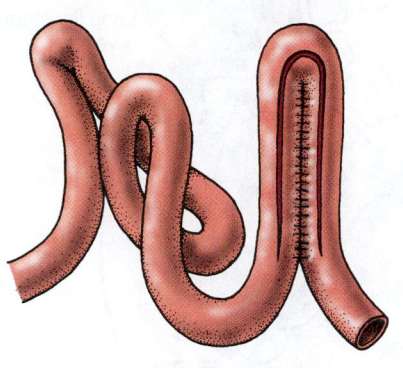 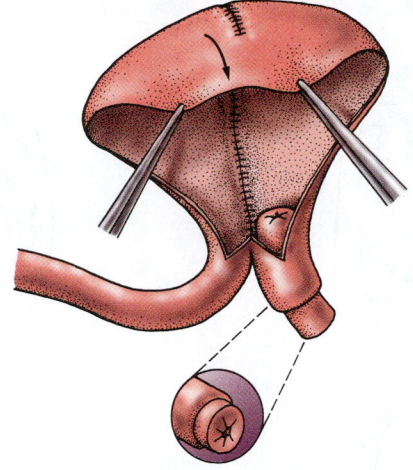 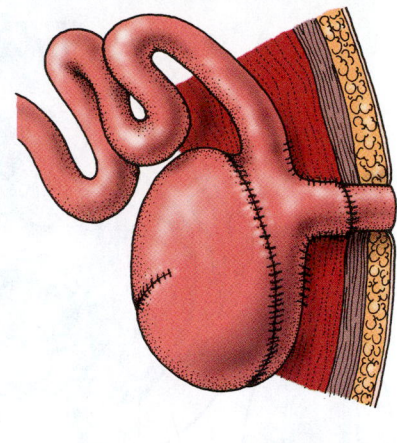

1. A reservoir, in which the client will retain stool until draining it, is constructed from a loop of ileum folded and sutured together, then cut.

2. A portion of the ileum is intussuscepted to form a nipple valve, and the upper part of the stitched and cut ileum is pulled down and sutured to form a pouch.

3. The nipple valve, which shuts tight against pressure from a filled pouch, is pulled through the stoma and sutured flush with the abdomen.

Figure 61-3 ■ The creation of a Kock's (continent) ileostomy.

minal ileum (Figure 61-3), where stool is stored in the pouch until the client drains it by using a catheter. The care of a Kock's ileostomy involves the connection of the pouch to the stoma, which is constructed with a nipple-like valve made from an intussuscepted portion of the ileum. The stoma is flush with the skin.

The nursing care of the client undergoing this procedure is similar to the care of the client undergoing a procto-colectomy with a permanent ileostomy (see the previous section). Immediately postoperatively, an indwelling Foley catheter is placed in the pouch, which is connected to low intermittent suction and irrigated as ordered.

Monitor the character and quality of **effluent** (drainage). Teach the client to drain the stoma. Initially the pouch holds only 50 to 75 mL; over time, the pouch capacity reaches 500 to 700 mL. When the pouch needs to be emptied, the client experiences a sensation of fullness. The client drains the pouch several times a day and wears a small dressing over the stoma to keep it moist and to protect clothing from the moist stoma. This procedure has several advantages. The client does not need to wear an external pouch for collection of stool and experiences minimal skin problems. Unfortunately, the need for frequent revisions and problems with leakage have made this procedure less desirable.

Total Colectomy with Ileoanal Anastomosis; Ileoanal Reservoir.

During a total colectomy with ileoanal anastomosis, the surgeon removes the colon and the rectum and sutures the ileum into the anal canal. Usually continence is excellent after this procedure, but up to 20% of clients will have some nocturnal leakage of stool. Care of the client undergoing this procedure is similar to the care of clients undergoing a colectomy. With an ileoanal anastomosis, perineal irritation is a common occurrence as a result of frequent, loose stools. The nurse or assistive nursing personnel should provide careful perineal care.

The creation of an **ileoanal reservoir,** also known as a **J pouch**, has become popular for clients with ulcerative coli-tis, especially young adults, because it spares the rectal sphincter and eliminates the need for an ostomy. During this procedure, the surgeon removes the colon and sutures the ileum into the rectal stump to form a reservoir. If residual rectal mucosa remains after either an ileoanal anastomosis or a reservoir procedure, proctoscopy is done at predetermined intervals to monitor for dysplasia.

Preoperative Care. The preoperative care for a client undergoing an ileoanal anastomosis is similar to that for a client undergoing an ileostomy. However, clients will not have an ostomy and therefore do not require consultation with an enterostomal therapist (ET).

Operative Procedures. Ileoanal anastomosis occurs in two stages (Figure 61-4). In the first stage the surgeon excises the rectal mucosa, performs an abdominal colectomy, constructs the reservoir or pouch to the anal canal, and creates a temporary loop ileostomy. The loop ileostomy is necessary to allow adequate healing of the internal pouch and all anastomosis sites and to allow for an increase in the capacity of the internal reservoir through fluid instillations. After 3 to 4 months the client returns to have the loop ileostomy closed. Stool formation resembles that in clients who have undergone a traditional ileostomy.

Postoperative Care. Provide the usual postoperative interventions for clients who have undergone abdominal surgery. All clients requiring surgical intervention for ulcerative colitis have an abdominal incision. Initially most clients are maintained on NPO status and a nasogastric (NG) tube is used for suction.

ACUTE PAIN; CHRONIC PAIN

NOC **PLANNING: EXPECTED OUTCOMES.** The client with ulcerative colitis is expected to take personal action to control pain. Indicators include that the client will be able to demonstrate consistently the ability to:

- Use preventive measures
- Use non-analgesic relief measures

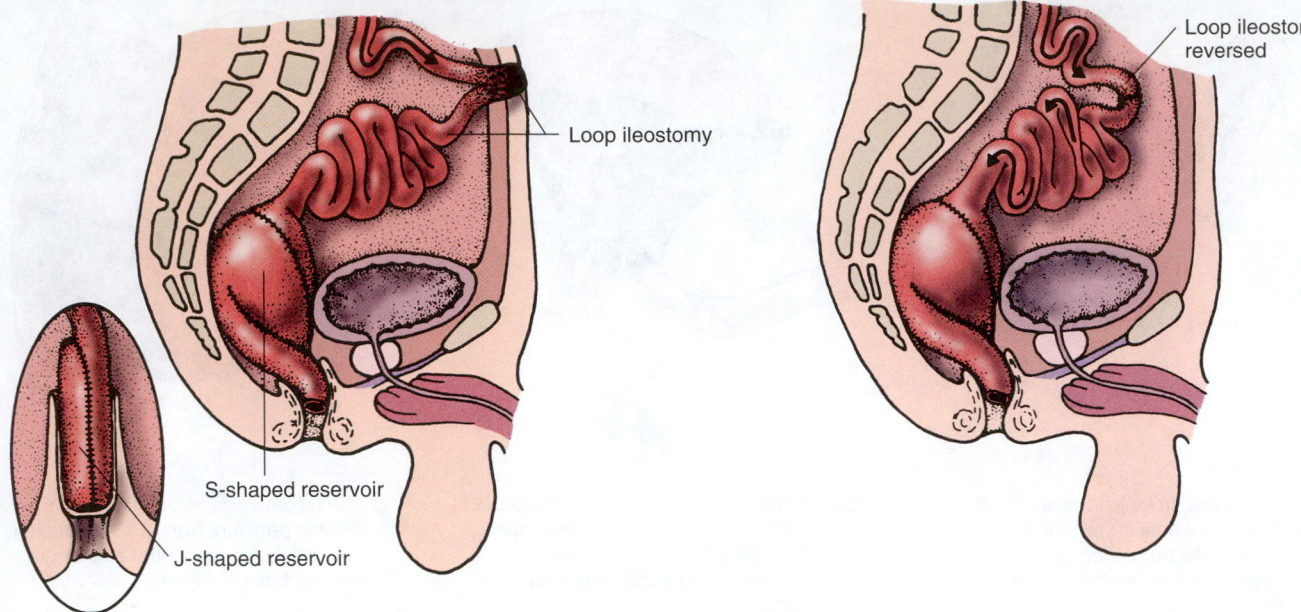

Loop ileostomy

Loop ileostomy reversed

S-shaped reservoir

J-shaped reservoir

Stage 1.
After removal of the colon, a temporary loop ileostomy is created and an ileoanal reservoir is formed. The reservoir is created in an S-shaped reservoir (using three loops of ileum) or a J-shaped reservoir (suturing a portion of ileum to the rectal cuff, with an upward loop).

Stage 2.
After the reservoir has had time to heal—usually several months—the temporary loop ileostomy is reversed, and stool is allowed to drain into the reservoir.

Figure 61-4 ■ The creation of an ileoanal reservoir.

- Report changes in pain symptoms to health care professional
- Use available resources
- Recognize associated symptoms of pain
- Report that pain is controlled

INTERVENTIONS. Pain control may be accomplished through pharmacologic and nonpharmacologic measures. The client's symptoms can cause physical discomfort, which can also contribute to emotional discomfort. The use of a variety of symptom-reducing interventions and supportive measures can provide increased comfort.

NIC **Pain Management.** The purpose of pain management is alleviation of pain or a reduction in pain to a level of comfort that is acceptable to the client (see Chart 61-3). The client with ulcerative colitis experiences abdominal pain and cramping, particularly with exacerbations of the disease. Increases in pain may also signal the development of complications such as peritonitis. Frequent bowel movements can cause skin irritation and increase the client's discomfort. The nurse performs a comprehensive pain assessment. With the client and the health care team, the nurse evaluates the effectiveness of past pain control measures that were used.

Assist the client in reducing or eliminating factors that can precipitate or increase the pain experience. Antidiarrheal medications may be prescribed to control diarrhea but must be used cautiously because they can precipitate toxic megacolon. The client may benefit from diet teaching and meal planning as a means of decreasing abdominal discomfort related to cramping and bloating. Excoriated skin can contribute to pain and discomfort. Scrupulous skin care prevents painful excoriation of the skin. Also teach the client to use nonpharmacologic measures (e.g., biofeedback, music therapy, guided imagery) as a means of pain modification (see Chapter 7).

Drug Therapy. Antidiarrheal medications are used to control diarrhea and thereby reduce the resulting discomfort. These must be used with caution because toxic megacolon can develop. **Toxic megacolon** is characterized by an enlarged colon, along with fever, leukocytosis, and tachycardia. The abdomen is often distended and tender; bowel elimination patterns differ from one person to another. The physician may prescribe anticholinergics, such as dicyclomine (Bentyl, Bentylol✦), before meals to provide relief from the pain and cramping that may occur with diarrhea. Opioids are used sparingly and cautiously because they can mask symptoms of life-threatening complications.

Diet Therapy. Dietary measures help to control symptoms and thereby promote relief from discomfort. Assess the client's needs for diet teaching, and evaluate the effects of implemented dietary measures on an ongoing basis.

Perineal Skin Care. Perineal skin can be irritated by frequent contact with loose stools and frequent cleaning, and it can cause discomfort. Explain special measures for skin care. For example, cleaning the perineal area with mild soap and warm water after each bowel movement keeps the skin free of any stool. Frequent sitz baths may be helpful, particularly after a bowel movement. The application of a thin coat of barrier creams, vitamin A and D ointment, aloe creams, or medicated foam applications may provide relief. Use of medicated wipes with witch hazel (e.g., Tucks) is soothing if the rectal area is tender or sensitive from the use of toilet tissue.

Various manufacturers of ostomies (e.g., Hollister and ConvaTec) produce a three-product system for skin care that may help prevent and heal perineal skin irritation, thus relieving discomfort. Such systems include a skin-cleaning solution, a moisturizing and healing cream, and a petroleum jelly–like barrier that prevents contact of moisture and stool with the skin.

POTENTIAL FOR GASTROINTESTINAL BLEEDING

PLANNING: EXPECTED OUTCOMES. The client with ulcerative colitis is expected to experience a reduction in or cessation of the gastrointestinal (GI) bleeding that accompanies chronic ulcerative colitis. The client is also expected to remain free of complications of the disease that can cause bleeding, such as perforation.

INTERVENTIONS. Primary responsibility is to monitor the client closely for signs and symptoms of GI bleeding resulting from acute disease or complications. All stools are monitored for blood, using both gross and occult examination. Monitor the client's hematocrit, hemoglobin, and electrolyte values for abnormalities as well as the client's vital signs. Observe the client for the development of fever, tachycardia, fluid volume depletion, electrolyte imbalances, and severe abdominal pain. Changes in mental status may be noted, especially among older adults.

If symptoms of GI bleeding are present, notify the health care provider immediately because surgical intervention may be necessary. Blood products may be necessary for clients with severe anemia. Prepare the client for transfusion by inserting a large-bore IV catheter for the administration of blood. Chapter 59 describes the management of GI bleeding in detail.

Community-Based Care

HOME CARE MANAGEMENT

The client with ulcerative colitis is managed at home but may require hospitalization during exacerbations. In addition, clients experiencing extraintestinal manifestations of the disease will require ongoing management of joint or skin problems. Clients with moderate to severe ulcerative colitis have more acute exacerbations than those with milder forms of the disease. Such clients may benefit from case manager services to coordinate and facilitate quality care in a cost-effective way.

For clients with ulcerative colitis, home care management focuses on managing symptoms and monitoring for complications. Instruct the client in measures to reduce or control abdominal pain, cramping, and diarrhea. Also teach the client and family members regarding symptoms that should be reported immediately to the health care provider. For clients returning home or transferring to nursing home or subacute care after surgery, ongoing respiratory care, incision care, ostomy care, and pain management are additional concerns.

HEALTH TEACHING

Educate the client about the nature of ulcerative colitis with regard to its acute episodes, remissions, and symptom management. Furthermore, emphasize that even though the cause is unknown, relapses can be resolved with proper health care.

CHART 61-4

CLIENT EDUCATION GUIDE
Ileostomy Care

Skin Protection
- Use a pectin-based skin barrier to protect your skin from contact with contents from the ostomy.
- Use skin care products, such as skin sealants and ostomy skin creams. If your skin continues to come into contact with ostomy contents.
- Watch your skin for any irritation or redness.

Pouch Care
- Empty your pouch when it is one third to one half full.
- Change the pouch during inactive times, such as before meals, before retiring at night, on waking in the morning, and 2 to 4 hours after eating.
- Change the entire pouch system every 3 to 7 days.

Diet
- Chew food thoroughly.
- Be cautious of high-fiber and high-cellulose foods. You may need to eliminate these from the diet if they cause severe problems (diarrhea, constipation, or blockage). Examples include popcorn, peanuts, coconut, Chinese vegetables, string beans, tough-fiber meats, shrimp and lobster, rice, bran, and skinned vegetables (tomatoes, corn, and peas).

Medications
- Avoid taking enteric-coated and capsule medications.
- Inform any health care provider who is prescribing medications for you that you have an ostomy. Before having prescriptions filled, inform your pharmacist that you have an ostomy.
- Do not take any laxative or enemas. You should usually have loose stool and should contact a physician if no stool has passed in 6 to 12 hours.

Symptoms to Watch for
- Report any drastic increase or decrease in drainage to your health care provider.
- If stomal swelling, abdominal cramping, or distention occurs or if ileostomy contents stop draining, do the following:
    Remove the pouch with faceplate.
    Lie down, assuming a knee-chest position.
    Begin abdominal massage.
    Apply moist towels to the abdomen.
    Drink hot tea.
    If none of these maneuvers is effective in resuming ileostomy flow or if abdominal pain is severe, call your health care provider right away.

Instruct the client about dietary measures to reduce bloating and cramping. The client needs to learn what foods are best tolerated, and adjust his or her diet accordingly. Teach about prescribed medications and medication side effects for which the client should remain alert. Clients taking immunosuppressive drugs should be taught to report signs of infection, such as sore throat, to the health care provider. Prepare written instructions for the client and family members about the signs of colonic dilation and perforation, and reiterate the importance of notifying the health care provider if these signs occur.

If the client has undergone a surgical diversion to manage colon effluent, you or the enterostomal therapist (ET) explains and demonstrates the required care. The client is encouraged to demonstrate self-care of the ileostomy. Also teach clients with an ileostomy to include adequate amounts of salt and water in their diets because the ileostomy promotes the loss of these elements. They will also be taught to be cautious in situations that promote profuse sweating or fluid loss, such as during strenuous physical activities, when environmental heat is excessive, and during episodes of diarrhea and vomiting. Chart 61-4 describes ileostomy care in detail.

A client with an ileostomy may have multiple concerns about management at home and about sexual and social adjustments. Considering possible sexual issues helps the client to identify and discuss these concerns with the sexual partner. Social situations may precipitate some anxieties related to decreased self-esteem and a disturbance in body image. Help the client explore possible concerns in addressing and resolving these potentially stressful events.

HEALTH CARE RESOURCES

If the client requires assistance with activities of daily living, the case manager or social worker may help to arrange the services of a home care aide. If the client is discharged from the hospital with an ileostomy, the case manager makes a referral to a home care agency. A home care nurse can provide assessment and guidance in integrating ostomy care into the client's lifestyle and possibly provide wound care, including the monitoring of wound healing (Chart 61-5). The client needs to know where to purchase ostomy supplies, along with the name, size, and manufacturer's order number. The ET or case manager contacts local and regional supply companies for prices and availability of supplies.

Identify the local ostomy support group by contacting the United Ostomy Association. A support group or the Crohn's and Colitis Foundation of America may be of assistance in obtaining supplies as well as providing education for ostomates. Inform the client and family or significant others of available ostomy outpatient clinics and ETs. If the

client agrees, a visit from an ostomate can be initiated or continued on an ambulatory care basis.

◆ Evaluation: Outcomes

Evaluate the care of the client with ulcerative colitis on the basis of the identified nursing diagnoses and collaborative problems. Expected outcomes may include that the client will:

- Have formed stools
- Take personal action to control pain

In addition, the client with an ileostomy can be expected to:

- Engage in self-care of the ileostomy
- Maintain peristomal skin integrity
- Demonstrate behaviors that integrate ostomy care into his or her lifestyle
- Verbalize signs and symptoms of stoma complications

❓ Critical Thinking Challenge

A 42-year-old woman with ulcerative colitis is placed on several drugs to manage her disease. Unfortunately, the medications are not successful and she requires a colectomy and ileostomy. Her husband recently left her, and she has no children. She also lost her job because she missed a lot of time from work because of her illness.

1. What discharge teaching will she require?
2. What support systems can you suggest for her after discharge from the hospital?
3. In your hospital, patient care technicians (PCTs) are allowed to provide ostomy care. Would you delegate health teaching about the client's ostomy to the PCT? Why or why not?

evolve For suggested answer guidelines, go to http://evolve.elsevier.com/Iggy/.

Crohn's Disease

PATHOPHYSIOLOGY

Crohn's disease is an idiopathic inflammatory disease of the small intestine (60%), the colon (20%), or both. It involves all layers of the bowel but most commonly involves the terminal ileum. It is a slowly progressive and recurrent disease with predominant involvement of multiple regions of the intestine with normal sections between.

Chronic, nonspecific inflammation of the entire intestinal tract characterizes the disease, with the terminal ileum the site most often affected. Eventually deep fissures and ulcerations develop and often extend through all bowel layers, predisposing the individual to the development of bowel fistulas. The result is severe diarrhea and malabsorption of vital nutrients. Chronic pathologic changes include thickening of the bowel wall, resulting in narrowing of the bowel lumen and strictures. In advanced disease, the bowel mucosa demonstrates nodular swelling (granulomas) intermingled with deep ulcerations.

The complications associated with Crohn's disease are similar to those of ulcerative colitis. As shown in Table 61-3, hemorrhage is more common in ulcerative colitis, but it can occur in Crohn's disease as well. Severe malabsorption by the small intestine is more common in clients with Crohn's disease. Rarely, cancer of the small bowel and colon develop but usually occurs after the disease has been present for 15 to 20 years. Fistula formation is a common complication of Crohn's disease. Fistulas can occur between segments of the intestine or

---

CHART 61-5

HOME CARE ASSESSMENT of
The Client with Inflammatory Bowel Disease

Assess gastrointestinal function and nutritional status, including the following:
- Abdominal cramping or pain
- Bowel elimination pattern, specifically frequency, characteristics and amount of stools, presence or absence of blood in stools
- Dietary and fluid intake and habits (include relationship of specific foods to cramping and stools)
- Weight gain or loss
- Signs and symptoms of dehydration
- Presence or absence of fever, rectal tenesmus, or urgency
- Bowel sounds
- Condition of perianal skin, including presence or absence of perianal fistula or abscess

Assess client's and family's coping skills, including the following:
- Current and ongoing stress level and coping style
- Availability of support system

Assess home environment, including the following:
- Adequacy and availability of bathroom facilities
- Opportunity for rest and relaxation

Assess ability to manage therapeutic regimen, including the following:
- Knowledge of medications
- Signs and symptoms to report
- Dietary management
- Availability of community resources
- Importance of follow-up care

manifest as cutaneous fistulas or perirectal abscesses. Fistulas can also extend from the bowel to other organs and body cavities, such as the bladder or vagina (Figure 61-5). Twenty to thirty percent of individuals with the disease will develop intestinal obstruction. Initially obstruction results from inflammation and edema. Over time, fibrosis develops and obstruction results secondary to a narrowing of the bowel.

Etiology and Genetic Risk

Mycobacterium paratuberculosis has been proposed as an environmental stimulus that could be implicated in the development of Crohn's disease because granulomas similar to those seen in individuals with pulmonary tuberculosis have been found on biopsy of the intestines of people with the disease. A genetic predisposition to the disease has also been found because the disease tends to cluster in families and appears equally in identical twins (Dooley et al., 2004). Fifteen percent of clients have first-degree relatives with inflammatory bowel disease (IBD). Family members develop the disease with similar patterns and similar age of onset. The most widely accepted cause of Crohn's disease is a combination of reasons—a defect in the immunoregulation of inflammation in the intestinal tract along with a genetic predisposition for the disease.

Incidence/Prevalence

More than one million people in the United States have the disease; peak incidence is between 15 and 40 years of age (Goldstein et al., 2004).

◆COLLABORATIVE MANAGEMENT
◆Assessment

HISTORY

Although the exact cause is not clear, Crohn's disease is aggravated by bacterial infection, inflammation, and smoking cessation. Therefore a detailed history assists in uncovering manifestations specific to the disease. A history of fever, abdominal pain, and loose stools is commonly seen in a client with Crohn's disease. Ask about recent unintentional loss of weight and the frequency, consistency, and presence of blood in the stool.

PHYSICAL ASSESSMENT/CLINICAL MANIFESTATIONS

Perform a thorough abdominal examination, assess for clinical manifestations of the disease, and evaluate the client's nutritional and hydration status. When performing an abdominal assessment, note findings that are consistent with those in acute appendicitis (e.g., tenderness, guarded movement, a palpable mass in the right lower quadrant).

On inspection of the abdomen, assess for distention, masses, or visible peristalsis. Inspection of the perianal area may reveal ulcerations or fissures. During auscultation, bowel sounds may be decreased or absent in the client with severe inflammation or obstruction. An increase in high-pitched or rushing sounds may be present over areas of narrowed bowel loops. Muscle guarding, masses, rigidity, or tenderness may be noted on palpation.

The clinical presentation of Crohn's disease can vary greatly from client to client. Most clients report diarrhea, abdominal pain, and low-grade fever. Fever is also commonly present with complications such as fistulas and severe inflammation. If the disease occurs in only the ileum, diarrhea occurs five or six times per day, often with a soft, loose stool. **Steatorrhea** (fatty diarrheal stools) is common. The stool may contain bright red blood, but this is a rare finding.

Abdominal pain from the inflammatory process is usually constant and is located in the right lower quadrant. Clients also experience periumbilical pain before and after bowel movements. If the lower colon is diseased, pain is often experienced in both lower abdominal quadrants.

Weight loss is experienced by about 80% of individuals with Crohn's disease. Clients often experience nutritional problems as a result of increased catabolism secondary to chronic inflammation, anorexia, malabsorption, or self-imposed dietary restrictions. The result is fluid and electrolyte imbalances and protein, iron, vitamin, and mineral deficiencies.

The marked inflammatory bowel changes decrease the small bowel's ability to absorb nutrients, which may be worsened by surgery and fistulas. Be acutely aware of the importance of detecting the clinical manifestations of peritonitis, bowel obstruction, and nutritional and fluid imbalances. Early detection of a change in the client's status helps to minimize these life-threatening complications.

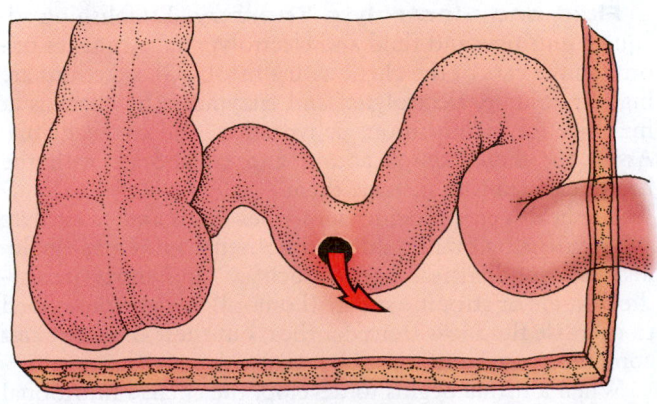

External enterocutaneous
(between skin and intestine)

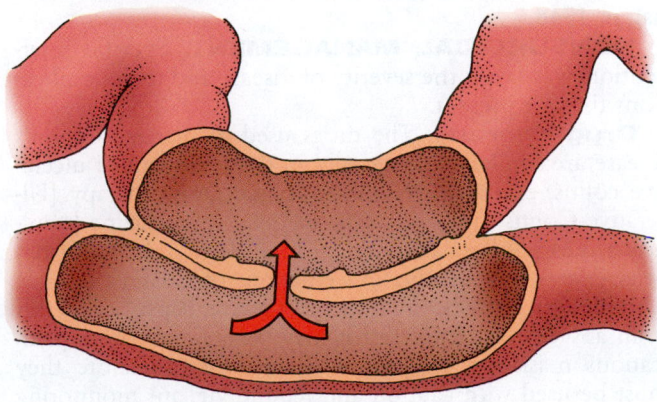

Enteroenteric
(between intestine and intestine)

Figure 61-5 ■ The types of fistulas that are complications of Crohn's disease.

PSYCHOSOCIAL ASSESSMENT

The client experiencing Crohn's disease needs a complete psychosocial assessment. The chronicity of the problem and the troublesome complications can greatly affect clients and their families. The assessment should be ongoing and should continuously reflect the client's status as well as the family's. Lifestyle changes are necessary to cope with such a disruptive and painful chronic illness. Assess the client's coping skill and identify support systems.

DIAGNOSTIC ASSESSMENT

The health care provider may order a number of laboratory studies for clients with Crohn's disease; however, no disease-specific tests are available to confirm the diagnosis. The results of laboratory tests often indicate the extent and severity of inflammation associated with the disease.

If bleeding is present, decreased hemoglobin and hematocrit values are likely. Serum levels of folic acid and cobalamin (vitamin B_{12} group) are generally low because of malabsorption, further contributing to anemia. Amino acid malabsorption may result in decreased albumin levels. An elevated erythrocyte sedimentation rate (ESR) is consistent with the presence of inflammation. White blood cells (WBCs) in the urine may indicate infection (pyuria), which may be caused by ureteral obstruction or an **enterovesical** (bowel to bladder) **fistula.** If significant diarrhea is present, the client will experience electrolyte losses, particularly potassium and magnesium.

The results of the contrast barium enema and upper gastrointestinal (GI) series often provide more specific diagnostic information. X-rays show narrowing, ulcerations, strictures, and fistulas consistent with Crohn's disease. In acute illness these tests are often deferred until the risk of perforation lessens.

Depending on which areas of the bowel are diseased, the sigmoidoscopic examination may not be diagnostic. If the rectosigmoid colon is involved, the physician may see ulcerations and inflamed mucosa, areas of fissure, fistula, and abscess formation of the perianal and perirectal areas.

Colonoscopy is used when other tests, especially the barium enema examination, have not led to a specific diagnosis.

◆ Interventions

Treatment of Crohn's disease is similar to that described earlier under Nonsurgical Management (Ulcerative Colitis), p. 1348.

NONSURGICAL MANAGEMENT. Specific interventions vary with the severity of disease and the complications that are present.

Drug Therapy. The drugs used to manage Crohn's disease are similar to those used in the treatment of ulcerative colitis, except for mesalamine (see Drug Therapy [Ulcerative Colitis], p. 1348). For example, sulfasalazine (Azulfidine, PMS-Sulfasalazine✦) 1.5 to 2 g twice daily PO has been effective in treating exacerbations of Crohn's disease. Although glucocorticoids can be effective, sepsis can result from abscesses or fistulas that may be present. These medications mask the symptoms of infection; therefore they must be used with caution and require vigilant monitoring by the nurse for signs of infection.

Metronidazole (Flagyl, Novonidazole✦) 250 to 500 mg three times daily PO has been helpful in clients with fistulas. Immunosuppressive therapy has been effective in clients with refractory disease or fistulas. Azathioprine (Imuran), an immunosuppressive agent, 50 mg daily for 12 months, may be instituted. After that time the health care provider may attempt to withdraw the drug, but long-term therapy may be needed in some cases. Methotrexate (Rheumatrex) may also be given to suppress immune activity.

Because a defect in the immunoregulation of inflammation may be implicated in the development of Crohn's disease, neutralization of a cytokine (specifically, tumor necrosis factor) may prove useful in decreasing bowel inflammation. Infliximab (Remicade), a monoclonal antibody form of antitumor necrosis factor alpha, has been approved for IV use at monthly intervals. The usual dose of 5 mg/kg has demonstrated efficacy in the treatment of active Crohn's disease and fistulas. Clients who have infections or those with hypersensitivity to murine proteins should not take this medication.

Nutritional Management. Long-standing nutritional deficits can have severe consequences for the client with Crohn's disease. Malnutrition can result in poor fistula and wound healing, loss of lean muscle mass, decreased immune system response, and increased morbidity and mortality. With severe exacerbations of the disease, the health care provider may recommend hospitalization to provide bowel rest and nutritional enhancement with total parenteral nutrition (TPN). For less severe exacerbations, the health care provider may prescribe an elemental diet using products such as Vivonex to induce remission. Elemental diets are absorbed in the jejunum and therefore permit the distal small intestine and colon to rest. Once remission is achieved, the health care provider usually prescribes a low-residue diet. Nutritional supplements, such as Ensure or Sustacal, can be added to provide nutrients and added calories. GI stimulants, such as caffeinated beverages and alcohol, should be avoided.

Complication Management. Fistulas (abnormal tract from intestine to skin or intestine to intestine) are common occurrences with acute exacerbations of Crohn's disease. Clients with fistulas often experience complications such as systemic infections, skin problems, malnutrition, and fluid and electrolyte imbalances. Treatment of the client with a fistula is multidimensional and includes nutrition and electrolyte therapy, skin care, and prevention of infection.

Fluid and Electrolyte Therapy. Establishing adequate nutrition and fluid and electrolyte balance takes priority in the care of the client with a fistula. GI secretions are high in volume, electrolytes, and enzymes. The client is at high risk for malnutrition, dehydration, and hypokalemia. Assess for these complications, and collaborate with the health care team to manage them.

The health care provider prescribes fluids and electrolyte replacement by oral liquids and nutrients as well as IV fluids. An antidiarrheal agent, such as diphenoxylate hydrochloride or atropine sulfate (Lomotil), may be prescribed to decrease fluid loss from diarrhea, but these drugs are not commonly used and must be given with caution.

When a fistula begins to develop, the client's nutritional status is usually compromised. After the fistula has developed, nutritional status worsens. The client requires at least 3000 calories daily to promote healing of the fistula. If the client cannot take adequate oral fluids and nutrients, the physician may prescribe TPN. In collaboration with the dietitian, do the following:

- Carefully monitor the client's tolerance to diet
- Assist the client in selecting high-calorie, high-protein, high-vitamin, low-fiber meals
- Offer enteral supplements, such as Ensure and Vivonex
- Record food intake for accurate calorie counts

Skin Care. Proteolytic enzymes and bile contribute to the problem of skin irritation and excoriation. Skin irritation needs to be prevented; this is usually accomplished through the use of skin barriers, application of pouches, and insertion of drains (Figure 61-6). By applying a pouch to the draining fistula, the risk of skin irritation is minimized and **effluent** (drainage) can be measured.

One approach to drainage management is to cover the area surrounding the fistula with barriers, such as Stomahesive or DuoDerm, and subsequently apply a wound drainage system over the fistula, securing it to the protective dressing. The skin adjacent to the fistula is cleaned with normal saline solution and gently patted dry.

Collaborate with the enterostomal therapist (ET) to provide wound management. Wound drainage must *never* be allowed to be in direct contact with skin without prompt cleaning because intestinal fluid enzymes are caustic.

Prevention of Infection. Clients with fistulas are at extremely high risk for intra-abdominal abscesses and sepsis. Intra-abdominal fistulas are treated with careful nursing interventions, containment of wound drainage, and antibiotic therapy. Observe for subtle signs of infection or sepsis, such as fever, abdominal pain, or a change in mental status.

Complementary and Alternative Therapies. Other options for disease management that are used to relax the client and soothe the GI tract include the following modalities:

- Naturopathy
- Herbs (e.g., ginger and peppermint oil)
- Acupuncture
- Hypnotherapy
- Ayurveda (a combination of diet, herbs, yoga, breathing exercises)

SURGICAL MANAGEMENT. Surgery for Crohn's disease is confined to those who have demonstrated failure on medical management or those who exhibit complications from the disease. Those who continue to have symptoms after long-term medical treatment and those with complications such as fistulas may undergo resection of the diseased area. Other indications include the following:

- Perforation
- Massive hemorrhage
- Intestinal obstruction (often caused by stricture)
- Abscesses
- Adenocarcinoma (rare)

In some cases the resection can be performed as minimally invasive surgery via laparoscopy. Both small bowel resection (usually the ileum) and ileocecal resections can be done using this procedure. The advantages of laparoscopic surgery over conventional open techniques include the following:

- Smaller incisions
- Less postoperative pain
- Quicker surgical recovery and return to usual lifestyle

Stricturoplasty may be performed for bowel strictures related to Crohn's disease. This procedure, which involves in-

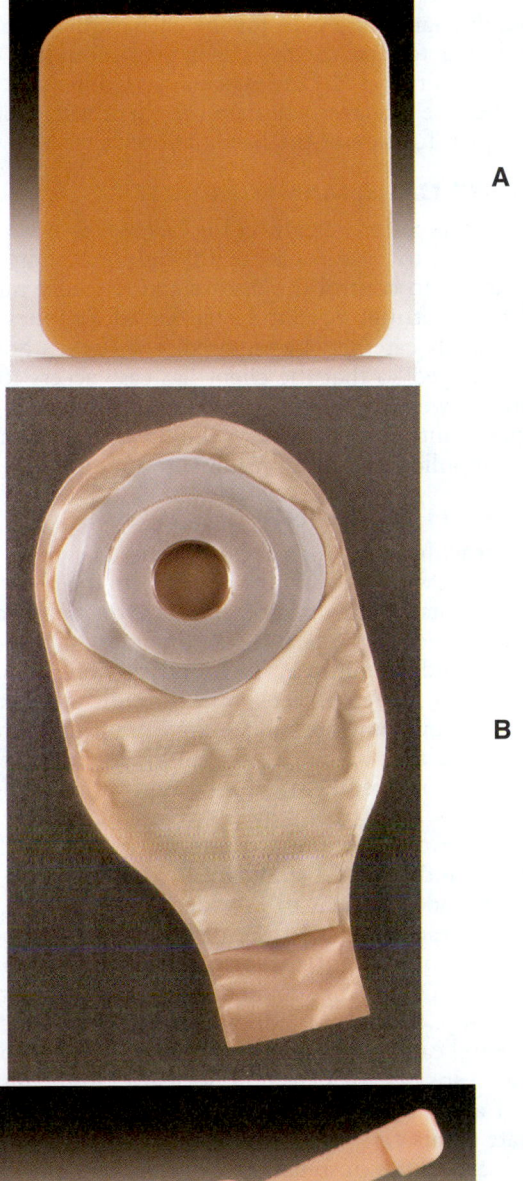

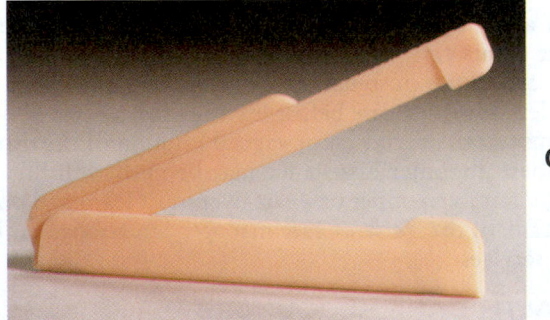

Figure 61-6 ■ Skin barriers, such as wafers **(A),** are cut to fit ⅛ inch around the fistula. A drainable pouch **(B)** is applied over the wafer and clamped **(C)** until the pouch is to be emptied. Effluent should drain into the bag and not contact the skin. (Courtesy ConvaTec, A Bristol-Myers Squibb Company, Skillman, NJ.)

cising along the length of the stricture and suturing the incised area on the horizontal plane, allows for an increase in the bowel diameter. Preoperative and postoperative care for each of these surgical procedures is similar to care for clients undergoing other types of abdominal surgery. (See Surgical Management [Ulcerative Colitis], p. 1350.)

Community-Based Care

The discharge care plan for the client with Crohn's disease is similar to that for the client with ulcerative colitis (see Community-Based Care [Ulcerative Colitis], p. 1353). You or the case manager will help the client with a draining fistula plan for care of the fistula at home.

HOME CARE MANAGEMENT

The interventions begun in the hospital to manage the disease need to be carried out to some extent in the home. Measures to control the disease and related symptoms and manage nutrition need to be reinforced. Supplies for wound and fistula care may be required. The client's home should be arranged so that the client has easy access to the bathroom as well as privacy to perform fistula care. To ensure adequate nutrition, the client should have easy access to a well-supplied kitchen of readily prepared foods.

HEALTH TEACHING

The teaching plan for Crohn's disease is similar to that for the client with ulcerative colitis. Inform the client about the usual course of the disease, symptoms of complications, and when to notify the health care provider. Medication teaching, including purpose, dose, and side effects, is incorporated into the teaching plan. In addition to other drugs, vitamin supplements, including monthly vitamin B_{12} injections may be needed due to the inability of the ileum to absorb nutrients. In collaboration with the dietitian, instruct the client to follow a low-residue, high-calorie diet and to avoid foods that cause discomfort, such as milk, gluten, and other GI stimulants.

Remind the client to provide for rest periods, especially during exacerbations of the disease. If stress appears to increase symptoms of the disease, stress management techniques or counseling should be recommended. For long-term follow-up, the client is educated regarding the increased risk of bowel cancer and the advisability of having a colonoscopy as a means of early detection of changes in the mucosa.

If a client has developed a fistula, explain and demonstrate fistula care. The client needs opportunities to practice the care in the hospital. Ideally the client should be independent in fistula care before leaving the hospital. However, because of the perirectal or vaginal location of the fistula or an obese abdomen, assistance may be needed. If this is the case, a family member or a caregiver must learn and practice the care, or the nurse or case manager can arrange for home care services.

HEALTH CARE RESOURCES

The client discharged to home after undergoing resection and anastomosis may require visits from a home care nurse to assess the surgical wound and monitor for complications. Assess the client's and his or her family's ability to monitor the progress of fistula healing and to watch for signs and symptoms of infection and sepsis. Home care nursing visits may also be appropriate for this purpose. A home care aide might be considered for clients who cannot meet their nutritional needs, who need help with meal preparation, and who need help in purchasing groceries.

If the client needs equipment for fistula care, such as skin barriers and wound drainage bags, the nurse or case manager contacts medical supply companies or local pharmacies to ascertain their availability and price. A support group sponsored by the United Ostomy Association or a local hospital in the community may also be available to assist the client and family with physical as well as psychosocial needs.

Diverticular Disease

Diverticula are congenital or acquired pouchlike herniations of the mucosa through the muscular wall of the small intestine or colon. **Diverticulosis** is the presence of many abnormal pouchlike herniations (diverticula) in the wall of the intestine. **Diverticulitis** is the term used to describe an inflammation of one or more diverticula.

PATHOPHYSIOLOGY

Diverticula can occur in any part of the small or large intestine, but they occur most commonly in the sigmoid colon (Figure 61-7). The musculature of the colon hypertrophies, thickens, and becomes rigid, and herniation of the mucosa and submucosa through the colon wall is seen. Diverticula seem to occur at points of weakness in the intestinal wall, often at areas where blood vessels interrupt muscular continuity. The muscle weakness develops as part of the aging process.

In and of themselves, diverticula cause few problems. If undigested food or bacteria become trapped in a diverticulum, however, blood supply to that area diminishes and bacteria invade the diverticulum. Diverticulitis results when the diverticulum perforates and a local abscess forms. The perforated diverticulum can also progress to an intra-abdominal perforation with generalized peritonitis.

Bleeding from diverticula can range from minor, localized bleeding to massive hemorrhage. Minor bleeding is often due to localized inflammation in areas of vascular granulation tissue at the base of the diverticulum. Hemorrhage can result when a blood vessel is eroded within a diverticulum. Inflammation secondary to recurrent diverticulitis can lead to narrowing of the bowel lumen, which may result in obstruction. Inflammation can also result in fistulas to other organs, such as the bladder and the vagina.

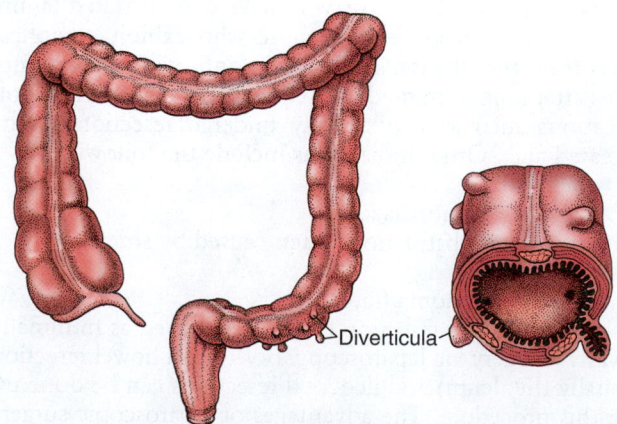

Figure 61-7 ■ Several abnormal outpouchings, or herniations, in the wall of the intestine, which are diverticula. These can occur anywhere in the small or large intestine but are found most often in the sigmoid, as shown in this figure. Diverticulitis is the inflammation of a diverticulum that occurs when undigested food or bacteria become trapped in the diverticulum.

Etiology

Diets with small amounts of fiber have been implicated in the development of diverticula in that they cause less bulky stool and possibly constipation. For diverticulosis and diverticulitis to occur, there must be an increase in intraluminal pressure and muscle contractions to move fecal material through the colon.

The etiologic factor in diverticulitis might be retained undigested food in diverticula, which compromises the blood supply to that area and facilitates bacterial invasion of the sac.

Incidence/Prevalence

The incidence of diverticulosis is difficult to determine, but it is estimated that millions of people are affected. Diverticulitis affects one third of adults over age 60 years, with more men than women affected. Although diverticulosis is common, only one of five people with this disease displays symptoms.

◆COLLABORATIVE MANAGEMENT
◆Assessment

HISTORY

Clients with diverticulosis are usually asymptomatic, and unless pain or bleeding develops, the condition may go undiagnosed or found incidentally on routine colonoscopy. Occasionally diverticulosis causes symptoms. For clients with uncomplicated diverticulosis, the nurse asks about a history of intermittent pain in the left lower quadrant and a history of constipation. If diverticulitis is suspected, the client is asked about a history of fever and abdominal pain. Inquire about recent bowel elimination patterns because constipation may develop as a result of intestinal inflammation. The client is also questioned about the presence of bleeding from the rectum.

PHYSICAL ASSESSMENT/CLINICAL MANIFESTATIONS

On physical examination of the client with uncomplicated diverticulosis, no clinical manifestations of the disorder may be present. Occasionally tenderness is elicited on abdominal palpation.

The client with diverticulitis has abdominal pain, most often localized to the left lower quadrant. The pain may be intermittent at first but becomes progressively steady. Occasionally pain may be suprapubic, or it may occur on one side. Abdominal pain is generalized if peritonitis has occurred. The client's temperature is elevated, ranging from a low-grade fever to 101° F (38.2° C), and may be accompanied by chills. Note any tachycardia secondary to fever. Nausea and vomiting are also commonly present.

On examination of the abdomen, observe for distention. Tenderness on palpation may be noted over the area involved (usually the left lower quadrant). The colon may be palpable. If localized peritoneal irritation is present, localized muscle spasm, guarded movement, and rebound tenderness are usually present. If generalized peritonitis is present, abdominal muscle spasm, guarding, and rebound tenderness are more diffuse.

If the perforated diverticulum is close to the rectum, the health care provider may palpate a tender mass during the rectal examination. Blood pressure checks may show orthostatic changes. If bleeding is massive, the client may have hypotension and dehydration that result in shock. If generalized peritonitis has occurred, sepsis and manifestations of hypotension and septic or hypovolemic shock can occur.

DIAGNOSTIC ASSESSMENT

For the client with uncomplicated diverticulosis, laboratory studies are not indicated. The client with diverticulitis, however, has an elevated white blood cell (WBC) count. Decreased hematocrit and hemoglobin values are noted if chronic or severe bleeding is present. In stool tests for occult blood, results are positive in 20% of clients (also called a fecal occult blood test [FOBT]). Urinalysis may show a few red blood cells (RBCs) if the left ureter is in proximity to a perforated diverticulum.

X-rays of the intestinal tract with barium contrast show diverticula. An upper gastrointestinal (GI) series shows diverticula of the small intestine, and barium enema examination shows diverticula of the large intestine. X-rays are not indicated for clients with uncomplicated diverticulosis because symptoms are usually minimal or nonexistent.

The client with diverticulitis usually does *not* undergo a barium enema examination in the acute phase of the illness because of the risk of rupture of the inflamed diverticulum. A barium enema examination may be completed after the client has been treated with antibiotics and the inflammation has resolved. A flat-plate film of the abdomen may reveal free air and fluid in the left lower quadrant, suggesting an abscess or free air under the diaphragm, indicating perforation. The health care provider may also order a computed tomography (CT) scan to diagnose an abscess or thickening of the bowel related to diverticulitis.

Ultrasonography, a noninvasive test, may reveal bowel thickening or an abscess. The physician may perform a sigmoidoscopy or colonoscopy *after the acute phase* of the illness, usually to rule out the presence of a tumor in the large intestine, particularly if the client has rectal bleeding. If the sigmoidoscope or colonoscope enters a diverticulum, however, the chances of perforating the diverticulum are high.

◆Interventions

Clients may be treated on an ambulatory care basis when symptoms are mild, with a temperature lower than 101° F (38.2° C) and a WBC count ranging from 13,000 to 15,000/mm³. The client who is an outpatient should be monitored for any prolonged or increased fever, abdominal pain, or blood in the stool.

Clients with moderate to severe diverticulitis usually require hospitalization. Clinical manifestations that suggest the need for admission are a temperature higher than 101° F (38.2° C), persistent abdominal pain for more than 3 days, or evidence of lower GI bleeding.

NONSURGICAL MANAGEMENT. For the client with diverticulitis, a combination of drug and diet therapy with rest to decrease inflammation and improve tissue perfusion is indicated. This plan is preferred for older adults and others with mild to moderate disease (Chart 61-6).

For clients with mild diverticulitis, the health care provider prescribes broad-spectrum antibiotics, such as metronidazole (Flagyl) plus trimethoprim/sulfamethoxazole (Bactrim, Septra) or ciprofloxacin (Cipro). A mild analgesic may be given for pain.

NURSING FOCUS on the OLDER ADULT
Diverticulitis

- Provide antibiotics, analgesics, and anticholinergics as prescribed. Observe older clients carefully for side effects of these drugs, especially confusion (or increased confusion), urinary retention or failure, and orthostatic hypotension.
- Do not give laxatives or enemas. Teach the client and the family about the importance of avoiding these measures.
- Encourage the client to rest and to avoid activities that may increase intra-abdominal pressure, such as straining and bending.
- While diverticulitis is active, provide a *low*-fiber diet (see Table 61-4). When the inflammation resolves, provide a *high*-fiber diet. Teach the client and family about these diets and when they are appropriate.
- Because older clients do not always experience the typical pain or fever expected, observe carefully for signs of active disease.
- Perform frequent abdominal assessments to determine distention and tenderness on palpation.
- Check stools for occult or frank bleeding.

The health care provider admits clients with more severe pain to the hospital and prescribes IV fluids to correct dehydration as well as IV antibiotics such as cefoxitin plus metronidazole. Anticholinergics may reduce intestinal hypermotility. For clients with moderate to severe diverticulitis, an opioid analgesic, such as meperidine hydrochloride (Demerol) or morphine sulfate, can alleviate pain.

Laxatives are avoided because they increase intestinal motility. Enemas are avoided because they increase intraluminal pressure. The nurse assesses the client for clinical manifestations of fluid and electrolyte imbalance on an ongoing basis.

Instruct the client to remain in bed during the acute phase of illness. He or she is advised to refrain from lifting, straining, coughing, or bending to avoid an increase in intra-abdominal pressure, which can result in perforation of the diverticulum.

During the acute phase of the illness, the client's diet is restricted to clear liquids. Clients who have more severe symptoms are admitted to the hospital and are kept on NPO status. A nasogastric (NG) tube is inserted if nausea, vomiting, or abdominal distention is severe. Administer IV fluids, as prescribed, for hydration. In collaboration with the dietitian, the client increases dietary intake slowly as symptoms subside. When inflammation has resolved and bowel function returns to normal, a fiber-containing diet is introduced gradually. If active diverticulitis recurs, fiber intake is stopped for the acute phase of the illness.

SURGICAL MANAGEMENT. The client with diverticulitis may need to undergo surgery for any of the following complications:

- Rupture of the diverticulum with subsequent peritonitis
- Pelvic abscess
- Bowel obstruction
- Fistula
- Persistent fever or pain after 4 days of medical treatment
- Uncontrolled bleeding

The surgeon performs emergency surgery if peritonitis, bowel obstruction, or pelvic abscess is present. Colon resection, with or without a colostomy, is the most common surgical procedure for clients with diverticular disease.

Preoperative Care. Preparation of the client for surgery depends on the severity of the condition. The surgery might be performed on an emergency basis, or it might be done with a few weeks' notice. The surgeon informs the client whether a temporary or permanent colostomy might be required.

If the client is *not* in the acute stage of diverticulitis, a thorough bowel preparation *may* be given, consisting of enemas and laxatives daily for 1 to 2 days before surgery. Because of the risk of perforation, however, the surgeon may forgo an aggressive bowel preparation. If the client has an acutely inflamed diverticulum or persistent fever and abdominal pain, the bowel preparation is most likely withheld.

For clients without acute inflammation, a well-structured preoperative diet is ordered. The client usually has a low-fiber diet for 4 to 5 days, followed by a full-liquid diet for 2 days, then a clear-liquid diet the evening before surgery.

Preoperative teaching may include information about the possible need for a colostomy. If a colostomy is a possible outcome, the enterostomal therapist (ET) or office nurse describes its function and purpose. The nurse need not discuss colostomy care in detail unless the client wishes this information at this time.

Operative Procedures. In a resection of the colon, the surgeon excises the portion that is inflamed or diseased and, if possible, creates an anastomosis of the colon to restore patency. Inflammation and infection, however, may preclude the feasibility of an anastomosis. If this is the case, the surgeon may perform a colostomy. Select clients may be candidates for colostomy closure and anastomosis after the bowel has been allowed to rest for 3 to 6 months.

Postoperative Care. The immediate physical care for clients undergoing a colon resection for diverticulitis is the same as that for clients undergoing abdominal surgery (see Chapter 22).

The client has a drain in place at the abdominal incision site for 2 to 3 days. If a colostomy has been performed, the stoma may be covered with petroleum gauze dressing because the colostomy does not drain for approximately 2 days, or a colostomy bag may be placed over the stoma. If the stoma is visible, monitor for color and integrity. The stoma should be pinkish to cherry red without retraction or prolapse into the abdomen.

The client is maintained on NPO status with a possible NG tube in place for 2 to 3 days after a colon resection, with or without a colostomy. When peristalsis returns, remove the NG tube, according to the health care provider's order, and introduce clear liquids *slowly. Gradually,* the diet is advanced to solids, depending on the return of peristalsis and bowel function.

If the client has had a colostomy created, it should begin functioning in 2 to 4 days. Most clients who undergo surgery and colostomy formation for diverticulitis have a sigmoid colostomy because the sigmoid colon is the most common site of diverticulitis. Drainage from a sigmoid colostomy initially consists of loose stool, but eventually the stool becomes formed. A tight seal around the stoma is essential to avoid contact of feces with the skin. Colostomy care is detailed in Chapter 60.

If a colostomy has been performed, give the client an opportunity to express feelings about the ostomy. Discuss these feelings with the client, acknowledging that anger and depression are normal responses. When the client is physically able, encourage him or her to look at the stoma and touch the apparatus.

Community-Based Care

The length of hospitalization for clients with diverticulitis ranges from 3 days to longer than a week, depending on the response to medical treatment and the need for surgery. Discharge plans vary according to the treatment.

HOME CARE MANAGEMENT

For the client with diverticulitis who has responded to medical treatment, home care focuses on proper diet. Assess the client's ability to obtain and prepare the recommended high-fiber foods. The client who has required surgical intervention has the added responsibilities of incision care and possibly colostomy care, with some temporary limitations placed on activities.

HEALTH TEACHING

All clients with diverticular disease require education regarding a high-fiber diet. For clients with diverticulosis, an increase in dietary fiber can regulate bowel function and bring about partial relief of symptoms. The nurse and dietitian encourage the client with diverticulosis to eat a diet high in cellulose and hemicellulose types of fiber. These substances can be found in wheat bran, whole-grain breads, and cereals. The client should ingest at least 25 to 35 g of fiber per day. This requirement can be derived from four slices of 100% whole-wheat bread and a 3-ounce serving of all-bran cereal. Teach the client to eat fresh fruits and vegetables with high-fiber content to add bulk to stools.

The client who is not accustomed to eating high-fiber foods should add them to the diet gradually to avoid flatulence and abdominal cramping. If the client cannot tolerate the recommended fiber requirement, a bulk-forming laxative, such as psyllium hydrophilic mucilloid (Metamucil), can be taken to increase fecal size and consistency. An adequate intake of fluids will help to prevent the bloating that may accompany a high-fiber diet. The client should also avoid alcohol because it irritates the bowel. Clients are instructed to avoid foods containing seeds or indigestible material that may block a diverticulum, such as nuts, corn, popcorn, cucumbers, tomatoes, figs, strawberries, and caraway seeds. In collaboration with the dietitian, the nurse teaches the client that dietary fat intake should not exceed 30% of the total daily caloric intake.

Clients should *avoid all fiber* when they have symptoms of *diverticulitis* because high-fiber foods are irritating. As diverticulitis resolves, fiber can gradually be added until progression to a high-fiber diet is once again obtained. The client who has undergone surgery is usually taking solid food by the time of discharge from the hospital.

Explain the usual disease course and factors that can exacerbate the disease to the client. Follow-up with the health care provider approximately 1 month after resolution of symptoms is recommended, and a repeat flexible sigmoidoscopy or barium enema may be preformed at that time.

Clients who have had abdominal surgery need oral and written instructions on incision care and the signs and symptoms to report to the health care provider. These are similar to the instructions given to clients after other types of abdominal surgery. Provide instructions on colostomy care for clients who have a temporary or permanent colostomy.

Instruct clients *with any type of diverticular disease,* orally and in writing, about the manifestations of acute diverticulitis, including fever, abdominal pain, and bloody, mahogany, or tarry stools. The client should be advised to avoid the use of laxatives (other than bulk-forming types) and enemas. All clients can also benefit from avoiding the activities that increase intra-abdominal pressure, such as straining at stool, bending, or lifting heavy objects.

Reassure clients with diverticulosis that this disorder need not cause problems if a proper diet is followed. The client is informed that this illness does not commonly recur and that with proper diet and elimination patterns, recurring episodes and potential complications can be avoided.

The client with a colostomy has special needs with regard to the alteration in body image and loss of body function. Encourage the client to verbalize concerns about body image.

HEALTH CARE RESOURCES

Clients who have undergone surgery may need assistance with incision and colostomy care. The nurse or case manager arranges for a home care nurse to assess wound healing and proper functioning of the ostomy and the appliance. If the client is interested, the nurse can arrange for a visit from an ostomy volunteer or an enterostomal therapist (ET). For information about other ostomy resources, instruct the client to contact the United Ostomy Association.

❓ *Critical Thinking Challenge*

A middle-aged man is informed that his colonoscopy revealed moderate diverticulosis and several polyps, which were removed. His mother died of colon cancer last year, and he is very nervous about his chances for cancer. He has had gastroesophageal reflux disease (GERD) and irritable bowel syndrome (IBS) for longer than 10 years and currently takes Metamucil daily.

1. Is this client a candidate for drug therapy? Why or why not?
2. What dietary modifications and restrictions should he follow and why? (Keep his GERD and IBS in mind also.)
3. What other health teaching does he need?

evolve For suggested answer guidelines, go to http://evolve.elsevier.com/Iggy/.

ANORECTAL ABSCESS

PATHOPHYSIOLOGY

Anorectal abscess is a localized induration and fluctuance caused by inflammation of the soft tissue near the rectum or anus. It is most often the result of obstruction of the ducts of glands in the anorectal region by feces, foreign bodies, or trauma. Stasis of obstructing contents occurs and causes infection that spreads into adjacent tissue. Most abscesses begin as cryptitis (a pocket of infection in an anal crypt).

The client may experience rectal pain as the first symptom. There may be no clinical manifestations at the time of the first physical assessment, but local swelling, erythema, and tenderness on palpation are apparent within a few days after the onset of pain. If the abscess becomes chronic, discharge, bleeding, and pruritus (itching) may exist. Fever occurs if larger abscesses are present.

BEST PRACTICE for
Promoting Perineal Comfort

- Keep the perineal area clean with mild soap.
- Pat the perineal area dry instead of rubbing it.
- Provide warm sitz baths, or apply warm compresses to the area.
- If the area is acutely inflamed, apply cold packs.
- Provide a chair cushion or a soft, inflatable ring for the seated client. For the older or debilitated client, monitor the skin carefully to prevent pressure sores.
- Use absorbent pads for drainage, if any, and change them often.
- Use premoistened wipes for cleaning the perineal area after a bowel movement.
- Use witch hazel wipes (e.g., Tucks) to relieve pain.
- Give bulk-forming agents, such as psyllium mucilloid (Metamucil), as prescribed, to reduce pain associated with defecation.
- Apply a topical anesthetic cream to the perineal area, as prescribed.
- Give oral analgesics, as prescribed, for pain relief.
- Do not administer enemas or give potent laxatives.

◆ COLLABORATIVE MANAGEMENT

Anorectal abscesses are managed by surgical incision and drainage. The physician can often incise simple perianal and ischiorectal abscesses using a local anesthetic. For clients with more extensive abscesses, a regional or general anesthetic may be needed. Systemic antibiotics are given only for clients who are immunocompromised, are diabetic, have valvular disease or a prosthetic valve, or have extensive subcutaneous fat. Incision and drainage in these clients are performed after antibiotic therapy.

Nursing interventions are focused on helping the client to maintain comfort and optimal perineal hygiene (Chart 61-7). Encourage the use of warm sitz baths, analgesics, bulk-producing agents, and stool softeners during the perioperative period until healing occurs. Emphasize the importance of ongoing perineal hygiene after all bowel movements and the maintenance of a regular bowel pattern with a high-fiber diet.

ANAL FISSURE

PATHOPHYSIOLOGY

An **anal fissure** is a common anorectal condition of particular concern because of the degree (if acute) of discomfort and disability. First-degree fissures are associated with diarrhea or constipation; second-degree fissures are associated with another disorder (e.g., Crohn's disease, tuberculosis, leukemia, or neoplasm) or with trauma (e.g., from a foreign body, childbirth, or perirectal surgery).

◆ COLLABORATIVE MANAGEMENT

An acute anal fissure is superficial and resolves spontaneously or heals quickly with conservative treatment. Chronic fissures recur, and surgical treatment may be needed. Pain during and after defecation and bleeding noted outside the stool are the most common symptoms. Other clinical manifestations associated with chronic fissures are pruritus, urinary frequency or retention, dysuria, and **dyspareunia** (painful intercourse).

The health care provider makes the diagnosis by inspecting and stretching the perianal skin. If the client is having pain at the time of the examination, diagnostic testing is usually limited to inspection. If the client is not in severe pain, a digital examination and possibly a sigmoidoscopy are performed. When painless or multiple fissures are present, the physician may perform a barium enema and sigmoidoscopy to rule out an associated inflammatory bowel disorder.

Management of an acute fissure is typically nonsurgical, with interventions aimed at local, symptomatic pain relief and softening of stools to reduce trauma to the area. Warm sitz baths and analgesia are recommended along with the use of bulk-producing agents, such as psyllium hydrophilic mucilloid (Metamucil), which help to minimize pain associated with defecation. Topical anti-inflammatories (Hydrocortisone creams and suppositories) or opiate suppositories (opium and belladonna suppositories) are helpful if spasms are severe.

Explain the appropriate pain control measures to the client. When nonsurgical management is initiated, instruct the client to notify the health care provider if pain is not relieved within a few days. If fissures do not respond to medical management within several days to weeks, surgical excision of the fissure with a local anesthetic may be necessary. Teach the client who undergoes surgery to continue with the same pain management and bowel regimen, including sitz baths, analgesics, and bulk-forming agents. He or she is reminded to report any drainage or bleeding from the rectum to the health care provider.

ANAL FISTULA

An anal fistula, or *fistula in ano*, is an abnormal tract leading from the anal canal to the perianal skin. Most anal fistulas result from anorectal abscesses, which are caused by obstruction of anal glands (see Anorectal Abscess, p. 1361). Fistulas can also be associated with tuberculosis, Crohn's disease, or cancer.

The client with an anal fistula has pruritus (itching), purulent discharge, and tenderness or pain that is worsened by bowel movements. The physician uses a proctoscope to identify the source of symptoms and to locate the fistula. Because fistulas do not heal spontaneously, surgery is necessary. To perform a **fistulotomy,** the surgeon incises the tissue overlying the tract and performs curettage (scraping) of the base. The incision site heals by secondary intention. In a client with a high fistula, a special surgical technique is necessary because important sphincters are often affected. Postoperatively the nurse instructs the client about sitz baths, analgesics, and the use of bulk-producing agents or stool softeners to minimize pain.

PARASITIC INFECTION

PATHOPHYSIOLOGY

Parasites can enter and invade the gastrointestinal (GI) tract and cause infections leading to varying degrees of illness. Parasites commonly enter through the mouth by means of fecal-oral transmission from the following:

- Contaminated food or water
- Oral-anal sexual practices
- Contact with feces from a contaminated person

Common **parasites** that cause infection in humans are *Entamoeba histolytica*, which causes amebiasis (amebic dysentery); *Giardia lamblia*, which causes giardiasis; and *Cryptosporidium*.

Infection with *Entamoeba histolytica*

Humans are the only known hosts for *E. histolytica* (also known as amebiasis). This organism occurs in cysts and trophozoites (sporozoan parasites). Trophozoites die rapidly after they leave the body in stool. Cysts, however, can remain viable in the right type of environment for weeks or months. Humans who eliminate cysts are infectious. Flies have been found to be vectors for transmission of the cysts, and transmission is increased in areas that use human excrement for fertilizer. Transmission occurs by the fecal-oral route.

Amebiasis occurs worldwide, but it is most prevalent and most severe in tropical areas. Prevalence rates are as high as 40% in areas with poor sanitation, crowding, and poor nutrition. Amebiasis causes 40,000 to 100,000 deaths annually worldwide. The disease causes less severe symptoms and often goes undiagnosed in temperate climates. The organism may occur in 5% of some populations in the United States.

E. histolytica either feeds on bacteria in the intestine or invades and ulcerates the mucosa of the large intestine. The parasite can be limited to the GI tract (intestinal amebiasis), or it can extend outside the intestines (extraintestinal amebiasis). People can have intestinal amebiasis without having any symptoms, or symptoms can range from mild to severe.

Infection with *Giardia lamblia*

G. lamblia is a protozoal parasite that causes superficial invasion, destruction, and inflammation of the mucosa in the small intestine. Like *E. histolytica*, *G. lamblia* has a trophozoite and cysts form, and cysts can transmit the organism. Humans are hosts to this organism, but beavers and dogs may be reservoirs for infection. *G. lamblia* is transmitted by the fecal-oral route. Giardiasis is a well-recognized problem in travelers, campers, male homosexuals, and immunosuppressed people.

Modes of transmission are similar to those for amebiasis; in the United States, however, giardiasis is much more prevalent and is the most common parasitic infection. Giardiasis affects only the intestinal system, causing acute diarrhea, chronic diarrhea, or malabsorption syndrome. The acute phase usually is self-limiting, lasting days or weeks. The chronic phase can last for years. Diarrhea is usually mild in both forms, but it can be severe. As stools increase in frequency, they become more watery, greasy, frothy, and malodorous with mucus. Weight loss and weakness are also common. Malabsorption can occur with diarrhea that continues for longer than 3 weeks. Manifestations result from malabsorption of fat, protein, vitamin B_{12}, and lactase deficiency.

Infection with *Cryptosporidium*

Cryptosporidium is another parasitic infestation transmitted by the fecal-oral route that is manifested by diarrhea. This infection commonly occurs in immunosuppressed clients, particularly those with human immunodeficiency virus (HIV). (See Chapter 25 for a discussion of HIV infection.)

◆COLLABORATIVE MANAGEMENT
◆Assessment

A thorough history can provide information about potential sources of exposure to parasitic infection. A history of travel to parts of the world where such infections are prevalent increases suspicion for infection with parasites. GI symptoms related to travel may be delayed as long as 1 to 2 weeks after the return home. A diet history is especially helpful if several people become ill. Common water supplies may be infected with *Giardia* or *Cryptosporidium*. Trichinosis should be considered if the client has ingested pork products.

Mild to moderate *E. histolytica* infestation causes clinical manifestations, including the daily passage of several strongly odoriferous stools, possibly with mucus but without blood, accompanied by abdominal cramping, flatulence, fatigue, and weight loss.

Clients experience characteristic remissions and recurrences. Severe amebic dysentery is manifested by frequent, more liquid, and odoriferous stools with mucus *and* blood. Fever up to 105° F (40° C), **tenesmus** (painful straining to defecate), generalized abdominal tenderness, and vomiting can also occur. The ulcerations characteristic of invading amebiasis that occur in the colon can cause pain, bleeding, and obstruction. Ulcerations can also be localized in the rectum, resulting in formed stool with blood. Complications are rare but include appendicitis and bowel perforation.

Extraintestinal amebiasis can occur without symptoms of intestinal infection. The most common form is amebic liver abscess, which causes symptoms of fever, pain, and an enlarged liver. The abscess can rupture, and death can result if the infection is not treated and complications occur.

The diagnosis of *amebiasis* is made by examination of stool for parasites. Because *E. histolytica* is difficult to detect, serial stool examinations are needed if the disease is suspected. The use of sigmoidoscopy may detect ulcerations in the rectum or colon. Exudate obtained during sigmoidoscopic examination is studied for the parasite. The white blood cell (WBC) count can be as high as 20,000/mm³ when severe dysentery is present.

The diagnosis of *giardiasis* is also confirmed by stool examination for parasites. Because organisms may not be detected for at least 1 week after symptoms appear, multiple stool samples should be examined. Duodenal aspirate can also be examined for the parasite.

Infection with *Cryptosporidium* is usually self-limiting in individuals who are not immunocompromised. Drug therapy for clients with immunosuppression may consist of paromomycin 500 to 750 mg four times daily.

◆Interventions

Interventions for Amebiasis. Treatment for all types of amebiasis mandate the use of amebicide drugs. The physician commonly prescribes metronidazole (Flagyl, Novonidazole✷) and diloxanide furoate (Entamide) or diloxanide furoate and tetracycline hydrochloride (Sumycin) followed by chloroquine. Clients with severe dysentery require IV fluids for replacement and maintenance of fluid volume and possibly opiates, such as diphenoxylate hydrochloride and atropine sulfate (Lomotil), to control bowel motility. Clients with extraintestinal amebiasis or severe dehydration are hospitalized. Clients with asymptomatic, mild, or moderate disease are treated as outpatients with drug therapy. For all clients, at least three stools are examined for parasites at 2- to 3-day intervals, starting 2 to 4 weeks after drug therapy has been completed.

Interventions for Giardiasis. Treatment for giardiasis is drug therapy. Metronidazole is the drug of choice, and the usual dose, is 250 mg three times daily PO for 5 days. Tinidazole (Fasigyn) can be used as an alternative. Stools are examined 2 weeks after treatment is begun to assess for eradication.

Explain modes of transmission and means to avoid the spread of infection and recurrent contact with parasitic organisms. Clients are taught that they can transmit the infection to others until amebicides effectively kill the parasites. The nurse instructs clients to do the following:

- Avoid contact with stool
- Keep toilet areas clean
- Wash their hands meticulously with an antimicrobial soap after bowel movements
- Maintain personal hygiene
- Avoid stool from dogs and beavers

The client is also advised to avoid sexual practices who allow rectal contact until drug therapy is completed. Inform the client that all household and sexual contacts should undergo stool examinations for parasites. If the water supply is suspected as the source, a sample is obtained and sent for analysis. Multiple infections are common in households, often as a result of contaminated water supplies. Well water and water from areas with inadequate or no filtration equipment can be sources of contamination.

HELMINTHIC INFESTATION

Helminths are wormlike animals; they are often parasitic and capable of causing infectious disease in humans. There are many species of helminths, which for purposes of classification are divided into three general categories:

- Roundworms (nematodes)
- Flukes (trematodes)
- Tapeworms (cestodes)

Helminths can cause various degrees of gastrointestinal (GI) symptoms in humans. Most often they enter the human body through the skin or via the oral route with ingestion of food, water, or other substances contaminated with worms. Some helminths gain access to the human body via insects, such as flies and mosquitoes. Helminths that are typically transmitted via insects are limited to tropical areas, however, and are not discussed here. Flukes (trematodes), which are passed to humans via snail-contaminated water, are also limited to tropical and subtropical areas outside the United States and are not discussed here.

Roundworms

Roundworms are commonly the cause of helminthic infections in the United States and worldwide. These infections include enterobiasis, trichinosis, and hookworm.

Enterobiasis

Enterobiasis ("pinworm infection") is caused by *Enterobius vermicularis* and is the most common helminthic infection in the United States. It is transmitted by oral ingestion of contaminated food, drink, or fomites. The most common clinical manifestations of infection include nocturnal perianal pruritus, vaginitis, insomnia, and restlessness.

The client may have vague GI symptoms, such as abdominal pain, nausea, vomiting, and diarrhea. However, many infected clients have no symptoms. Diagnosis is made when eggs of the helminth are found on the perianal skin or on cellulose tape that has been applied to the perianal skin.

Treatment of enterobiasis includes meticulous handwashing techniques after defecation and before meals to prevent spread of the worms to others. Drug therapy is indicated for all clients with symptoms and in some clients who are infected but are not symptomatic. Household cohabitants of an infected client may be treated with drug therapy even if they are asymptomatic. Pyrantel pamoate (Antiminth, Combantrin❋) or mebendazole (Vermox, Nemasol❋) is given orally in one dose, repeated at 2 and 4 weeks.

Infection with pinworms is curable and is not usually associated with complications; however, recurrences are common.

Trichinosis

Trichinosis is another helminthic disease caused by roundworms. The incidence in the United States is 50 to 100 cases annually, but many mild or asymptomatic cases are not diagnosed because the person is usually asymptomatic. *Trichinella spiralis,* which lives in the intestine of humans, pigs, bears, and rats, causes trichinosis. The organism is usually transmitted to people who ingest undercooked pork or pork products. Ingestion of other meats, such as ground beef, can also promote transmission if a meat grinder has been used for both beef and pork. Following ingestion, the larvae, encased in cysts, are released by the digestive action of acid and pepsin. Incubation is 12 hours to 28 days after ingestion. Clinical manifestations range from none to severe; death rarely results.

During the first week after infection, diarrhea results from the invasion of the gut by large numbers of the parasite. Abdominal pain, nausea, and vomiting may follow. During the second week, the larvae begin to invade the muscle, instigating a hypersensitivity reaction characterized by fever, periorbital and facial edema, and subconjunctival hemorrhage. Occasionally a rash or dyspnea develops. Two to three weeks after infection, symptoms of myositis, myalgia, and muscle weakness develop, particularly in the lower back, neck, jaw, biceps, and extraocular muscles. Vague muscle pain and malaise characterize the convalescence phase, which can last several months.

A diagnosis of trichinosis is confirmed by a history of ingestion of raw or undercooked meat. White blood cell (WBC) and eosinophil counts are elevated for 2 weeks after meat is ingested. Biopsy of skeletal muscle shows larvae of the *Trichinella* organism. Worms are rarely seen in feces.

During the first week after infection, the client is treated with oral mebendazole. During the stage of muscle invasion, he or she must be hospitalized to receive high doses of corticosteroids.

Hookworms

Hookworms are also roundworms. They differ from pinworms and *Trichinella* in that they initially enter the human body through the skin. Hookworm disease is caused by either *Ancylostoma duodenale* or *Necator americanus.*

Hookworms infect a quarter of the world's population, but the disease is rare in areas outside the tropics or in areas with little rain. Worms are infective outside the body in warm, moist soil for up to 1 week. Transmission occurs when larvae penetrate through the skin. The organism can migrate to pulmonary capillaries via the bloodstream and enter alveoli. Cilia carry the organisms up the respiratory tree to the pharynx and the mouth, where they are swallowed and enter the GI tract. Hookworms probably also enter the GI tract when a person ingests contaminated food.

Early symptoms of hookworm disease include a pruritic, erythematous, raised vesicular inflammation of the skin. Infection in the GI tract may produce no symptoms, or it may cause anorexia, diarrhea, or mild abdominal and epigastric discomfort. Bleeding and anemia may occur when worms suck blood at sites of attachment in the GI tract. If blood loss is severe, the client may have symptoms of iron deficiency anemia, such as pallor, hair thinning, deformed nails, pica, and shortness of breath.

Diagnosis of hookworm infection is based on the presence of ova (eggs) in the feces. Occult blood is often present in the stool. There may be a low hemoglobin concentration and hematocrit value or a low serum iron level and high iron-binding capacity, indicating hypochromic microcytic anemia. The WBC counts and eosinophil counts are elevated.

All clients with symptoms receive iron therapy and a diet high in protein and vitamins for at least 3 months after anemia is corrected. Pyrantel pamoate (Antiminth) or mebendazole (Vermox) is given for a complete recovery. Severe hookworm disease can cause malabsorption and protein loss, necessitating nutritional support in addition to other treatments.

Tapeworms

Five types of tapeworms (cestodes) may infect humans: tapeworms found in cattle, fish, dogs, pigs, and rodents. Tapeworm infections generally cause either no symptoms or only occasional GI upset, such as nausea, diarrhea, or abdominal pain.

Transmission of tapeworms occurs when a person ingests undercooked beef, raw fish, or other contaminated food or water or accidentally swallows infected lice or fleas from dogs. People can also accidentally ingest arthropods, such as cockroaches, in stored foods or cereals.

The diagnosis of tapeworm infestation is made by laboratory examination of eggs found in the stool (test of stool for ova and parasites). Clients are treated with medications for this type of infection.

When caring for clients with helminths, follow standard precautions or body substance precautions when in contact with any stool. All clients are taught to wash their hands after defecating and before eating. They should avoid ingesting undercooked beef, fish, or pork and drinking water that might be contaminated. After petting dogs, clients should take care to keep their mouth closed and wash their hands. All stored foods should be kept tightly closed to avoid contamination by cockroaches and other insects.

FOOD POISONING

Foodborne illnesses are a common problem, with 6.5 cases occurring in the United States every year (Van Benden et al., 1999). Food poisoning has been linked to as many as 9000 deaths per year in the United States. Food poisoning results when a person ingests infectious organisms in food. Unlike gastroenteritis, food poisoning is not directly communicable from person to person, and incubation periods are shorter. Like gastroenteritis, it causes diarrhea, nausea, and vomiting. You can differentiate food poisoning from gastroenteritis by obtaining a thorough history of common food intake in clients who have common symptoms of acute diarrhea, nausea, and vomiting.

The common types of food poisoning are caused by pathogens and include the following (Table 61-5):
- Gram-negative *Salmonella*
- *Staphylococcal aureus*
- *Escherichia coli*
- Botulism

All cases of botulism and salmonellosis need to be reported to the local health department. Cases of staphylococcal and *E. coli* food poisoning are reported if epidemic outbreaks occur.

Salmonellosis

Salmonellosis is a bacterial infection caused by the *Salmonella* organism. It can be transmitted by the "five Fs": flies, fingers, food, feces, and fomites.

Incubation is 8 to 48 hours after the person has ingested the contaminated food or liquid. Symptoms usually last for 3 to 5 days and include fever with or without chills, nausea, vomiting, cramping abdominal pain, and diarrhea, which may be bloody.

Salmonellosis is usually self-limiting, but bacteremia with localization in joints or bone may occur. The definitive diagnosis is made by stool culture. Treatment is symptomatic, and drug therapy is not usually indicated unless bacteremia occurs; in that case, the physician prescribes antibiotics.

Clients may be carriers of the bacterium for up to 1 year. The nurse instructs all clients with *Salmonella* gastroenteritis and their contacts to wash their hands before meals and after defecating to avoid transmission of the organism. The treatment for *Salmonella* infection is controversial because antibiotics tend not to shorten the illness. In some studies,

---

TABLE 61-5 Common Types of Food Poisoning

Staphylococcal Infection
- Caused by contaminated meats and dairy products
- Can be transmitted by human carriers
- Causes abrupt onset of vomiting and diarrhea without fever

***Escherichia coli* Infection**
- Caused by meat contaminated with animal feces
- Causes abrupt vomiting, diarrhea, abdominal cramping, and fever

Botulism
- Commonly associated with improperly canned foods, especially fruits and vegetables
- Nausea, vomiting, diarrhea, and weakness progressing to paralysis
- Diplopia, dysphagia, and dysarthria

Salmonellosis
- Caused by contaminated food or drink but can be transmitted by the fecal-oral route
- Fever, nausea, vomiting, abdominal cramping, and diarrhea lasting for 3 to 5 days

quinolones have been effective, but these are usually reserved for individuals with severe manifestations of the illness.

Staphylococcal Infection

Staphylococcus is associated with 25% of reported food poisoning outbreaks. *Staphylococcus* is found in meats and dairy products and can be transmitted by carriers of the organism. For staphylococcal food poisoning to occur, there must be contamination of food and a period of time (hours) during which the organisms multiply. This can take place during the slow cooling of food after it is cooked.

Symptoms of staphylococcal food poisoning include an abrupt onset of vomiting, abdominal cramping, and diarrhea. The person usually has symptoms 2 to 4 hours after ingesting the contaminated food. There is no fever, but the client is weak.

A diagnosis can be made when stool culture yields 100,000 enterotoxin-producing staphylococci; however, symptoms rarely last more than 24 hours, and people do not always seek medical attention. Antimicrobial drug therapy is not usually indicated unless an agent produces progressive systemic involvement. Parenteral fluids may be necessary if fluid volume is grossly depleted.

Escherichia coli Infection

E. coli is not usually associated with food poisoning. Since 1992, however, there have been several outbreaks of *E. coli* food poisoning in the United States. Enterohemorrhagic strains of *E. coli* produce cytotoxins that cause outbreaks of hemorrhagic colitis and hemolytic-uremic syndrome. Treatment of the client with *E. coli* food poisoning includes IV fluids and antibiotic therapy.

Botulism

Botulism is a paralytic disease resulting from ingestion of a toxin in food contaminated with *Clostridium botulinum*. Botulism is most commonly associated with home-canned foods, particularly vegetables, fruits, condiments and, less commonly, meat and fish. It can be associated with commercially prepared products and with products not adequately heated to destroy toxins before they are eaten.

Incubation is usually 18 to 36 hours. After this time, symptoms occur; illness may be mild or severe, with paralysis, respiratory failure, and death. Initial symptoms include diplopia, dysphagia, and dysarthria.

Weakness can progress rapidly from the neck to the arms, thorax, and legs. Paralytic ileus, severe constipation, and urinary retention can also occur. Nausea, vomiting, and abdominal pain may occur before or after the onset of paralysis.

The diagnosis is made on the basis of the client's history and a stool culture of *C. botulinum*. The serum may be positive for toxins.

Treatment with trivalent botulism antitoxin (ABE) is given as soon as the diagnosis is made if the client is not hypersensitive to it. The physician may lavage the stomach to stop absorption of toxin. All clients are hospitalized to observe for and treat respiratory paralysis. Nothing is given orally until swallowing and respiratory difficulties pass. The physician prescribes IV fluids as needed. If respiratory paralysis occurs, tracheostomy and mechanical ventilation are implemented. If ventilation can be maintained, the client can survive with no neurologic deficits after the illness.

To prevent botulism, teach clients the importance of discarding cans of food that are punctured or swollen or that have defective seals. Containers for home-canned foods must be sterilized by boiling for 20 minutes to destroy *C. botulinum* spores before canning.

GET READY for the NCLEX Examination!

KEY POINTS

Safe Effective Care Environment

- Recognize that perforation (rupture) of the appendix requires prompt intervention and can result in peritonitis.
- Be alert for GI bleeding in the client with chronic inflammatory bowel disease (IBD).
- Prioritize care for clients with IBD according to their major nursing diagnoses: diarrhea and acute or chronic pain or both.
- Be aware that clients with Crohn's disease are at high risk for malnutrition as a result of an inability to absorb nutrients via the small intestine.

Health Promotion and Maintenance

- Teach individuals ways to prevent transmission of gastroenteritis as stated in Chart 61-2.
- Teach clients with chronic IBD to avoid gastrointestinal stimulants, such as alcohol and caffeine; each client's response to foods differs.
- Teach clients taking immunosuppressive agents, such as 6-mercaptopurine, that these medications can cause decreased blood cell count, infection, and other adverse effects typical of this class of medications.
- Teach clients how to provide ileostomy care, paying particular attention to skin care; the effluent has a high enzyme content that can easily cause severe skin excoriation (see Chart 61-4).
- Consult with an ET nurse for ileostomy teaching and care.
- Instruct clients with diverticulosis about diet modifications, such as avoiding nuts, foods with seeds, and GI stimulants.
- Teach clients with diverticulosis to eat a high-fiber diet; diverticulitis requires a low-fiber diet.
- Instruct clients with anorectal disorders to use sitz baths, bulk-forming agents (such as Metamucil), and stool softeners to decrease pain.

Psychosocial Integrity

- Be aware that all inflammatory bowel diseases (acute and chronic) are very disruptive to one's daily routine; chronic IBD requires a lifetime of modifications.
- Recognize that having an ileostomy impacts the client's body image and self-esteem; assess for coping strategies that the client has previously used and identify personal support systems to assist in coping and acceptance of loss.

Physiological Integrity

- Assess for the classic clinical manifestations of appendicitis, which include abdominal pain, nausea and vomiting, and abdominal tenderness upon palpation (McBurney's point); some clients also have leukocytosis.

- Assess for the key features of peritonitis as listed in Chart 61-1.
- Assess for signs and symptoms of dehydration in clients who have inflammatory bowel disease.
- Administer antidiarrheal medications, as prescribed, to decrease stools and therefore prevent dehydration in clients with inflammatory bowel diseases.
- Be aware that there are two types of chronic inflammatory bowel disease (IBD): ulcerative colitis (UC) and Crohn's disease; both have similarities but also have differences (see Table 61-2).
- Monitor for complications of UC as listed in Table 61-3.
- Provide nursing interventions for clients with IBD as listed in Chart 61-3.
- Administer 5-aminosalicylic acid drugs, as prescribed (e.g., Pentasa and Dipentum), to decrease inflammation in clients with UC; most of these same drugs are also used for Crohn's disease management.
- Administer corticosteroids and 6-mercaptopurine, as prescribed, for both UC and Crohn's disease; infliximab (Remicade) is used primarily for Crohn's but may be useful for those with UC in selected cases.
- Observe for gastrointestinal bleeding in clients with diverticular disease.
- Be aware that gastrointestinal problems, including diarrhea, may also be caused by parasites and helminths.

ADDITIONAL STUDY RESOURCES

Go to your Student CD-ROM for Review Questions for the NCLEX Examination.

evolve Go to http://evolve.elsevier.com/Iggy/ for Integrated Management of Care Questions for the NCLEX Examination.

SELECTED BIBLIOGRAPHY

Asterisk indicates a classic or definitive work on this subject.

Bernstein, C., et al. (2000). Direct hospital costs for patients with inflammatory bowel disease in a Canadian tertiary care university hospital. *American Journal of Gastroenterology, 95*(3), 677-683.

Casellas, F., et al. (2000). Impact of surgery for Crohn's disease on health-related quality of life. *American Journal of Gastroenterology, 95*(1), 177-181.

Cohen, R., et al. (2000). The cost of hospitalization for Crohn's disease. *American Journal of Gastroenterology, 95*(2), 524-530.

*Delco, F., & Sonnenberg, A. (1999). Commonalities in the time trends of Crohn's disease and ulcerative colitis. *American Journal of Gastroenterology, 94*(8), 2172-2176.

Dooley, T.P., et al. (2004). Regulation of gene expression in inflammatory bowel disease and correlation with IBD drugs: Screening by DNA microassays. *Inflammatory Bowel Disease, 10*(1), 1-14.

Goldstein, E.S., Marion, J.F., & Present, D.H. (2004). 6-mercaptopurine is effective in Crohn's disease without concomitant steroids. *Inflammatory Bowel Disease, 10*(2), 79-84.

Joachim, G. (2002). An assessment of social support in people with inflammatory bowel disease. *Gastroenterology Nursing, 25*(6), 246-252.

*Klonowski, E., & Masoodi, J. (1999). The patient with Crohn's disease. *RN, 62*(3), 32-37.

*Martin, F. (1997). Ulcerative colitis. *American Journal of Nursing 97*(8), 38-39.

*Mikula, C. (1999). Anti-TNF alpha: New therapy for Crohn's disease. *Gastroenterology Nursing, 22*(6), 245-248.

*Mishkin, S. (1997). Dairy sensitivity, lactose malabsorption, and elimination diets in inflammatory bowel disease. *American Journal of Clinical Nutrition, 65*(2), 564-567.

*Northouse, L.L., et al. (1999). The concerns of patients and spouses after the diagnosis of colon cancer: A qualitative analysis. *Journal of Wound, Ostomy, and Incontinence Nursing, 26*(1), 8-17.

*Norton, B. (1998). Crohn's disease: A review of medical, surgical and nutritional management. *ADVANCE for Nurse Practitioners, 6*(9), 42-50.

*Olmstead, J. (1998). Evaluation and management of the patient with ulcerative colitis. *Gastroenterology Nursing, 21*(4), 176-180.

Pearson, C. (2004). Inflammatory bowel disease. *Nursing Times, 100*(9), 86-90.

*Rayhorn, N. (1999). Understanding inflammatory bowel disease. *Nursing 99, 29*(12), 57-61.

Tanaka, M., Miyawaki, I., & Kazuma. K. (2003). A study of relationships between self-evaluation of physical condition and perception of life in ulcerative colitis patients. *Gastroenterology Nursing, 26*(3), 115-124.

*Van Benden, C., et al. (1999). Multiple outbreak of *Salmonella enterica* serotype Newport infections due to contaminated alfalfa sprouts. *Journal of the American Medical Association, 281*(2), 158-162.

*Worley, J. (1999). Diagnosis and management of inflammatory bowel disease. *Journal of the American Academy of Nurse Practitioners, 11*(1), 23-31.

Interventions for Clients with Liver Problems

MADELEINE B. MURPHY

 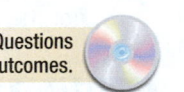
The liver is the largest and one of the most vital internal organs, performing more than 400 functions and affecting every system in the body. When the liver cannot perform its complex activities, hepatic failure results. Liver diseases range in severity from mild hepatic inflammation to chronic end-stage cirrhosis.

CIRRHOSIS

Cirrhosis is extensive scarring of the liver, usually caused by a chronic irreversible reaction to hepatic inflammation and necrosis. The disease typically develops insidiously and has a prolonged, destructive course.

The most common causes for cirrhosis in the United States are alcoholic liver disease and hepatitis C. Worldwide, hepatitis B is the leading cause.

PATHOPHYSIOLOGY

Cirrhosis is characterized by diffuse fibrotic bands of connective tissue that distort the liver's normal architecture. Inflammation caused by either toxins or disease results in extensive degeneration and destruction of **hepatocytes** (liver cells). As cirrhosis develops, the tissue becomes nodular. These nodules can block bile ducts and normal blood flow throughout the liver. Flow alterations in the vascular system

and lymphatic bile duct channels result from compression caused by the proliferation of fibrous tissue. In early disease, the liver is usually enlarged, firm and hard. As the pathologic process continues, the liver shrinks in size.

Complications of Cirrhosis

Common problems and complications associated with hepatic cirrhosis depend on the amount of damage sustained by the liver. In **compensated cirrhosis**, the liver has significant scarring but is still able to perform essential functions without causing significant symptoms.

In **decompensated cirrhosis**, liver function is significantly impaired with obvious manifestations of liver failure.

The loss of hepatic function contributes to the development of metabolic abnormalities. Hepatic cell degeneration may lead to the following:

- Portal hypertension
- Ascites
- Bleeding esophageal varices
- Coagulation defects
- Jaundice
- Portal-systemic encephalopathy (PSE) with hepatic coma
- Hepatorenal syndrome
- Spontaneous bacterial peritonitis

PORTAL HYPERTENSION

Portal hypertension, a persistent increase in pressure within the portal vein, is a major complication of cirrhosis. It results from increased resistance to or obstruction of the flow of blood through the portal vein and its tributaries. The blood meets resistance to flow and seeks collateral venous channels around the high-pressure area.

Blood flow backs into the spleen, causing splenomegaly. Veins in the esophagus, stomach, intestines, abdomen, and rectum become dilated. Portal hypertension can result in ascites, esophageal varices, prominent abdominal veins (caput medusae), and hemorrhoids.

ASCITES

Ascites is the accumulation of free fluid within the peritoneal cavity. Increased hydrostatic pressure from portal hypertension causes this fluid to leak into the peritoneal cavity. The accumulation of plasma protein, primarily albumin, in the peritoneal fluid reduces the amount of circulating plasma protein in the blood. When this decrease is combined with the inability of the liver to synthesize albumin because of impaired hepatocyte functioning, the effective serum colloid osmotic pressure is decreased in the circulatory system.

The decrease of effective intravascular circulation from massive ascites may cause renal vasoconstriction, triggering the renin-angiotensin system. This results in sodium and water retention, which increases hydrostatic pressure and the intravascular volume, which perpetuates the cycle of ascites.

BLEEDING ESOPHAGEAL VARICES

As a result of portal hypertension, the blood backs up from the liver and enters the esophageal and gastric vessels that carry it into the systemic circulation. **Esophageal varices** occur when fragile, thin-walled esophageal veins become distended from increased pressure. The potential for varices to bleed depend upon their size; size is determined by direct endoscopic observation. Varices occur most often in the distal esophagus but can also be present in the stomach.

Bleeding esophageal varices represent a life-threatening medical emergency. There can be significant blood loss, resulting in shock from hypovolemia. The bleeding may be manifested by **hematemesis** (vomiting blood) or **melena** (black, tarry stools). Loss of consciousness may precede any observed bleeding. Variceal bleeding can occur spontaneously with no precipitating factors. However, any activity that increases abdominal pressure may increase the likelihood of a variceal bleed. Clients with this problem should be advised against heavy lifting and vigorous physical exercise. There is no clear evidence that poorly chewed food, medications, or refluxed gastric acid cause variceal bleeding.

Clients with portal hypertension may also have **portal hypertensive gastropathy**. This complication can occur with or without the presence of esophageal varices. Slow gastric mucosal bleeding occurs, which may result in chronic slow blood loss, occult positive stools, and anemia.

COAGULATION DEFECTS

With cirrhosis, there is a decrease in the synthesis of bile in the liver; this prevents the absorption of fat-soluble vitamins (e.g., vitamin K). Without vitamin K, clotting factors II, VII, IX, and X are not produced in sufficient quantities, and the client is susceptible to bleeding and easy bruising. These abnormalities are manifested in abnormal prothrombin times (prolonged or elevated).

Splenomegaly (enlarged spleen) results from the backup of blood into the spleen. The enlarged spleen destroys platelets, causing thrombocytopenia (low serum platelet count). Thrombocytopenia is often the first clinical sign that a client has liver dysfunction.

JAUNDICE

Jaundice in clients with hepatic cirrhosis is caused by one of two mechanisms: hepatocellular disease or intrahepatic obstruction (Table 62-1). Hepatocellular jaundice develops because the liver cells cannot effectively excrete bilirubin. This decreased excretion results in excessive circulating bilirubin levels. Intrahepatic obstructive jaundice results from edema, fibrosis, or scarring of the hepatic bile channels and bile ducts, which interferes with normal bile and bilirubin excretion.

PORTAL-SYSTEMIC ENCEPHALOPATHY

Portal-systemic encephalopathy (PSE) is also known as **hepatic encephalopathy** and **hepatic coma** in the later stages. It is a clinical disorder seen in hepatic failure and cirrhosis. PSE is manifested by neurologic symptoms and is characterized by an altered level of consciousness, impaired thinking processes, and neuromuscular disturbances. Encephalopathy may be acute and reversible with early intervention.

The exact mechanisms causing hepatic encephalopathy are not clearly understood but most likely are the result of the shunting of portal venous blood into the central circulation so that the liver is bypassed. As a result, toxic substances absorbed by the intestine are not broken down or detoxified and may lead to metabolic abnormalities, most significantly elevated serum ammonia. Elevated ammonia levels are usually cited as the cause of hepatic encephalopathy. However, ammonia levels are not a clear indicator of the presence of encephalopathy. Some clients may have significant impairment without dramatic elevations of serum ammonia, and elevations of ammonia can occur without evidence of encephalopathy.

TABLE 62-1 Laboratory Diagnostic Differentiation of Jaundice

Test	Hepatocellular Jaundice	Obstructive Jaundice	Hemolytic Jaundice
Serum bilirubin			
Indirect (unconjugated)	Increased	Slightly increased	Increased
Direct (conjugated)	Increased	Moderately increased	Normal
Urine bilirubin	Increased	Increased	None
Urobilinogen			
Stool	Normal to decreased	None	Increased
Urine	Normal to increased	None	Increased

TABLE 62-2 Stages of Portal-Systemic Encephalopathy

Stage I Prodromal
- Subtle manifestations that may not be recognized immediately
- Personality changes
- Behavior changes (agitation, belligerence)
- Emotional lability (euphoria, depression)
- Impaired thinking
- Inability to concentrate
- Fatigue, drowsiness
- Slurred or slowed speech
- Sleep pattern disturbances

Stage II Impending
- Continuing mental changes
- Mental confusion
- Disorientation to time, place, or person
- Asterixis (see Figure 62-3)

Stage III Stuporous
- Progressive deterioration
- Marked mental confusion
- Stuporous, drowsy but arousable
- Abnormal electroencephalogram tracing
- Muscle twitching
- Hyperreflexia
- Asterixis

Stage IV Comatose
- Unresponsiveness, leading to death in 85% of clients progressing to this stage
- Unarousable, obtunded
- Response to painful stimulus
- No asterixis
- Positive Babinski's sign
- Muscle rigidity
- Fetor hepaticus (characteristic liver breath—musty, sweet odor)
- Seizures

PSE may develop insidiously in clients with chronic liver disease and go undetected until the late stages. Symptoms develop rapidly in acute liver dysfunction. Four stages of development have been identified: prodromal, impending, stuporous, and comatose (Table 62-2). The client's symptoms may gradually progress to coma or fluctuate among the four stages.

Factors that may precipitate PSE include the following:
- High-protein diet
- Infections
- Hypovolemia (deficient fluid volume)
- Hypokalemia (deficient serum potassium)
- Constipation
- Gastrointestinal (GI) bleeding (causes a large protein load in the intestines)
- Drugs (e.g., hypnotics, opioids, sedatives, analgesics, diuretics)

PSE may also occur after paracentesis or shunting procedures. The prognosis depends on the severity of the underlying cause, the precipitating factors, and the degree of liver dysfunction.

HEPATORENAL SYNDROME

The development of **hepatorenal syndrome** indicates a poor prognosis for the client with hepatic failure. It is often the cause of death in clients with cirrhosis. Progressive oliguric renal failure associated with hepatic failure results in functional impairment of kidneys with normal anatomic

TABLE 62-3 Common Causes of Cirrhosis

- Alcoholic liver disease	- Drugs and toxins
- Viral hepatitis	- Biliary disease
- Autoimmune hepatitis	- Metabolic/genetic causes
- Steatohepatitis	- Cardiovascular disease

and morphologic features. This syndrome is manifested by the following:
- A sudden decrease in urinary flow
- Elevated blood urea nitrogen and creatinine levels, with abnormally decreased urine sodium excretion
- Increased urine osmolarity

Hepatorenal syndrome often occurs after clinical deterioration from GI bleeding or the onset of PSE. It may also complicate other liver diseases, including acute hepatitis and fulminant liver failure.

SPONTANEOUS BACTERIAL PERITONITIS

Clients with cirrhosis and ascites may develop acute spontaneous bacterial peritonitis (SBP). Those who are particularly susceptible are clients with very advanced liver disease. This may be the result of low concentrations of proteins; proteins normally provide some protection against bacteria.

The bacteria responsible for SBP are typically from the bowel and reach the ascitic fluid after transmigrating through the bowel wall and transversing the lymphatics. Clinical manifestations vary, but may include fever, chills, and abdominal pain and tenderness. However, symptoms can also be minimal with only mild or vague complaints in the absence of fever. Worsening encephalopathy and increased jaundice may also be present without abdominal complaint.

The diagnosis of SBP is made when a sample of ascitic fluid is obtained by paracentesis for cell counts and culture. An ascitic fluid leukocyte count of more than 250 polymorphonuclear (PMN) leukocytes can be the basis for treatment.

Etiology

Cirrhosis can occur as a result of many factors and diseases. Table 62-3 lists the most common etiologies, which are described in the following sections.

ALCOHOL

Alcohol has a direct toxic effect on the hepatocytes and causes liver inflammation (**alcoholic hepatitis**). The liver becomes enlarged, with cellular degeneration and infiltration by fat, leukocytes, and lymphocytes. Over time, the inflammatory process decreases and the destructive phase increases. Early scar formation is caused by fibroblast infiltration and collagen formation. Damage to liver tissue progresses as a result of malnutrition and repeated exposure to the alcohol. If alcohol is withheld, the fatty infiltration and inflammation is reversible. If alcohol abuse continues, widespread scar tissue formation and fibrosis infiltrate the liver as a result of cellular necrosis.

The amount of alcohol necessary to cause cirrhosis varies widely from person to person and there are gender differences. In women, it may take as few as two to three drinks per day over a minimum of 10 years. In men, perhaps six drinks per day over the same time period may be needed to cause disease. However, there are other individuals, both male and female, who consume far more alcohol per day over a period of several years without ever developing cirrhosis.

VIRAL HEPATITIS

Hepatitis C is an infectious bloodborne illness that usually causes chronic disease. Inflammation caused by infection over time leads to progressive scarring of the liver. It usually takes decades for cirrhosis to develop, although alcohol use in combination with hepatitis C may accelerate the process.

Hepatitis B is the most common cause of cirrhosis worldwide. Hepatitis B also causes inflammation and low-grade damage over decades that can ultimately lead to cirrhosis. The role that concomitant use of alcohol plays in hepatitis B cirrhosis is not as clear as that of hepatitis C cirrhosis.

Hepatitis D is another virus that infects the liver, but only in people who already have hepatitis B (see later discussion on hepatitis in this chapter).

AUTOIMMUNE HEPATITIS

Unlike viral hepatitis, this is not an infectious disease. For reasons not clearly understood, the host's immune system produces a high level of circulating autoantibodies, causing inflammation of the liver. This chronic inflammation can lead to fibrosis and eventual cirrhosis.

STEATOHEPATITIS

Frequently referred to as "fatty liver," **steatohepatitis** occurs when fat and cholesterol deposits in the liver cause chronic inflammation. Over time, this inflammation may cause liver damage, or fibrosis and eventual cirrhosis. Obesity and elevated lipid profile are risk factors for steatohepatitis. This complication is discussed as a separate health problem later in this chapter.

DRUGS AND TOXINS

Medications, herbal supplements, and environmental exposure to toxins may damage the liver so significantly that cirrhosis occurs. Sometimes the development of cirrhosis occurs decades after the initial exposure.

BILIARY DISEASE

Biliary cirrhosis develops as a result of chronic biliary obstruction, bile stasis, inflammation, or diffuse hepatic fibrosis. The most common causes of biliary cirrhosis are primary biliary cirrhosis and primary sclerosing cholangitis. Both of these forms of biliary cirrhosis may also present as secondary to either stones or strictures affecting the common bile duct.

Primary biliary cirrhosis (PBC) is a disease, probably with an immunologic basis, that involves the slow progressive destruction of small intrahepatic ducts, resulting in cholestasis. The disease usually affects middle-aged women. One of the most common presenting features is an asymptomatic elevation of the alkaline phosphatase.

Primary sclerosing cholangitis (PSC) is an illness that is characterized by diffuse inflammation and fibrosis that involves the biliary system. It has the potential to cause cirrhosis because this process leads to a narrowing and eventual obliteration of the intrahepatic bile ducts. There is a strong association between PSC and inflammatory bowel disease. This disease predominantly affects men.

METABOLIC/GENETIC CAUSES

There are many metabolic and genetic disorders that can cause cirrhosis of the liver:

- **Hemachromatosis**, which is characterized by excessive iron storage
- **Wilson's disease**, a disorder of copper metabolism
- **Alpha₁ antitrypsin deficiency**, which may cause an abnormal accumulation of antitrypsin and produce inflammatory activity
- **Cystic fibrosis,** which can cause cirrhosis from intrahepatic bile duct plugging

CARDIOVASCULAR DISEASE

Vascular (cardiac) cirrhosis is associated with severe right-sided heart failure. The liver becomes enlarged, is congested with venous blood, and appears edematous and dark in color. The liver serves as a reservoir for large amounts of venous blood that the failing heart cannot pump back into the systemic circulation. The increase in hepatic volume and pressure causes severe venous congestion. The decrease in nourishing blood flow to the liver results in hepatic cell necrosis and fibrosis.

UNKNOWN CAUSES

Cryptogenic cirrhosis is a diagnosis given when no known etiology for liver disease can be demonstrated by serologic testing, liver biopsy, or diagnostic scanning. Cryptogenic cirrhosis occurs in about 10% of clients with cirrhosis.

Incidence/Prevalence

The incidence of cirrhosis is not well known, although the number of deaths from all liver diseases is about 43,000 per year in the United States.

> ### CULTURAL CONSIDERATIONS
> Deaths from chronic liver disease and cirrhosis are about four times more prevalent among Native Americans/American Indians and Alaskan Natives than among the general U.S. population. The cause of increased death rates is not known but may be related to a lack of health care access.

◆ COLLABORATIVE MANAGEMENT
◆ Assessment
HISTORY

It is important to obtain historical data from clients with suspected cirrhosis, including age, gender, race, and employment history, especially history of exposure to harmful chemical toxins. Keep in mind that all exposures are important regardless of how long ago they occurred. Determine whether there has ever been a needle stick injury. Sexual history may be important in determining an infectious cause for liver disease.

Elicit whether there is a family history of alcoholism and/or liver disease in the family. Ask the client to describe his or her alcohol intake, including the amount consumed during a given period of time. Is there a history of drug use? Oral? Intravenous (IV)? Intranasal? For clients previously or currently in an alcohol or drug recovery program, how long have they been in sobriety? What does their participation consist of in the treatment program? This information is sensitive and many times difficult for the client to answer.

Be sure to establish with the client why you are asking these questions and accept them in a nonjudgmental manner. For many people, the behaviors causing the liver disease occurred years before the onset of their current illness and they are regretful and often embarrassed.

Ask the client about previous medical conditions, such as an episode of jaundice or acute viral hepatitis, biliary tract disorders, viral infections, blood transfusions, autoimmune disorders, obesity, altered lipid profile and a history of heart failure or respiratory disorders.

PHYSICAL ASSESSMENT/CLINICAL MANIFESTATIONS

Because cirrhosis has an insidious onset, many of the early manifestations are vague and nonspecific. The client may report the following:

- Fatigue
- Significant change in weight
- Gastrointestinal (GI) symptoms
- Abdominal pain and liver tenderness (both of which may be ignored by the client)
- Pruritus

Hepatic function abnormalities are often detected when a physical examination or laboratory tests are completed for an unrelated illness or problem. It is not uncommon for a client with *compensated cirrhosis* to be completely unaware that there is a liver problem. The first sign of cirrhosis may present before the onset of symptoms when routine laboratory tests, presurgical evaluations, or life and health insurance assessments show abnormalities. These tests could indicate abnormal hepatic function or thrombocytopenia, prompting a more thorough diagnostic workup.

The development of late signs of advanced cirrhosis may cause the client to seek medical treatment. GI bleeding, jaundice, ascites, and spontaneous bruising indicate deteriorating hepatic function and represent complications of cirrhosis.

Thoroughly assess the client with liver dysfunction or hepatic failure, because it affects every body system (Figure 62-1). The clinical picture and course vary from client to client depending on the severity of hepatic failure. An inspection may reveal the following:

- Obvious yellowing of the skin (jaundice) and the sclerae (icterus)
- Dry skin

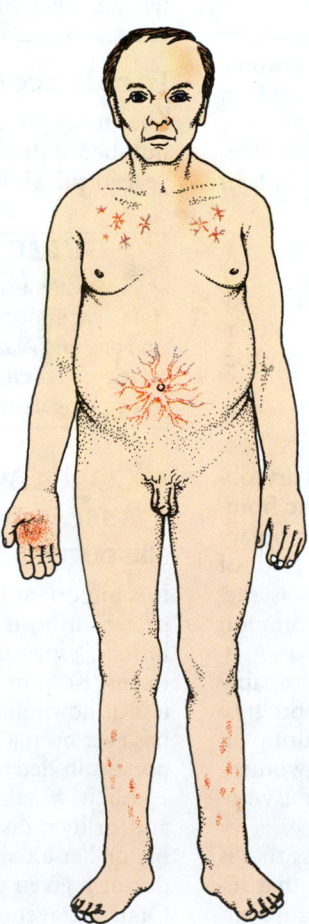

NEUROLOGIC FINDINGS
Asterixis
Paresthesias of feet
Peripheral nerve degeneration
Portal-systemic encephalopathy
Reversal of sleep-wake pattern
Sensory disturbances

GASTROINTESTINAL (GI)
FINDINGS
Abdominal pain
Anorexia
Ascites
Clay-colored stools
Diarrhea
Esophageal varices
Fetor hepaticus
Gallstones
Gastritis
Gastrointestinal bleeding
Hemorrhoidal varices
Hepatomegaly
Hiatal hernia
Hypersplenism
Malnutrition
Nausea
Small nodular liver
Vomiting

RENAL FINDINGS
Hepatorenal syndrome
Increased urine bilirubin

ENDOCRINE FINDINGS
Increased aldosterone
Increased antidiuretic hormone
Increased circulating estrogens
Increased glucocorticoids
Gynecomastia

IMMUNE SYSTEM DISTURBANCES
Increased susceptibility to infection
Leukopenia

CARDIOVASCULAR FINDINGS
Cardiac dysrhythmias
Development of collateral circulation
Fatigue
Hyperkinetic circulation
Peripheral edema
Portal hypertension
Spider angiomas

PULMONARY FINDINGS
Dyspnea
Hydrothorax
Hyperventilation
Hypoxemia

HEMATOLOGIC FINDINGS
Anemia
Disseminated intravascular
    coagulation
Impaired coagulation
Splenomegaly
Thrombocytopenia

DERMATOLOGIC FINDINGS
Axillary and pubic hair changes
Caput medusae
Ecchymosis
Increased skin pigmentation
Jaundice
Palmar erythema
Pruritus
Spider angiomas

FLUID AND ELECTROLYTE
DISTURBANCES
Ascites
Decreased effective blood volume
Dilutional hyponatremia or
    hypernatremia
Hypocalcemia
Hypokalemia
Peripheral edema
Water retention

Figure 62-1 ■ The clinical picture of a client with liver dysfunction. Manifestations vary according to the progression of the disease. Early manifestations are noted in color.

- Rashes
- Purpuric lesions, such as **petechiae** (round, pinpoint, red-purple lesions) or **ecchymosis** (large purple, blue, or yellow bruises)
- Warm and bright red palms of the hands (palmar erythema)
- Vascular lesions with a red center and radiating branches, known as "**spider angiomas**" (telangiectasias, spider nevi, or vascular spiders), on the nose, cheeks, upper thorax, and shoulders
- Peripheral dependent edema of the extremities and sacrum

ABDOMINAL ASSESSMENT. Usually *massive* ascites can be detected as a distended abdomen with bulging flanks. The umbilicus may protrude, and dilated abdominal veins (caput medusae) may radiate from the umbilicus. Ascites can cause physical problems; for example, orthopnea and dyspnea from increased abdominal distention can interfere with lung expansion. The client may have difficulty maintaining an erect body posture, and problems with balance may affect walking. Inspect and palpate for the presence of inguinal or umbilical hernias, which are likely to develop in clients with ascites because of increased intra-abdominal pressure.

Minimal ascites is often more difficult to detect. Advanced assessment techniques, such as the percussion test for shifting dullness and the presence of a fluid wave, may be performed by the health care provider.

When performing an assessment of the abdomen, keep in mind that **hepatomegaly** (liver enlargement) occurs in 60% of all cases of early cirrhosis. As the liver deteriorates it may become hard and small. The advanced practice nurse or other health care provider palpates the right upper quadrant for hepatomegaly below the costal (rib cage) border. The presence of hepatomegaly may be determined by percussing for dullness over the enlarged liver.

Measure the client's abdominal girth to evaluate the progression of ascites (Figure 62-2). To measure abdominal girth, the client lies flat while the nurse pulls a tape measure

around the largest diameter of the abdomen. The girth is measured at the end of exhalation. Mark the abdominal skin and flanks to ensure the same tape measure placement on subsequent readings.

OTHER PHYSICAL ASSESSMENTS. Assess nasogastric (NG) tube drainage (if present), vomitus, and stool for the presence of blood. This may be indicated by frank blood in the excrement or by a positive result of an *o*-toluidine test for occult blood content (Hema-Check, Hematest). Gastritis, stomach ulceration, or oozing esophageal varices may be responsible for the presence of blood (**melena).**

Note the presence of **fetor hepaticus**, which is the distinctive breath odor of chronic liver disease and portal-systemic encephalopathy (PSE) and is characterized by a fruity or musty odor. Fetor hepaticus results from the inability of the damaged liver to metabolize and detoxify mercaptan, which is produced by bacterial degradation of methionine, a sulfurous amino acid.

Amenorrhea may occur in women, and men may exhibit testicular atrophy, **gynecomastia** (enlarged breasts), and impotence as a result of inactive hormones and certain diuretics. Clients with problems of the hematologic system caused by hepatic failure may have bruising, petechiae (small, purplish hemorrhagic spots on the skin), and an enlarged spleen.

Continually assess the client's neurologic functioning. Subtle changes in mentation and personality often progress to coma, a late complication of PSE. Monitor for **asterixis** (liver flap or flapping tremor), a coarse tremor characterized by rapid, nonrhythmic extensions and flexions in the wrists and fingers. Figure 62-3 illustrates the technique used to elicit asterixis during physical assessment.

PSYCHOSOCIAL ASSESSMENT

The client with hepatic cirrhosis may undergo subtle or obvious personality, cognitive, and behavior changes, such as agitation and belligerence. He or she may experience sleep pattern disturbances or may exhibit signs of emotional lability, euphoria, or depression. A psychosocial assessment identifies needs and helps guide client care.

Repeated hospitalizations are common for clients with cirrhosis. It is a life-altering chronic disease, impacting not only the client, but immediate and extended family members as well. There are significant emotional, physical, and

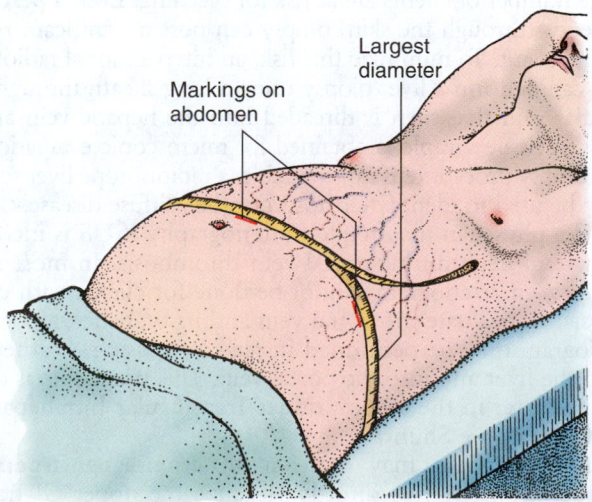

Figure 62-2 ■ How to measure abdominal girth. With the client supine, bring the tape measure around the client and take a measurement at the level of the umbilicus. Before removing the tape, mark the client's abdomen along the sides of the tape on the client's flanks (sides) and midline to ensure that later measurements are taken in the same place.

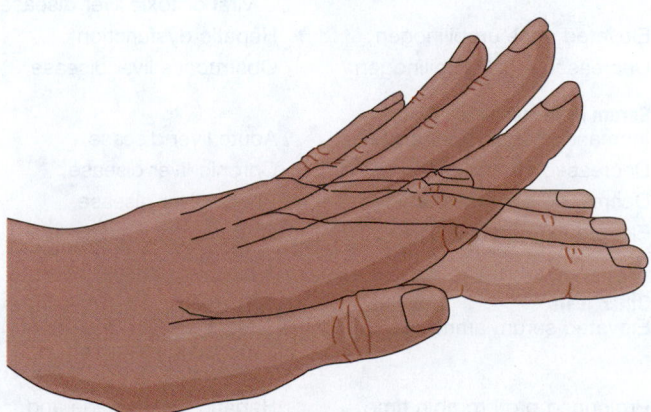

Figure 62-3 ■ To elicit asterixis (flapping tremor), have the client extend the arm, dorsiflex the wrist, and extend the fingers. Observe for rapid, nonrhythmic extensions and flexions.

financial changes. Substance abuse may continue in the face of deteriorating health. It is important, whenever possible, to use resources available to these individuals and their families. Social workers, substance abuse counselors, and mental health/behavioral health professionals should be involved in client management.

LABORATORY ASSESSMENT

Characteristic abnormalities are common in laboratory studies of clients with liver disease (Table 62-4). Serum levels of aspartate aminotransferase (AST), alanine aminotransferase (ALT), and lactate dehydrogenase (LDH) may be elevated because these enzymes are released into the blood during hepatic inflammation. However, as the liver deteriorates, the hepatocytes may be unable to create an inflammatory response and the AST and ALT may be normal.

Alkaline phosphatase levels are sensitive to mild extrahepatic or intrahepatic biliary obstruction and therefore may increase in clients with cirrhosis. Total serum bilirubin levels also rise. Indirect bilirubin levels increase in clients with cirrhosis because of the inability of the failing liver to excrete bilirubin. Therefore bilirubin is present in the urine (urobilinogen) in increased amounts. Fecal urobilinogen concentration is decreased in clients with biliary tract obstruction. These clients exhibit light- or clay-colored stools.

Total serum protein and albumin levels are decreased in clients with severe or chronic liver disease as a result of decreased synthesis by the liver. Prothrombin time (PT/INR) is prolonged because the liver decreases the synthesis of prothrombin. The platelet count is low, resulting in a characteristic thrombocytopenia of cirrhosis. Anemia may be reflected by an altered complete blood count (CBC), with decreased hemoglobin and hematocrit values. The white blood cell (WBC) count may also be decreased. Ammonia levels may be elevated in clients with advanced liver disease. Serum creatinine may be elevated as well due to deteriorating kidney function.

RADIOGRAPHIC ASSESSMENT

Plain x-rays of the abdomen may show hepatomegaly, splenomegaly, or massive ascites. A computed tomography (CT) scan may be requested if the diagnosis is more complex and ultrasound is not definitive.

OTHER DIAGNOSTIC ASSESSMENTS

Ultrasound (US) of the liver is often the first assessment for an individual with suspected liver disease to detect ascites, hepatomegaly, and splenomegaly. It can also determine the presence of biliary stones or biliary duct obstruction. Liver US is useful in detecting portal vein thrombosis and evaluating whether portal blood flow is from the portal vein into liver (normal flow) or vice versa.

Magnetic resonance imaging is another test used to diagnose and treat the client with liver disease. It can reveal mass lesions, giving additional specific information about their character. This information is helpful in determining whether the condition is malignant or benign.

Most clients being assessed for liver disease require biopsies to determine the exact pathology and the extent of disease progression. This procedure can be problematic because a large number of clients are at risk for bleeding. Even a **percutaneous** (through the skin) biopsy can pose a significant risk to the client. To minimize this risk, an interventional radiologist can perform a liver biopsy using a long sheath through a jugular vein that then is threaded into the hepatic vein and liver. A tissue sample is obtained for microscopic evaluation. If a biopsy procedure is not desirable, a radioisotope liver scan may be used to identify cirrhosis or other diffuse disease.

The physician may request arteriography if US is inconclusive in determining portal vein thrombosis. In most instances, an arteriogram cannot be done for clients with cirrhosis. To evaluate the portal vein and its branches, a portal venogram may be performed instead by passing a catheter into the liver and into the portal vein. This procedure is described later in the section under Transjugular Intrahepatic Portal-Systemic Shunt.

The physician may perform an **esophagogastroduodenoscopy** (EGD) to directly visualize the upper GI tract and to detect the presence of bleeding or oozing esophageal varices, stomach irritation and ulceration, or duodenal ulceration and bleeding. EGD is performed by introducing a flexible tube into the mouth, esophagus, and stomach while the client is under conscious sedation. A camera attached to

TABLE 62-4	Assessment of Abnormal Laboratory Findings in Liver Disease
Abnormal Finding	**Significance**
Serum Enzymes	
Elevated serum aspartate aminotransferase (AST)	Hepatic cell destruction, hepatitis (most specific indicator)
Elevated serum alanine aminotransferase (ALT)	Hepatic cell destruction, hepatitis
Elevated lactate dehydrogenase (LDH)	Hepatic cell destruction
Elevated serum alkaline phosphatase	Obstructive jaundice, hepatic metastasis
Bilirubin	
Elevated serum total bilirubin	Hepatic cell disease
Elevated serum direct conjugated bilirubin	Hepatitis, liver metastasis
Elevated serum indirect unconjugated bilirubin	Cirrhosis
Elevated urine bilirubin	Hepatocellular obstruction, viral or toxic liver disease
Elevated urine urobilinogen	Hepatic dysfunction
Decreased fecal urobilinogen	Obstructive liver disease
Serum Proteins	
Increased serum total protein	Acute liver disease
Decreased serum total protein	Chronic liver disease
Decreased serum albumin	Severe liver disease
Elevated serum globulin	Immune response to liver disease
Other Tests	
Elevated serum ammonia	Advanced liver disease or portal-systemic encephalopathy (PSE)
Prolonged prothrombin time (PT) or INR	Hepatic cell damage and synthesis of prothrombin

INR, International Normalized Ratio.

the scope permits direct visualization of the mucosal lining of the upper gastrointestinal tract. This test is discussed in detail in Chapter 56.

◆Analysis

COMMON NURSING DIAGNOSES AND COLLABORATIVE PROBLEMS

The most common nursing diagnosis for clients with cirrhosis is Excess Fluid Volume related to edema (portal hypertension).

The following are the primary collaborative problems for clients with cirrhosis:

1. Potential for Hemorrhage
2. Potential for Portal-Systemic Encephalopathy (PSE)

ADDITIONAL NURSING DIAGNOSES AND COLLABORATIVE PROBLEMS

In addition to the common nursing diagnoses and collaborative problems, clients with cirrhosis may have one or more of the following:

- Risk for Imbalanced Nutrition: Less Than Body Requirements related to inability to ingest or digest food due to biologic factors
- Ineffective Breathing Pattern related to decreased diaphragmatic excursion and pressure on the diaphragm from ascites
- Chronic Pain related to abdominal pressure
- Risk for Infection related to inadequate secondary defenses (leukopenia)
- Risk for Impaired Skin Integrity related to pruritus and altered nutritional state
- Ineffective Coping related to a high degree of threat (chronic and potentially fatal disease)
- Sexual Dysfunction related to altered hormonal function and decreased libido
- Disturbed Body Image related to biophysical changes (distended abdomen and skin lesions)

Additional collaborative problems include the following:

- Potential for Drug Toxicity
- Potential for Hypokalemia

◆Planning and Implementation

EXCESS FLUID VOLUME

NOC **PLANNING: EXPECTED OUTCOMES.** The client with cirrhosis is expected to have water balance in the intracellular and extracellular compartments of the body. Indicators include that the client will have:

- Noncompromised blood pressure
- Noncompromised peripheral pulses
- Noncompromised mean arterial pressure
- 24-hour intake and output balance
- Stable body weight
- Moist mucous membranes
- Noncompromised serum electrolytes
- Noncompromised hematocrit
- Noncompromised urine specific gravity

INTERVENTIONS. Fluid accumulations are minimal during the early stages of ascites, and therefore interventions are aimed at preventing the accumulation of additional fluid and mobilizing the existing fluid collection. Nonsurgi-cal treatment measures usually control ascites. If respiratory or abdominal functioning is compromised, surgical measures may be necessary. (See the Concept Map for chronic liver failure on p. 1376.)

NONSURGICAL MANAGEMENT. Supportive measures to control abdominal ascites include diet therapy, drugs, paracentesis, and comfort measures. The client's fluid and electrolyte status is also carefully monitored.

Diet Therapy. The health care provider usually places the client with abdominal ascites on a low sodium diet as an initial means of controlling fluid accumulation in the abdominal cavity. The amount of daily sodium intake restriction typically varies from 500 mg to 2 g. In collaboration with the dietitian, explain the purpose of the diet and advise the client and family to read the sodium content labels on all food and beverages. Table salt should be completely excluded. The absence of salt in low-sodium diets is distasteful to most people, so the dietitian suggests alternative flavoring additives such as lemon, vinegar, parsley, oregano, and pepper. Remind the client that seasoned and salty food is an acquired taste; in time he or she will become used to the decrease in dietary sodium.

The health care provider may limit the client's fluid intake if serum sodium levels fall. The kidneys retain sodium, and dilutional hyponatremia results, primarily from excessive fluid volume. IV and oral fluids are restricted to 1000 to 1500 mL/day in an effort to reverse the fluid overload and raise the serum sodium level. Calculate the permitted amount of oral fluids on the basis of the ordered IV intake. However, *it is not necessary for a client with ascites and a normal serum sodium to have fluid restriction.*

In general, clients with cirrhosis are malnourished and have multiple dietary deficiencies. Vitamin supplements, such as thiamine, folate, and multivitamin preparations, are typically added to the IV fluids because of the inability of the liver to store vitamins. Oral vitamins are given when IV fluid administration is discontinued.

Drug Therapy. The health care provider usually prescribes a diuretic to reduce fluid accumulation and to prevent cardiac and respiratory impairment. Monitor the effect of diuretic therapy by assessing intake and output, weighing the client daily, measuring abdominal girth, documenting peripheral edema, and assessing electrolyte levels. Serious electrolyte imbalances, such as hypokalemia (decreased potassium) and hyponatremia (decreased sodium), may accompany diuretic therapy. (See Chapter 16 for a discussion of electrolyte imbalances.) Depending on the diuretic selected, the provider may prescribe an oral or IV potassium supplement. Many clinicians prescribe a combination of furosemide (Lasix) and spironolactone (Aldactone) as a combination diuretic therapy for the treatment of ascites. Because of their different mechanisms of action, they are utilized for maintenance of sodium and potassium balance.

Keep in mind that all clients with ascites have the potential to develop SBP (spontaneous bacterial peritonitis). In some individuals, the presentation can be with very mild symptoms of low-grade fever and loss of appetite. In others, there may be abdominal pain, fever, rigors, and change in mental status.

Paracentesis. Abdominal **paracentesis** may be indicated if dietary restrictions and drug administration fail to control ascites (Chart 62-1). The procedure is performed at the bedside. The physician inserts a trocar catheter into the abdomen to remove and drain ascitic fluid from the peri-

CONCEPT MAP Cirrhosis

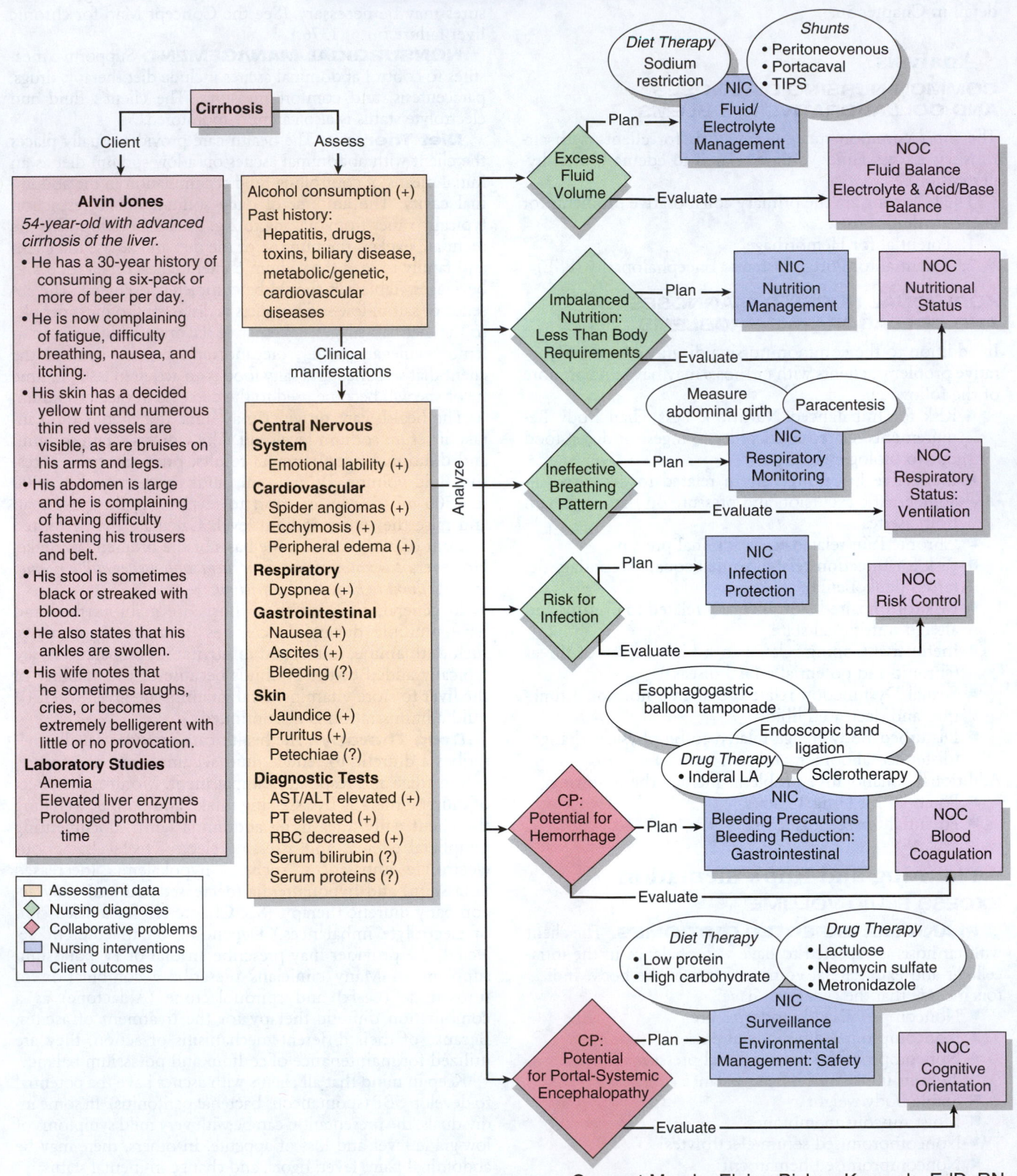

Cirrhosis

Client | Assess

Alvin Jones

54-year-old with advanced cirrhosis of the liver.

• He has a 30-year history of consuming a six-pack or more of beer per day.

• He is now complaining of fatigue, difficulty breathing, nausea, and itching.

• His skin has a decided yellow tint and numerous thin red vessels are visible, as are bruises on his arms and legs.

• His abdomen is large and he is complaining of having difficulty fastening his trousers and belt.

• His stool is sometimes black or streaked with blood.

• He also states that his ankles are swollen.

• His wife notes that he sometimes laughs, cries, or becomes extremely belligerent with little or no provocation.

Laboratory Studies
Anemia
Elevated liver enzymes
Prolonged prothrombin time

☐ Assessment data
◇ Nursing diagnoses
◆ Collaborative problems
☐ Nursing interventions
☐ Client outcomes

Alcohol consumption (+)
Past history:
Hepatitis, drugs, toxins, biliary disease, metabolic/genetic, cardiovascular diseases

Clinical manifestations

Central Nervous System
Emotional lability (+)
Cardiovascular
Spider angiomas (+)
Ecchymosis (+)
Peripheral edema (+)
Respiratory
Dyspnea (+)
Gastrointestinal
Nausea (+)
Ascites (+)
Bleeding (?)
Skin
Jaundice (+)
Pruritus (+)
Petechiae (?)
Diagnostic Tests
AST/ALT elevated (+)
PT elevated (+)
RBC decreased (+)
Serum bilirubin (?)
Serum proteins (?)

Analyze

Diet Therapy
Sodium restriction

Shunts
• Peritoneovenous
• Portacaval
• TIPS

Excess Fluid Volume

Plan → **NIC** Fluid/Electrolyte Management

Evaluate → **NOC** Fluid Balance Electrolyte & Acid/Base Balance

Imbalanced Nutrition: Less Than Body Requirements

Plan → **NIC** Nutrition Management

Evaluate → **NOC** Nutritional Status

Measure abdominal girth | Paracentesis

Ineffective Breathing Pattern

Plan → **NIC** Respiratory Monitoring

Evaluate → **NOC** Respiratory Status: Ventilation

Risk for Infection

Plan → **NIC** Infection Protection

Evaluate → **NOC** Risk Control

Esophagogastric balloon tamponade

Endoscopic band ligation

Drug Therapy
• Inderal LA

Sclerotherapy

CP: Potential for Hemorrhage

Plan → **NIC** Bleeding Precautions Bleeding Reduction: Gastrointestinal

Evaluate → **NOC** Blood Coagulation

Diet Therapy
• Low protein
• High carbohydrate

Drug Therapy
• Lactulose
• Neomycin sulfate
• Metronidazole

CP: Potential for Portal-Systemic Encephalopathy

Plan → **NIC** Surveillance Environmental Management: Safety

Evaluate → **NOC** Cognitive Orientation

Concept Map by Elaine Bishop Kennedy, EdD, RN

CHART 62-1

BEST PRACTICE for
The Client with Paracentesis

- Explain the procedure and answer client questions.
- Obtain vital signs, including weight.
- Ask the client to void.
- Position the client in bed with the head of the bed elevated.
- Monitor vital signs per protocol or physician's orders.
- Measure the drainage and record accurately.
- Describe the collected fluid.
- Label and send the fluid for laboratory analysis; document in the client record that specimens were sent.
- After the physician removes the catheter, apply a dressing to the site; assess for leakage.
- Maintain bedrest per protocol.
- Weigh the client after the paracentesis; document in the client record weight both before and after paracentesis.

CHART 62-2

NIC INTERVENTION ACTIVITIES for
The Client with Cirrhosis

Fluid/Electrolyte Management: *Regulation and prevention of complications from altered fluid and/or electrolyte levels*
- Obtain laboratory specimens for monitoring of altered fluid and electrolyte levels (e.g., hematocrit, BUN, protein, sodium, and potassium levels), as appropriate.
- Keep an accurate record of intake and output.
- Weigh client daily and monitor trends.
- Monitor for signs and symptoms of fluid retention.
- Monitor vital signs, as appropriate.
- Administer prescribed supplemental electrolytes, as appropriate.

Bleeding Precautions: *Reduction of stimuli that may induce bleeding or hemorrhage in at-risk clients*
- Monitor the client closely for hemorrhage.
- Monitor for signs and symptoms of persistent bleeding (e.g., check all secretions for frank or occult blood)
- Monitor coagulation studies, including prothrombin time (PT), partial thromboplastin time (PTT), fibrinogen, fibrin degradation/split products, and platelet counts, as appropriate.
- Monitor orthostatic vital signs, including blood pressure.
- Use electric razor, instead of straight-edge, for shaving.
- Use soft toothbrush or toothettes for oral care.
- Avoid injections (IV, IM, or SC), as appropriate.
- Protect the client from trauma, which may cause bleeding.

Neurologic Monitoring: *Collection and analysis of client data to prevent or minimize neurologic complications*
- Monitor level of consciousness.
- Monitor level of orientation.
- Monitor recent memory, attention span, past memory, mood, affect, and behaviors.
- Monitor vital signs: temperature, blood pressure, pulse, and respirations.

NIC intervention activities selected from Dochterman, J.M., & Bulechek, G.M. (Eds.). (2004). *Nursing interventions classification (NIC)* (4th ed.). St. Louis: Mosby. No part of this work is to be altered without prior written permission from the Publisher.
BUN, Blood urea nitrogen; *SC,* subcutaneous.

toneal cavity. This procedure is also done using ultrasound for added safety. In some situations, a short-term ascites drain catheter may be placed while the client is awaiting surgical intervention.

Once a primary treatment modality for ascites, paracentesis is more commonly used as a diagnostic tool to examine ascitic fluid. If SBP is suspected, ascitic fluid is withdrawn (10 to 20 mL) and sent for cell count and culture. If the client is symptomatic for infection, the physician may prescribe antibiotics while awaiting the culture results.

Paracentesis is also used as a palliative measure to relieve abdominal pressure because ascites may cause severe respiratory and abdominal distress. To relieve acute symptoms, the physician slowly drains the ascitic fluid (usually 1 to 3 L). Hypovolemia with a fluid volume deficit may occur with rapid fluid removal because these clients have adjusted to the excessive fluid volume in the abdomen. *Rapid, drastic removal of ascitic fluid leads to decreased abdominal pressure, which may contribute to vasodilation and shock.* Observe for impending signs of shock, such as hypotension and tachycardia, from fluid shifts during and immediately after the procedure.

Some physicians prescribe an albumin or other volume replacer infusion during paracentesis to avoid depleting the intravascular space and to avoid hypotension.

Repeated paracentesis procedures are discouraged because of the increased incidence of protein depletion, hypovolemia, and electrolyte imbalances. A low-sodium diet and diuretics are preferred as ways to control ascites.

Comfort Measures. Excessive ascitic fluid volume in the abdomen may cause the client to experience respiratory difficulty. Dyspnea may develop as a result of increased intra-abdominal pressure, which limits thoracic expansion and diaphragmatic excursion. The nurse or assistive nursing personnel elevates the head of the bed to at least 30 degrees or as high as the client wishes in an effort to minimize shortness of breath. The client is encouraged to sit in a chair. This upright position, with his or her feet elevated to discourage dependent ankle edema, often relieves dyspnea.

To weigh the client, the nurse or assistive nursing personnel uses a standard upright bedside scale if the client can stand. Weighing on a bed scale necessitates that the client lie flat; this supine position can cause the client to feel increasingly short of breath and can increase anxiety.

NIC Fluid/Electrolyte Management. Fluid and electrolyte imbalances are common as a result of the disease or treatment. Laboratory tests, such as blood urea nitrogen (BUN), serum protein, hematocrit, and electrolytes help determine fluid and electrolyte status. Nursing intervention activities are listed in Chart 62-2.

SURGICAL MANAGEMENT. When medical management fails to control ascites, the physician may choose surgical intervention to divert ascites into the venous system by creating a shunt. Clients with ascites are poor surgical risks. The **peritoneovenous shunt** has a pressure-sensitive one-way valve allowing ascitic fluid to flow from the abdominal cavity to the superior vena cava. Complications associated with this procedure include infection and thrombosis of the shunt. The **portacaval shunt** may also result in improvement in ascites (Figure 62-4). If symptoms return after placement of a shunt, a nuclear medicine examination called a peritoneal shunt evaluation may be requested. A radiologist injects a radioisotope tracer into the ascitic fluid in the abdomen or directly into the valve of the shunt. If functioning normally, the tracer should be seen in the shunt within about 10 minutes.

More recently, the **TIPS (transjugular intrahepatic portalsystemic shunt)** nonsurgical procedure has been the used to control refractory ascites and to reduce variceal bleeding. This procedure is described under the Interventions section for Potential for Hemorrhage on p. 1379.

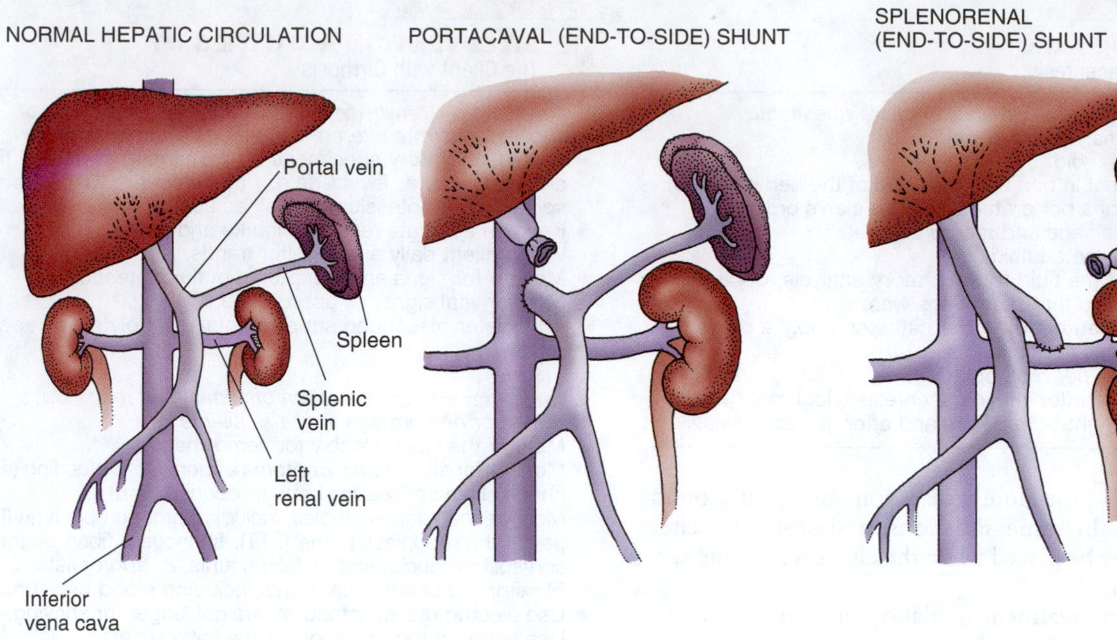

NORMAL HEPATIC CIRCULATION   PORTACAVAL (END-TO-SIDE) SHUNT   SPLENORENAL (END-TO-SIDE) SHUNT

Figure 62-4 ■ Surgical shunting diverts portal venous blood flow from the liver to decrease portal and esophageal pressure.

The client with cirrhosis has many underlying medical problems; an optimal physical state is desired before surgery is performed. Electrolyte imbalances are corrected, and abnormal coagulation is treated with the administration of fresh frozen plasma and vitamin K. Packed red blood cells are made available for transfusion, because these clients have bleeding tendencies.

Provide the usual postoperative care for a client undergoing abdominal surgery (see Chapter 22). Remain aware that the ascitic fluid is routed into the venous system, resulting in vascular volume expansion and hemodilution. Vital signs are monitored carefully; an increase in blood pressure reflects an increase in vascular volume. If the client has a central venous or pulmonary artery catheter in place, determine whether pressure is elevated. Breath sounds are auscultated for the presence of crackles, which indicates excessive lung fluid. A diuretic, such as furosemide (Lasix), is usually prescribed to rid the body of excessive fluid. Note any abnormal results of coagulation studies (prothrombin time [PT] and partial thromboplastin time [PTT]). The nurse or assistive nursing personnel measures the client's weight, abdominal girth, and urine output each shift to determine the effectiveness of the shunting procedure.

POTENTIAL FOR HEMORRHAGE

PLANNING: EXPECTED OUTCOMES. The client is expected to not have bleeding episodes. However, if the client experiences hemorrhage, it is expected to be controlled through medical and nursing interventions.

INTERVENTIONS. During the acute phase of bleeding, early interventions are based on identifying the source of bleeding and initiating treatment to halt it. Because massive esophageal bleeding can cause rapid blood loss, emergency interventions are initiated. If the client is a known alcoholic with a history of variceal bleeding, measures to treat the esophageal varices are initiated and therefore valuable time is not wasted looking for another source of bleeding.

NONSURGICAL MANAGEMENT. The role of drug therapy is to *prevent* bleeding in clients where varices are present. If bleeding occurs, the health care team intervenes quickly to control it by providing interventions, such as gastric intubation, balloon tamponade, blood products, endoscopic band ligation, or endoscopic injection sclerotherapy. After the acute bleeding episode has been controlled, the client may require a transjugular intrahepatic portal-systemic shunt (TIPS) to decrease portal hypertension, thereby decreasing the risk of further variceal bleeding. The client is managed in the critical care unit.

Drug Therapy. To *prevent* the incidence of esophageal hemorrhage, the client with esophageal varices may be placed on a nonselective beta-blocking agent such as the long-acting form of propranolol (Inderal LA). The client is started on a low dose that is increased every 3 to 5 days until the heart rate is about 55 beats/min. By decreasing heart rate and the hepatic venous pressure gradient, the chance of bleeding may be reduced.

Gastric Intubation. The client's reports of hematemesis or melena should be rapidly investigated. A nasogastric tube is placed when GI bleeding is known or suspected and gastric lavage is performed until the fluid returned is clear. **Lavage** is the introduction of saline or water into the nasogastric tube to achieve vasoconstriction of the bleeding gastric ulceration or varices. When lavage is unsuccessful, more aggressive therapy is indicated.

Esophagogastric Balloon Tamponade. If hematemesis has occurred because of bleeding esophageal varices, gastric lavage has been unsuccessful, and emergent endoscopy is not available, the physician usually inserts an esophagogastric tamponade tube. This is a temporary measure to avoid the complications of hemorrhage.

The classic method of treating bleeding esophageal varices is by compressing the bleeding vessels with an esophagogastric tube, such as the Sengstaken-Blakemore tube (Blakemore tube), which has two balloons. This type of tube is also referred to as a **tamponade tube.** When inflated, the large esophageal balloon compresses the esophagus. The smaller gastric balloon helps anchor the tube and exerts pressure against bleeding varices in the distal esophagus and the cardia of the stomach. A third lumen terminates in the stomach and is connected to suction, allowing the aspiration of gastric contents and blood. A Salem sump tube is used in conjunction with the Sengstaken-Blakemore tube and is placed in the proximal esophagus to enable clearing of collected esophageal secretions, saliva, and blood.

Before the physician inserts the tube, the nurse should inspect it and inflate and deflate the balloons to check for integrity and leaks. Each lumen is identified and labeled to prevent errors in adding or removing pressure and air volume.

The physician typically anesthetizes the client's nose and oropharynx, introduces the tube, and gently inserts it into the stomach. Alert clients who can follow directions to take sips of water through a straw. Often, though, these clients are encephalopathic and unable to cooperate, requiring soft restraints or sedation. After tube placement is verified, the stomach is aspirated and irrigated. The balloon is inflated with the recommended volume of air. The correct lumens are clamped, and the tube is then pulled back gently until the correct resistance is felt. Assist the physician in securing the tube and applying traction, which provides additional tamponading pressure. This is accomplished through various traction devices. One method is to secure it to an overbed traction apparatus and applying a 1-pound (0.45-kg) traction weight. Inflation of the balloon should be monitored using a manometry device at the bedside.

The most serious complications of esophageal tamponade are aspiration and airway occlusion. Aspiration of blood and gastric contents may lead to pneumonia. Airway occlusion and asphyxia can occur from tube displacement. It is imperative to monitor the client's respiratory status. Asphyxia can be prevented by tube deflation and extraction. It is standard practice to have surgical scissors at the bedside of these clients so that in an emergency, all tube lumens can be quickly cut distally to the bifurcation points to allow for removal.

Placement of the tamponade tube should halt variceal bleeding. After bleeding is controlled, the traction is released, and esophageal pressure is gradually decreased. The gastric balloon is deflated, and the tube is removed. Another tube should be kept at the bedside for potential reinsertion if bleeding recurs.

Blood Transfusions. Massive hemorrhage necessitates replacement by blood products. Blood is drawn to identify the client's blood type. Until the blood is available, administer IV fluids or colloid (plasma) volumes, as prescribed, into large-bore IV access routes to maintain blood pressure.

Give packed red blood cells and fresh frozen plasma (per physician order and agency policy) to replace blood volume and clotting factors. The physician and the nurse monitor trends in hemoglobin and hematocrit levels, and additional blood products are transfused as indicated.

Endoscopic Procedures. Esophageal varices may be treated with **endoscopic band ligation.** This involves the application of small "O" bands around the base of the varices to cut off blood supply. The client is unaware of the bands and they cause no discomfort. An IV infusion of the drug octreotide may be given to the client with bleeding esophageal varices before the procedure to reduce blood flow.

Injection **sclerotherapy** may also be employed to stop variceal bleeding. This is also done through an endoscopic procedure. The varices are injected with a sclerosing agent via a catheter. There is potential for this procedure to cause mucosal ulceration, which could result in further bleeding. Because of the lower potential for treatment-related side effects, band ligation is typically used for long-term obliteration.

Transjugular Intrahepatic Portal-Systemic Shunt. Insertion of a transjugular intrahepatic portal-systemic shunt (TIPS) is a nonsurgical procedure performed in larger interventional radiology departments. This procedure is done for clients who have not responded to other modalities for hemorrhage or intractable ascites. If time permits, clients have an ultrasound to assess vein anatomy and patency. The client receives moderate IV sedation or heavy general anesthesia for this procedure. The radiologist places a large sheath into the jugular vein and places it into a hepatic vein. A needle is guided through the sheath and pushed through the liver into the portal vein. A balloon enlarges this tract and a metal stent keeps it open. Most clients have an ultrasound Doppler study of the liver after the TIPS procedure to record the blood flow through the shunt.

Serious complications of a TIPS are not common. Clients are discharged in 2 to 4 days and are followed up with ultrasounds for the first year after the shunt is placed. About one third of clients with a TIPS need to be re-ballooned once during the first year as an ambulatory care procedure.

SURGICAL MANAGEMENT. Traditional portal-systemic shunts are considered a last resort intervention for clients with portal hypertension and bleeding esophageal varices. Surgical bypass shunting procedures decrease portal hypertension by diverting a portion of the portal vein blood flow from the liver.

Recurrent esophageal variceal bleeding after a portal-systemic shunt is not uncommon and may indicate the return of elevated portal pressures caused by a thrombosed (clotted) shunt. A rapid reaccumulation of abdominal fluid may also suggest a failed shunt. Continue to measure the client's abdominal girth and report sudden girth increases to the physician. Be alert for the development of post-shunt encephalopathy, because it is common in clients receiving either a shunt or TIPS procedure (see care measures for portal-systemic encephalopathy [PSE] in the next section).

Monitor the client closely for hemorrhage. Coagulation studies, including prothrombin time (PT), partial thromboplastin time (PTT), platelet count, and International Normalized Ratio (INR), are also monitored carefully. Chart 62-2 lists additional interventions for clients at risk for bleeding.

Other techniques that are being used are electrocautery, cryoablation, and laser procedures via laparoscopic surgery.

Critical Thinking Challenge

You are the nurse for a middle-aged client with cirrhosis caused by alcoholic liver disease. You go into the client's room and find the client in the bathroom vomiting what appears to be hematemesis (blood in the vomitus).

1. What actions will you take immediately?
2. In what order of priority should you implement these interventions?
3. How can you differentiate between a gastrointestinal bleed and an esophageal bleed?

evolve For suggested answer guidelines, go to http://evolve.elsevier.com/Iggy/.

POTENTIAL FOR PORTAL-SYSTEMIC ENCEPHALOPATHY

PLANNING: EXPECTED OUTCOMES. It is expected that the nurse report and document findings for clients who exhibit early signs of portal-systemic encephalopathy (PSE).

INTERVENTIONS. The mechanisms that produce portal systemic encephalopathy are not completely clear, but ammonia probably plays a significant role. The poorly functioning liver cannot convert ammonia and other byproducts of metabolism to a less toxic form. They are carried by the circulatory system to the brain where there is interference with normal cerebral function. The aim of PSE management is to halt this process.

Because ammonia is formed in the gastrointestinal (GI) tract by the action of bacteria on protein, nonsurgical treatment measures to decrease ammonia production include dietary limitations and drug therapy to reduce bacterial breakdown. Collaborate with the dietitian and physician to plan and implement these treatment measures.

Diet Therapy. The client with cirrhosis has increased nutritional requirements. In general, the client needs high-carbohydrate, moderate-fat, and high-protein foods. However, the diet is often modified for clients who have elevated serum ammonia levels and exhibit the signs of PSE.

The diet for a client with PSE or elevated ammonia levels usually includes low-protein foods and simple carbohydrates. There have been suggestions that vegetable protein is preferred over animal protein for this population. It is important to include family members or significant others in nutritional counseling. The client is often weak and unable to remember complicated guidelines. Brief, simple directions regarding dietary do's and don'ts are recommended. Keep in mind any financial or cultural limitations when discussing food choices.

When a client with cirrhosis experiences GI bleeding, it can result in the formation of increased amounts of ammonia as intestinal bacteria attempt to metabolize the blood cells. GI bleeding may precipitate hepatic coma (stage IV of PSE). These clients are maintained on nothing by mouth (NPO) status with a nasogastric (NG) tube or an esophageal tamponade tube, depending on the source of the bleeding.

Drug Therapy. Medications are used sparingly because they are difficult for the failing liver to metabolize. In particular, opioid analgesics, sedatives, and barbiturates should be restricted, especially for the client with a history of encephalopathy.

Several types of drugs, however, can eliminate or reduce ammonia levels in the body. These include lactulose, neomycin sulfate, and metronidazole.

Lactulose. The health care provider prescribes lactulose to promote the excretion of ammonia in the stool. Lactulose, a disaccharide with high molecular weight, is a viscous, sticky, sweet-tasting liquid that is administered either orally or by NG tube. The purpose is to obtain a laxative effect; cleansing the bowels rids the intestinal tract of the toxins that contribute to encephalopathy. The drug is prescribed to the client who has manifested signs of PSE, regardless of the stage.

Lactulose retention enemas may be necessary when the client cannot tolerate oral administration or when liquids are contraindicated in the upper GI tract.

Lactulose creates an acidic environment in the bowel by keeping ammonia in its ionized state; this decreases the pH of the colon from 7 to 5. A decreased pH causes ammonia to leave the circulatory system and move into the colon, which reverses the normal passage of ammonia from the colon to the bloodstream.

The desired effect of the drug is production of two to five soft stools per day and a decrease in client confusion caused by PSE. During the acute phase of PSE, 20 to 30 g of lactulose is administered at 4-hour intervals until stools are achieved; the dosage is then decreased to three or four times daily.

Observe for response to lactulose. The client may complain of intestinal bloating and cramping. Serum ammonia levels may be monitored but do not always correlate with symptoms. Hypokalemia and dehydration may result from excessive stools.

Neomycin Sulfate. Neomycin sulfate (Mycifradin), a broad-spectrum antibiotic, is given to act as an intestinal antiseptic. It destroys the normal flora in the bowel, diminishing protein breakdown and decreasing the rate of ammonia production. Maintenance doses of neomycin are given orally, but may also be administered as a retention enema. Long-term use has the potential for renal toxicity and, therefore, it is used with caution.

Metronidazole. Metronidazole (Flagyl, Novonidazole✱) is a broad-spectrum antibiotic with similar action to neomycin, but it has less potential for renal toxicity. It is used both as a single agent or in combination with lactulose for treatment and prophylaxis of PSE.

NIC **Neurologic Monitoring.** The nurse or assistive nursing personnel continually assesses for changes in level of consciousness and orientation (see Chart 62-2). An individualized neurologic assessment is developed for each client and includes the assessment of simple tasks such as name writing, bilateral hand grasping, and serial subtractions and additions. Continually assess for the presence of asterixis (liver flap) and fetor hepaticus (liver breath). These signs suggest worsening encephalopathy.

> ### Critical Thinking Challenge
>
> You are caring for a client in the prodromal stage of portal systemic encephalopathy (PSE).
> 1. In planning care, which common medications are hepatotoxic and should be avoided?
> 2. What type of dietary restrictions might be ordered?
> 3. How will you maintain the client's safety?
> 4. For what signs and symptoms indicating worsening PSE will you be observing?
>
> _evolve_ For suggested answer guidelines, go to http://evolve.elsevier.com/Iggy/.

Community-Based Care

If the client with hepatic cirrhosis survives life-threatening complications, he or she is usually discharged to the home or to a long-term care facility after treatment measures have combated the acute medical problems. A home care referral may be needed if the client is discharged to the home. These chronically ill clients are often readmitted, and community-based care is aimed at preventing rehospitalization. The client may benefit from hospice care. A case manager is often needed to coordinate interdisciplinary care.

CHART 62-3

CLIENT EDUCATION GUIDE
Cirrhosis

Diet Therapy
- Consume a diet that adheres to the guidelines set by your physician, nurse, or dietitian.
- If you have excessive fluid in your abdomen, follow the low-sodium diet prescribed for you.
- Eat small, frequent meals that are nutritionally well balanced.
- Include in your diet daily supplemental liquids (e.g., Ensure or Ensure Plus) and a multivitamin; low-protein supplements are available if needed.

Drug Therapy
- Take the diuretics or preventive beta blocker prescribed for you. If you experience muscle weakness, irregular heartbeat, or light-headedness, contact your health care provider right away.
- Take the medication prescribed for you that helps prevent gastrointestinal bleeding.
- Take the lactulose syrup as prescribed to maintain three to five bowel movements every day.
- Do *not* take any other medication unless specifically prescribed by your health care provider.

Alcohol Abstinence
- Do not consume any alcohol.
- Seek support services for help if needed.

HOME CARE MANAGEMENT

The nurse, case manager, client, and family or significant other should identify any physical adaptations needed to prepare the client's home for convalescence. The client's rest area needs to be close to a bathroom, because diuretic therapy increases the frequency of urination. If the client has difficulty reaching the toilet, additional equipment (e.g., urinals, bedpans, and bedside commodes) is necessary. Special, adult-sized incontinence pads or briefs may be helpful if the client has an altered mental status and has urinary incontinence.

Initial home activity may be limited for the client who has undergone surgical intervention. If the client experiences shortness of breath from massive ascites, elevating the head of the bed and maintaining the client in a semi-Fowler's to high Fowler's position may help alleviate respiratory distress. Alternatively, a reclining chair with a foot elevator may be used.

HEALTH TEACHING

The client is discharged to the home setting with an individualized teaching plan (Chart 62-3) that covers diet therapy, drug therapy, and alcohol abstinence.

DIET THERAPY. In collaboration with the dietitian, and in keeping with the client's financial and cultural status, provide dietary instructions. The client with portal-systemic encephalopathy (PSE) must avoid high-protein foods at home to decrease the incidence of progressive neurologic dysfunction. If the client's nutritional intake is decreased after discharge, multivitamin supplements and supplemental liquid feedings (e.g., Ensure, Boost) are usually needed.

DRUG THERAPY. The client is often discharged while receiving diuretics. Provide instructions regarding the health care provider's prescription for the diuretic. Teach the client

about side effects of therapy, such as hypokalemia. The client may need to take a potassium supplement.

If the client has had problems with bleeding from gastric ulcers, the provider may prescribe an H_2-receptor antagonist agent or proton pump inhibitor. Clients who have had episodes of SBP (spontaneous bacterial peritonitis) may be on a daily maintenance antibiotic. Because many of these individuals have alienated relatives over the years because of substance abuse, it may be necessary to help the client identify a friend, neighbor, or person in their recovery group to assist with medications.

Families and significant others should be informed about how to recognize signs of PSE and be instructed that it is necessary and safe to increase the daily lactulose at the first sign of encephalopathy. The health care provider should also be contacted. Clients and family members are reminded that constipation, bleeding, and infections may lead to PSE. They should also understand that PSE is usually reversible.

Advise the client to avoid all over-the-counter medications and to consult the physician for follow-up medical care. Remind the client and family to notify the physician immediately if any gastrointestinal (GI) bleeding is noted so that re-evaluation can be initiated quickly.

ALCOHOL ABSTINENCE. One of the most important aspects of ongoing care for the nurse to stress is the need to avoid alcohol and illicit drugs (see Chapter 8). By avoiding alcohol and drugs, the client:
- Prevents further fibrosis of the liver from scarring
- Allows the liver to heal and regenerate
- Prevents gastric and esophageal irritation
- Reduces the incidence of bleeding
- Prevents other life-threatening complications

HEALTH CARE RESOURCES

The client with chronic cirrhosis may require a home care nurse. The home care nurse can also monitor the effectiveness of drug therapy or the surgical shunt in controlling ascites. The encephalopathic client may need to be monitored for compliance with medications. For the individual recovering from bacterial peritonitis, home infusion of antibiotics may be needed. Individual and group therapy sessions may be arranged to assist clients in dealing with alcohol abstinence if they are too ill to attend a formal treatment program. The nurse may refer the client and family to self-help groups, such as Alcoholics Anonymous and Al-Anon. The client may also desire spiritual support. Finances are frequently a problem for the chronically ill client and family; social support and community services need to be identified. The American Liver Foundation is an excellent source for more information about liver disease.

◆ Evaluation: Outcomes

Evaluate the care of the client with cirrhosis on the basis of the identified nursing diagnoses and collaborative problems. The expected outcomes include that the client will:
- Experience a decrease in or no ascites
- Have electrolytes within normal limits (WNL)
- Have blood pressure WNL
- Not experience hemorrhage or will be managed immediately if bleeding occurs
- Not experience PSE or will be managed immediately if PSE occurs

- Avoid the development of SBP (spontaneous bacterial peritonitis)
- Have the optimal quality of life possible

Specific indicators for these outcomes are listed for each nursing diagnosis and collaborative problem under the Planning and Implementation section (see earlier).

HEPATITIS

PATHOPHYSIOLOGY

Hepatitis is the widespread inflammation of liver cells. *Viral* hepatitis is the most prevalent type and can be either acute or chronic. **Viral hepatitis** results from an infection caused by one of five major categories of viruses:

- Hepatitis A virus (HAV)
- Hepatitis B virus (HBV)
- Hepatitis C virus (HCV)
- Hepatitis D virus (HDV)
- Hepatitis E virus (HEV)

Hepatitis F and G have also been identified but are uncommon.

Liver injury with inflammation can also develop after exposure to a number of pharmacologic and chemical agents by inhalation, ingestion, or parenteral (IV) administration. **Toxic and drug-induced hepatitis** can result from exposure to hepatotoxins (e.g., industrial toxins, alcohol, and medications).

Hepatitis may also occur as a secondary infection during the course of infections with other viruses, such as Epstein-Barr, herpes simplex, varicella-zoster, and cytomegalovirus.

After the liver has been exposed to causative agents (e.g., a virus), it becomes enlarged and congested with inflammatory cells, lymphocytes, and fluid, resulting in right upper quadrant pain and discomfort. As the disease progresses, the liver's normal lobular pattern becomes distorted as a result of widespread inflammation, necrosis, and hepatocellular regeneration. This distortion increases pressure within the portal circulation, interfering with the blood flow into the hepatic lobules. Edema of the liver's bile channels results in intrahepatic obstructive **jaundice** (yellowing of the skin).

Classification of Hepatitis and Etiologies

VIRAL HEPATITIS

The five types of acute viral hepatitis vary by mode of transmission, manner of onset, and incubation periods (Table 62-5).

HEPATITIS A. The causative agent of **hepatitis A**, hepatitis A virus (HAV), is a ribonucleic acid (RNA) virus of the enterovirus family. HAV is characterized by a mild course similar to that of a typical viral syndrome and often goes unrecognized. It is spread via the fecal-oral route by the oral ingestion of fecal contaminants. Sources of infection include contaminated water, shellfish caught in contaminated water, and food contaminated by food handlers infected with HAV. The virus may also be spread by oral-anal sexual activity. The incubation period of hepatitis A is usually 15 to 50 days. The disease is usually not life threatening, but its course may be more severe in individuals older than 40 years of age. Hepatitis A can also complicate pre-existing liver disease.

Many people have had hepatitis A and do not know it. The course is similar to that of a gastrointestinal illness and the disease and recovery are usually uneventful.

HEPATITIS B. The **hepatitis B** virus (HBV) is not transmitted like HAV. It is a double-shelled particle containing deoxyribonucleic acid (DNA) composed of a core antigen (HBcAg), a surface antigen (HBsAg), and another antigen found within the core (HBeAg) that circulates in the blood. HBV may be spread through the following modes of transmission:

- Unprotected sexual intercourse with an infected partner (heterosexual and homosexual)
- Sharing needles
- Accidental needle sticks or injuries from sharp instruments (primarily in health care workers)
- Blood transfusions (that have not been screened for the virus)
- Hemodialysis
- Maternal-fetal route

The clinical course of hepatitis B may be varied. Symptoms usually occur within 25 to 180 days of exposure and include the following:

- Anorexia, nausea, and vomiting
- Fever
- Fatigue
- Right upper quadrant pain
- Dark urine with light stool
- Joint pain
- Jaundice

Blood tests confirm the disease, although about 40% of people with hepatitis B have no symptoms.

Most adults who get hepatitis B recover, clear the virus from their body, and develop immunity. However, up to 10% of clients with the disease do not develop immunity become carriers. **Hepatitis carriers** can infect others even though they are not sick and demonstrate no obvious signs of hepatitis B. Chronic carriers are at high risk for cirrhosis and liver cancer.

HEPATITIS C. The causative virus of **hepatitis C (HCV)** is an enveloped, single-stranded RNA virus. Transmission is blood to blood. The rate of sexual transmission is very low, and it is rarely transmitted from mother to fetus.

HCV is most commonly spread by:

- Illicit IV drug needle sharing (highest incidence)
- Blood, blood products, or organ transplants received before 1992
- Needle stick injury with HCV-contaminated blood (health care workers at high risk)
- Tattoos (unsanitary tattoo equipment)
- Intranasal cocaine use (sharing of intranasal cocaine)

The disease is **not** transmitted by casual contact or by intimate household contact. However, those infected are advised not to share razors, toothbrushes or pierced earrings, because there may be microscopic blood on these items.

The incubation period for HCV is 21 to 140 days, with an average incubation period of 7 weeks. Acute infection and illness is not common. Most individuals are completely unaware that they have been infected. They are asymptomatic and not diagnosed until many months or years after the initial exposure when an abnormality is detected during a routine laboratory evaluation or when symptoms of liver impairment appear. Unlike with hepatitis B, most people infected with hepatitis C do not clear the virus and a chronic infection develops.

HCV usually does its damage over decades by causing a chronic inflammation in the liver that eventually causes the

TABLE 62-5   Differential Features of the Five Types of Viral Hepatitis

Hepatitis A	Hepatitis B	Hepatitis C	Hepatitis D	Hepatitis E
Synonyms				
Infectious hepatitis	Serum hepatitis	Non-A, non-B hepatitis		Epidemic non-A, non-B hepatitis or enterically transmitted hepatitis
Diagnosis of Acute Disease				
Anti-HAV IgM in serum	HBsAg in serum	Anti-HCV in serum	Anti-HDV in serum	Anti-HEV in serum
Incubation Period				
15-50 days	48-180 days	14-180 days	14-56 days	15-64 days
High-Risk Groups				
More common in young children and institutional settings	All age-groups affected, especially drug addicts and health care workers	All ages of drug users Persons with hemophilia	Drug addicts Persons with hepatitis B	Persons living in underdeveloped countries
Season				
Fall and early winter	All year	All year	All year	All year
Transmission				
Usually by oral-fecal route among persons living in close contact; ingestion of contaminated water or contaminated shellfish	Primarily blood; drug abuse, sexual contact, mother to child at birth	Primarily blood; drug abuse, sexual contact (rarely), mother to child at birth	Co-infects with hepatitis B; nonpercutaneous; close personal contact	Oral-fecal route; transmitted principally by contaminated water
Clinical Findings				
Majority of type A infections (mild and anicteric); symptoms similar to those of influenza	Changes similar to those of hepatitis A Fatigue, anorexia, low-grade fever, abdominal discomfort, arthralgias, rashes, enlarged and tender liver, light stools, dark urine, jaundice Elevated serum AST and ALT levels (early), hyperbilirubinemia, abnormal liver function test results	Changes similar to those of hepatitis A Tends to have more severe symptoms; sometimes necessitates hospitalization for extended periods	Changes similar to those of hepatitis A, but symptoms often more severe than those in hepatitis A and hepatitis B Often asymptomatic	Resembles hepatitis A
Virus in Feces?				
Yes	Not infectious	Not identified	Not identified	Possible
Virus in Serum?				
Anti-HAV in serum during acute phase and incubation period is rare	HBsAg is in serum throughout the clinical course	Anti-HVC test is about 95% reliable; often takes up to 8 weeks to show antibody	Anti-HDV in serum	
Nosocomial Problem?				
No	Yes	Yes	Yes	No
Mortality				
Less frequent	More frequent, chronic form can be fatal	More frequent, chronic form can be fatal	Increased	Unknown

Anti-HAV, Antibody to HAV; *IgM,* immunoglobulin M; *HBsAg,* hepatitis B surface antigen; *anti-HCV,* antibodies to HCV; *anti-HDV,* antibodies to HDV; *anti-HEV,* antibodies to HEV; *AST,* aspartate aminotransferase; *ALT,* alanine aminotransferase.

hepatocytes (liver cells) to scar. This scarring may progress to cirrhosis. Concomitant use of alcohol hastens the progression to cirrhosis. Those infected with hepatitis C and in whom cirrhosis has developed are at risk for development of liver cancer.

Hepatitis C–induced cirrhosis is the leading indication for liver transplantation in the United States (National Institutes of Health Consensus Development Conference Statement, 2002). Unfortunately, the newly transplanted liver often becomes reinfected with the virus.

HEPATITIS D. **Hepatitis D** (delta hepatitis, or HDV) is caused by a defective RNA virus that needs the helper function of HBV. HDV co-infects with HBV and needs its presence for viral replication. Hepatitis D can co-infect a client with HBV or can occur as a superinfection in a client with chronic HBV. Superinfection usually develops into chronic

HDV. The incubation period is about 14 to 56 days. As with HBV, the disease is transmitted primarily by parenteral routes.

HEPATITIS E. The **hepatitis E** virus (HEV) was originally identified by its association with waterborne epidemics of hepatitis in the Indian subcontinent. Since then, it has occurred in epidemics in Asia, Africa, the Middle East, Mexico, and Central and South America. Many large outbreaks have occurred after heavy rains and flooding.

In the United States, hepatitis E has been found only in travelers returning from these endemic areas. The non-enveloped, single-stranded RNA virus is transmitted via the fecal-oral route, and the clinical course resembles that of hepatitis A. HEV has an incubation period of 15 to 64 days. There is no evidence at this time of a chronic form of HEV.

TOXIC AND DRUG-INDUCED HEPATITIS

Chemicals that are inhaled or swallowed can damage the liver. Prescription medications, over-the-counter (OTC) medications, herbals supplements, industrial solvents, pollutants, and even mushrooms have all been implicated as causes of hepatitis.

Complications of Hepatitis

Failure of the liver cells to regenerate, with progression of the necrotic process, results in a severe acute and often fatal form of hepatitis known as **fulminant hepatitis.** Hepatitis is considered to be chronic when liver inflammation lasts longer than several months (usually defined as 6 months). **Chronic hepatitis** usually occurs as a result of hepatitis B or C. Superimposed infection with hepatitis D (HDV) in clients with chronic HBV may also result in chronic hepatitis. As mentioned earlier, chronic hepatitis can lead to cirrhosis and liver cancer.

Incidence/Prevalence

Each year about 250,000 people in the United States become infected with hepatitis A. However, only a small portion of these cases is reported. Hepatitis B and C are much more of a concern, though, because of their connection to cirrhosis and liver cancer. Although exact numbers are not known, it is estimated that about 200 million people worldwide have the hepatitis C virus (HCV), making this type of hepatitis the most common type. In the United States, the rate of HCV is increasing among young adults, Hispanics, and war veterans who used IV drugs, experienced needle sticks, or had tattoos. About 3.9 million people in the United States have been exposed to HCV and about 3 million have chronic liver disease, making HCV very costly in dollars and quality of life (Centers for Disease Control and Prevention, 2002) (see the Resource Management box above).

Deaths from liver disease have been estimated at 43,000 per year, but that number is predicted to increase by 60% or more in the next decade. This increase will require a major increase in transplantations and lead to many more deaths.

HEALTH PROMOTION/ILLNESS PREVENTION

Measures for preventing hepatitis A (HAV) include the following:

- Proper handwashing
- Avoiding contaminated food or water

RESOURCE MANAGEMENT

HEPATITIS C

Cost of Care

- An estimated 3.9 million Americans, nearly 2% of the population, are chronically infected with hepatitis C.
- The cost of hepatitis C infections and related diseases is more than $600 million per year.
- More than half of the liver transplants performed in the United States are for hepatitis C. The average first-year cost for a liver transplant exceeds $200,000.
- From the year 2010 through 2019, the projected cost in direct medical expenses is $10.7 billion, with 165,900 deaths due to chronic liver disease and 27,200 deaths due to hepatocellular carcinoma.

Implications for Nursing

Nurses are at high risk for getting hepatitis C and becoming part of these statistics. As these costs rise, health care will be impacted further from this disease. Nurses must strive to disseminate information about this disease to prevent others from obtaining it and to help reduce costs.

Data from Wong, J.B., et al. (2000). Estimating future hepatitis C morbidity, mortality, and costs in the United States. *American Journal of Public Health, 90*(10), 1562-1569.

- Receiving the HAV vaccine before traveling to areas where the disease is common (e.g., Mexico, Caribbean)
- Receiving immune globulin within 14 days if exposed to the virus

For hepatitis B (HBV) prevention, a vaccine can provide protection against the disease. There is no vaccine yet available for the other types of viral hepatitis. HBV vaccine is now recommended as part of the routine schedule of childhood vaccinations in the United States. It is also recommended for the following:

- Infants born to HBV-infected mothers
- People who have unprotected sexual intercourse with more than one partner
- People with any chronic liver disease
- People who are exposed to blood or body fluids in the workplace, including health care workers, firefighters, and police
- People who live in close living accommodations, such as college dormitories, correctional institutions, and long-term care facilities

Case reporting to local health departments for all types of *viral* hepatitis is mandatory (reporting is usually the responsibility of the laboratory). Additional measures to prevent viral hepatitis for health care workers and others in contact with infected clients are listed in Charts 62-4 and 62-5.

◆COLLABORATIVE MANAGEMENT
◆Assessment
HISTORY

In any client who presents with the manifestations of acute hepatitis, it is important to obtain a focused history. First, ask the client whether he or she has had known exposure to a person with hepatitis. The client should also be asked about the following:

- Exposure to either inhaled or ingested chemical
- Use of herbal supplement
- Use of any new prescribed medication
- Recent ingestion of shellfish

(see Chapter 29)

CHART 62-4

BEST PRACTICE for
Prevention of Viral Hepatitis in Health Care Workers

- Use standard precautions to prevent the transmission of disease between clients or between clients and health care staff (see Chapter 29).
- Eliminate needles and other sharp instruments by substituting needleless systems. (Needle sticks are the major source of hepatitis B transmission in health care workers.)
- Take the hepatitis B vaccine (Heptavax-B, Recombivax HB), which is given in a series of three injections. This vaccine also prevents hepatitis D.
- For postexposure prevention of hepatitis A or B, seek medical attention immediately for immunoglobulin (Ig) administration.
- Report all cases of hepatitis to the local health department.

CHART 62-5

CLIENT EDUCATION GUIDE
Health Promotion/Illness Prevention of Viral Hepatitis

- Maintain adequate sanitation and personal hygiene. Wash your hands before eating and after using the toilet.
- Drink water treated by a water purification system.
- If traveling in underdeveloped or nonindustrialized countries, drink only bottled water. Avoid food washed or prepared with tap water, such as raw vegetables, fruits, and soups.
- Use adequate sanitation practices to prevent the spread of the disease between family members.
- Do not share bed linens, towels, eating utensils, or drinking glasses.
- Do not share needles for injection, body piercing, or tattooing.
- Do not share razors, nail clippers, toothbrushes, or WaterPiks.
- Use a condom during sexual intercourse or abstain from this activity.
- Cover cuts or sores with bandages.
- If ever infected with hepatitis, never donate blood, body organs, or other body tissue.

- Exposure to a possibly contaminated water source
- Employment
- Recent foreign travel
- Sexual activities with men, women, or both, and whether it was protected or unprotected
- Injectable drug use
- For health care workers, recent needle stick exposure
- Recent body piercing or tattooing
- Close living accommodations, such as military barracks, correctional institutions, and overcrowded dormitories, long-term facilities, or employment in any such setting

For the client who presents with few or no symptoms of liver disease but who has had an abnormality detected by a laboratory evaluation (e.g., an elevated ALT or AST level), the history may need to include additional questions regarding the following:

- Blood or blood products received before 1992
- Military service or other travel to a foreign country
- Place of birth (United States or other country) and parents' place of birth
- Sharing of needles or cocaine straw at any time in the past
- Sexual history

- History of alcohol use (how many drinks each day or week)

PHYSICAL ASSESSMENT/CLINICAL MANIFESTATIONS

Assess whether the client is experiencing the following:
- Abdominal pain
- Changes in skin or eye color
- **Arthralgia** (joint pain)
- **Myalgia** (muscle pain)
- Diarrhea/constipation
- Changes in color of urine or stool
- Fever
- Lethargy
- Malaise
- Nausea/vomiting
- Pruritus

Lightly palpate the right upper abdominal quadrant to assess for liver tenderness. The client may report right upper quadrant pain with jarring movements. Inspect the skin, sclerae, and mucous membranes for the presence of jaundice. The client may present for medical treatment only after jaundice appears, believing that other vague symptoms are related to an influenza-like syndrome.

Jaundice in hepatitis results from intrahepatic obstruction and is caused by edema of the liver's bile channels. Dark urine and clay-colored stools are often reported by the client. If possible, obtain a urine and stool specimen for visual inspection and laboratory analysis. The client may also report pruritus (itching) and may have skin abrasions from scratching.

PSYCHOSOCIAL ASSESSMENT

Viral hepatitis has various presentations, but for most infected individuals, the initial course is mild with few symptoms. It is the long-term complications of fibrosis and cirrhosis that cause the more serious problem. This is especially true for clients who have HBV and HCV infection.

When the presentation is dramatic with jaundice and significant impairment of liver function, the client is acutely ill and needs supportive care.

Emotional problems for affected clients often center on their feeling sick and fatigued. General malaise, inactivity, and vague complaints contribute to depression and despondency. These clients worry about the long-term effects and complications. They often feel guilty and are remorseful about decisions made that caused the disease. These feelings are most likely to occur when the source of infection is from drug abuse.

Infectious diseases such as hepatitis continue to have a social stigma. The client may feel embarrassed by the isolation and hygiene precautions that are imposed in the hospital and continue to be necessary at home. This embarrassment may cause the client to limit social interactions. Self-imposed visitor restrictions may be instituted by the client out of fear of spreading the virus to family and friends.

Family members are sometimes afraid of contracting the disease and may distance themselves from the client. Allow the client and family to verbalize these feelings and explore the reasons for these fears. The nurse also plays an important role in educating client and family members about modes of transmission. It is essential to dispel any misconceptions that would contribute to the client's isolation.

Clients may be unable to return to work for several weeks during the acute phases of illness. The loss of wages and the cost of hospitalization for a client without insurance coverage may produce great anxiety and financial burden for the client and the family.

LABORATORY ASSESSMENT

The presence of hepatitis A, B, and C is usually indicated by acute elevations in levels of liver enzymes, indicating liver cellular damage, and by specific serologic markers.

SERUM LIVER ENZYMES. Levels of alanine aminotransferase (ALT) and aspartate aminotransferase (AST) levels may rise into the thousands in acute or fulminant cases of hepatitis. Alkaline phosphatase levels may be normal or elevated. Serum total bilirubin levels are elevated and are consistent with the clinical appearance of jaundice. Elevated levels of bilirubin are also present in the urine.

SEROLOGIC MARKERS/ENZYME ASSAYS. The presence of *hepatitis A* is established when hepatitis A virus (HAV) antibodies (anti-HAV) are identified in the blood. Ongoing inflammation of the liver by HAV is evidenced by the presence of immunoglobulin M (IgM) antibodies, which persist in the blood for 4 to 6 weeks. Previous infection is indicated by the presence of immunoglobulin G (IgG) antibodies. These antibodies persist in the serum and provide permanent immunity to HAV.

The presence of the *hepatitis B* virus (HBV) is established when serologic testing confirms the presence of hepatitis B antigen-antibody systems in the blood. HBV is a double-shelled DNA virus consisting of an inner core and an outer shell. Antigens located on the surface (shell) of the virus (HBsAg) and IgM antibodies to hepatitis B core antigen (anti-HBc IgM) are the most significant serologic markers. The presence of these markers establishes the diagnosis of hepatitis B. The client is considered infectious as long as HBsAg (hepatitis B surface antigen) is present in the blood. Persistence of this serologic marker after 6 months or longer indicates a carrier state or chronic hepatitis. HBsAg levels normally decline and disappear after the acute hepatitis B episode. The presence of antibodies to HBsAb (hepatitis B surface antibody) in the blood indicates recovery and immunity to hepatitis B. Keep in mind that people who have been vaccinated against HBV have a positive HBsAb because they also have immunity to the disease.

Enzyme-linked immunosorbent assay (ELISA) is the initial screening test for clients suspected of being infected with *hepatitis C* virus (HCV). It is also the most commonly used enzyme test for HCV antibodies (anti-HCV). The antibodies can be detected within 4 weeks of the infection (Pagana & Pagana, 2002). A more specific assay called the recombinant immunoblot assay (RIBA) has been used as a confirmatory test. These tests confirm that the client has been exposed to HCV and has developed the antibody. To confirm the presence of actual circulating virus, the HCV polymerase chain reaction (PCR) RNA test is used. This confirms active virus and can quantify the viral load.

The presence of *hepatitis D* virus (HDV) can be confirmed by the identification of intrahepatic delta antigen or, more often, by a rise in the hepatitis D virus antibodies (anti-HDV) titer. This increase can be seen within a few days of infection (Pagana & Pagana, 2002).

Hepatitis E virus (HEV) testing is usually reserved for travelers in whom hepatitis is present but the virus cannot be detected. The presence of the hepatitis E antibodies (anti-HEV) is found in individuals infected with the virus.

OTHER DIAGNOSTIC ASSESSMENTS

Liver biopsy is also used to confirm the diagnosis of hepatitis. Characteristic changes help the pathologist distinguish among a virus, drug, toxin, fatty liver, and other disease. It is usually performed on in an ambulatory care setting and performed percutaneously (through the skin) after a local anesthetic is given. If coagulation is abnormal, however, it may be done using either a CT guided or transjugular route.

◆Interventions

The client with viral hepatitis can be mildly or acutely ill depending on the severity of the inflammation. Most clients are not hospitalized, although older adults and those with dehydration may be admitted for a short-term stay. Some clients are hospitalized during administration of potent medications to treat hepatitis B or C. The plan of care for all clients with viral hepatitis is based on measures to rest the liver, promote cellular regeneration, and prevent complications (see the Plan of Care on pp. 1387 to 1390).

NONSURGICAL MANAGEMENT. During the acute stage of viral hepatitis, interventions are aimed at resting the inflamed liver to promote hepatic cell regeneration. Rest is an essential intervention to reduce the liver's metabolic demands and increase its blood supply. Treatment is generally supportive.

Physical Rest. Assess the client's response to activity and rest periods. Strict bedrest may be indicated during the early icteric phase of hepatitis. The client is usually tired and expresses feelings of general malaise. Complete bedrest is usually not required, but rest periods alternating with periods of activity are indicated and are often sufficient to promote hepatic healing. Individualize the client's plan of care and change it as needed to reflect the severity of symptoms, fatigue, and the results of liver function tests and enzyme determinations. Teach the client to adhere to scheduled rest periods. Activities such as self-care and ambulating are gradually added to the activity schedule as tolerated.

Psychological Rest. Emotional and psychological rest is essential for the client. Because bedrest and inactivity can produce anxiety, the client should include diversional activities.

Diet Therapy. A special diet is usually not required. The diet should be high in carbohydrates and calories with moderate amounts of fat and protein. Small, frequent meals are often preferable to three standard meals. Ask the client about food preferences, because favorite foods are tolerated better than randomly selected foods. Encourage the client to select foods that are appealing. High-calorie snacks may be needed.

The health care provider typically prescribes supplemental vitamins. If caloric intake is low, the client may need supplemental commercial feedings, such as Ensure or Boost.

≡PLAN of CARE   MEDICAL DIAGNOSIS: HEPATITIS

NURSING DIAGNOSIS NO. 1   ■   Fatigue

	Expected Outcomes	Nursing Interventions	Rationales
RELATED FACTORS Disease states Malnutrition **DEFINING CHARACTERISTICS** Energy: Lack of Rest requirements: Increased Inability to maintain usual routines Increase in physical complaints	Denies fatigue No verbal report or observation of being lethargic or listless Denies feeling tired Denies an increase in rest requirements No verbal report or observation of lack of energy	**NIC Energy Management** **D** Monitor the client for evidence of excess physical and emotional fatigue. **D** Monitor nutritional intake. **D** Reduce physical discomforts. **D** Arrange physical activities (e.g., avoid activity immediately after meals). Encourage alternate rest and activity periods. Assist the client to schedule rest periods and avoid care activities during scheduled rest periods. Teach activity organization and time management techniques (e.g., assigning priority to activities to accommodate energy levels, establishing realistic activity goals). Instruct the client/significant other to recognize the signs and symptoms of fatigue. **Other Interventions** Consider the use of complementary and alternative therapies. **Continuing Care Considerations** Collaborate with the client/family and the rehabilitation team.	Extended periods of inactivity may place the client at risk for excessive fatigue when carrying out desired activities. Monitoring nutritional intake ensures that the client has adequate energy resources. Physical discomforts could interfere with cognitive function and self-monitoring/regulation of activity. Arranging physical activities reduces competition for oxygen supply to vital body functions. This avoids extended periods of either activity or exercise. Rest periods should help restore client energy levels. Activity organization and time management techniques are used to prevent fatigue. Symptoms of undue fatigue require a reduction in activity. Complementary and alternative therapies may be used to cope with chronic disease and disability, especially if chronic pain is a problem. Effective interdisciplinary interventions facilitate the client's ability to manage his or her life.

NURSING DIAGNOSIS NO. 2   ■   Nausea

	Expected Outcomes	Nursing Interventions	Rationales
RELATED FACTORS Irritation to the gastrointestinal system Stimulation of neuropharmacologic mechanisms **DEFINING CHARACTERISTICS** Verbal reports of "nausea" or being "sick to stomach"	Denies nausea No verbal report or observation of vomiting	**NIC Nausea Management** Assess nausea, including frequency, duration, severity, and precipitating factors. If possible, use an established nausea assessment tool.	Performing a complete assessment of nausea using tools such as Self-Care Journal, Visual Analog Scales, Duke Descriptive Scales, and Rhodes Index of Nausea and Vomiting (INV) Form 2 can better monitor the client's nausea patterns.

D Indicates tasks that can be delegated to unlicensed assistive nursing personnel at the discretion of the nurse.

Continued

PLAN of CARE   MEDICAL DIAGNOSIS: HEPATITIS—*cont'd*

NURSING DIAGNOSIS NO. 2 ■ Nausea—*cont'd*

Expected Outcomes	Nursing Interventions	Rationales
	Identify factors (e.g., medication and procedures) that may cause or contribute to nausea.	Identifying the source of nausea permits using strategies to prevent or diminish nausea.
	Ensure that effective antiemetic drugs are given, when possible.	Antiemetics are given to prevent nausea.
	D Control environmental factors such as aversive smells, sound, and unpleasant visual stimulation.	Environmental factors may evoke nausea.
	Encourage the use of nonpharmacologic techniques, as well as other nausea control measures, before nausea occurs or increases.	The use of nonpharmacologic techniques helps the client to control nausea and may amplify the relief obtained by other control measures.
	Inform other health care professionals and family members of any nonpharmacologic strategies being used by the client with nausea.	Health care professionals and family members can support the use of nonpharmacologic strategies and encourage their use.
	D Use frequent oral hygiene unless it stimulates nausea.	Frequent oral hygiene may promote comfort by removing unpleasant tastes from the mouth.
	D Encourage the client with nausea to eat small amounts of food that are appealing to him or her.	Foods that are appealing to the client with nausea are less likely to trigger nausea.
	Instruct in high-carbohydrate and low-fat food, as appropriate.	High-carbohydrate and low-fat food is absorbed more quickly in the intestinal tract and is less likely to add bulk, which might trigger nausea.
	D Give cold and clear liquid and odorless and colorless food, as appropriate.	Cold beverages are less likely to have an odor that may trigger nausea.
	Provide information about the causes of the nausea and how long it will last.	The client may believe that the nausea is not going to improve and may not understand why the nausea is occurring.
	Other Interventions	
	D Encourage supplemental commercial feedings, such as Ensure or Boost.	Commercial food supplements increase calories and are easy to ingest.
	Continuing Care Considerations	
	Collaborate with the client/family to monitor the client's weight and amount of nausea.	Continuing nausea is debilitating and significantly decreases the client's quality of life. Continuing therapy is essential to maintain nutrition.

D Indicates tasks that can be delegated to unlicensed assistive nursing personnel at the discretion of the nurse.

▤ PLAN of CARE   MEDICAL DIAGNOSIS: HEPATITIS—cont'd

NURSING DIAGNOSIS NO. 3 ■ Ineffective Health Maintenance

	Expected Outcomes	Nursing Interventions	Rationales
RELATED FACTORS Ineffective family coping Lack of material resources Lack of ability to make deliberate and thoughtful judgments Ineffective individual coping **DEFINING CHARACTERISTICS** Knowledge: Demonstrated lack regarding basic health practices Reported or demonstrated inability to take responsibility for meeting basic health practices in any or all functional pattern areas History of lack of health-seeking behaviors	Able to accurately perform needed health care tasks No verbal report or observation of lack of equipment, financial, and/or other resources No verbal report or observation of failure to adhere to treatment plan Keeps medical appointments Practices basic health maintenance activities	**NIC Health System Guidance** Inform the client of appropriate community resources and contact persons. Identify and facilitate communication among health care providers and the client/family, as appropriate. Give written instructions for the purpose and location of posthospitalization/outpatient activities, as appropriate. Provide a report to posthospital caregivers, as appropriate. **NIC Support System Enhancement** Identify the degree of family support. Determine the support systems currently used. Determine barriers to using support systems. Monitor the current family situation. Assess community resource adequacy to identify strengths and weaknesses. Refer to a community-based promotion/prevention/treatment program, as appropriate. Provide services in a caring and supportive manner. Involve the family/significant others/friends in the care and planning. Explain to concerned others how they can help.	Clients and their families may not know what resources are available or how to contact the appropriate agencies or services. Faulty communication may increase the time delays for service or foster distrust among the health care providers, client, and family. Written instructions provide clear information to which the client can refer for memory assistance. Posthospital caregivers need information about the client's current condition and changes in status in order to provide appropriate care. Family support is not guaranteed, even with proximity. Identify what the client is currently doing for support and the client's satisfaction with the amount of support. This intervention assists the client and family in identifying methods to overcome barriers as needed. The strain of providing emotional and financial support may stress family bonds. Understanding the strengths and weaknesses of available community resources permits realistic expectations of assistance from those sources. A community-based promotion/prevention/treatment program may provide the client/family with essential services and emotional support. Clients and their families deal with health status changes in individual ways; these ways need to be recognized in a caring manner. The involvement of family, significant others, and friends in the care and planning for the client shares the burden and builds bonds from shared experiences. Giving concerned others concrete suggestions for assistance provides them with guidance and provides the client with necessary aid.

Continued

PLAN of CARE MEDICAL DIAGNOSIS: HEPATITIS—*cont'd*

NURSING DIAGNOSIS NO. 3 ■ Ineffective Health Maintenance—*cont'd*

Expected Outcomes	Nursing Interventions	Rationales
	NIC **Other Interventions** Teach the client and family about the care necessary to manage the health state.	Lack of knowledge will render efforts at health maintenance less effective.
	Assist the client/family to identify areas in which they need help and to whom or where they might go to get the help they need.	Clients/families are not always able to ask for help when aid is needed, either because they do not recognize the need or do not know how to secure aid.
	Continuing Care Considerations Refer the family to appropriate counseling services.	Families in distress may be unable to provide essential support to a family member with a health maintenance problem.

Drug Therapy. Medications are used sparingly for clients with acute hepatitis to allow the liver to rest. An antiemetic to relieve nausea may be prescribed.

For clients with chronic hepatitis B and C, a number of drugs are being used, including antiviral medications and immunomodulators. Lamivudine (Epivir-HBV) and adefovir dipivoxil (Hepsera) are oral antiviral drugs given to destroy the hepatitis B virus in clients with chronic disease. Both of these medications can cause renal toxicity and granulocytopenia. A number of types of interferon, immunomodulating drugs, are being administered to treat both hepatitis B and C. Research on other possible drugs for hepatitis B is ongoing.

The most common treatment for hepatitis C is a combination of subcutaneous interferon (peginterferon alfa-2a [Pegasys]) and oral ribavirin. The length of treatment is dependent upon genotype, or strain of hepatitis. There are several different genotypes; most Americans who have hepatitis C are genotype 1. This genotype usually requires 48 weeks of treatment. Genotypes 2 and 3 have a better response rate and usually only need 24 weeks of treatment. The goal of treatment is to have a negative HCV PCR RNA level and to sustain a negative level after treatment has ended. Response rates vary, but in general, clients who are young, have a low viral load, and have minimal scarring on liver biopsy have a better chance of clearing the virus and remaining free of hepatitis C after treatment has ended.

Critical Thinking Challenge

You are the nurse caring for a 52-year-old man recently diagnosed with chronic hepatitis C. He denies any high-risk behavior but admits to getting a tattoo in Vietnam. How will you reply to his following questions?

1. "Could I have gotten this by a tattoo?"
2. "Could my wife and children have hepatitis?"
3. "How could I not have known I had hepatitis?"
4. "What is the treatment for hepatitis C?"

evolve For suggested answer guidelines, go to http://evolve.elsevier.com/Iggy/.

Community-Based Care

Home care management varies according to the type of hepatitis and whether the disease is acute or chronic. A primary focus in any case is preventing the spread of the infection. For hepatitis transmitted by the fecal-oral route, careful handwashing and sanitary disposal of feces are important. Standard precautions are used for hepatitis transmitted percutaneously and permucosally. Education is therefore very important. If the nurse and or assistive personnel are not sure about modes of transmission or precautions that need to be taken once the client is home and in the community, then the advice of hospital-based infection control personnel or infectious disease specialist should be sought. These experts can also suggest resources for the client and family.

Teach the client and the family to observe measures to prevent infection transmission (see Chart 62-5). In addition, instruct the client with viral hepatitis to avoid alcohol and check with the health care provider before taking any medication or vitamin, supplement, or herbal preparation.

The client must determine patterns for rest on the basis of physical tolerance of increased activity. Encourage the client to increase activity gradually to prevent fatigue. The client should eat small, frequent meals of high-carbohydrate and low-fat foods (Chart 62-6).

FATTY LIVER (STEATOHEPATITIS)

A **fatty liver** is caused by the accumulation of fats in and around the hepatic cells. Causes include the following:

- Diabetes mellitus
- Obesity
- Elevated lipid profile

Fatty infiltration of the liver may result from faulty fat metabolism in the liver and the mobilization of fatty acids from adipose tissue. Many clients with a fatty liver are asymptomatic. The most common and typical finding is asymptomatic elevation of alanine aminotransferase (ALT) and aspartate aminotransferase (AST).

CLIENT EDUCATION GUIDE
Viral Hepatitis

- Avoid all medications, including over-the-counter drugs, such as acetaminophen (Tylenol, Exdol✳), unless prescribed by your physician.
- Avoid all alcohol.
- Rest frequently throughout the day, and get adequate sleep at night.
- Eat small, frequent meals with a high-carbohydrate, low-fat content.
- Avoid sexual intercourse until antibody testing results are negative.
- Follow the guidelines for preventing transmission of the disease (see Chart 62-5).

KEY FEATURES of
Liver Trauma

- Right upper quadrant pain with abdominal tenderness
- Abdominal distention and rigidity
- Guarding of the abdomen
- Increased abdominal pain exaggerated by deep breathing and referred to the right shoulder (Kehr's sign)
- Indicators of hemorrhage and hypovolemic shock:
  Hypotension
  Tachycardia
  Tachypnea
  Pallor
  Diaphoresis
  Cool, clammy skin
  Confusion or other change in mental state

Magnetic resonance imaging, ultrasound, and nuclear medicine examinations can be used to confirm excessive fat in the liver. A percutaneous biopsy can provide the same information. Interventions are aimed at removing the underlying cause of the infiltration. Weight loss, glucose control, and improving cholesterol and triglyceride levels may help.

HEPATIC ABSCESS

PATHOPHYSIOLOGY

Although hepatic abscesses are uncommon, they carry a high mortality rate. **Liver abscesses** occur when the liver is invaded by bacteria or protozoa. These organisms destroy the liver tissue, producing a necrotic cavity filled with infective agents, liquefied liver cells and tissue, and leukocytes. The infectious necrotic tissue walls off the abscess from the healthy liver.

A **pyogenic liver abscess** occurs when bacteria invade the liver. Infecting organisms include *Escherichia coli* and *Klebsiella, Enterobacter, Salmonella, Staphylococcus,* and *Enterococcus* species. A pyogenic abscess is generally solitary and confined to the right lobe, but occasionally abscesses are multiple. The usual cause is acute cholangitis, which occurs as a complication of cholelithiasis. Pyogenic liver abscesses may also result from liver trauma, abdominal peritonitis, and sepsis, or an abscess can extend to the liver after pneumonia or bacterial endocarditis.

The protozoan *Entamoeba histolytica* causes an **amebic hepatic abscess**, which may occur after amebic dysentery. These abscesses usually occur in the form of a single abscess in the right hepatic lobe.

◆COLLABORATIVE MANAGEMENT

Clients with hepatic abscesses are generally quite ill. On occasion, an abscess is not diagnosed until autopsy. In clients with a pyogenic liver abscess, the onset of symptoms is usually sudden. Amebic abscesses cause a more insidious onset of symptoms. Common complaints include the following:

- Right upper abdominal pain with a palpable, tender liver
- Anorexia
- Weight loss

- Nausea and vomiting
- Fever and chills
- Shoulder pain
- Dyspnea
- Pleural pain if the diaphragm is involved

A hepatic abscess is usually diagnosed by contrast-enhanced computed tomography (CT) scan or ultrasound. These abscesses are usually drained under CT or ultrasound guidance. Specimens may be sent for laboratory analysis so that the optimal antibiotic can be selected.

LIVER TRAUMA

PATHOPHYSIOLOGY

The liver is the most common organ to be injured in clients with penetrating trauma of the abdomen (e.g., gunshot wounds, stab wounds, and rib fractures) and is the second most commonly injured organ in clients who have blunt abdominal trauma. Liver damage or injury should be suspected whenever any upper abdominal or lower chest trauma is sustained. The liver is often injured by steering wheels in vehicular accidents. Common injuries to the liver include simple lacerations, multiple lacerations, avulsions (tears), and crush injuries.

◆COLLABORATIVE MANAGEMENT
◆Assessment

The liver is a highly vascular organ and receives about 29% of the body's cardiac output. When hepatic trauma occurs, blood loss can be massive. The client may exhibit signs of hemorrhagic shock (Chart 62-7).

An ultrasound or CT scan of the abdomen is often done to determine the presence of a hematoma. A decreased hematocrit may confirm suspected blood loss. Clinical manifestations include right upper quadrant pain with abdominal tenderness, distention, guarding, and rigidity. Abdominal pain exaggerated by deep breathing and referred to the right shoulder may indicate diaphragmatic irritation.

◆Interventions

When hepatic and other abdominal organ trauma is confirmed, a surgeon performs an exploratory laparotomy to identify and control the source and type of bleeding. Minor surgical interventions, such as suture placement, wound packing, decompression, or a combination of these procedures, are often performed to halt bleeding. Liver lobe resection is required in some extensive liver injuries. This procedure may be done using laparoscopy.

Clients with hepatic trauma require the administration of multiple blood products, packed red blood cells, and fresh frozen plasma, as well as massive volume infusion to maintain adequate hydration. Postoperatively, the client with hepatic trauma is admitted to a critical care unit. The nurse monitors the client for persistent bleeding. Complete blood count and coagulation studies must be closely monitored for trends in changes.

CANCER OF THE LIVER

PATHOPHYSIOLOGY

Primary hepatic cancer, or hepatocellular carcinoma (HCC), is one of the most common tumors in the world. It is more prevalent in regions of Asia and Africa where the annual incidence is up to 500 cases per 100,000 people.

In the United States, the incidence of HCC is increasing. In 1975 to 1977, age-adjusted incidence rates were 1.4 cases of HCC per 100,000 people. The age-adjusted incidence rates of HCC for 1999-2000 was 3.1 persons per 100,000 population. The fastest rising rates have been observed in men between 45 and 55 years of age, especially African-American men (Velazquez et al., 2003).

Chronic infection with HBV and HCV frequently lead to cirrhosis, which is a risk factor for developing hepatocellular carcinoma. It is important to remember that cirrhosis from any cause, including alcoholic liver disease, increases the risk for HCC.

◆ **COLLABORATIVE MANAGEMENT**

The most common complaint is abdominal discomfort. Elevated serum alpha-fetoprotein and alkaline phosphatase are also common. Ultrasound and contrast-enhanced computed tomography (CT) are both useful in detecting metastasis. If the primary tumor site is not known, a CT- or ultrasound-guided liver biopsy can confirm the diagnosis.

Surgical management may be indicated for clients with a lesion confined to one liver lobe and may be performed through a laparoscope. Liver lobe resection has been successful in achieving survival rates of up to 5 years.

Unfortunately, 75% of clients are not candidates for surgical excision because their tumors are unresectable. The liver cannot tolerate high doses of radiation, so radiation treatments are not an option. Other approaches include hepatic artery embolization and chemotherapy (chemoembolization), alcohol ablation, and ultrasound-guided cryoablation. A newer device uses a radiofrequency (RF) generator as a heat source to "burn" a tumor in a percutaneous procedure. This procedure, called RF ablation, is done using CT or ultrasound guidance.

Chemotherapy may be administered by a surgically implanted infusion pump, which enables controlled infusion. It may also be given in a catheter-directed method. The interventional radiologist places a catheter into the hepatic tumor that supplies the tumor and injects a mixture of chemotherapy and contrast agent into the tumor. This procedure has the unique effect of depositing chemotherapeutic drugs directly into the tumor and blocking further blood flow into the tumor for weeks. Liver transplantation may also be used to treat liver cancer.

LIVER TRANSPLANTATION

Liver transplantation has become a common operation worldwide. The client with end-stage liver disease or acute liver failure who has not responded to conventional medical or surgical intervention is a potential candidate for liver transplantation. Liver transplantation may also be considered for the client with a primary malignant neoplasm of the liver.

The client for potential transplantation undergoes extensive physiologic and psychological assessment and evaluation by physicians and transplant coordinators to identify contraindications to the procedure. Clients who are not considered candidates for transplantation are those with the following:
- Severe cardiovascular instability with advanced cardiac disease
- Severe respiratory disease
- Active alcohol and/or substance abuse
- Metastatic malignant disease
- Inability to follow instructions regarding medications and self-care

Liver transplantation has become the most effective treatment for clients with an increasing number of acute and chronic liver diseases. Inclusion and exclusion criteria may vary among transplantation centers and are continually revised as treatment options change and surgical techniques improve.

Donor livers are obtained primarily from trauma victims who have not had liver damage. They are distributed through a nationwide program, the United Network of Organ Sharing (UNOS). This system distributes donor livers on the basis of regional considerations and recipient acuity. Candidates with the highest level of acuity receive highest priority.

The donor liver is transported to the surgery center in a cooled saline solution that preserves the organ for up to 8 hours. The diseased liver is removed through an incision made in the upper abdomen. The new liver is carefully put in its place and is attached to the client's blood vessels and bile ducts. The procedure can take up to 12 hours to complete and requires a highly specialized team and large volumes of fluid and blood replacement.

Living donors have also been used. This is done on a voluntary basis after careful psychological and physiologic preparation and testing. The donor's liver is resected (usually removal of one lobe) and implanted into the recipient after removal of the diseased liver. In both the donor and the recipient, the liver regenerates and grows in size to meet the demands of the body.

PATHOPHYSIOLOGY

Although liver transplantations are commonly done, complications can occur. Some problems can be medically managed, whereas others require removal of the transplant. The two most common complications are acute graft rejection and infection.

Acute Graft Rejection

The success of all transplantations has greatly improved since the introduction in 1980 of cyclosporine (cyclosporin A), an immunosuppressant drug. Now there are several other antirejection medications used, such as FK-506, Cell-Cept, Prograf, Imuran, sirolimus, and prednisone.

Clinical manifestations of rejection may include tachycardia, fever, right upper quadrant or flank pain, decreased bile pigment and volume, and increasing jaundice. Laboratory findings include elevated serum bilirubin, rising ALT and AST levels, elevated alkaline phosphatase levels, and increased prothrombin time/International Normalized Ratio (INR).

Transplant rejection is treated aggressively with immunosuppressive medication. As with all rejection treatments, the client is at a greater risk for infection. If therapy is not effective, a rapid deterioration of liver function occurs. Multisystem organ failure, including respiratory and renal involvement, develops along with diffuse coagulopathies and portal-systemic encephalopathy (PSE). The only alternative for treatment is emergency retransplantation.

Infection

Infection is another potential threat to the transplanted graft and the client's survival. Immunosuppressant therapy, which must be used to prevent and treat organ rejection, significantly increases the client's susceptibility to and risk for infection. Other risk factors include the presence of multiple tubes and intravascular lines, immobility, and prolonged anesthesia.

In the early post-transplantation period, common infections include pneumonia, wound infections, and urinary tract infections. Opportunistic infections usually develop after the first postoperative month and include cytomegalovirus, mycobacterial infections, and parasitic infections. Latent infections such as tuberculosis and herpes simplex may be reactivated.

The physician prescribes broad-spectrum antibiotics for prophylaxis during and after surgery. Obtain culture specimens from all lines and tubes and collect specimens for culture at predetermined time intervals as dictated by the agency's policy. If an infection is detected, the physician prescribes organism-specific anti-infective agents.

Other Complications

The biliary anastomosis is susceptible to breakdown, obstruction, and infection. If leakage occurs or if the site becomes necrotic or obstructed, an abscess can form or peritonitis, bacteremia, and cirrhosis may develop. Other potential complications include the following:

- Hemorrhage
- Hepatic artery thrombosis
- Fluid and electrolyte imbalances
- Pulmonary atelectasis
- Acute renal failure
- Chronic graft rejection
- Psychological maladjustment

Transplant complications cause clients to be very anxious. The nurse and other members of the health care team assure the client that these problems are common and usually successfully treated.

EVIDENCE-BASED PRACTICE for Nursing

What is the psychosocial experience of clients who receive a liver transplant?

Forsberg, A., Backman, L., & Moller, A. (2002). Experiencing liver transplantation: A phenomenological approach. *Journal of Advanced Nursing, 32*(2), 327.

The aim of this study was to investigate the subjective experience of the meaning of having a liver transplant. Seven categories emerged from interviews of 12 clients who volunteered for the study:

- Facing the inevitable
- Recapturing the body
- Emotional chaos
- Leaving the experts
- Family and friends
- Threat of graft rejection
- Honoring the donor

Social support was found to be essential for recovery. Meeting other transplant survivors helped to deal with the identity crisis of suddenly feeling totally unique.

Level of Evidence: 6—The research serves as a small pilot study that should be replicated to better understand the needs of the client undergoing transplantation.

Critique. The study population consisted of nine women and three men. A more balanced gender number may have changed the selected categories. The race/ethnic origin of the subjects is assumed to be white. It is difficult to generalize study findings, and additional study is needed using more diverse and larger groups.

Implications for Nursing. The authors believe that the clinical implications from this study are that interventions such as client education and social and mental support are important tools to optimize both self-care capacity and the ability to maintain a healthy perception of identity after liver transplantation. Nurses should also keep in mind how stressful it may be for the client to leave the hospital after receiving a transplant. "Leaving the experts" was identified as a significant milestone.

◆ COLLABORATIVE MANAGEMENT

Care of the client undergoing liver transplantation requires an interdisciplinary team approach. Receiving a transplant has a major psychosocial impact on the client. Forsberg and colleagues found seven themes that emerged from their research on clients who received liver transplants (see the Evidence-Based Practice for Nursing box above).

After the client is identified as a candidate and a donor organ is procured, the actual liver transplantation surgical procedure usually takes 8 hours. The length of the procedure can vary greatly.

In the immediate postoperative period, the client who has undergone liver transplantation is managed in the critical care unit and requires aggressive monitoring and care. The nurse assesses for signs and symptoms of complications of surgery and immediately reports their occurrence to the physician (Table 62-6).

Monitor the client's temperature and report elevations, increased abdominal pain, distention, and rigidity, which are indicators of peritonitis. Nursing assessment also includes monitoring for a change in neurologic status that could indicate encephalopathy from a nonfunctioning liver. Signs of coagulopathy (e.g., continuous bloody oozing from a catheter, drain, and incision sites; petechiae; or ecchymosis) are reported to the physician immediately because they can indicate impaired function of the transplanted liver.

TABLE 62-6 Assessment and Prevention of Common Postoperative Complications Associated with Liver Transplantation

Assessment	Prevention
Acute Graft Rejection Occurs from the 4th to 10th postoperative day Manifested by tachycardia, fever, right upper quadrant (RUQ) or flank pain, diminished bile drainage or change in bile color, or increased jaundice Laboratory changes: (1) increased levels of serum bilirubin, transaminases, and alkaline phosphatase: (2) prolonged prothrombin time	Prophylaxis with immunosuppressant agents, such as cyclosporine Early diagnosis to treat with more potent antirejection drugs, such as muromonab-CD3 (OKT3)
Infection Can occur at any time during recovery Frequent cultures of tubes, lines, and drainage Manifested by fever or excessive, foul-smelling drainage (urine, wound, or bile); other indicators depend on location and type of infection Early removal of invasive lines Good handwashing	Antibiotic prophylaxis Early diagnosis and treatment with organism-specific anti-infective agents
Hepatic Complications (Bile Leakage, Abscess Formation, Hepatic Thrombosis) Manifested by decreased bile drainage, increased RUQ abdominal pain with distention and guarding, nausea or vomiting, increased jaundice, and clay-colored stools Laboratory changes: increased levels of serum bilirubin and transaminases	Keep T-tube in dependent position and secure to client; empty frequently, recording quality and quantity of drainage. Report manifestations to physician immediately. May necessitate surgical intervention.
Acute Renal Failure Caused by hypotension, antibiotics, cyclosporine, acute liver failure, or hypothermia Indicators of hypothermia: shivering, hyperventilation, increased cardiac output, vasoconstriction, and alkalemia Early indicators of renal failure: changes in urine output, increased BUN and creatinine levels, and electrolyte imbalance	Monitor all drug levels with nephrotoxic side effects. Prevent hypotension. Observe for early signs of renal failure and report them immediately to the physician.

BUN, Blood urea nitrogen.

GET READY for the NCLEX Examination!

KEY POINTS

Safe Effective Care Environment

- Monitor the client with cirrhosis for bleeding and neurologic changes as described in Chart 62-2.
- For the client who has an esophagogastric tube, ensure airway patency because the tube may become displaced.
- Use standard precautions for all clients, especially for clients with hepatitis.
- Take precautions to prevent needle sticks or injury from other sharp instruments.
- Observe for hypovolemic shock from hemorrhage in the client with liver trauma.

Health Promotion and Maintenance

- Follow the guidelines listed in Chart 62-4 to prevent viral hepatitis in the workplace.
- Teach clients to take precautions to prevent viral hepatitis in the community as described in Chart 62-5.
- For clients with viral hepatitis, instruct them to follow the guidelines listed in Chart 62-6.

Psychosocial Integrity

- Recognize that clients with cirrhosis have mental and emotional changes due to portal systemic-encephalopathy (PSE).

- Be aware that clients with cirrhosis and/or chronic hepatitis may feel guilty about their disease because of past habits such as drug and alcohol abuse.
- Be aware that family members and friends may fear getting the disease from the client, causing client isolation.
- Encourage clients with cirrhosis and/or chronic hepatitis to verbalize their feelings.
- Be aware that clients having liver transplantation have major concerns about the possibility of complications, such as organ rejection.

Physiological Integrity

- Be aware that there are many causes of cirrhosis in addition to alcohol abuse (see Table 62-3).
- Monitor laboratory values of clients suspected of or diagnosed with cirrhosis of the liver as listed in Tables 62-1 and 62-4.
- Observe for clinical manifestations of portal-systemic encephalopathy (PSE) as listed in Table 62-2.
- Assess for manifestations of cirrhosis as shown in Figure 62-1.
- Provide care for the client having a paracentesis as described in Chart 62-1.
- Administer medications to decrease ammonia levels (which cause PSE) in clients with cirrhosis, such as lactulose, neomycin sulfate, and metronidazole.
- Differentiate the five major types of hepatitis as outlined in Table 62-5.

- Be aware that clients with chronic viral hepatitis often acquire cirrhosis and cancer of the liver.
- Recognize that potent immunomodulators, such as the interferons, and antivirals are being used to treat hepatitis B and C.
- Observe the client having a liver transplantation for complications, such as those described in Table 62-6.

ADDITIONAL STUDY RESOURCES

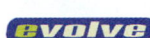 Go to your Student CD-ROM for Review Questions for the NCLEX Examination.

Go to http://evolve.elsevier.com/Iggy/ for Integrated Management of Care Questions for the NCLEX Examination.

SELECTED BIBLIOGRAPHY

Asterisk indicates a classic or definitive work on this subject.

Banasik, J. (2001). Diagnosing alpha 1 antitrypsin deficiency. *The Nurse Practitioner, 26*(1), 58-67.

Bockhold, K.M. (2000). Who's afraid of hepatitis C? *American Journal of Nursing, 100*(5), 26-31.

Centers for Disease Control and Prevention. (2002). *Hepatitis fact sheet.* Available at http://www.cdc.gov/ncidod/diseases/hepatitis.htm.

Compton, P. (2002). Caring for the alcohol dependent patient. *Nursing2002, 32*(12), 58-63.

DeCarlis, L., et al. (2003). Surgical treatment of hepatocellular cancer in the era of hepatic transplantation. *Journal of American College of Surgeons, 196*(6), 887-897.

Dougherty, A.S., & Dreher, H.M. (2001). Hepatitis C: Current treatment strategies for an emerging epidemic. *MEDSURG Nursing, 10*(1), 9-13.

Freeman, A.J., et al. (2003). Predicting progression to cirrhosis in chronic hepatitis C virus infection. *Journal of Viral Hepatitis, 10*(4), 285-293.

Hepatitis Liver Cirrhosis/HCC. Available at http://www.extremehealthusa.com/hepatitis.html.

Hilsabeck, R., et al. (2002). Neuropsychological impairment in patients with chronic hepatitis C. *Hepatology, 35*(2), 440-446.

Iosue, K. (2002). Chronic hepatitis C: Latest treatment options. *The Nurse Practitioner, 27*(4), 32-49.

Ma, Y., et al. (2002). Antibodies to conformational epitopes of soluble liver antigen define a severe form of autoimmune liver disease. *Hepatology, 35*(3), 658-664.

National Institutes of Health Consensus Development Conference Statement. *Management of hepatitis C: 2002.* June 10-12, 2002, Washington, DC: National Institutes of Health.

Ohata, K., et al. (2003). Hepatic steatosis is a risk factor for hepatocellular carcinoma in patients with chronic hepatitis C virus infection. *Cancer, 97*(12), 3036-3043.

Pagana, K., & Pagana, T. (2002). *Mosby's manual of diagnostic and laboratory tests* (2nd ed.). St. Louis: Mosby.

Portal hypertension-New treatments. (March 2, 2004). Available at http://www.ccspublishing.com/journals5a/portal_hypertension.htm.

*Starzl, T., et al. (1997). Liver transplantation. *Gastroenterology, 112*(1), 288-291.

Velazquez, R., et al. (2003). Prospective analysis of risk factors for hepatocellular carcinoma in patients with liver cirrhosis. *Hepatology, 37*(3), 520-527.

Wong, J.B., et al. (2000). Estimating future hepatitis C morbidity, mortality, and costs in the United States. *American Journal of Public Health, 90*(10), 1562-1569.

Yeung, E., Wong, F.S. (2002). The management of cirrhotic ascites. *Medscape General Medicine, 4*(4), 8. Review. No abstract available.

Interventions for Clients with Problems of the Biliary System and Pancreas

DONNA D. IGNATAVICIUS

LEARNING OUTCOMES

After studying this chapter, you should be able to:

1. Identify the common causes of cholecystitis and cholelithiasis (gallbladder disease).
2. Interpret diagnostic test results associated with gallbladder disease.
3. Compare postoperative care of clients undergoing a traditional cholecystectomy with that of clients undergoing a laparoscopic cholecystectomy.
4. Develop a community-based teaching plan for clients with gallbladder disease, including care of a T-tube.
5. Compare and contrast the pathophysiology of acute and chronic pancreatitis.
6. Interpret common assessment findings associated with acute pancreatitis and those associated with chronic pancreatitis.
7. Prioritize nursing care for clients with acute pancreatitis and clients with chronic pancreatitis.
8. Explain the use and precautions associated with enzyme replacement for chronic pancreatitis.
9. Develop a postoperative plan of care for clients undergoing a Whipple procedure.
10. Construct a discharge plan for care of clients with pancreatic cancer in the community.
11. Discuss the psychosocial needs of the client with pancreatic cancer and associated nursing interventions.

Go to your Student CD-ROM for Review Questions for the NCLEX Examination keyed to these Learning Outcomes.

Disorders of the biliary system and pancreas begin as single-organ processes, but the inflammatory response may extend to other organs if the primary disorder is not treated. This occurs because of the anatomic proximity of the liver, gallbladder, and pancreas and because the flow of bile from the liver through the biliary (gallbladder) ductal system may be impeded. Inflammation of the gallbladder, liver, or pancreas is caused by obstruction in the biliary system from gallstones, edema, stricture, or tumors. For example, gallstones impacted in the cystic duct cause cholecystitis; gallstones lodged in the ampulla of Vater impede the flow of bile and pancreatic secretions, which can result in pancreatitis.

BILIARY DISORDERS

Cholecystitis

PATHOPHYSIOLOGY

The two most common problems that occur within the biliary tree are stone formation (cholelithiasis) and associated chronic inflammation (cholecystitis). Cholecystitis may be either acute or chronic.

Acute Cholecystitis

Acute **cholecystitis** (inflammation of the gallbladder) usually develops in association with **cholelithiasis** (gallstones).

Either condition may occur singly, but most often they occur together.

Acalculous cholecystitis (inflammation occurring in the absence of gallstones) is typically associated with biliary stasis caused by any condition that affects the regular filling or emptying of the gallbladder. For example, a decrease in blood flow to the gallbladder or anatomic problems such as twisting or kinking of the gallbladder neck or cystic duct can result in pancreatic enzyme reflux into the gallbladder, causing inflammation.

Acute **calculous cholecystitis** usually follows obstruction of the cystic duct by a stone (calculus), which creates the inflammatory response. This response may be the result of a mechanical, chemical, or bacterial process. When the gallbladder is inflamed, trapped bile is reabsorbed and acts as a chemical irritant to the gallbladder wall; that is, the bile has a toxic effect. The presence of bile, in combination with impaired circulation, edema, and distention of the gallbladder, causes ischemia of the gallbladder wall. The result is tissue sloughing with necrosis and gangrene. Perforation (rupture) of the gallbladder wall may eventually occur. If the perforation is small and localized, an abscess may form. **Peritonitis**, infection of the peritoneum, may result if the perforation is large.

PATHOLOGIC CHANGES

The exact pathophysiology of gallstone formation is not clearly understood, but abnormal metabolism of cholesterol and bile salts plays an important role in their formation. Contributing factors may include the following:

- Supersaturation of bile with cholesterol
- Excessive bile salt losses
- Decreased gallbladder-emptying rates
- Changes in bile concentration or bile stasis within the gallbladder

Gallstones may lie dormant within the gallbladder or may move to other areas of the biliary tree as the gallbladder empties and refills with bile. They may migrate and lodge within the gallbladder neck, cystic duct, or common bile duct, causing obstruction (Figure 63-1). Gallstones interfere with or totally obstruct normal bile flow from the gallbladder to the duodenum, causing vascular congestion as a result of impeded venous return. Edema and congestion occur and contribute to the initial inflammatory process. When bile cannot flow from the gallbladder, the stasis of bile and local irritation from the gallstones lead to cholecystitis.

Cholangitis, usually associated with **choledocholithiasis** (common bile duct stones), involves infection of the bile ducts. *Ascending* **cholangitis** (inflammation of the biliary tree) occurs after bacterial invasion of the ducts. Bacterial invasion can lead to life-threatening *suppurative* cholangitis when symptoms are not recognized quickly and pus accumulates in the ductal system.

TYPES OF GALLSTONES

The gallbladder provides an excellent environment for the production of gallstones. In particular, the gallbladder only occasionally mixes its normally abundant mucus with its highly viscous, concentrated bile. The constant temperature within the gallbladder also contributes to stone formation by delaying bile emptying, causing biliary stasis.

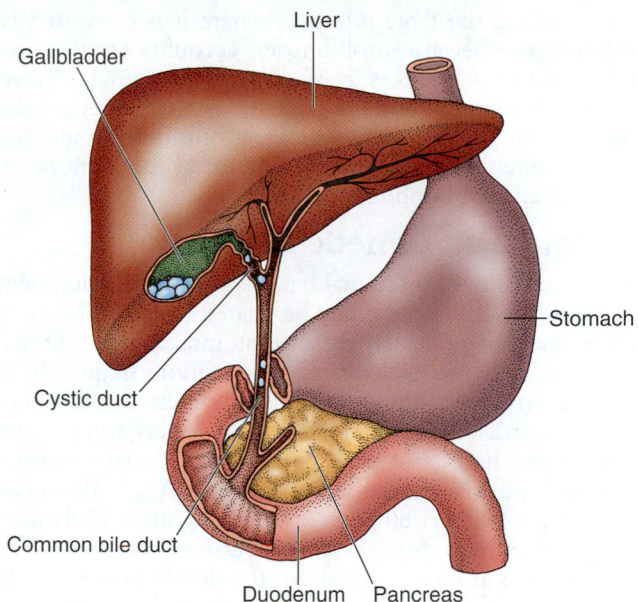

Figure 63-1 ■ Gallstones within the gallbladder and obstructing the common bile and cystic ducts.

Gallstones are composed of substances normally found in bile, such as cholesterol, bilirubin, bile salts, calcium, and various proteins. They are classified as either cholesterol stones or pigment stones. Cholesterol calculi form as a result of metabolic imbalances of cholesterol and bile salts. They are the most common type found in people in the United States, accounting for 90% of all gallstones, and generally originate from the gallbladder.

Chronic Cholecystitis

Chronic cholecystitis results when repeated episodes of cystic duct obstruction result in chronic inflammation. Calculi are almost always present. In chronic cholecystitis, the gallbladder becomes fibrotic and contracted, which results in decreased motility and deficient absorption.

Pancreatitis and cholangitis can occur as complications of cholecystitis. These problems result from the backup of bile throughout the biliary tract. Bile obstruction leads to jaundice.

Jaundice (yellow discoloration of the skin and mucous membranes) and **icterus** (yellow discoloration of the sclerae) can occur in clients with acute cholecystitis but is most commonly seen in clients with the chronic form of the disease. Impeded or obstructed bile flow caused by edema of the ducts or gallstones contributes to *extrahepatic* **obstructive jaundice**. Jaundice in cholecystitis may also be caused by direct liver involvement. Inflammation of the liver's bile channels or bile ducts may cause *intrahepatic* obstructive jaundice, resulting in an increase in circulating levels of bilirubin, the principal pigment of bile.

When the concentration of bilirubin in the blood increases to greater than 2.5 mg/dL, jaundice occurs (Pagana & Pagana, 2002). In a person with obstructive jaundice, the normal flow of bile into the duodenum is blocked, allowing excessive bile salts to accumulate in the skin. This accumulation of bile salts leads to **pruritus** (itching) or a burning sensation. The bile flow blockage also prevents bilirubin from reaching the large intestine, where it is converted to urobilinogen. Because urobilinogen accounts for the normal brown color of feces, clay-colored stools result. Water-soluble bilirubin is normally excreted by the kidneys in the urine. When an excess of circulating bilirubin occurs, the urine becomes dark and foamy because of the kidneys' effort to clear the bilirubin.

Etiology and Genetic Risk

There appears to be a familial tendency in the development of cholelithiasis, but this may be related to familial dietary habits (excessive dietary cholesterol intake) and familial sedentary lifestyles. Gallstones are seen more frequently in obese clients, probably as a result of impaired fat metabolism or increased cholesterol. Cholesterol-lowering drugs, which lower cholesterol levels in the blood, actually increase the amount of cholesterol secreted in bile. Age is also a factor, with people over 60 years of age being more likely than younger people to develop stones. Persons with type I diabetes are also at increased risk for the development of gallstones and cholecystitis because they generally have higher levels of fatty acids (triglycerides).

Cholesterol is increased following rapid weight loss, when the liver excretes extra cholesterol into bile. The ingestion of low-calorie or liquid protein diets also increases the susceptibility to gallstone development. These diets cause the liberation of cholesterol from tissues; the cholesterol is excreted as crystals in bile. Alcohol abuse may contribute to the formation of pigment stones, but alcohol in moderate amounts appears to reduce the formation of cholesterol stones. Cholelithiasis is seen with hemolytic blood disorders, with bowel disease such as Crohn's disease, and after gastric bypass surgery as a treatment of morbid obesity.

Cholecystitis is triggered by a number of other processes and health problems. In addition to the formation of gallbladder calculi, causes of acute cholecystitis include the following:

- Trauma
- Inadequate blood supply
- Prolonged anesthesia and surgery
- Adhesions
- Edema
- Neoplasms (tumors)
- Diabetes mellitus
- Cardiac events
- Long-term fasting
- Prolonged dehydration
- Gallbladder trauma
- Prolonged immobility
- Excessive opioid use
- Hormone replacement therapy

Incidence/Prevalence

More than 20 million persons in the United States have gallbladder disease, resulting in over 500,000 surgeries each year. Gallstones are very common, with about 20% of the U.S. population being affected. Native Americans/American Indians, particularly the Pima Indians of Arizona, have an unusually high incidence of gallstones, with Mexican Americans and white individuals following (Everhart et al., 1999). A high incidence of biliary tract disease and cholecystitis occurs in people with a sedentary lifestyle, a familial tendency

to biliary disease, obesity, or diabetes mellitus. Middle-aged white women have a high incidence of gallbladder disease, but the exact cause is unknown.

✹ WOMEN'S HEALTH CONSIDERATIONS

Women who are between 20 and 60 years of age are twice as likely to develop gallstones as men. Obesity is a major risk factor for gallstone formation, especially in women. Pregnancy tends to worsen gallstone formation. Pregnancy, as well as drugs such as estrogen and birth control pills, especially the older oral contraceptives, alter hormone levels and delay muscular contraction of the gallbladder, causing a decreased rate of bile emptying. The incidence of gallstones is higher in women who have had multiple pregnancies. Combinations of causative factors increase the incidence of stone formation, especially in women. For example, an obese pregnant woman or an obese woman taking birth control pills may be at higher risk.

◆COLLABORATIVE MANAGEMENT
◆Assessment

PHYSICAL ASSESSMENT/CLINICAL MANIFESTATIONS

Clients with acute cholecystitis frequently present with pain, although clinical manifestations vary in intensity and frequency (Chart 63-1).

Ask assistive nursing personnel to obtain the client's height, weight, and vital signs, and assess gender, age, race, and ethnic group. Ask about food preferences and determine whether excessive fat and cholesterol are included in the diet. The client is asked whether any foods are not tolerated. Question whether any of the following gastrointestinal (GI) symptoms occur in relation to the intake of fatty food: **flatulence** (gas), **dyspepsia** (indigestion), **eructation** (belching), anorexia, nausea, vomiting, and abdominal pain or discomfort.

Ask the client to describe the pain, including its intensity and duration, precipitating factors, and any measures that relieve it. The pain may be described as indigestion of varying intensity, ranging from a mild, persistent ache to a steady, constant pain in the right upper abdominal quadrant. The pain may radiate to the right shoulder or scapula.

CHART 63-1

KEY FEATURES of
Cholecystitis

- Episodic or vague upper abdominal pain or discomfort that can radiate to the right shoulder
- Pain triggered by a high-fat or high-volume meal
- Anorexia
- Nausea or vomiting
- Dyspepsia
- Eructation
- Flatulence
- Feeling of abdominal fullness
- Rebound tenderness (Blumberg's sign)
- Fever
- Jaundice, clay-colored stools, dark urine, steatorrhea (most common with chronic cholecystitis)

The abdominal pain of chronic cholecystitis may be vague and nonspecific. The usual pattern of more acute pain is episodic. Clients often refer to these episodes as "gallbladder attacks."

The severe pain of **biliary colic** is produced by obstruction of the cystic duct of the gallbladder. When a stone is moving through or is lodged within the duct, tissue spasm occurs in an effort to mobilize the stone through the small duct. This intense pain may be so severe that it is accompanied by tachycardia, pallor, diaphoresis, and **prostration** (extreme exhaustion).

Ask the client to describe his or her daily activity or exercise routines to determine whether his or her lifestyle is sedentary. Question whether there is a family history of gallbladder disease, because there is a familial tendency for biliary tract diseases. If the client is female, determine whether hormone replacement therapy (HRT) is being taken, because this therapy may contribute to biliary disorders.

Because of gallbladder tenderness, it is difficult to use abdominal palpation and percussion in assessment of the client with acute cholecystitis. With right subcostal palpation, pain increases with deep inspiration **(Murphy's sign)**. Guarding and rigidity, as well as rebound tenderness **(Blumberg's sign)**, are reliable indicators of peritoneal irritation.

Assessment for rebound tenderness and deep palpation are reserved for physicians and advanced practice nurses. To elicit rebound tenderness, the health care provider pushes his or her fingers deeply and steadily into the client's abdomen, then quickly releases the pressure. Pain that results from the rebound of the palpated tissue may indicate peritoneal inflammation. Deep palpation below the liver border in the right upper quadrant may reveal a sausage-shaped mass, representing the distended, inflamed gallbladder. Percussion over the posterior rib cage intensifies localized abdominal pain.

CONSIDERATIONS FOR OLDER ADULTS

Older adults and clients with diabetes mellitus have atypical manifestations, including the absence of pain and fever. Localized tenderness may be the only presenting sign. The older client may become acutely confused (delirium).

In *chronic* cholecystitis, clients may have insidious symptoms and may not seek medical treatment until late symptoms such as jaundice, clay-colored stools, and dark urine result from an obstructive process. Jaundice may also be seen as yellowing of the skin, sclerae, and oral mucous membranes. **Steatorrhea** (fatty stools) occurs because fat absorption is decreased owing to the lack of bile. Bile is needed for the absorption of fats and fat-soluble vitamins in the intestine. As with any inflammatory process, the client may have an elevated temperature of 99° to 102° F (37° to 39° C), tachycardia, and dehydration from fever and vomiting.

DIAGNOSTIC ASSESSMENT

There are no laboratory tests specific for gallbladder disease. A differential diagnosis must rule out other diseases that may cause similar symptoms, such as peptic ulcer disease, gastroesophageal reflux disorder, and pancreatitis. Serum levels of alkaline phosphatase, aspartate aminotransferase (AST), and lactate dehydrogenase (LDH) may be elevated, indicating abnormalities in liver function. The direct (conjugated) and indirect (unconjugated) serum bilirubin levels are elevated if an obstructive process is present. An increased white blood cell (WBC) count with a left shift on the differential count indicates inflammation. If there is pancreatic involvement, serum amylase and lipase levels are elevated.

Calcified gallstones are easily visualized on abdominal x-ray. Stones that are not calcified cannot be seen.

Ultrasonography of the right upper quadrant is the best diagnostic test for cholecystitis and has largely replaced the older cholecystogram. It is safe, accurate, and painless. Acute cholecystitis is evidenced by edema of the gallbladder wall and pericholecystic fluid, both of which are determined by the ultrasound. The health care provider may also order an upper GI radiographic series to rule out other causes of abdominal pain, such as gastritis and peptic ulcer disease.

A hepatobiliary scan can be performed to visualize the gallbladder and determine patency of the biliary system. The pretest fasting period for this scan can be as short as 4 hours, making it preferable to a diagnostic study that would require a longer fasting time. Visualization of the gallbladder excludes the diagnosis of acute cholecystitis with a high degree of certainty (Fischbach, 2004).

◆Interventions

Nonsurgical treatment measures prescribed during the acute phase of cholecystitis are directed at resting the inflamed gallbladder to reduce the inflammatory process and relieve pain. Because of the risk for sepsis and perforation, however, acute cholecystitis is generally managed surgically.

NONSURGICAL MANAGEMENT. Two thirds of gallstones are asymptomatic, or silent (Howard & Fromm, 1999). Asymptomatic stones are usually managed conservatively with no medical or surgical intervention. Acute pain occurs when the gallstones partially or totally obstruct the cystic or common bile duct.

Diet Therapy. In general, the client must adhere to a low-fat diet to prevent further pain of biliary colic. If gallstones are causing an obstruction of bile flow, the health care provider may prescribe replacement of fat-soluble vitamins (such as vitamins A, D, E, and K) and the administration of bile salts to facilitate digestion and vitamin absorption. Food and fluids are withheld if nausea and vomiting occur.

Drug Therapy. Pain caused by acute obstruction with gallstones necessitates opioid analgesia with meperidine hydrochloride (Demerol). Older clients should not be given Demerol, because it can cause acute confusion, seizures, or nausea (see Chapter 7). Morphine is usually not used, because it is thought to cause biliary spasm and constrict the sphincter of Oddi. Antispasmodic or anticholinergic drugs, such as atropine and dicyclomine (Bentyl, Lomine✱), may be given to relax smooth muscles and decrease ductal tone and spasm. The health care provider prescribes antiemetics to control nausea and vomiting.

Percutaneous Transhepatic Biliary Catheter Insertion. The physician may insert a **percutaneous transhepatic biliary catheter** under fluoroscopic guidance. This procedure decompresses obstructed extrahepatic ducts so that bile can flow. It is primarily used for inoperable hepatic, pancreatic, or bile duct carcinoma. It may be a nonsurgical alternative for the treatment of biliary obstruction caused by gallstones and hepatic dysfunction associated with obstructive jaundice and biliary sepsis in high-risk candidates. Nursing care associated with this treatment is outlined in Chart 63-4.

SURGICAL MANAGEMENT. The usual surgical treatment of clients with acute and chronic cholecystitis is **cholecystectomy**, the removal of the gallbladder. Two operative procedures are available to the surgeon for performing a cholecystectomy: the laparoscopic cholecystectomy and, less often, the traditional open approach cholecystectomy.

Laparoscopic Cholecystectomy. Laparoscopic cholecystectomy, a minimally invasive surgery (MIS), is considered the "gold standard," and is performed much more often than the traditional open cholecystectomy. The advantages of MIS versus the open technique include the following:

- Complications are not common.
- The death rate is very low (i.e., <0.1%).
- Bile duct injuries are rare.
- Client recovery is faster.
- Postoperative pain is less severe.

Preoperative Care. The laparoscopic procedure is commonly done on an ambulatory care basis in a same-day surgery suite. The surgeon explains the procedure; the nurse answers questions and reinforces the physician's instructions. There is no special preoperative preparation for the client. However, the physician typically orders the usual preoperative laboratory tests and requires the client to be on NPO (nothing by mouth) status before the surgery. Chapter 20 describes general preoperative care for the client undergoing anesthesia.

Operative Procedures. The surgeon makes a very small midline puncture at the umbilicus. The abdominal cavity is insufflated with 3 to 4 L of carbon dioxide. Gasless laparoscopic cholecystectomy using abdominal wall lifting devices is a more recent innovation. This technique results in improved pulmonary and cardiac function. A trocar catheter is inserted, through which a laparoscope is introduced. The laparoscope is attached to a video camera, and the abdominal organs are viewed on a monitor. The surgeon makes several small punctures through which to introduce laparoscopic forceps to manipulate the gallbladder. The gallbladder is dissected from the liver bed and the cystic artery and duct are closed. The surgeon mobilizes the gallbladder, aspirates the bile and crushes any large stones, and then extracts the gallbladder through the umbilical port.

Postoperative Care. Removing the gallbladder with the laparoscopic technique reduces the risk of wound complications. Some clients have a problem with "free air pain" from carbon dioxide retention in the abdomen. Teach about the importance of early ambulation to promote absorption of the carbon dioxide. Far less opioid analgesia is necessary after the laparoscopic procedure than following the open procedure.

The client is usually discharged from the hospital or surgery center within 1 day. Following laparoscopic surgery, the client can return to usual activities, including work, much sooner than if an open cholecystectomy had been done. Most clients are able to resume usual activities within 1 to 3 weeks.

Traditional Cholecystectomy. Use of the traditional surgical approach has markedly declined during the past decade. The client undergoing this surgery is usually hospitalized for several days following the procedure.

Preoperative Care. The surgical nurse provides the usual preoperative care and teaching in the operating suite on the day of surgery (see Chapter 20).

Operative Procedures. The surgeon not only removes the gallbladder through a right subcostal incision but also often explores the biliary ducts for the presence of stones. If the common bile duct is explored, the surgeon typically inserts a T-tube drain to ensure patency of the duct. Trauma to the common bile duct stimulates inflammation, which can impede bile flow and contribute to bile stasis. In addition, the surgeon usually inserts a drainage tube, such as a Jackson-Pratt (JP) drain. This drainage tube is positioned in the gallbladder bed to prevent fluid accumulation. The drainage is usually serosanguinous (serous fluid mixed with blood) and is stained with bile in the first 24 hours postoperatively.

Postoperative Care. Postoperative incisional pain relief after a traditional cholecystectomy is usually achieved with meperidine hydrochloride (Demerol) using a patient-controlled analgesia (PCA) pump. Older adults should not receive this medication because its toxic metabolite can cause seizures and other mental status changes. The client participates in coughing and deep breathing exercises more readily when pain is minimized.

Antiemetics may be necessary for clients with episodes of postoperative nausea and vomiting. Administer the antiemetic early, as prescribed, to prevent retching associated with vomiting and thus decrease the incidence of pain related to muscle straining.

Provide care for the incision, the surgical drain, and the T-tube. The surgeon typically removes the surgical dressing and drain within 24 to 48 hours after surgery. The T-tube, however, may remain in place for 6 weeks or longer. Chart 63-2 highlights the important nursing care activities associated with the T-tube system.

The client usually receives nothing by mouth (NPO) until the client is fully awake postoperatively. Gradually advance the diet from clear liquids to solid foods as tolerated. Within a day or two, the client resumes the ingestion of solid foods and is discharged to home.

The amount of fat allowed in the client's diet after a cholecystectomy depends on his or her tolerance of fat. In the early postoperative period, if bile flow is reduced, a low-fat diet may reduce discomfort and prevent nausea. For most clients, a special diet is not required. Advise the client to eat nutritious meals and avoid excessive intake of fat. If the client is obese, recommend a weight reduction program. Collaborate with the physician and the dietitian in planning the appropriate diet.

Community-Based Care

HOME CARE MANAGEMENT

After a traditional cholecystectomy, clients may need short-term assistance with procuring foods, preparing meals, performing dressing changes, and caring for the T-tube. Clients who have undergone traditional gallbladder surgery may also need transportation to follow-up appointments with the health care provider. The surgeon typically allows these clients to return to their usual activities 4 to 6 weeks after surgery.

HEALTH TEACHING

Following a cholecystectomy, discharge teaching for the client and the family may include the following:

- Pain management
- Diet therapy
- Wound, drain, and incision care
- Activity restrictions

CHART 63-2

BEST PRACTICE for
Care of the Client with a T-Tube

- Keep the drainage system below the level of the gallbladder. Maintain the client in the semi-Fowler's position.
- Assess the amount, color, consistency, and odor of drainage initially every 2 to 4 hours, then every 8 hours after the first 24 hours. In the immediate postoperative period, expect bloody drainage, which changes to green-brown bile. Bile output is about 400+ mL/day with a gradual decrease in amount. Report bile drainage amounts in excess of 1000 mL/day to the physician.
- Collect and administer excess bile output to the client by the nasogastric tube (uncommon), or give synthetic bile salts, such as dehydrocholic acid (Decholin).
- Report sudden increases in bile output after a normally decreasing output pattern is established. (The hospital-based nurse does not normally observe this, because it occurs 9 to 10 days postoperatively, but this information should be included in client discharge teaching.)
- Assess for foul odor and purulent drainage, which indicate infection or extensive inflammation. Report changes in drainage to the physician.
- Inspect the skin around the T-tube insertion site for signs of inflammation, including redness, swelling, and erythema, and observe for frank bile leakage. Keep the dressing dry. (Use the hospital's procedure and provide drain care and dressing change per protocol. The site is usually cleaned and the dressing changed daily.)
- *Never* irrigate, aspirate, or clamp a T-tube without a physician's order.
- Assess the drainage system for pulling, kinking, or tangling of tubing, especially when the client is positioned toward the right side. Assist the client with early turning and ambulation. Drape and secure the section of the T-tube emerging from the stab wound over a small roll of gauze taped to the client's skin to help prevent its lumen from occluding as a result of pressure.
- When the client is allowed to eat, clamp the T-tube for 1 to 2 hours (per physician's orders) before and after meals. Assess the client's response to determine tolerance of food.
- Teach client to observe stools for return of brown color 7 to 10 days postoperatively.

TABLE 63-1 Foods for Clients with Cholecystitis or Cholelithiasis to Avoid

Foods High in Cholesterol/Fat	Gas-Forming Vegetables
Dairy Products	■ Cabbage
■ Whole milk	■ Onions
■ Ice cream	■ Broccoli
■ Butter	■ Cauliflower
■ Cream	■ Sauerkraut
■ Cheese	■ Radishes
	■ Cucumbers
Other Foods	■ Beans
■ Fried, fatty foods	
■ Rich pastries	
■ Gravies	
■ Nuts	
■ Chocolate	
■ Egg yolks	
■ Avocado	

CHART 63-3

CLIENT EDUCATION GUIDE
Home Care for the Client with a T-Tube

- Coil the drainage tubing and secure it to your abdomen by taping or using a belt with Velcro fasteners. Keep the drainage bag below the level of the T-tube.
- Wear loose-fitting clothes.
- Wear older clothes to prevent ruining good-quality clothes.
- If staining occurs, soak the garment in a solution of detergent, baking soda, and bleach.
- Take showers instead of baths.
- Avoid heavy lifting and strenuous activity.
- Remove the dressing around the T-tube every day. Hold the tube in place and clean the skin around the tube. Apply a precut dressing around the catheter and tape it in place.
- Empty the drainage bag at the same time each day. Allow the bile to flow from the bag's spout; do not disconnect the system.
- The physician may advise you to clamp the T-tube for 1 to 2 hours before and after meals. Otherwise, keep the T-tube unclamped.
- Observe the amount, color, and odor of the drainage. Report any change in drainage, abdominal pain, nausea, or vomiting to your physician.
- Inspect the wound for signs of infection, including redness, swelling, warmth, abdominal firmness, pain, and purulent drainage at the tube site. Take your temperature, and report a temperature of 100° F (37° C) or greater to your physician.
- Return to the health care provider as scheduled for follow-up.

- Complication recognition
- Health care follow-up

During postoperative teaching and discharge planning, include a supportive spouse, family member, or significant other to provide reinforcement of information and to assist the client in adhering to the treatment plan.

Diet therapy for the client who has undergone a cholecystectomy is based on his or her tolerance of fats. The nurse or dietitian consults with the client to develop a nutrition program that includes nutritious, well-balanced meals that include the client's preferences, when possible. If the client has a poor tolerance of fats, a low-fat diet is developed and a list of foods to avoid is provided (Table 63-1). The dietitian may provide printed menu-planning guidelines. Some clients need to maintain a low-fat diet for 6 months or longer. They are advised to add fatty foods to the diet slowly and as tolerated.

If the client has problems tolerating three large meals a day, suggest trying smaller, more frequent meals. If the client is obese, a weight reduction diet is recommended and teaching is tailored to provide appropriate dietary guidelines.

Clients are leaving the hospital sooner after traditional open gallbladder surgery than they did in the past. Because

a T-tube is usually left in place for several weeks, clients are sent home with the drainage systems intact. Instruct the client and one or more family members to inspect the incision wound and the T-tube drainage site for inflammation. Signs and symptoms include redness, swelling, warmth, extreme tenderness, excessive drainage, and increased incisional pain. Any of these findings should be reported to the health care provider. The nurse provides oral and written instructions for drainage tube care (Chart 63-3).

Provide information to the client and family about the potential for **postcholecystectomy syndrome,** in which the clinical manifestations of biliary tract disease occur following cholecystectomy in a small percentage of clients. Postcholecystectomy syndrome is caused by residual or recurring calculi, inflammation, or stricture of the common bile duct.

Remind the client to report symptoms of biliary tract disease, including jaundice of the skin or sclera, darkened urine, light-colored stools, pain, fever, or chills, to the physician or nurse practitioner.

The client with cholecystitis who either refuses or postpones surgery must be instructed on the signs of potential complications of chronic cholecystitis, including fever, recurrent abdominal pain, and jaundice. If these signs occur, the client should notify the health care provider for prompt medical care.

HEALTH CARE RESOURCES

For clients at home with a T-tube or for those older adults who cannot manage self-care, a home care nurse may be needed to provide support and follow-up nursing care and teaching. The nurse assesses the client's adaptation to the treatment plan and evaluates wound healing and the integrity of the T-tube drainage system. The need for further wound and skin care interventions is also determined.

Critical Thinking Challenge

An older morbidly obese woman is admitted to the same-day surgical department where you work for a laparoscopic cholecystectomy. She has had severe episodic pain for several months following ingestion of fatty and spicy foods. Her history states that she has type 2 diabetes and has multiple lower extremity varicosities for which she has undergone two surgical procedures. The client stands all day for 6 days a week because she runs and cooks for a small, but busy restaurant in the local community.

1. The client is especially at risk for what postoperative complications?
2. What interventions should you implement to decrease these problems when she returns from the operating suite?
3. What discharge teaching will she need?

evolve For suggested answer guidelines, go to http://evolve.elsevier.com/Iggy/.

Cancer of the Gallbladder

PATHOPHYSIOLOGY

Primary cancer of the gallbladder is rare and is more common in women than in men. Adenocarcinoma and squamous cell carcinoma of the gallbladder account for the majority of gallbladder cancers, and may be hereditary in a small percentage of clients. They typically infiltrate the liver and ducts, as well as the gallbladder. These rare gallbladder carcinomas appear more frequently in clients with pre-existing chronic cholecystitis and cholelithiasis.

The diagnosis of gallbladder cancer is difficult. Early symptoms, when present, are insidious in onset and similar to those of chronic cholecystitis and cholelithiasis. Characteristic manifestations include the following:

- Anorexia
- Weight loss
- Nausea
- Vomiting
- General malaise
- Jaundice
- Hepatosplenomegaly
- Chronic, progressively severe epigastric or right upper quadrant pain

A moderately tender, irregularly shaped mass may be palpated. Gallbladder carcinoma is typically discovered during

CHART 63-4

BEST PRACTICE for
The Client with a Transhepatic Biliary Catheter

- Change the catheter dressing twice a week or more often if it is wet. Be extremely careful not to allow the catheter to pull out during the dressing change. Apply hydrogen peroxide and antibiotic ointment to the site.
- Check the chart for radiology orders on drainage bag instructions. Be very careful regarding sterile technique when emptying and changing the bag. Do not raise the bag above the insertion site and teach this precaution to the client.
- Do not irrigate or flush the catheter without specific orders to do so.
- Assess the client for decreasing jaundice. Stools should change from clay color to normal brown, and urine should change from dark to straw color. Monitor serum bilirubin test results for decreasing levels.
- Assess the client for fever, chills, and hypotension; report these findings to the physician.
- Inspect the catheter for the presence of blood, and notify the physician immediately if any is present.
- Inspect the catheter for patency.
- Affix the bag to the client's gown (not to the bed).
- Provide discharge instructions to the client or a family member, including:
  Dressing care
  Signs of catheter malfunction, infection, and dislodgment
  Outpatient and diagnostic testing appointments

other procedures for diagnosis of suspected cholecystitis or during cholecystectomy.

◆COLLABORATIVE MANAGEMENT

The prognosis for the client with cancer of the gallbladder is poor. Three treatments are used: surgery, radiation therapy, and chemotherapy. Surgical intervention, when performed, is usually extensive. Nursing care is similar to that for clients who have a cholecystectomy or Whipple procedure, depending on the extent of disease. (These procedures are described elsewhere in this chapter.) A bile drainage tube (transhepatic biliary catheter) may be inserted to relieve symptoms such as jaundice and itching (Chart 63-4).

PANCREATIC DISORDERS

Acute Pancreatitis

PATHOPHYSIOLOGY

Acute pancreatitis is a serious and, at times, life-threatening inflammatory process of the pancreas. This process is caused by a premature activation of pancreatic enzymes that destroy ductal tissue and pancreatic cells, resulting in autodigestion and fibrosis of the pancreas. The pathologic changes occur in variable degrees. The severity of pancreatitis depends on the extent of inflammation and tissue destruction. Pancreatitis can range from mild involvement evidenced by edema and inflammation to **necrotizing hemorrhagic pancreatitis (NHP).** NHP affects about 20% of clients with pancreatitis and is characterized by diffusely bleeding pancreatic tissue with fibrosis and tissue death.

The pancreas is unusual in that it functions as both an exocrine gland and an endocrine gland. The primary endocrine disorder is diabetes and is discussed in Chapter 68. The exocrine function of the pancreas is responsible for secreting enzymes that assist in the breakdown of starches,

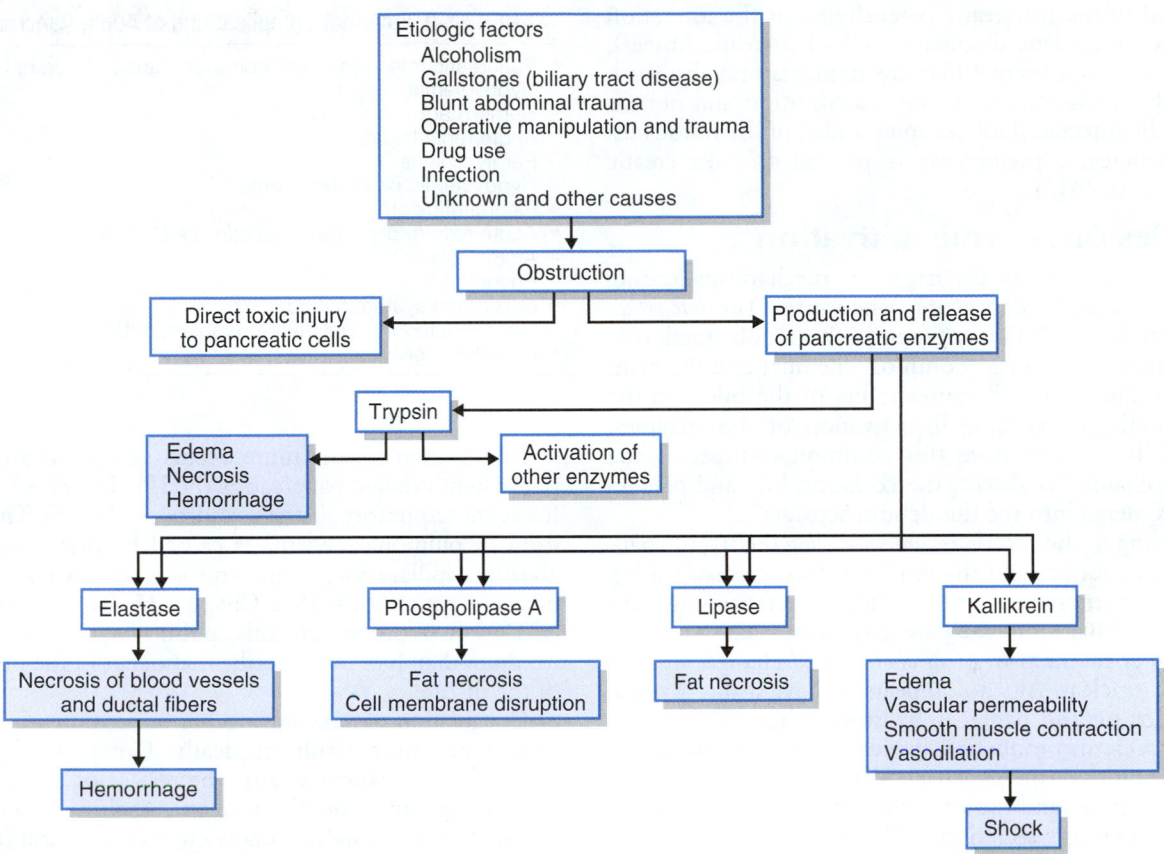

Figure 63-2 ■ The process of autodigestion in acute pancreatitis.

proteins, and fats. These enzymes are normally secreted in the inactive form and become activated once they enter the intestine. Early activation (i.e., activation within the pancreas rather than the intestinal lumen) results in the inflammatory process of pancreatitis. Direct toxic injury to the pancreatic cells and the production and release of pancreatic enzymes (trypsin, elastase, phospholipase A, lipase, and kallikrein) result from the obstructive damage. Following pancreatic duct obstruction, increased pressure within the pancreas and the pancreatic ducts may contribute to ductal rupture, allowing spillage of trypsin and other enzymes into the pancreatic parenchymal tissue. In acute pancreatitis, four major pathophysiologic processes occur: lipolysis, proteolysis, necrosis of blood vessels, and inflammation.

Lipolysis

The hallmark of pancreatic necrosis is enzymatic fat necrosis of the endocrine and exocrine cells of the pancreas caused by the enzyme lipase. Fatty acids are released during this lipolytic process and combine with ionized calcium to form a soaplike product. The initial rapid lowering of serum calcium levels is not readily compensated for by the parathyroid gland. Because the body needs ionized calcium and cannot use bound calcium, hypocalcemia occurs.

Proteolysis

The pathogenesis of pancreatitis involves **autodigestion** of the pancreatic parenchyma by the enzymes normally produced by the pancreas (Figure 63-2). **Trypsin** is the key element that activates all other proteolytic enzymes involved

in autodigestion. The agent that triggers the premature activation of trypsin to trypsinogen has not been identified and is being investigated. Proteolysis involves the splitting of proteins by hydrolysis of the peptide bonds, resulting in the formation of smaller polypeptides. Proteolytic activity may lead to thrombosis and gangrene of the pancreas. Pancreatic destruction may be localized and confined to one area or may involve the entire organ.

Necrosis of the Blood Vessels

Elastase is activated by trypsin and causes elastic fibers of the blood vessels and ducts to dissolve. The necrosis of blood vessels results in bleeding, ranging from minor bleeding to massive hemorrhage of pancreatic tissue. Another pancreatic enzyme, kallikrein, causes the release of vasoactive peptides, bradykinin, and a plasma kinin known as kallidin. These substances contribute to vasodilation and increased vascular permeability, further compounding the hemorrhagic process. This massive destruction of blood vessels by necrosis may lead to generalized hemorrhage with blood escaping into the retroperitoneal tissues. The client with hemorrhagic pancreatitis is critically ill, and extensive pancreatic destruction and shock may lead to death. The majority of deaths in clients with acute pancreatitis result from irreversible shock.

Inflammation

The inflammatory stage occurs when leukocytes cluster around the hemorrhagic and necrotic areas of the pancreas. A secondary bacterial process may lead to suppuration (pus formation) of the pancreatic parenchyma or the formation of an abscess (see later discussion under Pancreatic Abscess, p. 1412). Infected lesions that are mild may be absorbed. When infected lesions are severe, calcification and fibrosis occur. If the infected fluid becomes walled off by fibrous tissue, a pancreatic pseudocyst is formed (see Pancreatic Pseudocyst, p. 1412).

Theories of Enzyme Activation

Several theories explain the triggering mechanisms leading to enzyme activation in acute pancreatitis. The *bile reflux* ("common channel") theory proposes that an obstruction of the common channel (the common bile duct and the main pancreatic duct channel) causes reflux of the bile into the pancreatic tissue, resulting in activation of the enzymes. Not all biliary tracts have this common channel. If the common channel is absent, the common bile and pancreatic ducts merge into the duodenum separately.

According to the *hypersecretion-obstruction* theory, the pancreatic duct ruptures and the resulting disruption or tearing of the cell membrane allows pancreatic secretions and enzymes to leak back into the parenchymal tissue.

The exact mechanism of *alcohol-induced* changes in pancreatitis is unclear. Alcohol appears to have a direct metabolic effect on the pancreas by stimulating hydrochloric acid and secretin production, which in turn stimulates exocrine functions of the pancreas. Alcohol also causes edema of the duodenum and the ampulla of Vater, obstructing the flow of pancreatic secretions. Alcohol may decrease the tone of the sphincter of Oddi and cause sphincter spasm and duodenal reflux.

According to the fourth theory, reflux of duodenal contents can occur from biliary tract disease, gallstones in the bile duct (causing the sphincter of Oddi to dilate), or a generalized loss of tone caused by alcohol ingestion. Duodenal contents can enter the pancreatic duct through the weakened sphincter, activating the pancreatic enzymes.

The generalized abdominal pain of acute pancreatitis is related to peritoneal irritation. Ductal release of digested proteins and lipids into the peripancreatic tissues, along with stretching of the pancreatic tissue, causes the seepage of these substances into the mesentery. The resultant peritonitis stimulates the sensory nerves, contributing to intense pain in the back and flanks.

Complications of Acute Pancreatitis

Acute pancreatitis may result in severe, life-threatening complications (Table 63-2). Jaundice occurs from swelling of the head of the pancreas, which impedes bile flow through the common bile duct. The bile duct may also be compressed by calculi or a pancreatic pseudocyst. The resulting total bile flow obstruction causes severe jaundice. Transient hyperglycemia occurs as a result of the release of glucagon, as well as the decreased release of insulin due to damage to the pancreatic islet cells. Total destruction of the pancreas may occur, leading to type 1 diabetes.

Left lung pleural effusions frequently develop in the client with acute pancreatitis. Amylase effusions probably occur when exudate containing pancreatic enzymes passes from the peritoneal cavity into the pleural cavity via the transdiaphragmatic lymph channels. Atelectasis and pneumonia may also occur, especially in older clients.

TABLE 63-2 Potential Complications of Acute Pancreatitis
▪ Pancreatic infection (most common cause of death)
▪ Hypovolemia
▪ Hemorrhage
▪ Acute renal failure
▪ Paralytic ileus
▪ Hypovolemic or septic shock
▪ Pleural effusion
▪ Acute respiratory distress syndrome (ARDS)
▪ Atelectasis
▪ Pneumonia
▪ Multiorgan system failure
▪ Disseminated intravascular coagulation (DIC)
▪ Diabetes mellitus

Multisystem organ failure occurs as a sequela to necrotizing hemorrhagic pancreatitis (NHP). The client is at risk for acute respiratory distress syndrome (ARDS). This severe form of pulmonary edema is caused by disruption of the alveolar-capillary membrane and is a serious complication of acute pancreatitis. (See Chapter 35 for a discussion of ARDS.) In acute pancreatitis, pulmonary failure accounts for more than half of all deaths that occur in the first 7 days of the disease.

Coagulation defects are another major potential complication and may result in death. Complex physiologic changes in the pancreas cause the release of necrotic tissue and enzymes into the bloodstream, resulting in altered coagulation. Disseminated intravascular coagulation (DIC) involves hypercoagulation of the blood, with consumption of clotting factors and the development of microthrombi.

Shock in acute pancreatitis results from peripheral vasodilation from the released vasoactive substances and the retroperitoneal loss of protein-rich fluid from proteolytic digestion. Hypovolemia may result in decreased renal perfusion and acute renal failure. Paralytic (adynamic) ileus results from peritoneal irritation and seepage of pancreatic enzymes into the abdominal cavity.

Etiology and Genetic Risk

In many cases, the cause of pancreatitis is not known. Many factors can produce injury to the pancreas. The most commonly cited factors are excessive alcohol ingestion and biliary tract disease, with gallstones accounting for almost half of the cases of obstructive pancreatitis. Older adults with pancreatitis typically have biliary obstruction. Iatrogenic acute pancreatitis may occur as a result of trauma from surgical manipulation after biliary tract, pancreatic, gastric, and duodenal procedures, such as cholecystectomy, the Whipple procedure, and partial gastrectomy. The trauma may also originate as a complication of the diagnostic procedure endoscopic retrograde cholangiopancreatography (ERCP).

Other etiologic factors include the following:

▪ Trauma: external (blunt trauma) or operative
▪ Pancreatic obstruction: tumors, cysts, or abscesses; abnormal organ structure
▪ Metabolic disturbances: hyperlipidemia, hyperparathyroidism, or hypercalcemia
▪ Renal disturbances: failure or transplantation
▪ Familial, inherited pancreatitis
▪ Penetrating gastric or duodenal ulcers, resulting in peritonitis

- Viral infections, such as coxsackievirus B infection
- Toxicities of drugs, including opiates, sulfonamides, thiazides, steroids, and oral contraceptives (The exact mechanism by which these and other drugs cause pancreatitis is unknown.)

Incidence/Prevalence

Pancreatic attacks are especially common during holidays and vacations when alcohol ingestion is usually high, especially in men. Women are affected most often after cholelithiasis and biliary tract disturbances. In addition, acute pancreatitis is the most common complication of endoscopic retrograde cholangiopancreatography (ERCP).

Death occurs in about 10% of clients with acute pancreatitis, but with early diagnosis and treatment, mortality can be reduced. Death occurs at a higher rate in older adults and in clients with postoperative pancreatitis. The prognosis for recovery is usually favorable for pancreatitis associated with biliary tract disease and poor if pancreatitis accompanies alcoholism. Mortality rises as high as 60% when necrosis and hemorrhage occur.

HEALTH PROMOTION/ILLNESS PREVENTION

In view of the causes of pancreatitis, individuals who drink alcohol should do so in moderation to prevent alcohol-related health problems, such as pancreatitis. Gallbladder disease, especially when triggered by gallstones, should be treated promptly to avoid complications.

To help reduce the incidence of acute pancreatitis in ERCP, several antisecretory agents may be given. The most widely investigated drugs used for this purpose are somatostatin and its analogue octreotide. These drugs appear to have anti-inflammatory and cytoprotective properties. SecreFlo (injectable secretin) and diclofenac have also been used with success. They are most useful during ERCP when measuring pressures of the sphincter of Oddi.

◆ COLLABORATIVE MANAGEMENT
◆ Assessment

HISTORY

Most often, the client indicates that he or she needs relief from abdominal pain. Ask whether the abdominal pain occurs when ingesting alcohol or eating a high-fat meal. Information about alcohol usage should be obtained, including the amount of alcohol consumed during what period of time (i.e., years of consumption, how much usually consumed over a particular period). Because of the familial connection, the client is questioned about a family or personal history of alcoholism, pancreatitis, or biliary tract disease. Determine whether any abdominal surgical interventions, such as cholecystectomy, or diagnostic procedures, such as ERCP, have been performed recently.

Assess for the presence of other medical problems known to cause pancreatitis, including peptic ulcer disease, renal failure, vascular disorders, hyperparathyroidism, and hyperlipidemia. Inquire about recent viral infections. Ask the client or family member/significant other to list all prescription and over-the-counter (OTC) drugs taken recently.

PHYSICAL ASSESSMENT/CLINICAL MANIFESTATIONS

The diagnosis of pancreatitis is made on the basis of the clinical presentation combined with the results of diagnostic studies—both laboratory and radiologic. Clinical manifestations of acute pancreatitis vary widely and depend on the severity of the inflammation. Typically, a client is diagnosed after presenting with abdominal pain that localizes in the epigastrium; this is the most frequent symptom. Assess the intensity and quality of pain. The client often states that the pain had a sudden onset, is located in the mid-epigastric area or the left upper quadrant, and radiates to the back, left flank, or left shoulder. The pain is described as intense, **boring** (feeling that it is going through the body), and continuous, and is worsened by lying in the supine position. Often the client finds relief by assuming the fetal position (with the knees drawn up to the chest and the spine flexed) or when sitting upright and bending forward. The client may report weight loss resulting from nausea and vomiting.

When performing an abdominal assessment, you may find the following on inspection:
- Generalized jaundice
- Gray-blue discoloration of the abdomen and periumbilical area **(Cullen's sign)**
- Gray-blue discoloration of the flanks **(Turner's sign)**, caused by pancreatic enzyme leakage to cutaneous tissue from the peritoneal cavity

Listen for bowel sounds; absent or decreased bowel sounds usually indicate paralytic (adynamic) ileus. On light palpation, note abdominal tenderness, rigidity, and guarding as a result of peritonitis. A palpable mass may be found if a pancreatic pseudocyst is present. Pancreatic ascites creates a dull sound on percussion.

Assistive nursing personnel take and record vital signs frequently to assess for elevated temperature, tachycardia, and decreased blood pressure. Use these data to determine whether complications are occurring. Respiratory complications, such as left lung pleural effusions, atelectasis, and pneumonia, are common in clients with acute pancreatitis. Auscultate the lung fields for adventitious sounds or decreased aeration and observe respirations for dyspnea or orthopnea.

Significant changes in vital signs may indicate the life-threatening complication of shock. Hypotension and tachycardia may result from pancreatic hemorrhage, excessive fluid volume shifting, or the toxic effects of abdominal sepsis from enzyme damage. Observe the client for changes in behavior and sensorium that may be related to alcohol withdrawal, hypoxia, or impending sepsis with shock (see Chapter 8).

PSYCHOSOCIAL ASSESSMENT

Excessive alcohol intake, particularly in men, is the most frequent cause of acute pancreatitis. Therefore tactfully explore the client's alcohol intake history. You and the client should discuss the intake of alcohol and the reasons for overindulging. Ask him or her when increased drinking episodes occur, in particular, whether binges occur during holidays, vacations, or weekends or revolve around particular activities, such as television viewing. The client is also questioned about any recent traumatic event that may have contributed to increased alcohol consumption, such as the death of a family member or a job loss.

TABLE 63-3 Causes of Laboratory Diagnostic Abnormalities in Acute Pancreatitis

Abnormal Finding	Cause
Cardinal Diagnostic Tests	
Increased *serum* amylase	Pancreatic cell injury
Elevated *serum* lipase	Pancreatic cell injury
Elevated *serum* trypsin	Pancreatic cell injury
Elevated *serum* elastase	Pancreatic cell injury
Other Diagnostic Tests	
Elevated serum glucose	Pancreatic cell injury, resulting in impaired carbohydrate metabolism; decreased insulin release
Decreased serum calcium and magnesium	Fatty acids combined with calcium; seen in fat necrosis
Elevated bilirubin	Hepatobiliary obstructive process
Elevated alanine aminotransferase	Hepatobiliary involvement
Elevated leukocyte count	Inflammatory response

LABORATORY ASSESSMENT

Diagnostic laboratory abnormalities are found in clients with acute pancreatitis (Table 63-3). Amylase testing is quickly obtained and inexpensive. However, a variety of pancreatic and nonpancreatic disorders can cause increased serum levels. In clients with pancreatitis, amylase levels usually increase within 12 to 24 hours and remain elevated for 3 to 4 days. Persistent elevations may be an indicator of pancreatic abscess or pseudocyst. Lipase is considered more *specific* in the diagnosis of acute pancreatitis, and serum levels remain elevated for up to 2 weeks. Because serum lipase levels stay elevated for such a long time, the health care provider may find this test useful in diagnosing clients who are not examined until several days after the initial onset of symptoms. Trypsin testing is probably the most accurate serum indicator for acute pain, but is not widely available. Elastase has not proven to be better than lipase or trypsin in assisting the diagnosis of acute pancreatitis.

If pancreatitis is accompanied by biliary dysfunction (biliary pancreatitis), serum bilirubin and alkaline phosphatase levels are usually elevated. A sensitive indicator of biliary obstruction in acute pancreatitis is serum alanine aminotransferase (ALT). A threefold or greater rise in concentration offers a 95% probability that the diagnosis of acute biliary pancreatitis is correct. Elevated white blood cell (WBC) count and serum glucose levels are also common in acute pancreatitis.

Decreased serum calcium and magnesium levels are seen with fat necrosis. Calcium levels may fall and remain decreased for 7 to 10 days. Calcium levels that consistently remain below 8 mg/dL are associated with a poor prognosis.

RADIOGRAPHIC ASSESSMENT

A gas-filled duodenum (secondary to obstruction) on abdominal x-ray may support a diagnosis of pancreatitis. A chest x-ray may reveal elevation of the left side of the diaphragm or pleural effusion. Contrast-induced computed tomography (CT) provides a reliable diagnosis of acute pancreatitis. This noninvasive technique may be used to rule out pancreatic pseudocyst or ductal calculi.

OTHER DIAGNOSTIC ASSESSMENTS

In the client with severe pancreatitis, ultrasonography (US) and magnetic resonance imaging (MRI) of the pancreas help confirm an initial clinical impression, assess for the degree of inflammatory resolution, and reveal common bile duct dilation from obstruction or gallstones. US may be performed at the bedside.

◆ Analysis

COMMON NURSING DIAGNOSES AND COLLABORATIVE PROBLEMS

The following are priority nursing diagnoses for clients with acute pancreatitis:
1. Acute Pain related to biologic and injury agents (pancreatic inflammation and enzyme leakage)
2. Imbalanced Nutrition: Less Than Body Requirements related to the inability to ingest food and absorb nutrients

ADDITIONAL NURSING DIAGNOSES AND COLLABORATIVE PROBLEMS

In addition to the common nursing diagnoses, clients with acute pancreatitis may have one or more of the following:
- Nausea related to pancreatic disease
- Risk for Deficient Fluid Volume related to abnormal and normal routines
- Risk for Infection related to necrotic pancreatic tissue
- Ineffective Breathing Pattern related to the complications of pleural effusion or acute respiratory distress syndrome (ARDS)
- Risk for Activity Intolerance related to generalized weakness
- Disturbed Sleep Pattern related to pain

The client with pancreatitis may also have the following collaborative problems:
- Potential for Hyperglycemia
- Potential for Hemorrhage
- Potential for Hypovolemic or Septic Shock
- Potential for ARDS
- Potential for Paralytic Ileus
- Potential for Multisystem Organ Failure

◆ Planning and Implementation

ACUTE PAIN

PLANNING: EXPECTED OUTCOMES. The client with acute pancreatitis is expected to verbalize a decrease in or absence of abdominal pain, as evidenced by a pain scale measurement.

INTERVENTIONS. Abdominal pain is the prominent symptom of pancreatitis. The main focus of nursing care is aimed at reducing discomfort and pain by the use of interventions that decrease gastrointestinal (GI) tract activity, thus decreasing pancreatic stimulation. Pain assessment to measure the effectiveness of these interventions is a vital nursing activity (see Chapter 7).

NONSURGICAL MANAGEMENT. The health care team initially attempts to achieve pain relief with nonsurgical interventions, which include fasting, drug therapy, and comfort measures. If the client has a life-threatening complication or requires frequent monitoring, he or she is admitted to an intensive care unit.

NIC INTERVENTION ACTIVITIES for
The Client with Acute Pancreatitis

Analgesic Administration: *Use of pharmacologic agents to reduce or eliminate pain*
- Determine pain location, characteristics, quality, and severity before medicating client.
- Check medical order for drug, dose, and frequency of analgesic prescribed.
- Choose the appropriate analgesic or combination of analgesics when more than one is prescribed.
- Choose the IV route, rather than IM, for frequent pain medication injections, when possible.
- Attend to comfort needs and other activities that assist relaxation to facilitate response to analgesia.
- Administer analgesics around-the-clock to prevent peaks and troughs of analgesia, especially with severe pain.
- Administer adjuvant analgesics and/or medications when needed to potentiate analgesia.
- Consider use of continuous infusion, either alone or in conjunction with bolus opioids, to maintain serum levels.
- Institute safety precautions for those receiving narcotic analgesics, as appropriate.
- Correct misconceptions/myths client or family members may hold regarding analgesics, particularly opioids (e.g., addiction and risks of overdose).
- Evaluate the effectiveness of analgesic at regular frequent intervals after each administration, but especially after the initial doses, also observing for any signs and symptoms of untoward effects (e.g., respiratory depression, nausea and vomiting, dry mouth, and constipation).
- Document response to analgesic and any untoward effects.
- Implement actions to decrease untoward effects of analgesics (e.g., constipation and gastric irritation).
- Collaborate with the health care provider if drug, dose, route of administration, or interval changes are indicated, making specific recommendations based on equianalgesic principles.

Pain Management: *Alleviation of pain or a reduction in pain to a level of comfort that is acceptable to the client*
- Perform a comprehensive assessment of pain to include location, characteristics, onset/duration, frequency, quality, intensity or severity of pain, and precipitating factors.
- Observe for nonverbal cues of discomfort, especially in those unable to communicate effectively.
- Ensure that client receives attentive analgesic care.
- Consider cultural influences on pain response.
- Determine the impact of the pain experience on quality of life (e.g., sleep, appetite, activity, cognition, mood, relationships, performance of job, and role responsibilities).
- Evaluate, with the client and the health care team, the effectiveness of past pain control measures that have been used.
- Control environmental factors that may influence the client's response to discomfort (e.g., room temperature, lighting, noise).
- Reduce or eliminate factors that precipitate or increase the pain experience (e.g., fear, fatigue, monotony, and lack of knowledge).

- Consider the client's willingness to participate, ability to participate, preference, support of significant others for method, and contraindications when selecting a pain relief strategy.
- Select and implement a variety of measures (e.g., pharmacologic, nonpharmacologic, interpersonal) to facilitate pain relief, as appropriate.
- Provide the person optimal pain relief with prescribed analgesics.
- Implement the use of patient-controlled analgesia (PCA), if appropriate.
- Use pain control measures before pain becomes severe.
- Verify level of discomfort with client, note changes in the medical record, inform other health professionals working with the client.
- Evaluate the effectiveness of the pain control measures used through ongoing assessment of the pain experience.
- Institute and modify pain control measures on the basis of the client's response.
- Promote adequate rest/sleep to facilitate pain relief.
- Notify the health care provider if measures are unsuccessful or if current complaint is a significant change from client's past experience of pain.
- Inform other health care professionals/family members of nonpharmacologic strategies being used by the client to encourage preventive approaches to pain management.
- Use a multidisciplinary approach to pain management, when appropriate.
- Consider referrals for client, family, and significant others to support groups, and other resources, as appropriate.
- Provide accurate information to promote family's knowledge of and response to the pain experience.
- Incorporate the family in the pain relief modality, if possible.
- Monitor client satisfaction with pain management at specified intervals.

Patient-Controlled Analgesia (PCA) Assistance: *Facilitating client control of analgesic administration and regulation*
- Collaborate with health care providers, client, and family members in selecting the type of narcotic to be used.
- Ensure that client is not allergic to analgesic to be administered.
- Teach client and family to monitor pain intensity, quality, and duration.
- Teach client and family to monitor respiratory rate and blood pressure.
- Teach client and family members how to use the PCA device.
- Teach client and family members the action and side effects of pain-relieving agents.
- Document client's pain, amount and frequency of drug dosing, and response to pain treatment in a pain flow sheet.
- Recommend a bowel regimen to avoid constipation.
- Consult with clinical pain experts for a client who is having difficulty achieving pain control.

Fasting. To rest the pancreas and reduce pancreatic enzyme secretion, food and fluids are withheld in the acute period. The health care provider prescribes intravenous (IV) fluid administration to maintain hydration. IV replacement of calcium and magnesium may also be needed.

Nasogastric drainage and suction is reserved for clients who have continuous vomiting or biliary obstruction. Gastric decompression prevents gastric digestive juices from flowing into the duodenum. Because paralytic (adynamic) ileus is a common complication of acute pancreatitis, pro-

longed nasogastric intubation may be necessary. Assess frequently for the presence of bowel sounds, including before the nasogastric (NG) tube is removed.

Drug Therapy. To decrease pain, the primary drug class used is the opioid class of drugs. Other drugs may also be prescribed.

NIC *Analgesic Administration.* Pain management for acute pancreatitis typically begins with the administration of opioids by means of patient-controlled analgesia (PCA) or the intermittent intramuscular method (Chart 63-5). Meperidine

(Demerol) is the traditional drug of choice for relieving abdominal pain associated with acute pancreatitis. It has been thought that meperidine causes less incidence of spasm of the smooth musculature of the pancreatic ducts and the sphincter of Oddi than do other analgesics such as morphine.

However, the limitations and adverse drug reactions related to meperidine are well known (Waitman & McCaffery, 2001). Other options that have been used successfully to manage acute pain in clients with pancreatitis include transdermal fentanyl and epidural morphine with bupivacaine (Stevens, Esler, & Asher, 2002).

In mild pancreatitis, the pain usually subsides in 2 to 4 days; however, with severe acute pancreatitis, the abdominal pain and tenderness may persist for up to 2 weeks. The dosages and intervals of medication administration are individualized according to the severity of the disease and the symptoms.

Other Drugs. Anticholinergics, such as atropine (Urised), glucagons, calcitonin (Calcimar), histamine receptor antagonists (e.g., ranitidine [Zantac]), and protease inhibitors are indicated to decrease vagal stimulation, decrease GI motility, and inhibit pancreatic secretions. However, these drugs can cause unwanted side effects for older adults and have not been proven to alter clinical outcomes. Antibiotics may be used, but they are primarily indicated for clients with acute necrotizing pancreatitis. Common drugs used include cefuroxime (Zinacef), ceftazidime (Ceptaz), and imipenem cilastin (Primaxin).

Comfort Measures. Helping the client to assume the fetal position (with the legs drawn up to the chest) may decrease the abdominal pain of pancreatitis.

If the client has an NG tube in place, remind assistive nursing personnel to implement frequent oral hygiene measures to keep mucous membranes moist and free of inflammation or crusting. Because of the drying effect of medication and the absence of oral fluids, the mouth and oral cavity may be extremely dry, resulting in considerable discomfort.

Lowering the client's anxiety level may also substantially reduce pain. Provide thorough explanations of procedures. The client is encouraged to express the emotions and responses he or she is experiencing. Provide reassurance and offer diversional activities, such as television, music, and reading material, and encourage visitors to direct attention away from the pain.

Endoscopic Retrograde Cholangiopancreatography (ERCP). If pancreatitis was caused by gallstones, an ERCP with a **sphincterotomy** (opening of the sphincter of Oddi) may be performed on an urgent or emergent basis. If this procedure is not successful, surgery is required.

SURGICAL MANAGEMENT. Surgical intervention for acute pancreatitis is usually not indicated. However, if an ERCP is not successful in removing gallstones, a laparoscopic cholecystectomy is performed, as described under Surgical Management (Cholecystitis) on p. 1400.

Complications of pancreatitis, such as pancreatic pseudocyst and abscess, may also require surgical intervention. Laparoscopy (minimally invasive surgery [MIS]) may be performed for drainage of an abscess or pseudocyst. For clients who are high surgical risks, pseudocysts or abscesses can be treated by percutaneous drainage under computed tomography (CT) guidance.

Preoperative Care. In addition to general preoperative care measures, an NG tube may be inserted. The client is frequently in pain, a factor that inhibits the learning process. Provide preoperative teaching in a manner that takes the client's comfort level into account. Postoperative reminders may be needed to reinforce the preoperative learning. Teach the client having external drainage of the pseudocyst to expect a pancreatic drainage tube and explain its care during the postoperative period. Internal drainage via laparoscopy does not require an external tube and allows the client a faster recovery. Be certain that the client knows how to promote respiratory function by turning, coughing, deep breathing, and splinting the incision.

Operative Procedures. A laparoscopic **pseudocystojejunostomy** or **pseudocystogastrostomy** may be performed to drain a pseudocyst into the jejunum or stomach. Less often, an abscess or pseudocyst is incised and drained externally, drainage tubes are inserted, sutured in place, and connected to low suction to prevent further tissue erosion. An open approach, or laparotomy, may be used for this procedure.

Postoperative Care. The client having MIS typically spends less time in the hospital, requires less intense care, and recovers more quickly than those having open surgeries. If present, monitor drainage tubes for patency by assessing for kinks in the tubes and maintaining the ordered drain suction pressure and system integrity. Record the output amount from the drain and describe the character of the drainage. A sump type of drain is usually inserted. Ascertain that the drain is functioning, as indicated by the presence of a hissing noise from the sump lumen.

Provide meticulous skin care and dressing changes. Monitor for the first signs of redness or skin irritation because pancreatic enzyme drainage is particularly excoriating to the skin. Skin barriers, such as a Stomahesive wafer around the drainage tube, are applied to repel drainage from the skin. Collaborate with an enterostomal therapist (ET) for measures to promote skin integrity, such as the use of individualized ostomy appliances and the application of topical agents.

IMBALANCED NUTRITION: LESS THAN BODY REQUIREMENTS

NOC **PLANNING: EXPECTED OUTCOMES.** The client with acute pancreatitis is expected to have nutrients that are available to meet metabolic needs. Indicators include that the client will have normal:

- Nutrient intake
- Fluid intake
- Weight-height ratio
- Hematocrit
- Hydration

INTERVENTIONS. The client is maintained on NPO status in the early stages of pancreatitis. Antiemetics for nausea and vomiting are prescribed as needed. Clients who have severe pancreatitis and are unable to eat for 7 to 10 days should receive nutritional support in the form of total parenteral nutrition (TPN) (see Chapter 64) or total enteral nutrition (TEN). TEN has been shown to produce fewer episodes of glucose elevation and other complications associated with TPN, and to be as effective in maintaining nutritional status (Scolapio et al., 1999).

When food is tolerated during the recovery phase, the health care provider generally orders small, frequent, moderate- to high-carbohydrate, high-protein, low-fat meals. Foods should be bland with little spice; GI stimulants such as caffeine-containing foods (tea, coffee, cola, and chocolate), as well as alcohol, should be avoided.

To boost caloric intake, commercial liquid nutritional preparations, such as Ensure, supplement the diet. If caloric intake is less than desired, an NG tube may be required for additional nutrition via enteral feedings. The health care provider may also prescribe fat-soluble and other vitamin and mineral replacement supplements.

> ### Critical Thinking Challenge
>
> A middle-aged man is admitted to your medical unit with a diagnosis of acute pancreatitis. He has been admitted three other times for hepatic cirrhosis and has been treated for alcoholism for 15 years. Today he is complaining of excruciating abdominal pain that is "boring right through him." He has been nauseated and anorexic for over a week. His wife states that he just won't listen to her and she's very frustrated about his continued drinking; she is considering a divorce after he leaves the hospital.
>
> 1. What is his priority nursing diagnosis at this time?
> 2. What interventions will he need first?
> 3. How will you assess his nutritional status at this time?
> 4. What should you say to his wife who is so distraught about her husband's continued drinking despite his health problems?

evolve For suggested answer guidelines, go to http://evolve.elsevier.com/Iggy/.

Community-Based Care
HOME CARE MANAGEMENT

Home care preparation should be individualized for each client's circumstances. Some clients with acute pancreatitis may be severely weakened from their acute illness and need to confine activity to one floor, limiting stair climbing and other strenuous activities until they regain their strength.

HEALTH TEACHING

Education needs to be started early in the hospitalization period—as soon as the acute episodes of pain have subsided. Assess the client's and family members' or significant others' knowledge of the disease.

The goals of discharge planning and education are to avoid further episodes of pancreatitis and prevent progression to a chronic disease. Instruct the client to abstain from drinking alcohol to prevent further pain attacks and extension of inflammation and pancreatic insufficiency. The client is told that if alcohol is consumed, pain will be experienced, and further autodigestion of the pancreas will lead to chronic pancreatitis and chronic pain.

Teach the client to notify the health care provider after discharge to home if acute abdominal pain or biliary tract disease (as evidenced by jaundice, clay-colored stools, or darkened urine) occurs. These signs and symptoms are possible indicators of complications or disease progression.

HEALTH CARE RESOURCES

Clients with acute pancreatitis require visits by a home care nurse if the hospital course was complicated. In these cases, home care may be needed for wound care and assistance

with activities of daily living (ADLs). The client requires medical follow-up with the primary care physician or nurse practitioner for monitoring of the disease process. For clients with alcoholism, provide information about groups such as Alcoholics Anonymous (AA). Family members may attend support groups such as Al-Anon and Alateen.

◆ Evaluation: Outcomes

Evaluate the care of the client with acute pancreatitis on the basis of the identified nursing diagnoses and collaborative problems. The expected outcomes include that the client will:

- Experience an alleviation of or reduction in abdominal pain, as indicated by self-report
- Have adequate nutrients available to meet metabolic demand

Specific indicators for these outcomes are listed for each nursing diagnosis under the Planning and Implementation section (see earlier).

Chronic Pancreatitis
PATHOPHYSIOLOGY

Chronic pancreatitis is a progressive, destructive disease of the pancreas, characterized by remissions and exacerbations (recurrence). Inflammation and fibrosis of the tissue contribute to pancreatic insufficiency and diminished function of the organ. Chronic pancreatitis usually develops after repeated episodes of alcohol-induced acute pancreatitis. It may also be associated with chronic obstruction of the common bile duct. The disease may develop in the absence of a known acute disorder. Relief of pain, prevention of recurrence of attacks, prevention of complications, and nutritional support are the principal interventions.

Types of Chronic Pancreatitis

Alcohol-induced chronic pancreatitis is also known as **chronic calcifying pancreatitis (CCP).** Protein precipitates that plug the ducts and lead to ductal obstruction, atrophy, and dilation characterize CCP. As the protein plugging becomes diffuse, the epithelium of the ducts undergoes histologic changes, resulting in metaplasia (cell replacement) and ulceration. This inflammatory process causes fibrosis of the pancreatic tissue. Intraductal calcification and marked pancreatic parenchymal destruction develop in the late stages. Cystic sacs containing pancreatic secretions and enzymes form on the pancreas. The organ becomes hard and firm as a result of acinar cell atrophy and pancreatic insufficiency.

Chronic obstructive pancreatitis develops from inflammation, spasm, and obstruction of the sphincter of Oddi. Inflammatory and sclerotic lesions occur in the head of the pancreas and around the ducts, causing an obstruction and backflow of pancreatic secretions (see Complications of Acute Pancreatitis, p. 1404).

Pathologic Changes

Pancreatic insufficiency in chronic pancreatitis is characterized by the loss of exocrine function. Pancreatic exocrine secretion is divided into two components: aqueous bicarbonate and enzymes.

The aqueous component neutralizes the duodenal contents and pancreatic enzymes that are essential to normal digestion and absorption. Most clients with chronic pancreatitis have a decreased output of pancreatic secretion and bicarbonate. Pancreatic enzyme secretion must be reduced by more than 80% to produce steatorrhea resulting from severe malabsorption of fats. These characteristic stools are pale, bulky, and frothy and have an offensive odor. The action of colonic bacteria on unabsorbed lipids and proteins is responsible for the foul odor. On inspection of the stools, the fat content is visible. In severe chronic pancreatitis, stool fat output may exceed 40 g/day.

Fat malabsorption also contributes to weight loss and muscle wasting (a decrease in muscle mass) and leads to general debilitation of the client. Protein malabsorption results in a "starvation" edema of the feet, legs, and hands caused by decreased levels of circulating albumin.

The loss of pancreatic endocrine function is responsible for the development of frank diabetes mellitus in clients with chronic pancreatic insufficiency. (See Chapter 68 for a complete discussion of diabetes mellitus.)

The client with chronic pancreatitis may have pulmonary complications, such as pleuritic pain, pleural effusions, and pulmonary infiltrates. Pancreatic ascites may impede diaphragmatic excursion and decrease lung expansion, resulting in impaired ventilation. In the ill client with chronic pancreatitis, acute respiratory distress syndrome (ARDS) may develop.

Etiology

The cause of chronic calcifying pancreatitis is persistent excessive alcohol intake that results in repeated episodes of acute pancreatitis. The most common cause of chronic obstructive pancreatitis is cholelithiasis and biliary tract disease, which results in persistent inflammation. Other etiologic factors include pancreatic pseudocyst, postoperative ductal scarring, and cancer of the pancreas or duodenum. All of these factors can produce obstruction of the pancreatic duct. Interestingly, chronic pancreatitis is a risk factor for pancreatic cancer (McCance & Huether, 2002). Prolonged starvation and prolonged use of parenteral feedings for nutritional support can result in pancreatic atrophy, causing pancreatic insufficiency as well.

Incidence/Prevalence

Most clients with chronic pancreatitis are alcoholics (McCance & Huether, 2002). Alcohol-induced pancreatitis is predominantly found in men, but the incidence in women is increasing. In women, chronic pancreatitis occurs more commonly among those with biliary tract disease (cholecystitis and cholelithiasis). The age at occurrence of chronic pancreatitis is variable but is usually between 45 and 60 years.

◆COLLABORATIVE MANAGEMENT
◆Assessment

Clinical manifestations of chronic pancreatitis differ from those of an acute inflammation, although, as with acute pancreatitis, abdominal pain is the major clinical manifestation (Chart 63-6). The client with chronic pancreatitis typically describes the pain as a continuous burning or gnawing dullness with periods of acute exacerbation. The pain is intense and relentless. The frequency of acute exacerbations may increase as the pancreatic fibrosis develops.

CHART 63-6

KEY FEATURES of
Chronic Pancreatitis

- Intense abdominal pain (major clinical manifestation) that is continuous and burning or gnawing
- Abdominal tenderness
- Ascites
- Possible left upper quadrant mass (if pseudocyst or abscess is present)
- Respiratory compromise manifested by adventitious or diminished breath sounds, dyspnea, or orthopnea
- Steatorrhea; clay-colored stools
- Weight loss
- Jaundice
- Dark urine
- Polyuria, polydipsia, polyphagia (diabetes mellitus)

Perform the same abdominal assessment as for clients with acute pancreatitis, but the findings may not be as significant. Abdominal tenderness is less intense. A mass may be palpated in the left upper quadrant, which is indicative of a pancreatic pseudocyst or abscess. Massive pancreatic ascites may be present, producing dullness on abdominal percussion. Because respiratory complications can accompany the condition, the nurse auscultates the lung fields for adventitious sounds or decreased aeration and observes for dyspnea or orthopnea.

Ask the client to collect a random stool specimen, if able, or ask him or her to describe the stools. The specimen may show the presence of steatorrhea (foul-smelling fatty stools that may increase in volume as pancreatic insufficiency progresses and lipase production decreases). The client may also experience weight loss, muscle wasting, jaundice, dark urine, and the manifestations of diabetes mellitus, such as polyuria, polydipsia, and polyphagia.

In chronic pancreatitis, significant laboratory findings include normal or moderately elevated serum amylase and lipase levels. Obstruction of the intrahepatic bile duct can cause elevated serum bilirubin and alkaline phosphatase levels. Transient elevations in serum glucose levels are common and can be detected by blood glucose monitoring, both fasting and nonfasting.

The only definitive diagnostic test for chronic pancreatitis is the identification of calcification of pancreatic tissue in a biopsy specimen. Pancreas ultrasonography is also a helpful diagnostic tool, especially to reveal pseudocysts. Endoscopic retrograde cholangiopancreatography (ERCP) may reveal ductal system abnormalities, such as calcification and strictures, or it may delineate the presence of pancreatic pseudocyst.

◆Interventions

The focus of caring for the client with chronic pancreatitis is to manage pain, assist in maintaining a sufficient nutritional intake, and prevent recurrence.

NONSURGICAL MANAGEMENT. Nonsurgical interventions primarily include drug and diet therapy.

Drug Therapy. The major intervention for the pain of chronic pancreatitis is drug therapy. In addition, teach the client to avoid ingesting irritating substances that can precipitate pain.

NIC *Analgesic Administration.* Medicate the client as prescribed according to the assessment of the level and intensity of pain and evaluate the effectiveness of the drug intervention (see Chart 63-5). Opioid analgesia with meperidine hydrochloride (Demerol) is most frequently used, but opioid dependency may become a problem. Non-opioid analgesics may be tried to relieve pain. (See Chapter 7 for other interventions for chronic pain.)

If drug dependency becomes a problem, behavior modification programs and drug and alcohol counseling will be necessary. The health care provider may need to admit these clients to drug and alcohol dependency programs.

Enzyme Replacement. Pancreatic enzymes are essential dietary supplements (Chart 63-7). These are given with meals or snacks to aid in digestion and absorption of fat and protein. Drugs such as pancreatin (Donnazyme, Creon) and pancrelipase (Cotazym, Cotazym-65B✲, Viokase, or Pancrease) are prescribed in capsule, tablet, or powder form and contain amylase, lipase, and protease. Teach the client to take these medications immediately before or during meals with a glass of water. Donnazyme should not be broken, crushed, or chewed because it has an enteric coating. At the client's request, mix the powder form in applesauce or fruit juice to make it more palatable. Enzyme preparations should not be mixed with foods containing proteins, because the enzymatic action dissolves the food into a watery substance. Advise the client to wipe his or her lips with a wet towel to prevent the skin irritation and breakdown that residual enzymes can cause. Remind the client not to inhale the enzymatic powder while preparing to take it.

The dosage of pancreatic enzymes depends on the severity of the malabsorption and maldigestion. Record the number and consistency of stools per day to monitor the effectiveness of enzyme therapy. If pancreatic enzyme treatment is effective, the stools should become less frequent and less fatty.

Insulin Therapy. If the client has diabetes, the health care provider prescribes insulin or oral hypoglycemic agents for glucose control. Clients maintained on total parenteral nutrition (TPN) are particularly susceptible to labile glucose levels and may require regular insulin additives to the solution. Closely monitor blood glucose levels so that hyperglycemia is controlled and insulin or diabetic shock is prevented. Check finger stick blood glucose or sugar (FSBG or FSBS) levels every 2 to 4 hours.

Other Drugs. The health care provider may also prescribe histamine receptor antagonists, such as ranitidine hydrochloride (Zantac), to decrease gastric acid. Gastric acid destroys the lipase needed to break down fats. Controlling the acidity of the stomach with H_2 blockers or proton pump inhibitors, or neutralizing stomach acid with oral sodium bicarbonate may enhance the effectiveness of the non–enteric-coated enzyme therapy. Subcutaneous octreotide (Sandostatin), a growth hormone similar to somatostatin, is used by some physicians if pain and diarrhea persist.

Diet Therapy. Protein and fat malabsorption results in significant weight loss and decreased muscle mass in the client with chronic pancreatitis. Therefore the nutritional interventions for acute pancreatitis are also relevant for the chronic phase of pancreatitis. The client often limits food intake to avoid the recurrent pain, which is exacerbated by eating. For this reason, nutrition maintenance is often difficult to achieve, and clients are provided with TPN or total enteral nutrition (TEN), including vitamin and mineral replacement.

CHART 63-7

CLIENT EDUCATION GUIDE
Enzyme Replacement for the Client with Chronic Pancreatitis

- Take pancreatic enzymes before or with meals and snacks.
- Administer pancreatin after antacid or H_2 blockers; decreased pH inactivates drug.
- Tell the client to swallow the tablets without chewing to minimize oral irritation.
- Mix the powder form in applesauce or fruit juice at client's request.
- Do not mix enzyme preparations in protein-containing foods.
- Have the client wipe his or her lips after taking enzymes to avoid skin irritation.
- Do not crush enteric-coated preparations.
- Follow up on all scheduled laboratory testing. (Pancrelipase can cause an increase in uric acid levels.)

For long-term dietary management, the client needs an increased number of calories, up to 4000 to 6000 calories/day, to maintain weight. Foods high in carbohydrates and protein also assist in the healing process. Foods high in fat are avoided because they cause or increase diarrhea.

SURGICAL MANAGEMENT. Surgery is not a primary intervention for the treatment of chronic pancreatitis. However, it may be indicated for intractable abdominal pain, incapacitating relapses of pain, or complications such as abscesses and pseudocysts.

The underlying pathologic changes determine the procedure indicated. Using laparoscopy, the surgeon incises and drains an abscess or pseudocyst. Laparoscopic cholecystectomy or choledochotomy (incision of the common bile duct) may be indicated if biliary tract disease is an underlying cause of pancreatitis. If the pancreatic duct sphincter is fibrotic, the surgeon performs a sphincterotomy (incision of the sphincter) to enlarge it. Endoscopic sphincterotomy may be used for clients who are poor surgical candidates.

In some cases, laparoscopic distal pancreatectomy may be appropriate for resection of the distal pancreas. This procedure is discussed later under Surgical Management (Pancreatic Carcinoma), p. 1415.

In a few cases, pancreas transplantation may be done. However, this procedure is performed most often for clients with severe, uncontrolled diabetes. Chapter 68 discusses pancreas transplantation.

Community-Based Care
HOME CARE MANAGEMENT

The care of the client with pancreatitis usually involves a case manager or discharge planner. A community-based case manager may continue to follow the client while he or she requires health care in the home or other community-based setting.

Clients with chronic pancreatitis are usually discharged to home, but some may require care in a long-term care setting. If the client is discharged to home, the activity area should be limited to one floor until he or she regains strength and can increase activity. Toilet facilities must be easily accessible because of chronic steatorrhea and frequent defecation. If toilet facilities are not available in the immediate rest area, a bedpan or bedside commode is obtained for the home.

HEALTH TEACHING

Because there is no known cure for chronic pancreatitis, client and family education is aimed at preventing further acute exacerbations of this chronic disease, providing long-term care, and promoting health maintenance (Chart 63-8).

DIET THERAPY. Instruct the client to avoid known precipitating factors, such as the ingestion of caffeinated beverages and alcohol. The dietitian elicits the participation of the family or significant other in diet planning and food preparation. Diet teaching focuses on eating bland, low-fat, frequent meals and avoiding rich, fatty foods. The nurse and dietitian stress the importance of dietary compliance and the need for increased nutritional intake to prevent acute exacerbations of this chronic illness. Written instructions on diet and pancreatic enzyme replacement therapy are essential.

Remind the client and family members or significant others on the importance of adhering to the pancreatic enzyme replacement treatment. The client must take the prescribed enzymes with meals and snacks to aid in the digestion of food and promote the absorption of fats and proteins. Teach the client to take the enzymes before or at the beginning of the meal and to report to the health care provider any increase in the occurrence of foul-smelling, frothy, fatty stools; abdominal distention; and cramping so that pancreatic enzyme replacement may be increased as needed. The client should report any skin excoriation or breakdown so that therapeutic interventions to promote skin integrity can be instituted.

SKIN CARE. The frequency of defecation (whether continent or incontinent) poses challenging skin care problems. Instruct the client to keep his or her skin dry and free of the abrasive fatty stools, which are excoriating to the skin. The skin should be cleaned thoroughly after each stool and a soothing emollient, such as Sween, applied. To prevent breakdown and maintain skin integrity, a skin barrier may be needed. Many products on the market, such as zinc oxide cream, actively repel stool from the skin.

DRUG THERAPY. The client and family members must be able to state the desired effect of the prescribed drugs, the schedule for drug administration, and potential side effects. Provide written guidelines as reinforcement.

If the client develops diabetes mellitus as a result of chronic pancreatitis from endocrine dysfunction, management of elevated glucose levels after discharge from the hospital may necessitate oral hypoglycemic agents or insulin injections. If this is the case, the client and the family require in-depth teaching concerning diabetes, its signs and symptoms, medical management, insulin administration, dietary management, urine and blood glucose monitoring, and general care information. (See Chapter 68 for a discussion of diabetes.)

HEALTH CARE RESOURCES

Chronic illnesses are devastating for families. The high costs of medical insurance, medical treatment, and drug therapy cause serious financial problems. Often the client with chronic pancreatitis is unable or unwilling to work. Case management to coordinate care and manage resources should be instituted during hospitalization and continue throughout the course of the illness.

The client may require home visits by nurses and a dietitian, depending on the severity of the chronic health problems and home maintenance and support needs. The home care nurse assesses the client for pain management, compliance with dietary guidelines and alcohol abstinence, the effectiveness of pancreatic enzyme therapy, and psychosocial adaptation to a chronic illness.

Refer the client to a counselor or a self-help group, such as Alcoholics Anonymous, if appropriate.

Pancreatic Abscess

PATHOPHYSIOLOGY

Pancreatic abscesses are the most serious complication of pancreatitis. If untreated, they are always fatal. After surgery, the recurrence rate is higher than 30%. The abscesses form from collections of purulent liquefaction of the necrotic pancreas.

Pancreatic abscesses occur after severe acute pancreatitis, exacerbations of chronic pancreatitis, or biliary tract surgery. The development of either a single abscess or multiple abscesses results from extensive inflammatory necrosis of the pancreas that is readily invaded by infectious organisms such as *Escherichia coli, Klebsiella, Bacteroides, Staphylococcus,* and *Proteus.* They can erode through the retroperitoneum into the bowel mesentery, the mediastinum, the pleural space, or the pelvis.

◆COLLABORATIVE MANAGEMENT

Clients with pancreatic abscesses often appear more seriously ill than clients with pseudocysts. Clinical manifestations are similar; however, the temperature in clients with abscesses may spike to as high as 104° F (40° C). Blood cultures are helpful in revealing the infective organism. Pleural effusions commonly accompany these abscesses. Ultrasonography and computed tomography (CT) cannot differentiate between pancreatic pseudocysts and abscesses.

Drainage via the percutaneous method or laparoscopy should be performed as soon as possible to prevent sepsis. Antibiotic treatment alone does not resolve the abscess. Mortality remains as high as 60%, even after surgical drainage. Many clients require multiple drainage procedures for recurrent abscesses.

Pancreatic Pseudocyst

PATHOPHYSIOLOGY

Pancreatic pseudocysts develop as a complication of acute or chronic pancreatitis and are caused by alcoholism, biliary

---

CHART 63-8

CLIENT EDUCATION GUIDE
Prevention of Exacerbations of Chronic Pancreatitis

- Avoid things that make your symptoms worse, such as drinking caffeinated beverages.
- Avoid alcohol ingestion; refer to self-help group for assistance.
- Avoid nicotine.
- Eat bland, low-fat, high-protein, moderate-carbohydrate meals; avoid gastric stimulants, such as spices.
- Eat small meals and snacks high in calories.
- Take the pancreatic enzymes that have been prescribed for you with meals.
- Rest frequently; restrict your activity to one floor until you regain your strength.

tract disease, or abdominal or surgical trauma. They develop in 10% to 20% of all people with pancreatitis, and mortality is reported at about 10%.

Pancreatic pseudocysts, or false cysts, are so named because, unlike true cysts, they do not have an epithelial lining. They are encapsulated saclike structures that form on or surround the pancreas. The pseudocyst wall is inflamed, vascular, and fibrotic. It may contain up to several liters of straw-colored or dark-brown viscous fluid, the enzymatic exudate of the pancreas.

◆COLLABORATIVE MANAGEMENT

A pseudocyst can be palpated as an epigastric mass in about 50% of cases. The primary presenting symptom is epigastric pain radiating to the back. Other common clinical manifestations include abdominal fullness, nausea, vomiting, and jaundice.

Pseudocysts are diagnosed, and their growth and resolution monitored, by serial pancreatic ultrasonographic examination or CT.

Complications of pseudocyst formation include the following:

- Hemorrhage
- Infection
- Obstruction of the bowel, biliary tract, or splenic vein
- Abscess
- Fistula formation
- Pancreatic ascites

Pseudocysts may spontaneously resolve, or they may rupture and produce hemorrhage. Surgical intervention is necessary if the pseudocyst does not resolve within 6 weeks or if complications develop. To accomplish internal drainage, via laparoscopy, the surgeon creates an opening (ostomy) between the pseudocyst and the stomach (**pseudocystogastrostomy**) or the jejunum (**pseudocystojejunostomy**). To provide external drainage, the surgeon inserts a sump drainage tube to remove pancreatic secretions and exudate. Pancreatic fistulas are common after surgery, and skin breakdown from corrosive pancreatic enzymes in clients who have external drainage presents a major nursing care challenge (see earlier discussion under Postoperative Care [Acute Pancreatitis], p. 1408).

Insulinoma

Insulinoma is the most common type of neuroendocrine pancreatic tumor, even though it is rare. As the name implies, these tumors are typically benign tumors of the islets of Langerhans that cause excessive insulin secretion and subsequent hypoglycemia (low serum glucose). Endoscopic ultrasonography is usually done to locate the tumor.

Management includes removal of the tumor, usually via laparoscopic distal pancreatectomy. Nursing care associated with this surgery is described later under Pancreatic Carcinoma on pp. 1415 to 1417.

Pancreatic Carcinoma

PATHOPHYSIOLOGY

Cancer of the pancreas is one of the leading causes of cancer-related mortality, accounting for 2% to 3% of the new cancer cases each year. It is difficult to diagnose early be-

cause the pancreas is hidden and surrounded by other organs. The cost of care is almost $3 billion annually in the United States. Treatment has limited results, and 5-year survival rates are extremely low (American Cancer Society, 2004).

Pancreatic tumors usually originate from epithelial cells of the pancreatic ductal system. If the tumor is discovered in the early stages, the tumor cells may be localized within the glandular organ; however, this is highly unlikely. Most often, the tumor is discovered in the late stages of development and may be a well-defined mass or it is diffusely spread throughout the pancreas.

The tumor may be a primary cancer, or it may result from metastasis from cancers of the lung, breast, thyroid, kidney, or skin. Primary tumors are generally adenocarcinomas and grow in well-differentiated glandular patterns. They grow rapidly and spread to surrounding organs (stomach, duodenum, gallbladder, and intestine) by direct extension and invasion of lymphatic and vascular systems. This highly metastatic lesion may eventually invade the lung, peritoneum, liver, spleen, and lymph nodes.

Clinical manifestations depend on the site of origin or metastasis. The head of the pancreas is the most common site of pancreatic carcinoma. The tumors are usually small lesions with poorly defined margins. Jaundice results from tumor compression and obstruction of the common bile duct and from gallbladder dilation, causing the organ to enlarge.

Carcinomas of the body and tail of the pancreas are usually large and invade the entire tail and body. These tumors may be palpable abdominal masses, especially in the thin client. Through metastatic spread via the splenic vein, metastasis to the liver may cause **hepatomegaly** (enlargement of the liver up to two to three times its normal size). Carcinomas of the body and tail spread more extensively than do pancreatic head carcinomas, with invasion of the retroperitoneum, vertebral column, spleen, adrenal glands, colon, or stomach. Regardless of where it originates, pancreatic cancer spreads rapidly through the lymphatic and venous systems to other organs.

Venous thromboembolism is a common complication of pancreatic carcinoma. Necrotic products of the pancreatic tumor are believed to have thromboplastic properties, resulting in the blood's hypercoagulable state. Additionally, the client is at high risk due to decreased mobility and extensive surgical manipulation.

Etiology and Genetic Risk

The exact cause of pancreatic carcinoma is unknown. High-risk populations are those in their sixth to eighth decades of life and those with a personal history of smoking. About 10% of those with pancreatic cancer have an inherited risk. Mutations in certain oncogenes have been identified. Mutations have also been revealed in tumor suppressor genes, such as p16, p53, and BRCA2—the same mutation that makes some women susceptible to breast and ovarian cancer (Hahn et al., 2003).

A newly identified human pancreatic carcinoma cell line, FAMPAC, has a complex molecular pattern of mutations (Eisold et al., 2004). Clients with diabetes mellitus or chronic pancreatitis are slightly more at risk for pancreatic cancer, which may represent another genetic link. Research continues to explore the genetic origins of familial pancreatic cancer.

Incidence/Prevalence

About 30,000 people develop pancreatic cancer each year, and an equal number of people die of the disease each year (American Cancer Society, 2004). Fewer than 20% of persons diagnosed with pancreatic cancer survive longer than 1 year after diagnosis and less than 5% survive for 5 years (Konner & O'Reilly, 2002).

◆ COLLABORATIVE MANAGEMENT
◆ Assessment

PHYSICAL ASSESSMENT/CLINICAL MANIFESTATIONS

Pancreatic cancer often presents in an insidious, vague manner. The presenting symptoms depend somewhat on the location of the tumor. The first clue to the presence of pancreatic carcinoma may be the appearance of jaundice, which is actually a late sign (Chart 63-9). Jaundice appears as the initial sign in most cases because the gallbladder and liver are commonly involved. As the tumor spreads, the green-gold skin color associated with obstructive jaundice progressively worsens. On noting the jaundice, ask the client whether the color of the stool and urine has changed. As a result of the obstructive process, the stool is clay colored and the urine is dark and frothy. Inspect the skin for dryness and scratch marks, indicating pruritus from jaundice. Assess the sclerae for icterus and the mucous membranes for signs of jaundice.

By the time jaundice appears, the pancreatic carcinoma is usually in an advanced stage. The enlarged gallbladder and liver may be palpable. In advanced cases of pancreatic carcinoma, the tumor may be felt as a firm, fixed mass in the left upper abdominal quadrant or epigastric region.

The most common complaint, often misinterpreted by even the client, is fatigue. This fatigue is described as a diminished energy level and an increased need for rest disproportionate to the level of activity. The client notices an inability to perform usual physical or intellectual activities.

Question the client about abdominal pain, which may be described as a vague, constant dullness in the upper abdomen and nonspecific in nature. Pain, a common early complaint in clients with pancreatic carcinoma, is also present in the advanced stages of the disease. Pain may be related to eating or activity.

In addition, question whether the client is experiencing pain in other areas of the body. Referred back pain may be caused by pressure on the nerve plexus. Some clients have leg or calf pain with swelling and redness as a result of deep vein thrombosis or thrombophlebitis, a complication of pancreatic carcinoma.

Obtain the client's weight to determine the extent of weight loss and whether it has occurred rapidly. The client is questioned about food intake and intolerances. Anorexia accompanied by early satiety, nausea, flatulence, and vomiting is common. Gastrointestinal (GI) bleeding may develop from esophageal or gastric varices caused by the tumor pressing on the portal vein. A new diagnosis of diabetes is found in some clients.

In addition to the focused history, perform a general abdominal assessment. In particular, observe for distention and swelling, which may indicate **ascites** (abdominal fluid). Percussion over the ascitic abdomen elicits dullness. Pancreatic ascites occurs in the advanced stages of the disease process.

DIAGNOSTIC ASSESSMENT

There are no specific blood tests to diagnose pancreatic carcinoma. Serum amylase and lipase levels, as well as alkaline phosphatase and bilirubin levels, are elevated. The degree of elevation depends on the acuteness or chronicity of the pancreatic and biliary damage. Elevated carcinoembryonic antigen (CEA) levels occur in 80% to 90% of clients with pancreatic carcinoma. This test may provide early information about the presence of tumor cells. Other tumor markers, such as CA 19-9 and CA 242, have been found to be useful serologic tests for monitoring a proven diagnosis and for continuing surveillance for potential spread or recurrence. A recent study by Louhimo and colleagues (2004) found that serum HCG beta and CA 72-4 are the strongest independent prognostic indicators for pancreatic cancer.

Computed tomography (CT) can confirm the presence of a tumor and can differentiate the tumor from a cyst. Pancreatic ultrasonography (US) does not distinguish pancreatic carcinoma from other pancreatic disorders; however, it is an excellent test for identifying recurrence of the disease (Tanaka et al., 2004). Endoscopic retrograde cholangiopancreatography (ERCP) visualization and cytologic study of aspirate provide the most definitive diagnostic data. An alternative to ERCP is a percutaneous transhepatic biliary cholangiogram with placement of a percutaneous transhepatic biliary drain (PTBD). This drain decompresses the blocked biliary system by draining bile, either internally or externally. Aspiration of pancreatic ascitic fluid by abdominal paracentesis may reveal malignant cells and elevated amylase levels.

◆ Interventions

Management of the client with pancreatic carcinoma is geared toward preventing tumor spread and decreasing pain. These measures are not curative, only palliative. The cancers are often metastatic and recur despite treatment.

NONSURGICAL MANAGEMENT. As in other types of cancer, chemotherapy or radiation is used to relieve pain. (See Chapter 28 for general nursing interventions associated with these treatment modalities.)

Drug Therapy. To keep the pain under control, the client takes high doses of opioid analgesics (usually morphine) as prescribed and uses other comfort measures before

---

CHART 63-9

KEY FEATURES of
Pancreatic Carcinoma

- Jaundice
- Clay (light) colored stools
- Dark urine
- Abdominal pain: usually vague, dull, or nonspecific that radiates into the back
- Weight loss
- Anorexia
- Nausea or vomiting
- Glucose intolerance
- Splenomegaly (enlarged spleen)
- Flatulence
- Gastrointestinal bleeding
- Ascites (abdominal fluid)
- Leg or calf pain (from thrombophlebitis)
- Weakness and fatigue

the pain escalates and reaches a peak. Because of the poor prognosis, drug dependency is not a consideration. Chapter 7 describes the care of the client with chronic cancer pain in detail.

Chemotherapeutic interventions for pancreatic carcinoma have had limited success. Combining agents has been more successful than single-agent chemotherapy. 5-fluorouracil (5-FU), a typically used drug, is an antimetabolite that interferes with deoxyribonucleic acid (DNA) synthesis in rapidly dividing cells. The following are other drugs that are commonly used:

- Mitomycin (Mutamycin)
- Gemcitabine (Gemzar)
- Docetaxel (Taxotere)
- Cisplatin (Platinol)

The major benefit of these drugs to the client is pain management, with shrinkage of tumor size and prolonged survival being of secondary benefit.

Radiation Therapy. Intensive external beam radiation therapy to the pancreas may offer pain relief by shrinking tumor cells, alleviating obstruction, and improving food absorption; it does not improve survival rates. Implantation of radioactive iodine (^{125}I) seeds, in combination with systemic or intra-arterial administration of floxuridine (FUDR), has also been used. The client may experience discomfort during and after the radiation treatments. Supportive nursing interventions for the relief of symptoms are indicated.

Biliary Stent Insertion. For clients experiencing biliary obstruction who are high surgical risks, **biliary stents** placed percutaneously (through the skin) can ensure patency to relieve pain. Stents are devices made of plastic or metal materials that keep the ducts of the biliary system open. Using another approach, self-expandable stents may be inserted endoscopically to relieve obstruction.

SURGICAL MANAGEMENT. Complete surgical resection of the pancreatic tumor offers the individual with pancreatic cancer the only effective treatment, but the surgery is only possible in a small percentage of cases. Recent technologic advances have expanded the role of **minimally invasive surgery (MIS)** via laparoscopy in the staging, palliation, and resection of pancreatic malignancies. The surgery selected depends on the purpose of the surgery and stage of the disease. For example, if the client experiences biliary obstruction, a laparoscopic procedure to relieve the obstruction, such as a cholecystojejunostomy, is performed. This procedure diverts bile drainage into the jejunum. Less often, a **distal pancreatectomy** to remove tumors in the tail of the pancreas is done. The spleen may also be removed as part of this surgery.

For extensive metastasis, the surgeon may perform either a total pancreatectomy or the Whipple procedure (pancreaticoduodenectomy). These procedures have traditionally been done using an open surgical approach, but new advances in laparoscopic technology using a hand-assist device is beginning to replace the conventional method. At this time, this new technology is not available for some surgeons because they are not yet trained in how to perform this exciting new technique. Therefore the traditional, open surgical approach remains the most common method of performing the Whipple procedure.

Preoperative Care. The client with pancreatic carcinoma is a poor surgical risk because of malnutrition and debilitation. Specific care depends on the type of surgical approach being used. A nasogastric (NG) tube for decompression may be inserted, and the administration of IV fluids or total parenteral nutrition (TPN) is typically started before surgery.

Tube Feedings. As long as intestinal function is adequate, the client may be maintained nutritionally with enteral tube feedings. When tube feedings are tolerated, a small-lumen silicone feeding tube, such as a Dobbhoff tube, is inserted to avoid the complications of larger-lumen tubes, such as sinusitis and nasal irritation. Commercially prepared products chosen by the health care provider or dietitian provide specific nutrients. Feedings are given by bolus or continuous infusion, depending on the client's tolerance and residual volumes.

Often, in the late stages of pancreatic carcinoma or during the Whipple procedure, the physician inserts a small catheter into the jejunum (**jejunostomy**) so that enteral feedings may be given. This feeding method is preferred to prevent reflux and to facilitate absorption. Feedings are initiated in low concentrations and volumes and are gradually increased as tolerated. Provide feedings by means of a pump to maintain a constant volume and assess for diarrhea frequency as a means of measuring tolerance (see Chapter 64).

Total Parenteral Nutrition. For optimal nutrition, hyperalimentation by TPN may be necessary in addition to tube feedings or as a single measure to provide nutrition. When central venous access is required, a Hickman catheter or other type of catheter may be necessary. Meticulous IV line care is an important nursing measure to prevent catheter sepsis. Sterile dressing changes and site observation are extremely important (see Chapter 17). Additional nursing care measures for the client receiving TPN are given in Chapter 64. Monitor nutrition indicators such as serum prealbumin and albumin.

For the laparoscopic procedure, no bowel preparation is needed. However, either approach requires that the client have nothing by mouth (NPO) at least 6 to 8 hours before surgery. Surgeon preference and agency policy dictates the preferred protocol for preoperative preparation.

Operative Procedures. The **Whipple procedure (radical pancreaticoduodenectomy)** involves extensive surgical manipulation and is used to treat cancer of the head of the pancreas. The procedure entails removal of the proximal head of the pancreas, the duodenum, a portion of the jejunum, the stomach (partial or total **gastrectomy**), and the gallbladder, with anastomosis of the pancreatic duct (**pancreaticojejunostomy**), the common bile duct (**choledochojejunostomy**), and the stomach (**gastrojejunostomy**) to the jejunum (Figure 63-3). In addition, the surgeon may remove the spleen (**splenectomy**).

Postoperative Care. In addition to routine postoperative care measures, the client who has undergone an open radical pancreaticoduodenectomy requires intensive nursing care and is usually admitted to a surgical critical care unit. Assess for multiple potential complications of the open Whipple procedure as listed in Table 63-4.

The primary benefit of MIS is the client's fast postoperative recovery and less pain when compared to traditional open procedures. The client having the laparoscopic Whipple surgery or distal pancreatectomy is also less at risk for severe complications, but some problems have occurred. For clients

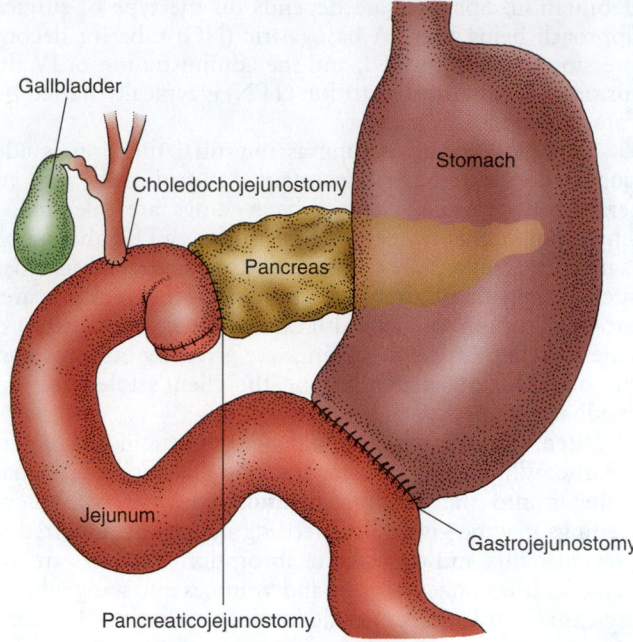

Figure 63-3 ■ The three anastomoses that constitute the Whipple procedure: choledochojejunostomy, pancreaticojejunostomy, and gastrojejunostomy.

TABLE 63-4 Potential Complications of the Whipple Procedure

Cardiovascular Complications
- Hemorrhage at anastomosis sites with hypovolemia
- Myocardial infarction
- Heart failure
- Thrombophlebitis

Pulmonary Complications
- Atelectasis
- Pneumonia
- Pulmonary embolism
- Acute respiratory distress syndrome
- Pulmonary edema

Gastrointestinal Complications
- Adynamic (paralytic) ileus
- Gastric retention
- Gastric ulceration
- Bowel obstruction from peritonitis
- Pancreatitis
- Hepatic failure
- Thrombosis to mesentery

Wound Complications
- Infection
- Dehiscence
- Fistulas: pancreatic, gastric, and biliary

Metabolic Complications
- Unstable diabetes mellitus
- Renal failure

---

having this procedure, observe for and implement preventive measures for the following surgical complications:

- Diabetes (Check blood glucose often.)
- Hemorrhage (Monitor pulse, blood pressure, skin color, and mental status.)

- Wound infection (Monitor temperature and wounds for redness and induration [hardness].)
- Bowel obstruction (Check bowel sounds and stools.)
- Intra-abdominal abscess (Monitor temperature and client's complaint of severe pain.)

Gastrointestinal Drainage Monitoring. If an NG tube is present, the monitoring of gastrointestinal (GI) drainage and tube patency is an important aspect of postoperative nursing care. In open approaches, drainage tubes are strategically placed during surgery to remove drainage and secretions from the area and to prevent stress on the anastomosis sites. Assess the tubes and drainage devices for stress or kinking and maintain the tubes in a dependent position. Check the suction pressure gauge frequently to maintain the desired suction level. Most often, Salem sump tubes are used and connected to low continuous suction (80 mm Hg or less) to maintain drain patency.

Monitor the drainage for color, consistency, and amount. The drainage should be serosanguineous; the appearance of clear, colorless, bile-tinged drainage or frank blood with an increase in output may indicate disruption or leakage of an anastomosis site. Most of the disruptions of the anastomosis site occur within 7 to 10 days after surgery. Hemorrhage can occur as an early or late complication.

If the NG tube is obstructed, instill air first. If this method does not keep the drainage lumen open, irrigation with 10 to 20 mL of normal saline is gently performed. If the problem continues, notify the physician for additional interventions.

The development of a fistula (an abnormal passageway) is the *most common and most serious* postoperative complication. Biliary, pancreatic, or gastric fistulas result from partial or total breakdown of an anastomosis site. The secretions that drain from the fistula contain bile, pancreatic enzymes, or gastric secretions, depending on which anastomosis site is ruptured. These secretions, particularly pancreatic fluid, are corrosive and irritating to the skin, and internal leakage causes a chemical peritonitis. Peritonitis (inflammation and infection of the peritoneum) necessitates treatment with multiple antibiotics. *If you suspect any postoperative complications resulting from MIS or open surgical approaches, call the physician immediately and provide assessment findings that support your concerns.*

Positioning. Place the client in the semi-Fowler's position to reduce stress on the suture line and anastomosis site as well as to optimize lung expansion. Stress on the gastric suture line of an open surgical procedure can be minimized by maintaining NG tube drainage at a low suction level to keep the remaining stomach (if a partial gastrectomy is done) or the jejunum (if a total gastrectomy is done) free of excessive fluid buildup and pressure. The NG tube also reduces stimulation of the remaining pancreatic tissue.

Assessment of Fluids and Electrolytes. Because the *open* Whipple procedure is extensive and can take 6 to 10 hours to complete, maintaining fluid and electrolyte balance can be difficult. Clients tend to experience significant intraoperative blood loss and postoperative bleeding. The intestine is exposed to air for long periods, and evaporation of fluid occurs. Significant losses of fluid and electrolytes occur from NG and other drainage tubes. In addition, these clients are usually malnourished and have low serum levels of protein and albumin, which maintain colloid osmotic pressure within the circulating system. Reduction in the serum osmotic pressure makes the client susceptible to third spacing of body fluids, with fluid moving from the intravascular to the interstitial space, resulting in shock. These problems are less likely to occur when MIS is used. Therefore, when possible, the trained surgeon prefers to perform laparoscopic Whipple procedures to shorten operating time and prevent the many complications that can occur.

Closely monitor vital signs for decreased blood pressure and increased heart rate, decreased vascular pressures with a pulmonary artery catheter (Swan-Ganz catheter), and decreased urine output to detect early signs of hypovolemia and prevent shock. Be alert for pitting edema of the extremities, dependent edema in the sacrum and back, and an intake that far exceeds output. Nutritional repletion via TPN helps promote the shift of fluid from the interstitial space back into the intravascular space.

Maintenance of ordered IV fluid volume replacement is important. Monitor hemoglobin and hematocrit values to assess for blood loss and the need for blood transfusions. Electrolyte values are reviewed for decreased serum levels of sodium, potassium, chloride, and calcium. IV fluid concentrations must be altered to correct these electrolyte imbalances. The physician orders replacement of electrolytes as needed.

Glucose Monitoring. Immediately after the Whipple procedure, the client may have transient hyperglycemia or hypoglycemia as a result of stress and surgical manipulation of the pancreas. Most of the endocrine cells (islets of Langerhans, responsible for insulin and glucose secretion) are located in the body and tail of the pancreas. In most clients, up to half of the gland remains, and diabetes does not develop; however, a large number of clients are diabetic before surgery. Monitor glucose levels frequently during the early postoperative period and administer insulin injections, as prescribed.

Critical Thinking Challenge

An older adult with a family history of pancreatic cancer is admitted to the intensive care unit where you work following a Whipple procedure for metastatic disease. He is alert but has acute delirium; he is unable to answer your questions. A head-to-toe assessment reveals that his breathing is very shallow. His color is normal, but his oxygen saturation is only 88%.

1. What are your priorities for his care at this time?
2. Why do you think he is acutely confused?
3. What complications is this client at risk for, in view of his age? How will you try to prevent them?
4. With what other members of the health care team might you collaborate?
5. Would you delegate his care to a licensed practical nurse at this time? Why or why not?

evolve For suggested answer guidelines, go to http://evolve.elsevier.com/Iggy/.

Community-Based Care

The client with pancreatic cancer is usually followed by a case manager, both in the hospital and in the home or other community-based setting. The role of the case manager is to ensure that the client receives cost-effective treatment and that his or her biopsychosocial needs are met.

HOME CARE MANAGEMENT

The stage of progression of pancreatic carcinoma and available home care resources dictate whether the client can be discharged to home or whether additional care is needed in a skilled nursing facility or with a hospice provider. Home care preparations depend on the client's physical and activity limitations and should be tailored to his or her needs. Coordinate care with the client and whoever will be providing care after discharge from the hospital—home care provider, hospice care provider, or extended care provider.

The client and family need emotional support to deal with issues related to this illness. Assist family members in ascertaining realistically and objectively the amount of physical care required for the client. The family members must be told that their own physical and emotional health is at risk during this stressful period and that supportive counseling is indicated. If the family does not have a religious affiliation or a spiritual leader (e.g., a minister or a rabbi) to provide support, suggest alternative counseling options. It is appropriate for the nurse to make the initial contact or appointment according to the client's or family's wishes.

HEALTH TEACHING

When the client is discharged to home, many of the care measures are palliative and aimed at providing relief of symptoms such as pain. Care measures and teaching information are similar to those for clients with chronic pancreatitis.

In many cases, the diagnosis of pancreatic cancer is made a few months before death occurs. The client needs time to adjust to the diagnosis, which is usually made too late for cure or prolonged survival. The nurse helps the client identify what needs to be done to prepare for death. For example, the client may want to write a will or see family members and friends whom he or she has not seen recently. The client needs to make specific requests for the funeral or memorial service known to family members or significant others. These actions help the client prepare for death in a dignified manner. Chapter 9 discusses anticipatory grieving and preparation for death in detail.

HEALTH CARE RESOURCES

Regular home care nursing and assistive nursing personnel visits are scheduled to assist the client and family by providing physical, psychological, and supportive care. Supply information about local hospice care (see Chapter 9) and cancer support groups.

GET READY for the NCLEX Examination!

KEY POINTS

Safe Effective Care Environment

- When caring for a client with a T-tube, do not place the drainage bag higher than the tube insertion site.
- Recognize that acute pain relief is the first priority for clients with acute pancreatitis.
- Be aware that clients with biliary and pancreatic disorders are at high risk for biliary obstruction, a serious and painful complication.
- Observe for and implement interventions to prevent life-threatening complications of the Whipple procedure as outlined in Table 63-4.

Health Promotion and Maintenance

- Teach clients having a cholecystectomy to avoid high-fat, high-cholesterol foods for several months following surgery; long-term food tolerances vary for each client.
- Provide health teaching for discharge with a T-tube as delineated in Charts 63-2 and 63-3.
- Teach clients about enzyme replacement therapy as described in Chart 63-7.
- Instruct clients about ways to prevent exacerbations of chronic pancreatitis as outlined in Chart 63-8.

Psychosocial Integrity

- Provide pain relief measures for clients with acute pancreatitis to reduce anxiety.
- Explore ways to decrease alcohol consumption in clients with pancreatitis who use excessive alcohol.
- Refer clients with pancreatic cancer for support services such as spiritual leaders and counselors.
- Help prepare the pancreatic cancer client and family for the death and dying process.

Physiological Integrity

- Be aware that autodigestion of the pancreas causes severe pain in clients with acute pancreatitis (see Figure 63-2).
- Monitor serum laboratory values, especially amylase and lipase, in clients with pancreatitis (see Table 63-3).
- Assess for common clinical manifestations of cholecystitis as listed in Chart 63-1.
- For clients with acute pancreatitis, provide interventions as specified in Chart 63-5; do not administer meperidine (Demerol).
- Assess for common clinical manifestations of chronic pancreatitis as listed in Chart 63-6.
- Recognize that obese, middle-aged white women are most likely to have gallbladder disease.
- Assess clients with presenting clinical manifestations of pancreatic carcinoma as described in Chart 63-9.

ADDITIONAL STUDY RESOURCES

Go to your Student CD-ROM for Review Questions for the NCLEX Examination.

evolve Go to http://evolve.elsevier.com/Iggy/ for Integrated Management of Care Questions for the NCLEX Examination.

SELECTED BIBLIOGRAPHY

Asterisk indicates a classic or definitive work on this subject.

American Cancer Society. (2004). *Cancer facts and figures—2004.* Atlanta: Author.

*Barton-Burke, M. (1999). Gemcitabine: A pharmacologic and clinical overview. *Cancer Nursing, 22*(2), 176-183.

Cole, L. (2001). Unraveling the mystery of acute pancreatitis. *Nursing2001, 31*(12), 58-63.

*Cooper, A.D. (1999). Bile salts: Metabolic, pathologic, and therapeutic considerations. *Gastroenterology Clinics of North America, 28*(1), xi, 1-245.

Eisold, S., et al. (2004). Characterization of FAMPAC, a newly identified human pancreatic carcinoma cell line with a hereditary background. *Cancer, 100*(1), 1978-1986.

Enzinger, P.C., & Mayer, R.J. (2004). Gastrointestinal cancer in older patients. *Seminars in Oncology, 31*(2), 206-219.

*Everhart, J.E., et al. (1999). Prevalence and ethnic differences in gallbladder disease in the United States. *Gastroenterology, 177*(3), 632-639.

Fischbach, F. (2004). *A manual of laboratory and diagnostic tests* (7th ed.). Philadelphia: J. B. Lippincott.

Gavaghan, M. (2002). The pancreas—Hermit of the abdomen. *AORN Journal, 75*(6), 1110-1114, 1117, 1119.

Hahn, S.A., et al. (2003). BRCA2 germline mutations in familial pancreatic carcinoma. *Journal of the National Cancer Institute, 95*(3), 214-221.

Hale, A.S., Moseley, M.J., & Warner, S.C. (2000). Treating pancreatitis in the acute care setting. *Dimensions of Critical Care Nursing, 19*(4), 15-21.

*Howard, D.E., & Fromm, H. (1999). Nonsurgical management of gallstone disease. *Gastroenterology Clinics of North America, 28*(1), 133-144.

*Izbicki, J.R., et al. (1999). Surgical treatment of chronic pancreatitis and quality of life after operation. *Surgical Clinics of North America, 79*(4), 913-944.

Klein, A.P., et al. (2004). Prospective risk of pancreatic cancer in familial pancreatic cancer kindreds. *Cancer Research, 64*(7), 2634-2638.

Konner, J., & O'Reilly, E. (2002). Pancreatic cancer: Epidemiology, genetics, and approaches to screening. *Oncology (Huntington), 16*(12), 1615-22, 1631-1632.

*Levin, B. (1999). Gallbladder carcinoma. *Annals of Oncology, 10*(Suppl. 4), 129-130.

Lightner, A.M., et al. (2004). Pancreatic resection in the elderly. *Journal of the American College of Surgery, 198*(5), 697-706.

Louhimo, J., et al. (2004). Serum HCG beta and CA 72-4 are stronger prognostic factors than CEA, CA-19 and CA 242 in pancreatic cancer. *Oncology, 66*(2), 126-131.

McCance, K.L., & Huether, S.E. (2002). *Pathophysiology: The biologic basis for disease in adults and children* (4th ed.). Philadelphia: W. B. Saunders.

*McCormick, M.E. (1999). Endoscopic retrograde cholangiopancreatography. *American Journal of Nursing, 99*(2), 24HH-JJ.

*Norton, I.D., & Petersen, B.T. (1999). Interventional treatment of acute and chronic pancreatitis: Endoscopic procedures. *Surgical Clinics of North America, 79*(4), 895-911, xii.

Pagana, K.D., & Pagana, T.J. (2002). *Mosby's manual of diagnostic and laboratory tests.* St. Louis: Mosby.

Quillen, S.M. (2001). Identification of pancreatitis in the ambulatory setting. *Gastroenterology Nursing, 24*(1), 20-22.

*Runzi, M., & Layer, P. (1999). Nonsurgical management of acute pancreatitis: Use of antibiotics. *Surgical Clinics of North America, 79*(4), 759-765, xii.

*Sauter, P.K., & Coleman, J. (1999). Pancreatic cancer: A continuum of care. *Seminars in Oncology Nursing, 15*(1), 36-47.

Sawabu, N., et al. (2004). Serum tumor markers and molecular diagnosis in pancreatic cancer. *Pancreas, 28*(3), 262-267.

*Scolapio, J.S., Mahli-Chowla, N., & Ukleja, A. (1999). Nutrition supplementation in patients with acute and chronic pancreatitis. *Gastroenterology Clinics of North America, 28*(3), 695-707.

Stevens, M., Esler, R., & Asher, G. (2002). Transdermal fentanyl for the management of acute pancreatitis pain. *Applied Nursing Research, 15*(2), 102-110.

*Strasberg, S. (1999). Laparoscopic biliary surgery. *Gastroenterology Clinics of North America, 28*(1), 117-130.

Tanaka, S., et al. (2004). Periodic ultrasonography checkup for the early detection of pancreatic cancer: A preliminary report. *Pancreas, 28*(3), 268-272.

*Understanding gallstone formation. (1999). *Nursing, 29*(4), 14.

Waitman, J., & McCaffery, M. (2001). Meperidine: A liability. *American Journal of Nursing, 101*(1), 57-58.

Interventions for Clients with Malnutrition and Obesity

DONNA D. IGNATAVICIUS

LEARNING OUTCOMES

After studying this chapter, you should be able to:

1. Interpret findings of a nutritional assessment.
2. Explain the potential consequences and complications associated with malnutrition.
3. Describe the risk factors for malnutrition, especially for older adults.
4. Discuss the role of laboratory testing in the diagnosis of malnutrition.
5. Analyze assessment data to determine common nursing diagnoses for the client with malnutrition.
6. Identify expected outcomes for clients who are malnourished.
7. Describe the nursing care of clients receiving total enteral nutrition (TEN).
8. Prioritize nursing care for clients receiving total parenteral nutrition (TPN).
9. Identify complications associated with TEN and TPN.
10. Explain the potential consequences and complications associated with obesity.
11. Discuss the multiple causes of obesity.
12. Identify the role of drug therapy in the management of obesity.
13. Develop a postoperative teaching plan for clients having bariatric surgery.

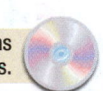

Go to your Student CD-ROM for Review Questions
for the NCLEX Examination keyed to these Learning Outcomes.

Nutrition plays a major role in promoting and maintaining health. Nutritional health not only contributes to positive care outcomes but also saves health care dollars. As part of a comprehensive health assessment, include nutritional screening to identify clients who have nutritional deficits or are at risk for developing nutritional deficits.

NUTRITION STANDARDS TO PROMOTE HEALTH

Dietary Recommendations

Several national standards are available for planning and evaluating nutrition. The standard most widely accepted in the United States is the Recommended Dietary Allowance (RDA). The RDA establishes recommendations for energy intake, protein, vitamins, and minerals for a healthy population. Healthy adults require about 1800 calories/day and 0.8 g of protein/kg of body weight to meet basal energy needs.

The RDA can be used to estimate the adequacy of nutrient intake over time. If a client does not meet 100% of the RDA, it is incorrect to assume that he or she is nutritionally deficient. The risk of inadequate intake for any nutrient is not presumed to be increased until less than 70% of the RDA is consumed. It is also incorrect to assume that all clients in a specific population who meet 100% of the RDA are not at risk for malnutrition.

The Food and Nutrition Board (FNB), with the involvement of Health Canada, has recommended that Dietary Reference Intakes (DRI) replace the RDA. The first DRI released recommended the intake of nutrients related to bone health (Food and Nutrition Board, 1997). The established standard of Canada, the Recommended Nutrient Intake (RNI), is similar to that of the United States.

The role of diet and nutrition in disease has been a subject of interest for many years. The current focus is on

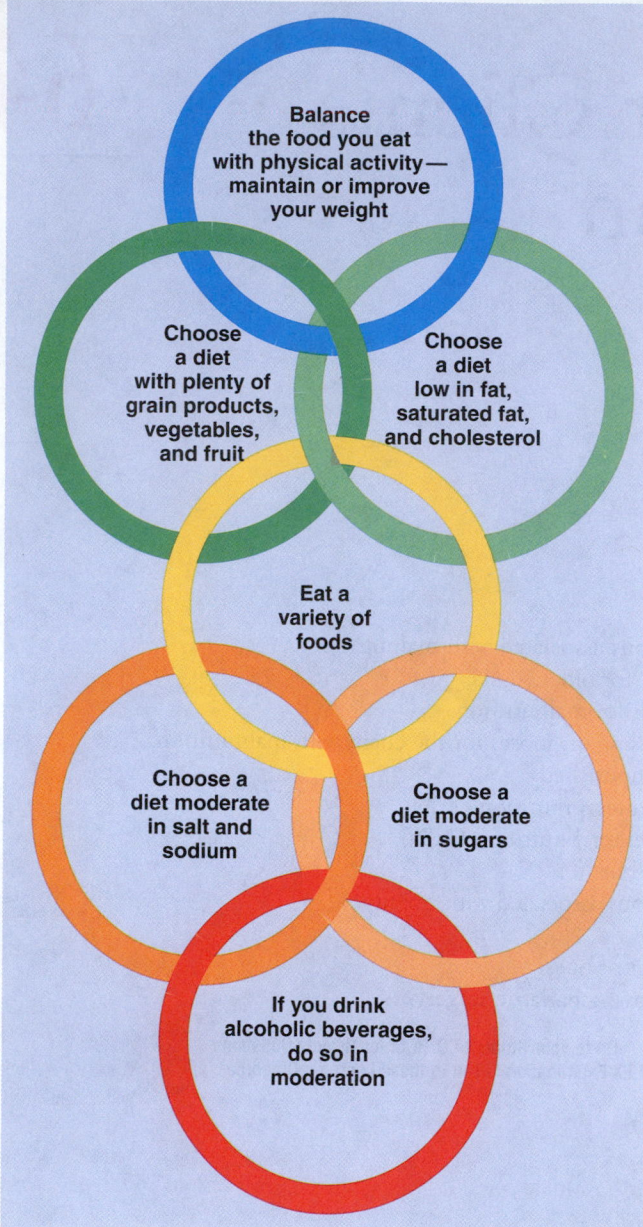

Figure 64-1 ■ Dietary guidelines developed by the U.S. Department of Agriculture and the U.S. Department of Health and Human Services.

TABLE 64-1   Nutrition Recommendations for Canadians

- The sodium content of the Canadian diet should be reduced.
- The Canadian diet should include no more than 5% of total energy as alcohol, or two drinks daily, whichever is less.
- The Canadian diet should contain no more caffeine than the equivalent of four cups of regular coffee per day.
- Community water supplies containing less than 1 mg/L of fluoride should be fluoridated to that level.
- The Canadian diet should provide energy consistent with the maintenance of body weight within the recommended range.
- The Canadian diet should include essential nutrients in amounts specified in the Recommended Nutrient Intake.
- The Canadian diet should include no more than 30% of energy as fat (33 g/1000 kcal or 39 g/5000 kJ) and no more than 10% as saturated fat (11 g/1000 kcal or 13 g/5000 kJ).
- The Canadian diet should provide 55% of energy as carbohydrates (138 g/1000 kcal or 165 g/5000 kJ) from a variety of sources.

From Communications/Implementation Committee, Minister of National Health and Welfare. (1990). *Action towards healthy eating: Canada's guidelines for healthy eating and recommended strategies for implementation.* Cat. No. H39-166/1990E. Ottawa: Branch Publications Unit.

fee per day as well as adding fluoride to community water supplies to a level of 1 mg/L.

Food Pyramids

The USDA developed the **Food Guide Pyramid** in 1992 to translate food recommendations into a practical graphic format (Figure 64-2). A pyramid format was chosen to communicate three key dietary principles: variety, moderation, and proportionality. The pyramid design emphasizes building the diet on a base of grains, fruits, and vegetables. Moderate quantities of lean meats, protein sources, and dairy products are added, and the intake of fats and sweets is limited. Table 64-2 suggests the daily servings of each food group and clarifies the size of a serving. Adhering to this pattern results in a nutritionally adequate intake if a variety of foods is chosen.

A variety of vegetarian diet patterns is being adopted by increasing numbers of people for health, environmental, and moral reasons. In general, vegetarians are leaner than those who consume meat. The **lacto-vegetarian** eats milk, cheese, and dairy foods but avoids meat, fish, poultry, and eggs. The **lacto-ovo-vegetarian** also includes eggs. The **vegan** eats only foods of plant origin. Vegans can develop megaloblastic anemia as a result of vitamin B_{12} deficiency. Vegans should include a daily source of vitamin B_{12} in their diets, such as a fortified breakfast cereal, fortified soy beverage, or meat analogue. All vegetarians should ensure that they get adequate amounts of calcium, iron, zinc, and vitamins D and B_{12}. Well-planned vegetarian diets can provide adequate nutrition. The **Vegetarian Food Pyramid,** endorsed by the Vegetarian Resource Group, can assist vegetarians with daily food choices (Figure 64-3).

A third pyramid has recently been developed to reflect the current trend toward low-carbohydrate ("low-carb") diets, such as the Atkins and South Beach diets. The **Atkins pyramid** emphasizes building the diet on protein sources and vegetables rather than on grains, fruits, and vegetables as in the USDA-approved pyramid. Moderate quantities of fruits, dairy products, and nuts are added, and whole grain foods are limited. Refined carbohydrates are the least desirable foods, such as pasta, cakes, and white bread.

health promotion and the prevention of disease. In 1995 the Dietary Guidelines for Americans were revised by the U.S. Department of Agriculture (USDA) and the U.S. Department of Health and Human Services (DHHS). These seven guidelines emphasize the importance of selecting foods to maintain a healthful diet with balance, moderation, and variety (Figure 64-1). One of the most noticeable changes from previous editions occurs in the weight guideline. For the first time, diet and physical activity were emphasized in the second guideline with the goal of maintaining or improving body weight.

The Nutrition Recommendations for Canadians (Table 64-1) are similar to the Dietary Guidelines for Americans. In addition, they recommend limiting the caffeine content of the diet to no more than the equivalent of four cups of cof-

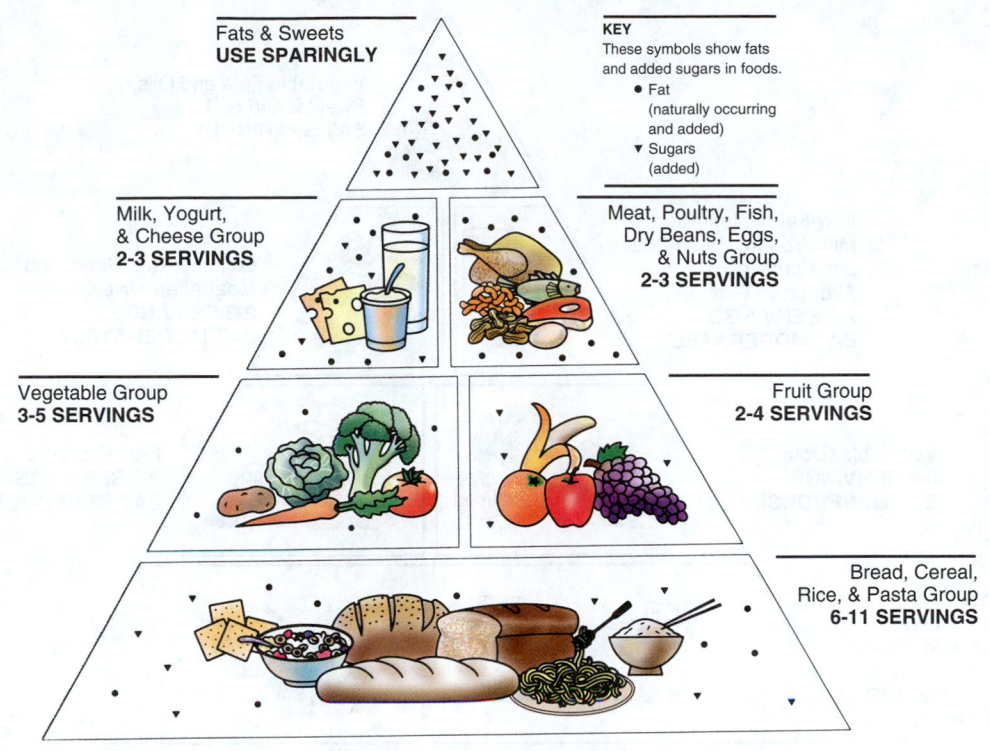

Figure 64-2 ■ The U.S. Department of Agriculture Food Guide Pyramid.

TABLE 64-2 Serving Sizes for Each Food Group

With the Food Guide Pyramid, what counts as a "serving" may not always be a typical "helping" of what you eat. The following are some examples of servings.

Bread, Cereal, Rice, and Pasta
6 to 11 servings recommended
Examples of one serving:
- 1 slice of bread
- 1 oz ready-to-eat cereal
- ½ c cooked cereal, rice, or pasta

Vegetables
3 to 5 servings recommended
Examples of one serving:
- 1 c raw leafy vegetables
- ½ c other vegetables, cooked or chopped raw
- ¾ c vegetable juice

Fruits
2 to 4 servings recommended
Examples of one serving:
- 1 medium apple, banana, or orange
- ½ c chopped, cooked, or canned fruit
- ¾ c fruit juice

Milk, Yogurt, and Cheese
2 to 3 servings recommended
Examples of one serving:
- 1 c milk or yogurt
- 1½ oz natural cheese
- 2 oz processed cheese

Meat, Poultry, Fish, Dry Beans, Eggs, and Nuts
2 to 3 servings recommended
Examples of one serving:
- 2 to 3 oz cooked lean meat, poultry, or fish
- ½ c cooked dry beans or 1 egg = 1 oz of lean meat
- 2 tbsp peanut butter or ⅓ c nuts = 1 oz of meat

How Much Is an Ounce of Meat?
Here is a handy guide for determining the weight of meat, chicken, fish, or cheese:
- 1 oz = the size of a matchbox
- 3 oz = the size of a deck of cards
- 8 oz = the size of a paperback book

Modified from Nutrition and your health: Dietary guidelines for Americans. (1995). *Home and Garden Bulletin No. 232* (4th ed.). Washington, D.C.: U.S. Department of Agriculture, U.S. Department of Health and Human Services.

CULTURAL CONSIDERATIONS

None of the food pyramids takes into account dietary preferences of diverse ethnic groups. For example, for individuals of Hispanic descent, tortillas, beans, and rice may be preferred over pasta, risotto, and potatoes. Therefore health teaching about diet should incorporate these variations (also see Chapter 6).

Some individuals have food allergies or intolerances. For instance, lactose intolerance (lactose is found in milk and milk products) is a relatively common condition that occurs in a number of ethnic groups. It is found more often in Mexican Americans and black individuals as well as in some Native American/American Indian tribes, Asian Americans, and Ashkenazic Jews. A small percentage of white individuals are also lactose intolerant. The cause of **lactose intolerance** is an insufficient amount of the lactase enzyme, which converts lactose into absorbable glucose.

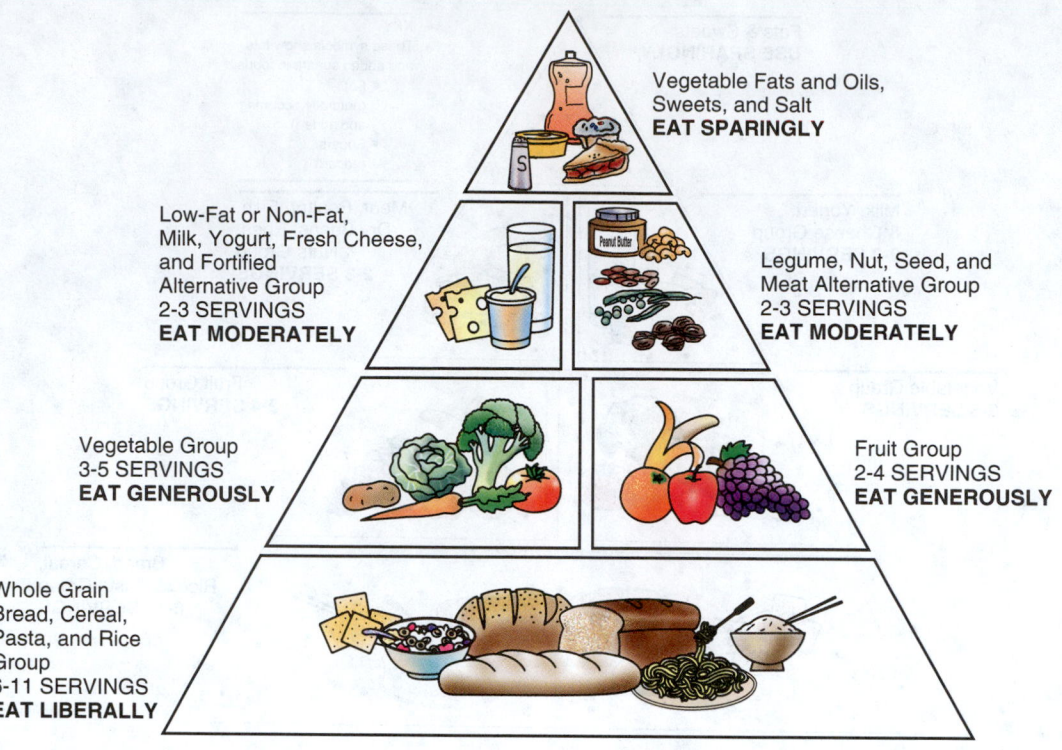

Figure 64-3 ■ Food pyramid for a vegetarian diet. (Courtesy The Health Connection, Hagerstown, MD.)

NUTRITIONAL ASSESSMENT

Malnutrition and obesity are common nutrition problems that occur as progressive changes within the client. When nutritional deficiencies or excesses develop, the body adapts through the use of homeostatic mechanisms. As the intake moves farther from the accepted range, however, the body accommodates by reducing functional levels or changing the status or size of the affected body compartments. The nutritional status of a client can be determined by the presence or absence of these adaptations.

Nutritional status reflects the balance between nutrient requirements and nutrient intake. Factors that affect nutrient requirements include disease, infection, and psychological stress. Nutrient intake is influenced by disease, eating behaviors, economic factors, emotional stability, medication, and disease.

Nutrition care is a major interdisciplinary outcome for malnutrition and obesity. Evaluation of food intake is an important part of total client assessment. Assessment of nutritional status in-

dietitian collaborate to identify clients at risk for nutritional problems.

Initial Nutritional Screening

Not every client needs a complete nutritional assessment, but it is important to identify clients at risk for nutritional problems through screening. An **initial nutritional screening** provides an inexpensive, quick way of determining which clients need more extensive nutritional assessment by the health care provider and dietitian.

The initial nutritional screening includes visual inspection, measured height and weight, weight history, usual eating habits, ability to chew and swallow, and any recent changes in appetite or food intake. Questions that may identify clients at risk for nutritional problems can be incorporated into the history and physical assessment (Chart 64-1).

The Mini Nutritional Assessment (MNA), which has been tested worldwide, provides a reliable, rapid assessment for clients in the community as well as in any health care setting (Stechmiller, 2003). The tool consists of six screening questions and, if needed, a follow-up set of more in-depth questions and arm and calf measurements. It can be completed in about 10 minutes; a low score indicates malnutrition or a risk for malnutrition (Figure 64-4).

Anthropometric Measurements

Anthropometric measurements are noninvasive methods of evaluating nutritional status. These measurements include height and weight and assessment of body fat.

BEST PRACTICE for
Initial Nutrition Screening Assessment

General
- Does the client have any conditions that cause nutrient loss, such as malabsorption syndromes, draining abscesses, wounds, fistulas, or protracted diarrhea?
- Does the client have any conditions that increase the need for nutrients, such as fever, burn, injury, sepsis, or antineoplastic therapies?
- Has the client been on NPO status for 3 days or more?
- Is the client receiving a modified diet or a diet restricted in one or more nutrients?
- Is the client being enterally or parenterally fed?
- Does the client describe food allergies, lactose intolerance, or limited food preferences?
- Has the client experienced a recent, unexplained weight loss?
- Is the client taking medications, either prescription, over-the-counter, or herbal/natural products?

Gastrointestinal
- Does the client complain of nausea, indigestion, vomiting, diarrhea, or constipation?
- Does the client exhibit glossitis, stomatitis, or esophagitis?
- Does the client have difficulty chewing or swallowing?
- Does the client have a partial or total gastrointestinal obstruction?
- What is the client's state of dentition?

Cardiovascular
- Does the client have ascites or edema?
- Is the client able to perform activities of daily living?
- Does the client have heart failure?

Genitourinary
- Does fluid input approximately equal fluid output?
- Does the client have an ostomy?
- Is the client hemodialyzed or peritoneally dialyzed?

Respiratory
- Is the client receiving mechanical ventilatory support?
- Is the client receiving oxygen via nasal prongs?
- Does the client have chronic obstructive pulmonary disease (COPD) or asthma?

Integumentary
- Does the client have nail or hair changes?
- Does the client have rashes or dermatitis?
- Does the client have dry or pale mucous membranes or decreased skin turgor?
- Does the client have pressure areas on the sacrum, hips, or ankles?

Extremities
- Does the client have pedal edema?
- Does the client exhibit cachexia?

Modified with permission of Ross Products Division, Abbott Laboratories, Columbus, OH.
NPO, Nothing by mouth.

MEASUREMENT OF HEIGHT AND WEIGHT

Height and weight provide a baseline determination of nutritional status. Be sure to obtain accurate measurements because clients who report their own measurements tend to overestimate height and underestimate weight. For clients who cannot stand, use a wheelchair or bed scales. Subsequent measurements may indicate an early change in nutritional status. Assistive nursing personnel often perform this activity.

Height

Clients should be measured and weighed while wearing minimal clothing and no shoes. Determine the client's height in inches or centimeters using the measuring stick of a weight scale if the client can stand. The client should stand erect and look straight ahead, with the heels together and the arms at the sides.

CONSIDERATIONS FOR OLDER ADULTS

Some older adults may have difficulty standing erect, and their actual height may be less than their height on recall. If height cannot be measured directly, it should be estimated by arm span or with use of a knee-height caliper, which provides a more precise height estimate.

Weight

The nurse or assistive nursing personnel weighs ambulatory clients with an upright balance-beam scale. Nonambulatory clients can be weighed with a movable wheelchair balance-beam scale or a bed scale. The manufacturer should calibrate weight scales twice yearly to ensure accurate readings. For daily or sequential weights, obtain the weight at the same time each day, if possible. Conditions such as congestive heart failure and renal disease cause weight gain; dehydration causes weight loss. *Weight is the most reliable indicator of fluid gain or loss.*

Normal weights for adult men and women are shown in the Metropolitan Life tables (Table 64-3). The latest U.S. Department of Agriculture (USDA) and U.S. Department of Health and Human Services (DHHS) Dietary Guidelines contain weight guidelines that emphasize both weight maintenance and weight loss. The same healthy weight guideline applies to all adults. Older adults are no longer permitted a higher weight standard. The weight range appears in the guidelines as a chart with three categories: healthy weight, moderate overweight, and severe overweight (Figure 64-5). Either the Metropolitan Life tables or the New Weight Guidelines from the USDA and the DHHS may be used for comparison with a client's height and weight. Some health care professionals prefer the Metropolitan Life tables because they consider body-build differences by gender.

Changes in body weight can be expressed by three different formulas:

1. Weight as a percentage of ideal body weight (IBW):

$$\%IBW = \frac{Current\ weight \times 100}{Ideal\ weight}$$

2. Current weight as a percentage of usual body weight (UBW):

$$\%UBW = \frac{Current\ weight \times 100}{Usual\ weight}$$

3. Change in weight:

$$Weight\ change = \frac{Usual\ weight - Current\ weight}{Usual\ weight} \times 100$$

NESTLÉ NUTRITION SERVICES

Mini Nutritional Assessment (MNA)

Last name:	First name:	Sex:	Date:

Age:	Weight, kg:	Height, cm:	I.D. Number:

Complete the screen by filling in the boxes with the appropriate numbers.
Add the numbers for the screen. If score is 11 or less, continue with the assessment to gain a Malnutrition Indicator Score.

Screening

A Has food intake declined over the past 3 months due to loss of appetite, digestive problems, chewing or swallowing difficulties?
0 = severe loss of appetite
1 = moderate loss of appetite
2 = no loss of appetite ☐

B Weight loss during last 3 months
0 = weight loss greater than 3 kg (6.6 lbs)
1 = does not know
2 = weight loss between 1 and 3 kg (2.2 and 6.6 lbs)
3 = no weight loss ☐

C Mobility
0 = bed or chair bound
1 = able to get out of bed/chair but does not go out
2 = goes out ☐

D Has suffered psychological stress or acute disease in the past 3 months
0 = yes   2 = no ☐

E Neuropsychological problems
0 = severe dementia or depression
1 = mild dementia
2 = no psychological problems ☐

F Body Mass Index (BMI) (weight in kg) / (height in m)²
0 = BMI less than 19
1 = BMI 19 to less than 21
2 = BMI 21 to less than 23
3 = BMI 23 or greater ☐

Screening score (subtotal max. 14 points) ☐ ☐
12 points or greater   Normal – not at risk – no need to complete assessment
11 points or below   Possible malnutrition – continue assessment

Assessment

G Lives independently (not in a nursing home or hospital)
0 = no   1 = yes ☐

H Takes more than 3 prescription drugs per day
0 = yes   1 = no ☐

I Pressure sores or skin ulcers
0 = yes   1 = no ☐

J How many full meals does the patient eat daily?
0 = 1 meal
1 = 2 meals
2 = 3 meals ☐

K Selected consumption markers for protein intake
• At least one serving of dairy products (milk, cheese, yogurt) per day?   yes ☐   no ☐
• Two or more servings of legumes or eggs per week?   yes ☐   no ☐
• Meat, fish or poultry every day   yes ☐   no ☐
0.0 = if 0 or 1 yes
0.5 = if 2 yes
1.0 = if 3 yes ☐.☐

L Consumes two or more servings of fruits or vegetables per day?
0 = no   1 = yes ☐

M How much fluid (water, juice, coffee, tea, milk...) is consumed per day?
0.0 = less than 3 cups
0.5 = 3 to 5 cups
1.0 = more than 5 cups ☐.☐

N Mode of feeding
0 = unable to eat without assistance
1 = self-fed with some difficulty
2 = self-fed without any problem ☐

O Self view of nutritional status
0 = views self as being malnourished
1 = is uncertain of nutritional state
2 = views self as having no nutritional problem ☐

P In comparison with other people of the same age, how does the patient consider his/her health status?
0.0 = not as good
0.5 = does not know
1.0 = as good
2.0 = better ☐.☐

Q Mid-arm circumference (MAC) in cm
0.0 = MAC less than 21
0.5 = MAC 21 to 22
1.0 = MAC 22 or greater ☐.☐

R Calf circumference (CC) in cm
0 = CC less than 31   1 = CC 31 or greater ☐

Assessment (max. 16 points) ☐ ☐.☐

Screening score ☐ ☐

Total Assessment (max. 30 points) ☐ ☐.☐

Malnutrition Indicator Score

17 to 23.5 points   at risk of malnutrition ☐

Less than 17 points   malnourished ☐

Ref.: Guigoz Y, Vellas B and Garry PJ. 1994. Mini Nutritional Assessment: A practical assessment tool for grading the nutritional state of elderly patients. *Facts and Research in Gerontology.* Supplement #2:15-59.
Rubenstein LZ, Harker J, Guigoz Y and Vellas B. Comprehensive Geriatric Assessment (CGA) and the MNA: An Overview of CGA, Nutritional Assessment, and Development of a Shortened Version of the MNA. In: "Mini Nutritional Assessment (MNA): Research and Practice in the Elderly". Vellas B, Garry PJ and Guigoz Y , editors. Nestlé Nutrition Workshop Series. Clinical & Performance Programme, vol. 1. Karger, Bâle, in press.

Figure 64-4 ■ The Mini Nutritional Assessment (MNA).

TABLE 64-3 Metropolitan Life Height and Weight Tables

Height*		Weight†			Height*		Weight†		
Feet	Inches	Small Frame	Medium Frame	Large Frame	Feet	Inches	Small Frame	Medium Frame	Large Frame
Men					**Women**				
5	2	128-134	131-134	138-150	4	10	102-111	109-121	118-131
5	3	130-136	133-143	140-153	4	11	103-113	111-123	120-134
5	4	132-138	135-145	142-156	5	0	104-115	113-126	122-137
5	5	134-140	137-148	144-160	5	1	106-118	115-129	125-140
5	6	136-142	139-151	146-164	5	2	108-121	118-132	128-143
5	7	138-145	142-154	149-168	5	3	111-124	121-135	131-147
5	8	140-148	145-157	152-172	5	4	114-127	124-138	134-151
5	9	142-151	148-160	155-176	5	5	117-130	127-141	137-155
5	10	144-154	151-163	158-180	5	6	120-133	130-144	140-159
5	11	146-157	154-166	161-184	5	7	123-136	133-147	143-163
6	0	149-160	157-170	164-188	5	8	126-139	136-150	146-167
6	1	152-164	160-174	168-192	5	9	129-142	139-153	149-170
6	2	155-168	164-178	172-197	5	10	132-145	142-156	152-173
6	3	158-172	167-182	176-202	5	11	135-148	145-159	155-176
6	4	162-176	171-187	181-207	6	0	138-151	148-162	158-179

Reprinted courtesy of Metropolitan Life Insurance Company, 1983.
*Shoes with 1-inch heels.
†Weight in pounds. Men: allow 5 pounds of clothing. Women: allow 3 pounds of clothing

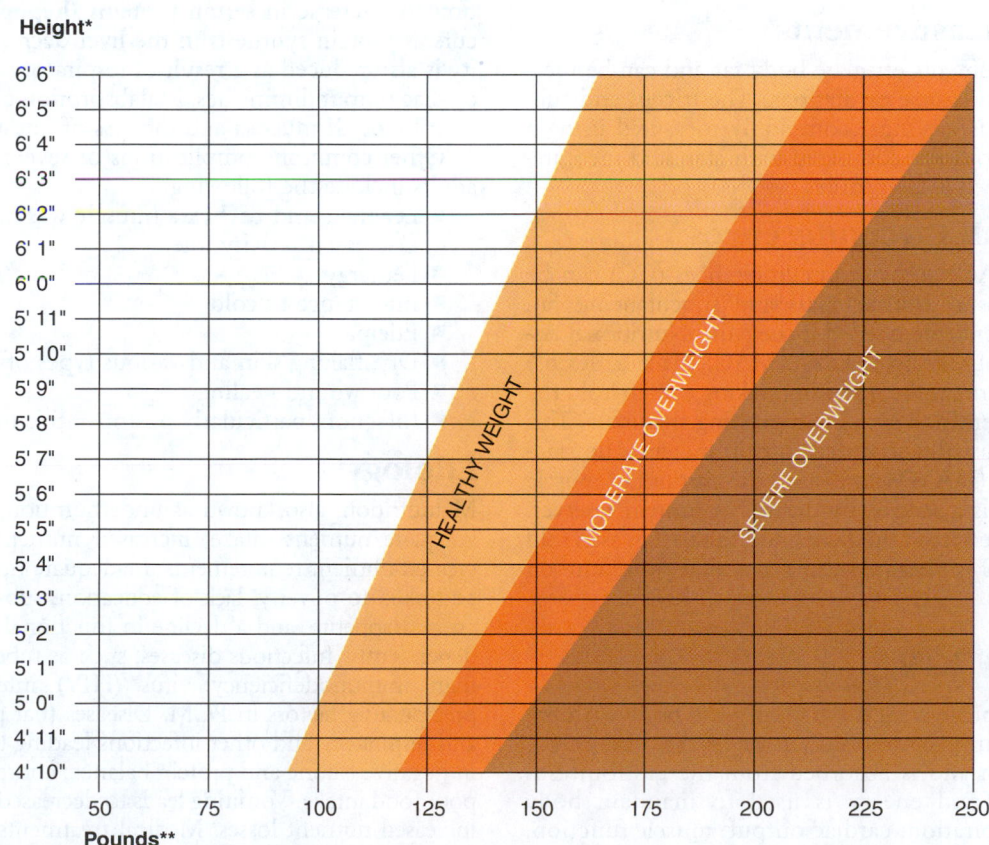

* Without shoes.
** Without clothes. The higher weights apply to people with more
   muscle and bone, such as many men.

Figure 64-5 ■ The U.S. Department of Agriculture and the U.S. Department of Health and Human Services guidelines for determining proper weight or degree of obesity. (Redrawn from http://www.nalusda.gov/fnic/Dietry/9dietgui.htm.)

An involuntary weight loss of 10% at any time significantly affects nutritional status. Weights may need to be taken daily, several times a week, or weekly for monitoring status and the effectiveness of nutritional support.

ASSESSMENT OF BODY FAT

Body Mass Index

The **body mass index (BMI)** is a measure of nutritional status that does not depend on frame size. The BMI indirectly estimates total fat stores within the body by the relationship of weight to height. Therefore an accurate height is as important as an accurate weight.

A simple calculation for estimating BMI can be programmed into handheld computers or calculators:

$$BMI = \frac{Weight\ (lb)}{Height\ (inches)^2} \times 703$$

BMI can also be determined using a nomogram. The least risk of malnutrition is associated with scores between 20 and 25. BMIs above and below these values are associated with increased health risks. Older adults should have a BMI between 24 and 27.

Skin Fold Measurements

Skin fold measurements estimate body fat and can be measured by either the nurse or dietitian. The triceps and subscapular skin folds are most commonly measured using a special caliper. Both are compared with standard measurements and recorded as percentiles.

Arm and Calf Circumferences

The midarm (MAC) and calf circumferences (CC) can be obtained to measure muscle mass and subcutaneous fat. These measurements are needed if the Mini Nutritional Assessment tool is used. To measure MAC, place a flexible tape around the arm at the midpoint, taking care to hold the tape firmly but gently to avoid compressing the tissue. This measurement is usually recorded in centimeters. The midarm muscle mass (MAMM) measures the amount of muscle in the body and is a sensitive indicator of protein reserves. It can be computed from the MAC and the triceps skin fold measure. The CC is obtained using a similar procedure on the calf.

MALNUTRITION

Carbohydrates, protein, and fat supply the body with energy. Under healthy conditions, most of this energy undergoes digestion and is absorbed from the gastrointestinal (GI) tract. Food energy is used to maintain body temperature, respiration, cardiac output, muscle function, protein synthesis, and the storage and metabolism of food sources.

Energy balance refers to the relationship between energy expended and energy stored. When energy expended exceeds energy intake, energy stores are used to supply the deficit; this results in weight loss. Body proteins are used for energy when calorie intake is insufficient. The body attempts to meet its calorie requirements even if it is at the expense of protein needs.

PATHOPHYSIOLOGY

Many severely ill or hospitalized clients experiencing trauma are at risk for **protein-calorie malnutrition (PCM),** also known as protein-energy malnutrition (PEM). PCM may present in three forms: marasmus, kwashiorkor, and marasmic-kwashiorkor. **Marasmus** is generally a calorie malnutrition in which body fat and protein are wasted. Serum proteins are often preserved. **Kwashiorkor** is a lack of protein quantity and quality in the presence of adequate calories. Body weight is more normal, and serum proteins are low. **Marasmic-kwashiorkor** is a combined protein and energy malnutrition. This problem often presents clinically when metabolic stress is imposed on a chronically starved client. The outcome of unrecognized or untreated PCM is often dysfunction or disability and increased morbidity and mortality.

Malnutrition is a multinutrient problem because foods that are good sources of calories and protein are also good sources of other nutrients. In the malnourished client, protein catabolism exceeds protein intake and synthesis, resulting in negative nitrogen balance, weight loss, decreased muscle mass, and weakness.

The functional ability of the liver, heart, lungs, GI tract, and immune system diminishes in the client with malnutrition. A decrease in serum proteins **(hypoproteinemia)** occurs as protein synthesis in the liver decreases. Vital capacity is also reduced as a result of respiratory muscle atrophy; cardiac output diminishes. Malabsorption occurs because of atrophy of GI mucosa and the loss of intestinal villi.

Other common complications of severe malnutrition in adults include the following:

- Leanness and **cachexia** (muscle wasting)
- Decreased activity tolerance
- Lethargy
- Intolerance to cold
- Edema
- Dry, flaking skin and various types of dermatitis
- Poor wound healing
- Infection, particularly postoperative infection

Etiology

Malnutrition, also known as undernutrition, results from inadequate nutrient intake, increased nutrient losses, and increased nutrient requirements. Inadequate nutrient intake can be linked to poverty, lack of education, substance abuse, decreased appetite, and a decline in functional ability to eat independently. Infectious diseases, such as tuberculosis and human immunodeficiency virus (HIV) infection, are also precipitating factors in PCM. Diseases that produce diarrhea and respiratory and other infections leading to anorexia result in negative calorie and protein balance; anorexia then leads to poor food intake. Vomiting leads to decreased absorption with increased nutrient losses. Medical treatments such as chemotherapy can also cause malnutrition. In addition, catabolic processes increase nutrient requirements and metabolic losses.

Inadequate nutrient intake can also result when a person is admitted to the hospital or nursing home (Cowan et al., 2004; Dudek, 2000). Many clients increase their nutritional risk during their hospitalization and therefore need to be frequently reassessed. For example, decreased staffing may not allow time for clients who need to be fed, especially older adults, who may eat slowly (Anderson, 2000). Many diagnostic tests, surgery, and unexpected medical complications require a period of having nothing by mouth (NPO) or anorexia.

> ### CONSIDERATIONS FOR OLDER ADULTS
>
> Unrecognized dysphagia is a common problem in nursing homes and can cause malnutrition, dehydration, and aspiration pneumonia. A nursing study by Kayser-Jones and Pengilly (1999) found that 45 of 82 residents in one nursing home had some degree of dysphagia (difficulty swallowing) ranging from mild to profound. Only 10 of the 45 residents had been referred for dysphagia evaluation by a speech-language pathologist.

Acute PCM may develop in clients who were adequately nourished before hospitalization if they experience starvation while in a catabolic state from infection, stress, or injury. *Chronic* PCM can occur in clients who have cancer, end-stage renal or hepatic disease, or chronic neurologic disease.

Eating disorders, such as anorexia nervosa and bulimia nervosa, also lead to malnutrition. **Anorexia nervosa** is a self-induced starvation resulting from a fear of fatness, even though the client is underweight. **Bulimia nervosa** is characterized by episodes of binge eating in which the client ingests a large amount of food in a short time. The binge eating is followed by some form of purging behavior, such as self-induced vomiting or excessive use of laxatives and diuretics. If not treated, death can result from starvation, infection, or suicide. Information about eating disorders can be found in textbooks on mental/behavioral health nursing.

Incidence/Prevalence

In a review of eight studies with more than 1347 hospitalized adults, 40% to 55% were determined to be malnourished or at risk for malnutrition, and up to 12% were severely malnourished (Dudek, 2000). Malnourished clients heal more slowly, suffer more complications, and have a higher mortality rate. Surgical clients with a likelihood of malnutrition were two to three times more likely to experience minor and major complications and excess mortality. Length of hospitalization in malnourished medical-surgical clients can be extended, which clearly increases health care costs.

◆COLLABORATIVE MANAGEMENT
◆Assessment
HISTORY

Review the medical history to determine the diagnosis, the possibility of increased metabolic needs or nutritional losses, chronic disease, recent surgery of the GI tract, drug and alcohol abuse, and recent significant weight loss. Each of these conditions can contribute to malnutrition. For older adults, explore mental status deterioration and note poor eyesight or hearing, diseases affecting major organs, constipation or incontinence, and slowed reactions. Review prescription and over-the-counter medications (including herbal and natural supplements) and physical disabilities (Chart 64-2).

For clients who live independently, the nurse or occupational therapist may assess the performance of instrumental activities of daily living (IADLs). Functional status can best be evaluated for institutionalized clients by assessing their performance of activities of daily living (ADLs). When func-

> ### CHART 64-2
> #### NURSING FOCUS on the OLDER ADULT
> #### Risk Assessment for Malnutrition
>
> - Recognize that clinical manifestations of malnutrition may not be apparent because they are similar to physiologic changes associated with aging (e.g., dry skin, decreased muscle tone, dry hair).
> - Assess body weight and compare it with the usual body weight or ideal body weight.
> - Be aware that multiple chronic diseases, especially gastrointestinal disorders such as malabsorption syndromes, predispose the client to malnutrition.
> - Assess the client's financial ability to buy healthy food.
> - Assess the client's physical and mental ability to prepare food.
> - Inspect the client's oral cavity for the presence of teeth or dentures, gum disease, or oral lesions that could affect food intake.
> - Review the client's medications, including prescription and over-the-counter (OTC) drugs. Many drugs interact with food or cause anorexia or nausea.
> - Use the Mini Nutritional Assessment.

tional status is evaluated with nutritional status, there appears to be a strong predictability of infections and complications among institutionalized adults. Chapter 10 describes functional assessment in detail.

Interview the client to obtain information about his or her usual daily food intake, eating behaviors, change in appetite, and recent weight changes. Ask the client to describe the usual foods eaten daily and the times of meals and snacks. The dietitian can more thoroughly analyze the diet, if necessary, based on the initial nutritional screening.

Explore changes in eating habits as a result of illness, and record any change in appetite, taste, and weight loss. A weight loss of 5% or more in 30 days, a weight loss of 10% in 6 months, or a weight that is below ideal body weight is significant for malnutrition.

Difficulty or pain in chewing or swallowing is also assessed. Ask the client whether any foods are avoided and why. The occurrence of nausea, vomiting, heartburn, or any other symptoms of discomfort with eating is also recorded. Finally, the client is asked about dental health problems, including the presence of dentures. Dentures or partial plates that do not fit well interfere with food intake.

PHYSICAL ASSESSMENT/CLINICAL MANIFESTATIONS

Assess for manifestations of various nutrient deficiencies (Table 64-4). Inspect the client's hair, eyes, oral cavity, nails, and musculoskeletal and neurologic systems. The condition of the skin, including any reddened or open areas, is observed. The previously described anthropometric measurements may also be obtained. The nurse or assistive nursing personnel monitors all food and fluid intake, observes the client at mealtime, and notes any mouth pain or difficulty in chewing or swallowing. A 3-day caloric intake may be collected and then calculated by the dietitian.

PSYCHOSOCIAL ASSESSMENT

The psychosocial history provides information about the client's economic status, occupation, educational level, living and cooking arrangements, and mental status. Determine

TABLE 64-4 Manifestations of Nutrient Deficiencies

Sign/Symptom	Potential Nutrient Deficiency
Hair	
Alopecia	Zinc, essential fatty acids
Easy pluckability	Protein, essential fatty acids
Lackluster hair	Protein, zinc
"Corkscrew" hair	Vitamin C, vitamin A
Decreased pigmentation	Protein, copper
Eyes	
Xerosis of conjunctiva	Vitamin A
Corneal vascularization	Riboflavin
Keratomalacia	Vitamin A
Bitot's spots	Vitamin A
Gastrointestinal Tract	
Nausea, vomiting	Pyridoxine
Diarrhea	Zinc, niacin
Stomatitis	Pyridoxine, riboflavin, iron
Cheilosis	Pyridoxine, iron
Glossitis	Pyridoxine, zinc, niacin, folic acid, vitamin B_{12}
Magenta tongue	Riboflavin
Swollen, bleeding gums	Vitamin C
Fissured tongue	Niacin
Hepatomegaly	Protein
Skin	
Dry and scaling	Vitamin A, essential fatty acids, zinc
Petechiae/ecchymoses	Vitamin C, vitamin K
Follicular hyperkeratosis	Vitamin A, essential fatty acids
Nasolabial seborrhea	Niacin, pyridoxine, riboflavin
Bilateral dermatitis	Niacin, zinc
Extremities	
Subcutaneous fat loss	Calories
Muscle wastage	Calories, protein
Edema	Protein
Osteomalacia, bone pain, rickets	Vitamin D
Arthralgia	Vitamin C
Hematologic	
Anemia	Vitamin B_{12}, iron, folic acid, copper, vitamin E
Leukopenia, neutropenia	Copper
Low prothrombin time, prolonged clotting time	Vitamin K, manganese
Neurologic	
Disorientation	Niacin, thiamine
Confabulation	Thiamine
Neuropathy	Thiamine, pyridoxine, chromium
Paresthesia	Thiamine, pyridoxine, vitamin B_{12}
Cardiovascular	
Congestive heart failure, cardiomegaly, tachycardia	Thiamine
Cardiomyopathy	Selenium

Used with permission of Ross Products Division, Abbott Laboratories, Columbus, OH.

whether financial resources are adequate for providing the necessary food. If resources are inadequate, the social worker may refer the client to available community services. Chapter 5 discusses nutrition in older adults in more detail.

LABORATORY ASSESSMENT

Laboratory tests supply objective data that can support subjective data and identify preclinical deficiencies. However, they must be carefully interpreted with regard to the total client; an isolated value may yield an inaccurate conclusion.

HEMATOLOGY. A low hemoglobin level may indicate anemia, recent hemorrhage, or hemodilution caused by fluid retention. Hemoglobin may also be low secondary to conditions such as low serum albumin, infection, catabolism, or chronic disease. High hemoglobin levels may indicate hemoconcentration or dehydration, or they may be secondary to liver disease.

Low hematocrit levels may reflect anemia, hemorrhage, excessive fluid, renal disease, or cirrhosis. High hematocrit levels may indicate dehydration or hemoconcentration.

PROTEIN STUDIES. Serum albumin, thyroxine-binding prealbumin, and transferrin can be measured in the laboratory. Serum albumin indicates the body's protein status but is not sensitive enough to detect early changes in nutritional status. The normal serum albumin level for men and women is greater than 3.5 g/dL.

Thyroxine-binding **prealbumin (PAB)** provides a more sensitive indicator of protein deficiency because of its short half-life of 2 days. Depending on the laboratory test used, the normal PAB range is 17 to 40 mg/dL. PAB can also assess improvement in nutritional status with refeeding; levels can increase by 1 mg/dL daily with adequate nutritional support.

Although not used as commonly, serum **transferrin,** an iron-transport protein, can be measured directly or calculated as an indirect measurement of total iron-binding capacity (TIBC). It has a short half-life of 8 to 10 days and therefore is also a more sensitive indicator of protein status than is albumin.

SERUM CHOLESTEROL. Cholesterol levels normally range between 160 and 200 mg/dL in adult men and women. Values are typically low with malabsorption, liver disease, pernicious anemia, terminal stages of cancer, or sepsis. A cholesterol level below 160 mg/dL has been identified as a possible indicator of malnutrition.

OTHER LABORATORY TESTS. Total lymphocyte count (TLC) can be used to assess immune function. Malnutrition suppresses the immune system and leaves the client more vulnerable to infection. When a client is malnourished, the TLC is usually decreased to below 1500 mm³ (Bender et al., 2000).

Critical Thinking Challenge

An older adult was admitted to your unit following a colon resection secondary to cancer. He is a type 2 diabetic and had a coronary artery bypass graft 5 years ago. On admission he was 10 pounds less than ideal body weight. His primary language is German, and he speaks very few English words. Since surgery 2 days ago, his blood glucose levels have been very high and unstable, and he has experienced several episodes of atrial fibrillation. He has refused to eat since surgery because, his wife says, he does not like the food.

1. What risk factors does this client have for malnutrition?
2. What further nutritional assessment should you perform?
3. What laboratory tests would be appropriate for him at this time?
4. What could you suggest at this time to increase his food intake?

evolve For suggested answer guidelines, go to http://evolve.elsevier.com/Iggy/.

◆Analysis

COMMON NURSING DIAGNOSES AND COLLABORATIVE PROBLEMS

The most common diagnosis for the client with malnutrition is Imbalanced Nutrition: Less Than Body Requirements related to inability to ingest or digest food or absorb nutrients due to biologic, psychological, or economic factors.

ADDITIONAL NURSING DIAGNOSES AND COLLABORATIVE PROBLEMS

In addition to the common nursing diagnosis, clients with malnutrition may have one or more of the following:

- Risk for Impaired Skin Integrity related to alterations in nutritional state
- Risk for Infection related to malnutrition
- Risk for Disturbed Body Image related to biophysical changes from weight loss

Some clients with malnutrition are at risk for collaborative problems such as the following:

- Anemia
- Immunocompromised State
- Multisystem Failure

◆Planning and Implementation

IMBALANCED NUTRITION: LESS THAN BODY REQUIREMENTS

NOC PLANNING: EXPECTED OUTCOMES. The client with malnutrition is expected to have nutrients available to meet metabolic needs. Indicators include that the client will have no deviation from normal range in the following:

- Nutrient intake
- Fluid intake
- Energy
- Weight-height ratio
- Hematocrit
- Muscle tone
- Hydration

INTERVENTIONS. The preferred route for feeding is through the GI tract because it enhances the immune system and is safer, easier, less expensive, and more physiologically sound (Chart 64-3).

NIC Nutrition Management. In collaboration with the health care provider and dietitian, provide high-calorie, high-protein foods (e.g., milkshakes, cheese and crackers). A feeding schedule of six small meals benefits many clients. If the client has difficulty chewing or is **edentulous** (toothless), a pureed or dental soft diet may facilitate food intake.

Malnourished ill clients often need to be encouraged to eat. The nurse or assistive nursing personnel provides a quiet environment, which is conducive to eating. Some clients, especially older adults, may take a long time to eat even small quantities of food.

Restorative feeding programs help nursing home residents who need special assistance. These residents eat in a separate dining area so that time and attention can be given to them. Chart 64-4 offers additional interventions to increase nutritional intake for older adults in any setting.

Drug Therapy. Medications may be given to some clients to stimulate appetite. For example, cyproheptadine (Periactin), an antihistamine, may be prescribed for clients

CHART 64-3

NIC INTERVENTION ACTIVITIES for
The Client with Malnutrition

Nutrition Management: *Assisting with or providing a balanced dietary intake of foods and fluids*
- Ascertain client's food preferences.
- Determine, in collaboration with dietitian as appropriate, number of calories and type of nutrients needed to meet nutrition requirements.
- Encourage increased intake of protein, iron, and vitamin C, as appropriate.
- Offer snacks (e.g., frequent drinks, fresh fruits/fruit juice), as appropriate.
- Adjust diet to client's lifestyle, as appropriate.
- Weigh client at appropriate intervals.
- Encourage client to wear properly fitted dentures and/or obtain dental care.
- Assist client in receiving help from appropriate community nutritional programs, as needed.

NIC intervention activities selected from Dochterman J.M., & Bulechek, G.M. (Eds.). (2004). *Nursing intervention classification (NIC)* (4th ed.). St Louis: Mosby. No part of this work is to be altered without prior written permission from the Publisher.

CHART 64-4

NURSING FOCUS on the OLDER ADULT
Promoting Nutritional Intake

- Observe the client during meals for food intake.
- Ask the client about food likes and dislikes.
- Encourage self-feeding, or feed the client slowly.
- Create an environment that is conducive to eating and socialization and relaxation, if possible.
- Decrease distractions, such as environmental noise from television, music, or other people.
- Provide adequate, nonglaring lighting.
- Keep away from offensive or medicinal odors.
- Keep eye contact with the client during the meal.
- Serve snacks with activities, especially in long-term care settings.
- Document the percentage of food eaten at each meal and snack.
- Ensure that meals are visually appealing, appetizing, and properly prepared.
- Review the client's medication profile, and discuss with the health care provider the use of drugs that might be suppressing appetite.
- If the client is depressed, be sure that the depression is treated by the health care provider.

who are underweight, especially those with eating disorders. Megestrol acetate (Megace), an antineoplastic drug, may be used to increase appetite in clients who have cachexia, acquired immunodeficiency syndrome (AIDS), or unexplained weight loss. The mechanism for how these drugs work to increase appetite is unknown.

Partial Enteral Nutrition. The dietitian calculates the nutrients required daily and translates these requirements into meals for the client. If the client cannot ingest sufficient nutrients as food, **partial enteral nutrition (PEN)** with fortified medical nutritional supplements (MNSs) (e.g., Boost, Ensure, or Carnation Instant Breakfast) may be given, especially for older adults. Many commercial enteral products are available. For clients with medical diagnoses such as liver and renal disease or diabetes, special products that meet their needs are also available. The client must enjoy the taste of the product for acceptability and optimal intake.

Nutritional supplements are supplied as liquid formulas, powders, bars, and puddings in a variety of flavors. They come in different degrees of sweetness and are also available as modular supplements that provide single nutrients. Examples of modular supplements are Polycose for carbohydrates and ProPac for protein. Carbohydrate modulars are useful only if additional calories are needed. Protein modulars are indicated when metabolic stress causes a need for higher protein intake.

CONSIDERATIONS FOR OLDER ADULTS

Supplements used in acute care, long-term care, and home care are costly. In addition, older adults may refuse them, and the supplements are then wasted. Bender at al. (2000) found that a more successful alternative to having the MNS distributed by food service or nursing assistant staff in the nursing home was to have the supplements delivered by nurses during their usual medication passes. In this study, the nurses gave 60 mL or more of the MNS at least four times a day with the clients' medications. The subjects increased weight and had fewer pressure ulcers, thus making the program very cost-effective.

The nurse or assistive nursing personnel maintains a daily calorie count and fluid intake to assess whether the client can meet the goals of nutritional therapy. The dietitian usually asks the nursing staff to keep the food intake record for at least three consecutive days. Accurate daily or weekly weights are also essential, depending on the amount of depletion.

Total Enteral Nutrition. Clients often cannot meet the goals of nutritional therapy through their usual oral intake because of increased metabolic demands or a decreased ability to eat. Therefore enteral tube feeding may be necessary to supplement oral intake or to provide total nutritional support.

Candidates for Total Enteral Nutrition. Clients likely to receive **total enteral nutrition (TEN)** can be divided into three groups:

- Clients who can eat but cannot maintain adequate nutrition by oral intake of food alone
- Clients who have permanent neuromuscular impairment and cannot swallow
- Clients who do not have permanent neuromuscular impairment but are critically ill and cannot eat because of their condition

Clients in the first group are often older adults or clients receiving cancer treatment who cannot meet their calorie and protein needs (see the Legal/Ethical Issues box above). Clients in the second group usually have permanent swallowing problems and require some type of feeding tube for delivery of the enteral product on a long-term basis. Examples of conditions that can cause permanent swallowing problems are strokes, severe head trauma, and advanced multiple sclerosis. Clients in the third group receive enteral nutrition for as long as their illness lasts. The feeding is discontinued when the client's condition improves and he or she can eat again. TEN is contraindicated for clients with diffuse peritonitis, severe pancreatitis, intestinal obstruction, intractable vomiting or diarrhea, and paralytic ileus.

LEGAL/ETHICAL ISSUES

TOTAL ENTERAL NUTRITION FOR OLDER ADULTS

Total enteral nutrition provides a client's total daily nutrient and fluid requirements. In some cases, this artificial nutrition and hydration may not be desired by the older adult. For example, some clients have advance directives stating that they do not want to be kept alive by artificial nutrition and hydration if certain conditions exist. However, questions arise when clients are not able to make their wishes known.

For many years it was believed that withholding food and fluids would cause discomfort. Recent cancer research indicates that clients who do not eat and drink do not suffer and in fact may be more comfortable if food and fluids are withheld. The decision to feed is complex, and there is no clear right or wrong answer. To compound this dilemma, medical complications (e.g., aspiration, pressure ulcers) are common in older adults who are tube fed.

When clinicians are making decisions about the desirability of tube feedings in these cases, the focus should be on achieving consensus by doing the following:

- Reviewing what is known about tube feedings, especially their risks and benefits
- Reviewing the medical facts about the client
- Investigating any available evidence that would help understand the client's wishes
- Obtaining the opinions of all stakeholders in the situation
- Delaying any action until consensus is achieved

Types of Enteral Products. Many commercially prepared enteral products are available. An appropriate combination of carbohydrates, fat, vitamins, minerals, and trace elements is available in liquid form. Differences among products allow the dietitian to select the right formula for each client. An order from the health care provider is required for enteral nutrition, but the dietitian usually makes the recommendation and computes the amount and type of product needed for each client.

Methods of Administration of Total Enteral Nutrition. Total enteral nutrition is administered as "tube feedings" through one of the available GI tubes, either via a **nasoenteric tube (NET)** or an **enterostomal tube.** It can be used in the client's home or any health care setting.

Types of Tubes. A NET is any feeding tube inserted nasally and then advanced into the GI tract. Commonly used NETs include the **nasogastric (NG) tube** and the **nasoduodenal tube (NDT).** A nasojejunal tube (NJT) is also available but is used less often than the other NETs. The NDTs and NJTs are usually indicated for critically ill clients at risk for aspiration or delayed stomach emptying. The NETs are used for delivering short-term enteral feedings because they are easy to use and are safer for the client at risk for aspiration *if* the tip of the tube is placed below the pyloric sphincter of the stomach. Small-bore polyurethane or silicone tubes from 8 to 12 Fr external diameter are preferred over large-bore plastic or latex tubes. The smaller tubes are more comfortable and are less likely to cause complications such as nasal irritation, sinusitis, tissue erosion, and pulmonary compromise.

Enterostomal feeding tubes are used for clients who need long-term enteral feeding. The most common types are gastrostomies and jejunostomies. The physician directly accesses the GI tract using various surgical, endoscopic, and laparoscopic techniques.

A **gastrostomy** is a stoma created from the abdominal wall into the stomach, through which a short feeding tube

CHART 64-5

BEST PRACTICE for
Tube Feeding Care and Maintenance

- If nasogastric or nasoduodenal feeding is ordered, use a soft, flexible, small-bore feeding tube (smaller than 12 Fr). The initial placement of the tube should be confirmed by x-ray study. Secure the tube with tape or a commercial attachment device after applying a skin protectant; change the tape regularly.
- Check tube placement by x-ray study when the correct position of the tube is in question; an x-ray study is the only reliable method. Checking the pH of the aspirant is the preferred method for rechecking placement after an x-ray.
- If a gastrostomy or jejunostomy tube is used, assess the insertion site for signs of infection or excoriation (e.g., excessive redness, drainage). Rotate the tube 360 degrees each day, and check for in-and-out play of about ¼ inch (0.5 cm). If the tube cannot be moved, notify the health care provider immediately because the retention disk may be embedded in the tissue. Cover the site with a dry sterile dressing, and change the dressing at least once a day.
- Check and record the residual volume every 4 hours by aspirating stomach contents into a syringe. If residual feeding is obtained, check the health care provider's order for the appropriate intervention (usually to slow or stop the feeding for a time).
- Check the feeding pump to ensure proper mechanical operation.
- Ensure that the prescribed enteral product is infused at the prescribed rate (mL/hr).
- Change the feeding bag and tubing every 24 hours; label the bag with the date and time of the change. Use an irrigation set for no more than 24 hours.
- For continuous or cyclic feeding, add only 4 hours of product to the bag at a time to prevent bacterial growth; a closed system may be used for 24 hours.
- Wear clean gloves when changing or opening the feeding system or adding product; wear sterile gloves for critically ill or immunocompromised clients.
- Do not use blue (or any color) food dye in formula because it does not prevent aspiration and can cause serious complications (Maloney et al., 2002).
- To prevent aspiration, keep the head of the bed elevated at least 30 degrees during the feeding and at least 1 hour after the feeding for bolus feeding; maintain semi-Fowler's position for clients receiving cyclic or continuous feeding.
- Monitor laboratory values, especially blood urea nitrogen (BUN), serum electrolytes, hematocrit, prealbumin, and glucose.
- Monitor for complications of tube feeding, especially diarrhea.
- Monitor and carefully record the client's weight and intake and output.

CHART 64-6

BEST PRACTICE for
Maintaining a Patent Feeding Tube

- Flush the tube with 30 to 60 mL of water (amount usually prescribed by the health care provider or dietitian):
  At least every 4 hours during a continuous tube feeding
  Before and after each intermittent tube feeding
  Before and after medication administration (use warm water)
  After checking residual volume
- If the tube becomes clogged, use 30 mL of water for flushing, applying gentle pressure with a 50-mL piston syringe.
- Avoid the use of carbonated beverage, except for existing clogs *when water is not effective*. Do not use cranberry juice.
- Whenever possible, use liquid medications instead of crushed tablets unless liquid forms cause diarrhea.
- Do not mix medications with the feeding product. Crush tablets as finely as possible and dissolve in warm water. *(Check to see which tablets are safe to crush. For example, do not crush slow-acting [SA] or slow-release [SR] medications.)*
- Consider use of automatic flush feeding pump such as Flexiflo, Quantum, or Kangaroo.

is inserted by the physician. The gastrostomy may require a small abdominal incision, or it may be placed endoscopically; these tubes are called **percutaneous endoscopic gastrostomy (PEG)** or dual-access gastrostomy-jejunostomy (PEG/J) tubes. The PEG does not require general anesthesia and is more secure and more durable than traditional gastrostomies. An alternative to either device is the **low-profile gastrostomy device (LPGD).** The LPGD is available with a firm or balloon-style internal bumper or retention disk. An antireflux valve keeps GI contents from leaking onto the skin. This device is less irritating to the skin, longer lasting, and more cosmetically pleasing, and it allows greater client independence. However, skin-level devices do not allow easy access for checking residuals.

Jejunostomies are used less often than gastrostomies. A **jejunostomy** is used for long-term feedings when it is desirable to bypass the stomach, such as with gastric disease,

upper GI obstruction, and abnormal gastric or duodenal emptying.

Types of Feedings. Tube feedings are administered by bolus feeding, continuous feeding, and cyclic feeding. **Bolus feeding** is an intermittent feeding of a specified amount of enteral product at specified times during a 24-hour period, typically every 4 hours. This method can be accomplished manually or by infusion through a mechanical pump or controller device. A more popular method of tube feeding is continuous enteral feeding. **Continuous feeding** is similar to IV therapy in that small amounts are continuously infused (by gravity drip or by a pump or controller device) over a specified time. The most commonly seen type, **cyclic feeding,** is the same as continuous feeding except the infusion is stopped for a specified time in each 24-hour period, usually 6 to 10 or more hours ("down time"). Down time typically occurs in the morning to allow bathing, treatments, and other activities.

Infusion rates for cyclic feedings (and to some extent for intermittent bolus feeding) vary with the total amount of solution to be infused, the specific composition of the product, and the response of the client to the procedure. The health care provider and dietitian usually decide the type, rate, and method of tube feeding as well as the amount of additional water needed. If the client can swallow small amounts of food, he or she may also eat orally while the tube is in place.

The nurse is responsible for the care and maintenance of the feeding tube and the enteral feeding. Chart 64-5 lists best practices for the client receiving enteral nutrition (Padula et al., 2004).

Complications of Total Enteral Nutrition. The nurse is responsible for the prevention, assessment, and management of complications associated with tube feeding. Some complications of therapy result from the type of tube used to administer the feeding, and other complications result from the enteral product itself. The most common problem associated with feeding tubes is the development of a clogged tube. Chart 64-6 lists best practices for maintaining a patent tube.

Aspiration. A less common but more serious complication is dislodgment of the tube, which can cause aspiration.

Several techniques should be used to confirm proper placement. *An x-ray is the most accurate confirmation method and should always be done on initial tube insertion.* After the initial placement is confirmed, check the placement before each intermittent feeding or at least every 4 to 8 hours during continuous or cyclic feeding.

The traditional auscultatory method is *not* reliable, especially for clients with small-bore tubes. In this method, the nurse instills 20 to 30 mL of air into the tube while listening over the stomach with a stethoscope. *The resulting whooshing sound that results does not guarantee correct tube placement!* Instead, aspirate a sample of the GI content, observe its color, and test its pH. When aspirating fluid, wait at least 1 hour after medication administration, and then flush the tube with 20 mL of air to clear it. Collect the aspirate and test with pH paper. The pH of gastric fluid ranges from 0 to 4.0. If the tube has migrated down into the intestines, the pH will be between 7.0 and 8.0. If the tube is in the lungs, the pH will be greater than 6.0 (Metheny et al., 1998). The pH may also be as high as 6 if the client takes certain medications, such as H_2 blockers (e.g., ranitidine [Zantac] and famotidine [Pepcid]). Because these drugs affect pH, research using bilirubin testing is ongoing as perhaps a more reliable and valid method for predicting tube location (Metheny, Smith, & Stewart, 2000; Metheny & Stewart, 2002).

Fluid Excess. Clients receiving enteral nutrition therapy are at an increased risk for fluid imbalances. Clients who receive this therapy are often older or debilitated and may also have cardiac or renal problems. Fluid imbalances associated with enteral nutrition are usually related to the body's response to increased serum osmolarity, but fluid overload can also occur.

Increased Osmolarity. Osmolarity is the amount or concentration of particles dissolved in solution. This concentration exerts a specific osmotic pressure within the solution. Normal osmolarity of extracellular fluid (ECF) ranges between 270 and 300 mOsm. Enteral feeding products range in osmolarity from isotonic (about 300 mOsm) to extremely hypertonic (600 mOsm). Electrolytes (including sodium) contribute to this hypertonicity, but more of the osmolarity is determined by the concentration of proteins and sugar molecules in the enteral product. Even when the product is isotonic, the ECF can become hyperosmolar unless some hypotonic fluids are also administered to the client. This situation is most likely to develop in clients who are unconscious, unable to respond to the thirst reflex, on fluid restrictions, or receiving hyperosmotic enteral preparations.

An increase in the osmolarity of the plasma increases the osmotic pressure of the plasma. Because this increased osmolarity is largely a result of extra glucose and proteins (which tend to remain in the plasma rather than move to interstitial spaces), the plasma osmotic pressure (water-pulling pressure) is increased. In this situation, intracellular and interstitial water moves into and expands the plasma volume. This volume expansion results in an increased renal excretion of water (among clients with normal renal function) and leads to osmotic dehydration. If clients do not have normal renal and cardiac function, expansion of the plasma volume can lead to circulatory overload and the formation of pulmonary edema, especially in older adults. Assess for signs and symptoms of circulatory overload, and collaborate

with the dietitian and physician in planning the correct amount of fluid to be provided to the client.

Dehydration. Excessive diarrhea may develop when hyperosmolar enteral preparations are delivered quickly. This situation can also lead to dehydration through excessive water loss. Consult with the health care provider and dietitian for recommendations to prevent diarrhea.

First the dietitian usually changes the feeding to a more iso-osmolar formula. Most of these formulas can be started full strength but slowly at 15 to 20 mL/hr. The rate is gradually increased as the client tolerates and as the expected nutritional outcome is achieved.

If diarrhea continues, the client should be evaluated for *Clostridium difficile* or other infectious organisms. Contamination can occur because of repeated and often faulty handling of the feeding solution and system. Some researchers recommend that clean gloves be used when changing systems and adding product. Sterile gloves may help to prevent infection in critically ill or immunocompromised clients. Tubes with medication ports also minimize contamination by preventing opening the feeding system to administer medications (Padula et al., 2004).

In some cases, diarrhea may be the result of liquid medications, such as elixirs and suspensions that have a very high osmolarity. Examples include acetaminophen, digoxin, furosemide, phenytoin, and potassium chloride. Clients receiving multiple liquid medications need to be evaluated to determine whether their drug regimen can be changed to prevent diarrhea. Diluting these liquids may also be an option.

Electrolyte Imbalances. Depending on the client's state of health, certain electrolyte imbalances can be avoided. This is achieved by the use of enteral preparations containing lower concentrations of the electrolytes that the client cannot handle well.

In addition to the client's specific electrolyte imbalances, the two most common electrolyte imbalances associated with enteral nutrition therapy are hyperkalemia and hypernatremia. Both of these conditions may be related to hyperglycemia-induced hyperosmolarity of the plasma and the resultant osmotic diuresis. Electrolyte imbalances are discussed in detail in Chapter 16.

Parenteral Nutrition. When a client cannot effectively use the GI tract for nutrition, parenteral nutrition therapy may maintain or improve his or her nutritional status. This form of IV therapy differs from standard IV therapy in that *all* nutrients (carbohydrates, proteins, fats, vitamins, minerals, and trace elements) can be delivered to the client. One liter of fluid containing 5% dextrose, which is often used as standard IV therapy, provides only 170 kcal. A hospitalized client typically receives 3 or 4 L a day, for a total number of calories ranging between 500 and 700 a day. This calorie intake is not sufficient when the client requires IV therapy for a prolonged period and cannot eat an adequate diet or has increased calorie needs for tissue repair and building.

Parenteral nutrition (**hyperalimentation,** or "hyperal") is subdivided into two categories:
- Partial parenteral nutrition, or peripheral parenteral nutrition
- Total parenteral nutrition, or central parenteral nutrition

As suggested by the names, these categories differ by the site of administration and the content of the solutions.

Partial Parenteral Nutrition. **Partial parenteral nutrition (PPN)** provides nutritional support to clients who are unable or unwilling to take a feeding via the GI tract. It is typically used when a client has a prolonged postoperative ileus or when placement of a central IV line is not advised. It is used when nutritional support is needed for less than 14 days. The client should be able to tolerate large fluid volumes and have readily accessible peripheral veins.

Usually PPN is delivered through a cannula or catheter in a large distal vein of the arm. Two types of solutions are commonly used in various combinations for PPN: lipid (fat) emulsions and amino acid dextrose solutions.

Most lipid emulsions (20%) are isotonic, but the tonicity of commercially prepared amino acid dextrose solutions ranges from 300 mOsm to nearly 1200 mOsm. Amino acid dextrose solutions are considered more stable than the lipid emulsions, and therefore additives (e.g., vitamins, minerals, electrolytes, and trace elements) tend to be mixed with the amino acid dextrose solutions. The amino acid dextrose solution must be delivered through an in-line filter. Lipids and amino acid dextrose solutions are administered by a pump or controller device for accuracy and constancy in delivery rate.

Most PPN products are a *mixture* of lipids (10% or 20% fat emulsion) and an amino acid dextrose (usually 10%) solution. This mixture of three types of nutrients is referred to as a 3:1, total nutrient admixture (TNA), or triple-mix solution.

Total Parenteral Nutrition. When the client requires intensive nutritional support for an extended time, the health care provider prescribes centrally administered **total parenteral nutrition (TPN)**. TPN is delivered through access to central veins, usually the subclavian or internal jugular veins. Central venous catheters and associated nursing care are described in detail in Chapter 17.

Total parenteral nutrition solutions contain higher concentrations of dextrose and proteins, usually in the form of synthetic amino acids or protein hydrolysates (3% to 5%). These solutions are hyperosmotic (three to six times the osmolarity of normal blood). The base solutions are available as commercially prepared solutions. The hospital or community pharmacist adds components (specific electrolytes, minerals, trace elements, and insulin) according to the client's nutritional needs. This therapy provides needed calories and spares body proteins from catabolism for energy requirements.

The TPN solutions should be administered with an infusion pump. The osmolarity of the fluid and the concentrations of the specific components make controlled delivery essential.

Complications of Parenteral Nutrition. Clients receiving PPN or TPN are at risk for a wide variety of serious and potentially life-threatening complications. Complications may result from the PPN and TPN solutions or from the central venous catheter. The following discussion is limited to the complications of PPN and TPN that involve fluid or electrolyte balance. Complications of IV cannulas and central venous catheters are discussed in Chapter 17.

Fluid Imbalances. Clients receiving PPN or TPN are at increased risk for fluid imbalance. Not only is fluid delivered directly into the venous system, but the extreme hyperosmolarity of the solutions stimulates fluid shifts between body fluid compartments.

The hyperosmolarity of parenteral nutrition solutions is caused by their amino acid and dextrose concentrations. Increased dextrose causes hyperglycemia. As a result, some of the dextrose moves into the interstitial and intracellular spaces, where it is metabolized. However, dextrose remains in the plasma volume when the solutions are administered too rapidly, without enough insulin coverage, or in the presence of hyponatremia and hypokalemia. The result is a shift of water from the interstitial and intracellular spaces into the plasma. Expansion of the plasma volume together with hyperglycemia can cause osmotic diuresis and lead to serious dehydration and hypovolemic shock. If the client has an accompanying cardiac or renal dysfunction, the situation can lead to overhydration, congestive heart failure, and pulmonary edema.

Monitor for these complications by taking daily weights and by recording accurate intake and output while the client is receiving parenteral nutrition. Serum glucose and electrolyte values are also monitored (Chart 64-7). Any major changes or abnormalities are reported to the health care provider.

Electrolyte Imbalances. Clients receiving either PPN or TPN are at an increased risk for many different electrolyte imbalances, depending on the electrolyte composition of the solution and whether a fluid imbalance occurs. The health care provider usually orders daily determinations of serum electrolyte levels to detect these imbalances. The risk of metabolic and electrolyte complications is reduced when the rate of administration is carefully controlled and clients are closely monitored for response to treatment. Potassium and sodium imbalances are common among clients receiving PPN and TPN, especially when insulin is also administered as part of the therapy. Calcium imbalances, especially hypercalcemia, are associated with PPN and TPN, although immobility may play more of a role than the actual parenteral therapy in the development of this imbalance.

Effects of Medication. No specific drug therapy for malnutrition has been established, although multivita-

---

CHART 64-7

BEST PRACTICE for
Care and Maintenance of Total Parenteral Nutrition

- Check each bag of total parenteral nutrition (TPN) solution for accuracy by comparing it with the physician's order.
- Monitor the IV pump for accuracy in delivering the prescribed hourly rate.
- If the TPN solution is temporarily unavailable, give 10% dextrose/water (D/W) or 20% D/W until the TPN solution can be obtained.
- If the TPN administration is not on time ("behind"), do not attempt to "catch up" by increasing the rate.
- Monitor the client's weight daily or according to agency protocol.
- Monitor serum electrolytes and glucose daily or per agency protocol. (Some agencies require finger stick blood sugars [FSBSs] every 4 hours, especially if the client is receiving insulin. Urine testing for ketones may also be ordered.)
- Monitor and carefully record the client's intake and output.
- Assess the client's IV site for signs of infection or infiltration (see Chapter 17).
- Change the IV tubing every 24 hours or per agency protocol.
- Change the dressing around the IV site every 48 to 72 hours or per agency protocol.

mins and an iron preparation may be prescribed to treat or prevent anemia. Carefully review the client's medications because of food-medication interactions. Medications can affect nutritional status, and the foods ingested can affect the efficacy of medications.

Community-Based Care

Malnourished clients can be cared for in a variety of settings, including the acute care hospital, transitional care unit, nursing home, or their own home. Malnutrition is often diagnosed when the client is admitted to the acute care hospital or as a consequence of events that occur after hospitalization, such as poor wound healing or sepsis. If the client is severely compromised, he or she may require admission to a traditional nursing home for either transitional or long-term care and be followed by a case manager. If adequate home support is available, the client may be discharged to home in the care of a family member, significant other, or other caregiver. Home care nurses may be needed to monitor and direct the care.

HEALTH TEACHING

The dietitian instructs the malnourished client and the family about high-calorie, high-protein diet and nutritional supplements. The pharmacist reviews any parenteral solutions with the client and family or significant others.

Reinforce the importance of adhering to the diet, and review any medications the client may be taking. If the client takes an iron preparation, teach the importance of taking the medication immediately before or during meals. Caution the client that iron tends to cause constipation. For the older adult already susceptible to constipation, emphasize the importance of measures for prevention, including adequate fiber intake, adequate fluids, and exercise.

Some clients are discharged to home with enteral or parenteral nutrition. Teach the family or other caregiver how to continue these therapies. Remind caregivers to consider also the psychosocial aspects of these alternative methods for nutrition. For example, the caregiver can bring the enteral product, napkin, and funnel to the client on a decorative tray to make the feeding experience more elegant and "normal." Moving the feeding equipment out of view of the client when it is not in use is another consideration (Nickel, 2004).

HOME CARE MANAGEMENT

The malnourished client needs a variety of resources at home to continue aggressive nutrition support. If the client can consume food by the oral route, the case manager or other discharge planner determines whether his or her financial resources are adequate for providing the necessary food and nutrition supplements. If the hospital provides ambulatory nutrition counseling services, the client is scheduled for follow-up after discharge for assessment of weight gain.

HEALTH CARE RESOURCES

The malnourished client discharged to home on enteral or parenteral nutrition support needs the specialized services of a home nutrition therapy team. This team generally consists of the physician, nurse, dietitian, pharmacist, and social worker. Several commercial companies supply these services to clients in addition to the feeding supplies and formulas.

◆ Evaluation: Outcomes

Evaluate the care of the malnourished client on the basis of the identified nursing diagnoses and collaborative problems. The primary expected outcome is that the client has available nutrients to meet metabolic demands. Specific indicators for this outcome are listed for the nursing diagnosis under the Planning: Expected Outcomes section (see earlier).

OBESITY

PATHOPHYSIOLOGY

Obesity, like cancer, is not just one disease but rather many conditions with varying causes. The terms **obesity** and **overweight** are often used interchangeably, but they refer to different health problems. Overweight is an increase in body weight for height compared with a reference standard, such as the Metropolitan Life height and weight tables (see Table 64-3) or 10% greater than ideal body weight (IBW). However, this weight may not reflect excess body fat. It is possible for well-developed athletes to appear overweight because of increased muscle mass; in such cases the proportion of muscle to fat is greater than average.

An obese person weighs at least 20% above the upper limit of the normal range for ideal body weight. **Morbid obesity** refers to a weight that has a severely negative effect on health—usually more than 100% above IBW or a body mass index (BMI) greater than 40.

Obesity refers to an excess amount of body fat. It is possible to be obese at a weight that is within normal range according to a reference standard. The normal amount of body fat in *men* is between 15% and 20% of body weight. For *women,* the normal amount is 18% to 32%.

A number of chemicals in the body affect appetite and fat metabolism. Some of the most common ones that are thought to play a role in obesity include the following:

- **Leptin,** a hormone that is released by fat cells and possibly by gastric cells; it also acts on the hypothalamus to control appetite
- **Insulin,** a hormone that controls the metabolism of glucose, fat, and protein
- **Resistin,** a hormone produced by fat cells that creates resistance to insulin activity
- **Agouti-related protein,** a protein controlled by leptin that regulates calorie consumption
- **Wnt-10b,** a protein that inhibits fat cell formation
- **Cholecystokinin,** a hormone that stimulates digestive juices and may work with leptin to increase or decrease appetite
- **PYY,** a hormone that indicates stomach fullness and helps to limit food intake

Additional research is needed to determine the exact mechanisms by which these substances work together to cause weight gain.

Obesity Indexes

To establish the percentage of IBW, the height and weight of the client are compared with the midpoint of the desirable weight for a medium frame of the client's height and gender in the Metropolitan Life height and weight tables (see Table 64-3). The body mass index (BMI), as described previously on p. 1426, is a measure of heaviness and is only an indirect indicator of body fat. It reflects the combined effects of body build, proportions, lean body mass, and body fat. However, BMI has exhibited substantial correlations with fat mass for adult men and women and has been validated as a risk factor for cardiovascular disease. As a general rule, a BMI of 30 or more indicates obesity and an increased risk for health problems. A BMI of 27 to 30 indicates overweight. Arm and calf circumference and skin-fold measurements more completely define body composition and adiposity (described earlier).

The distribution of excess body fat rather than the degree of obesity has been used to predict increased health risks. For example, in premenopausal women, the waist circumference (WC) is a stronger predictor of coronary artery disease (CAD) than is the BMI. Lofgren et al. (2004) found that women with a WC greater than 88 cm had the highest risk for biomarkers of CAD.

The waist-to-hip ratio (WHR) is also a predictor of CAD. This measure differentiates a predominantly peripheral lower body obesity from a central upper body obesity. A WHR of 0.95 or greater in men (0.8 or greater in women) indicates android obesity with excess fat at the waist and abdomen; this pattern carries the greatest health risk. Excessive abdominal fat may also enhance the risk for gallbladder disease.

Complications of Obesity

The major complications of obesity include the following:

- Diabetes mellitus
- Hypertension
- **Hyperlipidemia** (increased serum lipids)
- CAD
- Obstructive sleep apnea
- Obesity hypoventilation syndrome
- Depression and other mental health/behavioral health problems
- Urinary incontinence
- **Cholelithiasis** (gallbladder stones)
- Chronic back pain
- Early osteoarthritis
- Decreased wound healing

Obese people are also more susceptible to infections and infectious diseases than are thinner people.

Etiology and Genetic Risk

The causes of obesity involve complex interrelationships of many environmental, genetic, and behavioral factors. A number of causes of both human and animal obesity have been identified.

The first cause is dietary obesity associated with *high-fat and high-cholesterol diets*. Data repeatedly suggest that obesity is associated with diet when it contains a significant amount of saturated fat, which increases low-density lipoproteins (LDL-C). Trans-fat (trans-fatty acids) and cholesterol also contribute significantly. By contrast, monosaturated and polysaturated fats are healthy fats.

Trans-fat is made when food manufacturers add hydrogen to vegetable oil, a process known as hydrogenation. This process increases the food's shelf life and flavor. Large amounts of trans-fat can be found in vegetable shortening, commercial cookies, snack foods, and French fries. For many years, food labels have included amounts of total fat, saturated fat, and cholesterol content per serving. However, the amount of trans-fat has not been revealed. Manufacturers will be required to publish the amount of trans-fat in their foods starting in 2006.

Physical inactivity has been identified as another cause. The major identified barriers to increasing physical activity include a lack of time or decreased mobility associated with prolonged illness. Regular exercise is associated with lower death rates for adults of any age. It also increases lean muscle, decreases body fat, aids in weight control, and enhances psychological well-being. Regular exercise can also decrease the risk of falling in older adults (see Chapter 5).

The third major cause of obesity is *drug treatment*. Some prescribed medications contribute to weight gain when they are taken on a long-term basis. Drugs that promote obesity include the following:

- Corticosteroids
- Estrogens and certain progestins
- Nonsteroidal anti-inflammatory drugs
- Antihypertensives
- Antidepressants and other psychoactive drugs
- Antiepileptic drugs
- Certain oral hypoglycemics

Familial and genetic factors play a very important role in obesity. When both parents are overweight, about 80% of their children will be overweight. If neither parent is overweight, fewer than 10% of the children will be overweight. In studies of identical twins, nonidentical twins, and parent-sibling relationships, about 50% of the difference in body fatness is transmitted to children and about 50% of this amount is genetically controlled.

Genetic composition may predispose some people, but not others, to obesity. Researchers have identified the **ob gene** in mice, which helps to regulate energy balance. Leptin, the hormone encoded by the *ob* gene, appears to send a message to the brain that the body has stored enough fat; this message serves as a signal to stop eating. In some obese individuals, other gene mutations have been identified, including an abnormality of the melano-cortin-4 receptor that inhibits appetite in families with a history of obesity. Other genetic factors have been associated with uncommon diseases, such as the Prader-Willi syndrome.

A small number of obese individuals have disorders of the neuroendocrine system. Examples include injury to the hypothalamus, Cushing's disease, polycystic ovary failure, hypogonadism, growth hormone deficiency, and insulinoma.

Incidence/Prevalence

More than one third of the U.S. population is obese, and another third is overweight. About 6% to 10% of adults are morbidly obese (Gallagher, 2004). The total cost (medical cost and lost productivity) of obesity is more than $100 billion each year. In 2000, more than 100 million adults in the United States were overweight or obese.

HEALTH PROMOTION/ILLNESS PREVENTION

Obesity is a major public health problem and is associated with many complications, including death. As a result of this increasing problem, the Healthy People 2010 agenda addresses the need to reduce the proportion of children, adolescents, and adults who are obese. Nurses can help meet this goal through education and role modeling (see the Meeting Healthy People 2010 Objectives box above).

◆COLLABORATIVE MANAGEMENT
◆Assessment
HISTORY

In collaboration with the dietitian, collect the following information about the client:

- Economic status
- Usual food intake
- Eating behavior
- Cultural background
- Attitude toward food
- Appetite
- Chronic diseases
- Medications
- Physical activity
- Family history of obesity

A diet history usually incorporates a 24-hour recall of food intake and the frequency with which foods are consumed. The adequacy of the diet can be rapidly evaluated by comparing the amount and types of foods consumed daily with the Dietary Guidelines for Americans (see Figure 64-1). Gross inadequacies for specific nutrients can be identified using this approach. The dietitian can provide a more detailed analysis of dietary intake.

PHYSICAL ASSESSMENT/CLINICAL MANIFESTATIONS

Obtain an accurate height and weight. The dietitian then calculates the percentage of ideal body weight (% IBW) and the body mass index (BMI). The dietitian may also do the following:

- Measure the waist circumference
- Calculate the waist-hip ratio
- Determine arm and calf circumferences

Examine the skin of the obese client for reddened or open areas. Lift skin-fold areas, such as pendulous breasts and abdominal apron (also called a **panniculus**), to observe for *Candida* (yeast) or other infections and excoriations. Infection of the panniculus is referred to as **panniculitis.**

PSYCHOSOCIAL ASSESSMENT

Obtain a psychosocial history to determine the client's circumstances and emotional factors that might prevent successful therapy or that might be worsened by therapy. Interview the client to determine his or her perception of current weight. Some clients do not view weight as a problem, which affects treatment and outcome. Others experience low self-esteem and have a disturbed body image.

Explore the client's past history to assess the following:

- Cause and duration of weight gain
- Family history of obesity
- Past attempts at weight reduction and outcomes
- Effects of obesity on lifestyle
- Effects of obesity on social interactions
- History of mental health/behavioral health problems, such as depression
- Effects of obesity on intimate relationships, especially sexuality

Obese men often experience erectile dysfunction, which can cause or worsen depression (Esposito et al., 2004).

Ask about the following:

- Current reasons for wanting to lose weight
- Stressors (e.g., home, employment, personal, financial, or community) that might prevent success
- Exercise patterns
- Current medications
- Perceptions of self-worth

The diet history provides a detailed analysis of the client's eating habits. As a member of the health care team, evaluate the data to coordinate an interdisciplinary approach that incorporates diet, exercise, behavior modification, and psychological support.

◆Interventions

Weight is lost only when energy expended is greater than intake. Weight loss may be accomplished by dietary modification with or without the aid of drugs and in combination with a regular exercise program. Clients who are candidates for surgical treatment include those with the following:

- Repeated failure of nonsurgical interventions
- A BMI equal to or greater than 40
- Weight more than 100% above IBW (i.e., morbidly obese)

NONSURGICAL MANAGEMENT. Various diet approaches and medications have attempted to help obese clients achieve permanent weight loss.

Diet Programs. Modalities for helping people lose weight include fasting, very-low-calorie diets, balanced and unbalanced low-energy diets, and novelty diets.

Fasting. Short-term fasting programs have not been successful in treating morbidly obese clients, and prolonged fasting does not produce permanent benefits. Most clients regain the weight that was lost by this method. In addition, the risks associated with fasting (e.g., severe ketosis) require close medical supervision.

Very-Low-Calorie Diets. Very-low-calorie diets generally provide 200 to 800 calories/day. Two types of these diets include the *protein-sparing modified fast* and the *liquid formula diet.*

The protein-sparing modified fast provides protein of high biologic value (1.5 g/kg of desirable body weight daily) within a limited number of calories. The diet produces rapid weight loss while preserving lean body mass. The liquid-formula diet provides between 33 and 70 g of protein daily.

Both diets require an initial cardiac evaluation, supervision by an interdisciplinary health team with monitoring by a physician, nutrition counseling by a registered dietitian, and supplementation with vitamins and minerals. These diets are only one part of a weight reduction program. Clients who are following these diets should receive nutrition education, psychological counseling, exercise, and behavior therapy. Comparable weight losses have been achieved with both diets, but most clients do not sustain the weight loss and regain the weight.

Balanced and Unbalanced Low-Energy Diets.
Nutritionally balanced diets generally provide 1200 calories/day with a conventional distribution of carbohydrate, protein, and fat. Vitamin and mineral supplements may be necessary if energy intakes fall below 1200 calories for women and 1800 calories for men. This diet provides conventional foods that are economical and easy to obtain; thus the goal of weight loss is facilitated, and that loss is hopefully maintained. For example, Weight Watchers is an organization that provides education about nutritionally balanced diets based on a point system and weekly group support meetings

Unbalanced low-energy diets, such as the low-carbohydrate diet (e.g., Atkins or South Beach diet), restrict one or more nutrients. As described earlier, protein and vegetables are encouraged, but carbohydrates and fat foods are not. Although they remain controversial in the medical community, these diets are extremely popular. Scientific outcome data have been conflicting. However, a study by Yancy et al. (2004) found that compared with a low-fat diet, a low-carbohydrate diet had better participant retention and greater weight loss. Serum triglyceride levels decreased more and HDL-C levels increased more with the low-carb diet versus the low-fat diet.

Novelty Diets.
Novelty diets, such as the grapefruit and Hollywood diet, are often nutritionally *inadequate*. This type of diet implies that a certain food or liquid increases metabolic rate or accelerates the oxidation of body fat. Weight loss is achieved because energy is restricted by food choice, but clients do not sustain weight loss after terminating the diet.

Diet Therapy.
Diet recommendations for each client should be developed through close interaction between the client, physician, and dietitian. The diet should meet the client's needs and habits and should be realistic.

The dietitian develops a diet plan and instructs the client. At a minimum, the diet should do the following:

- Have a scientific rationale
- Be nutritionally adequate for all nutrients except energy
- Have a low risk-benefit ratio
- Be practical and conducive to long-term success

Calorie estimates are easily calculated. Resting metabolic rate is determined using a gender-specific formula that incorporates the appropriate activity factor. This figure reflects the total calories needed daily for maintaining current weight. To encourage a weight loss of 1 pound (2.2 kg) a week, the dietitian subtracts 500 calories each day. To encourage a weight loss of 2 pounds (4.4 kg) a week, the dietitian subtracts 1000 calories each day. The amount of weight lost varies with the client's food intake, level of

physical activity, and water losses. A reasonable goal of 5% to 10% loss of body weight has been shown to improve glycemic control and reduce cholesterol and blood pressure, and these benefits continue if the weight loss is sustained.

Exercise Program.
A major intervention for obesity is to increase the type and amount of daily exercise to create a calorie deficit along with modification of eating habits. For most people, adding exercise to a diet intervention produces more weight loss than just dieting alone. More of the weight lost is fat, which preserves lean body mass. An increase in exercise can produce a reduction in the waist-hip ratio.

Increasing and maintaining physical activity levels are important in maintaining weight loss. Many overweight or obese clients are so unfit that it may take several months of conditioning before they can exercise sufficiently to achieve weight loss.

The physical therapist or exercise physiologist or assistant first obtains a clinical exercise and health history. It is important to determine the client's current exercise pattern and exercise habits over a lifetime. The client should understand the importance of an exercise component in a weight loss program. The client's desire to participate in an exercise program and his or her preferred types of exercise is also ascertained.

The health care provider may evaluate the client by an exercise stress test. Not all clients need a stress test, but those with chronic disease may need the results to assist with individual exercise recommendations. Clients are counseled about unusual signs and symptoms during exercise (e.g., chest pain) and what to do if they occur. The physical therapist or exercise physiologist first emphasizes the importance of exercising consistently and then stresses the duration, intensity, and frequency.

A minimal-level workout should be developed for the client so that consistency can be achieved. The goal for the client is to maintain a lifetime of increased physical activity. The client is apt to be less fatigued and discouraged with a low-intensity, short-duration program. Sedentary clients are encouraged to increase their activity by walking 30 to 40 minutes daily (15 to 20 minutes per mile) or the equivalent. The activity may be performed all at once or divided over the course of the day. Remind the client to exercise only under the supervision of the physician. All members of the interdisciplinary team should provide encouragement and support for any increase in physical activity. Structured national programs with support staff, such as Curves, may be helpful for some clients. They typically offer diet counseling as well as cardiovascular and muscle-toning activities.

Drug Therapy.
A BMI of 30 or a BMI of 27 with comorbidities is one indicator for the use of drug therapy. **Anorectic drugs** suppress appetite, which reduces food intake and over time may result in weight loss. These drugs play a valuable role in a comprehensive weight reduction program but should be used only as part of such a program. Currently available drugs to treat obesity act on either the noradrenergic or serotonergic systems in the central nervous system. The most commonly used anorectic drug for the treatment of obesity is sibutramine (Meridia). Sibutramine is an anorectic drug that inhibits the reuptake of serotonin (which enhances satiety [feeling full when eating]) and nor-

epinephrine (which raises the metabolic rate). The usual dosage is 10 mg every day, which may be increased to 15 mg daily after 4 weeks or decreased to 5 mg daily, depending on the client's response. Adverse effects include dry mouth, constipation, and insomnia.

Orlistat (Xenical) is a different type of drug that inhibits lipase and leads to partial hydrolysis of triglycerides. Because fats are only partially digested and absorbed, calorie intake is decreased. The usual dosage is 120 mg three times daily with each main meal containing fat. Most clients taking orlistat experience GI symptoms that include loose stools, abdominal cramps, and nausea. Therefore this drug should be used with caution and limited to adults between 18 and 75 years of age. Treatment is usually not extended beyond 12 months.

A new drug is in the final stages of testing. Rimonabant (Acomplia) is the first of a new class of medications that reduces cravings for both food and smoking. It works by inhibiting a receptor found in a newly described physiologic system called the endocannabinoid system. Minor GI side effects may occur when the drug is first used, but these annoyances resolve after the first few weeks.

Behavioral Treatment. Behavioral treatment of obesity consists of various strategies to change daily eating habits to achieve weight loss. This ongoing process should produce a change in behavior. Self-monitoring techniques include keeping a record of foods eaten (food diary), exercise patterns, and emotional and situational factors. Stimulus control involves controlling the external cues that promote overeating. Reinforcement techniques are used to self-reward the behavior change. Cognitive restructuring involves modifying negative beliefs by learning positive coping self-statements.

Complementary and Alternative Therapies. Many other complementary and alternative therapies have been tested and used for obesity in both adults and children. These modalities aim to suppress appetite and therefore limit food intake to lose weight:

- Acupuncture
- Acupressure
- Ayurvedic (a combination of holistic approaches)
- Hypnosis

Descriptions of most of these methods can be found in Chapter 4.

SURGICAL MANAGEMENT. At any weight, some clients opt to improve their appearance by having a variety of cosmetic procedures to reduce the amount of adipose tissue in selected areas of the body. A typical example of this type of surgery is **liposuction,** which can be done in a physician's office. Whereas the client's appearance is improved, if weight gain continues, the fatty tissue will return. This procedure is not a solution for individuals who are morbidly obese.

Clients who do not respond to traditional dietary intervention may be considered for a major surgical procedure aimed at producing permanent weight loss. Clients with a body mass index (BMI) of 40 or greater or a BMI of 35 or greater along with additional risk factors should be considered for surgery.

Two major types of procedures may be performed for obesity:

- **Panniculectomy,** which is removal of any panniculus, most often the abdominal apron

- **Bariatric surgery,** which is surgical reduction of gastric capacity

For most clients, a panniculectomy is a safe, complication-free procedure that is usually done as a follow-up to bariatric surgery. Meticulous wound care is the priority for postoperative nursing care (Gallagher & Gates, 2003).

Most bariatric procedures today are of two types: gastric restrictive surgery and gastric restriction combined with malabsorption surgery, which offers the best results (Barrow, 2002). Every year, more than 100,000 individuals in the United States have these procedures, and that number is increasing. Many clients have minimally invasive surgery via laparoscopy. The decision of whether the client is a candidate for the laparoscopic procedure is based on weight, body build, history of abdominal surgery, and co-existing medical complications. With either approach, clients must agree to modify their lifestyle and follow stringent protocols to lose weight and keep the weight off. Following bariatric surgery, many clients no longer experience complications of obesity, such as diabetes mellitus, hypertension, depression, or sleep apnea.

Preoperative Care. Preoperative care is similar to that for any client undergoing abdominal surgery (see Chapter 20). However, obese clients are at increased surgical risks of pulmonary and thromboembolitic complications, as well as death. The primary role of the nurse is to reinforce health teaching in preparation for surgery.

Operative Procedures. Gastric restriction surgeries allow for normal digestion without the risk of nutritional deficiencies. As seen in Figure 64-6, for the **vertical banded gastroplasty,** the surgeon places a vertical line of staples to create a small stomach pouch to which a band is connected to provide an outlet to the small intestine. **Circumgastric banding** limits stomach size by placing an inflatable band around the fundus of the stomach. The band can be inflated or deflated through a subcutaneous port to change the size of the stomach as the client loses weight.

When gastric resection is combined with malabsorption surgery, the client's stomach, duodenum, and part of the jejunum is bypassed so that fewer calories can be absorbed. This procedure is commonly called a **gastric bypass** or **Roux-en-Y gastric bypass.**

Postoperative Care. Postoperative care depends on the type of surgical approach—the open conventional approach or minimally invasive technique (laparoscopy). Although many clients have laparoscopic surgery, they are considered as having major abdominal surgery along with all its risks. However, these clients usually require less than 24 hours in the hospital; some may need 1 to 2 days. Clients with open procedures may need 4 to 5 days to recover. All clients experience some degree of pain, but it is usually less severe when laparoscopy is used. Clients may use patient-controlled analgesia for the first day. All clients receive oral opioid analgesia as prescribed.

Care of the bariatric surgical client is similar to that for any client having abdominal or laparoscopic surgery. However, special bariatric equipment and accommodations, including an extra-wide bed and additional personnel for moving the client, are needed for both the surgical suite and postoperative care units. Beds must be wide enough to allow the client to turn. Bed rails should not be touching the body because they can cause pressure areas. Pressure be-

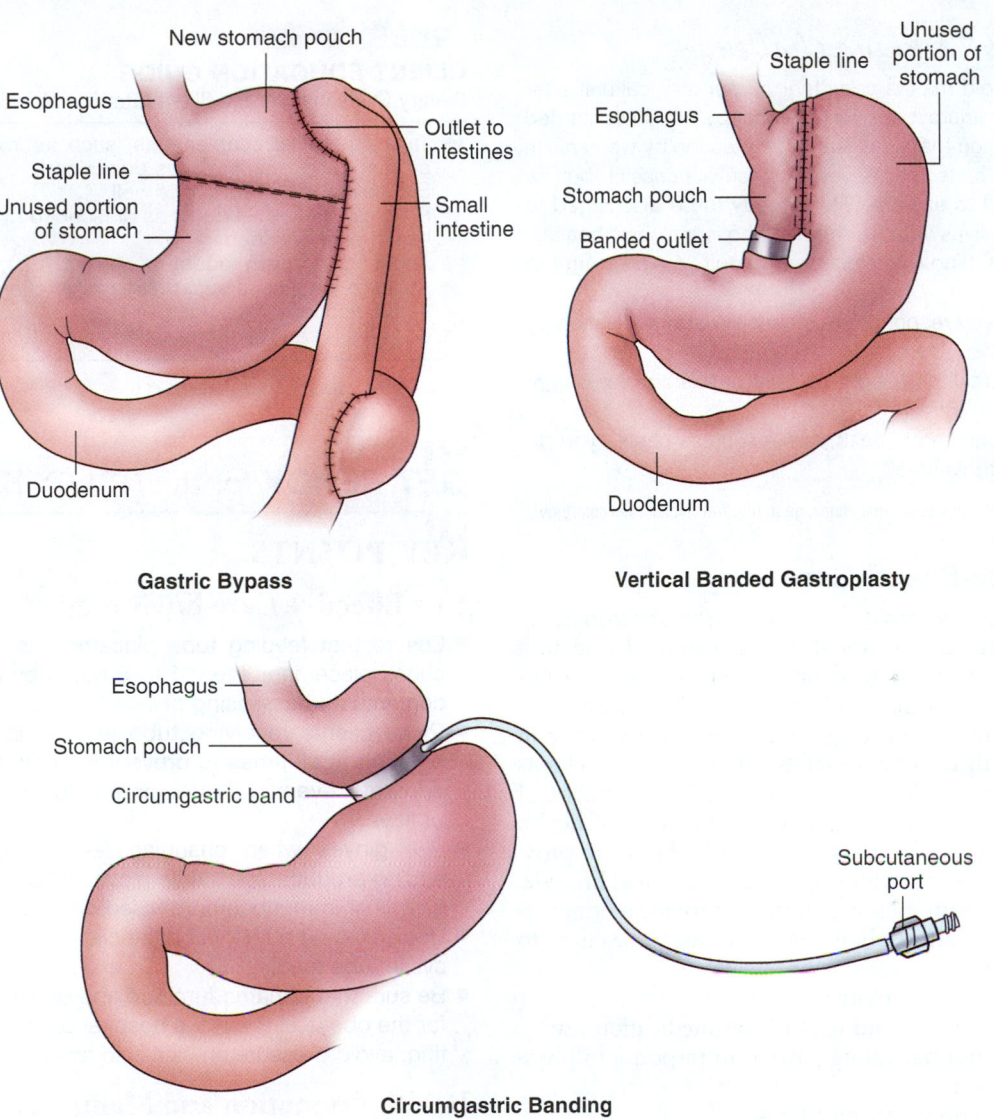

Gastric Bypass

Vertical Banded Gastroplasty

Circumgastric Banding

Figure 64-6 ■ Bariatric surgical procedures.

tween skin folds, as well as tubes and catheters, can also cause skin breakdown. Monitor the skin in these areas, and keep it clean and dry.

Some clients have a nasogastric (NG) tube put in place, especially after open surgical procedures. In gastroplasty procedures, the NG tube drains both the proximal pouch and the distal stomach. Closely monitor the tube for patency. *Never reposition the tube, because its movement can disrupt the suture line!* The NG tube is removed on the second or third day if the client has bowel sounds and is passing flatus. Clear liquids are introduced slowly if the client can tolerate water, and 1-ounce cups are used for each serving. Pureed foods, juice, and soups thinned with broth, water, or milk are added to the diet 24 to 48 hours after clear liquids are tolerated. Typically, the client can increase the volume to 1 ounce over 5 minutes or until satisfied, but the diet is limited to liquids or pureed foods for 6 weeks. The client then progresses to regular food, with an emphasis on nutrient-dense foods. Nausea, vomiting, or discomfort occurs if too much liquid is ingested.

In addition to the postoperative complications typically associated with abdominal surgery, bariatric clients have special needs and risks. Implement measures to prevent these complications:

■ Apply an abdominal binder to prevent wound dehiscence.
■ Place the client in semi-Fowler's position, or use continuous positive airway pressure (CPAP) ventilation at night to improve ventilation and decrease risk of sleep apnea.
■ Observe skin areas and folds for redness, excoriation, or breakdown to treat these problems early.
■ Use absorbent padding between folds to prevent pressure areas, particularly from tubes and catheters.
■ In collaboration with the dietitian, provide six small feedings to prevent dehydration.
■ Observe for signs and symptoms of **dumping syndrome** (caused by food entering the small intestine instead of the stomach) after gastric bypass, such as tachycardia, nausea, diarrhea, and abdominal cramping.

Critical Thinking Challenge

A 35-year-old man is admitted to your surgical unit after undergoing a gastric bypass via laparoscopy. He is not married and confides in you that he is fearful of rejection by women. He has tried many diets that have not been successful, but he never really liked to exercise. He is ready to be discharged to home, where he lives with his mother who is in "poor" health.

1. What diet teaching does this client require for discharge to home?
2. How should you respond to his concern about rejection by women?
3. What will you tell him about the role of exercise for weight loss?
4. What community and health care resources should you direct him to at this time?

evolve For suggested answer guidelines, go to http://evolve.elsevier.com/Iggy/.

Community-Based Care

Obese clients can be cared for in a variety of settings, including the acute care hospital and transitional care unit (particularly following surgery) or in their own home. Obesity is a chronic, lifelong problem. Diets, drug therapy, exercise, and behavior modification can produce short-term weight losses with reasonable safety. However, most clients who do lose weight often regain the weight. Treatment of obesity should focus on the long-term reduction of health risks and medical problems associated with obesity, improving quality of life, and promoting a health-oriented lifestyle. Interdisciplinary team members need to provide a nonjudgmental, supportive atmosphere that encourages the client to do the following:

- Increase physical activity
- Decrease fat intake and reliance on medication use
- Establish a normal eating pattern in response to physiologic hunger
- Address psychological problems

Frequent, long-term ambulatory care follow-up coordinated by a case manager is essential for successful treatment.

The most important features of client education for any obese client focus on health-related behavior patterns. In collaboration with the dietitian, counsel the client on a healthful eating pattern. The physical therapist or exercise physiologist recommends an appropriate exercise program. A psychologist may recommend cognitive restructuring approaches that help alter dysfunctional eating patterns. For clients who have surgery, additional modifications are needed (Chart 64-8).

Bariatric surgery results in a major lifestyle change as well as a variety of emotions. During weight loss, the client may become depressed or anxious. Some clients experience a "hibernation phase" for about a month after surgery because of physical and emotional adjustments (Gallagher, 2004). Plastic surgery, such as panniculectomy, may be performed after weight is stabilized, usually in about 12 to 15 months.

The chances for success in a weight control program are enhanced if additional support is available. Provide the client with a list of available community resources, such as Overeaters Anonymous and the American Obesity Association. For surgical clients, the American Society of Bariatric Surgery may be helpful.

CHART 64-8

CLIENT EDUCATION GUIDE
Dietary Guidelines for the Client After Bariatric Surgery

- Take nutritional supplements, such as iron, multivitamins, calcium, and vitamin B_{12} as prescribed.
- Eat slowly and chew foods well.
- Progress dietary amounts as prescribed by the dietitian and health care provider.
- Avoid high-protein foods.
- Avoid foods high in sugar (especially refined sugar) and fat.
- Avoid alcoholic beverages.
- Observe for and report signs and symptoms of dehydration.

GET READY for the NCLEX Examination!

KEY POINTS

Safe Effective Care Environment

- Ensure that feeding tube placement is verified by x-ray; check placement every 4 to 8 hours by aspirating gastric contents and assessing pH.
- Place clients receiving tube feeding in a semi-Fowler's position at all times to prevent aspiration; check residual contents every 4 hours or as designated per agency policy.
- Use gloves when changing feeding system tubing or adding product; use sterile gloves when working with critically ill or immunocompromised clients.
- Use a feeding pump when the client receives continuous or cyclic tube feeding.
- Be sure that bariatric furniture and equipment are available for the obese client in the hospital or other health care setting; avoid pressure on skin-fold areas.

Health Promotion and Maintenance

- For clients receiving enteral or parenteral nutrition at home, teach family members or other caregivers how to provide nutrition while avoiding complications.
- Teach clients who are undernourished to eat high-protein, high-calories foods and nutritional supplements.
- Instruct obese clients about the importance of health care provider–approved exercise for weight reduction.
- Provide health teaching about dietary guidelines after bariatric surgery as outlined in Chart 64-8.

Psychosocial Integrity

- Be aware that some obese clients may not view their weight as a problem and are therefore unlikely to be part of a weight reduction plan.
- Recognize that obesity can cause depression or anxiety, low self-esteem, and a disturbed body image.
- Be aware of legal and ethical issues related to tube feeding older adults with chronic or terminal illness.

Physiological Integrity

- Provide a nutritional screening for all inpatient clients (Charts 64-1 and 64-2); review serum prealbumin, hemoglobin, and hematocrit levels. Identify clients at nutritional risk, and refer to a dietitian.

- Assess clients with severe malnutrition for common complications, such as edema; cachexia; lethargy; and dry, flaking skin.
- Implement interventions to promote nutritional intake in older adults as specified in Chart 64-4.
- Provide nursing interventions for managing nutrition as listed in Chart 64-3.
- Provide care for clients receiving total enteral nutrition as described in Charts 64-5 and 64-6.
- Provide care for clients receiving total parenteral nutrition as specified in Chart 64-7.
- Recognize that many individuals are following low-carbohydrate rather than low-fat diets to lose weight.
- Recall that normal body mass index (BMI) for adults should be between 20 and 25; older adults should have a BMI between 24 and 27. A BMI of 27 to 30 indicates overweight, over 30 indicates obesity, and 40 and greater indicates morbid obesity.
- Recall that obesity causes early onset of many chronic illnesses, such as osteoarthritis, diabetes mellitus, hypertension, and coronary artery disease. Pulmonary problems, such as obstructive sleep apnea, delayed wound healing, and infections are also common.
- Remember that bariatric surgery includes gastric restriction procedures or gastric bypass; a panniculectomy may be performed to remove skin folds, especially the abdomen, once weight is stabilized.
- Provide postoperative care for clients having bariatric surgery including applying an abdominal binder, placing the client in semi-Fowler's position and using CPAP to increase ventilation, monitoring for skin breakdown and pressure, and observing for complications, such as dumping syndrome in clients who have a gastric bypass. Tachycardia, nausea, diarrhea, and abdominal cramping are common manifestations of dumping syndrome.

ADDITIONAL STUDY RESOURCES

Go to your Student CD-ROM for Review Questions for the NCLEX Examination.

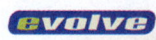 Go to http://evolve.elsevier.com/Iggy/ for Integrated Management of Care Questions for the NCLEX Examination.

SELECTED BIBLIOGRAPHY

Asterisk indicates a classic or definitive work on this subject.

*Ammon, P.K. (1999). Individualizing the approach to treating obesity. *Nurse Practitioner, 24*(2), 27-31, 36-38, 41-43.

Anderson, E.B. (2000). Facilitating quality of life through nutrition. *Advance for Nurses (DC/Baltimore), 2*(11), 17-18, 30.

Barrow, C.J. (2002). Roux-en-Y gastric bypass for morbid obesity. *AORN Journal, 76*(4), 595-604.

Bender, S., et al. (2000). Malnutrition: Role of the TwoCal® HN Med Pass Program. *MEDSURG Nursing, 9*(6), 284-296.

*Bowers, S. (1999). Nutrition support for malnourished, acutely ill adults. *MEDSURG Nursing, 8*(3), 145-166.

Bowers, S. (2000). All about tubes: Your guide to enteral feeding devices. *Nursing 2000, 30*(12), 41-48.

Cammon, S.A., & Hackshaw, H.S. (2000). Are we starving our patients? *American Journal of Nursing, 100*(5), 43-47.

Cowan, D.T., et al. (2004). Nutritional status of older people in long term care settings: Current status and future directions. *International Journal of Nursing Studies, 41*(3), 225-237.

Dudek, S.G. (2000). Malnutrition in hospitals: Who's assessing what patients eat? *American Journal of Nursing, 100*(4), 36-43.

Edwards, S.J., & Metheny, N.A. (2000). Measurement of gastric residual volume: State of the science. *MEDSURG Nursing, 9*(3), 125-128.

*Epley, D. (1999). Nutritional assessment in home care patients. *Home Care Provider, 4*(3), 102-105.

Esposito, K., et al. (2004). Effect of lifestyle changes on erectile dysfunction in obese men: A randomized controlled trial. *Journal of the American Medical Association, 291*(24), 2978-2984.

*Fairburn, C.G., & Cooper, Z. (1996). New perspectives on dieting and behavioural treatments for obesity. *International Journal of Obesity, 20* (suppl 1), S9-S13.

Fellows, L.S., et al. (2000). Evidence-based practice for enteral feedings: Aspiration prevention strategies, bedside detection, and practice change. *MEDSURG Nursing, 9*(1), 27-32.

*Food and Nutrition Board, Institute of Medicine, National Academy of Sciences. (1997). *Dietary reference intakes: Calcium, phosphorus, magnesium, vitamin D, and fluoride.* Washington, D.C.: National Academy Press.

*Food and Nutrition Board, National Research Council/National Academy of Sciences. (1989). *Recommended dietary allowances* (10th ed.). Washington, D.C.: National Academy Press.

Gallagher, S. (2004). Taking the weight off with bariatric surgery. *Nursing 2004, 34*(3), 58-63.

Gallagher, S., & Gates, J.L. (2003). Obesity, panniculitis, panniculectomy, and wound care: Understanding the challenges. *Journal of Wound, Ostomy, and Continence Nursing, 30*(6), 334-341.

*Grindel, C.G., & Costello, M.C. (1996). Nutrition screening: An essential assessment parameter. *MEDSURG Nursing, 5*(3), 145-156.

Holland, D.E., et al. (2001). How to creatively meet care needs of the morbidly obese. *Nursing Management, 32*(6), 39-41.

Kohn-Keeth, C. (2000). How to keep feeding tubes flowing freely. *Nursing 2000, 30*(3), 58-59.

Lofgren, I., et al. (2004). Waist circumference is a better predictor than body mass index of coronary heart disease risk in overweight premenopausal women. *Journal of Nutrition, 134*(5), 1071-1076.

Mackie, S.B. (2001). PEGs and ethics. *Gastroenterology Nursing, 24*(3), 138-142.

Maloney, J., et al. (2002). Food dye use in enteral feedings: A review and a call for a moratorium. *Nutrition and Clinical Practice, 17*, 169-181.

McGinnis, C. (2002). Parenteral nutrition focus: Nutrition assessment and formula composition. *Journal of Infusion Nursing, 25*(1), 54-64.

Metheny, N.A. & Titler, M.G. (2001). Assessing placement of feeding tubes. *American Journal of Nursing, 101*(5), 36-45.

Metheny, N.A. & Stewart, B.J. (2002). Testing feeding tube placement during continuous tube feedings. *Applied Nursing Research, 15*(4), 254-258.

Metheny, N.A., Smith, L., & Stewart, B.J. (2000). Development of a reliable and valid bedside test for bilirubin and utility for improving prediction of feeding tube location. *Nursing Research, 49*(6), 302-309.

Metheny, N.A., Schallom, M.E., & Edwards, S.J. (2004). Effect of gastrointestinal motility and feeding tube site on aspiration risk in critically ill patients: A review. *Heart and Lung, 33*(3), 131-145.

*Metheny, N.A., et al. (1998). Testing feeding tube placement: Auscultation vs. pH method. *American Journal of Nursing, 98*(5), 37-43.

Metheny, N.A., et al. (2002). Efficacy of dye-stained enteral formula in detecting pulmonary aspiration. *Chest, 122*(1), 276-281.

Mion, L.C., & O'Connell, A. (2003). Parenteral hydration and nutrition in the geriatric patient: Clinical and ethical issues. *Journal of Infusion Nursing, 26*(3), 144-152.

Nickel, K. (2004). Comparing voices. Tube feeding: Literature versus the textbook. *American Journal of Nursing, 104*(7), 65.

*Nutrition and your health: Dietary guidelines for Americans. (1995). *Home and Garden Bulletin No. 232* (4th ed.). Washington,

D.C.: U.S. Department of Agriculture and U.S. Department of Health and Human Services.

Padula, C.A., et al. (2004). Enteral feedings: What the evidence says. *American Journal of Nursing, 104*(7), 62-64, 66-69.

Payer, M., Ypungberg, B., & Pfister, S. (2003). Panniculectomy—An option for people who are morbidly obese. *AORN Journal, 77*(4), 782-794.

*Rotkoff, N. (1999). Care of the morbidly obese patient in a long-term care facility. *Geriatric Nursing, 20*(6), 309-313.

Schwarte, A. (2001). Ethical decisions regarding nutrition and the terminally ill. *Gastroenterology Nursing, 24*(1), 29-33.

Stechmiller, J.K. (2003). Early nutritional screening of older adults: A review of nutritional support. *Journal of Infusion Nursing, 26*(3), 170-177.

*Vegetarian food pyramid. (1994). *Vegetarian Journal, 13,* 21.

Voelker, M. (2004). Assessing quality of life in gastric bypass clients. *Journal of Perianesthesia Nursing, 19*(2), 89-101.

Wilson, J.A., & Clark, J.J. (2003). Obesity: Impediment to wound healing. *Critical Care Nursing Quarterly, 26*(2), 119-132.

Woodward, B. (2003). Bariatric surgery options. *Critical Care Nursing Quarterly, 26*(2), 89-100.

Yancy, W.S., et al. (2004). A low-carbohydrate, ketogenic diet versus a low-fat diet to treat obesity and hyperlipidemia: A randomized, controlled trial. *Annals of Internal Medicine, 140*(10), 769-777.

PROBLEMS of REGULATION and METABOLISM

Management of Clients with Problems of the Endocrine System

Assessment of the Endocrine System

M. LINDA WORKMAN

Go to your Student CD-ROM for Review Questions
for the NCLEX Examination keyed to these Learning Outcomes.

The endocrine system is made up of glands in many tissues and organs in a variety of body areas (Figure 65-1). A key feature of all endocrine glands is the secretion of hormones. **Hormones** are natural chemicals that exert their effects on specific tissues known as **target tissues.** Target tissues are usually located some distance from the endocrine gland, with no direct physical connection between the endocrine gland and its target tissue. For this reason endocrine glands are called "ductless" glands and must use the blood to transport secreted hormones to the target tissues. Endocrine glands include the following:

- Pituitary gland
- Adrenal glands
- Thyroid gland
- Islet cells of the pancreas
- Parathyroid glands
- Gonads

The endocrine system works with the nervous system to regulate overall body function, known as **neuroendocrine regulation.** Many interactions must occur between the endocrine system and all other body systems to ensure that each system maintains a constant normal balance (**homeostasis)** in response to environmental changes. For example,

neuroendocrine control of other body systems keeps the internal body temperature at or near 98.6° F (37° C), even when environmental temperatures are lower or higher. Other neuroendocrine actions help keep the serum sodium level between 136 and 145 mEq/L (mmol/L), regardless of whether a person eats 2 g or 12 g of sodium per day.

Table 65-1 lists the specific hormones secreted by various endocrine glands. Hormones travel through the blood to all body areas but exert their actions only on target tissues. Hormones recognize their target tissues and exert their actions by binding to receptor sites on or within the target tissue cells. In general, each receptor site type is specific for only one hormone. Hormone-receptor actions work in a "lock and key" manner in that only the correct hormone (key) can bind to and activate the receptor site (lock) (Figure 65-2). Binding a hormone to its receptor causes the target tissue to change its activity. In this way, hormones produce specific responses even though they circulate throughout the body. Table 65-2 lists the key features of hormones.

Disorders of the endocrine system are related to either an excess or a deficiency of a specific hormone or to a defect at its receptor site. The onset of these disorders can be either slow and insidious or abrupt and life threatening.

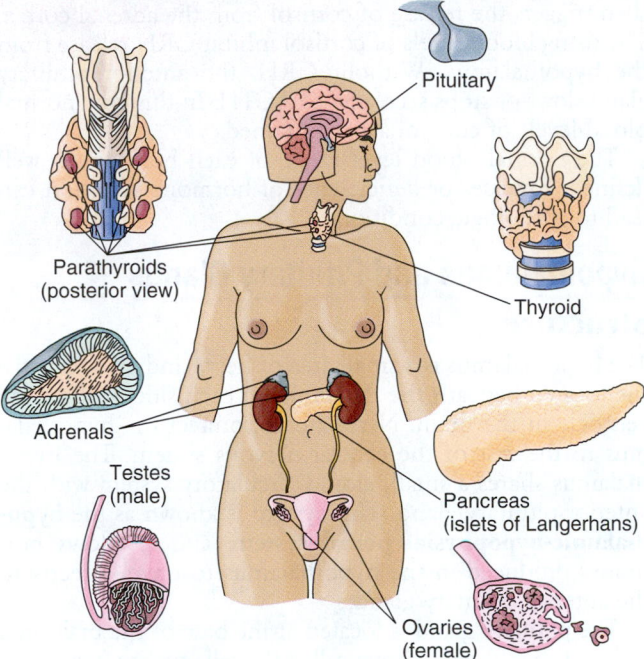

Figure 65-1 ■ The endocrine system.

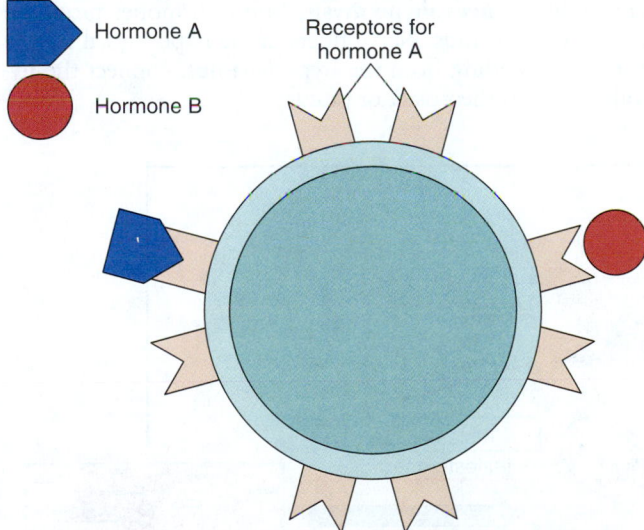

Figure 65-2 ■ "Lock and key" hormone-receptor binding. Hormone A fits and binds to receptor sites, causing a change in cell action. Hormone B does not fit or bind to receptor sites; no change in cell action results.

TABLE 65-1	Principal Hormones of the Endocrine Glands
Gland	**Hormones**
Hypothalamus	Corticotropin-releasing hormone (CRH)
	Thyrotropin-releasing hormone (TRH)
	Gonadotropin-releasing hormone (GnRH)
	Growth hormone–releasing hormone (GHRH)
	Growth hormone–inhibiting hormone (somatostatin GHIH)
	Prolactin-inhibiting hormone (PIH)
	Melanocyte-inhibiting hormone (MIH)
Anterior pituitary	Thyroid-stimulating hormone (TSH)
	Adrenocorticotropic hormone (ACTH, corticotropin)
	Luteinizing hormone (LH)
	Follicle-stimulating hormone (FSH)
	Prolactin (PRL)
	Growth hormone (GH)
	Melanocyte-stimulating hormone (MSH)
Posterior pituitary	Vasopressin (antidiuretic hormone [ADH])
	Oxytocin
Thyroid	Triiodothyronine (T_3)
	Thyroxine (T_4)
	Calcitonin
Parathyroid	Parathyroid hormone
Adrenal cortex	Glucocorticoids (cortisol)
	Mineralocorticoids (aldosterone)
Ovary	Estrogen
	Progesterone
Testes	Testosterone
Pancreas	Insulin
	Glucagon
	Somatostatin

TABLE 65-2 **Common Key Features of Hormones**

- All hormones exert their effects at low blood concentrations.
- Receptors on or within target tissues are needed for *all* hormones to exert an effect.
- Most hormones (except for thyroid and adrenal medullary hormones) are not stored to any great extent and must be produced as needed.
- Hormones in the blood are bound to plasma proteins.
- Only free hormones (those not bound to plasma proteins) can bind to their receptor sites.
- Most hormones cause target tissues to increase or decrease their activity by changing gene activity either directly or indirectly. Exceptions are hormones that alter membrane permeability.
- The activity of most hormones is of short duration.
- Continued hormone activity requires continued production and secretion.
- The clearance of secreted hormones occurs through cellular uptake, enzymatic breakdown, gastrointestinal excretion, or urinary excretion.

ANATOMY AND PHYSIOLOGY REVIEW

The control of cellular function by any hormone depends on a series of reactions working through **negative feedback control mechanisms.** Hormone secretion is dependent on the need of the body for the final action of that hormone. When a body condition starts to move away from the normal range and a specific action or response is needed to correct this change, secretion of the hormone capable of caus-

ing the correcting action or response is stimulated until the need (demand) is met. As the correction occurs, hormone secretion decreases (and may halt). This type of control for hormone synthesis is "negative feedback" because the hormone causes the opposite action of the initial condition change.

An example of a simple negative feedback hormone response is the control of insulin secretion. When blood glucose levels start to rise above normal, the hormone insulin is secreted. Insulin increases glucose uptake by the cells, causing a decrease in blood glucose levels. Thus the action of insulin (decreasing blood glucose levels) is the opposite of the condition that stimulated insulin secretion (elevated blood glucose levels).

Some hormones that use negative feedback mechanisms have more complex interactions. These interactions involve a series of reactions in which more than one endocrine gland, as well as the final target tissues, is stimulated. In such a situation, the first hormone in the series may have another endocrine gland as its target tissue. For this type of mechanism to maintain homeostasis, the following series of interactions must occur:

- The central nervous system receives and reacts to various stimuli transmitted to the hypothalamus.
- The hypothalamus responds to the stimuli with the production and release of either releasing or inhibiting factors, which are transported to the pituitary.
- In the pituitary gland, the releasing or inhibiting factors either stimulate or inhibit the release of specific hormones.
- The anterior pituitary hormones then control the secretion of hormones in target organs or tissue (Figure 65-3).

One example of this complex control is the interaction of the hypothalamus and the anterior pituitary with the adrenal cortex. Low blood levels of cortisol stimulate the secretion of corticotropic-releasing hormone (CRH) in the hypothalamus. CRH stimulates the anterior pituitary gland to secrete adrenocorticotropic hormone (ACTH). ACTH then triggers the release of cortisol from the adrenal cortex. The rising blood levels of cortisol inhibit CRH release from the hypothalamus. Without CRH, the anterior pituitary gland slows or stops secretion of ACTH. In this way, normal blood levels of cortisol are maintained.

The normal blood level range of each hormone is well defined. Excesses or deficiencies of hormone secretion can lead to pathologic conditions.

Hypothalamus and Pituitary Glands

Structure

The hypothalamus is a small area of nerve and glandular tissue located beneath the thalamus on each side of the third ventricle in the brain. Nerve fibers connect the hypothalamus to the rest of the central nervous system. The hypothalamus shares a small, closed circulatory system with the anterior pituitary gland. This system is known as the **hypothalamic-hypophysial portal system,** and it allows hormones produced in the hypothalamus to travel directly to the anterior pituitary gland.

The pituitary gland is located at the base of the brain in a valley of the sphenoid bone called the sella turcica (see Figure 65-1). The oval pituitary gland is about 1 cm in diameter and is divided into two lobes (Figure 65-4). The anterior lobe, or **adenohypophysis,** makes up about 70% of the gland. The posterior lobe, or **neurohypophysis,** stores hormones produced in the hypothalamus. Nerve fibers in the hypophysial stalk, a structure extending from the hypothalamus, connect the hypothalamus to the posterior pituitary.

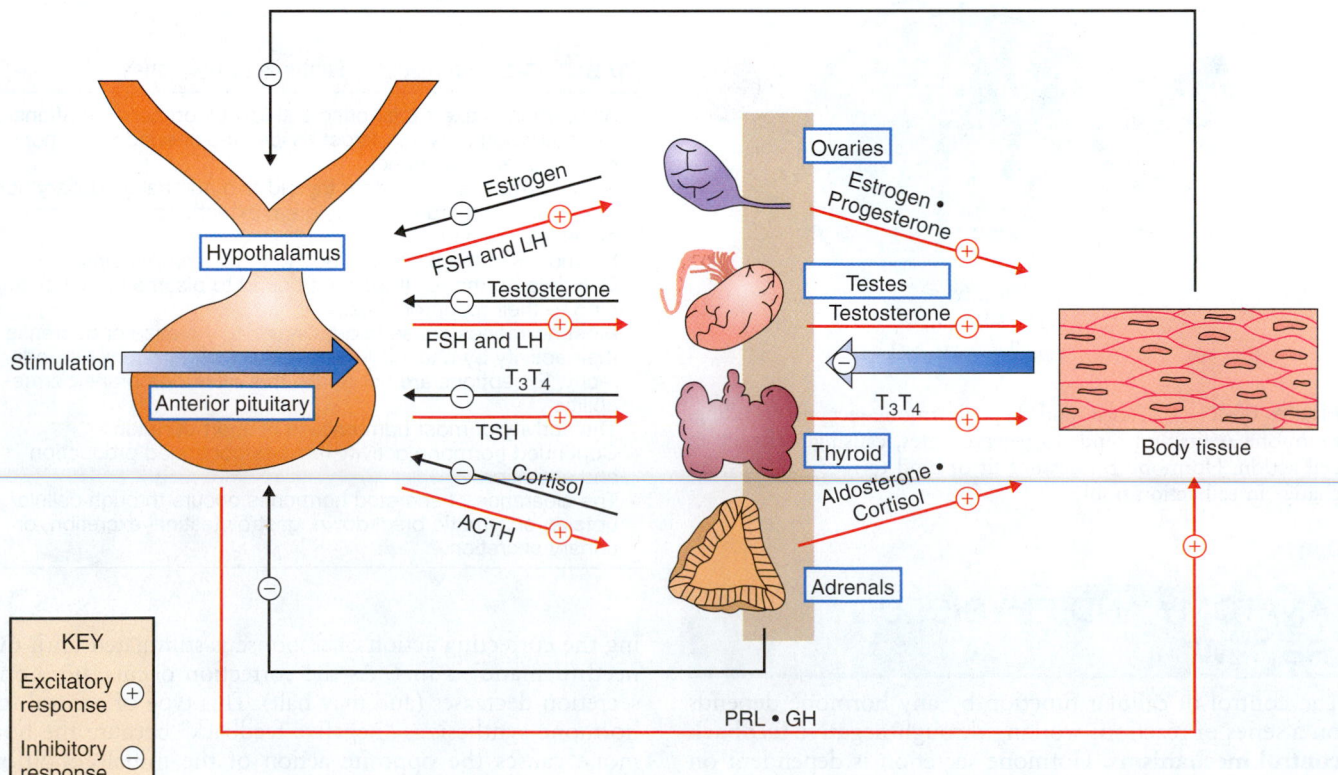

Figure 65-3 ■ The feedback system of the hypothalamic-pituitary-target gland axis. *ACTH,* Adrenocorticotropic hormone; *TSH,* thyroid-stimulating hormone; *T₃,* triiodothyronine; *T₄,* thyroxine; *FSH,* follicle-stimulating hormone; *LH,* luteinizing hormone; *PRL,* prolactin; *GH,* growth hormone.

Function

The hypothalamus has both endocrine and nonendocrine functions. The endocrine function is to produce regulatory hormones (see Table 65-1). Some of these hormones are released into the blood and travel to the anterior pituitary, where they either stimulate or inhibit the release of anterior pituitary hormones.

In response to the releasing hormones of the hypothalamus, the anterior pituitary secretes **tropic hormones**, which stimulate other endocrine glands. Other anterior pituitary hormones, such as prolactin, produce their effect directly on final target tissues (Table 65-3).

The hormones of the posterior pituitary, vasopressin (antidiuretic hormone [ADH]) and oxytocin, are produced in the hypothalamus and sent through the nerve tracts that connect the hypothalamus with the posterior pituitary. These hormones are stored in the nerve endings of the posterior pituitary and are released into the blood when needed.

Other conditions or substances can affect the release of hormones from the pituitary gland (Table 65-4). Drugs, diet, lifestyle, and pathologic conditions can increase or decrease pituitary hormone secretion.

Gonads

The **gonads** are the male and female reproductive endocrine glands. Male gonads are the testes, and female gonads are the ovaries. Although these glands are formed before birth and are present at birth, their function does not begin until puberty.

During puberty in the male, the increased secretion of gonadotropins (luteinizing hormone [LH] and follicle-stimulating hormone [FSH]) from the anterior pituitary gland stimulates maturation of the testes, production of testosterone, and maturation of the external genitalia. During puberty in the female, increased secretion of the same gonadotropins stimulates ovarian maturation, estrogen production, ovulation, and maturation of the external genitalia. The function of the testes and ovaries is detailed in Chapter 76.

Adrenal Glands

The adrenal glands are vascular, tent-shaped organs on the top of each kidney (see Figure 65-1). The adrenal gland has an outer portion (**cortex**) and an inner portion (**medulla**); each area has independent functions. The hormones of the adrenal glands have effects throughout the body.

ADRENAL CORTEX
Structure

The adrenal cortex makes up about 90% of the adrenal gland and has cells divided into three zones or layers (Figure 65-5). **Mineralocorticoids** are produced in the zona glomerulosa and help control the body's sodium and potassium content. Glucocorticoids, androgens, and estrogens are produced in the zona fasciculata and zona reticularis. The hormones produced and secreted by the cortex are often called **adrenal steroids** or **corticosteroids.**

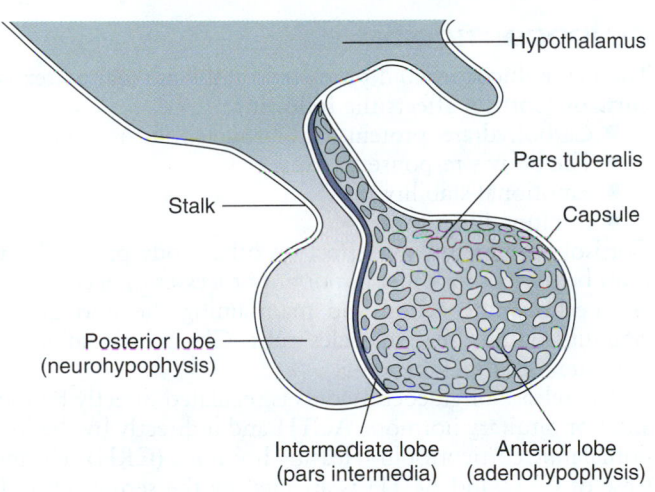

Figure 65-4 ■ The pituitary gland.

Labels: Hypothalamus, Pars tuberalis, Capsule, Anterior lobe (adenohypophysis), Intermediate lobe (pars intermedia), Posterior lobe (neurohypophysis), Stalk

TABLE 65-3 Pituitary Hormones: Target Tissues and Subsequent Actions

Hormone	Target Tissue	Actions
Anterior Pituitary		
TSH (thyroid-stimulating hormone)	Thyroid	Stimulates synthesis and release of thyroid hormone
ACTH (adrenocorticotropic hormone, corticotropin)	Adrenal cortex	Stimulates synthesis and release of corticosteroids and adrenocortical growth
LH (luteinizing hormone)	Ovary	Stimulates ovulation and progesterone secretion
	Testes	Stimulates testosterone secretion
FSH (follicle-stimulating hormone)	Ovary	Stimulates estrogen secretion and follicle maturation
	Testes	Stimulates spermatogenesis
PRL (prolactin)	Mammary glands	Stimulates breast milk production
GH (growth hormone)	Bone and soft tissue	Promotes growth through lipolysis, protein anabolism, and insulin antagonism
MSH (melanocyte-stimulating hormone)	Melanocytes	Promotes pigmentation
Posterior Pituitary*		
Vasopressin (antidiuretic hormone [ADH])	Kidney	Promotes water reabsorption
Oxytocin	Uterus and mammary glands	Stimulates uterine contractions and ejection of breast milk

*These hormones are synthesized in the hypothalamus and are stored in the posterior pituitary gland. They are transported from the hypothalamus to the posterior pituitary while bound to neurophysins.

Function

MINERALOCORTICOIDS

The adrenal cortex maintains life-sustaining physiologic activities. **Aldosterone,** the chief mineralocorticoid produced by the adrenal cortex, maintains extracellular fluid volume.

TABLE 65-4 Factors Affecting Secretion/Release of Selected Pituitary Hormones

Vasopressin
Potential Causes of Increased Secretion
- Congestive heart failure
- Hemorrhage
- Diuretics
- Opioids
- Chlorpropamide
  Diabinese
  Novo-Propamide ✱
- Cyclophosphamide
- Vincristine
- Nicotine
- Stress
- Hypoxia

Potential Causes of Decreased Secretion
- Alcohol consumption
- Phenytoin

Growth Hormone
Potential Causes of Increased Secretion
- High-protein diet
- Deep sleep
- Hypoglycemia
- Fasting
- Estrogen
- Glucagon
- Dopamine

Potential Causes of Decreased Secretion
- REM (rapid eye movement) sleep
- Hyperglycemia
- Obesity
- Hypothyroidism

Prolactin
Potential Causes of Increased Secretion
- Stress
- Nipple manipulation
- Estrogen
- Dopamine antagonists
- Chlorpromazine
  Thorazine
  Chlorpromanyl ✱

Potential Causes of Decreased Secretion
- Dopamine
- Hyperthyroidism

Oxytocin
Potential Causes of Increased Secretion
- Nipple manipulation
- Orgasm
- Extracellular fluid hypertonicity

Potential Causes of Decreased Secretion
- Stress
- Opioids

Data from Wilson, J., et al. (Eds.). (1998). *William's textbook of endocrinology* (9th ed.). Philadelphia: W.B. Saunders.

It promotes sodium and water reabsorption and potassium excretion in the kidney tubules. Aldosterone secretion is regulated by the renin-angiotensin system, serum potassium ion concentration, and adrenocorticotropic hormone (ACTH).

Renin is produced by the juxtaglomerular cells of the renal afferent arterioles. Its release is triggered by a decrease in extracellular fluid volume, which can occur from blood loss, sodium loss, or posture changes. Renin converts renin substrate (formerly called angiotensinogen), a plasma protein made in the liver, to angiotensin I. Angiotensin I is converted by a converting enzyme to form angiotensin II, the active form of angiotensin. In turn, angiotensin II stimulates the secretion of aldosterone. Chapters 14 (Figure 14-8), 15 (Figure 15-2), and 72 further describe the renin-angiotensin system. Aldosterone causes the kidney to reabsorb sodium and water to bring the plasma volume and osmolarity back to normal.

Serum potassium level also controls aldosterone secretion. The adrenal cortex secretes aldosterone when the serum potassium level increases above normal by as little as 0.1 mEq/L.

GLUCOCORTICOIDS

The main glucocorticoid produced by the adrenal cortex is **cortisol.** Cortisol affects the following:
- Carbohydrate, protein, and fat metabolism
- The body's response to stress
- Emotional stability
- Immune function

Cortisol has a permissive effect on other body processes. It must be present for other important processes to occur, such as catecholamine action and maintaining the normal excitability of the heart muscles cells. Glucocorticoid functions are listed in Table 65-5.

The release of glucocorticoids is regulated directly by the anterior pituitary hormone ACTH and indirectly by the hypothalamic corticotropin-releasing hormone (CRH). The release of CRH and ACTH is affected by the serum level of free cortisol, the normal sleep-wake cycle, and stress.

As described earlier, when blood cortisol levels are low, the hypothalamus secretes CRH, which triggers the pituitary to release ACTH. Then ACTH triggers the adrenal cortex to se-

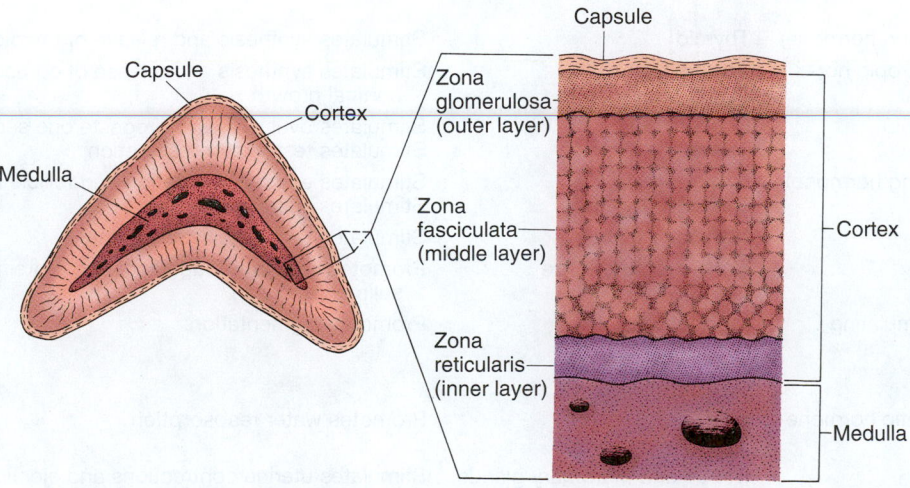

Figure 65-5 ■ The structural detail of the adrenal gland.

crete cortisol. Conversely, adequate or elevated blood levels of cortisol *inhibit* the release of CRH and ACTH. This inhibitory effect is an example of a negative feedback system.

Glucocorticoid release peaks in the morning and reaches its lowest level 12 hours after each peak. Emotional, chemical, or physical stress increases the release of glucocorticoids.

SEX HORMONES

Small amounts of androgens and estrogens are secreted by the adrenal cortex in both genders. Adrenal secretion of these hormones is usually not significant because the **gonads** (ovaries and testes) secrete much larger amounts of estrogens and androgens. In women, however, the adrenal gland is the major source of androgens. Women who have adrenal insufficiency or who have had surgical removal of the adrenals may need a small amount of testosterone replacement.

ADRENAL MEDULLA
Structure

The adrenal medulla is actually a sympathetic nerve ganglion that has secretory cells. Stimulation of the sympathetic nervous system results in the release of adrenal medullary hormones, the **catecholamines** (which includes epinephrine and norepinephrine). These hormones travel to all areas of the body through the blood and exert their effects on target cells. The adrenal medullary hormones are not essential for life but play a role in the physiologic stress response.

Function

The adrenal medulla secretes norepinephrine (NE) and epinephrine, in proportions of 15% and 85%, respectively. The effects of these hormones vary according to the specific receptor in the cell membranes of the target tissue.

These receptors are of two types: alpha adrenergic and beta adrenergic. Both types of receptors are further classified as alpha$_1$- and alpha$_2$-receptors and beta$_1$-, beta$_2$-, and beta$_3$-receptors. NE acts mainly on alpha-adrenergic receptors, and epinephrine most often stimulates beta-adrenergic receptors.

Catecholamines exert their actions on many target organs. Table 65-6 lists the effects of these hormones on body tissues and organs.

Activation of the sympathetic nervous system, which then releases adrenal medullary catecholamines, is an important part of the body's response to stress. Catecholamines are secreted in small amounts at all times to maintain homeostasis. Severe stress triggers increased secretion of catecholamines. This sympathetic activation results in the "fight-or-flight" response, a state of heightened physical and emotional awareness.

TABLE 65-5 Functions of Glucocorticoid Hormones

- Maintain blood glucose level by increasing hepatic gluconeogenesis and inhibiting peripheral glucose use
- Increase lipolysis, releasing glycerol and free fatty acids
- Increase protein catabolism
- Degrade collagen and connective tissue
- Increase the number of polymorphonuclear leukocytes released from bone marrow
- Exert anti-inflammatory effects that decrease the migration of inflammatory cells to sites of injury
- Maintain behavior and cognitive functions

Thyroid Gland
Structure

The thyroid gland is in the anterior neck, directly below the cricoid cartilage (Figure 65-6). It has two lobes joined by a thin strip of tissue (isthmus) in front of the trachea.

The thyroid gland has a rich blood supply, and the right lobe is slightly larger than the left lobe. It is composed of follicular and parafollicular cells. Follicular cells produce the thyroid hormones **thyroxine (T$_4$)** and **triiodothyronine (T$_3$)**.

TABLE 65-6 Catecholamine Receptors and Effects of Adrenal Medullary Hormone Stimulation on Selected Organs and Tissues

Organ or Tissue	Receptors	Effects
Heart	Beta$_1$	Chronotropic action
		Inotropic action
Blood vessels	Alpha	Vasoconstriction
	Beta$_2$	Vasodilation
Gastrointestinal tract	Alpha	Increased sphincter tone
	Beta	Decreased motility
Kidney	Beta$_2$	Increased renin release
Bronchioles	Beta$_2$	Relaxation; dilation
Bladder	Alpha	Sphincter contractions
	Beta$_2$	Relaxation of detrusor muscle
Skin	Alpha	Increased sweating
Fat cells	Beta	Increased lipolysis
Liver	Alpha	Increased gluconeogenesis and glycogenolysis
Pancreas	Alpha	Decreased glucagon and insulin release
	Beta	Increased glucagon and insulin release
Eyes	Alpha	Dilation of pupils

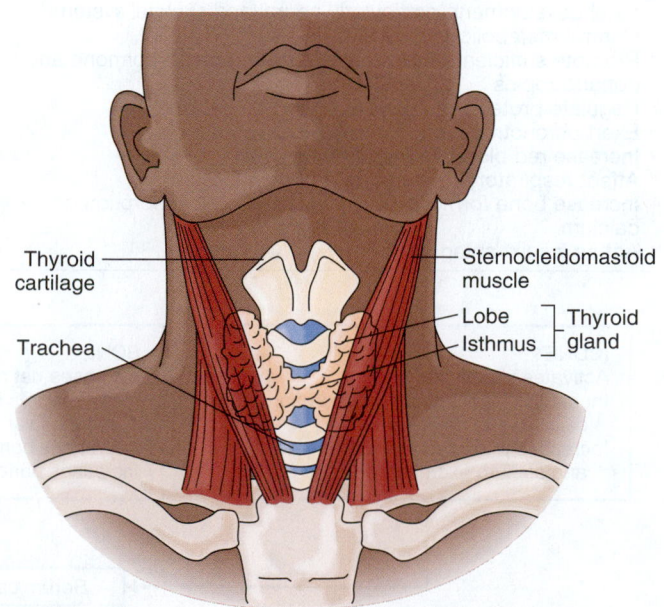

Thyroid cartilage

Trachea

Sternocleidomastoid muscle

Lobe ⎤ Thyroid
Isthmus ⎦ gland

Figure 65-6 ■ Anatomic location of the thyroid gland.

Parafollicular cells produce and secrete **thyrocalcitonin** (calcitonin), which helps to regulate serum calcium levels.

Function

CONTROL OF METABOLISM

Both T_3 and T_4 increase metabolism, which causes an increase in oxygen use and heat production in all tissues. The two hormones differ in structure, but their functions are the same. Most circulating T_4 and T_3 is bound to plasma proteins. The proportion of bound hormone is in balance with the free hormone. The free hormone moves into the cell, where it binds to its receptor in the cell nucleus. Once in the cell, T_4 is converted to T_3, the most active thyroid hormone. The conversion of T_4 to T_3 is impaired by stress, starvation, dyes, beta blockers, amiodarone, corticosteroids, and propylthiouracil (PTU). Cold temperatures increase the conversion. Table 65-7 lists thyroid hormone functions.

The secretion of the thyroid hormones T_3 and T_4 is controlled by the hypothalamic-pituitary-thyroid gland axis, or feedback mechanism. The hypothalamus secretes thyrotropin-releasing hormone (TRH). TRH triggers the anterior pituitary gland to secrete thyroid-stimulating hormone (TSH), which then stimulates the thyroid gland to make and release thyroid hormones. If thyroid hormone levels are high, TSH release is inhibited; if low, TSH release is increased. This is an example of a negative feedback system. Cold and stress are two factors that cause the hypothalamus to secrete TRH, which then stimulates the anterior pituitary to secrete TSH.

Thyroid hormone production involves a series of steps. Dietary intake of protein and iodine is needed to produce thyroid hormones. Iodine is absorbed from the intestinal tract as iodide. The thyroid gland withdraws iodide from the blood and concentrates it. After iodide is in the thyroid, it enters into a series of reactions to form T_4 and T_3. These hormones bind to thyroglobulin and are stored in the follicular cells of the thyroid gland. With stimulation, T_4 and T_3 break off from thyroglobulin and are released into the blood. They enter many cells, bind to the nucleus, and turn on genes important in metabolism. Thus the presence of T_4 and T_3 directly regulate basal metabolic rate (BMR).

CALCIUM AND PHOSPHOROUS BALANCE

Calcitonin (also called thyrocalcitonin, or TCT) is another hormone produced in the thyroid gland. Calcitonin lowers serum calcium and serum phosphorous levels by reducing bone resorption (breakdown). It works in opposition to parathyroid hormone (PTH).

The serum calcium level determines calcitonin secretion. Low serum calcium levels suppress the release of calcitonin; elevated serum calcium levels increase its secretion. Other factors that increase calcitonin release are pregnancy, a high-calcium diet, and an increased secretion of gastrin.

Parathyroid Glands

Structure

The parathyroid glands consist of four small glands located close to, embedded in, or attached to the back surface of the thyroid gland (see Figure 65-1). The chief cells of the parathyroid glands produce and secrete PTH.

Function

Parathyroid hormone regulates calcium and phosphorous metabolism by acting on bone, kidney, and the intestinal tract (Figure 65-7). Bone is the main storage site of calcium. PTH increases bone resorption, thus increasing serum calcium. In the kidneys, PTH activates vitamin D, which then increases the absorption of calcium and phosphate from the intestines. In the kidney tubules, PTH allows calcium to be reabsorbed and put back into the blood.

Serum calcium level is the major controlling factor of PTH secretion. PTH secretion decreases when serum calcium levels are high, and it increases when serum calcium levels are low. Serum phosphorous levels also affect PTH secretion, most likely because of the effect on serum calcium levels. PTH and calcitonin work together to maintain a normal level of ionic calcium in the blood and extracellular fluid.

Pancreas

Structure

The pancreas lies behind the stomach and has endocrine and exocrine functions. The islets of Langerhans areas perform the endocrine functions of the pancreas (Figure 65-8). About one million islet cells are found throughout the pancreas.

TABLE 65-7 Functions of Thyroid Hormones

- Fetal development, particularly neural and skeletal systems
- Control metabolic rate of all cells
- Promote sufficient pituitary secretion of growth hormone and gonadotropins
- Regulate protein, carbohydrate, and fat metabolism
- Exert chronotropic and inotropic cardiac effects
- Increase red blood cell production
- Affect respiratory rate and drive
- Increase bone formation and decrease bone resorption of calcium
- Act as insulin antagonists

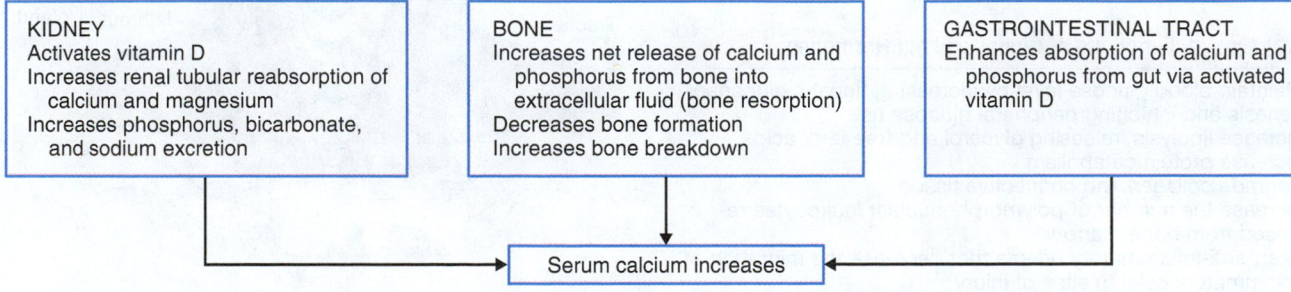

KIDNEY	BONE	GASTROINTESTINAL TRACT
Activates vitamin D Increases renal tubular reabsorption of calcium and magnesium Increases phosphorus, bicarbonate, and sodium excretion	Increases net release of calcium and phosphorus from bone into extracellular fluid (bone resorption) Decreases bone formation Increases bone breakdown	Enhances absorption of calcium and phosphorus from gut via activated vitamin D

Serum calcium increases

Figure 65-7 ■ Effects of parathyroid hormone on target organs.

The islets have three distinct cell types: alpha cells, which secrete glucagon; beta cells, which secrete insulin; and delta cells, which secrete somatostatin. Glucagon and insulin affect carbohydrate, protein, and fat metabolism. Somatostatin, which is secreted not only in the pancreas but also in the intestinal tract and the brain, inhibits the release of glucagon and insulin from the pancreas. It also inhibits the release of gastrin, secretin, and other gastrointestinal (GI) peptides.

Function

The exocrine function of the pancreas involves the secretion of digestive enzymes through ducts that empty into the duodenum (see Chapter 56). The main endocrine function of the pancreas is to regulate blood glucose (sugar).

Glucagon is a hormone that increases blood glucose levels. It is triggered by decreased blood glucose levels and increased blood amino acid levels. Together with epinephrine, growth hormone (GH), and cortisol, glucagon maintains blood glucose levels. In the liver (the main target organ of glucagon), it causes **glycogenolysis** (the conversion of glycogen to glucose). Glucagon also enhances amino acid transport from muscle and promotes **gluconeogenesis** (the conversion of amino acids to glucose). In fat metabolism, glucagon enhances **lipolysis** (fat breakdown) and ketone formation.

Insulin, an **anabolic** hormone (one that stimulates growth), promotes the movement and storage of carbohydrate (CHO), protein, and fat (Table 65-8). Insulin lowers blood glucose levels by enhancing glucose movement across cell membranes in many tissues. Basal levels of insulin are secreted continuously to control metabolism. Insulin secretion rises in response to an increase in blood glucose levels. CHO is the major stimulus for insulin secretion; amino acids trigger a lower-level response. More information on insulin is presented in Chapter 68.

Endocrine Changes Associated with Aging

The effects of aging on the endocrine system vary widely. The three endocrine tissues most commonly observed to have reduced function with aging include the gonads, the thyroid gland, and the endocrine pancreas. It is difficult to distinguish normal from abnormal endocrine activity because of the following other age-related variables:

- Acute and chronic illnesses
- Alterations in diet, activity, and lean body mass-fat ratio
- Disturbances in sleep patterns
- Decreased metabolic clearance rate of hormones
- Increased use of multiple drugs that may affect hormone function

It is important to consider these factors when assessing the older adult with endocrine dysfunction.

Encourage the older adult client to participate in regular screening examinations, including fasting and postprandial blood glucose checks, calcium level determinations, and thyroid function testing. Chart 65-1 lists the endocrine changes that occur in the older adult.

ASSESSMENT TECHNIQUES

History

Use a systems approach to obtain the history of clients with a suspected endocrine problem. This approach can be difficult because of the variety and combination of clinical manifestations. Identify the client's response to actual or perceived changes, and discuss the potential diagnostic and treatment plan. Chart 65-2 presents some assessment questions based on Gordon's Functional Health Patterns. Although endocrine problems can disturb any health pattern, the patterns most commonly affected are Nutritional-Metabolic, Activity, Elimination, Sleep-Rest, and Sexuality-Reproductive. These data are combined with physical, psychosocial, and laboratory findings for a complete assessment of endocrine function.

DEMOGRAPHIC DATA

The age and gender of the client provide baseline assessment data. Certain disorders are more common in older than in younger clients, such as diabetes mellitus, loss of ovarian function, and decreased thyroid function.

Manifestations of endocrine disorders can be gender related, such as the sexual effects of hyperpituitarism and hypopituitarism (see Chapter 66).

FAMILY HISTORY AND GENETIC RISK

Ask the client about any family history of obesity, growth or development difficulties, diabetes mellitus, infertility, or

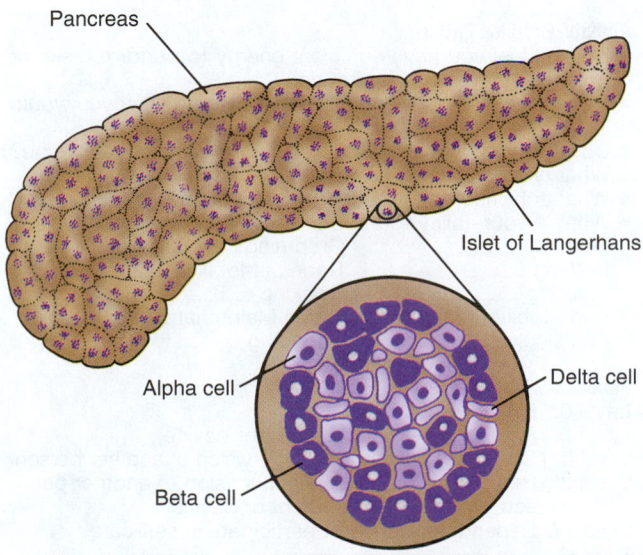

Figure 65-8 ■ The islets of Langerhans of the pancreas.

TABLE 65-8 Anabolic Effects of Insulin

Effects on Liver
- Promotes glycogen synthesis and storage
- Inhibits glycogenolysis, gluconeogenesis, and ketogenesis
- Increases triglyceride synthesis

Effects on Muscle
- Promotes protein synthesis
- Increases amino acid transport
- Promotes glycogenesis

Effects on Fat
- Increases fatty acid synthesis
- Promotes triglyceride storage
- Decreases lipolysis

CHART 65-1

NURSING FOCUS on the OLDER ADULT
Changes in the Endocrine System Related to Aging

Physiologic Change	Nursing Interventions	Rationales
Decreased antidiuretic hormone (ADH)	Assess for diluted urine and polyuria. Monitor fluid intake and output. Encourage fluid intake unless contraindicated.	Ongoing assessment helps to detect early signs of complications. A sufficient fluid intake may help prevent dehydration.
Decreased ovarian function	Teach the client the signs and symptoms of estrogen deficiency. Promote exercise and calcium intake.	The client's ability to cope with changes may be enhanced with knowledge. Sufficient exercise and calcium intake delay bone loss and prevent osteoporosis.
Decreased glucose tolerance	Identify at-risk clients by obtaining a family history of diabetes mellitus and obesity. Assess for greater-than-ideal body weight or body mass index, little physical exercise, frequent yeast infections, polydipsia, polyuria. Teach the client the signs and symptoms of hyperglycemia.	Identification of at-risk clients helps in early detection of complications and conditions such as diabetes. Knowledge helps to improve the client's ability to recognize hyperglycemia.
Decreased peripheral metabolism	Assess for signs and symptoms of hypothyroidism, especially constipation, lethargy, dry skin, and mental deterioration.	Ongoing assessment helps to differentiate hypothyroidism from the clinical features of aging.

CHART 65-2

Endocrine Assessment
USING GORDON'S FUNCTIONAL HEALTH PATTERNS

Nutritional-Metabolic Pattern
- What is your typical daily food intake? Describe a day's meals, snacks, and vitamins.
- How much salt do you typically add to your food? Do you use salt substitutes?
- How is your appetite?
- Do you have any difficulty chewing or swallowing?
- What is your typical daily fluid intake? What types of fluids (water, juices, soft drinks, coffee, tea)? How much?
- Have you had any recent change in your weight? Weight gain? Weight loss? How much?
- Have you noticed a change in the tightness of your rings or shoes? Tighter? Looser?
- Have you noticed any change in thirst?

Elimination Pattern
- What is your usual bowel elimination pattern? Frequency? Character? Discomfort? Laxatives?
- What is your usual urinary elimination pattern? Frequency? Amount? Color? Odor? Control?
- Have you noticed a change in the amount of urine?
- Do you have any problem with excessive perspiration?
- Do you have any other type of drainage?

Sleep-Rest Pattern
- Do you have any difficulty falling asleep when you go to bed?
- Is there a change in the number of hours you sleep per night?
- Do you take any medication to help you sleep?
- About how many times do you awaken during the night?
- Do you have any difficulty getting back to sleep?
- Are you bothered by nightmares or vivid dreams?
- Do you have difficulty awakening in the morning?
- Do you feel generally rested and ready for daily activities after sleep?
- Do you take scheduled naps or rest periods during the day?
- Do you find yourself falling asleep at work or at home while reading or watching television?
- Have you noticed any difficulty in your ability to concentrate?

Sexuality-Reproductive Pattern
- Are you sexually active?
- Are you satisfied with your level of sexual activity?
- Do you participate in sex as often as you would like?
- Do you participate in sex as often as your partner would like?
- Have you noticed a change in your interest in having sex over the past year?

Female:
- At what age did menstruation start?
- How regular are your periods?
- Do you have any pain, cramping, or clotting during your periods?
- Have you ever been pregnant? What was the outcome of the pregnancy(ies)?
- Do you use contraceptives? What type? Have you had any problems with your chosen method of contraception?

Activity-Exercise Pattern
- Do you feel you have sufficient energy to perform tasks or routines that are required of you?
- Do you feel you have sufficient energy to do what you would like to do?
- Do you exercise? How often? For how long each time? What type(s) of exercise do you perform?
- What activities do you perform in your spare time?
- What is your ability to perform the following tasks?

Feeding _____	Grooming _____
Bathing _____	General Mobility _____
Toileting _____	Cooking _____
Bed Mobility _____	Home Maintenance _____
Dressing _____	Shopping _____

Functional Levels Code
Level 0: Full self-care
Level I: Requires use of equipment or device
Level II: Requires assistance or supervision of another person
Level III: Requires assistance or supervision of another person and use of equipment or device
Level IV: Dependent; does not participate in self-care

Based on Gordon, M. (2002). *Manual of nursing diagnosis* (10th ed.). St. Louis: Mosby.

thyroid disorders. These problems may have an autosomal dominant, recessive, or cluster pattern of inheritance.

PERSONAL HISTORY

Assess the client for a history of endocrine dysfunction, manifestations that could indicate an endocrine disorder, and hospitalizations. Ask asked about past and current drugs, such as hydrocortisone, levothyroxine, oral contraceptives, and antihypertensive agents.

DIET HISTORY

Nutritional changes or GI tract disturbances may reflect many different endocrine problems. Ask about a history of nausea, vomiting, and abdominal pain. An increase or decrease in food or fluid intake may also indicate specific disorders. For example, diabetes insipidus triggers excessive thirst, and adrenal hypofunction triggers salt craving. Hunger and thirst may also be increased in diabetes mellitus. Rapid changes in weight without diet changes can signal the onset of a number of endocrine disorders, including diabetes mellitus and thyroid problems.

SOCIOECONOMIC STATUS

Because the client's socioeconomic status is a sensitive issue, explore with the client whether his or her resources are adequate for a healthy diet, needed drugs, and consistent health care follow-up. It may be appropriate to involve social service and home care agencies at an early stage.

CURRENT HEALTH PROBLEMS

Focus on the client's reason for seeking health care, asking questions such as the following:

- Did the symptoms occur gradually, or was the onset sudden?
- Has the client been treated for this problem in the past?
- How have the current symptoms affected the activities of daily living (ADLs)?

Such questions provide clues to specific endocrine disorders. Also explore changes in energy levels, elimination patterns, sexual and reproductive functions, and physical features.

Energy Levels

Changes in energy levels occur with many endocrine problems, especially thyroid problems (see Chapter 67) and adrenal problems (see Chapter 66). Ask the client about any change in ability to perform ADLs and assess the client's current energy level. For instance, has the client been sleeping longer, or does he or she have fatigue or generalized weakness?

Elimination

Elimination is also affected by the endocrine system. Identify the client's past pattern of elimination to determine deviations from the normal routine. Ask about the amount and frequency of urination. Does he or she urinate frequently in large amounts? Does the client wake during the night to urinate (**nocturia**), or is pain present with urination (**dysuria**)? Information about the frequency of bowel movements and their consistency and color may provide clues to problems in fluid balance or metabolic rate (i.e., thyroid function).

Sex and Reproduction

Sexual and reproductive functions are greatly affected by endocrine disturbances. Ask women about any changes in the menstrual cycle, such as increased flow, duration, and frequency of menses; pain or excessive cramping; or a recent change in the regularity of menses. Ask men whether they have experienced impotence. Question both men and women about a change in libido or any fertility problems.

Physical Appearance

Discuss any changes that the client perceives in physical features. Overt changes are identified during the physical assessment, but clients may be able to describe some of the more subtle changes. Ask the client about changes in the following:

- Hair texture and distribution
- Facial contours and eye protrusion
- Voice quality
- Body proportions
- Secondary sexual characteristics

For example, you might ask a man whether he is shaving less often or a woman if she has noticed an increase in facial hair. These changes may be associated with pituitary, thyroid, parathyroid, or adrenal dysfunction.

? Critical Thinking Challenge

The client is a 44-year-old woman who tells you that she feels fatigued, although she goes to bed early. She says that she awakens frequently and has a hard time getting back to sleep. Some of the physical changes she has noticed over the past 6 months include a thinning of her pubic hair and a weight gain of about 15 lbs. Her periods have become less predictable and vary in amount of flow from scant to heavy. A home pregnancy test indicates that she is not pregnant.

1. Which endocrine glands or tissues should be assessed for causing the problems she has noticed?
2. What questions could you ask to try and quantify her sense of fatigue?
3. Are there any questions you should ask about the information she has already provided?

evolve For suggested answer guidelines, go to http://evolve.elsevier.com/Iggy/.

Physical Assessment

INSPECTION

An endocrine problem can change physical features because of its effect on growth and development, regulation of sex hormone levels, fluid and electrolyte balance, and the body's use of nutrients. Different clinical findings can occur with multiple endocrine disorders or with nonendocrine problems.

Use a head-to-toe approach to inspect the client. Observe the client's general appearance, and assess height, weight, fat distribution, and muscle mass in relation to age. It is important to remember that heredity and age rather than a health problem may be responsible for some physical features (e.g., short stature).

When examining the head, focus on abnormalities of facial structure, features, and expression, such as the following:

- Prominent forehead or jaw
- Round or puffy face

- Dull or flat expression
- Exophthalmos (protruding eyeballs and retracted upper lids)

Check the lower half of the neck for a visible enlargement of the thyroid gland. Normally the thyroid tissue cannot be observed. The isthmus may be noticeable when the client swallows. Jugular vein distention may be seen on inspection of the neck and can indicate fluid overload (see Chapter 15).

Skin changes may reflect a specific endocrine dysfunction. Observe skin color, and look for areas of pigment loss (hypopigmentation) or hyperpigmentation. Fungal skin infections, slow wound healing, bruising, and petechiae are often seen in clients with adrenal hyperfunction. Skin infections, foot ulcers, and slow wound healing are common among clients with diabetes mellitus. In secondary hypofunction of the adrenal glands, the skin over the finger joints, elbows, and knees, as well as any scar tissue, may show increased pigmentation due to increased levels of ACTH and melanocyte-stimulating hormone.

Vitiligo (patchy areas of pigment loss with increased pigmentation at the edges) is seen with primary hypofunction of the adrenal glands and is due to autoimmune destruction of melanocytes in the skin. Areas of pigment loss most often occur on the face, neck, and extremities. Mucous membranes may have large areas of uneven pigmentation. Document the location, color, distribution, and size of skin color changes and lesions.

Inspect the client's fingernails for malformation, thickness, or brittleness, all of which may suggest thyroid gland problems. Examine the extremities and the base of the spine for edema, which suggests a fluid and electrolyte imbalance.

Inspection of the trunk can show signs of specific endocrine dysfunction. Check for any abnormalities in chest size and symmetry. Truncal obesity, supraclavicular fat pads, and a "buffalo hump" may indicate adrenocortical excess. Hormonal imbalance may also change secondary sexual characteristics. Inspect the breasts of both men and women for size, symmetry, pigmentation, and discharge. **Striae** (reddish purple "stretch marks") on the breasts or abdomen are often seen with adrenocortical excess.

Assess the client's hair distribution for indications of endocrine gland dysfunction. Changes can include **hirsutism** (excessive growth of body hair, especially on the face, chest, and the linea alba of the abdomen of women), excessive hair loss, or changes in hair texture.

Examination of the genitalia may reveal a dysfunction in hormone secretion. Observe the size of the scrotum and penis or of the labia and clitoris in relation to standards for the client's age. The distribution and quantity of pubic hair are often affected in hypogonadism.

PALPATION

The thyroid gland and the testes can be examined by palpation. Chapters 76 and 79 discuss examination of the testes. The thyroid gland is palpated for size, symmetry, general shape, and the presence of nodules or other irregularities.

Palpate the thyroid gland by standing either behind or in front of the client (Figure 65-9); the posterior approach may be easier. Asking the client to swallow sips of water during the examination helps the clinician palpate the thyroid gland.

Ask the client to sit and to lower the chin. Using the posterior approach, place the thumbs of both your hands on the back of the client's neck, with the fingers curved around to the

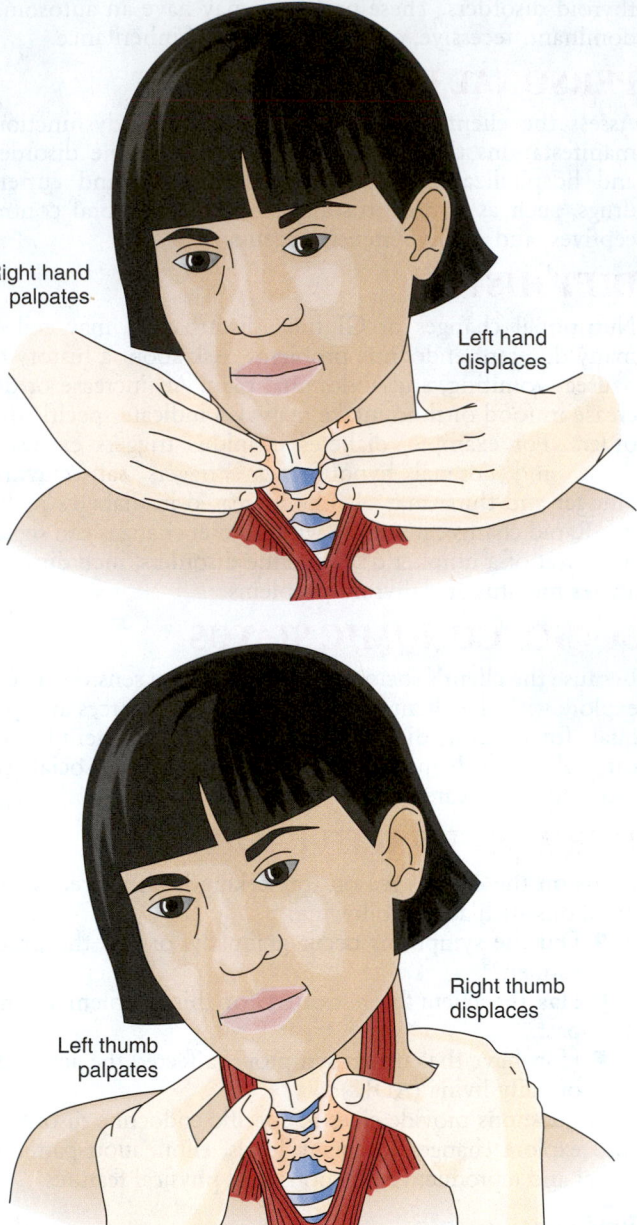

Figure 65-9 ■ Palpation of the thyroid gland.

front of the neck on either side of the trachea. Ask the client to swallow, and then locate the isthmus of the thyroid as you feel it rising. Identify the anterior surface of the thyroid lobe. To examine the right lobe, proceed in the following way:

- Turn the client's head to the right
- Displace the thyroid cartilage to the right with the fingers of your left hand
- Palpate the right lobe with your right hand

Reverse this procedure to examine the left lobe.

AUSCULTATION

Auscultate the client's chest to establish baseline vital signs and to assess cardiac rate and rhythm. Some endocrine problems induce dysrhythmias. Many endocrine disturbances can cause dehydration and volume depletion. Therefore document any difference in the client's blood pressure and pulse in the lying, standing, or sitting positions (orthostatic vital signs).

If an enlarged thyroid gland is palpated, auscultate the area of enlargement for bruits. Hypertrophy of the thyroid gland causes an increase in vascular flow, which may result in bruits.

Psychosocial Assessment

Information obtained from the history and physical examination may help to identify psychosocial problems. Assess the client's coping skills, support systems, and health-related beliefs.

A number of endocrine disorders affect the client's perception of self. For example, body features can change significantly in disorders of the pituitary, adrenal, and thyroid glands. Infertility, impotence, and other changes in sexual function may result from endocrine dysfunction. Ask about any difficulty in coping with such changes.

Clients with endocrine problems may require lifelong drugs and follow-up care. Assess the client's readiness to learn and his or her ability to carry out specific self-management skills. Clients may also face financial difficulties resulting from a prolonged medical regimen or loss of employment. A referral to social service agencies may be needed.

Diagnostic Assessment
LABORATORY TESTS

For the client with possible endocrine dysfunction, laboratory tests are an essential part of the diagnostic process. The specialized testing for specific disorders is described in Chapters 66 to 68. Best practices for the collection of specimens for general endocrine testing are listed in Chart 65-3.

Stimulation/Suppression Tests

Measurement of specific hormone levels does not always distinguish between the normal and the abnormal. The wide normal range for some hormones makes it necessary to trigger responses by stimulation or suppression tests.

For the client who might have underactivity of an endocrine gland, a stimulus may be provided to determine whether the gland is capable of normal hormone production. This method is called *stimulation testing*. Measured amounts of selected hormones are given to stimulate the target gland to maximal production. Hormone levels are then measured and compared with expected normal values. Failure of the hormone level to rise with stimulation indicates hypofunction.

Suppression tests are used when hormone levels are high or in the upper range of normal. Failure of suppression of hormone production during testing indicates hyperfunction. (See the specific tests in Chapters 66 and 67.)

Assays

An assay measures the level of a specific hormone in blood or other body fluid. Some assays are indirect, such as the radioimmunoassay. In this test, radioactively labeled amounts of hormone (antigen) compete with unlabeled hormones from the plasma or serum for antibody binding sites. Various techniques measure the amount of unbound and bound hormone. The unbound hormone is the active hormone.

CHART 65-3

BEST PRACTICE for
Endocrine Testing

- Explain the procedure to the client.
- Emphasize the importance of taking a medication prescribed for the test on *time*. Tell the client to set an alarm if the medication is to be taken during the night.
- Instruct the client to begin the urine collection (whether for 2, 4, 8, 12, or 24 hours) by emptying his or her bladder. Tell the client *not* to save the urine specimen that begins the collection. The timing for the urine collection begins after this specimen. To end the collection, the client empties his or her bladder at the end of the timed period and adds that urine to the collection.
- Make sure that the preservative has been added to the collection container at the beginning of the collection, if necessary. Tell the client of its presence in the container.
- Check your laboratory's method of handling hormone test samples. Blood samples drawn for certain hormones (e.g., catecholamines) must be placed on ice and taken to the laboratory immediately.
- If you are drawing blood samples from a line, clear the intravenous (IV) line thoroughly. Do not use a double- or triple-lumen line to obtain samples; contamination or dilution from another port is possible.

Other hormone assay methods include immunometric assays, chromatographic assays, and mass spectrometry. An immunometric assay uses a large antibody with a component that "captures" the hormone and a second component that creates a signal when the antibody binds to the hormone (antigen). Chromatographic assays separate molecules in the serum by size, light absorption, and other properties. Each hormone has very specific properties that allow it to separate from other blood substances and form a unique bandwidth. Mass spectrometry methods also allow individual hormones to separate from other serum molecules based on the amount (mass) and charge of individual components. On a graph these separate hormones each show as a unique "spike" pattern. Many different hormone concentrations can be analyzed at the same time by this method.

Urine Tests

Hormone levels and the metabolites of specific hormones in the urine are often measured to determine endocrine function. Because many of the endocrine hormones are secreted in a pulsatile fashion, measurement of a specific hormone in a 24-hour urine collection better reflects the overall function of certain glands, such as the adrenal gland. Teach the client how to collect a 24-hour urine sample (see also Chart 65-3).

Certain hormones require additives in the container at the beginning of the collection. Instruct the client not to discard the preservative from the container and to use caution when handling it because some solutions are caustic. Remind the client that this collection is timed for *exactly* 24 hours. Instruct the client to avoid taking any unnecessary drugs during endocrine testing because some drugs can interfere with the laboratory assays.

Tests for Glucose

Tests for functions of the islet cells of the pancreas are indirect; they measure the *result* of pancreatic islet cell function. Blood glucose values and the oral glucose tolerance test help to diagnose diabetes mellitus. The glycosylated hemoglobin (HbA$_{1C}$) value reveals the *average* blood glucose level over a period of 2 to 3 months. Its primary use is in assessing overall control of glucose level in diabetes mellitus. (See Chapter 68 for a full discussion of diabetes mellitus.)

RADIOGRAPHIC EXAMINATIONS

Anterior, posterior, and lateral skull x-rays may be used to visualize the sella turcica. Erosion of the sella turcica indicates invasion of the wall from an abnormal growth.

Magnetic resonance imaging (MRI) with contrast is the most sensitive method of imaging the pituitary gland, although computed tomography (CT) scans can also be used to evaluate it. The thyroid, parathyroid glands, ovaries, and testes are evaluated by ultrasound. In addition, CT scans are used to evaluate the adrenal glands, ovaries, and pancreas.

OTHER DIAGNOSTIC TESTS

Needle biopsy is a relatively safe and quick outpatient procedure used to indicate the composition of thyroid nodules. It is used to determine whether surgical intervention is needed.

Critical Thinking Challenge

The 44-year-old client with fatigue, menstrual changes, weight gain, and loss of pubic hair is scheduled to have blood drawn for follicle-stimulating hormone (FSH) levels, thyroid hormone levels, and blood glucose levels; an ultrasound of the ovaries; a 24-hour urine collection for estradiol beta-17 levels, and a CT scan of the head. In addition, she is to return for a glucose tolerance test. She is very anxious about the tests and the results.

1. How should you prepare her physically for each test?
2. What special instructions should you provide for the 24-hour urine test?
3. The client is very concerned about pain and modesty. What reassurances can you provide for the level of pain expected?
4. Is the client's modesty at risk with any of these procedures? If so, how? What precautions can be taken to reduce exposure?

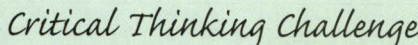 For suggested answer guidelines, go to http://evolve.elsevier.com/Iggy/.

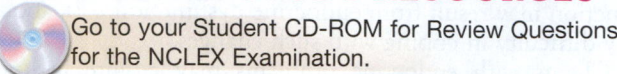

GET READY for the NCLEX Examination!

KEY POINTS

Safe Effective Care Environment

- Use good handwashing technique and precautions to reduce the spread of infection to any client who is taking exogenous corticosteroids or who has a problem that increases corticosteroid production.

Health Promotion and Maintenance

- Teach all clients that abusing hormones or steroids can have an adverse effect on endocrine function.

Psychosocial Integrity

- Explain all diagnostic procedures, restrictions, and follow-up care to the client scheduled for tests.
- Allow the client to express fears or concerns about a change in appearance or a reduction in fertility.
- Ask family members about changes in the client's personality or behavior.

Physiological Integrity

- Ask the client about other family members with endocrine disorders because some endocrine problems have a genetic component.
- Ask the client what prescribed and over-the-counter drugs are taken on a regular basis because some drugs can alter endocrine function (see Table 65-4).

ADDITIONAL STUDY RESOURCES

Go to your Student CD-ROM for Review Questions for the NCLEX Examination.

Go to http://evolve.elsevier.com/Iggy/ for Integrated Management of Care Questions for the NCLEX Examination.

SELECTED BIBLIOGRAPHY

Berne, R., et al. (2004). *Physiology* (5th ed.). St. Louis: Mosby.

Ebersole, P., Hess, P., & Luggen, A. (2004). *Toward healthy aging: Human needs and nursing response* (6th ed.). St. Louis: Mosby.

Gordon, M. (2002). *Manual of nursing diagnosis* (10th ed.). St. Louis: Mosby.

Holcomb, S. (2003). Detecting thyroid disease, part 1. *Nursing 2003, 33*(8), 32cc1-32cc4.

Holcomb, S. (2003). Detecting thyroid disease, part 2. *Nursing 2003, 33*(9), 32cc1-32cc4.

Jarvis, C. (2004). *Physical examination and health assessment* (4th ed.). Philadelphia: W.B. Saunders.

Klee, G. (2003). Laboratory techniques for recognition of endocrine disorders. In P.R. Larsen, et al. (Eds.). *Williams' textbook of endocrinology* (10th ed., pp. 65-79). Philadelphia: W.B. Saunders.

Lamberts, S. (2003). Endocrinology and aging. In P.R. Larsen, et al. (Eds.). *Williams' textbook of endocrinology* (10th ed., pp. 1287-1301). Philadelphia: W.B. Saunders.

Larsen, P.R., et al. (Eds.). (2003). *Williams' textbook of endocrinology* (10th ed., pp. 65-79). Philadelphia: W.B. Saunders.

Melmed, S., & Kleinberg, D. (2003). Anterior pituitary. In P.R. Larsen, et al. (Eds.). *Williams textbook of endocrinology* (10th ed., pp. 177-279). Philadelphia: W.B. Saunders.

Pagana, K., & Pagana, T. (2002). *Mosby's manual of diagnostic and laboratory tests* (2nd ed.). St. Louis: Mosby.

Robinson, A., & Verbalis, J. (2003). Posterior pituitary gland. In P.R. Larsen, et al. (Eds.). *Williams' textbook of endocrinology* (10th ed., pp. 281-329). Philadelphia: W.B. Saunders.

Interventions for Clients with Pituitary and Adrenal Gland Problems

M. LINDA WORKMAN

LEARNING OUTCOMES

After studying this chapter, you should be able to:

1. Compare the common clinical manifestations associated with pituitary hypofunction and pituitary hyperfunction.
2. Interpret clinical changes and laboratory data to determine the effectiveness of therapy for pituitary hypofunction.
3. Identify the teaching priorities for the client taking hormone replacement therapy for pituitary hypofunction.
4. Prioritize nursing care for the client immediately after a transsphenoidal hypophysectomy.
5. Interpret clinical changes and laboratory data to determine the effectiveness of therapy for pituitary hyperfunction.
6. Compare the problems associated with oversecretion and undersecretion of antidiuretic hormone on blood and on urine volumes and blood and urine osmolarities.
7. Describe the mechanisms of action, side effects, and nursing implications for pharmacologic management of diabetes insipidus.
8. Interpret clinical changes and laboratory data to determine the effectiveness of interventions for diabetes insipidus.
9. Develop a community-based teaching plan for the client with diabetes insipidus.
10. Interpret clinical changes and laboratory data to determine the effectiveness of interventions for SIADH.
11. Develop a community-based teaching plan for the client with SIADH.
12. Compare the clinical manifestations of Cushing's syndrome and Addison's disease.
13. Interpret clinical changes and laboratory data to determine the effectiveness of interventions for Cushing's syndrome.
14. Develop a community-based teaching plan for the client with Cushing's syndrome or disease.
15. Describe the mechanisms of action, side effects, and nursing implications for pharmacologic management of adrenal insufficiency.
16. Interpret clinical changes and laboratory data to determine the effectiveness of therapy for adrenal insufficiency.
17. Develop a community-based teaching plan for the client with adrenal insufficiency.
18. Prioritize nursing interventions for the client experiencing acute adrenal insufficiency.

Go to your Student CD-ROM for Review Questions
for the NCLEX Examination keyed to these Learning Outcomes.

Pituitary and adrenal gland problems can be caused by, or can cause, oversecretion or undersecretion of one or more hormones. At times, the correct amount of hormone may be produced but cannot be used because of receptor site failure.

Hormones secreted from the anterior pituitary gland regulate growth, metabolism, and sexual development. These functions are affected when the pituitary gland secretes too much or too little of one or more hormones. The posterior pituitary gland secretes **vasopressin** (antidiuretic hormone [ADH]).

Posterior pituitary problems result in fluid and electrolyte imbalance. The adrenal gland produces and secretes hormones that influence homeostasis and are life sustaining. The effects of these endocrine problems occur throughout the body and may induce psychological, as well as physical, changes. Nursing care for the client with pituitary or adrenal gland disorders includes assessment, client education, evaluation of client response to therapy, and providing support.

A complete history and physical examination are performed to detect specific clinical findings. The client also often undergoes many diagnostic tests and relies on the nurse for specific instructions and explanations. Surgical intervention may be indicated. The client often needs lifelong hormone replacement therapy. Physical and emotional support is critical.

Disorders of the Pituitary Gland

DISORDERS OF THE ANTERIOR PITUITARY GLAND

The anterior pituitary gland (adenohypophysis) controls growth, metabolic activity, and sexual development through the actions of the following hormones:

- Growth hormone (GH; somatotropin)
- Prolactin (PRL)
- Thyrotropin (thyroid-stimulating hormone [TSH])
- Corticotropin (adrenocorticotropic hormone [ACTH])
- Follicle-stimulating hormone (FSH)
- Luteinizing hormone (LH)
- Melanocyte-stimulating hormone (MSH)

Disorders of hormones secreted by the anterior pituitary gland can result from problems arising within the anterior pituitary gland itself (primary pituitary dysfunction) or from problems in the hypothalamus that change anterior pituitary function (secondary pituitary dysfunction). In either case, one or more hormones may be undersecreted (pituitary hypofunction) or oversecreted (pituitary hyperfunction).

Hypopituitarism
PATHOPHYSIOLOGY

A person with hypopituitarism has a deficiency of one or more anterior pituitary hormones, resulting in metabolic problems and sexual dysfunction. Decreased production of *all* of the anterior pituitary hormones is an extremely rare condition known as panhypopituitarism.

More commonly, there is a marked decrease in the secretion of one hormone and a lesser decrease in the other hormones. Deficiencies of adrenocorticotropic hormone (ACTH) and thyroid-stimulating hormone (TSH) are the *most* life threatening because they result in a corresponding decrease in the secretion of vital hormones from the adrenal and thyroid glands. Adrenal gland hypofunction is discussed on pp. 1470 to 1473; hypothyroidism is discussed in Chapter 67.

Deficiency of the gonadotropins (luteinizing hormone [LH] and follicle-stimulating hormone [FSH]—hormones that

TABLE 66-1   Causes of Hypopituitarism
Causes of Primary Hypopituitarism
■ Pituitary tumor (adenomas, granulomas, meningiomas)
■ Partial or total surgical hypophysectomy
■ Radiation of the brain
■ Infarction following systemic shock
■ Metastatic cancer
■ Trauma
Causes of Secondary Hypopituitarism
■ Infection
■ Trauma
■ Brain tumor

stimulate the ovaries and testes to produce sex hormones) changes sexual function in both men and women. In men, gonadotropin deficiency results in testicular failure, with decreased testosterone production from the Leydig cells and decreased or absent spermatogenesis. Decreased testosterone levels in men cause sterility. In women, gonadotropin deficiency results in ovarian failure, amenorrhea, and infertility.

Growth hormone (GH) deficiency changes tissue growth patterns indirectly. GH itself has little effect on tissues and cells. Rather, the presence of GH stimulates the liver to produce substances known as somatomedins. These somatomedins, especially somatomedin C (insulin-like growth factor-1 [IGF-1]), then enhance growth activities in cells and tissues. Somatomedin C is responsible for bone and cartilage growth and maintenance.

GH deficiency may be a result of decreased GH production, failure of the liver to produce somatomedins, or a failure of the cells or tissues to respond to the somatomedins. GH deficiency in children leads to short stature and other manifestations of growth retardation. GH deficiency in adults does not affect height but does increase the rate of bone destructive activity, leading to thinner, more fragile bones (osteoporosis).

The cause of hypopituitarism varies. Benign or malignant pituitary tumors can compress and destroy pituitary tissue. Pituitary function can be impaired by severe malnutrition or rapid loss of body fat, such as in people with anorexia nervosa (a disorder in which people see themselves as overweight and eat so little that starvation results). Shock or severe hypotension reduces blood flow to the pituitary gland, leading to hypoxia and infarction. Other causes of hypopituitarism are listed in Table 66-1. Idiopathic hypopituitarism is an isolated hormone deficiency with an unknown cause.

Postpartum hemorrhage is the most common cause of pituitary infarction, which results in decreased hormone secretion. This clinical problem is known as Sheehan's syndrome. The pituitary gland normally enlarges during pregnancy, and when hypotension results from hemorrhage, ischemia and necrosis of the gland occur. Usually this condition develops immediately after delivery, although some cases have occurred several years later.

◆ COLLABORATIVE MANAGEMENT
◆ Assessment

Changes in physical appearance and target organ function occur with deficiencies of specific pituitary hormones (Chart 66-1). Gonadotropin (LH and FSH) deficiency results in the

CHART 66-1

KEY FEATURES of
Pituitary Hypofunction

Deficient Hormone	Clinical Manifestations
Anterior Pituitary Hormones	
Growth hormone (GH)	Decreased bone density Pathologic fractures Decreased muscle strength Increased serum cholesterol levels
Gonadotropins (luteinizing hormone [LH], follicle-stimulating hormone [FSH])	Women: ■ Amenorrhea ■ Anovulation ■ Low circulating estrogen levels ■ Breast atrophy ■ Loss of bone density ■ Decreased axillary and pubic hair ■ Decreased libido ■ Fine facial wrinkles Men: ■ Decreased facial hair ■ Decreased ejaculate volume ■ Reduced muscle mass ■ Loss of bone density ■ Decreased body hair ■ Decreased libido ■ Impotence ■ Fine facial wrinkles
Thyrotropin	Decreased circulating TSH levels
Thyroid-stimulating hormone [TSH]	Decreased circulating thyroid hormone levels Weight gain Intolerance to cold Scalp alopecia Hirsutism Menstrual abnormalities Decreased libido Slowed cognition Lethargy
Adrenocorticotropic hormone (ACTH)	Decreased serum cortisol levels Pale, sallow complexion Malaise and lethargy Anorexia Postural hypotension Headache Hypoglycemia Hyponatremia Decreased axillary and pubic hair (women)
Posterior Pituitary Hormones	

Vasopressin (antidiuretic hormone [ADH])	Diabetes insipidus
	■ Greatly increased urine output
	■ Low urine specific gravity (<1.005)
	■ Hypovolemia
	   Hypotension
	   Dehydration
	■ Increased plasma osmolarity
	■ Increased thirst
	■ Output does not decrease when fluid intake decreases

Data from Melmed, S., & Kleinberg, D. (2003). Anterior pituitary. In P.R. Larsen, et al. (Eds.). *Williams textbook of endocrinology* (10th ed., pp. 281-329). Philadelphia: W. B. Saunders, and from Robinson, A., & Verbalis, J. (2003). Posterior pituitary gland. In P.R. Larsen, et al. (Eds.). *Williams textbook of endocrinology* (10th ed., pp. 177-279). Philadelphia: W. B. Saunders.

loss of or change in secondary sex characteristics in men and women. While assessing the male client, look for facial and body hair loss. Ask about episodes of impotence and decreased libido (sex drive). Women may report **amenorrhea** (absence of menstrual periods), **dyspareunia** (painful intercourse), **infertility** (difficulty becoming pregnant), and decreased libido. While examining the female client, check for dry skin, breast atrophy, and a decreased amount or absence of axillary and pubic hair.

Neurologic manifestations of hypopituitarism due to tumor growth often first occur as changes in vision. Assess the client's visual acuity, especially peripheral vision, for changes or loss. Temporal headaches are a common finding. Other manifestations may include **diplopia** (double vision) and ocular muscle paralysis, limiting eye movement.

Laboratory findings vary widely with hypopituitarism. Some pituitary hormone levels may be measured directly. Often, however, the *effects* of the hormones, rather than their actual levels, are assessed. Basal levels of triiodothyronine (T_3) and thyroxine (T_4) from the thyroid, as well as testosterone and estradiol from the gonads, are measured easily. If levels of one or all of these hormones are low or in the low-normal range, further evaluation is necessary. Levels of pituitary gonadotropins (LH and FSH) and TSH are sufficient if function of the target organ is apparent. Function of LH and FSH is assessed by observing for the presence of secondary sexual characteristics; function of TSH is assessed by measuring circulating levels of thyroid hormones. ACTH levels may be normal or low, and prolactin (PRL) levels are low to high.

Some tests for pituitary function involve injecting agents that are known to stimulate secretion of specific pituitary hormones and then measuring the response. Such tests are called **stimulation tests**. For example, insulin injection in people with normal pituitary function causes an increased release of GH and ACTH. The stimulation test for either GH or ACTH assessment involves injecting the client with regular insulin (0.05 to 1 units/kg of body weight) and checking the circulating levels of GH and ACTH. The stimulation test for TSH involves injecting thyrotropin-releasing hormone (TRH) and measuring the blood levels of thyroid hormones. The stimulation test for LH and FSH involves giving gonadotropin-releasing hormone (GnRH). In people with no pituitary problems, this injection results in a peak release of LH and FSH within 15 to 45 minutes after the injection. Stimulation testing for PRL is the same as for TSH.

Pituitary problems may cause changes in the sella turcica (the bony nest where the pituitary gland rests) that can be seen with skull x-rays. Changes may include enlargement, erosion, and calcifications as a result of pituitary tumors. Computed tomography (CT) and magnetic resonance imaging (MRI) can more distinctly define bone or soft-tissue lesions. An angiogram may be used to rule out the presence of an aneurysm or congenital vascular malformations before any surgical intervention.

◆Interventions

Management of the adult with hypopituitarism focuses on replacement of deficient hormones. Older clients or those with a chronic disease often require a lower amount of hormone replacement. Men who have gonadotropin deficiency receive sex steroid replacement therapy with **androgens** (testosterone). The most effective route of androgen replacement is intramuscular (IM), although use of transdermal testosterone patches is increasing. Instruct the client in self-administration. Therapy begins with high-dose testosterone and is continued until **virilization** (presence of male secondary sex characteristics) is achieved. Maximal effects of treatment include increases in penis size, libido, muscle mass, bone size, and bone strength. Chest, facial, pubic, and axillary hair growth also increases, and the voice deepens. Clients usually report improved self-esteem and body image after therapy is initiated. The dose may then be decreased, but therapy continues throughout life.

Androgen therapy is avoided in men with prostate cancer. Side effects of testosterone therapy include **gynecomastia** (the development of breast tissue in men), acne, baldness, and prostate enlargement.

Achieving fertility in these clients is difficult and requires additional parenteral testosterone therapy and injections of human chorionic gonadotropin (hCG). Teach the client about the course of additional therapy and provide emotional support because the outcome of fertility treatment is uncertain.

Women who have gonadotropin deficiency receive hormone replacement with a combination of estrogen and progesterone. The risk for hypertension or thrombosis (formation of blood clots in deep veins) is increased with estrogen therapy, especially among women who smoke. Emphasize measures to reduce risk and the need for regular health visits. For women who wish to become pregnant, clomiphene citrate (Clomid) may be given to induce ovulation. Gonadotropin-releasing hormone (GnRH) and human chorionic gonadotropin (hCG) are used to stimulate ovulation when therapy with clomiphene citrate fails.

Adult clients with GH deficiency may be treated with injections of GH, although this treatment is rare.

Hyperpituitarism

PATHOPHYSIOLOGY

Hyperpituitarism is hormone oversecretion that occurs with pituitary tumors or hyperplasia. Tumors occur most often in the anterior pituitary cells that produce growth hormone (GH), prolactin (PRL), and adrenocorticotropic hormone (ACTH). Overproduction of PRL also may occur in response to tumors that overproduce GH and ACTH. Hypersecretion of ACTH may occur with increased secretion of melanocyte-stimulating hormone (MSH).

The most common cause of hyperpituitarism is a pituitary adenoma, a benign tumor. Adenomas are classified by size, invasiveness, and the hormone secreted. An invasive pituitary adenoma involves a portion or all of the sella turcica. When the sella turcica is not involved, the adenoma is "enclosed."

As an adenoma gets larger and compresses brain tissue, neurologic symptoms, as well as endocrine symptoms, may occur. Such symptoms may include visual changes, headache, and increased intracranial pressure.

PRL-secreting tumors are the most common type of pituitary adenoma. Excessive PRL inhibits the secretion of gonadotropins and sex hormones in men and women, resulting in galactorrhea (breast milk production), amenorrhea, and infertility.

Overproduction of GH results in **gigantism** (Figure 66-1) or **acromegaly** (Figure 66-2). The onset of the disease may be gradual with slow progression, and changes may remain unnoticed for years before diagnosis of the disorder. Early detection and treatment are essential to prevent irreversible changes in the soft tissues, such as those of the face, hands, feet, and skin. These changes are, to a certain extent, reversible after treatment, but skeletal changes are permanent.

In the client with gigantism, the onset of GH hypersecretion occurs *before* puberty, which causes rapid proportional growth in the length of all bones. In the client with acromegaly, excessive GH secretion occurs *after* puberty and produces increased skeletal thickness, hypertrophy of the skin, and enlargement of many visceral organs, such as the liver and heart.

Bone thinning and bone cell overgrowth occur slowly. Degeneration of joint cartilage and hypertrophy of ligaments, vocal cords, and eustachian tubes are common. Nerve entrapment occurs because of tissue overgrowth and myelin loss in peripheral nerves. Because GH is an insulin **antagonist** (blocks the action of insulin), **hyperglycemia** (elevated blood glucose levels) is also common.

Excess ACTH overstimulates the adrenal cortex. The result is excessive production of glucocorticoids, mineralocorticoids, and androgens, which leads to the development of Cushing's disease (see Hypercortisolism [Cushing's Syndrome], p. 1474).

Etiology and Genetic Risk

Most cases of hyperpituitarism result from hormone-secreting adenomas arising from one pituitary cell type. Hyperpituitarism can also be caused by hypothalamic problems in which excessive amounts of releasing hormones are produced and then overstimulate the normal pituitary gland.

Genetic Considerations

Adenomas can develop in clients without a family history or as part of a syndrome known as multiple endocrine neoplasia (MEN). This familial disorder, inherited as an autosomal dominant trait, may include parathyroid and pancreatic tumors.

Incidence/Prevalence

Hyperpituitarism is a rare disorder. The most common tumors are prolactinomas, followed by GH-producing adenomas. Tumors secreting gonadotropin or thyroid-stimulating hormone (TSH) are the least common. About 70% of all pituitary tumors secrete one or more hormones.

◆ COLLABORATIVE MANAGEMENT
◆ Assessment

HISTORY

The manifestations of hyperpituitarism vary, depending on which hormone is produced in excess. Obtain data about the client's age, gender, and family history. Ask the client about any change in hat, glove, ring, or shoe size. Fatigue and lethargy are common. The client with high GH levels may have backache and **arthralgias** (joint pain) from bone changes. Ask specifically about headaches and changes in vision.

The client with hypersecretion of PRL often reports difficulties in sexual functioning. Ask women about menstrual changes (e.g., amenorrhea, irregular menses, and difficulty in becoming pregnant) and about decreased libido or dyspareunia (painful intercourse). Men may report decreased libido and impotence.

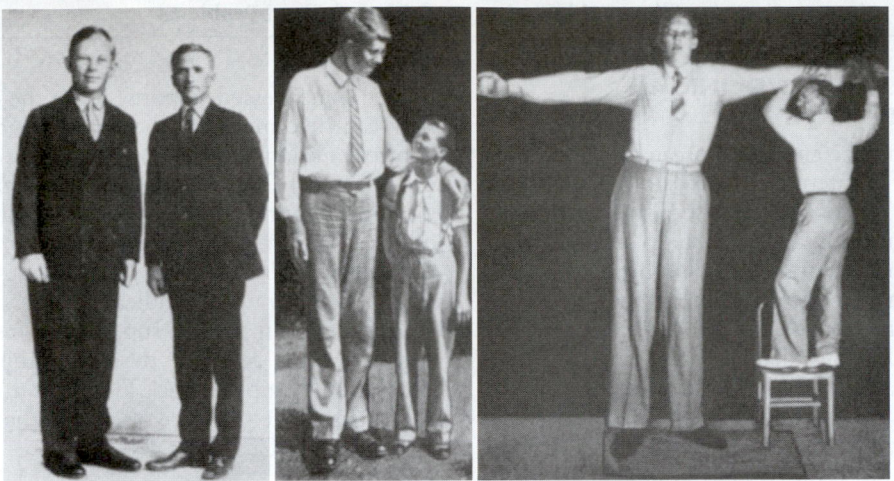

Figure 66-1 ■ The clinical features of growth hormone excess. Robert Wadlow, the "Alton giant," weighed 9 pounds at birth but grew to 30 pounds by the time he was 6 months old. By his first birthday, he had reached 62 pounds. At the time of his death at age 22 from cellulitis of the feet, he was 8 feet 11 inches tall and weighed 475 pounds. Wadlow's family members (left) were normal height and weight.

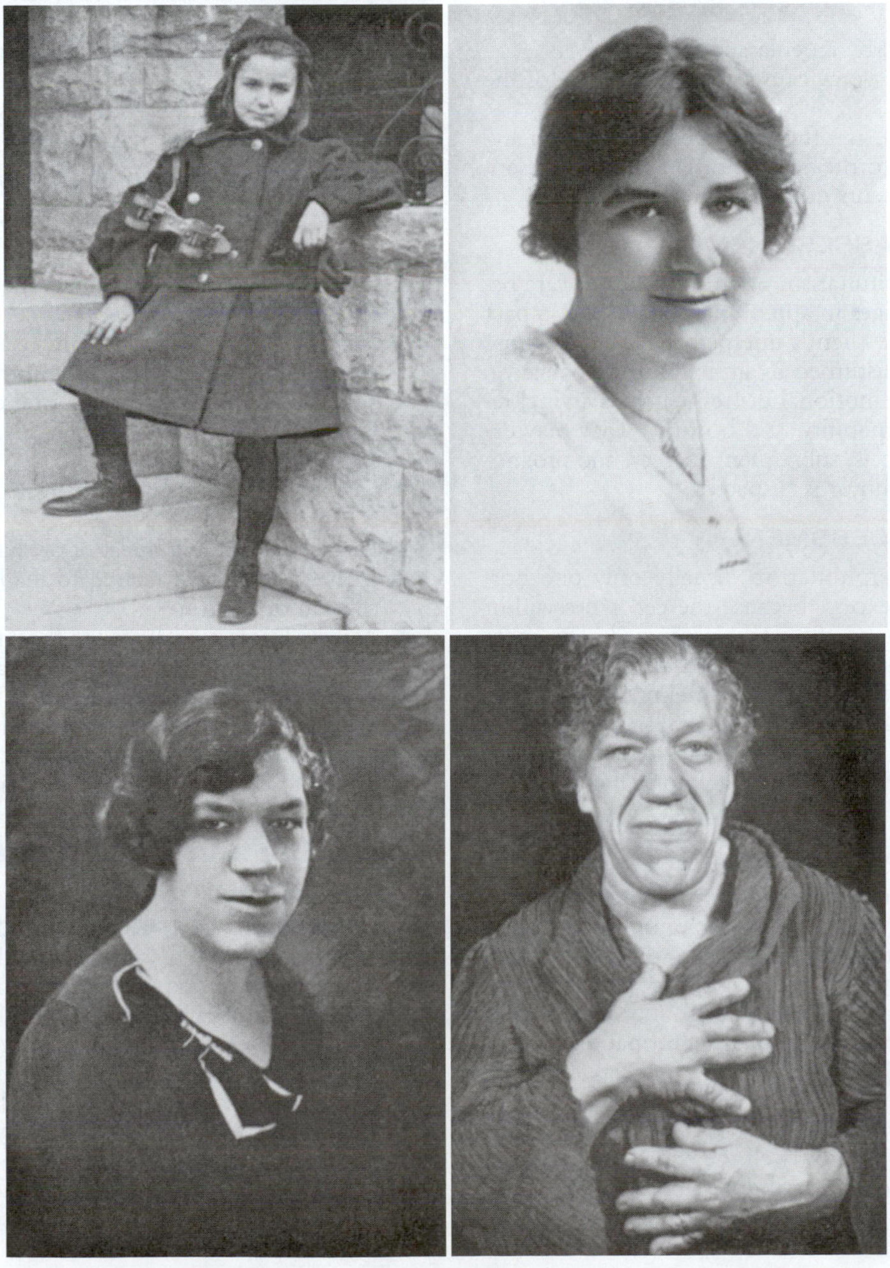

Figure 66-2 ■ The progression of acromegaly.

PHYSICAL ASSESSMENT/CLINICAL MANIFESTATIONS

Some changes in appearance and target organ function occur with excesses of specific anterior pituitary hormones (Chart 66-2). Initial manifestations of GH hypersecretion are changes in the facial features, including increases in lip and nose sizes and a prominent brow ridge; and increases in head, hand, and foot sizes. **Prognathism**, a projection of the jaw beyond the facial features, becomes marked. Assess the client for difficulty in chewing and for dentures that no longer fit. Arthritic changes causing joint pain and decreased mobility may also be noted. Fingers and toes may be thick with an arrowhead shape at the tips. At onset, acromegaly causes increased metabolism and strength. As the disease progresses, these manifestations are replaced with lethargy and weakness.

Assess the client's vision for any changes related to compression of the optic nerves. The client may also have increased perspiration and oil secretion on the skin. Other prominent features include the following:

- Organomegaly (cardiac or hepatic)
- Hypertension
- Dysphagia caused by an enlarged tongue
- Deepening of the voice caused by hypertrophy of the larynx

Hypersecretion of PRL is often observed, along with hypogonadism and galactorrhea. Galactorrhea may be present in either gender but occurs more often in women.

PSYCHOSOCIAL ASSESSMENT

The client with hyperpituitarism often seeks health care because of dramatic changes in appearance. Assess the impact of these changes on the client's interpersonal relationships.

In clients who are disturbed by an inability to conceive, identify symptoms of emotional distress, such as crying, reports of depression, irritability, and hostility. They may express fear of the diagnosis, subsequent surgery, and prognosis, especially when a tumor is suspected.

LABORATORY ASSESSMENT

In a person with hyperpituitarism, usually only one hormone is produced in excess, because the cell types within the pituitary gland are so discretely organized. The most common hormones produced in excess are PRL, ACTH, and GH. Tumors producing TSH, luteinizing hormone (LH), or follicle-stimulating hormone (FSH) are rare. Elevated levels of any of these hormones warrant evaluation. Elevations of LH and FSH, however, are normal in the postmenopausal woman.

RADIOGRAPHIC ASSESSMENT

Radiographic assessment of the client with hyperpituitarism is identical to that for a client with hypopituitarism. Skull x-rays are used to identify abnormalities of the sella turcica. Computed tomography (CT) and magnetic resonance imaging (MRI) can define soft-tissue lesions, and angiography can rule out an aneurysm or vascular malformations.

OTHER DIAGNOSTIC ASSESSMENTS

Rather than just measuring the blood level of a specific hormone, some tests measure how well the endocrine gland responds to stimulation changes. Suppression tests help diagnose hyperpituitarism. These tests involve giving agents that induce a suppressed response from the pituitary gland, and they can determine whether the normal negative feedback control mechanisms for hormonal regulation are intact. For example, high blood glucose levels suppress the release of GH. In a suppression test, 100 g of oral glucose or 0.5 g/kg of body weight is given intravenously (IV). GH levels are measured serially for up to 120 minutes. GH levels that do not fall below 5 ng/mL indicate a positive (abnormal) result.

Another example of a suppression test is the giving of IV cortisol in the form of dexamethasone (Decadron). This drug should suppress ACTH. When ACTH production continues in the presence of dexamethasone, the client may have pituitary Cushing's disease.

◆ Analysis

COMMON NURSING DIAGNOSES AND COLLABORATIVE PROBLEMS

The following are priority nursing diagnoses for clients with hyperpituitarism with excesses of prolactin (PRL) and growth hormone (GH):

1. Disturbed Body Image related to illness or illness treatment
2. Sexual Dysfunction related to disease (related to loss of libido, infertility, impotence)

ADDITIONAL NURSING DIAGNOSES AND COLLABORATIVE PROBLEMS

In addition to the common nursing diagnoses, clients with excessive prolactin or growth hormone also may have one or more of the following:

- Acute Pain and Chronic Pain related to compression of tissues by tumor (e.g., discomfort, headache), backache, or arthralgia secondary to the effects of excessive GH levels or to dyspareunia secondary to excessive PRL levels
- Fear related to a perceived threat of death from an intracranial tumor
- Anxiety related to a threat of or change in health status
- Ineffective Coping related to inadequate level of perception of control
- Activity Intolerance related to the effects of excessive GH levels (e.g., pain or discomfort, lethargy, and weakness)
- Disturbed Sensory Perception (Visual) related to altered sensory reception, transmission, or integration
- Deficient Knowledge (diagnosis and treatment regimen) related to unfamiliarity with information resources

◆ Planning and Implementation

DISTURBED BODY IMAGE

NOC **PLANNING: EXPECTED OUTCOMES.** The client with hyperpituitarism is expected to have a sense of congruence between body reality, body ideal, and body presentation. Indicators include that the client consistently or often demonstrates the following behaviors:

- Adjustment to changes in body function
- Willingness to use strategies to enhance appearance
- Willingness to touch affected body part
- A positive internal picture of self

INTERVENTIONS. The goals of therapy for the client who has hyperpituitarism are to return hormone levels to

CHART 66-2

KEY FEATURES of
Pituitary Hyperfunction

Excess Hormone	Clinical Manifestations
Anterior Pituitary Hormones	
Prolactin (PRL)	Hypogonadism (loss of secondary sexual characteristics)
	Decreased gonadotropin levels
	Galactorrhea
	Increased body fat
	Increased serum prolactin levels
Growth hormone (GH)	Acromegaly
	■ Thickened, oily skin (facial)
	■ Thickened lips
	■ Folding of the scalp skin
	■ Deepening of the voice
	■ Enlarged hands and feet
	■ Increasing head size
	■ Protrusion of the lower jaw
	■ Joint enlargement and pain (knees, hips, and shoulders)
	■ Kyphosis and backache
	■ "Barrel chest"
	■ Excessive sweating (especially of the hands, feet, head, and face)
	■ Coarse facial features
	■ Tufting of the fingertips
	■ Hyperglycemia
	■ Airway narrowing, sleep apnea
	■ Enlarged heart, lungs, and liver
Adrenocorticotropic hormone (ACTH)	Cushing's disease (pituitary)
	■ Elevated plasma cortisol levels
	■ Weight gain
	■ Truncal obesity
	■ "Moon face"
	■ Extremity muscle wasting
	■ Loss of bone density
	■ Hypertension
	■ Hyperglycemia
	■ Purple striae
	■ Acne
	■ Thin, easily damaged skin
	■ Hyperpigmentation
Thyrotropin (thyroid-stimulating hormone [TSH])	Elevated plasma TSH levels
	Elevated plasma thyroid hormone levels
	Weight loss
	Tachycardia
	Heat intolerance
	Increased gastrointestinal (GI) motility
	Fine tremors
Gonadotropins (luteinizing hormone [LH], follicle-stimulating hormone [FSH])	Men:
	■ Elevated LH and FSH levels
	■ Hypogonadism or hypergonadism
	Women:
	■ Normal LH and FSH levels
	(The most common clinical manifestations in men and women are related to the physical presence of a tumor rather than to excessive hormone secretion.)
Posterior Pituitary Hormones	
Vasopressin (antidiuretic hormone [ADH])	Syndrome of inappropriate antidiuretic hormone (SIADH)
	■ Decreased urine output
	■ Increased urine osmolarity
	■ Increased plasma volume
	■ Decreased plasma osmolarity
	■ Weight gain
	■ Hyponatremia
	■ Nonpitting edema
	■ Central nervous system (CNS) changes (confusion, seizures)

Data from Melmed, S., & Kleinberg, D. (2003). Anterior pituitary. In P.R. Larsen, et al. (Eds.). *Williams textbook of endocrinology* (10th ed., pp. 281-329). Philadelphia: W. B. Saunders, and from Robinson, A., & Verbalis, J. (2003). Posterior pituitary gland. In P.R. Larsen, et al. (Eds.). *Williams textbook of endocrinology* (10th ed., pp. 177-279). Philadelphia: W. B. Saunders.

normal or near normal, reduce or eliminate headache and visual disturbances, prevent complications, and reverse as many of the body changes as possible.

NONSURGICAL MANAGEMENT. Encourage the client to express concerns and fears about his or her altered physical appearance. Help the client identify personal strengths and positive characteristics, reinforcing each client's uniqueness and importance.

Galactorrhea, gynecomastia, and reduced sexual functioning can disturb body image and personal identity. Reassure the client that treatment may reverse some of these problems. Encourage the client to discuss his or her feelings.

Drug Therapy. Drug therapy may be used alone or in combination with surgery and/or radiation. The most common drugs used are dopamine agonists, especially bromocriptine mesylate (Parlodel) and cabergoline (Dostinex). These drugs stimulate dopamine receptors in the brain and inhibit the release of many pituitary hormones, most specifically GH and PRL. In most cases, small tumors decrease until the pituitary gland is of normal size. Large pituitary tumors usually decrease to some extent. In clients with acromegaly, bromocriptine reduces GH levels and decreases tumor size, especially when GH levels remain high after surgery or before the full effect of radiation therapy has occurred.

Side effects of bromocriptine include **orthostatic** (postural) hypotension, gastric irritation, nausea, headaches, abdominal cramps, and constipation. Give bromocriptine with a meal or a snack to reduce some of these side effects. Treatment starts with a low dose and is gradually increased until the desired level (usually 7.5 mg/day) is reached. *If pregnancy occurs, the drug is stopped immediately.*

Other agents used for acromegaly are the somatostatin analogues, especially octreotide (Sandostatin), and a growth hormone receptor blocker, pegvisomant (Somavert). Octreotide inhibits GH release through negative feedback. Pegvisomant blocks growth hormone (GH) receptor activity and production of insulin-like growth factor (IGF). Although these therapies are effective, a disadvantage is that they must be given as an injection on a daily or weekly schedule. A major side effect is gallbladder disease. Pegvisomant may cause an increase in tumor size.

Radiation Therapy. Radiation therapy is not useful in the immediate management of acute hyperpituitarism. These therapy regimens take a long time to complete, and several years may pass before a therapeutic effect can be seen. Side effects of radiation therapy include hypopituitarism, optic nerve damage, reduced coordinated eye movement, and visual field defects. Use of the gamma knife procedure is increasing the accuracy of radiation therapy.

SURGICAL MANAGEMENT. Surgical removal of the pituitary gland and tumor (**hypophysectomy**) is the most common treatment for hyperpituitarism.

Preoperative Care. Explain that hypophysectomy decreases hormone levels, relieves headaches, and may reverse changes in sexual functioning. Body changes, organ enlargement, and visual changes are not usually reversible. Explain that because nasal packing is present for 2 to 3 days after surgery, it will be necessary to breathe through the mouth, and a "mustache" dressing ("drip" pad) will be placed under the nose. Instruct the client not to brush teeth, cough, sneeze, blow the nose, or bend forward after surgery. These activities can open the muscle graft, increase intracra-

nial pressure, and delay healing of the incision. Nasal and oral mucous membrane swab specimens for bacterial culture and sensitivity are obtained before surgery because the surgery can move organisms from these areas into the blood and cause systemic infection.

Operative Procedures. A transsphenoidal approach to the pituitary gland is most commonly used (Figure 66-3). Transsphenoidal hypophysectomy is microscopic surgery performed with the client under general anesthesia and in a semi-sitting position. The surgeon makes an incision just above the upper lip and reaches the pituitary gland through the sphenoid sinus. After the gland is removed, a muscle graft is taken, often from the thigh, to support the area and prevent leakage of cerebrospinal fluid (CSF). Nasal packing is inserted after the incision is closed. A mustache dressing is then applied. If the tumor cannot be reached by this approach, a craniotomy may be indicated (see Chapter 48).

Postoperative Care. Monitor the client's neurologic response and document any changes in vision, mental status, altered level of consciousness, or decreased strength of the extremities. Observe the client for complications (e.g., transient diabetes insipidus).

In a client with diabetes insipidus, urine specific gravity is low and urine output is excessive. Monitor the intake of IV fluid, urge fluid intake in response to thirst, and give vasopressin as indicated. A Foley catheter may be inserted for accurate measuring of urine output, and daily weights are taken.

Teach the client to report any postnasal drip, which might indicate leakage of CSF. Keep the head of the bed elevated after surgery. Assess nasal drainage for quantity, quality, and the presence of glucose (which indicates that the fluid is CSF). A light yellow color at the edge of the clear drainage on the dressing is called the "halo sign" and indicates CSF. If the client has persistent, severe headaches, CSF fluid may have leaked into the sinus area. Most CSF leaks resolve with bedrest. If the CSF leak persists, the physician may perform a spinal tap to reduce CSF pressure. Surgical intervention is rarely necessary.

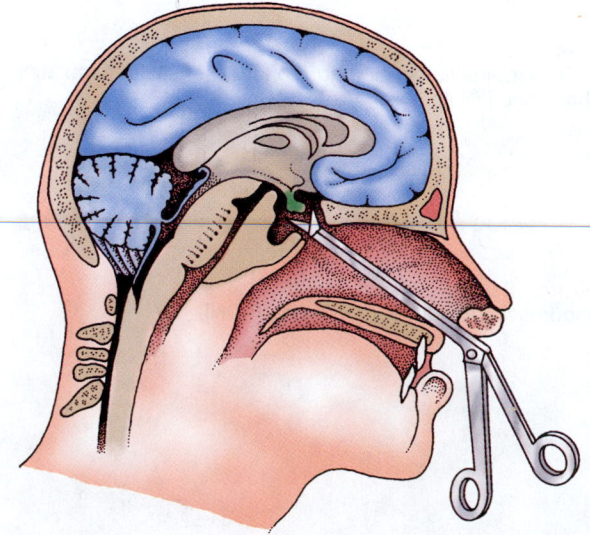

Figure 66-3 ■ The transsphenoidal surgical approach to the pituitary gland. Selective adenomectomy leaves normal pituitary tissue undisturbed.

Teach the client to avoid coughing early after surgery because it increases pressure in the incision area and may lead to a CSF leak. Remind the client to perform deep breathing exercises hourly while awake to prevent pulmonary problems. Clients may also have mouth dryness from mouth breathing. Perform frequent oral rinses and apply petroleum jelly to dry lips.

Infection can occur after surgery. Specifically assess for manifestations of meningitis, such as headache, fever, and nuchal (neck) rigidity. The surgeon may prescribe antibiotics, analgesics, and antipyretics.

If the entire pituitary gland has been removed, thyroid hormones and glucocorticoids must be replaced. Best practices for care after surgery are listed in Chart 66-3.

SEXUAL DYSFUNCTION

NOC **PLANNING: EXPECTED OUTCOMES.** The client with hyperpituitarism is expected to achieve a personally desired level of sexual expression and performance. Indicators include client consistently or often demonstrating the following:

- Expresses sexual interest
- Attains sexual arousal
- Adapts sexual techniques as needed

INTERVENTIONS. Identify the specific problems that the client is experiencing. Encourage the client to discuss any effect that sexual dysfunction has had on his or her sexual partner. Drug therapy with bromocriptine can decrease prolactin (PRL) levels in clients with PRL-secreting tumors. After PRL levels are decreased, gonadotropin function often returns to normal. Clients may have sexual dysfunction from gonadotropin deficiency and need hormone replacement (discussed earlier under Interventions [Hypopituitarism], p. 1459).

Community-Based Care

HOME CARE MANAGEMENT

Clients who have advanced acromegaly may have arthritic changes. Assess the degree of mobility impairment and identify appropriate adaptations, such as the use of ambulatory aids (cane or walker) and the accessibility of bathroom facilities.

After treatment, the client with hyperpituitarism needs daily self-management regimens and frequent checkups. The client may also need to develop strategies to reduce stress. Perform a focused assessment during the first several home visits to a client who has undergone a hypophysectomy (Chart 66-4). Review drug regimens and manifestations of infection and cerebral edema with the family.

HEALTH TEACHING

After a transsphenoidal hypophysectomy, advise the client to avoid activities that might interfere with healing. Bending over from the waist to pick up objects or tie shoes must be avoided because this position increases intracranial pressure (ICP). Teach the client to bend the knees and then lower the body to pick up fallen objects. ICP also increases when the client strains to have a bowel movement. Suggest techniques to prevent constipation, such as eating high-fiber foods, drinking plenty of fluids, and using stool softeners or laxatives. Activities that increase ICP should be avoided for up to 2 months after surgery.

The client must avoid toothbrushing for about 2 weeks after surgery until the incision has healed. Frequent mouth care (every 4 to 6 hours) with mouthwash and daily flossing provides adequate oral hygiene. Numbness in the area of

---

CHART 66-3

BEST PRACTICE for
The Client After Hypophysectomy

- Monitor the client's neurologic status hourly for the first 24 hours, then every 4 hours.
- Monitor fluid balance, especially for output greater than intake, because transient diabetes insipidus can occur.
- Encourage the client to maintain pulmonary hygiene through deep breathing exercises.
- Instruct the client *not* to cough, blow the nose, or sneeze.
- Instruct the client to use dental floss and oral mouth rinses because brushing the teeth is not permitted until the incision heals sufficiently.
- Instruct the client to avoid bending at the waist for any reason, because this position increases intracranial pressure.
- Monitor the nasal drip pad for the type and amount of drainage. The presence of the halo sign may indicate a CSF leak.
- Monitor bowel movements to prevent constipation and subsequent "straining."
- Teach the client self-administration of the prescribed hormones.

CSF, Cerebrospinal fluid.

CHART 66-4

HOME CARE ASSESSMENT of
The Client Who Has Undergone Transsphenoidal Hypophysectomy for Hyperpituitarism

Assess cardiovascular status:
- Vital signs, including apical pulse, pulse pressure, presence or absence of orthostatic hypotension, and the quality/rhythm of peripheral pulses.

Assess cognition and mental status:
- Level of consciousness
- Orientation to time, place, and person
- Accurate reading of a seven-word sentence containing no words longer than three syllables

Assess condition of operative site:
- Observe nasal area for drainage.
  If present, note color, clarity, and odor.
  Test clear drainage for the presence of glucose.

Assess neuromuscular status:
- Reactivity of patellar and biceps reflexes
- Oral temperature
- Handgrip strength
- Steadiness of gait
- Visual fields
- Distant and near visual acuity
- Pupillary responses to light

Assess renal system:
- Observe urine specimen for color, odor, cloudiness, and amount.

Ask about:
- Headaches or visual disturbances
- Ease of bowel movements
- 24-hour fluid intake and output
- 24-hour diet recall
- 24-hour activity recall
- Over-the-counter and prescribed medications taken

Assess client's understanding of illness and adherence with treatment:
- Signs and symptoms to report to health care provider
- Medication plan (correct timing and dose)

the incision and a decreased sense of smell are expected after surgery and usually last 3 to 4 months. Advise the client to use a mirror to check the gums for bleeding, because reduced sensation increases the risk for injury.

After a hypophysectomy, hormone replacement with vasopressin may be needed to maintain fluid balance (see later discussion under Interventions [Diabetes Insipidus], p. 1467). If the anterior portion of the pituitary gland is removed, instruct the client in cortisol, thyroid, and gonadal hormone replacement. Teach the client to report the return of any symptoms of hyperpituitarism immediately to the primary health care provider.

HEALTH CARE RESOURCES

The client with decreased mobility related to acromegaly or who has had recent surgery may require a home care aide or nurse to help maintain activities of daily living (ADLs). The client with hyperpituitarism must have hormone levels monitored at regular intervals to detect tumor recurrence. Regularly scheduled follow-up with the health care team is essential.

◆Evaluation: Outcomes

Evaluate the care of the client with hyperpituitarism on the basis of the identified nursing diagnoses and collaborative problems. The expected outcomes include that the client will:

- ■ Experience an improvement in body image
- ■ Achieve a personal desired level of sexual functioning

Specific indicators for these outcomes are listed for each nursing diagnosis under the Planning and Implementation section (see earlier).

DISORDERS OF THE POSTERIOR PITUITARY GLAND

Disorders of the posterior pituitary gland (**neurohypophysis**) are related to a deficiency or excess of the hormone vasopressin (antidiuretic hormone [ADH]). Diabetes insipidus occurs with ADH deficiency, and the syndrome of inappropriate antidiuretic hormone (SIADH) occurs with ADH excess.

Diabetes Insipidus

PATHOPHYSIOLOGY

Diabetes insipidus (DI) is a water metabolism problem caused by an ADH deficiency (either a decrease in ADH synthesis or an inability of the kidneys to respond to ADH). ADH deficiency results in the excretion of large volumes of dilute urine. Without ADH, distal kidney tubules and collecting ducts remain impermeable to water. Water is excreted as urine rather than being absorbed in these areas, which leads to **polyuria** (excessive water loss through urination) and dehydration.

Dehydration caused by this massive diuresis increases plasma osmolarity, which stimulates the osmoreceptors to relay a sensation of thirst to the cerebral cortex. Thirst promotes increased fluid intake and aids in maintaining water homeostasis. If the thirst mechanism is poor or absent, or if

the person is unable to obtain water, dehydration becomes more severe.

ADH deficiency is classified as nephrogenic, drug-related, primary, or secondary, depending on whether the problem is caused by insufficient production of ADH or an inability of the kidney to respond to the presence of ADH.

Nephrogenic diabetes insipidus is an inherited disorder. The renal tubules do not respond to the actions of ADH, which results in poor water reabsorption by the kidney. The actual amount of hormone produced is not deficient.

Primary diabetes insipidus is caused by a defect in the hypothalamus or pituitary gland, resulting in a lack of ADH production or release. Secondary diabetes insipidus can result from tumors within or adjacent to the hypothalamus or pituitary gland, head trauma, infectious processes, surgical procedures (hypophysectomy), or metastatic tumors, usually from the lung or the breast. Less often, it is caused by brain hemorrhage, brain disease, or cerebral aneurysm, which reduce ADH production.

Drug-related diabetes insipidus is caused by lithium carbonate (Eskalith, Lithobid, Carbolith✦) and demeclocycline (Declomycin). These drugs can interfere with the response of the kidneys to ADH.

◆COLLABORATIVE MANAGEMENT
◆Assessment

Most manifestations of DI are related to dehydration (Chart 66-5). The key manifestations are an increase in the frequency of urination and excessive thirst. Ask about a history of any known etiologic factors, such as recent surgery, head trauma, or drug use (e.g., lithium). Although increased fluid

---

CHART 66-5

KEY FEATURES of
Diabetes Insipidus

Cardiovascular Manifestations
- ■ Hypotension
- ■ Decreased pulse pressure
- ■ Tachycardia
- ■ Peripheral pulses weak, easily obliterated
- ■ Hemoconcentration
     Increased hemoglobin
     Increased hematocrit
     Increased BUN

Renal/Urinary Manifestations
- ■ Increased urine output
     Dilute, low specific gravity
     Hypo-osmolar

Integumentary Manifestations
- ■ Poor turgor
- ■ Dry mucous membranes

Neurologic Manifestations
- ■ Increased sensation of thirst
     Irritability*
     Decreased cognition*
     Hyperthermia*
     Lethargy to coma*
     Ataxia*

BUN, Blood urea nitrogen.
*Occurs when access to water is limited and rapid dehydration results.

intake prevents serious dehydration and volume depletion, the client who is deprived of fluids or who cannot increase oral fluid intake may develop shock from fluid loss. Manifestations of dehydration, such as poor skin turgor and dry or cracked mucous membranes or skin, may be present in varying degrees. (See Chapter 15 for further discussion of dehydration.)

Water loss produces changes in blood and urine tests. The initial step in diagnosis is to measure a 24-hour fluid intake and output. The amount of the client's food and fluid is not restricted during this measurement. Urine output must be more than 4 L during this period for diabetes insipidus to be diagnosed. The amount of urine excreted in 24 hours may vary from 4 to 30 L/day. Urine is dilute with a low specific gravity (less than 1.005) and low osmolarity (50 to 200 mOsm/kg). Dehydration and hypertonic saline tests are also used for diagnosis of the disorder (Table 66-2).

◆ Common Nursing Diagnoses and Collaborative Problems

Nursing diagnoses and collaborative problems that may apply to clients with diabetes insipidus include the following:

- Deficient Fluid Volume related to excessive fluid loss or inadequate fluid intake
- Decreased Cardiac Output related to decreased plasma volume
- Impaired Oral Mucous Membrane related to inadequate oral secretions
- Potential for Dysrhythmias

◆ Interventions

Medical management is aimed at controlling manifestations with drug therapy (Chart 66-6). If only a partial deficit of ADH is present, effective control can be achieved with oral chlorpropamide (Diabinese, Novo-Propamide✱). This drug increases the action of existing ADH and possibly has a stimulating effect on the production of ADH in the hypothalamus.

When ADH deficiency is severe, ADH is replaced in amounts sufficient to maintain water balance. Desmopressin acetate (DDAVP) is a synthetic form of vasopressin given intranasally in a metered spray and is the drug of choice. Chart 66-7 lists some NIC interventions for nasal drugs. The frequency of dosing varies with client responses. Each metered spray delivers 10 mcg, and the client with mild DI may need only one to two doses in 24 hours. For the client with more severe DI, one to two metered doses two to three times daily may be needed. Lypressin (Diapid) is a short-acting form of the drug and is given by nasal spray or subcutaneously when an immediate response is needed. Injections last only 3 to 6 hours. During severe dehydration, ADH may be given IV or IM. Ulceration of the mucous membranes, allergy, a sensation of chest tightness, and pulmonary inhalation of the spray may occur with use of the intranasal preparations. If side effects occur, or if the client has an upper respiratory infection, subcutaneous vasopressin is used.

Nursing management is aimed at the early detection of dehydration and maintaining adequate hydration. Interventions include accurately measuring fluid intake and output, checking urine specific gravity, and recording the client's weight daily.

Urge the client to drink fluids in an amount equal to urine output. If fluids are given IV, ensure the patency of the access catheter and accurately monitor the amount infused hourly.

The client with permanent DI requires lifelong vasopressin therapy. Assess the client's ability to follow instructions and participate in health care. Teach the client that polyuria and polydipsia are signals for the need for another dose. *Teach all clients taking vasopressin to weigh themselves daily to identify weight gain.* Emphasize the importance of using the same scale and weighing at the same time of day while wearing a similar amount of clothing. If weight gain occurs, instruct the client to notify the health care provider. Clients with DI should wear a medical alert bracelet identifying the disorder and the drugs.

TABLE 66-2 Care of the Client Undergoing Special Tests for Diabetes Insipidus

Nursing Interventions	Rationales
Dehydration Test	
Obtain baseline vital signs; then check them hourly.	Assessment permits detection of changes, especially postural hypotension and tachycardia.
Deprive the client of fluid. Observe the client for adherence to fluid restriction.	Fluid restriction must be maintained for test results to be of diagnostic importance.
Measure urine output, specific gravity, and osmolarity hourly.	Urine testing results determine whether testing can proceed.
Weigh the client hourly.	Testing can proceed if urine osmolarity stabilizes for three samples and 3% weight loss is noted.
Give 5 units of aqueous vasopressin (subcutaneously), as prescribed. Continue hourly urine measurements.	Vasopressin triggers—and ongoing assessment detects—changes in urine specific gravity and osmolarity. Specific gravity and osmolarity decrease with primary and secondary diabetes insipidus. No response is seen with nephrogenic diabetes insipidus.
Hypertonic Saline Test (to Stimulate Release of ADH)	
Administer a normal water load to the client, followed by infusion of hypertonic saline. Measure urine output hourly.	The procedure detects ADH release. A sudden decrease in urine output is a sign of ADH release.

ADH, Antidiuretic hormone.

CHART 66-6

DRUG THERAPY for
Diabetes Insipidus

Drug	Usual Dosage	Nursing Interventions	Rationales
Lypressin (Diapid)	4-8 sprays (5-10 pressor units) (nasal spray) in divided doses	Monitor for upper respiratory tract infections or allergy.	The effectiveness of nasal sprays is affected by upper respiratory tract infections.
Desmopressin (DDAVP)	0.1-0.4 mL in single or divided dose (nasal spray)	Teach the client the proper method of administration. Instruct the client to sit upright when spraying.	Some clients may have difficulty with measuring and inhaling. An upright position promotes effective absorption in the nasal mucosa.
Aqueous vasopressin [1](Pitressin)	5-20 units in divided doses (SC, IM, or nasal spray)	Instruct the client to hold his or her breath when using nasal spray. Monitor the client's intake and output. Have the client space fluid intake during waking hours. Monitor the client frequently (every 3-4 hr) for a recurrence of symptoms. Monitor the client's weight.	Holding one's breath prevents nasal spray from entering the lungs and potentially causing pneumonia. Intake and output measurement helps to guide dosage regulation. Extra fluid intake at night can cause nocturia. Monitoring detects the need for additional doses of these short-acting medications. Water retention can be detected by weight gain.
[2]Chlorpropamide (Diabinese, Novo-Propamide✹)	125-250 mg PO every other day *Older adults:* 100-125 mg PO every other day	Monitor the client for signs and symptoms of hypoglycemia.	Hypoglycemia is a potentially severe side effect.
Indomethacin (Indocin, Indameth✹)	25-50 mg PO three times daily	Teach client to observe for bruising and for bleeding gums. Drug should be discontinued before surgery or dental work.	Disrupts platelet activity. Excessive bleeding could result.

[1]**Med Error Alert!** *Do not confuse with Pitocin, an oxytocic hormone used to induce labor.*

[2]**Med Error Alert!** *Do not confuse with chlorpromazine, an antiemetic, or with chlorothiazide, a diuretic.*

SC, Subcutaneous; *SIADH,* syndrome of inappropriate antidiuretic hormone.

Critical Thinking Challenge

The client is your neighbor, a 34-year-old man who is being treated for gastroesophageal reflux disease with omeprazole (Prilosec) daily for this problem. He also has bipolar disorder for which he takes lithium. During the fall pollen season, he uses over-the-counter Benadryl and also takes ibuprofen occasionally for muscle and joint aches. He tells you that he thinks he may have diabetes mellitus or prostate problems like his father because he has to get up at least five times per night to urinate. In addition, he tells you that he is constantly thirsty and drinks a lot of water and coffee.

1. How are diabetes mellitus and diabetes insipidus similar and how are they different?
2. Which of this client's drugs could contribute to manifestations of diabetes insipidus?
3. Is his father's history of diabetes mellitus or prostate problems important in this client's health consideration?

evolve For suggested answer guidelines, go to http://evolve.elsevier.com/Iggy/.

CHART 66-7

NIC INTERVENTION ACTIVITIES for
The Client with Diabetes Insipidus

Medication Administration: Nasal: *Preparing and giving medications via nasal passages*
- Instruct client to blow nose gently prior to administration of nasal medication, unless contraindicated.
- Instruct client to remain upright and to not tilt head backward when nasal spray is administered.
- Insert nozzle into nostril and squeeze bottle quickly and firmly when nasal spray is administered.
- Instruct client not to blow nose for several minutes after administration.
- Monitor client to determine response to medication.

NIC intervention activities selected from Dochterman, J.M., & Bulechek, G.M. (Eds.). (2004). *Nursing interventions classification (NIC)* (4th ed.). St. Louis: Mosby. No part of this work is to be altered without prior written permission from the Publisher.

Syndrome of Inappropriate Antidiuretic Hormone

PATHOPHYSIOLOGY

The **syndrome of inappropriate antidiuretic hormone (SIADH)** occurs when vasopressin (antidiuretic hormone [ADH]) is secreted even when plasma osmolarity is low or normal. A decrease in plasma osmolarity normally inhibits ADH production and secretion. SIADH is also known as the Schwartz-Bartter syndrome. SIADH is also discussed in Chapter 28 as a complication of cancer and cancer therapy. SIADH occurs with many pathologic conditions and specific drugs. Table 66-3 lists common causes of SIADH.

In SIADH, the feedback mechanisms that regulate ADH do not function properly. ADH continues to be released even when plasma is hyposmolar. Water is *retained*, which results in dilutional **hyponatremia** (a decreased serum sodium level) and expansion of the extracellular fluid volume. The increase in plasma volume causes an increase in the glomerular filtration rate and inhibits the release of renin and aldosterone. The combined effect is an increased sodium loss in urine, leading to greater hyponatremia.

◆ COLLABORATIVE MANAGEMENT
◆ Assessment

HISTORY

Ask the client about his or her medical history, which may reveal conditions that occur with the development of SIADH. Information about the following conditions should be obtained:

- Recent head trauma
- Cerebrovascular disease
- Tuberculosis or other pulmonary disease
- Cancer
- All past and current drug use

PHYSICAL ASSESSMENT/CLINICAL MANIFESTATIONS

The early manifestations of SIADH are related to water retention. Gastrointestinal (GI) disturbances, such as loss of appetite, nausea, and vomiting, may occur first. Weigh the client and document any recent weight gain. In clients with SIADH, free water (not salt) is retained and dependent edema is not usually present, even though water is retained.

Water retention, hyponatremia, and fluid shifts affect central nervous system function, especially when the serum sodium level drops below 115 mEq/L. The client may have lethargy, headaches, hostility, disorientation, and a change in level of consciousness. Manifestations can progress from lethargy and headaches to decreased responsiveness, seizures, and coma. Assess deep tendon reflexes, which are often decreased.

Vital sign changes include tachycardia (caused by the increased fluid volume) and hypothermia (caused by central nervous system disturbance). Chapter 16 presents other findings that occur with hyponatremia.

DIAGNOSTIC ASSESSMENT

Water retention changes both plasma and urine osmolarity. Urine volume decreases and urine osmolarity increases. Plasma volume increases and plasma osmolarity decreases. Elevated urine sodium levels and specific gravity reflect increased urine concentration. Serum sodium levels are decreased, often as low as 110 mEq/L, because of fluid retention and sodium loss.

Radioimmunoassay of ADH can diagnose SIADH when ADH levels are inappropriately elevated when plasma osmolarity is normal or decreased.

◆ Interventions

Interventions to treat SIADH focus on restricting fluid intake, promoting the excretion of water, replacing lost sodium, interfering with the action of ADH, and preventing injury.

Fluid Restriction. Fluid restriction is essential because fluid intake further dilutes the plasma sodium levels. In some cases, fluid intake may be kept as low as 500 to 600 mL/24 hr. Dilute tube feedings with a solution other than plain water, and use saline to irrigate GI tubes. Mix drugs to be given by GI tube with saline.

Measure intake, output, and daily weights to assess the degree of fluid restriction needed. A weight gain of 2 pounds or more per day or a gradual increase over several days is cause for concern. A 1-kg weight increase is equal to a 1000-mL fluid retention (1 kg = 1 L). The client is uncomfortable during fluid restriction. Keep mucous membranes moist by offering frequent oral rinsing (remind the client not to swallow the rinses).

Drug Therapy. Diuretics may be used to treat SIADH, particularly if heart failure results from fluid overload. Be aware of the diuretic effects on sodium loss. Sodium loss can be potentiated, further contributing to the problems caused by SIADH.

Hypertonic saline (i.e., 3% sodium chloride [3% NaCl]) is often used to treat SIADH. Give IV saline cautiously because it may add to existing fluid overload and promote heart failure. If the client needs routine IV fluids, a saline solution rather than a water solution is prescribed.

Drugs such as lithium carbonate (Eskalith, Lithobid, Carbolith❋) and demeclocycline (Declomycin) may help treat SIADH. Lithium is seldom used because of its toxicity; demeclocycline is used more commonly.

Providing a Safe Environment. Observe for and document changes in the client's neurologic status. Assess for subtle changes, such as muscle twitching, before they

---

TABLE 66-3 Conditions Causing the Syndrome of Inappropriate Antidiuretic Hormone

Malignancies	CNS Disorders
■ Small cell carcinoma of the lung	■ Trauma
■ Pancreatic, duodenal, and GU carcinomas	■ Infection
■ Thymoma	■ Tumors (primary or metastatic)
■ Hodgkin's lymphoma	■ Strokes
■ Non-Hodgkin's lymphoma	■ Porphyria
	■ Systemic lupus erythematosus
Pulmonary Disorders	**Drugs**
■ Viral and bacterial pneumonia	■ Exogenous ADH
■ Lung abscesses	■ Chlorpropamide
■ Active tuberculosis	■ Vincristine
■ Pneumothorax	■ Cyclophosphamide
■ Chronic lung diseases	■ Carbamazepine
■ Mycoses	■ Opioids
■ Positive-pressure ventilation	■ Tricyclic antidepressants
	■ General anesthetics

ADH, Antidiuretic hormone; *CNS,* central nervous system; *GU,* Genitourinary.

progress to seizures or coma. Check orientation to time, place, and person every 2 hours because disorientation or confusion may be present. Reduce environmental noise and lighting to prevent overstimulation.

Flow sheets with continuing information about the level of consciousness, motor and sensory neurologic assessments, and laboratory data are helpful in detecting neurologic trends. The frequency of neurologic checks depends on the client's status. For the client with SIADH who is hyponatremic but alert, awake, and oriented, neurologic checks every 4 hours are sufficient. For the client who has had a change in level of consciousness, perform neurologic checks at least every hour. Inspect the environment every shift, making sure that basic safety measures, such as siderails being securely in place, are observed.

Disorders of the Adrenal Gland

ADRENAL GLAND HYPOFUNCTION

PATHOPHYSIOLOGY

Production of adrenocortical steroids may decrease as a result of inadequate secretion of adrenocorticotropic hormone (ACTH), dysfunction of the hypothalamic-pituitary control mechanism, and dysfunction of adrenal gland tissue. Manifestations may develop gradually or occur quickly with stress. In acute adrenocortical insufficiency (**adrenal crisis**), life-threatening manifestations may appear without warning.

Loss of the adrenal medulla, which produces **catecholamines** (dopamine, norepinephrine, and epinephrine), does not upset the maintenance of homeostasis. This is because catecholamines are also released from other areas in the sympathetic nervous system.

However, insufficiency of adrenocortical steroids causes problems through the loss of aldosterone and cortisol action. Impaired secretion of cortisol results in decreased **gluconeogenesis** (making glucose from proteins) along with depletion of liver and muscle glycogen, leading to **hypoglycemia** (low blood glucose levels). The glomerular filtration rate and gastric acid production decrease, leading to reduced urea nitrogen excretion, causing anorexia and weight loss.

Reduced aldosterone secretion causes potassium, sodium, and water imbalances. Potassium excretion is decreased, causing hyperkalemia. Sodium and water excretion is increased, causing hyponatremia and hypovolemia. Potassium retention also promotes reabsorption of hydrogen ions, which can lead to acidosis.

Low adrenal androgen levels decrease the body, axillary, and pubic hair, especially in women, because the adrenals produce most of the androgens in females. The severity of symptoms is related to the degree of hormone deficiency.

Acute adrenal insufficiency, or **Addisonian crisis**, is a life-threatening event in which the need for cortisol and aldosterone is greater than the available supply. Often, acute insufficiency occurs in response to a stressful event (e.g., surgery, trauma, or severe infection), especially when the adrenal hormone output is already reduced. The problems of acute adrenal insufficiency are almost the same as that of

chronic insufficiency. In clients with acute adrenal crisis related to bilateral adrenal hemorrhage, however, sodium and potassium levels may be normal because the time between the event and the presentation may be too short for a change in electrolyte composition to occur. Unless intervention is initiated promptly, however, sodium levels fall and potassium levels rise rapidly. More severe hypotension results from the blood volume depletion that occurs with the loss of aldosterone. Best practices for emergency care of clients with acute adrenal insufficiency are listed in Chart 66-8.

Adrenal insufficiency is classified as primary or secondary. Causes of primary and secondary adrenal insufficiency are listed in Table 66-4. One of the most common causes of secondary adrenal insufficiency is the sudden cessation of long-term, high-dose glucocorticoid therapy. This therapy suppresses production of glucocorticoids through negative feedback by causing atrophy of the adrenal cortex. Glucocorticoid drugs must be withdrawn gradually to allow for pituitary production of ACTH and activation of adrenal cells to produce cortisol.

◆ COLLABORATIVE MANAGEMENT
◆ Assessment

HISTORY

While taking a history from the client with possible adrenal insufficiency, ask questions about manifestations and factors that cause adrenal hypofunction. Ask about any change in activity level, because lethargy, fatigue, and muscle weak-

---

CHART 66-8

BEST PRACTICE for
Emergency Care of the Client with Acute Adrenal Insufficiency

EMERGENCY CARE

Hormone Replacement
- Start rapid infusion of normal saline or dextrose 5% in normal saline.
- Initial dose of hydrocortisone sodium succinate (Solu-Cortef) is 100 to 300 mg or dexamethasone 4 to 12 mg as an IV bolus.
- Infuse additional 100 mg of hydrocortisone sodium succinate by continuous IV drip over the next 8 hours.
- Give hydrocortisone 50 mg IM concomitantly every 12 hours.
- Initiate an H_2 histamine blocker (e.g., ranitidine) IV for ulcer prevention.

Hyperkalemia Management
- Administer insulin (20 to 50 units) with dextrose (20 to 50 mg) in normal saline to shift potassium into cells.
- Administer potassium binding and excreting resin (e.g., Kayexalate).
- Give loop or thiazide diuretics.
- Avoid potassium-sparing diuretics.
- Initiate potassium restriction.
- Monitor intake and output.
- Monitor heart rate, rhythm, and ECG for manifestations of hyperkalemia (slow heart rate, block, tall peaked T-waves, fibrillation, asystole).

Hypoglycemia Management
- Administer IV glucose.
- Administer glucagon, as needed.
- Maintain IV access.
- Monitor blood glucose level hourly.

ECG, Electrocardiogram.

TABLE 66-4	Causes of Primary and Secondary Adrenal Insufficiency

Primary Causes
- Idiopathic (autoimmune) disease*
- Tuberculosis
- Metastatic cancer
- Fungal lesions
- AIDS
- Hemorrhage
- Gram-negative sepsis (Waterhouse-Friderichsen syndrome)
- Adrenalectomy
- Abdominal radiation therapy
- Drugs (mitotane) and toxins

Secondary Causes
- Pituitary tumors
- Postpartum pituitary necrosis (Sheehan's syndrome)
- Hypophysectomy
- High-dose pituitary radiation
- High-dose whole-brain radiation

*Most common cause.

CHART 66-9

KEY FEATURES of
Adrenal Insufficiency

Neuromuscular Manifestations
- Muscle weakness
- Fatigue
- Joint/muscle pain

Gastrointestinal Manifestations
- Anorexia
- Nausea, vomiting
- Abdominal pain
- Bowel changes (constipation/diarrhea)
- Weight loss
- Salt craving

Integumentary Manifestations
- Vitiligo
- Hyperpigmentation

Cardiovascular Manifestations
- Anemia
- Hypotension
- Hyponatremia
- Hyperkalemia
- Hypercalcemia

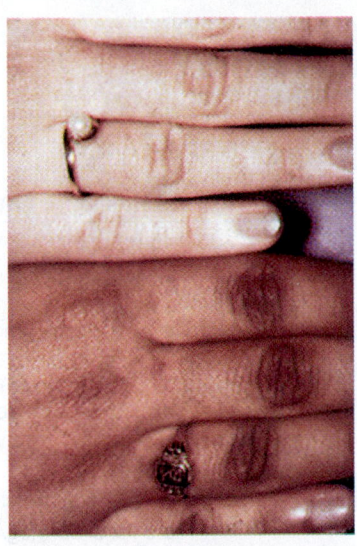

Figure 66-4 ■ The increased pigmentation seen in primary adrenocortical insufficiency.

PSYCHOSOCIAL ASSESSMENT

Depending on the degree of imbalance, clients may appear lethargic, depressed, confused, and even psychotic. Observe the client and check his or her orientation to person, place, and time. Families may report that the client has a decreased energy level, experiences wide mood swings, and is forgetful.

DIAGNOSTIC ASSESSMENT

Laboratory findings include low serum cortisol, low fasting blood glucose, low sodium, elevated potassium, and increased serum blood urea nitrogen (BUN) levels (Chart 66-10). In primary disease, the eosinophil count and ACTH level are elevated. Plasma cortisol levels do not rise during stimulation tests.

Urinary 17-hydroxycorticosteroids are the glucocorticoid metabolites, and 17-ketosteroid levels reflect the adrenal androgen metabolites. Both levels are in the low or low-normal range in adrenal hypofunction. Table 66-5 lists drugs that can interfere with test results.

Skull x-rays, computed tomography (CT), magnetic resonance imaging (MRI), and arteriography may help determine the cause of pituitary problems leading to adrenal insufficiency.

Noninvasive procedures of the adrenal gland, such as CT scans without dye, may show atrophy of the gland. CT scans may help determine adrenal hypofunction.

An ACTH stimulation test is the most definitive test for adrenal insufficiency. A rapid ACTH stimulation test may be performed on an outpatient basis. ACTH 0.25 to 1 mg is given IV, and plasma cortisol levels are obtained at 30-minute and 1-hour intervals. In primary insufficiency, the cortisol response is absent or markedly decreased; in secondary insufficiency, it is increased.

A longer ACTH stimulation test uses a continuous infusion of 50 units of ACTH in saline for 24 hours or an 8-hour infusion daily for 4 to 5 days, with simultaneously collected 24-hour urine samples. Levels of urinary 17-hydroxycorticosteroids and urinary free cortisol are also measured. In primary adrenal insufficiency, the response is low or absent; in

---

ness are often present. Include questions about salt intake because salt craving often occurs with hypofunction.

Gastrointestinal (GI) problems, such as anorexia, nausea, vomiting, diarrhea, and abdominal pain, often occur. Ask about weight loss during the past months. Women may have menstrual changes related to weight loss, and men may report impotence.

Ask whether the client has had radiation to the abdomen or head. Document medical problems (e.g., tuberculosis or previous intracranial surgery) and all past and current drugs, especially steroids, anticoagulants, opioids, or cytotoxic drugs.

PHYSICAL ASSESSMENT/CLINICAL MANIFESTATIONS

The manifestations of adrenal insufficiency vary, and the severity is related to the degree of hormone deficiency (Chart 66-9). In clients with primary insufficiency, plasma ACTH and melanocyte-stimulating hormone (MSH) levels are elevated because of the loss of the adrenal-hypothalamic-pituitary feedback system. Elevated MSH levels result in areas of increased pigmentation (Figure 66-4). In primary autoimmune disease, areas of decreased pigmentation may occur because of destruction of pigment-producing cells in the skin (melanocytes). Body hair may also be decreased. In secondary disease, there is no change in skin pigmentation.

Assess for manifestations of hypoglycemia (e.g., sweating, headaches, tachycardia, and tremors) and volume depletion (postural hypotension and dehydration). **Hyperkalemia** (elevated blood levels of potassium) can cause dysrhythmias with an irregular heart rate and result in cardiac arrest.

CHART 66-10

LABORATORY PROFILE
Adrenal Gland Assessment

Test	Normal Range for Adults	Significance of Abnormal Findings	
		Hypofunction of the Adrenal Gland	Hyperfunction of the Adrenal Gland
Sodium	136-145 mEq/L	Decreased	Increased
Potassium	3.5-5.0 mEq/L	Increased	Decreased
Glucose	70-115 mg/dL *Older adults:* slightly increased	Normal to decreased	Normal to increased
Calcium	9-10.5 mg/dL (total) 4.5-5.6 mg/dL (ionized) *Older adults:* slightly decreased	Increased	Decreased
Bicarbonate	21-28 mEq/L	Increased	Decreased
BUN	10-20 mg/dL *Older adults:* may be slightly higher	Increased	Normal
Cortisol	6 AM to 8 AM 5-23 mcg/dL or 138-635 SI units (nmol/L) 4 PM to 6 PM 3-16 mcg/dL or 83-359 SI units (nmol/L)	Decreased	Increased

BUN, Blood urea nitrogen; *SI*, System Internationale.

TABLE 66-5 Drugs That Interfere with Tests for Urinary 17-Hydroxycorticosteroids and Urinary 17-Ketosteroids

- Acetaminophen
- Acetazolamide
- Acetylsalicylic acid
- Amphetamines
- Ascorbic acid
- Barbiturates
- Calcium gluconate
- Carbon disulfide
- Chloral hydrate
- Chlordiazepoxide
- Chlormerodrin
- Chlorothiazide
- Chlorpromazine
- Chlorthalidone
- Colchicine
- Corticotropin
- Cortisone
- Dexamethasone
- Diazepam
- Digitoxin
- Digoxin
- Diphenhydramine
- Diphenylhydantoin
- Erythromycin
- Estrogens
- Fructose
- Glutethimide
- Hydralazine
- Iodides
- Medroxyprogesterone
- Meperidine
- Meprobamate
- Metyrapone
- Mitotane
- Morphine
- Nalidixic acid
- Oral contraceptives
- Paraldehyde
- Penicillin
- Pentazocine
- Perphenazine
- Phenobarbital
- Phenothiazines
- Phenylbutazone
- Promazine
- Propoxyphene
- Quinidine
- Quinine
- Reserpine
- Secobarbital
- Spironolactone
- Testosterone
- Vitamin K

secondary insufficiency, the value for 17-hydroxycortico-steroids fails to rise above 20 mg per total volume.

Common Nursing Diagnoses and Collaborative Problems

Nursing diagnoses that may apply to clients with adrenal gland hypofunction include the following:
- Decreased Cardiac Output related to decreased vascular volume and hyperkalemia

- Risk for Injury related to hypoglycemia
- Fatigue related to disease state

Interventions

Nursing interventions aim to promote fluid balance and monitor for fluid deficit (Chart 66-11). Weigh the client daily and record intake and output. Assess vital signs every 1 to 4 hours, depending on the client's condition and the presence of dysrhythmias or postural hypotension. Monitor laboratory values to identify hemoconcentration (e.g., increased hematocrit or BUN). Chapter 15 discusses fluid volume deficit in detail.

Cortisol and aldosterone deficiencies are corrected by replacement therapy. Hydrocortisone corrects glucocorticoid deficiency (Chart 66-12). Therapy replacement regimens vary. Generally, divided doses are given, with two thirds given in the morning and one third in the late afternoon to mimic the normal release of this hormone. Although most clients do well on this regimen, some may not tolerate the dosage or may need more.

An additional mineralocorticoid hormone, such as fludrocortisone (Florinef), may be needed to maintain electrolyte balance (especially sodium and potassium). Dosage adjustment may be needed, especially in hot weather, when more sodium is lost because of excessive perspiration. *Salt restriction or diuretic therapy should not be started without considering whether it might lead to an adrenal crisis.*

Critical Thinking Challenge

The client is a 60-year-old woman who was taking 80 mg of oral prednisone daily for 10 weeks because of a severe pulmonary problem. Her pulmonary problem has resolved and she tapered down her prednisone dose by 10 mg daily for 8 days. It has now been 10 days since her last dose. She is brought to the emergency department by her family who say that she is too weak to walk, has poor memory, and seems confused. They tell you about her prednisone therapy. On admission, her

CHART 66-11

NIC **INTERVENTION ACTIVITIES for**
The Client with Adrenal Insufficiency

Electrolyte Management: Hyperkalemia: *Promotion of potassium balance and prevention of complications resulting from serum potassium levels higher than desired*
- Administer electrolyte-binding and electrolyte-excreting resins (e.g., Kayexalate) as prescribed, if appropriate.
- Monitor lab values for changes in oxygenation or acid-base balance, as appropriate.
- Administer prescribed medications to shift potassium into the cell (e.g., 50% dextrose and insulin, sodium bicarbonate, calcium chloride, and calcium gluconate), as appropriate.
- Avoid potassium-sparing medications (e.g., spironolactone [Aldactone] and triamterene [Dyrenium]), as appropriate.
- Maintain potassium restrictions.
- Administer prescribed diuretics, as appropriate.
- Monitor fluid status, including intake and output, as appropriate.
- Monitor potassium levels after diuresis.
- Monitor cardiac manifestations of hyperkalemia (e.g., decreased cardiac output, heart blocks, peaked T waves, fibrillation, or asystole).
- Respond to cardiac arrest.

Hypoglycemia Management: *Preventing and treating low blood glucose levels*
- Determine recognition of hypoglycemia signs and symptoms.
- Monitor blood glucose levels, as indicated.
- Monitor for signs and symptoms of hypoglycemia (e.g., shakiness, tremor, sweating, nervousness, anxiety, irritability, impatience, tachycardia, palpitations, chills, clamminess, light-headedness, pallor, hunger, nausea, headache, tiredness, drowsiness, weakness, warmth, dizziness, faintness, blurred vision, nightmares, crying out in sleep, paresthesias, difficulty concentrating, difficulty speaking, incoordination, behavior change, confusion, coma, seizure).
- Provide simple carbohydrate, as indicated.
- Administer glucagon, as indicated.
- Maintain IV access, as appropriate.
- Instruct client and significant others on signs and symptoms, risk factors, and treatment of hypoglycemia.
- Instruct client to have simple carbohydrate available at all times.
- Instruct client to obtain and carry/wear appropriate emergency identification.

NIC intervention activities selected from Dochterman, J.M., & Bulechek, G.M. (Eds.). (2004). *Nursing interventions classification (NIC)* (4th ed.). St. Louis: Mosby. No part of this work is to be altered without prior written permission from the Publisher.

CHART 66-12

DRUG THERAPY for
Hypofunction of the Adrenal Gland

Drug	Usual Dosage	Nursing Interventions	Rationales
Cortisone	25-50 mg PO either once daily in AM or daily in divided doses	Instruct the client to take the drug with meals or a snack.	Gastrointestinal irritation can occur.
Hydrocortisone (Cortef, Hycort ✽)	20-50 mg PO either once daily in AM or daily in divided doses	Instruct the client to report the following signs or symptoms of excessive drug therapy:	Cushing's syndrome, which indicates a need for dosage adjustment, can occur.
Prednisone (Winpred ✽)	5-10 mg PO either once daily in AM or daily in divided doses	■ Rapid weight gain ■ Round face ■ Fluid retention	
Fludrocortisone (Florinef)	0.05-0.2 mg PO daily	Instruct the client to report illness, such as: ■ Severe diarrhea ■ Vomiting ■ Fever	Other conditions may indicate a need for dosage change. The usual daily dosage may not be adequate during periods of illness or severe stress.
Med Error Alert! *Drug name is similar to prednisolone, another corticosteroid that is 4 to 5 times more potent than prednisone.*		Monitor the client's blood pressure. Instruct the client to report weight gain or edema.	Hypertension is a potential side effect. Sodium-related fluid retention is possible.

vital signs are T 97; P 58, thready, with some "dropped" beats; R 14 and shallow; BP 92/50.

1. Should this client be seen in the emergency department or should she be told to make an appointment with either her primary care physician or her pulmonologist?
2. What other assessment data should you obtain?
3. What is the probable cause of this client's manifestations?
4. Should this client be started on oxygen? Why or why not?
5. Should an IV line be started on this client? If so, what fluid should you use?

evolve For suggested answer guidelines, go to http://evolve.elsevier.com/Iggy/.

ADRENAL GLAND HYPERFUNCTION

The adrenal gland may oversecrete just one hormone or all adrenal hormones. Hypersecretion by the adrenal cortex results in hypercortisolism (e.g., **Cushing's disease** or **Cushing's syndrome**), **hyperaldosteronism** (excessive mineralocorticoid production), or excessive androgen production.

Hyperstimulation of the adrenal medulla caused by a tumor (**pheochromocytoma**) results in excessive secretion of catecholamines, of which 80% is epinephrine and the remainder is norepinephrine.

Hypercortisolism (Cushing's Disease)
PATHOPHYSIOLOGY

Cushing's disease exaggerates the normal actions of glucocorticoids, causing widespread problems. Excessive stimulation of adrenocorticotropic hormone (ACTH) of either pituitary or ectopic origin causes adrenocortical hyperplasia, which disrupts normal hormone secretion rhythms. The client's endocrine tissues are less responsive to releasing hormones, especially prolactin (PRL), thyrotropin, and gonadotropin. Many clients also have abnormal sleep patterns. These changes are due to excessive amounts of glucocorticoids.

The client with Cushing's disease has problems in nitrogen, carbohydrate, and mineral metabolism. An increase in total body fat results from slow turnover of plasma fatty acids. This fat is redistributed to produce the typical body pattern of truncal obesity, "buffalo hump," and "moon face" (Figure 66-5). Increases in the breakdown of tissue protein and an increase in urine nitrogen excretion also occur, resulting in decreased muscle mass, thin skin, and bone density loss.

High levels of corticosteroids kill lymphocytes and shrink organs containing lymphocytes, such as the liver, the spleen, and the lymph nodes. Eosinophils and macrophages are reduced. Although the number of neutrophils may be increased, the reduction of cytokines makes these cells less active. Thus protection of the inflammatory and immune responses is reduced.

In most cases, increased androgen production causes acne, **hirsutism** (increased hair growth), and occasionally clitoral hypertrophy. Increased androgen production can also interrupt the normal hormone feedback mechanism for the ovary, decreasing the ovary's production of estrogens and progesterone. **Oligomenorrhea** (scant or infrequent menses) occurs as a result.

Cushing's disease or syndrome is a group of clinical problems caused by an excess of cortisol, secreted by the adrenal cortex (**endogenous** [Cushing's disease) or given for another clinical disorder (**exogenous** or **iatrogenic** [Cushing's syndrome]). Table 66-6 lists causes of cortisol excess. Women are more likely than men to develop Cushing's disease. Clients of either gender are at equal risk for Cushing's syndrome as a result of chronic use of exogenous corticosteroids.

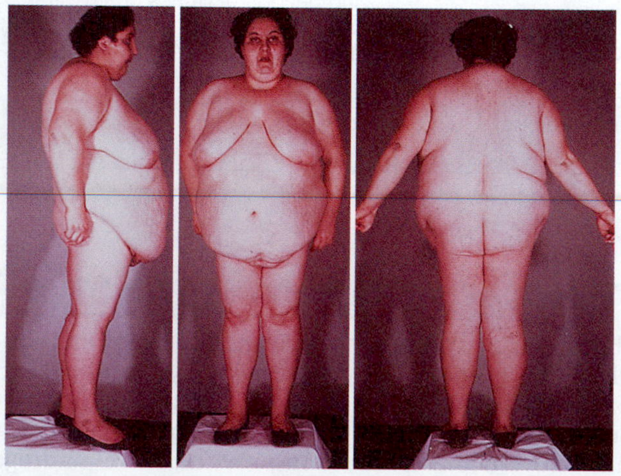

◆COLLABORATIVE MANAGEMENT
◆Assessment
HISTORY

The client with hypercortisolism has many changes because of the widespread effect of excessive cortisol levels. Ask about changes in activity or sleep patterns, fatigue, and muscle weakness. Ask about bone pain or a history of fractures because osteoporosis is common in hypercortisolism. Ask about a history of frequent infections and easy bruising, which suggest hypercortisolism. Women may report a cessation of menses. Gastrointestinal (GI) problems include ulcer formation from increased hydrochloric acid secretion and decreased production of protective gastric mucous.

Check the client's medical history. Steroid or alcohol abuse can induce the manifestations of Cushing's syndrome.

PHYSICAL ASSESSMENT/CLINICAL MANIFESTATIONS

The client with hypercortisolism has specific physical changes (see Figure 66-5 and Chart 66-13). Observe the client's general appearance. Changes in fat distribution may result in fat pads on the neck, back, and shoulders ("buffalo hump"); an enlarged trunk with thin arms and legs; and a round face ("moon face"). Other changes include muscle wasting and weakness.

Inspect for skin changes resulting from increased blood vessel fragility, such as bruises, thin or translucent skin, and wounds that have not healed. Reddish purple **striae** ("stretch marks") are often present on the abdomen, thighs, and upper arms because of the degradative effect of cortisol on collagen.

Excessive cortisol secretion may result in acne and a fine coating of hair over the face and body. In women, look for the presence of hirsutism, clitoral hypertrophy, and male pattern balding related to androgen excess.

Elevated blood glucose levels are common. Hypertension may occur from water and sodium retention.

Figure 66-5 ■ The typical appearance of a client with Cushing's disease or syndrome. Note truncal obesity, moon face, buffalo hump, thinner arms and legs, and abdominal striae. (From Jarvis, C. [2000]. Physical examination and health assessment [3rd ed.]. Philadelphia: W. B. Saunders, p. 210. Reprinted with permission.)

TABLE 66-6 Conditions Causing Increased Cortisol Secretion

Endogenous Secretion (Cushing's Disease)
- Bilateral adrenal hyperplasia*
- Pituitary adenoma increasing the production of ACTH (pituitary Cushing's disease)
- Malignancies: carcinomas of the lung, gastrointestinal tract, pancreas
- Adrenal adenomas or carcinomas

Exogenous Administration (Cushing's Syndrome)
- Therapeutic use of ACTH or glucocorticoids—most commonly for treatment of:
    Asthma
    Autoimmune disorders
    Organ transplantation
    Cancer chemotherapy
    Allergic responses
    Chronic fibrosis

ACTH, Adrenocorticotropic hormone.
*Most common cause.

The client with chronic hypercortisolism is immunosuppressed. The excess cortisol reduces the number of circulating lymphocytes, inhibits maturation of macrophages, reduces antibody synthesis, and inhibits production of cytokines and inflammatory chemicals (e.g., histamine). Not only are these clients at greater risk for infection, they may not have the expected inflammatory manifestations (fever, purulent exudate, redness in the affected area) when an infection is present.

PSYCHOSOCIAL ASSESSMENT

Hypercortisolism can result in emotional lability. Ask about mood swings, irritability, confusion, or depression. The client may have neurotic or psychotic behavior as a result of high blood cortisol levels.

DIAGNOSTIC ASSESSMENT

Plasma cortisol levels are high in clients with hypercortisolism. Blood for cortisol assays is obtained at the same time of day because levels vary throughout the day. Further diagnostic testing is performed to confirm the diagnosis of hypercortisolism, because an increase in cortisol levels is also seen in acute illness and trauma. Plasma ACTH levels vary,

depending on the cause of hypercortisolism. In ectopic (ACTH-producing) syndromes, ACTH levels are elevated. In primary Cushing's disease or when Cushing's syndrome results from chronic steroid use, ACTH levels are very low. Additional laboratory findings include the following:

- Increased blood glucose level
- Decreased lymphocyte count
- Increased sodium level
- Decreased serum calcium level
- Decreased serum potassium level

Urine is tested to measure levels of free cortisol and the metabolites of cortisol and androgens (17-hydroxycorticosteroids and 17-ketosteroids). Instruct the client to save *all* urine for 24 hours. In Cushing's disease, levels of urine cortisol, 17-ketosteroids, and 17-hydroxycorticosteroids are all elevated, as are urine calcium, potassium, and glucose levels.

X-rays, computed tomography (CT) scans, magnetic resonance imaging (MRI), and arteriography may identify lesions of the adrenal or pituitary glands, lung, GI tract, or pancreas.

The *overnight dexamethasone suppression test* is an initial screening test for Cushing's disease. Instruct the client not to take drugs, especially phenytoin (Dilantin) or phenobarbital, for at least 2 days before the test. Normally, plasma cortisol levels are lower than 5 mg/dL. Higher levels indicate that further testing is needed.

For the *3-day, low-dose* dexamethasone suppression test, the client must take no drugs for at least 2 days before the test (if possible) and have no stressful procedures (e.g., barium enema, myelogram, or an intense physical therapy session) performed during the test. Table 66-5 lists drugs that interfere with testing. A baseline 24-hour urine sample is collected on day 1. Dexamethasone 0.5 mg is given every 6 hours on days 2 and 3, during which time 24-hour urine collections are taken. The 24-hour urine collections are tested for 17-ketosteroids, 17-hydroxycorticosteroids, creatinine, and urine cortisol. Normally, urinary 17-hydroxycorticosteroid excretion and cortisol levels are suppressed by dexamethasone, and Cushing's disease is ruled out. If these levels are not suppressed, a higher-dose dexamethasone test is performed.

The *high-dose* (8-mg) dexamethasone suppression test distinguishes between bilateral adrenocortical hyperplasia (e.g., Cushing's disease) and an adrenocortical neoplasm as the cause of hypercortisolism. This test can be performed as an overnight test or a 2-day test and uses higher doses of dexamethasone. In the overnight test, the client with Cushing's disease has a reduced plasma cortisol level that is less than 50% of baseline. This test is more reliable than the 2-day high-dose test.

◆ Common Nursing Diagnoses and Collaborative Problems

Nursing diagnoses that may apply to clients with Cushing's disease or Cushing's syndrome include the following:

- Disturbed Body Image related to illness
- Fatigue related to sleep deprivation
- Excess Fluid Volume related to excess water and sodium reabsorption
- Risk for Infection related to immunosuppression and inadequate primary defenses

---

CHART 66-13

KEY FEATURES of
Hypercortisolism (Cushing's Disease/Syndrome)

General Appearance
- Fat redistribution
  - Moon face
  - Buffalo hump
  - Truncal obesity
- Weight gain

Cardiovascular Manifestations
- Hypertension
- Increased risk for thromboembolic events
- Frequent dependent edema
- Capillary fragility
  - Bruising
  - Petechiae

Musculoskeletal Manifestations
- Muscle atrophy (most apparent in extremities)
- Osteoporosis (bone density loss)
  - Pathologic fractures
  - Decreased height with vertebral collapse
  - Aseptic necrosis of the femur head
  - Slow or poor healing of bone fractures

Skin Manifestations
- Thinning skin ("paper-like" appearance, especially on the back of the hands)
- Striae
- Increased pigmentation (with ectopic or pituitary production of ACTH)

Immune System Manifestations
- Increased risk for infection
- Decreased immune function
  - Decreased circulating lymphocytes
  - Decreased production of immunoglobulins (antibodies)
- Decreased inflammatory responses
  - Decreased eosinophil count
  - Slight increase in neutrophil count but activity is reduced
- Decreased production of proinflammatory cytokines, histamine, and prostaglandins
- Manifestations of infection/inflammation may be masked

- Risk for Injury related to poor wound healing and bone density loss
- Deficient Knowledge (Illness and Treatment) related to lack of interest in learning and unfamiliarity with information resources
- Imbalanced Nutrition: More Than Body Requirements related to excess intake in relation to metabolic need as a result of appetite stimulation by cortisol

◆Interventions

Goals of treatment for hypercortisolism are the reduction of plasma cortisol levels, removal of tumors, prevention of complications, and restoration of normal or acceptable body appearance.

NONSURGICAL MANAGEMENT. Weigh the client daily and monitor intake and output to assess hydration status. Fluid intake restriction is sometimes needed to maintain fluid balance.

Drug Therapy. Most clients with endogenous hypercortisolism undergo surgery. Drugs that interfere with adrenocorticotropic hormone (ACTH) production or adrenal hormone synthesis, however, may be used for temporary relief. Mitotane (Lysodren) is an adrenal cytotoxic agent used for inoperable adrenal tumors. Aminoglutethimide (Elipten, Cytadren) and metyrapone (Metopirone) use different pathways to decrease cortisol production. For clients with hypercortisolism from increased ACTH production, cyproheptadine (Periactin) may be used because it interferes with ACTH production. Assess the client for therapy effectiveness and side effects or toxicity.

Radiation Therapy. Radiation may be used to treat hypercortisolism caused by pituitary adenomas. However, radiation is not always effective and often destroys normal tissue. Observe for any changes in the client's neurologic status, such as headache, elevated blood pressure or pulse, disorientation, or changes in pupil size or reaction. The client may have skin dryness, redness, flushing, or alopecia at the radiation site. Review these possible side effects with the client. Chapter 48 discusses radiation therapy to the head.

SURGICAL MANAGEMENT. The surgical treatment of adrenocortical hypersecretion depends on the cause of the disease. When adrenal hyperfunction is due to increased pituitary secretion of ACTH, removal of a pituitary adenoma may be attempted. In many instances, a total **hypophysectomy** (surgical removal of the pituitary gland) is needed. Hypophysectomy is performed via the transsphenoidal or transfrontal craniotomy route. (See earlier discussion of hypophysectomy on pp. 1464-1465; see also Chapter 48 for nursing care of clients undergoing a craniotomy.) If hypercortisolism is caused by adrenal tumors, a partial or complete **adrenalectomy** (removal of the adrenal gland) may be needed.

Preoperative Care. Electrolyte imbalances are corrected before surgery. Continue to monitor blood potassium, sodium, and chloride levels. Dysrhythmias from potassium imbalance may occur, and cardiac monitoring is needed. Hyperglycemia is controlled before surgery, and blood glucose levels are monitored.

The client with hypercortisolism is at risk for complications such as infections and fractures. Prevent infection with handwashing and aseptic technique. Decrease the risk for falls by raising bed siderails and encouraging the client to ask for assistance when getting out of bed. A high-calorie, high-protein diet is prescribed before surgery.

Glucocorticoid preparations are given before surgery. The client continues to receive glucocorticoids during surgery to prevent adrenal crisis because the removal of the tumor results in a sudden drop in cortisol levels. Before surgery, discuss the care needs for after surgery and the need for long-term drug therapy.

Operative Procedures. A unilateral adrenalectomy is performed when one gland is involved. A bilateral adrenalectomy is needed when ectopic ACTH-producing tumors cannot be treated by other means or when both adrenal glands are diseased.

Surgery can be abdominal or through the lateral flank. Abdominal surgery causes a higher degree of illness and risk. The flank approach is preferred because the abdominal cavity is not entered and complications are reduced. A laparoscopic adrenalectomy may reduce complications after surgery.

Postoperative Care. After an adrenalectomy, the client is usually sent to a critical care unit. Immediately after surgery, assess the client every 15 minutes for shock (e.g., hypotension, a rapid, weak pulse, and a decreasing urine output) due to possible insufficient glucocorticoid replacement. Monitor ongoing vital signs and other hemodynamic variables (central venous pressure, pulmonary wedge pressure), intake and output, daily weights, and serum electrolyte levels.

After a bilateral adrenalectomy, clients require lifelong glucocorticoid replacement, starting immediately after surgery. In unilateral adrenalectomy, glucocorticoid replacement continues until the remaining adrenal gland increases hormone production. This therapy may be needed for up to 2 years after surgery.

Preventing Complications. The client who has hypercortisolism is at risk for injury from skin breakdown, bone fractures, and gastrointestinal (GI) bleeding. Prevention of such injuries is a major nursing care focus.

Skin Breakdown. Assess the client's skin for reddened areas, excoriation, breakdown, and edema. If mobility is decreased, turn the client every 2 hours and pad bony prominences.

Instruct the client to avoid activities that can result in skin trauma. To reduce tissue injury, teach the client to use a soft toothbrush and an electric shaver. Instruct clients to keep the skin clean and to dry it thoroughly after washing. Excessive dryness can be prevented by using a moisturizing lotion.

Adhesive tape often causes skin breakdown. Use tape sparingly and use caution when removing it. After venipuncture or arterial puncture, the client may have increased bleeding because of blood vessel fragility. Exert pressure over the site for longer than normal to prevent bleeding and bruising.

Pathologic Fractures. Hypercortisolism causes bone density loss and osteoporosis. Teach the client about safety issues and dietary needs. The client is at risk for fractures as a result of minor falls or bumps. When helping the client to move in bed, use a lift sheet instead of grasping him or her. Instruct the client to call for help when ambulating. Review the use of ambulatory aids (walkers or canes), if needed. Keep rooms free of extraneous objects that might cause a fall.

Consult with a dietitian to counsel the client about diet therapy. A high-calorie diet is prescribed that includes items from all of the major food groups and increased amounts of calcium and vitamin D. Generous amounts of milk, cheese, yogurt, and green leafy and root vegetables add calcium. Advise the client to avoid caffeine and alcohol, which increase the risk for GI ulcers and may promote bone density loss.

Gastrointestinal Bleeding. Interventions aim to reduce gastric irritation, usually through drug therapy. Drug therapy involves agents that protect the GI mucosa and those that decrease the secretion of hydrochloric acid.

AGENTS PROTECTING THE GASTROINTESTINAL MUCOSA. Antacids buffer stomach acids and protect the GI mucosa. Teach the client that these drugs should be taken on a regular schedule, rather than on an as-needed basis.

AGENTS INHIBITING THE SECRETION OF HYDROCHLORIC ACID. Some agents block the H_2-receptor site in the gastric mucosa. When histamine binds to this receptor site, a series of actions occur that release hydrochloric acid. Drugs that block the H_2-receptor site include cimetidine (Tagamet, Peptol✲, Novo-Cimetine✲), ranitidine (Zantac, Apo-Ranitidine✲), famotidine (Pepcid), and nizatidine (Axid). Omeprazole (Losec✲, Prilosec) and esomeprazole (Nexium) inhibit the gastric proton pump and prevent the formation of hydrochloric acid.

PREVENTION OF IRRITATION. Encourage the client to reduce or eliminate habits that contribute to gastric irritation, such as consuming alcohol or caffeine, smoking, and fasting. Discuss other prescribed and over-the-counter drugs that the client may be taking. Nonsteroidal anti-inflammatory drugs (NSAIDs) and drugs that contain aspirin or other salicylates can cause gastritis and intensify GI bleeding.

CLIENT EDUCATION. Lifelong hormone replacement is needed after bilateral adrenalectomy. Teach the client and family about adherence with the drug regimen and its side effects (Chart 66-14). Wearing a medical alert bracelet is essential.

Hyperaldosteronism
PATHOPHYSIOLOGY

In clients with hyperaldosteronism, increased secretion of aldosterone results in mineralocorticoid excess. Primary hyperaldosteronism (Conn's syndrome) results from excessive

---

CHART 66-14

CLIENT EDUCATION GUIDE
Cortisol Replacement Therapy

- Take your medication in divided doses, the first dose in the morning and the second dose between 4 and 6 PM.
- Take your medication with meals or snacks.
- Weigh yourself daily.
- Increase your dosage as directed for increased physical stress or severe emotional stress, including surgery, dental work, influenza, fever, pregnancy, and family problems.
- Never skip a dose of medication. If you have persistent vomiting or severe diarrhea and cannot take your medication by mouth for 24 to 36 hours, call your physician. If you cannot reach your physician, go to the nearest emergency department. You may need an injection to take the place of your usual oral medication.
- Always wear your medical alert bracelet or necklace.
- Make regular visits for health care follow-up.
- Learn how to give yourself an intramuscular injection of hydrocortisone.

---

secretion of aldosterone from one or both adrenal glands. Most often, this is caused by an adrenal adenoma. In a person with secondary hyperaldosteronism, the excessive secretion of aldosterone is caused by high levels of angiotensin II that are stimulated by high plasma renin levels. Causes of high renin levels include renal hypoxemia and the use of thiazide diuretics.

Increased aldosterone levels affect the renal tubules and cause sodium retention with potassium and hydrogen ion excretion. Hypernatremia, hypokalemia, and metabolic alkalosis result. Sodium retention increases blood volume, which raises blood pressure and suppresses renin production. The elevated blood pressure may cause strokes and renal damage. Peripheral edema rarely occurs because of the "renal escape mechanism," in which the kidney decreases sodium reabsorption. However, no compensatory mechanism exists to stop or reverse potassium loss. (See Chapter 16 for discussion of electrolyte imbalances.)

◆ COLLABORATIVE MANAGEMENT
◆ Assessment

Problems from hypokalemia and elevated blood pressure are the most common issues of the client with hyperaldosteronism. The client may have headache, fatigue, muscle weakness, **nocturia** (excessive urination at night), and loss of stamina. **Polydipsia** (excessive fluid intake) and **polyuria** (excessive urine output) occur less frequently. **Paresthesias** (sensations of numbness and tingling) may occur if potassium depletion is severe. The client may have visual changes related to hypertension.

The diagnosis of hyperaldosteronism is made on the basis of laboratory studies, x-rays, and imaging with CT or MRI. Serum potassium levels are decreased, and sodium levels are elevated. Plasma renin levels are low; aldosterone levels are high. Increased hydrogen ion loss leads to metabolic alkalemia (elevated blood pH). Urine has a low specific gravity and high aldosterone levels.

◆ Interventions

Surgery is the most common treatment for early stage hyperaldosteronism. One or both adrenal glands may be removed. Surgery is not performed, however, until the client's potassium levels are normal. Drugs used to increase potassium levels include spironolactone (Aldactone, Novospiroton✲, Sincomen✲), a potassium-sparing diuretic and aldosterone antagonist. Potassium supplements may be prescribed to increase potassium levels before surgery. The client may also benefit from a low-sodium diet before surgery, but sodium restriction is not needed after surgery because aldosterone levels should return to normal.

The client who has undergone a unilateral adrenalectomy may need temporary glucocorticoid replacement. Replacement is lifelong if both adrenal glands are removed. Glucocorticoids are given before surgery to prevent adrenal crisis. The client receiving long-term replacement therapy should wear a medical alert bracelet. (See the discussion of adrenalectomy under Hypercortisolism [Cushing's syndrome], p. 1476, for more discussion of care after surgery and client education.)

When surgery cannot be performed, spironolactone therapy is continued to control hypokalemia and hypertension. *Because spironolactone is a potassium-sparing diuretic, hyperkalemia can occur in clients who have impaired renal function or excessive potassium intake.* Advise the client to avoid potassium supplements and foods rich in potassium (see Chart 16-6). Hyponatremia can occur with spironolactone therapy and the client may need increased dietary sodium. Instruct the client to report symptoms of hyponatremia, such as dryness of the mouth, thirst, lethargy, or drowsiness. Teach clients to report any additional side effects of spironolactone therapy, including gynecomastia, diarrhea, drowsiness, headache, rash, **urticaria** (hives), confusion, erectile dysfunction, hirsutism, and amenorrhea.

Pheochromocytoma

PATHOPHYSIOLOGY

Pheochromocytoma is a catecholamine-producing tumor that arises in chromaffin cells. These tumors usually occur as a single lesion in the right adrenal gland, although they can be bilateral or in the abdomen. Pheochromocytomas are most often benign, but about 10% are malignant. The tumors produce and store catecholamines.

Pheochromocytomas release epinephrine and norepinephrine (NE). Excessive epinephrine and NE stimulate alpha receptors and beta receptors and can have wide-ranging adverse effects mimicking the action of the sympathetic division of the autonomic nervous system.

The cause is unknown but some pheochromocytomas occur with inherited disorders such as neurofibromatosis and multiple endocrine neoplasia (MEN) syndromes. These tumors are rare and occur slightly more often in women. They can occur at any age but appear most commonly in clients between 40 and 60 years of age.

◆COLLABORATIVE MANAGEMENT
◆Assessment

The client often has intermittent episodes of hypertension or attacks that vary in length from a few minutes to several hours. During these episodes, the client has severe headaches, palpitations, profuse diaphoresis, flushing, apprehension, or a sense of impending doom. Pain in the chest or abdomen, with nausea and vomiting, can also occur. Increased abdominal pressure, urination, and vigorous abdominal palpation, can provoke a hypertensive crisis. Drugs, such as tricyclic antidepressants, droperidol, glucagon, metoclopramide, phenothiazines, and naloxone can induce a hypertensive crisis in ~~e~~ client with pheochromocytoma. Foods or beverages high ~~i~~ ~~ty~~ramine (e.g., aged cheese, red wine) also induce hyper~~tension~~. The client may also report heat intolerance, weight ~~loss, and~~ ~~t~~remors.

~~Diagnosti~~c tests include 24-hour urine collections for ~~vanillylmandeli~~c acid (VMA) (a product of catecholamine ~~metabolism), me~~tanephrine, and catecholamines, all of ~~which indicate~~ the presence of a pheochromocytoma. ~~Guidelines for VM~~A testing are listed in Chart 66-15. ~~These lev~~els are elevated after the client has ~~an attack.~~ The clonidine suppression test ~~distinguishes p~~heochromocytoma when the ~~results are incon~~sistent. When oral cloni~~dine (Catapres~~ ~~■~~) is given to a person ~~without pheochromocyt~~oma, the clonidine

CHART 66-15

BEST PRACTICE for
Vanillylmandelic Acid Testing

- Describe the test to the client and explain that his or her participation is needed for accurate test results.
- Instruct the client on the special vanillylmandelic acid (VMA)–restricted diet that starts 2 or 3 days before the 24-hour urine collection.
- Restricted foods include those containing caffeine (coffee, tea, cola, and chocolate or cocoa), certain fruits (citrus fruits and bananas), vanilla-containing foods, and licorice. Check your laboratory for a more inclusive food list.
- Confer with the physician about which medications should not be given during the 3- or 4-day test. Medications usually withheld include aspirin and antihypertensive agents.
- Be aware that strenuous physical activity, stress, and starvation can increase VMA levels; monitor, intervene, and teach the client as appropriate.
- Instruct the client about how to collect an accurate 24-hour urine sample: the collection is started with an empty bladder, and then all urine formed over the next 24 hours is collected in one container. At the end of the 24-hour period, the client voids and adds that urine to the collection.
- Obtain a urine collection container with preservative from the laboratory. Check with the laboratory about keeping the collection on ice.
- When the collection is complete, send the urine to the laboratory promptly.
- Help the client understand the test results; normal VMA excretion in 24 hours is 2 to 7 mg, or 10 to 35 µmol.

suppresses catecholamine release and reduces the serum catecholamine levels. This response is not seen in the client who has a pheochromocytoma.

Catecholamine stimulation tests, such as with glucagon, can help diagnose a pheochromocytoma; however, the danger of uncontrolled hypertension and effects on the heart limit the usefulness of this type of testing.

MRI or CT scans can precisely locate tumors in the adrenal gland. After diagnosis, computed tomography (CT) scans of the chest and abdomen may be used to locate any other tumors.

◆Interventions

Surgery is the main treatment for a pheochromocytoma. One or both adrenal glands are removed (depending on whether the tumor is bilateral). After surgery, focus on promoting adequate tissue perfusion, nutritional needs, and comfort measures.

Hypertension is the hallmark of the disease. Monitor the blood pressure regularly and place the cuff consistently on the same arm, with the client in lying and standing positions. Identify stressors that may lead to a hypertensive crisis and attempt to reduce them. Instruct the client not to smoke, drink caffeine-containing beverages, or change position suddenly. *Do not palpate the abdomen because this action could cause a sudden release of catecholamines and severe hypertension.* Provide a diet rich in calories, vitamins, and minerals.

The client often benefits from hydration before surgery because decreased blood volume increases the risk for hypotension during and after surgery. Assess the client's hydration status and report manifestations of dehydration or fluid overload.

Provide a calm, restful environment for the client who has a severe headache. Instruct the client to limit activity. A private, darkened room helps promote rest. If the client is sleeping, avoid interruptions if possible.

The client's blood pressure is stabilized with alpha-adrenergic blocking agents before surgery because of the increased risk for severe hypertension during surgery. Anesthetic agents and touching of the tumor during surgery can cause a catecholamine release. Short-acting alpha-adrenergic blockers are given by IV bolus or drip for a hypertensive crisis. Phenoxybenzamine (Dibenzyline) produces long-acting alpha-adrenergic blockade and is often used for management of hypertension before surgery. It is also used for management of the client who is not a candidate for surgery.

The drug dosages are adjusted for 2 to 3 weeks before surgery until blood pressure is controlled and hypertensive attacks do not occur. The blood volume expands, and blood pressure in the supine position returns to normal.

Beta-adrenergic blocking agents are avoided in clients with a pheochromocytoma until after alpha-adrenergic blockade is in effect, because these drugs may cause a rebound rise in blood pressure. After alpha-adrenergic blockade, low doses of propranolol (Inderal, Detensol✱) or labetalol (Trandate) may be used to treat tachycardia and dysrhythmias. Other drugs used for blood pressure control before surgery include calcium channel blockers, such as nicardipine (Cardene) and agents that suppress catecholamine synthesis such as metyrosine (Demser).

Nursing care after surgery is similar to that for the client who has undergone an adrenalectomy (see Hypercortisolism [Cushing's Syndrome], p. 1474). Closely monitor the client for hypotension (from the sudden decrease in catecholamine levels) and for hypovolemia. Hemorrhage and shock are possible, and plasma expanders or fluids may be needed. Monitor vital signs, as well as fluid intake and output. If opioids are given, check for their effect on blood pressure.

Tumors may be inoperable because of the client's other medical conditions. Treatment then is medical, with alpha-adrenergic and beta-adrenergic blocking agents, because the tumors do not respond well to chemotherapy or radiation therapy. For clients who are medically managed, self-measurement of blood pressure with home monitoring equipment is essential.

GET READY for the NCLEX Examination!

KEY POINTS

Safe Effective Care Environment

- Handle all clients with bone density loss carefully, using lift sheets whenever possible.
- Teach the client and family about the clinical manifestations of infection and when to seek medical advice.
- Use good handwashing techniques before providing any care to a client who is immunocompromised from hypercortisolism.

Health Promotion and Maintenance

- Teach all people about the hazards of using any unprescribed hormonal or steroid agents.

Psychosocial Integrity

- Allow the client the opportunity to express fear or anxiety regarding a change in health status.
- Explain all diagnostic procedures, restrictions, and follow-up care to the client scheduled for tests.
- Allow clients who experience a change in physical appearance to mourn this change.

Physiological Integrity

- Ensure that hormone replacement drugs are given as close to the prescribed times as possible.
- Use bleeding precautions for clients who have hypercortisolism.
- Teach clients who have permanent endocrine hypofunction the proper techniques and timing of hormone replacement therapy.
- During the immediate period after a transsphenoidal hypophysectomy, teach the client to avoid activities that increase intracranial pressure (e.g., bending at the waist, straining to have a bowel movement, coughing).
- Measure intake and output accurately on clients who have either diabetes insipidus or syndrome of inappropriate antidiuretic hormone (SIADH).
- Teach clients with diabetes insipidus the proper way to self-administer vasopressin nasal spray.
- Teach the client with diabetes insipidus the manifestations of dehydration.
- Instruct the client with adrenal insufficiency to wear a medical alert bracelet and to carry simple carbohydrates with them at all times.
- Do not palpate the abdomen of a client who has a pheochromocytoma.

ADDITIONAL STUDY RESOURCES

Go to your Student CD-ROM for Review Questions for the NCLEX Examination.

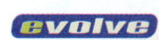 Go to http://evolve.elsevier.com/Iggy/ for Integrated Management of Care Questions for the NCLEX Examination.

SELECTED BIBLIOGRAPHY

Ackley, B., & Ladwig, G. (2002). *Nursing diagnosis handbook: A guide to planning care* (5th ed.). St. Louis: Mosby.

Carson, P. (2000). Emergency: Adrenal crisis. *American Journal of Nursing, 100*(7), 49-50.

Castiglione, V. (2000). Emergency: Hyperkalemia. *American Journal of Nursing, 100*(1), 55-56.

Daub, K. (2002). Pheochromocytoma, up close and personal. *Nursing2002, 32*(3), 32hn1-32hn4.

Dluhy, R., Lawrence, J., & Williams, G. (2003). Endocrine hypertension. In P.R. Larsen, et al. (Eds.), *Williams textbook of endocrinology* (10th ed., pp. 551-585). Philadelphia: W. B. Saunders.

Dochterman, J., & Bulechek, G. (Eds.). (2004). *Nursing interventions classification (NIC)* (4th ed.). St. Louis: Mosby.

Ebersole, P., Hess, P., & Luggen, A. (2004). *Toward healthy aging: Human needs and nursing response* (6th ed.). St. Louis: Mosby.

Facts and Comparisons. (2004). *Drug facts and comparisons* (58th ed.). St. Louis: Author.

Goldberg, M. (2000). The diagnostic challenge—Hyperaldosteronism caused by bilateral adrenal hyperplasia. *Emergency Medicine, 32*(3), 55-56.

Holcomb, S. (2002). Stopping the cascade of diabetes insipidus. *Nursing2002, 32*(3), 32cc1-32cc6.

Kearney, K. (2000). Emergency: Adrenal crisis. *American Journal of Nursing, 100*(7), 49-50.

Langfeldt, L., & Cooley, M. (2003). Syndrome of inappropriate antidiuretic hormone secretion in malignancy: Review and implications for nursing management. *Clinical Journal of Oncology Nursing, 7*(4), 425-430.

Larsen, P.R., et al. (Eds.). *Williams textbook of endocrinology* (10th ed.). Philadelphia: W. B. Saunders.

LoBuono, C. (2001). Managing geriatric endocrine disorders. *Patient Care for the Nurse Practitioner, 4*(11), 26-36.

McCance, K., & Huether, S. (2002). *Pathophysiology: The biologic basis for disease in adults and children* (4th ed.). St. Louis: Mosby.

McConnell, E. (2002). Myths and facts about Addison's disease. *Nursing2002, 32*(8), 79.

Melmed, S., & Kleinberg, D. (2003). Anterior pituitary. In P.R. Larsen, et al. (Eds.), *Williams textbook of endocrinology* (10th ed., pp. 177-279). Philadelphia: W. B. Saunders.

Moorhead, S., Johnson, M., & Maas, M. (Eds.). (2004). *Nursing outcomes classification (NOC)* (3rd ed.). St. Louis: Mosby.

Mosso, L., et al. (2003). Primary hyperaldosteronism and hypertensive disease. *Hypertension, 42*(1), 161-165.

Nayback, A. (2000). Hyponatremia as a consequence of acute adrenal insufficiency and hypothyroidism. *Journal of Emergency Nursing, 26*(2), 130-133.

Pagana, K., & Pagana, T. (2002). *Mosby's manual of diagnostic and laboratory tests* (2nd ed.). St. Louis: Mosby.

Reincke, M. (2000). Subclinical Cushing's syndrome. *Endocrinology and Metabolism Clinics of North America, 29*(1), 43-56.

Robinson, A., & Verbalis, J. (2003). Posterior pituitary gland. In P.R. Larsen, et al. (Eds.), *Williams textbook of endocrinology* (10th ed., pp. 281-329). Philadelphia: W. B. Saunders.

Sachse, D. (2001). Acromegaly. *American Journal of Nursing, 101*(11), 69-74.

Stewart, P. (2003). The adrenal cortex. In P.R. Larsen, et al. (Eds.), *Williams textbook of endocrinology* (10th ed., pp. 491-551). Philadelphia: W. B. Saunders.

Interventions for Clients with Problems of the Thyroid and Parathyroid Glands

M. LINDA WORKMAN

LEARNING OUTCOMES

After studying this chapter, you should be able to:

1. Compare the common clinical manifestations of hyperthyroidism with those of hypothyroidism.
2. Explain the pathophysiology of Graves' disease.
3. Describe the mechanisms of action, side effects, and nursing implications for pharmacologic management of hyperthyroidism.
4. Interpret clinical changes and laboratory data to determine the effectiveness of interventions for hyperthyroidism.
5. Prioritize nursing care for the client during the first 24 hours after a total thyroidectomy.
6. Explain the pathophysiology of Hashimoto's thyroiditis.
7. Identify teaching priorities for the client taking thyroid hormone replacement therapy.
8. Interpret clinical changes and laboratory data to determine the effectiveness of interventions for hypothyroidism.
9. Compare the clinical manifestations of hyperparathyroidism with those of hypoparathyroidism.
10. Prioritize nursing care for the client during the first 24 hours after a parathyroidectomy.
11. Interpret clinical changes and laboratory data to determine the effectiveness of interventions for parathyroid problems.

Go to your Student CD-ROM for Review Questions
for the NCLEX Examination keyed to these Learning Outcomes.

Hormones from the thyroid and parathyroid glands affect overall metabolism, electrolyte balance, and excitable membrane activity. Therefore problems of either thyroid or parathyroid function usually have widespread effects and manifestations. With mild disturbances, the problems are subtle. With more severe disturbances, the problems may be life threatening.

THYROID DISORDERS

Hyperthyroidism

PATHOPHYSIOLOGY

Excessive thyroid hormone secretion leads to **hyperthyroidism.** The manifestations of hyperthyroidism are called **thyrotoxicosis.** Thyroid hormones affect metabolism in all body organs. Increased thyroid function produces many different manifestations. Hyperthyroidism can be temporary or permanent, depending on the cause.

In hyperthyroidism the normal feedback control over thyroid hormone secretion fails. Because thyroid hormones stimulate most body systems, excessive thyroid hormones produce hypermetabolism and increased sympathetic nervous system activity. Many of the manifestations are caused by the body's response to the demands of hypermetabolism (Chart 67-1).

Thyroid hormones directly stimulate the heart. The resulting increased heart rate and stroke volume cause increased cardiac output and blood flow.

Elevated thyroid hormone levels affect protein, lipid, and carbohydrate metabolism. Protein **synthesis** (buildup) and **degradation** (breakdown) are increased. Breakdown ex-

CHART 67-1

KEY FEATURES of
Hyperthyroidism

Skin Manifestations
- Diaphoresis (excessive sweating)
- Fine, soft, silky hair (body)
- Smooth, warm, moist skin
- Thinning of scalp hair

Pulmonary Manifestations
- Shortness of breath with or without exertion
- Rapid, shallow respirations
- Decreased vital capacity

Cardiovascular Manifestations
- Palpitations
- Chest pain
- Increased systolic blood pressure
- Widened pulse pressure
- Tachycardia
- Dysrhythmias

Gastrointestinal Manifestations
- Weight loss
- Increased appetite
- Increased stools
- Hypoproteinemia

Musculoskeletal Manifestations
- Muscle weakness
- Muscle wasting

Neurologic Manifestations
- Blurred or double vision
- Eye fatigue
- Corneal ulcers or infections
- Increased tears
- Injected (red) conjunctiva
- Photophobia
- Eyelid retraction, eyelid lag*
- Globe lag*
- Hyperactive deep tendon reflexes
- Tremors
- Insomnia

Metabolic Manifestations
- Increased basal metabolic rate
- Heat intolerance
- Low-grade fever
- Fatigue

Psychological/Emotional Manifestations
- Decreased attention span
- Restlessness
- Irritability
- Emotional lability
- Manic behavior

Reproductive Manifestations
- Amenorrhea
- Decreased menstrual flow
- Increased libido

Other Manifestations
- Goiter
- Wide-eyed (startled) appearance*
- Decreased total white blood cell count
- Enlarged spleen

*Present in Graves' disease only.

TABLE 67-1 Causes of Hyperthyroidism

Cause	Mechanism
Graves' disease (toxic diffuse goiter)	Autoimmune in nature. Antibodies (TSH-Ab) bind to TSH receptors and keep them activated, increasing the size of the gland and increasing the production of thyroid hormones.
Toxic multinodular goiter	Multiple thyroid nodules, resulting in thyroid hyperfunction.
Thyroid adenoma	Uncontrolled secretion of T_3 and T_4 from benign thyroid tumor.
Pituitary hyperthyroidism	Pituitary adenoma resulting in excessive TSH secretion.
Thyroiditis (radiation-induced)	T_3 and T_4 secretion increased before destruction of gland. Hyperthyroid state usually transient.
T_3 thyrotoxicosis	Increase in thyroid secretion of T_3. Cause unknown.
Factitious hyperthyroidism	Ingestion of excessive amounts of thyroid hormone.
Jod-Basedow phenomenon (iodine induced)	Administration of iodine to an individual with endemic goiter, resulting in excessive production of thyroid hormone.
Thyroid carcinoma	Uncommon, usually occurs with large follicular carcinomas.
Tumors elsewhere in the body	Secrete TSH or thyroid hormones (T_3 and T_4) mimicking hyperthyroid activity.

T_3, Triiodothyronine; T_4, thyroxine; *TSH*, thyroid-stimulating hormone.

ceeds buildup, causing a net loss of protein known as a **negative nitrogen balance.** Glucose tolerance is decreased, and the client has **hyperglycemia** (elevated blood glucose levels). Fat metabolism is increased, and body fat decreases. Although the client has an increased appetite, food intake does not meet energy demands, and the client loses weight. With prolonged hyperthyroidism, the client has chronic nutritional deficiency.

Thyroid hormones are produced in response to the stimulation hormones secreted by the hypothalamus and anterior pituitary glands. Thus oversecretion of thyroid hormones changes the secretion of hormones from the hypothalamus and anterior pituitary gland. In addition, thyroid hormones have some influence over sex hormone production in both men and women. Women have menstrual problems and decreased fertility. Both men and women with hyperthyroidism have an increased libido (sexual urge or interest).

Etiology and Genetic Risk

Hyperthyroidism has many causes (Table 67-1), the most common cause of which is **Graves' disease,** also called toxic diffuse goiter. The client with Graves' disease usually has hyperthyroidism, a **goiter** (enlargement of the thyroid gland), **exophthalmos** (abnormal protrusion of the eyes), and **pretibial myxedema** (dry, waxy swelling of the front surfaces of the lower legs). *Not all clients with a goiter have hyperthyroidism.*

Graves' disease is an autoimmune disorder in which antibodies are made and attach to the thyroid stimulating hormone (TSH) receptor sites on the thyroid tissue. When these antibodies, known as thyroid-stimulating immunoglobulins (TSIs), bind to the thyroid gland, the gland increases in size and overproduces thyroid hormones.

Genetic Considerations

Although no specific gene or gene mutation has been identified as a cause of Graves' disease, its high incidence among family members suggests a genetic component for risk. The pattern of inheritance appears to be familial clustering and may involve mutations in different genes. The risk for Graves' disease is increased in people who have other autoimmune disorders such as type 1 diabetes mellitus and pernicious anemia.

Hyperthyroidism caused by multiple thyroid nodules is termed **toxic multinodular goiter.** The nodules may be enlarged thyroid tissues or adenomas. These clients usually have had a goiter for years. The overproduction of thyroid hormones is usually milder than that seen in Graves' disease, and the client does not have exophthalmos or pretibial edema.

Hyperthyroidism also can be caused by excessive use of thyroid replacement hormones. This type of problem is called **exogenous hyperthyroidism.**

A condition called thyroid storm or thyroid crisis can occur when hyperthyroidism is untreated or poorly controlled or when the client is severely stressed. This condition is an extreme state of hyperthyroidism in which all manifestations are more severe and life threatening.

Incidence/Prevalence

Hyperthyroidism is a common endocrine disorder. Graves' disease can occur at any age but is diagnosed most often in women between 20 and 40 years of age. Toxic multinodular goiter usually occurs after the age of 50 and affects women four times as often as men.

◆COLLABORATIVE MANAGEMENT
◆Assessment
HISTORY

The client may have noticed many changes and problems because hyperthyroidism affects all body systems. Record age, gender, and usual weight. The client may report a recent weight loss, an increased appetite, and an increase in the number of bowel movements per day.

A hallmark of hyperthyroidism is heat intolerance. The client may have **diaphoresis** (increased sweating) even when environmental temperatures are comfortable for others. He or she often wears lighter clothing in cold weather. The client may also report palpitations or chest pain as a result of the cardiovascular effects. Ask about changes in breathing patterns because dyspnea (with or without exertion) is common.

Visual changes may be the earliest problem the client notices, especially ophthalmopathy with Graves' disease (Figure 67-1). Ask the client about changes in vision, such as blurring or double vision and tiring of the eyes.

Ask whether the client has noticed a change in energy level or in the ability to perform activities of daily living (ADLs). Fatigue, weakness, and insomnia are common.

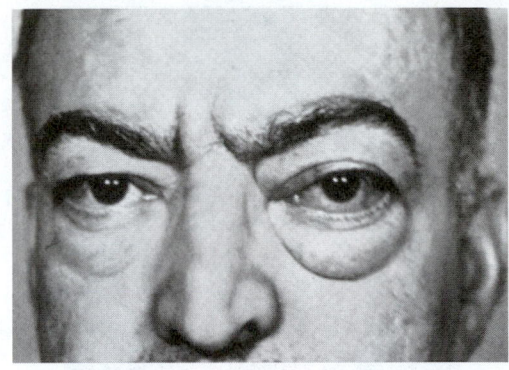

Figure 67-1 ■ Ophthalmopathy. The client has proptosis.

Family and friends may report that the client has become irritable or depressed.

Ask women about changes in menses because amenorrhea or a decreased menstrual flow is common. Initially both men and women may have an increase in libido.

Explore the client's medical history. Previous thyroid surgery or radiation therapy to the neck is important because some people remain hyperthyroid after surgery or are resistant to radiation therapy. Ask about past and current drugs, especially the use of thyroid hormone replacement or antithyroid drugs.

PHYSICAL ASSESSMENT/CLINICAL MANIFESTATIONS

Observe the client's general appearance. Two types of **ophthalmopathy** (abnormal eye appearance or function) are common with hyperthyroidism: eyelid retraction (eyelid lag) and globe (eyeball) lag. In eyelid lag, which occurs in all forms of thyrotoxicosis, the upper eyelid fails to descend when the client gazes slowly downward. In globe lag, the upper eyelid pulls back faster than the eyeball when the client gazes upward. During assessment ask the client to look down and then up, and document the response.

Infiltrative ophthalmopathy, which leads to exophthalmos, is common in clients with Graves' disease (Figure 67-2). The wide-eyed or "startled" look is due to edema in the extraocular muscles and increased fatty tissue behind the eye, which pushes the eyeball forward. Pressure on the optic nerve may impair vision. Swelling and shortening of the muscles may cause problems with focusing. If the eyelid fails to close completely and the eye is unprotected, the eye may become overdry and develop corneal ulcers or infection. Observe the client's eyes for excessive tearing and a bloodshot appearance, and ask about sensitivity to light (**photophobia).**

Observe the size and symmetry of the thyroid gland. Palpate the thyroid gland to assess the presence of a mass or general enlargement. In goiter, a generalized thyroid enlargement, the thyroid gland may increase to four times its normal size (Figure 67-3). Goiters are classified by size (Table 67-2). Bruits (turbulence from increased blood flow) may be heard with a stethoscope. (See Chapter 65 for a discussion of thyroid palpation and auscultation.)

The cardiac problems of hyperthyroidism include increased systolic blood pressure, tachycardia, and other dysrhythmias. Usually the diastolic pressure is decreased, causing a widened pulse pressure.

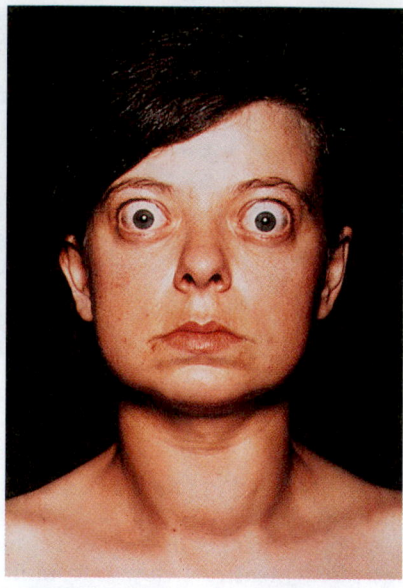

Figure 67-2 ■ Exophthalmos.

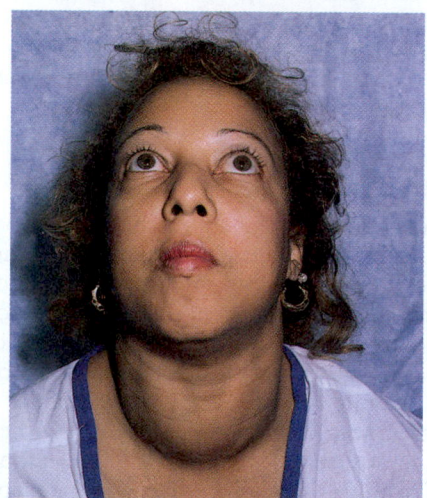

Figure 67-3 ■ Goiter.

TABLE 67-2	Goiter Classification
Goiter Grade	**Description**
0	No palpable or visible goiter.
1	Mass is not visible with neck in the normal position.
	Goiter can be palpated and moves up when the client swallows.
2	Mass is visible as swelling when the neck is in the normal position.
	Goiter is easily palpated and is usually asymmetric.

resin uptake (T_3RU), and thyroid-stimulating hormone (TSH). Antibodies to TSH (TSH-RAb) are measured to determine the presence of Graves' disease. Laboratory changes in hyperthyroidism are listed in Chart 67-2.

OTHER DIAGNOSTIC ASSESSMENTS

THYROID SCAN. The thyroid scan evaluates the position, size, and functioning of the thyroid gland. Radioactive iodine (RAI [^{123}I]) is given by mouth, and the uptake of iodine by the thyroid gland (RAIU) is measured. The half-life of ^{123}I is short, and radiation precautions are not needed. Pregnancy, however, should be ruled out before the scan is performed.

Normally the thyroid has an uptake of 5% to 35% of the given dose when measured at 24 hours. RAIU is increased in clients with hyperthyroidism.

Assess whether the client has undergone procedures or has taken drugs that might affect the results of the scan. Procedures that use iodine-containing dye (e.g., renography) should not be performed for at least 4 weeks before a thyroid scan is done. Any drug that contains iodine should be discontinued for 1 week before the scan.

ULTRASONOGRAPHY. Ultrasonography of the thyroid gland can determine its size and the composition of any masses or nodules. This procedure takes about 30 minutes to perform. Reassure the client that it is painless.

ELECTROCARDIOGRAPHY. An electrocardiogram (ECG) usually shows tachycardia. Other ECG changes with hyperthyroidism include atrial fibrillation and changes in P and T waveforms.

◆ Common Nursing Diagnoses and Collaborative Problems

Nursing diagnoses and collaborative problems that may apply to the client with hyperthyroidism include the following:

■ Imbalanced Nutrition: Less Than Body Requirements related to inadequate intake in relation to metabolic needs
■ Hyperthermia related to increased metabolic rate
■ Fatigue related to sleep deprivation
■ Potential for Hypertension and Cardiac Failure

Inspect the client's hair and skin. Fine, soft, silky hair and smooth, moist skin are common with hyperthyroidism. The client may have muscle weakness, hyperactive deep tendon reflexes, or tremors. Observe gross motor movements for tremors, especially of the hands. Reflexes may be hyperactive. The client may appear extremely restless, irritable, and fatigued.

PSYCHOSOCIAL ASSESSMENT

The client with hyperthyroidism often has wide mood swings, irritability, decreased attention span, and manic behavior. Mild to severe hyperactivity often leads to fatigue because of the inability to sleep well. Ask the client whether he or she has been crying or laughing inappropriately or has had difficulty concentrating. Family members often report these changes in mental or emotional status.

LABORATORY ASSESSMENT

Testing for hyperthyroidism includes measurement of the following blood values: triiodothyronine (T_3), thyroxine (T_4), T_3

Critical Thinking Challenge

One of the nurses on your med-surg unit is having a difficult time getting along with her co-workers. She has become very critical of others and very defensive when anyone suggests that her performance is less than perfect. Recently she was passed over for the assistant director position. You have noticed that she

CHART 67-2

LABORATORY PROFILE
Thyroid Function

Test	Normal Range for Adults	Significance of Abnormal Findings	
		Hyperthyroidism	Hypothyroidism
Serum T_3	70-205 ng/dL, or 1.2-3.4 SI units	Increased	Decreased
Serum T_4	4-12 mcg/dL, or 51-154 SI units	Increased	Decreased
Free T_4 index	0.8-2.4 ng/dL, or 10-31 SI units	Increased	Decreased
T_3 resin uptake	24%-34% (varies with different laboratories)	Increased	Decreased
TRH stimulation test	Doubling of baseline TSH 30 min after IV injection of 500 mcg TRH (women have greater response)	Little or no TSH response	Delayed or poor TSH response in secondary hypothyroidism (pituitary failure) Elevated two or more times the normal in primary hypothyroidism (thyroid gland failure)
Thyroid suppression test	N/A	Fails to suppress RAIU or T_4 levels	No change in RAIU or T_4 levels
TSH stimulation test (thyroid stimulation test)	>10% in RAIU or >1.5 mcg/dL	N/A (test differentiates primary from secondary hypothyroidism)	No response in primary hypothyroidism Normal response in secondary hypothyroidism
Thyroid antibodies (antithyroglobulan antibody)	Titer <1:100	High titer of antithyroglobulin antibodies	Increased titers
Thyrotropin receptor antibodies (TSH-RAb)	Titer <130% of basal activity	High titers indicate Graves' disease	No response
TSH	2-10 μU/mL or 2-10 SI units	Low in Graves' disease High in secondary or tertiary hyperthyroidism	High in primary disease Low in secondary or tertiary disease

N/A, Not applicable; *RAIU*, radioactive iodine uptake; *SI*, Système Internationale; T_3, triiodothyronine; T_4, thyroxine; *TRH*, thyrotropin-releasing hormone; *TSH*, thyroid-stimulating hormone.

---

has lost weight and is about 10 lbs underweight for her height. Her eyes seem to bulge a little. When you ask her if she is feeling okay, she tells you that she thinks she is losing her mind, that she is having a hard time getting to sleep at night, and that she seems to overreact to everything. She bursts into tears and says, "Nobody likes me. I don't even like myself anymore." You escort her down to employee health. Her vital signs there are as follows: T 99.4; P 102, slightly irregular; R 32; BP 130/68.

1. What questions about her health should you ask?
2. What additional questions should you ask related to her weight?
3. What diagnostic tests do you anticipate will be requested?
4. Is drug abuse a possible cause of her manifestations of hyperthyroidism?

evolve For suggested answer guidelines, go to http://evolve.elsevier.com/Iggy/.

◆ Interventions

Because Graves' disease is the most common form of hyperthyroidism, the interventions discussed in the following sections include those specific for the problems that occur with Graves' disease. The goals of management are to decrease the effect of thyroid hormone on cardiac function and to reduce thyroid hormone secretion.

NONSURGICAL MANAGEMENT. Monitor the client's apical pulse, BP, and temperature at least every 4 hours. Instruct the client to report immediately any palpitations, dyspnea, vertigo, or chest pain.

Encourage the client to rest. Keep the environment as quiet as possible. Use frequent bed linen changes, sponge baths, and a cool environment to decrease discomfort caused by diaphoresis and heat intolerance.

Drug Therapy. The most commonly used antithyroid drugs are the thioamides, including propylthiouracil (PTU), methimazole (Tapazole), and carbimazole (Neo-Mercazole✱), which block thyroid hormone production (Chart 67-3). The response to these drugs is delayed because the client may have large amounts of stored thyroid hormones that continue to be released. Other drugs are needed to control the cardiac manifestations until hormone production and release are reduced.

Iodine preparations decrease blood flow through the thyroid gland. This action reduces the production and release of thyroid hormone. Improvement usually occurs within 2 weeks, but weeks may be needed before metabolism returns to normal. This treatment can result in hypothyroidism, and the client must be closely monitored for the need for drug regimen changes.

Lithium carbonate also inhibits thyroid hormone release. However, its use is limited because of side effects such as depression, diabetes insipidus, tremors, nausea, and vomiting. Lithium may be used for a client who cannot tolerate other antithyroid drugs.

Beta-adrenergic blocking drugs, such as propranolol (Inderal, Detensol✱), relieve diaphoresis, anxiety, tachycardia, and palpitations.

CHART 67-3

DRUG THERAPY for Hyperthyroidism

Drug	Usual Dosage	Nursing Interventions	Rationales
Propylthiouracil (PTU, Propyl-Thyracil ✱)	100-150 mg PO three times daily	Give at 8-hr intervals around the clock.	Spreading out dosage helps maintain suppression of hormone.
Methimazole (Tapazole)	5-15 mg PO three times daily	Monitor vital signs. Weigh the client weekly. Observe for sore throat, fever, headache, and skin eruptions.	Changes in vital signs or weight and appearance or other signs and symptoms may indicate adverse reactions, which may necessitate discontinuation of drug use.
Carbimazole (Neo-Mercazole ✱)	10-15 mg twice daily	Instruct the client to avoid crowds and sick people.	Drug reduces immune and inflammatory responses.
Iodine products Strong iodine (Lugol's) solution Saturated solution of potassium iodide (SSKI) Potassium iodide tablets, solution, and syrup	Dosage varies, depending on the type of iodine prescribed, the manufacturer, and the form supplied (tablet, solution, or syrup)	Give in fruit juice or water. Observe for fever, rash, metallic taste, sore mouth, severe GI distress, and burning mouth and throat. Instruct the client to take tablets after meals.	Giving in fruit juice or water improves taste. Signs of iodism may necessitate discontinuation drug use. Taking after meals enhances absorption.
Lithium carbonate (Lithobid, Carbolith ✱ Lithizine ✱)	Individualized 900-1200 mg PO daily in divided doses	Observe for signs of hypothyroidism. Instruct the client to drink 10-12 glassfuls of fluid per day. Instruct the client to maintain normal sodium intake.	Signs of hypothyroidism may indicate drug-induced thyroid enlargement. Extra fluid intake helps to prevent dehydration. Reduced sodium intake can cause retention of the drug.
Dexamethasone (Decadron)	2 mg q6h	Instruct client to avoid crowds and sick people.	Drug reduces immune and inflammatory responses.
Propranolol (Inderal, Detensol ✱) ⚠️**Med Error Alert!** Do not confuse Inderal with Toradol, an anti-inflammatory agent.	20-80 mg four times daily in divided doses	Weigh the client daily. Measure intake and output. Instruct the client to take the drug with food. Instruct the client to avoid smoking. Monitor the client's pulse.	Increased weight and decreased output may indicate congestive heart failure. Taking the drug with food enhances absorption. The drug's effect is reduced by smoking. Tachycardia is a sign of hyperthyroidism.

GI, Gastrointestinal.

Radioactive Iodine Therapy. *Radioactive iodine (RAI) therapy is not used in pregnant women because* [131]*I crosses the placenta and can damage the fetal thyroid gland.* The client with hyperthyroidism may receive RAI in the form of oral [131]I. The dosage depends on the thyroid gland's size and sensitivity to radiation. The thyroid gland picks up the RAI, and some of the cells that produce thyroid hormone are destroyed by the local radiation. Because the thyroid gland stores thyroid hormones to some degree, the client may not have complete symptom relief until 6 to 8 weeks after RAI therapy. Additional drug therapy for hyperthyroidism is still needed during the first few weeks after RAI treatment.

RAI therapy is performed on an outpatient basis. One dose may be sufficient, although some clients need a second or third dose. The radiation dose is low enough that radiation precautions are not needed. Reassure the client that the radioactivity is quickly eliminated. The degree of thyroid destruction is variable. Some clients become hypothyroid as a result of treatment. This problem may occur within a few weeks, or it may take several years to develop. The client then needs lifelong thyroid hormone replacement. All clients who have undergone RAI therapy should be monitored regularly for changes in thyroid function.

SURGICAL MANAGEMENT. Antithyroid drugs and RAI therapy are now the most common treatments for clients with hyperthyroidism. Surgery to remove all or part of the thyroid gland may be needed for clients who have a large goiter causing tracheal or esophageal compression or who do not have a good response to antithyroid drugs. Removal of all (**total thyroidectomy**) or part (**subtotal thyroidectomy**) of the thyroid tissue decreases the production of thyroid hormones. After a total thyroidectomy, clients must take lifelong thyroid hormone replacement.

Preoperative Care. If possible the client is treated with drug therapy first and returns to near-normal thyroid function (**euthyroid**) before thyroid surgery. The euthyroid state is achieved with antithyroid drugs that decrease the secretion of thyroid hormones. Iodine preparations are used to decrease thyroid size and vascularity, thereby reducing the risk for hemorrhage and the potential for thyroid storm during surgery.

Hypertension, dysrhythmias, and tachycardia must be controlled before surgery. The client with hyperthyroidism is often not at an optimal weight and may need to follow a high-protein, high-carbohydrate diet for days or weeks before surgery.

Instruct the client to perform coughing and deep-breathing exercises. Teach the client how to support the neck when coughing or moving. Placing both hands behind the neck when moving reduces the strain on the suture line. Explain that hoarseness may be present for a few days as a result of endotracheal tube placement during surgery.

Clients often fear thyroid surgery, perhaps because the incision is on the neck. Reassure the client by calmly explaining the surgery and the care after surgery. Answer any questions the client and family have.

Operative Procedures. A thyroidectomy is performed with the client under general anesthesia. The client's neck is extended, and the surgeon makes a "collar" incision just above the clavicle. The parathyroid glands and recurrent laryngeal nerves are avoided to reduce the risk for complications and injury.

With a subtotal thyroidectomy, the remaining thyroid tissues are sutured to the trachea. With a total thyroidectomy, the parathyroid glands are left with an intact blood supply, but the entire thyroid gland is removed.

Postoperative Care. Monitor vital signs every 15 minutes until the client is stable and then every 30 minutes. Increase or decrease the monitoring of vital signs based on changes in the client's condition.

Assess the client's level of discomfort. Use sandbags or pillows to support the head and neck. Place the client, while he or she is awake, in a semi-Fowler's position. When positioning the client, decrease tension on the suture line by avoiding neck extension. Give prescribed pain medications as needed.

Humidifying the air promotes easier respiration and thins respiratory secretions. Assist the client to cough and deep-breathe every 30 minutes to 1 hour. Suction oral and tracheal secretions when necessary.

Thyroid surgery can cause hemorrhage, respiratory distress, parathyroid gland injury (resulting in **hypocalcemia** [low serum calcium levels] and **tetany** [hyperexcitability of nerves and muscles]), damage to the laryngeal nerves, and thyroid storm. Remain alert to the potential for complications and identify manifestations early.

Hemorrhage. Hemorrhage is most likely to occur during the first 24 hours after surgery. Inspect the neck dressing and behind the client's neck for blood. A drain may be present and have a moderate amount of serosanguineous drainage. Hemorrhage may also be seen as bleeding at the incision site or as respiratory distress caused by tracheal compression.

Respiratory Distress. Respiratory distress can result from swelling or tetany. Laryngeal **stridor** (harsh, high-pitched respiratory sounds) is heard in acute respiratory obstruction. Keep emergency tracheostomy equipment in the client's room. Check that oxygen and suctioning equipment are nearby and in working order. In some instances, nurses are instructed to remove clips or sutures when medical assistance is not immediately available and swelling at the surgical site is obstructing the airway.

Hypocalcemia and Tetany. The parathyroid glands can be damaged or their blood supply impaired during thyroid surgery. Hypocalcemia and tetany result when parathyroid hormone (PTH) levels decrease. Ask the client about any tingling around the mouth or of the toes and fingers. Assess for muscle twitching as signs of calcium deficiency. Calcium gluconate or calcium chloride for intravenous (IV) use must

---

CHART 67-4

BEST PRACTICE for
Emergency Care of the Client During Thyroid Storm

EMERGENCY CARE

- Maintain a patent airway and adequate ventilation.
- Give antithyroid drugs as prescribed: propylthiouracil (PTU, Propyl-Thyracil✲), 300 to 900 mg daily; methimazole (Tapazole), up to 60 mg daily.
- Administer sodium iodide solution, 2 g IV daily as prescribed.
- Give propranolol (Inderal, Detensol✲), 1 to 3 mg IV as prescribed. Give slowly over 3 minutes; the client should be connected to a cardiac monitor, and a central venous pressure catheter should be in place.
- Give glucocorticoids as prescribed: hydrocortisone, 100 to 500 mg IV daily; prednisone, 4 to 60 mg IV daily; or IM dexamethasone 2 mg every 6 hours.
- Monitor continually for cardiac dysrhythmias.
- Monitor vital signs every 30 minutes.
- Provide comfort measures, including a cooling blanket.
- Give nonsalicylate antipyretics as prescribed.
- Correct dehydration with normal saline infusions.
- Give aspirin or other antipyretic.
- Apply cooling blanket or ice packs to reduce fever.

---

be available in an emergency situation. (For information on the later signs of hypocalcemia, see Postoperative Care [Hyperparathyroidism], p. 1495, and Assessment [Hypoparathyroidism], p. 1495. The care of clients with hypocalcemia is discussed in Chapter 16.)

Laryngeal Nerve Damage. Hoarseness and a weak voice may occur if the laryngeal nerve is injured during surgery. Assess the client's voice at 2-hour intervals, and document any changes. Reassure the client that hoarseness is usually temporary.

Thyroid Storm. **Thyroid storm** or **thyroid crisis** is a life-threatening event that occurs in clients with uncontrolled hyperthyroidism and is usually caused by Graves' disease. Manifestations of crisis develop quickly. Thyroid storm is often triggered by stressors such as trauma, infection, diabetic ketoacidosis, and pregnancy. Other conditions that can lead to thyroid storm include vigorous palpation of the goiter, exposure to iodine, and radioactive iodine (RAI) therapy. Although thyroid storm after surgery is rare because clients receive antithyroid drugs, beta blockers, and iodides before thyroid surgery, it can still occur.

The manifestations of thyroid storm are caused by excessive thyroid hormone release, which dramatically increases metabolic rate. *Key manifestations include fever, tachycardia, and systolic hypertension.* The client may have gastrointestinal problems such as abdominal pain, nausea, vomiting, and diarrhea. Often the client with thyroid storm is very anxious and has tremors. As the crisis progresses, he or she may become restless, confused, psychotic, and may have seizures, leading to coma. *Even with treatment, thyroid storm has a mortality rate of 25%.*

Emergency measures to prevent death vary with the intensity and type of specific symptoms. After the cause has been identified, interventions focus on maintaining airway patency, providing adequate ventilation, reducing fever, and stabilizing the hemodynamic status. Chart 67-4 outlines the best practices for emergency management of thyroid storm.

INFILTRATIVE OPHTHALMOPATHY. Treatment for hyperthyroidism does not correct the eye and vision problems of Graves' disease. Treatment of infiltrative ophthalmopathy is symptomatic. Instruct the client with mild symptoms to elevate the head of the bed at night and to use artificial tears. If **photophobia** (sensitivity to light) is present, dark glasses or eye patches are often helpful. For the client who cannot close the eyelids completely, recommend gently taping the lids closed with nonallergenic tape. These actions prevent irritation and injury. If pressure behind the eye continues and forces the eye forward, blood supply to the eye can be compromised, leading to ischemia and blindness.

In severe cases short-term steroid therapy is prescribed to reduce swelling and halt the infiltrative process. Prednisone (Deltasone, Winpred✣) is given in high doses (often 120 mg daily) at first and then is tapered down according to the client's response. Explain the need to reduce the prednisone gradually, and review its side effects with the client.

Diuretics may be prescribed to decrease edema around the eye. Surgical intervention (orbital decompression) may be needed if loss of sight or damage to the eyeball is possible.

HEALTH TEACHING. Review with the client the manifestations of hyperthyroidism and instruct him or her to report an increase or recurrence of symptoms. Teach the client about the manifestations of hypothyroidism (discussed in the next section) and the need for thyroid hormone replacement. Reinforce the need for regular follow-up because hypothyroidism can occur several years after radioactive iodine therapy.

If the client has had surgery, the surgeon usually removes the sutures on the third or fourth postoperative day. Instruct the client to inspect the incision area and to report redness, tenderness, drainage, or swelling the health care provider.

The discharged client may continue to have mood changes as a result of hyperthyroidism. Explain the reason for mood swings to the client and family and reassure them that it will decrease with continued treatment.

Critical Thinking Challenge

The nurse with manifestations of hyperthyroidism is diagnosed as having Graves' disease. She has an iodine allergy and undergoes a partial thyroidectomy. You are caring for her about 12 hours after surgery. She puts on her call light, and when you come into the room she is sweating and anxious. She tells you that she feels "jittery" and that her heart is racing. She also tells you that she feels like she has a lump in her throat.

1. What should you do first?
2. What is the most likely cause of her current manifestations?

evolve For suggested answer guidelines, go to http://evolve.elsevier.com/Iggy/.

Hypothyroidism

PATHOPHYSIOLOGY

The manifestations of hypothyroidism (Chart 67-5) are the result of decreased metabolism from low levels of thyroid hormones. Hypothyroidism can occur anytime throughout the life span.

Thyroid cells may fail to produce sufficient levels of thyroid hormones (THs) for several reasons. Sometimes the cells themselves are damaged and no longer function normally. Other times the thyroid cells are functional, but the person does not ingest enough of the substances needed to make

---

CHART 67-5

KEY FEATURES of
Hypothyroidism

Skin Manifestations
- Cool, pale or yellowish, dry, coarse, scaly skin
- Thick, brittle nails
- Dry, coarse, brittle hair
- Decreased hair growth, with loss of eyebrow hair
- Poor wound healing

Pulmonary Manifestations
- Hypoventilation
- Pleural effusion
- Dyspnea

Cardiovascular Manifestations
- Bradycardia
- Dysrhythmias
- Enlarged heart
- Decreased activity tolerance
- Hypotension

Metabolic Manifestations
- Decreased basal metabolic rate
- Decreased body temperature
- Cold intolerance

Musculoskeletal Manifestations
- Muscle aches and pains
- Delayed contraction and relaxation of muscles

Neurologic Manifestations
- Slowing of intellectual functions
  Slowness or slurring of speech
  Impaired memory
  Inattentiveness
- Lethargy or somnolence
- Confusion
- Hearing loss
- Paresthesia (numbness and tingling) of the extremities
- Decreased tendon reflexes

Psychological/Emotional Manifestations
- Apathy
- Depression
- Paranoia
- Withdrawal

Gastrointestinal Manifestations
- Anorexia
- Weight gain
- Constipation
- Abdominal distention

Reproductive Manifestations
Women
- Changes in menses (amenorrhea or prolonged menstrual periods)
- Anovulation
- Decreased libido

Men
- Decreased libido
- Impotence

Other Manifestations
- Periorbital edema
- Facial puffiness
- Nonpitting edema of the hands and feet
- Hoarseness
- Goiter (enlarged thyroid gland)
- Thick tongue
- Increased sensitivity to opioids and tranquilizers
- Weakness, fatigue
- Decreased urine output
- Anemia
- Easy bruising
- Iron deficiency
- Folate deficiency
- Vitamin B_{12} deficiency

thyroid hormones, especially iodide and tyrosine. When the production of thyroid hormones is too low or absent, the blood levels of TH are very low and the client has a decreased metabolic rate. This lowered metabolism causes the hypothalamus and anterior pituitary gland to make stimulatory hormones, especially thyroid-stimulating hormone (TSH), as compensation. The TSH binds to thyroid cells and causes the thyroid gland to enlarge, forming a goiter.

Most tissues and organs are affected by the low metabolic rate caused by hypothyroidism. Cellular energy is decreased, and metabolites build up. The metabolites are compounds of proteins and sugars called glycosaminoglycans. These compounds build up inside cells, which increases the mucous and water, forms cellular edema, and changes organ texture. The edema is mucinous (called **myxedema**) rather than edema caused by water alone (Figure 67-4). This edema changes the client's appearance. Nonpitting edema forms everywhere, especially around the eyes, in the hands and feet, and between the shoulder blades. The tongue thickens and edema forms in the larynx, making the voice husky. General physiologic function is decreased.

Myxedema coma is a rare, serious complication of untreated or poorly treated hypothyroidism. The decreased metabolism causes the heart muscle to become flabby and the chamber size to increase. The result is decreased cardiac output and decreased perfusion to the brain and other vital organs. The decreased perfusion makes the already slowed cellular metabolism worse, resulting in tissue and organ failure. *The mortality rate for myxedema coma is extremely high, and this condition is considered a life-threatening emergency.* Myxedema coma can be caused by a variety of events or conditions (Table 67-3).

Etiology

Most cases of hypothyroidism in the United States occur as a result of thyroid surgery and radioactive iodine (RAI) treatment of hyperthyroidism. Worldwide, hypothyroidism is common in areas where the soil and water have little natural iodide, causing endemic goiter. (This problem was common in the Midwest region of the United States before io-

dide was added to table salt and before saltwater fish was widely available.) Hypothyroidism is also caused by a variety of other conditions (Table 67-4).

Incidence/Prevalence

Hypothyroidism occurs most often in women between 30 and 60 years of age. Women are affected 7 to 10 times more often than men (McCance & Huether, 2002). An association exists between the development of hypothyroidism and diabetes mellitus.

◆ COLLABORATIVE MANAGEMENT
◆ Assessment
HISTORY

A decrease in thyroid hormones produces many manifestations related to decreased metabolism. The client often reports an increase in time spent sleeping, sometimes up to 14 to 16 hours daily. Generalized weakness, anorexia, muscle aches, and paresthesias may also be present. Constipation is common. The client often has cold intolerance. Ask whether more blankets at night or sweaters and extra clothing in warm weather have been needed.

Both men and women with hypothyroidism may report a decrease in libido. Women may have had difficulty becoming pregnant or have changes in menses (heavy, prolonged bleeding or amenorrhea). Men can have problems with impotence and infertility.

TABLE 67-3	Conditions or Events Precipitating Myxedema Coma
■ Acute illness ■ Anesthesia ■ Surgery ■ Hypothermia ■ Chemotherapy ■ Sedatives/opioids	■ Rapid withdrawal of thyroid medications ■ Untreated hypothyroidism ■ Inadequately treated hypothyroidism

TABLE 67-4	Causes of Hypothyroidism

Primary Causes
Decreased Thyroid Tissue
- Surgical removal of the thyroid
- Radiation-induced thyroid destruction
- Autoimmune thyroid destruction
- Congenital thyroid agenesis
- Congenital thyroid hypoplasia
- Congenital thyroid dysgenesis
- Cancer (thyroidal or metastatic)

Decreased Synthesis of Thyroid Hormone
- Endemic iodine deficiency
- Excessive exposure to iodine
- Medications
  Lithium
  Phenylbutazone
  Propylthiouracil
  Sodium or potassium perchlorate
  Aminoglutethimide

Secondary Causes
Inadequate Production of Thyroid-Stimulating Hormone
- Pituitary tumors, trauma, infections, or infarcts
- Congenital pituitary defects
- Hypothalamic tumors, trauma, infections, or infarcts

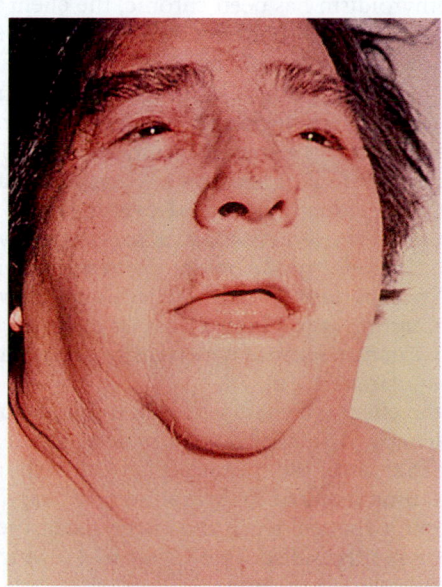

Figure 67-4 ■ Myxedema.

Ask the client about current or previous use of drugs, such as lithium, aminoglutethimide, sodium or potassium perchlorate, thiocyanates, or cobalt. All these drugs can impair thyroid hormone production.

PHYSICAL ASSESSMENT/CLINICAL MANIFESTATIONS

Observe the client's overall appearance. Figure 67-4 shows the typical appearance of an adult with hypothyroidism. Common changes include coarse features, edema around the eyes and face, a blank expression, and a thick tongue. The client's overall muscle movement is slow.

PSYCHOSOCIAL ASSESSMENT

Hypothyroidism causes many problems in psychosocial functioning. Depression is the most common reason for seeking medical attention. Family members often bring the client for the initial evaluation. The client may be too lethargic, apathetic, or drowsy to recognize changes in his or her condition. Families may report that the client is withdrawn. Assess the client's attention span and memory, both of which can be impaired by hypothyroidism.

LABORATORY ASSESSMENT

Laboratory findings for hypothyroidism are the opposite of those for hyperthyroidism. Triiodothyronine (T_3) and thyroxine (T_4) serum levels are decreased. TSH levels are high in primary hypothyroidism but can be decreased or near-normal in clients with secondary hypothyroidism (see Chart 67-2).

🤔 Critical Thinking Challenge

The client is a 78-year-old woman. She has resided in a nursing home for the past 3 years because a stroke paralyzed her left side and she is unable to care for herself. She does talk, although her speech is slow and sometimes she uses the wrong word to describe something. For several weeks you have noted that her speech is becoming less understandable and that she is sleeping more. Today the nursing assistant tells you that the client's heart rate is 34 beats/min and her temperature is 96.2°F. She also tells you that the client had trouble opening her eyes and swallowing.

1. What should you do first?
2. Should oxygen be applied? Why or why not?
3. What indications do you have that the changes in her health status are not related to her stroke?

evolve For suggested answer guidelines, go to http://evolve.elsevier.com/Iggy/.

◆ Analysis

COMMON NURSING DIAGNOSES AND COLLABORATIVE PROBLEMS

The following are priority nursing diagnoses for clients with hypothyroidism:
1. Decreased Cardiac Output related to altered heart rate and rhythm as a result of decreased myocardial metabolism
2. Ineffective Breathing Pattern related to decreased energy, obesity, and fatigue
3. Disturbed Thought Processes related to impaired brain metabolism and edema

The major collaborative problem is the Potential for Myxedema Coma.

ADDITIONAL NURSING DIAGNOSES AND COLLABORATIVE PROBLEMS

In addition to the common nursing diagnoses and collaborative problems, clients with hypothyroidism may have one or more of the following:
- Imbalanced Nutrition: More Than Body Requirements related to excessive intake in relation to metabolic need
- Hypothermia related to decreased metabolic rate
- Constipation related to decreased motility of the gastrointestinal tract
- Disturbed Body Image related to illness
- Deficient Knowledge of condition, diagnosis, and treatment related to cognitive limitation

Additional collaborative problems for clients with hypothyroidism are Potential for Paralytic Ileus and Potential for Cardiomyopathy.

◆ Planning and Implementation

DECREASED CARDIAC OUTPUT

NOC **PLANNING: EXPECTED OUTCOMES.** The client with hypothyroidism is expected to have cardiovascular function that is either not compromised or mildly compromised. Indicators include that the client:
- Maintains heart rate above 60 beats/min
- Maintains blood pressure within normal limits for his or her age and general health
- Has no dysrhythmias, peripheral edema, or neck vein distension

INTERVENTIONS. NIC interventions for the client with hypothyroidism are listed in Chart 67-6. The client with hypothyroidism can have decreased blood pressure, bradycardia, and dysrhythmias. Monitor blood pressure, heart rate, and rhythm, and observe closely for signs of shock, such as hypotension, decreasing urine output, and changes in mental status.

If hypothyroidism has been chronic, the client may have cardiovascular disease. *Instruct the client to report episodes of chest pain or discomfort immediately.*

The client with hypothyroidism requires lifelong thyroid hormone replacement. Synthetic hormone preparations are usually prescribed; the most common is levothyroxine sodium (Synthroid, T_4, Eltroxin✦). Therapy is started with low doses and gradually increased over a period of weeks. *The client with more severe symptoms of hypothyroidism is started on the lowest dose of thyroid hormone replacement.* This caution is especially important when the client has known cardiac problems. Starting at too high a dose or increasing the dose too rapidly can cause severe hypertension, heart failure, and myocardial infarction.

Assess the client for chest pain and dyspnea during initiation of therapy. The final dosage is determined by blood levels of TSH and the client's physical responses. The dosage and time required for symptom relief vary with each client. Monitor for and teach the client about the manifestations of hyperthyroidism (see Chart 67-1), which can occur with replacement therapy.

CHART 67-6

NIC INTERVENTION ACTIVITIES for
The Client with Hypothyroidism

Respiratory Monitoring: *Collection and analysis of client data to ensure airway patency and adequate gas exchange*
- Monitor rate, rhythm, depth, and effort of respirations.
- Note chest movement, watching for symmetry, use of accessory muscles, and supraclavicular and intercostal muscle refractions.
- Monitor breathing patterns for bradypnea.
- Monitor for diaphragmatic muscle fatigue (paradoxical motion).
- Note changes in Sao_2 and Svo_2, end tidal CO_2 and ABG values, as appropriate.
- Monitor client's ability to cough effectively.
- Monitor for dyspnea and events that decrease and worsen it.

Shock Prevention: *Detecting and treating a client at risk for impending shock.*
- Monitor temperature and respiratory status.
- Monitor circulatory status: BP, skin color, skin temperature, heart sounds, heart rate and rhythm, presence and quality of peripheral pulses, and capillary refill.
- Monitor for signs of inadequate tissue oxygenation.
- Monitor for apprehension, increased anxiety, and changes in mental status.
- Monitor intake and output.
- Administer oxygen and/or mechanical ventilation, as appropriate.
- Administer antiarrhythmic agents, as appropriate.

Hypothermia Treatment: *Rewarming and surveillance of a client whose core body temperature is below 35° C.*
- Monitor client's temperature, using a low-recording thermometer if necessary.
- Place on a cardiac monitor, as appropriate.
- Cover with warmed blankets, as appropriate.
- Administer heated oxygen, as appropriate.
- Monitor vital signs, as appropriate.
- Monitor skin color and temperature.
- Monitor intake and output.
- Avoid giving IM or subcutaneous medications during the hypothermic state.
- Give client warm oral fluids, if alert and able to swallow.
- Teach client to consume a caloric intake sufficient to maintain a normal body temperature.
- Emphasize the importance of wearing warm, protective clothing when going into a cold environment.

NIC intervention activities selected from Dochterman J.M., & Bulechek, G.M. (Eds.). (2004). *Nursing interventions classification (NIC)* (4th ed.). St. Louis: Mosby. No part of this work is to be altered without prior written permission from the Publisher.
Sao_2, Arterial oxygen saturation; Svo_2, venous oxygen saturation.

INEFFECTIVE BREATHING PATTERN

PLANNING: EXPECTED OUTCOMES. The client with hypothyroidism is expected to have respiratory function be not compromised or only mildly compromised. Indicators include the following:
- Maintenance of SpO_2 of at least 88%
- Absence of cyanosis
- Maintenance of cognitive orientation

INTERVENTIONS. Observe and record the rate and depth of respirations. Auscultate the lungs for any problems, such as a decrease in breath sounds. If hypothyroidism is severe, the client may have such severe respiratory distress that ventilatory support is required. Severe respiratory distress often occurs with myxedema coma.

Sedating a client with hypothyroidism can make respiratory difficulties worse and is avoided, if possible. When se-

CHART 67-7

BEST PRACTICE for
Emergency Care of the Client During Myxedema Coma

EMERGENCY CARE
- Maintain a patent airway.
- Replace fluids with IV normal or hypertonic saline.
- Give levothyroxine sodium IV as prescribed.
- Give glucose IV as prescribed.
- Give corticosteroids as prescribed.
- Check the client's temperature hourly.
- Monitor blood pressure hourly.
- Cover the client with warm blankets.
- Monitor for changes in mental status.
- Turn every 2 hours.
- Institute aspiration precautions.

dation is needed, the dosage is reduced because hypothyroidism increases sensitivity to these drugs. Assess the client receiving sedation for respiratory adequacy.

DISTURBED THOUGHT PROCESSES

PLANNING: EXPECTED OUTCOMES. The client with hypothyroidism is expected to have thought processes not compromised or only mildly compromised with correction of the hypothyroidism. Indicators include that the client:
- Demonstrates immediate memory
- Communicates clearly and appropriately for age and ability
- Is attentive during conversations

INTERVENTIONS. Observe for and record the presence and severity of lethargy, drowsiness, memory deficit, poor attention span, and difficulty communicating. These problems should decrease with thyroid hormone treatment, and mental awareness usually returns to normal levels within 2 weeks. Orient the client to person, place, and time, and explain all procedures slowly and carefully. Provide a safe environment.

Family members may have difficulty coping with the client's behavior. Encourage them to accept the mood changes and mental slowness as manifestations of the disease. Remind the family that these problems should improve with therapy.

MYXEDEMA COMA

Any client with hypothyroidism who has any other health problem or who is newly diagnosed is at risk for myxedema coma. Factors leading to myxedema coma are listed in Table 67-3. Problems that often occur with this condition include the following:
- Coma
- Respiratory failure
- Hypotension
- Hyponatremia
- Hypothermia
- Hypoglycemia

Untreated myxedema coma leads to shock, organ damage, and death. Assess the client with hypothyroidism every shift for changes that indicate increasing severity, especially changes in mental status.

Treatment is instituted quickly according to the client's manifestations and without waiting for laboratory confirmation. Best practices for emergency care of the client with myxedema coma are listed in Chart 67-7.

CHART 67-8

NURSING FOCUS on the OLDER ADULT
Thyroid Problems

Teach the client the following facts about changes in the thyroid gland related to aging:
- The thyroid gland decreases in size with increasing age.
- Thyroid hormone secretion decreases with age, but the hormone level remains stable because cellular clearance of the hormone also decreases with age.
- The basal metabolic rate decreases with age, usually as a result of decreased activity. This decrease changes the body composition from predominantly muscular to predominantly fatty.
- Older clients require lower doses of replacement thyroid hormone. Too large a dose may adversely affect the heart muscle.

CONSIDERATIONS FOR OLDER ADULTS

Metabolic rate and production of thyroid hormone both decrease with advancing age (Chart 67-8), particularly among people older than 80 years of age. Until recently, however, data regarding normal levels of T_3 and T_4 were established only for adults between the ages of 20 and 30 years. By such criteria, older people with T_3 and T_4 levels 15% to 20% below "normal levels" (established for a younger population) were considered to have hypothyroidism and therapy with thyroid hormone was initiated. In fact many of these clients were not truly hypothyroid, and therapy caused pseudohyperthyroidism, stressing many tissues and organs. Daily thyroid hormone therapy decreases the activity of the anterior pituitary gland and the thyroid gland, creating actual hypothyroidism. Health care providers need to assess more than just laboratory data to determine hypothyroidism in the older adult.

Community-Based Care

Hypothyroidism is usually a chronic condition. Clients with hypothyroidism are managed on an outpatient basis and may reside anywhere. Clients in acute care settings, subacute care settings, and rehabilitation centers may have long-standing hypothyroidism in addition to other acute or chronic health problems. Ensure that whoever is responsible for overseeing the client's daily care is aware of the condition and understands its treatment.

HOME CARE MANAGEMENT

The client with hypothyroidism does not usually require changes in the home unless cognition has decreased to the point that he or she poses a danger to himself or herself. Activity intolerance and fatigue may necessitate one-floor living for a short time. If manifestations have not improved before discharge, discuss the need for extra heat or clothing because of cold intolerance. The client who has a decreased attention span may need help with the drug regimen. Discuss this issue with the family and client, and develop a plan for drug therapy. One person should be clearly designated as responsible for drug preparation and delivery so that doses are neither missed nor duplicated.

HEALTH TEACHING

The most important educational need for the client with hypothyroidism is about hormone replacement therapy and its side effects. Emphasize the need for lifelong drugs, and

CHART 67-9

HOME CARE ASSESSMENT of
The Client with Thyroid Dysfunction

Assess cardiovascular status.
- Vital signs, including apical pulse, pulse pressure, presence or absence of orthostatic hypotension, and the quality and rhythm of peripheral pulses
- Presence or absence of peripheral edema
- Weight gain or loss

Assess cognition and mental status.
- Level of consciousness
- Orientation to time, place, and person
- Accurately reading a seven-word sentence containing no words greater than three syllables
- Can the client count backward from 100 by threes?

Assess condition of skin and mucous membranes.
- Moisture of skin, most reliable on chest and back
- Skin temperature and color

Assess neuromuscular status.
- Reactivity of patellar and biceps reflexes
- Oral temperature
- Handgrip strength
- Steadiness of gait
- Presence or absence of fine tremors in the hand

Ask about the following:
- Sleep in the past 24 hours
- Client warm enough or too warm indoors
- 24-hour diet recall
- 24-hour activity recall
- Over-the-counter and prescribed medications taken
- Last bowel movement

Assess client's understanding of illness and adherence with treatment.
- Manifestations to report to health care provider
- Medication plan (correct timing and dose)

---

review the manifestations of both hyperthyroidism and hypothyroidism. Instruct the client to wear a medical alert bracelet. Teach the client and family when to seek medical interventions for dosage adjustment. Instruct the client not to take any over-the-counter (OTC) drugs because thyroid hormone preparations interact with many other drugs. Older clients may need additional information about the effects of aging on the thyroid gland (see Chart 67-8).

Advise the client to eat a well-balanced diet with adequate fiber and fluid intake to prevent constipation. Caution clients that use of fiber supplements may interfere with the absorption of thyroid hormone. Remind the client about the importance of adequate rest. Encourage family members to voice their concerns to the health care provider.

Assist the family in understanding that the time required for resolution of hypothyroidism varies. During this time the client may continue to have mental dullness or slowness. Teach the family to orient the client often and to explain everything clearly and simply.

HEALTH CARE RESOURCES

Immediately after returning home, the client may need a support person to stay and provide more attention than could be given by a visiting nurse or home care aide. Contact with the health care team is needed for follow-up and identification of potential problems. The client taking thyroid drugs may have manifestations of hypothyroidism if the dosage is inadequate or manifestations of hyperthyroidism if the dose is too high. Perform a focused assessment at every home visit to the client under treatment for thyroid dysfunction (Chart 67-9).

◆ **Evaluation: Outcomes**

Evaluate the care of the client with hypothyroidism on the basis of the identified nursing diagnoses and collaborative problems. The expected outcome is that the client will:

- Maintain normal cardiovascular function
- Maintain adequate respiratory function
- Experience improvement in thought processes

Specific indicators for these outcomes are listed for each nursing diagnosis and collaborative problem under the Planning and Implementation section (see earlier).

Thyroiditis
PATHOPHYSIOLOGY

Thyroiditis is an inflammation of the thyroid gland. There are three types: acute, subacute, and chronic. Chronic thyroiditis (Hashimoto's disease) is the most common type.

Acute thyroiditis is caused by bacterial invasion of the thyroid gland. Manifestations include pain, neck tenderness, malaise, fever, and **dysphagia** (difficulty swallowing). It usually resolves with antibiotic therapy.

Subacute or granulomatous thyroiditis results from a viral infection of the thyroid gland after a cold or other upper respiratory infection. Manifestations include fever, chills, dysphagia, and muscle and joint pain. Pain can radiate to the ears and the jaw. The thyroid gland feels hard and enlarged on palpation. Thyroid function can remain normal, although hyperthyroidism or hypothyroidism may develop.

Chronic thyroiditis (Hashimoto's disease) is a type of hypothyroidism that affects women more often than men, most often clients in their 30s to 50s. Hashimoto's disease is an autoimmune disorder. The thyroid becomes invaded with antithyroid antibodies and lymphocytes, causing thyroid tissue destruction. When large amounts of the gland are destroyed, serum thyroid hormone levels are low and secretion of thyroid-stimulating hormone (TSH) is increased.

◆ **COLLABORATIVE MANAGEMENT**

The manifestations of Hashimoto's disease are dysphagia and painless enlargement of the gland. Diagnosis is based on circulating antithyroid antibodies and needle biopsy of the thyroid gland. Serum thyroid hormone levels, TSH levels, and radioactive iodine uptake (RAIU) vary with disease stage.

The client is given thyroid hormone to prevent hypothyroidism and to suppress TSH secretion, which decreases the size of the thyroid gland. Surgery (subtotal thyroidectomy) is needed if the goiter does not respond to thyroid hormone, is disfiguring, or compresses other structures.

Nursing interventions focus on promoting comfort and teaching the client about hypothyroidism, drugs, and surgery (see Surgical Management [Hyperthyroidism], pp. 1486 to 1487.)

Thyroid Cancer
PATHOPHYSIOLOGY

The four distinct types of thyroid cancer are papillary, follicular, medullary, and anaplastic. The initial manifestation of thyroid cancer is a single, painless lump or nodule in the thyroid gland. Additional manifestations depend on the presence and location of **metastasis** (spread of cancer cells).

Papillary carcinoma, the most common type of thyroid cancer, occurs most often in younger women. It is a slow-growing tumor that can be present for years before spreading to nearby lymph nodes. When the tumor is confined to the thyroid gland, the chance for cure is good with a partial or total thyroidectomy.

Follicular carcinomas are about 25% of all thyroid cancers. They occur most often in older clients. The cancer invades blood vessels and spreads to bone and lung tissue. It can adhere to the trachea, neck muscles, great vessels, and skin, resulting in **dyspnea** (difficulty breathing) and **dysphagia** (difficulty swallowing). When the tumor involves the recurrent laryngeal nerves, the client may have a hoarse voice. The prognosis is fair when metastasis is minimal at diagnosis.

Medullary carcinoma accounts for 5% to 10% of all thyroid cancers and is most common in clients older than 50 years of age. This tumor often occurs as part of multiple endocrine neoplasia (MEN) type II, a familial endocrine disorder. The tumor usually secretes calcitonin, adrenocorticotropic hormone (ACTH), prostaglandins, and serotonin.

Anaplastic carcinoma is a rapid-growing, aggressive tumor that directly invades nearby structures. Manifestations include stridor (harsh, high-pitched respiratory sounds), hoarseness, and dysphagia. The prognosis is poor.

◆ **COLLABORATIVE MANAGEMENT**

Surgery is the treatment of choice for papillary, follicular, and medullary carcinomas. A total thyroidectomy is usually performed with a nodal neck dissection if regional lymph nodes are involved. The physician prescribes suppressive doses of thyroid hormone for 3 months after surgery. A radioactive iodine uptake (RAIU) study is performed after drugs are withdrawn. If there is RAI uptake, the client is treated with **ablative** (enough to destroy the tissue) amounts of RAI. If thyroid cancer does not respond to RAI, a course of chemotherapy is initiated.

PARATHYROID DISORDERS
Hyperparathyroidism
PATHOPHYSIOLOGY

The parathyroid glands maintain calcium and phosphate balance (Figure 67-5). Serum calcium level is normally maintained within a narrow range; phosphate levels vary more widely. Increased levels of parathyroid hormone (PTH) act directly on the kidney, causing increased kidney reabsorption of calcium and increased phosphate excretion. These processes cause **hypercalcemia** (excessive calcium) and **hypophosphatemia** (inadequate phosphate) in the client with hyperparathyroidism.

In bone, excessive PTH levels increase bone resorption (bone loss of calcium) by decreasing **osteoblastic** (bone production) activity and increasing **osteoclastic** (bone destruction) activity. This process releases calcium and phosphate into the blood and reduces bone density. With chronic calcium excess, as in long-standing hypercalcemia, calcium is deposited in soft tissues.

Although the exact triggering mechanisms are unknown, primary hyperparathyroidism results when one or more parathyroid glands do not respond to the normal feedback of serum calcium. The most common cause is a

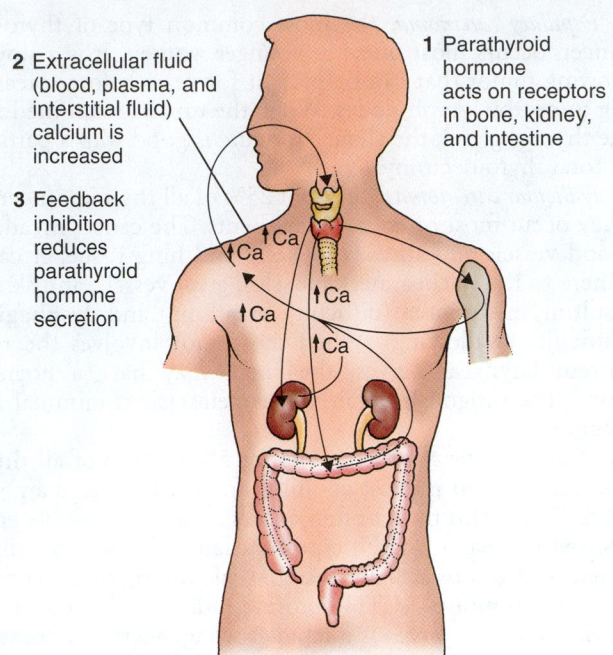

2 Extracellular fluid
(blood, plasma, and
interstitial fluid)
calcium is
increased

3 Feedback
inhibition
reduces
parathyroid
hormone
secretion

1 Parathyroid
hormone
acts on receptors
in bone, kidney,
and intestine

Figure 67-5 ■ The physiologic actions of parathyroid hormone.

TABLE 67-5 Causes of Parathyroid Dysfunction

Causes of Hyperparathyroidism
- Parathyroid adenoma
- Parathyroid carcinoma
- Congenital hyperplasia
- Neck trauma or radiation
- Vitamin D deficiency
- Chronic renal failure with hypocalcemia
- Parathyroid hormone-secreting carcinomas of the lung, kidney, or gastrointestinal tract

Causes of Hypoparathyroidism
- Surgical or radiation-induced thyroid ablation
- Parathyroidectomy
- Congenital dysgenesis
- Idiopathic (autoimmune) hypoparathyroidism
- Hypomagnesemia

---

benign tumor in one parathyroid gland. Table 67-5 lists other causes of hyperparathyroidism.

◆COLLABORATIVE MANAGEMENT

◆Assessment

Ask the client about any bone fractures, recent weight loss, arthritis, or psychological distress. Determine whether the client has received radiation treatment to the head or neck. The client with long-standing disease may have a waxy pallor of the skin and bone deformities in the extremities and back.

Manifestations of hyperparathyroidism may be related either to the effects of excessive PTH or to the effects of the accompanying hypercalcemia.

High levels of PTH cause **renal calculi** (kidney stones) and deposits of calcium in the soft tissue of the kidney. Bone lesions are due to an increased rate of bone destruction and may result in pathologic fractures, bone cysts, and osteoporosis.

Gastrointestinal manifestations (e.g., anorexia, nausea, vomiting, epigastric pain, constipation, weight loss) are common, particularly when serum calcium levels are high. Elevated serum gastrin levels are caused by hypercalcemia and lead to peptic ulcer disease. Fatigue and lethargy may be present and become more severe as the serum calcium levels increase. When serum calcium levels are greater than 12 mg/dL, the client may have psychosis with mental confusion, which leads to coma and death if left untreated. (See Chapter 16 for more information about hypercalcemia.)

Serum PTH, calcium, and phosphate levels and urine cyclic adenosine monophosphate (cAMP) are the most commonly used laboratory tests to detect hyperparathyroidism (Chart 67-10). X-rays may show kidney stones, calcium deposits, and bone lesions, such as cysts or fractures. Loss of bone density occurs in the client with chronic hyperparathyroidism. Other diagnostic tests include arteriography, computed tomography (CT), venous catheterization of the thyroid veins with sampling of the blood for PTH levels, and ultrasonography. Explain the procedures and care for the client undergoing diagnostic tests.

◆Interventions

NONSURGICAL MANAGEMENT
Diuretic and Fluid Therapy. The most common therapy for reducing serum calcium levels in clients who are not candidates for surgery is hydration and furosemide (Lasix, Uritol✱), a diuretic that increases kidney excretion of calcium. IV saline in large volumes also promotes renal calcium excretion.

Monitor cardiac function and intake and output every 2 to 4 hours during hydration therapy. Continuous cardiac monitoring may be needed. Closely monitor serum calcium levels, and immediately report any precipitous drop to the physician. Sudden drops in calcium levels may cause tingling and numbness in the muscles.

Drug Therapy. When hydration and furosemide cannot reduce hypercalcemia, or if it is necessary to discontinue IV fluids, other drugs can help to reduce the manifestations of hyperparathyroidism, especially those related to hypercalcemia.

Phosphates. Oral phosphates inhibit bone resorption and interfere with calcium absorption. IV phosphates are used only when serum calcium levels must be lowered rapidly.

Calcitonin. Calcitonin decreases the release of skeletal calcium and increases the kidney excretion of calcium. Calcitonin is not effective when used alone because of its short duration of action. Its therapeutic effects are greatly enhanced if given along with glucocorticoids.

Calcium Chelators. Some drugs lower calcium levels by binding (chelating) calcium, which reduces the levels of free calcium. Mithramycin, a cytotoxic agent, is the most effective and potent calcium chelator used to lower serum calcium levels. In most clients a single IV dose of 10 to 15 mg/kg of body weight by slow infusion can lower serum calcium levels within 48 hours. However, the toxic effects limit its use to two or three doses. Thrombocytopenia (decreased circulating platelets and an increased tendency to bleed) and kidney and liver toxicity can result after only one dose. Liver function studies, blood urea nitrogen and creatinine, complete blood count (CBC), and serum calcium levels are closely monitored

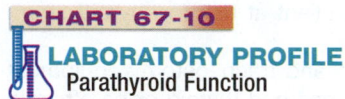

CHART 67-10
LABORATORY PROFILE
Parathyroid Function

Test	Normal Range for Adults	Significance of Abnormal Findings	
		Hyperthyroidism	**Hypothyroidism**
Serum calcium	Total: 9.0-10.5 mg/dL or 2.25-2.75 SI units Ionized (active): 4.64-5.28 mg/dL or 1.16-1.32 SI units	Increased in primary hyperparathyroidism	Decreased
Serum phosphate	3.0-4.5 mg/dL or 0.97-1.45 SI units *Older adults:* May be slightly lower	Decreased	Increased
Serum parathyroid hormone	C-terminal 50-330 pg/mL	Increased	Decreased

SI, Système Internationale.

in the client receiving mithramycin. Another calcium chelator is penicillamine (Cuprimine, Pendramine).

SURGICAL MANAGEMENT. Surgical management of hyperparathyroidism involves a parathyroidectomy.

Preoperative Care. Before surgery the client is stabilized and calcium levels are decreased to near normal. If mithramycin has been used to lower serum calcium levels, studies to determine bleeding and clotting times are needed, as is a CBC to determine bone marrow function.

Advise the client that coughing and deep-breathing exercises should be performed after surgery and that talking may be painful for the first day or two. Teach about neck support by having the client place both hands behind the neck to assist in elevating the head.

Operative Procedures. Using general anesthesia and with the client's neck hyperextended, the surgeon makes a transverse incision in the lower neck. All four parathyroid glands are examined for enlargement. If only one gland on a side is enlarged, a frozen section is done on both glands. If a tumor is present on one side but the other side is normal, the surgeon removes the tumor and leaves the remaining gland intact.

Postoperative Care. Observe the client for respiratory distress, which may occur from compression of the trachea by hemorrhage or swelling of neck tissues. Ensure that emergency equipment, including suction, oxygen, and tracheostomy equipment, is at the bedside. If severe swelling occurs, the surgeon may need to remove clips from the incision to preserve the airway. Monitor vital signs, identify any change in status, and check the neck dressing for abnormal amounts of drainage or bleeding. A small amount (1 to 5 mL) of drainage is normal.

The remaining glands, which may have atrophied as a result of PTH overproduction, require several days to several weeks to return to normal function. A hypocalcemic crisis can occur during this critical period. Check serum calcium levels immediately after surgery and every 4 hours thereafter until calcium levels stabilize. Monitor for manifestations of hypocalcemia, such as tingling and twitching in the extremities and face. Check for Trousseau's and Chvostek's signs, either of which signal potential tetany (see Chapter 16).

Damage to the recurrent laryngeal nerve can occur. Assess the client for changes in voice patterns and hoarseness.

When hyperparathyroidism is due to **hyperplasia** (tissue overgrowth), three glands plus half of the fourth gland are usually removed. If all four glands are removed, a small portion of a gland may be implanted in the forearm, where it produces PTH and maintains calcium homeostasis. If all these maneuvers fail, the client will need lifelong treatment with calcium and vitamin D because the resulting hypoparathyroidism is permanent.

Hypoparathyroidism
PATHOPHYSIOLOGY

Hypoparathyroidism is a rare endocrine disorder in which parathyroid function is decreased. Problems are directly related to a lack of parathyroid hormone (PTH) secretion or to decreased effectiveness of PTH on target tissue. Whether the problem is a lack of PTH secretion or an ineffectiveness of PTH on tissues, the result is the same: hypocalcemia.

Iatrogenic hypoparathyroidism, the most common form, is caused by the removal of all parathyroid tissue during total thyroidectomy or by deliberate surgical removal of the parathyroid glands.

Idiopathic hypoparathyroidism can occur spontaneously. The exact cause is unknown, but an autoimmune basis is suspected in many clients. Hypoparathyroidism may occur with other autoimmune disorders such as adrenal insufficiency, hypothyroidism, diabetes mellitus, pernicious anemia, and vitiligo.

Hypomagnesemia (decreased serum magnesium levels) may also cause hypoparathyroidism. Hypomagnesemia is seen in alcoholics and in clients with malabsorption syndromes, chronic renal disease, and malnutrition. It causes impairment of PTH secretion and may interfere with the effects of PTH on the bones and kidneys.

◆ COLLABORATIVE MANAGEMENT
◆ Assessment

Ask about any head or neck surgery or radiation therapy because these treatments may cause hypoparathyroidism. Assess whether the client has any manifestations of hypoparathyroidism, which may range from mild tingling and numbness to tetany. Tingling and numbness around the mouth or in the hands and feet reflect mild to moderate hypocalcemia. Severe muscle cramps, carpopedal spasms, and seizures (with no loss of consciousness or incontinence) reflect a more severe hypocalcemia. The client or caregiver may notice mental changes ranging from irritability to psychosis.

The physical assessment may show excessive or inappropriate muscle contractions that cause finger, hand, and elbow flexion; this can signal an impending attack of tetany. Check for Chvostek's sign and Trousseau's sign; positive responses indicate potential tetany. Bands or pits may encircle the crowns of the teeth, which indicates a loss of calcium from the teeth and causes enamel loss.

Diagnostic tests for hypoparathyroidism include electroencephalography (EEG), blood tests, and computed tomography (CT). EEG changes revert to normal with correction of hypocalcemia. Serum calcium, phosphate, magnesium, vitamin D, and urine cyclic adenosine monophosphate (cAMP) levels may be used in the diagnostic workup for hypoparathyroidism (see Chart 67-10). The CT scan can show brain calcifications, which indicate chronic hypocalcemia.

◆ Interventions

Management of hypoparathyroidism focuses on correcting hypocalcemia, vitamin D deficiency, and hypomagnesemia. For clients with acute and severe hypocalcemia, IV calcium is given as a 10% solution of calcium chloride or calcium gluconate over 10 to 15 minutes. Acute vitamin D deficiency is treated with calcitriol (Rocaltrol), 0.5 to 2 mg daily. Acute hypomagnesemia is corrected with 50% magnesium sulfate in 2-mL doses (up to 4 g daily) either intramuscularly or intravenously (IV). Long-term oral therapy for hypocalcemia involves the intake of calcium, 0.5 to 2 g daily, in divided doses.

Long-term therapy for vitamin D deficiency is 50,000 to 400,000 units of ergocalciferol daily. The dosage is adjusted to keep the client's calcium level in the low-normal range (slightly hypocalcemic), enough to prevent symptoms of hypocalcemia. It must also be low enough to prevent increased urine calcium levels, which can lead to stone formation.

Nursing management includes teaching about the drug regimen and interventions to reduce anxiety. Instruct the client to eat foods high in calcium but low in phosphorus. Milk, yogurt, and processed cheeses are avoided because of their high phosphorus content. *Stress that therapy for hypocalcemia is lifelong.* Advise the client to wear a medical alert bracelet. With adherence to the prescribed drug and diet regimen, the calcium level usually remains high enough to prevent a hypocalcemic crisis.

GET READY for the NCLEX Examination!

KEY POINTS

Safe Effective Care Environment

- Use a gait belt when assisting a client with muscle weakness to walk.
- Collaborate with the dietitian to teach clients about diets that are restricted in calcium or phosphate.
- Use a lift sheet to move or reposition a client with hypocalcemia.

- Keep the environment of a client at risk for thyroid storm cool, dark, and quiet.
- Keep emergency suctioning and tracheostomy equipment in the room of a client who has had thyroid or parathyroid surgery.

Health Promotion and Maintenance

- Teach all clients to take drugs as prescribed, especially diuretics, antihypertensives, and cardiac drugs.
- Include the person who prepares the client's meals when teaching about dietary electrolyte restrictions.

Psychosocial Integrity

- Be accepting of client behavior.
- Help clients and family members understand that changes in cognition and behavior are usually temporary.
- Allow the client who has a permanent change in appearance (such as exophthalmia) to mourn about the change.
- Assess clients who have a sudden change in cognition for electrolyte imbalances.
- Determine the client's food preferences and dislikes when planning an electrolyte-restricted diet.

Physiological Integrity

- Monitor the hydration status of clients who have hypercalcemia.
- Teach clients that hormone replacement therapy for hypothyroidism is lifelong.
- Teach clients to use clinical manifestations, such as the number of bowel movements per day and the ability to sleep, as indicators of therapy effectiveness and when the dose of thyroid hormone replacement may need to be adjusted.
- Assess the bowel sounds; deep tendon reflexes; heart rate, rhythm and quality; and hand grasps to evaluate the client's responses to therapy for an electrolyte imbalance.

ADDITIONAL STUDY RESOURCES

Go to your Student CD-ROM for Review Questions for the NCLEX Examination.

Go to http://evolve.elsevier.com/Iggy/ for Integrated Management of Care Questions for the NCLEX Examination.

SELECTED BIBLIOGRAPHY

Abbas, A., & Lichtman, A. (2003). *Cellular and molecular immunology* (5th ed.). Philadelphia: W.B. Saunders.

Ackley, B., & Ladwig, G. (2002). *Nursing diagnosis handbook: A guide to planning care* (5th ed.). St. Louis: Mosby.

American Cancer Society. (2005). *Cancer facts and figures 2005.* Report No. 00-300M-No. 5008.05. Atlanta: Author.

Dahlen, R. (2002). Managing patients with acute thyrotoxicosis. *Critical Care Nurse*, 22(1), 62-69.

Davies, T., & Larsen, P.R. (2003). Thyrotoxicosis. In P.R. Larsen, et al. (Eds.). *Williams' textbook of endocrinology* (10th ed., pp. 374-422). Philadelphia: W.B. Saunders.

Dochterman, J., & Bulechek, G. (Eds.). (2004). *Nursing interventions classification (NIC)* (4th ed.). St. Louis: Mosby.

Ebersole, P., Hess, P., & Luggen, A. (2004). *Toward healthy aging: Human needs and nursing response* (6th ed.). St. Louis: Mosby.

Elliott, B. (2000). Diagnosing and treating hypothyroidism. *The Nurse Practitioner*, 25(3), 92-105.

Facts and Comparisons. (2004). *Drug facts and comparisons* (58th ed.). St. Louis: Author.

Germano, T. (2001). The parathyroid gland and calcium-related emergencies. *Topics in Emergency Medicine, 23*(4), 51-56.

Holcomb, S. (2003). Detecting thyroid disease, part 1. *Nursing 2003, 33*(8), 32cc1-32cc4.

Holcomb, S. (2003). Detecting thyroid disease, part 2. *Nursing 2003, 33*(9), 32cc1-32cc4.

Husein, M., et al. (2002). Predicting calcium status post thyroidectomy with early calcium levels. *Otolaryngology-Head and Neck Surgery, 127*(4), 289-293.

Klee, G. (2003). Laboratory techniques for recognition of endocrine disorders. In P.R. Larsen, et al. (Eds.). *Williams' textbook of endocrinology* (10th ed., pp. 65-79) Philadelphia: W.B. Saunders.

Klein, I., & Ojamaa, K. (2001). Thyroid hormone and the cardiovascular system. *New England Journal of Medicine, 344*(7), 501-509.

Kumrow, D., & Dahlen, R. (2002). Thyroidectomy: Understanding the potential for complications. *MEDSURG Nursing, 11*(5), 228-235.

Kuritzky, L. (2001). Hypothyroidism. *The American Journal for Nurse Practitioners, 5*(5), 26-39.

Larsen, P.R., & Davies, T. (2003). Hypothyroidism and thyroiditis. In P.R. Larsen, H.M., et al. (Eds.). *Williams' textbook of endocrinology* (10th ed., pp. 423-455). Philadelphia: W.B. Saunders.

Larsen, P.R., et al. (2003). Thyroid physiology and diagnostic evaluation of patients with thyroid disorders. In P.R. Larsen, et al. (Eds.). *Williams' textbook of endocrinology* (10th ed., pp. 331-373). Philadelphia: W.B. Saunders.

Larsen, P.R., et al. (Eds.). (2003). *Williams' textbook of endocrinology* (10th ed.). Philadelphia: W.B. Saunders.

Li, T-M. (2002). Hypothyroidism in elderly people. *Geriatric Nursing, 23*(2), 88-93.

Malchiodi, L. (2002). Emergency: Thyroid storm. *American Journal of Nursing, 102*(5), 33-35.

McCance, K., & Huether, S. (2002). *Pathophysiology: The biologic basis for disease in adults and children* (4th ed.). St. Louis: Mosby.

Mead, M. (2000). Thyroid function tests. *Practice Nurse, 19*(6), 283.

Michalek, A., Mahoney, M., & Calebaugh, D. (2000). Hypothyroidism and diabetes mellitus in an American Indian population. *Journal of Family Practice, 49*(7), 638-640.

Moorhead, S., Johnson, M., & Maas, M. (Eds.). (2004). *Nursing outcomes classification (NOC)* (3rd ed.). St. Louis: Mosby.

Nussbaum, R., McInnes, R., & Willard, H. (2001). *Thompson & Thompson: Genetics in medicine* (6th ed.). Philadelphia: W.B. Saunders.

Pagana, K., & Pagana, T. (2002). *Mosby's manual of diagnostic and laboratory tests* (2nd ed.). St. Louis: Mosby.

Schlumberger, M.-J., Filetti, S., & Hay, I. (2003). Nontoxic goiter and thyroid neoplasia, In P.R. Larsen, et al. (Eds.). *Williams' textbook of endocrinology* (10th ed., pp. 457-490). Philadelphia: W.B. Saunders.

Schori-Ahmed, D. (2003). Thyroid disease: Defenses gone awry. *RN, 66*(6), 38-43.

Waltman, P., Brewer, J., & Lobert, S. (2004). Thyroid storm during pregnancy: A medical emergency. *Critical Care Nurse, 24*(2), 74-79.

Interventions for Clients with Diabetes Mellitus

M. ELAINE MCLEOD

LEARNING OUTCOMES

After studying this chapter, you should be able to:

1. Compare the age of onset, clinical manifestations, and pathologic mechanisms of type 1 and type 2 diabetes mellitus.
2. Identify clients at risk for type 2 diabetes mellitus.
3. Explain the effects of insulin on carbohydrate, protein, and fat metabolism.
4. Evaluate laboratory data to determine whether the client is using the prescribed dietary, medication, and exercise interventions for diabetes.
5. Explain the effect of aerobic exercise on blood glucose levels.
6. Describe the significance of ketone bodies in the urine of a diabetic client.
7. Discuss the dietary requirements of clients taking Humalog insulin before meals.
8. Identify eating habits and patterns that place the diabetic client at increased risk for hypoglycemia and hyperglycemia.
9. Compare the mechanisms of action of the sulfonylureas, meglitinide analogs, biguanides, alpha glucosidase inhibitors, and thiazolidinediones as antidiabetic agents.
10. Explain the effect of hypertension on the development of diabetic nephropathy and diabetic retinopathy.
11. Identify clients at risk for hypoglycemia.
12. Prioritize nursing interventions for the client with mild to moderate hypoglycemia and moderate to severe hypoglycemia.
13. Identify clients at risk for diabetic ketoacidosis (DKA).
14. Prioritize nursing interventions for clients with DKA.
15. Identify clients at risk for hyperglycemic-hyperosmolar nonketotic syndrome (HHNS).
16. Prioritize nursing interventions for clients with HHNS.
17. Use laboratory data and clinical manifestations to determine the effectiveness of the interventions for DKA and HHNS.
18. Describe the steps required for subcutaneous insulin administration.
19. Describe the correct technique to use when mixing different types of insulin in the same syringe.
20. Compare the clinical manifestations of hyperglycemia and hypoglycemia.
21. Perform foot assessment and foot care for the client with diabetes.

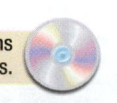

Go to your Student CD-ROM for Review Questions
for the NCLEX Examination keyed to these Learning Outcomes.

Diabetes mellitus is a common chronic disease requiring lifelong behavioral and lifestyle changes. It is best managed with a team approach to empower the client to successfully manage the disease. As part of the team, the nurse plans, organizes, and coordinates care among the various health disciplines involved; provides care and education; and promotes the client's health and well-being.

Diabetes is a major public health problem worldwide. Its complications cause many devastating health problems. The financial cost of diabetes is discussed in the Resource Management box on p. 1499. In the United States, diabetes is the leading cause of new cases of blindness, end-stage renal disease requiring dialysis or transplantation, and foot or leg amputations. Many people with diabetes are undiagnosed. Many who are diagnosed have unacceptably high blood glucose levels.

RESOURCE MANAGEMENT

DIABETES MELLITUS

Cost of Care

- Although people diagnosed with diabetes comprise 4% of the U.S. population, almost $1 out of every $5 spent on health care is for a person with diabetes.
- The annual cost of diabetes in medical expenses and lost workdays increased from $98 billion in 1997 to $132 billion in 2002.
- The per capita annual costs of health care for people with diabetes rose from $10,000 in 1997 to $13,242 in 2002—an increase of more than 3%. Health care costs for clients without diabetes amounted to $2560 in 2002.
- In 2002, the direct cost of diabetes was estimated to be $91.8 billion—19% of total personal health care costs.
- In 2002, about $40.3 billion dollars was spent for inpatient hospital care, $13.8 billion for nursing home care, and $10 billion for office visits.
- In 2002, indirect costs of diabetes was estimated to be $39.8 billion.
- In 2002, diabetes accounted for a loss of nearly 88 million disability days.
- In 2002, 176,000 cases of permanent disability were caused by diabetes at a cost of $7.5 billion.

Implications for Nursing

If costs related to diabetes are to be reduced, attention must be directed to the prevention and treatment of chronic complications of diabetes. Therapies are available to reduce the incidence of blindness, medications are available to reduce the incidence of kidney and coronary artery disease, and regular sensory evaluation of the feet can reduce the incidence of amputation. The challenge for the nurse is to assist the diabetic client in achieving and maintaining meticulous blood glucose control so that long-term complications are prevented.

Data from American Diabetes Association. (2003). Reviews: Economic costs of diabetes in the U.S. in 2002. *Diabetes Care*, *26*(3), 917-932, and from American Association of Diabetes Educators. Diabetes facts and statistics. Available at http://www.aadenet.org/GeneralDiabetesInfo/GovStats.html.

TABLE 68-1   Classification of Diabetes Mellitus

Type 1 Diabetes
- Primary beta cell destruction leading to absolute insulin deficiency
  Autoimmune process
  Idiopathic

Type 2 Diabetes
- Ranges from insulin resistance with an insulin deficiency to secretory deficit with insulin resistance

Other Specific Types (Conditions Resulting in Hyperglycemia)
- Genetic defects of beta cell function
- Genetic defects in insulin action
- Diseases of the exocrine pancreas: pancreatitis, trauma, neoplasia, cystic fibrosis, hemochromatosis
- Endocrinopathies: acromegaly, Cushing's disease glucagonoma, pheochromocytoma, hyperthyroidism, aldosteronoma
- Drug- or chemical-induced conditions (from use of pentamidine, nicotinic acid, glucocorticoids, thyroid hormone, diazoxide, beta-adrenergic agonists, thiazides, Dilantin, interferon-alpha, other drugs)
- Infections: congenital rubella, cytomegalovirus
- Uncommon forms of immune-related diabetes
- Other genetic syndromes associated with diabetes: Down syndrome, Klinefelter syndrome, Turner's syndrome, Huntington disease, and others

Gestational Diabetes Mellitus (GDM)
- Carbohydrate intolerance with onset or first recognized during pregnancy
- Children of mothers with GDM are at greater risk for neonatal mortality, congenital malformation, and macrosomia (large body size).
- Children of mothers with GDM have an increased risk of obesity and impaired glucose tolerance in late adolescence and young adulthood.
- Clients with GDM are at high risk for developing diabetes after pregnancy.
- Diagnosis is based on the results of a 100-g oral glucose tolerance test during pregnancy.

Data from American Diabetes Association. (2003). Committee report: Report of the Expert Committee on the Diagnosis and Classification of Diabetes Mellitus. *Diabetes Care*, *26*(Suppl. 1), 5-20, and American Diabetes Association. (2000). Position statement: Gestational diabetes mellitus. *Diabetes Care*, *26*(Suppl. 1), 103-105.

Studies confirm that **glycemic** (blood glucose) control reduces complications of diabetes. Treatment of hypertension and **hyperlipidemia** (high blood fat levels) is essential to prevent complications of diabetes.

The nurse's challenge is to help the client with diabetes achieve and maintain lifestyle changes that prevent long-term complications by keeping blood glucose levels as close to normal as possible. New insulins, oral antidiabetic drugs, and tools are available to help clients achieve normal glucose levels.

PATHOPHYSIOLOGY

Classification of Diabetes

For all types of diabetes mellitus, the main feature is chronic **hyperglycemia** (high blood glucose level) resulting from problems with insulin secretion, insulin action, or both. The disease is classified by the underlying problem causing a lack of insulin and the severity of the insulin deficiency. Table 68-1 outlines the types of diabetes.

The Endocrine Pancreas

The endocrine portion of the pancreas has about 1 million small glands, the islets of Langerhans, scattered through the gland. The islet cells are only a small portion of the gland. Most of the gland has digestive functions. Two types of islet cells are important to glucose control. Alpha cells produce glucagon; beta cells produce insulin. **Glucagon** is a major "counterregulatory" hormone that has actions opposite those of insulin. It causes the release of glucose from cell storage sites whenever blood glucose levels are low. Insulin allows body cells to use and store carbohydrate, fat, and protein.

Insulin Physiology

Insulin is a protein made up of 51 amino acids in two peptide chains: an alpha chain and a beta chain. Preproinsulin is produced initially. This protein is a precursor molecule. It is inactive and must be made smaller before becoming the active hormone insulin. Preproinsulin is cut by enzymes to **proinsulin** (a precursor that includes the alpha and beta chains of the insulin molecule) and an additional fragment, the C-peptide chain. Proinsulin is converted in the beta cells into equal amounts of insulin and C-peptide (Figure 68-1). C-peptide levels are used to measure the rate that beta cells secrete insulin.

Insulin allows glucose in the blood to move into cells to make energy. Thus, insulin is like a key to open cell membranes to glucose. Insulin starts by binding to insulin receptors on the cell membranes. The liver is the first major organ

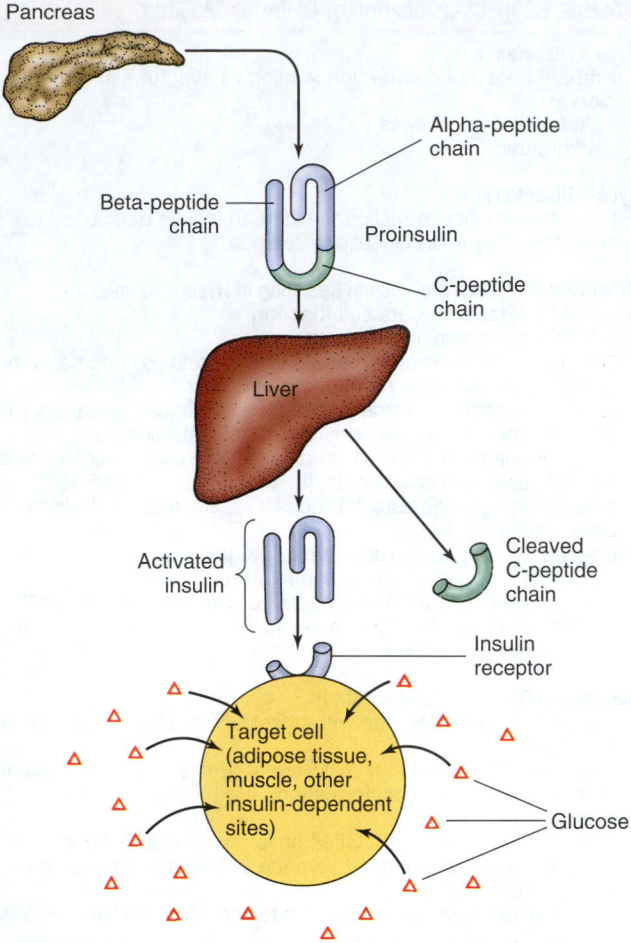

Figure 68-1 ■ Proinsulin, secreted by and stored in the beta cells of the islets of Langerhans in the pancreas, is transformed by the liver into activated insulin. Insulin attaches to receptors on target cells, where it promotes glucose transport into the cells through the cell membranes.

TABLE 68-2 Physiologic Response to Insufficient Insulin
■ Decreased glycogenesis (conversion of glucose to glycogen)
■ Increased glycogenolysis (conversion of glycogen to glucose)
■ Increased gluconeogenesis (formation of glucose from non-carbohydrate sources, such as amino acids and lactate)
■ Increased lipolysis (breakdown of triglycerides to glycerol and free fatty acids)
■ Increased ketogenesis (formation of ketones from free fatty acids)
■ Proteolysis (breakdown of protein with amino acid release in muscles)

to be reached by insulin in the blood. In the liver, insulin promotes the production and storage of glycogen **(glycogenesis)** at the same time that it inhibits glycogen breakdown into glucose **(glycogenolysis)**. Insulin increases protein and lipid (fat) synthesis. Insulin inhibits tissue breakdown by inhibiting liver glycogenolysis, **ketogenesis** (conversion of fats to acids), and **gluconeogenesis** (conversion of proteins to glucose). In muscle, insulin promotes protein and glycogen synthesis. In fat cells, insulin promotes triglyceride storage. Overall, insulin keeps blood glucose levels from becoming too high and helps keep blood lipid levels in the normal range.

The pancreas secretes about 40 to 50 units of insulin daily directly into liver circulation in a two-step manner. Insulin is secreted at low levels during fasting **(basal insulin secretion)** and at increased levels after eating **(prandial)**. An early burst of insulin secretion occurs within 10 minutes of eating. This is followed by an increasing insulin release that lasts as long as hyperglycemia is present.

Glucose Homeostasis

Glucose is the main fuel for central nervous system (CNS) cells. Because the brain cannot produce or store much glucose, it needs a continuous supply from circulation. Fatty

acids can be used as fuel when glucose is not available. The circulating fuels of glucose and free fatty acids are stored inside cells as glycogen in the liver and muscles and as triglyceride in fat cells. Fat, in the form of triglyceride, is the most efficient means of storing energy. Fat has 9 calories of stored energy per gram. Protein and carbohydrate have only 4 calories per gram. Although protein can be used as fuel during starvation, it is not used for fuel under normal conditions.

The combined actions of insulin and counterregulatory hormones (discussed in the next section) keep blood glucose levels in the range of 68 to 105 mg/dL (3.6 to 5.8 mmol/L) to support brain functions. When glucose levels fall, insulin secretion stops and glucagon is released. Glucagon causes the release of glucose from the liver. Liver glucose is made through **glycogenolysis** (breakdown of glycogen to glucose) and **gluconeogenesis.** When liver glucose is unavailable, **lipolysis** (breakdown of fat) and **proteolysis** (breakdown of amino acids) provide fuel for energy.

Counterregulatory hormones increase blood glucose by actions opposite those of insulin when more energy is needed. Glucagon is the main counterregulatory hormone. Other hormones that increase blood glucose levels are epinephrine, norepinephrine, growth hormone, and cortisol.

Absence of Insulin

Insulin is needed to move glucose into most body tissues. The lack of insulin in diabetes, from either a lack of production or a problem with insulin use at its cell receptor, prevents some cells from using glucose for energy. Without insulin, the body enters a serious state of breaking down body fat and protein. Levels of counterregulatory hormones increase in an attempt to make glucose from other sources. Table 68-2 outlines the body's response to insufficient insulin.

Without insulin, glucose builds up in the blood, causing **hyperglycemia** (high blood glucose levels). Hyperglycemia causes fluid and electrolyte imbalances, leading to the classic symptoms of diabetes: polyuria, polydipsia, and polyphagia.

Polyuria (frequent and excessive urination) results from an osmotic diuresis caused by excess glucose in the urine. As a result of diuresis, sodium, chloride, and potassium are excreted in the urine, and water loss is severe. Dehydration results and **polydipsia** (excessive thirst) occurs. Because the cells receive no glucose, cell starvation triggers **polyphagia** (excessive eating). Despite eating vast amounts of food, the person remains in starvation until insulin is available to move glucose into the cells.

With insulin deficiency, fats break down, releasing free fatty acids. Conversion of fatty acids to **ketone bodies** (small acids) provides a backup energy source. Because ketone bodies, or "ketones," are abnormal breakdown products of fatty acids, they may accumulate in the blood when insulin is not available. This accumulation causes metabolic acidosis.

The dehydration that occurs with diabetes leads to **hemoconcentration** (increased blood concentration), **hypovolemia** (decreased blood volume), **hyperviscosity** (thick, concentrated blood), **hypoperfusion** (decreased circulation) of tissues, and poor tissue oxygenation **(hypoxia)**. Hypoxic cells do not metabolize glucose efficiently, the Krebs cycle is blocked, and lactic acid increases, causing more acidosis. Restoring tissue perfusion and oxygenation by giving insulin halts lactic acid production.

The excess acids caused by absence of insulin increase hydrogen ion (H^+) and carbon dioxide (CO_2) levels in the blood. These products trigger the respiratory control areas of the brain to increase the rate and depth of respiration in an attempt to excrete more carbon dioxide and acid. This type of breathing is known as **Kussmaul respiration**. Acetone is exhaled, giving the breath a "fruity" odor. When the lungs can no longer offset acidosis, the pH drops. Arterial blood gas studies show a metabolic acidosis (decreased pH with decreased arterial bicarbonate [HCO_3^-] levels) and compensatory respiratory alkalosis (decreased partial pressure of arterial carbon dioxide [$PaCO_2$]) (see Chapter 19).

Insulin lack causes potassium depletion. Because of the increased fluid loss with hyperglycemia, excessive potassium is excreted in the urine, leading to low serum potassium levels. However, high serum potassium levels may occur in acidosis because of the shift of potassium from inside the cells to the blood and other extracellular fluids. Serum potassium levels in diabetes, then, may be low **(hypokalemia)**, high **(hyperkalemia)**, or normal, depending on hydration, the severity of acidosis, and the client's response to treatment. Chapters 18 and 19 discuss acid-base balance and acidosis in more detail.

Acute Complications of Diabetes

Three glucose-related emergencies can occur in clients with diabetes: diabetic ketoacidosis (DKA) caused by lack of insulin and ketosis; hyperglycemic-hyperosmolar-nonketotic syndrome (HHNS) caused by insulin deficiency and profound dehydration; and hypoglycemia from too much insulin or too little glucose. All three problems require emergency treatment and can be fatal if treatment is delayed or incorrect. These problems and their interventions are described later.

Chronic Complications of Diabetes

Diabetes mellitus can lead to health problems and early death because of changes in large blood vessels **(macrovascular)** and small blood vessels **(microvascular)** in tissues and organs. Complications result from poor tissue circulation and cell death. Macrovascular complications, including coronary heart disease, cerebrovascular disease, and peripheral vascular disease, lead to increased early death among those with diabetes. Microvascular complications of blood vessel structure and function lead to **nephropathy** (kidney dysfunction), **neuropathy** (nerve dysfunction), and **retinopathy** (vision problems). Three theories have been used to explain these diabetic vascular complications:

- Chronic hyperglycemia causes irreversible structural changes resulting in basement membrane thickening and organ damage.

- Glucose toxicity directly or indirectly affects functional cell integrity.
- Chronic ischemia in microcirculatory branches causes connective tissue hypoxia and microischemia.

Chronic high blood glucose levels are the main cause of microvascular complications and allow premature development of macrovascular complications (Bell, 2002). Macrovascular complications in people with type 2 diabetes seem more related to hypertension, a sedentary lifestyle, high blood lipid levels, and smoking than to hyperglycemia. Obesity is also important for people with type 2 diabetes. About 80% of clients with type 2 diabetes are obese, and cardiovascular events account for most of their deaths.

The National Diabetes Data Group of the National Institutes of Health estimates that type 2 diabetes starts 9 to 12 years before the disorder is diagnosed. During this time of no treatment, complications develop. Up to 21% of clients have retinopathy at the time of diagnosis (American Diabetes Association [ADA], 2003e). Many older diabetic clients have no classic signs of high blood glucose levels, and the diagnosis is made when the person seeks treatment for another illness or for complications of diabetes.

The Diabetes Control and Complications Trial (DCCT), a study involving 29 medical centers and more than 1400 people with type 1 diabetes, showed that hyperglycemia is a critical factor for long-term diabetic complications. Intensive therapy with blood glucose levels as close to normal as possible delays the onset and progression of retinopathy, nephropathy, and neuropathy. Additional studies show that intensive therapy with lowered blood glucose levels reduced the onset of retinopathy, nephropathy, and neuropathy in clients with type 2 diabetes. A strong relationship exists between risks for microvascular complications and blood glucose levels. For every percentage point decrease in HbA1c, a 35% reduction in the risk for kidney and eye complications has been shown (ADA, 2003j).

MACROVASCULAR COMPLICATIONS

CARDIOVASCULAR DISEASE. Cardiovascular disease (CVD) is the most common complication of diabetes mellitus. Diabetic clients have a two to three times greater risk for CVD compared to nondiabetic clients. This excess risk occurs in both type 1 and type 2 diabetes, affects women more than men, and is influenced by ethnicity. More than 50% of clients with diabetes have some degree of CVD at the time of diagnosis. Complications of atherosclerosis cause about 80% of deaths in clients with diabetes and 75% of hospitalizations for diabetic complications (Spanheimer, 2001).

Myocardial infarction (MI) is the leading cause of death among clients with diabetes. They tend to have extensive coronary artery disease, cardiomyopathy, and abnormal blood clotting. Left ventricular dysfunction with heart failure and fatal dysrhythmias are common in diabetic clients after MI. Heart failure occurs in up to 50% of diabetic clients after MI (Tang & Young, 2001).

Diabetes is a major cardiovascular risk factor. Furthermore, clients with type 2 diabetes are more likely to have the risk factors of obesity, hypertension, dyslipidemia (excessive blood levels of cholesterol and other fats), and a sedentary lifestyle—a combination of factors known as "metabolic syndrome" (see later discussion). Renal disease, indicated by albumin in the urine, increases the risk for coronary heart disease and mortality from MI (Watkins, 2003).

Cardiovascular disease rates can be reduced through management of hyperglycemia, hypertension, and hyperlipidemia. The American Diabetes Association (ADA) recommends that blood pressure be maintained below 130/80 mm Hg and that low-density lipoprotein (LDL) cholesterol be kept below 100 mg/dL [<2.60 mmol/L] (ADA, 2003r). The American Heart Association recommends replacing saturated fat with monounsaturated fat (Safeer & Cornell, 2000).

CEREBROVASCULAR DISEASE. Diabetes damages cerebrovascular arterial circulation and is a risk factor for stroke. Hypertension, hyperlipidemia, nephropathy, peripheral vascular disease, and alcohol and tobacco abuse, along with diabetes, further increase the risk for stroke (Ingall, 2000).

Diabetes affects stroke outcomes as well. Elevated blood glucose levels at the time of the stroke may lead to greater brain injury and higher mortality (Beckman et al., 2002).

MICROVASCULAR COMPLICATIONS

EYE AND VISION COMPLICATIONS. Legal blindness (a corrected visual acuity of 20/200 or less) is 25 times more common in people with diabetes. In the United States, diabetic retinopathy is the most frequent cause of new blindness among adults 20 to 74 years of age. Retinopathy is strongly related to the duration of diabetes. After 20 years of diabetes, nearly all clients with type 1 diabetes and 78% of those with type 2 diabetes have some degree of retinopathy (Skyler, 2001).

The cause and progression of diabetic retinopathy are related to problems that block retinal blood vessels and cause them to leak, leading to retinal hypoxia. **Nonproliferative diabetic retinopathy (NPDR)** (Figure 68-2) causes structural problems in retinal vessels, but growth of new blood vessels is not stimulated. There are areas of poor retinal circulation, edema, hard fatty deposits in the eye, and retinal hemorrhages. **Microaneurysms** (small capillary wall dilations in retinal vessels) form throughout the eye. They leak fluid and blood into the retina, causing retinal edema and hard exudates. Other retinal problems include retinal hemorrhages, nerve fiber atrophy from hypoxia, and venous beading. **Ve-**nous beading is the abnormal appearance of retinal veins in which areas of swelling and constriction along a segment of vein resemble links of sausage. Venous beading occurs in areas of retinal ischemia and is a predictor of proliferative diabetic retinopathy (PDR). NPDR develops slowly and rarely causes blindness. Clients with severe NPDR have a 45% chance of developing proliferative diabetic retinopathy (Franz, 2001).

Proliferative diabetic retinopathy (PDR) is the growth of new retinal blood vessels (**neovascularization**). When retinal circulation is poor and hypoxia develops, retinal cells secrete a "growth factor" that stimulates formation of new blood vessels in the eye. These new vessels are thin, fragile, and bleed easily. They lead to eye hemorrhage and more vision loss (Figure 68-3). Fibrous tissue bands, developing along with new blood vessels, cause retinal detachment and permanent vision loss. Chapter 50 discusses treatment of retinal problems.

Retinopathy is linked to fasting blood glucose levels above 129 mg/dL. Hyperglycemia and hypertension increase the rate of retinopathy development in clients with type 1 diabetes. Intensive diabetes management to obtain **near-euglycemic** (near-normal blood glucose) levels prevents or delays diabetic retinopathy (ADA, 2003e).

Vision loss also occurs from macular degeneration, corneal scarring, and changes in lens shape or clarity. Hyperglycemia may cause blurred vision, even with eyeglasses. Hypoglycemia may cause double vision. Cataracts occur at a younger age and progress faster among people with diabetes. Open-angle glaucoma also is more common in clients with diabetes. The management of cataracts and glaucoma are the same as for nondiabetic clients (see Chapter 50).

CONSIDERATIONS FOR OLDER ADULTS

The older client with diabetic retinopathy also has visual changes from aging. As a result, the older diabetic client's ability to perform self-care may be more seriously affected than that of a younger person with diabetes (see Chapter 50). The ability to discriminate among blues, greens, and violets decreases with normal aging. This problem makes performing visual blood glucose monitoring more difficult.

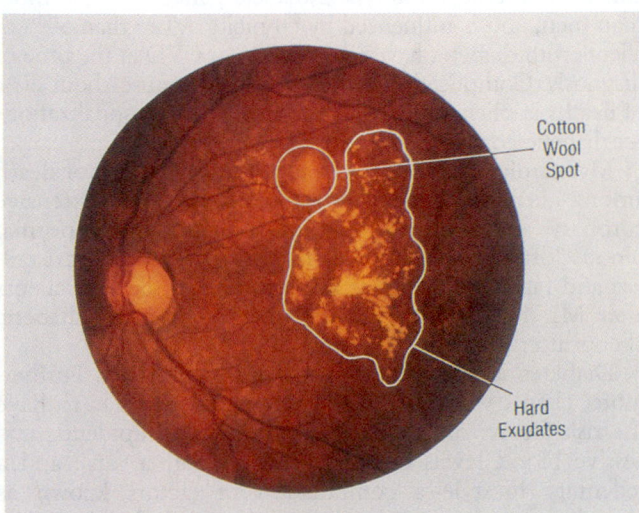

Figure 68-2 ■ Select ophthalmic changes seen in nonproliferative diabetic retinopathy (NPDR).

Cotton Wool Spot

Hard Exudates

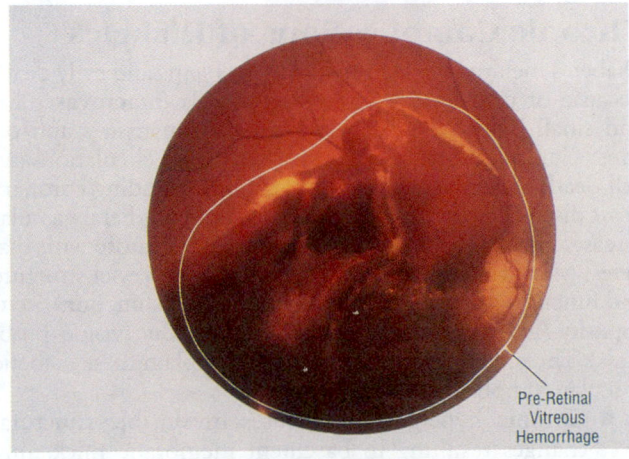

Figure 68-3 ■ Ophthalmic hemorrhage that is possible with proliferative diabetic retinopathy.

Pre-Retinal Vitreous Hemorrhage

DIABETIC NEUROPATHY. Neuropathy is a progressive deterioration of nerves that results in loss of nerve function. It is a common complication of diabetes and often involves all parts of the body. Damage to sensory nerve fibers results in either pain or loss of sensation. Damage to motor nerve fibers results in muscle weakness. Damage to nerve fibers in the autonomic nervous system results in widespread loss of many functions.

Diabetic neuropathy can be focal or diffuse, each with different causes, rates of progression, and treatments. The most common neuropathies in diabetes are diffuse. They involve widespread nerve function loss, have a slow onset, affect both sides of the body, involve motor and sensory nerves, progress slowly, and are permanent. Diffuse neuropathies include autonomic nerve dysfunction. Late complications include foot ulcers and deformities.

Focal neuropathies affect a single nerve or nerve group. They usually are caused by an acute ischemic event (ischemic neuropathy) or by the physical trapping of a nerve (entrapment neuropathy). Both types lead to nerve damage or nerve death. Ischemic neuropathies occur when the blood supply to a nerve or group of nerves is disrupted. The symptoms begin suddenly, affect only one side of the body or body area, and are self-limiting in duration. Recovery time varies. Entrapment neuropathies stem from compression of a nerve in a body compartment or between tissues. Symptoms begin gradually and can occur anywhere. They may be bilateral, having a waxing and waning course without spontaneous recovery. An example of focal entrapment neuropathy is carpal tunnel syndrome.

Hyperglycemia leads to neuropathy through blood vessel changes that cause nerve hypoxia. Both the axon and its myelin sheath are damaged by reduced blood flow, resulting in blocked nerve impulse transmission. Excessive glucose is converted to sorbitol, which accumulates in nerves. The increased sorbitol also impairs motor nerve conduction. Common diabetic neuropathies are listed in Table 68-3. Autonomic nervous system neuropathy leads to problems in cardiovascular, gastrointestinal (GI), and urinary function. Keeping blood glucose levels in the normal range delays the onset and reduces the severity of diabetic neuropathies.

The cardiovascular problems of **orthostatic** (postural) hypotension and **syncope** (brief loss of consciousness) increase the risk for falls. In addition, the neuropathy can mask the pain of MI. Common GI symptoms from diabetic neuropathy are **dysphagia** (difficulty swallowing), heartburn, nausea and vomiting, and bowel elimination problems. Diarrhea caused by diabetes is chronic, may be severe, and often occurs at night. Constipation, the most common GI symptom, is intermittent and may alternate with bouts of diarrhea. **Gastroparesis** (delay in gastric emptying) is a cause of hypoglycemia. Loss of nerve input to the bladder results in incomplete emptying, which leads to urinary infection and kidney problems.

DIABETIC NEPHROPATHY. Nephropathy is pathologic change in the kidney that reduces kidney function and leads to renal failure. Diabetes mellitus is the leading cause of end-stage renal disease (ESRD) and renal failure in the United States. Diabetic nephropathy affects 20% to 30% of those with type 1 diabetes 20 years after onset. Although less than 20% of clients with type 2 diabetes have nephropathy, about 60% of the clients with ESRD have type 2 diabetes (Skyler, 2001). Native Americans/American Indians, Hispanics (especially Mexican Americans), and African Americans have much

---

TABLE 68-3 Features of Diabetic Neuropathy

	Complication	Manifestation
Diffuse Neuropathies		
Distal symmetric polyneuropathy	Sensory alterations	Paresthesias: burning/tingling sensations, starting in toes and moving up legs Dysesthesias: burning, stinging, or stabbing pain Anesthesia: loss of sensation
	Motor alterations in intrinsic muscles of foot	Foot deformities: high arch, claw toes, hammertoes; shift of weight bearing to metatarsal heads and tips of toes
Autonomic neuropathy	Anhidrosis	Drying, cracking of skin
	Gastroparesis	Delayed gastric emptying, constipation, nausea, anorexia
	Diabetic diarrhea	Diarrhea and bowel incontinence
	Neurogenic bladder	Atonic bladder, urinary retention
	Impotence	Erectile dysfunction
	Loss of cardiac reflexes	Orthostatic hypotension, resting tachycardia
	Defective counterregulation	Loss of warning signs of hypoglycemia
Focal Neuropathies		
Focal ischemia	Thoracolumbar radiculopathy with sensory and reflex loss	Pain radiating across back, side, and front of chest or abdomen
	Cranial nerve palsies, third and sixth nerves	Sudden diplopia or ptosis; eye pain
	Amyotrophy	Pain; asymmetric weakness; wasting of iliopsoas, quadriceps, and adductor muscles
Entrapment neuropathies	Median nerve	Carpal tunnel syndrome
	Popliteal nerve/knee	Footdrop
	Posterior tibial nerve at tarsal tunnel	Tarsal tunnel syndrome: sensory impairment in sole of foot; weakness of intrinsic muscles of foot; burning pain and paresthesias at ankle and plantar surface

TABLE 68-4 Differentiation of Type 1 and Type 2 Diabetes

Features	Type 1	Type 2
Former names	Juvenile-onset diabetes Ketosis-prone diabetes Insulin-dependent diabetes mellitus (IDDM)	Maturity-onset diabetes Ketosis-resistant diabetes Non–insulin-dependent diabetes mellitus (NIDDM)
Age at onset	Usually under 30 yr of age, occurs at any age	Peaks in 50s; may occur earlier
Symptoms	Abrupt onset, thirst, weight loss	Frequently none; thirst, fatigue, visual blurring, vascular or neural complications
Etiology	Viral infection	Not known
Pathology	Pancreatic beta cell destruction	Insulin resistance Dysfunctional pancreatic beta cell
Antigen patterns	HLA-DR4, HLA-DR3	None
Antibodies	ICAs present at diagnosis	None
Endogenous insulin and C-peptide	None	Low, normal, or high
Inheritance	Recessive	Dominant, multifactorial
Nutritional status	Usually nonobese	60% to 80% obese
Insulin	All dependent on insulin	Required for 20% to 30%
Sulfonylurea therapy	None	Effective for most clients
Medical nutrition therapy	Mandatory	Mandatory

ICAs, Islet cell antibodies.

higher risks for developing ESRD than non-Hispanic whites. Keeping blood glucose levels in the normal range can delay the onset of nephropathy and, in some cases, may prevent it.

Risk factors for diabetic nephropathy include a 10- to 15-year history of diabetes, diabetic retinopathy, poor blood glucose control, uncontrolled hypertension, and genetic predisposition (Sweny, 2002). In addition, clients with diabetes who also produce excess collagen (such as people who form keloid scars) are at greater risk for developing diabetic nephropathy.

The earliest clinical sign of nephropathy is **microalbuminuria** (very small amounts of albumin in the urine). Annual testing for microalbuminuria is recommended for clients who have had type 1 diabetes for at least 5 years and in all clients with type 2 diabetes (ADA, 2003r).

Chronic high blood glucose levels cause hypertension in kidney blood vessels and excess kidney perfusion. The increased pressure damages the kidney in many ways. The blood vessels become more leaky, especially in the glomerulus. This leakiness allows filtration of larger particles (including albumin and other proteins), which then form deposits in the kidney tissue and blood vessels. Deposits narrow the vessels, decreasing kidney oxygenation and leading to kidney cell hypoxia and cell death. These processes worsen over time. Blood vessels in the glomerulus become scarred and unable to filter urine from the blood, leading to renal failure.

Renal damage is also related to increased mean arterial blood pressure in diabetic clients with cardiovascular disease. Both systolic and diastolic hypertension greatly speed the progression of diabetic nephropathy.

MALE ERECTILE DYSFUNCTION. Erectile dysfunction (ED) is the inability to achieve or maintain a penile erection sufficient for satisfactory sexual performance. ED occurs at a higher rate and an earlier age among men with diabetes as compared with the general population. About half of diabetic men have ED. This occurs 10 to 15 years earlier than in the general population (Paty & Hirsch, 2000). In diabetes, ED is related to poor blood glucose control, obesity, hypertension, heavy cigarette smoking, and the presence of other chronic microvascular and macrovascular complications.

ED may be caused by neuropathy, vascular disease, psychological factors, or endocrine disorders. Autonomic neuropathy or vascular changes are responsible for persistent ED in diabetes. Chapter 79 discusses erectile function problems in depth.

Etiology and Genetic Risk
TYPE 1 DIABETES

Type 1 diabetes is an autoimmune disorder in which beta cells are destroyed in a genetically susceptible person (Table 68-4). The immune system fails to recognize normal body cells as "self" and takes destructive actions against them. In type 1 diabetes, immune system cells and cell products attack and destroy insulin-secreting cells in the islets. Although the exact cause of a person's normal body cells being attacked by immune system cells is not known, people with certain tissue types are more likely to develop autoimmune diseases, including type 1 diabetes. Specifically, people who have the tissue types HLA-DR3 or HLA-DR4 are at an increased risk for type 1 diabetes. Certain viral infections, such as mumps, congenital rubella, and coxsackievirus infection, appear to trigger autoimmune destruction of pancreatic beta cells.

Indicators or markers of immune damage to insulin-producing cells (a key feature of type 1 diabetes) are the presence of blood antibodies directed against the beta cells themselves or against substances made by beta cells. Most clients with type 1 diabetes have islet cell antibodies (ICAs), insulin autoantibodies (IAAs), autoantibodies to glutamic acid decarboxylase (GAD), or autoantibodies to tyrosine phosphates. Circulating ICA and IAA may be present before manifestations of type 1 diabetes develop.

Genetic Considerations

Risk for type 1 diabetes is determined by inheritance of the HLA-DR3 and HLA-DR4 genes. However, although inheritance of these genes increases the risk, most people with these genes do not develop type 1 diabetes. Development of the disease is an interactive effect of genetic predisposition and exposure to certain environmental factors. The risk for type 1 diabetes in the general population ranges from 1 in 400 to 1 in 1000. The risk greatly increases for those who have at least one parent with diabetes (from 1 in 20 to 1 in 50) (Franz, 2001). It is unclear why some genetically susceptible people develop diabetes and others do not.

TYPE 2 DIABETES AND METABOLIC SYNDROME

Type 2 diabetes is a progressive disorder in which the pancreas makes less insulin over time. Clients with type 2 diabetes have a reduced ability of most cells to respond to insulin (**insulin resistance**), poor control of liver glucose output, and decreased beta-cell function, eventually leading to beta-cell failure. Most people with type 2 diabetes are obese adults. With the increased rate of obesity occurring in younger people, the age of onset for type 2 diabetes is also decreasing. The specific causes of type 2 diabetes are not known. Both insulin resistance and beta-cell failure have many genetic and nongenetic causes. Heredity plays a major role in the development of type 2 diabetes. Offspring of clients with type 2 diabetes have a 15% chance of developing the disease and a 30% risk of having impaired glucose tolerance. Specific gene defects have been identified in certain groups with high incidence rates of type 2 diabetes. Pima Indians have a 50% prevalence of type 2 diabetes (Franz, 2001).

Metabolic syndrome, also called **syndrome X,** is a group of disorders with insulin resistance as a main feature. Other features of the syndrome include obesity (particularly with excessive fat tissue around the waist and abdomen, giving the person a round, "apple-like" shape), low levels of physical activity, hypertension, and high blood levels of cholesterol. The syndrome is not a single disease but is a collection of related health problems thought to represent a gene-environment interaction. A genetic predisposition to type 2 diabetes increases the risk for the other metabolic syndrome health problems when compounded by obesity and a sedentary lifestyle. Any one of these health problems increases the rate of atherosclerosis and the risk for stroke, coronary heart disease, and early death. Together with metabolic syndrome, these health problems greatly increase the risk for potentially lethal cardiovascular complications. Although metabolic syndrome does not respond readily to drug therapy for any one of the health problems, lifestyle changes (e.g., getting regular aerobic exercise, achieving an ideal body weight) can reduce the insulin resistance and diabetic manifestations, reduce the high blood levels of cholesterol, and lower blood pressure.

Incidence/Prevalence

Diabetes mellitus is the seventh leading cause of death in the United States, where it affects 17 million people, or 6.2% of the population. In the United States, the incidence of diabetes is rising—up 49% from 1990 to 2000, with projections indicating a 165% increase by the year 2050. An additional 5.9 million people are unaware they have the disease (Lachuk et al., 2002).

About 90% of diabetic persons have type 2 diabetes. Diagnosed diabetes is most common among middle-aged and older adults, affecting about 6% of people 45 to 64 years of age and 11% of those over 65 years of age. About 10% of clients diagnosed with diabetes are older than 70 years of age. After 40 years of age, new-onset diabetes is usually type 2. The prevalence of diabetes is similar for men and women. Although type 2 diabetes is a disease of middle-aged and older adults, recent surveys show an increase of the disorder in childhood and adolescence as a result of obesity (El-Kebbi et al., 2003).

Because the prevalence of obesity is rising in the United States, diabetes will become even more common. Body mass index (BMI) is one of the strongest indicators of diabetes. Among clients diagnosed with diabetes, 68% have a BMI of at least 27 kg/m², and 46% have a BMI of at least 30 kg/m². Risk for diabetes increases dramatically as the degree of overweight increases.

HEALTH PROMOTION/ILLNESS PREVENTION

The fact that diabetes is a common disorder and causes many preventable but devastating complications makes the disease a major public health problem. The U.S. government has identified control of diabetes and its complications as a major focus for health promotion activities (see the Meeting Healthy People 2010 box on p. 1506).

No interventions are successful in preventing type 1 diabetes. Health promotion for clients with type 1 diabetes focuses on controlling hyperglycemia to reduce its long-term complications.

Type 2 diabetes can be prevented or delayed by weight loss and increased physical activity. Strategies to reduce the cardiovascular risk factors of tobacco use, hypertension, and high blood lipid levels also reduce the incidence of type 2 diabetes and its long-term complications. Drug therapy is not recommended for routine use to prevent diabetes (ADA, 2003t).

CULTURAL CONSIDERATIONS

Diabetes is a significant health problem for African Americans, Native Americans/American Indians, and Mexican Americans. The prevalence rates for this disease are 1.6 and 1.9 times higher, respectively, than the rate for white individuals. The increase in obesity and sedentary lifestyles in the U.S. population is the probable cause of this growing problem (El-Kebbi, 2003). The American Diabetes Association (ADA) has identified individuals who should be tested for diabetes in Table 68-5.

Racial and ethnic differences affect clinical outcomes for diabetic clients. The prevalence of hypertension in diabetic clients is at least twice the rate of nondiabetic clients, with non-Hispanic whites and African Americans having the highest prevalence. Microvascular complications of the eyes, nerves, and kidneys are more common in African Americans and Native Americans/American Indians with diabetes than in non-Hispanic whites with diabetes (Harris, 2001).

Meeting HEALTHY PEOPLE 2010 Objectives

DIABETES MELLITUS

Objective 18.4: _Reduce the diabetes death rates (diabetes as the underlying cause) to no more than 12.0 per 100,000 persons._

- Encourage all people to have a yearly screening physical examination that includes blood testing for diabetes.
- Inform all clients who have a sedentary lifestyle and who are overweight about the risk factors for and complications of diabetes.
- Assist diabetic clients who smoke to reduce or quit smoking.
- Instruct clients with diabetes mellitus to achieve and maintain body weight within 5 pounds of identified ideal weight for age and body size.
- Provide one-to-one educational sessions, group education sessions, and printed and videotape information on diabetes treatment and care to clients diagnosed with diabetes.
- Educate clients about the specific medications prescribed to manage their disease.
- Demonstrate the use of the diet strategy individually planned for the client with diabetes.
- Encourage all clients with diabetes to participate in an individualized education program at least 3 days per week.
- Assist those clients with diabetes who also have hypertension to understand the importance of adhering to the prescribed drug therapies for both health problems.
- Instruct clients with diabetes to obtain annual vaccinations against influenza.
- Teach clients with diabetes to maintain adequate hydration, especially when any other illness is present.
- Participate in mass screenings to identify people with undiagnosed type 2 diabetes among the general population.
- Develop culturally sensitive and literacy-appropriate education materials targeted to high-risk minority populations.

Objective 18.9: _Reduce the frequency of foot ulcers in persons with diabetes._

- Include foot assessment whenever caring for a client with diabetes.
- Include sensory testing of the feet for all people with diabetes.
- Instruct the client with diabetes about proper foot care.
- Teach the client with diabetes the importance of always wearing protective footwear whenever the client is out of bed.
- Show the client the proper type of footwear to prevent foot injury.
- Find resources for those diabetic clients who are unable to afford properly fitting shoes.
- Teach the client how to monitor the circulatory status of his or her feet.
- Encourage the client to see a podiatrist twice a year.
- Refer the client with foot lesions to a wound management specialist.
- Encourage the client with diabetes who smokes to reduce or quit smoking.

Objective 18.23 _Increase to 52% the proportion of persons with diabetes who have received formal diabetes education._

- Evaluate the diabetes education materials and programs currently in place at your institution for currency, literacy, cultural sensitivity, and adequacy.
- Identify resources within your agency and community for diabetes education and support.
- Meet with the diabetes educator at your agency and establish means for collaboration and referral.
- If a diabetes educator is not available at your agency, work with existing personnel to enhance diabetes knowledge and awareness.
- Assist in policy-making decisions within your agency to develop a formalized teaching plan for all clients with diabetes, regardless of whether the clients are newly diagnosed or have had diabetes for a long time.
- Develop and offer diabetes education programs within your community in a variety of settings.

Critical Thinking Challenge

You are caring for a 31-year-old man who has had type 1 diabetes for 8 years. He runs 5 miles three times per week, is about 10 pounds overweight, and is relatively healthy. His blood pressure is 138/88 and his urine is negative for microalbumin. He is newly married and works as an editor for a local newspaper. He worries about whether or not he should have children and whether they will have diabetes. His 58-year-old mother had a myocardial infarction 2 years ago. The client is concerned that he is doomed to an early death by heart attack or renal failure and that he may end up having a foot or leg amputated.

1. Explain the genetic influence for type 1 diabetes.
2. Is this client's family history of MI important? Why or why not?
3. How could this client reduce his risk for or delay complications?

evolve For suggested answer guidelines, go to http://evolve.elsevier.com/Iggy/.

◆ **COLLABORATIVE MANAGEMENT**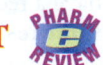
◆ **Assessment**

HISTORY

Ask questions about risk factors and symptoms related to diabetes. The client's age is important because type 2 diabetes is more common in older people, especially among African Americans and Mexican Americans. Ask women how large their children were at birth because many women who develop type 2 diabetes had gestational diabetes or were glucose intolerant during pregnancy. These women often have given birth to infants weighing 9 pounds or more.

Assessing weight and weight change is important because excess weight and obesity are risk factors for type 2 diabetes. The client with type 1 diabetes often has weight loss with increased appetite during the weeks before diagnosis. For both types of diabetes, clients usually have fatigue, polyuria, and

---

TABLE 68-5 Major Risk Factors for Type 2 Diabetes

Testing for diabetes should be considered in individuals 45 years of age and older, particularly in those with a BMI greater than 25 kg/m². If normal, it should be repeated at 3-year intervals.

Testing should be considered at a younger age or be carried out more frequently in individuals who are overweight (BMI >25 kg/m²) and have additional risk factors:

- Have a first-degree relative with diabetes
- Are habitually physically inactive
- Are members of a high-risk ethnic population (e.g., African American, Hispanic American, Native American/American Indian, Asian American, or Pacific Islander).
- Deliver a baby weighing more than 9 pounds or have been diagnosed with GDM
- Are hypertensive (>140/90 mm Hg)
- Have a high-density lipoprotein cholesterol (HDL) level less than 35 mg/dL (0.90 mmol/L) and/or a triglyceride level greater than 250 mg/dL (2.82 mmol/L)
- Have polycystic ovary syndrome
- Have IFG or IGT on previous testing
- Have a history of vascular disease

Data from American Diabetes Association. (2003). Committee report: Report of the Expert Committee on the Diagnosis and Classification of Diabetes Mellitus. _Diabetes Care_ _26_(Suppl. 1), 5-20.

BMI, Body mass index, _IFG,_ impaired fasting glucose; _IGT,_ impaired glucose tolerance.

polydipsia. Ask clients about recent major or minor infections. In particular, ask women about frequent vaginal yeast infections. Ask all clients whether they have noticed that small skin injuries become infected more easily or take longer to heal.

Explore the family history for parents and siblings with diabetes. If the client has one or more relatives with diabetes, it is important to determine whether these relatives use insulin or control their disease with diet, exercise, or oral antidiabetic drugs.

LABORATORY ASSESSMENT

BLOOD TESTS. Blood glucose values are used to diagnose diabetes. The nurse, the client, or a family member monitors the ongoing status of the disease by performing capillary blood glucose testing using a blood glucose meter. The physician and the nurse assess the overall result of treatment through review of glycosylated hemoglobin (hemoglobin A1c [HbA1c]) and fructosamine levels.

Instructions for blood glucose testing are listed in Chart 68-1. The American Diabetes Association (ADA) defines normal blood glucose values in Chart 68-2. ADA criteria for diagnosing adult diabetes mellitus are listed in Table 68-6.

FASTING BLOOD GLUCOSE TEST. Fasting blood glucose test results are most accurate when the blood is obtained by venipuncture. The client should fast for at least 8 hours (water is permitted). Draw the blood before insulin or oral antidiabetic agents have been taken. Diabetes is diagnosed when two separate test results exceed 126 mg/dL (7 mmol/L) (ADA, 2003a).

ORAL GLUCOSE TOLERANCE TEST. The oral glucose tolerance test (OGTT) is the most sensitive test for diagnosing diabetes, although it is not routinely used except in gestational diabetes. The test is inconvenient to clients, costly, and time consuming compared with the fasting blood glucose measure. Before the test, review instructions from Chart 68-1 with the client. Carbohydrate restriction or bedrest before the test alters glucose tolerance. The client drinks a beverage containing a glucose load of 75 g, and blood samples are collected at 30-minute intervals for 2 hours. A diagnosis of diabetes is made if the blood glucose is greater than 200 mg/dL (11.1 mmol/L) at 120 minutes.

GLYCOSYLATED HEMOGLOBIN ASSAYS. Blood glucose permanently attaches to hemoglobin. The higher the blood glucose level is over time, the more glycosylated hemoglobin becomes. Thus glycosylated hemoglobin

---

CHART 68-1

CLIENT EDUCATION GUIDE
Blood Glucose Testing

Fasting Plasma Blood Glucose
- Do not eat any food or drink any liquid for at least 8 hours.

Oral Glucose Tolerance Test
- Eat a balanced diet with carbohydrate intake of at least 150 g for a minimum of 3 days while maintaining normal physical activity.
- Carbohydrate restriction, bedrest, acute illness, and certain drugs interfere with the test. Phenytoin (Dilantin), anovulatory drugs, diuretics, nicotinic acid, and glucocorticoids adversely affect results.
- The test is performed in the morning after a 10- to 12-hour fast.
- A fasting blood sample is obtained.
- You will be asked to drink 300 mL (75 g) of a flavored beverage within 5 minutes of the fasting blood sample.
- Blood samples are drawn at 30-minute intervals for 2 hours.
- During the test, you will remain at rest and not be able to smoke or drink liquids.
- Report any signs suggesting hypoglycemia, such as weakness, dizziness, nervousness, and confusion.

TABLE 68-6   Criteria for the Diagnosis of Type 2 Diabetes

Symptoms of diabetes plus casual blood glucose concentration greater than 200 mg/dL (11.1 mmol/L). *Casual* is defined as any time of day without regard to time since last meal. The classic symptoms of diabetes include polyuria, polydipsia, and unexplained weight loss.
Or
Fasting plasma glucose greater than 126 mg/dL (7.0 mmol/L). *Fasting* is defined as no caloric intake for at least 8 hr.
Or
2-hr plasma glucose greater than 200 mg/dL during an oral glucose tolerance test. The test should be performed using a glucose load containing the equivalent of 75 g glucose dissolved in water.

NOTE: Each test must be confirmed, on a subsequent day, under similar circumstances.

Data from American Diabetes Association. (2003). Committee report: Report of the Expert Committee on the Diagnosis and Classification of Diabetes Mellitus. *Diabetes Care*, *26*(Suppl. 1), 5-20.

CHART 68-2

LABORATORY PROFILE
Blood Glucose Values

Test	Normal Range for Adults	Significance of Abnormal Results
Fasting blood glucose test	<110 mg/dL (6.1 mmol/L) *Older adults:* Levels rise 1 mg/dL per decade of age.	Levels >110 mg/dL (6.1 mmol/L) but <126 mg/dL (7.0 mmol/L) indicate impaired fasting glucose (IFG). Levels >126 mg/dL (7.0 mmol/L) obtained on at least two occasions are diagnostic of diabetes, even in older adults.
Glucose tolerance test (2-hr postload result)	<140 mg/dL (7.8 mmol/L)	Levels >140 mg/dL (7.8 mmol/L) and <200 mg/dL (11.1 mmol/L) indicate impaired glucose tolerance (IGT). Levels >200 mg/dL (11.1 mmol/L) indicate provisional diagnosis of diabetes.
Glycosylated hemoglobin (hemoglobin A1c [HbA1c]) test	4%-6%	Levels >8% indicate poor diabetic control and need for adherence to regimen or changes in therapy.

Data from American Diabetes Association. (2003). Committee report: Report of the Expert Committee on the Diagnosis and Classification of Diabetes Mellitus. *Diabetes Care*, *26*(Suppl. 1), 5-20, and the American Diabetes Association. (2003). Position statement: Tests of glycemia in diabetes. *Diabetes Care*, *26*(Suppl. 1), 106-108.

(HbA1c) is a good indicator of the average blood glucose levels. Measurement of HbA1c shows the average blood glucose level during the previous 120 days—the life span of red blood cells. HbA1c testing is used to assess long-term glycemic control, as well as to predict the risk for complications. Unlike the fasting blood glucose test, HbA1c test results are not altered by eating habits the day before the test. HbA1c testing is performed at diagnosis and at specific intervals to evaluate the treatment plan. Hemolysis, blood loss, and pregnancy all increase red blood cell turnover and reduce HbA1c levels. Triglycerides and bilirubin interfere with the assay, leading to overestimation of HbA1c levels in clients with hypertriglyceridemia. HbA1c testing is recommended at least twice yearly in clients who are meeting treatment goals and have stable blood glucose control. Quarterly assessment is recommended for clients whose therapy has changed or who are not meeting glycemic goals (ADA, 2003r).

GLYCOSYLATED SERUM PROTEINS AND ALBUMIN. Serum proteins and albumin become increasingly glycosylated with elevated blood glucose levels in the same way that hemoglobin does. However, because proteins and albumin turn over in 14 days, compared with 120 days for red blood cells, an assay of glycosylated serum proteins can indicate blood glucose control over a shorter period. These measures are useful when tight control of blood glucose levels is needed (e.g., pregnancy) or for follow-up of treatment changes. Available tests are called GSA (glycosylated serum albumin), GSP (glycosylated serum protein), and fructosamine.

URINE TESTS

URINE TESTING FOR KETONES. Ketones are a waste product of fat metabolism. Their presence in urine may indicate impending ketoacidosis. The ADA recommends testing urine for ketones during acute illness or stress, when blood glucose levels consistently exceed 300 mg/dL (16.7 mmol/L), during pregnancy, or when any symptoms of ketoacidosis are present (ADA, 2003s). Ketone testing is recommended for diabetic clients following a weight loss program.

URINE TESTING FOR RENAL FUNCTION. The presence of urine protein without renal symptoms may indicate microvascular changes in the kidney. Urine albumin excretion rates of 20 to 200 g/min (30 to 300 mg/hr) indicate microalbuminuria. Even minor elevations of albumin excretion are linked to increased mortality.

Once clinical proteinuria has been detected, kidney function (e.g., glomerular filtration rate) is assessed by creatinine clearance tests (see Chapter 72). In clients with nephropathy, a rise in serum creatinine levels is related to both poor blood glucose control and hypertension.

URINE TESTING FOR GLUCOSE. Blood glucose may be measured indirectly by urine testing for glucose, although this method is less precise than blood testing. Fluid intake, urine concentration, time since last voiding, and certain drugs affect the results.

OTHER DIAGNOSTIC ASSESSMENTS

Although not commonly used, other tests can help determine whether a client has type 1 or type 2 diabetes. Type 1 diabetes is an autoimmune disease with the presence of autoantibodies to proteins. Measuring levels of islet cell antibodies (ICAs) is an indicator of type 1 diabetes. Measurement of C-peptide levels indicates beta secretory function of the pancreas. C-peptide levels correlate well with insulin levels and are used to diagnose type 1 diabetes.

◆ Analysis

COMMON NURSING DIAGNOSES AND COLLABORATIVE PROBLEMS

The following are priority nursing diagnoses for clients with diabetes:

1. Risk for Injury related to hyperglycemia
2. Risk for Delayed Surgical Recovery related to endocrine and vascular effects of diabetes
3. Risk for Injury related to sensory alterations (diabetic neuropathy)
4. Chronic Pain related to peripheral nerve dysfunction (diabetic neuropathy)
5. Risk for Injury related to disturbed sensory perception: visual (diabetic retinopathy)
6. Ineffective Tissue Perfusion (Renal) related to impaired transport of oxygen across capillary membranes

The following are primary collaborative problems:

1. Potential for Hypoglycemia
2. Potential for Diabetic Ketoacidosis
3. Potential for Hyperglycemic-Hyperosmolar Nonketotic Syndrome and Coma

ADDITIONAL NURSING DIAGNOSES AND COLLABORATIVE PROBLEMS

In addition to the common nursing diagnoses and collaborative problems, clients with diabetes may have one or more of the following:

- Imbalanced Nutrition: More Than Body Requirements related to an imbalance of food intake and physical activity, lack of knowledge, and ineffective coping skills
- Risk for Deficient Fluid Volume related to fluid shifts, failure of regulatory mechanisms, hyperglycemic diuresis, polyuria, vomiting, diarrhea, decreased oral intake, and dehydration
- Impaired Oral Mucous Membrane related to microvascular circulatory changes and uncontrolled blood glucose levels
- Deficient Knowledge about diabetes management related to a lack of familiarity with information resources about disease, diet, exercise, drugs, weight control, and foot care
- Impaired Urinary Elimination and Urinary Retention (with Overflow Incontinence) related to diabetic neuropathy
- Constipation related to diabetic neuropathy
- Diarrhea related to diabetic neuropathy
- Risk for Impaired Skin Integrity related to decreased circulation, increased blood glucose levels, decreased mobility, and decreased sensation
- Risk for Infection related to increased blood glucose levels, decreased tissue perfusion, inadequate primary defenses, and the effects of chronic disease
- Risk for Infection related to wounds, urinary tract infection, intravenous (IV) access site, or oral mucous membranes
- Risk for Ineffective Sexuality Patterns (Male) related to autonomic neuropathy, decreased circulation, or psychological problems
- Risk for Ineffective Sexuality Patterns (Female) related to the stressors of diabetes
- Sexual Dysfunction related to impotence, impaired lubrication, painful intercourse with the changes in neu-

rologic control of the genitalia, the effects of actual or perceived limitations imposed by the disease or therapy, and altered self-concept

- Situational Low Self-Esteem related to an inability to deal with the self-care demands of the diabetic regimen
- Anxiety related to diagnosis of diabetes, potential complications of diabetes, and self-care regimens
- Fear related to diagnosis of diabetes, potential complications of diabetes, and self-care regimens
- Ineffective Coping and Compromised Family Coping related to a chronic disease, a complex self-care regimen, and decreased social support
- Powerlessness related to the complications of diabetes (blindness, amputations, renal failure, and neuropathy)
- Social Isolation related to visual impairment or blindness
- Noncompliance with self-care related to the complexity and duration of the prescribed regimen
- Ineffective Health Maintenance related to insufficient knowledge of diet restriction, weight control, weight maintenance, benefits and risks of exercise, self-monitoring of blood glucose, medications, sick-day care, foot care, hypoglycemia, and available resources

Planning and Implementation

The management of diabetes mellitus is complicated and involves considerable client cooperation and education. The Concept Map on p. 1510 highlights care issues for the client with type 2 diabetes mellitus.

RISK FOR INJURY RELATED TO HYPERGLYCEMIA

NOC **PLANNING: EXPECTED OUTCOMES.** The client with diabetes is expected to manage diabetes mellitus and prevent disease progression by maintaining blood glucose levels in the expected range. Indicators are that the client consistently demonstrates the following behaviors:

- Performs treatment regimen as prescribed
- Follows recommended diet
- Demonstrates correct procedure for blood glucose testing
- Monitors blood glucose
- Treats symptoms of hyperglycemia
- Seeks health care if blood glucose levels fluctuate outside of recommended parameters
- Follows recommended activity level
- Uses drugs as prescribed
- Maintains optimum weight

INTERVENTIONS

NONSURGICAL MANAGEMENT. Nonsurgical management of diabetes mellitus involves dietary interventions, blood glucose monitoring, a planned exercise program, and in some instances, medications to lower blood glucose levels. The nurse, together with the client, physician, dietitian, pharmacist, and in some cases, physical therapist, plans, organizes, and delivers care.

The American Diabetes Association (ADA) has proposed the following treatment goals for glycosylated hemoglobin (HbA1c) and blood glucose levels (ADA, 2003r):

- HbA1c levels should be maintained at 7% or below.
- The majority of premeal (**preprandial**) blood glucose levels should be 80 to 120 mg/dL (4.4 to 6.7 mmol/L).

- Blood glucose values at bedtime should be between 100 and 140 mg/dL (5.6 to 7.8 mmol/L).

Drug Therapy. Antidiabetic drugs are indicated when a client with type 2 diabetes does not have blood glucose control with diet changes, regular exercise, and stress management. See Table 68-7 for the cost of diabetes medications.

Oral Therapy. Oral agents are prescribed after dietary control has proven insufficient or if the client is highly symptomatic.

Sulfonylurea Agents. Sulfonylurea agents are used only for clients with some remaining pancreatic beta-cell function. These drugs stimulate insulin secretion (which reduces liver glucose output and increases cell uptake of glucose) and enhance the number or sensitivity of cell receptor sites for interaction with insulin. These drugs differ in strength, overall effects, metabolism, and risk for complications (Chart 68-3).

Hypoglycemia is the most serious complication of sulfonylurea therapy. Hypoglycemic episodes are more likely to occur with chlorpropamide (Diabinese, Novo-Propamide✱) because of its long duration of action. Underweight older clients with cardiovascular, liver, or kidney impairment are more susceptible to hypoglycemia.

Other less common side effects include leukopenia, thrombocytopenia, hemolytic anemia, allergic skin reactions, and gastrointestinal (GI) effects (nausea, epigastric fullness, heartburn). In addition, many drugs can potentiate or interfere with sulfonylureas (Table 68-8 on p. 1516).

Meglitinide Analogs. Repaglinide (Prandin) has actions and adverse effects similar to those of sulfonylureas. The drug is taken before meals and has a rapid onset with a limited duration of action. Adverse effects include hypoglycemia, GI disturbances, upper respiratory tract infection, arthralgia or back pain, and headache.

Nateglinide (Starlix) lowers blood glucose by triggering insulin secretion via interaction with the adenosine triphosphate (ATP)-sensitive potassium channel on pancreatic beta cells. The drug is rapidly absorbed and stimulates insulin secretion within 20 minutes of ingestion. It is taken just before meals to control mealtime hyperglycemia and improves overall glycemic control in clients with type 2 diabetes. The major adverse effect is hypoglycemia. Clients who skip meals should also skip their scheduled dose of Starlix to reduce the risk for hypoglycemia.

Biguanides. Metformin (Glucophage) lowers glucose by decreasing liver glucose release and decreasing cellular insulin resistance. It does not stimulate insulin release. When given alone, it does not cause hypoglycemia. It should not be given to anyone with renal disease and elevated blood creatinine levels. It should be withheld for 48 hours before and after using contrast material and surgical procedures requiring anesthesia (Slagle, 2002).

Metformin can cause lactic acidosis in diabetic clients with renal insufficiency and should not be used in conditions that decrease drug clearance, such as renal insufficiency, liver disease, alcoholism, severe congestive heart failure, or in clients older than 80 years of age (Bell, 2002). The symptoms of lactic acidosis are often nonspecific. Teach the client to report symptoms of fatigue, unusual muscle pain, difficulty breathing, unusual or unexpected stomach discomfort, dizziness, light-headedness, or irregular heartbeats

Text continued on p. 1516.

CONCEPT MAP Diabetes Mellitus—Type 2

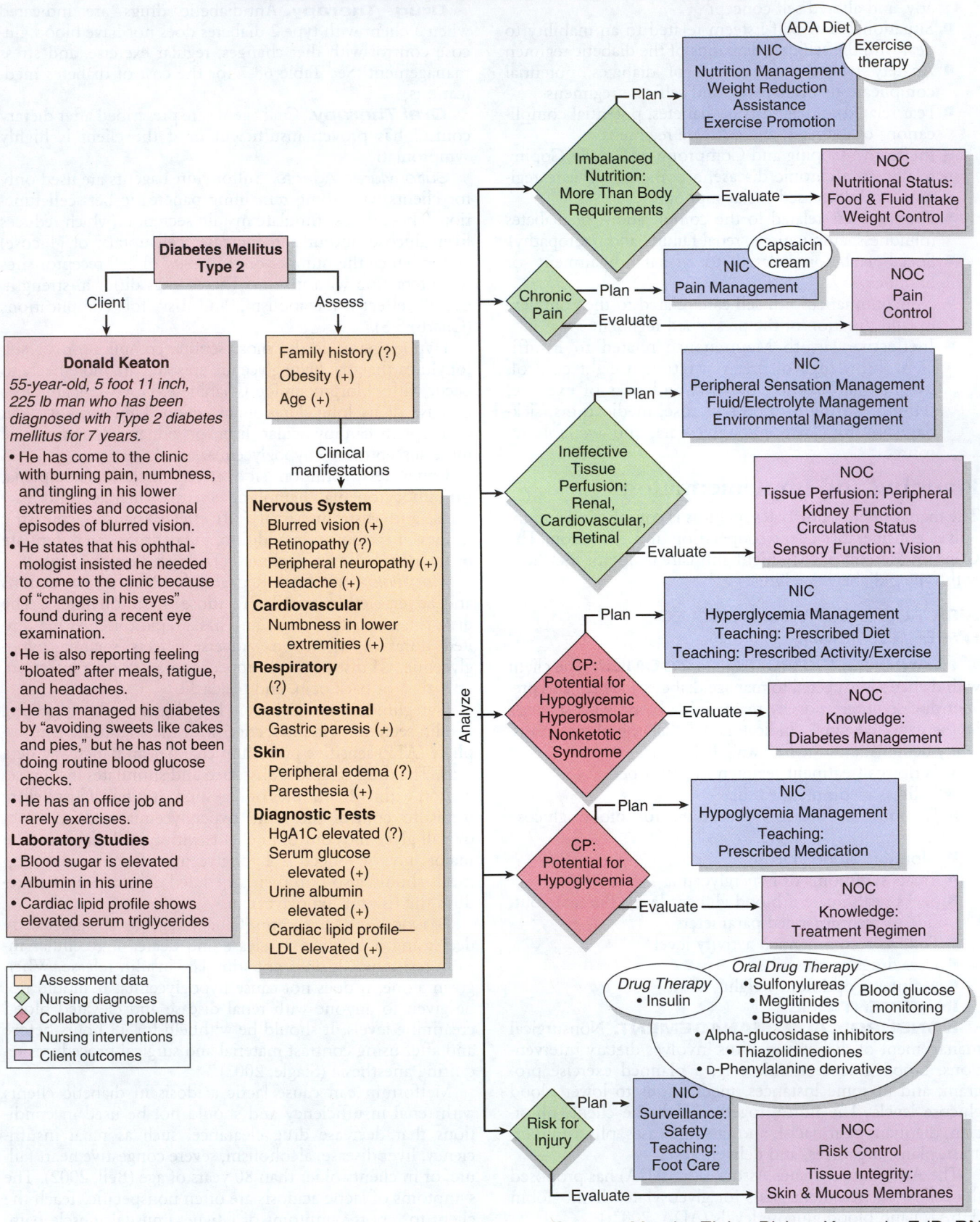

NIC
Nutrition Management
Weight Reduction
Assistance
Exercise Promotion

ADA Diet

Exercise therapy

Imbalanced Nutrition: More Than Body Requirements

NOC
Nutritional Status:
Food & Fluid Intake
Weight Control

Chronic Pain

Plan → **NIC** Pain Management — Capsaicin cream

Evaluate →

NOC
Pain Control

Diabetes Mellitus Type 2

Client → **Donald Keaton**
55-year-old, 5 foot 11 inch, 225 lb man who has been diagnosed with Type 2 diabetes mellitus for 7 years.
• He has come to the clinic with burning pain, numbness, and tingling in his lower extremities and occasional episodes of blurred vision.
• He states that his ophthalmologist insisted he needed to come to the clinic because of "changes in his eyes" found during a recent eye examination.
• He is also reporting feeling "bloated" after meals, fatigue, and headaches.
• He has managed his diabetes by "avoiding sweets like cakes and pies," but he has not been doing routine blood glucose checks.
• He has an office job and rarely exercises.
Laboratory Studies
• Blood sugar is elevated
• Albumin in his urine
• Cardiac lipid profile shows elevated serum triglycerides

Assess → Family history (?)
Obesity (+)
Age (+)

Clinical manifestations

Nervous System
  Blurred vision (+)
  Retinopathy (?)
  Peripheral neuropathy (+)
  Headache (+)
Cardiovascular
  Numbness in lower extremities (+)
Respiratory
  (?)
Gastrointestinal
  Gastric paresis (+)
Skin
  Peripheral edema (?)
  Paresthesia (+)
Diagnostic Tests
  HgA1C elevated (?)
  Serum glucose elevated (+)
  Urine albumin elevated (+)
  Cardiac lipid profile— LDL elevated (+)

Analyze →

Ineffective Tissue Perfusion: Renal, Cardiovascular, Retinal

Plan → **NIC**
Peripheral Sensation Management
Fluid/Electrolyte Management
Environmental Management

Evaluate → **NOC**
Tissue Perfusion: Peripheral
Kidney Function
Circulation Status
Sensory Function: Vision

CP: Potential for Hypoglycemic Hyperosmolar Nonketotic Syndrome

Plan → **NIC**
Hyperglycemia Management
Teaching: Prescribed Diet
Teaching: Prescribed Activity/Exercise

Evaluate → **NOC**
Knowledge: Diabetes Management

CP: Potential for Hypoglycemia

Plan → **NIC**
Hypoglycemia Management
Teaching: Prescribed Medication

Evaluate → **NOC**
Knowledge: Treatment Regimen

Drug Therapy
• Insulin

Oral Drug Therapy
• Sulfonylureas
• Meglitinides
• Biguanides
• Alpha-glucosidase inhibitors
• Thiazolidinediones
• D-Phenylalanine derivatives

Blood glucose monitoring

Risk for Injury

Plan → **NIC**
Surveillance:
Safety
Teaching:
Foot Care

Evaluate → **NOC**
Risk Control
Tissue Integrity:
Skin & Mucous Membranes

Legend:
☐ Assessment data
◇ Nursing diagnoses
◇ Collaborative problems
☐ Nursing interventions
☐ Client outcomes

Concept Map by Elaine Bishop Kennedy, EdD, RN

TABLE 68-7 Cost of Diabetes Medications

Medications	Specific Product	Size	Price*
Humulin insulins	Humulin R	100 units/mL, 10-mL vial	$26.56
	Humulin N	100 units/mL, 10-mL vial	$26.56
	Humulin L	100 units/mL, 10-mL vial	$26.56
	Humulin U	100 units/mL, 10-mL vial	$26.56
	Humulin R U-500	500 units/mL, 20 mL vial	$191.09
	Humulin N Pen	100 units/mL, 3 mL, #5	$78.54
	Humulin 70/30 pen	70 units - 30 units/mL, 3 mL, #5	$78.54
Humalog insulin	Insulin lispro	100 units/mL, 10-mL vial	$50.09
	Humalog pen	100 units/mL, 3 mL cartridge, #5	$100.80
Novolin insulins (Novo Nordisk)	Novolin R	100 units/mL, 10-mL vial	$25.30
	Novolin N	100 units/mL, 10-mL vial	$25.30
	Novolin L	100 units/mL, 10-mL vial	$26.65
	70/30	70 units - 30 units/mL, 10-mL vial	$25.30
NovoLog insulin	Insulin aspart	100 units/mL, 10-mL vial	$50.09
Combination insulins	Humulin 50/50	50 units - 50 units/mL, 10-mL vial	$26.56
	Humulin 70/30	70 units - 30 units/mL, 10-mL vial	$26.56
	Novolin 70/30	70 units - 30 units/mL, 10-mL vial	$50.09
	Humalog mix 75/25	75 units - 25 units/mL, 10-mL vial	$50.09
Lantus	Insulin glargine	100 units/mL, 10-mL vial	$46.99
Iletin insulins	Iletin II Regular pork	100 units/mL, 10-mL vial	$47.98
	Iletin II NPH pork	100 units/mL, 10-mL vial	$47.98
	Iletin II Lente pork	100 units/mL, 10-mL vial	$47.98
Oral agents	Chlorpropamide	100 mg, # 100	$18.37
		250 mg, # 100	$38.85
	Glipizide	5 mg, # 100	$6.99
		10 mg, # 100	$9.44
	Glyburide	1.5 mg, # 100	$25.50
		3 mg, # 100	$32.02
	Glimepiride	1 mg, # 100	$28.62
		4 mg, # 100	$87.47
	Metformin	500 mg, # 100	$70.35
	Repaglinide	0.5 mg, # 100	$92.96
		2 mg, # 100	$92.96
	Acarbose	100 mg, # 100	$74.22
	Pioglitazone	15 mg, # 90	$276.89
		30 mg, # 90	$426.71
	Rosiglitazone	4 mg, # 100	$256.09
		8 mg, # 100	$473.84

Data from *2002 Drug Topics Red Book*. (2002). Montvale, NJ: Medical Economics Company.
*Average wholesale price.

CHART 68-3

DRUG THERAPY for
Diabetes Mellitus: Oral Blood Glucose Lowering Agents

Drug	Dosage and Duration	Nursing Interventions	Rationales
First-Generation Sulfonylurea Agents			
Acetohexamide (Dymelor, Dimelor✱)	*Usual:* 0.25-1.5 g daily *Maximum:* 1.5 g daily *Duration:* 12-24 hr	Instruct client in measures to prevent and treat hypoglycemia. Caution clients to avoid drinking alcohol when taking acetohexamide.	Older, debilitated, or malnourished clients are more susceptible to hypoglycemia with acetohexamide. Disulfiram-like reaction may occur when alcohol is consumed with acetohexamide. Symptoms include flushing of face, pulsating headache, sweating, confusion, and slurred speech. Severe reaction can cause sudden death.
Chlorpropamide (Diabinese, Novo-Propamide✱)	*Usual:* 100-500 mg q24h (take with breakfast) *Maximum:* 500 mg daily *Duration:* 24-60 hr	Instruct client in measures to prevent and treat hypoglycemia. Monitor weight and intake and output patterns. Caution clients to avoid drinking alcohol when taking chlorpropamide.	Chlorpropamide is associated with a high incidence of hypoglycemia. Blood glucose lowering effects can persist for long after drug is discontinued. Chlorpropamide may potentiate antidiuretic hormone secretion and result in the syndrome of inappropriate antidiuretic hormone secretion (SIADH). Alcohol, even in small amounts, can cause a disulfiram-like reaction.

Continued

CHART 68-3

DRUG THERAPY for
Diabetes Mellitus: Oral Blood Glucose Lowering Agents—*cont'd*

Drug	Dosage and Duration	Nursing Interventions	Rationales
Tolazamide (Tolinase)	*Usual:* 100-500 mg q24h (take with meals) *Maximum:* 2000 mg daily *Duration:* 12-24 hr	Administer with meals. Caution clients to avoid drinking alcohol when taking tolazamide.	Taking with meals helps to avoid gastrointestinal upset. Alcohol, even in small amounts, can cause a disulfiram-like reaction.
Tolbutamide (Orinase, Mobenol✽)	*Usual:* 750-1500 mg/ 12-24hr *Maximum:* 3000 mg daily *Duration:* 6-10 hr	Administer 30 min before meals. Instruct client in measures to prevent and treat hypoglycemia. Caution clients to avoid drinking alcohol when taking tolbutamide.	Taking 30 min before meals gives the best reduction in postmeal hyperglycemia. Symptoms of a hypoglycemic reaction in an older client receiving a beta blocker may be masked. Teach family to observe for subtle signs of hypoglycemia. Alcohol, even in small amounts, can cause a disulfiram-like reaction.
Second-Generation Sulfonylurea Agents			
Glipizide		Administer 30 min before meals.	Absorption of glipizide is delayed by food.
(Glucotrol)	*Usual:* 2.5-5 mg q12-24h (30 min before meals) *Maximum:* 40 mg daily *Duration:* 12-24 hr	Instruct client in measures to prevent and treat hypoglycemia.	Hypoglycemia is more likely to occur with insufficient caloric intake.
(Glucotrol XL)	*Usual:* 5-20 mg daily *Maximum:* 40 mg daily *Duration:* 24 hr	Instruct clients taking Glucotrol XL that tablets must be swallowed whole and never crushed or chewed.	Glucotrol XL is designed to be slowly absorbed from the gastrointestinal tract. Crushing or chewing the tablet alters absorption of the drug.
Glyburide		Administer with first main meal.	Administration with food helps reduce gastrointestinal side effects.
(DiaBeta Micronase✽)	*Usual:* 1.25-20 mg daily with meals (single or divided doses) *Maximum:* 20 mg daily *Duration:* 24 hr	Instruct client in measures to prevent and treat hypoglycemia.	Hypoglycemia is more likely to occur with insufficient caloric intake.
(Glynase PresTabs)	*Usual:* 0.75-12 mg daily (divide doses >6 mg) *Maximum:* 12 mg daily *Duration:* 24 hr		
Glimepiride (Amaryl)	*Usual:* 1-4 mg once daily *Maximum:* 8 mg daily *Duration:* 24 hr	Administer with first main meal. Instruct client in measures to prevent and treat hypoglycemia.	Debilitated or malnourished clients and clients with impaired renal or hepatic function are more sensitive to blood glucose–lowering effects of glimepiride.
Meglitinide Analogs			
Repaglinide (Prandin)	*Usual:* 0.5-4 mg daily *Maximum:* 16 mg daily *Duration:* Less than 4 hr	Administer 30 min before meals. Instruct client to omit medication when skipping a meal. Instruct client to add a dose if an extra meal is eaten. Instruct client in measures to prevent and treat hypoglycemia. Store at 15°-30° C (59°-86° F) in a tightly closed container and protect from moisture and heat.	Taking drug 30 min before meals gives the best reduction in postmeal hyperglycemia. Drug reduces the risk of hypoglycemia. Duration of action of repaglinide is 4 hr. A dose of medication needs to be available for each meal eaten. Older, debilitated, or malnourished clients are more susceptible to hypoglycemia with repaglinide. Proper storage prevents deterioration of the drug.
Nateglinide (Starlix)	*Usual:* 60-120 mg before meals *Maximum:* Optimal dose not determined *Duration:* 4 hr	Administer 1-30 min before meals. Instruct client to omit medication when skipping a meal. Instruct client to add a dose if an extra meal is eaten.	Stimulates rapid secretion of insulin to reduce increases in blood glucose levels that occur soon after eating. Drug reduces the risk of hypoglycemia. Duration of action of nateglinide is 4 hr. A dose of medication needs to be available for each meal eaten.

CHART 68-3

DRUG THERAPY for
Diabetes Mellitus: Oral Blood Glucose Lowering Agents—*cont'd*

Drug	Dosage and Duration	Nursing Interventions	Rationales
Biguanides Metformin		Administer with food.	Slow titration adjustment and administration with food reduces gastrointestinal side effects.
(Glucophage)	*Starting dose:* 500 mg twice daily or 850 mg once daily with meals. *Maintenance dose:* Individualized *Maximum:* 2550 mg daily in divided doses	Monitor renal function. Withhold metformin for 48 hr before use of iodinated contrast materials used in certain radiographic studies. Monitor cardiopulmonary status throughout therapy.	Renal impairment increases the risk of lactic acidosis. Metformin is contraindicated in renal disease (serum creatinine >1.5 mg/dL in males, >1.4 mg/dL in females). Iodinated contrast materials can alter renal function and increase the risk for lactic acidosis. Metformin therapy is restarted when renal function has returned to normal. Conditions associated with hypoxia increase the risk for lactic acidosis.
(Glucophage XR [extended release])	*Starting dose:* 500 mg daily with largest meal *Maintenance dose:* Individualized *Maximum:* 2000 mg daily	Instruct the client taking metformin to report symptoms of lactic acidosis: malaise, unusual muscle pain, respiratory distress, increasing somnolence, and abdominal distress. Instruct clients taking metformin to report any illness that causes severe vomiting, diarrhea, or fever. Instruct clients taking Glucophage XL that tablets must be swallowed whole and never crushed or chewed.	Onset of lactic acidosis is subtle and accompanied by nonspecific symptoms. Precipitating events for lactic acidosis include hypoxemia, dehydration, and sepsis. Glucophage XL is designed to be slowly absorbed from the gastrointestinal tract. Crushing or chewing the tablet alters absorption of the drug.
Alpha-Glucosidase Inhibitors Acarbose (Precose)	*Usual:* 50-100 mg three times daily *Maximum:* 100 mg three times daily *Duration:* 2-4 hr	Instruct client to take with the first bite of each of the three main meals. Monitor renal function. Monitor for abdominal pain, diarrhea, and flatulence. Monitor liver function tests. Emphasize need to report symptoms of unexplained nausea, vomiting, abdominal pain, fatigue, anorexia, or dark urine. Instruct clients receiving acarbose and other hypoglycemic medications to treat hypoglycemia with glucose tablets, glucose gel, or low-fat milk. Instruct client to store the medication according to manufacturer's directions.	Acarbose must be taken at the beginning of a meal to be fully effective. Drug may accumulate in clients with renal dysfunction; drug not recommended for clients with serum creatinine >2 mg/dL. Gastrointestinal side effects are very common. Symptoms can be reduced by slow titration adjustment of dose. Acarbose is associated with an elevation in serum transaminase levels. Acarbose does not cause hypoglycemia when given alone. Hypoglycemia caused by other agents should be treated with oral dextrose. Sucrose (table sugar or candy bars) will not reverse symptoms of hypoglycemia due to the actions of acarbose. Remove from foil wrapper immediately before administration to prevent deterioration of acarbose.
Miglitol (Glyset)	*Usual:* 50 mg three times daily *Maximum:* 100 mg three times daily *Duration:* 2-4 hr	Instruct client to take with the first bite of each main meal. Monitor renal function. Monitor for abdominal pain, diarrhea, and flatulence.	Miglitol must be taken at the beginning of a meal to be fully effective. Drug may accumulate in clients with renal dysfunction; drug is not recommended for clients with serum creatinine >2 mg/dL. Gastrointestinal side effects are very common. Symptoms can be reduced by slow adjustment of dose.

Continued

CHART 68-3

DRUG THERAPY for
Diabetes Mellitus: Oral Blood Glucose Lowering Agents—*cont'd*

Drug	Dosage and Duration	Nursing Interventions	Rationales
Miglitol (Glyset)—*cont'd*		Monitor liver function tests. Emphasize need to report symptoms of unexplained nausea, vomiting, abdominal pain, fatigue, anorexia, or dark urine.	Miglitol is associated with an elevation in serum transaminase levels.
		Instruct clients receiving miglitol and other hypoglycemic medications to treat hypoglycemia with glucose tablets, glucose gel or low-fat milk. Treat hypoglycemia symptoms with dextrose.	Miglitol does not cause hypoglycemia when given alone. Hypoglycemia caused by other agents should be treated with oral dextrose. Sucrose (table sugar or candy bars) will not reverse symptoms of hypoglycemia due to the actions of miglitol.
Thiazolidinediones Pioglitazone (Actos)	*Starting dose:* 500 mg daily with largest meal *Usual:* 15 to 30 mg daily with or without food *Maximum:* 45 mg daily	Emphasize need for liver function tests as recommended. Emphasize need to report symptoms of unexplained nausea, vomiting, abdominal pain, fatigue, anorexia, or dark urine.	Rare cases of liver failure have occurred with pioglitazone. Liver function tests are measured at the start of therapy and at regular times thereafter.
		Advise women of childbearing age to use adequate contraception.	Administration of pioglitazone with certain oral contraceptives may reduce the plasma concentration of the oral contraceptive.
		Monitor weight and assess for edema.	Major side effects are fluid retention, weight gain, and congestive heart failure.
Rosiglitazone (Avandia)	*Usual:* 4 mg daily with or without food *Maximum:* 8 mg daily	Emphasize need for liver function tests as recommended. Emphasize need to report symptoms of unexplained nausea, vomiting, abdominal pain, fatigue, anorexia, or dark urine.	Rare cases of liver failure have occurred with rosiglitazone. Liver function tests are measured at the start of therapy and at regular times thereafter.
		Advise women of childbearing age to use adequate contraception.	Administration of rosiglitazone with certain oral contraceptives may reduce the plasma concentration of the oral contraceptive.
		Monitor weight and assess for edema.	Major side effects are fluid retention, weight gain, and congestive heart failure.
Fixed Combinations Glucovance (Glyburide and metformin) 1.25 mg/250 mg 2.5 mg/500 mg 5 mg/500 mg	*Initial therapy:* 1.25 mg/250 mg once or twice daily with meals *Maintenance:* Individualized *Maximum:* 20 mg glyburide and 2000 mg metformin daily *Previously treated clients:* 2.5 mg/500 mg or 5 mg/500 mg twice daily with meals. *Maintenance:* Individualized *Maximum:* 20 mg glyburide and 2000 mg metformin daily	Give in divided doses with meals. Instruct client in measures to prevent and treat hypoglycemia. Monitor renal and hepatic function.	Slow adjustment and administration with food minimizes hypoglycemia and gastrointestinal effects. Hypoglycemia can occur in clients with insufficient oral intake, excess exercise, or alcohol intake, or those who are older and debilitated. Renal or hepatic impairment increases blood levels of both drugs and increases the risk of hypoglycemia and lactic acidosis. Metformin is contraindicated in renal disease (serum creatinine >1.5 mg/dL in males, >1.4 mg/dL in females).

CHART 68-3

DRUG THERAPY for
Diabetes Mellitus: Oral Blood Glucose Lowering Agents—*cont'd*

Drug	Dosage and Duration	Nursing Interventions	Rationales
Avandamet (Rosiglitazone and metformin) 1 mg/500 mg 2 mg/500 mg 4 mg/500 mg	*Previously on metformin alone*: add 4 mg daily to current regimen *Previously on rosiglitazone alone*: add metformin 1000 mg to current regimen *Maximum*: 8 mg rosiglitazone and 2000 mg metformin daily	Give in divided doses with meals. Monitor renal and hepatic function.	Slow adjustment and administration with food minimizes hypoglycemia and gastrointestinal effects. Rare cases of liver failure have occurred with rosiglitazone. Liver function tests are measured at the start of therapy and at regular times thereafter. Metformin is contraindicated in renal disease (serum creatinine >1.5 mg/dL in males, >1.4 mg/dL in females).
		Monitor weight and assess for edema.	Major side effects are fluid retention, weight gain, and congestive heart failure.
		Monitor cardiopulmonary status throughout therapy. Instruct the client taking metformin to report symptoms of lactic acidosis: malaise, unusual muscle pain, respiratory distress, increasing somnolence, and abdominal distress.	Conditions associated with hypoxia increase the risk for lactic acidosis. Onset of lactic acidosis is subtle and accompanied by nonspecific symptoms.
		Instruct clients taking metformin to report any illness that causes severe vomiting, diarrhea, or fever.	Precipitating events for lactic acidosis include hypoxemia, dehydration, and sepsis.
		Instruct client in measures to prevent and treat hypoglycemia. Advise women of childbearing age to use adequate contraception.	Older, debilitated, or malnourished clients are more susceptible to hypoglycemia. Administration of rosiglitazone with certain oral contraceptives may reduce the plasma concentration of the oral contraceptive.
Metaglip (Glipizide and metformin) 2.5 mg/250 mg 2.5 mg/500 mg 5 mg/500 mg	*Initial therapy*: 2.5 mg/250 mg once or twice daily with meals. *Maintenance*: Individualized *Maximum*: 20 mg glipizide and 2000 mg metformin daily *Previously treated clients*: 2.5 mg/500 mg or 5 mg/500 mg twice daily with meals *Maintenance*: Individualized *Maximum*: 20 mg glipizide and 2000 mg metformin daily	Give in divided doses with meals. Instruct client in measures to prevent and treat hypoglycemia. Monitor renal and hepatic function.	Slow adjustment and administration with food minimizes hypoglycemia and gastrointestinal effects. Hypoglycemia can occur in clients with insufficient oral intake, excess exercise, or alcohol intake, or in those who are older and debilitated. Renal or hepatic impairment increases blood levels of both drugs and increases the risk of hypoglycemia and lactic acidosis. Metformin is contraindicated in renal disease (serum creatinine >1.5 mg/dL in males, >1.4 mg/dL in females).

TABLE 68-8 Drug Interactions with Sulfonylurea Agents

Potentiate Hypoglycemia	Worsen Hyperglycemia
Allopurinol (Zyloprim)	Amphetamines
Ammonium chloride	Asparaginase (Elspar)
Androgens (testosterone [Testoderm])	Bumetanide (Bumex)
Angiotensin-converting agents (captopril [Capoten], enalapril [Vasotec])	Calcium channel blockers (diltiazem, nifedipine)
Anticoagulants, oral (warfarin)	Cholestyramine (Questran)
Antifungal azoles, systemic (fluconazole [Diflucan], miconazole [Monistat])	Chlorthalidone (Hygroton)
Barbiturates	Clonidine (Catapres)
Beta-adrenergic blocking agents (atenolol, propranolol)	Corticosteroids (prednisone)
Bromocriptine	Corticotropin (adrenocorticotropin hormone)
Calcium channel blockers (verapamil)	Danazol (Danocrine)
Clofibrate (Atromid-S)	Diazoxide, parenteral (Hyperstat)
Disopyramide (Norpace)	Dextrothyroxine (Choloxin)
Ethanol	Diuretics, thiazide (hydrochlorothiazide)
Fenfluramine (Pondimin)	Estrogen (Estrace, Premarin)
Fluoroquinolone anti-infectives (ciprofloxacin)	Estrogen-progesterone-containing oral contraceptives (Brevicon, Depo-Provera, Estrostep)
Guanethidine (Ismelin)	Furosemide (Lasix)
Histamine H_2 antagonists (cimetidine [Tagamet], ranitidine [Zantac])	Gemfibrozil (Lopid)
Monoamine oxidase (MAO) inhibitors (phenelzine [Nardil])	Glucagon
Methyldopa (Aldomet)	Isoniazid (INH)
NSAIDs (indomethacin [Indocin], ibuprofen [Advil])	Lithium (Lithobid)
Octreotide (Sandostatin)	Morphine (morphine sulfate)
Probenecid (Benemid, Probalan)	Nicotinic acid (Nicolar)
Pyridoxine (vitamin B_6)	Pentamidine (pentamidine isethionate)
Quinidine (quinidine gluconate)	Phenothiazines (prochlorperazine [Compazine], trifluoperazine [Stelazine])
Quinine (quinine sulfate)	Phenytoin (Dilantin)
Sulfinpyrazone (Anturane)	Rifampin (Rifadin)
Sulfonamides (trimethoprim/sulfamethoxazole [Bactrim], sulfisoxazole [Gantrisin])	Salicylates (large doses)
Tetracycline	Thyroid hormones (liothyronine [Cytomel], levothyroxine [Levothroid, Synthroid])

to the primary care provider. Instruct clients to take metformin with meals to reduce GI effects. Caution against excessive alcohol intake because alcohol increases the risk for lactic acidosis.

Alpha-Glucosidase Inhibitors. Alpha-glucosidase inhibitors reduce hyperglycemia after meals by slowing intestinal digestion and absorption of carbohydrate. These agents inhibit enzymes in the intestinal tract, delaying carbohydrate digestion. The prolonged digestion time reduces the rate of glucose absorption and lowers blood glucose levels. Total glucose absorption is unchanged, and there is no weight loss or gain. The most common side effects are flatulence, diarrhea, and abdominal discomfort. There are two drugs in this class. Acarbose (Precose) is well tolerated when started at a low dose (25 mg once daily to three times daily with meals) and increased slowly. At higher doses, poor carbohydrate absorption can occur. Miglitol (Glyset) should be taken three times daily with the first bite of each main meal.

Alpha-glucosidase inhibitors do not cause hypoglycemia unless given with sulfonylureas or insulin. Because alpha-glucosidase inhibitors delay carbohydrate absorption and interfere with the conversion of complex sugars to glucose, many of the standard products used to treat hypoglycemia result in a delayed blood glucose response (see Chart 68-14). Alpha-glucosidase inhibitors do not inhibit absorption of glucose or lactose. Instruct clients to use oral glucose tablets, glucose gel, or low-fat milk to treat hypoglycemia. Severe hypoglycemia may require glucose infusion or glucagon injection.

Thiazolidinedione Antidiabetic Agents. Thiazolidinediones enhance insulin action, thus promoting glucose utilization in peripheral tissues. They are known as "insulin sensitizers" and include rosiglitazone (Avandia) and pioglitazone (Actos). These drugs improve sensitivity to insulin in muscle and fat tissue and inhibit gluconeogenesis. They can be used with a sulfonylurea or insulin to improve blood glucose control because their mechanisms of action are different. Clients taking these drugs should have periodic liver function studies performed because of the potential liver damage.

All drugs in this class have effects on serum lipid levels. Other side effects of these drugs include infection, headache, peripheral edema, and pain. They can reduce the effectiveness of oral contraceptives. About 15% of clients taking these drugs gain weight. Ensure that these clients receive instructions about following a low-sodium diet.

Combination Agents. Some oral agents combine drugs with different mechanisms of action. Glucovance, for example, combines glyburide with metformin. Combining drugs with different mechanisms of action may be highly effective in maintaining desired blood glucose control. Some clients may need a combination of oral agents and insulin to control blood glucose levels.

Drug Administration. Drugs are started at the lowest effective dose and increased every 1 to 2 weeks until the client reaches acceptable blood glucose control or the maximum dosage. If the maximal dosage does not control blood glucose levels, a different oral agent is used. Insulin therapy is indicated when blood glucose cannot be controlled after the use of two or three different oral agents.

Antidiabetic drugs are not a substitute for dietary modification and exercise. Teach the client about the need for continuing dietary restrictions and regular exercise while taking antidiabetic drugs. To avoid adverse drug interactions, teach the client to consult with the primary care provider or pharmacist before using any over-the-counter drugs.

Drug Selection. The choice of oral antidiabetic drug is based on cost, the client's ability to manage multiple drug doses, and the client's age and response to the drugs. Sulfonylureas are less expensive than other oral antidiabetic agents, can be taken once daily, and have few side effects. Metformin (Glucophage) can have more GI side effects than sulfonylureas. Acarbose must be taken before each meal.

Beta-cell function in type 2 diabetes often declines over time, reducing the effectiveness of some oral antidiabetic drugs. The treatment regimen for the client with type 2 diabetes may eventually require insulin therapy either alone or with oral agents.

Insulin Therapy. Insulin therapy is needed for type 1 diabetes and is used frequently for type 2 diabetes. The safety of insulin therapy in older clients may be affected by reduced vision, mobility and coordination problems, and decreased memory. There are many types of insulin and regimens, all aimed at achieving normal blood glucose levels.

TABLE 68-9 Insulin Preparations

Type	Source
Insulin Analog	
■ Humalog (Lilly)	DNA technology
■ Insulin aspart (Novo Nordisk)	DNA technology
■ Insulin glulisine (Aventis)	DNA technology
Short-Acting Insulin	
Insulin injection (regular crystalline insulin):	
■ Iletin II R (Lilly)	Pork (purified)
Insulin human injection (regular human insulin):	
■ Humulin R (Lilly)	DNA technology
■ Novolin R (Novo Nordisk)	DNA technology
■ Velosulin BR (Novo Nordisk)	Semisynthetic
■ Velosulin BR (Novo Nordisk)	DNA technology
Concentrated Insulin	
Insulin injection (regular crystalline insulin):	
■ Iletin II U-500 (Lilly)	Pork (purified)
Intermediate-Acting Insulin	
Isophane insulin suspension (NPH insulin):	
■ Iletin II (Lilly)	Pork (purified)
■ Humulin N (Lilly)	DNA technology
■ Novolin N (Novo Nordisk)	DNA technology
Insulin zinc suspension (Lente insulin):	
■ Iletin II (Lilly)	Pork (purified)
■ Humulin L (Lilly)	DNA technology
■ Novolin L (Novo Nordisk)	DNA technology
Fixed-Combination Insulin	
■ Humulin 50/50 (Lilly)	DNA technology
■ Humulin 70/30 (Lilly)	DNA technology
■ Novolin 70/30 (Novo Nordisk)	DNA technology
■ Humalog Mix 75/25	DNA technology
Long-Acting Insulin	
■ Humulin U (Lilly)	DNA technology
■ Insulin glargine (Aventis)	DNA technology

Types of Insulin. Insulin is obtained from animal sources (beef or pork pancreas), combined animal sources and semisynthetic human insulin, and synthetic human insulin (made through recombinant DNA technology). There are differences in strength and onset of action between human and animal-source insulins. Thus, dose and timing need adjustment when a client changes from one type of insulin to another. Human insulin has a more rapid onset of action, a shorter peak action, and a shorter duration of action than animal-source insulin. Human insulin is preferred for pregnant women or women considering pregnancy, clients with allergies or resistance to animal-source insulins, clients beginning insulin therapy, and clients who use insulin intermittently (ADA, 2003k).

Rapid-, short-, intermediate-, and long-acting forms of insulin can be injected separately and some can be mixed in the same syringe. Insulin is available in 100 units/mL (U-100) and 500 units/mL (U-500). U-500 is used only in rare cases of insulin resistance. U-500 and all analogs are the only insulins that need a prescription.

Teach the client that the insulin types, the injection technique, the site of injection, and the individual response can all affect the absorption, onset, degree, and duration of insulin activity. Reinforce that changing insulins may affect blood glucose control and should be done only under careful supervision (ADA, 2003k). Table 68-9 reviews the types and sources of insulin preparations, and Table 68-10 outlines the time activity of subcutaneous human insulin.

Insulin Regimens. Insulin regimens try to duplicate the normal release pattern of insulin from the pancreas. The pancreas produces a constant (basal) amount of insulin that balances liver glucose production with glucose use and maintains normal blood glucose levels between meals. The pancreas also produces additional (prandial) insulin, stimulated by food, that prevents blood glucose elevations after meals. The insulin dose required for blood glucose control varies among clients. A usual starting dose is between 0.5 and 1 unit/kg of body weight per day. For multiple-dose regimens or continuous subcutaneous insulin infusion (CSII), basal insulin makes up about 40% to 50% of the total daily dosage, with the remainder divided into premeal doses of regular insulin. Dosage adjustments are based on the results of blood glucose monitoring. Because the rate of absorption is slowed by increasing the dosage, adjustments in dosage should be made no more than every 3 to 4 days.

Basal insulin coverage can be provided by NPH insulin. Humulin U Ultralente insulin provides a lower basal rate and may be used instead of NPH insulin for a client with frequent hypoglycemic episodes. Insulin glargine (Lantus), a long-acting insulin analog, is available for once-daily injection for basal insulin coverage. The client determines the effect of long-acting insulin by monitoring fasting blood glucose values. Insulin protocols (regimens or programs) are shown in Figure 68-4.

SINGLE DAILY INJECTION PROTOCOL. Many clients inject insulin only once daily. This protocol may include only intermediate-acting insulin or combined short- and intermediate-acting insulin. A single dose of intermediate-acting insulin may not match the blood insulin level with food intake. When fasting glucose levels are elevated, a multiple-injection protocol should be considered.

TWO-DOSE PROTOCOL. Combinations of short- and intermediate-acting insulin are injected twice daily. Two thirds of the daily dose is given before breakfast and one third before the evening meal. At first, intermediate-acting and regular insulin are usually given in a 2:1 ratio, and the evening (or bedtime) dose is given in a 1:1 ratio. Changes in these ratios are based on results of blood glucose monitoring.

THREE-DOSE PROTOCOL. A combination of short- and intermediate-acting insulin is given before breakfast, short-acting insulin is given before the evening meal, and intermediate-acting insulin is given at bedtime. Giving intermediate-acting insulin at bedtime lowers fasting and after-breakfast blood glucose levels. This schedule avoids nighttime hypoglycemia but may not provide enough coverage for the noon meal (Franz, 2001).

FOUR-DOSE PROTOCOL. Giving short-acting insulin 30 minutes before meals allows the greatest amount of insulin to be present during the time of greatest insulin need. Basal insulin is provided by twice-daily injection of intermediate-acting insulin or a once daily injection of long-acting insulin. Injection of premeal short-acting insulin based on anticipated carbohydrate intake allows some clients with diabetes to have more flexibility in meal timing and size. Insulin lispro should be given within 15 minutes of eating a meal; action usually peaks in 30 to 90 minutes. Because this dura-

TABLE 68-10 Time Activity of Subcutaneous Human Insulin

Preparation	Brand	Onset (hr)	Peak (hr)	Duration (hr)
Rapid Acting				
Insulin aspart injection	NovoLog	0.25	1-3	3-5
Insulin lispro injection	Humalog	0.25	0.5-1.5	3-4
Insulin glulisine injection	Apidra	0.3	0.5-1.5	5
Short Acting				
Regular human insulin injection	Humulin R	0.5	2-4	6-8
	Novolin R	0.5	2.5-5	8
Buffered regular human insulin injection	Velosulin BR	0.5	1-3	8
Intermediate Acting				
Human insulin isophane suspension	NPH	1.5	4-12	24
Human insulin zinc suspension	Lente	2.5	7-15	22
Long Acting				
Human insulin extended zinc suspension	Ultralente	4-6	8-20	28
Insulin glargine injection	Lantus	2-4	None	24
Combination Insulin				
70% Insulin aspart protamine suspension/30% insulin aspart injection	NovoLog Mix 70/30	0.25	1-4	24
75% Insulin lispro protamine suspension/25% insulin lispro injection	Humalog Mix 75/25	0.25	1-2	24
70% Human insulin isophane suspension (NPH)/30% human insulin injection (regular)	Humulin 70/30	0.5	2-12	24
	Novolin 70/30	0.5	2-12	24
50% Human insulin isophane suspension (NPH)/50% human insulin injection (regular)	Humulin 50/50	0.5	3-5	24

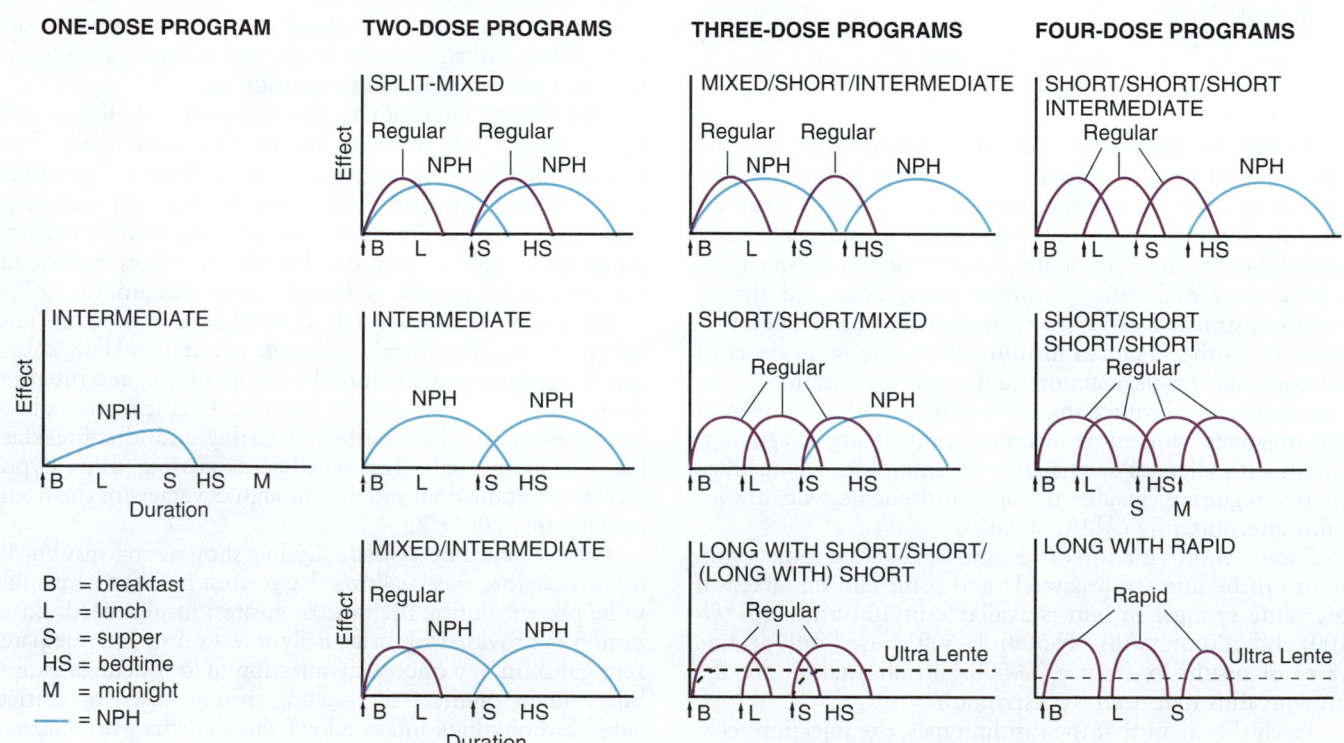

Figure 68-4 ■ Insulin regimens. One injection a day of short-acting or intermediate-acting insulin may be enough to control blood glucose levels. However, split doses (two, three, or four injections of the daily dose) or split mixed doses (a mixture of short-acting and longer acting insulins) may give better control.

tion of action is short, the client taking insulin lispro also needs longer-acting insulin for basal insulin requirements.

COMBINATION THERAPY. A combination of oral agents and intermediate-acting insulin is given to clients with type 2 diabetes who do not have blood glucose control with oral agents alone. Obese clients with higher fasting C-peptide levels are still making some insulin and may be more likely to respond to combination therapy than to single therapy.

INTENSIFIED THERAPY REGIMENS. Intensified regimens are a basal dose of intermediate-acting or long-acting insulin and a bolus dose of short-acting or rapid-acting insulin designed to bring the next blood glucose value into the target range. The client's blood glucose patterns determine insulin dosage. Frequency of blood glucose monitoring is based on the timed action of short- and intermediate-acting insulins and may occur as often as eight times daily. Blood glucose testing 1 to 2 hours after meals and within 10 minutes before the next meal helps determine the adequacy of the bolus dose. The client determines the effects of basal insulin by monitoring pre-evening meal and fasting blood glucose values. Blood glucose values at 3 AM detect nighttime hypoglycemia and indicate adequacy of both short- and intermediate-acting insulin doses.

Clients on intensified insulin regimens need extensive education to achieve target blood glucose values. They need to know how to adjust insulin doses and understand nutrition therapy to maintain dietary flexibility and target blood glucose values. Clients must also be able to perform accurate blood glucose monitoring so that therapy decisions can be based on accurate data.

Pharmacokinetics of Insulin. The action of insulin to move glucose into the cells after insulin injection depends on physical factors and injection techniques.

INJECTION SITE. Figure 68-5 shows common insulin injection sites. The site of injection affects the speed of insulin absorption. Absorption is fastest in the abdomen, followed by the deltoid, thigh, and buttocks. Rotating injection sites prevents lipohypertrophy (increased fat deposits in the skin) or lipoatrophy (loss of fatty tissue, leaving an uneven appearance). Rotation *within* one anatomic site is preferred to rotation from one site to another to prevent day-to-day changes in absorption. The abdomen (except for a 2-inch radius around the navel) is the preferred site because it provides the most rapid insulin absorption.

ABSORPTION RATE. Insulin properties affect its absorption. The longer the duration of action, the more unpredictable is absorption. Ultralente has less consistent absorption than shorter-acting insulins. The larger the dose of insulin, the more prolonged the absorption. Factors that increase blood flow from the injection site, such as local application of heat, massage of the area, and exercise of the injected area, increase insulin absorption. Scarred sites often become favorite injection sites because they are less sensitive to pain. Areas of lipohypertrophy usually slow the rate of insulin absorption (ADA, 2003k).

INJECTION DEPTH. Injections are made into the subcutaneous tissue. Most clients lightly grasp a fold of skin and inject at a 90-degree angle. Aspiration for blood is not necessary. A thin person may need to pinch the skin and inject at a 45-degree angle to avoid intramuscular (IM) injection. IM injection has a faster absorption and is not recommended for routine insulin use (ADA, 2003k). Assess the

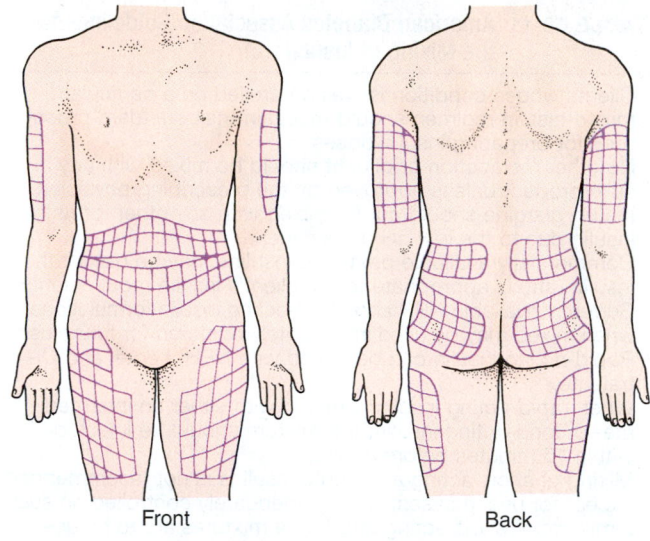

Figure 68-5 ■ Common insulin injection sites.

Front   Back

older client's ability to inject insulin and arrange for assistance when self-care is no longer possible.

TIME OF INJECTION. Injecting regular insulin 30 minutes before meals provides a greater amount of plasma free insulin at mealtime. Eating within a few minutes after (or before) injecting short-acting insulin reduces the ability of insulin to prevent rapid rises in blood glucose after meals and may increase the risk for delayed hypoglycemia (Kissin & Katzeff, 2002). Humalog (insulin lispro), NovoLog (insulin aspart), and insulin glulisine (Apidra) should be given 5 to 15 minutes before a meal.

MIXING INSULINS. Caution clients that mixing different types of insulin can change the timing of peak action. Mixtures of short- and intermediate-acting insulins produce a more normal blood glucose response in some clients than does a single dose. The response to mixed insulin may differ from the response to the same insulins given separately.

When rapid-acting (Humalog or NovoLog) or short-acting (regular) insulin is mixed with a longer-acting insulin, draw the shorter-acting dose into the syringe first. This procedure prevents contamination of the shorter-acting insulin vial with the longer-acting insulin. Short-acting and NPH insulins may be used immediately when mixed, or they may be stored (ADA, 2003k). *Insulin glargine (Lantus) must not be diluted or mixed with any other insulin or solution.* Mixing clouds the solution and makes the onset of action and peak effect time less predictable. Follow American Diabetes Association (ADA) guidelines for mixing insulins (Table 68-11).

Complications of Insulin Therapy. Hypoglycemia from insulin excess has many causes. Its effects and treatment are discussed later under Potential for Hypoglycemia, p. 1539.

Lipoatrophy is a loss of fat tissue in areas of repeated injection that results from an immune reaction to impurities in beef or pork insulin. Treatment consists of injection of human insulin at the edge of the atrophied area. **Lipohypertrophy** is an increased swelling of fat that occurs at the site of repeated insulin injections. The overlying skin has decreased sensitivity, and the area can become large and unsightly. Treatment consists of rotating the injection site among different body areas (White & Hirsch, 2000). Instruct

TABLE 68-11   American Diabetes Association Guidelines for the Mixing of Insulins

- Clients whose condition is well controlled on a particular mixed-insulin regimen should maintain their standard procedure for preparing insulin doses.
- No other medication or diluent should be mixed with any insulin product unless approved by the prescribing physician.
- Insulin glargine should not be mixed with any other forms of insulin due to the low pH of its diluent.
- Commercially available premixed insulins may be used if the insulin ratio is appropriate to the client's insulin requirements.
- Currently available NPH and short-acting insulin formulations when mixed may be used immediately or stored for future use.
- Rapid-acting insulin can be mixed with NPH, Lente, and Ultralente.
- When rapid-acting insulin is mixed with either an intermediate- or long-acting insulin, the mixture should be injected within 15 minutes before a meal.
- Mixing of short-acting and Lente insulins is not recommended except for use in cases already adequately controlled on such a mixture. If short-acting and Lente mixtures are to be used, the client should standardize the interval between mixing and injection.
- Phosphate-buffered insulins (e.g., NPH) should not be mixed with Lente insulins.
- Insulin formulations may change; therefore, the manufacturer should be consulted when their recommendations appear to conflict with the American Diabetes Association guidelines.

Data from American Diabetes Association. (2003). Position statement: Insulin administration. *Diabetes Care 26*(Suppl. 1), 121-124.

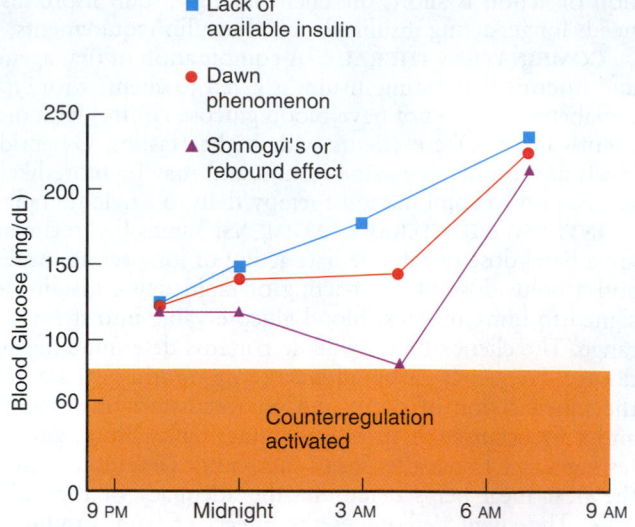

Figure 68-6 ■ Three blood glucose phenomena in diabetic clients.

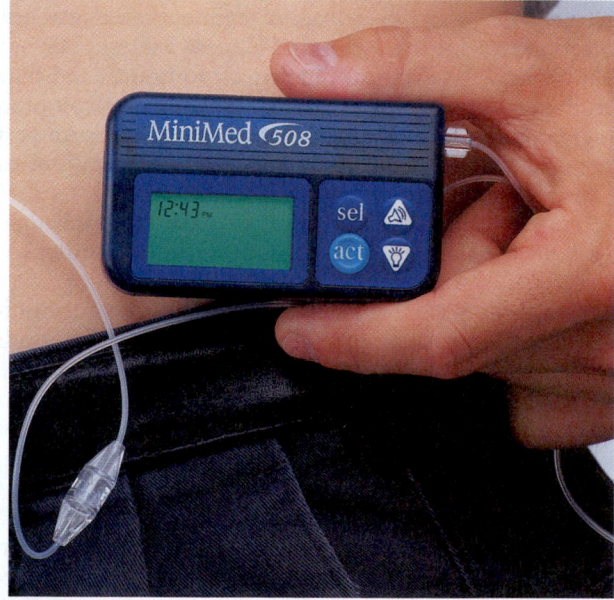

Figure 68-7 ■ External insulin pump. (Courtesy Medtronic MiniMed, Inc., Northridge, CA.)

clients who take insulin to rotate injection sites to prevent lipohypertrophy.

Two conditions of fasting hyperglycemia can occur (Figure 68-6). **Dawn phenomenon** results from a nighttime release of growth hormone that causes blood glucose elevations at about 5 to 6 AM. Dawn phenomenon is treated by providing more insulin for the overnight period (e.g., giving the evening dose of intermediate-acting insulin at 10 PM). **Somagyi's phenomenon** is morning hyperglycemia from the effective counterregulatory response to nighttime hypoglycemia. Somagyi's phenomenon is treated by ensuring adequate dietary intake at bedtime and evaluating the insulin dose and exercise programs to prevent conditions that lead to hypoglycemia. Both phenomena are diagnosed by blood glucose monitoring during the night. Help identify these problems and educate the client and family about management.

Alternative Methods of Insulin Administration. Many methods of insulin delivery are available in addition to traditional intermittent subcutaneous injections.

CONTINUOUS SUBCUTANEOUS INFUSION OF INSULIN. Continuous subcutaneous infusion of a basal dose of insulin (CSII) with increases in insulin at mealtimes is more effective in controlling blood glucose levels than a multiple-injection schedule. CSII allows for flexibility in meal timing, because if a meal is skipped, the mealtime dose of insulin is not given. CSII is given by an externally worn pump containing a syringe and reservoir with rapid- or short-acting insulin and is connected to the client by an infusion set. Teach the client to adjust the amount of insulin received based on data from blood glucose monitoring. Both Humalog (lispro) and NovoLog (insulin aspart) are appropriate for insulin infusion pumps (Figure 68-7).

Skin infections occur when the infusion site is not cleaned or the needle is not changed every 3 days. When the client is receiving rapid-acting insulin and has normal blood glucose levels, stopping the infusion quickly results in hyperglycemia. CSII may lead to more frequent and more severe ketoacidosis than other methods of insulin delivery. Ketoacidosis is related to inexperience in using the pump, infection, accidental cessation of insulin infusion, infusion set obstruction, or mechanical pump problems. Buffered insulin may be used to prevent precipitation of insulin crystals in the catheter. Stress the importance of regular testing for ketones.

Clients using CSII need intensive education. Because of the risk for hypoglycemia or hyperglycemia, the client must perform all the following functions to ensure accurate insulin delivery. Teach the client to operate the pump, adjust the settings, and respond appropriately to alarms. Removing

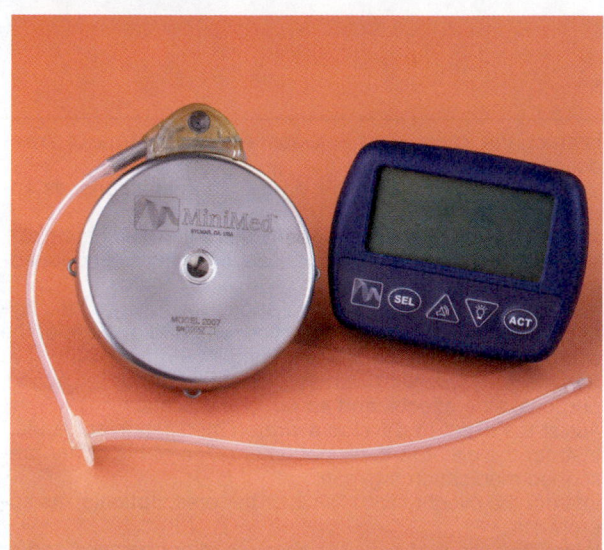

Figure 68-8 ■ Internal insulin pump. (Courtesy Medtronic MiniMed, Inc., Northridge, CA.)

the pump for any length of time can result in hyperglycemia. Provide supplemental insulin schedules for times when the pump is not operational. CSII is more costly than traditional insulin injections, and not all costs are covered by insurance.

IMPLANTED INSULIN PUMPS. Pumps are implanted in the peritoneal cavity, where insulin is absorbed by local blood vessels in a manner similar to that of natural insulin release (Figure 68-8). The pump is surgically implanted in a subcutaneous pocket in the lower abdomen. The pump reservoir is refilled with U-400 insulin every 1 or 2 months. Complications of implanted insulin pumps (IIPs) are catheter blockage, inflammation in the subcutaneous pocket, and mechanical pump failure. Because mechanical problems with the pump, catheter, and insulin delivery remain, the implantable pump is not widely available.

INJECTION DEVICES. In addition to traditional insulin syringes, injection devices include a needleless system and a pen-type injector. With a needleless device, the needle is replaced by an ultrathin liquid stream of insulin forced through the skin under high pressure. Insulin given by jet injection is absorbed at a faster rate, with a resulting shorter duration of action. Cost is a primary drawback to this system (Clarke, 2002).

Pen-type injectors hold small, lightweight, prefilled insulin cartridges. The injectors are easy to carry and make intensive therapy with multiple injections easier. These devices allow greater accuracy than traditional insulin syringes, especially when measuring doses smaller than 5 units (Robertson, Glazer, & Campbell, 2000). Discuss how to maintain the insulin cartridges at an appropriate temperature when using this device away from home. Be cautious when recommending pen-type injectors for visually or neurologically impaired clients. These devices are not meant for independent use by visually impaired people (Fleming, 2000).

NEW TECHNOLOGY. Inhaled insulin is currently under development. The insulin is contained in a pellet that is vaporized in an inhaler or delivered as a dry powder inhaled through a mouthpiece. These systems deliver insulin with a particle size of less than 5 micrometers in diameter able to reach deep lung tissues with a slow, deep inhalation by means of a handheld nebulizer. These particles quickly dissolve in the alveoli and pass into circulation. Systems are being developed to deliver both rapid-acting and long-acting insulins. Pulmonary insulin delivery appears to be safe and effective (White & Campbell, 2001).

Transdermal (through the skin) patch delivery of insulin is being tested. This method is predictable but slower than delivery by injection (Robertson, Glazer, & Campbell, 2000).

Client Education: Prescribed Medication. Provide specific instructions about insulin therapy. Chart 68-4 lists NIC activities for self-medication.

STORAGE. Refrigerate insulin not in use to maintain potency, prevent exposure to sunlight, and inhibit bacterial growth. Insulin in use may be kept at room temperature for up to 28 days to limit irritation at the injection site, which cold insulin may cause.

To prevent loss of drug potency, teach the client to avoid exposing insulin to temperatures below 36° F (2.2° C) or above 86° F (30° C) or to excessive shaking. Insulin lispro (Humalog) and insulin glargine (Lantus) should be stored in a refrigerator (2° to 8° C [36° to 46° F]). Neither type of insulin should be allowed to freeze. If refrigeration is not possible, the vial or cartridge of insulin lispro can be left unrefrigerated for up to 28 days, as long as it is kept as cool as possible (not above 86° F [30° C]) and away from direct heat and light. Discard any unused insulin after 28 days.

Instruct the client to always have a spare bottle of each type of insulin used. A slight loss in potency may occur after the bottle has been in use for more than 30 days even when the expiration date has not passed. When refrigerated, prefilled syringes are stable up to 30 days. If possible, store syringes in the upright position, needle pointing upward, so that insulin particles do not clog it. Teach clients to roll predrawn syringes between their hands before using. The effect of premixing insulins on blood glucose control is assessed by examining blood glucose levels.

DOSE PREPARATION. The person giving the insulin inspects the insulin before each use for changes (e.g., clumping, frosting, precipitation, or change in clarity or color) that may signal loss in potency. Rapid-, short-acting, and glargine insulins should be clear, and all other types of insulin should be uniformly cloudy after gently rolling the vial between the hands. If potency is questionable, another vial of the same type of insulin should be used.

SYRINGES. Standard insulin administration involves injection with syringes marked in insulin units. Insulin syringes are available in 1-mL (100-U), $\frac{1}{2}$ mL (50-U), and $\frac{3}{10}$ mL (30-U) sizes. The unit scale on the barrel of the syringe differs with the syringe size and manufacturer. Insulin syringe needle gauges are measured in 28 gauge, 29 gauge, and 30 gauge and in lengths of $\frac{1}{2}$ inch and $\frac{5}{16}$ inch. Short needles are not used for obese clients because of variability of insulin absorption. To ensure accurate insulin measurement, instruct the client to always buy the same type of syringes. Charts 68-5 and 68-6 review instructions for drawing up a single insulin injection and for mixing regular and NPH insulin in the same syringe.

Manufacturers of disposable syringes and pen needles recommend that needles be used only once. Reuse of an insulin

CHART 68-4

NIC   **INTERVENTION ACTIVITIES for**
The Diabetic Client with Hyperglycemia

Hyperglycemia Management: *Preventing and treating above normal blood glucose levels*
- Monitor blood glucose levels, as indicated.
- Monitor for signs and symptoms of hyperglycemia: polyuria, polydipsia, polyphagia, weakness, lethargy, malaise, blurring of vision, or headache.
- Monitor urine ketones, as indicated.
- Monitor ABG, electrolyte, and betahydroxybutyrate levels, as available.
- Monitor orthostatic blood pressure and pulse, as indicated.
- Administer insulin, as prescribed.
- Encourage oral fluid intake.
- Monitor fluid status (including intake and output), as appropriate.
- Maintain IV access, as appropriate.
- Administer IV fluids, as needed.
- Administer potassium, as prescribed.
- Consult physician if signs and symptoms of hyperglycemia persist or worsen.
- Identify possible causes of hyperglycemia.
- Anticipate situations in which insulin requirements will increase (e.g., intercurrent illness).
- Restrict exercise when blood glucose levels are >250 mg/dL, especially if urine ketones are present.
- Instruct client and significant others on prevention, recognition, and management of hyperglycemia.
- Encourage self-monitoring of blood glucose levels.
- Instruct on urine ketone testing, as appropriate.
- Instruct client and significant others on diabetes management during illness, including use of insulin and/or oral agents, monitoring fluid intake, carbohydrate replacement, and when to seek health professional assistance, as appropriate.
- Provide assistance in adjusting regimen to prevent and treat hyperglycemia (e.g., increasing insulin or oral agent), as indicated.

Teaching: Prescribed Medication: *Preparing a client to safely take prescribed medications and monitor for their effects*
- Instruct the client to recognize distinctive characteristics of the medication(s), as appropriate.
- Inform the client of both the generic and brand names of each medication.
- Instruct the client on the purpose and action of each medication.
- Instruct the client on the dosage, route, and duration of each medication.
- Instruct the client on the proper administration/application of each medication.
- Evaluate the client's ability to self-administer medications.
- Instruct the client to perform needed procedures before taking a medication (e.g., check pulse, glucose), as appropriate.
- Inform the client what to do if a dose of medication is missed.
- Inform the client of consequences of not taking or abruptly discontinuing medication(s), as appropriate.
- Instruct the client on which criteria to use when deciding to alter the medication dosage/schedule, as appropriate.
- Instruct the client on possible adverse effects of each medication.
- Instruct the client how to relieve and/or prevent certain side effects, as appropriate.
- Instruct the client on appropriate actions to take if side effects occur.
- Instruct the client on the signs and symptoms of overdosage/underdosage.
- Inform the client of possible drug-food interactions, as appropriate.
- Instruct the client how to properly store the medication(s).
- Instruct the client on the proper care of devices used for administration.
- Instruct the client on proper disposal of needles and syringes at home, as appropriate, and where to dispose of the sharps container in his or her community.
- Provide the client with written information about the action, purpose, side effects, and so on, of medication.
- Assist the client to develop a written medication schedule.
- Instruct the client to carry documentation of his or her prescribed medication regimen.
- Instruct the client how to fill his or her prescription(s), as appropriate.
- Inform the client of possible changes in appearance and/or dosage when filling generic medication prescription(s).
- Warn the client of the risks associated with taking expired medication.
- Determine the client's ability to obtain required medications.
- Provide information on medication reimbursement, as appropriate.
- Provide information on cost savings programs/organizations to obtain medications and devices, as appropriate.
- Provide information on medication alert devices and how to obtain them.
- Reinforce information provided by other health care team members, as appropriate.
- Include the family/significant others, as appropriate.

Teaching: Prescribed Diet: *Preparing a client to correctly follow a prescribed diet*
- Appraise the client's current level of knowledge about prescribed diet.
- Determine the client's/significant other's feelings/attitude toward prescribed diet and expected degree of dietary compliance.
- Instruct the client on the proper name of the prescribed diet.
- Explain the purpose of the diet.
- Instruct the client about how to keep a food diary, as appropriate.
- Instruct the client on allowed and prohibited foods.
- Inform the client of possible drug-food interactions, as appropriate.
- Assist the client to accommodate food preferences into the prescribed diet.
- Assist the client in substituting ingredients to conform favorite recipes to the prescribed diet.
- Instruct the client about how to read labels and select appropriate foods.
- Observe the client's selection of foods appropriate to prescribed diet.
- Instruct the client about how to plan appropriate meals.
- Provide written meal plans, as appropriate.
- Reinforce information provided by other health care team members, as appropriate.
- Refer client to dietitian/nutritionist, as appropriate.
- Include the family/significant others, as appropriate.

NIC intervention activities selected from Dochterman, J.M., & Bulechek, G.M. (Eds.). (2004). *Nursing interventions classification (NIC)* (4th ed.). St. Louis: Mosby. No part of this work is to be altered without prior written permission from the Publisher.
ABG, Arterial blood gas.

CHART 68-5

CLIENT EDUCATION GUIDE
Subcutaneous Insulin Administration

- Wash your hands.
- Inspect the bottle for the type of insulin and the expiration date.
- Gently roll the bottle of intermediate-acting insulin in the palms of your hands to mix the insulin.
- Clean the rubber stopper with an alcohol swab.
- Remove the needle cover and pull back the plunger to draw air into the syringe. The amount of air should be equal to the insulin dose. Push the needle through the rubber stopper and inject the air into the insulin bottle.
- Turn the bottle upside down and draw the insulin dose into the syringe.
- Remove air bubbles in the syringe by tapping on the syringe or injecting air back into the bottle. Redraw the correct amount.
- Make certain the tip of the plunger is on the line for your dose of insulin. Magnifiers are available to assist in measuring accurate doses of insulin.
- Remove the needle from the bottle. Recap the needle if the insulin is not to be given immediately.
- Select a site within your injection area that has not been used in the past month.
- Clean your skin with an alcohol swab. Lightly grasp an area of skin and insert the needle at a 90-degree angle.
- Push the plunger all the way down. This will push the insulin into your body. Release the pinched skin.
- Pull the needle straight out quickly. Do not rub the place where you gave the shot.
- Dispose of the syringe and needle without recapping in a puncture-proof container.

Data from American Diabetes Association. (2003). Position statement: Insulin administration. *Diabetes Care*, *26*(Suppl. 1), 121-124.

CHART 68-6

CLIENT EDUCATION GUIDE
How to Mix a Prescribed Dose of 10 Units of Regular Insulin and 20 Units of NPH Insulin

- Wash your hands.
- Inspect the bottle for the type of insulin and the expiration date.
- Gently roll the bottle of intermediate insulin in the palms of your hands to mix the insulin.
- Clean the rubber stopper with an alcohol swab.
- Inject 20 units of air into the NPH insulin bottle. The amount of air should be equal to the dose of insulin needed. Always inject air into the intermediate-acting insulin first. Withdraw the syringe.
- Inject 10 units of air into the regular insulin bottle. The amount of air is equal to the dose of insulin desired.
- Withdraw 10 units of regular insulin. Be sure that the syringe is free of air bubbles. Always withdraw the shorter-acting insulin first.
- Withdraw 20 units of NPH insulin with the same syringe, being careful not to inject any short-acting insulin into the bottle. (A total of 30 units should be in the syringe.)

Data from American Diabetes Association. (2003). Position statement: Insulin administration. *Diabetes Care*, *26*(Suppl. 1), 121-124.

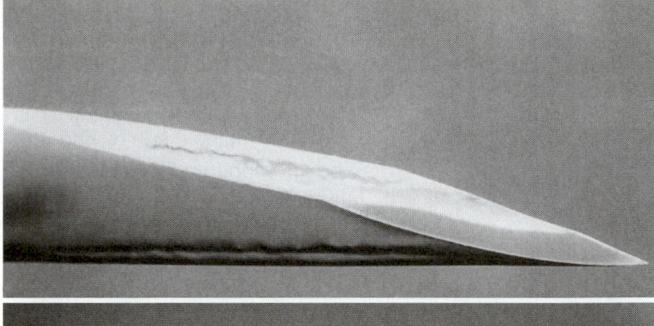
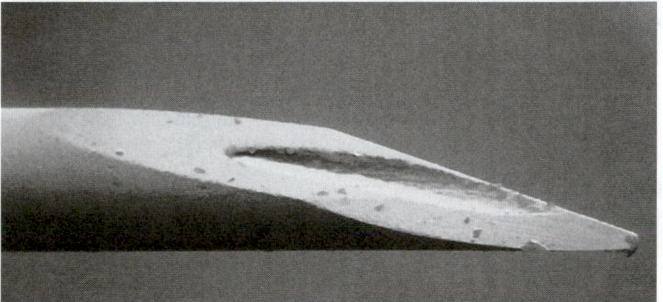
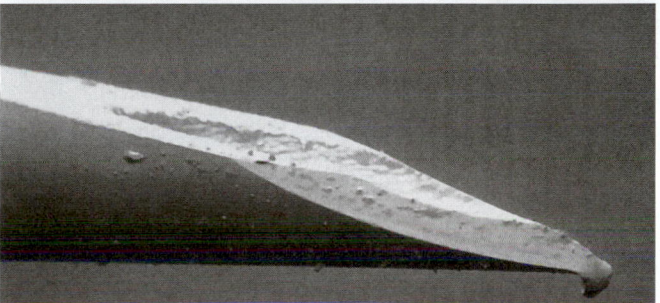
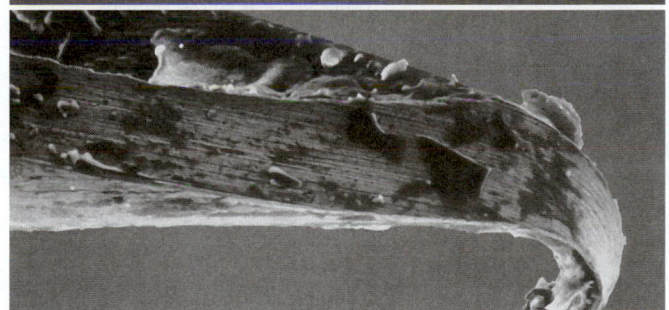

Figure 68-9 ■ Reuse of insulin needle. **A,** A new needle. **B,** A needle that has been used once. **C,** A needle that has been used twice. **D,** A needle that has been used six times. (Courtesy of BD Medical, Franklin Lakes, NJ.)

syringe and needle can compromise insulin sterility. Most insulins contain products that inhibit growth of bacteria commonly found on the skin. Some clients, however, have an increased risk of infection with syringe or needle reuse. A far more important reason to not reuse needles has arisen with the advent of new, smaller (30 and 31 gauge) needles. Even with one injection, the needle tip can become bent to form a hook, which can lacerate tissue or break off to leave needle fragments in the skin (Figure 68-9). Instruct the client to discard the syringe and needle after one use. The Environmental Protection Agency recommends that needles, syringes, lancets, and other sharp objects be placed in a hard-plastic or metal container with a screw-on lid or a tightly secured lid that is clearly marked "Not for Recycling" and discarded with other household trash (http://www.epa.gov/epaoswer/other/medical).

Client Education: Blood Glucose Monitoring. Self-monitoring of blood glucose levels (SMBG) provides information that allows the client to adjust therapy. Teach the client to use the prescribed formulas to (1) self-adjust diet, exercise, or pharmacologic therapy; (2) identify and properly treat hyperglycemia and hypoglycemia; and (3) improve decision making and problem solving. See Table 68-12 for costs of glucose monitors and strips.

TABLE 68-12 Blood Glucose Monitors

Meter	Features	Cost	Test strips (50)	Test Strips (100)
Bayer Diagnostics				
Ascensia ELITE	20 test memory with dates and times Easy to use meter with no buttons; turns on by inserting test strip Approved for multiple site testing	System: $39.95* (Rebate: $35.00)*	$36.99* (foil wrapped strips)	$64.99* (foil wrapped strips)
Ascensia DEX 2	Disk-based monitor eliminates need to handle strips 100-test memory with dates, times, and four daily averages Approved for multiple site testing Data management software available	System: $64.95* (Rebate: $55.00)	$37.99* (5 cartridges of 10 test strips)	$67.99* (10 cartridges of 10 tests each)
Ascensia ELITE XL	120-test memory with dates, times, and 14-day average Easy to use meter with no buttons; turns on by inserting test strip Approved for multiple site testing Advanced data management capability	System: $49.95* (Rebate: $45.00)	$36.99* (foil wrapped strips)	$64.99* (foil wrapped strips)
Lifescan				
One Touch Ultra	150-test memory and plasma values; 14- and 30-day averaging Approved for multiple site testing Advanced data management capability	System: $59.95* (Rebate: $30.00)	$39.49*	$71.44*
Medisense				
Precision QID	125-test memory Data management software available	System: $49.95* (Rebate: $20.00)	$39.44*	$70.99*
Precision Xtra	450-test memory Measures both blood glucose and ketone levels Advanced data management capability	System: $64.95* (Rebate: $20.00)*	$39.44* 8 ketone test strips: $27.95	$70.99*
Sof-Tact	A one-button automatic testing system: brings blood to skin surface, pricks the skin, draws the sample, and transfers it to the test strip with the push of a single button Stores up to 450 results with date and time Approved for multiple site testing Data management software available	Unit price: $195.99*	$39.44*	
Roche Diagnostics				
Accu-Chek Active	200-test memory with 7- and 14-day averaging of data Approved for multiple site testing Data management software available	Care Kit: $17.95*	$25.95*	
Accu-Chek Compact	Easy to use meter for clients with limited dexterity Clients insert a drum containing 17 test strips into the meter. It has a 100-test memory and reports highest, lowest, and average values Approved for multiple site testing Data management software available	System: $64.95* (Rebate $25.00)*	$ 39.99* (3 drums of 17 tests each)	$75.99* (6 drums of 17 tests each)
Accu-Chek Advantage	Easy to use meter, even for young children 100-test memory that stores the date and time for each test Data management software available	Meter: $49.99* (Rebate $25.00)*	Comfort Curve & Advantage strips $39.88*	Comfort Curve & Advantage strips $71.99*
Accu-Chek Complete	1000-test memory with date and time for each test Advanced data management capability	System: $97.95* (Rebate $25.00)	Comfort Curve & Advantage strips $39.88*	Comfort Curve & Advantage strips $71.99*
Accu-Chek Voicemate	Clear voice prompt to guide the visually impaired step-by-step through the blood glucose testing process using the Accu-Chek Advantage meter Insulin vial identification system for Lilly insulin Prescription required with visual impairment of 20/200 or greater for insurance reimbursement	System: $495.00*	Comfort curve strips $39.88*	Comfort Curve strips $71.99*

Pricing data for meters and strips from http://www.diabeticpromotions.com* and http://www.diabeticsupplies.com.

TABLE 68-12 Blood Glucose Monitors—*cont'd*

Meter	Features	Cost	Test strips (50)	Test Strips (100)
Therasense				
FreeStyle	250-test memory Approved for multiple site testing Data management software available	System: $64.95* (Rebate: $40.00)*	$38.99*	$68.95*
FreeStyle Tracker	2500-test memory Comprehensive data management system that combines a blood glucose meter, diabetes manager, and personal digital assistant (PDA) in one device Approved for alternate site testing	System: $299.00* (Rebate $75.00)*	Uses FreeStyle testing strips	

Pricing data for meters and strips from http://www.diabeticpromotions.com* and http://www.diabeticsupplies.com.

The American Diabetes Association (ADA) recommends SMBG for clients taking insulin or oral therapy. Assessment of blood glucose levels is very important for the following clients:

- Any diabetic client trying to keep glucose levels in the near-normal range
- Pregnant clients
- Clients with a tendency to develop severe ketosis or hypoglycemia
- Clients with hypoglycemic unawareness
- Clients undergoing intensive treatment programs, especially those using portable infusion devices, or taking multiple daily insulin injections

The principles of most self-monitoring systems are the same. The finger is pricked and a drop of blood is made to flow over a reagent pad on a testing strip. Meters measure blood glucose by using color reflectance or sensor technology. With reflectance meters, the glucose in a drop of blood reacts with an enzyme in the strip, changing the color of the strip. The meter reads the color of the strip and gives a number for the blood glucose value. Meters that use sensor technology measure small electrical currents produced by the interaction between the glucose in the blood and the chemicals on the strip (Peragallo-Dittko, 2002b). Clients can also perform visual blood glucose monitoring by comparing the color on a test strip with a color key on the vial.

There is some variation between glucose level in whole blood by SMBG systems and that measured by a clinical laboratory. The ADA has set the performance goal to be a total error of no more than 5% at glucose levels between 30 and 400 mg/dL (1.6 and 22.2 mmol/L) (Sacks et al., 2002). The accuracy of SMBG systems decreases at hypoglycemic and hyperglycemic levels. The overall performance of SMBG systems depends on the accuracy of the specific blood glucose meter, operator proficiency, and test strip quality. Results are influenced by the amount of blood on the strip; the meter's calibration to the strip currently in use; environmental conditions of altitude, temperature, and moisture; and client-specific conditions of hematocrit level, triglyceride level, and presence of hypotension.

Most meters indicate blood glucose results as a number, but some have voice readouts, memories that can be displayed, or graphic displays. A client's vision problems, including color blindness, determine the method of SMBG selected. Some models have large, bold display screens and simple, user-friendly procedures.

Teach the client to follow Centers for Disease Control and Prevention (CDC) guidelines for infection control during SMBG. The chances of becoming infected from blood glucose monitoring processes are reduced by handwashing before monitoring and by not reusing lancets. Instruct clients not to share their blood glucose monitoring equipment. Hepatitis B virus can survive in a dried state for at least 1 week. Infection can be spread by the lancet holder even when the lancet itself has been changed. Small particles of blood can stick to the device and infect multiple users. Regular cleaning of the meter is critical for infection control. Health care staff who perform blood glucose testing and family members who help with testing should wear gloves (American Association of Diabetes Educators, 2003b).

INTERPRETATION OF RESULTS. Accuracy of blood glucose measurements is reduced by errors in technique or by equipment failure. Data obtained from SMBG are evaluated with other measures of blood glucose levels (e.g., glycosylated hemoglobin, or hemoglobin A1c [HbA1c], values) or periodic laboratory blood glucose tests. Even when SMBG is performed correctly, the results are affected by hematocrit values (anemia falsely elevates glucose values; polycythemia falsely depresses them) and may be unreliable in the hypoglycemic or severe hyperglycemic ranges. Accuracy of the meter itself is also an issue. Even when highly trained personnel tested meters under optimal conditions, wide variation exists in accuracy and precision among capillary blood glucose monitoring devices. Laboratory glucose determinations are more accurate than SMBG.

FREQUENCY OF TESTING. The frequency of testing varies with the complexity of the drug schedules and the goals of therapy. Clients with unstable blood glucose levels, as well as those using intensive treatment regimens, require frequent monitoring. Clients using simple treatment regimens designed to prevent symptomatic hyperglycemia or clients with type 2 diabetes using oral agents need less frequent testing.

BLOOD GLUCOSE THERAPY GOALS. Work with the client to reach set goals for therapy. Target blood glucose levels are set individually for each client. The American Diabetes Association (ADA) recommends that clients with type 1 diabetes aim for hemoglobin A1c (HbA1c) values less than 7%, premeal glucose levels of 90 to 130 mg/dL (5.0 to 7.2 mmol/L), and postmeal glucose levels less than 180 mg/dL (10.0 mmol/L) (ADA, 2003r).

ACCURACY OF SELF-MONITORING OF BLOOD GLUCOSE LEVELS. All meters are reasonably accurate when the manufacturer's directions are followed. Results are technique dependent regardless of whether test strips are read visually or with a meter. Help the client select a meter based on cost of the meter and strips, ease of use, availability of repair and servicing, and ability to see color. Provide training, explain and demonstrate procedures, assess visual acuity, and check the client's ability to perform the procedure through a return demonstration. Assess color discrimination for those who do not use a blood glucose meter.

Common errors in SMBG involve failure to obtain a sufficient blood drop, poor storage of test strips, and not changing the code number on the meter to match the strip bottle code. Continued retraining of clients performing SMBG helps ensure accurate results because performance accuracy deteriorates over time.

ALTERNATE SITE TESTING. Blood samples for SMBG are usually obtained by pricking the fingertip, where blood glucose levels closely match arterial blood glucose levels. Some meters test blood glucose levels in the forearm, upper arm, abdomen, thigh, and calf. However, blood glucose levels from these alternate sites are not the same as those from the fingertip. Comparison studies indicate that these sites can vary by as much as 100 mg/dL from the fingertip. This variance is from circulation differences at times when blood glucose values are changing rapidly. Teach clients that there is a lag time for blood glucose levels between the fingertip and other sites when blood glucose levels are changing rapidly and that the fingertip reading is the only safe choice at those times.

Clients with a history of hypoglycemic unawareness should not test at alternative sites (Peragallo-Dittko, 2002). Alternative site testing is safe before a meal and 2 hours after a meal. Instruct the client to use only fingertip testing in the following situations:

- When hypoglycemic
- When risk for hypoglycemia is greater (at time of peak activity of basal insulin, or within 2 hours after injecting rapid-acting insulin)
- After exercise
- During an illness
- When blood glucose levels are changing rapidly (e.g., within 2 hours after a meal)
- Before driving

🔴 **CONSIDERATIONS FOR OLDER ADULTS**

Visual interpretation of blood glucose values is affected by normal age-related changes in color perception. The ability to discriminate shades of blue, violet, and green become less accurate, making performance of visual blood glucose monitoring more difficult. Also, older clients need more light to see things clearly. Placing a high-intensity light on the object or surface is more effective than increasing light for the entire room.

New Technology. Current methods of measuring blood glucose are not sufficiently adequate for adjusting insulin doses for clients receiving intense insulin therapy. Continuous blood glucose monitoring with an implanted sensor could allow more adequate insulin delivery and earlier detection of hypoglycemia (Gerritsen, 2000).

The GlucoWatch (Cygnus) sends a tiny electrical current through the skin to measure glucose from interstitial fluid just beneath the skin. It analyzes glucose every 20 minutes for up to 12 hours and appears best suited for detecting unsuspected hypoglycemia. The GlucoWatch is meant to supplement, not replace, finger stick tests. Insulin should only be given after confirming the results of the GlucoWatch with a finger stick test (Table 68-13).

The Continuous Glucose Monitoring System (Medtronic MiniMed) is a subcutaneous glucose sensor connected to an externally worn monitor. Blood glucose values, obtained every 5 minutes for up to 72 hours, are downloaded into computer for analysis. The data show blood glucose changes over the day, allowing more accurate adjustments in intensive insulin therapy.

Systems for obtaining blood without finger sticks are being developed. The Professional Lancette gets a drop of blood by vaporizing a pinpoint of skin on the finger with a laser beam.

Diet Therapy. Effective self-management of diabetes requires that the meal plan, education, and counseling programs be individualized for each client. A registered dietitian should be a member of the treatment team. The nurse, dietitian, client, and family work together on all aspects of the meal plan, which must be realistic and as flexible as possible.

Goals of Diet Therapy. Diet therapy focuses on the following goals:

- Keeping blood glucose and glycosylated hemoglobin levels as near normal as possible
- Having optimal serum lipid levels: low-density lipoprotein (LDL) cholesterol below 100 mg/dL (2.60 mmol/L), high-density lipoprotein (HDL) cholesterol above 40 mg/dL, and triglyceride levels below 150 mg/dL (1.7 mmol/L) (ADA, 2003l)
- Having a blood pressure consistently less than 130/80 mm Hg (ADA, 2003r)
- Ensuring adequate calories for achieving reasonable weight for adults, meeting increased metabolic needs during pregnancy and lactation, or promoting recovery from illness
- Preventing and treating the acute complications of hypoglycemic drugs, short-term illness, and exercise-related problems

TABLE 68-13 Cost of Blood Glucose Monitoring Products

Product	Cost	Cost of Supplies	Comments
Lasette	$495.00	Disposable cartridge: $12.90 for a two-pack system ($0.13 per test)	Cartridge is good for 120 uses. Battery is rechargeable, with 50 uses per charge.
GlucoWatch	$872.00	Auto sensor: $9.38	Auto sensor must be changed every 12 hr. Watch should last 2-3 yr.

Data from the following:
Lasette: Cell Robotics International (http://www.cellrobotics.com; http://www.diabeteswebsite.com; 800-846-0590); GlucoWatch: Automatic glucose biography (http://www.glucoewatch.com; 866-GLWATCH).

- Preventing and treating complications of diabetes (renal disease, neuropathy, and cardiovascular disease)
- Improving overall health through healthy food choices and physical activity
- Facilitating changes in eating habits that reduce insulin resistance and improve metabolic status
- Meeting the nutritional and psychosocial needs of older individuals
- Providing self-management education for clients treated with insulin or sulfonylureas for treatment and prevention of hypoglycemia, acute illness, and exercise related blood glucose problems
- For clients at risk for diabetes, encouraging food choices that facilitate moderate weight loss or at least prevent weight gain (ADA, 2003r)

Principles of Nutrition in Diabetes. The dietitian develops a meal plan based on the client's usual food intake. Day-to-day consistency in the timing and amount of food eaten helps control blood glucose. Clients receiving insulin therapy need to eat at consistent times that are coordinated with the timed action of insulin. Teach clients using intense insulin therapy to adjust premeal insulin to allow for timing and quantity changes in their meal plan (ADA, 2003f).

Protein. The usual protein intake (15% to 20% of total daily calories) is appropriate for diabetic clients with normal kidney function. In clients with microalbuminuria, reduction of protein to 10% of calories (0.8 g/kg) may slow progression of kidney failure (ADA, 2003f).

Fat and Carbohydrate. The amount of calories from fat and carbohydrates is based on individual goals. Of the remaining 80% to 90% of calories, less than 10% should be from saturated fat and up to 10% should be from polyunsaturated fat. Foods high in trans-fatty acids are avoided or severely limited. The remaining 60% to 70% of calories are from monounsaturated fat and carbohydrates (ADA, 2003f).

Further fat restrictions for clients with diabetes are determined by a dietitian based on specific lipid abnormalities. Adults with diabetes should be tested annually for lipid abnormalities. These tests include fasting serum cholesterol, triglyceride, high-density lipoprotein (HDL) cholesterol, and calculated LDL cholesterol levels (ADA, 2003l).

The percentage of calories obtained from carbohydrates is determined for each client. Various starches have different blood glucose responses. Emphasis is placed on the total amount of carbohydrate consumed each day rather than the source of the carbohydrate. Little scientific evidence supports the assumption that sugars are more rapidly absorbed than starches and cause blood glucose values to increase more rapidly.

Fiber. High-fiber diets improve carbohydrate metabolism and lower cholesterol levels. Teach the client to select foods with moderate to high amounts of dietary fiber (e.g., legumes, lentils, roots, leafy green vegetables, all types of whole-grain cereals, and fruits). Intake of 20 to 35 g of dietary fiber per day is ideal.

Teach the client that adding high-fiber foods to the diet gradually can reduce abdominal cramping, loose stools, and flatulence. An increase in fluid intake should accompany increased fiber intake. The nurse and the client should pay careful attention to blood glucose levels because hypoglycemia can result when dietary fiber intake increases significantly.

Nonnutritive Sweeteners. The use of products to enhance the taste of food while not disturbing blood glucose control is desirable. The FDA has approved four nonnutritive sweeteners for use: saccharin, aspartame, acesulfame K, and sucralose.

Fat Replacers. Fat replacers in foods create good-tasting, lower-fat foods but may increase carbohydrate content. Teach clients how to incorporate fat replacers into their meal plan. Guidelines regarding the use of fat replacers are as follows (ADA, 2001b):

- Fat replacer should be less than 20 calories or less than 5 g of carbohydrate per serving if it is a "free food."
- Limit fat replacer to three servings per day.
- From 6 to 10 g of carbohydrate per serving is one half of a carbohydrate choice.
- From 11 to 20 g of carbohydrate per serving is one carbohydrate choice.

Alcohol. Blood glucose levels are not affected by *moderate* use of alcohol when diabetes is well controlled. Teach clients using insulin that two alcoholic beverages for men and one for women can be ingested with, and in addition to, the usual meal plan. (One alcoholic beverage equals 12 ounces of beer, 5 ounces of wine, or 1.5 ounces of distilled spirits.) Because of the potential for alcohol-induced hypoglycemia, instruct the client to ingest alcohol only with or shortly after meals. Alcohol raises plasma triglycerides; thus, reducing or abstaining from alcohol is important for clients with hyperlipidemia. One alcoholic beverage is substituted for two fat exchanges when calculating caloric intake (ADA, 2003f).

Food Labeling. Nutrient and ingredient information help clients make good food and portion choices. For clients with diabetes, foods containing sucrose or other sugars are not restricted. These foods are used sparingly and substituted for other carbohydrates in the individual meal plan. Teach the client to use the food label to determine carbohydrate content.

Client Education: Prescribed Diet. No one meal plan is right for all clients with diabetes. Each client's nutrition recommendations are based on blood glucose monitoring results, total blood lipid levels, and glycosylated hemoglobin. These tests help to determine whether current meal and exercise patterns need adjustment or whether present habits need reinforcement. A specific dietary prescription is developed for each client.

Support and reinforce nutrition information provided by the dietitian. The diabetic client needs to understand how to make adjustments in food intake during illness, planned exercise, and social occasions (such as restaurant meals) where the usual time of eating is delayed. The client may be unable to follow the prescribed diet because of an inability to see, read, or understand printed materials. Share dietary information with the person who prepares the meals. The dietitian sees each client at least yearly to identify changes in lifestyle and make appropriate diet therapy changes. Some clients, such as those with weight control problems or low incomes, may need more frequent evaluation and counseling.

Meal-Planning Strategies. Many meal-planning approaches are available. Each approach emphasizes different aspects of nutrition.

EXCHANGE SYSTEM. The exchange system is based on three food groups: carbohydrates, meat and meat substitutes, and fat. The exchange list for meal planning assumes

TABLE 68-14 Exchange System of Medical Nutrition Therapy

Food Content	Carbohydrate (g)	Protein (g)	Fat (g)	Calories	Example
Carbohydrate					
Breads/grains	15	3	1 or less	80	1 slice bread ½ bagel ½ hamburger bun ½ cup corn ½ cup mashed potato
Fruit	15	0	0	60	1 small apple ½ medium banana ½ grapefruit
Milk					
Skim	12	8	0-3	90	1 cup skim milk (½%-1%)
Low-fat	12	8	5	120	1 cup 2% milk
Whole	12	8	5	150	1 cup whole milk
Other carbohydrates	15	Varies	Varies	Varies	Brownie, unfrosted (2-inch square) Fruit juice bar 1 tablespoon jelly, regular
Vegetables	5	2	0	25	Carrots, green beans, spinach, ½ cup cooked, 1 cup raw 1 large tomato
Meat or Meat Substitute					
Very lean	0	7	0-1	35	1 oz chicken (white meat, skinless), 1 oz fat-free cheese (1 g fat or less)
Lean	0	7	3	55	1 oz lean beef (trimmed rump roast), dark meat chicken (skinless), or salmon; ¼ cup cottage cheese (4.5% fat)
Medium-fat	0	7	5	75	1 oz ground beef, pork cutlet, lamb, or dark meat chicken with skin
High-fat	0	7	8	100	1 oz pork sausage, 1 tablespoon peanut butter, 1 oz American cheese
Fat	0	0	5	45	1 teaspoon butter or margarine, 1 strip bacon

that foods with similar nutrient content affect blood glucose levels similarly. Diets based on the exchange system produce predictable blood glucose responses. The client's prescription identifies how many items from each food group are to be eaten at a meal or snack. Table 68-14 provides an example of the exchange system of diet therapy.

CARBOHYDRATE COUNTING. Carbohydrate (CHO) counting is a simple approach to meal planning that uses label information of the nutritional content of packaged food items. Because fat and protein have little effect on postmeal blood glucose levels, CHO counting focuses on the nutrient that has the greatest impact on these levels. CHO counting uses total grams of carbohydrate, regardless of the food source. The dietitian determines the number of grams of carbohydrate to be eaten at each meal and snack and helps the client to make appropriate food choices. CHO counting is effective in achieving overall blood glucose control when carbohydrate intake is consistent from day to day.

Clients using intensive insulin or pump therapies can use CHO counting to determine insulin coverage. After the amount of insulin needed to cover the usual meal is determined, insulin may be added or subtracted for changes in carbohydrate intake. An initial formula of 1 unit of rapid-acting insulin for each 15 g of carbohydrate provides flexibility to meal plans. The client determines the grams of carbohydrate in a specific meal or snack by label reading or weighing and measuring of each item. The total grams of carbohydrate are used to calculate the bolus dose of insulin based on their individual insulin to carbohydrate ratio. See Table 68-15 for an example of carbohydrate counting.

SPECIAL CONSIDERATIONS FOR TYPE 1 DIABETES. A meal plan based on the client's usual food intake is developed, and insulin therapy is integrated into the usual eating and exercises patterns. To match the effects of insulin, the daily caloric intake is spread among three main meals and any between-meal or bedtime snacks. Blood glucose monitoring before and within 1 to 2 hours after meals determines whether the insulin/carbohydrate ratio is correct. For clients who are on fixed insulin regimens and do not adjust premeal insulin dosages, consistency of carbohydrate intake at each meal is important. Clients using intensified insulin therapy with multiple daily injections of insulin or an insulin pump have more flexibility in the choice and timing of meals and snacks. The need for between-meal or bedtime snacks is based on the peak action time of insulin and the need to prevent hypoglycemia. Additional carbohydrate may be needed before unplanned exercise to prevent exercise-related hypoglycemia.

Besides maintaining blood glucose levels within a target range, a second goal for clients with type 1 diabetes is to avoid gaining weight. Hyperinsulinemia (chronic high blood insulin levels) can occur with intensive treatment

TABLE 68-15 Carbohydrate Counting

	Food Source	Grams of Carbohydrates	Total	Insulin Dose* (1:15 ratio)
Breakfast	2 slices honey grain bread	32		
	¼ cup egg substitute	0		
	½ cup orange juice	15		
	1 Tablespoon lower-fat margarine	0	47	3
Lunch	2 oz tuna, canned in water	0		
	1 hamburger bun	30		
	Fat-free Pringles (#15)	15		
	1 Tablespoon reduced-fat mayonnaise	0		
	1 tomato and 1 lettuce slice	0		
	1 medium dill pickle	0		
	Sugar-free pudding made with fat-free milk	15	60	4
Supper	3 oz chicken breast, grilled	0		
	1 small (3 oz) baked potato	15		
	1 cup steamed broccoli	10		
	1 French roll	25		
	1 Tablespoon lower-fat margarine	0		
	2 Tablespoons reduced-fat sour cream	0		
	½ cup canned pineapple (in own juice)	15	65	4

*Insulin dosage has been rounded off to the nearest whole unit. Tenths of units of insulin can only be given with an insulin pump.

schedules and may result in weight gain. These clients may need to treat hyperglycemia by restricting calories rather than increasing insulin. Weight gain can be minimized by following the prescribed meal plan, getting regular exercise, and avoiding overtreatment of hypoglycemia.

SPECIAL CONSIDERATIONS FOR TYPE 2 DIABETES. Many clients with type 2 diabetes are overweight and insulin resistant. Diet therapy stresses lifestyle changes that reduce calories eaten and increase calories expended through physical activity. Many clients with diabetes also have abnormal blood fat levels (metabolic syndrome) and hypertension, making reductions of saturated fat, cholesterol, and sodium desirable. A moderate caloric restriction (250 to 500 calories less than average daily intake) and an increase in physical activity improves diabetic control and weight control. Decreases of more than 10% of body weight can result in significant improvement in glycosylated hemoglobin (hemoglobin A1c) (King & Wofford, 2000). Decreasing intake of cholesterol-raising fatty acids helps reduce the risk of cardiovascular disease.

When clients with type 2 diabetes need treatment with insulin, consistency in timing and carbohydrate content of meals is important. Division of the total daily calories into three meals or into smaller meals and snacks is based on individual preference.

CONSIDERATIONS FOR OLDER ADULTS

Older clients are at increased risk for malnutrition, hypoglycemia, and especially dehydration, a factor in the development of the hyperglycemic hyperosmolar nonketotic (HHNS) syndrome. Many factors contribute to malnutrition. Older clients who prepare their own food or have tooth loss or poorly fitting dentures may not eat enough food. Neuropathy with gastric retention or diarrhea compounds poor food intake. Impaired cognition and depression may disrupt self-care. Older clients may have a marginal food supply because of inadequate income, may have poor understanding of meal planning goals, or may live alone and have reduced incentive to prepare or eat proper meals. They may eat in restaurants or live in situations in which they have little control over meal preparation. Regular visits by home health nurses can assist older clients in following a diabetic meal plan.

A realistic approach to diet therapy is essential for the older diabetic client. Changing the eating habits of 60 to 70 years is very difficult. The nurse, dietitian, and client assess the client's usual eating patterns. Teach the older client taking antidiabetic drugs about the importance of eating meals and snacks at the same time every day, eating the same amount of food from day to day, and eating all food allowed on the diet.

Exercise Therapy. Regular exercise is an essential part of a diabetic treatment plan. Exercise has beneficial effects on carbohydrate metabolism and insulin sensitivity. It also improves the client's sense of well-being and reduces the risk for atherosclerosis (ADA, 2003n). Motivation to start an exercise program, especially among people who are sedentary, can be difficult. A large study indicated that gender differences rather than racial or ethnic differences were a better predictor of exercise success. (See the Evidence-Based Practice for Nursing Box on p. 1530.)

In the person without diabetes, glucose use during exercise is matched by glucose production by the liver; thus exercise does not induce hyperglycemia or hypoglycemia. The client with type 1 diabetes is unable to make these hormonal changes. Without an adequate insulin supply, cells are unable to use glucose. Low insulin levels trigger release of glucagon and epinephrine to increase hepatic glucose production, further raising blood glucose levels. In the absence of insulin, free fatty acids become the source of energy. Exercise in the client with uncontrolled diabetes results in further hyperglycemia and the formation of ketone bodies. Diabetic clients may have prolonged elevated blood glucose levels after vigorous exercise.

Exercise in the person with diabetes can cause hypoglycemia because of increased muscle glucose uptake and inhibited glucose release from the liver. Hypoglycemia can occur during exercise and for up to 24 hours after exercise. Replacement of muscle and liver glycogen stores, along with

EVIDENCE-BASED PRACTICE for Nursing

Do exercise practices among people with diabetes vary with ethnicity?

Wood, F. (2002). Ethnic differences in exercise among adults with diabetes. *Western Journal of Nursing Research, 24*(5), 502-515.

Exercise has been identified as an important strategy to reduce complications among adults who have diabetes. Previous studies of exercise patterns among adult Americans are largely confined to white men. This study sought to identify exercise patterns among men and women with diabetes from racially and ethnically diverse backgrounds. The study examined data previously collected by the National Health and Nutrition Examination Survey (NHANES) III Household Adult Data Files from 1988 through 1994. Sixteen questions from the original survey provided information about diabetes, gender, ethnicity/race, and exercise. Data obtained as responses to these 16 survey items were reanalyzed to compare exercise patterns among adults with diabetes from diverse ethnic backgrounds: African American, Hispanic American, and European American. Survey and interview data from 1614 adults with diabetes were examined. Fifty-nine percent (953) of the subjects were women, 41% (661) of the subjects were men. About half were over 56 years of age. Twenty-seven percent (448) were African American and 29% (505) were Hispanic American. This secondary analysis revealed that about one third of subjects did not engage in any form of regular exercise or physical activity. Rates and types of exercise were not statistically different among the three different ethnic/racial groups. Overall, men of all ethnicities were more physically active than women. Walking and gardening were the two most widely practiced forms of exercise or physical activity.

Level of Evidence: 3—Well-designed trial without randomization.

Critique. This secondary analysis used data collected from a large, cross-sectional sample that originally oversampled nonwhite individuals and people older than 60 years of age. The findings of this secondary analysis support the findings of other studies indicating little or no performance of regular physical activity in individuals older than 60 years of age.

Implications for Nursing. The benefits of mild to moderate exercise for clients with diabetes are well-documented. This study indicates that many people with diabetes of all ethnicities do not participate in any form of exercise. What is not known is why some individuals do not exercise. Providing information to clients with diabetes that exercise is beneficial is not sufficient. Nurses must assess each client's level of physical activity and determine what factors prevent the person from participating in regular physical exercise as well as what factors enhance participation in regular exercise. In this way, nurses can help individualize an exercise program for each client with the potential to increase overall participation in regular physical activity.

increased insulin sensitivity following exercise, causes insulin requirements to drop.

Benefits of Exercise. Regular, moderate-intensity exercise helps regulate blood glucose levels and lowers insulin requirements for clients with type 1 diabetes. It also improves control by increasing insulin sensitivity, enhancing cell uptake of glucose, and promoting weight loss.

Regular exercise decreases risk factors for cardiovascular disease. For clients with type 1 diabetes, exercise decreases most blood lipid levels and increases high-density lipoproteins (HDLs). Exercise decreases blood pressure and improves cardiovascular function. Regular vigorous physical activity prevents or delays type 2 diabetes by reducing body weight, insulin resistance, and glucose intolerance.

Risks Related to Exercise. Assess the diabetic client for risk for injury related to exercise. Prolonged hypo-

glycemia or hyperglycemia can occur, particularly after sustained high-intensity exercise.

Several complications of diabetes can be made worse by exercise. The client with proliferative retinopathy is advised to avoid the Valsalva maneuver (breath-holding while bearing down) and activities that increase blood pressure. Heavy lifting, rapid head motion, or jarring activities can cause eye hemorrhage or retinal detachment. Exercise may increase proteinuria in clients with diabetic nephropathy. The risk for foot and joint injury rises for clients with peripheral neuropathy. Autonomic neuropathy can cause orthostatic hypotension after exercise.

Screening Before Starting an Exercise Program. Advise a diabetic client to have a complete physical examination before starting an exercise program. Regular physical activity increases the risk for musculoskeletal injury and life-threatening cardiovascular events. The ability of the heart to respond to increasing levels of exercise on a treadmill, as well as the presence of other risk factors, forms the basis of the exercise prescription. For clients who are unable to perform vigorous exercise, the heart's ability to tolerate exercise is tested with cardiac stressor drugs (e.g., coronary vasodilators, dipyridamole thallium scans). The client needs to be carefully evaluated for vascular complications that may be worsened by exercise (ADA, 2003n).

Guidelines for Exercise. The client checks blood glucose levels before exercise. When levels exceed 250 mg/dL (13.8 mmol/L), the client tests the urine for ketones. The absence of urine ketones indicates that enough insulin is available for glucose transport and use, and that exercise should be effective in lowering blood glucose levels. When urine ketones are present, the client should **not** exercise. Ketones indicate that current insulin levels are not adequate and that exercise would elevate blood glucose levels.

Low-intensity aerobic exercise for longer durations is most effective in achieving desired health effects for clients with diabetes. These exercises require slow, submaximal effort, continue for more than 12 to 15 minutes, and moderately elevate the heart rate (above 50% of maximal rate). Such activities include walking briskly, running, jogging, stationary or regular bicycling, swimming, dancing, rowing, and cross-country skiing. These activities improve cardiac output.

For clients with type 1 diabetes, the aerobic exercise should last for 20 to 40 minutes and be performed 4 to 7 days per week. A 5- to 10-minute warm-up period with stretching and low-intensity exercise before exercise and a 5- to 10-minute cool-down period after exercise reduce the risk for dysrhythmias. Daily exercise increases total energy expenditure, helps weight loss, and improves blood glucose control.

Client Education: Exercise Promotion. Chart 68-7 lists NIC intervention activities for exercise. Instruct the client to wear shoes with good traction and cushioning and to examine the feet daily and after exercise. Discourage exercise in extreme heat or cold or during periods of poor blood glucose control. Advise the client to stay hydrated, especially during and after exercise in a warm environment.

Teach clients not to exercise within 1 hour of insulin injection or at the peak time of insulin action. Exercise can increase absorption of insulin from the injection site, increasing blood insulin levels. The risk for hypoglycemia increases when insulin is injected into an area that is exercised.

CHART 68-7

NIC INTERVENTION ACTIVITIES for
The Diabetic Client Needing to Increase Physical Activity

Exercise Promotion: *Facilitation of regular physical activity to maintain or advance to a higher level of fitness and health*
- Appraise individual's health beliefs about physical exercise.
- Encourage verbalization of feelings about exercise or need for exercise.
- Include family/caregivers in planning and maintaining the exercise program.
- Inform individual about health beliefs and physiologic effects of exercise.
- Instruct individual about appropriate type of exercise for level of health, in collaboration with physician and/or exercise physiologist.
- Instruct individual about desired frequency, duration, and intensity of the exercise program.
- Instruct individual about conditions warranting cessation of or alteration in the exercise program.
- Instruct individual on proper warm-up and cool-down exercises.
- Instruct the individual in techniques to avoid injury while exercising.
- Assist individual to develop an appropriate exercise program to meet needs.
- Assist individual to set short-term and long-term goals for the exercise program.
- Assist individual to schedule regular periods for the exercise program into weekly routine.
- Monitor individual's response to exercise program.
- Provide positive feedback for individual's efforts.

Vital Signs Monitoring: *Collection and analysis of cardiovascular, respiratory, and body temperature data to determine and prevent complications*
- Monitor blood pressure, pulse, temperature, and respiratory status, as appropriate.
- Monitor for and report signs and symptoms of hypothermia and hyperthermia.
- Monitor presence and quality of pulses.
- Monitor cardiac rhythm and rate.
- Monitor respiratory rate and rhythm (e.g., depth and symmetry).
- Monitor for abnormal respiratory patterns (e.g., Cheyne-Stokes, Kussmaul, Biot, apneustic, ataxic, and excessive sighing).
- Monitor skin color, temperature, and moistness.
- Identify possible causes of changes in vital signs.

NIC intervention activities selected from Dochterman, J.M., & Bulechek, G.M. (Eds.). (2004). *Nursing interventions classification (NIC)* (4th ed.). St. Louis: Mosby. No part of this work is to be altered without prior written permission from the Publisher.

Make sure clients engaging in exercise know the risk for hypoglycemia, and teach preventive measures. Clients taking oral drugs or insulin should monitor blood glucose levels to determine the effects of exercise. Teach the client that snacks containing rapidly absorbable carbohydrate may be eaten before and during exercise to maintain blood glucose levels within normal ranges. Extra carbohydrate may be needed for up to 24 hours after exercise to prevent hypoglycemia. The amount of additional carbohydrate is directed by the results of blood glucose monitoring. Instruct the client to decrease insulin dosage before planned exercise as directed.

Clients with type 1 diabetes should perform vigorous exercise only if blood glucose levels are 80 to 250 mg/dL (4.4 to 13.8 mmol/L) and no ketones are present in the urine. Advise the non-obese client who is taking insulin to have a carbohydrate-containing snack before exercise if at least 1 hour has elapsed since the last food was eaten or if high-intensity exercise is planned. There is no need for additional carbohydrate intake when the blood glucose level exceeds 100 mg/dL (5.6 mmol/L) before exercise and the planned activity is of low intensity and short duration. When vigorous activity of long duration is planned, the client should eat an additional 15 to 30 g of carbohydrate for every 30 to 60 minutes of exercise. Snacks such as fruit, fruit juice, bread products, and whole milk are effective in preventing hypoglycemia. Instruct the client to carry a simple sugar (hard candy) to eat if symptoms of hypoglycemia occur. Also instruct the client to carry identifying information about having diabetes.

CONSIDERATIONS FOR OLDER ADULTS

With age, the ability of the heart and lungs to deliver oxygen to tissues and organs declines. These changes may result more from a decline in muscle mass than to changes in cardiac output. Aerobic activities are important in maintaining muscle mass. Healthy older clients are able to maintain cardiac output by increasing stroke volume during exercise.

In the absence of retinopathy-related restrictions, strength (resistance) training for major muscles of the legs, arms, stomach, and trunk, performed two or three times weekly helps preserve muscle mass and minimizes general functional decline (Flood & Constance, 2002).

SURGICAL MANAGEMENT. Surgical interventions for diabetes mellitus include transplantation of all or part of the pancreas. Successful pancreas and islet cell transplantations are the only therapies that achieve blood glucose control by providing normal insulin secretion that responds to feedback regulation (Robertson et al., 2000). Clients' quality of life is improved when they no longer have to take insulin injections and are free of diabetic dietary restrictions.

Whole-Pancreas Transplantation. Improved surgical techniques and newer immunosuppressive therapies have improved pancreatic transplantation outcomes. The 1-year survival rate is above 90%, with more than 80% of clients remaining free of insulin injection and diet restrictions after 1 year (Cattral et al., 2000). The degree of tissue-type matching affects the results.

Pancreatic transplantation is performed in one of three ways: transplant of the pancreas alone (PTA), transplant of the pancreas after successful kidney transplant (PAK), and simultaneous pancreas and kidney transplant (SPK). The ideal procedure for diabetic clients with uremia is SPK. These clients are generally poor surgical candidates because of complications from the diabetes. The problems of diabetes must be severe enough to balance the toxicity of immunosuppressive drugs. Pancreatic transplant is only partially successful in reversing the long-term complications of diabetes (ADA, 2003m).

Operative Procedures. Most pancreatic transplants are from cadaver donors using a total pancreas still attached to the exit of the pancreatic duct. The pancreas is placed in the pelvis and the pancreatic duct outlet is attached to the urinary bladder. Endocrine hormones from the pancreas drain into systemic circulation and exocrine hormones drain into the urinary bladder (systemic venous-bladder). Pancreatic transplant is successful when the client no longer needs insulin therapy and all blood measures of glucose are normal.

Chronic loss of pancreatic secretions can cause dehydration and electrolyte imbalance, and drainage of exocrine hormones into the urinary bladder causes irritation. Some techniques allow drainage of endocrine hormones into the portal venous system and intestinal drainage of exocrine secretions (portal venous-enteric).

Rejection Management. A combination of drugs and antibodies are used to reverse rejection. (See Chapter 23 for a listing of agents used to prevent or treat transplant rejection.) Clients undergoing immunosuppressive therapy first receive drugs to prevent viral, bacterial, and fungal infection because of the risk for opportunistic infections.

In nearly 90% of rejections, kidney problems occur before pancreatic problems. An increase in serum creatinine indicates rejection of both the transplanted kidney and the pancreas. In clients with bladder drainage of pancreatic hormones, a decrease in the urine amylase level by 25% is an indication to treat rejection. High blood glucose levels are a later marker of rejection and usually indicate irreversible graft failure.

Long-Term Effects. Long-term immunosuppressive therapy increases the risk for infection, cancer, and atherosclerosis. The transplanted pancreas does not duplicate all the functions of a normal pancreas. When insulin drains into systemic rather than portal circulation, circulating insulin levels rise (hyperinsulinemia) and increase the risk for hypertension and macrovascular disease.

Complications. Complications are common in clients taking long-term immunosuppressive therapy. Pancreatic transplant complications include venous thrombosis, rejection, and infection. Monitor laboratory values, fluid and electrolyte status, physical manifestations, and changes in vital signs to identify possible complications. Early removal of IV and intra-arterial lines, use of sterile technique with dressing changes and catheter irrigations, strict handwashing by health care personnel, and good pulmonary hygiene all help prevent infection.

Pancreatic blood vessel thrombosis occurs in about 30% of clients after transplantation. Observe for and report any sudden drop in urine amylase levels, rapid increases in blood glucose, gross **hematuria** (bloody urine), and tenderness or pain in the graft area (iliac fossa).

Assess the client for manifestations of rejection. In acute rejection, decreased kidney function is indicated by increased serum creatinine, decreased urine output, hypertension, increased weight, graft tenderness, and fever. Proteinuria is often the first indicator of chronic graft rejection. Check for increased blood amylase, lipase, or glucose; decreased urine amylase; graft tenderness; hyperglycemia; and fever. It is especially important to assess for signs of infection and start appropriate treatment. Fever can signal both infection and rejection.

Monitor for side effects of the immunosuppressive drugs. Cyclosporine (Neoral) is toxic to the kidney. Signs of toxicity are elevated creatinine and decreased urine output. Monitor white blood cell counts daily, because azathioprine (Imuran) can suppress bone marrow function. Prednisone has many side effects, including elevated blood glucose levels. Common side effects of tacrolimus (Prograf) are hypertension, kidney toxicity, neurotoxicity, gastrointestinal (GI) toxicity, and glucose intolerance.

The client's quality of life improves as a result of freedom from the need for insulin, a less restricted lifestyle, and a return to a normal diet. You must stress, however, the poten-

tial need for insulin injections to treat hyperglycemia caused by immunosuppressive drugs.

Islet Cell Transplantation. Islet cell transplantation eliminates the need for insulin and provides protection from the complications of diabetes. Wider use of this procedure is hindered by the limited supply of beta cells available for transplantation and by problems caused by antirejection drugs. Islet cells from tissue-typed (HLA-matched) cadaver pancreas glands are injected into the portal vein. The new cells lodge in the liver and begin to function, secreting insulin and maintaining near perfect blood glucose control. Successful transplantation has occurred in a small number of clients, and this therapy is currently experimental (ADA, 2003m).

RISK FOR DELAYED SURGICAL RECOVERY

NOC **PLANNING: EXPECTED OUTCOMES.** The client with diabetes undergoing a surgical procedure is expected to recover completely without complications. Indicators include the following:

- Wound healing
- Absence of infection
- Maintenance of blood glucose levels within expected range
- Discharge readiness

INTERVENTIONS. Surgery is a physical and emotional stressor, and the diabetic client has a higher than average risk for complications. Acute stress increases the blood glucose levels. Counterregulatory hormones suppress insulin action, increasing the risk for ketoacidosis and metabolic acidosis. Fasting worsens ketoacidosis. Diuresis from hyperglycemia can cause severe dehydration and electrolyte loss.

Coronary artery disease, diabetic nephropathy, and autonomic neuropathy further increase the risk for surgical complications. Diabetic nephropathy complicates fluid management. Cardiac dysrhythmias may result from the combined effect of anesthesia and autonomic neuropathy. Autonomic neuropathy may cause paralytic ileus and urinary retention after surgery.

Blood glucose must be controlled to prevent hypoglycemia, diabetic ketoacidosis (DKA), and hyperglycemic-hyperosmolar nonketotic syndrome (HNNS). Blood glucose control is needed to reduce infection and promote wound healing. For best healing, the blood glucose level should be less than 200 mg/dL (11.1 mmol/L) (Franz, 2001).

Preoperative Care. Chlorpropamide (Diabinese) is stopped for at least 36 hours before surgery. Metformin (Glucophage) is stopped 48 hours before surgery and restarted only after renal function is normal. All other oral drugs are stopped the day of surgery. Insulin is adjusted based on blood glucose levels before surgery. IV access is used to maintain hydration, monitor blood glucose results, and allow insulin delivery.

Surgery for clients with type 1 diabetes is performed early in the day to cause the least disruption in blood glucose control. When surgery is performed later in the day, IV insulin is used to stabilize blood glucose levels. Withholding insulin can cause hyperglycemia, ketosis, and electrolyte problems. Monitor blood glucose often during the perioperative period to determine the need for additional insulin.

Plan ahead for pain control after surgery. Pain, a stressor, triggers the release of counterregulatory hormones, increasing blood glucose levels and insulin needs. Opioid analgesics slow gastrointestinal (GI) motility and alter blood glucose levels. The older client who receives opioids is more at risk for confusion, paralytic ileus, hypoventilation, and hypotension. Compared with IM opioids, patient-controlled analgesia (PCA) systems cause fewer respiratory complications and less confusion. (See Chapter 7 for pain interventions and Chapter 20 for general preoperative care.)

Intraoperative Care. The frequency of blood glucose assessment depends in part on the type of anesthetic agent used. Epidural anesthesia has little effect on glucose metabolism. During general anesthesia, glucose levels increase early and remain elevated through surgery. Surgery lasting 3 to 5 hours or longer leads to greater hyperglycemia, with these clients needing supplemental short-acting insulin.

The goal is to keep the glucose level between 140 and 200 mg/dL during surgery to prevent hypoglycemia. Levels below 200 mg/dL reduce the risk for wound infection. IV delivery of short-acting insulin in 5% to 10% glucose is recommended for all insulin-treated clients, as well as in clients with poorly controlled type 2 diabetes who are receiving general anesthesia. Larger than normal insulin doses may be needed during surgery because stress releases glucagon and epinephrine. Insulin/glucose infusion rates are based on hourly capillary glucose tests.

NIC intervention activities for vital sign monitoring are listed in Chart 68-7. Monitor the client's temperature; it may be lowered deliberately in some surgical procedures and inadvertently in others. Low operating room temperatures and large incisions also lower body temperature. Hypothermia decreases metabolic needs, depresses heart rate and contractility, causes vasoconstriction, and impairs insulin release, resulting in high blood glucose levels. Monitor arterial blood gas values for acidosis.

Postoperative Care. Continue glucose and insulin infusions, as prescribed, until the client is stable and can tolerate oral feedings. Supplemental short-acting insulin may be needed to control blood glucose levels until the client's usual drug regimen is restarted. Short-term insulin therapy may be needed after surgery for the client who usually uses oral agents alone. For the client receiving insulin therapy, the usual dosage may change until the stress of surgery subsides. To prevent insulin allergy, use only human insulin for short-term therapy.

Monitoring. Clients with autonomic neuropathy or vascular disease need close monitoring to avoid hypotension or respiratory arrest. Clients who take beta blockers for hypertension need close monitoring for hypoglycemia because these drugs mask hypoglycemia. Clients with **azotemia** (increased nitrogen waste products in the blood) may have problems with fluid management. Check central venous pressure or pulmonary artery pressure as needed.

Hyperkalemia (high blood potassium level) is common in clients with mild to moderate kidney failure and can lead to an acute cardiac dysrhythmia. In other clients, **hypokalemia** (low blood potassium level) may occur and be made worse by insulin and glucose given during surgery. Watch the client's cardiac rhythm and serum potassium values.

CARDIOVASCULAR MONITORING. Serial electrocardiograms (ECGs) are recommended for older diabetic clients, those with long-standing type 1 diabetes, and those with heart disease. Diabetic clients are at higher risk for myocardial infarction (MI) after surgery with a higher mortality rate. Changes in ECG or in potassium level may indicate a silent MI.

RENAL MONITORING. Monitoring fluid balance helps detect acute kidney failure. Diagnosis of renal impairment may require the use of x-ray studies using dyes, which may be nephrotoxic. Treatment of infections may require the use of nephrotoxic antibiotics. Ensure adequate hydration when these drugs are used. Watch for impending renal failure by assessing fluid and electrolyte status.

Nutritional Care. Using total parenteral nutrition (TPN) in diabetic clients can cause severe metabolic changes. Monitor blood glucose often to determine the need for supplemental short-acting insulin. After the insulin dose is stabilized, it can be added to the TPN solution and the frequency of capillary blood glucose monitoring decreased.

Returning to a normal meal plan as soon as possible after surgery promotes healing and metabolic balance. When oral foods are tolerated, make sure the client takes at least 150 to 200 g of carbohydrate daily to prevent hypoglycemia.

RISK FOR INJURY RELATED TO SENSORY ALTERATIONS

PLANNING: EXPECTED OUTCOMES. The client with diabetes is expected to identify factors that increase the risk for injury, practice proper foot care, and maintain intact skin on the feet. Indicators include that the client consistently demonstrates the following behaviors:

- Following preventive foot care practices
- Cleansing and inspecting the feet daily
- Wearing properly fitting shoes
- Avoiding walking in bare feet
- Trimming toenails properly
- Reporting non-healing breaks in the skin of the feet to the health care provider

INTERVENTIONS. Clients with diabetes need intensive teaching about foot care. Foot injury is the most common complication of diabetes leading to hospitalization. Diabetes is the leading cause of amputation worldwide. The overall risk for amputation is 15 times greater in diabetic clients than in nondiabetic clients. For clients with a previous amputation, the risk for amputation in the second leg is 10 to 20 times greater than among the general population. The 5-year mortality rate after leg or foot amputation ranges from 39% to 68%. Factors related to an increased risk for amputation include duration of diabetes, poor glucose control, and low levels of high-density lipoprotein (HDL) cholesterol.

Sensory neuropathy, ischemia, and infection are the leading causes of foot disease among clients with diabetes. Peripheral sensory neuropathy occurs in 60% to 90% of diabetic foot ulcers (Inlow, Orsted, & Sibbald, 2000). Loss of pain, pressure, and temperature sensation in the foot increases the risk for injury and ulceration. Impaired blood flow to the foot limits wound healing.

Claw toe deformity is common in diabetic neuropathy (Inlow, Orsted, & Sibbald, 2000). Toes are hyperextended, which increases pressure on the metatarsal heads ("ball" of the foot), resulting in ulceration. Thinning or shifting of the fat pad under the metatarsal heads decreases cushioning and increases areas of pressure. These changes predispose the client to callus formation, ulceration, and infection. Figure 68-10 shows hallux valgus (turning of the great toe), and Figure 68-11 shows a hammertoe.

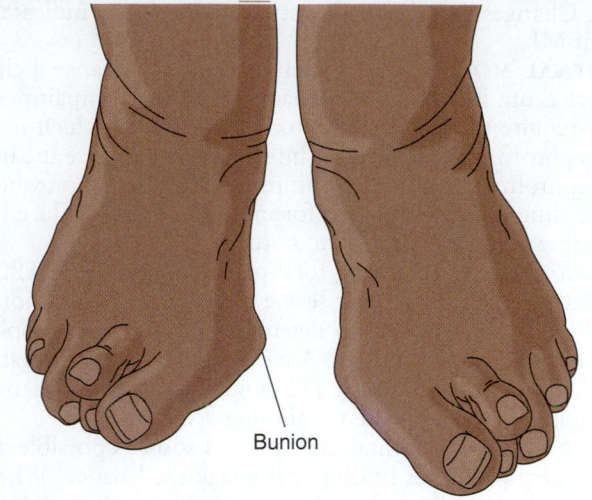

Figure 68-10 ■ The appearance of hallux valgus with a bunion.

Bunion

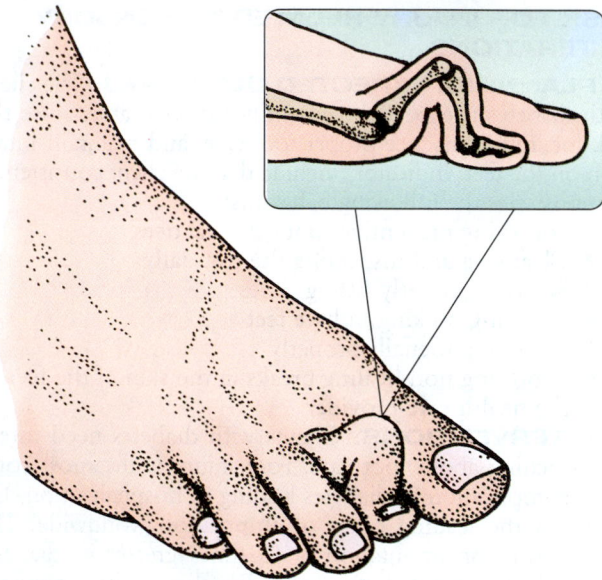

Figure 68-11 ■ Hammertoe of the second metatarsophalangeal (MTP) joint.

The Charcot foot is a type of diabetic foot deformity. The foot is warm, swollen, and painful. Walking collapses the arch, shortens the foot, and gives the foot a "rocker bottom" shape.

Sensory neuropathy may cause tingling or burning, but more often it produces numbness and reduced sensation. Neuropathy causes loss of normal sweating and skin temperature regulation, resulting in dry, thinning skin. Skin cracks and fissures increase the risk for infection.

Without sensation, the client does not notice physical, thermal, or chemical injuries to the foot and does not treat them. Foot injuries can be caused by walking barefoot, wearing ill-fitting shoes, sustaining thermal injuries from hot water (e.g., water bottles, heating pads, baths), or receiving caustic burns from over-the-counter corn treatments. Because the blood supply to the diabetic foot is poor, these injuries sometimes lead to amputation.

Ulcers result from continued pressure. Plantar ulcers (on the sole, usually the ball) are from standing or walking. Ul-

cers on the top or sides of the foot usually are from shoes. The increased pressure causes calluses. Ulcers usually form over or around the great toe, under the metatarsal heads, and on the tops of claw toes.

Broken skin increases the risk for infection. Skin tends to break in areas of pressure. Infection is common in diabetic foot ulcers and, once present, is difficult to treat. Infection also impairs glucose control, leading to higher blood glucose levels and reduced immune defense mechanisms. Decreased immune function further increases the risk for infection.

Prevention of High Risk Conditions. Neuropathy of the feet and legs can be delayed by keeping blood glucose levels as near normal as possible. Poor blood glucose control increases the risk for neuropathy and amputation. Intensive therapy reduces the risk for peripheral sensory neuropathy by 60%. Encourage smoking cessation to reduce the risk for vascular complications.

The risk for ulcers or amputation increases with duration of diabetes. Other risk factors are male gender; poor glucose control; and cardiovascular, retinal, or renal complications. Foot-related risks include poor gait and stepping mechanics, peripheral neuropathy, increased pressure (callus, erythema, hemorrhage under a callus, limited joint mobility, foot deformities, or severe nail pathology), peripheral vascular disease, and a history of ulcers or amputation (ADA, 2003p).

NIC Peripheral Sensation Management. The feet should be evaluated closely at least annually (ADA, 2003p). Chart 68-8 lists NIC intervention activities for peripheral sensation management and foot care, and Table 68-16 lists foot risk categories. The Evidence-Based Practice for Nursing box on p. 1536 supports the need for continued education on foot care practices.

Complete a full foot assessment as outlined in Chart 68-9. Sensory examination with Semmes-Weinstein monofilaments is the most practical measure of the risk for foot ulcers. The nylon monofilament is mounted on a holder standardized to exert a 10-g force. There is no agreement on the exact number of sites to test. A person who cannot feel the 10-g pressure at any point is at increased risk for ulcers. Perform the examination in the following way:

- Provide a quiet and relaxed setting. Ask the client to close his or her eyes during the test.
- Test the monofilament on the client's cheek so he or she knows what to expect.
- Test the sites noted in Figure 68-12.
- Apply the monofilament at a right angle to the skin surface.
- Apply enough force to bend the filament using a smooth, not jabbing motion (Figure 68-13).
- The approach, contact, and removal of the filament at each site should take 1 to 2 seconds.
- Apply the filament along the perimeter and **not** on an ulcer site, callus, scar, or necrotic tissue. Do not slide the filament across the skin or make repeated contact at the test site.
- Randomize the sequence of applying the filament throughout the examination. Have the client identify where the filament touched (*Feet Can Last a Lifetime*, 2001).

Footwear. All clients with any degree of peripheral neuropathy need to wear protective shoes. They must be fitted by an experienced shoe fitter, such as a certified podiatrist. The shoe should be $\frac{1}{2}$ to $\frac{5}{8}$ inch longer than the

CHART 68-8

NIC **INTERVENTION ACTIVITIES for**
The Diabetic Client with Reduced Sensation in the Lower Extremities

Peripheral Sensation Management: *Prevention or minimization of injury or discomfort in the client with altered sensation.*
- Monitor sharp/dull and/or hot/cold discrimination.
- Monitor for paresthesia: numbness, tingling, hyperesthesia, and hypoesthesia.
- Encourage client to use the unaffected body part to determine temperature of food, liquids, bathwater, and so on.
- Instruct client or family to monitor position of body parts while the client is bathing, sitting, lying, or changing position.
- Instruct client or family to examine skin daily for alteration in skin integrity.
- Monitor fit of bracing devices, prostheses, shoes, and clothing.
- Instruct client or family to use thermometer to test water temperature.
- Encourage use of gloves or other protective clothing over affected body part when body part is in contact with objects that—because of their thermal, textural, or other characteristics—may be potentially hazardous.
- Avoid or carefully monitor use of heat or cold, such as heating pads, hot water bottles, and ice packs.
- Encourage client to wear well-fitting, low-heeled, soft shoes.
- Check shoes, pockets, and clothing for wrinkles or foreign objects.
- Instruct client to use timed intervals, rather than presence of discomfort, as a signal to alter position.
- Protect body parts from extreme temperature changes.
- Discuss or identify causes of abnormal sensation or sensation changes.
- Instruct client to visually monitor position of body parts, if proprioception is impaired.

Foot Care: *Cleansing and inspecting the feet for the purposes of relaxation, cleanliness, and healthy skin*
- Inspect skin for irritation, cracking, lesions, corns, calluses, deformities, or edema.
- Inspect client's shoes for proper fit.
- Dry carefully between toes.
- Apply lotion.
- Clean nails.
- Apply moisture-absorbing powder, as indicated.
- Discuss with client usual foot care routine.
- Instruct client/family on the importance of foot care.
- Offer positive feedback about self-care foot activities.
- Monitor client's gait and weight distribution on feet.
- Monitor cleanliness and general condition of shoes and stockings.
- Instruct client to inspect inside of shoes for rough areas.
- Monitor hydration level of feet.
- Monitor for arterial insufficiency in lower legs.
- Monitor legs and feet for edema.
- Instruct client to monitor temperature of feet using the back of the hand.
- Instruct client in the importance of inspection, especially when sensation is diminished.
- Cut normal-thickness toenails when soft, using a toenail clipper and using the curve of the toe as a guide.
- Refer to podiatrist for trimming of thickened nails, as appropriate.

NIC intervention activities selected from Dochterman, J.M., & Bulechek, G.M. (Eds.). (2004). *Nursing interventions classification (NIC)* (4th ed.). St. Louis: Mosby. No part of this work is to be altered without prior written permission from the Publisher.

TABLE 68-16 Foot Risk Categories

Risk Categories	Management Categories
Risk Category 0	**Management Category 0**
■ Has disease that leads to insensitivity	■ Examine feet at each visit, at least four times per year
■ Has protective sensation	■ Foot clinic once a year
■ Has not had a plantar ulcer	■ Client education
Risk Category 1	**Management Category 1**
■ Does not have protective sensation	■ Examine feet at each visit, at least four times per year
■ Has not had a plantar ulcer	■ Foot clinic visit every 6 months
■ Does not have a foot deformity	■ Soft insoles
	■ Client education
Risk Category 2	**Management Category 2**
■ Does not have protective sensation	■ Examine feet at each visit, at least 4 times per year
■ Has not had a plantar ulcer	■ Foot clinic visit every 3-4 months
■ Does have a foot deformity	■ Custom-molded insoles
	■ Prescription footwear
	■ Client education
Risk Category 3	**Management Category 3**
■ Does not have protective sensation	■ Examine feet at each visit, at least four times per year
■ Has history of plantar ulcer	■ Foot clinic visit every 1 to 2 months
	■ Custom-molded insoles
	■ Prescription footwear
	■ Client education

From Gillis W. Long Hansen's Disease Center Rehabilitation Branch. (1992). *Foot screening: Care of the foot in diabetes: The Carville approach.* Carville, LA: Department of Health and Human Services.

longest toe. Heels should be less than 2 inches high. Shoes that are too tight damage tissue when worn for 4 hours or longer. Teach the client to change shoes by midday and again in the evening. Socks or stockings need to fit properly and be appropriate for the planned activity. Stockings should feel soft and have no thick seams, creases, or holes. They should pad the foot and absorb excess moisture. Teach clients to avoid tight stockings or those that have constricting bands. Clients with toe deformities should buy custom shoes with high, wide toe boxes and extra depth. Clients with severely deformed feet, such as Charcot feet, need specially molded shoes. All new shoes need a long break-in period with frequent inspection for irritation or blistering.

Foot Care. Teach clients about preventive foot care and the need for examination of the feet and legs at each visit to a health care provider. Identify clients with high-risk foot conditions and teach them about foot care. Explain problems caused by loss of protective sensation, the importance of monitoring the feet daily, proper care of the feet (including nail and skin care), and how to select appropriate footwear. Advise clients with neuropathy to break in new shoes slowly to reduce blisters (ADA, 2003p).

Teach clients to inspect their feet daily. Assess the client's ability to inspect all areas of the foot and to perform foot care. Teach family members how to inspect and care for client's feet if the client cannot (ADA, 2003p). Chart 68-10 lists foot care instructions.

Wound Care. The standards of care for diabetic ulcers are a moist wound environment, debridement of necrotic tissue, and elimination of pressure (off-loading).

EVIDENCE-BASED PRACTICE for Nursing

Rural-dwelling diabetics are at risk for foot ulcers

Neil, J.A. (2002). Assessing foot care knowledge in a rural population with diabetes. *Ostomy/Wound Management, 48*(1), 50-56.

This study follows a group of rural-dwelling individuals with diabetes who received education in foot care and foot wear management at some time during their illness. All of the participants had "diminished protective sensation" on Semmes-Weinstein monofilament testing. The purpose of the study was to evaluate foot care practices among rural persons with diabetes mellitus and diminished protective sensation. The study sample included 61 persons (average 46 years of age). At the time of the study, 24% to 39% of the participants had a foot ulcer. The participants were divided into two groups, those with ulcers, and those without foot ulcers. Subjects were interviewed to determine their foot cares practices. Foot care behaviors were determined by use of the Siriraj Foot-Care instrument, a previously validated tool on client knowledge of foot care.

Improper foot care practices were evident in a group of diabetic clients who already had foot ulcers as well as in those who were at high risk for developing ulcers. Reasons given for not performing foot care by subjects in the study were that they were unable to reach their feet or that they could not see their feet. Diabetic retinopathy and obesity were common in the study group. No statistical differences were found between the two groups on daily examination of their feet for reddened areas, blisters, corns, calluses, or open areas, for daily foot cleansing with warm water, or for nail cutting practices. Statistically significant differences were found in answers to questions about going barefoot. Those without ulcers were more likely to go barefoot inside the house. Poor foot care practices such as not adequately washing their feet, using knives or razor blades to trim nails, and going barefoot inside and outside the house were noted for both groups.

Level of Evidence: 6—Uncontrolled descriptive study.

Critique. The methods used were appropriate for this descriptive study.

Implications for Nursing. Nurses need to teach all clients with diabetes about appropriate foot care practices, especially for those clients identified at being at high risk for foot injury. The American Diabetes Association estimates that 50% of amputations are preventable. This study supports the work of others that indicates the need for frequent education for prevention of foot ulcers in people with diabetes mellitus.

CHART 68-9

FOCUSED ASSESSMENT of
The Diabetic Foot

Assess the client for risk of diabetic foot problems:
- History of previous ulcer
- History of previous amputation

Assess the foot for abnormal skin and nail conditions:
- Dry, cracked, fissured skin
- Ulcers
- Toenails: thickened, long nails; ingrown nails
- Tinea pedis; onychomycosis (mycotic nails)

Assess the foot for status of circulation:
- Symptoms of claudication
- Presence or absence of dorsalis pedis or posterior tibial pulse
- Prolonged capillary filling time (greater than 25 seconds)
- Presence or absence of hair growth on the top of the foot

Assess the foot for evidence of deformity:
- Calluses, corns
- Prominent metatarsal heads (metatarsal head is easily felt under the skin)
- Toe contractures: clawed toes, hammertoes
- Hallux valgus or bunions
- Charcot foot ("rocker bottom")

Assess the foot for loss of strength:
- Limited ankle joint range of motion
- Limited motion of great toe

Assess the foot for loss of protective sensation:
- Numbness, burning, tingling
- Semmes-Weinstein monofilament testing at 10 points on each foot

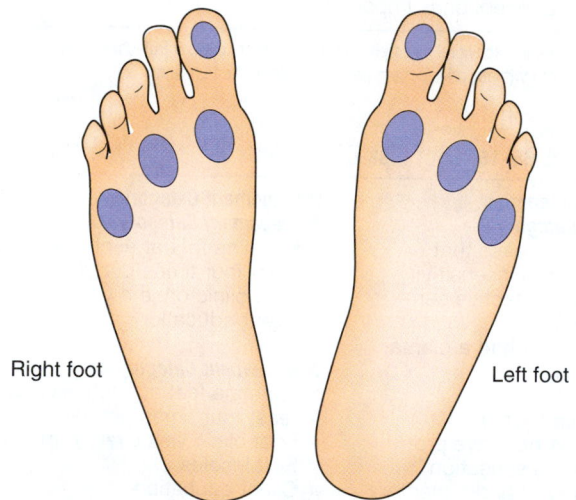

Right foot   Left foot

Figure 68-12 ■ Placement sites of monofilaments for testing of protective sensation.

Wound Environment. Dressings reduce or prevent infection, allow debridement, reduce wound pain, and stimulate granulation tissue. Many commercial products are available. Antiseptics such as povidone iodine, hydrogen peroxide, and chlorhexidine interfere with wound healing. Dressings that keep the wound moist are essential.

Debridement. Debridement removes dead tissues that support bacterial growth. It is accomplished with surgery, topical debriding agents, and dressings. Mechanical debridement, although helpful, can delay wound healing by removing newly formed tissue (Ayello, Cuddigan, & Kerstein, 2002).

Elimination of Pressure. Eliminating pressure on an infected area is essential to wound healing. Teach clients with foot ulcers to not wear a shoe on the foot while the ulcer is healing. Clients with poor sensation keep walking on an ulcer because it does not hurt. This results in pressure necrosis that delays healing and increases ulcer size. Pressure is reduced by specialized orthotic devices, custom-molded shoes inserts, or shoe adjustments that redistribute weight.

The best way to avoid weight-bearing is with a contact cast (Levin, 2002). Casting material is molded to the foot and leg

so pressure is spread along the entire surface of contact, thereby reducing vertical force. The almost complete elimination of motion of the total-contact cast reduces plantar shear forces. The cast is removed 24 to 48 hours after application and weekly thereafter until the ulcer is healed. *Teach the client that foot ulcers will recur unless weight is permanently redistributed.*

Growth Factors. Growth factors applied to wounds increase the rate of healing by stimulating new tissue and enhancing cell growth. This treatment has helped heal foot ulcers present for many months or even years. Because it is costly and based on having other aspects of diabetes controlled, growth factor therapy is usually performed in specialized treatment centers.

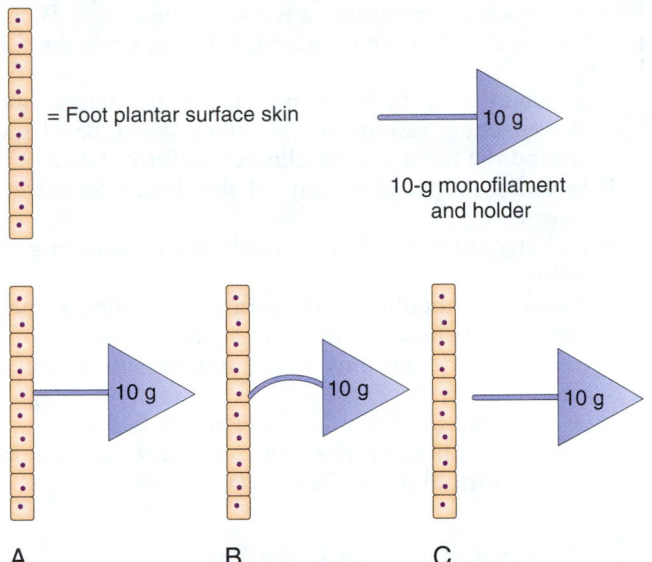

Figure 68-13 ■ Correct technique for sensation testing with 10-g monofilament. **A,** Apply monofilament to designated areas of the foot sole (intact skin, see Figure 68-12). **B,** Apply pressure to the filament until either the client states he or she can feel the pressure or until the filament bends (see p. 1534). **C,** Quickly remove the filament without sliding the filament or touching other areas of the foot.

CHRONIC PAIN

NOC PLANNING: EXPECTED OUTCOMES. The client with neuropathic pain is expected to experience relief of pain. Indicators include the following consistent behaviors:

- Using preventive measures
- Using available resources to increase comfort
- Reporting pain controlled.

INTERVENTIONS. NIC intervention activities to manage pain are listed in Chart 68-11. Maintaining normal blood glucose levels prevents neuropathy and relieves symptoms of acute nerve dysfunction. Anticonvulsants and antidepressants are often used to treat the pain of neuropathy. Drugs such as gabapentin (Neurontin) can reduce pain and improve quality of life (Bowker & Pfeifer, 2001). Tricyclic antidepressants, particularly amitriptyline hydrochloride (Elavil, Levate✱) and nortriptyline (Pamelor), also are used for neuropathic pain. Smaller doses are needed for analgesia than for antidepressant effects.

The burning of neuropathy may respond to capsaicin cream 0.075% (Axsain✱, Zostrix-HP). This drug reduces amounts of substance P, which is involved in pain transmission (see Chapter 7). Teach the client how to apply it four times daily for several weeks. Neuropathic pain may worsen for several days after therapy is started before improving.

RISK FOR INJURY RELATED TO DISTURBED SENSORY PERCEPTION: VISUAL

PLANNING: EXPECTED OUTCOMES. The client with diabetes is expected to be free of injury related to decreased visual acuity and to maintain current level of vision. Indicators include the following:

- No further reduction of visual fields
- No double vision

INTERVENTIONS.

Blood Glucose Control. Poor blood glucose control, proteinuria, diastolic hypertension, and long duration

---

CHART 68-10

CLIENT EDUCATION GUIDE
Foot Care Instructions

- Inspect your feet daily, especially the area between the toes.
- Wash your feet daily with lukewarm water and soap. Dry thoroughly.
- Apply moisturizing cream to your feet after bathing. Do not apply to the area between your toes.
- Change into clean cotton socks every day.
- Do not wear the same pair of shoes 2 days in a row, and wear only leather shoes.
- Check your shoes for foreign objects (nails, pebbles) before putting them on. Check inside the shoes for cracks or tears in the lining.
- Purchase shoes that have plenty of room for your toes. Buy shoes later in the day, when feet are normally larger. Break in new shoes gradually.
- Wear socks to keep your feet warm.
- Trim your nails straight across with a nail clipper. Smooth the nails with an emery board.
- See your physician or nurse immediately if you have blisters, sores, or infections. Protect area with a dry, sterile dressing. Do not use adhesive tape to secure dressing.
- Do not treat blisters, sores, or infections with home remedies.
- Do not smoke.
- Do not step into the bathtub without checking the temperature of the water with your wrist. Optimal temperature is 95° F (29.4° to 35° C).
- Do not use very hot or cold water. Never use hot water bottles, heating pads, or portable heaters to warm your feet.
- Do not treat corns, blisters, bunions, calluses, or ingrown toenails yourself.
- Do not go barefooted.
- Do not wear sandals with open toes or straps between the toes.
- Do not cross your legs or wear garters or tight stockings that constrict blood flow.
- Do not soak your feet.

---

of diabetes are risk factors for diabetic retinopathy and vision loss. Surgical intervention for retinal hemorrhage or new retinal blood vessel growth can reduce vision loss.

Only about 10% of all visually impaired clients are totally blind. The rest have reduced vision. Besides regular eye examinations to evaluate retinopathy, urge the diabetic client with impaired vision to have an optometrist or ophthalmologist assess the remaining vision and prescribe appropriate eyewear. A functional vision assessment, performed by a low-vision technician, rehabilitation teacher, or diabetes educator, determines the client's use of lighting, contrast, non-optical and low-vision devices, and large-print options. Included in this assessment is whether the client uses central or peripheral vision. Clients with macular edema have loss of central vision. This process causes difficulty seeing details, reading printed materials, preparing insulin syringes for injection, and self-monitoring blood glucose levels (SMBG).

Environmental Management. Not all visually impaired clients need special devices. Adjustments in lighting, contrast, color, distance, type size of printed materials, and eye movement often improve visual abilities. Instruct the client to supplement overhead fluorescent lighting with an incandescent lamp directed toward the workspace. Placing dark equipment against a white or yellow background (or vice versa) provides contrast to enhance vision. Coding objects such as vials of insulin with bright colors or with felt-tipped markers help identify the correct bottle. Bringing the blood glucose lancet or insulin syringe close to the eye

NIC **INTERVENTION ACTIVITIES for**
The Diabetic Client Experiencing Pain

Analgesic Administration: *Use of pharmacologic agents to reduce or eliminate pain*
- Determine pain location, characteristics, quality, and severity before medicating client.
- Check medical order for drug, dose, and frequency of analgesic prescribed.
- Attend to comfort needs and other activities that assist in relaxation to facilitate response to analgesia.
- Set positive expectations regarding the effectiveness of analgesics to optimize client response.
- Document response to analgesic and any untoward effects.
- Teach about the use of analgesics, strategies to decrease side effects, and expectations for involvement in decisions about pain relief.

Teaching: Individual: *Planning, implementation, and evaluation of a teaching program designed to address a client's particular needs*
- Establish rapport.
- Determine the client's learning needs.
- Appraise the client's current level of knowledge and understanding of content.
- Appraise the client's educational level.
- Appraise the client's cognitive, psychomotor, and affective abilities/disabilities.
- Determine the client's ability to learn specific information (i.e., developmental level, physiologic status, orientation, pain, fatigue, unfulfilled basic needs, emotional state, and adaptation to illness).
- Set mutual, realistic learning goals with the client.
- Identify learning objectives necessary to reach goals.
- Determine the sequence for presenting the information.
- Appraise the client's learning style.
- Select appropriate teaching method/strategies.
- Select appropriate educational materials.
- Tailor the content to the client's cognitive, psychomotor, and/or affective abilities/disabilities.
- Adjust instruction to facilitate learning, as appropriate.
- Provide an environment conducive to learning.
- Instruct the client, when appropriate.
- Evaluate the client's achievement of the stated objectives.
- Reinforce behavior, as appropriate.
- Correct information misinterpretations, as appropriate.
- Provide time for the client to ask questions and discuss concerns.
- Select new teaching methods/strategies, if previous ones were ineffective.
- Refer the client to other specialists/agencies to meet the learning objectives, as appropriate.
- Document the content presented, the written materials provided, and the client's understanding of the information or client behaviors that indicate learning on the permanent medical record.
- Include the family/significant others, as appropriate.

NIC intervention activities selected from Dochterman, J.M., & Bulechek, G.M. (Eds.). (2004). *Nursing interventions classification (NIC)* (4th ed.). St. Louis: Mosby. No part of this work is to be altered without prior written permission from the Publisher.

makes it easier to see. Suggest large type or bold print to ease reading. Teach the client to use peripheral vision.

Certain devices can help the client self-administer insulin independently. Some syringes may have a magnifier attached to the syringe. Other devices include preset dose gauges (which measure the space between the end of the syringe barrel and the plunger) to help the client draw up the correct amount of insulin by feeling this distance. Variable dose gauges draw insulin in variable and mixed doses of 1-, 2-, and 10-unit increments. The client sets the desired dose

by pressing a lever or turning a screw on the device. When teaching the client to use an adaptive device, stress the following:
- Differentiating between bottles of fast-acting and slower-acting insulin by wrapping a rubber band around the fast-acting insulin bottle, for instance
- Ensuring proper placement of the device on the syringe
- Holding the insulin bottle upright when measuring insulin
- Avoiding air bubbles in the syringe by pulling a small amount of insulin into the syringe, moving the plunger in and out three times, and measuring insulin on the fourth draw

Design a system to determine how many doses can be drawn from a bottle so the client does not inject air from an empty bottle instead of insulin (Williams, 2000).

Critical Thinking Challenge

The client has had type 2 diabetes for many years and now needs insulin for glucose control. He has severe vision impairment. His wife has normal vision, but does not want "to stick him with needles," either for glucose testing or giving insulin. He would like to be as independent as possible in his two-dose protocol. He also has arthritis in his dominant shoulder (right side) and cannot reach around behind him.
1. What role can the wife have in blood glucose monitoring and insulin delivery?
2. What procedures could this client perform safely by himself?
3. Should the wife be taught insulin injection techniques? Why or why not?

evolve For suggested answer guidelines, go to http://evolve.elsevier.com/Iggy/.

INEFFECTIVE TISSUE PERFUSION: RENAL

NOC **PLANNING: EXPECTED OUTCOMES.** The client with diabetes is expected to maintain a normal urine elimination pattern. Indicators include the following:
- Urine protein levels within normal limits
- 24-hour intake and output balance
- Blood urea nitrogen (BUN) and serum creatinine within the normal ranges
- Serum electrolytes within the normal ranges

INTERVENTIONS

Prevention. Tight control of blood glucose levels may slow renal disease in clients with type 1 diabetes. Control of hypertension also slows diabetic nephropathy and the complications of hypertensive nephropathy (ADA, 2003r).

Stress the need for yearly evaluation of kidney function according to American Diabetes Association (ADA) Standards of Care. Screening is performed by three methods: (1) random, spot urine collection to measure the albumin-creatinine ratio, (2) 24-hour urine collection to measure creatinine clearance, and (3) timed urine collection (e.g., 4 hours or overnight) (ADA, 2003r). Timed urine collections are not reliable in clients with neuropathy and incomplete bladder emptying. Random urine albumin/creatinine testing is recommended as the standard measurement of proteinuria in clients with diabetes (Loon, 2003). Explain the implications of the test and help the client collect the specimen if necessary.

Aggressive control of blood glucose and hypertension in diabetic clients without microalbuminuria can avoid nephropathy. Once microalbuminuria develops, treatment is aimed at controlling blood pressure and blood glucose, restricting dietary protein, avoiding nephrotoxic agents, promptly treating urinary tract infections (UTIs), and preventing dehydration.

Control of blood pressure and blood glucose levels requires the client's effort. Prescribed drugs must be taken according to schedules, and dietary restriction must be maintained. Teach diabetic clients about the roles of blood pressure and blood glucose levels in renal disease. Help the client maintain normal blood glucose levels and blood pressure levels below 130/80 mm Hg (ADA, 2003d). Stress the need for yearly screening for microalbuminuria.

Any UTI can lead to kidney infection and further reduce renal function. Explain the manifestations of UTI. Urge the client to take antibiotics exactly as prescribed, completing the course of treatment. Reinforce the need for follow-up urine cultures to reduce the risk of renal damage. Avoid indwelling urinary catheters when possible.

Drugs can affect renal function either through toxic effects on the kidney or by an acute but reversible reduction in function. The most common nephrotoxic drugs are antifungal agents (amphotericin B); aminoglycoside antibiotics such as amikacin (Amikin), streptomycin, kanamycin (Kantrex), gentamicin (Garamycin), and tobramycin (Tobrex); and nonsteroidal anti-inflammatory drugs such as ibuprofen (Advil) or naproxen (Aleve). Radiocontrast dyes can also affect renal function (Singri, Ahya, & Levin, 2003). To prevent accidental ingestion of nephrotoxic drugs, caution the client to check with a health care provider before taking over-the-counter or prescription drugs.

Diet Therapy. Clients with nephropathy should restrict dietary protein to 0.8 g/kg of body weight per day. Once the glomerular filtration rate (GFR) starts falling, further reducing protein to 0.6 g/kg may slow the decline in renal function (ADA, 2003d). Because lifelong dietary restrictions are difficult, provide ongoing teaching to encourage adherence.

NIC **Fluid/Electrolyte Management.** Fluid and electrolyte management can prevent more loss of renal function. NIC intervention activities for fluid and electrolyte management are listed in Chart 68-12. Avoiding dehydration is important for renal perfusion and function. Any illness that leads to dehydration or hypotension is treated with isotonic saline for volume replacement (Singri, Ahya, & Levin, 2003). Assess fluid balance, and use measures to prevent dehydration. The most common cause of dehydration in clients with diabetes is overuse of diuretics. Teach clients to report edema or symptoms of orthostatic hypotension and provide ongoing education to promote dietary goals.

Dialysis for clients with diabetes and renal failure is the same as for clients without diabetes (see Chapter 75). The dosage of insulin needs to be adjusted when dialysis starts.

POTENTIAL FOR HYPOGLYCEMIA

Central nervous system (CNS) function depends on a continuous supply of glucose in the blood. The brain cannot make glucose and stores only a few minutes' supply as glycogen. This needed supply is not maintained when blood glucose levels fall below critical levels.

The first defense against falling blood glucose levels in the nondiabetic client is decreased insulin secretion, de-

creased glucose use, and increased glucose production. Normally, insulin secretion decreases when blood glucose levels drop to about 83 mg/dL (4.5 mmol/L). Counter-regulatory hormones are activated at about 68 mg/dL (3.8 mmol/L), a level well above the threshold for symptoms of hypoglycemia. The main counterregulatory hormone is glucagon; epinephrine also becomes important in diabetic clients who are deficient in glucagon. Both glucagon and epinephrine raise blood glucose levels by stimulating liver glycogenolysis and gluconeogenesis. Epinephrine also limits insulin secretion.

Type 1 diabetes disrupts the body's response to hypoglycemia, a change that occurs within 1 to 5 years of diagnosis. Regulation of circulating insulin levels is lost because the insulin comes from an injection rather than from the pancreas. As blood glucose levels fall, insulin levels do not decrease. Over time, the pancreas loses its ability to secrete glucagon in response to hypoglycemia. After a few more years of type 1 diabetes, the response of epinephrine to falling blood glucose levels is also reduced. It does respond, but it takes a lower blood glucose level to become active. These problems dramatically increase the risk for severe hypoglycemia.

A second problem with long-standing type 1 diabetes is *hypoglycemic unawareness*. Clients no longer have the warning symptoms of impending hypoglycemia that should prompt them to take preventive action. Hypoglycemic unawareness occurs in about 25% of diabetic clients and about 50% of all clients who have had type 1 diabetes for 30 years or longer.

Symptoms of hypoglycemia are neuroglycopenic or neurologic. Neuroglycopenic symptoms occur when brain glucose gradually declines to a low level. Neurologic symptoms result from autonomic nervous activity triggered by a rapid decline in blood glucose (Table 68-17).

The blood glucose level at which symptoms of hypoglycemia occur varies among clients. Many have symptoms when blood glucose levels are well above 50 mg/dL (2.8 mmol/L), especially if the level dropped rapidly or they are used to chronic hyperglycemia. Thus, clinical criteria are used to categorize hypoglycemic severity rather than blood glucose levels. In mild hypoglycemia, the client remains alert and able to treat symptoms. In severe hypoglycemia, neurologic function is so impaired that the client needs another person's help.

PLANNING: EXPECTED OUTCOMES. The diabetic client is expected to have decreased episodes of hypoglycemia and remain oriented to person, place, and time, as indicated by a Glasgow Coma Scale score above 7.

INTERVENTIONS. Because symptoms of hypoglycemia commonly occur at levels above 50 mg/dL, a blood glucose level below 70 mg/dL requires an assessment (Franz, 2001) (Table 68-18; see Table 68-17).

NIC **Hypoglycemia Management.** NIC intervention activities for hypoglycemia appear in Chart 68-13. Monitor blood glucose levels before giving antidiabetic drugs, before meals, before bedtime, and when the client is symptomatic. All clients who take insulin or other antidiabetic drugs are at risk for hypoglycemia, especially if they are older, have liver or kidney impairment, or are taking drugs that enhance the effects of antidiabetic drugs. Proper client selection, drug dosage, and instructions are important factors in avoiding severe hypoglycemia. Hypoglycemia may be difficult to rec-

CHART 68-12

NIC **INTERVENTION ACTIVITIES for**
The Diabetic Client Experiencing Fluid and Electrolyte and Acid-Base Imbalances

Fluid/Electrolyte Management: *Regulation and prevention of complications from altered fluid and/or electrolyte levels*
- Monitor for abnormal serum electrolyte levels, as available.
- Obtain laboratory specimens for monitoring of altered fluid or electrolyte levels (e.g., hematocrit, BUN, protein, sodium, and potassium levels), as appropriate.
- Weigh client daily and monitor trends.
- Promote oral intake (e.g., provide oral fluids that are the client's preference, place in easy reach, provide a straw, and provide fresh water), as appropriate.
- Set an appropriate intravenous infusion (or blood transfusion) flow rate.
- Monitor laboratory results relevant to fluid balance (e.g., hematocrit, BUN, albumin, total protein, serum osmolarity, and urine specific gravity levels).
- Monitor hemodynamic status, including CVP, MAP, PAP, and PCWP levels, if available.
- Keep an accurate record of intake and output.
- Monitor for signs and symptoms of fluid retention.
- Monitor vital signs, as appropriate.
- Maintain intravenous solution containing electrolyte(s) at a constant flow rate, as appropriate.
- Monitor client's response to prescribed electrolyte therapy.
- Monitor for manifestations of electrolyte imbalance.
- Assess client's buccal membranes, sclera, and skin for indications of altered fluid and electrolyte balance (e.g., dryness, cyanosis, and jaundice).
- Consult physician if signs and symptoms of fluid and/or electrolyte imbalance persist or worsen.
- Administer prescribed supplemental electrolytes, as appropriate.
- Monitor for fluid loss (e.g., bleeding, vomiting, diarrhea, perspiration, and tachypnea).

Acid-Base Management: Metabolic Acidosis: *Promotion of acid-base balance and prevention of complications resulting from serum HCO_3 levels lower than desired.*
- Obtain ordered specimens for laboratory analysis of acid-base balance (e.g., ABG, urine, and serum levels), as appropriate.
- Monitor ABG levels for decreasing pH level, as appropriate.
- Maintain patent IV access.
- Monitor intake and output.
- Monitor determinants of tissue oxygen delivery (e.g., Pao_2, Sao_2, and hemoglobin levels and cardiac output) if available.
- Monitor for electrolyte imbalances associated with metabolic acidosis (e.g., hyponatremia, hyperkalemia or hypokalemia, hypocalcemia, hypophosphatemia, and hypomagnesemia), as appropriate.
- Monitor for decreasing bicarbonate from excessive nonvolatile acids (e.g., renal failure, diabetic ketoacidosis, tissue hypoxia, and starvation), as appropriate.
- Administer prescribed alkaline medications (e.g., sodium bicarbonate), as appropriate, based on ABG results.
- Prevent complications from excessive $NaHCO_3$ administration (e.g., metabolic alkalosis, hypernatremia, volume overload, decreased oxygen delivery, decreased cardiac contractility, and enhanced lactic acid production).
- Administer fluids as prescribed.
- Administer insulin and fluid hydration (isotonic and hypotonic) for diabetic ketoacidosis, causing metabolic acidosis, as appropriate.
- Institute seizure precautions.
- Monitor for CNS manifestations of metabolic acidosis (e.g., headache, drowsiness, decreased mentation, seizures, and coma), as appropriate.
- Monitor for cardiopulmonary manifestations of metabolic acidosis (e.g., hypotension, hypoxia, arrhythmias, and Kussmaul respiration), as appropriate.
- Monitor for GI manifestations of metabolic acidosis (e.g., anorexia, nausea, and vomiting), as appropriate.
- Provide comfort measures to deal with the GI effects of metabolic acidosis.
- Instruct the client and/or family on actions instituted to treat the metabolic acidosis.

NIC intervention activities selected from Dochterman, J.M., & Bulechek, G.M. (Eds.). (2004). *Nursing interventions classification (NIC)* (4th ed.). St. Louis: Mosby. No part of this work is to be altered without prior written permission from the Publisher.

ABG, Arterial blood gas; *BUN*, blood urea nitrogen; *CNS*, central nervous system; *CVP*, central venous pressure; *GI*, gastrointestinal; *MAP*, mean arterial pressure; *NaHCO₃*, sodium bicarbonate; *Pao₂*, partial pressure of arterial oxygen; *PAP*, pulmonary artery pressure; *PCWP*, pulmonary capillary wedge pressure; *Sao₂*, arterial oxygen saturation.

---

ognize in older clients and those who take beta-blocking drugs.

Diet Therapy. When the client is hypoglycemic, start carbohydrate replacement per physician prescription or standing protocols. If the client can swallow, give a liquid form of carbohydrate, although any source of carbohydrate can be used to treat hypoglycemia. Specific recommendations appear in Chart 68-14. The blood glucose level determines the form and amount of glucose used. Fluid is absorbed much more quickly from the gastrointestinal (GI) tract than solids. Concentrated sweet fluids, such as juice with sugar added or a soft drink, may slow absorption. Commercially available products provide predictable glucose absorption.

Drug Therapy. Glucagon given subcutaneously or IM and 50% dextrose given IV is the therapy for diabetic clients who cannot swallow. Glucagon converts liver glycogen to glucose but is not effective in severely starved clients. Take care

TABLE 68-17 Symptoms of Hypoglycemia

Neuroglycopenic Symptoms	Neurogenic Symptoms
- Warmth	- Adrenergic
- Weakness	Shaky/tremulous
- Fatigue	Heart pounding
- Difficulty thinking	Nervous/anxious
- Confusion	- Cholinergic
- Behavior changes	Sweaty
- Emotional lability	Hungry
- Seizures	Tingling
- Loss of consciousness	
- Brain damage	
- Death	

to prevent aspiration in clients receiving glucagon, because it often causes vomiting. Give 50% dextrose carefully to avoid extravasation. The effects of glucagon and dextrose are temporary. After the client responds, give a simple sugar followed by a small snack or meal. IV glucose is used to maintain mild

TABLE 68-18 Differentiation of Hypoglycemia and Hyperglycemia

Feature	Hypoglycemia	Hyperglycemia
Skin	Cool, clammy	Hot, dry*
Dehydration	Absent	Present
Perspiration	Profuse*	Absent
Respirations	No particular or consistent change	Rapid, deep*; Kussmaul type; acetone odor ("fruity" odor) to breath
Mental status	Anxious, nervous,* irritable, mental confusion,* seizures, coma	Varies from alert to stuporous, obtunded, or frank coma
Symptoms	Weakness,* double vision, blurred vision, hunger, tachycardia, palpitations	No specific symptoms for DKA Acidosis; hypercapnia; abdominal cramps, nausea and vomiting Dehydration: decreased neck vein filling, orthostatic hypotension, tachycardia, poor skin turgor
Glucose	50 mg/dL (2.8 mmol/L)	>250 mg/dL (13.8 mmol/L)
Ketones	Negative	Positive

DKA, Diabetic ketoacidosis.
*Classic symptoms.

CHART 68-13

NIC **INTERVENTION ACTIVITIES for**
The Diabetic Client Experiencing or at Risk for Hypoglycemia

Hypoglycemia Management: *Preventing and treating low blood glucose levels*
- Identify client at risk for hypoglycemia.
- Monitor blood glucose levels, as indicated.
- Monitor for signs and symptoms of hypoglycemia (e.g., shakiness, tremor, sweating, nervousness, anxiety, irritability, impatience, tachycardia, palpitations, chills, clamminess, light-headedness, pallor, hunger, nausea, headache, tiredness, drowsiness, weakness, warmth, dizziness, faintness, blurred vision, nightmares, crying out in sleep, paresthesias, difficulty concentrating, difficulty speaking, incoordination, behavior change, confusion, coma, seizure).
- Provide simple carbohydrate, as indicated.
- Provide complex carbohydrate and protein, as indicated.
- Administer glucagon, as indicated.
- Contact emergency medical services, as necessary.
- Administer intravenous glucose, as indicated.
- Maintain patent airway, as necessary.
- Maintain IV access, as appropriate.
- Protect from injury, as necessary.
- Review events prior to hypoglycemia to determine probable cause.
- Provide feedback regarding appropriateness of self-care management of hypoglycemia.
- Instruct client and significant others on signs and symptoms, risk factors, and treatment of hypoglycemia.
- Instruct client to have simple carbohydrates available at all times.
- Instruct client to obtain and carry/wear appropriate emergency identification.
- Instruct significant others on the use and administration of glucagon, as appropriate.
- Instruct on interaction of diet, insulin/oral agents, and exercise.
- Provide assistance in making self-care decisions to prevent hypoglycemia (e.g., reducing insulin/oral agents and/or increasing food intake for exercise).
- Encourage self-monitoring of blood glucose levels.
- Encourage ongoing telephone contact with diabetes care team for consultation regarding adjustments in treatment regimen.

NIC intervention activities selected from Dochterman, J.M., & Bulechek, G.M.(Eds.). (2004). *Nursing interventions classification (NIC)* (4th ed.). St. Louis: Mosby. No part of this work is to be altered without prior written permission from the Publisher.

CHART 68-14

CLIENT EDUCATION GUIDE
Treatment of Hypoglycemia at Home

For *mild* hypoglycemia (hungry, irritable, shaky, weak, headache, fully conscious; blood glucose usually less than 60 mg/dL [3.4 mmol/L]):
- Treat the symptoms of hypoglycemia with 10 to 15 g of carbohydrate. You may use one of the following:
  - Glucose tablets or glucose gel (dosage is printed on the package)
  - ½ cup of fruit juice
  - ½ cup of regular (nondiet) soft drink
  - 8 ounces of skim milk
  - 6 to 10 hard candies
  - 4 cubes of sugar
  - 4 teaspoons of sugar
  - 6 saltines
  - 3 graham crackers
  - 1 tablespoon of honey or syrup
- Retest blood glucose in 15 minutes.
- Repeat this treatment if symptoms do not resolve.
- Eat a small snack of carbohydrate and protein if your next meal is more than an hour away.

For *moderate* hypoglycemia (cold, clammy skin; pale; rapid pulse; rapid, shallow respirations; marked change in mood; drowsiness; blood glucose usually less than 40 mg/dL [2.2 mmol/L]):
- Treat the symptoms of hypoglycemia with 15 to 30 g of rapidly absorbed carbohydrate.
- Take additional food, such as low-fat milk or cheese, after 10 to 15 minutes.

For *severe* hypoglycemia (unable to swallow; unconsciousness or convulsions; blood glucose usually less than 20 mg/dL [1.0 mmol/L]):
Treatment administered by family members:
- Administer 1 mg of glucagon as intramuscular or subcutaneous injection.
- Administer a second dose in 10 minutes if the person remains unconscious.
- Notify a primary care provider immediately, and follow instructions.
- If still unconscious, transport the person to the emergency department.
- Give a small meal when the person wakes up and is no longer nauseated.

hyperglycemia. Diazoxide (Proglycem), an antidote to sulfonylurea-induced hypoglycemia, or octreotide (Sandostatin), which inhibits sulfonylurea-induced insulin release, may be needed if blood glucose levels cannot be maintained by infusion alone (Herbel & Boyle, 2000).

Evaluate response by monitoring blood glucose levels for several hours. Symptoms may persist for an hour or more after treatment. A target blood glucose level is 70 to 110 mg/dL (3.9 to 6.2 mmol/L).

Prevention Strategies. Teach the client how to prevent future episodes of hypoglycemia. Four common causes of hypoglycemia are (1) excess insulin, (2) deficient intake or absorption of food, (3) exercise, and (4) alcohol intake.

Insulin Excess. Even when insulin is injected correctly, variable absorption can cause hypoglycemia. Excess insulin also can be caused by lowered insulin resistance, which occurs with termination of pregnancy or resolution of an infection. Increased insulin sensitivity can occur with weight loss or exercise programs. Differences in insulin formulation can result in hypoglycemia. Instruct the client not to change insulin brands or change from animal-source to human insulin without medical supervision.

Deficient Food Intake. Inadequate or incorrectly timed meals can result in hypoglycemia. Changes in gastric absorption sometimes cause hypoglycemia in clients with delayed gastric emptying. This problem is more common in clients with diabetes of long duration, is more severe with solid than with liquid meals, and is made worse by illness or poor glucose control. Instruct the client about the importance of regularity in timing and quantity of food eaten.

Exercise. Blood glucose levels usually fall during exercise in a client with type 1 diabetes. Prolonged exercise increases cellular glucose uptake for several hours after exercise. Teach the client about blood glucose monitoring and carbohydrate consumption during exercise.

Alcohol. The main cause of alcohol-induced hypoglycemia is inhibited liver glucose production. Alcohol is more likely to cause hypoglycemia when fasting is prolonged and glycogen stores are depleted before drinking begins. Alcohol interferes with the counterregulatory response to insulin-induced hypoglycemia and impairs glycogen breakdown, making exercise-induced hypoglycemia more severe. Teach clients to ingest alcohol only with or shortly after eating a meal with enough carbohydrate to prevent hypoglycemia (ADA, 2003f). Caution clients to avoid excess alcohol at bedtime to prevent nighttime hypoglycemia.

Client Education. The cause of hypoglycemia may be subtle. At the onset of menses, a fall in hormone levels decreases insulin needs and contributes to hypoglycemia. When clients switch to a new bottle of insulin, hypoglycemia may occur because the fresh insulin has greater potency. Some clients have hypoglycemia when they change injection sites. Drugs such as propranolol (Inderal, Detensol✱) or other beta blockers mask warning signs and thus predispose clients to severe hypoglycemia. Some episodes of hypoglycemia occur without an obvious cause, and many are due to the erratic absorption of insulin, a problem for even the most careful client.

Help each diabetic client develop a personal treatment plan for hypoglycemia. Routinely taking 10 to 15 g of carbohydrate results in overtreatment of hypoglycemia in some clients and undertreatment in others. The exact glucose rise from a set amount of carbohydrate varies. Using the estimate that each 5 g of carbohydrate raises blood glucose about 20 mg/dL, a personal treatment plan can be developed. For example, the client may be directed to take the following (Farkas-Hirsch, 2000):

- 20 to 30 g of carbohydrate if the blood glucose level is 50 mg/dL (2.8 mmol/L) or less
- 10 to 15 g of carbohydrate if the blood glucose level is 51 to 70 mg/dL (2.9 to 3.9 mmol/L)

Use blood glucose monitoring results to revise or reinforce this plan.

Instruct the client to wear a medical alert bracelet and help the client obtain one. This bracelet is helpful if the client becomes hypoglycemic and is unable to provide self-care.

Teach the client and family about the manifestations of hypoglycemia. Emphasize that delaying a meal for more than 30 minutes raises the risk for hypoglycemia when using some insulin regimens. Instruct the client to keep a carbohydrate source nearby at all times.

Hypoglycemia is a major risk for clients receiving intensive insulin protocols who engage in exercise programs. Explain that nightmares or headaches on days after prolonged or severe exercise occur with hypoglycemia.

Establishing Treatment Plans. Blood glucose monitoring directs hypoglycemia treatment. Treatment continues until blood glucose levels reach and stay in the target range. Once blood glucose control is regained, the specific cause of each hypoglycemic episode must be determined and measures taken to prevent recurrence.

☝ CONSIDERATIONS FOR OLDER ADULTS

Older clients who take antidiabetic drugs are at increased risk for hypoglycemia. Age-related changes in liver and kidney function slow metabolism of these drugs, predisposing the client to prolonged and recurrent hypoglycemia. Older clients may have a delayed release of epinephrine in response to falling blood glucose levels and are less likely to notice and act on hypoglycemic symptoms. Physical symptoms such as confusion may make the older client unable to correct hypoglycemia.

Instruct the older diabetic client and family to monitor blood glucose values when symptoms such as unsteadiness, lightheadedness, poor concentration, trembling, or sweating occur. Assess eating patterns to make sure the client is eating sufficient foods at appropriate times. Encourage a client with a poor appetite to eat a small snack at bedtime to prevent hypoglycemia during the night.

When possible, an antidiabetic drug with low hypoglycemia potential is selected for older clients. The highest risk for severe or fatal hypoglycemia is among older adults taking glyburide (Dailey, 2002). Drug regimens that require meals to be eaten on time only increase the risk for hypoglycemia.

POTENTIAL FOR DIABETIC KETOACIDOSIS

Metabolic problems of diabetic ketoacidosis (DKA) are caused by a total or partial lack of insulin combined with the action of counterregulatory hormones (Figure 68-14). Laboratory diagnosis of DKA is shown in Table 68-19. DKA occurs in 2% to 5% of clients with type 1 diabetes and most often starts from infection. *Death occurs in 1% to 10% of these cases even with appropriate treatment.* Mortality is highest for older clients who also have infection, stroke, myocardial infarction, vascular thrombosis, intestinal obstruction, or pneumonia.

Polyuria, polydipsia, and polyphagia start before DKA. Central nervous system (CNS) depression changes consciousness from lethargy to coma. The client is dehydrated with severe fluid loss. Kussmaul respiration, pain, nausea, and vomiting occur. Initial serum s els may be low or normal. Initial potassium lev on how long DKA lasts before treatment. After therapy starts, serum potassium levels drop quickly.

TABLE 68-19 Differences Between Diabetic Ketoacidosis and Hyperglycemic-Hyperosmolar Nonketotic Syndrome

	Diabetic Ketoacidosis (DKA)	Hyperglycemic-Hyperosmolar Nonketotic Syndrome (HHNS)
Onset	Sudden	Gradual
Precipitating factors	Infection Other stressors Inadequate insulin dose	Infection Other stressors Poor fluid intake
Manifestations	Ketosis: Kussmaul respiration, "fruity" breath, nausea, abdominal pain Dehydration or electrolyte loss: polyuria, polydipsia, weight loss, dry skin, sunken eyes, soft eyeballs, lethargy, coma	Altered central nervous system function with neurologic symptoms Dehydration or electrolyte loss: same as for DKA
Laboratory Findings		
Serum glucose	>300 mg/dL (16.7 mmol/L)	>800 mg/dL (44.5 mmol/L)
Osmolarity	Variable	>350 mOsm/L
Serum ketones	Positive at 1:2 dilutions	Negative
Serum pH	<7.35	>7.4
Serum HCO_3	<15 mEq/L	>20 mEq/L
Serum Na	Low, normal, or high	Normal or low
Serum K	Normal; elevated with acidosis, low following dehydration	Normal or low
BUN	>20 mg/dL; elevated because of dehydration	Elevated
Creatinine	>1.5 mg/dL; elevated because of dehydration	Elevated
Urine ketones	Positive	Negative

BUN, Blood urea nitrogen; *HCO₃*, bicarbonate.

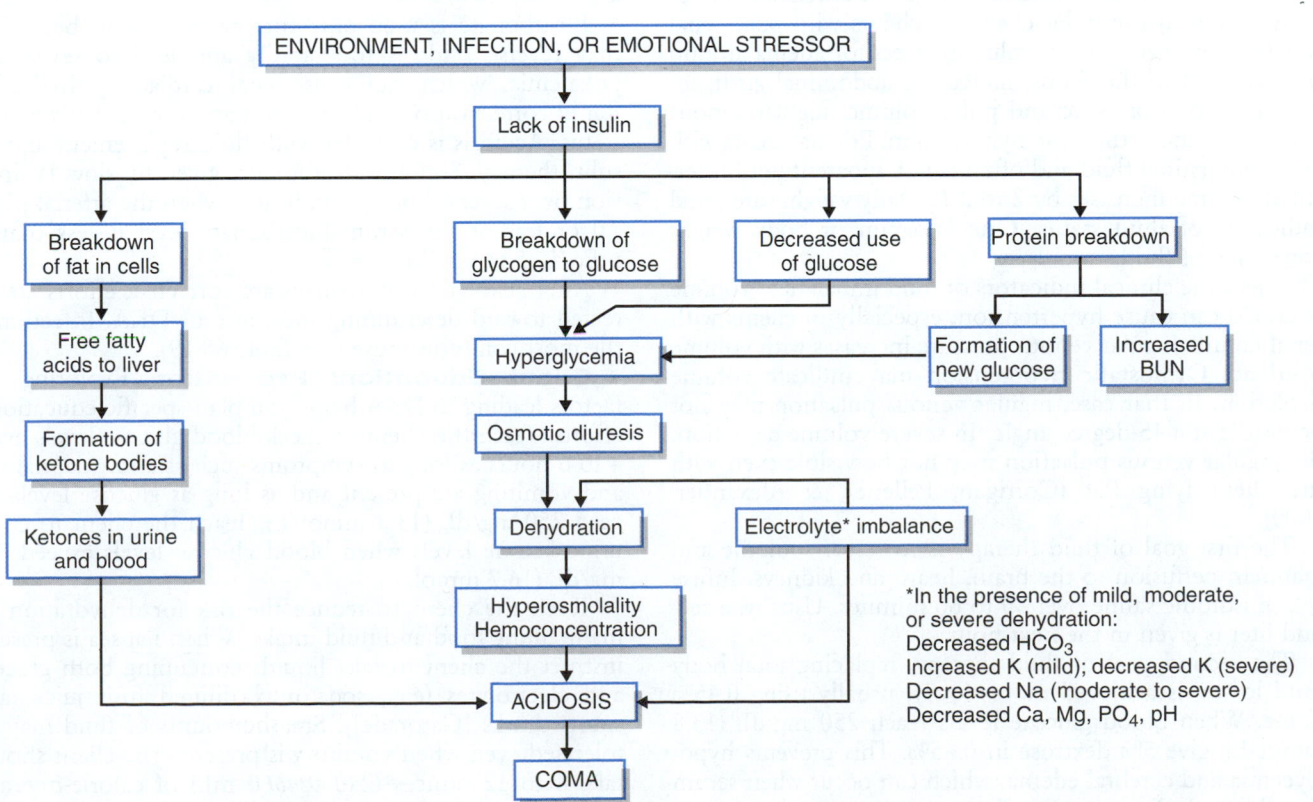

Figure 68-14 ■ The pathophysiologic mechanism of diabetic ketoacidosis.

NOC **PLANNING: EXPECTED OUTCOMES.** The client is expected to have few episodes of hyperglycemia and avoid diabetic ketoacidosis. Indicators include that the client consistently demonstrates the following behaviors:

- Maintains blood glucose levels within the target range
- Adjusts insulin doses to match eating patterns and blood glucose levels during illness
- Describes correct procedure for urine ketone testing
- Describes when to seek help from health care professional

INTERVENTIONS

Hyperglycemic Management. Monitor for manifestations of DKA (see Table 68-19 and Figure 68-14). *First assess the airway, level of consciousness, hydration status, electrolytes, and blood glucose level.* Early in treatment, check the client's blood pressure, pulse, and respirations every 15 minutes until stable. Record urine output, temperature, and mental status every hour. When a central venous catheter is present, assess central venous pressure every 30 minutes or as prescribed. After treatment starts and these values are stable, monitor and record vital signs every 4 hours. Use blood glucose values to assess therapy and determine when to switch from saline to dextrose-containing solutions.

Fluid and Electrolyte Management. *Closely assess the client's fluid status.* The kidneys are less able to respond to changes in pH or fluid and electrolyte balance, to concentrate urine, or to regulate blood osmolarity. The risk for kidney failure rises with age. Impaired bicarbonate reabsorption and acid excretion in poorly functioning renal tubules can lead to acidosis. Cardiovascular disease can cause fluid retention. The dehydrated client's lips and mouth may be dry, and the tongue furrowed. Temperature may be elevated. Age-related skin changes, such as loss of elasticity and dryness, make skin turgor an unreliable sign of dehydration in the older client. In clients with poor renal function and excess fluid volume, assess for edema around the eyes and in the limbs, increasing abdominal girth, increasing blood pressure and pulse volume, jugular venous distention, and orthostatic hypotension. Edema occurs with excess interstitial fluid and often is not apparent until interstitial volume increases by 2 to 3 L. Daily weights are good indicators of fluid status. One kilogram of body weight equals 1 L of fluid.

Check the clinical indicators of fluid imbalance. Volume overload can cause hypertension, especially in clients with renal failure. Jugular venous pressure increases with volume overload. Orthostatic hypotension may indicate volume depletion. In that case, jugular venous pulsation may not be visible at a 45-degree angle. In severe volume depletion, the jugular venous pulsation may not be visible even with the client lying flat (Corrigan, Pelletier, & Alexander, 2000).

The first goal of fluid therapy is to restore volume and maintain perfusion to the brain, heart, and kidneys. Infuse 1 L of isotonic saline over 30 to 60 minutes. Usually, a second liter is given in the next hour.

The second goal of fluid therapy, replacing total body fluid losses, is achieved more slowly, usually using 0.45% saline. When blood glucose levels reach 250 mg/dL (13.8 mmol/L), give 5% dextrose in 0.45%. This prevents hypoglycemia and cerebral edema, which can occur when serum osmolarity declines too rapidly.

During the first 24 hours of treatment, the client needs enough fluids to replace the actual volume deficit and ongoing losses. This may be as much as 6 to 10 L. Watch for signs of congestive heart failure and pulmonary edema. Central venous pressure may be monitored for older clients and those with myocardial disease.

Drug Therapy. The goal of insulin therapy is to lower serum glucose by about 75 to 150 mg/dL/hr. The best way to accomplish this goal is controversial. "Low-dose" insulin therapy results in less hypokalemia and hypoglycemia than a "high-dose" regimen. Although both IM and IV routes are used, continuous IV delivery of regular insulin is recommended because other routes have more erratic absorption. A steady-state level of insulin can be reached in 25 to 30 minutes. Effective blood insulin levels are reached quickly when an IV bolus dose is given at the start of the infusion. Usually, regular insulin is given in an initial IV bolus dose of 0.1 unit/kg, followed by an IV drip of 0.1 unit/kg/hr. Continuous insulin infusion is used because of the 4-minute half-life of IV insulin. Subcutaneous insulin is started when the client can take oral fluids and ketosis has stopped. Assess therapy effectiveness by hourly blood glucose measurements.

Acidosis Management. Regardless of the initial potassium value, there is a large total-body potassium deficit. With insulin therapy, serum potassium levels fall rapidly as potassium shifts into the cells. *Watch for signs of hypokalemia, including fatigue, malaise, confusion, muscle weakness, shallow respirations, abdominal distention or paralytic ileus, hypotension, and weak pulse.* An electrocardiogram (ECG) shows cardiac conduction changes related to potassium. Hypokalemia is a significant cause of death in the treatment of DKA. *Before giving IV potassium, make sure the client produces at least 30 mL/hr of urine.*

Bicarbonate is used only for severe acidosis because it may reverse acidosis too rapidly and lead to severe hypokalemia, which can cause fatal cardiac dysrhythmias. Rapid correction of acidosis can worsen the client's mental status. Acidosis is corrected with fluid replacement and insulin therapy. Sodium bicarbonate, given by slow IV infusion over several hours, is indicated when the arterial pH is 7.0 or less or the serum bicarbonate level is less than 5 mEq/L (5 mmol/L).

After acid-base disturbances are corrected, efforts are directed toward determining the cause of DKA. Infection is the most common cause (see Table 68-19).

Client Education: Prevention. Exploring the factors leading to DKA helps you plan specific educational efforts. Teach the client to check blood glucose levels every 4 to 6 hours as long as symptoms such as anorexia, nausea, and vomiting are present and as long as glucose levels exceed 250 mg/dL (13.8 mmol/L). Teach the client to check urine ketone levels when blood glucose levels exceed 300 mg/dL (16.7 mmol/L).

Teach the client to reduce the risk for dehydration by maintaining food and fluid intake. When nausea is present, instruct the client to take liquids containing both glucose and electrolytes (e.g., soda pop, diluted fruit juice, and sports drinks [Gatorade]). Small amounts of fluid may be tolerated even when vomiting is present. The client should take 8 to 12 ounces (240 to 360 mL) of calorie-free and caffeine-free liquids every hour while awake.

Liquids containing carbohydrate can be taken if the diabetic client cannot eat solid food. Ingesting at least 150 g of carbohydrate daily reduces the risk for starvation ketosis. After consulting a primary care provider, urge the client to take additional rapid-acting (lispro) or short-acting (regular) insulin based on blood glucose levels.

CHART 68-15

CLIENT EDUCATION GUIDE
Sick Day Rules

- Notify your health care provider that you are ill.
- Monitor your blood glucose at least every 4 hours.
- Test your urine for ketones when your blood glucose level is greater than 240 mg/dL (13.8 mmol/L).
- Continue to take insulin or oral antidiabetic agents.
- To prevent dehydration, drink 8 to 12 ounces of sugar-free liquids every hour that you are awake.
- Continue to eat meals at regular times.
- If unable to tolerate solid food because of nausea, consume more easily tolerated foods or liquids equal to the carbohydrate content of your usual meal.
- Call your primary care provider for any of the following danger signals:
  - Persistent nausea and vomiting
  - Moderate or large ketones
  - Blood glucose elevation after two supplemental doses of insulin
  - High (101.5° F [38.6° C]) temperature or increasing fever; fever for more than 24 hours
- Treat symptoms (e.g., diarrhea, nausea, vomiting, and fever) as directed by your primary care provider.
- Get plenty of rest.

Instruct the client to consult the primary care provider when the following problems occur:

- Blood glucose exceeds 250 mg/dL (13.8 mmol/L).
- Ketonuria lasts for more than 24 hours.
- The client cannot take food or fluids.
- Illness lasts more than 1 to 2 days.

Also instruct the client or family to detect hyperglycemia by performing SMBG whenever the client is ill. Illness can result in dehydration with DKA, hyperglycemic-hyperosmolar nonketotic syndrome, or both. The sooner the client seeks treatment, the less severe the metabolic alteration. The client should understand not to omit insulin therapy during illness. Chart 68-15 reviews guidelines for the ill client.

POTENTIAL FOR HYPERGLYCEMIC-HYPEROSMOLAR NONKETOTIC SYNDROME AND COMA

Hyperglycemic-hyperosmolar nonketotic syndrome (HHNS) is a hyperosmolar (increased blood osmolarity) state caused by hyperglycemia. The processes of HHNS are outlined in Figure 68-15. Although both HHNS and diabetic ketoacidosis (DKA) are caused by hyperglycemia, HHNS is different from DKA because of the absence of ketosis and the much higher blood glucose levels and blood osmolarity. Blood glucose levels may exceed 800 mg/dL (44.5 mmol/L) and blood osmolarity may exceed 350 mOsm/L. Other biochemical problems with HHNS also are more severe than those with DKA. Table 68-19 lists the differences between DKA and HHNS.

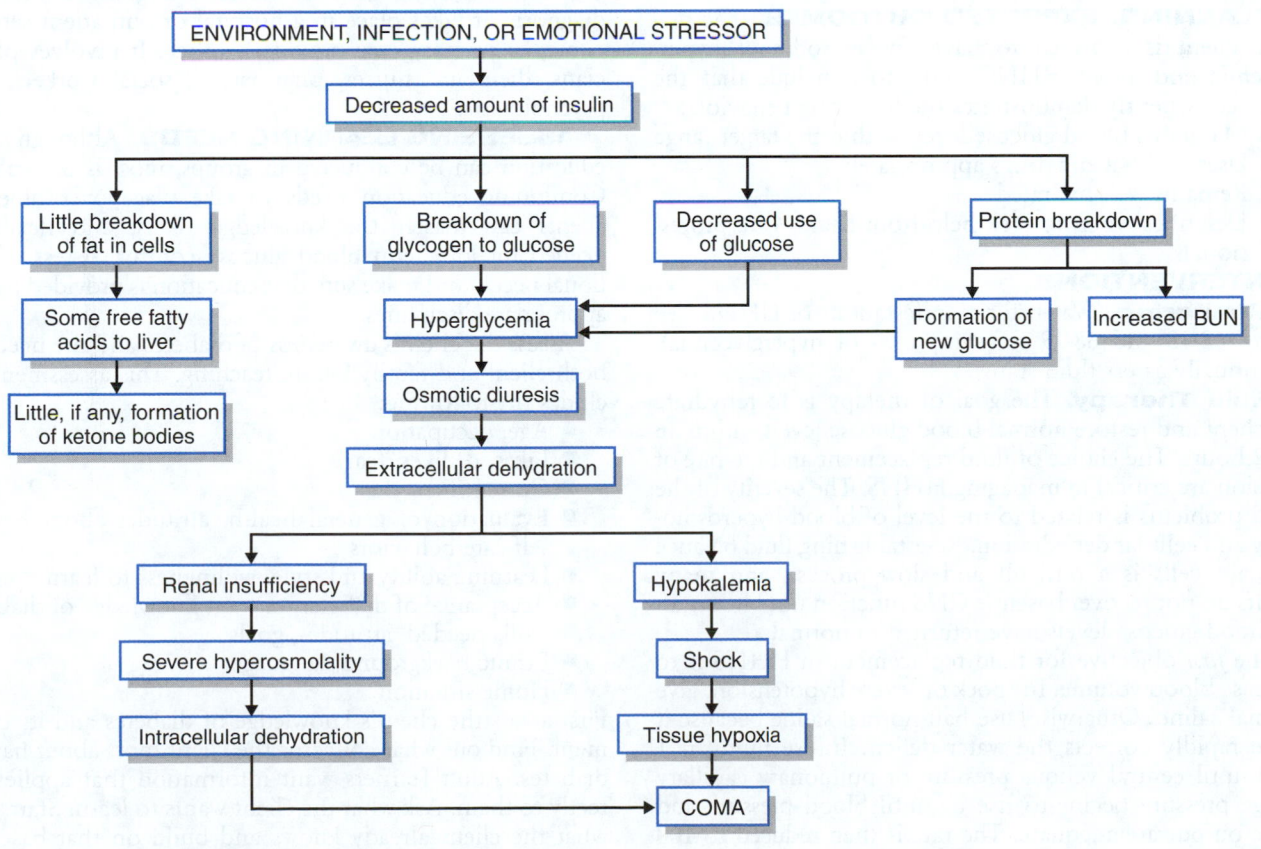

Figure 68-15 ■ The pathophysiologic mechanism of hyperglycemic-hyperosmolar nonketotic syndrome.

CONSIDERATIONS FOR OLDER ADULTS

HHNS occurs most often in older clients with type 2 diabetes mellitus, many of whom did not know that they had diabetes. Mortality rates in older clients are as high as 40% to 70%. The onset of HHNS is slow and may not be recognized. The older client often seeks medical attention later and is sicker than the younger client. HHNS does not occur in adequately hydrated people. Older diabetic clients are at greater risk for dehydration and HHNS because of age-related changes in thirst perception and poor urine-concentrating abilities.

Myocardial infarction, sepsis, pancreatitis, and stroke, and some drugs (glucocorticoids, diuretics, phenytoin [Dilantin], propranolol [Inderal], and calcium channel blockers) also may cause HHNS. Central nervous system (CNS) changes range from confusion to complete coma. Unlike DKA, clients with HHNS may have seizures, myoclonic jerking, and reversible paralysis.

The development of HHNS rather than DKA is related to residual insulin secretion. In HHNS, the client secretes just enough insulin to prevent ketosis but not enough to prevent hyperglycemia. The hyperglycemia of HHNS is more severe than that of DKA, greatly increasing the blood osmolarity and causing profound diuresis. Severe dehydration and electrolyte loss occur, and the client may lose 15% to 25% of body fluid. When dehydration is severe, glucose is not filtered into the urine, causing even greater hyperglycemia and hyperosmolarity. Impairment of the thirst center in the brain occurs, making it impossible for the client to drink enough fluid to prevent dehydration.

NOC   PLANNING: EXPECTED OUTCOMES. The diabetic client is expected to have few episodes of hyperglycemia and avoid HHNS. Indicators include that the client consistently demonstrates the following behaviors:

- Maintains blood glucose levels within the target range
- Uses antidiabetic drugs appropriately
- Remains well hydrated
- Describes when to seek help from health care professionals

INTERVENTIONS

Monitoring. Watch for manifestations of HHNS (see Tables 68-18 and 68-19 for symptoms of hyperglycemia). Continually assess fluid status.

Fluid Therapy. The goal of therapy is to rehydrate the client and restore normal blood glucose levels within 36 to 72 hours. The choice of fluid replacement and the rate of infusion are critical in managing HHNS. The severity of the CNS problems is related to the level of blood hyperosmolarity and cellular dehydration. Re-establishing fluid balance in brain cells is a difficult and slow process, and many clients do not recover baseline CNS function until hours after blood glucose levels have returned to normal.

The *first* objective for fluid replacement in HHNS is to increase blood volume. In shock or severe hypotension, give normal saline. Otherwise, use half-normal saline because it more rapidly corrects the water deficit. Infuse fluids at 1 L/hr until central venous pressure or pulmonary capillary wedge pressure begins to rise or until blood pressure and urine output are adequate. The rate is then reduced to 100 to 200 mL/hr. Half of the estimated water deficit is replaced in the first 12 hours, and the rest is given during the next 36

hours. Body weight, urine output, kidney function, and the presence or absence of pulmonary congestion and jugular venous distention determine the rate of fluid infusion. In clients with congestive heart failure, renal insufficiency, or acute kidney failure, monitor central venous pressure. *Assess the client hourly for signs of cerebral edema; abrupt changes in mental status, abnormal neurologic signs, and coma. Immediately report changes in the level of consciousness; changes in pupil size, shape, or reaction; or seizures.* Lack of improvement in level of consciousness may indicate inadequate rates of fluid replacement or reduction in plasma osmolarity. Regression after initial improvement may indicate a too rapid reduction in plasma osmolarity. A slow but steady improvement in CNS function is the best evidence that fluid management is satisfactory.

Continuing Therapy. IV insulin given at 10 units/hr is often needed to reduce blood glucose levels. Although fluid replacement reduces hyperglycemia, it cannot alone return blood glucose levels to normal. A reduction of blood glucose by 10% per hour is a reasonable goal (Delaney et al., 2000). Potassium loss occurs in HHNS, although not to the degree it does in DKA. Because of the initial low urine output (**oliguria**) or absent urine output (**anuria**), potassium replacement may not be needed at the start of therapy. Client education and interventions to minimize dehydration are similar to those for ketoacidosis.

Community-Based Care

HEALTH TEACHING

Education about blood glucose control begins at the time of diagnosis. It takes place in a hospital or outpatient setting, clinic, or primary care provider's office. It involves physicians, dietitians, nurses, pharmacists, social workers, and psychologists.

ASSESSING LEARNING NEEDS. Although some education can be conducted in groups, most is one-to-one. Continuing education needs to take place over time, so clients can master the knowledge, skills, and flexibility needed for long-term blood glucose control. Assess educational needs, and make sure that education is provided by the appropriate disciplines.

Assess the client's awareness of diabetes and the needs of both client and family before teaching. This assessment includes the following:

- Age, occupation
- Likes, dislikes, fears
- Current lifestyle
- Evaluation of general health, attitudes about health, self-care behaviors
- Learning ability and style, willingness to learn
- Acceptance of diabetes, current knowledge of diabetes
- Skills needed, attitudes, goals
- Ethnic background, language
- Home situation

First assess the client's knowledge of diabetes and its treatment. Find out what concerns the client most about having diabetes. Adult learners want information that applies directly to them. Ask what the client wants to learn. Start with what the client already knows and build on that base. To capture interest and motivate clients for learning, present material relevant to their first questions. Because they will be managing their own care after discharge, clients tend to focus on issues most important to them. Treatment measures that need to start soon after diagnosis may be of more interest to the client than long-term control.

The client's physical condition dictates the timing of teaching. When blood glucose levels are fluctuating, the client does not have the energy to learn complex information. Explaining that well-controlled blood glucose levels improve the sense of well-being can help the client accept the therapy plan. Use an informal teaching program until the client feels able to attend a formal class. Teach and observe the client's technique for injections and blood glucose monitoring.

Each client learns in an individual way. A successful diabetic education program combines several teaching methods. Some clients learn better when they read pamphlets. Others learn better when they watch videotapes. Learning improves when the equipment is handled, techniques are practiced, success is rewarded, and errors are corrected immediately.

ASSESSING PHYSICAL, COGNITIVE, AND EMOTIONAL LIMITATIONS. Assess the client's education and reading level to determine what level of information to present. Assess the client's ability to read printed information, insulin labels, and markings on syringes and equipment. Many clients with type 2 diabetes have **presbyopia** (age-related far-sightedness) and other visual difficulties made worse by blurred vision caused by fluctuating blood glucose levels. The client must be able to understand the printed material. Even highly educated clients do not want to read complicated information when they are sick. Much of the printed material from drug companies is printed at the sixth- or seventh-grade level. The International Diabetes Center prepares printed diabetic education material at the second- and third-grade levels. Develop creative teaching strategies for the client who cannot read.

Assess the client's ability to conceptualize. Adjusting insulin dosage based on blood glucose monitoring is a difficult concept and may not be appropriate for clients who cannot understand it. Managing drugs, exercise, and diet requires complex interpretation and behavior.

Assess manual dexterity for any physical limitations that may alter the teaching plan. A hand injury, tremors, or severe arthritis may require a change in insulin preparation.

Information is best learned when the client is ready. Clients with newly diagnosed diabetes are facing a life crisis. Some are motivated to learn information and are willing to change lifelong behaviors. Others may grieve the loss of their previous lifestyle and use denial as a means of coping. In this instance, the client may not be able to learn needed information right away.

EXPLAINING SURVIVAL SKILLS. The initial phase of diabetic education involves basic survival skills. The physical changes of diabetes and the relationship of diet, drugs, and exercise to overall control are important.

A dietitian provides the initial diet instruction. The client needs to understand what to eat, how much to eat, and when to eat. Stress the importance of eating on time and the dangers of skipping meals. The client must know how to maintain food intake during illness. Reinforce dietary instruction, answer questions, and refer questions to the dietitian or physician as indicated.

After being taught, the client should be able to identify the drugs needed to control blood glucose levels. If insulin is needed, the client must be able to prepare and give the dose accurately using sterile technique. The client must also be able to state when insulin is to be injected, where insulin is injected, and how insulin is stored. Stress the dangers of skipping doses. Carefully review drug interactions, especially with older clients taking oral antidiabetic drugs.

The client should be able to state a plan for regular physical activity. The client must be able to describe the relationship between exercise and blood glucose control and identify situations when activity should not be performed. Provide guidelines for additional carbohydrate intake to prevent hypoglycemia from excessive exercise.

The diabetic client also must be able to state the plan for monitoring blood glucose. The person doing the monitoring must be able to do the procedure accurately and understand the results. Explain when blood glucose should be monitored, acceptable ranges, and actions to take when results are out of these ranges. If the client cannot perform SMBG due to illness, ensure that a resource (e.g., home care agency, health clinic, or primary care provider's office) will be available to do the monitoring.

The most important part of diabetes education is to ensure that the client understands the significance, symptoms, causes, and treatment of hypoglycemia. The client must be able to state the causes of hypoglycemia and the activities needed to prevent it. He or she must be able to describe appropriate carbohydrates to have available and the need to notify the physician of hypoglycemic episodes.

The client also must understand the significance of hyperglycemia and its relationship to illness. The client must describe actions to take during illness and when to communicate with the primary care provider.

Most of this information is best retained when the client is ready to learn. Education is a challenge because clients tend to be hospitalized for shorter periods. All diabetic education may be provided in an outpatient setting, where contact with the client is limited. Important information must be squeezed into the time available. Many clients do not progress in self-management beyond the survival level because of psychological barriers.

COUNSELING. The major goal of in-depth counseling is to help the client become self-sufficient in diabetes management. Educational sessions with client and family are needed to individualize the diabetes regimen for their needs and abilities. Education is often provided by a team of a physician, nurse educator, dietitian, social worker, pharmacist, psychologist, and other health care professionals as needed. Education may occur in various outpatient settings.

Besides knowledge gained at the survival level, the client should be able to discuss the action of insulin in the body and the effects of insulin deficiency. The client should also be able to explain the effects of diet, drugs, and activity on blood glucose. He or she should be able to relate maintaining normal blood glucose levels to preventing complications. This includes relating changes in glucose level to the possible need for a change in insulin dosage.

The client must be able to describe the meal plan and explain the adjustments needed to meet diabetic diet requirements. He or she should state how food intake should be altered when eating out or increasing exercise. *The client must be able to list specific foods to be eaten to prevent and treat hypoglycemia, as well as adjustments to make when ill.*

The client must be able to prepare and give insulin accurately. He or she should be able to discuss the onset, peak, and duration of the insulin used. In reviewing insulin administration, stress the importance of injection site selection and rotation. Review adjustments in insulin based on SMBG results (when permitted by the physician) and explain that follow-up SMBG results are needed to evaluate the effects of additional insulin. The client should know how to protect insulin when traveling. For clients at risk for severe hypoglycemia, teach a family member to inject glucagon. If the client takes an oral diabetic drug, ask him or her to identify the drug and describe its prescribed schedule. The client must identify over-the-counter drugs with the potential to cause adverse interactions and the need to inform all care providers of the drug regimen.

Within health status–imposed physical limitations, the client should be able to perform desired physical activities. The client must state blood glucose levels that are safe for exercise, the frequency of SMBG during exercise, food required before exercise, and what food to have available during exercise. He or she should be aware of the risk for injury during exercise and explain the importance of protective footwear.

The goals of in-depth education are to help the diabetic client solve problems of blood glucose fluctuation through the use of SMBG. The client should be able to identify practices, such as travel (Chart 68-16), that cause blood glucose to fluctuate and to treat these problems with supplemental insulin, changes in activity, or changes in diet. Ask the client to demonstrate urine ketone testing and to describe when urine ketones should be measured.

The client must be able to describe a plan for periodic evaluation of blood glucose control by the primary care provider, as well as periodic dental and eye examinations. He or she must be able to perform foot care, wear properly fitting shoes, and describe hazards related to foot care. The client must be able to describe ways to reduce specific risk factors, such as cigarette smoking and hypertension.

The client must state that diabetes is a lifelong disease that requires lifestyle changes, describe the changes being made, and indicate those that need to be made. He or she should be able to identify stress-producing situations and discuss ways to reduce stress.

PSYCHOSOCIAL PREPARATION

The diagnosis of diabetes may represent a loss of control. All but a few clients lose flexibility. Life becomes ordered and routines must be followed. Certain events surrounding diabetes are predictable. Taking an insulin injection and not eating for several hours causes hypoglycemia. Poorly controlled diabetes leads to complications and premature death. Tight control of blood glucose levels prevents complications.

The stress of diabetes is in addition to the demands of normal daily life. The client must be able to integrate the demands of diabetes into daily and recreational schedules while keeping blood glucose stable.

You can assist in healthy psychological adaptation to diabetes by providing successful educational experiences. Mastery of blood glucose monitoring helps the client feel that he or she has control over the disease. Knowing the ef-

---

CHART 68-16

CLIENT EDUCATION GUIDE
Travel Tips for Diabetic Clients

Before traveling visit your primary care provider and diabetes educator.
- See your physician to make certain you do not have any other health problems.
- Obtain a letter from your physician (typed on office letterhead) that indicates you have diabetes and lists the medications you are taking.
- Obtain any needed immunizations or inoculations.
- Obtain prescriptions from your physician for your medications, including glucagon if you take insulin, and prescriptions for motion sickness, nausea and vomiting, and traveler's diarrhea.
- Develop a plan for changing strengths of insulin if you are traveling to a country that does not carry the type of insulin you use. Learn how to use a U-100 syringe to draw up U-40 insulin.
- Develop a plan for meal and medication adjustment across time zones. Eastbound travel will shorten the day, requiring a reduction in the amount of medication needed. Westbound travel may add an extra meal to the day and require additional medication.
- Obtain a list of foods from your diabetes educator that you can substitute for food served in restaurants or airplanes.

If you are traveling by air, train, or boat, call ahead and request special meals for individuals with diabetes.
- Plan for delays in eating.
- Eat something every 4 hours.
- Drink a glass of water every 2 hours to prevent dehydration.
- Do not assume that special meals will be available; substitute items you cannot eat with foods you have in your travel kit.

Notify airline and hotel personnel that you have diabetes.
- Always wear medical alert identification and keep your medical alert card in your wallet.

While traveling:
- Check your blood glucose level frequently.
- Do not engage in activities when blood glucose levels are lower than 65 mg/dL.
- Stretch and walk around every 2 hours to help your circulation.
- Check your feet frequently for blisters and sores. You may be doing more walking than usual.
- Take extra shoes with you, and plan to change shoes often when walking more than normal.
- Protect your skin against exposure to the sun. Drug-induced photosensitivity can occur with some oral hypoglycemic agents.

Always have your travel kit with you; do not check your kit along with the rest of your luggage. Include these items in your travel kit:
- Insulin bottles in boxes with prescription labels
- Twice as much medication and twice as many supplies as you think you will need (Pack medications separately from checked luggage.)
- Insulin stored in an insulated carrying case that will maintain temperatures according to the manufacturer's directions
- The letter from your physician (typed on office letterhead) that indicates you have diabetes and lists the medications you are taking
- A supply of fast-acting sugar (such as glucose tablets or gel, hard candy, and sugar cubes), as well as longer-acting foods (such as cheese and crackers and peanut butter and crackers)
- A self-monitoring diary

---

fects of extra activities, extra food, or extra insulin is helpful in learning to adjust the regimen.

Feeling a sense of control over the condition does much to promote a positive attitude about diabetes. Success in injecting insulin provides concrete evidence that he or she can mas-

FOCUSED ASSESSMENT of
The Insulin-Dependent Diabetic Client During a Home or Clinic Visit

Assess overall mental status, wakefulness, ability to converse. Take vital signs and weight:
- Fever could indicate infection.
- Are blood pressure and weight within target range? Why or why not?

Question client regarding any change in visual acuity; check current visual acuity.

Inspect oral mucous membranes, gums, and teeth.

Question client about injection areas used; inspect areas being used; assess whether client is using areas and sites appropriately.

Inspect skin for intactness, wounds that have not healed, new sores, ulcers, bruises, or burns; assess any previously known wounds for infection, progression of healing.

Question client regarding foot care.

Assess lower extremities and feet for peripheral pulses, lack of or decreased sensation, abnormal sensations, breaks in skin integrity, condition of toes and nails.

Question client regarding color and consistency of stools and frequency of bowel movements; assess abdomen for bowel sounds.

Review client's home health diary:
- Is blood glucose within targeted range? Why or why not?
- Is glucose monitoring being recorded often enough?
- Is the client's food intake adequate and appropriate? Why or why not?
- Is exercise occurring regularly? Why or why not?

Assess client's ability to perform self-monitoring of blood glucose.

Assess client's procedures for obtaining and storing insulin and syringes, cleaning equipment, disposing of syringes and needles.

Assess client's insulin preparation and injection technique.

---

ter the disease. Teach by breaking a task into small, achievable units to ensure mastery; for example, a client may begin learning how to inject insulin by first obtaining an accurate dose.

Devote as much teaching time as possible to insulin injection and blood glucose monitoring. Clients with newly diagnosed diabetes are often fearful of giving themselves injections. After this technique has been mastered, clients become less anxious and are able to attend to other tasks.

HOME CARE MANAGEMENT

Clients with diabetes self-manage their disease. Each day the client decides what to eat, whether to exercise, and whether to take prescribed drugs. Maintaining blood glucose control depends on the accuracy of self-management skills. The main role of the health care professional is to provide support and education and to empower the client to make informed decisions. Self-management education allows clients to identify their problems and provides techniques to help them make decisions, take appropriate actions, and alter these actions as needed.

Provide information about resources. The client must know whom to contact in case of emergency. Older adults who live alone must have daily telephone contact with a friend or neighbor. The client may also need help shopping and preparing meals. He or she may have limited access to transportation and may not have sufficient supplies of food, particularly in bad weather. Because of the likelihood of visual problems in older clients, they may need assistance in preparing insulin syringes for injection or in monitoring blood glucose. Make referrals to home care or public health

---

TABLE 68-20 Outcome Criteria for Diabetic Teaching

Before being discharged to home, the diabetic client or the significant other should be able to:
- Tell why insulin or an oral hypoglycemic agent is being prescribed.
- Name which insulin or oral hypoglycemic agent is being prescribed, and name the dosage and frequency of administration.
- Discuss the relationship between mealtime and the action of insulin or the oral hypoglycemic agent.
- Discuss plans to follow diabetic diet instructions.
- Prepare and administer insulin accurately.
- Test blood for glucose, or state plans for having blood glucose levels monitored.
- Test urine for ketones, and state when this test should be done.
- Verbalize how to store insulin.
- List symptoms that indicate a hypoglycemic reaction.
- Tell what carbohydrate sources are used to treat hypoglycemic reactions.
- Tell what symptoms indicate hyperglycemia.
- Tell what dietary changes are needed during illness.
- Verbalize when to call the physician or the nurse (frequent episodes of hypoglycemia, symptoms of hyperglycemia).
- Verbalize the procedures for proper foot care.

---

agencies as needed. Referral is especially important for older women who are insulin dependent. Chart 68-17 identifies areas for assessment during a home or clinic visit.

HEALTH CARE RESOURCES

A wide array of diabetic education material is available from drug companies. The American Diabetes Association (ADA) will refer a diabetic client to specific agencies or resources (phone 800-DIABETES [800-342-2383] in the United States; 800-BANTING [800-226-8464] in Canada). The American Association of Diabetes Educators can refer a diabetic client to a local certified diabetes educator (phone [800] TEAM-UP-4). Additional resources are listed in the bibliography.

? Critical Thinking Challenge

A 68-year-old client has had type 2 diabetes for several years. She has come to the clinic for a 6-month evaluation. During the interview, she complains of burning and tingling sensations in her feet and tells you that her feet are always cold. She keeps her feet warm with a hot water bottle. Examination of her feet reveals the skin to be very dry with deep cracks and fissures. Her feet are cold to the touch with calluses over the metatarsal heads. Her toenails are long and thickened. She has a history of an ulcer on the plantar surface of her left foot, which developed after she stepped on a sharp object on her kitchen floor.

1. List four parameters you would assess to determine the client's risk for foot injury.
2. Discuss three elements of education that are especially important for this client.
3. What referrals would you make for this client?

evolve For suggested answer guidelines, go to http://evolve.elsevier.com/Iggy/.

◆ Evaluation: Outcomes

Evaluate the care of the client with diabetes on the basis of the identified nursing diagnoses and collaborative problems. Outcome success for diabetic education is the ability of the client to maintain blood glucose levels within the normal range. General outcome criteria are listed on the next page and in Table 68-20. More specific outcomes are listed with each nursing diagnosis and collaborative problem. The expected outcomes include that the client will:

- Achieve blood glucose control
- Avoid acute and chronic complications of diabetes
- Have a satisfactory and complete postoperative recovery without complications
- Avoid injury
- Experience relief of pain
- Maintain optimal vision
- Maintain a urine elimination pattern in the expected range
- Have an optimal level of mental status functioning
- Have decreased episodes of hypoglycemia
- Have decreased episodes of hyperglycemia

Specific indicators for these outcomes are listed for each nursing diagnosis and collaborative problem under the Planning and Implementation section (see earlier).

GET READY for the NCLEX Examination!

KEY POINTS

Safe Effective Care Environment

- Use aseptic technique during all central line dressing changes or any invasive procedure.
- Use good handwashing techniques before providing any care to a client who has diabetes.
- Wash your hands before and after testing the client's blood glucose levels.

Health Promotion and Maintenance

- Encourage all people to maintain weight within an appropriate range.
- Encourage all people, including clients with diabetes, to participate regularly in exercise or physical activity appropriate to their health status.
- Teach the client and family about the clinical manifestations of infection and when to seek medical advice.
- Instruct clients with diabetes to wear a medical alert bracelet.
- Instruct clients not to share blood glucose monitoring equipment.
- Reinforce to all clients with diabetes that tight control over blood glucose levels reduces the risk for the vascular complications of diabetes.
- Remind the diabetic client to have yearly eye examinations by an ophthalmologist.
- Teach diabetic clients with peripheral neuropathy to use a bath thermometer to test water for bathing, to avoid walking barefoot, and to inspect their feet daily.
- Encourage all clients who smoke cigarettes to quit smoking.
- Help clients who want to stop smoking find an appropriate smoking cessation program.

Psychosocial Integrity

- Explore with the client what the diagnosis of diabetes means to him or her.
- Allow the client the opportunity to express fear or anxiety regarding the diagnosis of diabetes or the treatment regimen.
- Explain all procedures, restrictions, medications, and follow-up care to the client and family.

- Pace your education sessions to match the learning needs and style of the individual client.
- Use return demonstration strategies when teaching the client about medication regimen, insulin injection, blood glucose monitoring, and foot assessment.
- Refer clients newly diagnosed with diabetes to local resources and support groups.
- Assess clients' visual acuity and peripheral tactile sensation to determine needed adjustments in teaching self-medication and self-monitoring of blood glucose levels.

Physiological Integrity

- Teach the client about any drugs to be continued after discharge from the hospital.
- Instruct the client and family in the manifestations of complications and when to seek assistance.
- Instruct all clients with diabetes to avoid becoming dehydrated and to drink at least 3 L of water each day unless another medical condition requires fluid restriction.
- Instruct clients who are taking sulfonylurea antidiabetic agents, especially chlorpropamide, about an increased risk for hypoglycemic reactions.
- Teach clients who are taking metformin the clinical manifestations of lactic acidosis (fatigue, dizziness, difficulty breathing, stomach discomfort, irregular heartbeat).
- Warn the client not to take over-the-counter drugs with their oral antidiabetic drugs without consulting their primary care provider.
- When mixing different kinds of insulin together, draw the shorter-acting insulin into the syringe before drawing up the longer-acting insulin.
- Never dilute or mix insulin glargine with any other insulin or solution.
- Teach clients to rotate insulin injection areas within one site rather than to other sites, to prevent changes in absorption.
- Avoid injecting insulin within a 2-inch radius of the umbilicus.
- Avoid intramuscular insulin injection.
- Teach clients who experience Somagyi's phenomenon (early morning hyperglycemia) to ensure an adequate dietary intake at bedtime.
- Instruct the client to always carry a glucose source.
- Teach clients who exercise to test urine for ketone bodies if blood glucose levels are greater than 250 mg/dL before engaging in strenuous exercise.
- Instruct clients in foot care as outlined in Chart 68-10.

ADDITIONAL STUDY RESOURCES

Go to your Student CD-ROM for Review Questions for the NCLEX Examination.

Go to http://evolve.elsevier.com/Iggy/ for Integrated Management of Care Questions for the NCLEX Examination.

SELECTED BIBLIOGRAPHY

Asterisk indicates a classic or definitive work on this subject.

2002Drug topics red book. (2002). Montvale, NJ: Medical Economics Company.

Ahern, J. (2001). Site rotation. *Diabetes Forecast, 54*(4), 66-68.

American Association of Diabetes Educators. (2003a). Diabetes—Facts and Statistics. Available at http://www.aadenet.org/GeneralDiabetesInfo/GovStats.html.

American Association of Diabetes Educators. (2003b). Position statement: Educating providers and persons with diabetes to prevent transmission of bloodborne infections and avoid injuries from sharps. Available at http://www.aadenet.org.

American Association of Diabetes Educators. (2003c). Position statement: Special considerations for the education and management of older adults with diabetes. *The Diabetes Educator,* 29(1), 93-96.

American Diabetes Association. (2001a). Consensus statement: Postprandial blood glucose. *Diabetes Care,* 24(4), 775-778.

American Diabetes Association. (2001b). Position statement: Role of fat replacers in diabetes medical nutrition therapy. *Diabetes Care,* 24(Suppl. 1), 104-105.

American Diabetes Association. (2003a). Committee report: Report of the Expert Committee on the Diagnosis and Classification of Diabetes. *Diabetes Care,* 26(Suppl. 1), 5-20.

American Diabetes Association. (2003b). Position statement: Aspirin therapy in diabetes. *Diabetes Care,* 26(Suppl. 1) 87-88.

American Diabetes Association. (2003c). Position statement: Continuous subcutaneous insulin infusion. *Diabetes Care,* 26(Suppl. 1), 125.

American Diabetes Association. (2003d). Position statement: Diabetic nephropathy. *Diabetes Care,* 26(Suppl. 1), 94-98.

American Diabetes Association. (2003e). Position statement: Diabetic retinopathy. *Diabetes Care,* 26(Suppl. 1), 99-102.

American Diabetes Association. (2003f). Position statement: Evidence-based nutrition principles and recommendations for the treatment and prevention of diabetes and related complications. *Diabetes Care,* 26(Suppl. 1), 51-61.

American Diabetes Association. (2003g). Position statement: Gestational diabetes mellitus. *Diabetes Care,* 26(Suppl. 1), 103-105.

American Diabetes Association. (2003h). Position statement: Hyperglycemic crisis in patients with diabetes mellitus. *Diabetes Care,* 26(Suppl. 1), 109-117.

American Diabetes Association. (2003i). Position statement: Implications of the Diabetes Control and Complications Trial. *Diabetes Care,* 26(Suppl. 1), 25-27.

American Diabetes Association. (2003j). Position statement: Implications of the United Kingdom Prospective Diabetes Study. *Diabetes Care,* 26(Suppl. 1), 28-32.

American Diabetes Association. (2003k). Position statement: Insulin administration. *Diabetes Care,* 26(Suppl. 1), 121-124.

American Diabetes Association. (2003l). Position statement: Management of dyslipidemia in adults with diabetes. *Diabetes Care,* 26(Suppl. 1), 83-86.

American Diabetes Association. (2003m). Position statement: Pancreas transplantation. *Diabetes Care,* 26(Suppl. 1), 120.

American Diabetes Association. (2003n). Position statement: Physical activity/exercise and diabetes mellitus. *Diabetes Care,* 26(Suppl. 1), 73-77.

American Diabetes Association. (2003o). Position statement: Prevention of type 1 diabetes mellitus. *Diabetes Care,* 26(Suppl. 1), 140.

American Diabetes Association. (2003p). Position statement: Preventive foot care in people with diabetes. *Diabetes Care,* 26(Suppl. 1), 78-79.

American Diabetes Association. (2003q). Position statement: Screening for type 2 diabetes. *Diabetes Care,* 26(Suppl. 1), 21-24.

American Diabetes Association. (2003r). Position statement: Standards of medical care for patients with diabetes mellitus. *Diabetes Care,* 25(Suppl. 1), 33-49.

American Diabetes Association. (2003s). Position statement: Tests of glycemia in diabetes. *Diabetes Care,* 26(Suppl. 1), 106-108.

American Diabetes Association. (2003t). Position statement: The prevention or delay of type 2 diabetes. *Diabetes Care,* 26(Suppl. 1), 62-69.

American Diabetes Association. (2003u). Position statement: Treatment of hypertension in adults with diabetes. *Diabetes Care,* 26(Suppl. 1), 80-86.

American Diabetes Association. (2003v). Reviews: Economic costs of diabetes in the U.S. in 2002. *Diabetes Care,* 26(3), 917-932.

American Dietetic Association. (2003). *Exchange lists for meal planning.* (2003). Chicago: Author.

Arauz-Pacheco, C., Parrott, M.A., & Raskin, P. (2002). The treatment of hypertension in adult patients with diabetes. *Diabetes Care,* 25(1), 134-147.

Ayello, E., Cuddigan, J., & Kerstein, M. (2002). Skip the knife: Debriding wounds without surgery. *Nursing2002,* 32(9), 58-63.

Bailes, B. (2002). Diabetes mellitus and its chronic complications. *AORN Journal,* 76(2), 265-282.

Barr, R.G., et al. (2002). Tests of glycemia for the diagnosis of type 2 diabetes mellitus. *Annals of Internal Medicine,* 137(4), 263-272.

Bartol, T. (2002). Putting a patient with diabetes in the driver's seat. *Nursing2002,* 32(2), 53-55.

Beckman, J.A., Creager, M.A., & Libby, P. (2002). Diabetes and atherosclerosis: Epidemiology, pathology and management. *Journal of the American Medical Association,* 287(19), 2570-2581.

Beebe, C., & O'Donnell, M. (2001). Educating patients with type 2 diabetes. *Nursing Clinics of North America,* 36(2), 375-386.

Begany, K. (2000). Over the counter drugs: What's safe to take? *Diabetes Self-Management.* 17(6), 46-52.

Bell, D.S.H. (2002). Chronic complications of diabetes. *Southern Medical Journal,* 95(1), 30-34.

Bergenstal, R., et al. (2000). Identifying variables associated with inaccurate self-monitoring of blood glucose: Proposed guidelines to improve accuracy. *The Diabetes Educator,* 26(6), 981-989.

Berkowitz, K. (2002). Lantus? or Lente? *American Journal of Nursing,* 102, 8, 55.

Bishop, M.L., & Duben-Engelkirk, J.L. (2000). *Clinical chemistry.* Philadelphia: Lippincott Williams & Wilkins.

Blonde, L. (2001). Optimizing therapy in type 2 diabetes. *Patient Care for the Nurse Practitioner,* 4(Suppl. Fall, 2001), 8-14.

Bode, B.W., Sabbah, H., & Davidson, P.C. (2001). What's ahead in glucose monitoring? *Postgraduate Medicine,* 109(4), 41-49.

Bodenheimer, T., et al. (2002). Patient self-management in chronic disease in primary care. *Journal of the American Medical Association,* 288(19), 2469-2475.

*Bowker, J.H., & Pfeifer, M.A. (2000). Levin and O'Neal's *the diabetic foot* (6th ed.). St. Louis: Mosby.

Buse, J.B., Sisca, T.S., & Menke, M. (Eds.). (2002). Diabetic ketoacidosis in the adult patient. Available at http://www.novonordisk.com.

Caballero, E., Habershaw, G.M., & Pinzur, M.S. (2000). Preventing amputation in patients with diabetes. *Patient Care for the Nurse Practitioner,* 3(9), 17-45.

Caffrey, R.M. (2003). Diabetes under control: Are all syringes created equal? *American Journal of Nursing,* 103(6), 46-49.

Cameron, B.L. (2002). Making diabetes management routine. *American Journal of Nursing,* 102(2), 26-33.

Canobbio, M.M. (2000). *Handbook of patient teaching.* St. Louis: Mosby.

Cattral, M.S., et al. (2000). Portal venous and enteric exocrine drainage versus venous and bladder exocrine drainage of pancreatic grafts. *Annals of Surgery,* 232(5), 688-695.

Chan, J.L., & Abrahamson, M.J. (2003). Pharmacologic management of type 2 diabetes mellitus: Rationale for rational use of insulin. *Mayo Clinic Proceedings,* 78(4), 459-468.

Chau, D., & Edelman, S. (2001). Clinical management of diabetes in the elderly. *Clinical Diabetes,* 19(4), 172-175.

Chu, N.V., & Edelman, S. (2001). Diabetes and erectile dysfunction. *Clinical Diabetes,* 19(1), 45-47.

Clark, W.L. (2000). Beta cell replacement and islet cell transplantation. *Diabetes Self-Management,* 17(1), 52-54.

Clarke, K. (2002). New insulin therapy: No needles needed. *Nursing2002,* 32(5), 49-51.

Colwell, J.A., et al. (2000). Strategies for managing diabetes. *Patient Care for the Nurse Practitioner,* 3(9), 2-16.

Conlon, P.C. (2001). A practical approach to type 2 diabetes. *Nursing Clinics of North America, 36*(2), 193-202.

Corrigan, A.M., Pelletier, G., & Alexander, M. (Eds.). (2000). *Core curriculum for intravenous nursing.* Philadelphia: J.B. Lippincott.

Creviston, T., & Quinn, L. (2001). Exercise and physical activity in the treatment of type 2 diabetes. *Nursing Clinics of North America, 36*(2), 243-272.

Crump, V. (2004). Hyperglycemic crisis: Regaining control. *RN, 67*(4), 23-28.

Cryer, P.E., & Childs, B.P. (2002). Negotiating the barrier of hypoglycemia in diabetes. *Diabetes Spectrum, 15*(1), 20-27.

Cunningham, M.A. (2001). Glucose monitoring in type 2 diabetes. *Nursing Clinics of North America, 36*(2), 361-374.

Dagogo-Jack, S., & Alberti, K.G. (2002). Management of diabetes mellitus in surgical patients. *Diabetes Spectrum, 15*(1), 44-48.

Dahmen, R., Haspels, B., Koomen, B., et al. (2001). Therapeutic footwear for the neuropathic foot. *Diabetes Care, 24*(4), 705-709.

Dailey, G. (2002). Hypoglycemia in elderly patients treated with oral agents. *Practical Diabetology, 21*(2), 7-14.

Daly, A., et al. (2003). Diabetes medical nutrition therapy: Practical tips to improve outcomes. *Journal of the American Academy of Nurse Practitioners, 15*(5), 206-211.

Deedwania, P.C. (2000). Hypertension and diabetes. *Archives of Internal Medicine, 160*(11), 1585-1594.

Delaney, M.F., Zisman, A., & Kettyle, W.M. (2000). Diabetic ketoacidosis and hyperglycemic hyperosmolar nonketotic syndrome. *Endocrinology and Metabolism Clinics of North America, 29*(4), 683-705.

Devlin, J.T. (2001). Exercise therapy in the management of diabetes. *Practical Diabetology, 20*(1), 38-44.

Diabetic foot disorders: A clinical practice guideline. (2000). Available at http://acfas.org/diabeticpg.html.

Dinsmoor, R.S. (2000a). High blood sugar after meals: Why it matters. *Diabetes Self-Management, 17*(4), 46-49.

Dinsmoor, R.S. (2000b). Insulin resistance at the root of type 2 diabetes. *Diabetes Self-Management, 17*(3), 38-41.

Donovan, D.S. (2001). Gaining control: A guide to aggressive management of monotherapy failure. *Consultations in Primary Care, 41*(13), 22-31.

Dowell, M., et al. (2004). Economic and clinical disparities in hospitalized patients with type 2 diabetes. *Journal of Nursing Scholarship, 36*(1), 66-72.

El-Kebbi, I.M., et al. (2003). Association of younger age with poor glycemic control and obesity in urban African Americans with type 2 diabetes. *Archives of Internal Medicine, 163*(1), 69-75.

Ellison, J.M., et al. (2001). Rapid changes in postprandial blood glucose produce concentration differences at finger, forearm, and thigh sampling sites. *Diabetes Care, 25*(6), 961-964.

Fain, J. (2002). Delivering insulin 'round the clock. *Nursing2002, 32*(8), 54-56.

Farkas-Hirsch, R. (2000). All about hypoglycemia. *Diabetes Self-Management, 17*(1), 21-27.

Feet can last a lifetime. (2001). Available at http://www.niddk.nih.gov.

Fleming, D. (2000). Mightier than the syringe. *American Journal of Nursing, 100*(11), 44-48.

Flood, L., & Constance, A. (2002). Diabetes & exercise safety. *American Journal of Nursing, 102*(6), 47-55.

*Franz, M. (Ed.). (2001). *A core curriculum for diabetes educators.* Chicago: American Association of Diabetes Educators.

Fritschi, C. (2001). Preventive care of the diabetic foot. *Nursing Clinics of North America, 36*(2), 303-320.

Funnell, M.M., & Barlage, D.L. (2000). Oral diabetes drugs. *Nursing2000, 30*(11), 34-39.

Funnell, M.M., & Barlage, D.L. (2004). Managing diabetes with "Agent Oral." *Nursing2004, 34*(3), 36-43.

Gavin, J.R. (2001). The pathophysiology of type 2 diabetes. *Patient Care for the Nurse Practitioner, 4*(Suppl. Fall, 2001) 4-7.

Gehling, E. (2000). Injecting insulin 101. *Diabetes Self-Management, 17*(5), 7-15.

Gerritsen, M. (2000). Problems associated with subcutaneously implanted glucose sensors. *Diabetes Care, 22*(2), 143-145.

Gonsalves, M.Y. Coordinating care for patients with type 2 diabetes. *Patient Care for the Nurse Practitioner, 3*(9), 15-36.

Green, M.F., Zarrintaj, A., & Green, B.T. (2002). Diabetic foot: Evaluation and management. *Southern Medical Journal, 95*(1), 95-101.

Gregg, E.W., et al. (2002). Is diabetes associated with cognitive impairment and cognitive decline among older women? *Archives of Internal Medicine, 160*(2), 174-180.

Harris, M.I. (2001). Racial and ethnic differences in health care access and health outcomes for adults with type 2 diabetes. *Diabetes Care, 24*(3), 454-459.

Herbel, G., & Boyle, P. (2000). Hypoglycemia: Pathophysiology and treatment. *Endocrinology and Metabolism Clinics of North America, 29*(4), 725-743.

Hunt, D. (2002). Using evidence in practice: Foot care in diabetes. *Endocrinology and Metabolism Clinics of North America, 31*(3), 603-611.

Ingall, T.J. (2000). Preventing ischemic stroke: Current approaches to primary and secondary prevention. *Postgraduate Medicine, 107*(6), 34-50.

Inlow, S., Orsted, H., & Sibbald, R.G. (2000). Best practices for the prevention, diagnosis and treatment of diabetic foot ulcers. *Ostomy Wound Management, 46*(11), 55-67.

Insulin delivery systems for the management of diabetes. (2002). Available at http://www.novonordisk.com.

Insulin: New products, new strategies. (2002). Available at http://www.novonordisk.com.

Jacober, S., & Sowers, J.R. (2001). Management of diabetes in patients undergoing surgery. *Practical Diabetology, 201*(42), 7-14.

Jungheim, K., & Koschinsky, T. (2002). Glucose monitoring at the arm. *Diabetes Care, 25*(6), 956-960.

Kim, R.P., Edelman, S.V., & Kim, D.K. (2001). Musculoskeletal complications of diabetes mellitus. *Clinical Diabetes, 19*(3), 132-135.

King, D.S., & Wofford, M.R. (2000). Obesity and new-onset diabetes mellitus. Available at http://www.drugtopics.com.

Kissin, A., & Katzeff, H. L. (2002). New insulin therapies for the management of diabetes mellitus. *Practical Diabetology, 21*(1), 14-20.

Kulkarni, K. (2003). Managing type 2 diabetes. Available at http://www.clinicianreviews.com.

Lachuk, L., McGee, K.H., & Voris, J.C. (2002). Current guidelines for managing diabetes mellitus. *Federal Practitioner, 20*(11), 54-61.

Laffel, L. (2000). Sick-day management in type 1 diabetes. *Endocrinology and Metabolism Clinics of North America, 29*(4), 707-723.

Lenhard, M.J., & Reeves, G.D. (2001). Continuous subcutaneous insulin infusion. *Archives of Internal Medicine, 161*(19), 2293-2300.

Levetan, C.S., & Magee, M.F. (2000). Hospital management of diabetes. *Endocrinology and Metabolism Clinics of North America, 29*(4), 745-770.

Levin, M. (2002). Management of the diabetic foot: Preventing amputation. *Southern Medical Journal, 95*(1), 10-20.

Loon, N.R. (2003). Diabetic kidney disease: Preventing dialysis and transplantation. *Clinical Diabetes, 21*(2), 55-62.

Lorig, K. (2001). *Patient education: A practical approach* (3rd ed.). London: Sage Publications.

Lower, J. (2002). Facing neuro assessment fearlessly. *Nursing2002, 32*(2), 58-64.

McCloskey, J.C., & Bulechek, G.M. (Eds.). (2000). *Nursing interventions classification (NIC)* (3rd ed.). St. Louis: Mosby.

McCormick, J.L., & Deeg, M.A. (2000). Pharmacologic treatment of dyslipidemia. *American Journal of Nursing, 100*(2), 55-60.

Meece, J., & Campbell, R.K. (2002). Insulin lispro update. *The Diabetes Educator. 28*(2), 269-277.

Mokdad, A.H., et al. (2000). Diabetes trends in the U. S.: 1990-1998. *Diabetes Care, 23*(9), 1278-1283.

Mudaliar, S., & Edelman, S.V. (2001). Insulin therapy in type 2 diabetes. *Endocrinology and Metabolism Clinics of North America, 30*(4), 935-982.

Nath, C., & Ponte, C.D. (2000). Lessons learned about insulin therapy. *Nursing 2000, 30*(11), 40-45.

National Task Force on the Prevention and Treatment of Obesity. (2000). Overweight, obesity and health risk. *Archives of Internal Medicine, 160*(7), 898-904.

Neil, J.A. (2002). Assessing foot care knowledge in a rural population with diabetes. *Ostomy/Wound Management, 48*(1), 50-56.

Nurse Practitioner's Prescribing Reference. (2003). New York: Prescribing Reference, Inc.

Paty, B.W., & Hirsch, I. (2000). Erectile dysfunction in diabetes. *Practical Diabetology, 19*(2), 16-23.

Peragallo-Dittko, V. (2002a). Alternate site testing. *Practical Diabetology, 21*(4), 48-49.

Peragallo-Dittko, V. (2002b). Blood glucose monitoring update. *Diabetes Self-Management, 19*(1), 46-52.

Peragallo-Dittko, V. (2000c). How accurate is your meter? *Diabetes Self-Management, 17*(5), 78-85.

Plodkowski, R.A., & Edelman, S. (2001). Pre-surgical evaluation of diabetic patients. *Clinical Diabetes, 19*(1), 92-95.

Quinn, L. (2001a). Diabetes emergencies in patients with type 2 diabetes. *Nursing Clinics of North America, 36*(2), 341-360.

Quinn, L. (2001b). Type 2 diabetes: Epidemiology, pathophysiology, and diagnosis. *Nursing Clinics of North America, 36*(2), 175-192.

Quinn, L. (2002a). Pharmacologic treatment of the critically ill patient with diabetes. *Critical Care Clinics of North America, 14*(1), 87-98.

Quinn, L. (2002b). Pharmacologic management of the patient with diabetes. *Nursing Clinics of North America, 36*(2), 217-242.

Rao, S.H. (2001). Treating to target: A rational approach based on pathophysiology. *Consultations in Primary Care, 41*(13), 14-21.

Reasner, C.A. (2002). Aggressive control of type 2 diabetes using oral agents. Available at http://www.cliniciansCME.com.

Rezabek, K.M. (2001). Medical nutrition therapy in type 2 diabetes. *Nursing Clinics of North America, 36*(2), 203-216.

Robertson, K.E., Glazer, N.B., & Campbell, R.K. (2000). The latest development in insulin injection devices. *The Diabetes Educator, 26*(1), 135-152.

Robertson, R.P., et al. (2000). Pancreas and islet transplantation for patients with diabetes. *Diabetes Care, 23*(1), 112-116.

Sacks, D.B., et al. (2002). Guidelines and recommendations for laboratory analysis in the diagnosis and management of diabetes mellitus. *Clinical Chemistry, 48*(3), 436-472.

Safeer, R.S., & Cornell, M.O. (2000). The emerging role of HDL cholesterol. *Postgraduate Medicine, 108*(7), 87-98.

Saleh, M., & Grunberger, G. (2001). Hypoglycemia: An excuse for poor glycemic control? *Clinical Diabetes, 19*(4), 161-167.

Sammer, C. (2001). How should you respond to hypoglycemia? *Nursing2001, 31*(7), 48-50.

Seley, J. (2003).Giving the fingers a rest: Alternative site testing eases blood glucose monitoring. *American Journal of Nursing, 103*(3), 73-77.

Seley, J.J. (2001). The role of insulin in type 2 diabetes. *Patient Care for the Nurse Practitioner, 4*(Suppl. Fall, 2001), 15-20.

Singri, N., Ahya, S., & Levin, M.L. (2003). Acute renal failure. *Journal of the American Medical Association, 289*(6), 747-751.

Skelly, A. (2002). Elderly patients with diabetes. *American Journal of Nursing, 102*(2), 15-16.

Skyler, J. (2001). Microvascular complications: Retinopathy and nephropathy. *Endocrinology and Metabolism Clinics of North America, 29*(4), 833-856.

Slagle, M. (2002). Medication update: Diabetes mellitus. *Southern Medical Journal, 95*(1), 50-55.

Spanheimer, R.G. (2001). Cardiovascular risk in diabetes. *Postgraduate Medicine, 109*(4), 26-36.

Stevens, R.B., Matsumoto, S., & Marsh, C.L. (2001). Is islet cell transplantation a realistic therapy for treatment of type 1 diabetes in the near future? *Clinical Diabetes, 19*(1), 51-60.

Strock, E. (2001). Strategies for patient care and education. *Consultations in Primary Care, 41*(13), 6-13.

Sweny, S. (2002). Toward a better understanding of diabetic nephropathy. *The Diabetes Educator, 28*(1), 72-75.

Tang, W.H.W., & Young, J.B. (2001). Cardiomyopathy and heart failure in diabetes. *Endocrinology and Metabolism Clinics of North America, 29*(4), 1031-1046.

Tkacs, N.C. (2002). Hypoglycemia unawareness. *American Journal of Nursing, 102*(2), 34-41.

Tripp-Reimer, T., et al. (2001). Cultural barriers to care: Inverting the problem. *Diabetes Spectrum, 14*(1), 13-22.

Umpierrez, G.E., Murphy, B.E., & Kitabchi, A.E. (2002). Diabetic ketoacidosis and hyperglycemic hyperosmolar syndrome. *Diabetes Spectrum, 15*(1), 28-36.

U.S. Environmental Protection Agency. (2005). Medical waste. Retrieved February 3, 2005 from http://www.epa.gov/epaoswer/other/medical.

Valentine, V. (2000). When diabetes affects the stomach. *Diabetes Self-Management, 17*(4), 52-56.

Valentine, V. (2002). Using a laser to make a point. *Nursing2002, 32*(110), 56-57.

Valk, G.D., Kriegsman, D.M.W., & Assendelft, W.J.J. (2002). Patient education for preventing food ulceration: A systematic review. *Endocrinology and Metabolism Clinics of North America, 31*(3), 634-658.

van Bijsterveld, O.O. (Ed.). (2000). *Diabetic retinopathy*. London: Martin Dunitz Ltd.

Vijan, S., & Hayward, R.A. (2003). Treatment of hypertension in type 2 diabetes mellitus: Blood pressure goals, choice of agents, and setting priorities in diabetes care. *Annals of Internal Medicine, 138*(7), 593-602.

Vinik, A.I., et al. (2003). Diabetic autonomic neuropathy. *Diabetes Care, 26*(5), 1553-1579.

Watkins, P.J. (2003). Cardiovascular disease, hypertension, and lipids. *British Medical Journal, 326*(7394), 874-976.

White, J.R., & Campbell, R.K. (2000). Dangerous and common drug interactions in patients with diabetes mellitus. *Endocrinology and Metabolism Clinics of North America, 29*(4), 789-803.

White, J.A., & Hirsh, I.R. (2000). Nonhypoglycemic drug reactions of agents used to treat diabetes. *Endocrinology and Metabolism Clinics of North America, 29*(4), 803-811.

White, J.R., & Campbell, R.K. (2001). Inhaled insulin: An overview. *Clinical Diabetes, 19*(1), 13-16.

Williams, A.S. (2000). Helpful odds and ends. *Diabetes Self-Management, 17*(2), 22-27.

Wilson, B.A., Shannon, M.T., & Stang, C.L. (2002). *Nurse's drug guide*. Upper Saddle River, N J: Prentice Hall.

Wilson, P.W.F. (2001). Diabetes mellitus and coronary artery disease. *Endocrinology and Metabolism Clinics of North America, 29*(4), 857-881.

Wood, F. (2002). Ethnic differences in exercise among adults with diabetes. *Western Journal of Nursing, 24*(5), 502-515.

INTERNET REFERENCES

U.S. Department of Health and Human Services, Bureau of Primary Health Care: The LEAP Program:
http://www.bphc.hsra.gov/leap

Centers for Disease Control and Prevention:
http://www.cdc.gov/health/diabetes.htm

Cell Robotics International:
  http://www.cellrobitics.com/perslasette.html
Diabeteswebsite.com:
  http://www.diabeteswebsite.com
U.S. Environmental Protection Agency:
  http://www.epa.gov/epaoswer/other/medical/dispose1.pdf
GlucoWatch: Automatic Glucose Biographer:
  http://www.glucowatch.com

National Institutes of Diabetes and Digestive and Kidney Diseases:
  http://www.niddk.nih.gov
Diabetes Prevention Program:
  http://www.gwu.edu/dpp/index.htmlvdoc
Discount Diabetic Supplies:
  http://www.diabeticpromotions.com
Diabetic Supplies.com:
  http://www.diabeticsupplies.com

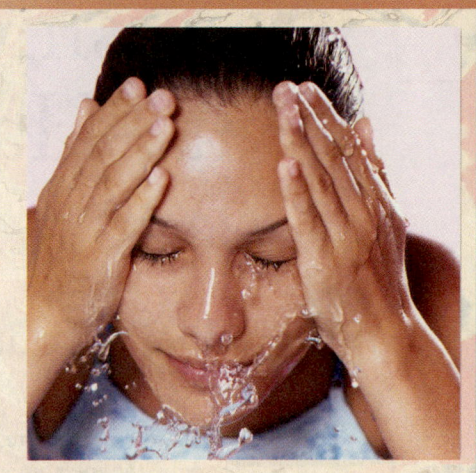

PROBLEMS of PROTECTION

Management of Clients with Problems of the Skin, Hair, and Nails

Assessment of the Skin, Hair, and Nails

JANICE CUZZELL • M. LINDA WORKMAN

The integumentary system is composed of the skin, hair, and nails. This system is the first line of defense in protecting the inner organs from the external environment. The skin is the largest organ of the body, and it plays a major role in homeostasis. Not only is it a barrier to organisms, but it also helps to regulate body temperature and maintains fluid and electrolyte balance. Changes in the skin can communicate information about a person's health and well-being.

Emotional stress, systemic disease, and skin injury or disease can alter the function, appearance, and texture of the skin. Therefore examine the skin for important clues about the client's health. Because the skin has many sensory receptors, the client can report subjective skin sensations that might indicate specific health problems. The sensory function of the skin allows the use of touch as a therapeutic intervention to provide comfort, relieve pain, and communicate caring.

ANATOMY AND PHYSIOLOGY REVIEW

Structure of the Skin

As shown in Figure 69-1, the skin has three layers: fat, dermis, and epidermis. Each layer has unique properties that contribute to the skin's ability to maintain its complex functions.

SUBCUTANEOUS FAT (ADIPOSE TISSUE)

The innermost layer of the skin, which lies over muscle and bone, is the site for fat formation and storage. Fat cells serve as an energy reserve in the event extra calories are needed to power the body. These cells also act as heat insulators for the body. They absorb shock and protect against injury by padding internal structures. Fat distribution varies with body area, age, and gender. Many blood vessels go through the fatty layer and extend into the dermal layer, forming capillary networks that supply nutrients and remove wastes.

DERMIS (CORIUM)

Above the fat layer lies the **dermis**, a layer of connective tissue that contains no cells. The dermis is composed of collagen and elastic fibers that are interwoven to give the skin both flexibility and strength.

Collagen, the main component of dermal tissue, is a protein formed by dermal cells called fibroblasts. Collagen production increases in areas of tissue injury and helps to form scar tissue. Fibroblasts also produce **ground substance**, a lubricant composed of protein and sugar groups that surrounds the dermal cells and fibers and contributes to the skin's normal suppleness and turgor.

The elasticity of the skin depends on both the amount and quality of the elastic fibers, which are scattered among the collagen fibers. The major component of the elastic fiber is **elastin.**

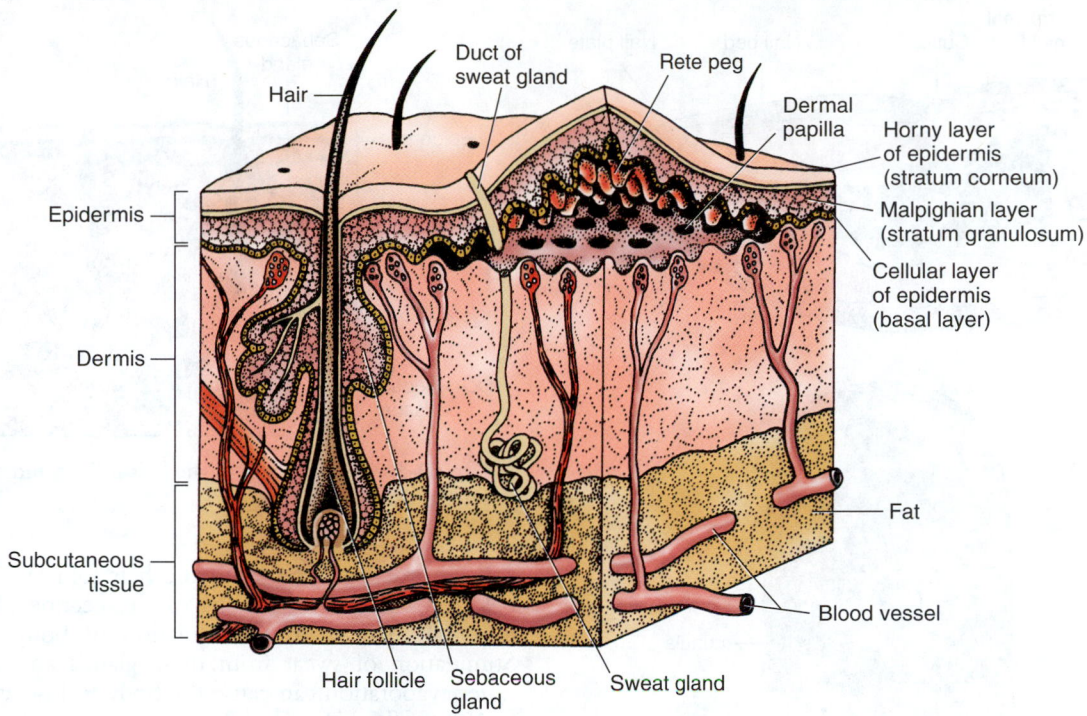

Figure 69-1 ■ Anatomy of the skin.

The dermis houses a network of capillaries and lymph vessels in which the exchange of oxygen and heat occurs. The dermis is also rich in sensory nerves that transmit the sensations of touch, pressure, temperature, pain, and itch.

EPIDERMIS

The outermost skin layer, the **epidermis,** is anchored to the dermis by fingerlike projections of dermal tissue **(dermal papillae).** The fingers of epidermal tissue that project into the dermis are called **rete pegs.** The epidermis is less than 1 mm thick, but it is the protective barrier between the body and the environment.

The epidermis does not have a separate blood supply. It receives its nutrients by diffusion from the many blood vessels in the dermal layer through a porous basement membrane at the dermal-epidermal junction. Attached to the basement membrane are the keratinocytes. The basal cells (those keratinocytes capable of cell division and located closest to the basement membrane) continuously divide to form new cells. Older keratinocytes are pushed upward to form the stratified layers of the epithelium **(malpighian layers).** As keratinocytes move toward the surface, they flatten and eventually die. The outermost skin layer, the **stratum corneum** (horny layer), is composed of these dead cells. **Keratin,** the protein produced by keratinocytes, makes the horny layer waterproof. A keratinocyte takes about 28 to 45 days to move from the basement membrane to the skin surface, where it is shed (exfoliated).

Vitamin D is activated in the epidermis by ultraviolet (UV) light. It is then distributed by the blood to other body areas.

Melanocytes are pigment-producing cells found at the level of the basement membrane in a ratio of about one melanocyte for every 10 keratinocytes. These cells give color to the skin and account for the racial differences in skin tone. Darker skin tones are not caused by increased numbers of melanocytes; rather, the size of the pigment granules (melanin) contained in each cell determines the color. Freckles, birthmarks, and age spots are caused by patches of melanin within the skin. UV light stimulates the production of melanin, which protects against the harmful effects of sun exposure. Melanin production increases locally in response to endocrine changes or inflammation. Specialized cells called Langerhans cells also are present in the epidermis. If the skin is damaged, these cells engulf any foreign substances (antigens) that invade the body. These cells then alert the immune system to the presence of the antigen.

Structure of the Skin Appendages
HAIR

Hair, a remnant of the thick protective pelt worn by most mammals, is mainly a cosmetic feature for modern humans. Hair growth varies with race, gender, age, and genetic predisposition. Individual hairs can differ in both structure and rate of growth, depending on body location.

Hair follicles are located in the dermal layer of the skin but are actually extensions of the epidermal layer (see Figure 69-1). Within each hair follicle, a round column of keratin forms the hair shaft. Hair keratin contains more sulfur than do skin cells, which toughens the hair shaft as it forms. Hair color is genetically determined by a person's rate of melanin production.

Hair growth occurs in cycles; a growth phase (anagen) is followed by a resting phase (telogen). Local and systemic stressors can alter the growth cycle and result in temporary hair loss. Permanent baldness, such as male pattern baldness, is genetic in origin and is seldom influenced by personal or environmental factors.

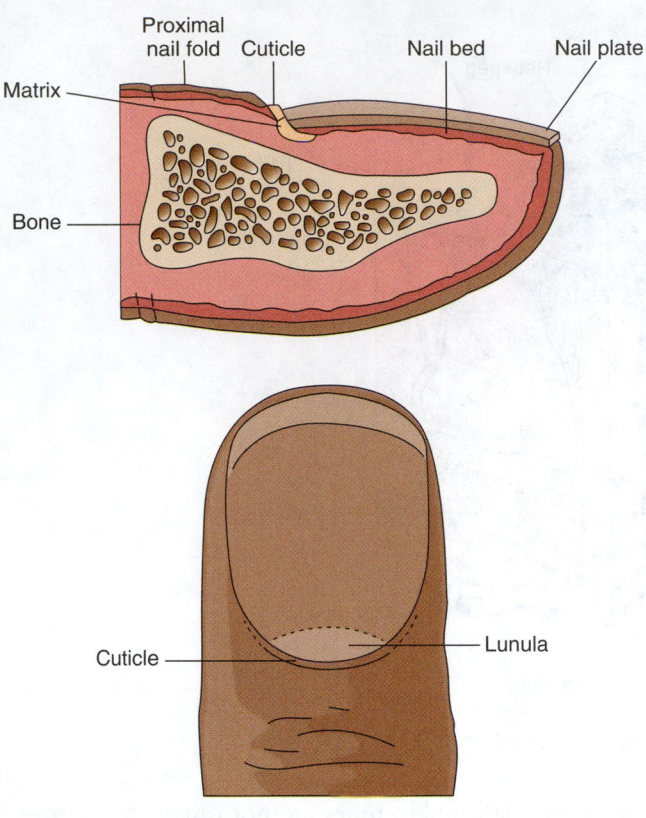

Figure 69-2 ■ Anatomy of the nail.

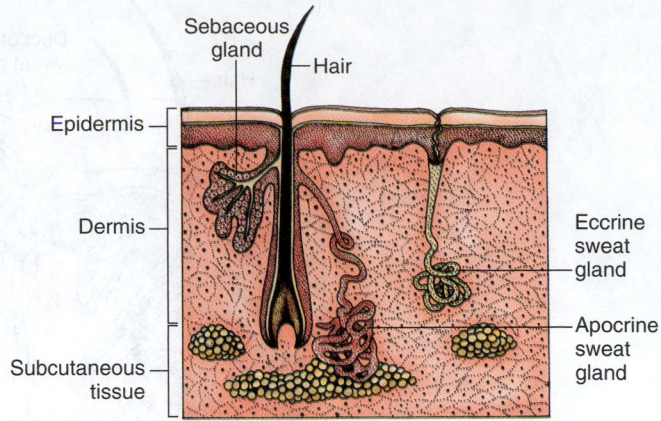

Figure 69-3 ■ Anatomy of the hair follicle and sebaceous and sweat glands.

NAILS

Well-groomed fingernails and toenails have cosmetic value and serve as useful tools with which to scrape and grasp. Like hair follicles, the nails are extensions of the keratin-producing epidermal layers of the skin.

The white crescent-shaped portion of the nail at the lower end of the nail plate **(lunula)** reflects the underlying nail matrix, where nail keratin is formed and nail growth begins (Figure 69-2). Unlike hair growth, which is cyclic, nail growth is a continuous but slow process. Total replacement of a fingernail requires 3 to 4 months. Total replacement of a toenail may take up to 12 months.

The **cuticle,** a layer of keratin at the nail fold, attaches the nail plate to the soft tissue of the nail fold. The nail body is translucent, and the pinkish hue reflects a rich blood supply beneath the nail surface. Nail growth and appearance are often altered during systemic disease or serious illness.

GLANDS

SEBACEOUS GLANDS. The sebaceous glands are distributed over the entire skin surface, except for the palms of the hand and soles of the feet. Most sebaceous glands are directly connected to the hair follicles (Figure 69-3). The sebaceous glands of the eyelids, nipple areolae, and genitalia are freestanding.

Sebaceous glands produce **sebum,** a mildly bacteriostatic, fat-containing substance. Sebum lubricates the skin and reduces water loss from the skin surface.

SWEAT GLANDS. The skin has two types of sweat glands: eccrine and apocrine. Eccrine sweat glands arise from the epithelial cells. They are found over the entire skin surface and are not associated with the hair follicle. The odorless, colorless, isotonic secretions of the eccrine glands are an important factor in the regulation of body temperature. Stimulation of sweat from these glands and the resultant water evaporation can cause the body to lose as much as 10 to 12 L of fluid in a single day.

Apocrine sweat glands are in direct contact with the hair follicle. They are found mostly in the axillae, perineal, nipple areolae, and periumbilicus body areas. The interaction of skin bacteria with the secretions of the apocrine glands causes the distinctive body odor.

Functions of the Skin

The skin is a complex organ responsible for the regulation of many body functions throughout the life span (Table 69-1). In addition to the skin's protective and regulatory functions, its location on the outside of the body makes it an important way to communicate a client's state of health and body image.

Skin Changes Associated with Aging

The process of aging begins at birth. As changes in physiology progress with aging, the skin also undergoes age-related changes in both structure and function (Chart 69-1). Figures 69-4 through 69-15 show some common age-related skin changes.

Individual differences exist in how quickly and to what degree the skin ages. Although genetic background, hormonal changes, and systemic disease may change the appearance of the skin over time, chronic sun exposure is the single most important factor leading to degeneration of the skin components (Figure 69-16).

ASSESSMENT TECHNIQUES

History

Before examining the skin, take an accurate history from the client so that actual and potential skin problems can be readily identified. Chart 69-2 lists the best practices for obtaining a history from a client with a skin problem. Begin by gathering information about skin changes and current skin care practices.

TABLE 69-1 Functions of the Skin

Epidermis	Dermis	Subcutaneous Tissue
Protection		
Keratin provides protection from injury by corrosive materials	Provides fibroblasts for wound healing.	Mechanical shock absorber.
Inhibits proliferation of microorganisms because of dry external surface	Provides mechanical strength. ■ Collagen fibers ■ Elastic fibers ■ Ground substance	Energy reserve.
Mechanical strength through intercellular bonds		
Homeostasis (Water Balance)		
Low permeability to water and electrolytes prevents systemic dehydration and electrolyte loss	Lymphatic and vascular tissues respond to inflammation, injury, and infection.	
Temperature Regulation		
Eccrine sweat glands allow dissipation of heat through evaporation of sweat secreted onto the skin surface	Cutaneous vasculature, through dilation or construction, promotes or inhibits heat conduction from the skin surface.	Fat cells act as insulators and assist in retention of body heat.
Sensory Organ		
Transmits a variety of sensations through the neuroreceptor system	Encloses an extensive network of nerve endings for relaying sensations to the brain.	Contains large pressure receptors.
Vitamin Synthesis		
7-Dehydrocholesterol is present in large concentrations in malpighian cells; photoconversion to vitamin D takes place	No function.	No function.
Psychosocial		
Body image alterations occur with many epidermal diseases, such as generalized psoriasis	Body image alterations occur with many dermal diseases, such as scleroderma.	Body image alterations may result from increases, decreases, and redistribution of body fat stores.

CHART 69-1

NURSING FOCUS on the OLDER ADULT
Changes in the Integumentary System Related to Aging

Physical Changes	Clinical Findings	Changes in Functional Ability
Epidermis		
Decreased thickness in epidermal layer	Increased skin transparency and fragility	
Decreased epidermal mitotic activity	Delayed wound healing	Decreased cell replacement
Decreased epidermal mitotic homeostasis	Skin hyperplasia, such as hyperkeratoses and skin cancers (especially in sun-exposed areas)	
Increased epidermal permeability	Increased susceptibility to irritant reactions	Decreased barrier function
Decreased number of Langerhans cells	Decreased cutaneous inflammatory response	Decreased injury response
Decreased number of active melanocytes	Increased sensitivity to sun exposure	
Hyperplasia of melanocytes at the dermal-epidermal junction (especially in sun-exposed areas)	Mottled hyperpigmentation and hypopigmentation (e.g., liver spots, age spots)	
Decreased vitamin D production	Increased susceptibility to osteomalacia	Decreased vitamin D production
Flattening of the dermal-epidermal junction	Increased susceptibility to shearing forces, with resultant blisters, purpura, skin tears, and pressure-related skin problems	
Dermis		
Decreased dermal blood flow	Increased susceptibility to dry skin (xerosis)	Decreased chemical clearance
Decreased vasomotor responsiveness	Increased thermoregulatory alterations (predisposition to heat stroke and hypothermia)	Decreased vascular responsiveness
Decreased dermal thickness	Paper-thin, transparent skin with an increased susceptibility to trauma	Decreased injury response
Degeneration of elastic fibers	Decreased tone and elasticity (wrinkles)	Body image alterations
Benign proliferation of capillaries	Cherry hemangiomas	
Abnormal nerve endings	Alterations in sensory perception	Decreased sensory perception

Continued

CHART 69-1

NURSING FOCUS on the OLDER ADULT
Changes in the Integumentary System Related to Aging—*cont'd*

Physical Changes	Clinical Findings	Changes in Functional Ability
Subcutaneous Layer		
Redistribution of adipose tissue	"Bags," cellulite, double chin, abdominal apron	Body-image alterations
Thinning of subcutaneous fat layer	Increased susceptibility to hypothermia	Decreased thermoregulation
	Decreased resistance to mechanical injury (especially pressure necrosis)	Decreased injury response
Hair		
Decreased number of hair follicles and rate of growth	Increased hair thinning	Decreased cell replacement
Decreased number of active melanocytes in follicle	Gradual loss of hair color (graying)	Body image alterations
Nails		
Decreased rate of growth	Increased susceptibility to fungal infections	Decreased cell replacement
Decreased blood flow beneath the nail bed	Longitudinal nail ridges	
Glands		
Decreased sebum production despite sebaceous gland hyperplasia	Increased size of pores (especially on nose); large comedones in malar region	Decreased sebum production
Decreased eccrine and apocrine gland activity	Increased susceptibility to dry skin	
	Decreased perspiration, leading to decreased cooling effect	Decreased sweat production
	Decreased need for antiperspirants	Decreased thermoregulation

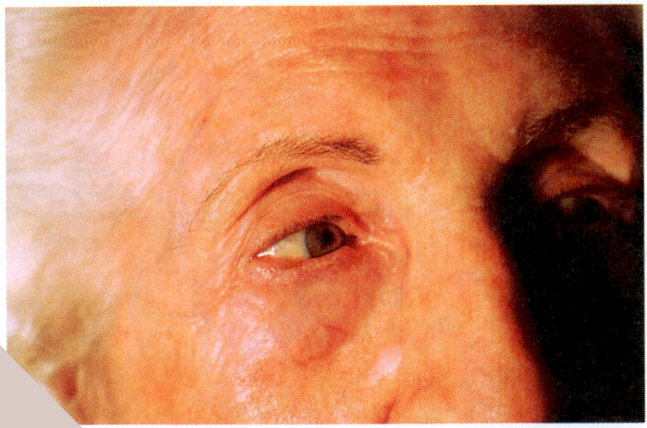

Figure 69-4 ■ Eyelid eversion.

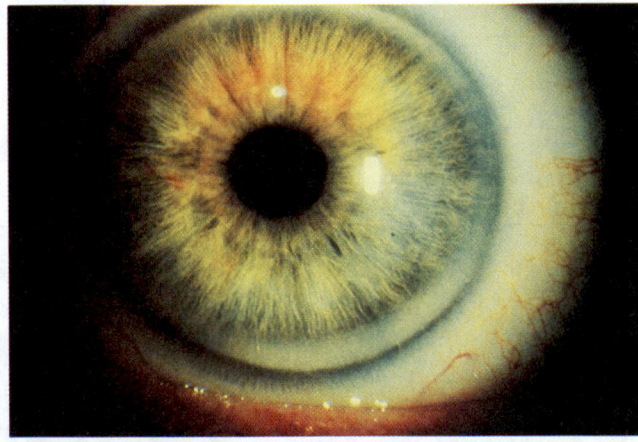

Figure 69-6 ■ Arcus senilis of the iris.

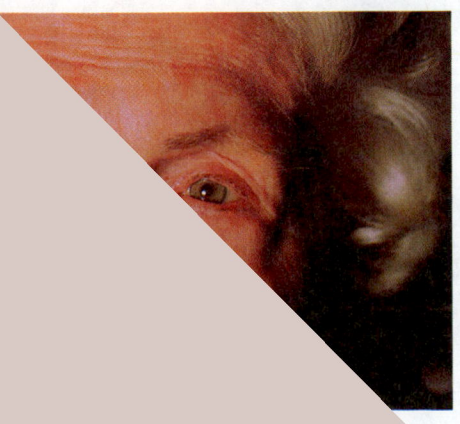

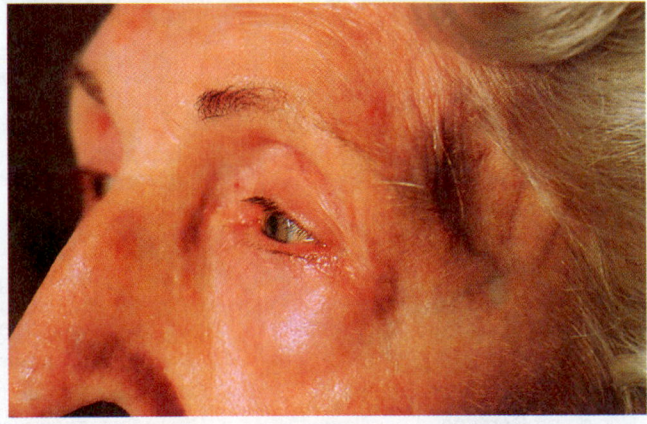

Figure 69-7 ■ Changes in the body contour: "bags" under the eyes.

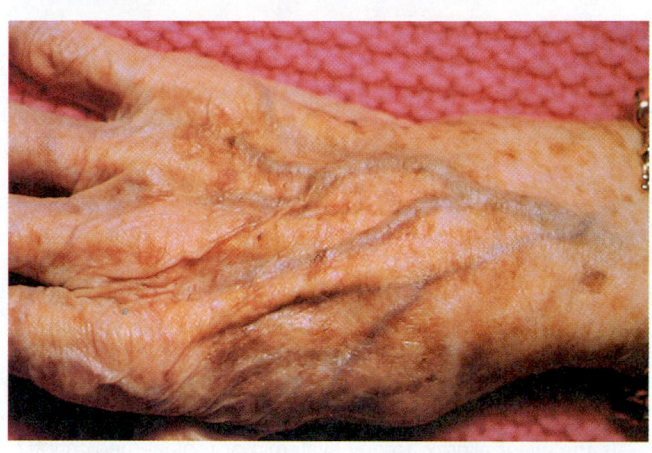

Figure 69-8 ■ Paper-thin, transparent skin.

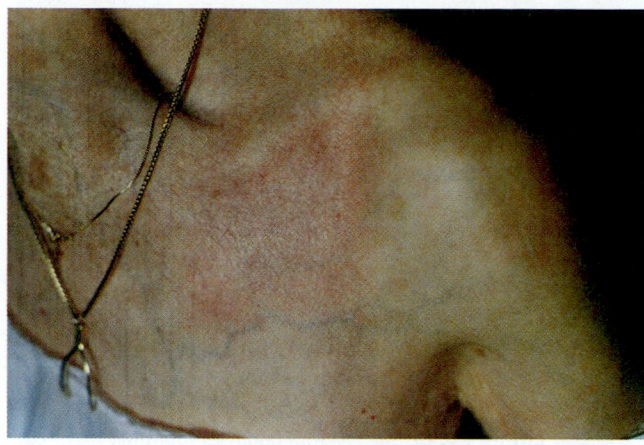

Figure 69-11 ■ Xerosis (dry skin).

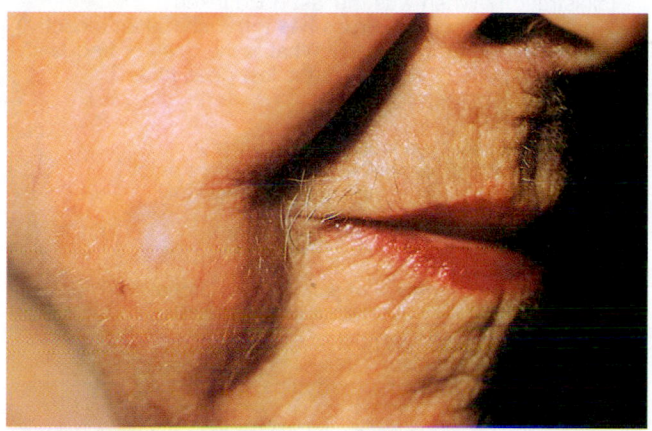

Figure 69-9 ■ Wrinkles.

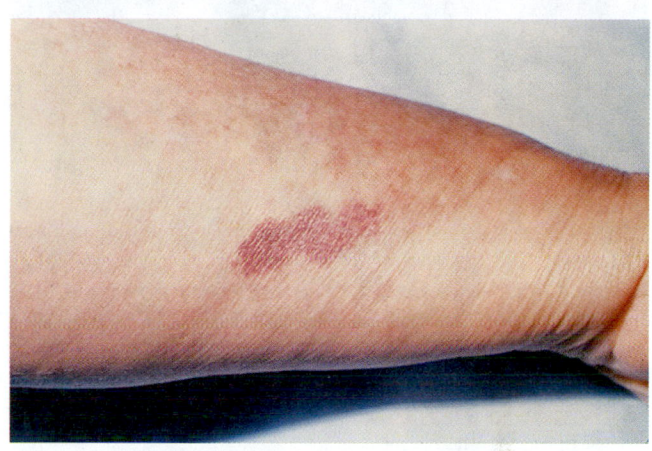

Figure 69-12 ■ Actinic purpura.

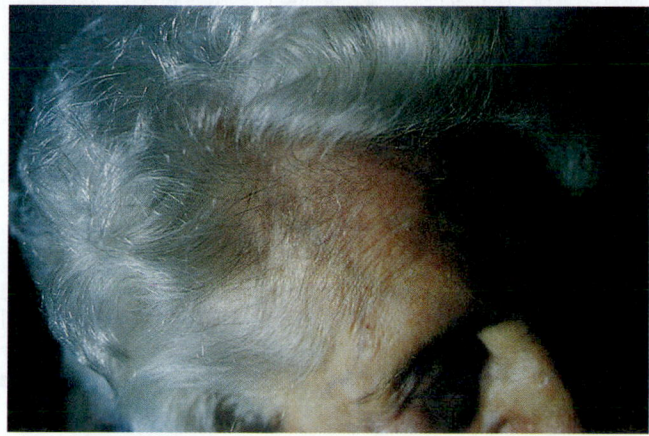

Figure 69-10 ■ Graying and thinning of the hair.

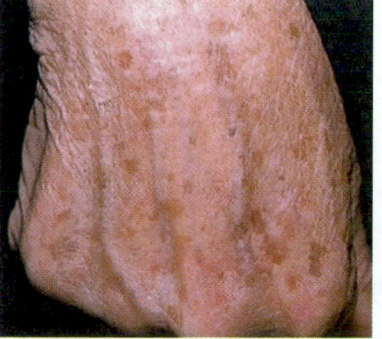

Figure 69-13 ■ Actinic lentigo (liver spots).

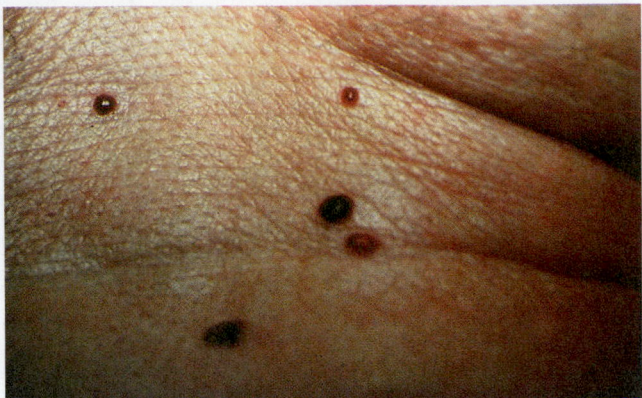

Figure 69-14 ■ Senile (cherry) angiomas.

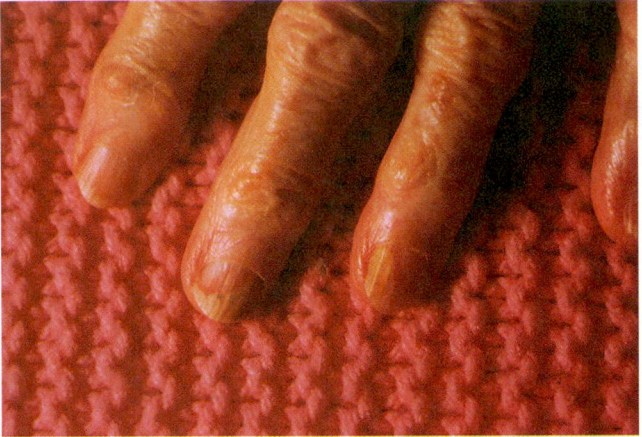

Figure 69-15 ■ Nail changes: longitudinal ridges and thickening.

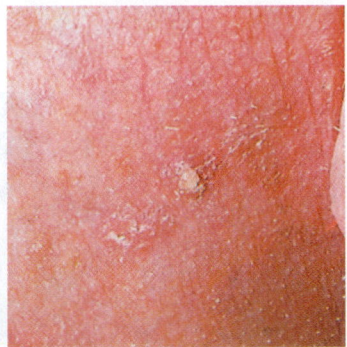

Figure 69-16 ■ Actinic (solar) keratosis.

DEMOGRAPHIC DATA

Obtain demographic data from clients with actual or potential skin disorders. Age is important because many changes in the integumentary system are normal manifestations of the aging process.

Race and nationality can also be important. Some variations in the appearance of skin are normal among clients of specific races and ethnicities but are abnormal for clients of other races or ethnicities.

Information regarding the client's occupation and hobbies can provide clues to chronic skin exposure to chemi-

---

CHART 69-2

BEST PRACTICE for
Obtaining an Accurate Nursing History of the Client with a Skin Problem

Medical-Surgical History
- Does the client have any current or previous medical problems?
- Has the client undergone any recent or previous surgical procedures?

Family History
- Is there any family tendency toward chronic skin problems?
- Do any members of the immediate family have recent skin complaints?

Medication History
- Is the client allergic to any systemic or topical medication? If so, have the client describe the reaction.
- What prescription drugs has the client taken recently? When was the drug started? What is the dose or frequency of administration? When was the last dose taken?
- What over-the-counter drugs has the client taken recently? When was the drug started? What is the dose or frequency of administration? When was the last dose taken?

Social History
- What is the client's occupation?
- What recreational activities does the client enjoy?
- Has the client traveled recently?
- What is the client's nutritional status?

Current Health Problem
- When did the client first notice the skin problem?
- Where on the body did the problem begin?
- Has the problem gotten better or worse?
- Has a similar skin condition ever occurred before? If so, have the client describe the typical course and how it was treated.
- Is the problem associated with any of the following: itching, burning, stinging, numbness, pain, fever, nausea and vomiting, diarrhea, sore throat, cold, stiff neck, new foods, new soaps or cosmetics, new clothing or bed linens, or stressful situations?
- Does anything seem to make the problem worse (e.g., sun exposure, medications, heat or cold, and menses)?
- Does anything seem to make the problem better?

---

cals, irritants, abrasive substances, and other environmental factors that can contribute to skin problems.

FAMILY HISTORY AND GENETIC RISK

Many skin disorders have a familial predisposition or can be inherited. Therefore explore any family tendency toward chronic skin problems. Ask about all immediate family members' current health status to identify a communicable disease that has been transferred between family members.

PERSONAL HISTORY

Take the client's medical history, including previous or current illnesses and surgical procedures. This information helps to determine whether skin changes are a manifestation of an underlying systemic disorder.

MEDICATION HISTORY

Skin reactions to systemic drugs are common. Ask the client about any recent use of prescription and over-the-counter (OTC) drugs (e.g., laxatives, antacids, and cold remedies). Determine when each drug was started, the dose and frequency of the drug, and the time the last dose was taken. A drug history also helps identify skin changes that result from the treatment of other health problems, such as the changes that occur with long-term steroid or anticoagulant therapy.

DIET HISTORY

Document the client's weight, height, body build, and food preferences. Poor nutrition, especially protein deficiencies, vitamin deficiencies, and obesity, can increase the client's risk for skin lesions and delay wound healing. Fat-free diets and chronic alcoholism can lead to vitamin deficiencies and related skin changes. Some skin diseases, such as chronic urticaria and acne, may be worsened by certain foods or food additives.

SOCIOECONOMIC STATUS

Ask the client about his or her social and economic background to identify environmental factors that might contribute to skin disease. Recent travel may be a source of skin infections or unusual lesions.

If the client is well tanned, ask about the amount of time spent in the sun and tanning booths and whether he or she has any skin problems from sun exposure.

Skin problems related to poor hygiene are common. Ask about living conditions, bathing practices, and the availability of running water.

CURRENT HEALTH PROBLEMS

If a skin problem is identified, obtain more information about the specific problem, such as the following:

- When did the client first notice the rash or skin change?
- Where on the body did the rash begin?
- Has the problem improved or become worse?

If a similar problem has occurred before, ask the client to describe the course of the skin lesion and how it was treated. Try to link the problem with specific symptoms, such as itching, burning, numbness, pain, fever, sore throat, stiff neck, or nausea and vomiting. Ask the client to identify anything that seems to make the problem better or worse.

Skin Assessment

INSPECTION

Skin changes may be related to specific skin diseases and may also reflect an underlying systemic disorder. By using skin assessment skills, you are in a unique position to identify clues about a client's state of health.

A thorough assessment of the skin is best performed with the client partially or completely undressed. Incorporate skin examination for actual or potential impairments into the routine part of daily care while bathing or assisting the client.

Inspect the client's skin surfaces in a well-lighted room; natural or bright fluorescent lighting enhances the visibility of subtle skin changes. Although no special equipment is needed, use a penlight for close inspection of lesions and to illuminate the mouth.

Assess each skin surface systematically, including the scalp, hair, nails, and mucous membranes. Give particular attention to the skin-fold areas. The moist, warm environment of skin folds can harbor organisms, such as yeast or bacteria. Observe and document the following features:

- Obvious changes in color and vascularity
- Presence or absence of moisture
- Edema
- Skin lesions
- Skin integrity

Check the cleanliness of the various body areas to determine whether the client's self-care activities need to be evaluated.

Color

Skin color is affected by a number of factors, including blood flow, oxygenation, body temperature, and pigment production. In addition to these factors, the wide variation in natural skin tones may require different techniques for clients who have darker skin. (See Cultural Considerations, p. 1571, for suggestions for assessing clients with darker skin.)

Describe changes in skin color by their appearance (Table 69-2). Document changes in color, and describe whether the changes are generalized or localized. Color changes can be seen most easily in the areas of least pigmentation, such as the oral mucosa, sclera, nail beds, and the palms and soles. Inspect these areas to help confirm more subtle color changes of general body areas.

Lesions

Skin disease is clinically described in terms of primary and secondary lesions (Figure 69-17). **Primary lesions** are an initial reaction to a problem that alters one of the structural components of the skin. **Secondary lesions** are changes in the appearance of the primary lesion. These changes occur with progression of an underlying disease or in response to a topical or systemic therapeutic intervention.

For example, acute dermatitis often occurs as primary vesicles with associated **pruritus** (itching). Secondary lesions in the form of crusts occur as the client scratches, the vesicles are opened, and the exudate dries. With chronic dermatitis, the skin often becomes **lichenified** (thickened) because of the client's continual rubbing of the area to relieve itching.

Describe lesions in terms of their color, size, location, and configuration. Document whether the lesions occur as isolated changes or are grouped and form a distinct pattern. Table 69-3 defines terms commonly used to describe lesions.

Assess each lesion for the following ABCD features that are associated with skin cancer:

A Asymmetry of shape
B Border irregularity
C Color variation within one lesion
D Diameter greater than 6 mm

A client who has a lesion with one or more of the ABCD features should be evaluated by a dermatologist or surgeon.

In describing the location of lesions, determine whether they are generalized or localized. If the lesions are localized, identify the specific body areas involved. This information is important because some diseases have a specific pattern of skin lesions. Involvement of only the sun-exposed areas of the body is important information when a possible cause is being considered. Rashes limited to the skin fold areas (e.g., on the axillae, beneath the breasts, in the groin) may reflect problems related to friction, heat, and excessive moisture.

TABLE 69-2 Common Alterations in Skin Color

Alteration	Underlying Cause	Location	Significance
White (pallor)	Decreased hemoglobin level Decreased blood flow to the skin (vaso-constriction)	Conjunctivae Mucous membranes Nail beds Palms and soles Lips	Anemia Shock or blood loss Chronic vascular compromise Sudden emotional upset Edema
	Genetically determined defect of the melanocyte (decreased pigmentation)	Generalized	Albinism
	Acquired patchy loss of pigmentation	Localized	Vitiligo, tinea versicolor
Yellow-orange	Increased total serum bilirubin level (jaundice)	Generalized Mucous membranes Sclera	Increased hemolysis of red blood cells Liver disorders
	Increased serum carotene level (carotenemia)	Perioral Palms and soles Ears and nose Absent in sclera and mucous membranes	Increased ingestion of carotene-containing foods (carrots) Pregnancy Thyroid deficiency Diabetes
	Increased urochrome level	Generalized Absent in sclera and mucous membranes	Chronic renal failure (uremia)
Red (erythema)	Increased blood flow to the skin (vasodilation)	Generalized	Generalized inflammation (e.g., erythroderma)
		Localized (to area of involvement)	Localized inflammation (e.g., sunburn, cellulitis, trauma, and rashes)
		Face, cheeks, nose, upper chest Area of exposure	Fever, increased alcohol intake Exposure to cold
Blue	Increase in deoxygenated blood (cyanosis)	Nail beds Mucous membranes Generalized	Cardiopulmonary disease Methemoglobinemia
	Bleeding from vessels into tissue: • Petechiae (1-3 mm) • Ecchymosis (>3 mm)	Localized Localized	Thrombocytopenia Increased blood vessel fragility
Reddish blue	Increased overall amount of hemoglobin Decreased peripheral circulation	Generalized Distal extremities, nose	Polycythemia vera Inadequate tissue perfusion
Brown	Increased melanin production	Localized (to area of involvement) Pressure points, areolae, palmar creases, and genitalia Face, areolae, vulva, and linea nigra	Chronic inflammation Exposure to sunlight Addison's disease Pregnancy; oral contraceptives (melasma)
	Café au lait spots (tan-brown patches) • <6 spots • >6 spots	Localized Generalized	Nonpathogenic Possible neurofibromatosis
	Melanin and hemosiderin deposits (bronze or grayish tan color)	Distal lower extremities Exposed areas or generalized	Chronic venous stasis Hemochromatosis

Edema

The presence of edema causes the skin to appear shiny, **taut** (tightly stretched), and paler than uninvolved skin. During skin inspection, document the location, distribution, and color of any areas of edema.

Skin elasticity is also affected by edema. Using moderate pressure, place the tip of the index finger against edematous tissue to determine the degree of indentation, or pitting (see Chapters 14 and 15).

Moisture

Examine skin for moisture content, noting the thickness and consistency of secretions. Normally, increased moisture in the form of sweat occurs with increased activity or elevated environmental temperatures. Dampness of skin fold areas is common because of decreased air circulation where the skin surfaces touch. Excess moisture can cause eventual skin breakdown in bedridden and debilitated clients.

Overly dry skin can be caused by factors such as a dry environment, poor skin lubrication, inadequate fluid intake, and the normal processes of aging. Dry skin usually has scaling of the stratum corneum. Dry skin may be especially marked in areas of limited circulation, such as the feet and lower legs. Dry skin becomes a problem for most adults during the winter months, when the air contains less moisture, and in the hospital environment, where humidity is often poorly controlled.

Vascular Markings

Vascular changes are classified as normal or abnormal, depending on the cause. Normal vascular markings include birthmarks, cherry angiomas (see Figure 69-14), spider angiomas, and venous stars (Table 69-4). Bleeding into the tissue is abnormal and results in purpuric lesions: petechiae and ecchymosis.

Petechiae are small, reddish purple lesions (<0.5 mm in di-

PRIMARY LESIONS

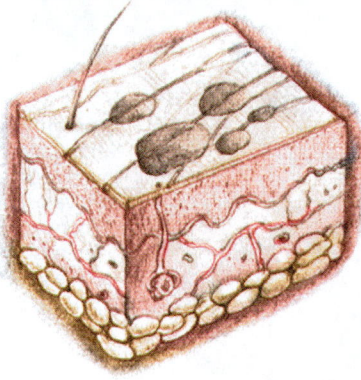

Macules (such as *freckles, flat moles, or rubella*) are flat lesions of less than 1 cm in diameter. Their color is different from that of the surrounding skin—most often white, red, or brown.

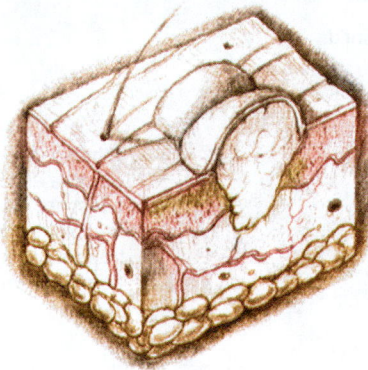

Nodules (such as *lipomas*) are elevated, marble-like lesions more than 1 cm wide and deep.

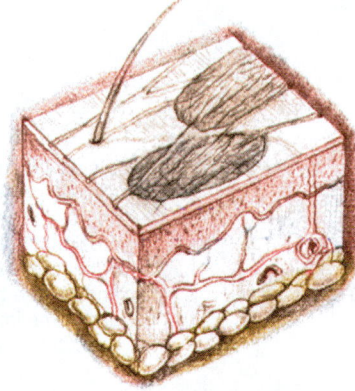

Patches (such as *vitiligo or café au lait spots*) are macules that are larger than 1 cm in diameter. They may or may not have some surface changes—either slight scale or fine wrinkles.

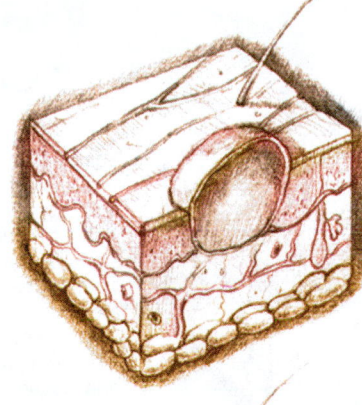

Cysts (such as *sebaceous cysts*) are nodules filled with either liquid or semisolid material that can be expressed.

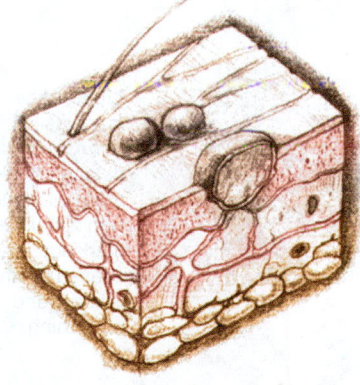

Papules (such as *warts* or *elevated moles*) are small, firm, elevated lesions less than 1 cm in diameter.

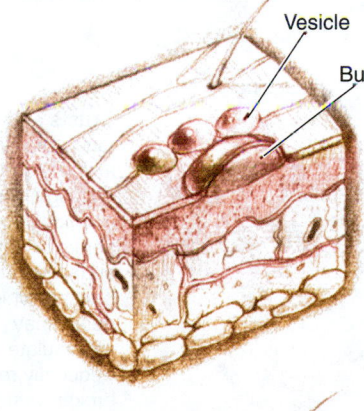

Vesicle

Bulla

Vesicles (such as in *acute dermatitis*) and **bullae** (such as *second-degree burns*) are blisters filled with clear fluid. Vesicles are less than 1 cm in diameter, and bullae are more than 1 cm in diameter.

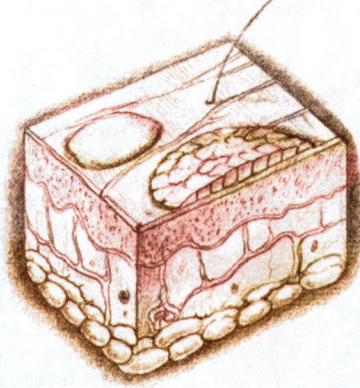

Plaques (such as in *psoriasis or seborrheic keratosis*) are elevated, plateau-like patches more than 1 cm in diameter that do not extend into the lower skin layers.

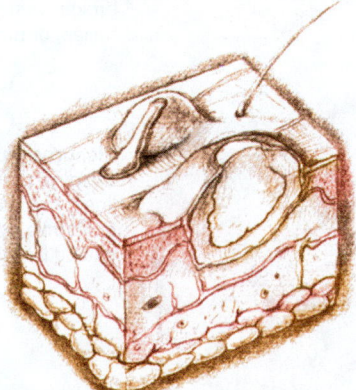

Pustules (such as in *acne* and *acute impetigo*) are vesicles filled with cloudy or purulent fluid.

Figure 69-17 ■ Classification of skin lesions.

Continued

PRIMARY
LESIONS—cont'd

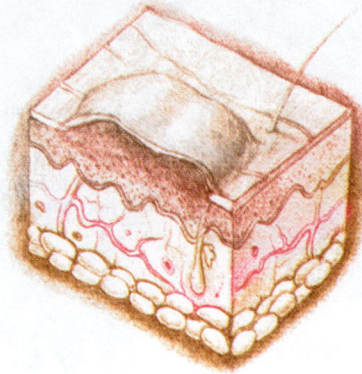

Wheals (such as *urticaria* and *insect bites*) are elevated, irregularly shaped, transient areas of dermal edema.

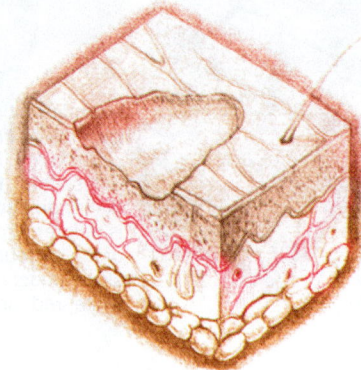

Erosions (such as in *varicella*) are wider than fissures but involve only the epidermis. They are often associated with vesicles, bullae, or pustules.

SECONDARY
LESIONS

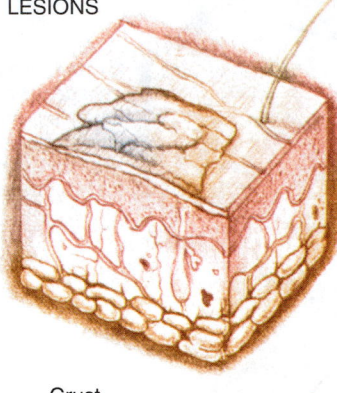

Scales (such as in *exfoliative dermatitis* and *psoriasis*) are visibly thickened stratum corneum. They appear dry and are usually whitish. They are seen most often with papules and plaques.

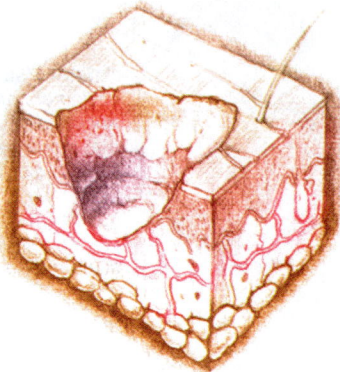

Ulcers (such as *stage 3 pressure sores*) are deep erosions that extend beneath the epidermis and involve the dermis and sometimes the subcutaneous fat.

Crust

Oozing

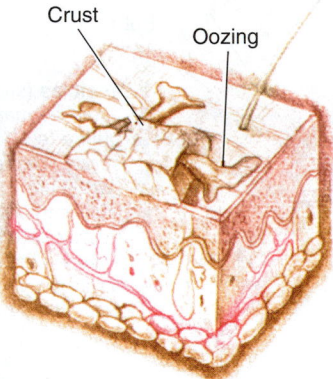

Crusts and oozing (such as in *eczema* and *late-stage impetigo*) are composed of dried serum or pus on the surface of the skin, beneath which liquid debris may accumulate. Crusts frequently result from broken vesicles, bullae, or pustules.

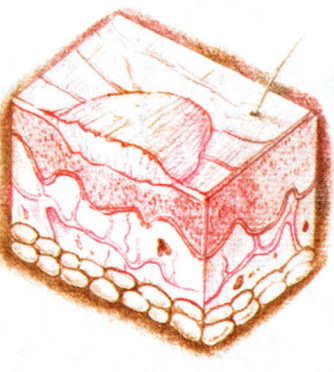

Lichenifications (such as in *chronic dermatitis*) are palpably thickened areas of epidermis with accentuated skin markings. They are caused by chronic rubbing and scratching.

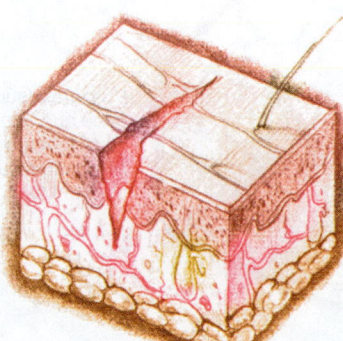

Fissures (such as in *athlete's foot*) are linear cracks in the epidermis, which often extend into the dermis.

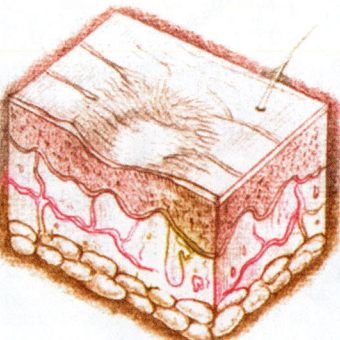

Atrophy (such as *striae* [stretch marks] and *aged skin*) is characterized by thinning of the skin surface with loss of skin markings. The skin is translucent and paper-like. Atrophy involving the dermal layer results in skin depression.

Figure 69-17, cont'd ■ Classification of skin lesions.

ameter) that do not fade or blanch when pressure is applied (Figure 69-18). They often indicate increased capillary fragility. Petechiae of the lower extremities often occur with stasis dermatitis, a condition commonly seen in clients with a history of chronic venous insufficiency.

Ecchymoses (bruises) are larger areas of hemorrhage that range in size from several millimeters to many centimeters. In older adults, bruising is common after minor trauma to the skin, especially on sun-exposed areas of the body. Certain drugs and low platelet counts lead to easy or excessive bruising. Anticoagulants and decreased numbers of platelets disrupt clotting action, resulting in ecchymosis.

Integrity

Thoroughly examine areas with actual breaks in skin integrity. For example, skin tears are a common finding in older people as a result of a flattening of the dermal-epidermal junction with aging. The thin, fragile skin is easily damaged by friction or shearing forces, especially if bruising is already present. Look for skin tears in the following areas:

- In areas where constricting clothing rubs against the skin
- On the upper extremities, where the skin is grasped when assisting a client to ambulate or change position

---

TABLE 69-3   Terms Commonly Used to Describe Skin Lesion Configurations

annular Ringlike with raised borders around flat, clear centers of normal skin
circinate Circular
circumscribed Well-defined with sharp borders
clustered Several lesions grouped together
coalesced Lesions that merge with one another and appear confluent
diffuse Widespread, involving most of the body with intervening areas of normal skin; generalized
linear Occurring in a straight line
serpiginous With wavy borders, resembling a snake
universal All areas of the body involved, with no areas of normal-appearing skin

---

- In areas where adhesive tapes or dressings have been applied and removed

Check for the presence of multiple abrasions or early pressure-related skin changes. These problems may signal previously unrecognized impairments in physical mobility or changes in sensory perception.

Describe breaks in skin integrity by their location, size, color, and distribution as well as by the presence of drainage or any signs of infection. The evaluation of partial-thickness and full-thickness wounds, including objective criteria that describe progress toward healing, is discussed in Chapter 70.

Cleanliness

Evaluate the cleanliness of the skin to gain information about self-care needs. Inspect the hair, nails, and skin closely for excessive soiling and offensive odor. Depending on a client's degree of self-care deficit, hard-to-reach areas (e.g., perirectal and inguinal skin folds, axillae, feet) may be less clean than other skin surface areas.

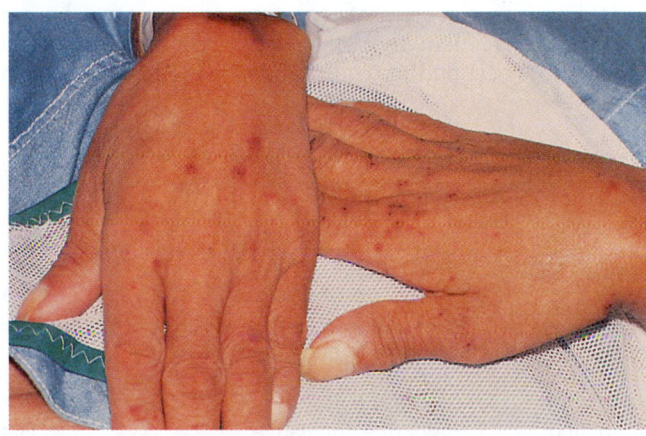

Figure 69-18 ■ Petechiae.

TABLE 69-4   Common Vascular Skin Lesions

Lesion	Clinical Findings	Location	Significance
Cherry angioma (senile angioma)	Bright to dusky red, dome-shaped papule 2-5 mm in diameter Adjacent lesions may vary in size and color Partial blanching on palpation	Chest and back	Normal skin change with aging
Spider angioma	Bright red, starlike lesion varying in size from small to 2 cm Center of "star" is sometimes raised and may pulsate when palpated	Face, neck, and upper trunk	Associated with liver disease, pregnancy (change in estrogen level), and vitamin B deficiency May be normal finding
Telangiectasia	Reddish blue linear or star-like lesion caused by enlargement of the superficial blood vessels	Face and trunk	Associated with sun exposure and prolonged alcohol intake May be seen in systemic scleroderma and after continued use of potent topical steroids
Venous star	Spider-like blue marking varying in size from small to several inches May have a "cascading" appearance Does not blanch with pressure	Legs (near veins) and anterior chest Face, scalp, and groin	Associated with increased pressure in superficial veins (varicose veins)
Port-wine stain	Large, dark-red to purple area of discoloration Does not blanch with pressure	Any body location Very common on the face and the back of the neck	Congenital abnormality If on the face, may be associated with neurologic disorders and ocular abnormalities

PALPATION

Skin inspection alone can be misleading. Use palpation to gather additional information about skin lesions, moisture, temperature, texture, and turgor (Table 69-5).

Palpation confirms the size of the lesions and determines whether they are flat or slightly raised. The consistency of larger lesions can vary from soft and pliable to firm and solid. Subtle changes, such as the difference between a fine **macular** (flat) rash and a **papular** (raised) rash, may best be determined by palpating with your eyes closed. Ask the client whether he or she has pain or tenderness during palpation of the skin.

In areas of excess dryness, rub your finger against the skin surface to determine the degree of flaking or scaling. Both generalized and localized changes in skin temperature can be detected by placing the back of a hand on the skin surface. Before assessing for changes in skin temperature, make certain to have warm hands. Cold hands interfere with accurate assessment and are uncomfortable for the client.

Palpate skin surfaces to assess texture, which differs according to body region and exposure to environmental irritants. For example, areas of long-term sun exposure have a rougher texture than that of protected skin surfaces. The client whose occupation requires repeated exposure to harsh soaps or chemicals may show skin changes related to this exposure. Increased skin thickness from scarring, lichenification, or edema usually decreases elasticity.

Turgor indicates the amount of skin elasticity. Skin turgor can be altered by a number of factors, including water content and aging. Gently pinch the client's skin between your thumb and forefinger and then release. If skin turgor is normal, the skin immediately returns to its original state when released. Poor skin turgor is evidenced by "tenting" of the skin, with a gradual return to the original state (see Chapter 14). Normal loss of elasticity with aging makes the assessment of skin turgor difficult in an older client. Assess skin turgor of an older client on the forehead or chest.

Hair Assessment

During the skin assessment, inspect and palpate the hair for cleanliness, distribution, quantity, and quality. Hair is normally found in an even distribution over most of the body surfaces, with the hair on the scalp, in the pubic region, and in the axillary folds thicker and coarser than hair on the trunk, arms, and legs. Although color and growth patterns vary widely, sudden or marked changes in hair characteristics may reflect an underlying disease process.

TABLE 69-5 Common Clinical Findings in Skin Palpation

Clinical Findings	Cause	Location	Examples of Predisposing Conditions
Edema			
Localized	Inflammatory response	Area of injury or involvement	Trauma
Dependent or pitting	Fluid and electrolyte imbalance Venous and cardiac insufficiency	Ambulatory: dorsum of foot and medial ankle Bedridden: buttocks, sacrum, and lower back	Congestive heart failure Renal disease Hepatic cirrhosis Venous thrombosis or stasis
Nonpitting	Endocrine imbalance	Generalized, but more easily seen over the tibia	Hypothyroidism (myxedema)
Moisture			
Increased	Autonomic nervous system stimulation	Face, axillae, skin folds, palms, and soles	Fever, anxiety, activity Hyperthyroidism
Decreased	Dehydration Endocrine imbalance	Buccal mucous membranes with progressive involvement of other skin surfaces	Fluid loss Postmenopausal status Hypothyroidism Normal aging
Temperature			
Increased	Increased blood flow to the skin	Generalized Localized	Fever, hypermetabolic states Inflammation
Decreased	Decreased blood flow to the skin	Generalized Localized	Impending shock, sepsis, anxiety Hypothyroidism Interference with vascular flow
Turgor			
Decreased	Decreased elasticity of the dermis (tenting when pinched)	Abdomen, forehead, or radial aspect of the wrist	Severe dehydration Sudden, severe weight loss Normal aging
Texture			
Roughness or thickness	Irritation, friction	Pressure points (e.g., soles, palms, elbows)	Calluses Chronic eczema Atopic skin diseases
	Sun damage Excessive collagen production	Areas of sun exposure Localized or generalized	Normal aging Scleroderma Keloids
Softness or smoothness	Endocrine disturbances	Generalized	Hyperthyroidism

As with skin changes, check any abnormal findings by obtaining an in-depth history of the circumstances surrounding any change.

How well the hair is groomed, including the cleanliness of areas of thicker hair growth, can confirm information already gathered about a client's social history and health care needs. If the client has intense itching or scratches continually, examine the scalp and pubis for lice and **nits** (lice eggs). Inspect the scalp for scaling, redness, lesions, excoriation, crusting, and tenderness.

Dandruff, an accumulation of patchy or diffuse white or gray scales that appear on the surface of the scalp, is common. Dandruff is mainly a cosmetic problem, but a very oily scalp can induce inflammatory changes with redness and itching. Severe inflammatory dandruff can extend to the eyebrows and the skin of the face and neck. *If severe dandruff is not treated, hair loss can occur.*

Although gradual hair loss occurs with aging, sudden asymmetric or patchy hair loss at any age is of concern. Assess the scalp for distribution and thickness of the hair, and document variations.

Hirsutism is excessive growth of body hair or hair growth in abnormal body areas. Increased hair growth across the face and chest in women is a sign of hirsutism. Hirsutism is one manifestation of hormonal imbalance. If hirsutism is present, look for changes in fat distribution and capillary fragility, which can occur in Cushing's disease, and for clitoral enlargement and deepening of the voice, which may indicate ovarian dysfunction.

Nail Assessment

Dystrophic (abnormal) nails may occur with a serious systemic illness or local skin disease involving the epidermal keratinocytes. Evaluate the fingernails and toenails for color, shape, thickness, texture, and the presence of lesions.

Many variations in color, texture, and grooming of the nails are influenced by factors unrelated to disease, such as occupation. When assessing the older adult, observe for minor variations associated with the aging process (see Figure 69-15), such as a gradual thickening of the nail plate, the presence of longitudinal ridges, or a yellowish gray discoloration.

Color

The color of the nail plate depends on many factors, including nail thickness and transparency, amount of red blood cells, arterial blood flow, and pigment deposits (Table 69-6). Figure 69-19 shows normal variations in nail color. Changes in color can be caused by external factors, such as the chemical damage that occurs with some occupations and in the long-term use of nail polish.

During examination, the client's fingers and toes should be free of any surface pressure that might interfere with local blood flow or alter the appearance of the digits. To differentiate between color changes attributable to the underlying vascular supply and those resulting from pigment deposition, blanch the nail bed to see whether a color change occurs with pressure. Do this by gently squeezing the end of the finger or toe, exerting downward pressure on the nail bed, and then releasing the pressure. Color caused by vascular alterations changes as pressure is applied and returns to the original state when pressure is released. Color caused by pigment deposition remains unchanged.

Shape

Nail shape may indicate early or late changes specific to systemic disease. For example, fingernail clubbing occurs with impaired gas exchange.

Evaluate the nail shape by examining the curve of the nail plate and surrounding soft tissue from all angles. Palpate the fingertips to define areas of sponginess, tenderness, or edema. Table 69-7 describes common variations in nail shape.

TABLE 69-6	Common Alterations in Nail Color	
Alteration	**Clinical Findings**	**Significance**
White	Horizontal white banding or areas of opacity	Chronic hepatic or renal disease (hypoalbuminemia)
	Generalized pallor of nail beds	Shock
		Anemia
		Early arteriosclerotic changes (toenails)
		Myocardial infarction
Yellow-brown	Diffuse yellow to brown discoloration	Jaundice
		Peripheral lymphedema
		Bacterial or fungal infections of the nail
		Psoriasis
		Diabetes
		Cardiac failure
		Staining from tobacco, nail polish, or dyes
		Long-term tetracycline therapy
		Normal aging (yellow-gray color)
	Vertical brown banding extending from the proximal nail fold distally	Normal finding in dark-skinned clients
		Nevus or melanoma of nail matrix in light-skinned clients
Red	Thin, dark-red vertical lines 1-3 mm long (splinter hemorrhages)	Bacterial endocarditis
		Trichinosis
		Trauma to the nail bed
		Normal finding in some clients
	Red discoloration of the lunula	Cardiac insufficiency
	Dark-red nail beds	Polycythemia vera
Blue	Diffuse blue discoloration that blanches with pressure	Respiratory failure
		Methemoglobinuria
		Venous stasis disease (toenails)

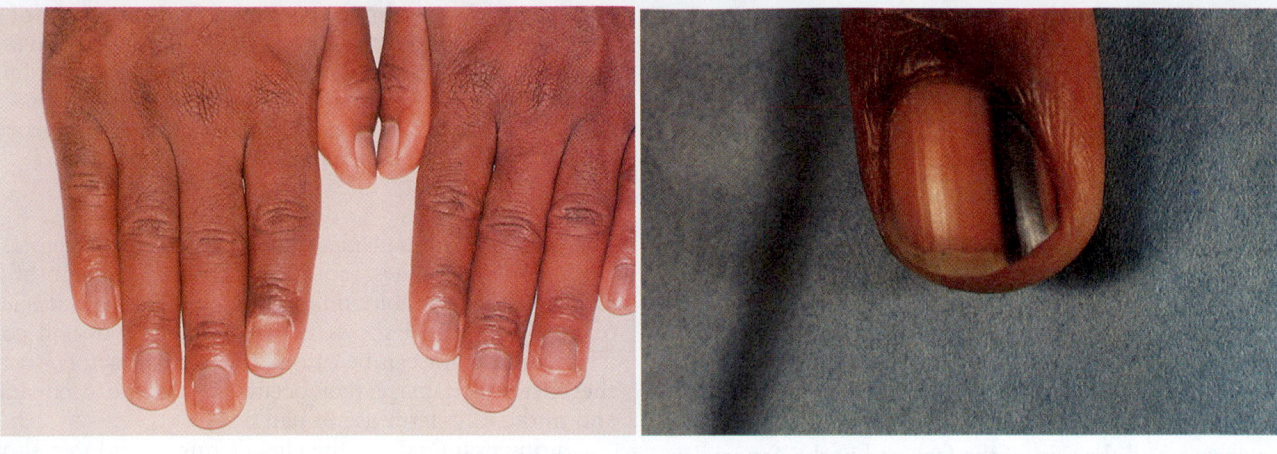

Figure 69-19 ■ **A,** Diffuse nail pigmentation. **B,** Linear nail pigmentation.

TABLE 69-7 Common Variations in Nail Shape

Nail Shape	Clinical Findings		Significance
Normal	Angle of 160 degrees between the nail plate and the proximal nail fold ■ Nail surface slightly convex ■ Nail base firm when palpated		Normal finding
Clubbing Early clubbing	Straightening of angle between the nail plate and the proximal nail fold to 180 degrees ■ Nail base spongy when palpated		Hypoxia Lung cancer
Late clubbing	Angle between the nail plate and the proximal nail fold exceeds 180 degrees ■ Nail base visibly edematous and spongy when palpated ■ Enlargement of the soft tissue of the fingertips gives a "drumstick" appearance when viewed from above		Prolonged hypoxia Emphysema Chronic obstructive pulmonary disease Advanced lung cancer
Spoon nails (koilonychia) Early koilonychia	Flattening of the nail plate with an increased smoothness of the nail surface		Iron deficiency (with or without anemia) Poorly controlled diabetes >15 yr in duration
Late koilonychia	Concave curvature of the nail plate		Local injury Psoriasis Chemical irritants Developmental abnormality
Beau's grooves	1-mm wide horizontal depressions in the nail plates caused by growth arrest (involves all nails)		Acute, severe illness Prolonged febrile state Isolated periods of severe malnutrition
Pitting	Small, multiple pits in the nail plate ■ May be associated with plate thickening and onycholysis ■ Most often involves the fingernails (several or all)		Psoriasis Alopecia areata

Thickness

The nail plate can thicken as a result of trauma, chronic dermatologic disease, or decreased arterial blood flow. In older clients, look for a "heaped-up" appearance of the toenails, which may occur with fungal infection (onychomycosis).

Consistency

Nail consistency is described as hard, soft, or brittle. Nail plates may become hard, with increased thickening. A warm-water soak or lubrication with petroleum jelly is required to soften the nail plates before they can be trimmed.

Soft nail plates, which are thin and bend easily with pressure, are associated with malnutrition, chronic arthritis, myxedema, and peripheral neuritis.

Brittle nails can split, as in the client with onychomycosis or advanced psoriasis. Splitting of the nail plate is also caused by repeated exposure to water and detergents, which damage the plate over time.

Lesions

Separation of the nail plate from the nail bed (onycholysis) creates an air pocket beneath the nail plate. The pocket first appears as a grayish white opacity. The color may change as dirt and keratin collect in the pocket, and the area begins to have a bad odor. Onycholysis is common with fungal infections and after trauma. Separation of the nail plate may also occur with psoriasis or as a result of prolonged contact with chemicals.

Inspect the soft-tissue folds around the nail plate for redness, heat, swelling, and tenderness. Inflammation of the skin around the nail (**acute paronychia**) usually occurs with a torn cuticle or an ingrown toenail. If acute paronychia occurs in an immunocompromised client, an opportunistic infection caused by the *Staphylococcus* organism is probable.

Chronic paronychia is more common and is an inflammation that persists for months. People at risk for chronic paronychia are men and women with frequent exposure to water, such as homemakers, bartenders, and laundry workers.

CULTURAL CONSIDERATIONS

Pallor, erythema, cyanosis, and other color changes reflective of the physical state are less visible in clients with naturally dark skin tones. Although physiologic processes are the same for both light-skinned and dark-skinned clients, the amount of skin pigmentation greatly alters how the skin appears in response to physiologic alterations. Consequently **assessment** skills to detect the more subtle color changes are needed. Become familiar with the normal appearance of a dark-skinned client's mucous membranes, nail beds, and skin tone so that variations from normal can be identified. Chart 69-3 lists specific assessment techniques for skin manifestations of health in people with dark skin.

Skin Assessment Techniques for Clients with Dark Skin

ASSESSMENT OF PALLOR IN DARK-SKINNED CLIENTS

To detect generalized pallor, inspect the mucous membranes for an ash-gray color. If the lips and the nail beds are not heavily pigmented, they appear paler than normal for that client. Use good lighting to assess for the absence of the underlying red tones that normally give heavily pigmented skin a healthy glow. With generalized decreased blood flow to the skin, brown skin appears yellow-brown, and very dark brown skin is ash gray.

ASSESSMENT OF CYANOSIS IN DARK-SKINNED CLIENTS

If impaired gas exchange is suspected, examine the lips, tongue, nail beds, conjunctivae, and palms and soles at regular intervals for subtle color changes. In a client with cyanosis, the lips and

---

CHART 69-3

BEST PRACTICE for
Assessing Changes in Dark Skin

Cyanosis
- Examine lips and tongue for gray color.
- Examine nail beds, palms, and soles, for blue tinge.
- Examine conjunctiva for pallor.

Inflammation
- Compare affected area with nonaffected area for increased warmth.
- Examine the skin of the affected area to determine whether it is shiny, taut, or pits with pressure.
- Compare the skin color of affected area to the same area on the opposite side of the body.
- Palpate the affected area and compare it with unaffected area to determine whether there is a difference in texture (affected area may feel hard or "woody").

Jaundice
- Check for yellow tinge to oral mucous membranes, especially the hard palate.
- Examine the sclera nearest to the iris rather than the corners of the eye.

Bleeding
- Compare the affected area with the same area on the unaffected body side for swelling or skin darkening.
- If the client has thrombocytopenia, petechiae may be present on the oral mucosa or conjunctiva.

---

tongue are gray, and the palms, soles, conjunctivae, and nail beds have a bluish tinge. To support these findings, assess for other obvious manifestations of hypoxia, including tachycardia, hypotension, changes in respiratory rate or rhythm, decreased breath sounds, changes in level of consciousness, and any increase in the amount or viscosity of secretions.

ASSESSMENT OF INFLAMMATION IN DARK-SKINNED CLIENTS

Use the back of your hand to palpate areas of suspected inflammation for the increased warmth that occurs when blood flow to the skin increases. With the fingertips, palpate for hardened areas deep in the tissue, which may give the skin a "woody" feeling. Inflamed skin is tender and edematous. If edema is extensive, the skin is taut and shiny.

Areas of the body where inflammation (e.g., inflammatory rash or cellulitis) has recently resolved appear darker than the normal skin tone. This change is due to stimulation of the melanocytes during the inflammatory process and to the increased pigment production that continues after inflammation subsides. More extensive injury to the skin with destruction of melanocytes (e.g., deep ulcer, full-thickness burn) may heal with color changes that are lighter than the normal skin tone. Unlike acute changes, chronic inflammatory changes seldom produce tenderness on palpation. If scar tissue is present, the skin may feel less supple, especially over the joints. If chronic inflammatory changes are suspected, ask the client about a history of skin problems in that area of the body.

ASSESSMENT OF JAUNDICE IN DARK-SKINNED CLIENTS

Jaundice in a client with dark skin is best assessed by inspecting the oral mucosa, especially the hard palate, for yellow discoloration. Inspection of the conjunctivae and adjacent sclera may be misleading because normal deposits of fat produce a yellowish hue that is visible in contrast to the dark skin around the eyes. Examine the sclera closest to the cornea for a more accurate determination of jaundice. The palms and soles of dark-skinned clients may appear yellow if they are callused; a callus should not be mistaken for jaundice.

ASSESSMENT OF SKIN BLEEDING IN DARK-SKINNED CLIENTS

Purpuric lesions may not be visible in areas of deep pigmentation. Areas of ecchymosis appear darker than normal skin; they may be tender and easily palpable, depending on whether hematoma is present. In most cases, the client relates a history of trauma to the area that confirms the assessment. Petechiae are rarely visible in dark skin and may be seen only in the oral mucosa and conjunctiva.

Psychosocial Assessment

Skin changes, especially when more visible skin surfaces (e.g., face, hair, hands) are involved, often affect a person's body image. Assess the client's body language for clues indicating a disturbance in self-concept. For example, the avoidance of eye contact or the use of garments to cover the affected areas communicates concern about physical appearance. Clients with chronic skin diseases often relate a history of social isolation related to a fear of rejection by others or a belief that the skin problem is contagious.

Skin changes linked to poor hygiene are common in clients from low socioeconomic backgrounds. Assess the client's overall appearance for excessive soiling, matted hair, body odor, or other self-care deficits. Confirm unsanitary living conditions by obtaining a social history. Clients may relate similar skin problems among family members, friends, and sexual contacts.

If skin problems related to poor hygiene are identified in older clients, also evaluate any physical limitations that might contribute to poor health maintenance. For example, visual or mobility problems can make it difficult for clients to see or reach skin surfaces to clean them.

? Critical Thinking Challenge

The client is a 73-year-old Hispanic woman who has hypertension and some degree of heart failure. Her lower legs are swollen and have reddish purple patches with a few small open areas. When you ask her how long these areas have been present, she tells you that they started in the wintertime and are very itchy. On closer inspection, you can see scratches around the open areas. She tells you she has been putting alcohol on the open areas to prevent infection.

1. What additional health history information should you obtain?
2. What further assessment of the skin problem should you perform?
3. Should she continue to use the alcohol? Why? Why not?

evolve For suggested answer guidelines, go to http://evolve.elsevier.com/Iggy/.

Diagnostic Assessment
LABORATORY TESTS

When a fungal, bacterial, or viral pathogen is suspected as the cause of certain skin changes, confirmation by microscopic examination is necessary.

Cultures for Fungal Infections

When superficial fungal (**dermatophyte**) infections are suspected, gently scrape scales from the skin lesions into a clean container and send to the laboratory for culture. Collect fingernail clippings and hair in a similar manner. Unfortunately waiting for culture results can delay treatment of a superficial fungal infection. For this reason the specimen is also treated with a potassium hydroxide (KOH) preparation and examined microscopically. Fungal infections show branched hyphae when viewed under a microscope after treatment with KOH. A positive KOH test often eliminates the need for a culture.

For deeper fungal infections, a piece of tissue is obtained for culture. The physician obtains the specimen by punch biopsy (see Skin Biopsy below). When a specimen is needed for cell analysis and special fungal stains, either two specimens are obtained or one biopsy tissue specimen is bisected before being sent to the laboratory.

Cultures for Bacterial Infections

Specimens for bacterial culture are obtained from intact primary lesions (bullae, vesicles, or pustules), if possible. Express material from the lesion, collect it with a cotton-tipped applicator, and place the material in a bacterial culture medium. For intact lesions, **unroofing** (lifting or puncturing of the outer surface) may be needed using a sterile small-gauge needle before the material can be easily expressed. If crusts are present, remove the crusts and swab the underlying exudate.

A biopsy of deep bacterial infections may be required to obtain a specimen for culture. If bacterial cellulitis is suspected, nonbacteriostatic saline can be injected deep into the tissue and aspirated; the aspirant is sent for culture.

Cultures for Viral Infections

Viral cultures are indicated if a herpes virus infection is suspected. A cotton-tipped applicator is used to obtain vesicle fluid from intact lesions. Unlike bacterial and fungal specimens, which can remain at room temperature until being transported to the laboratory, viral culture tubes are placed on ice immediately after the specimen is obtained and are transported to the laboratory as soon as possible.

OTHER DIAGNOSTIC TESTS

Skin Biopsy

A small piece of skin tissue is obtained for pathologic study to establish an accurate diagnosis or assess the effectiveness of an intervention. Before preparing the client, check with the physician to determine the number, location, and type of skin biopsies to be performed.

TYPES OF BIOPSIES

Depending on the size, depth, and location of the skin changes, the physician may perform a punch biopsy, shave biopsy, or scalpel excision (excisional biopsy).

PUNCH BIOPSY. The punch biopsy is the most common technique. A small circular cutting instrument, or punch, ranging in diameter from 2 to 6 mm is used. After the site is injected with a local anesthetic, a small plug of tissue is cut to the depth of the subcutaneous fat and removed with forceps and scissors. The site may be closed with one or two sutures if it is on the face or leg. Some physicians allow the biopsy site to heal without suturing.

SHAVE BIOPSY. A shave biopsy removes only the portion of the skin elevated above the surrounding tissue when injected with a local anesthetic. A scalpel or razor blade is moved parallel to the skin surface to remove the tissue specimen. Shave biopsies are usually indicated for superficial or raised lesions. Suturing is not necessary.

EXCISIONAL BIOPSY. In rare instances, larger or deeper specimens are obtained by excision with a scalpel. Deep incisions are made and then sutured after the specimen is removed. Unlike punch and shave biopsies, excisional biopsies involve more discomfort for the client while the site is healing.

CLIENT PREPARATION. Explain to the client what to expect. Emphasize that a biopsy is a minor procedure with few, if any, complications. If a punch or shave biopsy is planned, reassure the client that scarring is minimal because of the small size of the tissue removed. If an excisional biopsy is planned, tell the client that a scar similar to that of a healed surgical incision will result.

PROCEDURE. Establish a sterile field and assemble all needed supplies and instruments. Local anesthesia is provided by local infiltration using a small-gauge needle (no. 25) to reduce discomfort during injection. Although preparation of the biopsy site differs according to the physician's preference, the skin is simply wiped with alcohol in most cases.

The most uncomfortable time for the client is during the injection of a local anesthetic agent, which produces a burning or stinging sensation. Reassure the client that the discomfort will subside as the anesthetic takes effect. Talking the client through the procedure with a quiet voice, in combination with a gentle touch, has a calming effect.

After removal tissue specimens for routine pathologic study are placed directly in 10% formalin for fixation. Specimens for culture are placed in sterile saline solution. Bleeding of the biopsy site may be controlled by applying a topical hemostatic agent. If topical treatment does not stop the bleeding, suturing is considered.

FOLLOW-UP CARE. After bleeding is under control and any sutures have been placed, the site is covered with an adhesive bandage or a dry gauze dressing. Instruct the client to keep the dressing dry and in place for a minimum of 8 hours. Teach the client to clean the site daily after the dressing is removed. Tap water or saline can be used to remove any dried blood or crusts. An antibiotic ointment may be prescribed to reduce the risk for infection. The biopsy site may be left open unless a covering is preferred for cosmetic reasons or because the site is an area often soiled. Instruct the client to report any redness or excessive drainage. Sutures are usually removed 7 to 10 days after biopsy.

Wood's Light Examination

A handheld, long-wave length ultraviolet (black) light or Wood's light is sometimes used during physical examina-tion. Exposure of some skin infections with this light produces a specific color, such as blue-green or red, that can be used to identify the infection. Hypopigmented skin is more prominent when it is viewed under black light, which makes evaluation of pigment changes in fair-skinned clients easier.

Wood's light examination of the skin is always carried out in a darkened room. Reassure the client that no discomfort occurs with a Wood's light examination.

Diascopy

Diascopy is a noninvasive and painless technique that eliminates erythema caused by increased blood flow to the skin, thereby easing the inspection of skin lesions. A glass slide or lens is pressed down over the area to be examined, blanching the skin and revealing the shape of the lesions.

Skin Testing

If a client's rash might be an allergic contact dermatitis, patch testing may identify the allergen. The technique for skin testing for allergy is described in Chapter 26.

❓ Critical Thinking Challenge

The client is an 84-year-old white woman who has several slightly raised, bright red lesions on her upper back. They are smaller than 2 mm and are in a line with about 1 inch between the lesions. She tells you these lesions have been there for about 10 years and she is afraid that they might be skin cancer.

1. What additional questions should you ask this client about these lesions?
2. What additional physical assessment data should you obtain regarding these lesions?
3. Should these lesions be examined by a surgeon or dermatologist? Why or why not?

evolve For suggested answer guidelines, go to http://evolve.elsevier.com/Iggy/.

GET READY for the NCLEX Examination!

KEY POINTS

Safe Effective Care Environment

- Assist all clients with limited mobility to change positions at least every 2 hours while awake.
- Wash your hands before and after touching any skin lesions.
- Use standard precautions when providing care to a client who has any areas of nonintact skin.

Health Promotion and Maintenance

- Encourage all clients to reduce sun exposure and exposure to ultraviolet (UV) light.
- Teach clients how to examine all skin areas on a monthly basis for new lesions and changes to existing lesions. The client should keep a record or "body map" of skin lesions.
- Encourage all clients to bathe, shampoo the hair, and keep fingernails clean and trimmed on a regular basis.
- Teach all clients the ABCD method of evaluating a lesion for melanoma.

Psychosocial Integrity

- Allow the client the opportunity to express feelings about a change in body image that results from changes in the skin, hair, or nails.
- Explain all procedures, restrictions, medications, and follow-up care to the client and family.
- Check the cognitive function of any client whose hygiene of the skin, hair, and nails appears inadequate.
- Offer alternative therapies for reducing skin discomfort or itching, such as massage, music therapy, and guided imagery.

Physiological Integrity

- Document any known specific allergies that have skin manifestations.
- Keep skin-fold areas on clients clean and dry.
- Position clients who are confined to bed in a way that promotes air circulation to skin-fold areas.
- Ask any client who has started taking a newly prescribed or over-the-counter drug whether he or she has noticed any skin changes that occurred since starting the medication.

ADDITIONAL STUDY RESOURCES

Go to your Student CD-ROM for Review Questions for the NCLEX Examination.

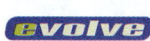 Go to http://evolve.elsevier.com/Iggy/ for Integrated Management of Care Questions for the NCLEX Examination.

SELECTED BIBLIOGRAPHY

Asterisk indicates a classic or definitive work on this subject.

American Cancer Society. (2005). *Cancer facts and figures 2005.* Report No. 00-300M-No. 5008.05. Atlanta: Author.

Carter, K., Dufour, L., & Ballard, C. (2004). Identifying secondary skin lesions. *Nursing 2004, 34*(1), 68.

Cole, J., & Gray-Miceli, D. (2002). The necessary elements of a dermatologic history and physical evaluation. *Dermatology Nursing, 14*(6), 377-383.

*Gaskin, F.C. (1986). Detection of cyanosis in the person with dark skin. *Journal of the National Black Nurses Association, 1*(1), 52-60.

Guyton, A., & Hall, J. (2000). *Textbook of medical physiology* (10th ed.). Philadelphia: W.B. Saunders.

Harris, J. (2000). A plan to promote the prevention and early detection of melanoma. *Dermatology Nursing, 12*(5), 329-333.

Jarvis, C. (2004). *Physical examination and health assessment* (4th ed.). Philadelphia: W.B. Saunders.

Lookingbill, D.P., & Marks, J.G., Jr. (2000). *Principles of dermatology* (3rd ed.). Philadelphia: W.B. Saunders.

Nussbaum, R., McInnes, R., & Willard, H. (2001). *Thompson & Thompson: Genetics in medicine* (6th ed.). Philadelphia: W.B. Saunders.

Pagana, K., & Pagana, T. (2002). *Mosby's manual of diagnostic and laboratory tests* (2nd ed.). St. Louis: Mosby.

Zulkowski, K. (2003). Protecting your patient's aging skin. *Nursing 2003, 33*(1), 84.

Interventions for Clients with Skin Problems

JANICE CUZZELL • M. LINDA WORKMAN

Go to your Student CD-ROM for Review Questions
for the NCLEX Examination keyed to these Learning Outcomes.
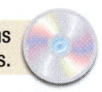

Skin problems are common, and often the cause is not known. In addition to direct skin functions, the skin reflects other body conditions. Thus skin problems may truly arise in the skin, or they may be a symptom of a systemic disease or injury. Drugs and other interventions for any health problem can trigger a skin response or reaction. Skin problems can interfere with the medical or surgical treatment of other conditions. Age-related skin changes and problems arising from immobility, chronic disease, debility, and change in immune function place the older client at an increased risk for skin damage.

MINOR SKIN IRRITATIONS

Dryness

PATHOPHYSIOLOGY

Dry skin (**xerosis**) is a common problem, especially in older clients. It is seen as a fine flaking of the **stratum corneum** (outermost skin layer), and it is usually worse on the lower legs. Generalized **pruritus** (itching) often occurs with dry skin. In clients with chronic skin conditions, unrelieved itching causes the client to scratch and rub the skin in an attempt to relieve the intense itching. These actions may result in secondary skin lesions, excoriations, **lichenification** (thickening), and infection.

Xerosis is worse in dry climates. Central heating and air-conditioning reduce the humidity in the air and increase skin dryness. Wind, cold, and sunlight also worsen the problem. Frequent bathing with harsh soap and hot water further dries the skin, especially if moisturizers are not applied after bathing.

◆COLLABORATIVE MANAGEMENT

Nursing interventions aim to rehydrate the skin and relieve itching. Bathing with moisturizing soaps, oils, and lotions may reduce dryness. Using soap only in soiled or skin-fold areas can also reduce dryness. A 20-minute soak in a warm bath, followed by application of an emollient cream or lotion, can rehydrate the skin and reduce itching. If the client cannot take a tub bath, wrap the trunk and extremities in warm, moist towels covered by plastic sheeting and additional blankets to prevent chilling. Always apply skin creams or lotions to slightly damp skin within 2 to 3 minutes after bathing.

Contrary to popular belief, the cream or lotion is *not* what makes the skin soft and supple. Water is the agent that softens the outer skin layers. Lubricating creams and lotions seal in the moisture provided by water, promoting suppleness and preventing flaking. Some skin lotions are **hydrophilic** (water seeking) and actually draw moisture from the skin, making the dryness worse if they are not applied directly to damp skin.

Teach clients and family members how to maintain healthy skin. Chart 70-1 lists practical ways to avoid drying the skin.

Pruritus

PATHOPHYSIOLOGY

Pruritus, or itching, is a distressing symptom that may or may not occur with skin disease. Pruritus is caused by stimulation of itch-specific nerve fibers at the dermal-epidermal junction. Physical or chemical agents either act directly on these nerve fibers or activate chemical mediators, such as histamine, which then act on the itch receptors.

Itching is a subjective symptom similar to pain. Thus the sensation varies among clients in location and severity. Regardless of the underlying cause, clients usually report that itching is worse at night. Other conditions that make itching worse include poor skin hydration, increased skin temperature, perspiration, and emotional stress.

◆COLLABORATIVE MANAGEMENT

Clients usually try to relieve itching by scratching or rubbing the skin, a response that further stimulates the itch receptors and causes a pattern referred to as the **"itch-scratch-itch" cycle.** When the skin lesions are present with itching, relief can usually be obtained by treatment of the underlying skin disorder with topical or systemic medications. Systemic diseases, such as liver and venous disorders, can also cause itching without skin lesions.

Plan care to promote comfort and prevent disruption of skin integrity that can result from vigorous scratching. Because dry skin worsens itching, emphasize proper bathing and skin lubrication techniques (see Chart 70-1). Encourage clients to keep the fingernails trimmed short, with rough edges filed, to reduce skin damage. Tell clients that wearing mittens or splints at night can help to prevent inadvertent scratching during sleep.

A cool sleeping environment along with a larger dose of sedating antihistamines at bedtime (when the side effect of drowsiness is welcome) may provide an uninterrupted night's sleep. Therapeutic baths **(balneotherapy)** with colloidal oatmeal preparations or tar extracts may give temporary relief (Table 70-1).

If antihistamines are prescribed, closely monitor the client's response to therapy so that the dosage can be adjusted as needed. The anti-inflammatory properties of topical steroid preparations are increased if the drug is applied to slightly damp skin.

CHART 70-1

CLIENT EDUCATION GUIDE
Prevention of Dry Skin

- Use a room humidifier during the winter months or whenever the furnace is in use.
- Take a complete bath or shower only every other day (wash face, axillae, perineum, and any soiled areas with soap daily).
- Use tepid water.
- Use a superfatted, nonalkaline soap instead of deodorant soap.
- Rinse the soap thoroughly from your skin.
- If you like bath oil, add the oil to the water at the end of the bath.
- Pat rather than rub skin surfaces dry.
- Avoid clothing that continuously rubs the skin, such as tight belts, nylon stockings, or pantyhose.
- Maintain a daily fluid intake of 3000 mL unless contraindicated for another medical condition.
- Do not apply rubbing alcohol, astringents, or other drying agents to the skin.
- Avoid caffeine and alcohol ingestion.

TABLE 70-1 Uses of Therapeutic Baths

Agents	Disease	Purpose
Antibacterial Baths		
Potassium permanganate (1:32,000; 1:64,000)	Infected eczema Pemphigus Multiple infected ulcerations	To lower skin bacterial load
Colloidal Baths		
Starch and baking soda (1 c. each per tub)	Atopic eczema	To relieve itching
Aveeno colloidal oatmeal (1 c. per tub)	Psoriasis	To soothe
Aveeno oilated colloidal oatmeal	Chickenpox	To lubricate
Emollient Baths*		
Bath oils; Alpha Keri Lubath	Any dry skin condition	To clean and hydrate the skin
Mineral oil		
Tar Baths*		
Bath oils with tar: Balnetar, Zetar, Polytar	Scaly dermatosis	To loosen scale
Coal tar concentrate (liquor carbonis, detergents)	Psoriasis	To relieve itching
	Eczema	To potentiate ultraviolet A or ultraviolet B light therapy

Modified from Rosen, T., Lanning, M.B., & Hill, M.J. (1983). *The nurse's atlas of dermatology.* Boston: Little, Brown & Co. Copyright 1983 by Theodore Rosen and Marilyn B. Lanning.
* For emollient and tar baths, add 3 to 6 capfuls of therapeutic agent per standard bathtub.

Sunburn

PATHOPHYSIOLOGY

Sunburn is a first-degree or superficial burn and a very common skin injury. Excessive exposure to ultraviolet (UV) light injures the dermis and dilates the capillaries, leading to redness, tenderness, edema, and occasional blister formation. When large areas of the body are sunburned, systemic symptoms, such as headache, nausea, and fever, are produced.

◆COLLABORATIVE MANAGEMENT

Redness (**erythema**) and pain begin within a few hours after sunburn has occurred and increase in intensity for 1 to 2 days before subsiding. Treatment is directed toward comfort and includes cool baths and soothing lotions, such as bland lubricants or refrigerated moisturizing lotions. Antibiotic ointments are used only if blistering of the skin causes infection. If pain is severe, topical corticosteroids may decrease the inflammation temporarily.

Urticaria

PATHOPHYSIOLOGY

Urticaria (hives) is the presence of white or red edematous papules or plaques of various sizes. Urticaria is usually caused by exposure to a specific substance (different for different people), which releases histamine in the dermal tissue, causing blood vessel dilation and leakage of plasma protein to form lesions or wheals. Unfortunately the exact cause of urticaria is rarely identified. The following factors are thought to cause urticaria: drugs, foods, infections, autoimmune diseases, malignancies, physical stimuli, and psychogenic responses.

◆COLLABORATIVE MANAGEMENT

Treatment is aimed at removal of the triggering substance and relief of symptoms. Because the skin reaction is caused by histamine release, antihistamines are helpful. Instruct the client to avoid overexertion, alcohol consumption, and warm environments, which contribute to blood vessel dilation and make the symptoms worse.

TRAUMA

PATHOPHYSIOLOGY

Skin trauma can vary from an aseptic surgical incision to a grossly infected, draining pressure ulcer with deep-tissue destruction. Injury to the skin starts a series of actions to repair the skin and re-establish this protective barrier.

Phases of Wound Healing

Wound healing occurs in three phases: the inflammatory, or "lag," phase; the fibroblastic, or connective tissue repair phase; and the maturation, or remodeling, phase. Table 70-2 lists the key events of normal wound healing. The length of each phase depends on the type of injury and whether the wound is healing by first, second, or third intention (Figure 70-1).

A wound without tissue loss, such as a clean laceration or a surgical incision, can be closed with sutures or staples. The wound edges are brought together with the skin layers lined up in correct anatomic position (**approximated**) and held in place until healing is complete. Because the wound can be easily closed and dead space eliminated, healing by **first intention** shortens the phases of tissue repair. Inflammation resolves quickly, and connective tissue repair is minimal, resulting in a thin scar.

Deeper tissue injuries or wounds with tissue loss, such as a chronic pressure ulcer or venous stasis ulcer, result in a cavity-like defect that requires gradual filling in of the dead space with connective tissue. This healing occurs by **second intention** and prolongs the repair process.

Wounds with a high risk for infection, such as surgical incisions that enter a nonsterile body cavity or traumatic wounds that occur under unclean conditions, may be intentionally left open for several days. After debris and exudate have been removed and inflammation has subsided, the wound is closed by first intention. This type of healing involves delayed primary closure (**third intention**) and results in a scar similar to that found in wounds that heal by first intention. As shown in Table 70-3, healing can be impaired by a number of factors.

Mechanisms of Wound Healing

When injury occurs, the body restores skin integrity through three processes: re-epithelialization, granulation, and wound contraction. The extent to which these processes contribute to tissue repair depends on the depth of injury and the extent of tissue loss.

PARTIAL-THICKNESS WOUNDS

Partial-thickness (superficial) wounds involve damage to the epidermis and upper layers of the dermis. These wound heal

---

TABLE 70-2 Normal Wound Healing

Inflammatory Phase
- Begins at the time of injury or cell death and lasts 3-5 days.
- Immediate responses are vasoconstriction and clot formation.
- After 10 minutes, vasodilation with increased capillary permeability and leakage of plasma (and plasma proteins) into the surrounding tissue.
- Migration of white blood cells (especially macrophages) into the wound.
- Clinical manifestations of local edema, pain, erythema, and warmth.

Fibroblastic Phase
- Begins about the fourth day after injury and lasts 2 to 4 weeks.
- Fibrin strands form a scaffold or framework.
- Mitotic fibroblast cells migrate into the wound, attach to the framework, divide, and stimulate the secretion of collagen.
- Collagen, together with ground substance, builds tough and inflexible scar tissue.
- Capillaries in areas surrounding the wound form "buds" that grow into new blood vessels.
- Capillary buds and collagen deposits form the "granulation" tissue in the wound, and the wound contracts.
- Epithelial cells grow over the granulation tissue bed.

Maturation Phase
- Begins as early as 3 weeks after injury and may continue for a year.
- Collagen is reorganized to provide greater tensile strength.
- Scar tissue gradually becomes thinner and paler in color.
- The mature scar is firm and inelastic when palpated.

The Process of Wound Healing

 Healing by First Intention

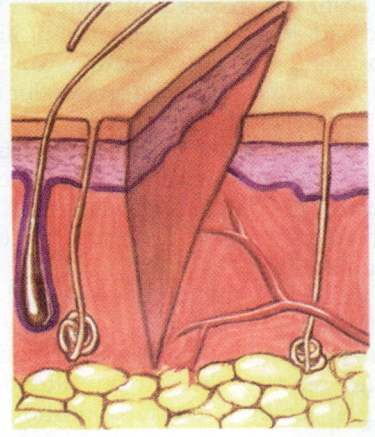

Clean incision

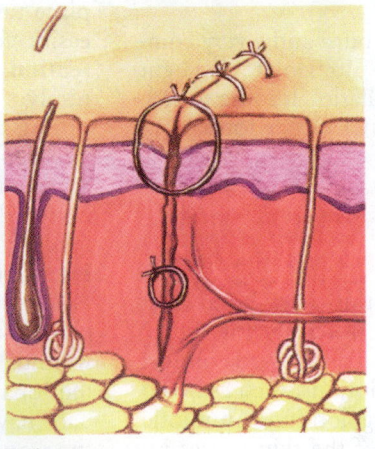

Early suture

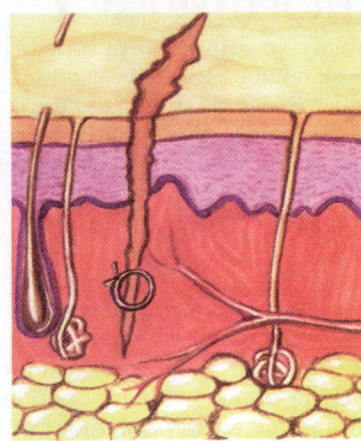

"Hairline" scar

An aseptically made wound with minimal tissue destruction and minimal tissue reaction begins to heal as the edges are approximated by close sutures or staples. No open areas or dead spaces are left to serve as potential sites of infection.

Healing by Second Intention (Granulation) and Contraction

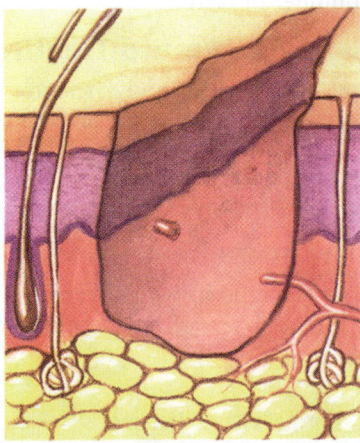

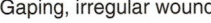

Gaping, irregular wound

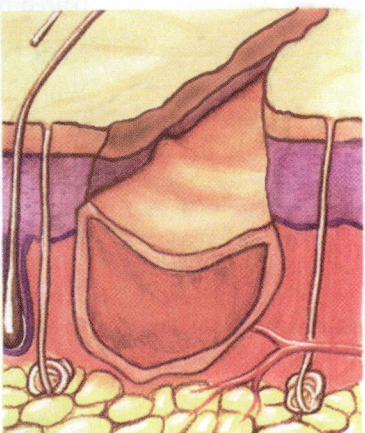

Granulation and contraction

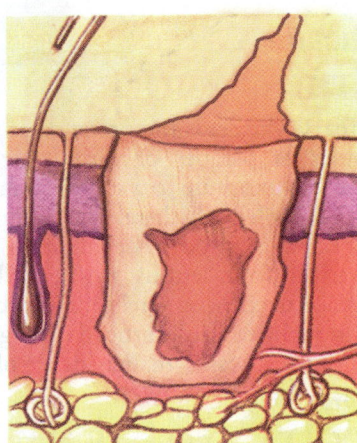

Growth of epithelium over scar

An infected or chronic wound or one with tissue damage so extensive that the edges cannot be smoothly approximated is usually left open and allowed to heal from the inside out. The nurse periodically cleans and assesses the wound for healthy tissue production. Scar tissue is extensive, and healing is prolonged.

Healing by Third Intention (Delayed Closure)

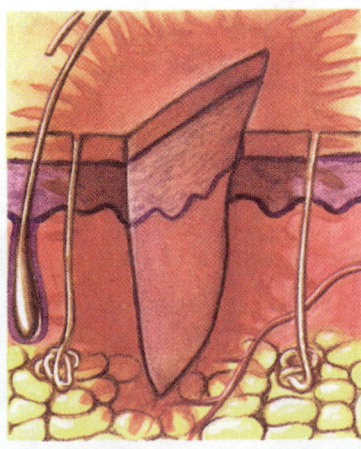

Infected wound

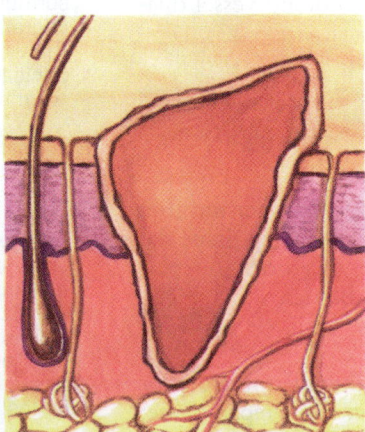

Granulation

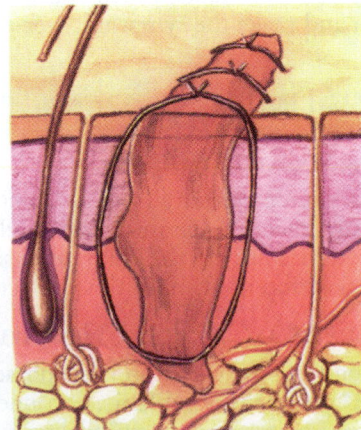

Closure with wide scar

A potentially infected surgical wound may be left open for several days. If no clinical signs of infection occur, the wound is then closed surgically.

Figure 70-1 ■ The process of wound healing.

TABLE 70-3   Causes of Impaired Wound Healing

Cause	Mechanism
Altered Inflammatory Response	
Local	
Arteriosclerosis	Reduced local tissue circula-
Diabetes	tion, resulting in ischemia,
Vasculitis	impaired leukocytic re-
Thrombosis	sponse to wounding, and
Venous insufficiency	increased probability of
Lymphedema	wound infection
Pharmacologic vasoconstriction	
Irradiated tissue	
Crush injuries	
Primary closure under tension	
Systemic	
Leukemia	Systemic inhibition of leuko-
Prolonged administration of	cytic response, resulting in
high-dose anti-inflamma-	impaired host resistance to
tory drugs	infection
■ Corticosteroids	
■ Aspirin	
Impaired Cellular Proliferation	
Local	
Wound infection	Prolonged inflammatory re-
Foreign body	sponse, which can result in
Necrotic tissue	low tissue oxygen tension
Repeated injury or irritation	and further tissue
Movement of wound (e.g.,	destruction
across a joint)	
Wound desiccation or maceration	
Systemic	
Aging	Impaired cellular proliferation
Chronic stress	and collagen synthesis
Nutritional deficiencies	Decreased wound contraction
■ Calories	
■ Protein	
■ Vitamins	
■ Minerals	
■ Water	
Impaired oxygenation	
■ Pulmonary insufficiency	
■ Heat failure	
■ Hypovolemia	
Cirrhosis	
Uremia	
Prolonged hypothermia	
Coagulation disorders	
Cytotoxic drugs	

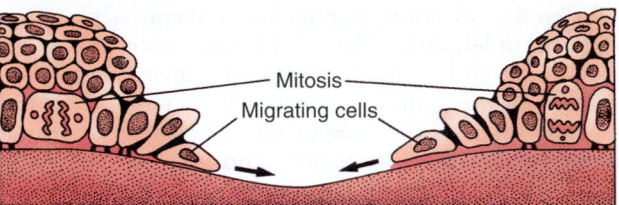

Skin cells at the edge of the wound begin multiplying and migrate toward the center of the wound.

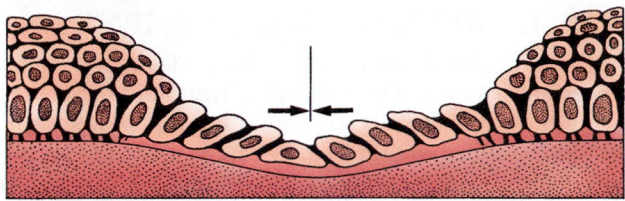

Once advancing epidermal cells from the opposite sides of the wound meet, migration halts.

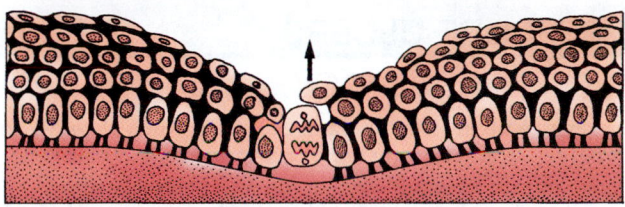

Epithelial cells continue to divide until the thickness of the new skin layer approaches normal.

Figure 70-2 ■ Re-epithelialization. (Modified from Swaim, S.F. [1980]. *Surgery of traumatized skin.* Philadelphia: W.B. Saunders.)

by **re-epithelialization,** the production of new skin cells by undamaged epidermal cells in the basal layer of the dermis and lining the epidermal appendages (Figure 70-2). Skin injury is followed immediately by local inflammation. The inflammatory response causes the formation of a fibrin clot and the release of chemical messengers (growth factors) that stimulate epidermal cell division (mitosis). New skin cells move into "cell-free" spaces on the wound surface, where the fibrin clot acts as a frame or scaffold to guide cell movement. Regrowth across the open area **(resurfacing)** is only one cell layer thick at first. As healing continues, the cell layer thickens and stratifies to resemble normal skin. A healed wound re-establishes the barrier properties of the skin with keratin production.

In a healthy client, healing of a partial-thickness wound by re-epithelialization takes about 5 to 7 days. This process occurs most rapidly in tissue that is hydrated, oxygenated, and has few organisms present.

FULL-THICKNESS WOUNDS

In deep partial-thickness and full-thickness wounds, damage extends into the lower layers of the dermis and underlying subcutaneous tissue. As a result most, if not all, the epithelial cells at the base of the wound have been destroyed and cannot replicate. Removal of the damaged tissue results in a defect that must be filled with scar tissue **(granulation)** for healing to occur. During the proliferative phase of healing, new blood vessels form at the base of the wound and fibroblastic cells begin moving into the wound space. Fibroblasts deposit new collagen to replace the damaged tissue.

Some of these fibroblasts take on the features of smooth-muscle cells and begin to pull the wound edges inward along the path of least resistance **(contraction)** (see Figure 70-1). This causes the wound to decrease in size at a uniform rate of about 0.6 to 0.75 mm/day. Complete closure of a wound by contraction depends on the mobility of the surrounding skin as tension is applied to it. If tension in the surrounding skin exceeds the counter force of wound contraction, healing will be delayed until undamaged epidermal cells at the wound edges are able to bridge the defect. Unlike re-epithelialization in partial-thickness wounds, which results in the return of a near-normal epithelial barrier, the bridging of epithelial cells across a large area of granulation tissue results in an unstable barrier. A venous leg ulcer is one example of a skin defect that heals poorly by contraction. Re-epithelialization of these chronic wounds often results in a thin epidermal barrier that is easily reinjured.

Re-epithelialization, granulation, and contraction do not continue indefinitely. Natural healing processes can slow down and even stop in the presence of infection, unrelieved pressure, or mechanical obstacles. For example, dead tissue not only supports the overgrowth of organisms, but it also obstructs collagen deposition and wound contraction. Therefore thorough wound debridement is necessary for healing to occur. In the case of chronic wounds, healing may cease spontaneously and without an obvious cause.

◆COLLABORATIVE MANAGEMENT

Treatment of skin trauma varies with the depth and circumstances of the injury. The focus of all treatment for any type of skin trauma is to enhance wound healing, prevent infection, and restore function to the area. Management for pressure ulcers presents interventions common to wound healing, as does treatment for burns (see Chapter 71).

PRESSURE ULCERS

PATHOPHYSIOLOGY

A **pressure ulcer** is tissue damage caused when the skin and underlying soft tissue are compressed between a bony prominence and an external surface for an extended period. Historically referred to as a decubitus ulcer, *pressure ulcer* is the term endorsed by the Agency for Healthcare Research and Quality (AHRQ). Although they commonly occur over the sacrum, hips, and ankles, pressure ulcers can occur on any body surface. For example, nasal cannula tubing that is too tight can cause pressure ulcers behind the ear or in the nares.

Tissue compression from pressure restricts blood flow to the skin, resulting in tissue anoxia and cell death. These ulcers commonly occur in people with limited mobility because they are unable to change their position to relieve pressure. Sensory impairment is also a contributing factor. Clients who are unable to feel or communicate the pain that occurs with unrelieved pressure are more likely to develop pressure ulcers. Once formed, these chronic wounds are slow to heal, resulting in increased morbidity and health care costs.

In addition to pressure, other factors may predispose a client to pressure ulcers. Friction and shear are mechanical forces that impair skin integrity and set the stage for skin breakdown. Excessive skin moisture, such as urinary incontinence, increases the risk for skin damage when mechanical forces are applied. Nutritional status is also a concern. Protein malnutrition not only makes normal tissue more prone to breakdown, but it also delays healing.

Mechanical Forces
PRESSURE

Pressure occurs as a result of gravity. Dependent tissues in contact with a fixed surface experience varying degrees of pressure. Pressure is determined by the amount of weight exerted at the point of contact, the distribution of weight at the point of contact, and the density of the contacting surface. Excessive or prolonged pressure can compress blood vessels at the point of contact, leading to ischemia, inflammation, and tissue necrosis. Pressure occurs when the client is positioned on a hard surface that does not diffuse the weight or when he or she remains in the same position too long.

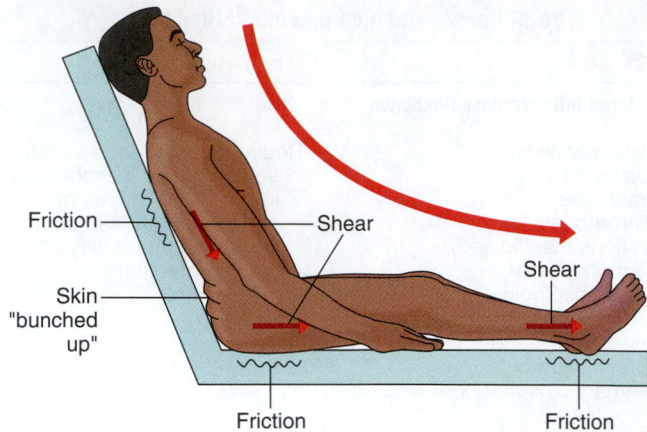

Figure 70-3 ■ Shearing forces pulling skin layers away from deeper tissue. The skin is "bunched up" against the back of the mattress while the rest of the bone and muscle in the area press downward on the lower part of the mattress. Blood vessels become kinked, obstructing circulation and leading to tissue death.

FRICTION

Friction occurs when surfaces rub the skin and irritate or directly pull off epithelial tissue. Such forces are generated when the client is dragged or pulled across bed linen.

SHEAR

Shear or shearing forces are generated when the skin itself is stationary and the tissues below the skin (such as fat and muscle) shift or move (Figure 70-3). The movement of the deeper tissue layers reduces the blood supply to the skin, leading to skin hypoxia, anoxia, ischemia, inflammation, and necrosis.

Gravity plays a role in the development of shearing forces. A shear injury usually occurs when a client is in bed in a semisitting position and gradually slides downward. Often the skin over the sacrum does not slide down at the same pace as the deeper tissues; thus the skin is mechanically "sheared," causing blood vessels to stretch and leading to soft-tissue ischemia, although no break in external skin integrity is observed.

> ### CONSIDERATIONS FOR OLDER ADULTS
> Older adults are at particular risk for pressure ulcers because of the presence of age-related skin changes. Progressive flattening of the dermal-epidermal junction predisposes older people to skin tears from mechanical shearing forces, such as the removal of adhesive tape and friction from tightly applied restraints. In addition, skin moisture and irritation from incontinence and friction over bony prominences can lead to partial-thickness skin destruction and early pressure ulcer formation. *If pressure is unrelieved, tissue destruction progresses to full-thickness injury.*

Incidence/Prevalence

Pressure ulcer development is a problem found among clients in the acute care setting, long-term care facility, and home care setting. Although client care has improved in many ways and new products are available for prevention and treatment, 3% to 14% of hospitalized clients still experience pressure ulcer formation.

CHART 70-2

NIC   **INTERVENTION ACTIVITIES for**
The Client at Risk for or with Pressure Ulcers

Pressure Ulcer Prevention: *Prevention of pressure ulcers for a client at high risk for developing them*
- Use an established risk assessment tool to monitor client's risk factors (e.g., Braden scale).
- Document skin status on admission and daily.
- Monitor any reddened areas closely.
- Remove excessive moisture on the skin resulting from perspiration, wound drainage, and fecal or urinary incontinence.
- Apply protective barriers, such as creams or moisture-absorbing pads, to remove excess moisture, as appropriate.
- Turn every 1 to 2 hours, as appropriate.
- Turn with care (e.g., avoid shearing) to prevent injury to fragile skin.
- Post a turning schedule at the bedside, as appropriate.
- Inspect skin over bony prominences and other pressure points when repositioning at least daily.
- Avoid massaging over bony prominences.
- Position with pillows to elevate pressure points off the bed.
- Keep bed linens clean, dry, and wrinkle free.
- Utilize specialty beds and mattresses, as appropriate.
- Use devices on the bed (e.g., sheepskin) that protect the individual.
- Moisturize dry, unbroken skin.
- Avoid hot water and use mild soap when bathing.
- Apply elbow and heel protectors, as appropriate.
- Facilitate small shifts of body weight frequently.
- Ensure adequate dietary intake, especially protein, vitamins B and C, iron, and calories, using supplements, as appropriate.
- Instruct family member/caregiver about signs of skin breakdown, as appropriate.

Pressure Ulcer Care: *Facilitation of healing in pressure ulcers*
- Describe characteristics of the ulcer at regular intervals, including size (L × W × D), stage (I-IV), location, exudate, granulation or necrotic tissue, and epithelialization.

- Monitor color, temperature, edema, moisture, and appearance of surrounding skin.
- Keep the ulcer moist to aid in healing.
- Cleanse the skin around the ulcer with mild soap and water.
- Debride ulcer, as needed.
- Cleanse the ulcer with the appropriate nontoxic solution, working in a circular motion from the center.
- Note characteristics of any drainage.
- Apply dressings, as appropriate.
- Monitor for signs and symptoms of infection in the wound.
- Position every 1 to 2 hours to avoid prolonged pressure.
- Use specialty beds and mattresses, as appropriate.
- Ensure adequate dietary intake.
- Monitor nutritional status.
- Teach individual or family member(s) wound care procedures.
- Initiate consultation services of the enterostomal therapy nurse, as needed.

Pressure Management: *Minimizing pressure to body parts*
- Place client on an appropriate therapeutic mattress/bed.
- Place client on a polyurethane foam pad, as appropriate.
- Refrain from applying pressure to the affected body part.
- Elevate injured extremity.
- Turn the immobilized client at least every 2 hours, according to a specific schedule.
- Facilitate small shifts of body weight.
- Monitor skin for areas of redness and breakdown.
- Use an established risk assessment tool to monitor client's risk factors (e.g., Braden scale).
- Monitor the client's nutritional status.
- Monitor for sources of pressure and friction.

NIC intervention activities selected from Dochterman, J.M., & Bulechek, G.M. (2004). *Nursing interventions classification (NIC)* (4th ed.). St. Louis: Mosby. No part of this work is to be altered without prior written permission from the Publisher.

HEALTH PROMOTION/ILLNESS PREVENTION

Pressure ulcers can be prevented if the risk is recognized and intervention begins early (Charts 70-2 and 70-3). Key health care team members for pressure ulcer prevention and management are the enterostomal therapist (ET), the certified wound specialist, and the registered dietitian (RD).

A pressure ulcer prevention program consists of two steps: (1) identification of high-risk clients and (2) implementation of aggressive intervention for prevention with the use of pressure relief or reduction devices. Many facilities do not recognize the value of preventing pressure ulcers through appropriate consultation, the use of pressure relief and pressure reduction products, and ensuring adequate nutrition. The costs of such prevention strategies is more than justified by the savings seen in comparison with the costs of interventions for care when actual ulceration is present (see the Resource Management box on p. 1582).

Risk identification and prevention measures must include education of the client and the caregiver. Documentation of risk assessment, prevention measures implemented, and education of all individuals involved in the care of the client at risk for pressure ulcer formation are key to the plan's success. Periodic reassessment of risk and continuing evaluation of the implemented plan are necessary as client conditions change.

Identification of High-Risk Clients

All clients admitted to a health care facility or home care agency should be assessed for pressure ulcer risk, as recommended by the AHRQ. The use of a risk assessment tool increases the chances of identifying those clients at greater risk for skin breakdown. The two risk assessment tools recommended by the AHRQ guidelines are the Norton Scale and the Braden Scale (Figure 70-4). Other factors to consider when determining the risk category for pressure ulcer formation are mental status, activity/mobility, nutritional status, and incontinence.

MENTAL STATUS/DECREASED SENSORY PERCEPTION

The client's mental status determines whether he or she is a partner in the prevention of pressure. When the client understands that turning and shifting of weight prevent tissue damage, the risk for pressure ulcers decreases. When he or she has a mental status problem because of stroke, head injury, organic brain disease, Alzheimer's disease, or other problem with cognition, the risk for pressure ulcer formation increases.

ACTIVITY/MOBILITY

The level of the client's independent mobility is a direct factor in the risk for pressure ulcer formation. Clients who

CHART 70-3

BEST PRACTICE for
Preventing Pressure Ulcers

Positioning
- Pad contact surfaces with foam, silicon gel, or air pads.
- Do not keep the head of the bed elevated above 30 degrees.
- Use a lift sheet to move client in the bed. Avoid dragging or sliding the client.
- When positioning a client on his or her side, do not position directly on the trochanter.
- Reposition an immobile client every 2 hours while in bed and every 1 hour while sitting in a chair.
- Do not place a rubber ring or doughnut under the client's sacral area.
- When moving an immobile client from a bed to another surface use a designated slide board well lubricated with talc.
- Place pillows or foam wedges between two bony surfaces.
- Keep the client's skin directly off plastic surfaces.
- Keep the client's heels off the bed surface.

Nutrition
- Ensure a fluid intake between 2000 and 3000 mL/day.
- Help the client maintain an adequate intake of protein and calories.

Skin Care
- Use moisturizers daily on dry skin, and apply when skin is damp.
- Keep moisture from prolonged contact with skin.
  Dry areas where two skin surfaces touch, such as the axilla and under the breasts.
  Place absorbent pads under areas where perspiration collects.
  Use moisture barriers on skin areas where wound drainage or incontinence occurs.
- Do not massage bony prominences.
- Humidify the room.

Skin Cleaning
- Clean the skin as soon as possible after soiling occurs and at routine intervals.
- Use a mild, heavily fatted soap.
- Use tepid rather than hot water.
- While cleaning, use the minimal scrubbing force necessary to remove soil.
- Gently pat rather than rub the skin dry.

RESOURCE MANAGEMENT

PRESSURE ULCER PREVENTION

Cost of Care
- Medicare reimbursement for medically complex residents of long-term care decreased from an average of $408 to $231 per day, beginning in 1997.
- Most residents with complex wounds and stage III or IV pressure ulcers fall into the category of medically complex.
- Pressure relief/reduction devices and appropriate dressing materials cost more than the available reimbursement.
- Many long-term care facilities made product choices based on cost alone.
- Use of pressure relief/reduction devices for prevention of pressure ulcers was limited.
- The number and severity of pressure ulcers among residents of long-term care facilities increased during this budget reduction period.

Implications for Nursing
An ounce of prevention may be worth tons rather than pounds of cure. Although on the surface, pressure relief/reduction devices, high protein diets, and appropriate dressing materials appear expensive, the actual cost in nursing hours, equipment, devices, and consumable supplies when caring for a client with even one pressure ulcer is far greater. Legislation signed in 1999 allows prevention costs as well as care costs to be justly reimbursed. Nurses need to consider pressure ulcer prevention in care setting as a number one priority of care.

Data from Motta, G. (2000). Reimbursement relief. *Continuing Care, 19*(4), 14-16.

to consume an adequate diet; and the need for vitamin, mineral, or protein supplementation. Nutrition is inadequate when the client's serum albumin level is lower than 3.5 mg/dL or the lymphocyte count is less than 1800/mm³. Other indicators of inadequate nutrition include a weight loss of 15% of total body weight or greater.

A positive nitrogen balance requires an intake of 30 to 35 calories per kilogram of body weight daily with a protein intake of 1.25 to 1.5 g/kg/day. Up to 2 g/kg/day of protein may be needed when nutritional deficits are severe or protein loss is ongoing. Vitamin supplementation is based on the client's nutritional status.

INCONTINENCE

Incontinence results in prolonged contact of the skin with such substances as urea, bacteria, yeast, and enzymes carried in urine and feces. These substances are irritants and lead to skin breakdown. Excessive moisture macerates intact skin, increasing the risk for breakdown. Daily inspection of the skin for any areas of redness or skin breakdown is a major part of pressure ulcer prevention. Maintenance of clean, intact skin also assists in the prevention process. The skin should be washed with a pH-balanced soap to maintain the normal acid level. Creams or lotions are used to lubricate and moisturize the skin. Barrier ointment protection is needed whenever incontinence is present. Absorbent pads or garments must be changed quickly with each incontinence episode to avoid prolonged skin contact with urine or feces. *Reddened areas are never massaged because this action can damage capillary beds and increase tissue necrosis.*

Pressure-Relieving Techniques

The cornerstone in the prevention (and treatment) of pressure ulcers is adequate pressure relief. A factor in pressure re-

have unimpaired mobility and can respond to physical sensation changes are at low risk for pressure ulcer formation. Any client, regardless of age, who requires assistance with turning and positioning or who is less aware of physical sensation changes is at high risk for pressure ulcer formation. A client who is confined to bed or a chair is at higher risk than a client who requires assistance with ambulation.

NUTRITIONAL STATUS

Nutritional status is a critical risk factor for pressure ulcer development. Intact skin and wound healing are dependent on a positive nitrogen balance and adequate serum protein levels. The client in a negative nitrogen balance not only heals more slowly but also is at greater risk for tissue destruction. In addition, draining wounds are a route of protein loss.

Adequate nutrition is critical in the prevention of pressure ulcer formation. A dietitian or nutrition specialist should be a part of the pressure reduction team or program.

Nutritional status assessment includes laboratory studies; evaluation of weight and weight change; ability of the client

Client's name _____ Evaluator's name _____ Date of assessment _____

Sensory perception Ability to respond meaningfully to pressure-related discomfort	**1. Completely limited** Unresponsive to painful stimuli (does not moan, flinch, or grasp) because of diminished level of consciousness or sedation OR limited ability to feel pain over most of body surface	**2. Very limited** Responds only to painful stimuli; cannot communicate discomfort except by moaning or restlessness OR has a sensory impairment that limits the ability to feel pain or discomfort over half of the body	**3. Slightly limited** Responds to verbal commands but cannot always communicate discomfort or need to be turned OR has some sensory impairment that limits ability to feel pain or discomfort in one or two extremities	**4. No impairment** Responds to verbal commands; has no sensory deficit that would limit ability to feel or voice pain or discomfort
Moisture Degree to which skin is exposed to moisture	**1. Constantly moist** Skin is kept moist almost constantly by perspiration, urine; dampness is detected every time the client is moved or turned	**2. Very Moist** Skin is often but not always moist; linen must be changed at least once a shift	**3. Occasionally moist** Skin is occasionally moist, requiring an extra linen change approximately once a day	**4. Rarely moist** Skin is usually dry; linen requires changing only at routine intervals
Activity Degree of physical activity	**1. Bedfast** Confined to bed	**2. Chairfast** Ability to walk severely limited or nonexistent; cannot bear own weight and must be assisted into chair or wheelchair	**3. Walks occasionally** Walks occasionally during the day but for very short distances, with or without assistance; spends the majority of each shift in bed or chair	**4. Walks frequently** Walks outside the room at least twice a day and inside the room at least once every 2 hours during waking hours
Mobility Ability to change or control body position	**1. Completely immobile** Does not make even slight changes in body or extremity position without assistance	**2. Very limited** Makes occasional slight changes in body or extremity position but unable to make frequent or significant changes independently	**3. Slightly limited** Makes frequent though slight changes in body or extremity position independently	**4. No limitations** Makes major and frequent changes in position without assistance
Nutrition Usual food intake pattern	**1. Very poor** Never eats a complete meal; rarely eats more than a third of any food offered; eats two servings or less of protein (meat or dairy products) per day; takes fluids poorly; does not take a liquid dietary supplement OR is NPO or maintained on clear liquids or IV for more than 5 days	**2. Probably inadequate** Rarely eats a complete meal and generally eats only about half of any food offered; protein intake includes only three servings of meat or dairy products per day; occasionally will take a dietary supplement OR receives less than optimal amount of liquid diet or tube feeding	**3. Adequate** Eats over half of most meals; eats a total of four servings of protein (meat, dairy products) each day; occasionally will refuse a meal, but will usually take a supplement if offered OR is receiving tube feeding or total parenteral nutrition, which probably meets most nutritional needs	**4. Excellent** Eats most of every meal; never refuses a meal; usually eats a total of four or more servings of meat and dairy products; occasionally eats between meals; does not require supplementation
Friction and shear	**1. Problem** Requires moderate to maximum assistance in moving; complete lifting without sliding against sheets is impossible; frequently slides down in bed or chair, requiring frequent repositioning with maximum assistance; spasticity, contractures, or agitation leads to almost constant friction	**2. Potential problem** Moves feebly or requires minimum assistance during a move; skin probably slides to some extent against sheets, chair, restraints, or other devices; maintains relatively good position in chair or bed most of the time but occasionally slides down	**3. No apparent problem** Moves in bed and in chair independently and has sufficient muscle strength to lift up completely during move; maintains good position in bed or chair at all times	

Total score _____

Scoring system: 15-16 = mild risk, 12-14 = moderate risk, <11 = severe risk

Figure 70-4 ■ The Braden Scale for predicting pressure ulcer risk. IV, Intravenous; NPO, nothing by mouth. (From Barbara Braden and Nancy Bergstrom. Copyright 1988. Reprinted with permission.)

lief is the **capillary closing pressure,** which is the amount of pressure needed to occlude skin capillary blood flow, in the area at risk. The normal capillary closing pressure ranges from 12 to 32 mm Hg. Any device used must provide pressure relief below the capillary closing pressure to prevent tissue ischemia. *Most devices have a standardized guaranteed pressure relief reading; however, these readings do not ensure that capillary blood flow for any given client is adequate. You must observe skin color, integrity, and temperature to determine capillary flow adequacy.*

Devices are classified according to whether they relieve pressure or merely reduce pressure. In addition, devices are further classified as dynamic or static. Dynamic systems alternate inflation and deflation of the device through the use of electricity. Static devices made of gel, water, foam, or air are in a constant state of inflation that distributes the client pressure load over a larger area and reduce the pressure any one area experiences.

Pressure relief/reduction products come in many forms, such as specialty beds, mattress replacements, overlays, and assistive devices. Choosing the correct product is important in the success of the prevention plan. The product selected is re-evaluated daily for effectiveness in reducing pressure, comfort, and elimination of "bottoming out," wherein the client's bony prominences sink into the mattress or cushion, causing him or her to have pressure even with the product in place.

PRESSURE-RELIEF DEVICES

Pressure-relief devices consistently reduce pressure below capillary closing pressure. These devices are recommended for clients who need the following:

- Prevention of skin breakdown because they cannot turn
- Prevention of extension of skin breakdown that has already occurred
- Promotion of healing for breakdown present on several turning surfaces

PRESSURE-REDUCTION DEVICES

Pressure-reduction devices lower pressure below that of a standard hospital mattress or chair surface but do not reduce pressure consistently below the capillary closing pressure. Such devices must be used along with a turning schedule.

POSITIONING

A good plan for positioning is the 30-degree rule. This plan ensures that the client is positioned and propped so that whatever part of the body is elevated is tilted back at least 30 degrees to the mattress rather than resting directly on a dependent bony prominence. This rule applies to side-lying as well as head-of-bed elevation positions. The client who must be elevated to a full 90 degrees because of respiratory difficulties should be tilted forward even more than 90 degrees, with pillows behind the back to keep pressure off of the sacral/coccyx area.

The client at risk for pressure ulcers in bed is also at risk while sitting. Carefully assess for proper wheelchair or regular chair cushioning. Consult with physical therapists and rehabilitation specialists for selection of these products.

Even with an appropriate mattress or cushion, the client must change or be helped to change positions periodically. Many facilities require turning and positioning every 2 hours. *However, pressure can occur in less time, and the actual turning or repositioning schedule for each client must be individualized.*

Use pillows and other positioning/padding devices to keep heels pressure-free at all times for high-risk clients. Assess heel positioning frequently to ensure that pressure is not redistributed to another high-risk area, such as the sides of the feet. Assess even more frequently when devices that hide the feet, such as boots, are used, especially if the client has a peripheral vascular problem.

◆COLLABORATIVE MANAGEMENT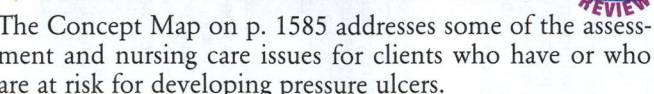

The Concept Map on p. 1585 addresses some of the assessment and nursing care issues for clients who have or who are at risk for developing pressure ulcers.

◆Assessment

HISTORY

When taking a history from the client with a pressure ulcer, identify the underlying cause of skin loss as well as factors that may impair healing. Ask about the specific circumstances of the skin loss. In general, clients with chronic pressure ulcerations usually have a history of delayed healing or recurrence of the ulcer after healing has occurred. Because pressure-related skin loss is common among severely debilitated clients, determine whether a client has any of the following contributing factors:

- Prolonged bedrest
- Immobility
- Incontinence
- Inadequate nutrition or hydration
- Altered mental status (decreased sensory perception)

PHYSICAL ASSESSMENT/CLINICAL MANIFESTATIONS

Inspect the entire body, including the back of the head, for areas of skin injury or pressure. Give special attention to bony prominences (such as the heels, sacrum, elbows, trochanter, posterior and anterior iliac spines) and areas that are vulnerable to excessive moisture. In addition, assess the client's general appearance for issues related to skin health. Such issues include body weight and the proportion of weight to height because obese persons as well as thin persons are at increased risk for pressure ulcer formation. Check overall cleanliness of the skin, hair, and nails. Determine whether any loss of mobility or range of joint motion has occurred.

WOUND ASSESSMENT

The appearance of pressure ulcers changes with the depth of the injury. Chart 70-4 lists the features of the four stages of pressure ulceration, and Figures 70-5 to 70-8 show examples.

Assess wounds for location, size, color, extent of tissue involvement, cell types in the wound base and margins, exudate, condition of surrounding tissue, and the presence of foreign bodies. Document this initial assessment to serve as a starting point for determining the intervention plan and its effectiveness. How often a wound is assessed is determined by the written policies and procedures at the facility or agency. Weekly documented assessment is the standard in many facilities. *However, also assess the wound at each dress-*

CONCEPT MAP Pressure Ulcer

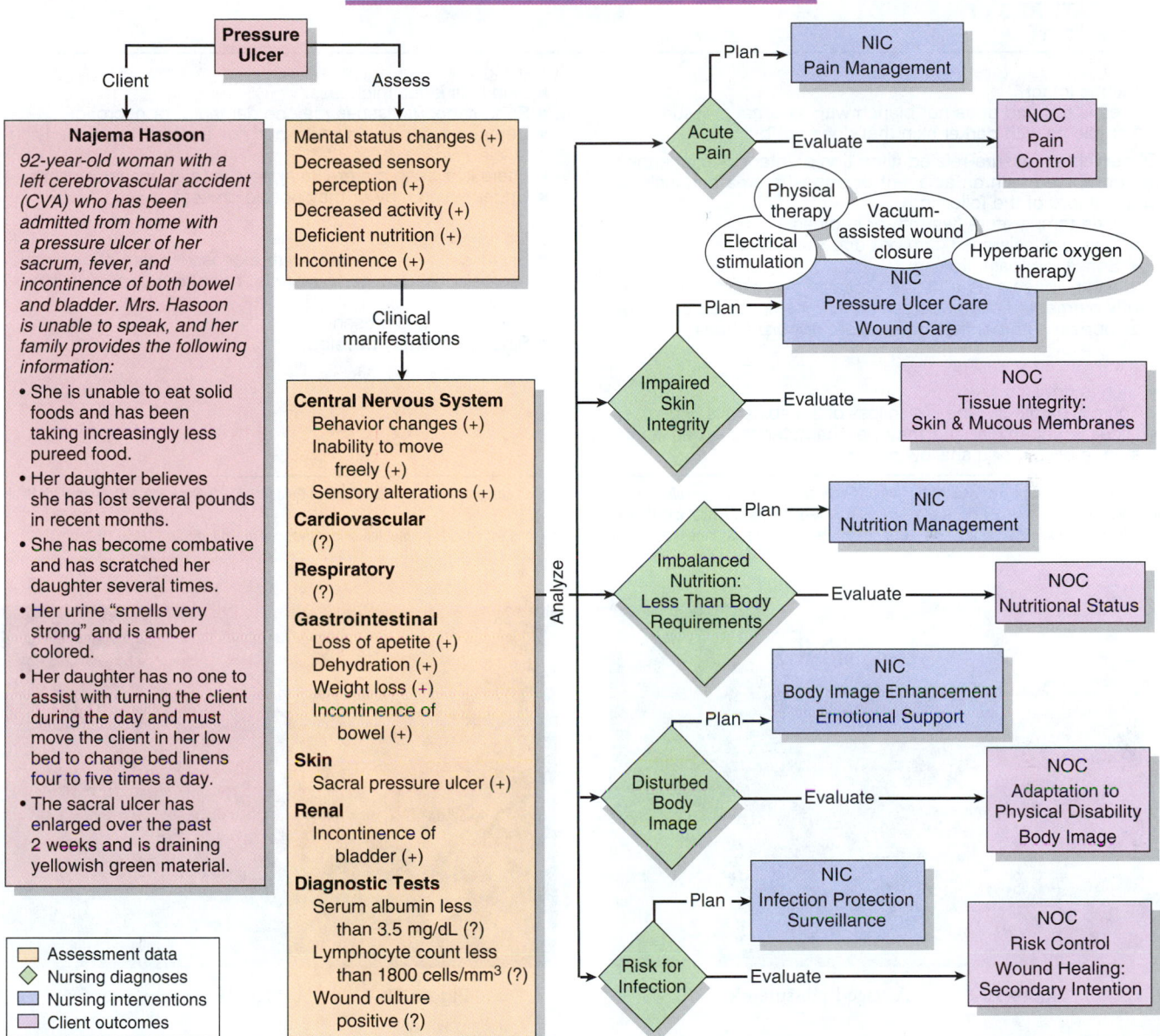

Concept Map by Elaine Bishop Kennedy, EdD, RN

ing change, comparing the existing wound features with those documented previously to determine the current state of healing or deterioration.

Record the location and size of the wound first. Wounds are sized by length, width, and depth using millimeters or centimeters. In standardizing wound size for documentation and communication purposes, assess the wound as a clock face with 12 o'clock in the direction of the client's head and 6 o'clock in the direction of the client's feet. Always measure the length from 12 o'clock to 6 o'clock and the width between 9 o'clock and 3 o'clock. Measure depth as the distance from the deepest portion of the wound base to the skin level. When all caregivers use this format, measurement is accurate and wound progress can be determined.

Inspect the wound margins for **cellulitis** (inflammation of the skin cells) extending beyond the area of injury. Progressive tissue destruction, seen as an increase in the size or

depth of the ulcer and increased wound drainage, usually indicates an impairment in the client's ability to resist infection if proper measures have been taken to relieve pressure.

Inspect the wound for the presence or absence of necrotic tissue. Because of the depth of tissue destruction, a full-thickness pressure ulcer is often covered by a layer of black, gray, or brown nonviable, denatured collagen called wound **eschar.**

In the early stages of wound healing, the eschar is dry, leathery, and firmly attached to the wound surface. As the inflammatory phase of wound healing begins and removal of wound debris progresses, the eschar starts to lift and separate from the tissue beneath. This nonliving eschar is a good breeding ground for bacteria normally found on the skin surface as well as those introduced by other means. As bacteria increase, they release enzymes, which softens necrotic tissue. This tissue becomes softer and more yellow.

CHART 70-4

KEY FEATURES of
Pressure Ulcers

Stage I
- Skin is intact.
- Area is red and does not blanch with external pressure.
- For clients with darker skin that does not blanch:*

Observable pressure-related alteration of intact skin; changes are compared with an adjacent or opposite area and include one or more of the following:
  - Skin temperature (warmth or coolness)
  - Tissue consistency (firm or boggy)
  - Sensation (pain, itching)

The ulcer appears as a defined area of persistent redness in lightly pigmented skin, whereas in darker skin tones, the ulcer may appear with persistent red, blue, or purple hues.

Stage II
- Skin is not intact.
- There is partial-thickness skin loss of the epidermis or dermis.
- Ulcer is superficial and may be characterized as an abrasion, a blister, or a shallow crater.

Stage III
- Skin loss is full thickness.
- Subcutaneous tissues may be damaged or necrotic.
- Damage extends down to but not through the underlying fascia.
- There is a deep crater-like appearance or eschar present.
- Undermining may or may not be present.

Stage IV
- Skin loss is full thickness with extensive destruction, tissue necrosis, or damage to muscle, bone, or supporting structures.
- Undermining is present.
- Sinus tracts may develop.

Data from U.S. Department of Health and Human Services. (1992). *Pressure ulcers in adults: Prediction and prevention.* Clinical Practice Guideline No. 3. Rockville, MD: Agency for Health Care Policy and Research, Public Health Service, U.S. Department of Health and Human Services.
* Data from Henderson, C., et al. (1997). Draft definition of stage I pressure ulcers: Inclusion of persons with darkly pigmented skin. *Advances in Wound Care, 10*(5), 16-19.

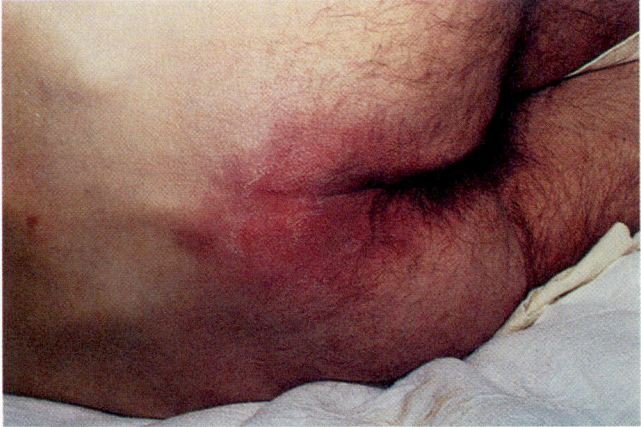

Figure 70-5 ■ A stage I pressure ulcer.

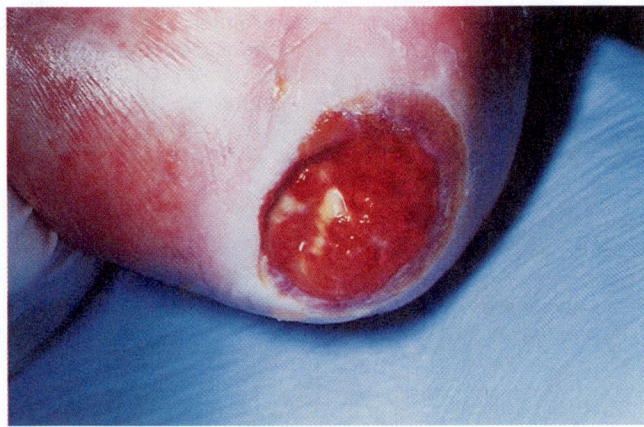

Figure 70-7 ■ A stage III pressure ulcer.

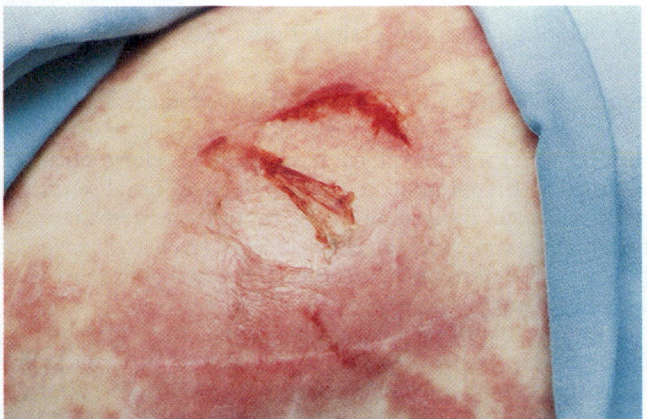

Figure 70-6 ■ A stage II pressure ulcer.

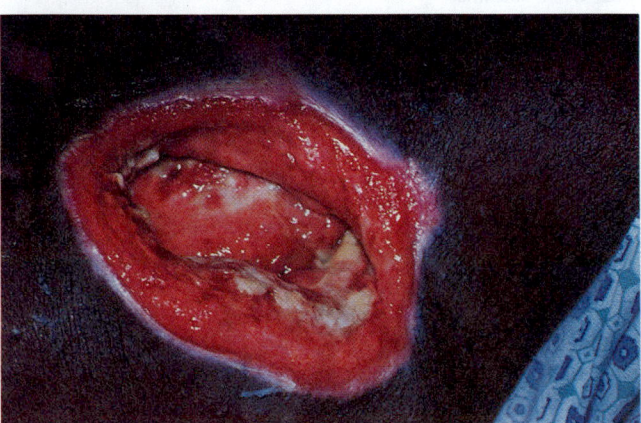

Figure 70-8 ■ A stage IV pressure ulcer.

TABLE 70-4   Types of Wound Exudate

Characteristics	Significance
Serosanguineous Exudate	
Blood-tinged amber fluid consisting of serum and red blood cells	Normal for first 48 hr after injury
	Sudden increase in amount precedes wound dehiscence in wounds closed by first intention
Purulent Exudate	
Creamy yellow pus	Colonization with *Staphylococcus*
Greenish blue pus causing staining of dressings and accompanied by a "fruity" odor	Colonization with *Pseudomona*
Beige pus with a "fishy" odor	Colonization with *Proteus*
Brownish pus with a "fecal" odor	Colonization with aerobic coliform and *Bacteroides* (usually occurs after intestinal surgery)

In the presence of bacterial colonization, wound exudate increases substantially; the color and odor of wound exudate indicate the major organism present. The features of wound exudate are listed in Table 70-4.

Beneath the separating dead tissue, granulation tissue appears. Early granulation is pale pink, progressing to a beefy red color as it grows and fills the wound. A wound with poor local arterial blood supply appears dry with pale, immature granulation tissue present. Venous obstruction causes an excessively moist ulcer surface with a deep red color (reflective of the deoxygenated blood beneath the ulcer surface).

Palpate the wound to determine the texture of the granulations. Healthy granulations have a slightly spongy texture. Pressure ulcers may involve more extensive tissue destruction than is first seen on inspection. Separation of the skin layers at the wound margins from the underlying granulation tissue is known as **undermining.** Inspect undermined areas for gradual filling with healthy granulations and for wound-healing progress. Palpate the bony prominences for deep hardening of the surrounding soft tissue, which often suggests tissue ischemia well beneath the surface of the skin.

After ischemia has occurred, continued pressure over the area of injury allows progression of tissue destruction from the deep tissue layers toward the surface. This "hidden" wound may first have a small opening in the skin with purulent drainage. If you observe such an opening, use a cotton-tipped applicator to probe gently for a much larger pocket of necrotic tissue beneath the opening.

PSYCHOSOCIAL ASSESSMENT

The client with pressure ulcers may have an altered body image. Ineffective coping patterns emerge as the client and family or significant others strive to adhere to changes in lifestyle that are needed for healing. In addition, chronic, slow-healing ulcers are often painful and costly to treat.

Assess the client's and family's knowledge of the treatment goals at each stage of the healing process as well as adherence to the prescribed treatment regimen. Also assess the client's skills in cleaning the wound and applying a dressing. Poor adherence to pressure ulcer care procedures may reflect an inability to accept the diagnosis or to cope with the pain,

cost, or potential scarring associated with prolonged healing. Depending on the client's activity level and the location of the ulcer, assistance of a family member or home care nurse may be needed to care for the pressure ulcer at home.

Explore with the client specific changes in activities of daily living (ADLs) that are needed to relieve pressure and promote healing. Promote increased activity whenever possible to enhance circulation to the affected tissue. Bedrest with elevation of the legs may be needed for healing when ulcers occur on the lower legs, especially for the client with poor venous blood flow and lower-leg edema. When the client is bedridden, frequent repositioning to relieve pressure (every 2 hours in bed, every 1 hour in a chair) can be labor intensive. In the home environment, repositioning, incontinence management, and dressing changes are often needed around the clock, disrupting family routines and contributing to stress.

LABORATORY ASSESSMENT

A wound that is exposed is always *contaminated* but is not always *infected.* **Contamination** is the presence of organisms without any clinical manifestation of infection. The normal immune defenses of the body keep the number of bacteria to a minimum and prevent infection. **Wound infection** is contamination with pathogenic organisms to the degree that growth and spread cannot be controlled by the body's immune defenses. Wounds that are inflamed, indurated, red, have an odor, and have moderate to heavy exudate should be cultured to identify the causative organism and determine its sensitivity to antibiotics. The presence of pus as exudate alone does not indicate an infection because pus formation occurs when necrotic tissue debrides and liquefies.

If wounds are extensive, if the client is severely immunocompromised, or if local blood supply to the wound is impaired, bacterial growth may exceed the body's ability to defend against invasion into deeper tissue layers. The result is deep wound infection and eventually bacteremia and **sepsis** (systemic infection).

Swab cultures are helpful only in identifying the types of bacteria present on the ulcer surface and may be misleading when trying to identify or quantify bacteria in deeper tissues. Tests such as quantitative wound biopsies allow the numbers of bacteria to be analyzed. Unfortunately these tests are time consuming, costly, and unavailable in many laboratories. Therefore clinical indicators of infection (cellulitis, progressive increase in ulcer size or depth, changes in the quantity and quality of exudate) and systemic signs of bacteremia are important criteria in the diagnosis and treatment of an infection.

OTHER DIAGNOSTIC ASSESSMENTS

Additional laboratory studies are performed on the basis of the suspected cause of the wound. For pressure ulcers to show progress toward healing, the factors contributing to delayed healing must be diagnosed and treated. For example, noninvasive and invasive arterial blood flow studies are indicated if arterial occlusion is suspected in delayed healing of a pressure ulcer on the heel or ankle. Blood tests to establish specific nutritional deficiencies are helpful in treating the debilitated, malnourished client with a pressure ulcer.

◆ Analysis

COMMON NURSING DIAGNOSES AND COLLABORATIVE PROBLEMS

The most common nursing diagnosis for clients with pressure ulcers is Impaired Skin Integrity related to vascular insufficiency and trauma. The most common collaborative problem is Risk for Infection and Wound Extension.

ADDITIONAL NURSING DIAGNOSES AND COLLABORATIVE PROBLEMS

In addition to the common nursing diagnoses and collaborative problems, clients with pressure ulcers may have one or more of the following:

- Acute Pain or Chronic Pain related to skin trauma, wound infection, and wound treatment
- Disturbed Body Image related to altered appearance
- Ineffective Coping related to the chronicity of the ulcer, alteration in body image, and changes in lifestyle required to promote healing
- Imbalanced Nutrition: Less Than Body Requirements related to inability to ingest food due to biologic, psychological, or economic factors
- Ineffective Tissue Perfusion (Peripheral) related to mechanical reduction of venous or arterial blood flow
- Deficient Knowledge (treatment) related to cognitive limitation or unfamiliarity with information resources

◆ Planning and Implementation

IMPAIRED SKIN INTEGRITY

NOC **PLANNING: EXPECTED OUTCOMES.** The client with a pressure ulcer is expected to experience complete wound healing and not experience the formation of new pressure ulcers. Indicators include the following:

- Presence of granulation, re-epithelialization, and scar tissue formation
- Decreased wound size
- Absence of new pressure ulcers

INTERVENTIONS. Wound care techniques for pressure ulcers vary according to each client's needs and the physician's preferences. Surgery with aggressive removal of necrotic tissue may be indicated for some clients, whereas a nonsurgical approach to ulcer debridement is preferred for an older client who has adequate defenses but is too ill or debilitated for surgery.

TABLE 70-5 Common Dressing Techniques for Wound Debridement

Technique	Mechanism of Action
Wet-to-dry saline-moistened gauze	Dry, necrotic debris is softened by the saline, allowing it to become more effectively entrapped in the interstices as the gauze dries and shrinks. Dressing may also entrap healing tissue.
Wet-to-damp saline-moistened gauze	As with the wet-to-dry technique, necrotic debris is mechanically removed but with less trauma to healing tissue.
Continuous wet gauze	The wound surface is continually bathed with a wetting agent of choice, promoting dilution of viscous exudate and softening of dry eschar.
Topical enzyme preparations	Proteolytic action on thick, adherent eschar causes breakdown of denatured protein and more rapid separation of necrotic tissue.
Moisture-retentive dressing	Spontaneous separation of necrotic tissue is promoted by autolysis.

NONSURGICAL MANAGEMENT. The NIC interventions for pressure ulcer prevention and management are listed in Chart 70-2. Nonsurgical intervention of pressure ulcers is often left to the discretion of the nurse, who collaborates with the physician to select a method of wound dressing on the basis of the identified goal of wound management.

Dressings. A properly designed dressing can speed healing by removing unwanted debris from the ulcer surface, protecting exposed healthy tissues, and creating a barrier between the body and the environment until the ulcer is closed. For a client with a draining, necrotic ulcer, the dressing must also remove excessive exudate and loose debris without damaging epithelial cells or newly formed granulation tissue. If necrosis is extensive and the eschar is thick, dead tissue must be surgically or chemically removed before further debridement with dressings will be effective. Depending on the dressing material used, dressings help to remove debris either through mechanical entrapment and detachment of dead tissue or by creating an environment that promotes self-digestion of dead tissues by the bacterial enzymes (autolysis) (Table 70-5).

After all the dead tissue has been removed, protection of any exposed vital structures, such as tendon, bone, and newly formed collagen, is critical to pressure ulcer care. The ideal environment for healing is a clean, *slightly* moist ulcer surface with minimal bacterial colonization. Heavy moisture from an excessively draining ulcer or a dressing that is too wet interferes with healing by promoting the growth of organisms and causing maceration of healthy tissue. Likewise, if a clean ulcer surface is exposed to air or if highly absorbent dressing materials are used for prolonged periods, the drying effect can dehydrate surface cells, form scabs, or convert the wound to a deeper injury.

Assess the ulcer for necrotic tissue and the quantity of exudate. Select a dressing material with properties that promote an optimal environment for healing (Table 70-6). For example, a material that does not stick to the wound surface and does not remove fragile epithelial cells when it is

TABLE 70-6   Commonly Used Dressing Materials

	Alginates	Biologic Dressings	Cotton Gauze Dressing	Foams	Hydrocolloidal Wafers	Hydrogel Dressing	Transparent Films
Indications	Absorption Protection	Debridement after eschar removal* Protection Test before skin grafts (pigskin and cadaver skin) Burns Dormant, nonhealing wounds that do not respond to other topical therapies	**Continuous Dry** Absorption Protection (nonadherent contact layer) **Continuous Wet** Delivery of topical agent Debridement (autolysis) Protection **Wet to Damp** Atraumatic mechanical debridement **Wet to Dry** Aggressive mechanical debridement	Absorption Protection	Debridement* Absorption Protection	Debridement* Absorption Protection	Debridement* (partial-thickness lesions) Secondary (cover) dressing
Advantages	Highly absorbent Biodegradable Easy application Nonadhesive Can be used as packing for deep wounds Can be used for infected wounds	Most "natural" wound covering Reduces pain Conforms to uneven wound surfaces Acts as a catalyst for healing Alternative to autograft	Readily available Good mechanical debridement *if used properly* Effective delivery of topical agents	Absorbent Insulates wound Easy application Nonadhesive (most products) Conforms to uneven wound surfaces	Absorbent Excludes bacteria Waterproof Reduces pain Easy application Easy to store	Absorbent Nonadhesive Reduce pain Conducive to use with topical agents Conforms to uneven wound surfaces Amorphous form can be used as a filler Easy to store	Wound visualization Good adhesion Waterproof Reduces pain Cost-effective Easy to store
Disadvantages	Requires secondary dressing to secure Can cause desiccation of tissue if drainage is minimal	Requires secondary dressing to secure Very expensive Skin substitutes require skill to apply	Delayed healing if used improperly Pain on removal Requires frequent dressing changes	Poor barrier function Requires secondary dressing to secure	Nontransparent Softening and loss of shape with pressure, heat, and friction Odor with dressing removal Expensive Requires use of "fillers" for deep, draining lesions	Poor barrier function Only partial wound visualization Requires secondary dressing to secure Can promote growth of *Pseudomonas* and other microorganisms	Difficult to apply properly Nonabsorbent Adhesive to normal and healing tissue Limited to superficial lesions
Dressing changes	When dressing is saturated (q3-5 days) or more frequently	Topical growth factors: Daily skin substitutes: Varies (similar to grafts)	Necrotic base: q4-6h Clean base: q12-24h	When dressing is saturated or more frequently	Necrotic base: q24h Clean base: on leakage of exudate	Necrotic base: q6-8h Clean base: q24h	Necrotic base: q24h Clean base: on leakage of exudate

*Use with caution in clients with leukopenia or vascular disease.

changed is the dressing of choice for protecting new tissue. Depending on the amount of drainage, select either a hydrophobic or a hydrophilic material:

- A **hydrophobic** (nonabsorbent, waterproof) material is useful when the wound is relatively free of drainage and the purpose is to protect the ulcer from external contamination.
- A **hydrophilic** (absorbent) material draws excessive drainage away from the ulcer surface, preventing maceration.

A variety of synthetic materials with hydrophilic and hydrophobic properties is available. Unlike cotton gauze dressings, these may be left intact for extended periods. Biologic and synthetic skin substitutes are available that can also prevent tissue dehydration and promote healing (see Chapter 71). However, the use of these products for chronic wounds is often cost prohibitive.

The frequency of dressing changes depends on the amount of necrotic material or exudate. Dry gauze dressings are changed when "strike through" occurs or when the outer layer of the dressing first becomes saturated with exudate. Gauze dressings used for debridement, such as those placed on a wound wet, allowed to dry, and then removed, are changed often enough to take off any loose debris or exudate, usually every 4 to 6 hours. Synthetic dressings are changed when exudate causes the adhesive seal to break and leakage to occur.

Before reapplying any dressing, gently clean the ulcer surface with saline or a nontoxic wound cleanser as prescribed. If an antibacterial cleanser is prescribed, dilute the agent to reduce tissue toxicity and then rinse and dry the surface thoroughly before applying the dressing.

Physical Therapy. The use of daily whirlpool treatments along with dressing changes for debridement can help remove dead tissue. The ulcerated area is immersed in warm tap water that contains an antibacterial cleansing agent. Continuous agitation of the water loosens the debris and washes away exudate and particulate matter. During treatment, clean the ulcer surface with a gauze pad. After treatment the therapist or certified wound specialist often uses instruments to trim away any obvious bits of dead tissue that are still loosely attached to the ulcer surface.

Drug Therapy. Clean, healthy granulation tissue has a blood supply and is capable of providing white blood cells and antibodies to the ulcer surface to combat infection. If extensive necrosis is present or if local tissue defenses are impaired, topical antibacterial agents are often needed to control bacterial growth. (Chapter 71 details the advantages and uses of topical antimicrobial agents.) In the absence of infection, antibiotics are avoided because of the danger of the development of resistant strains of bacteria.

Diet Therapy. Successful healing of pressure ulcers depends on adequate nutritional stores of calories, protein, vitamins, minerals, and water (Zulkowski & Albrecht, 2003). Nutritional deficiencies are common among older adults and chronically ill clients. Such deficiencies increase the risk for skin breakdown and delayed healing of wounds that are already present. Severe protein deficiency inhibits all stages of the healing process and impairs host defenses against bacterial invasion.

To promote healing, encourage the client to eat a well-balanced diet, emphasizing foods containing nutrients vital to cell growth and collagen synthesis (Table 70-7). If the client cannot eat sufficient amounts of food, nasogastric feedings and hyperalimentation via a central venous catheter may be needed to increase protein and caloric intake. Vitamin and mineral supplements are also indicated.

New Technologies. For chronic ulcers that remain open for months, new technologies have had some success. These include electrical stimulation, vacuum-assisted wound closure, and hyperbaric oxygen therapy.

Electrical Stimulation. Applying a low-voltage current to a wound area can increase blood vessel growth and promote granulation (Kloth, 2002). This treatment is usually performed by a certified wound care specialist. A single electrode can be applied directly to a wound through a sterile dressing, or multiple electrodes can be applied around a wound. When multiple electrodes are used, the positive and negative poles are arranged to allow the current to move through the wound area. Voltage intensities ranging from 50 to 150 are delivered in "pulses" that may cause the client to feel a "tingling" sensation. Usually electrical stimulation is performed for one hour each day five to seven times per week. This form of treatment is not used with clients who have a pacemaker or who have a wound over the heart.

Vacuum-Assisted Wound Closure. Vacuum-assisted wound closure has been used successfully to reduce or even close chronic ulcers by enhancing the formation of granulation tissue (Patel, Kinsey, Koperski-Moen, & Bungum, 2000). This technique requires that a suction tube be covered by a special sponge and sealed in place for 48 hours. During that time, continuous low-level negative pressure is applied through the suction tube. Duration of the treatment is determined by the wound's response.

Hyperbaric Oxygen Therapy. Hyperbaric oxygen (HBO) therapy is the administration of oxygen under high pressure, raising the tissue oxygen concentration (Leifer, 2001). This type of therapy is costly and usually reserved for life- or limb-threatening wounds such as burns, necrotizing soft tissue infections, brown recluse spider bites, osteomyelitis, and diabetic ulcers. The client is enclosed in a large chamber and exposed to 100% oxygen at pressures greater than normal atmospheric (sea level) pressure. Systemic oxygen enhances the ability of white blood cells to kill bacteria and reduce swelling. Treatment usually lasts from 60 to 90 minutes. Topical oxygen delivery devices are also available. These devices are applied directly over an open wound to promote local tissue oxygenation. Studies supporting the benefits of topical oxygen are limited, and more research in this area is needed.

SURGICAL MANAGEMENT. Surgical management of a pressure ulcer includes removal of necrotic tissue and skin grafting to close wounds that cannot heal by epithelialization and contraction.

Preoperative Care. Preoperative care is focused on preparing the ulcer to accept a skin graft. Monitor potential donor sites, taking care to maintain the integrity of the donor skin and to avoid minor injuries that may result in infection and graft loss.

Operative Procedures. The operative procedures used for surgical management of pressure ulcers include debridement and grafting. One or both of these procedures may be done.

Debridement, or sharp excision of thick, adherent wound eschar using a scalpel or scissors, may be performed

TABLE 70-7 Foods That Promote Wound Healing

Food	Function	Food	Function
Protein Sources Meat Fish Poultry Milk Cheese Eggs Soybeans Legumes Nuts Nutritional supplements	Maintenance and healing of body tissues Antibody production Energy	**Sources of Vitamin B$_{12}$** Liver Organ meats Muscle meats Fish Eggs Shellfish Milk Yogurt Cheese	Protein synthesis

Carbohydrate Sources
Whole grains (preferable
  to enriched because of
  higher nutritional and
  fiber content)
Enriched grain and cereal
  products
Fruit
Juices
Vegetables (especially
  starchy ones: corn,
  peas, potatoes)
Milk
Desserts and sweets
	Energy
	Sparing of protein (if diet does
	  not contain sufficient nonpro-
	  tein calories, protein from body
	  tissues will be broken down to
	  supply energy)
	Wound healing
		Sources of Vitamin B$_6$
		Meats
		Liver
		Some vegetables (includ-
		  ing potatoes)
		Wheat germ
		Wheat bran
		Whole-grain cereals and
		  breads
		Fish
		Brewer's yeast
		Dried beans
			Amino acid metabolism

Sources of Vitamin C
Berries
Broccoli
Brussels sprouts
Cabbage
Citrus fruits and juices
Green peppers
Kale
Melons
Spinach and dark green
  vegetables
Tomatoes
Vitamin C–enriched juices
	Collagen synthesis
	Immunity
		Folate Sources
		Liver
		Yeast
		Leafy vegetables
		Dried beans
		Green vegetables
		Nuts
		Fresh oranges
		Whole-wheat cereals and
		  breads
			Protein synthesis

Zinc Sources
Same as protein sources
Beef
Organ meat
Shellfish
Salmon
Poultry
Cheese
Whole grains
Dried beans
	Tissue repair (zinc-deficient diet
	  causes poor wound healing,
	  decreased ability to taste, and
	  poor appetite)
	Protein synthesis
		Water Sources
		Water
		Milk
		Juices
		Gelatin
		Tomatoes
		Citrus fruit
		Melons
		Vegetables
		Berries
		Broths
		Soups
		Tea
		Coffee
		Carbonated beverages
			Maintain condition of the skin
			  (dehydration can lead to tissue
			  breakdown, poor appetite, and
			  constipation)

Iron Sources*
Liver
Meat
Baked beans
Dried fruits
Legumes
Eggs
Dark-green leafy vegeta-
  bles
Blackstrap molasses
Whole-grain breads and
  cereals
	Cellular respiration
	Hemoglobin synthesis		

From Ross, R., & Noe, J. (1983). *Chronic problem wounds.* Boston: Little, Brown & Co.
* Iron cooking utensils add iron to the diet.

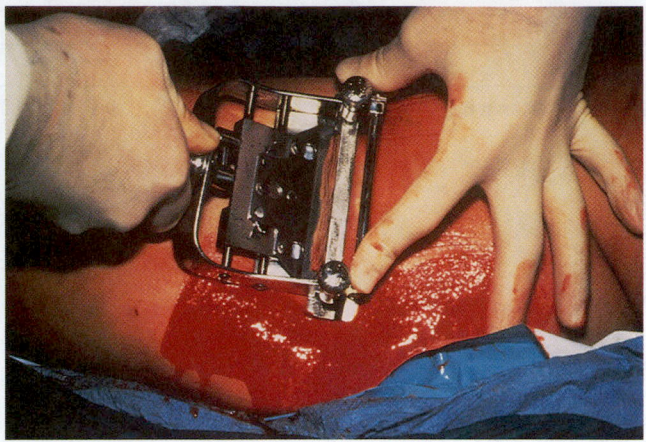

Figure 70-9 ■ Removal of a partial-thickness (split-thickness) skin graft.

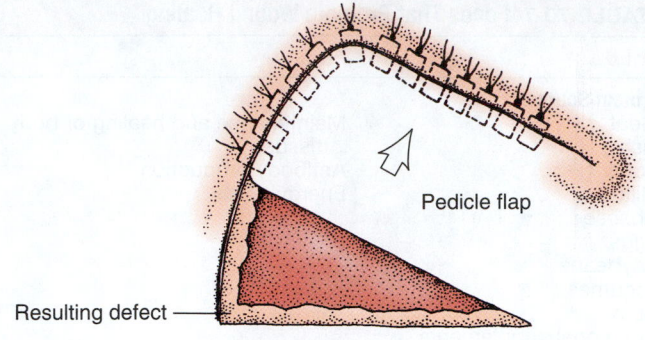

Figure 70-10 ■ A full-thickness pedicle flap of skin is separated and rotated to cover the wound. Blood vessels are left intact. The resultant defect is either primarily closed or covered with skin grafts. The flap is held in place with staples or sutures.

to hasten the removal of the dead tissue, a potential source of infection. Surgical debridement is indicated for severely immunosuppressed clients or those with large, full-thickness ulcers because of the extensive time required for spontaneous separation of eschar. The longer open wounds exist, the greater the risk for systemic sepsis or prolonged hospitalization. Depending on the size and depth of the ulcer and the projected blood loss, debridement can be performed at the bedside, in the treatment room, or in an operating room.

Grafting is used for wound closure when full-thickness ulcers are unable to close and when natural healing would result in loss of joint function, an unacceptable cosmetic appearance, or a high potential for wound recurrence. Successful skin grafting requires a clean and granulating or freshly excised ulcer bed. Partial-thickness (split-thickness) or full-thickness strips of skin are removed from the donor area (Figure 70-9), transferred to the ulcer, and sutured or stapled in place. Full-thickness free grafts and myocutaneous flaps are used to cover deep, massive ulcers or ulcers in which vital structures, such as bone or tendon, are exposed.

Unlike free grafts, a pedicle flap is a full-thickness flap of skin that is raised and rotated to cover the defect, with one edge of the flap still attached to the site of origin to provide a blood supply (Figure 70-10). Because all skin layers are removed, full-thickness donor sites are closed surgically or covered with additional split-thickness skin grafts. Partial-thickness donor sites heal spontaneously if infection is avoided.

Postoperative Care. Postoperative graft sites are immobilized with bulky cotton pressure dressings for 3 to 5 days to allow vascularization, or "take," of the newly grafted skin. Do not disturb the dressing, and encourage elevation and complete rest of the grafted area. Any activity that might cause movement of the dressing against the body and separation of the graft from the wound is prohibited.

After dressings are removed, monitor the graft for indications of failure to vascularize, nonadherence to the wound, or graft necrosis. If a pedicle flap has been used to cover the wound, inspect the edges of the flap at least every 4 hours for changes in color. A pale flap with delayed capillary filling when blanched may have inadequate arterial perfusion. A dusky color or sharp line of color change suggests inadequate venous or lymphatic drainage. Other techniques to monitor trends of blood flow in the graft, depending on

the graft's location, include pulse oximetry, Doppler ultrasonography, and transcutaneous oxygen determination.

Postoperative care of donor sites aims to protect the area from injury and infection until healing can occur and to promote comfort. A pressure dressing is usually placed over the donor area to promote hemostasis. After 24 to 48 hours, this outer dressing is removed, revealing a single wound contact layer of fine-mesh gauze or synthetic mesh material.

If the donor site is treated with dry exposure, promote air circulation to the wound by positioning the client to avoid pressure on the site and using an overbed cradle to tent the sheets. In the rare instance when heat lamps are prescribed, place the 60- to 100-watt bulb at least 2 feet from the wound to prevent thermal injury to the skin. After the dressing has dried and formed a "scab," keep the wound dry and undisturbed until healing is evident (at 10 to 14 days). As the donor site heals, the gauze and dried blood lift away from the new epithelium beneath. Trimming the separating gauze close to the skin surface reduces the chance of the client's catching the loose end of the dressing on an object and removing the still adherent gauze before healing is complete. Today most surgeons prefer to dress donor sites with moisture-retentive dressings, such as synthetic transparent films, instead of the traditional dry exposure method of treatment (see Table 70-6).

Because exposed donor sites are initially more painful than graft sites, give pain medication as prescribed and provide other comfort measures as needed. Reposition the client during the immediate period after surgery to promote comfort only if movement of the graft site can be avoided. Offer back rubs to help relieve muscle spasms that occur with reduced mobility. Pay attention to relieving pressure over unaffected bony prominences that may lead to additional ulcers.

Graft and donor sites on posterior body surfaces present a particular problem. For the graft or flap to become fully vascularized or for the donor sites to dry, the client must be immobilized in a side-lying or prone position for 7 to 10 days.

An alternative to this positioning is the use of special low-pressure or air-fluidized beds, which not only reduce ischemia of the graft or flap while the client is supine but also help prevent breakdown of intact skin. A major limitation to the use

TABLE 70-8 Monitoring the Wound

Variable	Frequency of Assessment	Rationale
Wounds Without Tissue Loss *Examples* Surgical incisions and clean lacerations closed primarily by sutures or staples		
Observations (Using First Postoperative Dressing Change as Baseline) Check for the presence or absence of increased: ■ Localized tenderness ■ Swelling of the incision line ■ Erythema of the incision line >1 cm on each side of wound ■ Localized heat	At least every 24 hr until sutures or staples are removed	To detect cellulitis (bacterial infections)*
Check for the presence or absence of: ■ Purulent drainage from any portion of the incision site ■ Localized fluctuance (from fluid accumulation) and tenderness beneath a *portion* of the wound when palpated	At least every 24 hr until sutures or staples are removed	To detect abscess formation related to presence of foreign body (suture material) or deeper would infection*
Check for the presence or absence of approximation (sealing) of wound edges with or without serosanguineous drainage	At least every 24 hr until sutures or staples are removed	To detect potential for wound dehiscence
Wounds with Tissue Loss *Examples* Partial- or full-thickness skin loss caused by pressure necrosis, vascular disease, trauma, etc., and allowed to heal by secondary intention		
Observations *Wound Size* Measure wound size at greatest length and width using a metric ruler or, for asymmetric ulcers, by tracing the wound onto a piece of plastic film or sheeting (plastic template). Compare all subsequent measurements against the initial measurement.	At least every week	To detect increase in wound size and depth secondary to infectious process
Ulcer Base Check for the presence or absence of: ■ Necrotic tissue (loose or adherent) ■ Presence or absence of foul odor from wound when dressing is changed Note the frequency of dressing changes or dressing reinforcements owing to drainage.	At least every 24 hr	To detect the need for debridement or the response to treatment (necrotic tissue) and to detect local wound infection (frequent dressing changes and foul odor)
Wound Margins Check for the presence or absence of: ■ Erythema and swelling extending outward >1 cm from wound margins ■ Increased tenderness at wound margins	At least every 24 hr or at each dressing change	To detect wound infection*
Systemic Response Check for the presence or absence of elevated body temperature, WBCs, or positive blood culture	As needed	To detect bacteremia

WBCs, White blood cells.
*The wounds of clients who are severely immunosuppressed or those wounds with compromised blood supply may not exhibit a typical inflammatory response to local wound infection.

of these beds is cost, which is usually outweighed by the potential for decreased morbidity and length of hospital stay.

RISK FOR INFECTION AND WOUND EXTENSION

NOC **PLANNING: EXPECTED OUTCOMES.** The client with a pressure ulcer is expected to remain free of wound infection or systemic sepsis. Indicators include that the client will have mild or no:

- White blood cell elevation
- Wound site culture colonization
- Purulent drainage
- Increase in wound size or depth

INTERVENTIONS. Closely monitor the ulcer's progress so that timely treatment with topical and systemic antibiotics can be started if ulcer deterioration occurs. Steps are taken to reduce introduction of pathogenic organisms to the ulcer through direct contact.

Monitoring Ulcer Progress. Monitoring the ulcer's appearance using objective criteria allows evaluation of the response to treatment and early recognition of infection. If an ulcer shows no progress toward healing within 3 weeks, the treatment plan should be re-evaluated. Table 70-8 outlines objectives of monitoring wounds with and without tissue loss. Clients who are at highest risk for infection are those who are older, have white blood cell disorders, are receiving steroid therapy, or have wounds with a compromised blood supply.

Prevention of Infection and Wound Extension. Complications of infection and wound extension are avoided by monitoring of the ulcer's progress and by prevention of new ulcer formation. Report the following signs to the physician:

- Sudden deterioration of the ulcer as evidenced by an increase in the size or depth of the lesion
- Changes in the color or texture of the granulation tissue
- Changes in the quantity, color, or odor of exudate

Also check for the classic signs of wound infection: increased redness, edema, purulent and malodorous drainage, and tenderness of the wound margins. These manifestations may occur with or without clinical signs of bacteremia, such as fever, an elevated white blood cell count, and positive blood cultures. Use appropriate interventions to prevent the formation of new pressure ulcers and to prevent early-stage ulcers from progressing to deeper wounds (Chart 70-3; see also Chart 70-2).

Maintaining a Safe Environment. Because of the variety of organisms in the hospital environment, keeping an ulcer totally free of bacteria is impossible. Optimal ulcer management is based on maintaining acceptably low levels of organisms through meticulous wound care and reducing contamination with pathogenic organisms. All personnel must use standard precautions to prevent direct contact with ulcer secretions and cross-contamination among clients. All personnel must practice thorough handwashing before and after dressing changes and properly dispose of soiled dressings and linens.

Community-Based Care

Clients with pressure ulcers may be in acute care, subacute care, long-term care, or home care settings. If pressure ulcer therapy requires hospitalization, most clients with pressure ulcers are discharged before complete wound closure is achieved. Discharge may be to the home setting or to a long-term care facility, depending on the degree of debilitation and other client factors.

HOME CARE MANAGEMENT

Care of the ulcer in the client's home is similar to care in the hospital. Most dressing supplies and pressure-relief devices can be easily obtained at the local pharmacy or medical supply store. If debridement of the ulcer is still needed, a handheld shower device or forceful irrigation of the wound with a 35-mL syringe and 19-gauge angiocatheter can be substituted for whirlpool therapy.

Clients with chronic pressure ulcers are often depressed about their debilitated state, which may affect their adherence to wound care measures. Many clients cannot change their own dressings because of distress over an altered body image or the pain of dressing removal. Others are dependent on family members or support personnel because of limited physical mobility or inability to reach the wound.

For some clients, drastic changes in daily activities are needed to promote healing. Clients with pressure ulcers on the legs may need frequent rest periods with leg elevation to avoid or reduce edema. Immobile clients with pressure ulcers require around-the-clock repositioning as often as every 2 to 4 hours to prevent further breakdown, which takes its toll on family members or caregivers. Explain the rationale for activity changes to the client and family and explore alternative ways of coping with these changes.

HEALTH TEACHING

Before the client is discharged, the client or person who will be performing the wound care should demonstrate facility in removing the dressing, cleaning the wound, and applying the dressing. When choosing a dressing to be used at home, consider the client's or caregiver's ability to apply the dressing properly. If the client's finances are limited, also address the cost of the dressing material. Some dressings may be easier to apply and less expensive than other materials. At times, the more expensive dressing materials that require less frequent changing may be preferred. Explain the manifestations of wound infection.

Encourage the client to eat a balanced diet with frequent high-protein snacks. Discuss diet preferences with the client, and suggest foods that promote wound healing (see Table 70-7). The health care provider may prescribe vitamin and mineral supplements if there are dietary deficiencies.

If the client is incontinent, emphasize the need to keep the skin clean and dry. If bowel and bladder training is not possible, discuss the use of absorbent underpads, briefs, and topical moisture barrier creams and ointments as a method to reduce skin exposure to urine and feces.

HEALTH CARE RESOURCES

A home care nurse may be needed to follow wound progress after the client is discharged. The hospital nurse provides details of ulcer size and appearance and any special wound care needs to the nurse in the home, who can then accurately judge changes in ulcer appearance. Chart 70-5 is guideline for a focused assessment of the client with pressure ulcers.

To reduce waste and to help decrease the overall cost of treatment, emphasize proper use of dressing materials. Clean tap water and nonsterile supplies are acceptable for treatment of chronic wounds in the home and are less costly than sterile products. Nonsterile dressing materials can often be purchased in bulk from a local medical supply store at reduced cost. However, items reused in the home can become contaminated with pathogens and pose a risk to some clients. (See the Evidence-Based Practice for Nursing box on p. 1595.) Stress the importance of proper cleaning of reused items and of handwashing when before touching any supplies.

The client with activity restrictions may need daily assistance from a home care aide. Consultation with a physical therapist may be appropriate to help the client and family or significant others continue rehabilitation efforts in the home.

Critical Thinking Challenge

Despite preventive care, the diabetic client with pneumonia developed a stage II pressure ulcer on her left heel. She is being discharged to home today. She has stated that she will keep her foot in the "down" position to relieve pressure on the heel.

1. Is keeping the foot in the down position a good strategy? Why or why not?

CHART 70-5

HOME CARE ASSESSMENT of
The Client at Risk for Pressure Ulcers

Assess cardiovascular status:
- Presence or absence of peripheral edema
- Hand-vein filling in the dependent position
- Neck-vein filling in the recumbent and sitting positions
- Weight gain or loss

Assess cognition and mental status:
- Level of consciousness
- Orientation to time, place, and person
- Can the client accurately read a seven-word sentence containing no words greater than three syllables?

Assess condition of skin:
- Assess general skin cleanliness.
- Observe all skin areas, paying particular attention to bony prominences and those areas in greatest contact with the bed and other firm surfaces.
- Measure and record any areas of redness or loss of integrity.
- If possible, photograph areas of concern.
- Note the presence or absence of skin tenting over the sternum or the forehead.
- Note the moistness of skin and mucous membranes.
- If wounds are present, remove dressings (noting condition of dressings), cleanse the wound, and compare with previous notations of wound condition.
    - Presence, amount, and nature of exudate
    - Use a ruler to measure wound diameter and depth
    - Amount (%) and type of necrotic tissue
    - Presence of granulation/epithelium
    - Presence or absence of cellulitis
    - Presence or absence of odor

Take the client's temperature.

Assess the client's understanding of illness and compliance with treatment:
- Manifestations to report to health care provider
- Mediation plan (correct timing and dose)
- Ambulation or positioning schedule
- Dressing changes/skin care
- Diet modifications (24-hour diet recall)

Assess the client's nutritional status:
- Change in muscle mass
- Lackluster nails, sparse hair
- Recent weight loss of more than 10% of usual weight
- Impaired oral intake
- Difficulty swallowing
- Generalized edema

---

2. What care techniques will you teach this client to help heal this ulcer? (You may want to review diabetic foot care in Chapter 68.)

evolve For suggested answer guidelines, go to http://evolve.elsevier.com/Iggy/.

◆ Evaluation: Outcomes

Evaluate the care of the client with a pressure ulcer on the basis of the identified nursing diagnoses and collaborative problems. The expected outcomes include that the client will:

- Experience wound healing by secondary intention as evidenced by granulation, epithelialization, and resolution of wound size
- Develop skin thickness in expected range at ulcer area
- Remain infection free

Specific indicators for these outcomes are listed for each nursing diagnosis and collaborative problem under the Planning and Implementation section (see earlier).

⬦ EVIDENCE-BASED PRACTICE for Nursing

Reuse of supplies increases contamination risk

Zwanziger, P., & Roper, S. (2002). Bacterial counts and types found on wound care supplies used in the home setting. *Journal of Wound, Ostomy, and Continence Nursing. 29*(2), 83-87.

The purpose of this prospective, descriptive study was to determine the length of time needed for wound care supplies left in the home setting to become contaminated. Homes of 17 clients with wounds were selected as study sites. The level of home cleanliness varied from filthy to clean. Forty-seven wound care supplies used by home care nurses, caregivers and clients were cultured before placement in the homes and recultured after 7 days in the home setting. New supplies were then cultured, placed in the homes, and recultured after 14 days. The supplies included scissors, plastic wound-measuring guides, plastic cleanser nozzles, forceps, normal saline irrigant, and gauze sponges, squares and strips. Caregivers and clients were instructed in the proper use and cleaning methods for the supplies.

Data collection occurred at 7 and 14 days. Data collectors used sterile gloves and appropriate containers to transport the study items to the laboratory for culture. Handling of the items for culture and culture techniques were within recommended guidelines to prevent accidental contamination.

Seventy-five percent of items had some degree of contamination after being in the home. Items left in the home for 14 days had greater numbers of bacterial colonies and more varieties of bacteria than did those left in the home for only seven days. Multiple use items, such as scissors and wound measuring devices, harbored some of the more virulent pathogens commonly associated with wound infection.

Level of Evidence: 6—Descriptive study.

Critique. The study was appropriately designed for the research questions. Although the use of the supplies and cleanliness of the homes varied, this condition is consistent with the reality of home care.

Implications for Nursing. Many protocols stress that clean technique rather than sterile technique can be used for wound care and dressing changes in the home because the home environment tends to harbor fewer pathogenic organisms than do acute care environments. However, such protocols may erroneously lead nurses, clients, and caregivers to believe that wound infections are not likely in the home setting. Reusing supplies and equipment for wound care requires appropriate cleaning to prevent serious wound infections. Nurses must ensure that caregivers and clients understand how microorganisms are transmitted from one object to another and how to properly use/clean/dispose of these items. Appropriate cleaning and storage of wound care supplies is critical to the objective of wound closure and infection prevention.

COMMON INFECTIONS

PATHOPHYSIOLOGY
Bacterial Infections

Bacterial skin lesions usually start at the hair follicle, where bacteria easily collect and grow in the warm, moist environment. **Folliculitis** is a superficial infection involving only the upper portion of the follicle and is usually caused by *Staphylococcus* (Figure 70-11). **Furuncles** (boils) are also caused by *Staphylococcus,* but the infection is much deeper in the follicle (Figure 70-12). **Cellulitis** is a generalized infection with either *Staphylococcus* or *Streptococcus* and involves the deeper connective tissue.

Minor skin trauma usually occurs before the appearance of folliculitis and furuncles and may or may not contribute

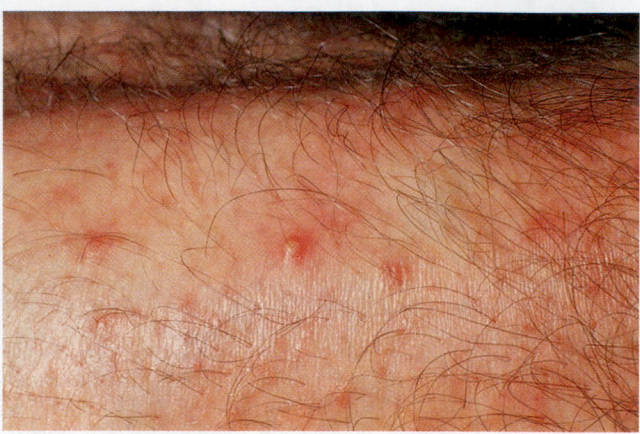

Figure 70-11 ■ Folliculitis.

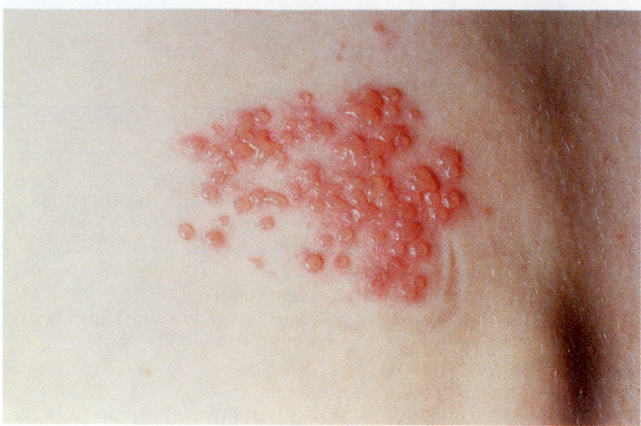

Figure 70-13 ■ Herpes simplex.

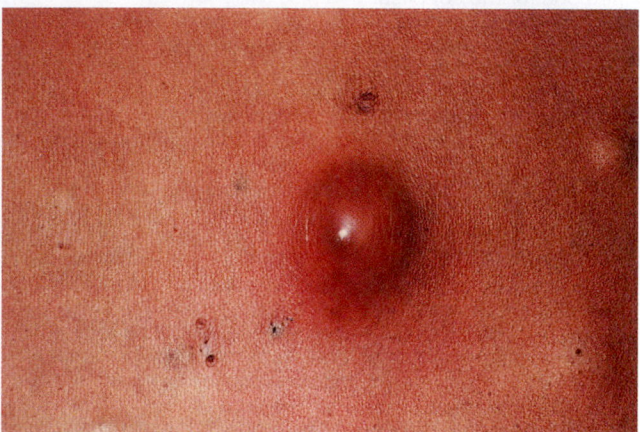

Figure 70-12 ■ A furuncle.

to the development of cellulitis. Clients may spread the infection to other parts of their bodies by scratching or rubbing the skin with fingernails that have organisms under them. Furuncles are more likely to occur in areas of heat and moisture, such as in the hair-bearing skin-fold areas. Cellulitis can occur as a result of secondary bacterial infection of an open wound, or it may be unrelated to skin trauma.

Viral Infections

HERPES SIMPLEX VIRUS

Herpes simplex virus (HSV) infection is the most common viral infection of adult skin. HSV infections are of two types. Type 1 (HSV 1) infections cause the classic recurring cold sore. The severity of the disease increases with age and is worse when the client is immunosuppressed. Genital herpes, caused by type 2 infection (HSV-2), is also recurrent (see Chapter 80).

After the first infection, the virus remains in the body in a dormant state in the nerve ganglia, and the client has no symptoms. Reactivation stimulates the virus to travel the pathway of sensory nerves to the skin, where lesions reappear. In healthy people, recurrence of HSV infection is triggered by physical or psychological stressors, such as sunburn, trauma, fever, menses, and fatigue. The virus can also be spread by direct contact between an actively infected per-

son and a susceptible host. *Autoinoculation,* or transfer of either viral type from one part of the body to another, is also possible.

The time span between episodes and the severity of each attack varies. Outbreaks of oral herpes simplex usually last 3 to 10 days. The client sheds virus and is contagious for the first 3 to 5 days. The client may have tingling or burning of the lip before any lesion is evident.

The most common clinical picture of HSV 1 infection is isolated or grouped vesicles on a red base (Figure 70-13). The infection can occur anywhere on the skin and may be spread by respiratory droplets or by direct contact with an active lesion or virus-containing fluid (such as saliva).

Herpetic whitlow is a form of herpes simplex infection occurring on the fingertips of medical personnel who have come in contact with viral secretions. This form of herpes can easily be spread to clients. Immunosuppressed clients are at increased risk for severe and persistent eruptions that can lead to life-threatening complications.

HERPES ZOSTER

Herpes zoster (shingles) is caused by reactivation of the dormant varicella-zoster virus in clients who have previously had chickenpox. The dormant virus resides in the dorsal root ganglia of the sensory cranial and spinal nerves. The lesions of herpes zoster infections are similar to those of herpes simplex, but they have a different distribution pattern (Figure 70-14). Multiple lesions occur in a segmental distribution on the skin area innervated by the infected nerve. Herpes zoster eruptions usually occur after several days of discomfort, which may vary from minor irritation and itching to severe, deep pain. The eruption usually lasts several weeks. **Postherpetic neuralgia,** pain persisting after the lesions have resolved, is a common complication in older clients.

Herpes zoster is a disease of immunosuppression, occurring most often and with greater severity in older people or in anyone who is immunosuppressed for any reason. The disorder can be accompanied by fever and malaise, often progressing to visceral involvement. Herpes zoster is contagious to people who have not previously had chickenpox.

Complications include full-thickness skin necrosis, Bell's palsy, or eye infection, and scarring if the virus is introduced into the eye.

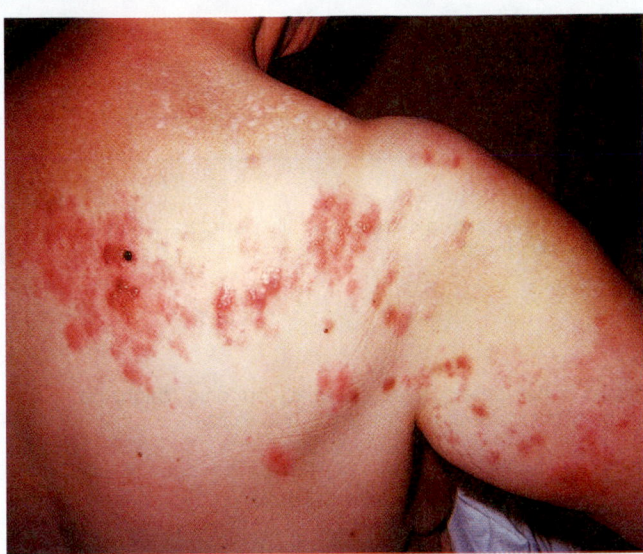

Figure 70-14 ■ Herpes zoster.

TABLE 70-9 Tinea Infections

Infection	Location
Tinea pedis	Feet (athlete's foot)
Tinea manus	Hands
Tinea cruris	Groin (jock itch)
Tinea corporis	Smooth skin surfaces (ringworm)
Tinea capitis	Scalp
Tinea barbae	Beard

Fungal Infections

Superficial fungal (dermatophyte) infections can differ in lesion appearance, anatomic location, and species of the infecting organism. The term *tinea* is used to describe dermatophytoses. Table 70-9 lists the anatomic locations of the various categories of infection.

Depending on the species, dermatophytes live mainly in the soil, on animals, and on humans. Superficial infection can start only if conditions are right for inoculation and maintenance of the organism in the outer layers of the skin.

Dermatophyte infections occur when the infecting organism comes in contact with impaired skin in a susceptible host. Most infections are spread by direct contact with infected humans or animals. Certain types of infections, such as tinea capitis and tinea corporis, can be transmitted by means of inanimate objects. For example, tinea capitis can be spread by the sharing of contaminated combs, brushes, hats, pillowcases, and similar objects from people with poor personal hygiene.

◆COLLABORATIVE MANAGEMENT
◆Assessment
HISTORY

The manifestations of the skin infection provide direction for questions and collection of data to confirm a suspected diagnosis. To differentiate among the possible causes of the lesions, concentrate on risk factors for each type of infec-

tion. If the location and appearance of lesions suggest a bacterial infection, explore any recent history of skin trauma as well as past or current staphylococcal or streptococcal infections. Ask whether fever and malaise are also present.

Lesions appearing on the lips, in the mouth, or in the genital region are more likely to be a possible viral infection. Ask about the following:

- A history of similar lesions in the same location
- Signs of burning, tingling, or pain
- Recent stress factors that may have precipitated the outbreak
- Recent contact with an infected person

Information that the same type of lesions has occurred before is important in helping to differentiate viral from bacterial lesions. If herpes zoster is suspected, ask whether the client has had chickenpox in the past and about a history of shingles.

The type of information you should ask a client with probable dermatophyte infection depends on the location of the lesions. If tinea corporis or tinea capitis is present, assess the social and environmental factors that may have contributed to infection, such as direct contact with an infected person, poor personal hygiene practices, or frequent contact with animals. If tinea cruris and tinea pedis are suspected, ask the client about the type and frequency of athletic activities.

PHYSICAL ASSESSMENT/CLINICAL MANIFESTATIONS

Because most skin infections are contagious, take precautions to prevent the spread of infection when performing a physical assessment. Chart 70-6 lists the manifestations of common skin infections.

LABORATORY ASSESSMENT

When pustules are present in bacterial infections, the infecting organism is confirmed by swab culture of the purulent material. Blood cultures may be helpful, especially if the client is showing clinical signs of bacteremia.

Viral infections are confirmed by *Tzanck's smear* and viral culture. Tzanck's smear is a cytologic examination in which cells from the base of a lesion are examined under a microscope. The presence of multinucleated giant cells confirms a viral infection, although the exact virus is not identified.

Fungal infections are confirmed by a potassium hydroxide (KOH) test. Scales from the lesions are scraped, prepared with KOH, and examined under a microscope. The presence of fungal hyphae confirms the diagnosis. In addition to a KOH test, a fungal culture may be needed. Occasionally a skin biopsy is performed to obtain organisms for identification.

◆Interventions

Most skin infections heal well with nonsurgical management. Surgery may be required when an infectious agent is present in deep tissue layers.

NONSURGICAL MANAGEMENT. Nursing interventions focus on meticulous skin care and prevention of infection spread. In some instances, drug therapy is needed.

Skin Care. Instruct clients with bacterial infections to bathe daily with an antibacterial soap. Instruct the client to remove any pustules or crusts gently so that topical drugs can be more easily absorbed. Teach the client to apply warm

KEY FEATURES of
Common Skin Infections

Clinical Manifestations	Distribution
Bacterial Infections	
Folliculitis	
Isolated erythematous pustules occur singly or in groups; hairs grow from centers of many of the lesions.	Areas of hair-bearing skin, especially buttocks, thighs, beard area, and scalp
Occasional papules are present.	
There is little or no associated discomfort.	
There is no residual scarring.	
Furuncle	
Small, tender erythematous nodules become pus filled and more tender over time.	Areas of hair-bearing skin, especially buttocks, thighs, abdomen, posterior neck regions, and axillae
Lesions may be single or multiple and also recurrent.	
Regional lymphadenopathy is sometimes present; fever is rare.	
Occasional scarring results.	
Cellulitis	
Localized area of inflammation may enlarge rapidly if not treated.	Lower legs, areas of persistent lymphedema, and areas of skin trauma (leg ulcer, puncture wound, and others)
Redness, warmth, edema, tenderness, and pain are present.	
On rare occasions, blisters are present.	
Cellulitis is often accompanied by lymphadenopathy and fever.	
Viral Infections	
Herpes Simplex	
Grouped vesicles are present on an erythematous base.	Type 1 classically on the face and type 2 on the genitalia, but either may develop in any area where inoculation has occurred; recurrent infections occur repeatedly in the same skin area
Vesicles evolve to pustules, which rupture, weep, and crust.	
Older lesions may appear as punched-out, shallow erosions with well-defined borders.	
Lesions are associated with itching, stinging, or pain.	
Secondary bacterial infection with necrosis is possible in immunocompromised clients.	
Herpes Zoster	
Lesions are similar in appearance to herpes simplex and also progress with weeping and crusting.	Anterior or posterior trunk following involved dermatome; face, sometimes involving trigeminal nerve and eye
Grouped lesions present unilaterally along a segment or skin following the pathway of a spinal or cranial nerve (dermatomal distribution).	
Eruption is preceded by deep pain and itching.	
Postherpetic neuralgia is common in older adults.	
Secondary infection with necrosis is possible in immunocompromised clients.	
Fungal Infections	
Dermatophytosis	
Annular or serpiginous patches are present with elevated borders, scaling, and central clearing.	Anywhere on the body
Itching is common.	
Lesions may be single or multiple.	
Candidiasis	
Erythematous macular eruption occurs with isolated pustules or papules at the border (satellite lesions).	Skin-fold areas: perineal and perianal region, axillae, beneath breasts, and between the fingers; under wet or occlusive dressings
Candidiasis is associated with burning and itching.	
Oral lesions (thrush) appear as creamy white plaques on an inflamed mucous membrane.	Lesions possibly present on the oral or vaginal mucous membranes
Cracks or fissures at the corners of the mouth may be present.	

compresses twice a day to furuncles or areas of cellulitis to increase comfort.

Applying astringent compresses, such as Burow's solution, to viral lesions for 20 minutes three times a day promotes crust formation and healing. Compresses also relieve the irritation and pain associated with herpetic infection. Instruct the client to avoid constricting garments that might rub the lesions and increase irritation.

Most superficial skin infections resolve more quickly if the involved skin is allowed to dry between treatments. Excessive moisture, especially if occluded by dressings, clothing, or bedding, promotes growth of organisms. If the client is bedridden, position him or her for optimal air circulation to the area and avoid occlusive dressings or garments.

Isolation Precautions. Take precautions to reduce the spread of pathogenic organisms to other people. For most superficial bacterial infections, proper handwashing prevents cross-contamination. However, when hospitalized clients are colonized with *Staphylococcus* that is resistant to antibiotic therapy, strict adherence to isolation procedures is necessary.

Of the dermatophyte infections, tinea capitis, tinea corporis, and tinea pedis are most easily transmitted to others. Instruct clients to avoid sharing personal items, such as hairbrushes, articles of clothing, or footwear. Repeated infections transmitted by dogs or cats may mean that clients might have to get rid of a family pet to control infections.

Drug Therapy. Commonly used topical drugs for the treatment of bacterial, viral, and fungal skin infections are listed in Chart 70-7.

Mild bacterial infections of the skin usually resolve with topical antibacterial treatment. Clients with extensive infections, especially if fever or lymphadenopathy is present, require systemic antibiotic therapy.

Acyclovir (Zovirax) or penciclovir (Denavir) is used for the treatment of viral infections. Topical treatment decreases the numbers of active virus on the skin surface and reduces pain in primary herpetic infections and localized lesions in immunocompromised clients. Topical treatment is of little benefit in recurrent infection. Intravenous (IV) administration is limited to severe primary infections and immunosuppressed clients with symptoms of systemic infection.

Topical antifungal agents are used for clients with dermatophyte and yeast infections. An imidazole cream is applied to the infected skin at least twice a day until the lesions have cleared. To prevent recurrence, therapy is usually continued for 1 to 2 weeks after clearing. In some instances, antifungal powders may also help to suppress fungal growth. For widespread or resistant fungal infections, systemic antifungal agents, such as ketoconazole (Nizoral), are given.

SURGICAL MANAGEMENT. Surgery is not usually performed for a superficial skin infection, except for incision and drainage of furuncles. In severely immunocompromised clients, superficial lesions can progress to full-thickness wounds requiring surgical excision.

CUTANEOUS ANTHRAX

PATHOPHYSIOLOGY

Cutaneous anthrax is an infection caused by the spores of the bacterium *Bacillus anthracis.* The infection can be confined to the skin, or it may be systemic. At first a raised vesicle appears on an exposed body area such as the head or arms. The lesion may itch and often resembles an insect bite. Within a few days, the center of the vesicle becomes hemorrhagic and sinks inward. An area of necrosis and ulceration begins. Usually this process is painless. The tissue around the wound swells and can become quite edematous. With necrosis an eschar forms. The two features that distinguish anthrax lesions from insect bites or other skin lesions are the fact that it is painless and that eschar forms regardless of treatment. Clients may have only one lesion, or there may be multiple lesions, usually in the same body area.

Some clients develop glandular symptoms with cutaneous anthrax. The entire area becomes edematous and tender. Fever and chills may be present, as may enlarged lymph nodes.

◆COLLABORATIVE MANAGEMENT

Diagnosis is made based on the appearance of the lesions, a culture that is positive for the organism, or the presence of anthrax antibodies in the client's blood. Cultures are most easily obtained in the vesicle stage. Once the eschar is formed, a biopsy may be needed for culture. Blood cultures should be obtained from clients who have a fever.

Oral antibiotics for 60 days are indicated for clients who have no edema, systemic symptoms, and the lesions are not located on the head or neck. The antibiotics of choice are ciprofloxacin (Cipro) or doxycycline (Doryx, Vibramycin). For clients who have a fever, have lesions on the head or neck, are pregnant, or have extensive edema, antibiotics are given intravenously and then followed by an oral course of 60 days.

PARASITIC DISORDERS

Parasitic skin disorders occur most often in clients with poor hygiene and substandard living conditions. Any client who shows obvious signs of a self-care deficit should be examined for these contagious parasitic infections.

Pediculosis

PATHOPHYSIOLOGY

Pediculosis is an infestation by human lice: *pediculosis capitis* (head lice), *pediculosis corporis* (body lice), and *pediculosis pubis* (pubic, or crab, lice). Human lice are oval and 2 to 4 mm long. The female louse lays hundreds of eggs, called *nits*, which are deposited at the hair shaft base in hair-bearing areas.

◆COLLABORATIVE MANAGEMENT

The most common symptom of pediculosis is itching (**pruritus**). Excoriation from scratching may or may not be present. In addition to causing discomfort, these parasites can also be carriers of disease such as typhus and recurrent fever.

◆Assessment

Pediculosis capitis occurs more commonly in women than in men, especially on the sides and back of the scalp. Itching, the result of biting of the scalp by the parasites, is intense. A secondary infection may also be present from scratching.

Because the louse is difficult to see, examine the scalp for visible white flecks, the nits of the female louse. Matting and crusting of the scalp along with a foul odor indicates a probable secondary infection.

Pediculosis corporis is caused by lice that live and lay eggs in the seams of clothing. The parasites also cause itching. The only visible sign of infestation may be excoriations on the trunk, abdomen, or extremities.

Pediculosis pubis causes intense itching of the vulvar or perirectal region. Pubic lice, which are more compact and crablike in appearance than body lice, can be contracted from infested bed linens or during sexual intercourse with an infected person. Although lice are usually found in the genital region, it can also infest the axillae, the eyelashes, and the chest.

◆Interventions

The treatment of pediculosis is chemical killing of the parasites with agents such as lindane (Bio-Well, Kwell, Kwellada)

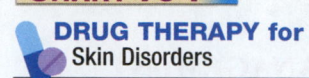
CHART 70-7

DRUG THERAPY for Skin Disorders

Drug	Usual Dosage	Nursing Interventions	Rationales
Antibacterial Drugs			
Ointments			
Neomycin sulfate Combination antibiotics (Neosporin, Bacitracin, Polysporin, Mycitracin)	Apply a thin layer to the affected area three times daily. Dressing is optional.	Gently clean affected areas with saline, half-strength peroxide, or tap water before applying ointments.	Atraumatic cleaning promotes healing by preventing further injury to skin cells. Cleaning helps to remove exudate, crusts, and residual medication and increases the effectiveness of therapy.
Gentamicin (Garamycin) Chloramphenicol (Chloromycetin)		Avoid rubbing ointment into skin. Apply with downward strokes in direction of hair growth.	Ointments can irritate hair follicles and lead to folliculitis.
Povidone-iodine (Betadine) Bactroban		Assess for worsening of problem in spite of topical therapy. Discontinue use if rash appears.	Client may become allergic to active ingredients, the ointment base, or added preservatives.
Creams			
Silver sulfadiazine (Silvadene, SSD, Flamazine ✱)	Apply in layer about $\frac{1}{16}$-inch thick to affected areas three times daily and PRN. Dressing is optional.	Assess for allergy to sulfa drugs. Gently clean affected areas with saline, half-strength hydrogen peroxide, or tap water before reapplying. If affected areas are left open without dressings, reapply cream PRN between cleanings to maintain a layer of cream at all times. Monitor white blood cell count for drop to <5000/mm³.	Use should be avoided in clients with a suspected or known sulfa allergy. Cleaning removes crusts, exudate, and caked-on medication while promoting percutaneous absorption of drug. Cream base melts with an increase in body or room temperature and is easily rubbed off with movement if left uncovered. Use of silver sulfadiazine over large skin surface areas has been associated with a transient leukopenia (cause unknown).
Antifungal Drugs			
Ointments and Creams			
Clotrimazole (Lotrimin, Mycelex, Canesten ✱)	Apply a thin layer to the affected area three times daily.	Teach the importance of thoroughly drying the skin before applying medication.	Moist environment promotes the growth of fungal organisms.
Nystatin (Mycolog II, Mycostatin, Nilstat)		Position bedridden clients for maximal air circulation to involved areas.	Increasing air circulation to the affected areas promotes drying.
Ciclopirox olamine (Loprox) Miconazole nitrate (Monistat-Derm 2%) Econazole (Spectazole, Ecostatin ✱) Tolnaftate (Tinactin) Haloprogin (Halotex ✱) Undecylenic acid (Desenex) Ketoconazole (Nizoral)		Emphasize wearing nonconstricting cotton garments to absorb perspiration.	Cream base is easily removed with perspiration, decreasing the effectiveness of therapy.
Powders			
Nystatin (Mycostatin) Tolnaftate (Zeasorb-AF 1%)	Apply a thin dusting of powder to the affected area three times daily.	Teach the client to thoroughly dry skin before applying powder.	In addition to discouraging the growth of fungal organisms, a dry skin surface minimizes caking of powder in skin fold areas.
Oral Preparations			
Nystatin (Mycostatin oral suspension, Nilstat oral suspension)	Rinse the mouth four times daily with 4-6 mL (400,000-600,000 units) and swallow.	Teach the client to coat the entire oral cavity with drug and hold the suspension in the mouth for several minutes before swallowing.	Effectiveness of drug is dependent on good contact of drug with mucous membrane surfaces.
Clotrimazole (Mycelex troche)	Take 1 troche five times daily.	Teach the client to let troche dissolve slowly in the mouth.	

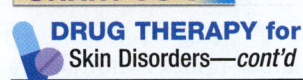

CHART 70-7

DRUG THERAPY for
Skin Disorders—*cont'd*

Drug	Usual Dosage	Nursing Interventions	Rationales
Anti-Inflammatory Drugs **Potent Fluorinated** **Steroid Preparations** Clobetasol propionate (Temovate 0.05%) Triamcinolone acetonide (Aristocort 0.5%, Kenalog 0.5%, Tria- derm✱ 0.5%) Amcinonide (Cyclocort 0.1%) Betamethasone dipro- pionate (Diprosone 0.05%, Betaderm✱ 0.5%) Diflorasone diacetate (Maxiflor 0.05%, Florone 0.05%) Halcinonide (Halog 0.025%) Fluocinonide (Lidex 0.05%, Top- syn gel✱ 0.05%, Lidemol✱ 0.05%, Topsyn✱ 0.05%) Fluocinolone acetonide (Synalar-HP 0.2%, Fluoderm✱ 0.2%) Desoximetasone (Topicort 0.25%) Betamethasone benzoate (Uticort 0.025%, Novobetamet✱ 0.025%)	Apply a small amount to affected areas no more than 4 times in 24 hr.	Teach the client to use the least amount of drug possible to cover the treatment site and to use the drug *only* under the direction of a physician. Never apply highly potent steroid preparations to the face, genital area, or skin fold areas.	Overuse of topical steroid preparations can cause serious side effects, including skin thinning (atrophy), superficial dilated blood vessels (telangiectasia), acne-like eruptions, and adrenal suppression. The incidence of side effects increases proportionately with the potency of the steroid and is most common with prolonged widespread use of the high-potency preparations. Absorption of topical steroids is much higher in these areas, and the associated side effects are more severe.
Medium-Potency Fluorinated Steroid Preparations Triamcinolone ace- tonide (Kenalog 0.025%, 0.1%; Aristocort 0.025%, 0.1%) Flurandrenolide (Cordran 0.5%, 0.025%) Fluocinolone ace- tonide (Fluonid 0.025%, Synalar 0.025%) Desoximetasone (Topicort LP 0.05%) Betamethasone valerate (Valisone 0.1%)		Teach the client to hydrate the skin before applying a topical steroid.	Skin hydration increases percutaneous absorption and maximizes the effectiveness of topical treatment.
Low-Potency Nonfluorinated Steroid Preparations Hydrocortisone 0.5%, 1.0%, 2.5% Desonide (Tridesilon) Hydrocortisone valerate (Westcort)		Teach the client to hydrate the skin before applying a topical steroid.	Skin hydration increases percutaneous absorption and maximizes the effectiveness of topical treatment.
Antiviral Drugs **Ointments** Acyclovir (Zovirax)	Apply to affected areas six times daily.	Teach the client to use topical acyclovir only under the direction of a physician for primary infections. Emphasize precautionary measures to prevent transmission of infection while the lesion is present.	Topical acyclovir has no proven clinical benefit in the prevention or treatment of recurrent infections. There is no evidence that topical treatment prevents transmission of infection.

or topical malathion (Ovide, Prioderm). In the case of pediculosis capitis, areas where the client's head has rested (such as on pillows or chair backs) are also treated. Clothing and bed linens should be washed in hot water or dry-cleaned. The use of a fine-toothed comb can help remove nits from an infested scalp but alone does not cure the infection. In all cases of louse infestation, social contacts are treated when possible.

Scabies
PATHOPHYSIOLOGY

Scabies is a contagious skin disease caused by mite infestations. Scabies infections are transmitted by close and prolonged contact with an infested companion or infested bedding. Infestation is common among clients with poor hygiene or crowded living conditions. The scabies mite is carried by pets and is found among schoolchildren and institutionalized older clients.

◆COLLABORATIVE MANAGEMENT

Scabies is manifested by curved or linear ridges in the skin. The itching is more intense than with pediculosis, and clients often report that the itching becomes unbearable at night.

The visible white skin ridges are formed by burrowing of the mite into the outer skin layers. Closely examine the skin between the fingers and on the palms and inner aspects of the wrists, where these ridges are most common. A hypersensitivity reaction to the mite results in excoriated erythematous papules, pustules, and crusted lesions on the elbows, nipples, lower abdomen, buttocks, thighs, and in the axillary folds. Male clients can also have excoriated papules on the penis.

Infestation is confirmed by taking a scraping of a lesion and examining it under the microscope for mites and eggs. Close contacts also should be examined for possible infestation.

Treatment involves the use of scabicides, such as lindane (Kwell, Kwellada) or topical sulfur preparations. Laundering of clothes and personal items is sufficient to eliminate the mites.

COMMON INFLAMMATIONS

PATHOPHYSIOLOGY

The inflammatory skin conditions have a variety of nonspecific manifestations, including severe itching, lesions with indistinct borders, and different distribution patterns. The cause of the eruption may or may not be identifiable. Inflammatory rashes can evolve from acute to chronic conditions.

Most inflammatory rashes are related to allergic immune responses. The responses may be triggered by external skin exposure to allergens or by exposure of the internal environment to allergens and irritants. The result is tissue destruction or skin changes induced by antibodies or cellular mediators of the immune system. (A more detailed description of these immune mechanisms is presented in Chapter 23.)

The specific cause of inflammatory rashes is not always known. When this is the case, the catch-all diagnosis of non-specific eczematous dermatitis, or *eczema*, is often used.

Contact dermatitis is an acute or chronic rash caused by either direct contact with an irritant substance, resulting in toxic injury to the skin, or by contact with an allergen, resulting in a cell-mediated immune reaction.

Atopic dermatitis is a chronic rash that occurs with respiratory allergies and atopic skin disease. The mechanism is unknown, but atopic dermatitis is made worse by factors that include dry or irritated skin, food allergies, chemicals, or stress. (Atopic reactions are described in Chapter 26.)

◆COLLABORATIVE MANAGEMENT
◆Assessment

Because all the inflammatory skin eruptions appear similar, data collected from the client are needed to identify the cause. Inflammatory skin problems differ from eczematous dermatitis in the chronicity of the disease, the distribution of lesions, and associated symptoms. Chart 70-8 lists the manifestations of many types of inflammatory skin conditions. Diagnosis is based on historical and clinical data.

◆Interventions

If the cause of the rash is identified, avoidance therapy is used to reverse the reaction and clear the rash. Even when the cause is unclear, certain irritants may cause the rash to worsen and increase discomfort. Additional interventions promote comfort through suppression of the inflammatory response.

Steroids. Topical, intralesional, or systemic steroids are prescribed to suppress inflammation. The vehicle used to deliver a topical steroid depends on the body area involved. Because a side effect of oral corticosteroids is adrenal suppression, clients receiving long-term therapy must taper their drug dosages rather than come to an abrupt halt.

Corticosteroids never cure. During active disease, these drugs reduce manifestations and relieve associated discomfort. Moisten dressings with warm tap water and place over topical steroids for short periods to increase absorption.

Oil-Based Products. Avoid applying oil-based ointments and pastes to the sweaty skin fold areas because maceration and blocking of pores may result in folliculitis. Instead, water-soluble creams are the vehicle of choice for these areas. Lotions and gels prevent matting of the hair and are more appropriate for hairy areas, such as the scalp. Stiff pastes are used to apply therapy to localized areas because this vehicle clings to the skin where it is applied and resists spreading to uninvolved skin.

Creams are used when the client has acute dermatitis with oozing and weeping. Chronic dermatitis responds more favorably to oil-based ointments that seal in moisture and help combat dryness and scaling.

Antihistamines. Antihistamines provide some relief of itching but may not keep the client totally symptom free. The sedative effects of antihistamines can be reduced if the client takes most of the daily dose near bedtime.

Compresses and Baths. Cool, moist compresses and lukewarm baths with bath additives have a soothing effect, decrease inflammation, and help to debride crusts and

CHART 70-8

KEY FEATURES of
Common Inflammatory Skin Conditions

Clinical Manifestations	Distribution
Nonspecific Eczematous Dermatitis Evolution of lesions from vesicles to weeping papules and plaques. Lichenification occurs in chronic disease. Oozing, crusting, fissuring, excoriation, or scaling may be present. Itching is common.	Anywhere on the body; localized eczema commonly involves the hands or feet
Contact Dermatitis Localized eczematous eruption with well-defined, geometric margins that are consistent with contact by an irritant or allergen. Usually seen in the acute form, but may become chronic if exposure is repeated. Allergy to plants (e.g., poison ivy or oak) classically occurs as linear streaks of vesicles or papules.	Cosmetic/perfume allergy: head and neck Hair product allergy: scalp Shoe/rubber allergy: dorsum of feet Nickel allergy: earlobes Mouthwash/toothpaste allergy: perioral region Airborne contact allergy (e.g., paint and ragweed): generalized
Atopic Dermatitis Hallmark in adults is lichenification with scaling and excoriation. Extremely itchy. Face involvement is seen as dry skin with mild to moderate erythema, perioral pallor, and skin folds beneath the eyes (Dennie-Morgan lines). Associated with linear markings on the palms.	Face, neck, upper chest, and antecubital and popliteal fossae
Drug Eruption Bright red erythematous macules and papules are found. Skin blisters in extreme cases. Lesions tend to be confluent in large areas. Moderately itchy. Fever is rare. Dehydration and hypothermia can occur with extensive involvement. Condition clears only after offending medication has been discontinued.	Generalized Involvement begins on trunk, proceeds distally (legs are the last to be involved)

scales. Colloidal oatmeal preparations, tar extracts, cornstarch, or oils are often added to baths to relieve itching (see Table 70-1).

PSORIASIS

PATHOPHYSIOLOGY

Psoriasis is a lifelong disorder that has exacerbations and remissions. Even though psoriasis cannot be cured, clients can usually achieve control of symptoms with proper treatment.

Psoriasis is a scaling disorder with underlying dermal inflammation. The problem involves an abnormality in the growth of epidermal cells in the outer skin layers. Normally cells at the basement membrane of the epidermis take about 27 days to reach the outermost layer, where they are shed. In a person with psoriasis, the rate of cell division is speeded up so that cells are shed every 4 to 5 days.

Etiology and Genetic Risk

Although the antigens responsible for psoriasis have yet to be identified, psoriasis appears to be an autoimmune reaction resulting from over stimulation of the immune system. Langerhans cells in the skin respond to the unknown antigen, leading to T-lymphocyte activation. These cells target the keratinocytes, causing increased cell division and plaque formation.

A genetic predisposition has been recognized in some cases; however, often there is no family history of the disease. Many environmental factors lead to outbreaks and influence the severity of clinical symptoms, but these vary from person to person. Triggering factors may be local or systemic. A psoriatic lesion may appear after skin trauma (Koebner's phenomenon in which a previously injured area is more susceptible to development of cancer or chronic skin problems), such as surgery, sunburn, or excoriation.

Clients with psoriasis seem to improve in warmer climates, where there is more exposure to sunlight. Systemic factors that can aggravate the disease include infections (severe streptococcal throat infection, *Candida* infection, upper respiratory tract infection), hormonal changes (during puberty and menopause), psychological stress, drugs (lithium, beta-blocking agents, indomethacin, antimalarials), obesity, and the presence of other diseases.

Some clients with psoriasis also develop a debilitating arthritis. Psoriatic arthritis may be mild or can lead to severe joint changes similar to those seen in rheumatoid arthritis. The association of arthritis with psoriasis strongly suggests that psoriasis is really a systemic connective tissue disorder rather than a simple skin disease. See Chapter 24 for more discussion of connective tissue disorders.

◆ COLLABORATIVE MANAGEMENT
◆ Assessment

HISTORY

In addition to collecting routine epidemiologic data, ask the client about any family history of psoriasis, including the age at onset, a description of the disease progression, and the pattern of recurrences. Ask the client to describe the current flare-up of psoriasis, including whether the onset was gradual or sudden, where the lesions first appeared, whether there have been any changes in severity over time, and whether fever and itching are present. Explore possible precipitating factors, including recent skin trauma, upper respiratory tract infection, recent surgeries, menopause status, past and current use of drugs, and recent stress. Ask about previous interventions and the effectiveness of each in reducing symptoms.

PHYSICAL ASSESSMENT/CLINICAL MANIFESTATIONS

The appearance of psoriasis and its course vary among clients. Typically during flare-ups of the disease, lesions thicken and extend to involve new areas of the body. As psoriasis responds to treatment, lesions become thinner with less scaling.

PSORIASIS VULGARIS. Psoriasis vulgaris is the most common type of psoriasis and presents as thick reddened papules or plaques covered by silvery white scales (Figure 70-15). Borders between the lesions and normal skin are sharply defined. Patches are less red and more moist in

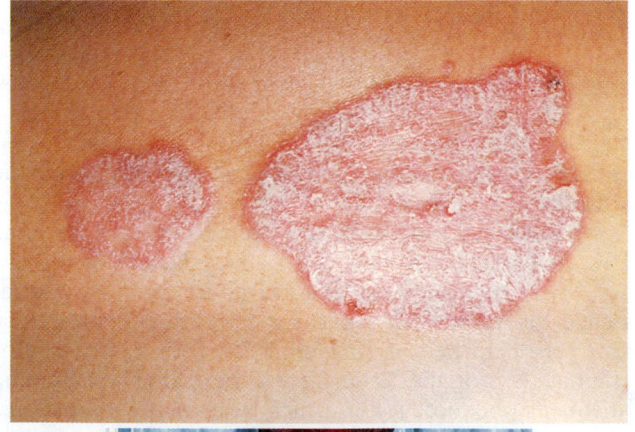

A

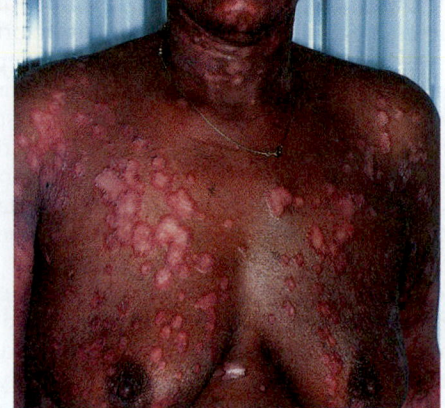

B

Figure 70-15 ■ **A,** Psoriasis vulgaris in a light-skinned client. **B,** Psoriasis vulgaris in a dark-skinned client.

skin fold areas because of sweat-induced maceration. Lesions are usually present in the same areas on both sides of the body. The more common sites are the scalp, elbows, trunk, knees, sacrum, and outside surfaces of the limbs. The facial skin is rarely affected. The client may have only a few isolated lesions, or the entire skin surface may be affected.

EXFOLIATIVE PSORIASIS. Exfoliative psoriasis (erythrodermic psoriasis) is an explosively eruptive and inflammatory form of the disease with generalized erythema and scaling that do not form obvious lesions. Examine for signs of dehydration and hypothermia or hyperthermia related to this severe inflammatory reaction. The increased blood vessel dilation and blood flow to the skin can reduce fluid volume through evaporative water loss from the skin surface.

◆ Common Nursing Diagnoses and Collaborative Problems

Nursing diagnoses that may apply to the client with psoriasis include the following:
- Disturbed Body Image related to altered appearance
- Ineffective Coping related to the chronicity of the disease and alteration in body image
- Deficient Knowledge (Treatment) related to lack of exposure or unfamiliarity of information resources
- Chronic Low Self-Esteem related to alteration in body image
- Social Isolation related to alteration in physical appearance.

◆ Interventions

The different approaches to therapy are based on the extent of disease, the client's distress, the physician's preference, and the response of the psoriasis to treatment. Clients must understand that no cure for psoriasis exists yet. Therapy is aimed at reducing cell proliferation and the inflammation.

Topical Therapy. The topical agents used to treat psoriasis are topical steroids, topical tar and anthralin preparations, and ultraviolet (UV) light.

Topical Steroids. Corticosteroids have anti-inflammatory actions. When they are applied to psoriatic lesions, they suppress cell division. The effectiveness of a topical steroid depends on its potency and ability to be absorbed into the skin. The more potent agents are used to treat clients with psoriasis.

A simple way to enhance the skin penetration of these drugs is to apply the steroid directly to the skin. Follow this step with warm, moist dressings and an occlusive outer wrap of plastic (film, gloves, booties, or similar garments). When large surface areas are involved, limit occlusive therapy to 12 hours per day because of the increased risk of local and systemic side effects.

Tar Preparations. When a tar preparation is applied to the skin, it suppresses cell division and reduces inflammation. Coal tar derived preparations are available as solutions, ointments, lotions, gels, and shampoos. The use of coal tar ointments is usually limited to inpatient care and specialized outpatient treatment clinics because these ointments are messy, cause staining, and have an unpleasant odor.

Topical therapy with anthralin (Anthraforte✳, Drithocreme, Lasan), a hydrocarbon similar in action to tar, also relieves chronic psoriasis. These drugs can be used alone or in combination with coal tar baths and UV light.

Apply high-potency anthralin, suspended in a stiff paste, to each lesion for short periods (not exceeding 2 hours). Anthralin is a strong irritant and can cause chemical burns. During therapy observe for local tissue reaction and prevent this drug from coming into contact with uninvolved skin. Anthralin is not used to treat acute, spreading psoriasis because it tends to induce Koebner's phenomenon (see Skin Cancer, p. 1608).

Newer topical therapy with calcipotriene (Dovonex) as a cream, ointment, or lotion is effective for many clients with mild to moderate psoriasis. This drug is a synthetic form of vitamin D that regulates skin cell division. Tazarotene (Tazorac), a vitamin A derivative primarily used for acne, has been helpful for treatment of psoriasis in clients who have lesions on less than 20% of the body surface. This drug is teratogenic (can cause birth defects) even when used topically. In addition, methotrexate delivered as a topical agent can help control psoriasis. Other immunosuppressive agents are being tested for effectiveness in a topical form.

Ultraviolet Light Therapy. Ultraviolet (UV) radiation is a physical agent commonly used as a topical treatment in many skin conditions, including psoriasis. Ultraviolet B (UVB) light, which produces more energy, is responsible for the obvious biologic effects of the sun, such as burning. Ultraviolet A (UVA) light emits a lower level of energy, requiring longer exposure time before cellular destruction occurs. Although the sun is an inexpensive source of UV radiation, better availability and intensity control occur with the use of artificial light sources. These sources include lamps or cabinets containing UV tubes. *The use of commercial tanning beds is not recommended for the client with psoriasis.*

Ultraviolet therapy is limited by the potency and distance of the source from the skin as well as the exposure time. Potency and distance remain constant, and the time of exposure is gradually increased to achieve a mild suntan effect without burning or tenderness. The client's skin type, ranging from fair to darkly pigmented, affects his or her risk for burning and determines the exposure times. Because of the extremely high intensity of most artificial UVB light sources, treatments are measured in seconds of exposure; clients must wear eye protection during treatment.

Teach clients to inspect the skin carefully each day for signs of overexposure. If clients have tenderness on palpation and have clinical signs of severe erythema or blister formation, notify the physician before therapy is resumed.

Psoralen and UVA (PUVA) treatments are more common on an outpatient basis (Figure 70-16). Clients ingest psoralen, a photosensitizing agent, 2 hours before exposure to UVA light. Because UVA light produces less energy than UVB light, the onset of erythema and skin darkening may be delayed as long as 96 hours after exposure. Treatments are limited to two or three times a week and are not given on consecutive days. Exposure is gradually increased until tanning occurs. As with UVB exposure, dosages are adjusted according to the erythema reaction of normal skin as well as the response of psoriatic lesions.

Observe for generalized redness with edema and tenderness. If these symptoms are present, treatment must be interrupted until they subside. Because of the strong photosensitizing properties of psoralen, clients must wear dark glasses during treatment and for the remainder of the day.

Long-term side effects of both UVB and PUVA therapies include premature aging of the skin, actinic keratosis, and an increased risk for skin cancer.

Systemic Therapy. Some clients have severe psoriasis that is resistant to topical therapy. In these instances, systemic treatment with a cytotoxic agent, such as methotrexate (Folex, Mexate), is warranted. Because of the liver-damaging side effects of methotrexate, liver studies are recommended before therapy is started and at least yearly thereafter. Small doses are usually effective in clearing the lesions. This treatment of last resort is avoided for clients who have liver damage, bone marrow suppression, or impaired renal function.

Because psoriasis has an autoimmune basis, some systemic agents that induce immunosuppression are used when lesions do not respond to other therapies. Such agents include cyclosporine (Sandimmune) and azathioprine (Imuran). The many health risks associated with these therapies must be considered along with the potential benefits.

A better understanding of the role of the immune system in the cause of psoriasis has led to biologic therapies to treat moderate to severe disease. This treatment is most successful for clients with moderate to severe plaque disease who are candidates for systemic therapy or phototherapy. Biologic agents alter the acquired immune response, thus preventing over stimulation of keratinocytes. Although precautions vary with the specific mechanism of action, these drugs induce immunosuppression, and clients are at an increased risk for infection.

Approved biologic agents include alefacept (Amevive) and efalizumab (Raptiva). Alefacept is given by intramuscular

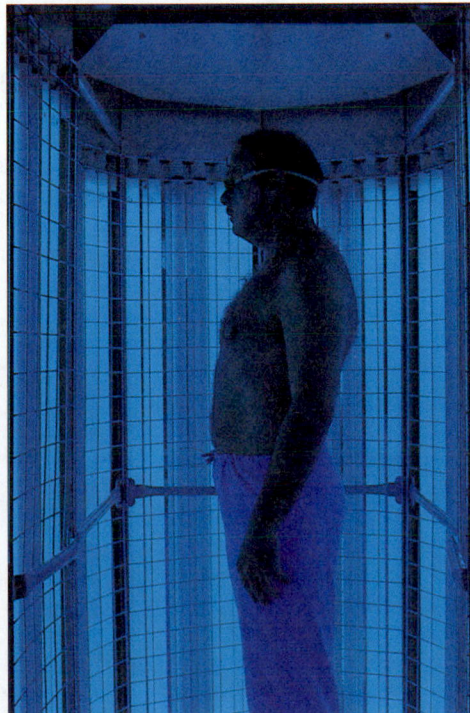

Figure 70-16 ■ A client receiving psoralen ultraviolet (PUVA) treatment. (Courtesy of the Department of Dermatology, Baylor College of Medicine, Houston, TX.)

(IM) injection weekly for 12 weeks. Efalizumab is given by subcutaneous injections once per week.

Emotional Support. Often clients' self-esteem suffers not only because of the presence of skin lesions but also because of the unpleasantness of some of the treatments. Tar not only looks dirty but also has a very unpleasant odor. Bed linens and pajamas become stained, further discouraging social interaction.

Encourage contact with other clients who have similar problems. Group discussions with family members or significant others can increase the socialization process.

The use of touch takes on an added significance for clients with psoriasis. For example, shake the client's hand during an introduction or place a hand on the client's shoulder when explaining a procedure. Do not wear gloves during these social interactions. Touch, more than any other gesture, communicates acceptance of the person and the skin problem.

BENIGN TUMORS

Cysts

PATHOPHYSIOLOGY

Cysts are firm flesh-colored nodules that contain liquid or semisolid material. Unlike cancerous growths, which are hard and firmly attached to underlying structures, a cyst moves and indents on palpation. Often there is a central pore through which the material can be expressed if the lesion is squeezed.

The most common cyst is an epidermal inclusion cyst. These growths are often asymptomatic and can be located anywhere, but they occur most often on the head and trunk (Figure 70-17). The most common cyst on the scalp is the sebaceous, or pilar, cyst.

◆COLLABORATIVE MANAGEMENT

If the client wants to have a cyst removed for appearance or any reason, surgical excision with primary closure is performed with a local anesthetic agent. The surgeon removes the entire cyst wall during excision to prevent recurrence.

A pilonidal cyst is a lesion of the sacral area that often has a sinus track extending into deeper tissue structures. As this cyst fills or becomes infected, it can become tender. An incision and drainage can be performed. Often the cyst is surgically removed and the area heals by second intention.

Seborrheic Keratoses

PATHOPHYSIOLOGY

Seborrheic keratoses are a common problem of older people. These benign epidermal neoplasms are gradually acquired after middle age and are often mistaken for actinic keratoses or pigmented skin cancers. These growths may occur anywhere but are more commonly found on the face, neck, upper trunk, and arms.

◆COLLABORATIVE MANAGEMENT

On inspection, seborrheic keratoses appear as multiple "pasted-on" papules or plaques ranging in color from flesh tones to brown or black (Figure 70-18). The surface of the lesion has a rough, greasy, wartlike texture on palpation.

Seborrheic keratoses are removed only for cosmetic reasons or if a lesion becomes irritated from friction. Cryosurgery or curettage with or without a local anesthetic is performed.

Keloids

PATHOPHYSIOLOGY

A keloid is overgrowth of a scar with an excessive accumulation of collagen and ground substance. Keloids are more common in darker-skinned people and often arise at sites of surgical incisions, burns, and ear piercing (Figure 70-19).

◆COLLABORATIVE MANAGEMENT

On physical examination, a keloid is an elevated, protruding lesion that extends beyond the edges of the original injury. These lesions can be cosmetically disfiguring. Treatment is difficult and not always successful. Because surgical excision alone can result in an even larger scar, surgery is usually combined with another form of therapy, such as intralesional steroid injections or low-dose radiotherapy. Pressure dressings or elastic garments worn over the skin for 1 year after excision or steroid injection may also help to keep the lesion flat.

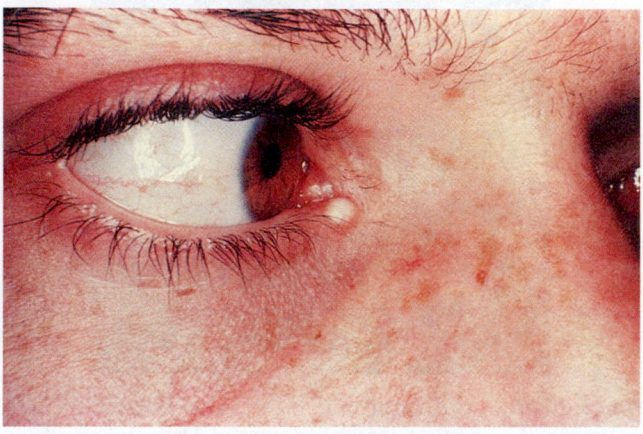

Figure 70-17 ■ An epidermal inclusion cyst.

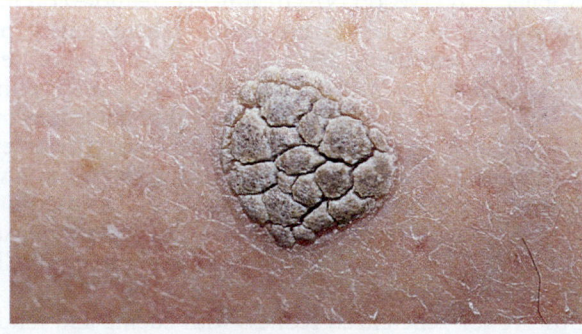

Figure 70-18 ■ Seborrheic keratosis. (From Lookingbill, D.P., & Marks, J.G. [2000]. *Principles of dermatology* [3rd ed.]. Philadelphia: W.B. Saunders.)

Nevi

PATHOPHYSIOLOGY

A **nevus,** or mole, is a benign growth of the pigment-forming cells. These lesions are classified according to their location within the layers of the skin.

◆COLLABORATIVE MANAGEMENT

Normal nevi have regular, well-defined borders and are uniform in color, ranging from light colors to dark brown (Figure 70-20). The lesion's surface may be rough or smooth. Because about 50% of malignant melanomas arise from moles, nevi with irregular or spreading borders and those with multiple colors should be considered highly suspicious. Other abnormal findings include sudden changes in the size of the lesion and complaints of itching or bleeding.

Unsightly nevi or those subject to repeated irritation or trauma can be removed. Biopsy of any suspicious lesions is performed to rule out malignancy.

Warts

PATHOPHYSIOLOGY

Warts, or **verrucae,** are small tumors caused by papillomavirus infection of the skin cells. They may occur singly or in groups and are classified according to their anatomic location.

Common warts are raised, flesh-colored papules with a rough surface (Figure 70-21). Although they may grow anywhere on the skin surface, they often occur on the hands and fingers.

Flat warts range in size from 2 to 4 mm. They appear as slightly elevated reddish brown or flesh-colored papules with flat tops and minimal scale. These warts often multiply and affect the hands and the face.

An often painful wart occurring on the bottom of the foot is the plantar wart. Plantar warts have a thick callus that, when removed, reveals tiny black dots (thrombosed capillaries).

◆COLLABORATIVE MANAGEMENT

The treatment of warts is aimed at destroying the skin cells containing the virus, a process that can be destructive and painful. Treatment modalities include surgical excision, electrodesiccation and curettage, and cryosurgery. Cryosurgery is usually preferred because a local anesthetic is not required and scarring is less likely. Topical caustic agents, including salicylic acid and lactic acid, are also used. These agents are painted onto the surface of the lesion and result in destruction of the cells and peeling of the infected skin area.

Hemangiomas

Hemangiomas (angiomas) are blood vessel tumors and are common benign tumors. The appearance varies from lesions that appear shortly after birth and gradually regress to those that are present at birth and gradually expand with growth.

Nevus flammeus is a congenital hemangioma involving the capillaries. These lesions are usually found on the face and the upper body. They are well-demarcated macular patches ranging in color from pink to bluish purple. Although nevus flammeus may gradually fade during the first years of life, a form of this neoplasm, the port-wine stain, grows with the child and remains unchanged in adult life. Port-wine stains usually occur as solitary lesions that vary in size.

The problem of nevus flammeus is cosmetic. Depending on the size of the lesion, surgical excision with or without skin grafting may be indicated. Treatment with laser therapy is also an alternative to surgery. Noninvasive treatment consists of masking the lesion by covering it with an opaque makeup.

Cherry hemangiomas are often seen in older adults. These lesions are small, dome-shaped papules ranging in color from red to purple (see Figure 69-14). Treatment is not indicated except when the client is unhappy with his or her appearance.

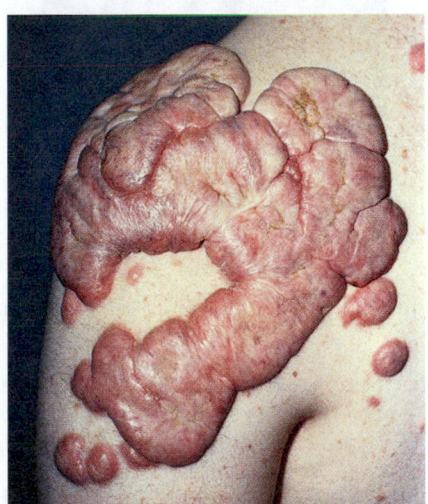

Figure 70-19 ■ A keloid.

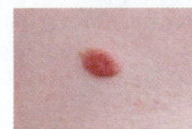

Figure 70-20 ■ A typical nevus (mole).

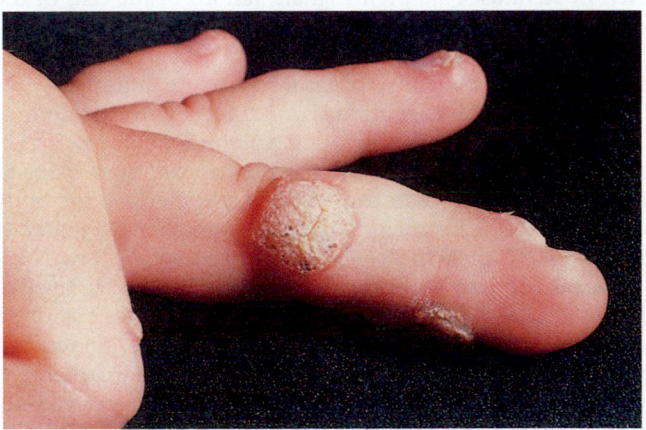

Figure 70-21 ■ A common wart.

TABLE 70-10   Common Skin Cancers

Clinical Manifestations	Distribution	Course
Actinic Keratosis (Premalignant) Small (1-10 mm) macule or papule with dry, rough, adherent yellow or brown scale Base may be erythematous Associated with yellow, wrinkled, weather-beaten skin Thick, indurated keratoses more likely to be malignant	Cheeks, temples, forehead, ears, neck, backs of hands, and forearms	May disappear spontaneously or reappear after treatment. Slow progression to squamous cell carcinoma is possible.
Squamous Cell Carcinoma Firm, nodular lesion topped with a crust or with a central area of ulceration Indurated margins Fixation to underlying tissue with deep invasion	Sun-exposed areas, especially head, neck, and lower lip Sites of chronic irritation or injury (e.g., scars, irradiated skin, burns, and leg ulcers)	Rapid invasion with metastasis via the lymphatics occurs in 10% of cases. Larger tumors are more prone to metastasis.
Basal Cell Carcinoma Pearly papule with a central crater and rolled, waxy borders Telangiectasias and pigment flecks visible on close inspection	Sun-exposed areas, especially head, neck, and central portion of face	Metastasis is rare. May cause local tissue destruction. 50% recurrence rate related to inadequate treatment.
Melanoma Irregularly shaped, pigmented papule or plaque Variegated colors, with red, white, and blue tones	Can occur anywhere on the body especially where nevi (moles) or birthmarks are evident Commonly found on upper back and lower legs Soles of feet and palms in dark-skinned individuals	Horizontal growth phase followed by vertical growth phase. Rapid invasion and metastasis with high morbidity and mortality.

SKIN CANCER

PATHOPHYSIOLOGY

Overexposure to sunlight is the major cause of skin cancer, although other factors are associated. Because sun damage is an age-related skin finding, screening for suspicious lesions is an important part of physical assessment of the older adult. The most common skin cancers are actinic or solar keratosis, squamous cell carcinoma, basal cell carcinoma, and melanoma. Table 70-10 lists common skin cancers.

Etiology and Genetic Risk

Actinic keratoses are premalignant lesions of the cells of the epidermis. These lesions are common in people with chronically sun-damaged skin (see Figure 69-16). Progression to squamous cell carcinoma may occur if lesions are untreated.

   Squamous cell carcinomas are cancers of the epidermis. They can invade locally and are potentially metastatic. Lesions on the ear, lip, and external genitalia are more likely to invade and spread than those found elsewhere on the body (Figure 70-22). Chronic skin damage from repeated injury or irritation also predisposes to this malignancy.

   Basal cell carcinomas arise from the basal cell layer of the epidermis (Figure 70-23). Early malignant lesions often go unnoticed, and although metastasis is rare, underlying tissue destruction can progress to include vital structures. Genetic predisposition and chronic irritation are risk factors; however, UV exposure is the most common cause.

   Melanomas are pigmented cancers arising in the melanin-producing epidermal cells (Figure 70-24). Risk factors include

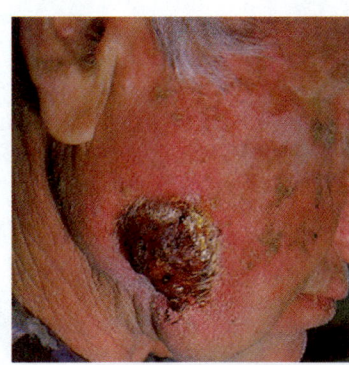

Figure 70-22 ■ Squamous cell carcinoma.

genetic predisposition, excessive exposure to UV light, and the presence of one or more precursor lesions that resemble unusual moles. *This skin cancer is highly metastatic, and a person's survival depends on early diagnosis and treatment.*

   Lighter skin and less pigmentation are genetically inherited traits. Additionally, a genetic mutation that is inherited in an autosomal-dominant pattern has been found for some cases of familial melanoma. The mutation occurs in a suppressor gene resulting in loss of tumor suppressor function. Two such mutated genes are *PTCH* and *CDKN2* (Nussbaum, McInnes, & Willard, 2001).

Incidence/Prevalence

The incidence of skin cancer is highest among light-skinned races and individuals older than 60 years of age (American Cancer Society, 2005). The incidence is higher among indi-

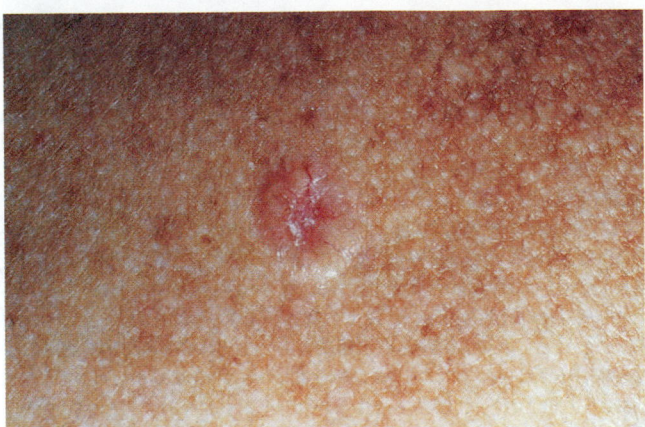

Figure 70-23 ■ Basal cell carcinoma.

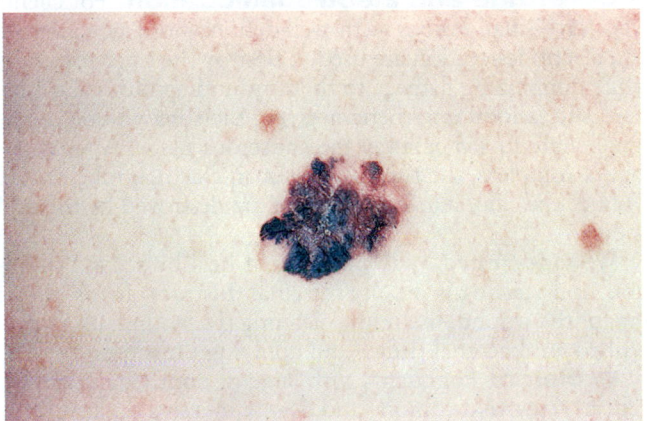

Figure 70-24 ■ Melanoma.

EVIDENCE-BASED PRACTICE for Nursing

Good role modeling requires knowing your risk!

Grubbs, L., & Tabano, M. (2000). Use of sunscreen in health care professionals. *Cancer Nursing, 23*(1), 164-167.

The purpose of this descriptive study was to examine the relationship between perceived risk for skin cancer and use of sunscreen among a convenience sample of 98 health care professionals living in a high sun exposure area of the United States. The health care professionals group was comprised of registered nurses, pharmacists, psychologists, nurse practitioners, and physicians. The level of education in this group was high with 63% having postgraduate or professional degrees. Most of the participants were white women.

The study involved completion of a questionnaire that included demographic and skin cancer risk assessment questions. A total of 90 questionnaires were returned (92% response rate). The perceived risk for skin cancer among this group was 50% low perceived risk, 44% high perceived risk, and 6% neutral. The actual risk for skin cancer, based on family history, burn history, and skin type was 7% low risk, 48% average risk, and 45% high risk. Statistical analysis confirmed that subjects at high risk and those at low risk had an accurate perception of actual risk. The subjects at average risk overwhelmingly reported their perceived risk as low. There was no relationship between perceived risk and consistent use of sunscreen.

Level of Evidence: 6—Correlational descriptive study.

Critique. The study was appropriately designed as a descriptive pilot study. Subject homogeneity limits the generalizability of the study results beyond this group.

Nursing Implications. Nurses and other health care professionals are perceived by the general public as role models of healthy behaviors. With a preventable cancer, such as skin cancer, nurses can have the greatest impact by the encouragement of prevention practices. An inaccurate perception of personal risk and inconsistent use of protective or preventive practices reduce this positive impact.

viduals who work outdoors and live at higher altitudes or lower latitudes. Occupational exposure to arsenic or other chemical carcinogens also increases risk. The incidence of melanoma has increased during the past 30 years, accounting for 2% of all cancers and 1% of all cancer deaths (American Cancer Society, 2005).

HEALTH PROMOTION/ILLNESS PREVENTION

The single most effective prevention strategy for skin cancer is avoiding or reducing skin exposure to sunlight. However, even when people understand the cause of skin cancer and the seriousness of the disease, preventive behaviors are not always practiced (see the Evidence-Based Practice for Nursing box above). Chart 70-9 lists methods of prevention that clients can use to reduce their risk for skin cancer.

◆ COLLABORATIVE MANAGEMENT
◆ Assessment

In addition to age and race, ask the client about any family history of skin cancer and any past surgery for removal of skin growths. Recent changes in the size, color, or sensation of any mole, birthmark, wart, or scar are also significant. Ask the client about which geographic regions he or she has lived in and where he or she currently resides. Obtain in-

CHART 70-9

CLIENT EDUCATION GUIDE
Prevention of Skin Cancer

- Avoid sun exposure between 11:00 AM and 3:00 PM.
- Use sunscreens with the appropriate skin protection factor for your skin type.
- Wear a hat, opaque clothing, and sunglasses when you are out in the sun.
- Examine your body monthly for possibly cancerous or precancerous lesions.
- Seek medical advice if you note any of the following:
  - A change in the color of a lesion, especially if it darkens or shows evidence of spreading
  - A change in the size of a lesion, especially rapid growth
  - A change in the shape of a lesion, such as a sharp border becoming irregular or a flat lesion becoming raised
  - Redness or swelling of the skin around a lesion
  - A change in sensation, especially itching or increased tenderness of a lesion
  - A change in the character of a lesion, such as oozing, crusting, bleeding, or scaling

formation about occupational and recreational activities in relation to sun exposure as well as any occupational history of exposure to chemical carcinogens (e.g., arsenic, coal tar, pitch, radioactive waste, radium). Ask whether any skin lesions are repeatedly irritated by the rubbing of clothes against them.

Skin that has been injured previously is at greater risk for cancer development, an effect known as *Koebner's phenomenon*. Ask the client if he or she has ever experienced a severe skin injury that resulted in a scar. Examine all scarred skin areas for the presence of potentially cancerous lesions.

The skin cancers vary in their appearance and distribution. Although most skin cancers appear in sun-exposed areas of the body, inspect the entire skin surface. Systematically examine the skin for any unusual lesions, particularly moles, warts, birthmarks, and scars. Also examine hair-bearing areas of the body, such as the scalp and genitalia. Palpate lesions to determine surface texture. Document the location, size, color, and surface features of all lesions and any subjective reports of tenderness or itching. Use the ABCD method of evaluating all lesions for possible melanoma (see Chapter 69).

Table 70-10 lists facts about common skin cancers. Punch, shave, or excisional biopsy of suspicious lesions is necessary to determine whether a skin lesion is benign or malignant.

◆ Interventions

Nonsurgical and surgical interventions are combined for the effective management of skin cancer. Treatment is determined by the size and severity of the malignancy, the location of the lesion, and the age and general health of the client.

NONSURGICAL MANAGEMENT

Drug Therapy. Topical chemotherapy with 5-fluorouracil cream is used for treatment of multiple actinic keratoses or for widespread superficial basal cell carcinoma that would require several surgical procedures to eradicate. Therapy is continued for several weeks, and the treated areas become increasingly tender and inflamed as the lesions crust, ooze, and erode. Prepare the client for an unsightly appearance during therapy, and reassure the client that the cosmetic result will be positive.

After treatment is discontinued, cool compresses and topical corticosteroid preparations help to decrease inflammation and promote comfort.

Systemic chemotherapeutic agents are used in the treatment of skin cancer, except when the prognosis is poor, as in advanced melanoma.

Drug therapy with interferon, a biological response modifier, is now an accepted treatment after surgery for melanomas that are at stage III or higher. The client is first started on high-dose (20,000,000 units/m²) interferon infusions daily for 5 days per week for 4 weeks after the surgical wound is well healed. Maintenance doses of 10,000,000 units/m² are continued three times per week for 1 year. The maintenance doses are given subcutaneously, and the client must learn to self-inject the drug.

Radiation Therapy. Radiation therapy for skin cancer is limited to older clients with large, deeply invasive basal cell tumors and to those who are poor risks for surgery. Malignant melanoma is resistant to radiation therapy; however, radiation therapy may be helpful for clients with metastatic disease when used in combination with systemic corticosteroids.

Immunotherapy. An experimental treatment available at some centers for clients with melanoma that has spread to distant sites is a melanoma vaccine. This treatment takes advantage of distinctive cell surface proteins found on some melanomas that can act like antigens. Although this therapy is new and as yet unapproved, it shows promise for melanoma.

SURGICAL MANAGEMENT. Surgical intervention ranges from local removal of small lesions, with minimal discomfort and positive cosmetic results, to massive excision of large areas of the skin.

Cryosurgery. Cryosurgery involves the local application of liquid nitrogen (−200° C) to isolated lesions, causing cell death and tissue destruction. Local anesthesia is seldom needed because most clients have only minor discomfort during the procedure. Prepare clients for swelling and increased tenderness of the treated area when the skin thaws. Tissue freezing is followed in 1 or 2 days by hemorrhagic blister formation. Instruct clients to clean the sites with hydrogen peroxide to prevent infection. A topical antibiotic may also be prescribed.

Curettage and Electrodesiccation. For clients who have small lesions with well-defined borders, curettage and electrodesiccation are used to destroy the cancerous cells while minimizing damage to the surrounding uninvolved tissue. After a local anesthetic is given, the surgeon uses a dermal curette to scrape away the cancerous tissue. After curettage is complete, the surgeon places an electric probe on the wound, and remnants of the tumor are destroyed by thermal energy.

Wounds created by this treatment heal by second intention, and scarring is usually minimal. Instruct clients in caring for the wound, including cleaning the wound, using prescribed antibacterial drugs, and applying dressings.

Excision. For clients with large or poorly defined skin cancers, recurrent tumors, and deeply invasive cancers, wide excision is used to remove the cancer. If the size and location of the lesion permit, surgical excision with primary closure is the preferred method. If the tumor has already been removed several times or if radiation therapy has damaged the surrounding skin, healing by second intention is indicated. This procedure allows the wound to be monitored for cancer recurrence. Skin grafts and flaps are used to repair large defects if tissue destruction is deep.

A specialized form of excision, Mohs' surgery, is used to treat basal and squamous cell carcinomas. The cancerous tissue is sectioned horizontally in layers, and each layer is examined histologically to determine the presence of residual tumor cells. Although the procedure is long and tedious, cure rates are high and there is less removal of healthy tissue compared with other surgical methods.

PLASTIC OR RECONSTRUCTIVE SURGERY

PATHOPHYSIOLOGY

The aim of plastic or reconstructive surgery is to correct functional defects and alter physical appearance (processes that influence a person's self-image). Plastic surgery is usually an elective procedure. Such intervention is sought by clients who cannot perform activities of daily living (ADLs) as a result of an anatomic problem or by those who are unsatisfied with their body image. In the United States the decision to undergo plastic surgery is often a response to social and cultural norms about beauty. Clients become self-conscious about scars, facial lesions, disproportionate anatomic features, or changes in physical features associated with aging. For some clients, severe trauma or extensive surgery causes functional problems that warrant surgical correction. For example, breast reconstruction is commonly performed after a mastectomy. This surgery not only serves an aesthetic purpose for some clients but also replaces lost anatomy and negates the need for a prosthesis.

Clients may request plastic surgery as a remedy for the normal changes in appearance that occur with aging. Loss of skin elasticity and changes in fatty tissue distribution are progressive and especially noticeable around the eyes, near the cheeks, and on the neck. Fine facial wrinkles around the eyes and mouth are one of the first signs of aging. These changes are followed by gradual stretching and downward displacement of the soft tissue of the lower two thirds of the face. Similar changes are seen as skin wrinkling and looseness on the arms, chest, abdomen, buttocks, and thighs. These changes are also seen after dramatic weight loss. Appearance of skin lesions associated with chronic sun exposure may trouble the aging client.

◆COLLABORATIVE MANAGEMENT
◆Assessment

HISTORY

When taking a history from a client who elects to have plastic surgery, use a nonjudgmental approach, and be careful not to assume the reason for surgery on the basis of physical appearance. Often what might appear to be unsightly to you is of little concern to the client, who wishes to change something else. Observe for any nonverbal communication that might establish the emotional state of the person or reveal feelings of embarrassment or guilt. Encourage the client to describe the problem, including why it is bothersome and what he or she expects as a result of the change. Ask about his or her health history and recent medical problems, including obesity and trauma, to predict the amount of surgery needed to correct the defect and potential complications.

PHYSICAL ASSESSMENT/CLINICAL MANIFESTATIONS

The client seeking plastic surgery may have changes in appearance ranging from minor to significant deformity. Depending on the location of the problem, the client may need to undress before the examination. Ensure privacy because the client may be embarrassed by the problem.

Begin the physical assessment by closely examining the area of involvement to determine the extent of the deformity or problem. Have the client assume different normal sitting and standing postures to provide better visibility of nonfacial defects. Document asymmetry of anatomic features, wrinkling or skin redundancy, scars or disfiguring skin marks, and obvious skin lesions.

PSYCHOSOCIAL ASSESSMENT

Address the client's expectations of plastic surgery. Often people who seek plastic surgery have unrealistic expectations or are uncertain about what they actually want. For example, the client with minor deformities who is seeking perfection is sure to be disappointed. The client who wants an operation mainly to please the spouse or partner is also a poor candidate. His or her psychological outlook before surgery should be positive if results are to be therapeutic.

◆Interventions

SURGICAL MANAGEMENT. Depending on the planned intervention, surgery is performed either in the outpatient setting with the client under local anesthesia or in the hospital. Most clients scheduled for plastic surgery have had consultations with their surgeon to discuss the planned intervention, possible complications, and postoperative expectations. The indications and complications of common cosmetic procedures are listed in Table 70-11.

Many plastic surgeons use photography both as a visual aid when discussing clients' problems and as a means of documenting before and after surgical intervention. Pictures taken of clients are confidential. Showing clients pictures of other clients is done only after proper consent is obtained.

Preoperative Care. Because of the large amount of blood loss associated with skin (particularly facial) surgery, instruct the client to avoid aspirin and other nonsteroidal anti-inflammatories for several weeks before and after the procedure. Immediate preoperative care is focused on collection of any routine laboratory test data required before general anesthesia and preparation of the operative site. In most cases, the procedure for shaving and washing the skin is dictated by the physician's preference.

Clients undergoing facial surgery, specifically **rhytidectomy** (face-lift), are often asked to wash their hair several times with antibacterial soap to decrease bacterial flora near the incision site. Instruct clients to remove any makeup and to avoid using face creams before surgery. If a **rhinoplasty** (reconstruction of the nose) is scheduled, explain the need for nasal packing and review mouth-breathing techniques.

Operative Procedures. Reconstructive procedures vary depending on the location, purpose, and extent of reconstruction. Ironically, in performing plastic surgery, the surgeon must make a wound to correct existing skin deformities.

Postoperative Care. Care after surgery focuses on monitoring for complications (see Chapter 22). Pressure dressings may be applied at the time of surgery and left in place for several days to control hemorrhage and edema formation. Check dressings and any nasal packing for bright red bleeding, and monitor changes in vital signs and level of consciousness indicating active hemorrhage.

Repeated swallowing followed by belching after rhinoplasty is a sign of postnasal bleeding and must be reported immediately to the surgeon. The client who has had breast surgery may have drains in place after surgery. Monitor the amount and color of drainage. Place the client who has had any facial reconstruction in a semi-Fowler's position to reduce edema and promote comfort.

Use additional comfort measures, such as the application of ice packs or cold compresses, as prescribed. Support garments are used after breast augmentation surgery to reduce edema and tension on the suture line from the weight of the breast tissue.

Monitor for wound infection and progress toward healing. Of particular concern are any areas of skin necrosis or eschar formation near the operative site, a complication from excessive tension on the suture line as a result of edema and blood vessel obstruction. Table 70-8 lists wound monitoring criteria.

TABLE 70-11 Common Plastic Surgery Procedures		
Description	**Indications**	**Complications**
Blepharoplasty Excision of bulging fat and redundant skin of the periorbital area with primary closure	Bags under the eyes	Hematoma Ectropion Corneal injury Visual loss (rare) Wound infection (rare)
Breast Augmentation (Augmentation Mammoplasty) Insertion of synthetic breast-shaped implants through a skin incision	Inadequate breast volume or contour	Hematoma or hemorrhage Wound infection (with gram-positive organisms) Phlebitis
Breast Reduction (Reduction Mammoplasty) Excision of excessive breast tissue and skin with primary closure	Hypertrophy of breast tissue caused by elevated hormone levels, endocrine abnormalities, or obesity Weight of large breasts can contribute to back pain	Hematoma or hemorrhage Nipple, areola, and skin flap necrosis Wound infection Fat necrosis Wound dehiscence
Dermabrasion Abrasive removal of the facial epidermis and portion of the dermis followed by healing by second intention	Moderate to severe acne scar Deep wrinkling Multiple actinic keratoses Hyperpigmentation (postinflammatory or after the use of estrogens)	Hypertrophic scarring Altered skin pigmentation Acne flare Wound infection (rare)
Rhinoplasty Removal of excessive cartilage and tissue from the nose with correction of septal defects if indicated	Disproportionate anatomy Post-traumatic nasal deformity Difficulty breathing through the nose	Hematoma or hemorrhage Ecchymosis and edema (temporary) Wound infection (with gram-positive organisms) Septal perforation Minor skin irritation
Rhytidectomy (Face Lift) Removal of excess skin and tissue from the face at the level of the hairline followed by primary closure	Excessive wrinkling or sagging of facial skin	Hematoma or hemorrhage Facial nerve damage (temporary or permanent) Wound infection Ecchymosis and edema (temporary) Skin necrosis Hair loss
Liposuction (Suction Lipectomy) Removal of subcutaneous fat from localized areas of accumulation such as the hips, abdomen, neck, and arms	Disproportionate distribution of adipose tissue	Hematoma Severe pain Infection Emboli Sagging of skin (if skin is not elastic enough to contract after fat removal)

Regardless of the planned procedure, inform the client to expect edema and discoloration of the operative site. Swelling and bruising alter the facial features and may not resolve for several weeks after surgery. Remind the client that the true results of surgery will not be visible until healing is complete, usually 6 months to a year or longer after surgery.

OTHER SKIN DISORDERS

Acne

PATHOPHYSIOLOGY

Acne is a red pustular eruption that affects the sebaceous glands of the skin. It is a common condition that, despite popular belief, is not confined to adolescents. Lesions result from increased sebum production, which is stimulated by androgenic hormones and obstruction of the sebaceous canal outlet. Debris collection promotes bacterial growth and rupture of the gland into the surrounding dermis with inflammation.

◆**COLLABORATIVE MANAGEMENT**

Acne is a progressive disorder that manifests as several types of skin lesions, including non-inflammatory **comedones** (blackheads and whiteheads), inflammatory papules, pustules, and cysts. These lesions are usually present only on the face and upper trunk (Figure 70-25).

Control of acne is possible, with spontaneous remission occurring over time. However, severe eruptions or chronic inflammation can lead to extensive scarring.

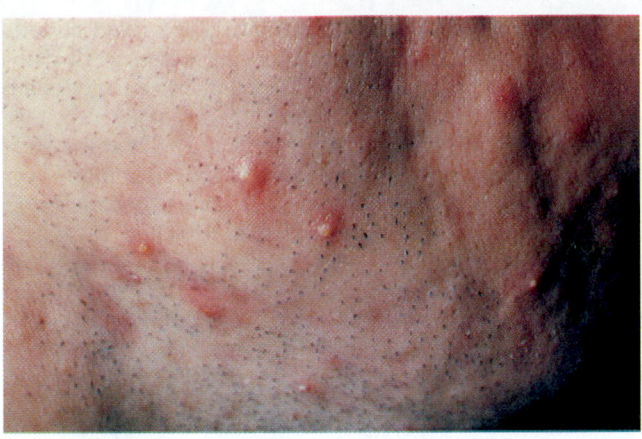

Figure 70-25 ■ Acne.

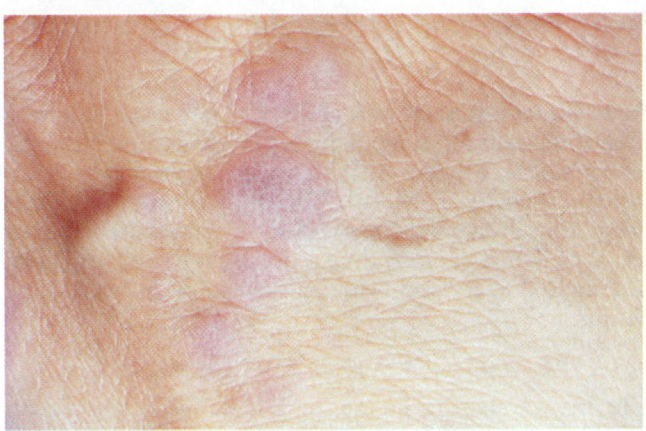

Figure 70-26 ■ Lichen planus.

For clients with superficial lesions, topical agents (retinoic acid, benzoyl peroxide, antibiotic solutions) are used. Systemic antibiotics are indicated for those with inflammatory disease. Clients with severe acne may have improvement after receiving isotretinoin (Accutane, Accutane Roche❋). Side effects include elevated liver function test results; dry, chapped skin; and depression in some clients. The most important concern, however, is the teratogenic effect of systemic retinoic acid. A pregnancy test is required before therapy, and strict birth control measures must be used during therapy.

Lichen Planus
PATHOPHYSIOLOGY
Lichen planus is a common skin disorder of purple, flat-topped papules that are itchy. Although viral infections and emotional stress may be possible causes, the actual etiology of lichen planus is not known. The course of the disease can be chronic, or it can resolve spontaneously.

◆COLLABORATIVE MANAGEMENT
Lesions of lichen planus are usually occur over the wrists and the inner surfaces of the forearms, but they may also be present on the lower legs, genitalia, and other body areas. Oral lesions may occur alone or with other skin changes. Unlike the skin lesions, oral lesions have a white lacelike appearance. These lesions usually occur on the oral mucosa and are often confused with thrush (Figure 70-26).

Treatment is determined by the symptoms. Topical steroids help to reduce inflammation, and antihistamines help to relieve itching. Systemic steroids may be prescribed when lesions are widespread, but long-term use is avoided because of the side effects.

Pemphigus Vulgaris
PATHOPHYSIOLOGY
Pemphigus vulgaris is a rare, chronic blistering disease with high morbidity and mortality. It is caused by an autoimmune disorder that occurs most often during middle and old age.

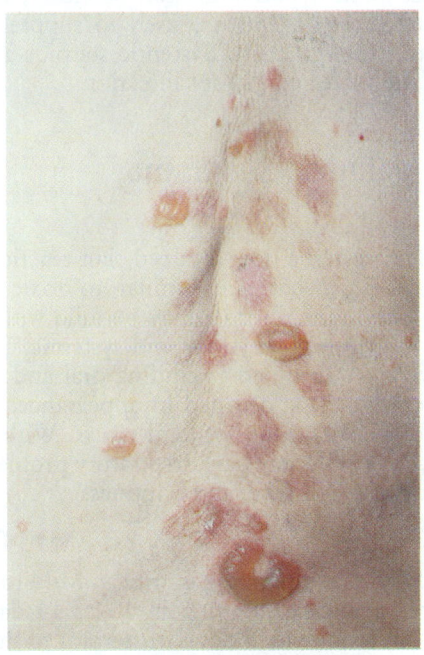

Figure 70-27 ■ Pemphigus vulgaris.

◆COLLABORATIVE MANAGEMENT
The acute lesions occur on normal-appearing skin or mucous membrane surfaces as fragile, flaccid bullae (Figure 70-27). Breaking the bullae leaves partial-thickness wounds that bleed, weep, and eventually form crusts.

Lesions can occur anywhere. The initial lesions usually occur on the oral mucosa, and later lesions form on the trunk. Spread of the disease is seen with the appearance of new lesions on the face and in skin-fold areas while older lesions are in the process of healing. Oral lesions are common and can make chewing and swallowing difficult.

Treatment of pemphigus vulgaris is aimed at suppressing the immune response that causes the blister formation. Systemic steroids and cytotoxic agents are used to bring about remission. Topical antibiotic creams or ointments are used to reduce bacterial infection of the unhealed lesions.

Toxic Epidermal Necrolysis

PATHOPHYSIOLOGY

Toxic epidermal necrolysis (TEN) is a rare acute drug reaction of the skin resulting in diffuse erythema and large blister formation. Mucous membranes are often involved, and systemic toxicity is evident. The most common causative drugs are sulfonamides, pyrazolones, barbiturates, and antibiotics. Removal of the drug is usually followed by gradual healing in 2 to 3 weeks, with widespread peeling of the epidermis.

◆COLLABORATIVE MANAGEMENT

The drug thought to be causing a toxic reaction is discontinued, and therapy is aimed at systemic support and prevention of secondary infection. Clients with TEN are often admitted to burn units, where fluid and electrolyte balance, caloric intake, and hypothermia can be closely monitored. Topical antibacterial agents are used to suppress bacterial growth until healing occurs. Systemic steroids are avoided because of the increased risk for infection.

Stevens-Johnson Syndrome

PATHOPHYSIOLOGY

This disorder is often a drug-induced skin reaction through an immunologic mechanism, similar to toxic epidermal necrolysis (TEN). The disorder may be mild with only skin involvement, or it may be severe and systemic. The skin lesions are widely distributed (including oral and respiratory mucous membranes) and varied in appearance. The client has a mix of vesicles, erosions, and crusts. With severe involvement, the client may have respiratory problems, excessive fluid loss, renal failure, and blindness.

◆COLLABORATIVE MANAGEMENT

Removal of the offending drug is critical. Mild forms of the disorder are usually self-limiting in 10 to 14 days. Severe manifestations require high doses of steroids to suppress the immune and inflammatory reactions. Supportive care may include fluid replacement, mechanical ventilation, and even renal replacement therapy.

Frostbite

PATHOPHYSIOLOGY

Cold injury of the skin depends on the intensity of the external temperature, the duration of exposure to cold temperatures, and the relative hypoxia of the tissues at the time of exposure. Cell death occurs as a result of poor tissue oxygenation owing to cold-induced blood vessel constriction. With continued exposure to the cold, vascular necrosis and gangrene result. Factors that increase the risk for cold injury are age, immobility, alcohol use, vascular disease, and psychiatric disorders.

◆COLLABORATIVE MANAGEMENT

Acute frostbite is treated in the hospital setting, with rapid and continuous rewarming of the tissue in a water bath (90° to 107° F [32° to 42° C]) for 15 to 20 minutes or until flushing of the skin occurs. Slow thawing or interrupted periods of warmth are avoided because this can increase cell damage. Thawing can cause considerable pain, and analgesics are needed.

After thawing, the wound is left exposed so that local tissue changes can be monitored. Blisters are left intact. With time, the degree of actual tissue destruction becomes evident as an eschar forms. After eschar has formed, local care of the wound is similar to that for skin trauma. Complications of cold injury include amputation, scarring, depigmentation, and thickened nail plates.

Leprosy

PATHOPHYSIOLOGY

Leprosy (Hansen's disease) is a chronic contagious, systemic mycobacterial infection of the peripheral nervous system with skin involvement. The clinical course of the disease is either progressive or self-limiting, depending on the immunologic status of the host. Hansen's disease is still found in the United States. Most cases are reported in Florida, Louisiana, Texas, New York, California, and Hawaii.

The exact mechanism of infection remains unknown. Studies suggest transmission via the airborne route, by insects, or through direct contact with skin lesions.

◆COLLABORATIVE MANAGEMENT

Manifestations of leprosy, including skin changes, are directly related to how resistant the client is to the mycobacteria:

- Localized (high-immunity) leprosy—one or two isolated, red, anesthetic, hairless plaques that are sometimes scaly
- Generalized (low-immunity) leprosy—widespread, faintly red macules, papules, nodules, and plaques
- Varying degrees of reduced skin sensation of the lesions are caused by peripheral nerve damage

Treatment is available on an outpatient basis. The aim is to control bacterial growth and reduce physical deformities. The drug of choice is dapsone (DDS; Avlosulfon), a sulfone with relatively few side effects that clients must take for life. In clients with sulfone-resistant disease, clofazimine (Lamprene) is indicated. This drug has a slow bactericidal effect on the organism that causes leprosy. Major side effects include skin discoloration (pink to brownish black) and abdominal discomfort.

NAIL DISORDERS

Ingrown Toenail

PATHOPHYSIOLOGY

Although seemingly a minor problem, an ingrown toenail **(unguis incarnatus)** can be troublesome. Pain and infection result when the edge of the nail plate grows into the soft pulp of the toe.

◆COLLABORATIVE MANAGEMENT

Management is aimed at controlling local infection while encouraging the nail edges to grow beyond the level of the pulp, where the nail plate can be trimmed. Teach clients to soak the foot in warm water (to which an antiseptic has been added) for 20 to 30 minutes. The softened nail plate then is gently lifted, and a small piece of gauze is inserted between the nail and the flesh on each side. This procedure is repeated twice daily until the nail has grown beyond the flesh so that it can be cut.

An ingrown toenail can be treated more aggressively with surgical removal of the nail plate. However, the pain of surgical removal can be severe, and recurrence is possible if the nail bed is not completely destroyed.

GET READY for the NCLEX Examination!

KEY POINTS

Safe Effective Care Environment

- Assist all clients with limited mobility to change positions at least every 2 hours while awake.
- Evaluate the pressure ulcer risk for all clients on admission and regularly thereafter.
- Be proactive in the use of pressure-relieving devices for any client who is identified to be at risk for pressure ulcer formation (i.e., requires prolonged bedrest, is an older adult, has some degree of immobility, is incontinent, has some degree of malnutrition, is dehydrated, has decreased sensory perception, or has an altered mental state).
- Wash your hands before and after touching any skin lesions.
- Use standard precautions when providing care to a client who has any areas of nonintact skin.
- Use a tongue depressor or gloved finger to remove topical medication from a jar or other type of open container.
- Do not reuse disposable supplies between clients.
- Use a lift sheet to move immobilized older clients rather than pulling or dragging them across bed linens.

Health Promotion and Maintenance

- Encourage all clients to reduce sun exposure and exposure to ultraviolet (UV) light.
- Teach clients how to examine all skin areas on a monthly basis for new lesions and changes to existing lesions. The client should keep a record or "body map" of skin lesions.
- Teach clients who have skin scarring from a previous skin injury to examine this area at least monthly for changes related to cancer development or chronic skin conditions (Koebner's phenomenon).
- Encourage all clients to bathe, shampoo the hair, and keep fingernails clean and trimmed on a regular basis.
- Teach all clients the ABCD method of evaluating a lesion for melanoma.
- Keep the skin of clients who are incontinent clean and dry.
- Ensure that female clients in their child-bearing years who are receiving isotretinoin therapy understand the teratogenic effects of this therapy and are using at least two forms of contraception during treatment.

Psychosocial Integrity

- Allow the client the opportunity to express feelings about a change in body image as a result of changes in the skin, hair, or nails.
- Explain all procedures, restrictions, medications, and follow-up care to the client and family.
- Touch the client who has skin problems to show acceptance.
- Ask the client who plans to have plastic surgery what he or she expects as a result of the surgery.

Physiological Integrity

- Keep skin-fold areas on clients clean and dry.
- Avoid applying oil-based ointments or pastes to skin fold areas.
- Ask any client who has started taking a newly prescribed drug whether he or she has noticed if any skin changes have occurred since starting the medication.
- Avoid rubbing any area of the skin that has been subjected to pressure.
- Encourage clients with itching to avoid scratching the skin.
- Teach clients to avoid using over-the-counter cortisone preparations on skin lesions until the cause has been identified.
- Teach clients who have a skin infection how to avoid spreading the infection to either other parts of their own bodies or to other people.
- Evaluate any open skin area on a client daily for size, depth, exudate, and presence of infection.

ADDITIONAL STUDY RESOURCES

Go to your Student CD-ROM for Review Questions for the NCLEX Examination.

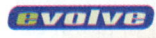   Go to http://evolve.elsevier.com/Iggy/ for Integrated Management of Care Questions for the NCLEX Examination.

SELECTED BIBLIOGRAPHY

Asterisk indicates a classic or definitive work on this subject.

Abbas, A., & Lichtman, A. (2003). *Cellular and molecular immunology* (5th ed.). Philadelphia: W.B. Saunders.

Ackley, B., & Ladwig, G. (2002). *Nursing diagnosis handbook: A guide to planning care* (5th ed.). St. Louis: Mosby.

American Academy of Dermatology. (2002). Actinic keratoses and skin cancer. *Dermatology Nursing, 14*(6), 397-399.

American Cancer Society. (2005). *Cancer facts and figures 2005.* Report No. 00-300M-No. 5008.05. Atlanta: Author.

Ayello, E. (2003). Predicting pressure ulcer sore risk. *Dermatology Nursing, 15*(1), 62, 65.

Ayello, E., Cuddigan, J., & Kerstein, M. (2002). Skip the knife: Debriding wounds without surgery. *Nursing 2002, 32*(9), 58-63.

Ayello, E., et al. (2004). Time heals all wounds. *Nursing 2004, 34*(4), 36-41.

Ayers, D.M. (2004). Melanoma. *Nursing 2004, 34*(4), 52-53.

Bamberg, R., Sullivan, P.K., & Conner-Kerr, T. (2002). Diagnosis of wound infections: Current culturing practices of U.S. wound care professionals. *Wounds, 14*(9), 314-327.

Baranoski, S. (2000). Skin tears: The enemy of frail skin. *Advances in Skin and Wound Care, 13*(3), 123-126.

Beitz, J. (2004). Anticoagulant-induced skin necrosis. *American Journal of Nursing, 104*(4), 31-32.

Bielan, B. (2000). What's your assessment? *Dermatology Nursing, 12*(5), 350-351.

Bruce, S. (2004). Radiation-induced xerostomia: How dry is your patient? *Clinical Journal of Oncology Nursing, 8*(1), 61-67.

Carter, K., Dufour, L., & Ballard, C. (2004). Identifying secondary skin lesions. *Nursing 2004, 34*(1), 68.

Clark, J. (2002). Wound repair and factors influencing healing. *Critical Care Nursing Quarterly, 25*(1), 1-12.

Cloote, H. (2000). Psoriasis. *Nursing Standard, 14*(45), 47-52.

Cole, J., & Gray-Miceli, D. (2002). The necessary elements of a dermatologic history and physical evaluation. *Dermatology Nursing, 14*(6), 377-383.

Cuzzell, J. (2002a). Wound assessment and evaluation of wound dressings - Confusion or choice? *Dermatology Nursing, 14*(3), 187-188, 191.

Cuzzell, J. (2002b). Wound assessment and evaluation: Wound documentation guidelines. *Dermatology Nursing, 14*(4), 265-266.

Cuzzell, J. (2002c). Wound healing: Translating theory into clinical practice. *Dermatology Nursing, 14*(4), 257-261.

Davidson, M. (2002). Sharpen your wound assessment skills. *Nursing 2002, 32*(10), 32hn1-32hn4.

DeBoer, S., & Zeglin, D. (2001). Necrotizing fasciitis. *American Journal of Nursing, 101*(4), 37-38.

Dochterman, J., & Bulechek, G. (eds). (2004). *Nursing interventions classification (NIC)* (4th ed.). St. Louis: Mosby.

Ebersole, P., Hess, P., & Luggen, A. (2004). *Toward healthy aging: Human needs and nursing response* (6th ed.). St. Louis: Mosby.

Facts and Comparisons. (2004). *Drug facts and comparisons* (58th ed.). St. Louis: Author.

Ferguson, M., et al. (2000). Pressure ulcer management: The importance of nutrition. *MEDSURG Nursing, 9*(4), 163-176.

Fink, A., & DeLuca, G. (2002). Necrotizing fasciitis: Pathophysiology and treatment. *Dermatology Nursing, 14*(5), 324-327.

Fishman, T. (2000). Wound assessment and evaluation. *Dermatology Nursing, 12*(3), 194-195.

Friedberg, E., Harrison, M., & Graham, I. (2002). Current home care expenditures for persons with leg ulcers. *Journal of Wound, Ostomy, and Continence Nursing, 29*(4), 186-192.

Gray, M., Ratliff, C., & Donovan, A. (2002). Tender mercies: Providing skin care for an incontinent patient. *Nursing 2002, 32*(7), 51-54.

Grubbs, L., & Tabano, M. (2000). Use of sunscreen in health care professionals. *Cancer Nursing, 23*(1), 164-167.

Hallett, C., Caress, A., & Luker, K. (2000). Wound care in the community setting: Clinical decision-making in context. *Journal of Advanced Nursing, 31*(4), 783-793.

Harris, J. (2000). A plan to promote the prevention and early detection of melanoma. *Dermatology Nursing, 12*(5), 329-333.

Harrison-Mackey, C., & Colquitt, E.C. (2001). The hidden culprit: Stevens-Johnson syndrome. *American Journal of Nursing, 101*(5), 24AA-24CC.

Hayes, J. (2003). Are you assessing for melanoma? *RN, 66*(2), 36-40.

Hess, C. (2000). Skin care basics. *Advances in Skin and Wound Care, 13*(3), 127-128.

Hilton, D., Williams, L., & Nesbitt, L. (2000). Systemic glucocortico-steroid therapy in dermatology. *Dermatology Nursing, 12*(4), 258-263.

Hockett, K. (2004). Stevens-Johnson syndrome and toxic epidermal necrolysis: Oncologic considerations. *Clinical Journal of Oncology Nursing, 8*(1), 27-30, 55.

Kaufman, M., & Pahl, D. (2003). Vacuum-assisted closure therapy: Wound care and nursing implications. *Dermatology Nursing, 15*(4), 317-325.

Kloth, L. (2002). How to use electrical stimulation for wound healing. *Nursing 2002, 32*(12), 17.

Lang, P. (2000). Dermatoses in African-Americans. *Dermatology Nursing, 12*(2), 87-98.

Lapka, D. (2000). Oncology today: Skin cancer. *RN, 63*(7), 32-39.

Leifer, G. (2001). Hyperbaric oxygen therapy. *American journal of Nursing, 101*(8), 26-34.

Leininger, S. (2002). The role of nutrition in wound healing. *Critical Care Nursing Quarterly, 25*(1), 13-21.

Levine, N. (2000). Exfoliative erythroderma: Skin biopsy is required to determine the cause of this pruritic eruption. *Geriatrics, 55*(8), 25.

Liao, D. (2003). Management of acne. *The Journal of Family Practice, 52*(1), 43-51.

Lindow, K., & Warren, C. (2001). Understanding rosacea. *American Journal of Nursing, 101*(10), 44-51.

Lookingbill, D.B., & Marks, J.G., Jr. (2000). *Principles of dermatology* (3rd ed.). Philadelphia: W.B. Saunders.

Markova, T. (2002). What is the most effective treatment for tinea pedis (athlete's foot)? *The Journal of Family Practice, 51*(1), 21.

McCance, K., & Huether, S. (2002). *Pathophysiology: The biologic basis for disease in adults and children* (4th ed.). St. Louis: Mosby.

McKay, S. (2000). Why we need to worry about warts. *RN, 63*(9), 68-72.

Moorhead, S., Johnson, M., & Maas, M. (Eds.). (2004). *Nursing outcomes classification (NOC)* (3rd ed.). St. Louis: Mosby.

Moss, R., Moss, C., & Broadway, D. (2000). Body contouring with ultrasound-assisted lipoplasty. *AORN Journal, 71*(2), 370-385.

Motta, G. (2000). Reimbursement relief. *Continuing Care, 19*(4), 14-16.

Novatnack, E., & Steven, S. (2002). HERPES: A bigger problem than you think. *RN, 65*(6), 31-38.

Nussbaum, R., McInnes, R., & Willard, H. (2001). *Thompson & Thompson: Genetics in medicine* (6th ed.). Philadelphia: W.B. Saunders.

Oprica, C., Emtestam, L., & Nord, C. (2002). Overview of treatments for acne. *Dermatology Nursing, 14*(4), 242-246.

Pagana, K., & Pagana, T. (2002). *Mosby's manual of diagnostic and laboratory tests* (2nd ed.). St. Louis: Mosby.

Palmissano, C., & Norman, R. (2000). Geriatric dermatology in chronic care and rehabilitation. *Dermatology Nursing, 12*(2), 116-123.

Patel, C., et al. (2000). Vacuum-assisted wound closure. *American Journal of Nursing, 100*(12), 45-48.

Peters, J. (2000). Toxic epidermal necrolysis. *Nursing Times, 96*(36), 43-44.

Pirrung, M. (2001). Management of toxic epidermal necrolysis. *Journal of Intravenous Nursing, 24*(2), 107-113.

Randolph, S. (2002). When candida turns deadly. *RN, 65*(3), 41-45.

Rapaport, M. (2000). Eyelid dermatitis. *Dermatology Nursing, 12*(5), 352-354.

Rayner, V. (2000). Cosmetic rehabilitation. *Dermatology Nursing, 12*(4), 267-271.

Rivera, E., Walsh, A., & Bradley, M. (2000). Using behavior modification to promote wound healing. *Home Healthcare Nurse, 18*(9), 579-586.

Roy, D., & Stotts, N. (2002). Targeting cellulitis. *Nursing 2002, 32*(12), 46-47.

Rudy, S., & Parham-Vetter, P. (2003). Percutaneous absorption of topically applied medication. *Dermatology Nursing, 15*(2), 145-152.

Schiech, L. (2002). Malignant cutaneous wounds. *Clinical Journal of Oncology Nursing, 6*(5), 305-312.

Scholl, D., & Langkamp-Henken, B. (2001). Nutrient recommendations for wound healing. *Journal of Intravenous Nursing, 24*(2), 124-132.

Sheppard, C., & Brenner, P. (2000). The effects of bathing and skin care practices on skin quality and satisfaction with an innovative product. *Journal of Gerontological Nursing, 25*(10), 36-45.

Sibbald, G., et al. (2000). Preparing the wound bed: Debridement, bacterial balance, and moisture balance. *Ostomy Wound Management, 46*(11), 14-35.

Stanley, W. (2003). Nailing a key assessment. *Nursing 2003, 33*(10), 50-51.

Stotts, N., & Hopf, H. (2003). The link between tissue oxygen and hydration in nursing home residents with pressure ulcers: Preliminary data. *Journal of Wound, Ostomy, and Continence Nursing, 30*, 184-190.

Thompson, J. (2003). Maximizing your pressure ulcer care. *RN, 66*(4), 16-24.

*U.S. Department of Health and Human Services. (1992a). *Pressure ulcers in adults: Prediction and prevention.* Clinical Practice Guideline No. 3. Rockville, MD: Agency for Health Care Policy and Research, Public Health Service, U.S. Department of Health and Human Services.

*U.S. Department of Health and Human Services. (1992b). *Preventing pressure ulcers: A patient's guide.* Clinical Practice Guideline No. 3. Rockville, MD: Agency for Health Care Policy and Research, Public Health Service, U.S. Department of Health and Human Services.

U.S. Preventive Services Task Force (2004). Counseling to prevent skin cancer: Recommendations and rationale. *American Journal of Nursing, 104*(4), 87-91.

Van Rijswijk, L. (2004). Wound wise: Moist dressings are better than dry ones. *American Journal of Nursing, 104*(2), 28-31.

Weiss, S., et al. (2003). Quality of life considerations in psoriasis treatment. *Dermatology Nursing, 15*(2), 120-127.

Wilson, J., & Clark, J. (2003). Obesity: Impediment to wound healing. *Critical Care Nursing Quarterly, 26*(2), 119-132.

Worley, C. (2004a). The wound healing process symphony: Part I. *Dermatology Nursing, 16*(1), 67, 72.

Worley, C. (2004b). The wound healing process symphony: Part II. *Dermatology Nursing, 16*(2), 179-180.

Young, M. (2003). Preparing dermatology nurses: Biologic therapies for psoriasis. *Dermatology Nursing, 15*(2), 413-423.

Zulkowski, K., & Albrecht, D. (2003). How nutrition and aging affect wound healing. *Nursing 2003, 33*(8), 70-71.

Zwanziger, P., & Roper, S. (2002). Bacterial counts and types found on wound care supplies used in the home setting. *Journal of Wound, Ostomy, and Continence Nursing, 29*(2), 83-87.

Interventions for Clients with Burns

TAMMY L. COFFEE

LEARNING OUTCOMES

After studying this chapter, you should be able to:

1. Identify burn clients at risk for inhalation injury.
2. Compare the clinical manifestations of superficial, partial-thickness, and full-thickness burn injuries.
3. Explain the expected clinical manifestations of neural and hormonal compensation during the emergent phase of burn injury.
4. Calculate the total body surface area (TBSA) involved in a burn injury.
5. Identify clients at risk for problems of oxygenation.
6. Prioritize nursing care for the client during the emergent phase of burn injury.
7. Use laboratory data and clinical manifestations to determine the effectiveness of fluid resuscitation during the emergent phase of burn injury.
8. Use the Parkland formula to establish the correct rate and timing of fluid replacement.
9. Describe methods to prevent infection from autocontamination and cross-contamination in clients with burn injuries.
10. Prioritize nursing care for the client during the acute phase of burn injury.
11. Explain the alteration of nutritional needs for the burn client during the acute phase of burn injury.
12. Evaluate wound healing in the client during the acute phase of burn injury.
13. Compare pain management strategies for clients in the emergent and acute phases of burn injury.
14. Describe the characteristics of infected burn wounds.
15. Explain the positioning and range-of-motion interventions for the prevention of mobility problems in the client with burns.
16. Prioritize nursing care for the client during the rehabilitation phase of burn injury.
17. Discuss the potential psychosocial problems associated with burn injury.
18. Develop a community-based teaching plan for the client recovering from a burn injury.
19. Identify populations at risk for burn injury and discuss preventive measures.

Go to your Student CD-ROM for Review Questions
for the NCLEX Examination keyed to these Learning Outcomes.

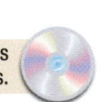

Clients who have burn injuries experience many physiologic, metabolic, and psychological changes. Burn injuries can range from a "sunburn" to complex injuries involving all layers of the skin. When the skin is injured, fluid loss and large inflammatory responses change the function of most body systems. The burn client needs comprehensive care for weeks to months in order to survive the injury, reduce complications, and return to his or her best possible functional status. A multidisciplinary team of health care providers is essential to ensure best care and client outcomes.

INTRODUCTION TO THE BURN PROBLEM

PATHOPHYSIOLOGY OF BURN INJURY

The tissue destruction caused by a burn injury leads to many local and systemic problems. Such problems include fluid and protein losses, sepsis, and changes in metabolic, endocrine, respiratory, cardiac, hematologic, and immune functioning. The extent of local and systemic problems is related to age, general health, extent of injury, depth of injury, and the specific body area injured. Even after healing, the burn injury results in late complications such as contracture formation and scarring. Therefore the prevention of infection and closure of the burn wound are vitally important. A lack of or delay in healing is a key factor for all systemic problems and causes much morbidity and mortality among clients who are burned.

Skin Changes Resulting from Burn Injury

ANATOMIC CHANGES

The skin is the largest organ of the body (see Chapter 69). Each of its two major layers, the epidermis and dermis, has several sublayers. The epidermis, the outer layer of skin, is a superficial layer of stratified epithelial cells about 0.15 mm thick (somewhat thinner in older adults). This layer can grow back after a burn injury because the epidermal cells surrounding sweat and oil glands and hair follicles extend into dermal tissue and regrow to heal partial-thickness wounds. Together, the sweat and oil glands and the hair follicles are the **dermal appendages.** The depth of the dermal appendages varies from one body area to another. The sweat and oil glands in the palm of the hand and the sole of the foot, for example, extend deep into the dermis. This allows for healing of fairly deep burns in these areas. The epidermis has no blood vessels. Nutrients to this layer are diffused from the second layer of skin, the dermis.

The basement membrane, a thin noncellular protein surface, separates the dermis from the epidermis. The dermis is sometimes called the "true skin" because it is not constantly shed and replaced. The dermis is thicker than the epidermis and ranges in thickness from 0.60 to 1.2 mm. The dermis is the thicker part of the skin and is made up of collagen, fibrous connective tissue, and elastic fibers. Within the dermis are the blood vessels, sensory nerves, hair follicles, lymph vessels, sebaceous glands, and sweat glands.

When burn injury occurs, the skin can regenerate as long as parts of the dermis are present. When the entire layer of dermis is burned, all epithelial cells and dermal appendages are destroyed, and the skin can no longer restore itself. The subcutaneous tissue, or superficial fascia, varies in thickness and lies below the dermis. With deep burns, the subcutaneous tissues may be damaged, leaving bones, tendons, and muscles exposed.

FUNCTIONAL CHANGES

The skin has many functions (see Table 69-1). The skin is a protective barrier against injury and microbial invasion from the environment. A burn injury breaks this barrier, greatly increasing the risk for infection.

The skin also helps maintain the delicate fluid and electrolyte balance essential for life. After a burn injury, massive fluid loss occurs through evaporation. Evaporate through burn-injured skin occurs four times as rapidly as from intact skin. The rate of evaporation is in proportion to the total body surface area (TBSA) burned and the depth of injury.

The skin is an excretory organ through sweating. Full-thickness burns destroy the sweat glands, reducing excretory ability.

The skin is the largest sensory organ of the body. Pain, pressure, temperature, and touch are sensed on the skin in normal daily activities, which allows a person to react to changes in the environment. All burn injuries are painful. With partial-thickness burns, nerve endings are exposed, increasing sensitivity and pain. With full-thickness burns, nerve endings are completely destroyed. At first these wounds are completely **anesthetic** (do not transmit sensation) when a sharp stimulus is applied. Despite this destruction, clients often have dull or pressure-type of pain in these areas.

Skin exposed to sunlight activates vitamin D. Partial-thickness burns reduce the activation of vitamin D. Activation of vitamin D is lost completely in full-thickness burns.

The skin helps determine physical identity. The skin's cosmetic quality is part of each person's unique appearance. With a change in appearance through a major burn, psychological problems may develop.

TEMPERATURE. The internal body temperature remains within a narrow range (about 84.2° to 109.4° F [29° to 43° C]) compared with the wide temperature changes in the external environment. Several processes normally adjust to wide differences in external temperature. Circulating blood both provides and dissipates heat efficiently. When heat is applied to the skin, the temperature of the immediate subdermal layer rises rapidly. As soon as the heat source is removed, compensatory processes quickly return the area to a normal temperature. If the heat source is not removed, or if it is applied at a rate that exceeds the skin's capacity to dissipate it, cells are destroyed.

The skin can tolerate temperatures up to 104° F (40° C) without injury. At temperatures of 158° F (71° C) and above, cell destruction is so rapid that even brief exposure damages the skin and subcutaneous levels. Figure 71-1 shows the relationship between temperature and exposure time for burn injury.

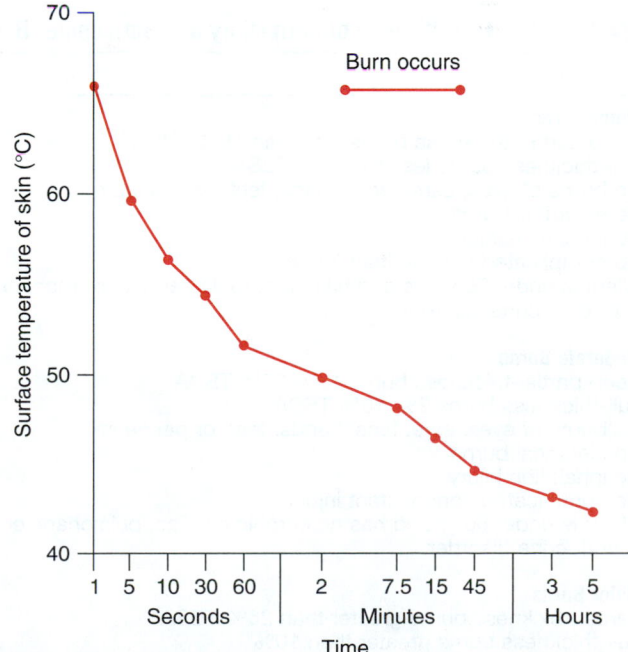

Figure 71-1 ■ Relationship between intensity of heat and the duration of exposure. Exposure for prolonged periods causes burns, even with milder temperatures. At more extreme temperatures, tissue damage results after only seconds. (Modified from Mortiz, A.R. [1947]. Studies of thermal injuries. II: The relative importance of time and surface temperature in causation of cutaneous burns. *American Journal of Pathology, 23,* 695.)

DEPTH OF BURN INJURY. The severity of a burn is determined by the extent of the body surface area involved and the depth of the burn. The degree of tissue damage is related to what agent caused the burn and to the temperature and duration of exposure to the heat source.

Differences in skin thickness in various parts of the body also affect burn depth. In areas where the skin is thin (e.g., eyelids, ears, nose, genitalia, tops of the hands and feet, fingers, and toes), a short exposure to high temperatures causes a deep burn injury. The skin is thinner in older adults, which predisposes them to increased burn severity, even at lower temperatures of shorter duration.

Burn wounds are classified as superficial-thickness wounds, partial-thickness wounds, full-thickness wounds, and deep full-thickness wounds. The partial-thickness wounds are further divided into superficial and deep subgroups. Table 71-1 lists the clinical differences of these burns.

The American Burn Association (ABA) describes burns as minor, moderate, or major depending on the depth, extent, and location of injury (Table 71-2). Figure 71-2 shows

TABLE 71-1   Classification of Burn Depth

Characteristic	Superficial	Partial-Thickness Superficial	Deep Partial-Thickness	Full-Thickness	Deep Full-Thickness
Color	Pink to red	Pink to red	Red to white	Black, brown, yellow, white, red	Black
Edema	Mild	Mild to moderate	Moderate	Severe	Absent
Pain	Yes	Yes	Yes	Yes and no	Absent
Blisters	No	Yes	Rare	No	No
Eschar	No	No	Yes, soft and dry	Yes, hard and inelastic	Yes, hard and inelastic
Healing time	3-5 days	~2 wk	2-6 wk	Weeks to months	Weeks to months
Grafts required	No	No	Can be used if healing is prolonged	Yes	Yes
Example	Sunburn, flash burns	Scalds, flames, brief contact with hot objects	Scalds; flames; prolonged contact with hot objects, tar, grease, chemicals	Scalds; flames; prolonged contact with hot objects, tar, grease chemicals, electricity	Flames, electricity, grease, tar, chemicals

TABLE 71-2   Classification of Burn Injury and Burn Center Referral Criteria

Characteristics	Comments
Minor Burns Deep partial-thickness burns less than 15% TBSA Full-thickness burns less than 2% TBSA No burns of eyes, ears, face, hands, feet, or perineum No electrical burns No inhalation injury No complicated concomitant injury Client is under 60 years and has no chronic cardiac, pulmonary, or endocrine disorder	Clients in this category should receive emergency care at the scene and be taken to a hospital emergency department. A special expertise hospital or designated burn center is not necessary.
Moderate Burns Deep partial-thickness burns 15%-25% TBSA Full-thickness burns 2%-10% TBSA No burns of eyes, ears, face, hands, feet, or perineum No electrical burns No inhalation injury No complicated concomitant injury Client is under 60 yr and has no chronic cardiac, pulmonary, or endocrine disorder	Clients in this category should receive emergency care at the scene and be transferred either to a special expertise hospital or to a designated burn center.
Major Burns Partial-thickness burns greater than 25% TBSA Full-thickness burns greater than 10% Any burn involving the eyes, ears, face, hands, feet, perineum Electrical injury Inhalation injury Client over 60 yr of age Burn complicated with other injuries (e.g., fractures) Client has cardiac, pulmonary, or other chronic metabolic disorders	Clients who meet *any one* of the criteria for a major burn should receive emergency care at the nearest emergency department and then be transferred to a designated burn center as soon as possible.

TBSA, Total body surface area.

the tissue layers involved with different depths of injury and describes the criteria for referral to a burn center.

SUPERFICIAL-THICKNESS WOUNDS. Of all burn types, superficial-thickness wounds have the least damage because the epidermis is the only part of the skin that is injured. The epithelial cells and basement membrane, needed for total regrowth, are present.

Superficial-thickness wounds are caused by prolonged exposure to low-intensity heat (e.g., sunburn) or short (flash) exposure to high-intensity heat. Redness with mild edema, pain, and increased sensitivity to heat occur as a result. Peeling of dead skin (**desquamation**) occurs for 2 to 3 days after the burn. The area heals rapidly in 3 to 5 days without a scar or other complication.

PARTIAL-THICKNESS WOUNDS. A partial-thickness wound involves the entire epidermis and varying depths of the dermis. Depending on the amount of dermal tissue damaged, partial-thickness wounds are further subdivided into superficial partial-thickness and deep partial-thickness injuries.

Superficial Partial-Thickness Wounds. Superficial partial-thickness wounds are caused by heat injury to the upper third of the dermis leaving a good blood supply. These wounds are red, moist, and **blanch** (whiten) when pressure is applied (Figure 71-3). The small vessels perfusing this area are injured, resulting in the leakage of large amounts of plasma, which in turn lifts off the heat-destroyed epidermis, causing blister formation. The blisters continue to increase in size after the burn as cell and protein breakdown occurs. When intact, the blister is a sterile environment, which can protect the wound from infection and water loss. Large or numerous blisters are opened to promote healing and prevent immunosuppression.

Superficial partial-thickness wounds increase pain sensation. Nerve endings are exposed, and any stimulation (touch or temperature change) causes intense pain. With standard care these burns heal in 10 to 21 days with no scar, but some minor pigment changes may occur.

Deep Partial-Thickness Wounds. Deep partial-thickness wounds extend deeper into the skin dermis, and fewer healthy cells remain. In these clients, blister formation does not usually occur because the dead tissue layer is so thick and sticks to underlying viable dermis that it does not readily lift off the surface. The wound surface is red and dry with white areas in deeper parts (dry because fewer

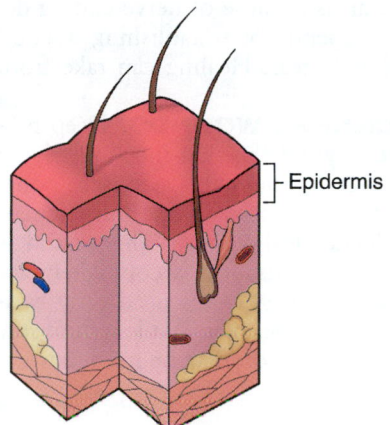

Superficial burns damage only the top layer of the skin—the epidermis. Healing occurs in 3-6 days.

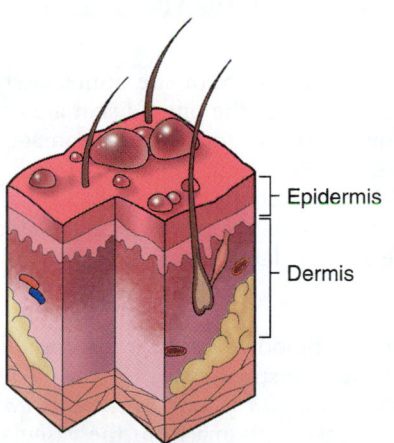

Superficial partial-thickness burns are those in which the entire epidermis and variable portions of the dermis layer of skin are destroyed. Uncomplicated healing occurs in 10-21 days.

Deep partial-thickness burns extend into the deeper layers of the dermis. Healing occurs in 2-6 weeks.

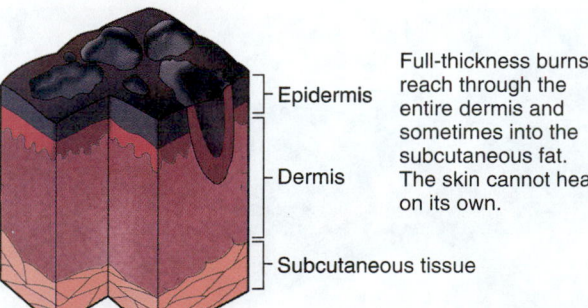

Full-thickness burns reach through the entire dermis and sometimes into the subcutaneous fat. The skin cannot heal on its own.

Figure 71-2 ■ The tissues involved in burns of various depths.

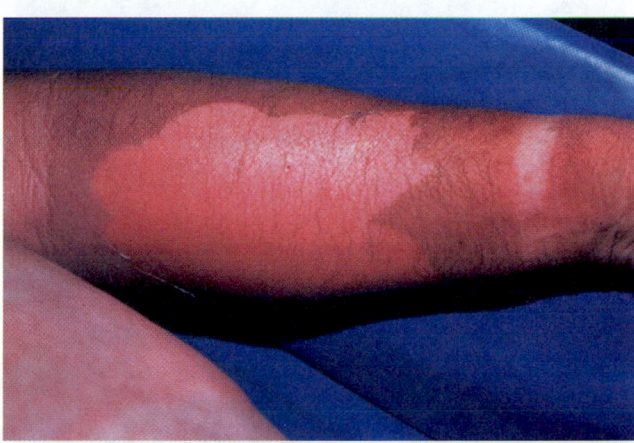

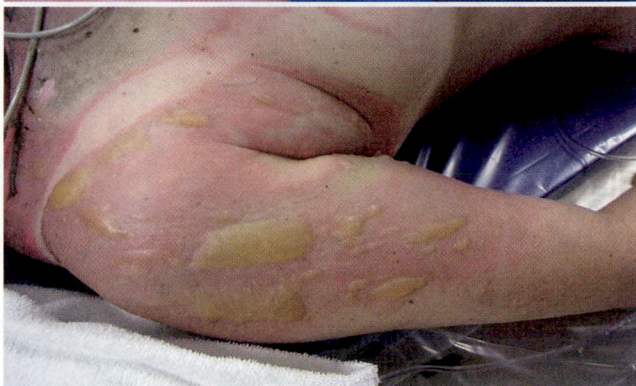

Figure 71-3 ■ The typical appearance of superficial partial-thickness burn injury.

blood vessels are patent). When pressure is applied to the burn, it may blanch slowly or not at all (Figure 71-4). Edema is moderate; pain is present to a lesser degree than with superficial burns because more of the nerve endings have been destroyed.

The blood supply to these areas is reduced by blood vessel constriction. Progression to deeper injury can occur from hypoxia and ischemia. Adequate hydration, nutrients, and oxygen are needed for regrowth of skin cells and prevention of conversion to deeper burns. Partial-thickness wounds can convert to full-thickness wounds when tissue damage increases with infection, hypoxia, or ischemia. Deep partial-thickness wounds generally heal in 3 to 6 weeks, but scar formation results. Surgical intervention with skin grafting can reduce healing time.

FULL-THICKNESS WOUNDS. A full-thickness wound occurs with destruction of the entire epidermis and dermis, leaving no residual epidermal cells to repopulate (Figure 71-5). This wound, therefore, does not re-epithelialize and whatever area of the wound is not closed by wound contraction (see Chapter 70) will require grafting.

The full-thickness injury has a hard, dry, leathery **eschar** (burn crust) that forms from coagulated particles of destroyed dermis. *The eschar is dead tissue; it must slough off or be removed from the burn wound before healing can occur.* The thick

particles often stick to the subcutaneous layer by collagen fibers, which makes eschar removal difficult. Edema is pronounced under the eschar in a full-thickness wound. When the injury completely surrounds an extremity or the thorax **(circumferential),** blood flow and chest movement for breathing may be reduced by tight eschar. **Escharotomies** (incisions through the eschar) or **fasciotomies** (incisions through eschar and fascia) may be needed to relieve pressure and allow normal blood flow and breathing (see Surgical Management [Ineffective Tissue Perfusion], p. 1634).

A full-thickness burn wound may be waxy white, deep red, yellow, brown, or black. Thrombosed vessels may be visible beneath the surface of the burn because the dermal blood vessels are heat coagulated, causing the burned tissue to be without a blood supply **(avascular).** Sensation is reduced or absent in these areas because of nerve ending destruction. Healing time depends on establishing a good blood supply in the injured areas. Healing can take from weeks to months.

DEEP FULL-THICKNESS WOUNDS. Deep full-thickness wounds extend beyond the skin into underlying fascia and tissues. These deep injuries damage muscle, bone, and tendons and leave them exposed. These burns occur with flame, electrical, or chemical injuries. The wound is blackened and depressed, and sensation is completely absent (Figure 71-6). All full-thickness burns need early excision and grafting. Grafting decreases pain and length of stay and accelerates recovery. Amputation may be needed when an extremity is involved.

Vascular Changes Resulting from Burn Injuries

Circulatory disruption occurs at the burn site immediately after a burn injury. Blood vessels to the burned skin are occluded, and blood flow decreases or ceases. Damaged macrophages within the tissues release chemicals (mediators) that at first cause blood vessel constriction. Blood vessel thrombosis may occur, causing necrosis, which can lead to deeper injuries in the already damaged areas.

FLUID SHIFT

After initial vasoconstriction, blood vessels near the burn dilate and leak fluid into the interstitial space (Figure 71-7). This fluid shift, also known as *third spacing* or *capillary leak syndrome,* is a continuous leak of plasma from the vascular

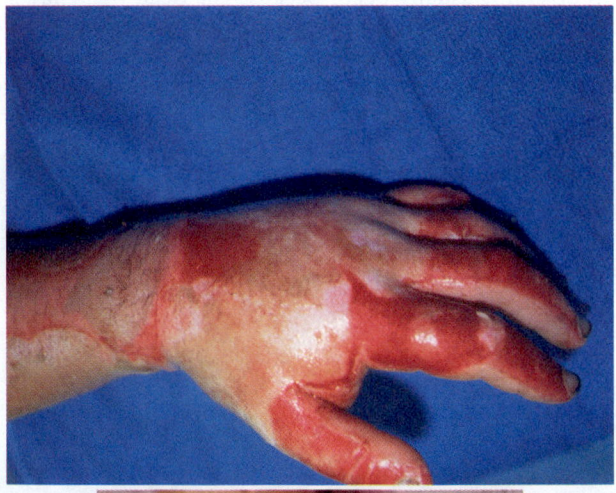

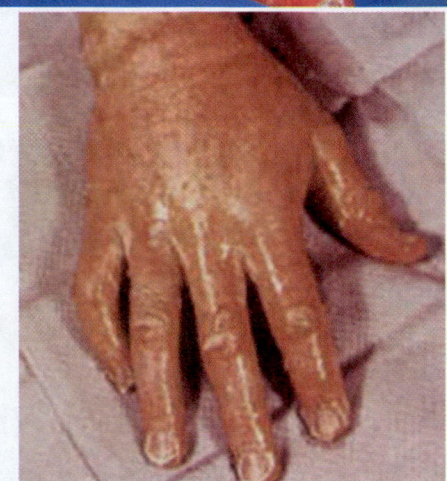

Figure 71-4 ■ The typical appearance of a deep partial-thickness burn injury.

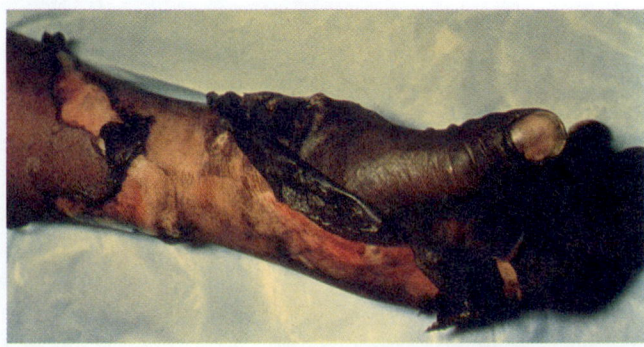

Figure 71-5 ■ The typical appearance of a full-thickness burn injury.

space into the interstitial space. The loss of plasma fluids and proteins decreases blood volume and blood pressure. Leakage of fluid and electrolytes from the vascular space continues, causing extensive edema, even in areas that were not injured. Fluid shift, with excessive weight gain, usually occurs in the first 12 hours after the burn and can continue for 24 to 36 hours.

The amount of fluid shifted depends on the extent and severity of injury. Capillary leak occurs in both burned and unburned area when tissue damage is extensive (i.e., greater than 20% to 30% total body surface area [TBSA]). Edema develops as plasma and electrolytes escape into the interstitial space. The proteins now in the interstitial space increase the movement of fluids out from the vascular space.

Profound imbalances of fluid, electrolytes, and acid-base occur as a result of the fluid shift and cell damage. These imbalances usually include hypovolemia, metabolic acidosis, **hyperkalemia** (elevated blood potassium levels), and **hyponatremia** (decreased blood sodium levels). Hyperkalemia occurs as a result of direct cell injury that releases large amounts of cellular potassium. Sodium is retained by the body as a result of the endocrine response to stress. Aldosterone secretion increases, leading to increased sodium reabsorption by the kidney. This sodium, however, quickly passes into the interstitial spaces of the burned area with the fluid shift; therefore despite the increased amount of sodium in the body, most of the sodium is trapped in the interstitial space, and a sodium deficit occurs in the blood. **Hemoconcentration** (elevated blood osmolarity, hematocrit, and hemoglobin) develops from vascular dehydration. Hemoconcentration increases blood viscosity, reducing flow through small vessels and increasing tissue hypoxia.

FLUID REMOBILIZATION

At about 24 hours after injury, the capillary leak stops and capillary integrity is restored. The diuretic stage begins at about 48 to 72 hours after the burn injury as capillary membrane integrity returns and edema fluid shifts from the interstitial spaces into the vascular space. Blood volume increases, leading to increased renal blood flow and diuresis unless renal damage has occurred. Body weight returns to normal over the next several days as edema subsides.

During this phase, **hyponatremia** (low blood sodium level) develops because of increased renal sodium excretion and the loss of sodium from wounds. **Hypokalemia** (low blood potassium level) results from potassium moving back into the cells and being excreted in urine output. Anemia often develops as a result of hemodilution, but it is generally not severe enough to require blood transfusions. Transfusions are needed if the client's hematocrit is less than 20% to 25% and the client has manifestations of hypoxia. Transfusions are given only when absolutely necessary. Protein continues to be lost from the wounds. Metabolic acidosis remains a possibility because of the loss of sodium bicarbonate in the urine and the increased fat metabolism secondary to decreased carbohydrate intake.

Cardiac Changes Resulting from Burn Injury

Heart rate increases and cardiac output decreases because of the initial fluid shifts and hypovolemia that occur after a burn injury. Cardiac output may remain low until 18 to 36 hours after the burn injury occurs. Cardiac output increases with fluid resuscitation and reaches normal levels before plasma volume is restored completely. Proper fluid resuscitation and support with adequate oxygenation prevent further complications.

Pulmonary Changes Resulting from Burn Injury

Direct injury to the lung from contact with flames rarely occurs. Rather, respiratory problems are caused by superheated air, steam, toxic fumes, or smoke. Such problems are a major

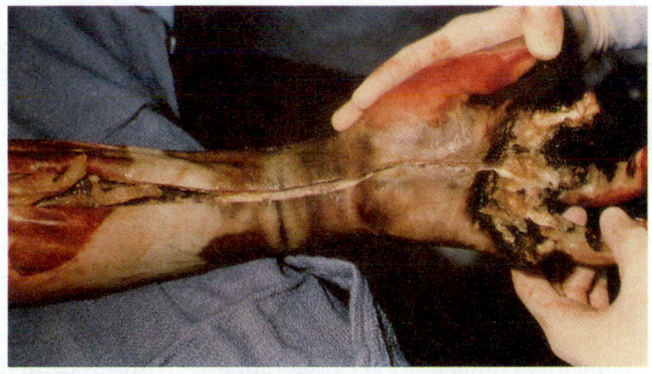

Figure 71-6 ■ The typical appearance of a deep full-thickness burn injury.

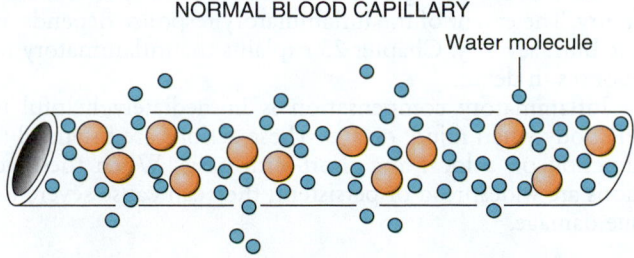

NORMAL BLOOD CAPILLARY

Water molecule

Water is the smallest molecule that can pass through the capillary pores.

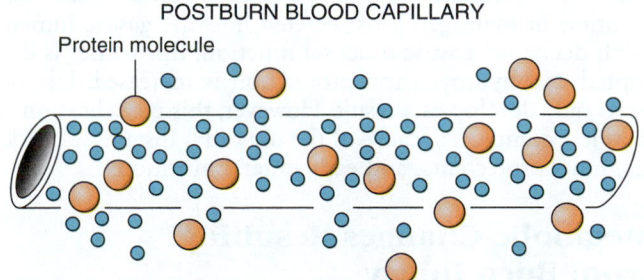

POSTBURN BLOOD CAPILLARY

Protein molecule

Permeability is drastically increased, which allows large molecules such as proteins to pass through the capillary pores easily.

Figure 71-7 ■ The capillary response to burn injury (early phase). This response is also known as "capillary leak syndrome."

cause of death in clients with burns. Respiratory failure with burn injuries can result from airway edema during fluid resuscitation, pulmonary capillary leak, circumferential chest burns that restrict chest movement, and carbon monoxide poisoning.

Respiratory damage from an inhalation injury can occur in the upper and major airways and the lung tissue. The upper airway is affected when inhaled smoke or irritants cause edema and obstruct the trachea. Irritants coming in contact with the upper airway cause a reflex closure of the vocal cords. This protective reflex decreases the amount of smoke and toxic gases entering the lungs. Although air is a poor conductor of heat, some heat does reach the upper airway, causing an inflammatory response that leads to edema of the mouth and throat with the potential of airway obstruction.

More airway injury is caused by chemicals and toxic gases (rather than heat) that are produced during combustion. The ciliated membranes lining the trachea normally trap bacteria and foreign materials. Smoke and combustion products slow this activity, which allows foreign particles to enter the bronchi. The lining of the trachea and bronchi may slough 48 to 72 hours after injury, enter the airway, narrow the tracheal lumen, and obstruct the lower airways.

Lung tissue injuries result from toxic irritant damage to the alveoli and capillaries. Leaking capillaries cause alveolar edema. This edema can occur immediately or as late as 1 week after the injury. The fluid that diffuses into the lung tissue spaces contains proteins that form fibrinous membranes and lead to respiratory distress. Progressive pulmonary failure develops with acute pulmonary insufficiency and infection.

Gastrointestinal Changes Resulting from Burn Injury

The fluid shifts and decreased cardiac output that occur after injury divert blood flow to the brain, heart, and liver. As a result, other organs, including the gastrointestinal (GI) tract, have decreased perfusion. Gastric mucosal integrity and motility are impaired. The sympathetic nervous system stress response increases secretion, especially of epinephrine and norepinephrine, which inhibit GI motility and reduce the flow of blood to the area. Peristalsis decreases, and a paralytic ileus may develop. Secretions and gases collect in the intestines and stomach, causing abdominal distention.

Curling's ulcer (acute ulcerative gastroduodenal disease) may develop within 24 hours after a severe burn injury because of reduced GI blood flow and mucosal damage. The mucosal membrane normally acts as a barrier to the absorption of hydrogen ions secreted into the gastric lumen. With decreased gastric mucosal function, this barrier is disrupted and hydrogen ion production is increased. Ulcerations may develop as a result. However, this complication is now less common because of the use of H_2 histamine blockers, mucoprotectants, and early enteral nutrition.

Metabolic Changes Resulting from Burn Injury

A serious burn injury greatly increases metabolism by increasing secretion of catecholamines, antidiuretic hormone, aldosterone, and cortisol. With this hypermetabolism, the client's oxygen and calorie needs are high.

The catecholamines activate the stress response. The increased production (and loss) of heat breaks down protein and fat (**catabolism**), rapidly uses glucose and calories, and increases urine nitrogen loss. The heat and water lost from the burn also increase metabolic and catabolic rates, which increase calorie needs. Depending on the extent of injury, the client's calorie needs double or triple normal energy needs. These increased rates peak 4 to 12 days after the burn and can remain elevated for months until all wounds are closed.

The hypermetabolic condition also increases core body temperature. The client loses heat through the burned skin because the protective barrier is lost. Core body temperature increases as a response to the adjustment in the hypothalamus. Central body temperature control changes to adapt to the hypermetabolic state and a low-grade fever commonly develops. Essentially what occurs is a "resetting" of the body's normal temperature-control system.

Immunologic Changes Resulting from Burn Injury

Burn injury disrupts the protective barrier of the skin, increasing the risk for infection. The injury activates the inflammatory response and often suppresses immune function (see Chapter 23). Antibody-mediated immunity and cell-mediated immunity are both suppressed. Topical and systemic antibiotics, general anesthesia, blood transfusion, and the stress of surgery further reduce immune function.

Compensatory Responses to Burn Injury

Any tissue injury is a threat to homeostasis and is a stressor. Two compensatory responses have immediate benefit: the inflammatory response and the sympathetic nervous system stress response. Together these responses cause changes that result in many of the manifestations seen in the first 2 to 3 days after a burn injury.

INFLAMMATORY COMPENSATION

Inflammatory compensation can be helpful by triggering healing in the injured tissues. It also is responsible for some of the serious problems that occur with the fluid shift. Inflammatory compensation causes blood vessels to leak fluid into the interstitial space and white blood cells to release chemicals that trigger local tissue reactions. These responses cause the massive fluid shift, edema, and hypovolemia that are seen in the **emergent phase** (first 48 hours) after a burn injury. The extent of the inflammatory response depends on the burn severity. Chapter 23 explains the inflammatory responses in detail.

Inflammatory compensation is immediately helpful to the body when injury occurs. These actions are intended to function on a local and short-term basis. When these actions are widespread or persistent, they can cause severe tissue damage.

SYMPATHETIC NERVOUS SYSTEM COMPENSATION

The sympathetic nervous system stress response occurs when any physical or psychological stressors are present. Changes caused by sympathetic compensation are most ev-

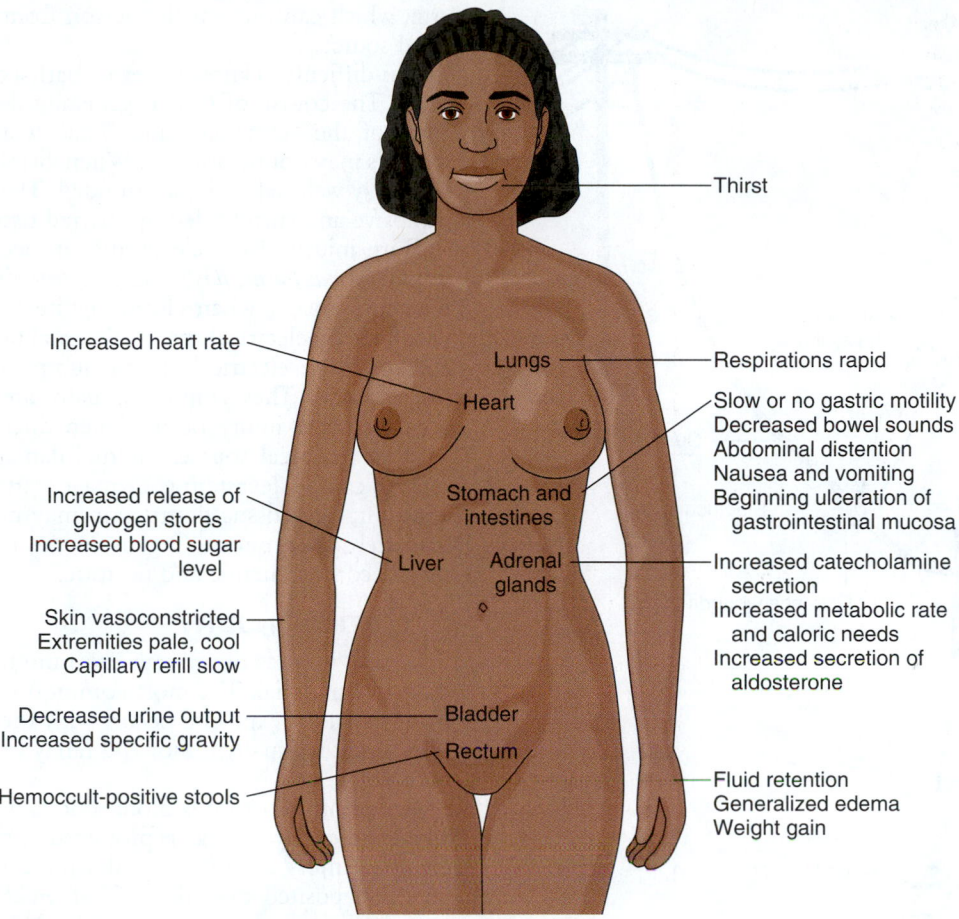

Thirst

Increased heart rate

Lungs

Heart

Respirations rapid

Slow or no gastric motility
Decreased bowel sounds
Abdominal distention
Nausea and vomiting
Beginning ulceration of
  gastrointestinal mucosa

Increased release of
glycogen stores
Increased blood sugar
level

Stomach and
intestines

Liver   Adrenal
glands

Increased catecholamine
  secretion
Increased metabolic rate
  and caloric needs
Increased secretion of
  aldosterone

Skin vasoconstricted
Extremities pale, cool
Capillary refill slow

Decreased urine output
Increased specific gravity

Bladder

Rectum

Fluid retention
Generalized edema
Weight gain

Hemoccult-positive stools

Figure 71-8 ■ The physiologic actions of the sympathetic nervous system compensatory responses to burn injury (early phase).

ident in the cardiovascular, respiratory, and gastrointestinal (GI) systems. Figure 71-8 shows the results of sympathetic nervous system stimulation.

Etiology of Burn Injury

Burn injuries are caused by dry heat (flame), moist heat (scald), contact with hot surfaces, chemicals, electricity, and ionizing radiation. The cause of the injury affects both the prognosis and the treatment.

DRY HEAT

Dry heat injuries are caused by open flame. The most common flame injuries occur in house fires and explosions. Ignited clothing from an open flame accounts for most of the injuries. Explosions usually result in flash burns because they produce a brief exposure to very high temperatures.

MOIST HEAT

Moist heat (scald) injuries are caused by contact with hot liquids or steam. Scald injuries are most common among older adults (Stone, Ahmed, & Evans, 2000). Hot liquid spills usually burn the upper, frontal surfaces of the body, whereas immersion scald injuries usually involve the lower body.

CONTACT BURNS

Hot metal, tar, and grease can cause full-thickness burns when they contact the skin. Hot metal injuries occur when

a body part contacts a hot surface, such as a space heater or iron. They also can occur in industrial settings from molten metals. Tar and asphalt temperatures usually are greater than 400° F, and serious deep injuries occur within seconds when the skin is immersed in or splashed with the agent. Hot grease injuries from cooking are usually deep because of the temperature of the grease.

CHEMICAL INJURY

Chemical burns occur as a result of accidents in homes or industry. They can also be the result of a deliberate assault on an individual. Tissue injury occurs when chemicals come in direct contact with the skin and epithelial tissues or are ingested. The severity of the injury depends on the duration of contact, the concentration of the chemical, the amount of tissue exposed, and the action of the chemical.

Alkalis found in oven cleaners, fertilizers, drain cleaners, and heavy industrial cleaners damage the tissue by causing tissues to liquefy and proteins to denature. This allows for deeper spread of the chemical and more severe burns. Acids found in bathroom cleaners, rust removers, chemicals for swimming pools, and industrial drain cleaners damage tissue by coagulating cells and proteins, which tends to limit the depth of tissue damage. Organic compounds are found in many chemical disinfectants and in gasoline. Organic compounds cause damage due to their fat solvent action. Once absorbed they can produce toxic effects on the kidneys and liver.

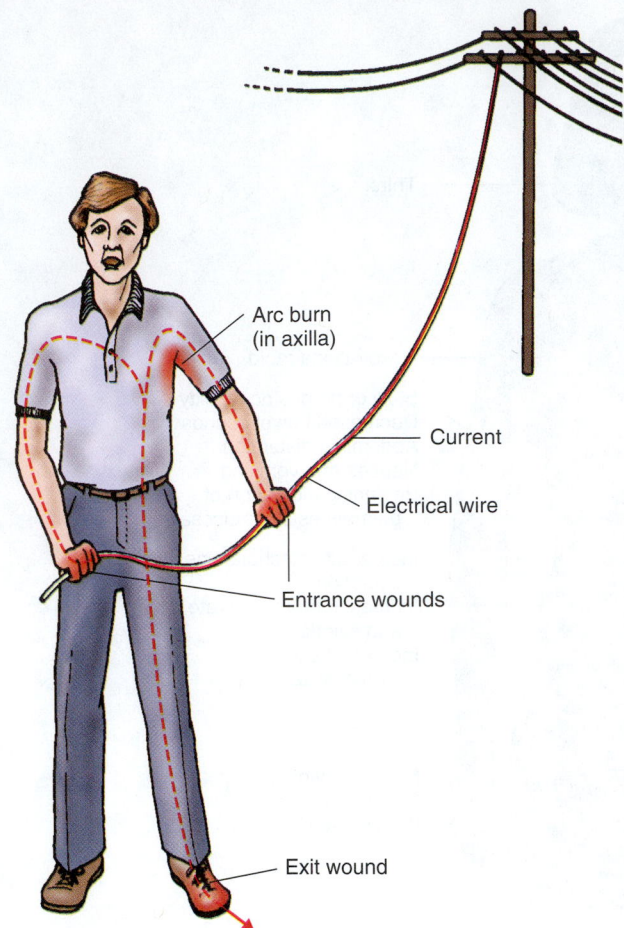

Figure 71-9 ■ The mechanism of electrical injury: Currents passing through the body follow the path of least resistance to the ground.

ELECTRICAL INJURY

An electrical injury is a burn occurring when an electrical current enters the body (Figure 71-9). Electrical injuries have been called the "grand masquerader" of burn injuries because small surface injuries may be associated with devastating internal injuries. Electrical injuries are divided into high and low voltage with high voltage being greater than 1000 volts. Tissue injury from electrical trauma results from electrical energy being converted to heat energy. The extent of injury depends on the type of current, the pathway of flow, the local tissue resistance, and the duration of contact. The skin is the most resistant organ; the greatest resistance is in the epidermis of the skin. At high voltages the difference in tissue resistance is clinically unimportant. Although various underlying tissues have different resistance to current flow, once skin resistance is overcome, the body acts as a conductor and current flows throughout the involved body part. Bone has a very high resistance because of its density. Current flows along the surface of the bone, and the heat generated damages adjacent muscle. As a result, deep muscle injury may be present even when superficial muscles appear normal or uninjured.

The longer the electricity is in contact with the body, the greater the damage. The duration of contact is increased by tetanic contractions of the strong flexor muscles in the fore-arm, which can prevent the person from releasing the electrical source.

It is difficult to know the exact path a current takes in the body. The course of flow is generally defined by the locations of the "entrance" and "exit" wounds. At first, the wounds may not be obvious. When visible, the entrance site is usually well defined and rounded. The exit site is usually explosive and surrounded by charred tissue.

Burn injuries from electricity can occur in one of three ways: *thermal burns, flash burns,* or *true electrical injury.* Thermal burns occur when clothes ignite from heat or flames produced by electrical sparks. External burn injuries can occur when the electrical current jumps, or "arcs," between two surfaces. These injuries usually are severe and deep. True electrical injury occurs when direct contact is made with an electrical source. Internal damage results, and the injuries can be devastating. Damage starts on the inside and goes out; deep-tissue destruction may not be apparent immediately after injury. Organs in the path of the current may become ischemic and necrotic.

RADIATION INJURY

Radiation injuries occur with exposure to large doses of radioactive material. The most common type of tissue injury from radiation exposure occurs with therapeutic radiation. This injury is usually minor and rarely causes extensive skin damage.

Radiation exposure is more serious in industrial settings where radioactive energy is produced or radioactive isotopes are used. Injury severity depends on the amount and type of energy deposited over time. Chapter 28 discusses the potential for tissue damage from alpha, beta, and gamma radiation. The severity of injury is determined by the type of radiation, distance from the source, duration of exposure, absorbed dose, and depth of penetration into the body.

Incidence/Prevalence of Burn Injury

The incidence of burn injuries in the United States has declined significantly in the past two decades. As of the early 1990s, the rate of reportable burn injuries in the United States had declined from 10 in 10,000 to 4.2 in 10,000.

An estimated 4500 fire and burn deaths occur each year. This total includes deaths from fires and motor vehicle or aircraft crashes, electricity, chemicals, hot liquids and substances, and any other sources of burn injury. Fire and burn deaths in the United States declined about 50% from 1971-1998. The death rate from burns has declined by 60%. Of the clients who seek medical attention, 45,000 are hospitalized each year. Half of the hospitalizations occur in the 125 specialized burn treatment centers. The average TBSA affected in burn victims admitted to a burn center is 14%. Fifty-four percent of burn center admissions are for burns affecting 10% or less TBSA, whereas 4% of admissions are for burns affecting greater than 60% TBSA.

Burns are the sixth leading cause of accidental death in the United States. Causes vary among different age-groups (Table 71-3). The highest risk is among those 75 years and older. Men are at slightly higher risk for fatal and nonfatal burn injuries.

Death from burn injuries decreases with appropriate intervention. Factors that increase the risk for death include age older than 60 years, a burn greater than 40% total body

TABLE 71-3 Percentage of Burn Injuries by Age in the United States

Age	Dry Heat (Flame)	Moist Heat (Scalds)	Contact	Chemical	Electrical	Ionizing Radiation
Birth-23 mo	10	72	15	1	2	<1
2-4 yr	34	54	8	1	3	<1
5-12 yr	70	23	4	1	2	<1
13-18 yr	69	20	5	2	4	<1
19-35 yr	56	26	10	4	4	<1
36-54 yr	44	33	13	4	6	<1
55 yr and older	73	21	4	1	1	<1

surface area (TBSA), and the presence of an inhalation injury. When a client has all three risk factors, the risk for mortality is 90%.

The successful treatment of burns can be attributed to many therapeutic advances including vigorous fluid resuscitation, early burn wound excision, improved critical care monitoring, early enteral nutrition, improved topical and systemic antibiotics, and the use of specialized burn centers.

EMERGENT PHASE OF BURN INJURY

OVERVIEW

Burns can be a devastating and dehumanizing injury. Events within the first hour after injury can make the difference between life and death for the client with a burn injury. Immediate care focuses on maintaining an open airway, ensuring adequate breathing and circulation, limiting the extent of injury, and maintaining the function of vital organs. Chart 71-1 outlines the emergency management of a burn injury.

The **emergent phase** is the first phase of a burn injury. It begins at the onset of injury and continues to about 48 hours. During this phase the injury is evaluated and the immediate problems of fluid loss, edema, and reduced blood flow are assessed. The goals of management during this period are to (1) secure the airway, (2) support circulation by fluid replacement, (3) keep the client comfortable with analgesics, (4) prevent infection through careful wound care, (5) maintain body temperature, and (6) provide emotional support.

◆ COLLABORATIVE MANAGEMENT
◆ Assessment

HISTORY

Knowledge of circumstances surrounding the burn injury is extremely valuable in the management of a burn victim. If possible, obtain information directly from the client. If this is not possible, ask significant others or witnesses. Ask questions that include the circumstances of the injury, the time and place of injury, and the source and cause of injury. Obtain a detailed description of how the burn occurred, and the events occurring from the time of injury until help arrived. Also obtain demographic data, health history (including pre-existing illness), drug use, any accompanying injuries, and pain information.

Demographic data include age, weight, and height. The rate of serious complications and death from burn injuries is increased among adults over 50 years of age. Chart 71-2 lists the age-related differences in the older adults' response to a burn injury. The client's preburn weight is used to cal-

CHART 71-1

BEST PRACTICE for
Emergency Management of Burns

General Management for All Types of Burns
- Assess for airway patency.
- Administer oxygen as needed.
- Cover the client with a blanket.
- Keep the client on NPO status.
- Elevate the extremities if no fractures are obvious.
- Obtain vital signs.
- Initiate an IV line and begin fluid replacement.
- Administer tetanus toxoid for prophylaxis.
- Perform a head-to-toe assessment.

Specific Management
Flame Burns
- Smother the flames.
- Remove smoldering clothing and all metal objects.

Chemical Burns
- Brush off any dry chemicals present on the skin or clothing.
- Remove the client's clothing.
- Ascertain the type of chemical causing the burn.
- Do not attempt to neutralize the chemical unless it has been positively identified and the appropriate neutralizing agent is available.

Electrical Burns
- At the scene, separate the client from the electrical current.
- Smother any flames that are present.
- Initiate cardiopulmonary resuscitation.
- Obtain an electrocardiogram (ECG).

Radiation Burns
- Remove the client from the radiation source.
- If the client has been exposed to radiation from an unsealed source, remove the client's clothing (using tongs or lead protective gloves).
- If the client has radioactive particles on his or her skin, send the client to the nearest designated radiation decontamination center.
- Help the client to bathe or shower.

culate fluid rates, energy requirements, and drug doses. The preburn weight often is referred to as "dry weight," because it represents the client's weight before edema begins to form. Calculations based on a weight obtained after fluid replacement is started are not accurate because of water-induced weight gain. Height is important in determining body surface area (**BSA**), which is used to calculate nutritional needs.

A health history, including any pre-existing illnesses, must be known for appropriate treatment to be given. Obtain information from the client specifically about his or her history of cardiac or renal impairment, chronic alcoholism, substance abuse, and diabetes mellitus; any of these problems

NURSING FOCUS on the OLDER ADULT
Age-Related Changes That Increase Mortality and Morbidity from Burns

- Older adults are at a higher risk for burn injury because of thinner skin, decreased mobility and reaction time, and visual and hearing impairment.
- The skin of an older adult person is thinner and more easily damaged than that of a younger person. Therefore burn injuries tend to be more extensive in older clients, even when exposure to causative agent is shorter.
- Healing time is slower in the older adult, which increases risk for infection and other complications.
- Cardiac impairment in the older client with burns limits the amount and type of fluids used in resuscitation. As a result, older clients are more likely to develop complications from hypovolemic shock and inadequate renal perfusion.
- The immune responses of the older client may be reduced, which increases the risk for infection and sepsis. In addition, the older adult may not have a fever when an infection is present.
- Decreased elasticity of the thoracic cage and decreased number and efficiency of alveoli make older adults more likely to develop hypoxia, hypoventilation, and atelectasis.
- Older adults are more likely to have pre-existing medical condition (e.g., diabetes mellitus, cardiovascular disorders, pulmonary or renal impairment, or immunosuppression) that may further compromise vital organ function or interfere with resuscitation and treatment.

TABLE 71-4 Factors Determining Inhalation Injury or Airway Obstruction

- Individuals who were injured in a closed space
- Clients with extensive burns or with burns of the face
- Intra-oral charcoal, especially on teeth and gums
- Clients who were unconscious at the time of injury
- Clients with singed hairs, nasal hairs, eyelids, or eyelashes
- Clients who are coughing up carbonaceous sputum
- Changes in voice such as hoarseness or brassy cough
- Use of accessory muscles or stridor
- Poor oxygenation or ventilation
- Edema, erythema, and ulceration of airway mucosa
- Wheezing, bronchospasm

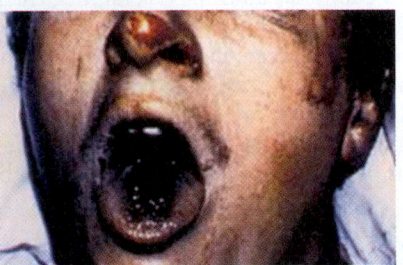

influence fluid resuscitation. The physiologic stress seen with a burn can make a latent disease process develop symptoms or worsen an active process. Obtain a drug history that includes allergies, current drugs, and immunization status from the client or family. Determine the dose and time the last drug was taken. Ask whether or not the client smokes or drinks alcohol daily; these factors can influence treatment and physical responses.

Other injuries are unusual but may occur at the time of the burn. The most common causes of associated injuries are falls and motor vehicle accidents. Such injuries increase the client's risk for complications or death. Determine whether additional injuries such as fractures, chest injuries, and abdominal trauma are causing pain or discomfort.

PHYSICAL ASSESSMENT/CLINICAL MANIFESTATIONS

Physical assessment findings in the emergent phase vary greatly from findings later in the course of the injury. Use a systematic approach to ensure that no problem is missed. The systems assessed first are those that can have immediate, life-threatening changes in function.

RESPIRATORY ASSESSMENT. Clients with major burn injuries and those with inhalation injury are at risk for respiratory problems. Respiratory manifestations common with a burn injury are listed in Table 71-4.

DIRECT AIRWAY INJURY. Inhalation injuries are present in 20% to 50% of the clients admitted to burn centers. The degree of inhalation damage depends on the fire source, temperature, environment, and types of toxic gases generated. Ask about the source of the fire, duration of exposure, and history of being in an enclosed space. Assess the respiratory system by visually inspecting the mouth, nose, and pharynx. Burns of the lips, face, ears, neck, eyelids, eye-

brows, and eyelashes are strong indicators that an inhalation injury may be present. Burns inside the mouth and singed nasal hairs indicate potentially serious injuries. Carbonaceous particles in the nose, mouth, and sputum along with edema of the nasal septum indicate smoke inhalation, as does a "smoky" smell to the client's breath.

A change in respiratory pattern may indicate a pulmonary injury. The client may:
- Become progressively hoarse
- Develop a brassy cough
- Drool or have difficulty swallowing
- Produce expiratory sounds that include audible wheezes, crowing, and stridor

Upper airway edema and inhalation injury are most common in the trachea and mainstem bronchi. Auscultation of these areas may reveal wheezes, which are a sign of obstruction. Clients with severe inhalation injuries may have such rapid obstruction that within a short time they cannot force air through the narrowed airways. As a result, the wheezing sounds disappear. *This finding indicates impending airway obstruction and demands immediate intubation.* Many clients are intubated when an inhalation injury is suspected rather than waiting until obstruction makes endotracheal or nasotracheal intubation difficult or impossible.

CARBON MONOXIDE POISONING. Carbon monoxide is one of the leading causes of death associated with fires. It is a colorless, odorless, tasteless gas released as oxygen is being consumed in the process of combustion. Inhalation injury is a risk for carbon monoxide poisoning.

Carbon monoxide is rapidly transported across the alveolar membrane and preferentially binds to hemoglobin in place of oxygen to form carboxyhemoglobin (COHb). In addition, CO causes the oxyhemoglobin dissociation curve to shift to the left, thereby impairing oxygen unloading at the tissue level. This shift results in a substantial reduction in oxygen delivery, given that 98% of the oxygen supplied to the tissues comes bound to hemoglobin. Even though the oxygen-carrying capacity of the hemoglobin is reduced,

TABLE 71-5 Physiologic Effects of Carbon Monoxide Poisoning

Carbon Monoxide Level	Physiologic Effects
1%-10% (normal)	Increased threshold to visual stimuli Increased blood flow to vital organs
11%-20% (mild poisoning)	Headache Decreased cerebral function Decreased visual acuity Slight breathlessness
21%-40% (moderate poisoning)	Headache Tinnitus Nausea Drowsiness Vertigo Altered mental state Confusion Stupor Irritability Decreased blood pressure, increased and irregular heart rate Depressed ST segment on ECG and dysrhythmias Pale to reddish purple skin
41%-60% (severe poisoning)	Coma Convulsions Cardiopulmonary instability
61%-80% (fatal poisoning)	Death

ECG, Electrocardiogram.

the partial pressure of arterial oxygen (PaO₂) is normal. The vasodilating action of carbon monoxide causes the "cherry red" color in these clients. Clinical manifestations vary with the concentration of COHb. Table 71-5 lists the effects of carbon monoxide poisoning.

THERMAL (HEAT) INJURY. Except for rare events such as steam inhalation, aspiration of scalding liquid or explosion occurring while a client is breathing very high concentrations of oxygen or flammable gases under pressure, thermal burns to the respiratory tract are limited to the upper airway above the glottis (nasopharynx, oropharynx, and larynx). The respiratory tract's heat exchange capability is so efficient that most damage occurs above the true vocal cords. Heat damage of the pharynx is often severe enough to produce upper airway obstruction, which can occur any time during resuscitation. In the unresuscitated client, supraglottic edema may be delayed in onset until fluid resuscitation is well underway. Early intervention with intubation may be preferred.

Inhaled steam can injure the lower respiratory tract because water holds heat better than does dry air. The respiratory tract down to the major bronchioles can be damaged by steam. Ulcerations, redness, and edema of the mouth and epiglottis are the first manifestations, with rapid edema formation progressing to upper airway obstruction. Stridor, hoarseness, and shortness of breath result.

SMOKE POISONING. Smoke poisoning, or chemical injury from the inhalation of combustion by-products, is the most common type of inhalation injury. Toxic by-products, especially hydrogen cyanide, are produced when plastics or home furnishings are burned. Cyanide binds to the cytochrome system, thereby inhibiting cell metabolism

and adenosine triphosphate (ATP) production. This problem disrupts cell function.

PULMONARY FLUID OVERLOAD. Pulmonary edema can result even when the lung tissues have not been damaged directly. Other damaged tissues release such large amounts of histamine and other inflammatory mediators causing capillary leak that even lung capillaries leak fluid into the pulmonary tissue spaces.

Circulatory overload from fluid resuscitation may cause left-sided heart failure. This problem creates such high hydrostatic pressure within pulmonary blood vessels that even more fluid is lost from the pulmonary vascular space into the tissue spaces. Excess lung tissue fluid makes gas exchange difficult. The client is short of breath and has dyspnea in the supine position. Crackles are heard on auscultation.

EXTERNAL FACTORS. In addition to pulmonary problems, clients with burn injuries may have breathing problems as a result of external factors. The most common external factor affecting breathing is tight eschar from deep circumferential chest burns. The eschar either restricts chest movement or compresses structures in the neck and throat to such an extent that ventilation is impaired. Inspect the client's chest for ease of respiration, amount of chest movement, rate of breathing, and effort required to breathe. Use pulse oximetry to assess breathing effectiveness in maintaining blood oxygen levels.

CARDIOVASCULAR ASSESSMENT. Changes in the cardiovascular system begin immediately after the burn injury and include shock from various causes. *Shock is a common cause of death in the emergent phase in clients with serious injuries.* See Chapter 40 for discussion of all types of shock.

At first, cardiac manifestations reflect hypovolemia and decreased cardiac output. Monitor the degree of edema and assess cardiac status by measuring central and peripheral pulses, blood pressure, capillary refill, and pulse oximetry. Noninvasive blood pressure readings are inaccurate in clients with large burns involving the upper extremities. Thus invasive monitoring may be needed for blood pressure measurement. At first, the client has tachycardia, decreased blood pressure, and decreased peripheral pulses. Peripheral capillary refill is slow or absent as tissue blood flow decreases. With fluid resuscitation, peripheral edema increases, as does the client's body weight.

Electrocardiographic (ECG) changes indicate electrical damage to the heart. These changes are most common with electrical burn injuries or with stress that induces a myocardial infarction. Obtain baseline ECG tracings at the time of admission to the hospital or burn center.

RENAL/URINARY ASSESSMENT. Changes in renal function with burn injury are related to decreased renal blood flow and to the presence of cellular debris. During the fluid shift of the emergent period, blood flow to the kidney may not be adequate for glomerular filtration. As a result, urine output is greatly decreased compared with intravenous (IV) fluid intake. The urine is highly concentrated and has a high specific gravity.

Other substances may be present in the blood that flows through the kidney. Destroyed red blood cells release hemoglobin and potassium. When muscle damage occurs from a major burn or electrical injury, a large oxygen-carrying protein called **myoglobin** is released from damaged muscle and

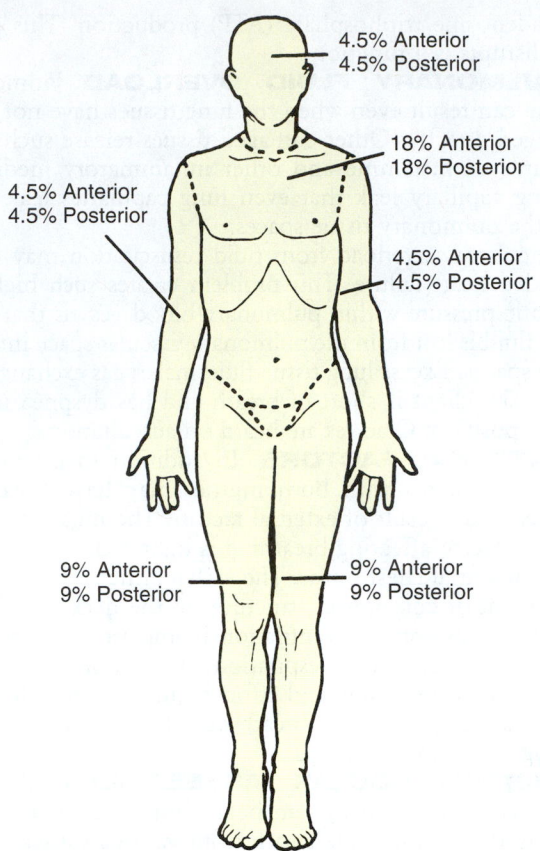

4.5% Anterior
4.5% Posterior

18% Anterior
18% Posterior

4.5% Anterior
4.5% Posterior

4.5% Anterior
4.5% Posterior

9% Anterior
9% Posterior

9% Anterior
9% Posterior

Figure 71-10 ■ The rule of nines for estimating burn percentage.

circulates to the kidney. Most damaged cells release proteins that form uric acid. All of these large molecules in the blood may precipitate in the kidney tubular system. This precipitation blocks kidney blood and urine flow and may cause renal failure.

Assess renal function by accurately measuring urine output and comparing this value with fluid intake. Urine output is decreased during the first 24 hours of the emergent phase. Fluid resuscitation is provided at the rate needed to maintain adult urine output at 30 to 50 mL or 0.5 mL/kg/hr. Assess response to fluid resuscitation by measuring urine specific gravity, blood urea nitrogen (BUN), serum creatinine, and serum sodium levels in addition to urine output. Examine the urine for color, odor, and the presence of particles or foam.

SKIN ASSESSMENT. Assess the skin to determine the size and depth of burn injury. The size of the injury is first estimated in comparison to the total body surface area (TBSA). For example, a burn that involves 40% of the TBSA is a 40% burn. The size of the injury is important not only for diagnosis and prognosis but also for calculating drug doses, fluid replacement volumes, and caloric needs.

Inspect the skin to identify injured areas and changes in color and appearance. Except with electrical burns, this initial size assessment usually can be made accurately with specific assessment tools and charts.

The most rapid method for calculating the size of a burn injury in adult clients whose weights are in normal propor-

tion to their heights is the *rule of nines* (Figure 71-10). With this method, the body is divided into areas that are multiples of 9%. Although the rule of nines is useful at the site of injury and in emergency departments, overestimation of the TBSA involved can easily occur.

The Lund-Browder and Berkow methods are more accurate for evaluating the size of the injury (Figure 71-11). These methods take into account changes in body surface area from birth through adulthood.

Because specific treatments are related to the depth of the burn injury, initial assessment of the skin includes estimations of burn depth. Criteria for depth of injury are based on appearance and associated characteristics (see Depth of Burn Injury, p. 1620).

GASTROINTESTINAL ASSESSMENT. Although the gastrointestinal (GI) tract usually is not directly injured (except in those with chemical burns), changes in GI function are expected in all burn clients. The decreased blood flow and sympathetic stimulation during the emergent phase causes reduced GI motility and paralytic ileus. Auscultate the abdomen to assess bowel sounds. Bowel sounds are commonly reduced or absent in a client with severe burns. Other manifestations include nausea, vomiting, and abdominal distention. Clients with burns of 25% TBSA or who are intubated generally require a nasogastric (NG) tube inserted to prevent aspiration and remove gastric secretions. Assess the tube for placement and patency after insertion. Because of the potential for ulcer formation in the GI tract, you must examine the stool and vomitus for the presence of gross blood or other material indicative of partially digested blood. Tests for the presence of occult blood are performed.

LABORATORY ASSESSMENT

Changes in laboratory test values are found in different phases of postburn recovery and reflect tissue damage or compensatory responses. However, other changes in specific laboratory findings may suggest complications.

During the emergent phase and before the start of fluid resuscitation, venous blood analysis reflects the fluid shift and direct tissue damage. Baseline laboratory test values and early postburn variations are listed in Chart 71-3.

Changes in the total white blood cell (WBC) count and differential count reflect immune function and inflammatory responses to the burn injury. The burn client's total WBC count, especially the neutrophil percentage, first rises and then drops rapidly, with a "left shift" (see Chapter 23) as the immune system becomes unable to sustain its defenses. If sepsis occurs, the total WBC count may be as low as 2000 cells/mm³.

Other laboratory tests that provide useful information about the burn client's status include urine electrolyte assays, urine cultures, liver enzyme studies, and clotting studies. Drug and alcohol screens are obtained if drug or alcohol intoxication is suspected.

CULTURAL CONSIDERATIONS

For African-American clients, a sickle cell preparation may be appropriate if sickle status is unknown. Trauma often triggers a sickle cell crisis in clients who have the disease and in those who carry the trait.

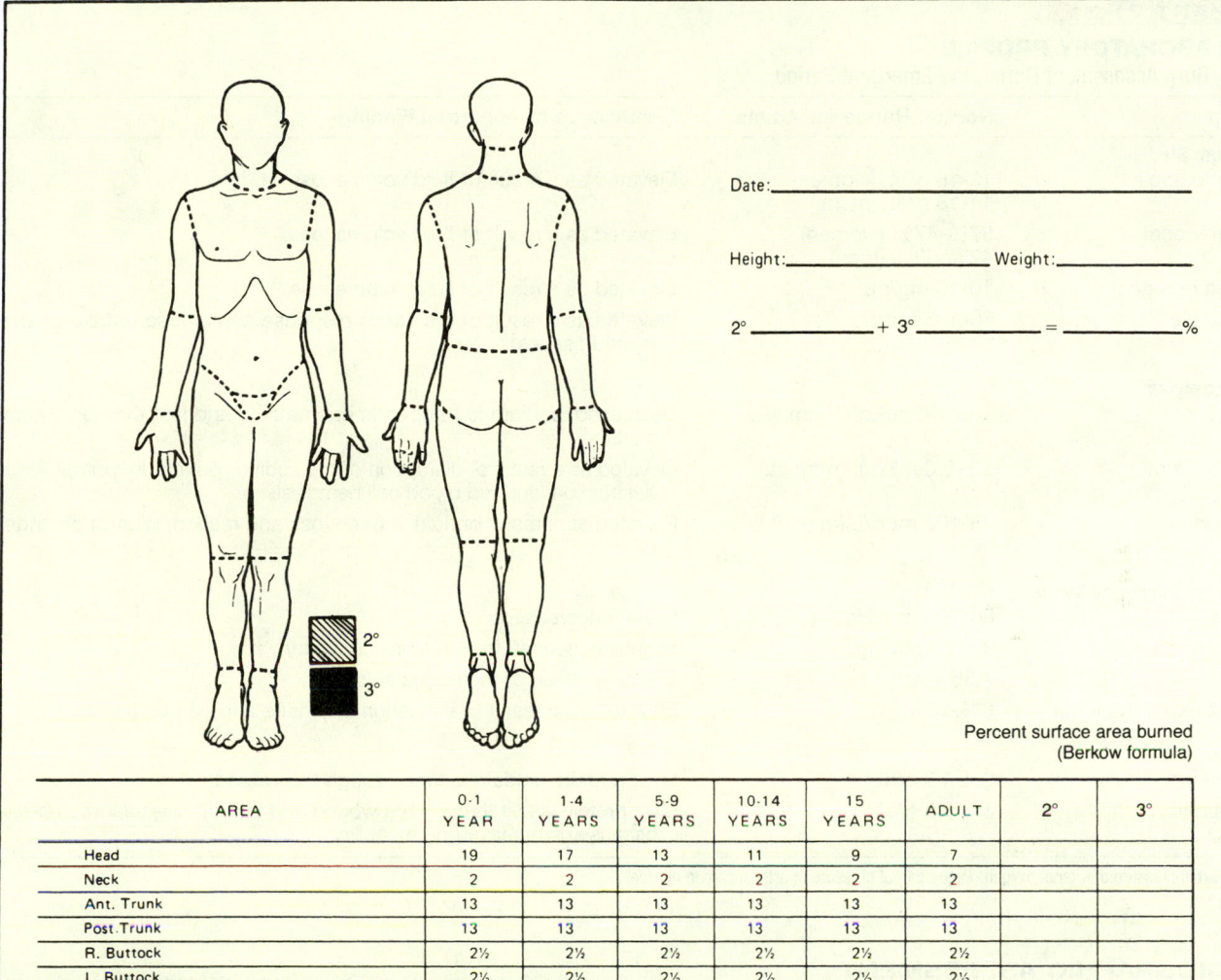

Date:_____

Height:_____ Weight:_____

2° _____ + 3° _____ = _____%

Percent surface area burned
(Berkow formula)

AREA	0-1 YEAR	1-4 YEARS	5-9 YEARS	10-14 YEARS	15 YEARS	ADULT	2°	3°
Head	19	17	13	11	9	7		
Neck	2	2	2	2	2	2		
Ant. Trunk	13	13	13	13	13	13		
Post. Trunk	13	13	13	13	13	13		
R. Buttock	2½	2½	2½	2½	2½	2½		
L. Buttock	2½	2½	2½	2½	2½	2½		
Genitalia	1	1	1	1	1	1		
R. U. Arm	4	4	4	4	4	4		
L. U. Arm	4	4	4	4	4	4		
R. L. Arm	3	3	3	3	3	3		
L. L. Arm	3	3	3	3	3	3		
R. Hand	2½	2½	2½	2½	2½	2½		
L. Hand	2½	2½	2½	2½	2½	2½		
R. Thigh	5½	6½	8	8½	9	9½		
L. Thigh	5½	6½	8	8½	9	9½		
R. Leg	5	5	5½	6	6½	7		
L. Leg	5	5	5½	6	6½	7		
R. Foot	3½	3½	3½	3½	3½	3½		
L. Foot	3½	3½	3½	3½	3½	3½		
TOTAL								

Figure 71-11 ■ Estimation of the extent of burn injury by the Berkow method. *Ant.*, Anterior; *Post.*, posterior; *R.*, right; *L.*, left; *R.U.*, right upper; *L.U.*, left upper; *R.L.*, right lower; *L.L.*, left lower.

CHART 71-3

LABORATORY PROFILE
Burn Assessment During the Emergent Period

Test	Normal Range for Adults	Significance of Abnormal Findings
Serum Studies		
Hemoglobin	12-16 g/dL (women) 14-18 g/dL (men)	Elevated as a result of fluid volume loss
Hematocrit	37%-47% (women) 42%-52% (men)	Elevated as a result of fluid volume loss
Urea nitrogen	10-20 mg/dL	Elevated as a result of fluid volume loss
Glucose	70-105 mg/dL	Elevated as a result of the stress response and altered uptake across injured tissues
Electrolytes		
Sodium	136-145 mEq/L (mmol/L)	Decreased; sodium is trapped in edema fluid and lost through plasma leakage
Potassium	3.5-5.0 mEq/L (mmol/L)	Elevated as a result of disruption of the sodium-potassium pump, tissue destruction, and red blood cell hemolysis
Chloride	98-106 mEq/L (mmol/L)	Elevated as a result of fluid volume loss and reabsorption of chloride in urine
Arterial Blood Gas Studies		
Pao_2	80-100 mm Hg	Slightly decreased
$Paco_2$	35-45 mm Hg	Slightly increased from respiratory injury
pH	7.35-7.45	Low as a result of metabolic acidosis
Carboxyhemoglobin	0%-10%	Elevated as a result of inhalation of smoke and carbon monoxide
Other		
Total protein	6.4-8.3 g/dL	Low; protein exudate is lost through the wound
Albumin	3.5-5.0 g/dL	Low; protein is lost through the wound and through vascular membranes because of increased permeability

Pao_2, Partial pressure of arterial oxygen; $Paco_2$, partial pressure of arterial carbon dioxide.

RADIOGRAPHIC ASSESSMENT

Standard x-rays and scans do not provide direct assessment data about the burn wound. These assessments are not performed unless other trauma is suspected.

OTHER DIAGNOSTIC ASSESSMENTS

In addition to routine laboratory tests, specific studies of involved organs are performed. For example, when burn injuries involve the eye, an ophthalmic evaluation detects corneal damage (see Chapters 49 and 50 for specific eye and vision evaluation procedures).

Specific diagnostic studies are performed when deep organ trauma is suspected. Such studies include IV renograms, computed tomography (CT), ultrasonography, bronchoscopy, and magnetic resonance imaging (MRI).

Critical Thinking Challenge

The client is a 57-year-old woman admitted directly to the burn center after being rescued from a house fire. She apparently was reading in bed and fell asleep while smoking. Following rescue from the burning house, she was given oxygen, 12 L/min through nasal prongs. She has partial-thickness burns on her face and anterior neck. Full-thickness circumferential burns are present on the upper trunk and both upper limbs. Estimated TBSA burn is 41%. The client is disoriented and complaining of shortness of breath as well as pain in the face and neck area. Further assessment reveals a hoarse, productive cough of carbonaceous sputum and carbon deposits on the tongue and throughout the oral pharynx. The client has a 20-gauge IV line in the left hand.

1. Is this client at risk for an inhalation injury? Why or why not?
2. What initial consideration must be given in moving the client from the stretcher to the bed?
3. Once the client is found to have an adequate airway and level of consciousness, what is your next priority?

evolve For suggested answer guidelines, go to http://evolve.elsevier.com/Iggy/.

◆Analysis

A burned client has dramatic changes not only in the directly damaged tissues but also in many other body systems. During the course of the illness, most burn clients experience all of the common and many of the additional nursing diagnoses listed in the following sections.

COMMON NURSING DIAGNOSES AND COLLABORATIVE PROBLEMS

The following are priority nursing diagnoses for clients with burn injuries in the emergent phase who have sustained a burn injury greater than 25% of the total body surface area (TBSA):

1. Decreased Cardiac Output related to altered stroke volume from an increase in capillary permeability
2. Deficient Fluid Volume related to active fluid volume loss, electrolyte imbalance, and inadequate fluid resuscitation

3. Ineffective Tissue Perfusion (Cerebral, Cardiopulmonary, Renal, Gastrointestinal, and Peripheral) related to hypovolemia from extravascular fluid shifts, decreased cardiac output, constriction of eschar, and edema
4. Ineffective Breathing Pattern related to respiratory distress from upper airway edema, pulmonary edema, airway obstruction, or pneumonia
5. Acute Pain and Chronic Pain related to biologic injury, damaged or exposed nerve endings, debridement, dressing changes, invasive procedures, and donor sites

The following are primary collaborative problems:
1. Potential for Pulmonary Edema
2. Potential for Acute Respiratory Distress Syndrome (ARDS)

ADDITIONAL NURSING DIAGNOSES AND COLLABORATIVE PROBLEMS

In addition to the common nursing diagnoses and collaborative problems, clients with burn injuries in the emergent phase may have one or more of the following:

- Excess Fluid Volume related to massive IV fluid administration
- Risk for Ineffective Thermoregulation related to trauma, hypermetabolism, and a loss of the protective barrier
- Disturbed Sensory Perception (Visual, Auditory, and Tactile) related to periorbital edema or ulcerations, hospital environment, noise, infections, and dressings
- Anxiety related to threat of death, initial burn trauma, situational crisis, painful procedures, unfamiliar environment, separation from significant others, and loss of control
- Fear related to pain, knowledge deficit, therapeutic procedures, hospitalization, separation, and social re-entry

◆ Planning and Implementation

DECREASED CARDIAC OUTPUT; DEFICIENT FLUID VOLUME; INEFFECTIVE TISSUE PERFUSION

NOC **PLANNING: EXPECTED OUTCOMES.** With appropriate intervention, the client is expected to have cardiac output restored to normal. Indicators include that the client should:

- Have normal or only mildly compromised blood pressure and heart rate
- Have normal or only mildly compromised peripheral pulses
- Have normal or only mildly compromised oxygen saturation, partial pressure of arterial oxygen (PaO$_2$), partial pressure of arterial carbon dioxide (PaCO$_2$), and arterial pH

INTERVENTIONS. Interventions are aimed at increasing blood fluid volume, supporting compensatory mechanisms, and preventing complications. Chart 71-4 lists some NIC intervention activities for the burn client with decreased cardiac output, deficient fluid volume, and ineffective tissue perfusion. Nonsurgical management is often sufficient for achieving these aims. Surgical management is required most often for full-thickness burns.

NONSURGICAL MANAGEMENT. Fluid volume and tissue blood flow are restored through IV fluid therapy, plasma exchange therapy, and drug therapy.

CHART 71-4

NIC **INTERVENTION ACTIVITIES for**
The Burn Client with Decreased Cardiac Output, Deficient Fluid Volume, and Ineffective Tissue Perfusion

Fluid Monitoring: *Collection and analysis of client data to regulate fluid balance*
- Monitor serum and urine electrolyte values, as appropriate.
- Monitor blood pressure, heart rate, and respiratory status.
- Monitor orthostatic blood pressure and change in cardiac rhythm, as appropriate.
- Monitor weight.
- Keep an accurate record of intake and output.
- Note presence or absence of vertigo on rising.
- Monitor color, quantity, and specific gravity of urine.

Fluid Resuscitation: *Administering prescribed intravenous fluids rapidly*
- Obtain and maintain a large-bore IV.
- Administer IV fluids, as prescribed.
- Monitor hemodynamic response.
- Monitor oxygen status.
- Monitor for fluid overload.
- Monitor output of various body fluids (e.g., urine and nasogastric drainage, and chest tube drainage)
- Monitor BUN, creatinine, total protein, and albumin levels.
- Monitor for pulmonary edema and third spacing.

Fluid Management: *Promotion of fluid balance and prevention of complications resulting from abnormal or undesired fluid levels*
- Administer IV therapy, as prescribed.
- Give fluids, as appropriate.
- Distribute the fluid intake over 24 hours, as appropriate.

NIC intervention activities selected from Dochterman, J.M., & Bulechek, G.M. (Eds.). (2004). *Nursing interventions classification (NIC)* (4th ed.). St. Louis: Mosby. No part of this work is to be altered without prior written permission from the Publisher. *BUN*, blood urea nitrogen.

IV Fluid Therapy. Infusion of IV fluids is needed to maintain sufficient blood volume for normal cardiac output, mean arterial pressure, and tissue oxygenation. Clients with burns involving 15% to 20% of the TBSA require IV fluid resuscitation. Many formulas for calculating fluid requirements exist. Table 71-6 lists the formulas commonly used for the therapy of adult clients. Although the types and amounts of electrolytes, crystalloids, and colloids vary, the purpose of all of these formulas is to prevent shock by maintaining adequate circulating blood fluid volume. The optimal formula and infusion schedules remain controversial.

Resuscitation for a severe burn requires large fluid loads in a short time to maintain blood flow to vital organs. The Parkland formula recommends that half of the calculated fluid volume for 24 hours be given in the first 8 hours after injury. The other half is given over the next 16 hours for a total of 24 hours. Fluid boluses are avoided because they increase capillary pressure and worsen edema. In the second 24-hour period after a burn injury, the volume and content of the IV fluids are based on the client's specific fluid volume and electrolyte imbalances and his or her response to treatment.

Fluid replacement formulas are calculated from the time of injury and not from the time of arrival at the hospital. For example, if a burn injury occurred at 8 AM but the client was not admitted to the hospital until 10 AM, the first 8-hour period would be completed at 4 PM, or 8 hours after the injury. Thus if resuscitation was delayed by 2 hours until admission

TABLE 71-6 Common Fluid Resuscitation Formulas for the First 24 Hours After a Burn Injury

	Formula	Solution	Rate of Administration
Modified Brooke	0.5 mL/kg/% TBSA burn 1.5 mL/kg/% TBSA burn	Protenate or 5% albumin in isotonic saline Lactated Ringer's without dextrose	½ given in first 8 hr ½ given in next 16 hr
Parkland (Baxter)	4 mL/kg/% TBSA burn for 24-hr period	Crystalloid only (lactated Ringer's)	½ given in first 8 hr ½ given in next 16 hr
Monafo		Crystalloid (hypertonic saline: sodium = 250 mEq/L)	Adjust to maintain urine output of 30 mL/hr
Modified Parkland	4 mL/kg/% TBSA burn + 15 mL/m² of TBSA	Crystalloid only (lactated Ringer's)	½ given in first 8 hr ½ given in next 16 hr
Winski	2 mL/kg/% burn + maintenance fluid	Crystalloid only (lactated Ringer's)	½ given in first 8 hr ½ given in next 16 hr

to the hospital, calculated fluids would need to be given over the next 6-hour period rather than an 8-hour period. All burn resuscitation formulas are used as *guides*. The client's response to therapy determines exact fluid requirements. No single formula has been found to provide superior results over another.

The management of extensive burns may require placement of a large-bore central venous catheter so that massive fluid loads can be given. Peripheral lines are less useful because they become dislodged or fluid flow is cut off when massive peripheral edema compresses the IV catheter.

Plasma Exchange Therapy. Shock may persist in the postburn period despite adequate fluid resuscitation. The cause of this persistent shock is unknown, but toxic serum factors have been suggested. Plasma exchange therapy is used in some burn centers for clients with massive burns who fail to respond from burn shock with fluid resuscitation.

The plasma exchange process either removes the client's plasma and replaces it with fresh frozen plasma (**plasmapheresis**) or removes the client's blood and replaces it with whole blood (**exchange transfusion**). Plasma exchange can decrease the amount of required fluid and increase urine output, thus helping those clients who do not respond to conventional fluid therapy.

Monitoring. Monitor client responses to determine the adequacy of fluid resuscitation for hydration and adequate blood perfusion of the brain, heart, and kidneys. Urine output is the most common and most sensitive noninvasive assessment parameter for cardiac output and tissue perfusion (see Chapters 15 and 40). Regardless of the total amount of fluid calculated as needed to meet the fluid requirements of the client, the amount of fluid given depends on how much IV fluid per hour is needed to maintain the hourly urine output at 0.5 mL/kg (about 30 mL/hr). Adjustment of the IV fluid rate on the basis of urine output plus serum electrolyte values is known as the **titration** of fluid. *In clients with burns larger than 35% TBSA, the use of urine output and vital signs to guide resuscitation may be insufficient. Invasive monitoring of cardiac and pulmonary function is necessary to ensure optimal fluid resuscitation.*

Burn clients often develop severe hypovolemic shock and need invasive cardiac monitoring. Vital parameters such as central venous pressure, pulmonary artery pressures, and cardiac output are obtained on a frequent to continuous basis. Monitor the electrocardiographic (ECG) activity of

clients who have sustained large burns. Nonburn-related dysrhythmias, such as atrial fibrillation, are often present in older clients.

Drug Therapy. A common mistake in treatment is giving diuretics to increase urine output rather than changing the amount and rate of fluid administration. *Diuretics do not increase cardiac output; they actually decrease circulating volume and cardiac output by pulling fluid from the circulating blood volume to enhance diuresis.* This effect reduces blood flow to other vital organs (especially the heart, lungs, and brain) and greatly increases the risk for severe hypovolemic shock. Therefore diuretics are not generally used to improve urine output for burn clients. An exception is the client with a burn injury caused by electrical energy. Muscle and deep tissue damage release large protein molecules (myoglobin), which precipitate in and obstruct the renal tubules. Although the diuretic mannitol (Osmitrol) is often used in this situation, it should always be given after adequate urine output has been established.

In older clients or those with cardiac disease, a complicating factor in reduced cardiac output may be heart failure or myocardial infarction. Drugs that increase cardiac output, such as dopamine (Intropin), or that strengthen the force of myocardial contraction, such as digoxin (Lanoxin), may be used along with fluid therapy.

SURGICAL MANAGEMENT. The surgical procedure for the treatment of inadequate tissue perfusion is *escharotomy*. An incision through the burn eschar relieves pressure caused by the constricting force of circumferential burns on the extremity or chest and improves circulation. If the pressure is not relieved, arterial compression can occur with a loss of blood flow to the extremity leading to ischemia and possible necrosis. Incisions are made along sides of the extremity and extend into the subcutaneous tissue (Figures 71-6 and 71-12). This procedure relieves the tourniquet effect of the eschar. If tissue pressure remains elevated after escharotomy, a *fasciotomy* (a deeper incision extending through the fascia) may be needed.

Escharotomies and fasciotomies are often performed at the bedside. No anesthesia is needed for escharotomy because nerve endings have been destroyed by the burn injury, but sedation and analgesia are given to reduce anxiety. Assure the client that he or she will be made as comfortable as possible during the procedure. Remove the dressings and thoroughly cleanse the areas to be incised. After the procedure, apply topical antimicrobial agents and dressings to the

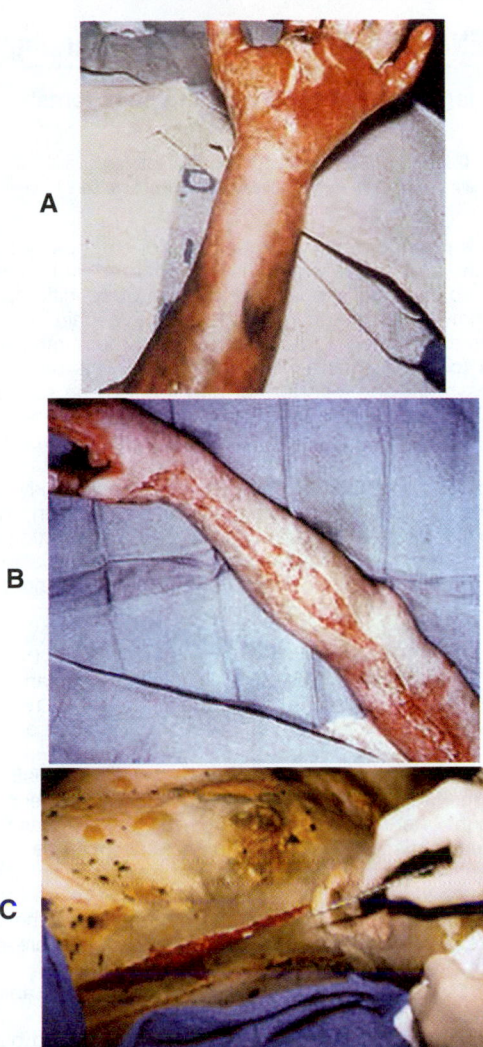

Figure 71-12 ■ Escharotomy to release circumferential burn eschar and improve circulation to a distal extremity or to improve ventilation. **A,** Tight circumferential eschar restricting swelling as edema forms in the tissue beneath the eschar. Edema compresses blood vessels, which inhibits blood flow to the distal extremity. **B,** An escharotomy incision allows outward swelling of edematous tissues. Restricted blood flow through the vessels to the distal extremity is relieved. **C,** An anterior axillary incision is made bilaterally to relieve respiratory distress.

area. Carefully monitor escharotomy sites for bleeding. Fasciotomies generally require large doses of narcotics or anesthesia for pain management.

INEFFECTIVE BREATHING PATTERN

NOC **PLANNING: EXPECTED OUTCOMES.** With proper intervention, the client is expected to maintain a patent airway and have an effective breathing pattern. Indicators include that the client should have either mildly compromised or not compromised oxygen saturation, PaO_2, $PaCO_2$, and arterial pH.

INTERVENTIONS. Interventions are aimed at supporting normal pulmonary function and preventing pulmonary problems. Specific plans for pulmonary management depend on the cause of the breathing problem and the status of the respiratory tract.

NONSURGICAL MANAGEMENT. Interventions include airway maintenance, promotion of ventilation, monitoring gas exchange, oxygen therapy, drug therapy, positioning, and deep breathing.

Airway Maintenance. Maintenance of the airway begins at the burn scene in an unconscious client and may involve only a chin lift or a head tilt maneuver. Upper airway edema becomes pronounced 8 to 12 hours after the beginning of fluid resuscitation. These clients often require nasal or oral intubation if crowing, stridor, or dyspnea is present.

A bronchoscopy is performed to examine the vocal cords and airways of clients at risk for obstruction. Clients with severe smoke inhalation or poisoning may require a bronchoscopy on admission and routinely thereafter for examination of the respiratory tract, deep suctioning of the lungs, and removal of sloughing necrotic tissue. Assess the endotracheal tube hourly to ensure patency and location in intubated clients.

Other causes of airway obstruction are excessive secretions and sloughed tissue from damaged lungs. Suction as indicated based on clinical assessment or clinician order. Vigorous endotracheal or nasotracheal tube suctioning is performed after chest physiotherapy and aerosol treatments. Clients report that deep endotracheal suctioning is extremely painful. Therefore suctioning the endotracheal tube often requires increased analgesia or sedation.

Promotion of Ventilation. Respiration depends on skeletal muscle movement of the chest for ventilation. Chest movement can be restricted by tight dressings that cover the neck, chest, and abdomen. Observe the client for ease of respiratory movements and loosen tight dressings as needed to assist with ventilation.

Monitoring Gas Exchange. Monitor the effectiveness of gas exchange by using laboratory tests (e.g., arterial blood gas, carboxyhemoglobin levels) and by assessing for cyanosis, disorientation, and increased pulse rate. Other data to monitor in critically ill clients include chest x-ray, pulmonary artery catheters, and central venous pressure measurement.

The possibility of cyanide poisoning is considered in clients involved in house fires. An elevated plasma lactate level is a useful indicator of cyanide toxicity in clients who do not have severe burns.

Oxygen Therapy. Management of impaired breathing patterns includes giving humidified oxygen by face mask, cannula, or hood. Arterial oxygenation less than 60 (PaO_2 <60 mm Hg) is an indication for intubation and mechanical ventilation. Keep emergency airway equipment at or near the client's bedside. This equipment must include oxygen, masks, cannulas, manual resuscitation bags, laryngoscope, endotracheal tubes, and equipment for tracheostomy. Chapter 35 addresses specific nursing actions for clients during mechanical ventilation.

Drug Therapy. When pneumonia or other pulmonary infections impair breathing, antibiotics are prescribed. Drug selection is based on known culture and sensitivity reports or on the specific microflora common to that burn unit. Impaired breathing from cardiac failure and increased pulmonary pressures may be treated with drugs that improve cardiac output and enhance urine output.

When a client's activity during mechanical ventilation severely compromises respiratory mechanics, it may be necessary to use a paralytic drug, such as atracurium (Tracrium) or vecuronium (Norcuron). This situation is often referred to as "bucking" the ventilator. Paralytic agents remove all breathing control from the client, making mechanical ventilation easier. *These drugs do not prevent the client from seeing and hearing or from experiencing fear, pain, and loss of control. Any client receiving neuromuscular blockade drugs must also receive agents for sedation, analgesia, and antianxiety unless clinically contraindicated.* Extreme care must be taken to ensure that all alarms are operative and that clients are checked frequently, because the client cannot call for help if he or she becomes extubated.

Positioning and Deep Breathing. To improve breathing patterns and oxygenation, turn the client frequently and assist him or her out of bed to a chair as much as possible. Teach the client to use coughing and deep breathing exercises. Encourage the client to use incentive spirometry every 2 hours while awake. Chest physiotherapy may be helpful to mobilize lung secretions, depending on the client's clinical condition and the clinician's prescription.

SURGICAL MANAGEMENT. A tracheostomy may be needed when long-term intubation is expected. A tracheostomy increases the risk for infection in burn clients even more than in nonburned clients. Emergency tracheostomies are performed when an airway becomes occluded and oral or nasal intubation cannot be achieved.

Other surgical procedures for improving the burn client's breathing pattern include inserting chest tubes and performing an escharotomy. Chest tubes are used to re-expand the lung when a pneumothorax or hemothorax has occurred (see Chapters 33 and 35). Tight eschar on the neck, chest, or abdomen can restrict respiratory movement. Escharotomies (described on p. 1634) can relieve this restriction and permit greater respiratory movement.

ACUTE PAIN; CHRONIC PAIN

The pain with burn injuries is both chronic and acute. Many factors contribute to burn pain and may be altered to reduce pain perception. Pain from the actual injury is worse when painful procedures are performed. Many nursing procedures needed by burn clients increase pain. Accurate assessment of the client's pain before and during procedures is an essential part of pain management. Visual analog scales and pain assessment scales that use color or faces have been used successfully to assess pain in the client with burns (see the Evidence-Based Practice for Nursing box at right).

NOC **PLANNING: EXPECTED OUTCOMES.** The pain level of a client with a burn injury is expected to be alleviated or reduced. Indicators include that the client should rarely demonstrate the following behaviors:

■ Report pain
■ Moan and cry
■ Make facial expressions of pain
■ Lose his or her appetite

INTERVENTIONS. The plan for pain management is tailored to the client's tolerance for pain, coping mechanisms, and physical status.

NONSURGICAL MANAGEMENT. Interventions for the client having pain include drug therapy, complementary therapy measures, and environmental manipulation.

Drug Therapy. Opioid and non-opioid analgesics, such as morphine sulfate, hydromorphone (Dilaudid), and fentanyl, are given often. However, these drugs rarely offer

---

EVIDENCE-BASED PRACTICE for Nursing

Pain management—Are we meeting our clients' goals?

Carrougher, G.J., et al. (2003). Comparison of patient satisfaction and self-reports of pain in adult burn-injured patients. *Journal of Burn Care and Rehabilitation, 24*(1), 1-8.

Health care providers place a great deal of emphasis on pain assessment and management in hospitalized burn clients. Current medical practices include the use of specific opioids and adjunctive treatment to obtain effective pain management. Pain assessment tools have provided the nurse with information to guide treatment effectiveness. This study took pain assessment one step further and focused on evaluating whether the treatments used to prevent and treat burn-related pain met the client's analgesic goals. Background, procedural pain, and treatment goals were assessed in 84 clients.

In addition to obtaining pain scores, twice-weekly client self-reports of worst and average procedural pain, background pain, treatment goals, and overall satisfaction with pain management plans were assessed. Data were also collected regarding type and amount of analgesia and nonpharmacologic adjunct therapy.

Sixty-seven of the participants were male and 17 were female. A total of 351 assessments were performed on these 84 clients. The mean age was 36.9, 85% white, mean TBSA 13.3%, and average length of hospital stay was 18 days. Eighty percent of the burns were a result of a scald or flame injury.

The results of this study indicated that client satisfaction with pain management is highest in those who experience the least amount of burn care pain. The opposite result was found in treatment satisfaction being the highest in those whose pain experiences most closely matched treatment analgesics goals. Reasons stated for this outcome may be related to the high pain scores reported during procedures. When the average pain scores were analyzed, the researchers were more successful in meeting the clients' goals.

Level of Evidence: 3—Well-designed trial without randomization (cohort study).

Critique. The authors of this study have brought to our attention another aspect of pain management. As they stated, pain assessment is more than just asking for a number. No data were provided regarding the percentage of partial- or full-thickness burn of the wound. The study could have been strengthened by correlating the size of burn and degree of satisfaction with pain management. There is a need for further studies of this type.

Implications for Nursing. Managing pain related to burn injuries continues to be a challenge for health care professionals. To achieve effective pain management, the nurse must not only accurately assess the level of pain but also obtain client self-reports and evaluate the individualized treatment goals with the pain regimen.

more than moderate relief during acutely painful procedures, and they depress respiratory function and reduce intestinal motility.

During the emergent postburn phase, the IV route is used for giving opioid drugs because of problems with absorption from the muscle and stomach. When these drugs are given by the intramuscular or subcutaneous route, they remain in the spaces and do not relieve pain. In addition, when edema is present, cumulative doses are rapidly absorbed when the fluid shift is resolving. This delayed absorption can result in lethal blood levels of analgesics.

Anesthetic agents, such as ketamine (Ketalar), pentobarbital sodium (Nembutal, Novopentobarb✱), and nitrous oxide, also reduce pain. Use strict protocols when giving these agents to prevent serious complications.

Complementary and Alternative Therapy. Complementary and alternative therapy measures include relaxation techniques, meditative breathing, guided imagery, music therapy, massage, and healing or therapeutic touch. Hypnosis and autohypnosis can be used by lucid, cooperative clients under the direction of trained therapists. Therapeutic touch, acupuncture, and acupressure are used to a limited extent for burn clients; the results are variable. Nontraditional and complementary therapy types of pain intervention are detailed in Chapter 7.

Environmental Change. You can increase the client's comfort by providing a quiet environment, using nonpainful tactile stimulation, and increasing the client's control. Sleep deprivation increases the client's discomfort. Increasing sleep or rest time in a quiet environment helps reduce the adverse effects of sleep deprivation, replenishes catecholamine stores, helps prevent critical care unit psychosis, and restores the diurnal effects of endorphins. Health care providers need to ensure that most procedures are performed during the client's waking hours.

Tactile stimulation can reduce pain. Help the client change positions every 2 hours to reduce pressure on any specific area, improve circulation to painful areas, and ease pain. Massage nonburn areas to reduce pain transmission and stimulate endorphin release. Apply heat and maintain warm room temperatures to prevent shivering.

To reduce anxiety and increase feelings of confidence and independence, encourage the client to participate in pain control measures. For example, make a contract with the client that specifies how long a painful procedure will last. This helps clients deal with the pain for that particular period. Patient-controlled analgesia (PCA) also reduces pain in burned clients. Important issues and techniques for the best use of PCA include the following: give an initial bolus of 5 to 10 mg of morphine (or equivalent drug), increasing the PCA dose as needed to achieve pain relief, and plan for a change in dosing regimens at night (e.g., giving a bolus dose at bedtime).

SURGICAL MANAGEMENT. Early surgical excision of the burn wound is used in many burn centers (see Surgical Excision, p. 1642). Early excision under anesthesia reduces the pain from daily debridement at the bedside or during hydrotherapy.

POTENTIAL FOR PULMONARY EDEMA

PLANNING: EXPECTED OUTCOMES. With intervention, the client with a burn injury is expected to be free of pulmonary edema.

INTERVENTIONS. Pulmonary edema can arise from lung injury or from fluid resuscitation and myocardial overload. Even a young healthy person can become fluid overloaded. These clients usually receive digoxin or other drugs to improve left ventricular function and prevent or treat pulmonary edema. Diuretics, a mainstay of therapy for pulmonary edema from other causes, may or may not be used in the emergent phase depending on the client's blood volume and renal function.

POTENTIAL FOR ACUTE RESPIRATORY DISTRESS SYNDROME

PLANNING: EXPECTED OUTCOMES. The client with a burn injury is expected to:

- Not experience acute respiratory distress
- Have arterial blood gases (ABGs) within normal limits
- Maintain normal lung compliance

INTERVENTIONS. Clients who develop acute respiratory distress syndrome (ARDS) as a result of burn injury require thorough assessments and interventions. The interventions are aimed at increasing lung compliance and improving PaO₂ (partial pressure of arterial oxygen) levels.

In collaboration with the physician and respiratory therapist, give positive end-expiratory pressure (PEEP) to augment the decreased lung volume by providing a continuous positive pressure in the airways and alveoli. This procedure enhances the diffusion of oxygen across the alveolar-capillary membrane. PEEP can be combined with intermittent mandatory volume (IMV) to enhance its effectiveness.

Assess and document the client's response so that needed ventilator changes can be made. Document and report any signs of respiratory distress or change in respiratory patterns. Monitor pulse oximetry and arterial blood gas (ABG) levels to assess changes in respiratory status.

Neuromuscular blocking agents (atracurium) can be used in clients receiving mechanical ventilation to reduce oxygen consumption (see the discussion of specific nursing care under Drug Therapy [Ineffective Breathing Pattern], p. 1635).

> ### ⁇ Critical Thinking Challenge
>
> The client who sustained a 41% TBSA burn (36% full-thickness) injury described earlier is started on fluid resuscitation. You notice that her urine is becoming darker and has a high specific gravity.
>
> 1. Do you expect that this client needs more fluid for resuscitation as a person who has only a partial-thickness burn? Why or why not?
> 2. What should be your first action upon viewing the change in the character of this client's urine?
> 3. What additional drugs or adjustments in resuscitation should you expect to be prescribed?
>
> *evolve* For suggested answer guidelines, go to http://evolve.elsevier.com/Iggy/.

ACUTE PHASE OF BURN INJURY

OVERVIEW

The acute phase of burn injury begins about 36 to 48 hours after injury and lasts until wound closure is complete. During this phase, a multidisciplinary approach to care is needed. Care is directed toward continued assessment and maintenance of the cardiovascular and respiratory systems, as well as toward gastrointestinal and nutritional status, burn wound care, pain control, and psychosocial interventions.

◆ COLLABORATIVE MANAGEMENT
◆ Assessment

PHYSICAL ASSESSMENT/CLINICAL MANIFESTATIONS

CARDIOPULMONARY ASSESSMENT. In the acute phase of burn injury, the cardiovascular and respiratory systems are assessed for maintaining these systems and treating or preventing potential complications. At this time, the client may develop pneumonia that can result in respiratory failure requiring mechanical ventilation. Although cardiovascular problems should be resolved, the client is at risk for infection and sepsis, which affect cardiovascular function. The interventions used in the emergent phase also may be needed for these new problems.

NEUROENDOCRINE ASSESSMENT. The increased metabolic demands placed on the body after a severe burn injury can severely deplete nutritional stores. Weigh the client daily without dressings or splints and compare it to his or her preburn weight. A 2% loss of body weight indicates a mild deficit. A 10% or greater weight loss is important and requires the evaluation and modification of calorie intake. For very accurate calorie requirements, indirect calorimetry may be used. This method determines kilocalories of energy expenditure by measuring oxygen consumption (VO_2) and carbon dioxide production (VCO_2). Measurements are taken while the client is at rest and preferably at least 30 minutes after the most recent dressing changes or other stressful procedures. Indirect calorimetry often is performed shortly after admission and at least once each week until the wounds are closed.

TABLE 71-7   Local and Systemic Signs of Infection

Local Signs
- Conversion of a partial-thickness injury to a full-thickness injury
- Ulceration of healthy skin at the burn site
- Erythematous, nodular lesions in uninvolved skin and vesicular lesions in healed skin
- Edema of healthy skin surrounding the burn wound
- Excessive burn wound drainage
- Pale, boggy, dry, or crusted granulation tissue
- Sloughing of grafts
- Wound breakdown after closure
- Odor

Systemic Signs
- Altered level of consciousness
- Changes in vital signs (tachycardia, tachypnea, temperature instability, hypotension)
- Increased fluid requirements for maintenance of a normal urine output
- Hemodynamic instability
- Oliguria
- Gastrointestinal dysfunction (diarrhea, vomiting, abdominal distention, paralytic ileus)
- Hyperglycemia
- Thrombocytopenia
- Change in total white blood cell count (above normal or below normal)
- Metabolic acidosis
- Hypoxemia

IMMUNE ASSESSMENT. The client with a burn injury is at risk for infection as a result of open wounds and reduced immune function. Burn wound sepsis is a serious complication of burn injury, and infection is the leading cause of death during the acute phase of recovery. Continually assess the client for signs of local and systemic infections (Table 71-7), including changes in wound appearance, changes in neurologic and GI function, and subtle changes in vital signs. Monitor for the manifestations of gram-positive, gram-negative, and fungal infections (Table 71-8). Enforce meticulous handwashing by all health care personnel. Use aseptic technique in caring for wounds and during invasive monitoring to prevent infections.

MUSCULOSKELETAL ASSESSMENT. Clients with a burn injury are at risk for musculoskeletal problems as a result of other injuries, immobility, healing processes, and treatment. The musculoskeletal status is first evaluated on admission to the hospital or burn center and throughout the acute phase of injury. Assess active and passive range of motion for all joints, including the neck. Give special attention to joints within the burn area. Ranges and limitations are documented for future reference.

◆Analysis

During the acute phase of the burn injury, the client with a burn injury has resolution of some earlier problems, may have initial problems that extend into the acute phase, and may develop new problems.

COMMON NURSING DIAGNOSES AND COLLABORATIVE PROBLEMS

The following are priority nursing diagnoses for clients with burn injuries greater than 25% TBSA in the acute phase of recovery:

1. Impaired Skin Integrity related to burn wound, graft site, or donor site, and physical immobilization
2. Risk for Infection related to inadequate primary defenses (wounds), the presence of multiple invasive catheters, reduced immune function, and malnutrition
3. Imbalanced Nutrition: Less Than Body Requirements related to increased metabolic rate; reduced calorie intake; and increased urinary nitrogen losses
4. Impaired Physical Mobility related to open burn wounds, pain, and scars and contractures
5. Disturbed Body Image related to trauma, changes in physical appearance and lifestyle, as well as alterations in sensory and motor function

---

TABLE 71-8   Signs and Symptoms of Sepsis Caused by Different Organisms

Sign/Symptom	Gram-Positive	Gram-Negative	Fungal
Onset	Insidious, 2-6 days	Rapid, 12-36 hr	Delayed
Sensorium	Severe disorientation and lethargy	Mild disorientation	Mild disorientation
Ileus	Severe	Severe	Mild
Diarrhea	Rare	Severe	Occasional
Temperature	Hyperpyrexia	Hypothermia	Hyperpyrexia
Hypotension	Late	Early	Late
White blood cell count	Neutrophilia	Neutropenia	Neutrophilia
Platelets	Normal	Low	Low

The primary collaborative problem is Wound Care Management.

ADDITIONAL NURSING DIAGNOSES AND COLLABORATIVE PROBLEMS

In addition to the common nursing diagnoses and collaborative problems, clients with burn injuries in the acute phase may have one or more of the following:

- Anticipatory Grieving related to loss of significant others, loss of possessions, physical disfigurement, and changes in body image
- Disabled Family Coping related to loss of home, family, or significant others; crises resulting from burn injury; disturbances in normal functions; role changes; and prolonged hospitalization and rehabilitation
- Ineffective Coping related to situational crises, disfigurement, separation, and sensory overload
- Self-Care Deficits (Feeding, Bathing/Hygiene, Dressing/Grooming, Toileting) related to pain; contractures; and loss of function in the hands, extremities, and other body parts
- Sexual Dysfunction related to trauma; perineal, genital, and breast burns; immobility, fatigue, and depression; and disturbance in body image
- Disturbed Sleep Pattern related to pain, treatment regimen, and environmental noise
- Social Isolation related to the altered state of wellness, protective isolation treatment regimen, and alterations in physical appearance
- Deficient Knowledge (treatment regimen and healing process) related to unfamiliarity of information resources and cognitive limitation
- Potential for Pneumonia
- Potential for Septicemia

◆ Planning and Implementation

IMPAIRED SKIN INTEGRITY; WOUND CARE MANAGEMENT

NOC   PLANNING: EXPECTED OUTCOMES. With appropriate intervention, the client with a burn injury is expected to have no further loss of skin integrity and to have skin integrity restored. Indicators include that the client:

- Has presence of granulation, re-epithelialization, and scar tissue formation
- Has decreased wound size
- Has no new wounds

INTERVENTIONS. Interventions aim to preserve the integrity of nonburned skin, enhance wound healing of burned skin, and prevent complications.

NONSURGICAL MANAGEMENT. Nonsurgical burn wound management involves removing exudates and necrotic tissue, cleaning the area, stimulating granulation and revascularization, and applying dressings. Restoring skin, whether by natural healing or grafting, starts with the removal of eschar and other cellular debris from the burn wound. This removal is called **debridement**. Nonsurgical treatment allows debris removal through mechanical and enzymatic actions that separate eschar over time. The goal is to have the wound prepare itself for grafting and wound closure by a natural process.

Mechanical Debridement. Burn wounds are debrided and cleaned one to two times each day during **hydrotherapy** (the application of water for treatment). Nurses, unlicensed nursing personnel, and physical therapists perform hydrotherapy daily to debride and examine the wounds. Hydrotherapy can be performed by immersing the client in a tub, showering the client on a specially designed shower table, or washing only small areas of the wound at the bedside. Showering enhances wound inspection and allows water temperature to be kept constant.

Nurses and skilled technicians use forceps and scissors to remove loose, nonviable tissue during hydrotherapy. The care of intact blisters is controversial. At most burn units, small blisters are left alone because they serve as a protective barrier that promotes wound healing. Because the protein-filled fluid within blisters can cause some reduced immune function, many units open larger blisters. Washcloths or gauze sponges are used to debride soft "cheesy" eschar. During hydrotherapy, wash burn areas thoroughly and gently with mild soap or detergent and water. Then rinse these areas with room temperature water.

Enzymatic Debridement. Enzymatic debridement can occur naturally by autolysis or artificially by the application of exogenous agents. **Autolysis** is the disintegration of tissue by the action of the client's own cellular enzymes. This process is seldom used in North America for larger burns because it is slow and results in a prolonged hospital stay.

Topical enzyme agents, such as collagenase (Santyl), are used for rapid wound debridement. When these agents are applied directly to the burn wound in a once-a-day dressing change, the enzymes digest collagen in necrotic tissues. They require a moist environment within a specific pH range for activation. Polysporin powder is often used with this topical agent to prevent infection.

Dressing the Burn Wound. After burn wounds are cleaned and debrided, topical antibiotics are reapplied to prevent infection (see Risk for Infection, p. 1643). Some type of dressing is then applied to the burn wound. Burn dressings include standard wound dressings, biologic dressings, and synthetic dressings and artificial skin. (Table 71-9 describes the features of many types of dressings.)

Standard Wound Dressings. Standard wound dressings are multiple layers of gauze applied over the topical agents on the burn wound. The number of gauze layers depends on the following:

- Depth of the injury
- Amount of drainage expected
- Area injured
- Client's mobility
- Frequency of dressing changes

The gauze layers are held in place with roller-type gauze bandages applied in a distal to proximal direction or with circular net fabrics. Cover gauze dressings on the client's arms and legs with elastic wraps, especially if the client is ambulatory. Dressings are generally changed and reapplied every 8 to 24 hours after thoroughly cleaning the areas.

Biologic Dressings. Biologic wound dressings are often used for temporary wound coverage and closure. Biologic dressings are skin or membranes obtained from human tissue donors (homograft or allograft) or animals (heterograft or xenograft). When applied over open wounds, a biologic dressing rapidly adheres and promotes healing or prepares the wound for permanent skin graft coverage.

TABLE 71-9 Advantages and Disadvantages of Dressings and Dressing Systems for Burns

Product	Description	Action	Advantages	Disadvantages	Interventions
Acticoat	Prepackaged in sheets	Silver-coated antimicrobial Broad-spectrum coverage	Painless Change dressing every 3 days Effective against antibiotic-resistant *Pseudomonas*, vancomycin-resistant *Enterococcus* (VRE), methicillin-resistant *Staphylococcus aureus*, and fungi May be used in sulfa-allergic clients Provides moist (nonmacerating) wound coverage	Expensive May cause transient discoloration of tissue Known sensitivity to silver Not compatible with oil-based products	Must be moistened with sterile water before application. Dressings must be wetted down every 8 hours with sterile water. Use on partial-thickness wounds, grafts or donor sites. Do not combine with any other topical anti-microbial. Not compatible with magnetic resonance imaging procedures. Should not come into contact with electrodes or conductive gels during electronic measurements.
Accuzyme	Water insoluble Derived from fruit of papaya melon tree (Papain)	Enzymatic debrider Breaks down nonviable tissue	Harmless to viable tissue Once-a-day dressing	Painful Infection	Apply directly to wound. Cover with normal saline gauze. Use on deep-partial thickness wounds. Discontinue use when wound is free of eschar.
Xeroform	Petroleum-based gauze impregnated with 3% bismuth tribromophenate	Contains no antimicrobial action Encourages migration of epithelial cells	Acts as barrier dressing Prevents wound desiccation Prevents loss of body fluid Inexpensive	Allows bacterial growth due to minimal antibacterial properties	Use daily dressings. Use on clean partial-thickness burns or donor sites. Only place a single layer. Monitor for signs of infection.
Scarlet Red	Vaseline-impregnated gauze containing red dye	Encourages spread of epithelial cells at faster rate than Xeroform	Use on clean partial-thickness wounds or donor site Inexpensive	Promotes bacterial growth if infection is present No antimicrobials	Change daily or every other day. Apply single layer. Red dye permanently stains clothes, furniture, and the like. Dye on skin is not permanent. Monitor for signs of infection.
Mepitel	Pliable nonadherent dressing Fine mesh netting coated with silicone	Mild antimicrobial properties Provides protective barrier dressing to allow for epithelial growth	Pores allow for drainage of exudates Does not adhere to wound May use on grafts	Sensitivity/allergy reactions Provides no antimicrobial effect	May leave in place for 5 days when used with grafts. May apply topical solutions over Mepitel.

Biobrane	Biosynthetic skin substitute (nylon and Silastic membrane combined with collagen derivative)	Promotes epithelialization Physiologic barrier Allows water vapor to escape Adherence due to wound binding to collagen then by tissue growth into nylon fabric	One time application Visualization of wound progression through Biobrane Decreased pain medication required	Expensive Infection or wound conversion prohibits adherence Recommended application time within 6 hours of injury No antimicrobials	Use on clean partial-thickness wounds, donor sites, grafts. May not reapply once removed. Must apply dull side down. Monitor for infection and adherence. Once Biobrane is adherent, may change dressing every other day. Keep in place until wound is healed.
Transcyte	Human fibroblast-derived temporary skin substitute Contains human dermal matrix, growth factors, essential structural proteins Consists of polymer membrane and newborn human fibroblast cells cultured under aseptic conditions in vitro on nylon mesh	Provides physiologic barrier Accelerates re-epithelialization Provides tissue matrix	One time application Visualization of wound through Transcyte Decrease pain medication Apply within 24 hours of burn injury	Expensive Infection of wound conversion prohibits adherence No antimicrobials Use only on clean partial-thickness wounds	Monitor adherence to wound. Monitor for infection. Maintained frozen, must use within 2 hours after thawing.
Pigskin (xenograft, heterograft)	Biologic skin substitute Skin harvested from pigs, cryopreserved for long-term storage	Provides biologic covering of clean wounds	Decreases pain Prevents water, electrolyte, and protein losses Used on wounds as bridge to skin grafting	Infection No antimicrobials	Monitor for infection. Monitor for wound adherence. Remove dressing daily for inspection; replace if purulent drainage or nonadherent.
Homograft (allograft)	Skin harvested from human	Provides biologic covering of clean wounds	Decreases pain Prevents wound drying Promotes healing Remains adherent until rejection occurs or is surgically removed	Disease transmission Hypersensitivity reaction	Client eventually rejects skin. Monitor for infection and adherence. Use on newly excised wounds.
Alloderm	Cadaver skin in which the epidermis is removed and allogenic cells are removed.	Provides dermal base to excised wounds Thin graft placed over Alloderm	Requires thinner autograft to be harvested Used in extensive burns with limited donor tissue		Managed identical to skin grafts.
Integra	Biosynthetic dermal regeneration template	Dermal template for the formation of a neodermis within 14-21 days Consists of bovine collagen dermal layer and silicone epidermis	Used in extensive burns with limited donor tissue Potentially less scarring Requires thinner autografts to be harvested	Expensive Requires two-stage surgical procedure 14-21 days apart	Monitor for infection. Limit motion and friction. Monitor for adherence.

TABLE 71-10   Biologic Dressings

Uses
- Debridement of untidy wounds after separation of eschar
- Promotion of re-epithelialization of deep partial-thickness wounds
- Temporary coverage after excision of the burn wound
- Protection of granulation tissue between autografts
- Test graft before autografting

Advantages
- Early adherence to the wound
- Reduction of evaporative heat loss
- Reduction of evaporate water loss
- Prevention of desiccation of granulation tissue
- Reduction of exudate protein losses
- Reduction of pain
- Assistance in wound debridement
- Enhancement of healing with partial-thickness injuries
- Protection of exposed neovascular tissue
- Inhibition of bacterial proliferation

Disadvantages
- Early lysis resulting in bacterial proliferation
- Expensive
- Rejection responses
- Possible burn wound sepsis if applied over eschar
- Not readily available
- Storage (some may require refrigeration or freezing)
- Possible transmission of diseases, such as hepatitis

Biologic materials are used in healing partial-thickness and granulating full-thickness wounds that are clean and free of eschar. Table 71-10 outlines the advantages and disadvantages of biologic dressings. The type of biologic dressing selected depends on the type of wound to be covered and the availability of the material.

Homograft. A **homograft** or **allograft** is human skin obtained from a cadaver and provided through a skin bank. It is fresh or frozen; frozen skin is thawed in a warm bath of sterile normal saline before application. Disadvantages to the use of homografts are the high costs ($750 to $1000 per square foot) and the risk of transmitting a bloodborne infection.

Heterograft. A **heterograft** or **xenograft** is skin obtained from another species. Pigskin is the most common heterograft and is compatible with human skin. Pigskin is assessed daily for adherence and need for replacement.

Amniotic Membrane. Amniotic membrane is another form of biologic dressing used on burn wounds. Its large size, low cost, and availability have helped with its success. In full-thickness injuries, the amniotic membrane adheres to the wound. With partial-thickness areas, the amniotic membrane is effective as a dressing until epithelial cell regrowth occurs. The membrane requires frequent changes because it does not develop a blood supply and it disintegrates in about 48 hours.

Cultured Skin. Cultured skin can be grown from a small specimen of epidermal cells from an unburned portion of the client's body. The cells are grown in a laboratory to produce cell sheets that can be grafted on the client to generate a permanent skin surface. The length of time for culturing and growing the skin is prolonged, and the cell sheets are not durable. Take care when applying these sheets to ensure adherence and prevent sloughing. This process is very costly.

Artificial Skin. Artificial skin is an alternative approach to closure of the burn wound. This substance has two layers, a Silastic epidermis and a porous dermis made from bovine hide collagen and shark cartilage.

After the artificial skin is applied to a clean, excised wound surface, fibroblasts move into the collagen part of the artificial skin and create a structure similar to normal dermis. The artificial dermis slowly dissolves and is replaced with normal blood vessels and connective tissue (*neodermis*). The neodermis supports a standard autograft placed over it when the Silastic layer is removed.

Biosynthetic Wound Dressings. Biosynthetic wound dressings are a combination of biosynthetic and synthetic materials. Biobrane is commonly used and effective in the treatment of clean superficial partial-thickness burns such as scalds, as a covering for meshed autografts, and as donor site dressings.

Biobrane is made up of a nylon fabric that is partially embedded into a silicone film. Collagen is incorporated into both the silicone and nylon components. The nylon fabric comes into contact with the wound surface and forms an adherent bond until epithelialization has occurred. The porous silicone film allows exudates to pass through.

Synthetic Dressings. Synthetic dressings are made of solid silicone and plastic membranes (e.g., polyvinyl chloride and polyurethane). They may be substituted for standard or biologic dressings. Synthetic dressings are applied directly to the surface of a clean or surgically prepared wound and remain in place until they fall off or are removed. Because many of these dressings are transparent or translucent, the wound can be inspected without removing the dressing. Pain is reduced at the site because these agents also prevent contact of the wound with air. These dressings also are used to cover donor sites where skin was obtained for autografting.

Transparent film appears to be the best dressing for the care of donor site wounds. This dressing type promotes faster healing with low infection rates, minimal pain, and reduced cost (Rakel et al., 1998).

Another strategy to manage donor site pain is the topical application of lidocaine to donor harvest sites. The resulting analgesic effects reduce opioid requirements, lower pain scores, and do not cause systemic effects when used for small areas (less than 15% TBSA) (Jellish et al., 1999).

SURGICAL MANAGEMENT. Surgical management of burn wounds focuses on excision and wound covering. Surgical excision is performed early in the postburn period. Grafting may be performed throughout the acute phase as burn wounds are made ready and donor sites are available. Early grafting reduces the time clients are at risk for infection and sepsis.

Wound covering through autografting involves taking skin from an area of the client's intact, healthy skin and transplanting it to an excised burn wound.

Surgical Excision. Surgical excision is the most common treatment for full-thickness and deep partial-thickness wounds. The client is taken to the operating room within the first 5 days after injury and again as needed until all wounds are closed permanently.

The burn wound is excised by either a tangential or a fascial excision technique. In the tangential technique, the surgeon excises very thin layers of the necrotic burn surface until bleeding tissue is encountered. Bleeding indicates that a bed of healthy dermis or subcutaneous fat has been reached.

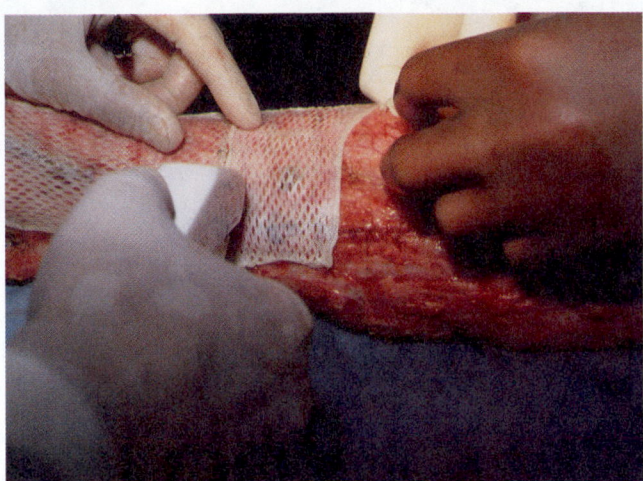

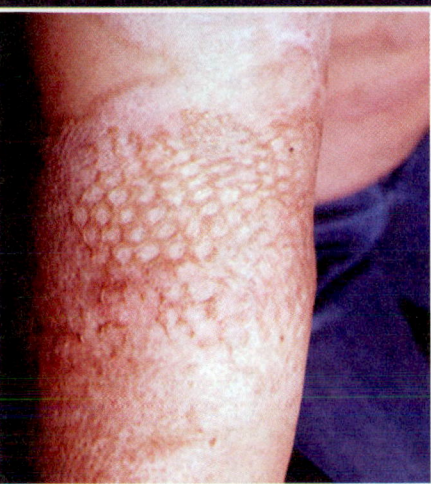

Figure 71-13 ■ The typical appearance of meshed autografts. **A,** Appearance during application of meshed autograft. **B,** Appearance of meshed autograft after healing.

In the fascial technique, the surgeon excises the burn wound to the level of superficial fascia. Fascial excision usually is reserved for very deep and extensive burns. Blood loss is minimal, and grafting is usually successful.

Wound Covering. Permanent skin coverage for large full-thickness injuries is achieved by applying an autograft. Skin for an autograft is taken from the client's own body. The surgeon removes a piece of skin from a remote unburned area of the body and transplants it to cover the burn wound. Skin grafts are generally of split thickness (0.015 inch) and a partial-thickness injury is formed at the site of surgical removal (the donor site). Grafts are placed either on a clean granulated bed or over a surgically excised area of burn (see also Chapter 70).

The availability of donor sites for larger burns is small. Clients with larger burns may have only 5% to 20% of healthy skin surface available to cover the 80% to 95% burned area. Coverage is accomplished in the following ways:

- Successive reharvesting of the available donor site. Time is allowed between harvests for healing.
- Meshing the split-thickness skin grafts (Figure 71-13) to allow a small graft to cover a larger area. Healing time is slower for a meshed graft because the skin must fill

in open meshed areas (interstices) as well as attach to the granulation bed.

RISK FOR INFECTION

Burn wound infection occurs through **autocontamination,** in which the client's own normal flora overgrows and penetrates the internal environment; and **cross-contamination,** in which organisms from elsewhere are transferred to the client.

NOC PLANNING: EXPECTED OUTCOMES. The client is expected to remain free from infection by cross-contamination and not develop septicemia. Indicators include that the client will exhibit only mild instances or none of the following manifestations:

- Foul-smelling discharge
- Fever
- Blood culture colonization
- Wound site colonization
- White blood cell count elevation

INTERVENTIONS. Interventions aim to prevent infection and remove infected tissue.

NONSURGICAL MANAGEMENT. Nonsurgical management consists of minimizing exposure of the burn client to exogenous organisms, reducing the risk for autocontamination, and recognizing the manifestations of infection early. Drug therapy, isolation therapy, and environmental manipulation are strategies for preventing and managing infection.

Drug Therapy for Infection Prevention. Burn wound conditions promote the growth of *Clostridium tetani* and all burn clients are at risk for this dangerous infection. Tetanus toxoid, 0.5 mL given IM, enhances acquired immunity to *C. tetani*. This agent is a routinely given when the client is admitted to the hospital. Tetanus immune globulin (human) (Hyper-Tet) injection is recommended when the client's history of tetanus immunization is not known.

The use of topical antimicrobial drugs is an important intervention for infection prevention in burn wounds. The goal of this therapy is to reduce bacterial growth into the wound and prevent systemic sepsis.

Topical antibiotics are applied by either the *open* or the *closed* technique. With the open technique, use either aseptic or clean methods to apply the drug directly to the burn wound without further dressing the wound. Clean the wound every 8 to 24 hours and apply fresh antimicrobial drugs. With the more common closed technique, dress the burn wound after applying the topical drugs.

Two of the more commonly used drugs are silver sulfadiazine (Silvadene, Flamazine✱) and mafenide acetate (Sulfamylon). Topical antimicrobial drugs are not applied to freshly grafted areas because they may inhibit cell growth. Chart 71-5 lists the features of various topical antimicrobial drugs.

Drug Therapy for Treatment of Infection. Systemic antibiotics are used when burn clients have symptoms of an actual infection, including septicemia. Broad-spectrum antibiotics are given until the results of blood cultures and sensitivity status are available. At that time, more specific antibiotics, including the aminoglycosides such as amikacin (Amikin) or gentamicin (Garamycin, Alcomicin✱) and cephalosporins such as cephalothin (Keflin) or ceftriaxone (Rocephin), are used. Because of increased metabolism,

CHART 71-5

DRUG THERAPY for

Burns

Agent	Description	Action	Advantages	Disadvantages	Interventions
Silver sulfadiazine (Silvadene, Thermazene)	Nontoxic salt of silver sulfadiazine in water-based cream	Binds to bacterial cell membranes and interferes with DNA synthesis	Does not cause hypochloremia, hyponatremia, electrolyte imbalance, or kidney disease Painless Wide-spectrum antimicrobial action against gram-positive and gram-negative organisms Long shelf life Delays eschar separation to a lesser degree than do many other topical drugs	Absorbed into eschar less than other drugs May cause rash, pruritus, burning, and leukopenia Not consistently effective for burns covering 60% of the body Not effective against *Pseudomonas*	Watch for signs of infection, such as soupiness of wound area. Watch for allergic reaction causing a drop in white blood cell count. Do not use if reaction to sulfonamide has occurred. Use on deep-partial or full-thickness wounds.
Collagenase (Santyl) with Polysporin powder	Topical enzymatic debriding agent with 250 collagenase units/g of white petroleum	Digests collagen in necrotic tissue	Painless Daily dressing changes No side effects Quick debridement action Easy to apply Not harmful to healthy tissue Specific only to nonviable tissue	Expensive	Apply once a day. Painless. Use on deep-partial wound with eschar. Monitor wounds for infection. May be used with barrier dressing such as Xeroform.
Mafenide acetate (Sulfamylon)	Soft, white, non-staining water-based cream Available in solution	Bacteriostatic action against many gram-positive and gram-negative organisms	Effective against *Pseudomonas* Long shelf life Excellent for treating electrical burns Penetrates thick eschar May use as a solution to wet down grafts or wounds	May lead to infection May cause metabolic acidosis, hyperpnea, and rash When applied, may cause pain that lasts 30-40 minutes	Premedicate for pain before application. Monitor blood gas and serum electrolyte levels. Monitor for infection.
Nitrofurazone (Furacin)	Cream, solution, or water-soluble ointment, or foam	Wide-spectrum anti-bacterial	Effective against *Staphylococcus aureus* and some antibiotic-resistant organisms Causes neither pain nor maceration	May cause contact dermatitis (rare) Messy to apply in cream form May cause renal problems if used in extensive burns	Observe carefully for signs of allergic reaction and evidence of superinfection.
Gentamicin sulfate (Garamycin, Gentamar)	Available as a cream or solution for topical use	Antibiotic action against organisms resistant to other drugs	Effective against *Pseudomonas* Does not cause pain	May have ototoxic and nephrotoxic effects May result in resistance by certain organisms	Use with caution in clients with decrease renal function. Monitor serum and urine creatinine clearance before and during treatment.
Polymyxin B-bacitracin	Topical cream	Wide-spectrum antimicrobial	Painless Effective against many gram-positive and gram-negative organisms Can be used on face Can be placed on healed grafts to lubricate	May cause urticaria, burning, and inflammation Does not penetrate eschar	Apply q2-8h to keep areas moist.

burn clients generally require a larger than normal dose of these drugs to maintain therapeutic blood levels. If aminoglycosides are used, serial peak and trough blood levels are monitored to determine the efficacy of treatment and evaluate potential ear and kidney toxicity.

Isolation Therapy. Some burn care philosophy believes that isolation therapy effectively reduces cross-contamination. However, methods of isolation are varied and controversial. Some burn centers practice virtually no isolation, whereas others use near-total sterile conditions. All isolation methods emphasize proper and consistent handwashing as the most effective technique for preventing infection transmission.

Environmental Management. All health care personnel wear gloves during all contact with open wounds. The use of sterile versus clean gloves for routine wound care varies by agency and is a matter of debate. Regardless of sterility, change gloves when handling wounds on different areas of the body and between handling old and new dressings.

The equipment on burn units is not shared among clients. Disposable items (e.g., pillows, syringes, and dishes) are used as much as possible. Assign to each client any equipment used in daily routine care (e.g., thermometers, blood pressure cuffs, and stethoscopes). Daily cleaning of the equipment and general housekeeping are essential for infection control. All equipment must be cleaned after use on one client and before use on another. Because *Pseudomonas* has been shown to sequester in plants, the presence of plants and flowers is prohibited. Some burn units do not permit clients to eat raw foods (such as salads, fruit, and pepper) to reduce exposure to organisms. Rugs and upholstered articles are difficult to clean and may harbor organisms; their use is also restricted.

Visitors are restricted when the client is immunosuppressed. Ill people, small children, and other clients should not come into direct contact with the burn client. Some burn units recommend that all visitors wear protective clothing (gowns, gloves, masks, and shoe and hair covers) in the room of the burn client, but no data support the effectiveness of this approach.

Secondary Prevention/Early Detection. Carefully monitor the burn wounds at each dressing change. Examine the wounds for the following signs of infection:

- Pervasive odor
- Color changes—focal, dark red, brown discoloration in the eschar
- Change in texture
- Purulent drainage
- Exudate
- Sloughing grafts
- Redness at the wound edges extending to nonburned skin

Laboratory cultures and biopsies are recommended. Quantitative biopsies of the eschar and granulation tissue are performed routinely and as needed to monitor the proliferation of organisms and are considered the gold standard for wound monitoring.

SURGICAL MANAGEMENT. Infected burn wounds with colony counts of or approaching 10^5 colonies per gram of tissue are life threatening, even with antibiotic therapy. Surgical excision of the burn wound may be necessary.

IMBALANCED NUTRITION: LESS THAN BODY REQUIREMENTS

NOC PLANNING: EXPECTED OUTCOMES. The client is expected to maintain adequate nutrient intake for meeting the body's calorie needs. Indicators include that the client should have mild or no deviations from the normal ranges of the following:

- Weight/height ratio
- Food intake
- Hematocrit and hemoglobin
- Serum albumin
- Blood glucose

INTERVENTIONS. Interventions aim to calculate the client's calorie needs and provide an adequate daily source of calories and nutrients that the client can ingest and metabolize.

Diet therapy begins with calculating the client's current daily calorie needs. Several formulas and charts are used for this calculation. Nutritional requirements for a client with a large burn area can exceed 5000 kcal/day. In addition to a high-calorie intake, the burn client requires a diet high in protein for wound healing. Collaborate with the dietitian and the client to plan additions to standard nutritional patterns.

Oral diet therapy may be delayed for several days after the injury until the GI tract is motile. Nasoduodenal tube feedings are often started soon after admission. Beginning enteral feedings early helps to decrease weight loss, gut atrophy, bacterial translocation, and sepsis. These feedings often are started within 4 hours of beginning fluid resuscitation. This type of supplement prevents nutritional deficits in severely burned clients.

Encourage clients who can eat solid foods to ingest as many calories as possible. Take the client's preferences into consideration for diet planning and food selection. Encourage clients to request food whenever they feel they can eat, not just according to the hospital's standard meal schedule. Offer frequent high-calorie, high-protein supplemental feedings. Keep an accurate calorie count for foods and beverages that are actually ingested by the client.

Clients who cannot swallow but who have adequate gastric motility may meet calorie and nutrition needs through enteral tube feedings (see Chapter 64). Parenteral nutrition may be given IV when the GI tract is not functional or when the client's nutritional needs cannot be met by oral and enteral feeding. This method is used as a last resort because it is invasive and can lead to infectious and metabolic complications.

IMPAIRED PHYSICAL MOBILITY

NOC PLANNING: EXPECTED OUTCOMES. The client with a burn injury is expected to regain and maintain an optimal ability to move purposefully. Indicators include that the client should be mildly compromised or not compromised in the following actions:

- Muscle movement
- Joint movement
- Walking
- Body positioning performance

INTERVENTIONS. Interventions aim to maintain the client's preburn range of joint motion and prevent contracture formation.

CHART 71-6

BEST PRACTICE for
Positioning to Prevent Contractures

Affected Body Part	Position of Function	Intervention
Head and neck	Hyperextension	No pillow. Place a towel roll under the client's neck or shoulder. Neck splint.
Posterior neck	Flexion	Have client turn the head from side to side.
Upper chest and chest	Shoulder retraction	Place client in supine position. Place a folded towel under the spine, between the scapulae.
Lateral trunk	Flexion to uninvolved side	Place the client supine with arm on the affected side up over the head.
Anterior shoulder	Abduction and external rotation	Maintain the upper arm at 90 degrees of abduction from the lateral aspect of the trunk.
Posterior shoulder	Slight flexion and interior rotation	Keep the arm slightly behind the midline.
Axilla	Abduction with 10-15 degree forward flexion and external rotation	Support the abducted arm with suspension from IV pole or bedside table. Axilla splint
Elbow	Extension and supination	Keep the joint in the extended position.
Wrist	30-45 degrees of extension	Use a splint.

Fingers
  MP joints
  PIP and DIP joints
	
	70-90 degrees of flexion
	Extended
		
		Use a splint.
		Use a splint.

Ankle	90 degrees of dorsiflexion	Use a padded footboard or splint with heels free of pressure.
Legs	15-20 degrees of abduction	Place small pillow between legs.
Hip	Extension and neutral rotation	Supine with lower extremity extended. Trochanter roll. Foam wedge along lateral aspect of thigh.

NONSURGICAL MANAGEMENT. Nonsurgical management includes positioning, range-of-motion exercises, ambulation, and pressure dressings.

Positioning. Positioning is critical for clients with burn injuries because the position of comfort for the client is often one of joint flexion, which predisposes him or her to contracture development. Maintain the client in a neutral body position with minimal flexion. Best practice for the prevention of contractures is listed in Chart 71-6. Splints and other conforming devices may assist in maintaining position. These devices are used most often on the joints of the hands, elbows, knees, neck, and axillae.

Range-of-Motion Exercises. Range-of-motion exercises are performed actively at least three times a day. If the client cannot move a joint actively, perform passive range-of-motion exercises. Give burned hands special attention. Encourage the client to perform active range-of-motion exercises for the hand, thumb, and fingers every hour while he or she is awake.

Ambulation. Ambulation is started as soon as possible after the fluid shifts have resolved. Clients with a variety of attached equipment (IV catheters, nasogastric tubes, electrocardiographic leads, extensive dressings) can ambulate with preparation and assistance. Ambulation is performed two or three times a day and progresses in length each time. Ambulation inhibits the loss of bone density, strengthens muscles, stimulates immune function, promotes ventilation, and prevents many complications.

Pressure Dressings. After the graft heals, pressure dressings are applied to help prevent contractures and tight hypertrophic scars, which can inhibit mobility. These dressings also inhibit venous stasis and edema formation in areas

with decreased lymphatic outflow. Pressure dressings may be elastic wraps or specially designed, custom-fitted, elasticized clothing that provide continuous pressure over the burned area. Figure 71-14 shows such garments. For best effectiveness, pressure garments must be worn at least 23 hours a day, every day, until the scar tissue is mature (12 to 24 months). Pressure garments cause some personal discomfort with itchiness and increased warmth. Reinforce to the client that wearing pressure garments is very beneficial in maintaining mobility and reducing scarring.

SURGICAL MANAGEMENT. Surgical management restores mobility rather than prevents immobility. Surgical release of contractures is most commonly performed in the neck, axilla, elbow flexion areas, and hand. Specific surgical procedures to improve movement vary for each client.

Nursing responsibilities after surgery include interventions to prevent contractures from reforming as well as the care of new grafts and suture lines. Constantly reinforce the need for the client to adhere to exercise and splinting regimens to prevent the recurrence of joint immobility.

DISTURBED BODY IMAGE

NOC **PLANNING: EXPECTED OUTCOMES.** Following intervention, the client with a burn injury is expected to have a positive perception of his or her own appearance and body functions. Indicators include that the client should consistently demonstrate the following behaviors:

- Willingness to touch the affected body part
- Adjustment to changes in body function
- Willingness to use strategies to enhance appearance and function

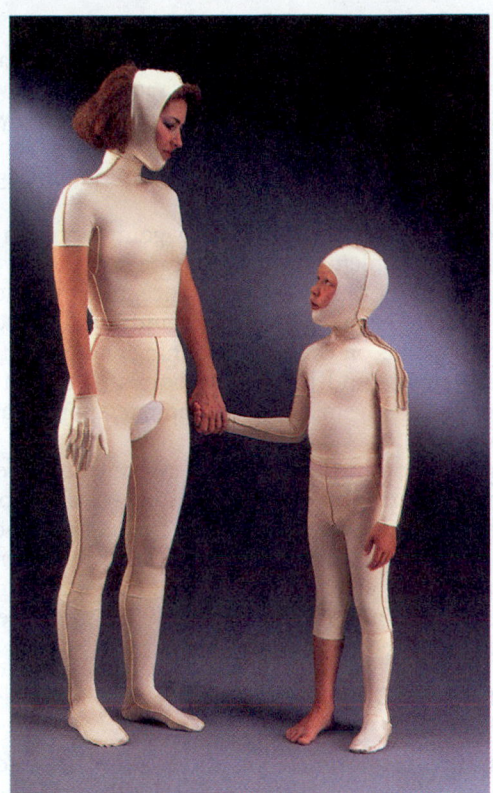

Figure 71-14 ■ Models wearing pressure garments. (Courtesy of Beiersdorf-Jobst, Inc., Charlotte, NC.)

- Successful progression through the grieving process
- Use of support systems

INTERVENTIONS. Nonsurgical and surgical interventions can assist clients who have body image disturbances as a result of burn injury.

NONSURGICAL MANAGEMENT. Understanding the stages of grief is helpful for the client, family, and health professionals. Assess which stage of grief the client is currently experiencing and help interpret his or her behaviors. The client often is unaware of or is confused by his or her feelings. Reassure the client that feelings of grief, loss, anxiety, anger, fear, and guilt are normal. The client may be grieving the loss of body parts, appearance, role identity, and social identity. Collaborate with other health care team members (e.g., psychologist, psychiatrist, social worker, or clergy or religious leader) in addressing these problems.

Accept the physical and psychological characteristics of the client. Present clients and families with realistic expected outcomes for the client's functional capacity and physical appearance. Provide information sessions and counseling for the family to help identify effective patterns of support. Facilitate client's use of these systems and the development of new support systems. Make referrals to support groups. To identify the effectiveness of such assistance and possible gaps in support, evaluate support resources throughout the course of illness.

Engaging in decision making and independent activities fosters feelings of self-worth, which are closely linked to body image. To this end, plan and encourage the client's active participation in self-care activities. Assist family members to understand that it is more beneficial for the client to perform these activities than to have them performed by someone else. Encourage families to include the client in family decision making to the same degree that he or she participated in this process before the injury.

SURGICAL MANAGEMENT. Reconstructive and cosmetic surgery can be performed for many years after the burn injury. Restoring function and improving appearance through surgical techniques often increase the client's feelings of self-worth and promote a positive body image. Many clients have unrealistic expectations of reconstructive surgery and envision an appearance identical or equal in quality to the preburn state. Teach the client and family about expected cosmetic outcomes.

？ *Critical Thinking Challenge*

The 57-year-old who sustained a 41% TBSA flame burn was grafted with split-thickness meshed grafts to her bilateral upper limbs and hands taken from her thighs. When performing the initial postoperative dressing, you note that the graft has a dusky appearance and that the edges of the graft are beginning to curl. The margins of the wound are firm and red with some purulent drainage. You also note a greenish blue color in the burned area next to the graft.

1. What is your first action?
2. Should range-of-motion exercises be performed to the upper extremities at this time? Why or why not?
3. What is the best position for the upper extremities and hands to prevent contractures?
4. What additional assessment data should you obtain about the graft and the surrounding burn wound?

evolve For suggested answer guidelines, go to http://evolve.elsevier.com/Iggy/.

REHABILITATIVE PHASE OF BURN INJURY

OVERVIEW

Although rehabilitation efforts are started from the time of admission, the technical rehabilitative phase begins with wound closure and ends when the client returns to the highest possible level of functioning. The emphasis during this phase is the psychosocial adjustment of the client, the prevention of scars and contractures, and the resumption of preburn activity, including resuming work, family, and social roles. This phase may take years or even a lifetime as clients adjust to permanent limitations that may not be apparent until long after the initial injury.

◆COLLABORATIVE MANAGEMENT

Although attention is placed first on the physical interventions for the burn injury, psychological care is equally important. Provide psychosocial support to the client and family throughout hospitalization but more extensively in the rehabilitative phase.

Information from the client and family aids in the assessment and diagnosis of psychological problems and allows treatment to be instituted. Explore the client's feelings about the burn injury. It is extremely difficult for clients to concentrate on the many tasks before them when obstacles such as guilt and grief are in the forefront.

TABLE 71-11   Needs to Address Before Discharge of the Client with Burns

- Early client assessment
- Financial assessment
- Evaluation of family resources
- Weekly discharge planning meeting
- Psychological referral
- Client and family teaching (home care)
- Designation of principal learners (specific family members or significant others who will help with care)
- Development of teaching plan
- Training for wound care
- Rehabilitation referral
- Home assessment (on-site visit)
- Medical equipment
- Public health nursing referral
- Evaluation of community resources
- Visit to referral agency
- Re-entry programs for school or work environment
- Nursing home placement
- Environmental interventions
- Auditory testing
- Speech therapy
- Prosthetic rehabilitation

Ask the client or family member whether there is a history of psychological problems. Assess and document the type of coping mechanisms the client has used successfully during times of stress to assist with a future plan of care. Also assess the client's family unit and the family members' history of interaction. Identify cultural and ethnic factors and take these into consideration when planning psychosocial interventions.

Throughout the hospitalization the client progresses through a variety of stages and exhibits many feelings, including denial, regression, and anger. Assess the client's feelings during each stage so appropriate plans of care can be developed and carried out.

Community-Based Care

Discharge planning for the client with a burn injury begins at the time of admission to the hospital or burn center. In most burn centers, the multidisciplinary team meets regularly to plan for discharge. In helping the client reach mutually established discharge goals, the team evaluates the progress of each discipline. Table 71-11 lists common discharge needs of the client with burns.

PSYCHOSOCIAL PREPARATION

During the recovery period and for some time after discharge from the hospital, clients with severe burn injuries are likely to have psychological problems that require intervention. Such problems include posttraumatic stress disorder, sexual dysfunction, and severe depression. Assistance is coordinated with the client, family, and health care team. Psychosocial assistance is best provided by a professional counselor with experience in helping burn clients.

One specific area to address with the client is the reaction of others to the sight of healing wounds and disfiguring scars. Clients with facial burns are especially subjected to stares and other reactions from the general public. Visits from friends and short public appearances before discharge may help the client begin adjusting to this problem. Community reintegration programs can assist the psychosocial and physical recovery of the client with serious burns.

HOME CARE MANAGEMENT

The client with severe burns is discharged from the acute care setting when life-threatening complications are resolved and minimal wound areas remain open. During the first weeks at home, the client usually needs at least daily wound care, physical therapy, nutritional support, symptom management, and drug therapy.

Although the client usually views going home in a positive light, the problems of physical care and the psychological stresses from changes in appearance, role, function, and lifestyle may overwhelm the client and family. Successful discharge depends on extensive planning and preparation of the client, family, and home environment through education and the involvement of appropriate support agencies and services.

Preparation for discharge includes assessment of the family and home care situation from physical and social perspectives. Consider the needs of the client when evaluating the home for cleanliness; access to bathing facilities, electricity, and running water; stairways; number of occupants; temperature control; and safety. If the burn injuries occurred in a house fire, a new residence may need to be established.

HEALTH TEACHING

Education about burn care and living with the consequences of burn injuries begins when the client is admitted to the hospital or burn center. A weekly plan for client education is outlined; the goal is progression toward independence for the client and family. Critical for this goal is teaching clients and family members to perform such care tasks as dressing changes. Allow clients and family members to first observe dressing changes, then to assist in performing the changes, and finally to change the dressings independently under your supervision.

Before discharge, all people who will be involved in the client's home care participate in discharge planning and teaching sessions. In addition to details about dressing changes, explain the following:

- Signs and symptoms of infection
- Drug regimens
- Proper use of prosthetic and positioning devices
- Correct application and care of pressure garments
- Comfort measures to reduce pruritus
- Dates for follow-up appointments

HEALTH CARE RESOURCES

The health care team evaluates the family in terms of capacity and willingness to assist in providing care to the client after discharge. A visiting nurse or case manager referral can assist the family with care problems arising at home. In addition, the visiting nurse can help the family determine what special equipment, supplies, or services will be needed. The frequency of home visits depends on the client's condition and the ability of family members to function as care providers. *It is imperative that the visiting nurse have extensive experience in providing burn care.* The home care nurse may need a brief visit to the client while in the hospital and observation of burn wound care.

The home care of a client after a serious burn often involves daily physical therapy and rehabilitation sessions at special centers. Address and resolve transportation problems before the client is discharged. In some instances, the burn center has arrangements for transportation. Some community volunteer agencies provide transportation by private car.

When rehabilitation is prolonged, the client may be discharged to a rehabilitation facility. Consult with the rehabilitation team and provide copies of the care and teaching plans used with the client.

? Critical Thinking Challenge

The 57-year-old client who sustained a flame injury and received skin grafting is being prepared for discharge. You notice that your client's appetite has decreased, she refuses to participate in her occupational therapy, and she complains of fatigue despite staying in her bed all day. Your assessment reveals that she is depressed.

1. Are these symptoms the client is experiencing part of the complex systemic response to burn injuries? Why or why not?
2. What resources or referrals would be most appropriate for this client at this time?
3. What other needs should be addressed before discharge?

evolve For suggested answer guidelines, go to http://evolve.elsevier.com/Iggy/.

◆ Evaluation: Outcomes

Evaluate the care of the client with a burn injury on the basis of the identified nursing diagnoses and collaborative problems. The expected outcomes include that the client should:

- Have cardiac output restored to normal
- Maintain adequate oxygenation and circulation to all vital organs
- Maintain a patent airway
- Have an effective breathing pattern
- Have pain alleviated or reduced
- Experience no further loss of skin integrity
- Have skin integrity restored without complications
- Remain free from infection by cross-contamination
- Not experience septicemia
- Maintain an adequate nutrient intake for meeting the body's calorie needs
- Regain and maintain an optimal ability to move purposefully
- Have a positive perception of his or her own appearance and body functions

Specific indicators for these outcomes are listed for each nursing diagnosis and collaborative problem under the Planning and Implementation section (see earlier).

GET READY for the NCLEX Examination!

KEY POINTS

Safe Effective Care Environment

- Use strict aseptic technique when caring for clients who have open burn wounds.
- Check ventilator alarms hourly for clients who are receiving paralytic drugs during mechanical ventilation.

Health Promotion and Maintenance

- Encourage all people to have and maintain home smoke detectors.

- Warn clients who smoke about not smoking in bed or when taking any substance that induces sedation (drugs or alcohol).
- Instruct clients who have reduced sensation in hands or feet to use a bath thermometer to check water temperature before bathing.
- Teach clients to avoid exposing the burned skin areas to the sun or to temperature extremes.

Psychosocial Integrity

- Allow clients time to grieve over a change in body image.
- Reassure clients that pain will be managed effectively.
- Explain all procedures to the client.
- Give analgesics, sedatives, and antianxiety drugs to clients receiving paralytic drugs during mechanical ventilation.
- Encourage the client to actively participate in pain control measures.
- Encourage the client to look at and touch burned areas.

Physiological Integrity

- Assess the burn client's airway and adequacy of breathing before assessing any other body system.
- Keep an endotracheal kit or tracheostomy kit at the bedside of any client with facial burns, burns inside the mouth, singed nasal hairs, or a "smoky" smell to the breath.
- Notify the physician immediately if the client with an inhalation injury becomes more dyspneic or audible wheezes disappear.
- Give half of the fluid volume calculated for the first 24 hours after burn injury in the first 8 hours postburn.
- Give prescribed opioid analgesics by the IV route during the emergent phase of burn recovery.
- Position clients to prevent contractures and promote joint function.
- Assist clients to ambulate several times each day as soon as the fluid shifts have resolved.
- Encourage clients to use the prescribed splints and pressure garments to prevent joint immobility.

ADDITIONAL STUDY RESOURCES

Go to your Student CD-ROM for Review Questions for the NCLEX Examination.

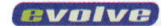 Go to http://evolve.elsevier.com/Iggy/ for Integrated Management of Care Questions for the NCLEX Examination.

SELECTED BIBLIOGRAPHY

Asterisk indicates a classic or definitive work on this subject.

Ackley, B., & Ladwig, G. (2002). *Nursing diagnosis handbook: A guide to planning care* (5th ed.). St. Louis: Mosby.

American Burn Association. (2002). U.S. trauma and burn statistics. Available at http://www.ameriburn.org.

Badger, J. (2001). Burns: The psychological aspects. *American Journal of Nursing, 101*(11), 38-44.

Carrougher, G., et al. (2003). Comparison of patient satisfaction and self-reports of pain in adult burn-injured patients. *Journal of Burn Care and Rehabilitation, 24*(1), 1-8.

*Covington, D., Wainwright, D., & Parks, D. (1996). Prognostic indicators in the elderly patient with burns. *Journal of Burn Care and Rehabilitation, 17*(3), 222-230.

Demling, R., & DeSanti, L. (2002). The rate of re-epithelialization across meshed skin grafts is increased with exposure to silver. *Burns, 28*(3), 264-266.

DiLuigi, K. (2001). Hydrofluoric acid burns. *American Journal of Nursing 101*(6), 24AAA-24DDD.

Dochterman, J., & Bulechek, G. (Eds). (2004). *Nursing interventions classification (NIC)* (4th Ed.). St. Louis: Mosby.

Ebersole, P., Hess, P., & Luggen, A. (2004). *Toward healthy aging: Human needs and nursing response* (6th ed.). St. Louis: Mosby.

Facts and Comparisons. (2004). *Drug facts and comparisons* (58th ed.). St. Louis: Author.

*Flynn, M. (1999). Identifying and treating inhalation injuries in fire victims. *DCCN: Dimensions of Critical Care Nursing, 18*(4), 18-23.

Gosain, A., & Gamelli, R. (2005). The role of the gastrointestinal tract in burn sepsis. *Journal of Burn Care and Rehabilitation, 26*(1), 85-91.

*Hansbrough, J., et al. (1995). Wound healing in partial-thickness burn wounds treated with collagenase ointment versus silver sulfadiazine cream. *Journal of Burn Care and Rehabilitation, 16*(3), 241-247.

Helvig, E. (2002). Managing thermal injuries within WOCN practice. *Journal of Wound Ostomy, and Continence Nursing, 29*(2), 76-82.

Hunt, J., et al. (2000). Occupation-related burn injuries. *Journal of Burn Care: Rehabilitator 21*(4), 327-332.

Iraniha, S., et al. (2000). Determination of burn depth with non-contact ultrasonography. *Journal of Burn Care and Rehabilitation, 21*(4), 333-338.

*Jellish, W.S., et al. (1999). Effect of topical local anesthetic application to skin harvest sites for pain management in burn patients undergoing skin-grafting procedures. *Annals of Surgery, 229*(1), 115-120.

Kagan, R., & Smith, S. (2000). Evaluation and treatment of thermal injuries. *Dermatology Nursing, 12*(5), 334-335, 338-344, 347-350.

Koschel, M.J. (2002). Where there's smoke, there may be cyanide. *American Journal of Nursing, 102*(8), 39-42.

Kraft, P. (2000). The osmotic shift. *Journal of Intravenous Nursing, 23*(4), 220-224.

*Kravitz, M., et al. (1989). A randomized trial of plasma exchange in the treatment of burn shock. *Journal of Burn Care and Rehabilitation, 10*(1), 17-26.

Lawrence, J., & Fauerbach, J. (2003). Personality, coping, chronic stress, social support and PTSD symptoms among adult burn survivors: A path analysis. *Journal of Burn Care and Rehabilitation, 24*(1), 63-72.

*Mayes, T., Gottschlich, M., & Warden, G. (1997). Clinical nutrition protocols for continuous quality improvements in the outcomes of patients with burns. *Journal of Burn Care and Rehabilitation, 18*(4), 365-368.

McCance, K., & Huether, S. (2002). Pathophysiology: The biologic basis for disease in adults and children (4th ed.). St. Louis: Mosby.

McGwin, G., et al. (2003). Long-term trends in mortality according to age among adult burn patients. *Journal of Burn Care and Rehabilitation, 24*(1), 21-25.

Milner, S., Mottar, R., & Smith, C. (2001). The burn wheel: An innovative method for calculating the need for fluid resuscitation in burned patients. *American Journal of Nursing, 101*(11), 35-37.

Moorhead, S., Johnson, M., & Maas, M. (Eds.). (2004). *Nursing outcomes classification (NOC)* (3rd ed.). St. Louis: Mosby.

*Moritz, A.R. (1947). Studies of thermal injuries: II. The relative importance of time and surface temperature in the causation of cutaneous burns. *American Journal of Pathology, 23,* 695.

Nanchalhal, J., Dover, R., & Otto, W. (2002). Allogeneic skin substitutes applied to burns patients. *Burns, 28*(3), 254-257.

*Nguyen, T.T., et al. (1996). Current treatment of severely burned patients. *Annals of Surgery, 223*(1), 14-25.

Pagana, K., & Pagana, T. (2002). *Mosby's manual of diagnostic and laboratory tests* (2nd ed.). St. Louis: Mosby.

*Rakel, B., et al. (1998). Split-thickness skin graft donor site care: A quantitative synthesis of the research. *Applied Nursing Research, 11*(4), 174-182.

Scholl, D., & Langkamp-Henken, B. (2001). Nutrient recommendations for wound healing. *Journal of Intravenous Nursing, 24*(2), 124-132.

Sheridan, R. (2000). Evaluating and managing burn wounds. *Dermatology Nursing, 12*(1), 17-28.

Sibbald, G., et al. (2000). Preparing the woundbed: Debridement, bacterial balance, and moisture balance. *Ostomy Wound Management, 46*(4), 14-35.

Stone, M., Ahmed, J., & Evans, J. (2000). The continuing risk of domestic hot water scalds to the elderly. *Burns, 26*(4), 347-350.

Wiebelhaus, P., & Hansen, S. (2001). What you should know about managing burn emergencies. *Nursing2001, 31*(1), 36-41.

*Winfrey, M., Cochran, M., & Hegarty, M. (1999). A new technology in burn therapy: Integra artificial skin. *Dimensions of Critical Care Nursing, 18*(1), 14-20.

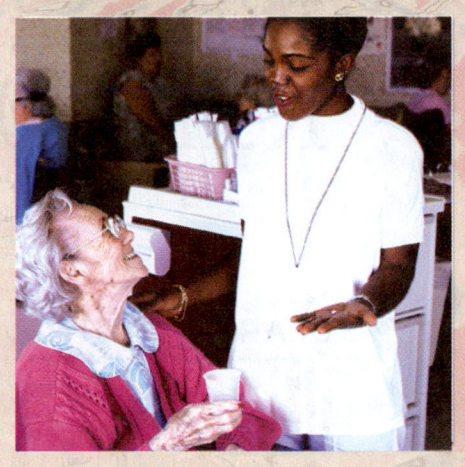

PROBLEMS of EXCRETION

Management of Clients with Problems of the Renal/Urinary System

Assessment of the Renal/Urinary System

CHRIS WINKELMAN

Kidneys help maintain health in several ways. Their primary role is to maintain body fluid volume and composition and to filter waste products for elimination. The kidneys also help regulate blood pressure, participate in acid-base balance, produce erythropoietin for red blood cell (RBC) synthesis, and metabolize vitamin D to an active form.

The renal system includes the kidneys and the entire urinary tract. The ureters, bladder, and urethra are the drainage route for the excretion of urine. Structural or functional problems in the kidney or urinary tract usually alter fluid, electrolyte, and acid-base balance.

Assessment of the client at risk for or with actual problems of the renal system begins with a history and physical assessment. Understanding the anatomy, physiology, and diagnostic tests of the renal system helps you in problem-solving about renal function in the clinical setting. It also assists you in teaching the client about the purpose of tests or procedures and in physically and emotionally preparing the client for assessment.

ANATOMY AND PHYSIOLOGY REVIEW

Kidneys

Structure

GROSS ANATOMY

Normally, two kidneys are located behind the peritoneum, not really in the abdominal cavity, one on either side of the spine (Figure 72-1). The adult kidney is 4 to 5 inches (11 to 13 cm) long, 2 to 3 inches (5 to 7 cm) wide, and about 1 inch (2.5 to 3 cm) thick. It weighs about 8 ounces (250 g). The left kidney is slightly longer and narrower than the right kidney. Kidney size is can be determined via ultrasound. Larger-than-usual kidneys may indicate renal obstruction or polycystic disease, whereas smaller-than-usual kidneys may indicate chronic renal disease.

Several layers of tissue surround the kidney, providing protection and support. On the outer surface of the kidney is a layer of fibrous tissue called the **renal capsule** (Figure 72-2). This capsule covers most of the kidney except the **hilum,** the area in which the renal artery and nerve plexus enter and the renal vein and ureter exit. The renal capsule is surrounded by layers of fat and connective tissue (Gerota's fascia).

Lying beneath the renal capsule are the two layers of functional kidney tissue, the cortex and the medulla. The **renal cortex,** or outer tissue layer, is covered by the renal capsule. The **medulla,** or medullary tissue, lies below the cortex in the shape of many fans. Each "fan" is called a **pyramid,** and there are 12 to 18 pyramids per kidney. The **renal columns** (columns of Bertin) are cortical tissue that dip down into the interior of the kidney and separate the pyramids.

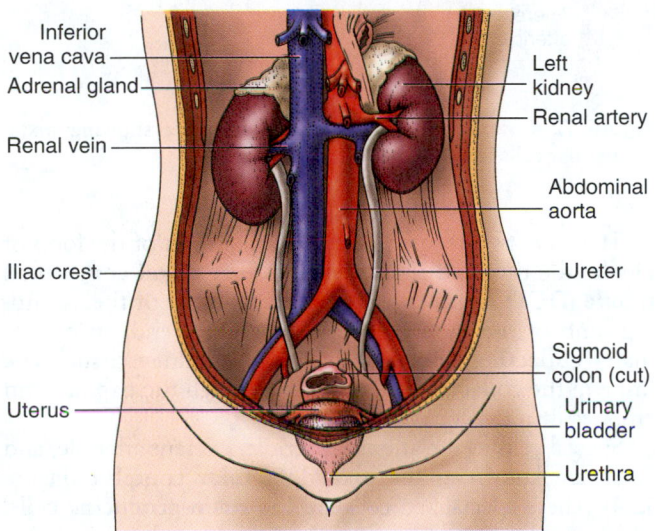

Figure 72-1 ■ Anatomic location of organs of the renal/urinary system.

The tip, or end, of each pyramid is called a **papilla.** The papillae drain urine into the collecting system. A cuplike structure called a **calyx** collects the urine at the end of each papilla. The calices join together to form the **renal pelvis,** which narrows to become the ureter.

The kidneys receive 20% to 25% of the total cardiac output. Renal blood flow per minute varies from about 600 to 1300 mL/min. The blood supply to each kidney comes from the **renal artery,** which branches from the abdominal aorta (Table 72-1). The renal artery divides into progressively smaller arteries, supplying all areas of the renal tissue **(parenchyma)** and the nephrons. The smallest arteries, the afferent arterioles, feed the nephrons directly to form urine.

Venous blood from the kidneys starts with the capillaries surrounding each nephron. These capillaries drain into progressively larger veins, with blood eventually returned to the inferior vena cava through the renal vein.

MICROSCOPIC ANATOMY

The **nephron** is the "working" unit of the kidney, and it is here that urine is actually formed from blood. There are

TABLE 72-1	The Sequence of Renal Blood Flow from the Renal Artery to the Renal Vein

1. Renal artery
2. Interlobar artery
3. Arcuate artery
4. Interlobular artery
5. Afferent arteriole
6. Glomerulus
7. Efferent arteriole
8. Peritubular capillaries or vasa recta
9. Stellate vein
10. Interlobular vein
11. Arcuate vein
12. Interlobar vein
13. Renal vein

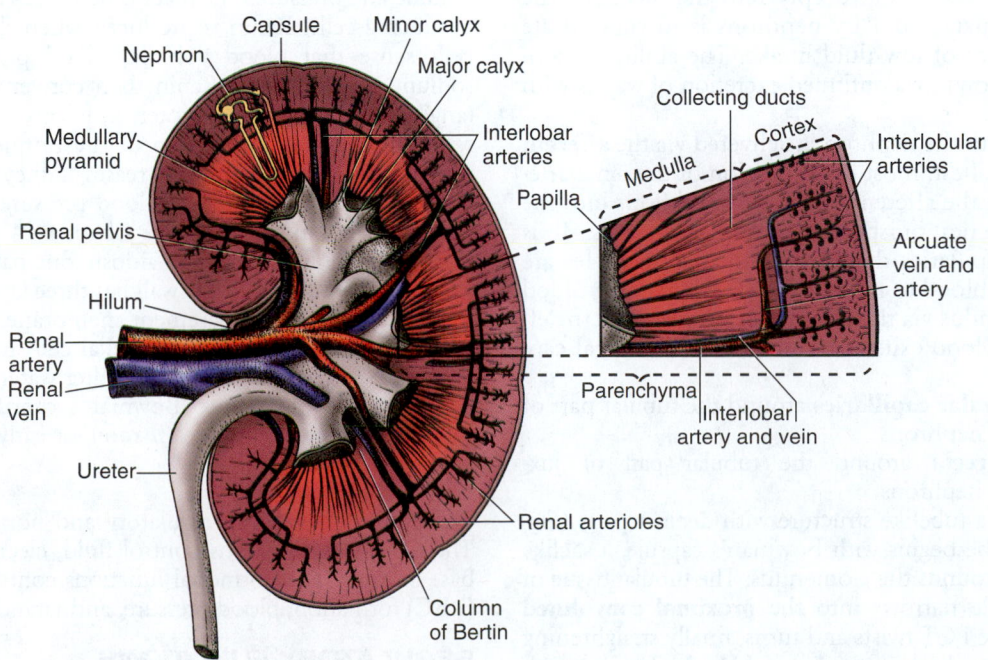

Figure 72-2 ■ Bisection of the kidney showing the major structures of the kidney.

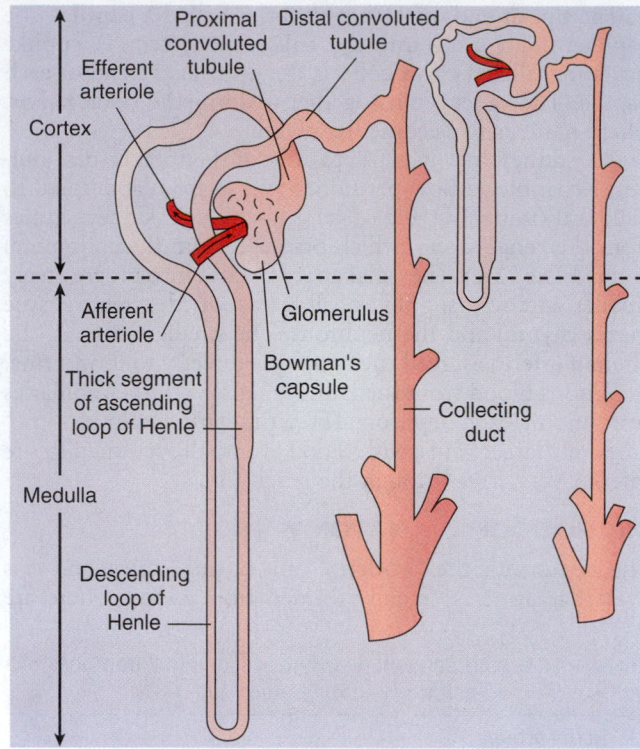

Figure 72-3 ■ Anatomy of the nephron, the functional unit of the kidney. Note that the particular nephron labeled here is a juxtamedullary nephron.

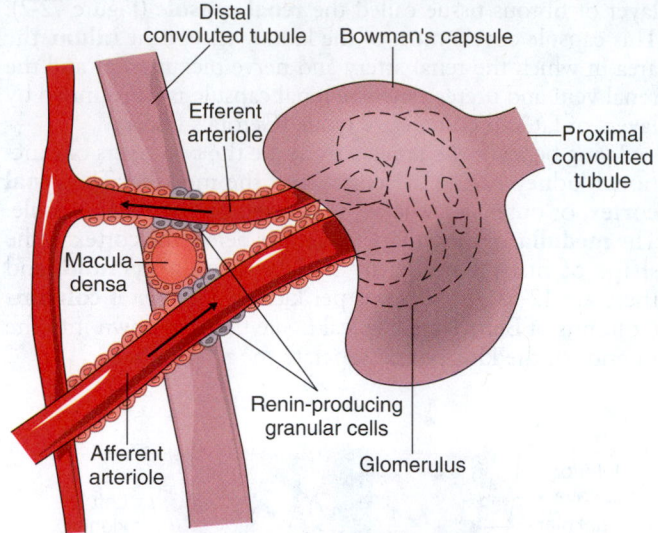

Figure 72-4 ■ The juxtaglomerular complex showing juxtaglomerular cells and the macula densa.

about 1 million nephrons per kidney, and each nephron separately makes urine from blood.

There are two types of nephrons: cortical nephrons and juxtamedullary nephrons. The cortical nephrons are short, with all parts located in the renal cortex. The juxtamedullary nephrons (about 20% of all nephrons) are longer, and their tubes and blood vessels dip deeply into the medulla. The purpose of the juxtamedullary nephrons is to concentrate urine during times of low fluid intake. The ability to concentrate urine allows for continued excretion of wastes with less fluid loss.

Blood supply to the nephron is delivered via the **afferent arteriole,** the smallest, most distal portion of the renal arterial system. From the afferent arteriole, blood flows into the **glomerulus,** a series of specialized capillary loops. It is through these capillaries that water and small particles are filtered from the blood to make urine. The remaining blood leaves the glomerulus via the **efferent arteriole.** From the efferent arteriole, blood exits into one of two additional capillary systems:

- The **peritubular capillaries** around the tubular part of the cortical nephrons
- The **vasa recta** around the tubular part of juxtamedullary nephrons

Each nephron is a tubelike structure with distinct parts (Figure 72-3). The tube begins with Bowman's capsule, a saclike structure that surrounds the glomerulus. The tubular tissue of Bowman's capsule narrows into the **proximal convoluted tubule (PCT).** The PCT twists and turns, finally straightening into the descending limb of the **loop of Henle.** The descending loop of Henle dips in the direction of the medulla but forms a hairpin loop and comes back up into the cortex.

There are two segments of ascending limb of the loop of Henle: the thin and thick segments. The **distal convoluted tubule (DCT)** forms from the thick segment of the ascending limb of the loop of Henle. The DCT ends in one of many **collecting ducts** located in the kidney tissue. The urine in the collecting ducts passes through the papillae and empties into the renal pelvis.

Special cells in the afferent arteriole, efferent arteriole, and DCT are known as the **juxtaglomerular complex** (Figure 72-4). These specialized cells are the **renin-producing cells,** which produce and store renin. **Renin** is a hormone that helps to regulate blood flow, glomerular filtration rate (GFR), and blood pressure. Renin is secreted when sensing cells in the DCT (called the **macula densa**) sense changes in blood volume and pressure. The macula densa lies next to the renin-producing cells. Renin is produced when the macula densa cells sense that blood volume, blood pressure, or blood sodium levels are low. Renin then converts renin substrate (angiotensinogen) into angiotensin I. This leads to a series of reactions that cause secretion of the hormone **aldosterone** (Figure 72-5). Aldosterone increases kidney reabsorption of sodium and water, restoring blood pressure, blood volume, and blood sodium levels. (See Chapter 14 for more discussion of the renin-angiotensin-aldosterone pathway).

The glomerular capillary wall has three layers (Figure 72-6): the endothelium, the basement membrane, and the epithelium. The endothelial and epithelial cells lining these capillaries are separated by pores that filter water and small particles from the blood into Bowman's capsule. This fluid is called the **filtrate** (also **ultrafiltrate**), or early urine.   ●

Function

The kidneys have both regulatory and hormonal functions. The regulatory functions control fluid, electrolyte, and acid-base balance. The hormonal functions control red blood cell (RBC) formation, blood pressure, and vitamin D activation.

REGULATORY FUNCTIONS

The kidney processes that maintain fluid, electrolyte, and acid-base balance are glomerular filtration, tubular reab-

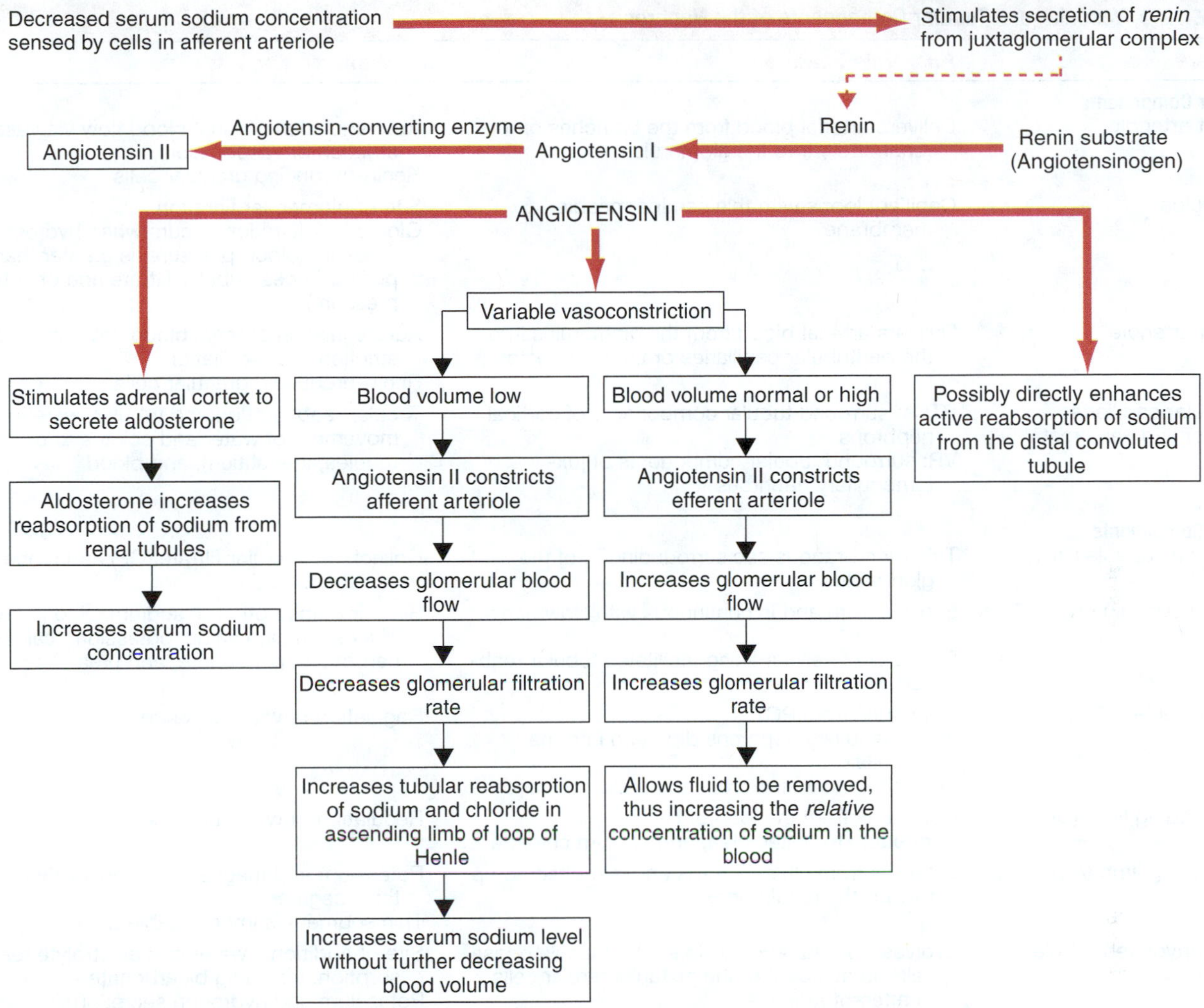

Decreased serum sodium concentration sensed by cells in afferent arteriole → Stimulates secretion of *renin* from juxtaglomerular complex

Renin

Angiotensin II ← Angiotensin-converting enzyme ← Angiotensin I ← Renin substrate (Angiotensinogen)

ANGIOTENSIN II

Variable vasoconstriction

| Stimulates adrenal cortex to secrete aldosterone | Blood volume low | Blood volume normal or high | Possibly directly enhances active reabsorption of sodium from the distal convoluted tubule |

Aldosterone increases reabsorption of sodium from renal tubules

Increases serum sodium concentration

Angiotensin II constricts afferent arteriole

Decreases glomerular blood flow

Decreases glomerular filtration rate

Increases tubular reabsorption of sodium and chloride in ascending limb of loop of Henle

Increases serum sodium level without further decreasing blood volume

Angiotensin II constricts efferent arteriole

Increases glomerular blood flow

Increases glomerular filtration rate

Allows fluid to be removed, thus increasing the *relative* concentration of sodium in the blood

Figure 72-5 ■ The role of aldosterone, renin substrate (angiotensinogen), angiotensin I, and angiotensin II in the renal regulation of water and sodium.

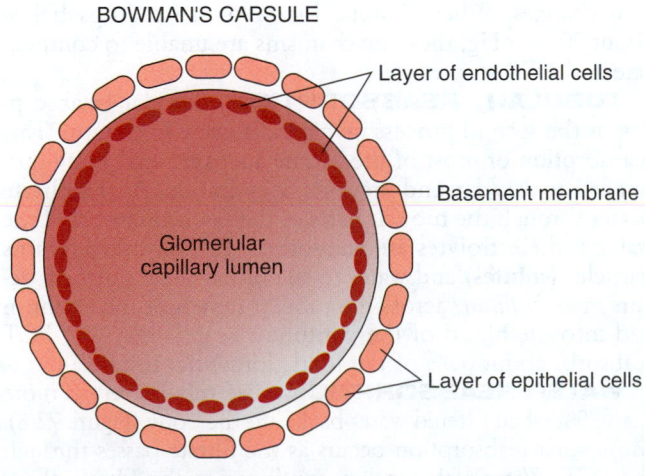

BOWMAN'S CAPSULE

Layer of endothelial cells

Basement membrane

Glomerular capillary lumen

Layer of epithelial cells

Figure 72-6 ■ Glomerular capillary wall.

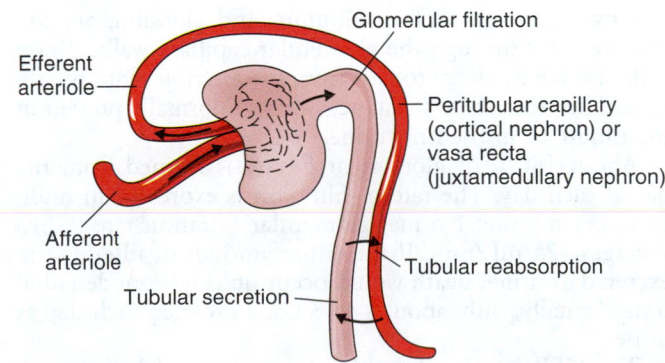

Glomerular filtration

Efferent arteriole

Peritubular capillary (cortical nephron) or vasa recta (juxtamedullary nephron)

Afferent arteriole

Tubular reabsorption

Tubular secretion

Figure 72-7 ■ Glomerular filtration, tubular reabsorption, and tubular secretion.

GLOMERULAR FILTRATION. Glomerular filtration is the first process in urine formation. As blood passes from the afferent arteriole into the glomerulus, water, electrolytes, and other small particles (e.g., creatinine, urea nitrogen, and glucose) are filtered across the glomerular membrane into the Bowman's capsule to form *glomerular* filtrate. As the filtrate enters the proximal convoluted tubule (PCT), it is called *tubular* filtrate.

sorption, and tubular secretion (Figure 72-7). These processes use filtration, diffusion, active transport, and osmosis. (See Chapter 14 for a review of these actions.) Table 72-2 lists the functions of nephron tubules and blood vessels.

TABLE 72-2 Vascular and Tubular Components of the Nephron

Structure	Anatomic Features	Physiologic Aspects
Vascular Components		
Afferent arteriole	Delivers arterial blood from the branches of the renal artery into the glomerulus	Autoregulation of renal blood flow via vasoconstriction or vasodilation Renin-producing granular cells
Glomerulus	Capillary loops with thin semipermeable membrane	Site of glomerular filtration Glomerular filtration occurs when hydrostatic pressure (blood pressure) is greater than opposing forces (tubular filtrate and oncotic pressure)
Efferent arteriole	Delivers arterial blood from the glomerulus into the peritubular capillaries or the vasa recta	Autoregulation of renal blood flow via vasoconstriction or vasodilation Renin-producing granular cells
Peritubular capillaries (PTCs) and vasa recta (VR)	PTCs: surround tubular components of cortical nephrons VR: surround tubular components of juxtamedullary nephrons	Tubular reabsorption and tubular secretion allow movement of water and solutes to or from the tubules, interstitium, and blood
Tubular Components		
Bowman's capsule (BC)	Thin membranous sac surrounding $\frac{7}{8}$ of the glomerulus	Collects glomerular filtrate (GF) and funnels GF into the tubule
Proximal convoluted tubule (PCT)	Evolves from and is continuous with Bowman's capsule Specialized cellular lining facilitates tubular reabsorption	Site for reabsorption of sodium, chloride, water, glucose, amino acids, potassium, calcium, bicarbonate, phosphate, and urea
Loop of Henle	Continues from PCT Juxtamedullary nephrons dip deep into the medulla Permeable to water, urea, and sodium chloride	Regulation of water balance
Descending limb (DL)	Continues from the loop of Henle Permeable to water, urea, and sodium chloride	Regulation of water balance
Ascending limb (AL)	Emerges from DL as it turns and is redirected up toward the renal cortex	Potassium and magnesium reabsorption in the thick segment Thin segment is impermeable to water
Distal convoluted tubule (DCT)	Evolves from AL and twists so the macula densa cells lie adjacent to the juxtaglomerular cells of afferent arteriole	Site of additional water and electrolyte reabsorption, including bicarbonate Potassium and hydrogen secretion
Collecting ducts	Collects formed urine from several tubules and delivers it into the renal pelvis	Receptor sites for antidiuretic hormone regulation of water balance

Large particles, such as albumin and globulin, are too large to filter through the glomerular capillary walls. Blood cells also are too large to pass from the arterioles into the filtrate. Therefore these substances are not normally present in the filtrate or in the final urine.

About 180 L of glomerular filtrate is formed from the blood each day. The rate of filtration is expressed in milliliters per minute. Normal glomerular filtration rate (GFR) averages 125 mL/min. If the entire amount of filtrate were excreted as urine, death would occur quickly from dehydration. Actually, only about 1 to 3 L are excreted each day as urine.

The GFR is related to blood pressure and blood flow. The ability of the kidneys to self-regulate renal blood pressure and renal blood flow keeps GFR constant. GFR is controlled by selectively constricting and dilating the afferent and efferent arterioles. When the afferent arteriole is constricted or the efferent arteriole is dilated, pressure in the glomerular capillaries falls and filtration decreases. When the afferent arteriole is dilated or the efferent arteriole is constricted, pressure in the glomerular capillaries rises and filtration increases. Through this process the kidney can maintain a constant GFR, even when systemic blood pressure changes. When systolic blood pressure drops below about 70 mm Hg, these mechanisms are unable to compensate and GFR stops.

TUBULAR REABSORPTION. Tubular reabsorption is the second process involved in urine formation. This reabsorption of most of the filtrate keeps normal urine output at 1 to 3 L/day and prevents dehydration. As the filtrate passes through the tubular parts of the nephron, most of the water and electrolytes are reabsorbed. Reabsorption returns particles (**solutes**) and water to the blood. Reabsorption occurs *from the filtrate* across the tubular lumen of the nephron and into the blood of the peritubular capillaries. The PCT reabsorbs about 65% of the total glomerular filtrate.

WATER REABSORPTION. The tubules return more than 99% of all filtered water back into the body (Figure 72-8). Most water reabsorption occurs as the filtrate passes through the PCT. Water reabsorption continues as the filtrate flows down the descending loop of Henle. The thin and thick segments of the ascending loop of Henle is *not* permeable to water and water reabsorption does not occur here.

The distal convoluted tubule (DCT) can be permeable to water, and some water reabsorption can occur as the filtrate continues to flow through the tubule. The membrane of the

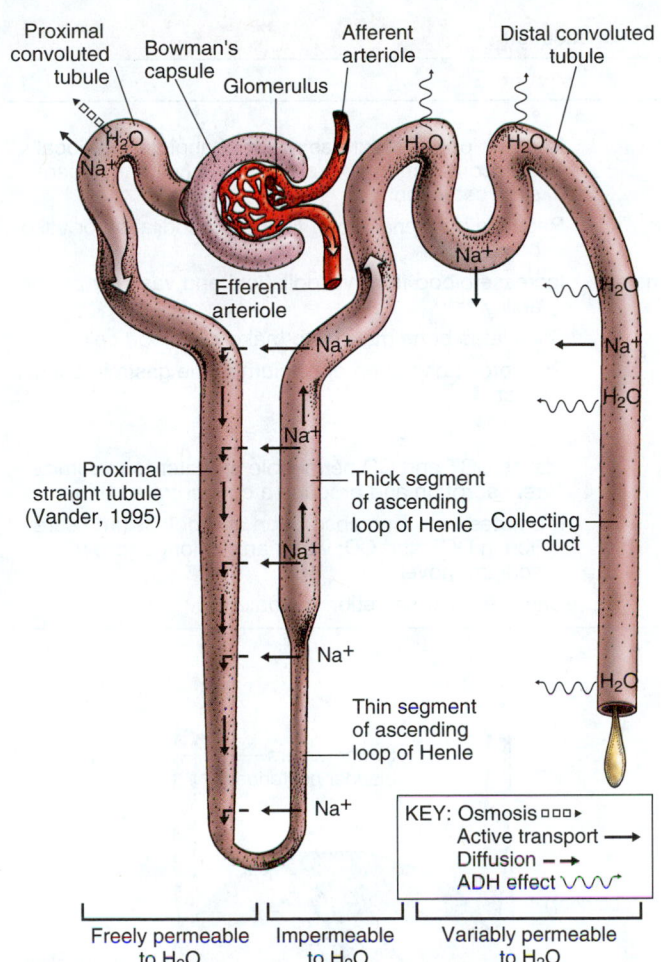

Figure 72-8 ■ Sodium and water reabsorption by the tubules of a cortical nephron.

DCT may be made more permeable to water through the action of the hormones **antidiuretic hormone (ADH)** and aldosterone. ADH increases membrane permeability to water and enhances water reabsorption. Aldosterone promotes the reabsorption of sodium in the DCT; water reabsorption occurs as a result of the movement of sodium (where sodium goes, water follows).

The ability of the kidneys to vary the volume or concentration of urine helps regulate total water balance regardless of water intake. In this way, the healthy kidney can prevent dehydration when fluid intake is low and prevent circulatory overload when fluid intake is excessive.

SOLUTE REABSORPTION. Some particles in the tubular filtrate are *returned to the blood.* This process is called **tubular reabsorption** and is selective. About 50% of all urea in the early urine is reabsorbed. On the other hand, no creatinine is reabsorbed.

Most sodium, chloride, and water reabsorption occurs in the PCT. The collecting ducts are the other site of sodium, chloride, and water reabsorption. Here reabsorption is caused by aldosterone. Potassium is also mostly reabsorbed in the PCT, with an additional 20% to 40% reabsorbed in the thick segment of the ascending loop of Henle.

Bicarbonate, calcium, and phosphate are mostly reabsorbed in the PCT. Bicarbonate reabsorption helps neutralize acids and maintain a normal blood pH. Blood levels of calcitonin and parathyroid hormone (PTH) (see Chapters 16 and 67) control calcium reabsorption and excretion.

The kidney reabsorbs some of the glucose filtered from the blood. However, there is a limit to how much glucose the kidney can reabsorb. This limit is called the **renal threshold** for glucose reabsorption or the **transport maximum** for glucose reabsorption. The usual renal threshold for glucose is about 220 mg/dL. This means that at a blood glucose level of 220 mg/dL or less, all glucose is reabsorbed and returned to the blood, with no glucose present in final urine. When blood glucose levels are greater than 220 mg/dL, some glucose stays in the filtrate and is present in the urine. Normally, almost all glucose and any filtered amino acids or proteins are reabsorbed and are not present in the urine.

TUBULAR SECRETION. Tubular secretion is the third process involved in urine formation. Like glomerular filtration, it allows substances to move *from the blood* into the early urine. During tubular secretion, substances move from the peritubular capillaries, across capillary membranes, and into the cells that line the tubules. From the cells, these substances are moved into the urine and are excreted from the body. Potassium (K^+) and hydrogen ions (H^+) are some of the substances moved in this way to maintain homeostasis of electrolytes and pH.

HORMONAL FUNCTIONS

The kidneys produce renin, prostaglandins, bradykinin, erythropoietin, and activated vitamin D (Table 72-3). Other kidney products, such as the kinins, change renal blood flow and capillary permeability. The kidneys also help break down and excrete insulin.

RENIN. As discussed earlier under Microscopic Anatomy (p. 1653), renin assists in blood pressure control. Renin is formed and released when there is a decrease in blood flow, volume, or pressure through the renal arterioles or when too little sodium is present in renal blood. These conditions are detected through the receptors of the juxtaglomerular complex.

Renin release causes the production of *angiotensin II* through a series of steps (see Figure 72-5). Angiotensin II increases systemic blood pressure through powerful blood vessel constricting effects and stimulates the release of aldosterone from the adrenal cortex. Aldosterone increases the reabsorption of sodium in the distal tubule of the nephron. Therefore more water is reabsorbed and blood pressure is increased because of increases in blood volume. When renal blood flow is reduced, this renin-angiotensin-aldosterone system of blood pressure control regulates pressures in the nephron as well as systemic blood pressure (see also Chapter 14).

PROSTAGLANDINS. Prostaglandins are produced in many tissues, including the kidney. Specific prostaglandins produced in the kidney are prostaglandin E_2 (PGE$_2$) and prostacyclin (PGI$_2$). These substances help regulate glomerular filtration, kidney vascular resistance, and renin production. PGE$_2$ acts on the distal tubule and collecting duct to increase sodium and water excretion.

BRADYKININ. The presence of angiotensin II, prostaglandins, and ADH stimulates the release of bradykinin in the kidney. **Bradykinin** dilates the afferent arteriole and increases capillary membrane permeability to some solutes. These actions maintain kidney blood flow and reabsorption even when other conditions cause systemic blood vessel constriction.

TABLE 72-3   Renal Hormone Production and Hormones Influencing Renal Function

	Site	Action
Renal Hormone Production		
Renin	Renin-producing granular cells	Raises blood pressure as result of angiotensin (local vasoconstriction) and aldosterone (volume expansion) secretion
Prostaglandins	Renal tissues	Regulate intrarenal blood flow by vasodilation or vasoconstriction
Bradykinins	Juxtaglomerular cells of the arterioles	Increase blood flow (vasodilation) and vascular permeability
Erythropoietin	Renal parenchyma	Stimulates bone marrow to make red blood cells
Activated vitamin D	Renal parenchyma	Promotes absorption of calcium in the gastrointestinal tract
Hormones Influencing Renal Function		
Antidiuretic hormone (ADH, vasopressin)	Released from posterior pituitary	Makes DCT and CD permeable to water to maximize reabsorption and produce a concentrated urine
Aldosterone	Released from adrenal cortex	Promotes sodium reabsorption and potassium secretion in DCT and CD; water and chloride follow sodium movement
Natriuretic hormones	Cardiac atria, brain	Cause tubular secretion of sodium

DCT, Distal convoluted tubule; *CD*, collecting ducts.

ERYTHROPOIETIN. Erythropoietin is produced and released in response to decreased oxygen tension in the renal blood supply. Erythropoietin triggers red blood cell (RBC) production in the bone marrow. When kidney tissue is nonfunctional, erythropoietin production decreases and the person becomes anemic.

VITAMIN D ACTIVATION. A series of steps are needed for vitamin D, a hormone, to become active. Some of these steps take place in the skin when it is exposed to ultraviolet light and then more processing occurs in the liver. From there, vitamin D is converted to its active form (1,25-dihydroxy-cholecalciferol) in the kidney. Activated vitamin D is needed to absorb calcium in the intestinal tract and to regulate calcium balance.

ers

re

as a single ureter, a hollow tube that connects
ith the urinary bladder. The ureter is about
diameter and about 12 to 18 inches (30

reter narrows in three areas:
the ureter, at the point at which
s the ureter, is a narrowing
junction (UPJ).

ends toward the abdom-

enters the bladder;
junction (UVJ).

short distance
gure 72-9).
mucous
uscle
ver

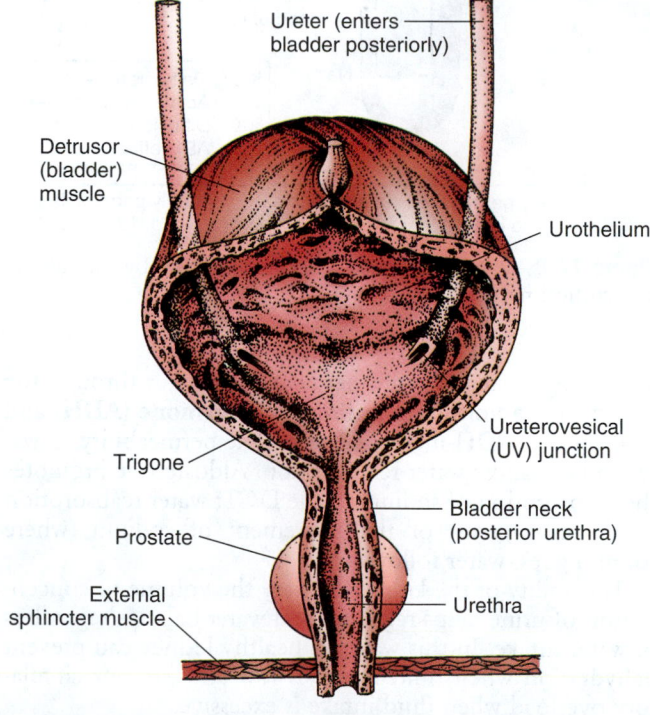

Figure 72-9 ■ Gross anatomy of the urinary bladder.

Labels: Ureter (enters bladder posteriorly); Detrusor (bladder) muscle; Urothelium; Trigone; Ureterovesical (UV) junction; Prostate; Bladder neck (posterior urethra); External sphincter muscle; Urethra

muscle fibers is controlled by several nerve pathways from the lower spinal cord.

Function

Contractions of the smooth muscle in the ureter move urine from the renal pelvis of the kidney to the bladder. Stretch receptors in the renal pelvis regulate this movement. For example, a large volume of urine in the renal pelvis triggers the stretch receptors, which respond by increasing ureteral contractions and peristalsis.

Urinary Bladder

Structure

The urinary bladder is a muscular sac. The upper surface lies next to the peritoneal cavity. In men, the bladder is in front of the rectum. In women, the bladder is in front of the vagina. The bladder lies directly behind the pubic bone.

The bladder is composed of the **body** (the rounded sac portion) and the **bladder neck** (posterior urethra), which connects to the bladder body. The bladder has three linings, an inner lining of epithelial cells (**urothelium**), middle layers of smooth muscle (**detrusor muscle**), and an outer lining. The **trigone** is an area on the posterior wall between the points of ureteral entry (ureterovesical junctions [UVJs]) and the urethra.

The **internal urethral sphincter** is the smooth detrusor muscle of the bladder neck and elastic tissue. The **external urethral sphincter** is skeletal muscle that surrounds the urethra.

In men, the external sphincter surrounds the urethra at the base of the prostate gland. In women, the external sphincter is at the base of the bladder. The pudendal nerve from the spinal cord controls the external sphincter.

Function

The bladder is a temporary urine storage site. The bladder also provides continence and enables voiding. The secretions of the bladder lining resist bacteria.

Continence is the ability to voluntarily control bladder emptying. Bladder continence occurs during bladder filling through the combination of detrusor muscle relaxation, internal sphincter muscle tone, and external sphincter contraction. As the bladder fills with urine, stretch sensations are transmitted to spinal sacral nerves S2 and S3.

MAINTAINING CONTINENCE

Continence is maintained by the interaction of the nerves that control the muscles of the bladder, bladder neck, urethra, and pelvic floor, as well as by factors that close the urethra. During bladder filling, the sympathetic nervous system fibers prevent detrusor muscle contraction. These control centers are located in the cerebral cortex, the brainstem, and the sacral part of the spinal cord. For urethral closure to be adequate for continence, the mucosal surfaces must be in contact and must be adhesive. Contact depends on the presence and proper function of the involved nerves and muscles. Adhesion depends on the adequate secretion of mucus-like substances.

MICTURITION

Micturition (voiding) is a reflex of autonomic control that triggers contraction of the detrusor muscle at the same time as relaxation of the external sphincter and the muscles of the pelvic floor. With detrusor muscle contraction, the UVJ of the ureter closes, and the normally round bladder assumes the shape of a funnel. Voiding is a voluntary act as the result of a learned response and is controlled by the cerebral cortex and the brainstem. Contraction of the external sphincter inhibits the micturition reflex and prevents voiding.

Urethra

Structure

The urethra is a narrow tube lined with mucous membranes and epithelial cells. The **urethral meatus,** or opening, is the end point of the urethra. In men, the urethra is about 6 to 8 inches (15 to 20 cm) long, with the meatus located at the tip of the penis. The male urethra has three sections:

- The prostatic urethra, which extends from the bladder to the prostate gland
- The membranous urethra, which extends to the wall of the pelvic floor
- The cavernous urethra, which is external and extends through the length of the penis

In women, the urethra is about 1 to 1.5 inches (2.5 to 3.75 cm) long and exits the bladder through the pelvic floor. The meatus lies slightly below the clitoris and directly in front of the vagina and rectum.

Function

The urethra is a tube for eliminating urine from the body. The passing of urine normally removes bacteria from the urethra.

Renal/Urinary System Changes Associated with Aging

RENAL CHANGES

Structural and functional changes occur in the kidney as a result of the aging process. These changes often have clinical significance. The kidney loses cortical tissue and gets smaller by 80 years of age. This cortical loss is caused by reduced renal blood flow. The medulla is not affected by aging, and the juxtamedullary nephron functions are preserved. However, the glomerular and tubular basement membranes thicken, reducing filtrating ability. Both the number of glomeruli and their surface areas decrease with aging. Tubule length also decreases.

Kidney function also changes with aging (Chart 72-1). Blood flow to the kidney decreases by about 10% per decade as blood vessels thicken. Glomerular filtration rate (GFR) decreases with age, especially after 45 years of age. By age 65, the GFR is about 65 mL/min (half the rate in a young adult). This decline is more rapid in clients with diabetes or hypertension.

Tubular changes with aging decrease the ability to concentrate urine, resulting in **nocturnal polyuria** (increased urination at night). The excretion and regulation of sodium, acids, and bicarbonate remain effective but are less efficient. Along with an age-related impairment in the thirst mechanism, these changes increase the risk for dehydration and **hypernatremia** (increased blood sodium levels) in the older adult (Brenner, 2000). Hormonal changes include a decrease in renin secretion, aldosterone levels, and activation of vitamin D.

CULTURAL CONSIDERATIONS

African Americans have more rapid age-related decreases in GFR than do white individuals (Brenner, 2000). The renal excretion of sodium is less effective in hypertensive African Americans who have high sodium intake, and the kidneys have about 20% less blood flow as a result of anatomic changes in small renal ves-

Continued

CHART 72-1

NURSING FOCUS on the OLDER ADULT
Changes in the Renal/Urinary System Related to Aging

Physiologic Change	Nursing Interventions	Rationales
Decreased glomerular filtration rate (GFR)	Monitor hydration status.	With aging, the ability of the kidneys to regulate water balance is decreased.
	Ensure adequate fluid intake.	The kidneys are less able to conserve water when necessary.
	Administer potentially nephrotoxic agents or drugs carefully.	Dehydration results in decreased renal blood flow and increases the nephrotoxic potential of many agents. Acute or chronic renal failure may result.
Nocturia	Ensure adequate nighttime lighting and a hazard-free environment.	Nocturia may occur from decreased renal concentrating ability associated with aging.
	Ensure the availability of a toilet, bedpan, or urinal.	The desire to maintain continence prompts individuals to seek the bathroom. Falls and injuries are common among older clients seeking bathroom facilities.
	Discourage excessive fluid intake for 2-4 hr before the client retires for the evening.	Excessive fluid intake at nighttime may increase nocturia.
	Evaluate medications and timing.	Some drugs increase urine output.
Decreased bladder capacity	Encourage the client to use the toilet, bedpan, or urinal at least q2h.	By emptying the bladder on a regular basis, urinary incontinence from overflow may be avoided.
	Respond as soon as possible to the client's indication of the need to void.	
Weakened urinary sphincter muscles and shortened urethra in women	Respond as soon as possible to the client's indication of the need to void.	A quick response may alleviate episodes of urinary stress incontinence.
	Provide thorough perineal care after each voiding.	The shortened urethra increases the potential for bladder infections.
		Good perineal hygiene may prevent skin irritations and urinary tract infection (UTI).
Tendency to retain urine	Observe the client for urinary retention (e.g., bladder distention) or urinary tract infection (e.g., dysuria, foul odor, confusion).	Urinary stasis may result in a UTI. UTIs may become bloodstream infections, resulting in septicemia or septic shock.
	Provide privacy, assistance, and voiding stimulants such as warm water over the perineum as needed.	Nursing interventions can help to initiate voiding.
	Evaluate medications for possible contribution to retention.	Anticholinergic drugs promote urinary retention.

sels and intrarenal responses to renin (Price et al., 2001; Shulman & Hall, 1991). Thus African American clients are at greater risk for renal failure than are white clients. Yearly health examinations should include urinalysis and checking for the presence of microalbuminuria.

URINARY CHANGES

Changes in the detrusor muscle elasticity lead to decreased bladder capacity and reduced ability to retain urine. The urge to void may cause immediate bladder emptying because the urinary sphincters lose muscle tone and often become weaker with age. In women, weakened muscles shorten the urethra and promote incontinence. In men, an enlarged prostate gland makes starting the urine stream difficult and may cause urinary retention.

ASSESSMENT TECHNIQUES

History

One way to assess renal and urologic function is to use Gordon's Functional Health Patterns (Gordon, 2002). The pat-

terns most related to the renal system are Nutritional/Metabolic and Elimination (Chart 72-2).

FAMILY HISTORY AND GENETIC RISK

The family history of the client with a suspected kidney or urologic problem is important because some disorders have a familial inheritance pattern. Ask the client whether his or her siblings, parents, parents' siblings, or grandparents have had renal problems. Past terms used for kidney disease include Bright's disease, nephritis, and nephrosis. Clients may use these terms to describe kidney disease as it was known by their parents or grandparents years ago. Adult polycystic kidney disease can occur in clients of either gender.

DEMOGRAPHIC DATA AND PERSONAL HISTORY

Age, gender, race, and ethnicity are important to assess in the client with any renal or urinary problem. A sudden onset of hypertension in clients older than 50 years of age suggests possible kidney disease. Clinical changes with adult polycystic kidney disease typically occur in clients in their

CHART 72-2

Renal/Urinary Assessment
USING GORDON'S FUNCTIONAL HEALTH PATTERNS

Nutritional/Metabolic Pattern
- What is your typical daily food intake? Describe a day's meals, snacks, and vitamins.
- How much salt do you typically add to your food? Do you use salt substitutes?
- How is your appetite?
- Have you experienced any nausea or vomiting?
- What is your typical daily fluid intake?
- What types of fluids do you drink (water, juices, soft drinks, coffee, tea)?
- How much fluid do you drink each day?
- Have you had any recent change in your weight? Weight gain? Weight loss? How much?
- Have you noticed a change in the tightness of your rings or shoes? Tighter? Looser?
- Have you noticed any skin changes lately? More dry? Less dry? Itchy?

Elimination Pattern
- What is your usual bowel elimination pattern? Frequency? Character? Discomfort? Laxatives?
- What is your usual urinary elimination pattern? Frequency? Amount? Color? Odor? Control?
- Have you noticed a change in the amount of urine?
- Do you have any problem with excessive perspiration?
- Do you have any other type of drainage?

Based on Gordon, M. (2002). *Manual of nursing diagnosis* (10th ed.). St. Louis: Mosby.

40s or 50s. In men older than 50 years of age, altered urine patterns accompany prostate disease.

Anatomic gender differences make some disorders worse or more common. For example, men rarely have urinary tract infections unless there are abnormalities, such as ureteral reflux or prostatic enlargement. Women have a shorter urethra and more commonly develop **cystitis** (bladder infection) because bacteria pass more readily into the bladder.

Ask the client about any previous renal or urologic problems, including tumors, infections, stones, or urologic surgery. A history of any chronic health problems, such as diabetes mellitus or hypertension, increases the risk for development of renal disease.

Identify all of the client's prescription drugs. Ask the client about the duration of drug use and whether there have been any recent changes in prescribed drugs. Drugs for diabetes mellitus, hypertension, cardiac disorders, hormonal disorders, cancer, arthritis, and psychiatric disorders are potential causes of renal dysfunction. Antibiotics, such as gentamicin (Garamycin, Cidomycin✶), may also cause sudden renal dysfunction.

Explore the use of over-the-counter (OTC) drugs or agents, including vitamin and mineral supplements and replacements, laxatives, analgesics, and nonsteroidal anti-inflammatory drugs (NSAIDs). Many of these drugs affect renal function. The long-term use of NSAIDs can seriously reduce renal function.

Ask the client about chemical exposures at the work place or with hobbies. Exposure to hydrocarbons (e.g., gasoline, oil), heavy metals (mercury, lead), and some gases (e.g., chlorine, toluene) can impair kidney function.

Specifically ask the client whether he or she has ever been told about the presence of protein or albumin in the urine. The question "Have you ever been told that your blood pressure is high?" may prompt a different response than "Do you have high blood pressure?" Ask women about health problems during pregnancy (e.g., proteinuria, high blood pressure, gestational diabetes, and urinary tract infections). Obtain information about the following:

- Chemical or environmental toxin exposure in occupational or other settings
- Recent travel to geographic regions that pose infectious disease risks
- Recent physical injuries
- Trauma
- Sexual contacts
- A history of altered patterns of urinary elimination

DIET HISTORY

Ask the client with known or suspected renal or urologic disorders about his or her usual diet and any recent changes in the diet. Note any excessive intake or omission of certain food categories. Ask about food and fluid intake. If the client has followed a diet for weight reduction, the details of the diet plan are important. A high-protein intake can result in temporary renal problems. Clients at risk for **calculi** (stone) formation who ingest large amounts of calcium-containing foods or have a poor fluid intake may form new stones.

Ask about any change in appetite or in the ability to discriminate tastes. These symptoms can occur with the accumulation of nitrogenous waste products from renal failure. Changes in thirst or fluid intake may also cause changes in urine output. Endocrine disorders may also cause changes in thirst, fluid intake, and urine output (see Chapter 65).

SOCIOECONOMIC STATUS

The client's socioeconomic status may influence health care practices. People with limited income or no health insurance often ignore physical problems or delay seeking health care because they lack the funds to pay for tests or treatment. They may also have difficulty following medical advice, having prescriptions filled, and keeping follow-up appointments.

Educational level may affect health-seeking practices and the client's understanding of a disease or its symptoms. Recurring urinary tract infections often result from inadequate or incomplete treatment, including lack of follow-up to ensure eradication. The lack of money to pay for antibiotics or nutritious foods may inhibit or delay recovery.

The client's health beliefs affect the approach to health and illness. Cultural background or religious affiliation may influence the belief system.

The language used by clients may be different from that used by the health care professional. Anatomic or medical terms may have no meaning for the client (Table 72-4). When obtaining a history, listen to and explore the terms used by the client. By using the client's own terms, you may help him or her to provide a more complete description of the problem. This technique may increase the amount of information obtained and decrease the client's discomfort when discussing bodily functions.

CURRENT HEALTH PROBLEM

The effects of renal failure result in changes in all body systems. Therefore document all of the client's current health problems. Encourage the client to describe all

TABLE 72-4 Commonly Used Renal and Urinary Terms

anuria Total urine output of less than 100 mL in 24 hours

azotemia Increased blood urea nitrogen and serum creatinine levels suggestive of renal impairment but without outward symptoms of renal failure

dysuria Discomfort or pain associated with micturition

frequency Feeling the need to void often, usually voiding small amounts of urine each time; may void every hour or even more frequently than hourly

hesitancy Difficulty in initiating the flow of urine, even when the bladder has sufficient urine to initiate a void and the sensation of the need to void is present

micturition The act of voiding

nocturia Awakening prematurely from sleep because of the need to empty the bladder

oliguria Decreased urine output; total urine output between 100 and 400 mL in 24 hours

polyuria Increased urine output; total urine output usually greater than 2000 mL in 24 hours

uremia Full-blown manifestations of renal failure; sometimes referred to as the uremic syndrome, especially if the cause of the renal failure is unknown

urgency A sudden onset of the feeling of the need to void immediately; may result in incontinence if the client is unable to locate or get to toileting facilities quickly

health concerns, because some renal disorders cause systemic problems or problems in other body systems. Recent upper respiratory problems, generalized muscle and joint pain, or gastrointestinal (GI) problems may be related to problems of kidney function.

Assess the kidney and urologic system specifically. Ask the client about any changes in the appearance (color, odor, clarity) of the urine, pattern of urination, ability to initiate or control voiding, and other unusual symptoms. Urine that is reddish, dark brown or black, greenish, or otherwise different from the usual yellowish, straw color usually prompts the client to seek health care assistance. Urine typically has a mild but distinct odor of ammonia. An increase in the intensity of color, a change in odor quality, or a decrease in urine clarity may suggest infection.

Ask the client about changes in urination patterns, such as **nocturia** (urination at night), frequency, or an increase or decrease in the amount of urine. The normal urine output for adults is 1 mL/kg/hr, or about 1500 to 2000 mL/day. The client usually does not know the exact amount of urine produced; a bladder diary may provide useful data. Also ask the following:

- If the client has difficulty initiating urine flow
- If a burning sensation or other discomfort occurs with urination
- If the force of the urine stream is decreased (in men)

Ask about any loss of urinary continence, especially when coughing, sneezing, or laughing. Clients may also report a persistent dribbling of urine.

The onset of pain in the flank, in the lower abdomen or pelvic region, or in the perineal area is often of great concern and usually prompts the client to seek assistance. Ask about the onset, intensity, and duration of the pain, its location, and its association with any activity or event.

Pain associated with renal or ureteral irritation is often severe and spasmodic. Pain that radiates into the perineal area, groin, scrotum, or labia is described as **renal colic.** Renal colic pain occurs with distention or spasm of the ureter,

such as in an obstruction or the passing of a stone. Renal colic pain may be intermittent or continuous and may be accompanied by pallor, diaphoresis, and hypotension. These general symptoms occur because of the location of the nerve tracts near or in the kidneys and ureters.

Because the kidneys are close to the GI organs and the nerve pathways are similar, GI manifestations may be part of the presenting history. These **renointestinal reflexes** often complicate the description of the renal problem.

Uremia results from the accumulation of nitrogenous waste products in the blood, a result of renal failure. Manifestations include anorexia, nausea and vomiting, muscle cramps, **pruritus** (itching), fatigue, and lethargy.

Physical Assessment

The physical assessment of the client with a known or suspected renal or urologic disorder includes general appearance, a general review of body systems, and specific structure and functions of the renal/urinary systems.

Assess the general appearance of the client and check for a yellowish skin color and the presence of any rashes, bruising, or other discoloration. The skin and tissues may show edema, which with renal disorders may be detected in the **pedal** (foot), **pretibial** (shin), sacral tissues, and around the eyes. Auscultate the lungs to determine whether fluid is present. Weigh the client and take his or her blood pressure as a baseline for later comparisons.

Assess the client's level of consciousness and level of alertness, recording any deficits in concentration, thought processes, or memory. Family members may report subtle changes. Such cognitive changes may be the result of accumulated waste products when renal disease is present.

ASSESSMENT OF THE KIDNEYS, URETERS, AND BLADDER

Assess the kidneys, ureters, and bladder during an abdominal assessment. Auscultate before percussion and palpation because these activities can enhance bowel sounds and obscure abdominal vascular sounds.

Inspection

Inspect the abdomen and the flank regions with the client in both the supine and the sitting position. Observe the client for asymmetry (e.g., swelling) or discoloration (e.g., bruising or redness) in the flank region, especially in the area of the **costovertebral angle (CVA).** The CVA is located between the lower portion of the twelfth rib and the vertebral column.

Auscultation

Listen for a bruit over each renal artery on the midclavicular line. A **bruit** is an audible swishing sound produced when the volume of blood or the diameter of the blood vessel changes. A bruit often occurs with blood flow through a narrowed vessel, as in renal artery stenosis.

Palpation

Renal palpation can help locate masses and areas of tenderness in or around the kidney. Lightly palpate the abdomen in all quadrants. Ask about areas of tenderness or discom-

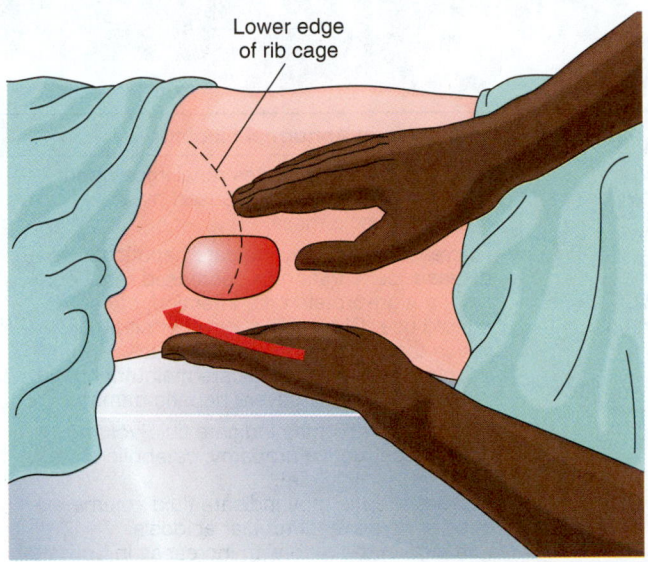

Lower edge of rib cage

Figure 72-10 ■ Advanced technique for palpation of the kidney.

fort and examine nontender areas first. The outline of the bladder may be seen as high as the umbilicus in clients with severe bladder distention. Special training and practice under the guidance of a qualified practitioner are necessary; therefore appropriate education is essential before attempting the procedure. If tumor or aneurysm is suspected, palpation may harm the client.

Because the kidneys are located deep and posterior, palpation is easier in thin clients who have little abdominal musculature. For palpation of the right kidney, the client assumes a supine position while you place one hand under the right flank and the other hand over the abdomen below the lower right part of the rib cage. Use the lower hand to raise the flank, and the upper hand to depress the abdomen as the client takes a deep breath (Figure 72-10). The left kidney is deeper and rarely palpable. A transplanted kidney is readily palpable in either the lower right or left abdominal quadrant. The kidney should feel smooth, firm, and nontender.

Percussion

A distended bladder sounds dull when percussed. After gently palpating to determine the outline of the distended bladder, begin percussion on the lower abdomen and continue in the direction of the umbilicus until dull sounds are no longer produced.

If the client identifies flank pain or tenderness, percuss the nontender flank first. Have the client assume a sitting, side-lying, or supine position, and then form one of your hands into a clenched fist. Place your other hand flat over the CVA of the client. Then quickly deliver a firm thump to your hand over the CVA area. Costovertebral tenderness often occurs with kidney infection or inflammation. Clients with inflammation or infection in the kidney or adjacent structures may describe their pain as severe or as a constant, dull ache.

ASSESSMENT OF THE URETHRA

Using a good light source and wearing gloves, inspect the urethra by examining the meatus and surrounding tissues. Record any unusual discharge such as blood, mucus, or purulent drainage. Inspect the skin and mucous membranes of

surrounding tissues, documenting the presence of lesions, rashes, or other abnormalities of the penis or scrotum or of the labia or vaginal opening. Urethral irritation is suspected when the client reports discomfort with urination.

Psychosocial Assessment

Concerns about the urologic system may evoke fear, anger, embarrassment, anxiety, guilt, or sadness in the client. Childhood learning often includes privacy with regard to urination habits. Urologic disorders may bring up forgotten memories of difficult toilet training and bedwetting or of childhood experiences of exploring one's body. The client may ignore symptoms or delay seeking health care because of emotional responses or cultural taboos about the urogenital area.

> ### ? Critical Thinking Challenge
>
> The client is a 67-year-old woman who has a change in mental status: she is lethargic and, when roused, not clearly able to state the correct place or time. Her daughter, with whom the client lives because of limited mobility due to rheumatoid arthritis, states that her mom was able to take care of herself and was quite alert 3 days ago. Since then she had a 2-day episode of "stomach flu" and this morning was not able to get out of bed, becoming increasingly confused. She has not voided for 24 hours. This woman is about 5 feet tall and weighs 95 pounds. The admitting diagnosis indicates that this woman is dehydrated, leading to decreased cerebral perfusion and mental status changes.
>
> 1. What personal or demographic data should you obtain?
> 2. How would you proceed in gathering physical assessment data?
> 3. Given this client's health problems, what drugs might she be taking that could affect kidney function or her hydration status?

evolve For suggested answer guidelines, go to http://evolve.elsevier.com/Iggy/.

Diagnostic Assessment
LABORATORY TESTS
Blood Tests
SERUM CREATININE

Serum creatinine is an end product of muscle and protein metabolism. Creatinine is filtered by the kidneys and excreted in the urine. Because muscle mass and metabolism are usually constant, the serum creatinine level is a good indicator of kidney function. Normal serum creatinine levels vary with age, gender, and body muscle mass. The normal serum creatinine level is slightly higher in men than in women (Chart 72-3). In general, men have a larger muscle mass than do women, but there are exceptions. Muscle mass and the amount of creatinine produced decrease with age. Because of decreased rates of creatinine clearance, however, the serum creatinine level remains relatively constant in older adults unless renal disease is present.

No common pathologic condition other than renal disease increases the serum creatinine level. The serum creatinine level does not increase until at least 50% of the renal function is lost, and therefore *any* elevation of serum creatinine values is important.

LABORATORY PROFILE
Renal Function Blood Studies

Test	Normal Range for Adults	Significance of Abnormal Findings
Serum creatinine	*Males:* 0.6-1.2 mg/dL (53-106 mmol/L) *Females:* 0.5-1.1 mg/dL (44-97 mmol/L) *Older adults:* may be decreased	An *increased level* indicates renal impairment. A *decreased level* may be caused by a decreased muscle mass.
Blood urea nitrogen (BUN)	10-20 mg/dL (3.6-7.1 mmol/L) *Older adults:* 60-90 yr: 8-23 mg/dL (2.9-8.2 mmol/L) Over 90 yr: 10-31 mg/dL (3.6-11.1 mmol/L)	An *increased level* may indicate hepatic or renal disease, dehydration or decreased renal perfusion, a high-protein diet, infection, stress, steroid use, GI bleeding, or other situations in which there is blood in body tissues. A *decreased level* may indicate malnutrition, fluid volume excess, or severe hepatic damage.
BUN/creatinine ratio	Mass ratio: 12:1 to 20:1 Mole ratio: 48.5:1 to 80.8:1	An *increased ratio* may indicate fluid volume deficit, obstructive uropathy, catabolic state, or a high-protein diet. A *decreased ratio* may indicate fluid volume excess or acute renal tubular acidosis. *No change* in the ratio with increases in both the BUN and creatinine levels indicates renal impairment.

Data from Pagana, K.D., & Pagana, T.J. (2002). *Mosby's manual of diagnostic and laboratory tests* (2nd ed.). St. Louis: Mosby.
GI, Gastrointestinal.

BLOOD UREA NITROGEN

Blood urea nitrogen (BUN) measures the renal excretion of urea nitrogen, a by-product of protein metabolism in the liver. Urea nitrogen is mostly produced from liver metabolism of food sources of protein. The kidneys filter urea nitrogen from the blood and excrete the nitrogenous waste in urine. BUN levels indicate the extent of renal clearance of this nitrogenous waste product.

Other factors influence the BUN level, and an elevation does not always mean renal disease is present (see Chart 72-3). For example, rapid cell destruction from infection or steroid therapy may elevate BUN level. In addition, blood is a protein. Blood in the tissues rather than in the blood vessels is reabsorbed as if it were a general protein. Thus reabsorbed blood protein is processed by the liver and increases BUN levels. This means that injured tissues can result in increased BUN levels even when kidney function is normal.

The liver must function properly to produce urea nitrogen. When liver and kidney dysfunction are both present, urea nitrogen levels are actually decreased because the liver failure limits urea production. The BUN level is not always elevated with kidney disease and is not the best indicator of kidney function. However, an elevated BUN level is highly *suggestive* of kidney dysfunction.

RATIO OF BLOOD UREA NITROGEN TO SERUM CREATININE

The BUN/creatinine ratio can help determine whether nonrenal factors, such as dehydration or poor renal perfusion, are causing the elevated BUN level rather than kidney damage. When blood volume is deficient (dehydration) or blood pressure is low, the BUN level rises more rapidly than the serum creatinine level. As a result, the ratio of BUN to creatinine is *increased*.

When both the BUN and serum creatinine levels increase at the same rate, the BUN/creatinine ratio remains normal. However, the elevated serum creatinine and BUN

levels suggest renal dysfunction that is not related to dehydration or poor perfusion.

Urine Tests

URINALYSIS

Urinalysis is a part of any complete physical examination but is particularly useful for clients with suspected kidney or urologic disorders (Chart 72-4). Ideally, the urine specimen is collected at the morning's first voiding. Specimens obtained at other times may not be adequately concentrated. The specimen may be collected by several techniques (Table 72-5).

COLOR, ODOR, AND TURBIDITY. Urine color comes from urochrome pigment. Color variations may result from increased levels of urochrome or other pigments, changes in the concentration or dilution of the urine, and the presence of drug metabolites in the urine. Urine smells faintly like ammonia and is normally clear without **turbidity** (cloudiness) or haziness.

SPECIFIC GRAVITY. The specific gravity of urine is density of urine compared to water. Density is related to the number of particles in a specific volume of urine. The specific gravity of urine ranges from 1.000 (the specific gravity of water) to greater than 1.035. In kidney disease, changes in specific gravity do not reflect systemic fluid volume. For example, dilute urine with a low specific gravity may occur in a dehydrated client who has a lack of nephron receptors for antidiuretic hormone (ADH).

An *increase* in specific gravity occurs with dehydration, decreased kidney perfusion, or the presence of ADH. (ADH production is normally increased with stress, surgery, anesthetic agents, and certain drugs such as morphine and oral antidiabetic agents.) In these situations the normal kidney response is to reabsorb water and decrease urine output. As a result, the urine produced is more concentrated.

A *decrease* in specific gravity occurs with increased fluid intake, diuretic administration, and diabetes insipidus. In

CHART 72-4

LABORATORY PROFILE
Urinalysis

Test	Normal Range for Adults	Significance of Abnormal Findings
Color	Pale yellow	*Dark amber* indicates concentrated urine. *Very pale yellow* indicates dilute urine. *Dark red or brown* indicates blood in the urine; brown also may indicate increased urinary bilirubin level, red may also indicate the presence of myoglobin. *Other color changes* may result from diet or medications.
Odor	Specific aromatic odor, similar to ammonia	*Foul smell* indicates possible infection, dehydration, or ingestion of certain foods or drugs.
Turbidity	Clear	*Cloudy urine* indicates infection, sediment, or high levels of urinary protein.
Specific gravity	Usually 1.005-1.030; possible range 1.000-1.030 (after 12-hr fluid restriction, >1.025) *Older adult*: Decreased because of decreased concentrating ability	*Increased* in decreased renal perfusion, inappropriate antidiuretic hormone secretion, or congestive heart failure. *Decreased* in chronic renal insufficiency, diabetes insipidus, malignant hypertension, diuretic administration, and lithium toxicity.
pH	Average: 6; possible range: 4.6-8	*Changes* are caused by diet, the administration of medications, infection, freshness of the specimen, acid-base imbalance, and altered renal function.
Glucose	<0.5 g/day (<2.78 mmol/L)	*Presence* reflects hyperglycemia or a decrease in the renal threshold for glucose.
Ketones	None	*Presence* reflects incomplete metabolism of fatty acids, as in diabetic ketoacidosis, prolonged fasting, anorexia nervosa.
Protein	0.8 mg/dL	*Increased amounts* may indicate stress, infection, recent strenuous exercise, or glomerular disorders.
Bilirubin (urobilinogen)	None	*Presence* suggests hepatic or biliary disease or obstruction.
Red blood cells (RBCs)	0-2 per high-power field	*Increased* amounts are normal with indwelling or intermittent catheterization or menses but may reflect tumor, stones, trauma, glomerular disorders, cystitis, or bleeding disorders.
White blood cells (WBCs)	*Males:* 0-3 per high-power field *Females:* 0-5 per high-power field	*Increased* amounts may indicate an infectious or inflammatory process anywhere in the renal/urinary tract, renal transplant rejection, fever, or exercise.
Casts	A few or none, composed of RBC or WBC, protein or tubular cell casts	*Increased amounts* indicate the presence of bacteria or protein, which is seen in severe renal disease and could also indicate urinary calculi.
Crystals	None	*Presence* of normal or abnormal crystals may indicate that the specimen has been allowed to stand.
Bacteria	<1000 colonies/mL	*Increased amounts* indicate the need for urine culture to determine the presence of urinary tract infection.
Parasites	None	*Presence* of *Trichomonas vaginalis* indicates infection, usually of the urethra, prostate, or vagina.
Leukoesterase	None	*Presence* suggests urinary tract infection
Nitrites	None	*Presence* suggests bacteria, usually *Escherichia coli*.

these situations, the normal kidney response is to excrete more water; thus urine output is increased. In kidney disease, the specific gravity decreases because the damaged kidneys reabsorb less water. The specific gravity does not vary with changes in plasma osmolarity (e.g., it becomes fixed).

pH. A pH value less than 7 is acidic, and a value greater than 7 is alkaline. Many factors influence urine acidity or alkalinity. A diet high in certain fruits and vegetables results in a more alkaline urine, whereas a high-protein diet produces a more acidic urine. The presence of *Escherichia coli* in the urine also results in an acidic urine.

Urine specimens become more alkaline when left standing unrefrigerated for more than 1 hour, if bacteria are present, or if a specimen is left uncovered. Alkaline urine increases cell breakdown; thus the presence of red blood cells may be missed on analysis. Ensure that urine specimens are

covered and delivered to the laboratory promptly or refrigerated. During acidosis or alkalosis, the kidneys, along with blood buffers and the lungs, normally respond to keep serum pH normal. Chapters 18 and 19 discuss acid-base balance and imbalance.

GLUCOSE. Glucose is filtered by the glomerulus and is reabsorbed in the proximal tubule of the nephron. When the blood glucose level rises above 220 mg/dL, the renal threshold for reabsorption is exceeded, and some glucose is present in the urine. Changes in the renal threshold for glucose occur in many clients, such as those with infection or those with long-standing diabetes mellitus. It is possible that their serum glucose level may be high (e.g., greater than 400 mg/dL), and glucose may still not be present in the urine.

KETONE BODIES. Ketone bodies are by-products of the incomplete metabolism of fatty acids. Three types of

TABLE 72-5 Collection of Urine Specimens

Nursing Interventions	Rationales
Voided Urine	
Collect the first specimen voided in the morning.	Urine is more concentrated in the early morning.
Send the specimen to the laboratory as soon as possible.	After urine is collected, cellular breakdown results in more alkaline urine.
Refrigerate the specimen if a delay is unavoidable.	Refrigeration delays the alkalinization of urine. Bacteria are more likely to multiply in an alkaline environment.
Clean-Catch Specimen	
Explain the purpose of the procedure to the client.	Correct technique is needed to obtain a valid specimen.
Instruct the client to self-clean before voiding.	Surface cleaning is necessary to remove secretions or bacteria from the urethral meatus.
Instruct the female client to separate the labia and use the sponges and solution provided to wipe with three strokes over the urethra. The first two wiping strokes are over each side of the urethra; the third wiping stroke is centered over the urethra (from front to back).	
Instruct the male client to retract the foreskin of the penis and to similarly clean the urethra, using three wiping strokes with the sponge and solution provided (from the head of the penis downward).	
Instruct the client to initiate voiding after cleaning. The client then stops and resumes voiding into the container. Only 1 ounce (30 mL) is needed; the remainder of the urine may be discarded into the commode.	A midstream collection further removes secretions and bacteria because urine flushes the distal portion of the internal urethra. An improperly collected specimen may result in inappropriate or incomplete treatment.
Ensure that the client understands the procedure.	The client's understanding and the nurse's assistance ensure proper collection.
Assist the client as needed.	
Catheterized Specimen	
For non-indwelling (straight) catheters:	The one-time passage of a urinary catheter may be necessary to obtain an uncontaminated specimen for analysis or to measure the volume of residual urine.
Avoid routine use.	
Follow the facility's procedures for catheterization technique.	These procedures minimize bacterial entry.
For indwelling catheters:	Collection of urine from an indwelling catheter or tubing is performed when clients have catheters for continence or long-term urinary drainage.
Apply a clamp to the drainage tubing, distal to the injection port.	Clamping allows urine to collect in the tubing at the location where the specimen is obtained.
Clean the injection port cap of the catheter drainage tubing with an appropriate antiseptic. Povidone-iodine solution or alcohol is acceptable.	Surface contamination is prevented by following the cleaning procedures.
Insert a sterile 5-mL syringe into the port and aspirate the quantity of urine required.	A minimum of 5 mL is needed for culture and sensitivity (C&S) testing.
Inject the urine sample into a sterile specimen container.	A sterile container is used for C&S specimens.
Remove the clamp to resume drainage.	
Properly dispose of the syringe.	
24-Hour Urine Collection	
Instruct the client thoroughly.	A 24-hr collection of urine is necessary to quantify or calculate the rate of clearance of a particular substance.
Provide written materials to assist in instruction.	Instructional materials for clients, signs, and so on remind clients and staff to ensure that the total collection is completed.
Place signs appropriately.	
Inform all personnel or family caregivers of test in progress.	
Check laboratory or procedure manual on proper technique for maintaining the collection (e.g., on ice, in a refrigerator, or with a preservative).	Proper technique prevents breakdown of elements to be measured.
On initiation of the collection, ask the client to void, discard the urine, and note the time. If a Foley catheter is in use, empty the tubing and drainage bag at the start time and discard the urine.	Proper techniques ensure that *all* urine formed within the 24-hr period is collected.
Collect all urine of the next 24 hr.	
Twenty-four hours after initiation, ask the client to empty the bladder and add that urine to the container.	
Do not remove urine from the collection container for other specimens.	Urine in the container is not considered a "fresh" specimen and may be mixed with preservative.

ketone bodies are acetone, acetoacetic acid, and beta-hydroxybutyric acid. Normally there are no ketones in urine. Ketone bodies are produced when fat is used instead of glucose for cellular energy. Ketones present in the blood are partially excreted in the urine.

PROTEIN. Protein, such as albumin, is not normally present in the urine. Levels greater than 300 mg/24 hr, or 200 mcg/min, are abnormal. Protein molecules are too large to pass through intact glomerular membranes. When glomerular membrane permeability is increased, protein molecules pass through and are excreted in the urine. Increased membrane permeability is caused by infection, inflammation, or immunologic problems. Some systemic problems cause production of abnormal proteins, such as globulin. These proteins are not detected by routine urinalysis, and require electrophoresis or other tests for detection.

A random finding of proteinuria followed by a series of negative (normal) findings does not imply renal disease. If infection is the cause of the **proteinuria** (protein in the urine), urinalyses after elimination of the infection should be negative for protein. Persistent proteinuria needs further investigation.

Microalbuminuria is the presence of albumin in the urine that is not measurable by a urine dipstick or usual urinalysis procedures. Specialized assays are used to quickly analyze a freshly voided urine specimen for microscopic levels of albumin. The normal microalbumin levels in a freshly voided specimen should range between 2.0 and 20 mg/mmol for men and between 2.8 and 28 mg/mmol for women. Higher levels indicate microalbuminuria and could mean the presence of very early kidney disease, especially in clients with diabetes mellitus. In 24-hour urine specimens, levels of 30 to 300 mg/24 hr, or 20 to 200 mcg/min, indicate microalbuminuria.

LEUKOESTERASE. Leukoesterase is an enzyme found in some white blood cells, especially neutrophils. When the number of these cells increases in the urine or they are lysed, the urine will contain measurable amounts of leukoesterase. The presence of leukoesterase and nitrites in the urine is a sensitive screen for assessing urinary tract infections. A normal reading is no leukoesterase in the urine. A positive test (+ sign) indicates increasing leukocytes in the urine.

NITRITES. Urine does not usually contain nitrites. Many types of bacteria, when present in the urine, convert nitrates (normally found in urine) into nitrites. A positive finding is associated with urinary tract infection.

SEDIMENT. Urine sediment is precipitated particles in the urine. These particles include cells, casts, crystals, and bacteria.

CELLS. Normally, urine contains few, if any, cells. Types of cells abnormally present in the urine include tubular cells (from the tubule of the nephron), epithelial cells (from the lining of the urinary tract), red blood cells (RBCs), and white blood cells (WBCs).

CASTS. Casts are structures formed around other particles. There may be casts of cells, bacteria, or protein. When cells, bacteria, or proteins are present in the urine, minerals and gelatinous materials clump around them and form a cast. Casts are described by the type of particle they have surrounded (e.g., RBC cast, WBC cast, tubular epithelial cast) or the stage of cast breakdown. Casts are described as "granular" (coarse or fine) and "waxy."

CRYSTALS. Urine crystals come from various mineral salts. These minerals may be a result of diet, drugs, or disease. Common salt crystals are formed from calcium, oxalate, urea, phosphate, magnesium, or other substances. Some drugs, such as the sulfates, can also form crystals.

BACTERIA. Bacteria in a urine sample multiply quickly, so the specimen must be analyzed promptly. Normally urine is sterile, but is easily contaminated by perineal bacteria during collection.

URINE FOR CULTURE AND SENSITIVITY

Urine is analyzed for the number and types of organisms present. Manifestations of infection and unexplained bacteria in a urine specimen are indications for urine culture and sensitivity testing. Bacteria from urine are placed in a medium with different antibiotics to determine which drugs are effective in killing or stopping the growth of the bacteria (**sensitivity**). In this way we can know which antibiotics are effective in killing the organisms (organisms are "sensitive") and which are not effective (organisms are "resistant"). A clean-catch or catheter-derived specimen is best for culture and sensitivity testing.

COMPOSITE URINE COLLECTIONS

Some urine collections are made for a specified number of hours (e.g., 24 hours) for more quantitative analysis of one or more substances. These collections are often used to measure urine levels of creatinine or urea nitrogen, sodium, chloride, calcium, catecholamines, or other components (Chart 72-5). For a composite urine specimen, *all* urine within the designated time frame must be collected (see Table 72-5). If other voided or catheterized specimens must be obtained while the collection is in progress, measure and record the amount collected but not added to the timed collection.

The urine collection may need to be refrigerated or stored on ice to prevent changes in the urine during the collection time. Follow the procedure from the laboratory for urine storage. The urine collection must be free from fecal contamination. Menstrual blood and toilet tissue also contaminate the specimen and can invalidate the results.

The collection of urine for a 24-hour period is often more difficult than it seems. With hospitalized clients, the cooperation of staff personnel, the client, family members, and visitors is essential. Placing signs in the bathroom, instructing the client and family, and emphasizing the need to save the urine are helpful.

CREATININE CLEARANCE

Creatinine clearance is a calculated measure of glomerular filtration rate. It is the best indication of overall kidney function. The amount of creatinine cleared from the blood (e.g., filtered into the urine) is measured in the total volume of urine excreted in a defined period. A urine specimen for a creatinine clearance test is usually collected for 24 hours, but it can be collected for shorter periods (e.g., 8 or 12 hours). The calculation compares the urine creatinine level with the blood creatinine level, and therefore a blood specimen or creatinine must also be collected.

The laboratory or care provider calculates the creatinine clearance. The client's age, gender, height, weight, diet, and activity level influence the expected amount of creatinine to be excreted. Thus these factors are considered when interpreting creatinine clearance test results.

The following formula is used to calculate creatinine clearance:

$$\text{Creatinine clearance} = U \times V/P \times T$$

where U is creatinine in urine (mg/dL), V is volume of urine (mL/24 hr), P is creatinine in plasma or blood (mg/dL), and T is time (minutes).

The rate of creatinine clearance is expressed as milliliters per minute per square meter of body surface area. The range

CHART 72-5

LABORATORY PROFILE
24-Hour Urine Collections

Component	Normal Range for Adults	Significance of Abnormal Findings
Creatinine	0.8-2 g/24 hr *Males:* 1-2 g/24 hr or 14-26 mg/kg/24 hr (124-230 μmol/kg/24 hr or 7.1-17.7 mmol/24 hr) *Females:* 0.6-1.8 g/24 hr or 11-20 mg/kg/24 hr (97-177 μmol/kg/24 hr or 5.3-15.9 mmol/24 hr) *Older adults:* 10 mg/kg/24 hr (88.4 μmol/kg/24 hr) at 90 yr	*Decreased amounts* indicate a deterioration in renal function caused by renal disease, shock, hypovolemia, or any condition affecting muscle. *Increased amounts* occur with infections, exercise, diabetes mellitus, and meat meals.
Urea nitrogen	12-20 g/24 hr (0.43-0.71 mmol/24 hr)	*Decreased amounts* occur when renal damage or liver disease is present. *Increased amounts* commonly result from a high-protein diet, dehydration, trauma, or sepsis.
Sodium	40-220 mEq/24 hr (40-220 mmol/24 hr)	*Decreased amounts* are seen in hemorrhage, shock, hyperaldosteronism, and prerenal acute renal failure. *Increased amounts* are common with diuretic therapy, excessive salt intake, hypokalemia, and acute tubular necrosis.
Chloride	110-250 mEq/24 hr (110-250 mmol/24 hr) *Older adults:* 95-195 mEq/24 hr (95-195 mmol/24 hr)	*Decreased amounts* are seen in certain renal diseases, malabsorption syndrome, pyloric obstruction, prolonged nasogastric tube drainage, diarrhea, diaphoresis, heart failure, and emphysema. *Increased amounts* are seen with hypokalemia, adrenal insufficiency, and massive diuresis.
Calcium	100-400 mg/24 hr (2.50-7.50 mmol/kg/24 hr)	*Decreased amounts* are often associated with hypocalcemia, hypoparathyroidism, nephrosis, and nephritis. *Increased amounts* are commonly seen with calcium renal stones, hyperparathyroidism, sarcoidosis, certain cancers, immobilization, and hypercalcemia.
Total catecholamines*	<100 mcg/24 hr (<591 mmol/24 hr)	*Increased amounts* occur with pheochromocytoma, neuroblastomas, stress, or strenuous exercise.
Protein	1-14 mg/dL (10-140 mg/L) or 50-80 mg/24 hr at rest	*Increased amounts* indicate glomerular disease, nephrotic syndrome, diabetic nephropathy, urinary tract malignancies, and irritations.

*Epinephrine and norepinephrine only; dopamine is not measured.

for normal creatinine clearance is 90 to 139 mL/min for adult males and 80 to 125 mL/min for females.

Creatinine clearance values are used to determine the client's current kidney function. Decreases in the creatinine clearance rate may require reducing drug doses and often signifies the need to further explore the cause of kidney deterioration.

URINE ELECTROLYTES

Urine samples can be analyzed for electrolyte levels (e.g., sodium and chloride). Normally the amount of sodium excreted in the urine is nearly equal to that consumed. Urine sodium levels of less than 10 mEq/L indicate that the tubules are able to conserve (reabsorb) sodium.

OSMOLARITY

Osmolarity measures the concentration of particles in solution. The particles in urine contributing to osmolarity include electrolytes, glucose, urea, and creatinine.

BLOOD/PLASMA OSMOLARITY. The kidneys excrete or reabsorb water to keep blood osmolarity in the range of 285 to 295 mOsm/L. Osmolarity is slightly higher in older adults (285 to 301 mOsm/L). When blood osmolarity is decreased, the release of antidiuretic hormone (ADH) is inhibited. Without ADH, the distal tubule and collecting ducts are *not* permeable to water. As a result, water is *excreted*, not reabsorbed, and blood osmolarity increases. When blood osmolarity increases, ADH is released. ADH increases the permeability of the distal tubule to water. Then water is reabsorbed, and blood osmolarity decreases.

URINE OSMOLARITY. Urine osmolarity can vary from 50 to 1400 mOsm/L, depending on the client's hydration status and kidney function. With average fluid intake, the range for urine osmolarity is 300 to 900 mOsm/L. Electrolytes, acids, and other wastes of normal metabolism are continually produced. These particles are the solute load that must be excreted in the urine on a regular basis. This is referred to as *obligatory solute excretion*. If the client loses excessive fluids, the renal response is to save water while excreting wastes by excreting small amounts of highly concentrated urine. Diet, drugs, and activity can change urine osmolarity. Thus urine with an increased osmolarity is concentrated urine with less water and more solutes. Urine with a decreased osmolarity is dilute urine with more water and fewer solutes.

Bedside Sonography/Bladder Scanners

The use of portable ultrasound scanners in the hospital and rehabilitation setting by nurses is a noninvasive method of estimating bladder volume. Bladder scanners are used to screen clients for postvoid residual volumes and to determine the need for intermittent catheterization based on the amount of urine in the bladder rather than the time between catheterizations. The scan does not require client preparation beyond an explanation of what to expect. There is no discomfort associated with the scan.

PROCEDURE. Explain the rationale for the procedure and share information about sensations commonly experienced during the procedure. For example, "This test will measure the amount of urine in your bladder. I will place a gel pad just above your pubic area, then place the probe that is a little bigger and heavier than a stethoscope on the gel."

Before scanning, select the male or female icon on the bladder scanner. Using the female icon allows the scanner software to subtract the volume of the uterus from any measurement. Use the male icon on all men and any woman who has undergone a hysterectomy.

Place an ultrasound gel pad right above the symphysis pubis (pubic bone) or moisten the round dome of the scan head area with 5 mL of conducting gel to improve ultrasound conduction. Use conducting gel on the scanner head for obese clients and those with heavy body hair in the area to be scanned. Place the probe midline over the abdomen about 1.5 inches (4 cm) above the pubic bone. Aim the scan head so the ultrasound is projected toward the expected location of the bladder, typically toward the client's coccyx. Press and release the scan button; the scan is complete with the sound of a beep and a volume is displayed. Two readings are recommended for best accuracy. An aiming icon on the portable bladder scanner indicates whether the bladder image is centered on the crosshairs of the scan head. If the crosshairs on the aiming icon are not centered on the bladder, the measured volume may not be accurate.

? Critical Thinking Challenge

The 67-year-old client described earlier has the following vital signs and laboratory data: T 98.4; P 112, thready, slightly irregular; R 30 and shallow; BP 98/50; oxygen saturation 95%; serum potassium 2.9 mEq/L; serum sodium 151 mEq/L; hematocrit 47%.
1. Which of these data support a diagnosis of dehydration?
2. What alterations in BUN, and creatinine do you anticipate?
3. What findings in a urinalysis would suggest a urinary tract infection?

evolve For suggested answer guidelines, go to http://evolve.elsevier.com/Iggy/.

RADIOGRAPHIC EXAMINATIONS

Radiographic and other procedures are used to diagnose abnormalities within the urinary system (Table 72-6). Explain the procedures thoroughly to the client, prepare the client, and provide follow-up care.

Kidney, Ureter, and Bladder X-rays

An x-ray of the kidneys, ureters, and bladder (KUB) is a plain film of the abdomen obtained without any specific client preparation. The KUB study shows gross anatomic features and obvious stones, strictures, calcifications, or obstructions in the urinary tract. This test identifies the shape, size, and relationship of the organs to other parts of the urinary tract. Other tests are needed to diagnose functional or structural problems.

There is no discomfort or risk from this procedure. Tell the client that the x-ray will be taken while the client is in a supine position. No specific follow-up care is needed.

Intravenous Urography

Other names for IV urography include excretory urography and (the older term) IV pyelography (IVP).

CLIENT PREPARATION. Before urography, assess the client (Chart 72-6), perform bowel preparation, and teach the client. Report allergy information to the physician. Contrast reactions can be minor (nausea and vomiting, urticaria, itching, sneezing), moderate (nephrotoxic effects, congestive heart failure, pulmonary edema), or severe (bronchospasm, anaphylaxis). If the diagnostic test must be performed in a client with a minor allergy to the contrast dye, drugs such as a steroid (prednisone or methylprednisolone), and an antihistamine (diphenhydramine hydrochloride [Benadryl, Allerdryl✳]) are prescribed before the procedure to reduce an allergic response. Explain the rationale for the procedure to the client.

Some preparations may be needed to ensure that urinary structures are not obscured by bowel contents. Some radiologists recommend a light evening meal or clear liquids, then fasting (NPO status) from midnight on the night before the procedure. Others recommend increased fluid intake to prevent dehydration up until the time of the procedure. Because some clients may vomit as a reaction to the IV contrast, some physicians prefer the client to remain on NPO status for a few hours before the procedure. Hydration with IV fluids may be prescribed.

A bowel preparation is prescribed to remove fecal contents, fluid, and air from the gut, any of which could obscure part of the outline of the kidneys, ureters, and bladder. Bowel preparation procedures vary but usually include the use of laxatives the day before the procedure. Enemas also may be prescribed but their use is controversial because some air and fluid can be retained.

CONSIDERATIONS FOR OLDER ADULTS

Bowel preparation procedures increase the risk for dehydration, especially in older adult clients. To help prevent dehydration, contact the testing department and ask that urograms be scheduled early in the day for older clients.

The contrast dye is potentially nephrotoxic. The risk for *contrast-induced renal failure* is greatest in clients who are older or dehydrated, who have some renal insufficiency (e.g., serum creatinine levels greater than 1.5 mg/dL), or who are also taking other nephrotoxic drugs. These clients need additional IV fluids before the procedure to maintain hydration and decrease the nephrotoxic risk. Acetylcysteine (an antioxidant) or fenoldopam (a dopamine-1 agonist) may be used to prevent contrast-induced nephrotoxic effects in radiologic procedures. Diuretics may be given immediately after the dye is injected to enhance dye excretion.

Instruct the client in the preparation procedures for the urogram and explain the procedure so that he or she knows what to expect (Chart 72-7). Intervene on behalf of the client to ensure that questions are answered *before* the procedure.

PROCEDURE. A radiopaque dye is injected intravenously with the client in a supine position. As blood (with

TABLE 72-6 Common Radiologic and Special Diagnostic Tests for Clients with Disorders of the Renal/Urinary System

Test	Purpose	Comments
Radiography of kidneys, ureters, and bladder (KUB) (plain film of abdomen)	To screen for the presence of two kidneys To measure kidney size To detect gross obstruction	
Excretory urography	To measure kidney size To detect obstruction To assess parenchymal mass	Radiopaque contrast media may cause an allergic (hypersensitivity) reaction in iodine-sensitive clients. Contrast agent is also hypertonic and increases the risk of acute renal failure in adults with serum creatinine levels greater than 1.5 mg/dL, diabetes mellitus, multiple myeloma, or dehydration. Nephrotoxic complications can be prevented by parenteral fluid administration, the use of mannitol, and daily monitoring of serum creatinine levels.
Nephrotomography	To assess various planes of kidney tissue for cysts, tumors, or calculi	Same as for excretory urogram.
Computed tomography (CT)	To measure kidney size To evaluate contour to assess for masses or obstruction	Contrast medium may provoke acute renal failure. See comments with excretory urography for high-risk clients and preventive measures related to contrast. May be performed without contrast medium and still obtain adequate visualization.
Cystography and cystoscopy	To identify abnormalities of the bladder wall and urethral and ureteral occlusions To treat small obstructions or lesions via fulguration, lithotripsy, or removal with a stone basket	Instrumentation of the urinary tract increases the risk of infection. Monitor for infection for 48-72 hr after the procedure.
Voiding cystourethrography (VCUG)	To outline bladder's contour and detect urinary reflux from vesicourethral junctions	The risk of infection is similar to that in cystography because urinary catheterization is necessary. Monitor for postprocedure infection.
Renal arteriography	To identify vascular abnormalities within each kidney and adjacent aorta	Contrast medium may provoke acute renal failure. See comments with excretory urography for high-risk clients and preventive measures related to contrast. Essential for diagnosis and treatment of some vascular abnormalities, such as renal artery stenosis. Monitor for bleeding after the procedure.
Ultrasonography (US)	To identify the size of the kidneys or obstruction in the kidneys or the lower urinary tract May detect tumors or cysts	Ultrasonography entails minimal risk to the client. Ultrasonography is a good alternative to excretory urography.
MAG3 study 99m	To assess renal function, structural abnormalities, renal failure, obstruction, and renal calculi	Radioactive material (technetium Tc mertiatide) is used for this test.
Intravenous pyelography (fluoroscopy)	To assess renal function, identify anomalies To image renal/urinary calculi (size, location, radiodensity) To screen for renal injury after trauma	Contraindicated during pregnancy (ionizing radiation is a risk to the fetus). Contrast dye can cause renal dysfunction. Colonic cleaning improves quality of image.
Magnetic resonance imaging (MRI)	Staging of cancers, similar to CT	Client must be able to lie still (motion can interfere with imaging).
Renal scan	Evaluation of renal blood flow Estimation of renal glomerular filtration rate Provides functional information without exposing the client to iodinated contrast dye	ACE inhibitors should be held for 48 hours before the test. ACE inhibitors may be given during the test, placing the client at risk for episodes of hypotension. Ensure adequate hydration for best results.

ACE, Angiotensin converting enzyme.

CHART 72-6

BEST PRACTICE for
Assessing the Client About to Undergo a Diagnostic Test
or Interventional Procedure Using Contrast Media

Before the procedure:
- Ask the client if he or she has ever had a reaction to contrast media. (Such a client has the highest risk for having another reaction.)
- Ask the client about a history of asthma. (Clients with asthma have been shown to be at greater risk for contrast reactions than the general public; when reactions do occur, they are more likely to be severe.)
- Ask the client about known hay fever or food or medication allergies, especially to seafood, eggs, milk, or chocolate. (Contrast reactions have been reported to be as high as 15% in these clients.)
- Ask the clients to describe any specific allergic reactions (e.g., hives, facial edema, difficulty breathing, bronchospasm).
- Assess for a history of renal insufficiency and for conditions that have been implicated in increasing the chance of developing renal failure after contrast media (e.g., diabetic nephropathy, class IV heart failure, dehydration, concomitant use of potentially nephrotoxic medications such as the aminoglycosides or NSAIDs, and cirrhosis).
- Ask the client if he or she is taking metformin (Glucophage). (Metformin must be discontinued at least 48 hours before any study using contrast media because the life-threatening complication of lactic acidosis, although rare, could occur.)
- Assess hydration status by checking blood pressure, heart and respiratory rates, mucous membranes, skin turgor, and urine concentration.
- Ask the client when he or she last ate or drank anything.

From Cohan, R.H., & Ellis, J.H. (1997). Iodinated contrast material in uroradiology. Choice of agent and management of complications. *Urologic Clinics of North America, 24*(3), 471-491. *NSAIDs,* Nonsteroidal anti-inflammatory drugs.

the dye) rapidly circulates into the kidney blood vessels and is filtered by the glomeruli, the dye is excreted in the urine. A series of x-rays are taken at various times after injection. Nephrotomograms may be taken at the same time as the urogram. Tomograms take images of different planes of tissue and show any abnormalities present at varying depths. The technologist then asks the client to empty the bladder and return for a few more x-rays. An outline of the kidneys, ureters, and bladder result as urine containing the dye is excreted.

The urogram provides information about the following:
- The number, size, shape, and location of the kidneys
- The adequacy of filling and the rate of excretion of contrast medium
- The number, size, location, appearance, and patency of the calices, pelves, and ureters
- The size, location, and nature of the urinary bladder

FOLLOW-UP CARE. After the urogram, monitor the client for altered renal function and other effects from the dye. Ensure adequate hydration by urging the client to take oral fluid or by giving IV fluids. Hydration reduces the risk for renal damage. Monitor blood creatinine levels to assess ongoing renal function.

Computed Tomography

CLIENT PREPARATION. Inform the client that a computed tomography (CT) scan provides three-dimensional information about the kidneys, ureters, bladder, and surrounding tissues. A CT scan is usually performed after other diagnostic procedures and can provide information about

CHART 72-7

CLIENT EDUCATION GUIDE
Excretory Urogram

- The urogram outlines your urinary tract and helps determine any problems there.
- Notify your nurse or physician if you have had any reactions (allergic or otherwise) to any food or drugs, especially shellfish (shrimp, scallops, crab, lobster, and so on) or iodine, or to x-ray "dyes" such as contrast media; if you have a history of asthma; or if you are taking metformin (Glucophage) or Glucovance.
- The day before the test, follow the instructions about changes in your diet and fluid intake to be sure that as much information as possible is gained from the test.
- After you start the bowel preparation, you may need to be close to toileting facilities. The preparation medications usually work quickly.
- You will be lying on an x-ray table with the x-ray machine above you for most of the procedure.
- A pressure band, similar to a large blood pressure cuff, may be placed around your stomach or abdomen to help obtain better x-rays.
- If you do not already have an IV access site, one will be started to give you the contrast agent.
- After the contrast is injected, you may feel a sense of warmth or heat as it travels throughout your body. You also may have a taste in your mouth that is sometimes described as metallic. These sensations last only a few seconds or minutes.
- When the pressure band is inflated, you may feel some tightness around your abdomen. The sensation is similar to the feeling on your arm when you have your blood pressure taken.
- A series of x-rays will be taken. You may be asked to empty your bladder and return to the table for more films. You also may be asked to have a standing film taken.
- After the test is completed, you are usually able to resume your normal activities and diet.
- You will not notice any change in the color or characteristics of your urine.
- Please do not hesitate to ask your nurse, physician, or x-ray technologist any question, no matter how slight the question may seem to you. It is important that you have as much understanding as possible.

tumors, cysts, abscesses, other masses, obstruction, and certain blood vessel abnormalities.

Some hospitals require clients having abdominal CT scans to be NPO for some period before the scan. For the scan using contrast, extra hydration may be needed before the test, especially if the client has reduced renal function. Ask about allergy to dyes and intervene as with IV urography.

PROCEDURE. The CT scan is performed in a special room, usually in the radiology department. An IV injection of radiopaque dye may be given before starting the imaging procedures. Dye use may be eliminated in clients at risk for contrast media-induced acute renal failure, but the images produced are less distinct.

FOLLOW-UP CARE. No special follow-up care is needed unless dye was used. In that case, the follow-up care is the same as for IV urography.

Cystography and Cystourethrography

CLIENT PREPARATION. Explain the procedure to the client. A urinary catheter is temporarily needed to instill contrast dye. The dye is needed to enhance x-ray visibility of the lower urinary tract.

PROCEDURE. In both cystography and cystourethrography, dye is instilled into the bladder via a urethral catheter. After bladder filling, x-rays are taken from the front, back, and side positions. For the voiding cystourethrogram (VCUG), the client is requested to void, and x-rays are taken during the voiding. A VCUG is obtained to determine whether a vesicoureteral reflux is present. The cystogram is often used in cases of trauma when urethral or bladder injury is suspected.

FOLLOW-UP CARE. Monitor for the development of infection as a result of catheter placement. In this test, the dye is not nephrotoxic because it does not enter the bloodstream. Encourage fluid intake to dilute the urine and reduce the burning sensation from catheter irritation after removal. Also monitor for changes in urine output because pelvic or urethral trauma may be present.

OTHER RENAL DIAGNOSTIC TESTS

Renal Arteriography (Angiography)

Indications for this test include suspected causes of decreased renal function such as renovascular hypertension, other vessel abnormalities, and bleeding from trauma.

CLIENT PREPARATION. Inform the client that this procedure is used to assess the arterial blood supply of the kidneys. A bowel preparation may be needed before the test if a barium study has been performed recently. A light evening meal is given, and the client is on NPO status until after the procedure. An IV may be placed before the procedure and fluids may be given to ensure adequate hydration because dye is used in this study.

Review the procedure with the client, answer questions, and review the drug regimen and blood study results as indicated. For example, review the medication record for drugs affecting blood clotting, such as heparin, Lovenox, warfarin (Coumadin, Warfilone✽), or aspirin. The client needs to sign an informed consent statement.

PROCEDURE. The injection of a radiopaque dye into the renal arteries requires entry into an artery, usually the femoral artery in the groin. After the client is sedated and the skin is prepared and draped, the radiologist injects a local anesthetic. An arterial puncture is then performed and the angiographic catheter is inserted.

Using fluoroscopy, the radiologist guides the catheter into the abdominal aorta and the renal artery. When the tip of the catheter is positioned at each renal artery, dye is injected and x-rays are taken. The speed of distribution of the dye and any areas of blood vessel narrowing are recorded. Arterial blockage is found when the dye fails to circulate within the kidney. **Extravasation** (infiltration) of dye into surrounding tissue indicates vessel rupture, which could be present after trauma.

FOLLOW-UP CARE. Bleeding from the catheter insertion site is the most common delayed complication of renal arteriography. Monitor the insertion site for bleeding or swelling. If the site bleeds or if a hematoma forms, hold manual, non-occlusive pressure on the entry site and notify the radiology department for an evaluation.

Monitor vital signs as per the physician's prescription or according to the agency's policy, usually every 15 minutes for 1 hour, then every 30 minutes for 2 hours, then every hour for 4 hours, and then every 4 hours. Check the temperature and color of the extremities and distal pulses. A sudden absence of pulses in the catheterized vessel may reflect hematoma formation or embolization.

The period of absolute bedrest (to prevent bleeding) after arteriography varies. Usually bedrest is maintained for 4 to 6 hours. Instruct the client about the importance of keeping the leg in a straight position for those 4 to 6 hours. A restraint may be used on the leg with the client's consent. Encourage ankle flexing and weight shifting to prevent deep vein thrombosis. If there is no evidence of bleeding after 4 to 6 hours, the client may be permitted to stand to void or may use a bedside commode.

Serum creatinine is measured for several days after the arteriogram to determine whether the test has affected kidney function. For some clients with renal insufficiency, the dye may cause an episode of acute renal failure severe enough to require short-term dialysis. Because the test is used to determine the need for interventions to restore kidney blood flow and preserve kidney function, many clients accept the risk of short-term dialysis to prevent the need for permanent dialysis. Urge clients to drink fluids after the procedure to enhance dye excretion.

Renal Biopsy

CLIENT PREPARATION. Explain that a kidney biopsy can help to determine a cause of for unexplained renal problems and to direct or change therapy. Most renal biopsies are performed **percutaneously** (through the skin and other tissues) using ultrasound or CT guidance. The client signs an informed consent. Clients are NPO for 4 to 6 hours before the procedure.

Because of the risk for postprocedure bleeding, coagulation studies such as platelet count, activated partial thromboplastin time (aPTT), prothrombin time (PT), and bleeding time are performed before surgery. A blood transfusion may be needed to correct anemia before biopsy. Hypertension and uremia increase the risk for bleeding and antihypertensive drugs or dialysis may be ordered before a biopsy.

PROCEDURE. In a percutaneous biopsy, the nephrologist or radiologist obtains tissue samples without an incision. Clients receive sedation and are monitored throughout the procedure. The client is placed in the prone position on the procedure table. The entry site is selected after taking preliminary images. The area is prepped and sterilely draped. A local anesthetic is injected and the physician then inserts the biopsy device into the tissues toward the kidney. Needle depth and placement is confirmed by ultrasound or CT. While the client holds his or her breath, the needle is advanced into the renal cortex. Samples are then taken with a spring-loaded coring biopsy needle and sent for pathologic analysis.

FOLLOW-UP CARE. After a percutaneous biopsy, the major risk is bleeding from the biopsy site. For 24 hours after the biopsy, monitor the dressing site, vital signs, urine output, hemoglobin level, and hematocrit. Even if the dressing is dry and there is no hematoma, the client could be bleeding from the site. An internal bleed is not readily visible but is suspected with flank pain, decreasing blood pressure, decreasing urine output, or other signs of hypovolemia or shock.

The client follows a plan of strict bedrest, lying in a supine position with a back roll for additional support for 2 to 6 hours after the biopsy. The head of the bed may be elevated, and the client may resume oral intake of food and fluids. After bedrest, the client may have limited bathroom privileges if there is no evidence of bleeding.

Monitor for hematuria, the most common complication of renal biopsy. Hematuria occurs microscopically in most clients, but 5% to 9% have gross hematuria. This problem usually resolves without treatment in 48 to 72 hours after the biopsy but can persist for 2 to 3 weeks. In rare cases, transfusions and surgery are required. There should be no obvious blood clots in the urine.

The client may have some local discomfort after the percutaneous renal biopsy. If aching originates at the biopsy site and begins to radiate to the flank and around the front of the abdomen, bleeding may have started or a perinephric hematoma is forming. This pattern of discomfort with bleeding occurs because blood in the tissues around the kidney increases pressure on local nerve tracts.

If bleeding occurs, IV fluid, packed red blood cells, or both may be needed to prevent shock. In general, a small amount of bleeding creates enough pressure to compress bleeding sites; this is called a "tamponade effect." If tamponade does not occur and bleeding is extensive, surgery for hemostasis or even nephrectomy may be needed. A hematoma in, on, or around the kidney may become infected, requiring treatment with antibiotics and surgical drainage.

If no bleeding occurs, the client can resume general activities after 24 hours. Instruct him or her to avoid lifting heavy objects, exercising, or performing other strenuous activities for 1 to 2 weeks after the biopsy procedure. Driving may also be restricted. Refer to Chapter 22 for general postoperative care for the client undergoing an open renal biopsy.

Renography (Kidney Scan)

CLIENT PREPARATION. Explain that a kidney scan is performed to provide general information about renal blood flow. A small amount of radioactive material, a radionuclide, is used. Reassure the client that there is no danger from the small amount of radioactive material present in the agent.

PROCEDURE. For a kidney scan, the radionuclide is injected intravenously. After injection, the radionuclide is absorbed into kidney tissue and gives off low-level radioactive emissions (scintillations). The amount of emission is measured by a scintillation counter. A special camera records the emissions and produces an image. At the same time, the rate and location of the emissions are recorded by computer, and information about renal blood flow, or glomerular filtration, is provided.

In some cases, captopril (Capoten), an antihypertensive drug, is given at the start of the procedure to change blood flow in the kidney. This procedure is a "captopril renal scan." The drug can cause severe hypotension during and after the procedure.

FOLLOW-UP CARE. If the client is able, urination into a commode is acceptable without risk from the small amount of radioactive material excreted. If the client is incontinent, change the bed linens promptly and wear gloves to maintain standard precautions. If captopril was used during the procedure, assess the client's blood pressure frequently. Caution the client to avoid rapid position changes and about the risk for falling as a result of orthostatic (positional) hypotension.

Ultrasonography

CLIENT PREPARATION. Inform the client that ultrasonography does not cause discomfort and is without risk. This test usually requires a full bladder. Ask the client to drink water, if needed, to help fill the bladder. This test applies sound waves to structures of different densities to produce images of the kidneys, ureters, and bladder and surrounding tissues. Ultrasonography allows assessment of kidney size, cortical thickness, and status of the calices. The test can identify obstruction in the urinary tract, tumors, cysts, and other masses without the use of nephrotoxic contrast material (dye).

PROCEDURE. The client undergoing renal ultrasound is usually placed in the prone position. Sonographic gel is applied to the skin over the back and flank areas to enhance sound wave conduction. A transducer in contact with and moving across the skin delivers sound waves and measures the echoes. Images of the internal structures are produced.

FOLLOW-UP CARE. Skin care to remove the gel is all that is needed after ultrasonography.

OTHER URINARY TRACT DIAGNOSTIC TESTS

Cystoscopy and Cystourethroscopy

CLIENT PREPARATION. Cystoscopy and cystourethroscopy are operative procedures and require completion of a preoperative checklist and a signed informed consent statement. The physician provides a complete description of and reasons for the procedure and the nurse reinforces this information. Cystoscopy may be performed for diagnosis or treatment. This test is used to examine for bladder trauma (cystoscopy) or urethral trauma (cystourethroscopy) and to identify causes of urinary tract obstruction. Cystoscopy may be used to remove bladder tumors or an enlarged prostate gland.

Cystoscopy may be performed under general or local anesthesia with sedation. The client's age, general health, and expected duration of the procedure are considered in the decision about anesthesia. A light evening meal may be eaten. Usually the client is NPO after midnight on the night before the cystoscopy. A bowel preparation with laxatives or enemas is performed the evening before the procedure.

PROCEDURE. The cystoscopy is performed in a designated cystoscopic examination room. If the procedure is performed in a surgical suite under general anesthesia, the usual surgical support personnel are present (see Chapter 21). This procedure is often performed in clinics, ambulatory surgery or short-procedure units, or a urologist's office.

Assist the client onto a table and, after sedation, place him or her in the lithotomy position. After the anesthesia is given and the area cleansed and draped, the urologist inserts a cystoscope through the urethra into the urinary bladder. This exam commonly includes the use of both the cystoscope and the urethroscope.

FOLLOW-UP CARE. After cystoscopic examination with general anesthesia, the client is returned to a postanesthesia care unit (PACU) or area. If local anesthesia and sedation were used, the client may be returned directly to the hospital room. Clients undergoing cystoscopic examinations as outpatients are transferred to an area for monitoring before discharge to home. Monitor the client for airway patency and breathing, changes in vital signs (including temperature), and changes in urine output. Also observe for the complications of bleeding and infection.

A catheter may or may not be present after cystoscopy. The client without a catheter has urinary frequency due to irritation from the procedure. The urine may be pink tinged, but gross bleeding is not expected. Bleeding or the presence of clots may obstruct the catheter and decrease urine output. Monitor urine output and notify the physician of obvious blood clots or a decreased or absent urine output. Irrigate the Foley catheter with sterile saline, if prescribed. Notify the physician if the client has a fever (with or without chills) or an elevated white blood cell (WBC) count, which suggests infection. Encourage the client to take oral fluids to promote adequate urine output (which helps prevent clotting) and to reduce the burning sensation on urination.

Retrograde Procedures

Retrograde means going against the normal flow of urine. A retrograde examination of the ureters and pelves (pyelogram), the bladder (cystogram), and the urethra (urethrogram) involves instilling dye into the lower urinary tract. Because the dye is instilled directly to obtain an outline of the structures desired, the dye does not enter the bloodstream. Therefore the client is not at risk for dye-induced acute renal failure or a systemic allergic response.

CLIENT PREPARATION. The client is prepared for retrograde procedures (retrograde pyelography, retrograde cystography, and retrograde urethrography) in the same way as for cystoscopy.

PROCEDURE. Retrograde x-rays are obtained during the cystoscopy. After placement of the cystoscope by the urologist, catheters are placed into each ureter, and contrast dye is instilled into each ureter and renal pelvis. The catheters are removed by the urologist, and x-rays are taken by the radiology technician to outline these structures as the dye is excreted. The procedure identifies obstruction or structural abnormalities.

For clients undergoing retrograde cystoscopy or urethrography, contrast dye is instilled similarly into the bladder or urethra. Cystography and urethrography identify structural problems, such as fistulas, diverticula, and tumors.

FOLLOW-UP CARE. After retrograde procedures, monitor the client for infection caused by placing instruments in the urinary tract. Because these procedures are performed during cystoscopic examination, follow-up care is the same as that for cystoscopy.

Urodynamic Studies

Urodynamic studies examine the processes of voiding and include the following:
- Tests of bladder capacity, pressure, and tone
- Studies of urethral pressure and urine flow
- Tests of perineal voluntary muscle function

These tests are often used along with voiding urographic or cystoscopic procedures to evaluate problems with urine flow.

CYSTOMETROGRAPHY

The purpose of a cystometrogram (CMG) is to determine how well the bladder wall (detrusor) muscle functions and how sensitive it is to stretching as the bladder fills. This test provides information about bladder capacity, bladder pressure, and voiding reflexes.

CLIENT PREPARATION. Explain the procedure and inform the client that a urinary catheter may be needed temporarily during the procedure.

PROCEDURE. Ask the client to void normally. Record the amount, rate of flow, and time of voiding. Insert a urinary catheter to measure the residual urine volume. The cystometer is attached to the catheter, and fluid is instilled via the catheter into the bladder. The point at which the client first notes a feeling of the urge to void and the point at which the client notes a strong urge to void are recorded. Bladder capacity and bladder pressure readings are recorded graphically. The client is asked to void when the bladder instillation is complete (about 500 mL). The residual urine after voiding is recorded, and the catheter is removed. Electromyography of the perineal muscles may be performed during the cystometric examination.

FOLLOW-UP CARE. As with any procedure that involves inserting instruments into the urinary tract, monitor for infection. Record the client's temperature, the character of the urine, and the amount of urine output.

URETHRAL PRESSURE PROFILE

A urethral pressure profile (also called a urethral pressure profilometry [UPP]) can provide information about the nature of urinary incontinence or urinary retention.

CLIENT PREPARATION. Explain the procedure and inform the client that a urinary catheter may be needed temporarily during the procedure.

PROCEDURE. A special catheter with pressure-sensing capabilities is inserted into the bladder. Variations in the pressure of the smooth muscle of the urethra are recorded as the catheter is slowly withdrawn.

FOLLOW-UP CARE. As with any study involving inserting instruments into the urinary tract, monitor the client for manifestations of infection.

ELECTROMYOGRAPHY

Electromyography (EMG) of the perineal muscles tests the strength of the muscles used in voiding. This information may help to identify methods of improving continence.

CLIENT PREPARATION. Inform the client that some temporary discomfort may accompany placement of the electrodes. Any discomfort is usually mild and of short duration.

PROCEDURE. In EMG of the perineal muscles, electrodes are placed in either the rectum or the urethra to measure muscle contraction and relaxation.

FOLLOW-UP CARE. After the completion of EMG, administer analgesics as prescribed to promote the client's comfort. Any discomfort is usually mild and of short duration.

URINE STREAM TEST

A urine stream test is used to evaluate pelvic muscle strength and the effectiveness of pelvic muscles in stopping the flow of urine. It is useful in assessing urinary incontinence.

CLIENT PREPARATION. Explain the procedure and reassure the client that efforts will be made to ensure privacy.

PROCEDURE. The client is asked to begin urinating. Three to five seconds after urination begins, the examiner gives the client a signal to stop urine flow. The length of time required to stop the flow of urine is recorded.

FOLLOW-UP CARE. Cleaning the perineal area, as after any voiding, is all that is necessary after the urine stream test.

❓ *Critical Thinking Challenge*

The client, a 62-year-old man with type 2 diabetes and benign prostatic hyperplasia (BPH), is scheduled to have an IV urogram. He asks you whether he should take his oral antidiabetic drugs in the morning before the procedure. He also asks if the procedure will be painful and if he can attend a baseball game the evening after the procedure.

1. Should this client take his usual antidiabetic medication before the procedure? Why or why not?
2. What will you tell this client about activity restrictions?
3. How will you reassure this client about pain management during and after the procedure?
4. What effect can the BPH have on this procedure?

evolve For suggested answer guidelines, go to http://evolve.elsevier.com/Iggy/.

GET READY for the NCLEX Examination!

KEY POINTS

Safe Effective Care Environment

- Use sterile technique when inserting a catheter or any other instrument into the urinary system.
- Use contact precautions with any client who has drainage from the genitourinary tract.

Health Promotion and Maintenance

- Teach clients the proper way to clean the perineal area after voiding, having a bowel movement, or after sexual intercourse.
- Encourage all clients to maintain an adequate fluid intake (minimum of 3 L/day unless another condition requires fluid restriction.
- Teach clients who come into contact with chemicals in their workplaces or for leisure time activities, to avoid direct skin or mucous membrane contact with these chemicals.

Psychosocial Integrity

- Pace your interview to match the learning needs and style of the individual client.
- Allow the client the opportunity to express fear or anxiety regarding tests of the renal and urinary tract or about a potential change in renal function.
- Assess the client's level of comfort in discussion issues related to elimination and the urogenital area.
- Explain all diagnostic procedures, restrictions, and follow-up care to the client scheduled for tests.
- Provide as much privacy as possible for clients undergoing examination or testing of the renal/urinary tract.
- Use language and terminology that the client can understand during discussions of renal/urinary assessment.

Physiological Integrity

- Ask the client about renal problems in any other members of the family because some problems have a genetic component.

- Ask the client whether or not any nephrotoxic medications have ever been used.
- Ask the client if he or she has ever had an allergic reaction to radiopaque contrast dye, shellfish, or iodine.
- Assess urine output closely after any procedure in which contrast dye is used intravenously.
- Assess the client for bleeding or manifestations of infection after any invasive test of renal/urinary function.

ADDITIONAL STUDY RESOURCES

Go to your Student CD-ROM for Review Questions for the NCLEX Examination.

Go to http://evolve.elsevier.com/Iggy/ for Integrated Management of Care Questions for the NCLEX Examination.

SELECTED BIBLIOGRAPHY

Asterisk indicates a classic or definitive work on this subject.

Aranout, M. (2001). Molecular genetics and the pathogenesis of autosomal dominant polycystic kidney disease. *Annual Review of Medicine, 52,* 93-123.

Beck, L.H. (2000). The aging kidney. Defending a delicate balance of fluid and electrolytes. *Geriatrics, 55*(4), 31-32.

Brenner, B.M. (Eds.). (2000). *Brenner & Rector's the kidney* (6th ed.). Philadelphia: W.B. Saunders.

*Driver, D.S. (1996). Renal assessment: Back to basics. *American Nephrology Nurses' Association Journal, 23*(4), 361-368.

*Duthrie, E.H., & Katz, P.R. (1998). *Practice of geriatrics* (3rd ed.). Philadelphia: W.B. Saunders.

Ebersole, P., Hess, P., & Luggen, A. (2004). *Toward healthy aging: Human needs and nursing response* (6th ed.). St. Louis: Mosby.

Gordon, M. (2002). *Manual of nursing diagnosis* (10th ed.). St. Louis: Mosby.

Guyton, A.C., & Hall, J.E. (2000). *Textbook of medical physiology* (10th ed.). Philadelphia: W.B. Saunders.

Jarvis, C. (2004). *Physical examination and health assessment* (4th ed.). Philadelphia: W.B. Saunders.

Lancaster, L.E. (Ed.). (2001). *Core curriculum for nephrology nursing* (4th ed.). Pitman, NJ: A.J. Janetti.

Little, C. (2000). Renovascular hypertension. *American Journal of Nursing, 100*(2), 46-51.

Kee, J.L. (2002). *Laboratory and diagnostic tests with nursing implications.* Upper Saddle River, NJ: Prentice-Hall.

Maddox, T.G. (2002). Adverse reactions to contrast material: recognition, prevention, and treatment. *American Family Physician, 66*(7), 1229-1231.

Manjunath, G., Sarnak, M.J., Levey, A.S. (2001). Estimating the glomerular filtration rate: Dos and don'ts for assessing kidney function. *Postgraduate Medicine, 110* (6), 55-62.

O'Farrell, B., et al. (2001). Evaluation of portable bladder ultrasound: Accuracy and effect on nursing practice in an acute care neuroscience unit. *Journal of Neuroscience Nursing, 33*(6), 310-319.

Price, D.A., et al. (2001). Renal perfusion and function in healthy African Americans. *Kidney International, 59*(3), 1037-1043.

Schaeffer, A.J. (2002). Infections and inflammations of the genitourinary tract. In P.C. Walsh, et al. (Eds.). *Campbell's urology.* Philadelphia: W.B. Saunders.

Shinopulos, N. (2000). Bedside urodynamic studies: Simple testing for urinary incontinence. *The Nurse Practitioner, 25*(6), 19-20, 22, 25-26, 28, 33-34, 37.

*Shulman, N.B., & Hall, W.D. (1991). Renal vascular disease in African-Americans and other racial minorities. *Circulation, 83*(4), 1477-1479.

Thompsom, E.J., & King, S.L. (2003). Acetylcysteine and fenoldopam: Promising new approaches for preventing effects of contrast nephrotoxicity. *Critical Care Nurse, 23*(3), 39-46.

U.S. Renal Data Systems. (2002). *USRDS 2002 annual data report.* Bethesda, MD: The National Institutes of Health, National Institute of Diabetes and Digestive and Kidney Diseases.

Vander, A.J,. & Navar, L.G. (2003) *Renal physiology* (6th ed.). New York, McGraw-Hill.

Walsh, P.C., Retik, A.B., & Vaughn, E. D. (Eds.). (2002). *Campbell's urology* (8th ed.). Philadelphia, W.B. Saunders

*Yucha, C., & Keen, M. (1996). Renal regulation of extracellular fluid volume and osmolality. *American Nephrology Nurses' Association Journal, 23*(5), 487-497.

Interventions for Clients with Urinary Problems

CHRIS WINKELMAN

LEARNING OUTCOMES

After studying this chapter, you should be able to:

1. Describe the clinical manifestations of cystitis.
2. Develop a community-based teaching plan for a person at risk for cystitis.
3. Describe nursing interventions to prevent urinary tract infections among hospitalized clients.
4. Compare the pathophysiology and manifestations of stress incontinence, urge incontinence, overflow incontinence, mixed incontinence, and functional incontinence.
5. Describe the mechanisms of action, side effects, and nursing implications for the management of a urinary tract infection with sulfonamide and fluoroquinolone antibiotics.
6. Describe the techniques used to assess pelvic floor strength in the client who is experiencing some incontinence.
7. Explain the proper application of exercises to strengthen pelvic floor muscles.
8. Explain the drug therapy for different types of incontinence.
9. Develop a community-based teaching plan for the client who must perform intermittent self-catheterization for incontinence.
10. Prioritize nursing care for the client with renal colic.
11. Describe the manifestations of urinary obstruction.
12. Describe the common clinical manifestations of bladder cancer.
13. Develop a community-based teaching plan for continuing care of clients who have a urinary diversion for bladder cancer.

Go to your Student CD-ROM for Review Questions
for the NCLEX Examination keyed to these Learning Outcomes.

Urinary problems affect the storage or elimination of urine. Both acute and chronic urinary problems are common and costly. More than 20 million people in the United States are treated annually for urinary tract infections, cystitis, kidney and ureter stones, or urinary incontinence (U.S. Renal Data Systems, 2002). Although life-threatening complications are rare with urinary problems, clients may have significant functional, physical, and psychosocial changes that reduce quality of life. Nursing interventions are directed toward prevention, detection, and management of urologic disorders.

INFECTIOUS DISORDERS

Infections of the urinary tract and kidneys are common, especially among women. Manifestations of urinary tract infection (UTI) account for more than 6.5 million health care visits annually in the United States, and 1.5 million hospital discharges involve a diagnosis of UTI (National Kidney and Urologic Diseases Information Clearinghouse, 2004). In the hospital, UTIs are the most prevalent nosocomial infection (Foxman, 2002). Total direct and indirect costs for adult urinary tract infections are estimated at $1.6 billion each year.

Urinary tract infections are described by their location in the tract. Acute infections in the lower urinary tract include urethritis (urethra), cystitis (bladder), and prostatitis (prostate gland). Acute **pyelonephritis** is an upper urinary tract (kidney) infection. The site of infection is important to know because site, along with the specific type of bacteria present, determines treatment. Several risk factors are associated with occurrence of UTIs (Table 73-1).

Cystitis

PATHOPHYSIOLOGY

Cystitis is an inflammation of the bladder. It can be caused by infection from bacteria, viruses, fungi, or parasites. Infectious cystitis is the most common of the UTIs. Noninfectious cystitis is caused by irritation from chemicals or

TABLE 73-1 Factors Contributing to Urinary Tract Infections

Factor	Mechanism	Interventions
Obstruction	Incomplete bladder emptying creates a continuous pool of urine where bacteria can grow, prevents flushing out of bacteria, and allows bacteria to ascend more easily to higher structures.	Relieve or bypass the obstruction to promote complete bladder emptying.
	Bacteria have a greater chance of multiplying the longer they remain in residual urine.	Increase liquids to dilute urine and encourage more frequent voiding.
	Overdistention of the bladder damages the mucosa and allows bacteria to invade the bladder wall.	Use intermittent catheterization to keep the bladder from becoming distended.
Stones (calculi)	Large stones can cause obstruction to urine flow.	Remove stones and/or treat the underlying condition that causes the stones to form.
	The rough surface of a stone irritates mucosal surfaces and creates a spot where bacteria can establish and grow.	
	Bacteria can live within stones and cause reinfection.	
Vesicoureteral reflux	Bacteria-laden urine is forced backward from the bladder up into the ureters and kidneys, where pyelonephritis can develop.	The affected ureters may be able to be surgically reimplanted in the bladder to eliminate the reflux.
	Reflux of sterile urine can cause renal scarring, which may promote renal dysfunction.	
Diabetes mellitus	Excess glucose in urine provides a rich medium for bacterial growth.	Maintain good glucose control in clients with diabetes.
	Peripheral neuropathy affects bladder innervation and leads to a flaccid bladder and incomplete bladder emptying.	
Characteristics of urine	Alkalotic urine promotes bacterial growth.	Acidify urine by taking vitamin C tablets, not citrus fruits. Such fruits make the urine alkaline.
	Concentrated urine promotes bacterial growth.	Increase urine dilution by increasing fluid intake.
Gender	Female clients are susceptible to periurethral colonization with coliform bacteria.	Explain the importance of perineal hygiene (wiping front to back) to prevent large amounts of coliform bacteria from remaining in the perineal area.
	Bladder displacement during pregnancy predisposes women to cystitis and the development of pyelonephritis.	Routine monitoring of pregnant women for UTIs prevents complications.
	A diaphragm or pessary that is too large can cause an obstruction to urine flow or trauma to the urethra.	Be sure diaphragms and pessaries are properly fitted.
Age	Obstruction may be caused by incomplete bladder emptying as a result of an enlarged prostate in men and cystocele and prolapse in women.	Do not rush older clients during toileting; provide regular and private toileting times to promote complete bladder emptying.
	Neuromuscular conditions that cause incomplete bladder emptying, such as Parkinson's disease and strokes, affect older adults more frequently.	Straight catheter for residual and Credé maneuver to promote more complete emptying.
	The use of anticholinergic medications in older adults contributes to delayed bladder emptying.	Monitor and report this medication side effect.
	Fecal incontinence contributes to poor perineal hygiene.	Promptly clean clients after episodes of incontinence.
	Hypoestrogenism in older women adversely affects the cells of the vagina and urethra, making them more susceptible to infections.	Give vaginal estrogen cream as directed to improve the health of the client's vaginal and urethral cells.
Sexual activity	Irritation of the perineum and urethra during intercourse can promote migration of bacteria from the perineal area to the urinary tract in some women.	Empty the bladder before and after intercourse.
		Drink 8 oz of fluid (especially water) after intercourse.
	Spermicides can alter vaginal pH, increasing potential numbers of pathogens.	Consider alternate method of birth control if experiencing repeated UTIs.
	Inadequate vaginal lubrication may exacerbate potential urethral irritation.	Use an artificial vaginal lubricant.
	Bacteria may be introduced into the man's urethra during anal intercourse or during vaginal intercourse with a woman who has a bacterial vaginitis.	Use a condom.

radiation. **Interstitial cystitis** is an inflammatory process of unknown etiology.

Infectious agents, most commonly bacteria, move up the urinary tract from the external urethra to the bladder. Less common, spread of infection through the blood and lymph fluid can occur. Once bacteria enter the urinary tract, several factors influence the outcome (Table 73-2).

Asymptomatic bacteriuria is common in older adults and is a benign condition. No studies have demonstrated a relationship between asymptomatic bacteriuria and progression

TABLE 73-2 Important Factors Influencing the Outcome of Urinary Tract Infection

Facilitating Aspects	Protective Aspects
Anatomy	
Females: Short length of the urethra and its proximity to the vagina and rectum facilitate colonization of coliform bacteria.	*Males:* Long length of the urethra and its distance from the rectum provide protection from colonization with coliform bacteria.
Males: With age, the prostate enlarges and may obstruct the normal flow of urine, producing stasis.	
Physiology	
Females: Pregnancy predisposes a woman to ureteral reflux and subsequent pyelonephritis; with age the decline in estrogen facilitates colonization of *Escherichia. coli.*	*Females:* Well-estrogenized mucosa in the urethra and trigone may inhibit bacterial colonization.
Males: With age, prostatic secretions lose their antibacterial characteristics and predispose to bacterial proliferation in the urine.	*Males:* Normal prostatic secretions inhibit bacterial growth.
	Both males and females: Mucin is produced by urothelial cells lining the bladder—this helps to maintain mucosal integrity and prevent cellular damage; mucin may also prevent bacteria from adhering to urothelial cells.
Trauma	
Females: Vaginal penetration with sexual intercourse may traumatize the urethra and bladder base, leading to postcoital (or honeymoon) cystitis; a vaginal diaphragm that is too large can place pressure on the urethra, causing trauma; vaginal childbirth can cause permanent damage to the urethra.	*Females:* Adequate lubrication, either natural or artificial, with intercourse may prevent any trauma.
Males: Sexually transmitted diseases may cause urethral strictures that obstruct the flow of urine and predispose to urinary stasis.	
Both males and females: Urethral instrumentation (such as catheterization) may disturb the urothelial surface and predispose to adherence of bacteria that would ordinarily not be pathogenic.	
Infectious Agent	
Some organisms are better able to adhere to host cells and secrete substances that induce inflammation.	A small inoculum (number of microorganisms) introduced into the body) is more easily flushed away by the flow of urine.

to acute infection or renal insufficiency in clients without other pathologic problems.

Etiology and Genetic Risk

UTIs, like other infections, are the result of interactions between a pathogen and the host. A high bacterial virulence is necessary to overcome usual strong host resistance. However, a compromised host is more likely to be infected with a pathogen that has a low virulence. Genetically, invading bacteria with special adhesions are more likely to cause ascending urinary tract infections (UTIs). Host genetic factors such as blood group secretor status and ability to generate bladder surface biofilms may influence the risk for UTI (Moore, Day, & Albers; 2002).

The most common organisms in infectious cystitis are from the intestinal tract. About 90% of UTIs are caused by *Escherichia coli.* Less common organisms include *Staphylococcus saprophyticus, Klebsiella pneumoniae,* and organisms from the *Proteus* and *Enterobacter* species (Moore, Day, & Albers, 2002).

In most cases, organisms first grow in the perineal area, then move into the urethra as a result of irritation, trauma, or catheterization of the urinary tract, and finally ascend to the bladder. Catheters are the most common predisposing factor for UTIs in the hospital setting. Within 48 hours of catheter insertion, bacterial colonization begins. About 50% of clients with indwelling catheters become infected within 1 week of catheter insertion.

The etiology of catheter-related infections varies between genders. Bacteria from a women's perineal area are more likely to ascend to the bladder by moving along the catheter. In men, bacteria tend to gain access to the bladder from inside the lumen of the catheter (Warren et al, 1999). Any break in the closed urinary drainage system allows bacteria to migrate through the urinary tract. Best practices to reduce the risk of catheter contamination are listed in Chart 73-1.

Organisms other than bacteria can cause cystitis. Fungal infections, such as those caused by *Candida,* can occur during long-term antibiotic therapy, because antibiotics change normal flora. Clients who are severely immunocompromised, are receiving corticosteroids or other immunosuppressive agents, or have diabetes mellitus or acquired immunodeficiency syndrome (AIDS) are at higher risk for fungal UTIs.

Viral and parasitic infections are rare and usually are transferred to the urinary tract from an infection at another site. For example, *Trichomonas,* a parasite found in the vagina, can also be found in the urine. Treatment of the vaginal infection (see Chapter 78) also resolves the UTI.

Noninfectious cystitis may result from chemical exposure, such as to drugs (e.g., cyclophosphamide [Cytoxan, Procytox❋]), from radiation therapy, and from immunologic responses, as with systemic lupus erythematosus (SLE).

Interstitial cystitis is a rare, chronic inflammation of the entire lower urinary tract (bladder, urethra, and adjacent pelvic muscles) that is not a result of infection. The condition affects women more often than men (in a 10:1 ratio), and the diagnosis is difficult to make. Manifestations are similar to those of infectious cystitis with more intense urgency and bladder pain. Results from urinalysis and urine

CHART 73-1

BEST PRACTICE for
Minimizing Catheter-Related Infection

- Avoid long-term use (>3 days) during active illness or perioperatively.
- Use aseptic routine when handling catheter devices; manipulation can promote an environment favorable to pathogens.
- Use strict sterile technique to insert the catheter (in the hospital setting); a break in technique can introduce pathogens into the urinary tract.
- Ensure that catheter tubing connections are sealed securely; disconnections can introduce pathogens into the urinary tract.
- Keep urine collection bags below the level of the bladder at all times; elevating the collection bag above the bladder causes reflux of pathogens from the bag into the urinary tract.
- Secure the catheter to the client's thigh (female) or lower abdomen (male); catheter movement can cause urethral friction and irritation.
- Perform daily catheter care by washing the perineum and proximal portion of the catheter with soap and water, drying gently (removes pathogens and reduces pathogenic population).
- Consider the use of silver-iodide coated catheters for clients requiring indwelling catheters for more than 3 to 5 days. This coating reduces bacterial colonization along the catheter.
- *Application of antiseptic solutions or antibiotic ointments to the perineal area of catheterized clients has not been demonstrated to have any beneficial effect.*

culture are negative for infection (Gray, Albo, & Huffstutler, 2002).

Although cystitis is not life threatening, infectious cystitis can lead to life-threatening complications, including pyelonephritis and sepsis. The risk for kidney tissue damage and subsequent kidney failure as a result of bacteria ascending from the bladder to the kidney is controversial. Severe kidney damage is a rare complication unless the client also has other predisposing factors, such as anatomic abnormalities, pregnancy, obstruction, reflux, calculi, or diabetes mellitus.

The spread of the infection from the urinary tract to the bloodstream is termed **urosepsis**. Sepsis from any source is a systemic infection that can lead to overwhelming organ failure, shock, and death. The most common cause of sepsis in the hospitalized client is a UTI (Warren et al., 1999). Sepsis has a high mortality and prolongs hospital stays (see Chapter 40).

Incidence/Prevalence

The incidence of UTI is second only to that of upper respiratory infections in primary care. Clients who have **frequency** (an urge to urinate frequently in small amounts), **dysuria** (pain or burning with urination), and **urgency** (the feeling that urination will occur immediately) account for more than 5 million health care visits annually. About 50% of these clients will have a confirmed UTI (National Kidney and Urologic Diseases Information Clearinghouse, 2004).

CONSIDERATIONS FOR OLDER ADULTS

The prevalence of UTIs varies with age and gender. Women of any age are more commonly affected with UTIs than men. In men 65 to 73 years old, the incidence of UTI is 3%; after 73 years of age, however, the incidence is 20%. In women, the prevalence of UTIs increases from 20% among all women to 50% in those older than 80 years of age. Skin and mucous

membrane changes from a lack of estrogen appear to account for much of the increased risk in older women. Prostate disease increases risk for UTIs in men.

◆ COLLABORATIVE MANAGEMENT
◆ Assessment

PHYSICAL ASSESSMENT/CLINICAL MANIFESTATIONS

Frequency, urgency, and dysuria are the common clinical manifestations of a urinary tract infection (UTI), but other manifestations may be present (Chart 73-2). Urine may be cloudy, foul smelling, or blood tinged. Risk factors for UTI are included in the assessment (see Table 73-1).

Before performing the physical assessment, ask the client to void so that the urine can be examined and the bladder emptied before palpation. Assess vital signs to help rule out sepsis. Inspect the lower abdomen and palpate the urinary bladder. Distention after voiding indicates incomplete bladder emptying.

Using standard precautions (see Chapter 29), record any skin lesions around the urethral meatus and vaginal opening. To help differentiate between a vaginal and a urinary tract infection, note whether there is any vaginal discharge (i.e., vaginal discharge and irritation are more indicative of vaginal infection). Women often report burning with urination when normal, acidic urine touches labial tissues that are inflamed or ulcerated by vaginal infections or sexually transmitted diseases (STDs). Maintain privacy with drapes during the examination.

The prostate is palpated by rectal examination for size, change in shape or consistency, and tenderness. The physician or advanced practice nurse performs the rectal prostate assessment.

LABORATORY ASSESSMENT

Laboratory assessment for a UTI is a urinalysis with testing for leukocyte esterase and nitrate. The combination of a positive leukocyte esterase and nitrate is 85% to 90% sensitive and 95% specific in the diagnosis of a UTI (Bass, Jarvis, and Mitchell, 2003). Although more time-consuming and expensive, a urinalysis can include a microscopic count of bacteria, white blood cells (WBCs), and red blood cells (RBCs). The presence of 100,000 colonies/mL or the presence of WBCs (**pyuria**) with RBCs (**hematuria**) indicate infection.

A urinalysis is performed on a clean-catch midstream specimen. If the client cannot produce a clean-catch specimen, you may need to obtain the specimen with a small-caliber (6 Fr) catheter. For a routine urinalysis, 10 mL of urine is required; smaller quantities are sufficient for culture.

A urine culture confirms the type of organism and the number of colonies. Urine culture is expensive and takes 48 hours to obtain results. It is indicated when the UTI is complicated, does not respond to usual therapy, or if the diagnosis is uncertain. A UTI is confirmed when there are more than 10^5 colony-forming units in the urine from any client. In clients who have UTI manifestations, as few as 10^3 colony-forming units may be diagnostic. Multiple types of organisms in low colony counts indicate a contaminated specimen.

CHART 73-2

KEY FEATURES of
Urinary Tract Infection

Common Clinical Manifestations
- Frequency
- Urgency
- Dysuria
- Hesitancy or difficulty in initiating urine stream
- Low back pain
- Nocturia
- Incontinence
- Hematuria
- Pyuria
- Bacteriuria
- Retention
- Suprapubic tenderness or fullness
- Feeling of incomplete bladder emptying

Rare Clinical Manifestations
- Fever
- Chills
- Nausea
- Vomiting
- Malaise
- Flank pain

Atypical Clinical Manifestations That May Occur in the Older Adult
- The only symptom may be something as vague as increasing mental confusion or frequent, unexplained falls.
- A sudden onset of incontinence or a worsening of incontinence may be the only symptom of an early UTI.
- Fever, tachycardia, tachypnea, and hypotension, even without any urinary symptoms, may be signs of urosepsis.
- Loss of appetite, nocturia, and dysuria are common symptoms.

UTI, Urinary tract infection.

Sensitivity testing follows culture results when complicating factors are present, such as stones or recurrent infection, or when the client is older.

Occasionally the serum WBC count may be elevated, with the differential WBC count showing a "left shift" (see Chapter 23). This shift indicates that the number of immature WBCs is increasing in response to the infection. As a result, the number of bands, or immature WBCs, is elevated. Left shift most often occurs with urosepsis and rarely occurs with uncomplicated cystitis.

OTHER DIAGNOSTIC ASSESSMENTS

The diagnosis of cystitis is based on the history, physical examination, and laboratory data. If urinary retention and obstruction of urine outflow are suspected, urography, abdominal sonography, or computed tomography (CT) may be needed to locate the site of obstruction or the presence of calculi. Voiding cystourethrography (see Chapter 72) is needed when vesicoureteral reflux is suspected.

Cystoscopy (see Chapter 72) may be performed when the client has recurrent UTIs (more than three or four a year). The urine is sterilized with antibiotic therapy before the procedure to reduce the risk for sepsis. Cystoscopy identifies abnormalities that increase the risk for cystitis. Such abnormalities include bladder calculi, bladder diverticula, urethral strictures, foreign bodies (such as sutures from previous surgery), and **trabeculation** (an abnormal thickening of the bladder wall caused by urinary retention and obstruction). Retrograde pyelography, along with the cystoscopic exami-

nation, shows outlines and images of the drainage tract. Areas of obstruction or malformation and the presence of reflux are then identified early.

Cystoscopy is needed to accurately diagnose interstitial cystitis. A urinalysis usually shows WBCs and RBCs but no bacteria. Common findings in interstitial cystitis are a small-capacity bladder, the presence of **Hunner's ulcers** (a type of bladder lesion), and small hemorrhages after bladder distention.

◆ Common Nursing Diagnoses and Collaborative Problems

Nursing diagnoses and collaborative problems that may apply to clients with cystitis include the following:
- Acute Pain related to bladder spasms
- Deficient Knowledge (risk factors for cystitis and drug regimen) related to information misinterpretation or unfamiliarity with information resources
- Urge Urinary Incontinence related to irritation of bladder stretch receptors causing spasm (e.g., bladder infection)
- Risk for Impaired Skin Integrity related to moisture from incontinence
- Risk for Sepsis

◆ Interventions

NONSURGICAL MANAGEMENT

Drug Therapy. Drugs used to treat bacteriuria and promote client comfort include urinary antiseptics or antibiotics, analgesics, and antispasmodics. Cure of a UTI is dependent on the antibiotic levels achieved in the urine (Chart 73-3). Antifungal agents are prescribed for fungal infections. Amphotericin B is most often given in daily bladder instillations, and ketoconazole (Nizoral) is usually given orally. Antispasmodic drugs decrease bladder spasm and promote complete bladder emptying.

Antibiotic therapy is used for bacterial UTIs (see Chart 73-3). Guidelines indicate that a 3-day course of trimethoprim/sulfamethoxazole or fosfomycin is effective in treating an uncomplicated, community-acquired UTI in women (Bass, Jarvis, & Mitchell, 2003). Single-dose therapy with long-acting fluoroquinolones is under investigation. The shorter courses increase adherence and reduce cost. Longer antibiotic treatment (7 to 21 days) is required for hospitalized clients, those with complicating factors, such as indwelling catheters or calculi, and those with diabetes or immunosuppression.

Long-term antibiotic therapy is recommended for chronic, recurring infections caused by structural abnormalities or calculi. Trimethoprim 100 mg daily may be used for long-term management of the older client with frequent UTIs. For women who have recurrent UTIs after intercourse, one low-dose tablet of trimethoprim (TMP) (Proloprim, Trimpex) or TMP/sulfamethoxazole (half- or single-strength Bactrim, Cotrim, Septra) or nitrofurantoin (Macrodantin, Nephronex✱, Novofuran✱) after intercourse is often recommended (McLaughlin & Carson, 2004). Estrogen used as an intravaginal cream may prevent recurrent UTIs in the postmenopausal woman; the benefits of systemic estrogen replacement therapy in preventing UTIs may not outweigh the risks of hormone replacement therapy for most clients (Maloney, 2002).

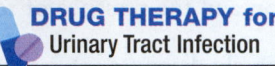

CHART 73-3

DRUG THERAPY for
Urinary Tract Infection

Drug	Usual Dosage	Nursing Interventions	Rationales
Antimicrobials			
Quinolones		Avoid use in pregnancy and in those under 18 yr.	Drug can interfere with cartilage formation in weight-bearing joints.
Ciprofloxacin (Cipro)	250 mg PO twice daily for 3 days with uncomplicated cystitis, for 7 days with complicated cystitis, and for 10-14 days with uncomplicated pyelonephritis	Avoid taking with aluminum- or magnesium-containing antacids. Give 1 hr before or 2 hr after food or drink. Avoid caffeinated beverages, and use with caution in clients receiving theophylline.	Food, calcium, and antacids interfere with drug adsorption. Quinolones prolong the half-life of caffeine and theophylline.
¹Lomefloxacin (Maxaquin)	400 mg PO daily for 3 days for uncomplicated cystitis, for 7 days for complicated cystitis, and for 10-14 days for uncomplicated pyelonephritis	As above. Avoid the sun.	As above. Drug causes photosensitivity.
²Levofloxacin (Levaquin)	250 mg PO daily for 3 days for uncomplicated cystitis, for 7 days for complicated cystitis, and for 10-14 days for uncomplicated pyelonephritis	As above. Avoid the sun.	As above. Drug causes photosensitivity.
Norfloxacin (Noroxin)	400 mg PO twice daily for 3 days for uncomplicated cystitis, for 7 days for complicated cystitis, and for 10-14 days for uncomplicated pyelonephritis	As above.	As above.
Ofloxacin (Floxin)	200 mg PO twice daily for 3 days for uncomplicated cystitis, for 7 days for complicated cystitis, and for 10-14 days for uncomplicated pyelonephritis	As above.	As above.
³Sparfloxacin (Zagam)	400 mg PO for 1 day, then 200 mg daily for 2 days for uncomplicated cystitis, for 7 days for complicated cystitis, and for 10-14 days for uncomplicated pyelonephritis	As above.	As above.

¹***Med Error Alert!*** *Do not confuse with Maxidex, a glucocorticoid, or Maxalt, an antimigraine agent.*

²***Med Error Alert!*** *Do not confuse with levothyroxine, a synthetic thyroid hormone.*

³***Med Error Alert!*** *Do not confuse with Zantac, an H₂ histamine blocker.*

CHART 73-3

DRUG THERAPY for
Urinary Tract Infection—*cont'd*

Drug	Usual Dosage	Nursing Interventions	Rationales
Antimicrobials—*cont'd*			
Penicillins		Inquire about penicillin allergy.	
Amoxicillin (Amoxil)	500 mg PO twice daily for 3 days	Give with food.	Food reduces GI upset.
Amoxicillin/ clavulanate (Augmentin, Clavulin ✱)	500 mg/125 mg PO twice daily for 3 days	Give with food.	Food reduces GI upset.
Cephalosporins		Inquire about allergy to cephalosporin or penicillin.	There is a 1% to 20% cross-reactivity between penicillin and cephalosporins.
Cefadroxil (Duricef)	1000 mg PO daily for 3 days for uncomplicated cystitis, or 1000 mg twice daily for 10 days for complicated cystitis		
⊕⁴Cefixime (Suprax)	400 mg PO daily for 3 days for uncomplicated cystitis, for 7 days for complicated cystitis, and for 10-14 days for uncomplicated pyelonephritis		
Fosfomycin (Monurol)	3 g PO (1 packet) as a single dose	Avoid use of GI drugs during dosing.	Drug is less effective if given with drugs that increase GI motility.
Sulfonamide			
Trimethoprim/ sulfamethoxazole (Bactrim, Septra, Sulfatrim Roubac ✱)	1 double-strength tablet (DS or 160/800 mg) for 3 or 10 days for uncomplicated cystitis, or single-strength PO (80/400 mg) after coitus for prophylaxis	Provide adequate fluid intake. Avoid ascorbic acid and ammonium chloride that acidify urine. Use with caution in clients with asthma, G6PD deficiency, or multiple allergies.	Sulfa can crystallize in acidic or concentrated urine. Sulfa allergies are relatively common; monitor client for potential reaction.
Urinary Antiseptic			
Nitrofurantoin (Macrobid Macrodantin, Nephronex ✱, Novofuran ✱)	*Macrobid:* 100 mg PO twice daily for 7 days *Macrodantin:* 100 mg PO four times daily for 7 days	Give with food or milk. Monitor for flulike symptoms in older clients and in those with pulmonary disease.	Food or milk decreases GI upset. Rare case of interstitial pneumonitis can occur in susceptible clients.
Analgesic			
Phenazopyridine (Pyridium, Urogesic, ⊕⁵Phenazo ✱)	100-200 mg PO three times daily for 2-3 days	Give with food. Advise client that urine will become red or orange. Help the client to understand the difference between a urinary analgesic and antibiotic.	Food helps reduce GI upset. Urine discoloration is normal. A complete dosing schedule is not necessary.
Antispasmodic			
Hyoscyamine (Anaspaz, Cystospaz-M, others)	0.125-0.5 PO three times daily and at bedtime	Assess for safety, constipation, and urinary retention.	Anticholinergics cause drowsiness, blurred vision, dry mouth, constipation, and urinary retention.

⊕⁴***Med Error Alert!*** *Do not confuse with Surfak, a stool softener.*
⊕⁵***Med Error Alert!*** *Do not confuse with pyridostigmine, an anticholinesterase.*

GI, Gastrointestinal; *G6PD,* glucose-6-phosphate dehydrogenase deficiency.

NIC **Urinary Elimination Management.** The goal is to maintain an optimal urinary elimination pattern. Nursing interventions for the management of cystitis are listed in Chart 73-4.

WOMEN'S HEALTH CONSIDERATIONS

Pregnant women with a bacterial UTI require vigorous intervention because of the tendency of simple cystitis to lead to acute pyelonephritis during pregnancy. Pyelonephritis in pregnancy can cause preterm labor and adversely affect the fetus.

Diet Therapy. The diet should include all food groups and include increased calories for the increased metabolism caused by infection. Urge clients to drink at least 2 to 3 L of fluid each day unless another condition requires fluid restriction. There is no evidence that additional fluid intake alters the course of a UTI (Gray, Albo, & Hufstutler, 2002). Although a critical review of the literature suggests that there is not enough evidence to routinely ingest cranberry products to prevent UTIs, one study suggests that 50 mL of concentrated cranberry juice consumed daily decreases bacterial adherence to the urinary tract, decreasing the incidence of UTIs in some clients. Cranberry juice must be consumed for 3 to 4 weeks to be effective (Jepson, Mihaljevic, & Craig, 2002; Kontiokari et al., 2001).

Other Pain Relief Measures. A warm sitz bath taken two or three times a day for 20 minutes may provide comfort and some relief of local symptoms. If burning with urination is severe or urinary retention occurs, instruct the client to sit in the sitz bath and urinate into the warm water.

SURGICAL MANAGEMENT. Surgery for cystitis treats the conditions that predispose to recurrent UTIs (e.g., removal of obstructions and repair of vesicoureteral reflux). Procedures may include cystoscopy (see Chapter 72) to identify and remove calculi or obstructions.

Community-Based Care

Assess the client's level of understanding of the problem. The client's knowledge about factors contributing to the development of cystitis is the basis on which further teaching interventions are planned.

Teach the client how to take prescribed drugs. Emphasize the need for correct spacing of doses throughout the day and the need to complete all of the prescribed drugs. If the drug will change the color of the urine, as it does with phenazopyridine (Pyridium, Urogesic, Phenazo✱), inform the client to expect this occurrence. Offer techniques for remembering the drug schedule, such as the use of a daily calendar or the association of drugs with usual activities (e.g., mealtimes).

Clients may associate symptoms of discomfort with sexual activities and have feelings of guilt and embarrassment. Frank and sensitive discussions with a woman who experiences frequent recurrences of UTI after sexual intercourse can help her find techniques to handle the problem (see Table 73-1). Explore with the woman the factors that contribute to her infections, such as diaphragm use and her general resistance to infection. Remind the client that vigorous cleaning of the perineum with harsh soaps and vaginal douching may irritate the perineal tissues and increase the risk for UTI. At the client's request, discuss the problem with the client and her partner to help them find ways of maintaining their intimate relationship. Chart 73-5 lists actions for preventing UTIs.

Critical Thinking Challenge

The client is a 22-year-old woman who comes to the clinic saying that she has to "pee" all the time and that it burns. She did not complete high school and currently works as a waitress at a truck stop. Her symptoms started 5 days ago and she says that she is so busy at work that she couldn't get off work to come to the clinic sooner. She uses street language to describe her symptoms and body areas. She also tells you that she is sexually active and uses a diaphragm for birth control. She is afraid that she may give this infection to her partner.

CHART 73-4

NIC **INTERVENTION ACTIVITIES for**
The Client with a Urinary Tract Infection

Urinary Elimination Management: *Maintenance of an optimum urinary elimination pattern*
- Monitor urinary elimination, including frequency, consistency, odor, volume, and color, as appropriate.
- Teach client signs and symptoms of urinary tract infection.
- Obtain midstream voided specimen for urinalysis, as appropriate.
- Refer to physician if signs and symptoms of urinary tract infection occur.
- Instruct client to respond immediately to urge to void, as appropriate.
- Teach client to drink eight ounces of liquid with meals, between meals, and in early evening.
- Assist client with development of toileting routine, as appropriate.

NIC intervention activities selected from Dochterman, J.M., & Bulechek, G.M. (Eds.). (2004). *Nursing interventions classifications (NIC)* (4th ed.). St. Louis: Mosby. No part of this work is to be altered without prior written permission from the Publisher.

CHART 73-5

CLIENT EDUCATION GUIDE
Preventing a Urinary Tract Infection

- Drink 1 to 3 L of fluid every day.
- Drink 300 mL of cranberry juice daily.
- Be sure to get enough sleep, rest, and nutrition daily.
- [For women] Clean your perineum (the area between your legs) from front to back.
- [For women] Avoid irritating substances, such as bubble bath, nylon underwear, and scented toilet tissue. Wear loose-fitting cotton underwear.
- [For women] Empty your bladder before and after intercourse.
- If you experience burning when you urinate, if you have to urinate frequently, or if you find it difficult to begin urinating, notify your physician or other health care provider right away, especially if you have a chronic medical condition (such as diabetes) or are pregnant.
- Empty your bladder as soon as you feel the urge to urinate.
- Empty your bladder regularly (e.g., every 4 hours), even if you do not feel the urge to urinate.
- You may try the following home therapies:
  Cranberry juice (pure) 50 mL daily.
  Apple cider vinegar, 2 tablespoons three times daily in juice.
  Vitamin C 500 mg daily to acidify the urine.
- To prevent recurrent infection:
  Take your medication as directed even after the symptoms go away.
  Schedule a follow-up appointment for 10 to 14 days after you finish taking your medication. At your follow-up visit, another urine sample may be taken for analysis or culture.

1. Should you use medical terminology during your assessment with this client? Why or why not?
2. What factors may have contributed to this client's infection?
3. What other assessment data should you obtain and why?
4. What is the risk that the client's infection could be passed on to her sexual partner?
5. What interventions will you teach her for comfort and treatment of this infection?
6. What interventions will you teach her for prevention of future episodes of cystitis?

evolve For suggested answer guidelines, go to http://evolve.elsevier.com/Iggy/.

Urethritis
PATHOPHYSIOLOGY

Urethritis is an inflammation of the urethra that causes symptoms similar to urinary tract infection (UTI). In men, manifestations of urethritis are burning or difficulty with urination and a discharge from the urethral meatus. The most common cause of urethritis in men is sexually transmitted diseases (STDs). These include gonorrhea or nonspecific urethritis caused by *Ureaplasma* (a gram-negative bacterium), *Chlamydia* (a sexually transmitted gram-negative bacterium), or *Trichomonas vaginalis* (a protozoan found in both the male and female genital tract).

In women, urethritis causes manifestations similar to those of bacterial cystitis. Urethritis is known by several other terms: *pyuria-dysuria syndrome, frequency-dysuria syndrome, trigonitis syndrome,* and *urethral syndrome.* Urethritis is most common in postmenopausal women and is probably caused by tissue changes related to low estrogen levels.

◆COLLABORATIVE MANAGEMENT
◆Assessment

Ask the client about a history of STD, painful or difficult urination, discharge from the penis or vagina, and discomfort in the lower abdomen. Urinalysis may show **pyuria** (white blood cells [WBCs]) without a large number of bacteria; however, results of urethral culture may indicate an STD. In women, the diagnosis may be made by exclusion when urinalysis and urethral culture are negative for bacteria and symptoms persist. In such cases, pelvic examination may reveal tissue changes from low estrogen levels in the vagina. Urethroscopy may show low estrogen changes with inflammation of urethral tissues.

◆Interventions

STDs are treated with antibiotic therapy. More information on STDs can be found in Chapter 80.

Postmenopausal women often have improvement in their urethral symptoms with the use of estrogen vaginal cream. Estrogen cream applied locally to the vagina increases the amount of estrogen in the urethra as well, and irritating symptoms are reduced.

NONINFECTIOUS DISORDERS
Urethral Strictures
PATHOPHYSIOLOGY

Urethral strictures are narrowed areas of the urethra. These problems may be caused by complications of an STD (usu-

ally gonorrhea) and from trauma during catheterization, urologic procedures, or childbirth. Strictures occur more often in men than in women. They may be a factor in other urologic problems, such as recurrent UTIs, urinary incontinence, and urinary retention.

◆COLLABORATIVE MANAGEMENT

The most common symptom of urethral stricture is obstruction of urine flow. Strictures rarely cause pain. Because urine stasis can result when flow is obstructed, the client with a stricture is at risk for developing a UTI and may have overflow incontinence. **Overflow incontinence** is the involuntary loss of urine when the bladder is overdistended. Assess the client for these two problems.

A urethral stricture is treated surgically. Dilation of the urethra (using a local anesthetic) is only a temporary measure, not a curative one. The best chance of long-term cure is with **urethroplasty,** surgical removal of the affected area with or without grafting to create a larger opening. The recurrence rate after surgery is still high, and most clients need repeated procedures.

Urinary Incontinence
PATHOPHYSIOLOGY

Continence (control over the time and place of urination) is unique to humans and some domestic animals. Continence is a learned behavior whereby a person can suppress the urge to urinate until a socially appropriate location is available (e.g., a toilet). Efficient bladder emptying (i.e., coordination between bladder contraction and urethral relaxation) is needed for continence.

Incontinence is an involuntary loss of urine severe enough to cause social or hygienic problems. Incontinence is *not* a normal consequence of aging or childbirth. Incontinence is stigmatizing and an underreported health problem. Many people suffer in silence, are socially isolated, and may be unaware that treatment is available. In addition, costs associated with incontinence are enormous for individuals and institutions.

Continence occurs when pressure in the urethra is greater than pressure in the bladder. For normal voiding to occur, the urethra must relax and the bladder must contract with enough pressure and duration to empty completely. Voiding should occur in a smooth and coordinated manner under a person's conscious control. Incontinence has several possible causes and can be either temporary or chronic (Table 73-3). Temporary causes usually do not involve a disorder of the urinary tract. The most common forms of urinary incontinence in adults are stress incontinence, urge incontinence, overflow incontinence, functional incontinence, and a mixed form.

Stress Incontinence

Stress incontinence is the most common type of incontinence. It is characterized by the loss of small amounts of urine during coughing, sneezing, jogging, or lifting. In the continent person, the urethra can be relaxed and tightened under conscious control because skeletal muscles of the pelvic floor surround it. When a person feels the urge to urinate, the conscious contraction of the urethra can override a bladder contraction if the urethral contraction is strong enough.

TABLE 73-3 Types of Urinary Incontinence

Type	Definition/Description	Cause	Clinical Manifestations
Stress incontinence	The involuntary loss of urine during activities that increase abdominal and detrusor pressure. Clients cannot tighten the urethra sufficiently to overcome the increased detrusor pressure; leakage of urine results.	Weakening of bladder neck supports; associated with childbirth. Intrinsic sphincter deficiency caused by such congenital conditions as epispadias (abnormal location of the urethra on the dorsum of the penis) or myelomeningocele. Acquired anatomic damage to the urethral sphincter (from repeated incontinence surgeries, prostatectomy, radiation therapy, and trauma).	Urine loss with physical exertion, cough, sneeze, or exercise. Usually only small amounts of urine are lost with each exertion. Normal voiding habits (≤8 times per day, 2 or fewer times per night). Postvoid residual usually ≤50 mL. Pelvic examination shows hypermobility of the urethra or bladder neck with Valsalva maneuvers.
Urge incontinence	The involuntary loss of urine associated with a strong desire to urinate. Clients cannot suppress the signal from the bladder muscle to the brain that it is time to urinate.	Unknown.	An abrupt and strong urge to void. May have loss of large amounts of urine with each occurrence.
Detrusor hyperreflexia (reflex incontinence)	The abnormal detrusor contractions result from neurologic abnormalities.	Central nervous system (CNS) lesions from stroke, multiple sclerosis, and parasacral spinal cord lesions. Local irritating factors such as caffeine, medications, or bladder tumor.	Postvoid residual <50 mL.
Overflow incontinence	The involuntary loss of urine associated with overdistention of the bladder when the bladder's capacity has reached its maximum. The urethra is obstructed, so it fails to relax sufficiently to allow urine to flow, resulting in incomplete bladder emptying or complete urinary retention, causing overflow incontinence.	Diabetic neuropathy; side effects of medication; after radical pelvic surgery or spinal cord damage; outlet obstruction. Causes external to the mechanism of the urethra: an enlarged prostate (male clients) and large genital prolapse (female clients). When the cause is intrinsic to the urethra, abnormal contraction of the skeletal muscle occurs, causing obstruction. This condition, called *detrusor dyssynergia*, is seen in clients with spinal cord injuries and multiple sclerosis.	Bladder distention, often up to the level of the umbilicus. Constant dribbling of urine.
Mixed incontinence	A combination of stress, urge, and overflow incontinence.	As with each separate disorder.	As with each separate disorder.
Functional incontinence	Leakage of urine caused by factors other than disease of the lower urinary tract.		Quantity and timing of urine leakage vary; patterns are difficult to discern.
Transient causes	Transient causes improve with treatment of the underlying condition.	Loss of cognitive functioning. Loss of awareness that urination is to occur in a socially acceptable place. Abnormal openings in the urinary tract, such as a fistula or diverticulum. Medications, such as sedatives, hypnotics, diuretics, anticholinergics, decongestants, antihypertensives, and calcium channel blockers. Diabetes insipidus or psychogenic polydipsia. Inability to get to toileting facilities. Direct bladder pressure or urethral obstruction.	Altered mental state, as in delirium, confusion, depression, dementia, sepsis, mental illness, or severe psychological stress. Urinary drainage noted from areas other than the urinary meatus. Some medications cause altered mental state; others cause increased urine production. Increased urine output. Restraints, restricted mobility. Constipation or fecal impaction.
Permanent causes	Permanent causes are organic but may be improved with treatment.	Cognitive impairment. Traumatic or surgical effects. Those factors contributing to stress incontinence, urge incontinence, and overflow incontinence. Structural or functional defects of the bladder or the sphincters. Injuries or diseases of the spinal cord, brainstem, or cerebral cortex (neurogenic bladder). Congenital defects, including exstrophy of the bladder (bladder turned "inside out") and spina bifida.	Clinical manifestations depend on the cause.

Clients who have *stress incontinence* cannot tighten the urethra enough to overcome the increased detrusor pressure. Stress incontinence is common after childbirth, when the pelvic muscles are stretched and weakened. The weakened pelvic floor allows mobility and displacement of the urethra during exertion. If the pelvic muscles are not strengthened, this condition continues. Low estrogen levels after menopause also contribute to stress incontinence. Vaginal, urethral, and pelvic floor muscles become thin and weak without estrogen.

Urge Incontinence

Bladder contractions are perceived as an urge to urinate. When the bladder is full, contraction of the smooth muscle fibers of the bladder detrusor muscle normally signals the brain that it is time to urinate. Continent persons override that signal and relax the detrusor muscle for the time it takes to locate a toilet. Those who suffer from urge incontinence cannot suppress the signal and leak large amounts of urine associated with a sudden, strong urge to void. Urge incontinence is also known as an "overactive bladder" or an unstable bladder. Overactivity may have no known cause or be the result of abnormal detrusor contractions related to other problems. Such problems include stroke, Parkinson's disease, multiple sclerosis, and spinal tumors or disease; UTI; benign prostatic enlargement; bladder irritability from concentrated urine or artificial sweeteners, caffeine, alcohol, and citric intake; use of diuretics and other drugs; nicotine; and atrophic vaginitis (Rigsby, 2003).

Mixed Incontinence

Many clients with urinary incontinence fall into the mixed category. Often urine loss is related to both stress and urge incontinence. The manifestations have aspects of more than one subtype. This category is more common in older women.

Overflow Incontinence

When the detrusor muscle fails to contract, the bladder becomes overdistended. Overflow incontinence (also known as "reflex incontinence") occurs when the bladder has reached its absolute maximal capacity and some urine must leak out to prevent bladder rupture. Causes for the underactive (acontractile) bladder may or may not be determined.

The urethra can be obstructed so that it fails to relax enough to allow urine flow. Incomplete bladder emptying or urinary retention due to urethral obstruction results in overflow incontinence.

Functional Incontinence

Factors other than the abnormal function of the bladder and urethra result in functional incontinence. A common factor is the loss of cognitive function in clients affected by dementia. To maintain continence, a person must be aware that urination needs to occur in a socially acceptable place; clients with dementia may not have that awareness.

Etiology and Genetic Risk

Incontinence may have temporary or permanent causes. Evaluation of the incontinent client means considering all possible causes, beginning with those that are temporary and correctable. Surgical and traumatic causes of urinary incontinence are related to procedures or surgery in the lower pelvic structures, areas that contain complex nerve pathways. Radical urologic, prostatic, and gynecologic procedures for treatment of pelvic cancers may result in urinary incontinence. Injury to segments S2 to S4 of the spinal cord may cause incontinence from impairment of normal nerve pathways.

Inappropriate bladder contraction may result from disorders of the brain and nervous system or from bladder irritation due to chronic infection, stones, chemotherapy, or radiation therapy. Failure of bladder contraction occurs with the autonomic neuropathy of diabetes mellitus and syphilis.

> ### CONSIDERATIONS FOR OLDER ADULTS
> Many factors contribute to urinary incontinence in older adults (Chart 73-6). An older person may have decreased mobility from disease, neurologic dysfunction, or musculoskeletal degeneration. In the hospital or extended care setting, mobility is limited when the older client is restrained or placed on bedrest. Vision and hearing impairments may also prevent the client from locating a call bell to notify the nurse or assistive personnel of the need to void. Assess for these factors and minimize them to prevent urinary incontinence.

Incidence/Prevalence

Incontinence is a major health problem that affects more than 13 million people of all ages in the United States (AHCPR, 1996); about 85% are women. It is most common in older adults, including 15% to 30% of community-dwelling older people and at least one half of all nursing home residents (AHCPR, 1996).

CHART 73-6

NURSING FOCUS on the OLDER ADULT
Factors Contributing to Urinary Incontinence*

Medications
- Central nervous system depressants, such as opioid analgesics, decrease the client's level of consciousness and the urge to void, and they contribute to constipation.
- Diuretics cause frequent voiding, often of large amounts of urine.
- Multiple medications can contribute to changes in mental status or mobility, and they can irritate the bladder.

Disease
- Cerebrovascular accidents and other neurologic disorders decrease mobility, sensation, or cognition.
- Arthritis decreases mobility and causes pain.
- Parkinson's disease causes muscle rigidity and an inability to initiate movement.

Depression
- Depression decreases the energy necessary to maintain continence.
- Decreased self-esteem and feelings of self-worth decrease the importance to the client of maintaining continence.

Inadequate Resources
- Clients who have glasses or use a cane, walker, or slippers may be afraid to ambulate.
- Products that help clients manage incontinence are often costly.
- No one may be available to assist the client to the bathroom or help with incontinence products.

*These factors are in addition to the physiologic changes of aging given in Chapter 5.

In adult clients under 65 years of age, urinary incontinence occurs twice as often in women as in men. Incontinence in women of this age may occur after one or more pregnancies. Men in this age group rarely experience incontinence unless they have prostate disease or a spinal cord injury.

◆COLLABORATIVE MANAGEMENT
◆Assessment

HISTORY

Effective screening includes asking clients to respond "always," "sometimes," or "never" to the following questions (Castina, Boyington, & Dougherty, 2002):

- Do you ever leak urine or water when you don't want to?
- Do you ever leak urine or water when you cough, laugh, or exercise?
- Do you ever leak urine or water on the way to the bathroom?
- Do you ever use pads, tissue, or cloth in your underwear to catch urine?

If any answer is always or sometimes, proceed with a focused assessment (AHCPR, 1996; Bates, 2002) (Chart 73-7). Incontinence may be underreported because health care professionals do not ask clients about urine loss. Do not assume that clients will volunteer the information without specifically being asked.

PHYSICAL ASSESSMENT/CLINICAL MANIFESTATIONS

Assess the abdomen to estimate bladder fullness, to rule out palpable hard stool, and to evaluate bowel sounds. With a physician's order, determine the amount of postvoid residual urine by portable ultrasound or catheterizing the client immediately after voiding. Urinary incontinence is confirmed by evaluating the force and character of the urine stream during voiding by the client. Asking the client to cough while wearing a perineal pad is useful in evaluating stress incontinence; a wet pad with forceful coughing may indicate stress incontinence. A cystometrogram (see Chapter 72) is used for diagnosis in most cases (Walsh et al., 2002).

For women, inspect the external genitalia to determine whether there is apparent urethral or uterine prolapse, **cystocele** (herniation of the bladder into the vagina), or rectocele. These conditions occur with pelvic floor muscle weakness. An advanced practice nurse puts on an examination glove and inserts two fingers into the vagina to assess the strength of these muscles. Strength is described as weak, adequate, or strong on the basis of the amount of pressure felt by the nurse as the client tightens her vaginal muscles. Describe and document the color, consistency, and odor of any secretions from the genitourinary orifices. The urine stream interruption test (see Chapter 72) is another method of determining pelvic muscle strength. For men, inspect the urethral meatus for any discharge.

A digital rectal examination is performed on both male and female clients. This examination provides information about the integrity of the nerve supply to the bladder. The examiner determines whether there is tactile sensation in the anorectal area by observing whether the rectal sphincter is relaxed or contracted on digital insertion. Because nerve supply to the bladder is similar to nerve supply to the rectum, the presence of tactile sensation and a rectal sphincter

CHART 73-7

FOCUSED ASSESSMENT of
The Client with Urinary Incontinence

Note the presence of risk factors for urinary incontinence:
- Age
- If female, menopausal status
- Neurologic disease
  - Parkinson's disease
  - Dementia
  - Multiple sclerosis
  - Stroke
  - Spinal injury
- Diabetes mellitus
- Childbirth
- Urologic procedures
- Medications
- Bowel patterns
- Stress/anxiety level

Detail the symptoms of urinary incontinence:
- Leakage
- Frequency
- Urgency
- Nocturia
- Sensation of full bladder before leakage

Obtain a 24-hour intake and output record:
- Time and amount of oral intake and continent voidings
- Time and estimated amount of incontinent leakages
- Activity around the time of leakage

Assess client's:
- Mobility
- Self-care ability
- Cognitive ability
- Communication patterns

Assess the environment for barriers to toileting:
- Privacy
- Restrictive clothing
- Access to toilet

Data from Mather, K. (2002). Nursing assistants' perceptions of their ability to provide continence care. *Geriatric Nursing, 23*(2), 76-81; and Agency for Health Care Policy and Research. (1996). *Urinary incontinence in adults: Acute and chronic management. Clinical practice guideline.* AHCPR Publication No. 96-0682. Rockville, MD: Agency for Health Care Policy and Research, Public Health Service, U.S. Department of Health and Human Services; http://www.ahcpr.gov/clinic/uhistory.html (Clinical Practice Guidelines Online: Urinary Incontinence Guideline: Real World Examples of Use).

that contracts suggest that the nerve supply to the bladder is intact. A fecal impaction may be discovered during rectal examination. The health care provider assesses for prostate enlargement in men.

LABORATORY ASSESSMENT

A urinalysis is useful to rule out infection. This test is the first step in the assessment of incontinent clients of any age. The presence of red blood cells (RBCs), white blood cells (WBCs), leukocyte esterase, or nitrites is an indication for culturing the urine. Any infection is treated before further assessment of incontinence.

RADIOGRAPHIC ASSESSMENT

Radiographic assessment is rarely needed unless surgery is being considered. Urography is the most useful for locating the kidneys and ureters. A voiding cystourethrogram (VCUG) may be performed to assess the size, shape, support, and function of the bladder. Problems identified by this test include obstruction (especially prostate obstruction in men), or postvoid residual (PVR). Assessment of PVR also can be made with a portable ultrasonographic bladder scanner.

OTHER DIAGNOSTIC ASSESSMENTS

Clients who have unusual symptoms, medical complications, or a history of failed incontinence surgery may need urodynamic studies to determine the cause of their incontinence. Such studies are not standardized procedures and may consist of any combination of the following tests:

- Cystourethroscopy to examine the inside of the bladder and urethra directly
- Cystometrogram (CMG) to measure the pressure inside the bladder as it fills
- Urethral pressure profilometry (UPP) to measure the pressure in the urethra in relation to the bladder pressure during various activities
- Uroflowmetry to measure rate and degree of bladder emptying

Testing may take several hours and more than one visit (see Chapter 72).

Electromyography (EMG) of the pelvic muscles may be a part of the urodynamic studies. A perineometer is a tampon-shaped instrument inserted into the vagina to measure the strength of pelvic muscle contractions. The graph shows the amplitude of muscle contraction to the client as a method of biofeedback.

Critical Thinking Challenge

The client is a 78-year-old woman who is being admitted to an assisted living environment. When you ask her what she needs help with and what she can do independently, she confides in you that she has trouble getting to the bathroom in time and has frequent "accidents." She states, "It seems my bladder is smaller than ever. When I have to go, I really have to go right then." She wears paper towels in her underwear to catch the urine before she wets her clothes. She says that she expected this to happen because her mother and sisters all had bladder problems when they got old. She also says "That's what happens when you have nine pound babies." She says she tries to drink very little so that she will remain dry.

1. What other questions should you ask?
2. What type or types of incontinence is she most likely to have from the information she has provided thus far?
3. Is this problem likely to be genetic? Why or why not?
4. Which nursing diagnoses would be priority for this client?

evolve For suggested answer guidelines, go to http://evolve.elsevier.com/Iggy/.

◆ Analysis

COMMON NURSING DIAGNOSES AND COLLABORATIVE PROBLEMS

The following are priority nursing diagnoses for clients with urinary incontinence:

1. Stress Urinary Incontinence related to weak pelvic muscles and structural supports
2. Urge Urinary Incontinence related to decreased bladder capacity, bladder spasms, diet, and neurologic impairment
3. Reflex Urinary Incontinence related to neurologic impairment
4. Functional Urinary Incontinence related to impaired cognition or neuromuscular limitations
5. Mixed or Total Urinary Incontinence related to many causes

ADDITIONAL NURSING DIAGNOSES AND COLLABORATIVE PROBLEMS

In addition to the common nursing diagnoses, clients with urinary incontinence may have one or more of the following:

- Social Isolation related to altered state of wellness or fear of embarrassment
- Risk for Impaired Skin Integrity related to excessive moisture from urinary excretions
- Disturbed Body Image related to odor, need to alter clothing selections, or need to wear protective briefs or supplies
- Risk for Infection related to increased environmental exposure to pathogens from retained or refluxing urine

◆ Planning and Implementation

Several interventions are useful for each type of incontinence. Collaborative management uses these interventions, as well as medication, surgical repair, and diet therapy (Newman & Palmer, 2003).

STRESS URINARY INCONTINENCE

NOC **PLANNING: EXPECTED OUTCOMES.** With appropriate therapy, the client with urinary incontinence is expected to develop urinary continence. Indicators include that the client rarely or never demonstrates the following actions:

- Urine leakage between voidings
- Urine leakage with increased abdominal pressure (e.g., sneezing, laughing, lifting)

INTERVENTIONS. Initial interventions for clients with stress incontinence include keeping a diary, behavioral interventions, and drugs. Surgery also may be an option if other interventions are not effective. Explain the purpose of a detailed diary in which the client records times of urine leakage, activities, and foods eaten. The diary is then used by the health care practitioner to plan and evaluate interventions. Collection devices, absorbent pads, and undergarments may be used during the sometimes lengthy process of assessment and treatment and by those clients who elect not to pursue further interventions.

NONSURGICAL MANAGEMENT. Drug therapy and behavioral interventions (primarily diet and exercise) for stress incontinence require the client's active participation for success; however, these efforts have had significant proven success (see the Evidence-Based Practice for Nursing box on p. 1690). Providing ongoing encouragement, clarification, and support is extremely valuable for maximizing the effects of all interventions.

Exercise Therapy. Pelvic floor (Kegel) exercises for women with stress incontinence strengthen the muscles of the pelvic floor (circumvaginal muscles). These muscles become strengthened, as any other skeletal muscle does, by frequent, systematic, and repeated contractions.

The most important step in teaching pelvic muscle exercises is to help the client become aware of which muscle to exercise. During the pelvic examination in women and the rectal examination in men or women, instruct the client to tighten the pelvic muscles around your fingers. Then provide feedback about the strength of the contraction. Biofeedback devices, such as electromyography (EMG) or perineometers (see earlier discussion under Other Diagnostic Assessments), measure the strength of contraction. Retention of a vaginal weight is also evidence that the client

EVIDENCE-BASED PRACTICE for Nursing

Low tech is effective when reinforced by nurses

Goode, P., et al. (2003). Effect of behavioral training with or without pelvic floor electrical stimulation on stress incontinence in women. *Journal of the American Medical Association, 290*(3), 345-352.

The purpose of this prospective randomized controlled clinical trial was to determine whether pelvic floor electrical stimulation (PFES) could increase the efficacy of behavioral training for continence improvement among community-dwelling women with stress incontinence. The sample consisted of 200 women between 40 and 78 years of age with stress incontinence or mixed incontinence in which stress incontinence was dominant. Incontinence was confirmed with clinical evaluation and urodynamic studies. The subjects were randomly assigned to one of three treatment groups. One group received 8 weeks of behavioral training for pelvic floor exercises, including four visits from a nurse practitioner. A second group received the same 8-week behavioral training and additionally used PFES. The third group did not receive nurse-guided behavioral training or PFES; these subjects used a self-administered behavior training booklet for performing pelvic floor exercises. All subjects used bladder diaries throughout the study period to document episodes of incontinence. Evaluation of change in incontinence was determined by data in the bladder diaries and changes in urodynamic study results.

Of the 200 subjects who began the study, 155 completed the study. The group using the self-administered program had the highest attrition rate (37.3%) and the group receiving behavioral training plus PFES had the lowest attrition rate (11.9%). A significant reduction in incontinence was found across all groups (52.5% to 71.9%). Although greatest reduction was seen in the group receiving behavioral training plus PFES, it was not significantly different from the group receiving only the behavioral training. The investigators concluded that pelvic floor exercises are effective in improving pelvic muscle tone and reducing stress incontinence. They also concluded that having nurses teach, reinforce, and monitor behavior activities is a key factor in improving adherence to the behavioral intervention.

Level of Evidence: 2—Properly designed randomized controlled trial of appropriate size.

Critique. The study was well designed and used multiple objective measures as well as subjective measures to determine outcome. A major strength is the number of subjects. The study could have been strengthened by having a fourth group of subjects with stress incontinence who did not receive an intervention during the 8 weeks, but did receive four visits by a nurse.

Implications for Nursing. Stress incontinence is a common and costly problem for middle-aged and older women. Consistently and correctly performing pelvic floor exercises can reduce the severity of stress incontinence for many women; however, improvement is not immediate and requires adherence to the regimen. Nurses can provide the encouragement and recognition of positive advances to help women continue this therapeutic regimen. Nurses should ask about the presence of stress incontinence in all female clients older than 40 years of age and instruct clients in the correct techniques for progressive pelvic floor exercise.

CHART 73-8

CLIENT EDUCATION GUIDE
Pelvic Muscle Exercises

- The pelvic muscles are composed of a sling of muscles that support your bladder, urethra, and vagina. Like any other muscles in your body, you can make your pelvic muscles stronger by alternately contracting (tightening) and relaxing them in regular exercise periods. By strengthening these muscles, you will be able to stop your urine flow more effectively.
- *To identify your pelvic muscles*, sit on the toilet with your feet flat on the floor about 12 inches apart. Begin to urinate, then try to stop the urine flow. Do not strain down, lift your bottom off the seat, or squeeze your legs together. When you start and stop your urine stream, you are using your pelvic muscles.
- *To perform pelvic muscle exercises*, tighten your pelvic muscles for a slow count of 10, then relax for a slow count of 10. Do this exercise 15 times while you are lying down, sitting up, and standing (a total of 45 exercises). Repeat, this time rapidly contracting and relaxing the pelvic muscles 10 times. This should take no more than 10 to 12 minutes for all three positions, or 3 to 4 minutes for each set of 15 exercises.
- Begin with 45 exercises a day in three sets of 15 exercises each. You will notice faster improvement if you can do this twice a day, or a total of 20 minutes each day. Remember to exercise in all three positions so your muscles learn to squeeze effectively despite your position. At first, it is helpful to have a designated time and place to do these exercises because you will have to concentrate to do them correctly. After you have been doing them for several weeks, you will notice improvement in your control of urine; however, many people report that improvement may take as long as 3 months.

---

has identified the proper muscle. The ability to start and stop the urine stream or stop the passage of flatus is evidence that the client has correctly identified the pelvic muscles.

Instructions for pelvic muscle exercises are given in Chart 73-8. Although improvement may take several months, most clients notice a positive change after 6 weeks. Teach clients to continue the exercises to maintain the improvement.

Diet Therapy. A diet plan for weight reduction is helpful for obese clients because stress incontinence is made worse by increased abdominal pressure from obesity. Instruct the client to avoid alcohol, nicotine, artificial sweeteners, citrus, and caffeine (bladder irritants). Refer the client to the dietitian as needed.

Drug Therapy. Because bladder pressure is greater than urethral resistance in clients with stress incontinence, drugs may be used to improve urethral resistance (Chart 73-9).

Estrogen is used to treat postmenopausal women with stress incontinence, although its exact mechanism of action is unknown. Estrogen may increase the blood flow and tone of the circumvaginal and periurethral muscles, thus improving the client's ability to contract those muscles during times of increased intra-abdominal stress.

Vaginal Cone Therapy. Vaginal cones are a set of five small, cone-shaped weights. They are of equal size but of varying weights and are used with pelvic muscle exercise. The woman inserts the lightest cone, labeled 1, into her vagina (Figure 73-1), with the string to the outside, for a 1-minute test period. If she can hold the first cone in place without its slipping out while she walks around, she proceeds to the second cone, labeled 2, and repeats the procedure. The client begins her treatment with the heaviest cone she can comfortably hold in her vagina for the 1-minute test period. Treatment periods are 15 minutes twice a day. When the client can comfortably hold the cone in her vagina for the 15-minute period, she progresses to the next heaviest weight. Treatment is completed with the cone labeled 5.

Weighted vaginal cones are helpful in strengthening the pelvic muscles and decreasing stress incontinence but may not help pelvic prolapse. Vaginal cones are available without prescription.

CHART 73-9

DRUG THERAPY for
Urinary Incontinence

Drug	Usual Dosage	Nursing Interventions	Rationales
Estrogen (Premarin, C.E.S.✱)	0.3-1.25 mg PO daily 1-2 g every other day per vagina	Report any unusual vaginal bleeding or calf pain.	Estrogen use can increase the risk of endometrial cancer and thrombophlebitis.
Anticholinergics/ antispasmodics Propantheline (Pro-Banthine, Propanthel✱)	7.5-30 mg PO three to four times daily	Check the client's intraocular pressure before starting the regimen.	Anticholinergics can increase intraocular pressure and are contraindicated in the presence of narrow-angle glaucoma.
Oxybutynin (Ditropan)	2.5-5 mg PO three to four times daily	Offer fluids and hard candy to moisten the mouth. Give the drug between meals.	Anticholinergics cause extreme dryness of the mouth. Food interferes with absorption of the drug.
(Ditropan XL) Dicyclomine hydrochloride (Bentyl, Di-Spaz, Bentylol✱, Formulex✱, Lomine✱)	5-15 mg PO daily 10-20 mg PO three times daily	Increase fluids and fiber in the client's diet.	Anticholinergics decreases GI motility and can cause constipation.
Tolterodine ⬇️¹(Detrol) (Detrol LA)	2 mg PO twice daily 4 mg PO daily	Warn the client to check that daily urine output is equal to intake.	Drug can cause urinary retention.
Tricyclic antidepressants Imipramine (Tofranil, Novo-Pramine✱)	25-100 mg PO daily	Administer the full dose at bedtime if possible and warn clients that dizziness may occur on arising in the morning.	Tricyclics have a high potential to cause postural hypotension.
Desipramine (Norpramin)	10-25 mg PO three times daily	Warn clients about other anticholinergic and alpha-adrenergic side effects.	Tricyclics have a combination of anticholinergic and alpha-adrenergic effects.
Nortriptyline ⬇️²(Pamelor)	10-25 mg PO three times daily		

⬇️¹*Med Error Alert!* Do not confuse with Detensol, a beta blocker.
⬇️²*Med Error Alert!* Do not confuse Pamelor with pamidronate, a drug used to prevent osteoporosis.

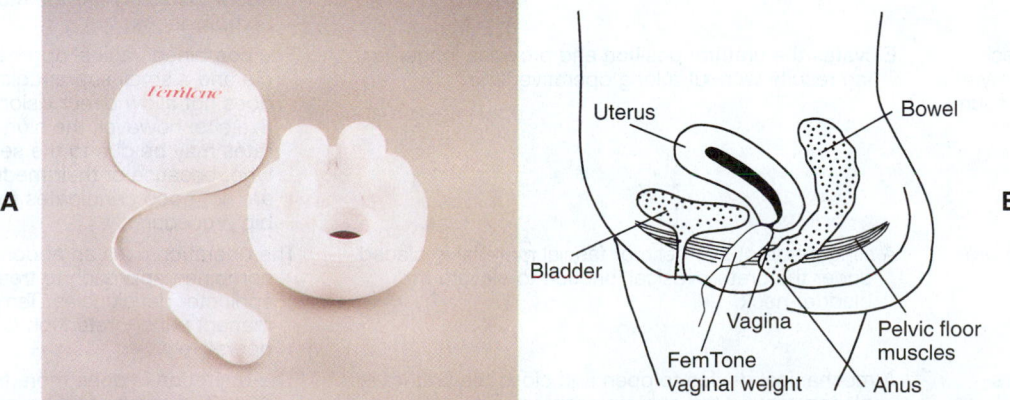

A

B

Uterus
Bowel
Bladder
Vagina
FemTone vaginal weight
Pelvic floor muscles
Anus

Figure 73-1 ■ **A,** FemTone vaginal weights, or cones. The number on the top of each cone represents increasing weight up to the heaviest cone, a 5. **B,** Diagram showing the correct positioning of a vaginal weight, or cone, in place. (**A** courtesy of ConvaTec, A Bristol-Meyers Squibb Company, a Division of E.R. Squibb & Sons, Inc., Princeton, NJ; **B** from ConvaTec. [1996]. FemTone vaginal weights: A training aid for pelvic floor exercises [brochure]. Princeton, NJ: Author.)

Other Therapy. Other interventions for stress incontinence include behavior modification, psychotherapy, and electrical stimulation devices to strengthen urethral contractions. Many intravaginal and intrarectal electrical stimulation devices have been used with varying degrees of success. More research is needed to determine the ideal level of stimulation and methods of reducing discomfort before electrical stimulation becomes a standard treatment for incontinence.

The Reliance insert is like a tiny tampon that the client inserts into the urethra. After insertion, the client inflates a tiny balloon, which rests at the bladder neck and prevents the flow of urine. To void, the client pulls a string to deflate the balloon and removes the device. The applicator is reusable, although the tampon part is disposed of after each void.

SURGICAL MANAGEMENT. Stress incontinence may be corrected by vaginal, abdominal, or retropubic surgeries. Success rates vary between 50% and 90% for most procedures, but these rates are difficult to evaluate because of the varying definitions of cure. Cure also may vary between short-term and long-term (over 5 years) results. Complications can be significant, with rates ranging from less than 2% for collagen or Siloxane injection to 50% for bladder neck suspension.

Preoperative Care. Teach the client about the procedure and clarify events surrounding the surgery. Extensive urodynamic testing (see Chapter 72) is often performed before surgery, and the need for such thorough assessment should be explained to the client.

Operative Procedures. The surgical procedures used for women include repositioning the urethra and bladder, changing the structure of the involved tissues, or inserting artificial devices to improve function (Table 73-4).

Postoperative Care. After surgery, assess for and intervene to prevent or detect complications. For prevention of movement or traction on the bladder neck, secure the urethral catheter with tape or a tube holder. If a suprapubic catheter is used instead of a urethral catheter, monitor the dressing for urine leakage and other drainage. Catheters are usually in place until the client can urinate easily and has postvoid residual urine of less than 50 mL. (See Chapters 20 and 22 for a discussion of general care before and after surgery.)

URGE URINARY INCONTINENCE

NOC **PLANNING: EXPECTED OUTCOMES.** The client with urinary incontinence is expected to use techniques to prevent or manage urge incontinence. Indicators include that the client often or consistently demonstrates the following behaviors:

- Responds to urge in a timely manner
- Gets to toilet between urge and passage of urine
- Avoids substances that stimulate the bladder (e.g., caffeine and alcohol)

INTERVENTIONS. Interventions for clients with urge incontinence or overactive bladder include behavioral

---

TABLE 73-4 Surgical Procedures for Stress Incontinence

Procedure	Purpose	Nursing Considerations
Anterior vaginal repair (colporrhaphy)	Elevates the urethral position and repairs any cystocele.	Because the operation is performed by vaginal incision, it is often done in conjunction with a vaginal hysterectomy. Recovery is usually rapid, and a urethral catheter is in place for 24-48 hr.
Retropubic suspension (Marshall-Marchetti-Krantz or Burch colposuspension)	Elevates the urethral position and provides longer-lasting results.	The operation requires a low abdominal incision and a urethral or suprapubic catheter for several days postoperatively. Recovery takes longer, and urinary retention and detrusor instability are the most frequent complications.
Needle bladder neck suspension (Pereyra or Stamey procedure)	Elevates the urethral position and provides longer-lasting results without a long operative time.	The combined vaginal approach with a needle and a small suprapubic skin incision does not allow direct vision of the operative site; however, the high complication rates may be due to the selection of clients who, because of their medical condition, are not good candidates for longer retropubic procedures.
Pubovaginal sling procedures	A sling made of synthetic or fascial material is placed under the urethrovesical junction to elevate the bladder neck.	The operation uses an abdominal, vaginal, or combined approach to treat intrinsic sphincter deficiencies. Temporary or permanent urinary retention is common postoperatively.
Artificial sphincters	A mechanical device to open and close the urethra is placed around the anatomic urethra.	The operation is done more frequently in men. The most common complications include mechanical failure of the device, erosion of tissue, and infection.
Periurethral injection of collagen or Siloxane	Implantation of small amounts of an inert substance through several small injections provides support around the bladder neck.	The procedure can be done in an ambulatory care setting and can be repeated as often as necessary. Certain compounds may migrate after injection; an allergy test to bovine collagen must be performed before implantation.

Data from Schultz, J.A., & Drutz, H.P. (1999). The surgical management of recurrent urinary stress incontinence. *Current Opinions in Obstetrics and Gynecology, 11*(5), 489-494; and Lighter, D.J., & Itano, N.M. (1999). Treatment options for women with stress urinary incontinence. *Mayo Clinic Proceedings, 74*(11), 1149-1156.

interventions and drugs (Newman & Giovannini, 2002). Surgery is not the recommended treatment of this condition. Collection devices and absorbent pads and undergarments may be used.

Drug Therapy. Because the hypertonic bladder contracts involuntarily in clients with urge incontinence, drugs that relax the smooth muscle and increase the bladder's capacity are prescribed (see Chart 73-9).

The most effective drugs are anticholinergics, such as propantheline (Pro-Banthine, Propanthel✱), and anticholinergics with smooth muscle relaxant properties, such as oxybutynin (Ditropan and Ditropan XL), tolterodine (Detrol and Detrol LA), and dicyclomine hydrochloride (Bentyl, Formulex✱, Spasmoban✱, Viscerol✱). This class of drugs has serious side effects and is used in conjunction with behavioral interventions. These drugs inhibit the nerve fibers that stimulate bladder contraction. Tricyclic antidepressants with anticholinergic and alpha-adrenergic agonist activity, such as imipramine (Tofranil, Novopramine✱), have been used successfully. The effectiveness of other drugs, such as flavoxate (Urispas) and the antihistamines, nonsteroidal anti-inflammatory agents, beta-adrenergic agonists, and calcium channel blockers, have yet to be determined.

Diet Therapy. Instruct the client to avoid foods that have a direct bladder-stimulating or diuretic effect, such as caffeine and alcohol. Spacing fluids at regular intervals throughout the day (e.g., 120 mL every hour or 240 mL every 2 hours) and limiting fluids after the dinner hour (e.g., only 120 mL at bedtime) help avoid fluid overload on the bladder and allow urine to accumulate at a steady pace.

Behavioral Interventions. Behavioral interventions for urge incontinence include bladder training, habit training, exercise therapy, and electrical stimulation.

NIC interventions for urinary bladder training and urinary habit training are listed in Chart 73-10. It can be difficult for clients to use these interventions because they involve a significant amount of client participation. Provide ongoing encouragement, clarification, and support to maxi-

---

CHART 73-10

NIC **INTERVENTION ACTIVITIES for**
The Client with Urinary Incontinence

Urinary Bladder Training: *Improving bladder function for those with urge incontinence by increasing the bladder's ability to hold urine and the client's ability to suppress urination*
- Determine ability to recognize urge to void.
- Keep a continence specification record for 3 days to establish voiding pattern.
- Establish interval of initial toileting schedule, based on voiding pattern.
- Establish beginning and ending time for toileting schedule, if not for 24 hours.
- Establish interval for toileting of not less than 1 hour and preferably not less than 2 hours.
- Toilet client or remind client to void at prescribed intervals.
- Provide privacy for toileting.
- Use power of suggestion (e.g., running water or flushing toilet) to assist client to void.
- Avoid leaving client on toilet for more than 5 minutes.
- Reduce toileting interval by one half hour if there are more than three incontinence episodes in 24 hours.
- Increase toileting interval by 1 hour if client has no incontinence episodes for 3 days until optimal 4-hour interval is achieved.
- Teach the client to consciously hold urine until the scheduled toileting time.
- Discuss daily record of continence with client to provide reinforcement.

Urinary Habit Training: *Establishing a predictable pattern of bladder emptying to prevent incontinence for persons with limited cognitive ability who have urge, stress, or functional incontinence.*
- Keep a continence specification record for 3 days to establish voiding pattern.
- Establish interval of initial toileting schedule, based on voiding pattern and usual routine (e.g., eating, rising, and retiring).
- Establish beginning and ending time for the toileting schedule, if not for 24 hours.
- Establish interval for toileting of preferably not less than 2 hours.
- Assist client to toilet and prompt to void at prescribed intervals.
- Provide privacy for toileting.
- Use power of suggestion (e.g., running water or flushing toilet) to assist client to void.

- Avoid leaving the client on toilet for more than 5 minutes.
- Reduce toileting interval by one half hour if there are more than two incontinence episodes in 24 hours.
- Maintain toileting interval if there are two or fewer incontinence episodes in 24 hours.
- Increase the toileting interval by one half hour if client has no incontinence episodes in 48 hours until optimal 4-hour interval is achieved.
- Discuss daily record of continence with staff to provide reinforcement and encourage compliance with toileting schedule.
- Maintain scheduled toileting to assist in establishing and maintaining voiding habit.
- Give positive feedback or positive reinforcement (e.g., 5 minutes of social conversation) to client when he/she voids at scheduled toileting times, and make no comment when client is incontinent.

Urinary Catheterization: *Intermittent: Regular periodic use of a catheter to empty the bladder*
- Teach client/family purpose, supplies, method, and rationale of intermittent catheterization.
- Teach client/family clean intermittent catheterization technique.
- Provide quiet private room for the procedure.
- Demonstrate procedure and have a return demonstration, as appropriate.
- Determine catheterization schedule based on comprehensive urinary assessment.
- Adjust frequency of catheterization to maintain output of 300 cc or less.
- Maintain client on prophylactic antibacterial therapy for 2 to 3 weeks at initiation of intermittent catheterization, as appropriate.
- Complete a urinalysis about every 2 weeks to 1 month.
- Establish a catheterization schedule based on individual needs.
- Maintain a detailed record of catheterization schedule, fluid intake, and output.
- Teach client/family signs and symptoms of urinary tract infection.
- Monitor color, odor, and clarity of urine.

NIC intervention activities selected from Dochterman, J.M., & Bulechek, G.M. (Eds.). (2004). *Nursing interventions classification (NIC)* (4th ed.). St. Louis: Mosby. No part of this work is to be altered without prior written permission from the Publisher.

mize the effects of all interventions. Behavioral interventions are often combined with drug therapy for maximal effect.

Bladder Training. Bladder training is an education program for the client that begins with a thorough explanation of the problem of urge incontinence. Instead of the bladder being in control of the client, the client learns to control the bladder. For the program to succeed, he or she must be alert, aware, and able to resist the urge to urinate.

Start a schedule for voiding, beginning with the longest interval that is comfortable for the client, even if the interval is only 30 minutes. Instruct the client to void every 30 minutes and to ignore any urge to urinate between the mandated intervals. Once the client is comfortable with the initial schedule, increase the interval by 15 to 30 minutes. Instruct the client to follow the new schedule until success is again achieved. As the interval increases, the bladder gradually tolerates more volume. Teach the client relaxation and distraction techniques to maximize success in the retraining. Provide positive reinforcement for maintaining the prescribed schedule.

Habit Training. Habit training (scheduled toileting) is a type of bladder training that is successful in reducing incontinence in cognitively impaired clients. To use habit training, caregivers assist the client in voiding at specific times (e.g., every 2 hours on the even hours). The goal is to get the client to the toilet before incontinence occurs. There is no effort to increase bladder capacity by gradually lengthening the voiding intervals.

Prompted voiding, a supplement to habit training, attempts to increase the client's awareness of the need to void and to prompt him or her to ask for toileting assistance. Habit training otherwise relies completely on a time schedule.

Exercise Therapy. Pelvic muscle exercises for urge incontinence have been helpful and are taught in the same way as for stress incontinence (see Chart 73-8). Improved urethral resistance helps the client overcome abnormal detrusor contractions long enough to get to the toilet.

Electrical Stimulation. Many different intravaginal and intrarectal electrical stimulation devices are available to treat both urge and stress incontinence.

REFLEX URINARY INCONTINENCE

NOC PLANNING: EXPECTED OUTCOMES. With appropriate intervention, the client with urinary incontinence is expected to achieve continence. Indicators include that the client often or consistently demonstrates the following behaviors:

- Recognizes the urge to void
- Maintains a predictable pattern of voiding
- Responds to urge in a timely manner
- Empties bladder completely
- Keeps urine volume in the bladder within normal limits to prevent bladder overdistention

INTERVENTIONS. Interventions for the client with reflex (overflow) incontinence caused by obstruction of the bladder outlet may include surgery to relieve the obstruction. The most common surgical procedures are prostate removal (see Chapter 79) and repair of genital prolapse (see Chapter 78). For overflow incontinence related to detrusor muscle weakness, the most effective method of treatment is intermittent catheterization. Behavioral interventions such as bladder compression and intermittent self-catheterization are the primary management techniques for urinary retention with overflow incontinence.

Drug Therapy. Drugs are prescribed for short-term management of urinary retention, often after surgery. They are not used in long-term management of overflow incontinence caused by a hypotonic bladder. The most commonly used drug is bethanechol chloride (Urecholine), an agent that increases bladder pressure.

Behavioral Interventions. The most common behavioral interventions are bladder compression and intermittent self-catheterization.

Bladder Compression. Techniques that promote bladder emptying include the Credé method, the Valsalva maneuver, double-voiding, and splinting.

In the Credé method, instruct the client in external compression of the urinary bladder or parasympathetic stimulation via tugging at pubic hair or massaging the genital area. These techniques manually assist the bladder in emptying. In the Valsalva maneuver, breathing techniques increase intrathoracic and intra-abdominal pressure. This increased pressure is then directed toward the bladder during exhalation. With the technique of double-voiding, the client empties the bladder and then, within a few minutes, attempts a second bladder emptying.

For women who have a large cystocele (prolapse of the bladder into the vagina), a technique called *splinting* both compresses the bladder and moves it into a better position. The woman inserts her fingers into her vagina, gently pushes the cystocele back into the vagina, and begins to urinate.

Intermittent Self-Catheterization. NIC interventions for intermittent urinary catheterization are listed in Chart 73-10. Teach intermittent self-catheterization to clients with long-term problems of incomplete bladder emptying. Self-catheterization is effective and can be learned fairly easily. The following points are important in teaching this technique:

- Proper handwashing and cleaning of the catheter reduce the frequency of infection.
- A small lumen and good lubrication of the catheter prevent urethral trauma.
- A regular schedule for bladder emptying prevents bladder overdistention and mucosal trauma.

Clients must be able to understand instructions and have the manual dexterity to manipulate the catheter. Caregivers or family members in the home can also be taught to perform straight catheterization using a clean (rather than sterile) technique with good outcomes.

FUNCTIONAL URINARY INCONTINENCE

NOC PLANNING: EXPECTED OUTCOMES. The client with functional urinary incontinence is expected to remain dry. Indicators include that the client often or consistently demonstrates the following behaviors:

- Uses urine containment or collection measures to ensure dryness
- Manages clothing independently

INTERVENTIONS. Causes of functional (or chronic intractable) incontinence vary greatly; some are reversible, and others are not. The focus of intervention is treatment of reversible causes. When incontinence is not reversible, urinary habit training (see Habit Training, p. 1694) is used to establish a predictable pattern of bladder emptying to prevent incontinence. A final strategy focuses on containment of the urine and protection of the client's skin. Nonsurgical interventions include applied devices, containment, and catheterization.

Applied Devices. Applied devices include intravaginal pessaries for women and penile clamps for men. The intravaginal pessary supports the uterus and vagina and helps maintain the correct position of the bladder. (See Chapter 78 for further discussion of pessaries.) The penile clamp is applied externally to compress the urethra and prevent leakage of urine.

The dangers of pessaries and penile clamps include damage to the tissues and infection from constant pressure in sensitive areas. Both devices require either that the client have manual dexterity or that a caregiver applies and removes the device. Instruct the client or caregivers in the use of these devices. Male clients may use an external collecting device, such as a condom catheter. Design of an effective external collecting device for women has not been as successful.

Containment. Absorbent pads and briefs are designed to collect urine and keep the client's skin and clothing dry. Many types and sizes of pads are available:

- Shields or liners inserted inside a panty
- Undergarments consisting of full-sized pads with waist straps
- Plastic-lined protective underpants with or without elastic legs
- Combination pad and pant systems
- Absorbent bed pads

A major concern with the use of protective pads is the risk that skin breakdown will occur. Materials and costs vary. Some are reusable; others are disposable. The disposal of these products raises ecologic concerns. Avoid use of the word "diaper" when discussing these adult protective pants, however, because of the usual association of diapers with babies.

Urinary Catheterization. Catheterization for control of incontinence may be intermittent or involve an indwelling catheter. Intermittent catheterization is preferred to an indwelling catheter because of the reduced risk for infection. Indwelling urinary catheters should be used temporarily and only when all other interventions have been unsuccessful. A long-term indwelling urinary catheter is appropriate for clients with skin breakdown who need a dry environment for healing, clients who are terminally ill and need comfort, and clients who are critically ill and require careful measurement of urine output.

MIXED OR TOTAL URINARY INCONTINENCE

Mixed or total urinary incontinence is a combination of two or more types of involuntary urine loss syndromes. For example, stress incontinence and urge incontinence often occur together in perimenopausal and postmenopausal women. For the client with mixed or total incontinence, combinations of assessment techniques (as discussed under each syndrome) are used. Interventions are similarly combined to promote continence. The problems and interventions for mixed incontinence are the same as they are for each specific type of incontinence separately. After identifying the specific types of incontinence experienced by the client with mixed incontinence, apply the appropriate nursing diagnoses, collaborative problems, interventions, and expected outcomes discussed earlier with each incontinence type.

Critical Thinking Challenge

Your older client in assistive living (previously described) is diagnosed with mixed stress and urge incontinence. Her en-

vironment has no barriers to toileting. She has been prescribed to take tolterodine (Detrol) for her urge incontinence. Additionally, she is to use vaginal cones for improving her pelvic floor muscles for the stress incontinence. She tells you she isn't sure she should be touching herself "down there."

1. What should you teach her about the effects and side effects of her newly prescribed drug?
2. How could she strengthen her pelvic floor muscles without touching herself?
3. How can you help evaluate this client's response to exercise and the prescribed drug to improve continence?

evolve For suggested answer guidelines, go to http://evolve.elsevier.com/Iggy/.

Community-Based Care

Community-based care for the client with urinary incontinence considers his or her personal, physical, emotional, and social resources. Important personal resources for self-care include mobility, vision, and manual dexterity. When planning care, consider who will be the primary caregiver and what factors may influence the effectiveness of the plan.

HOME CARE MANAGEMENT

Assess the home environment for barriers that impede access to the toileting facilities. Eliminate hazards that might slow walking or contribute to injury. These hazards might include small area rugs (throw rugs), tables or chairs with legs that extend into the walking area, slippery waxed or polished floors, and inadequate lighting.

If the client must climb stairs to reach a bathroom, handrails should be installed and stairs should be kept free of obstacles. Toilet seat extenders may help provide the right level of seating so that maximal abdominal pressure may be applied to encourage voiding. Portable commodes may be obtained for homes in which ambulatory access to toilets is impractical or impossible. Physical and occupational therapists are valuable resources for assisting with home care management.

HEALTH TEACHING

Teach the client and family about the cause of the specific type of incontinence and discuss available treatment options for its management. The teaching plan addresses the prescribed drugs (purpose, dosage, method and route of administration, and expected and potential side effects). Instruct the client and family about the importance of weight reduction and dietary modification to help control urinary incontinence.

When external devices or protective pads are needed, describe the possible options, discuss the advantages and disadvantages of each, and help the client make a selection that considers lifestyle and resources. For clients who will use intermittent catheterization or those with artificial urinary sphincters, demonstrate the correct technique to the client or caregiver. Evaluate return demonstrations for correct technique. Chart 73-11 also addresses teaching.

PSYCHOSOCIAL PREPARATION

The embarrassment of incontinence can be devastating to a client's self-esteem, body image, and interpersonal relationships. The unpredictability of incontinence creates anxiety. Clients are often embarrassed to seek help, and even when resources are identified, they may need assistance to feel

CLIENT EDUCATION GUIDE
Urinary Incontinence

- Maintain a normal body weight to reduce the pressure on your bladder.
- Do not try to control your incontinence by limiting your fluid intake. Adequate fluid intake is necessary for kidney function and health maintenance.
- If you have a catheter in your bladder, follow the instructions given to you about maintaining the sterile drainage system.
- If you are discharged with a suprapubic catheter in your bladder, inspect the entry site for the tube daily, clean the skin around the opening gently with warm soap and water, and place a sterile gauze dressing on the skin around the tube. Report any redness, swelling, drainage, or fever to your physician.
- Do not put anything into your vagina, such as tampons, medications, hygiene products, or exercise weights, until you check with your physician at your 6-week checkup after surgery.
- Do not have sexual intercourse until after your 6-week postoperative checkup.
- Do not lift or carry anything heavier than 5 lb or participate in any strenuous exercise until your physician gives you postoperative clearance. In some cases, this could be as long as 3 months.
- Avoid exercises, such as running, jogging, step or dance aerobic classes, rowing, cross-country ski or stair-climber machines, and mountain biking. Brisk walking without any additional hand, leg, or body weights is allowed. Swimming is allowed after all drains and catheters have been removed and your incision is completely healed.
- If Kegel exercises are recommended, ask your nurse for specific instructions.

comfortable in using the resources. Even buying supplies at a local store can be a threat to their privacy.

Accept and acknowledge the personal concerns of the client and caregiver. Never minimize the concerns or make them seem trivial. Help the client learn methods of controlling or managing the fear or anxiety. As the client learns the specifics of the plan that will allow control of urinary incontinence, the confidence to resume social interactions should return.

HEALTH CARE RESOURCES

Referral to home care agencies for help with personal care and to continence clinics that specialize in evaluation and treatment may be helpful. In many continence clinics, nurses collaborate with physicians and other health care professionals to evaluate and manage clients. The treatment plan is specific for each client; supplies and products are custom selected.

Clients may benefit from education and from the support of others who experience similar concerns. The National Association for Continence (NAFC) (http://www.nafc.org), Access to Continence Care and Treatment (http://www.well-web.com/INCONT/acct/contents.htm), and the Wound, Ostomy, and Continence Nurses (http://www.wocn.org) publish newsletters and educational materials written with simple, easy-to-understand explanations. The American Foundation for Urologic Disease (http://www.afud.com) provides information on several areas of bladder dysfunction. The Agency for Healthcare Research and Quality (AHRQ) has also published a caregiver guide (AHCPR Publication No. 96-0683) for the public that is available on the Internet or by calling (800) 358-9295. Local hospitals, in collaboration with the NAFC, may conduct local support groups.

◆ Evaluation: Outcomes

Evaluate the care of the client with urinary incontinence on the basis of the identified nursing diagnoses. The expected outcomes are that the client will:

- Describe the type of urinary incontinence experienced
- Demonstrate knowledge of proper use of medications and correct procedures for self-catheterization, use of the artificial sphincter, or care of an indwelling urinary catheter
- Demonstrate effective use of the selected exercise or bladder training program
- Select and use incontinence devices and products
- Have a reduction in the number of incontinence episodes

Specific indicators for these outcomes are listed for each nursing diagnosis under the Planning and Implementation section (see earlier).

Urolithiasis

PATHOPHYSIOLOGY

Urolithiasis is the presence of calculi (stones) in the urinary tract. Stones are often asymptomatic until they pass into the lower urinary tract, where they can cause excruciating pain. **Nephrolithiasis** is the formation of stones in the kidney. Formation of stones in the ureter is **ureterolithiasis.**

Urologic stones are caused by many metabolic disorders. However, the exact mechanism of stone formation is not entirely understood. Everyone excretes crystals in the urine at some time, but fewer than 10% of people form stones. About 75% of stones contain calcium as one part of the stone complex, which may be calcium oxalate or calcium phosphate. Struvite (15%), uric acid (8%), and cystine (3%) make up the less common stones.

Formation of stones seems to involve three conditions:

- Slow urine flow, resulting in supersaturation of the urine with the particular element (such as calcium) that first becomes crystallized and later becomes the stone
- Damage to the lining of the urinary tract (i.e., from crystals)
- Decreased inhibitor substances in the urine that would otherwise prevent supersaturation and crystal aggregation

High urine acidity (as with uric acid and cystine stones) or alkalinity (as with calcium phosphate and struvite stones) as well as drugs (as with triamterene, indinavir, and acetazolamide) contribute to stone formation.

One example of a metabolic problem causing stone formation begins when excessive amounts of calcium are absorbed through the intestinal tract (the most common cause of hypercalciuria). As blood circulates through the kidneys, the excess calcium is filtered into the urine, causing supersaturation of calcium in the urine. If fluid intake is inadequate, such as when a client is dehydrated, supersaturation is more likely to occur, and the risk for calcium combining with another compound to form a larger molecule increases. Calcium complexes often serve as a center for other deposits, and eventually a stone forms.

TABLE 73-5 Metabolic Defects That Commonly Cause Calculi

Metabolic Deficit	Etiology
Hypercalcemia Primary	Absorptive: increased intestinal calcium absorption Renal: decreased renal tubular excretion of calcium
Secondary	Resorptive: hyperparathyroidism, vitamin D intoxication, renal tubular acidosis, prolonged immobilization
Hyperoxaluria Primary	Genetic: autosomal recessive trait resulting in high oxalate production
Secondary	Dietary: excess oxalate from foods such as spinach, rhubarb, Swiss chard, cocoa, beets, wheat germ, pecans, peanuts, okra, chocolate, and lime peel
Hyperuricemia Primary	Gout is an inherited disorder of purine metabolism (20% of clients with gout have uric acid calculi)
Secondary	Increased production or decreased clearance of purine from myeloproliferative disorders, thiazide diuretics, carcinoma
Struvite	Made of magnesium ammonium phosphate and carbonate apatite; formed by urea splitting by bacteria, most commonly, *Proteus mirabilis;* needs an alkaline urine to form
Cystinuria	Autosomal recessive defect of amino acid metabolism that precipitates insoluble cystine crystals in the urine

Stones that form in the kidney and then pass into the ureter often lodge in the ureteropelvic angle, the aortoiliac bend, or the ureterovesical angle. When the stone occludes the ureter and blocks the flow of urine, the ureter dilates. Enlargement of the ureter is called **hydroureter**.

The pain associated with ureteral spasm is excruciating and may cause the client to go into shock from stimulation of nearby sympathetic nerves. In addition, **hematuria** (bloody urine) may result from damage to the urothelial lining. If the obstruction is not removed, urinary stasis can cause infection and impair kidney function on the side of the blockage. As the blockage persists, **hydronephrosis** (enlargement of the kidney caused by blockage of urine lower in the tract and filling of the kidney with urine) and permanent kidney damage may develop.

Etiology and Genetic Risk

The cause of urolithiasis is unknown. At least 90% of clients who form stones have a metabolic risk factor. Table 73-5 lists some metabolic defects that commonly cause stone formation.

A diet high in calcium is not believed to cause stones unless a metabolic defect or renal tubular defect already exists. Data suggest that a normal-calcium diet that is relatively low in animal protein, salt, or both may be effective in preventing stone formation. A low calcium diet does not prevent stone formation (Borghi et al., 2002). Urinary stasis, urinary retention, immobilization, and dehydration all contribute to a stone-forming environment. Except for the use of the

thiazides for calcium oxalate stones, diuretics can cause volume depletion and thus may promote the formation of stones.

Genetic Considerations

More than 30 genetic variations are associated with the formation of renal stones (Danpure, 2000). Single gene disorders are rare. More commonly, nephrolithiasis is a complex disease, with genetic variation in intestinal calcium absorption, renal calcium transport, or renal phosphate transport all associated with stone formation (Frick & Bushinsky, 2003).

Incidence/Prevalence

The incidence of stone disease is high and varies with geographic location, race, and family history. About 12% of adults will have at least one episode of renal stone disease. The incidence is higher in men; however, struvite stones are twice as common in women. Recurrence rates vary depending on the type of treatment. The recurrence rate of untreated calcium oxalate stones is 35% to 50% in 5 to 10 years. A higher recurrence of stones occurs in clients with a family history of stone disease and in those who had their first occurrence by age 25 years.

CULTURAL CONSIDERATIONS

The incidence of stone disease is most common in the southeastern United States, Japan, and Western Europe. Calcium stone disease is more common in men than in women and tends to occur in young adults or during early middle adulthood. Kidney stone disease occurs more often in younger adults than older adults and more commonly among white individuals. For clients in these higher-risk groups, nursing care should include teaching family members, as well as clients, about the manifestations of a stone and interventions to reduce stone formation.

◆COLLABORATIVE MANAGEMENT
◆Assessment

HISTORY

Ask the client about a personal or family history of urologic stones. Obtain a diet history, including fluid intake patterns. If the client has a history of stone formation, ask about past treatment, whether chemical analysis of the stone was performed, and what preventive measures are followed.

PHYSICAL ASSESSMENT/CLINICAL MANIFESTATIONS

The major manifestation of stones is severe pain, commonly called **renal colic.** Flank pain suggests that the stone is in the kidney or upper ureter. Flank pain that radiates abdominally or into the scrotum and testes or the vulva suggests that stones are in the ureters or bladder. Pain is most intense when the stone is moving or when the ureter is obstructed.

Renal colic begins suddenly and is often described as "unbearable." Nausea, vomiting, pallor, and diaphoresis often accompany the pain. A large stationary stone in the kidney (staghorn calculus), however, rarely causes much pain because it is not moving. Frequency and dysuria occur when a stone reaches the bladder. **Oliguria** (scant urine output) or **anuria** (absence of urine output) suggests obstruction, possibly at the bladder neck or urethra. *Urinary tract obstruction is an emergency and must be treated immediately to preserve kidney function.*

Examine the client to detect bladder distention. The client may appear pale, ashen, and diaphoretic, and suffer from excruciating pain. Vital signs may be moderately elevated with pain; body temperature and pulse are elevated with infection. Blood pressure may decrease if the severe pain causes shock.

LABORATORY ASSESSMENT

Urinalysis is performed in clients with suspected calculi. Hematuria is a common finding; blood may make the urine appear smoky or rusty. RBCs are usually caused by stone-induced direct trauma on the lining of the ureter, bladder, or urethra. WBCs and bacteria may be present as a result of urinary stasis. Increased turbidity and odor are manifestations of infection that may accompany urolithiasis Microscopic examination of the urine may identify crystals from which stones could form. Urinary pH is measured to determine acidity or alkalinity.

The serum WBC count is elevated with infection. Increases in the serum calcium, serum phosphate, or serum uric acid levels indicate excess minerals are present and may contribute to stone formation.

RADIOGRAPHIC ASSESSMENT

Stones are easily seen on x-rays of the kidneys, ureters, and bladder (KUB) (Figure 73-2), or on intravenous (IV) pyelograms, computed tomography (CT) scans, or magnetic resonance imaging (MRI) scans. Noncontrast helical CT has the highest sensitivity for the identification of urinary tract stones (Portis & Sudaram, 2001). These procedures confirm the presence and location of the stones.

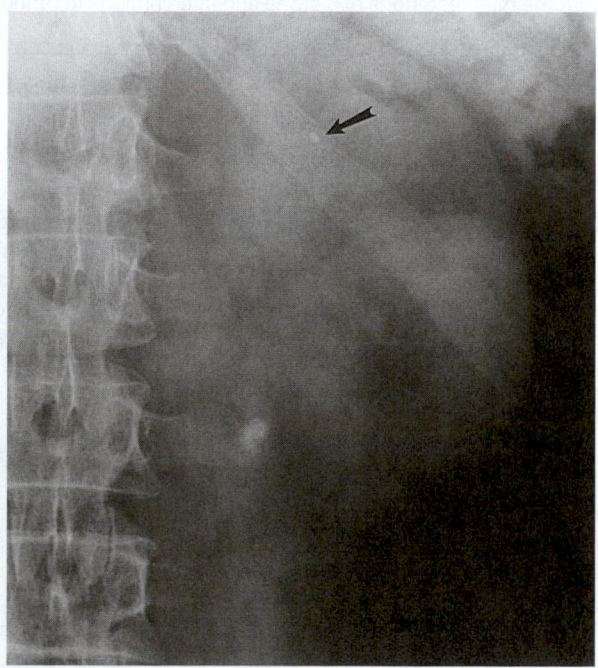

Figure 73-2 ■ Urinary stones on x-ray of the kidneys, ureters, and bladder (KUB). (From Pollack, H.M. [2000]. Clinical urography [2nd ed.] Philadelphia: W.B. Saunders.)

IV pyelography is useful for identifying whether urinary tract obstruction is present. However, because of the risk of acute renal failure induced by contrast dye, other diagnostic tests may be chosen for high-risk clients (older adults and clients with diabetes mellitus, multiple myeloma, or elevated serum creatinine levels). CT or MRI is needed to identify cystine or uric acid stones, neither of which can be seen on x-ray.

OTHER DIAGNOSTIC ASSESSMENTS

Renal ultrasonography creates images from sound waves. Structures of varying density are imaged. Solid structures, such as stones, are extremely dense; therefore the images of stones are clear. Small stones are harder to identify and locate.

◆ Common Nursing Diagnoses and Collaborative Problems

Nursing diagnoses that may apply to clients with urolithiasis include the following:

- Acute Pain related to presence of stone in the urinary tract
- Deficient Knowledge (risk factors for stone formation) related to information misinterpretation and unfamiliarity with information resources
- Fear related to potential recurrence of the stone
- Risk for Infection related to trauma of the ureter, bladder, or urethra lining
- Risk for Injury (renal) related to obstruction

◆ Interventions

Nursing interventions focus on pain management and prevention of infection and urinary obstruction. Most clients can expel the stone without invasive procedures. The most important factors regarding whether a stone will pass on its own are its composition, size, and location. The larger the stone and the higher up in the urinary tract it is, the less likely it is to be passed. Other interventions may be needed when the client does not pass the stone spontaneously (Portis & Sudaram, 2001) (Figure 73-3).

PAIN RELIEF MEASURES

Nonsurgical and surgical approaches are used to assist the client with a kidney stone in achieving an acceptable degree of pain relief.

NONSURGICAL MANAGEMENT. Nonsurgical measures to relieve pain include strategies to enhance stone passing as well as direct pain management.

Drug Therapy. Pain is usually most severe in the first 24 to 36 hours. Opioid analgesics are often needed to control the severe pain caused by stones in the urinary tract. Opioid agents, such as morphine sulfate (Statex✶), are often given IV to ensure prompt and adequate absorption. Nonsteroidal anti-inflammatory drugs (NSAIDs) such as ketorolac (Toradol) in the acute phase may be quite effective. The antiplatelet effects of NSAIDs are a contraindication to the use of extracorporeal shock wave lithotripsy.

Control of pain is more effective when drugs are given at regularly scheduled intervals or via a constant delivery system (e.g., skin patch) instead of as needed (PRN). Spasmolytic drugs, such as oxybutynin chloride (Ditropan) and propantheline bromide (Pro-Banthine, Propanthel✶), are important for the relief and control of pain (see Chart 73-9). Give the drugs and assess the response by asking the client to rate the discomfort on a rating scale.

Complementary and Alternative Therapy. Relaxation techniques, such as hypnosis and imagery, therapeutic or healing touch, and acupuncture, can relieve pain. Clients often have difficulty finding a comfortable position in which to relax. Thus assisting the client with positioning can often aid in relaxation. Breathing techniques, such as those used in childbirth, can also help clients relax.

Other Management Techniques. Avoiding overhydration and underhydration in the acute phase helps make the spontaneous passage of a stone less painful. Strain the urine to monitor for stone passage. Send any stone passed to the laboratory for analysis because preventive therapy is based on stone composition.

Lithotripsy. Lithotripsy, also known as extracorporeal shock wave lithotripsy (ESWL), is the use of sound, laser, or dry shock wave energies to break the stone into small fragments. The client receives conscious sedation and lies on a flat table with the lithotriptor aimed at the stone, which is located by fluoroscopy. A local anesthetic cream is applied to the skin site over the stone 45 minutes before the procedure. During the procedure, cardiac rhythm is monitored by electrocardiography (ECG), and the shock waves are delivered in synchrony with the R wave. About 500 to 1500 shock waves are applied in 30 to 45 minutes. Continuous ECG monitoring for dysrhythmia and fluoroscopic observation for stone destruction are maintained.

After lithotripsy, strain the urine to monitor the passage of stone fragments. Some bruising may occur on the flank of the affected side after extracorporeal shock wave lithotripsy (ESWL). Occasionally a stent is placed in the ureter before ESWL to ease passage of the stone fragments. Cystine stones are often resistant to ESWL.

SURGICAL MANAGEMENT. Minimally invasive surgical and open surgical procedures are indicated if uri-

nary obstruction occurs or if the stone is too large to be passed spontaneously.

Minimally Invasive Surgical Procedures. Minimally invasive surgical (MIS) procedures include stenting, retrograde ureteroscopy, and percutaneous ureterolithotomy and nephrolithotomy.

Stenting. A **stent** is a small tube that is placed in the ureter by ureteroscopy. The stent dilates the ureter and enlarges the passageway for the stone or stone fragments. This procedure prevents the passing stone from coming in contact with the ureteral mucosa, thereby reducing pain. A Foley catheter may be placed to facilitate passage of the stone through the urethra.

Retrograde Ureteroscopy. Retrograde ureteroscopy is an endoscopic procedure. The ureteroscope is passed through the urethra and bladder into the ureter. Once the stone is seen, it is removed using grasping baskets, forceps, or loops. Lithotripsy also can be performed through the ureteroscope. A Foley catheter may be placed to facilitate passage of the stone fragments through the urethra.

Percutaneous Ureterolithotomy and Nephrolithotomy. The client lies prone or laterally and receives local or general anesthesia. The physician identifies the ideal entry point with fluoroscopy and then passes a needle into the collecting system of the kidney. Once a tract has been made in the kidney, other equipment, such as an **intracorporeal** (inside the body) ultrasonic or laser lithotriptor, can be used to break up and remove the stone. An endoscope with a special attachment to grasp and extract the stone can be used. Often a nephrostomy tube is left in place at first to prevent the stone fragments from passing through the normal urinary tract.

Provide routine nephrostomy tube care and monitor the client for complications after the procedure. Complications include bleeding at the site or through the tube, pneumothorax, and infection.

Open Surgical Procedures. When other stone removal attempts have failed, or when risk of a lasting injury

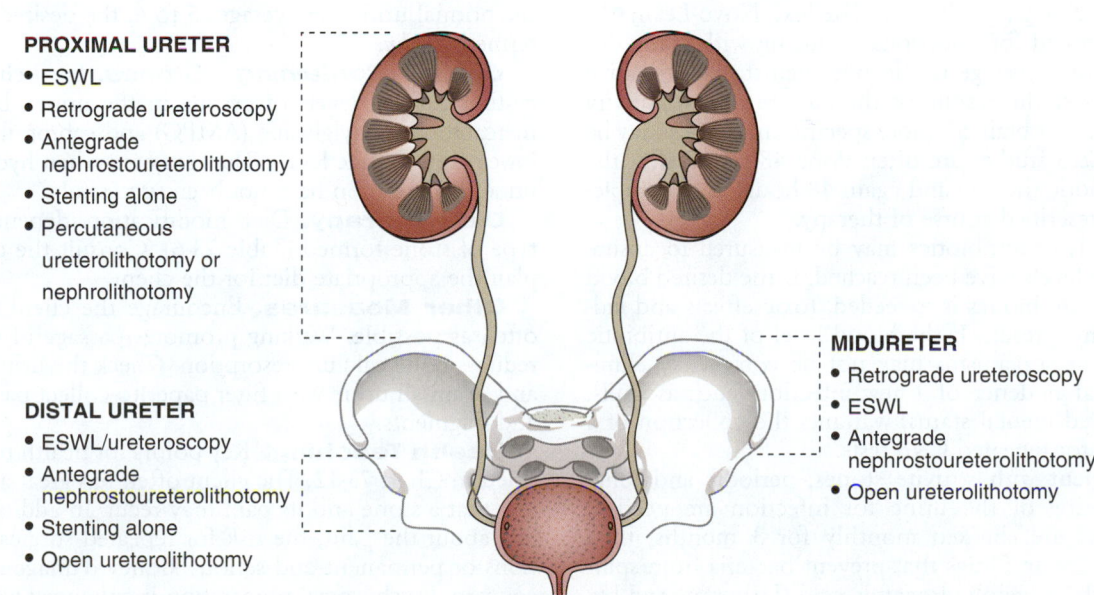

PROXIMAL URETER
- ESWL
- Retrograde ureteroscopy
- Antegrade nephrostoureterolithotomy
- Stenting alone
- Percutaneous ureterolithotomy or nephrolithotomy

DISTAL URETER
- ESWL/ureteroscopy
- Antegrade nephrostoureterolithotomy
- Stenting alone
- Open ureterolithotomy

MIDURETER
- Retrograde ureteroscopy
- ESWL
- Antegrade nephrostoureterolithotomy
- Open ureterolithotomy

Figure 73-3 ■ Treatment options for ureteral stones. (Modified from Singal, R.K., & Denstedt, J.D. [1997]. Contemporary management of ureteral stones. *Urologic Clinics of North America, 24*[1], 59-70.)

to the ureter or kidney is possible, an open ureterolithotomy (into the ureter), pyelolithotomy (into the kidney pelvis), or nephrolithotomy (into the kidney) procedure may be indicated. These procedures are used for a large or impacted stone.

Preoperative Care. Prepare the client for the selected procedure by explaining how, when, and where the procedure will be performed. Describe what the client can expect to see, hear, and feel before and after the procedure. The client is given nothing by mouth and also receives preoperative bowel preparation. (See Chapter 20 for routine care before surgery.)

Operative Procedures. The retroperitoneal area is entered through a large flank incision, as for nephrectomy (see Chapter 74), pyelolithotomy, or nephrolithotomy, and through a lower abdominal incision for ureterolithotomy. The urinary tract is entered surgically and the stone is removed. Before closure, tubes and drains may be placed (e.g., nephrostomy tube, ureteral stent, Penrose or other wound drainage device, and Foley catheter).

Postoperative Care. Follow routine procedures for assessment of the client who has received anesthesia. (See Chapter 22 for routine care after surgery.) Monitor the amount of bleeding from incisions and in the urine. Maintain adequate fluid intake. Strain the urine to monitor the passage of stone fragments. Teach the client how to prevent future stones through dietary changes.

PREVENTION OF INFECTION

Control of infections before invasive and noninvasive procedures is critical for the prevention of urosepsis. Interventions include giving appropriate antibiotics, either to eliminate an existing infection or to prevent new infections, and the maintenance of adequate nutrition and fluid intake. Because infection always occurs with struvite stone formation, the health care team plans for long-term infection prevention.

Drug Therapy. Broad-spectrum antibiotics, such as the aminoglycosides (e.g., gentamicin [Garamycin]) and cephalosporins (e.g., cephalexin [Keflex, Novo-Lexin✦]), are first prescribed for infections occurring with stone disease. The broad coverage is effective against gram-negative organisms. After the results of the culture and sensitivity (C&S) studies are obtained, more specific antibiotics may be prescribed. C&S studies are often done 48 hours after the start of antibiotic therapy and again 48 hours after completion of the prescribed course of therapy.

Blood levels of antibiotics may be measured to ensure that adequate levels have been reached. If the desired blood level of these antibiotics is exceeded, toxic effects and kidney damage may result. If the blood level of the antibiotic is not adequate, organisms may not be completely eliminated. Clinical evidence of a new infection (such as chills, fever, or altered mental status) warrants the collection of a urine sample for repeated C&S tests.

For the client with struvite stones, periodic and long-term monitoring of the urine for infection are needed. Urine cultures are checked monthly for 3 months, then quarterly for 1 year. Drugs that prevent bacteria from splitting urea, such as acetohydroxamic acid (Lithostat) and hydroxyurea (Hydrea), are often prescribed on a long-term basis for clients with struvite stones. Serum creatinine levels are monitored in clients receiving acetohydroxamic acid.

This drug is stopped if creatinine levels are above 2 mg/dL. Review interventions aimed at preventing urinary tract infection (UTI) (see Interventions [Cystitis], p. 1681).

Diet Therapy. The client's diet ideally includes adequate calorie intake with a balance of all food groups. Encourage a fluid intake of 2 to 3 L/day unless another condition requires fluid restriction.

PREVENTION OF OBSTRUCTION

Measures to prevent urinary obstruction by stones include a high intake of fluids (3 L/day or more) and careful measures of intake and output. A liberal but not excessive fluid intake helps prevent dehydration, promotes the flow of urine, and decreases the chance of crystals forming a stone. Interventions also depend on the type of stone. Drugs, diet modification, and fluid intake are the major strategies available.

Drug Therapy. Drug selection to prevent obstruction depends on what is promoting the formation of stones and the type of stone formed. Teach the client the reason for the drug and assess for side effects or adverse drug reactions.

Calcium-Containing Stones. Drugs to treat hypercalciuria (high levels of calcium in the urine) include thiazide diuretics (e.g., chlorothiazide [Diuril] or hydrochlorothiazide [HydroDIURIL, Urozide✦]), orthophosphate, and sodium cellulose phosphate. Thiazide diuretics promote calcium resorption from the renal tubules back into the body, thereby reducing urine calcium loads. Orthophosphates alter calcium-phosphorus metabolism, resulting in decreased urine saturation of calcium oxalate. Sodium cellulose phosphate reduces intestinal absorption of calcium.

Oxalate-Containing Stones. For clients with hyperoxaluria (high levels of oxalic acid in the urine), allopurinol (Zyloprim) and vitamin B_6 (pyridoxine) are used.

Uric Acid–Containing Stones. For clients with chronic gout, allopurinol helps prevent the formation of urate (uric acid) stones. To alkalinize the urine, drugs such as potassium citrate, 50% sodium citrate, and sodium bicarbonate are used. The desired urine pH is 6 to 6.5. Because the normal urine pH averages 5 to 6, the desired values are termed *alkaline*.

Cystine-Containing Stones. For clients with cystinuria (high levels of cystine in the urine), both alpha-mercaptopropionylglycine (AMPG) and captopril (Capoten) lower urine cystine levels. They are used when hydration and urine alkalinization have not been successful.

Diet Therapy. Diet modification depends on the type of stone formed (Table 73-6). Consult the dietitian to plan the appropriate diet for the client.

Other Measures. Encourage the client to walk as often as possible. Walking promotes passage of stones and reduces bone calcium resorption. Check the urine pH daily and strain all urine with filter paper to collect passed stones and fragments.

Health Teaching. Key points for health teaching are listed in Chart 73-12. The client often has great anxiety and fear that a stone and its pain may recur. In addition to anxiety about the pain, the risk for repeated surgical interventions or permanent and serious kidney damage is of major concern. Psychosocial preparation is enhanced when clients know what to expect and what actions to take if problems develop. Reassure the client that preventive and health promotion activities help prevent recurrence.

TABLE 73-6 Dietary Treatment for Renal Stones

Stone Type	Dietary Interventions	Rationales
Calcium oxalate	Avoid oxalate sources, such as spinach, black tea, and rhubarb (see also Table 73-5).	Reduction of urinary oxalate content may help prevent these stones from forming. Urinary pH is not a factor.
	Decrease sodium intake.	High sodium intake reduces renal tubular calcium reabsorption.
Calcium phosphate	Limit intake of foods high in animal protein to 5-7 servings per week and never more than 2 per day.	Reduction of protein intake reduces acidic urine and prevents calcium precipitation.
	Some clients may benefit from a reduced calcium intake (milk, other dairy products).	Reduction of urine calcium concentration may prevent calcium precipitation and crystallization.
	Decrease sodium intake.	High sodium intake reduces renal tubular calcium reabsorption.
Struvite (magnesium ammonium phosphate)	Limit high-phosphate foods, such as dairy products, red, and organ meats, and whole grains.	Reduction of urinary phosphate content may help prevent these stones from forming.
Uric acid (urate)	Decrease intake of purine sources, such as organ meats, poultry, fish, gravies, red wines, and sardines.	Reduction of urinary purine content may help prevent these stones from forming.
Cystine	Limit animal protein intake (as above).	Reduces urinary uric acid.
	Encourage oral fluid intake (500 mL every 4 hours while awake and 750 mL at night).	Increased fluid helps dilute the urine and prevents the cystine crystals from forming.

CHART 73-12

CLIENT EDUCATION GUIDE
Urinary Calculi

- Finish your entire prescription of antibiotics to ensure that you will not get a urinary tract infection.
- You may resume your usual daily activities.
- Remember to balance regular exercise with sleep and rest.
- You may return to work 2 days to 6 weeks after surgery, depending on the type of intervention, your personal tolerance, and your physician's directives.
- Depending on the type of stone you had, your diet may be restricted to prevent further stone formation.
- Remember to drink at least 3 L of fluid a day to dilute potential stone-forming crystals, prevent dehydration, and promote urine flow.
- Monitor urine pH as directed (possibly up to three times per day).
- Expect bruising after lithotripsy. The bruising may be quite extensive and may take several weeks to resolve.
- Your urine may be bloody for several days after surgery.
- Pain in the region of the kidneys or bladder may signal the beginning of an infection or the formation of another stone. Report any pain, fever, chills, or difficulty with urination immediately to your physician or nurse.
- Keep follow-up appointments to check on infection, have repeat cultures done, and so forth.

Urothelial Cancer
PATHOPHYSIOLOGY

Urothelial cancers are malignant tumors of the urothelium, the lining of transitional cells in the kidney, renal pelvis, ureters, urinary bladder, and urethra. Most urothelial cancers occur in the bladder. Consequently, the term *bladder cancer* is often used to describe this condition.

In the United States, about 73% of urinary tract cancers are transitional cell carcinomas of the bladder (American Cancer Society [ACS], 2005). The second most common site of urinary tract cancer is the kidney and renal pelvis (27%). Urothelial cancers are usually low grade, have multiple points of origin (**multifocal**), and are recurrent. Once the cancer spreads beyond the transitional cell layer, they are highly invasive and metastatic. Because of the multifocal and recurrent nature of this cancer, clients may have recurrence up to 10 years after being cancer free.

Table 73-7 shows the staging of bladder cancer. Tumors confined to the mucosa are treated by simple excision, whereas carcinoma in situ (CIS), or stage T_{is}, is treated with excision plus **intravesical** (inside the bladder) chemotherapy. Cancer that has spread beyond CIS is treated with more extensive surgery, often a radical **cystectomy** (removal of the bladder and surrounding tissue) with urinary diversion. Chemotherapy and radiation therapy are used in addition to surgery. If untreated, the tumor invades surrounding tissues, spreads to distant sites (liver, lung, and bone), and ultimately leads to death.

Exposure to toxins, especially chemicals used in the hairdressing, rubber, paint, electric cable, and textile industries, increases the risk for bladder cancer. The greatest risk factor for bladder cancer is tobacco use. Other risks include *Schistosoma haematobium* (a parasite) infection, excessive use of drugs containing phenacetin, and long-term use of cyclophosphamide (Cytoxan, Procytox✲).

About 54,300 new cases of bladder cancer are diagnosed each year in the United States and about 12,400 deaths occur each year from the disease (ACS, 2005). This cancer is rare in adults younger than age 40, and is most common after 60 years of age.

◆ COLLABORATIVE MANAGEMENT
◆ Assessment

PHYSICAL ASSESSMENT/CLINICAL MANIFESTATIONS

Ask about the client's perception of his or her general health. Document the gender and age of the client. Ask about active and passive exposure to cigarette smoke. To detect exposure to harmful environmental agents, ask the client to describe his or her occupation in detail. Also ask

TABLE 73-7 Staging of Bladder Cancer

Primary Tumor (T)

T_x	Primary tumor cannot be assessed
T_0	No evidence of primary tumor
T_{is}	Carcinoma in situ: "flat tumor"
T_1	Tumor invades submucosa (subepithelial connective tissue)
T_2	Tumor invades superficial muscle (inner half)
T_3	Tumor invades deep muscle or perivesical fat
T_{3a}	Tumor invades deep muscle (outer half)
T_{3b}	Tumor invades perivesical fat
T_4	Tumor invades any of the following: prostate, uterus, vagina, pelvic wall, abdominal wall
T_{4a}	Tumor invades prostate, uterus, vagina
T_{4b}	Tumor invades pelvic or abdominal wall

Lymph Node (N)

N_x	Regional lymph nodes cannot be assessed
N_0	No regional lymph node metastasis
N_1	Metastasis in a single lymph node, 2 cm or less in greatest dimension
N_2	Metastasis in a single lymph node, more than 2 cm but not more than 5 cm in greatest dimension, or multiple lymph nodes, none more than 5 cm in greatest dimension, pelvic only

Distant Metastasis (M)

M_x	Presence of distant metastasis cannot be assessed
M_0	No distant metastasis
M_1	Distant metastasis or nodes positive above aortic bifurcation

Modified from American Joint Committee on Cancer. (1992). In O.H. Beahrs (Ed.), *Manual for staging of cancer* (4th ed.). Philadelphia: Lippincott-Raven; and Bennett, J.C., & Plum, F. (Eds.). (2002). *Cecil textbook of medicine* (22nd ed.). Philadelphia: W.B. Saunders.

the client to describe any change in the color, frequency, or amount of urine and any abdominal discomfort.

Observe the overall appearance of the client, especially skin color and general nutritional status. Inspect, percuss, and palpate the abdomen for asymmetry, tenderness, and bladder distention.

Examine the urine for color and clarity. Hematuria is the major sign occurring with bladder cancer. It may be gross or microscopic and is usually painless and intermittent. Dysuria, frequency, and urgency are common when infection or obstruction is also present.

PSYCHOSOCIAL ASSESSMENT

Assess the client's emotions, including his or her response to a tentative diagnosis of bladder cancer, and note anxiety, fear, sadness, anger, or guilt. Early manifestations are painless, and many clients ignore hematuria because it is intermittent. Clients also may be reluctant to seek treatment because they suspect a sexually transmitted disease (STD). Consequently, they may have guilt or anger about their own delays in seeking medical attention.

Assess the client's methods of coping and the degree of support from family members. Social support may provide motivation and improve coping during convalescence.

DIAGNOSTIC ASSESSMENT

The only significant finding on a routine urinalysis is gross or microscopic hematuria. Cytologic testing on voided urine specimens is not usually helpful. Bladder-wash specimens and bladder biopsies are the most specific tests for cancer.

Cystoscopy with retrograde pyelography is usually performed to evaluate painless hematuria. A biopsy of a visible bladder tumor can be performed during cystoscopy. This is essential for staging and is usually performed in a day-surgery unit before admission to the hospital for treatment. IV pyelography may be used in the presence of hematuria. Excretory urography is useful in identifying obstructions, especially at the ureterovesical junction. Computed tomography (CT) scans show tumor invasion of surrounding tissues. Ultrasonography shows masses but is less valuable for tumor staging. Magnetic resonance imaging (MRI) may help to assess deep, invasive tumors.

◆ Common Nursing Diagnoses and Collaborative Problems

Nursing diagnoses that may apply to clients with bladder cancer include the following:

- Fear or Anxiety related to potential diagnosis of a malignant disease
- Disturbed Body Image related to surgery-induced changes in urinary habits, or changes in appearance from chemotherapy
- Risk for Infection related to invasive procedures or side effects of systemic chemotherapy
- Risk for Impaired Skin Integrity related to surgical incision or urinary diversion
- Risk for Social Isolation related to altered physical appearance, embarrassment, or odors

◆ Interventions

Therapy for the client with bladder cancer usually begins with surgical removal of the tumors for diagnosis and staging of disease. For tumors extending beyond the mucosa, surgery is followed by intravesical chemotherapy or immunotherapy. High-grade or recurrent tumors are treated with more radical surgery plus intravesical chemotherapy, radiotherapy, or both. Systemic chemotherapy is reserved for clients with distant metastases. (See Chapter 28 for general care of the client receiving chemotherapy or radiation therapy.)

NONSURGICAL MANAGEMENT. Prophylactic immunotherapy with intravesical instillation of bacille Calmette-Guérin (BCG), a compound used to vaccinate against tuberculosis in some countries, is used to prevent tumor recurrence of superficial cancers (stage T_1 or lower). This procedure is more effective than single-agent chemotherapy.

Multiagent chemotherapy is successful in prolonging life after distant metastasis has occurred but rarely results in a cure. Radiation therapy is also useful in prolonging life.

SURGICAL MANAGEMENT. The type of surgery for bladder cancer depends on the type and stage of the cancer and the client's general health. Complete bladder removal (cystectomy) with additional removal of surrounding muscle and tissue offers the best chance of a cure for large, invasive bladder cancers. Four alternatives are used after cystectomy: ileal conduit, continent pouch, bladder reconstruction also known as neobladder, and ureterosigmoidostomy (Oosterlinck et al., 2002).

Preoperative Care. Specific client education depends on the type and extent of the planned surgical procedure. Coordinate education before surgery with the surgeon

Ureterostomies divert urine directly to the skin surface through a ureteral skin opening (stoma). After ureterostomy, the client must wear a pouch.

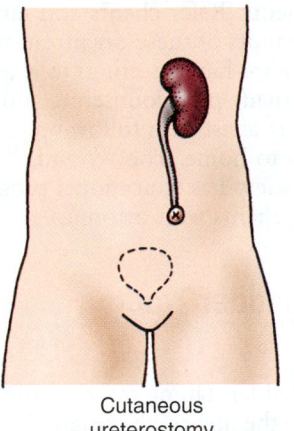

Cutaneous
ureterostomy

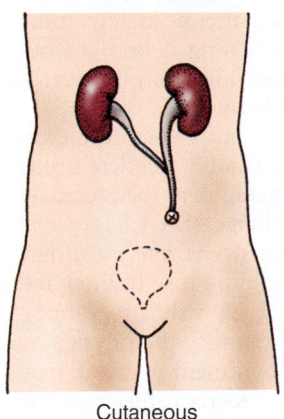

Cutaneous
ureteroureterostomy

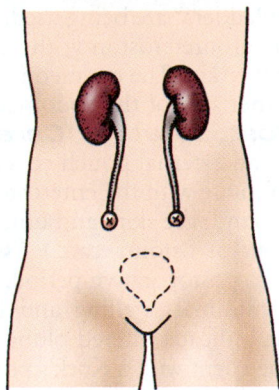

Bilateral cutaneous
ureterostomy

Conduits collect urine in a portion of the intestine, which is then opened onto the skin surface as a stoma. After the creation of a conduit, the client must wear a pouch.

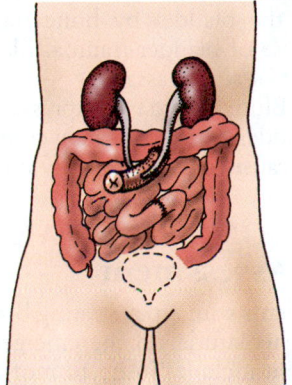

Ileal (Bricker's) conduit

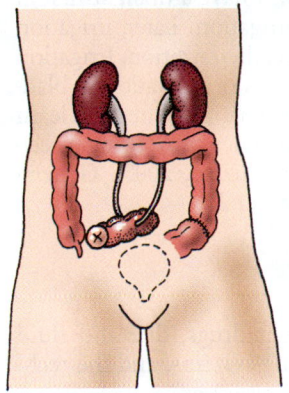

Colon conduit

Ileal reservoirs divert urine into a surgically created pouch, or pocket, that functions as a bladder. The stoma is continent, and the client removes urine by regular self-catheterization.

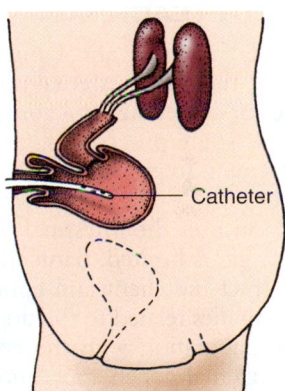

Catheter

Continent internal
ileal reservoir
(Kock's pouch)

Sigmoidostomies divert urine to the large intestine, so no stoma is required. The client excretes urine with bowel movements, and bowel incontinence may result.

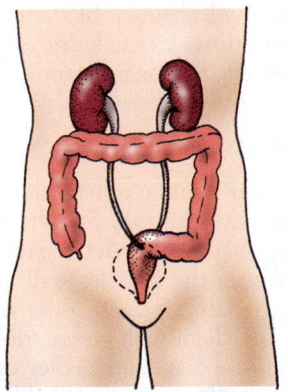

Ureterosigmoidostomy

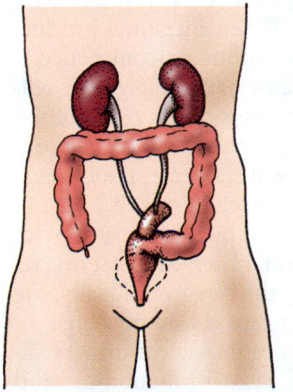

Ureteroiliosigmoidostomy

Figure 73-4 ■ Urinary diversion procedures used in the treatment of bladder cancer.

and enterostomal therapist. Discuss the type of planned urinary diversion and the selection of a site for the stoma. The goal is for the client to have a positive attitude about body image and a positive self-image. Use educational counseling to ensure understanding about self-care practices, methods of pouching, control of urine drainage, and management of odor.

The site selected for the stoma should be visible and avoid folds of skin, bones, and scar tissue. When possible, the client's waistline or belt area is avoided. Prepare the client for the number and type of drains that will be present after surgery. General care before surgery is discussed in Chapter 20.

Operative Procedures. Transurethral resection of the bladder tumor (TURBT) or partial cystectomy is performed for small, early, superficial tumors. In a partial (segmental) cystectomy, a portion of the bladder is removed. This procedure is used when there is only a single isolated bladder tumor.

When the entire bladder must be removed (complete **cystectomy**), the ureters are diverted into a collecting reservoir. Techniques for urinary diversion are shown in Figure 73-4. With an ileal conduit, the ureters are surgically placed in the ileum, and urine is collected in a pouch on the skin around the stoma. More often, continent reservoirs or "neobladders" are being used. With cutaneous ureterostomy or ureteroureterostomy, the ureter opening is brought out onto the skin. The cutaneous ureterostomies may be located on either side of the abdomen or side by side.

Postoperative Care. After cutaneous ureterostomy, an external pouch covers the ostomy to collect urine. Collaborate with the enterostomal therapist to focus care on the wound, the skin, and urinary drainage. (See Chapters 59 and 60 for ostomy care.) Assess the stoma every 8 hours early in postoperative period. It should be rose to brick red with minimal swelling and bleeding. A pale or cyanotic stoma indicates altered blood supply; notify the physician.

The client with a Kock's pouch, a continent reservoir, may have a Penrose drain and a plastic Medena catheter in the stoma. The drain removes lymphatic fluid or other secretions; the catheter ensures urine drainage so that suture lines may heal. The client with a neobladder will have a drain at first in the event the neobladder requires irrigation. Later, irrigation can be performed with intermittent catheterization. Irrigation is performed to ensure patency. There is no sensation of bladder fullness with a neobladder, so the client will need to learn new cues to void, such as prescribed times or noticing a feeling of neobladder pressure (Beitz & Zuzelo, 2003). General care after surgery is discussed in Chapter 22.

Community-Based Care

HEALTH TEACHING

Educate the client and family about drugs, diet and fluid therapy, the use of external pouching systems, and the technique for catheterizing a continent reservoir.

With some procedures, the client may need electrolyte replacement to prevent long-term deficits. Instruct the client to avoid foods that are known to produce gas if the urinary diversion uses the intestinal tract. When intestinal production of gas is limited, flatus will not induce incontinence.

Instruct the client and family about any changes in self-care activities related to the urinary diversion. In conjunction and collaboration with the enterostomal therapist, demonstrate external pouch application, local skin care, pouch care, methods of adhesion, and drainage mechanisms. If a Kock's pouch has been created, teach the client how to use a catheter to drain the pouch. For all instruction, observe at least one return demonstration by the client or the caregiver. Ideally, the client assumes responsibility for self-care before discharge.

Assist the client to prepare for the impact of urinary diversion on self-image, body image, sexual functioning, and self-esteem. Counseling provides information and support to reduce feelings of powerlessness.

Through discussions with the client about usual social situations, help the client gain control over new toileting practices. Men with a urinary diversion into the sigmoid colon need to learn the habit of sitting to urinate. For clients of either gender, promote confidence in social situations by encouraging frequent emptying of urinary collection devices before traveling or attending social functions. Resumption of sexual activity is a major concern for many clients, regardless of age. Address this topic openly and with sensitivity. Cystectomy causes impotence in men, but treatment is available (see Chapter 79).

HEALTH CARE RESOURCES

The United Ostomy Association and the American Cancer Society have educational materials that may be useful to clients. Refer clients and family members to local chapters or units of these organizations. In some areas, local support groups have meetings to assist others and to send visitors to provide peer counseling and support. Home care personnel may assist with follow-up, easing the transition from hospital to home. The Wound, Ostomy, and Continence Nurses Society has educational programs and a journal for the care of clients with ostomies.

Bladder Trauma

PATHOPHYSIOLOGY

Bladder trauma can be caused by penetrating or blunt injury to the lower abdomen. Penetrating injury may occur by stabbing, gunshot wound, or other trauma in which objects pierce the abdominal wall. A fractured pelvis with puncture of the bladder by bone fragments is the most common cause of bladder trauma. Bladder trauma may also be a result of sexual assault.

Blunt trauma compresses the abdominal wall and the bladder. A seat belt may compress the bladder hard enough to cause injury, especially if the bladder is full or distended.

◆ COLLABORATIVE MANAGEMENT
◆ Assessment

Clients with a penetrating bladder wound often have anuria or hematuria. In the emergency department, initial assessment includes inspection of the urinary meatus for blood.

Diagnostic tests include cystography and voiding cystourethrography (VCUG). If renal or ureteral trauma is suspected, IV urography is scheduled before cystography so that any leakage of bladder contrast medium does not mask the outlines of the kidneys or ureters. The cystogram shows whether there is a defect in bladder filling; the voiding cystourethrogram defines bladder emptying.

◆ Interventions

Bladder trauma, other than a simple contusion, requires surgical intervention. Stabilization of any fractures usually is done before bladder repair. Surgical interventions include repairing the bladder wall and peritoneal membrane. Usually, repairs of the bladder are closure procedures.

The client with an anterior bladder wall injury usually has a Penrose drain and a Foley catheter in place after surgery. The client with a posterior bladder wall injury has a Penrose drain and Foley or suprapubic catheter after surgery. In some instances, vaginal or rectal fistulas may also require repair.

Psychosocial support is critical for clients who have sustained traumatic injuries. Refer the client to counseling resources to assist in dealing with psychosocial issues.

▉ GET READY for the NCLEX Examination!

KEY POINTS

Safe Effective Care Environment

- Use sterile technique when inserting a catheter or any other instrument into the urinary system.

- Use contact precautions with any client who has drainage from the genitourinary tract.

Health Promotion and Maintenance

- Teach clients the proper way to clean the perineal area after voiding, having a bowel movement, or after sexual intercourse.
- Encourage all clients to maintain an adequate fluid intake (minimum of 2 L daily unless another condition requires fluid restriction).
- Instruct women who have stress incontinence the proper way to perform pelvic floor strengthening exercises.
- Teach clients who come into contact with chemicals in their workplaces or with leisure time activities to avoid direct skin or mucous membrane contact with these chemicals.

Psychosocial Integrity

- Pace your interview to match the learning needs and style of the individual client.
- Allow the client the opportunity to express fear or anxiety regarding a potential cancer diagnosis.
- Use a nonjudgmental approach in caring for clients with urinary incontinence.
- Avoid referring to protective pads or pants as "diapers."
- Recognize the need for the client undergoing cystectomy and urinary diversion to grieve about the body image change.
- Assess the client's level of comfort in discussing issues related to elimination and the urogenital area.
- During renal/urinary assessment, use language and terminology that is comfortable for the client.
- Refer clients to community resources and support groups.

Physiological Integrity

- Identify hospitalized clients at risk for urosepsis.
- Report immediately any condition that obstructs urine flow.
- Instruct clients with UTI to complete all prescribed antibiotic therapy even when symptoms of infection are absent.
- Avoid maintaining indwelling catheters long term in hospitalized clients.
- Teach clients the expected side effects and any adverse reactions to prescribed drugs.
- Assess the client's manual dexterity and cognitive awareness before teaching a regimen of intermittent self-catheterization.

ADDITIONAL STUDY RESOURCES

Go to your Student CD-ROM for Review Questions for the NCLEX Examination.

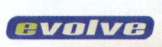
Go to http://evolve.elsevier.com/Iggy/ for Integrated Management of Care Questions for the NCLEX Examination.

SELECTED BIBLIOGRAPHY

Asterisk indicates a classic or definitive work on this subject.

*Agency for Health Care Policy and Research. (1996). (Reviewed 2001). *Urinary incontinence in adults: Acute and chronic management. Clinical practice guideline.* AHCPR Publication No. 96-0682. Rockville, MD: Agency for Health Care Policy and Research, Public Health Service, U.S. Department of Health and Human Services.

American Cancer Society. (2005). *Cancer facts and figures–2005.* Report No. 01-300M-No. 5008.05. Atlanta: Author.

Barkin, J. (2003). Interstitial cystitis: The great imposter! Epidemiology, etiology, diagnosis, and management. *Journal of Sexual and Reproductive Medicine, 3*(2), 57-64.

Bass, P.F., Jarvis, J.W., & Mitchell, C.K. (2003). Urinary tract infections. *Primary Care: Clinics in Office Practice, 30*(1), 1-16.

Bates, F. (2002). Assessment of the female patient with urinary incontinence. *Urologic Nursing, 22*(5) 305-314.

Beisel, B., Hale, W., & Graves, R., (2002). Does postcoital voiding prevent urinary tract infections in young women? *The Journal of Family Practice, 51*(11), 977.

Beitz, J., & Zuzelo, P. (2003). The lived experience of having a neobladder. *Western Journal of Nursing Research, 25*(3), 294-316.

Borghi, L., et al. (2002). Comparison of two diets for the prevention of recurrent stones in idiopathic hypercalciuria. *The New England Journal of Medicine, 346*(2), 77-84.

Castina, S., Boyington, A., & Dougherty, M. (2002). Urinary incontinence. *American Journal of Nursing 102*(8), 85-87.

Choe, J. (2002). Interstitial cystitis: Pelvic pain from the bladder. *The Clinical Advisor, 5*(11/12), 118-127.

Cohen, M., & Rothmann, M. (2001). Gemcitabine and cisplatin for advanced metastatic bladder cancer. *Journal of Clinical Oncology, 19*(4), 1229-1231.

Danpure, C.J. (2000). Genetic disorders and urolithiasis. *Urologic Clinics of North America, 27*(2), 1-16.

Diering, C., & Palmer, M. (2001). Professional information about urinary incontinence on the World Wide Web: Is it timely? Is it accurate? *Journal of Wound, Ostomy, and Continence Nursing, 28*(1), 55-62.

Dochterman, J., & Bulechek, G. (Eds.). (2004). *Nursing interventions classification (NIC)* (4th ed.). St. Louis: Mosby.

Foxman, B. (2002). Epidemiology of urinary tract infections: incidence, morbidity, and economic costs. *American Journal of Medicine, 113*(Suppl. 1A), 5S-13S.

Frick, K.K., & Bushinsky, D.A. (2003). Molecular mechanisms of primary hypercalciuria. *Journal of the American Society of Nephrology, 14*(4), 222-224.

Goode, P., et al. (2003). Effect of behavioral training with or without pelvic floor electrical stimulation on stress incontinence in women. *Journal of the American Medical Association, 290*(3), 345-352.

Gray, M. (2000a). Urinary retention management in the acute care setting, Part 1. *American Journal of Nursing, 100*(7), 40-48.

Gray, M. (2000b). Urinary retention management in the acute care setting, Part 2. *American Journal of Nursing, 100*(8), 36-44.

Gray, M. (2004). Stress incontinence in women. *Journal of the American Academy of Nurse Practitioners, 16*(5), 188-197.

Gray, M. (2003). Gender, race, and culture in research on UI. *American Journal of Nursing, 103*(Suppl. 3), 20-25.

Gray, M., & Krissovich, M. (2003). Does fluid intake influence the risk for urinary incontinence, urinary tract infection, and bladder cancer? *Journal of Wound, Ostomy, and Continence Nursing, 30,* 126-131.

Gray, M., Albo, M., & Huffstutler, S. (2002). Interstitial cystitis: A guide to recognition, evaluation, and management for nurse practitioners. *Journal of Wound Care, Ostomy, and Continence Nursing, 29*(2), 93-102.

Hay-Smith, E.J.C., et al. (2003). Pelvic floor training for urinary incontinence in women. *Cochrane Database of Systemic Reviews* (*www.gateway2.ovid.com*). Accessed June, 2003. Last updated January, 2003.

Hess, B. (2002). Nutritional aspects of Stone disease. *Endocrinology and Metabolism Clinics, 31*(4), 1-11.

Hruska, K. (2001). Renal calculi. In J.C. Bennett & F. Plum (Eds.), *Cecil textbook of medicine* (22nd ed.). Philadelphia: W.B. Saunders.

Ingelfinger, J. (2002). Diet and kidney stones. *The New England Journal of Medicine, 346*(2), 74-76.

Jepson, R.G., Mihaljevic, L., & Craig, J. (2002). Cranberries for preventing urinary tract infections. Cochrane Renal Group. *Cochrane Database of Systematic Reviews*. Accessed June, 2003.

Johnson, S. (2000). From incontinence to confidence. *American Journal of Nursing, 100*(2), 69-76.

Johnson, V. (2001). Effects of a submaximal exercise protocol to recondition the pelvic floor musculature. *Nursing Research, 50*(1), 33-41.

Kiel, R., & Nashelsky, M. (2003). Does cranberry juice prevent or treat urinary tract infection? *The Journal of Family Practice, 52*(2), 154-155.

Kincade, J., Peckous, B., & Busby-Whitehead, J. (2001). A pilot study to determine predictors of behavioral treatment completion for urinary incontinence. *Urologic Nursing, 21*(1), 39-44.

Kontiokari, T., et al. (2001). Randomised trial of cranberry-ligonberry juice and *Lactobacillus* GG drink for the prevention of urinary tract infection in women. *British Medical Journal, 332*, 1571-1573.

Lehmann, S., & Dietz, C. (2002). Double-J stents: They're not trouble free. *RN, 65*(1), 54-60.

Lekan-Rutledge, D., & Colling, J. (2003). Urinary incontinence in the frail elderly. *American Journal of Nursing, 103*(3 Suppl.), 36-46.

Lopez, R., Smith, P., & Thering, A. (2002). What are the indications for urodynamic testing in older adults with incontinence? *The Journal of Family Practice, 51*(12), 1077.

Lyons, S., & Specht, J. (2000). Prompted voiding protocol for individuals with urinary incontinence. *Journal of Gerontological Nursing, 20*(6), 5-13.

Maloney, C. (2002). Estrogen and recurrent UTI in postmenopausal women. *American Journal of Nursing, 102*(8), 44-53.

Maloney, C., & Cafiero, M. (2001). Non-invasive evaluation and treatment of bladder control problems in the primary care setting. *The American Journal for Nurse Practitioners, 5*(5), 42, 45-46, 49-50, 53-54.

Mather, K., & Bakas, T. (2002). Nursing assistants' perceptions of their ability to provide continence care. *Geriatric Nursing, 23*(2), 76-81.

McCance, K., & Huether, S. (2002). Pathophysiology: The biologic basis for disease in adults and children (4th ed.). St. Louis: Mosby.

McLaughlin, S.P., & Carson, C.C. (2004). Urinary tract infections in women. *Medical Clinics of North America, 88*(2), 417-429.

Miller, C. (2002). Anticholinergics: The good and the bad. *Geriatric Nursing, 23*(5), 286-287.

Miller, C. (2002). Recently approved and forthcoming drugs for elders. *Geriatric Nursing, 23*(1), 51-52.

Moore, K., Day, R., & Albers, M. (2002). Pathogenesis of urinary tract infections: A review. *Journal of Clinical Nursing, 11*(5), 568-574.

Moorhead, S., Johnson, M., & Maas, M. (Eds.). (2004). *Nursing outcomes classification (NOC)* (3rd ed.). St. Louis: Mosby.

Mueller, C., & Cain, H. (2002). Comprehensive management of urinary incontinence through quality improvement efforts. *Geriatric Nursing, 23*(2), 82-87.

National Kidney and Urologic Diseases Information Clearinghouse. (2004). *Kidney and urologic diseases statistics for the United States.* NIH Pub. No. 04-3895. Bethesda, MD. National Institutes of Health. Available at http://kidney.niddk.nih.gov/kudiseases/pubs/kustats/index.htm.

Newman, D. (2003). Stress urinary incontinence in women. *American Journal of Nursing, 103*(8), 46-55.

Newman, D., & Giovannini, D. (2002). Overactive bladder: A nursing perspective. *American Journal of Nursing, 102*(6), 36-46.

Newman, D.K., & Palmer, M.H. (2003). State of the science on urinary incontinence. *American Journal of Nursing, 103*(March Suppl.), 3-56.

Oosterlinck, W., et al. (2002). Guidelines on bladder cancer. *European Urology, 41*, 105-112.

Portis, A.J., & Sudaram, C.P. (2001). Diagnosis and management of kidney stones. *American Family Physician, 63*(7), 1329-1338.

*Resnick, M.I. (Ed.). (1997). Urolithiasis. *Urologic Clinics of North America, 24*(1), entire issue.

Rigsby, D. (2003). The overactive bladder. *Nursing Standard, 17*(39), 45-54.

Saint, S. (2000). Clinical and economic consequences of nosocomial catheter-related bacteriuria. *American Journal of Infection Control, 28*, 68-75.

Sampselle, C. (2003). Behavioral interventions in young and middle-age women. *American Journal of Nursing, 103*(Suppl. 3), 9-19.

Sampselle, C. (2003). Teaching women to use a voiding diary. *American Journal of Nursing, 103*(11), 62-64.

U.S. Renal Data Systems. (2002). *USRDS 2002 annual data report.* Bethesda, MD: The National Institutes of Health, National Institute of Diabetes and Digestive and Kidney Diseases.

Vaughn, D., & Malkowicz, S. (2001). Recent advances in bladder cancer chemotherapy. *Cancer Investigation, 19*(1), 77-85.

Walsh, P.C., et al. (2002). *Campbell's urology* (8th ed.). Philadelphia: W.B. Saunders.

*Warren, J.W., et al. (1999). Guidelines for antimicrobial treatment of uncomplicated acute bacterial cystitis and acute pyelonephritis in women. *Clinics in Infectious Disease, 29*(4), 745-758.

Wyman, J. (2003). Treatment of urinary incontinence in men and older women. *American Journal of Nursing, 103*(Suppl. 3), 26-35.

*Young-McCaughan, S. (1999). Invasive bladder cancer. In C. Miaskowski & P. Buchsel (Eds.), *Oncology nursing: Assessment and clinical care* (pp. 1055-1087). St. Louis: Mosby.

Interventions for Clients with Renal Disorders

CHRIS WINKELMAN

LEARNING OUTCOMES

After studying this chapter, you should be able to:

1. Prioritize nursing care for the client with polycystic kidney disease.
2. Describe the clinical manifestations of hydronephrosis.
3. Identify clients at risk for pyelonephritis.
4. Describe the mechanisms of action, side effects, and nursing implications for drug therapy for pyelonephritis.
5. Use laboratory data and clinical manifestations to determine the effectiveness of therapy for pyelonephritis.
6. Compare the pathophysiology and clinical manifestations of acute glomerular nephritis and nephrotic syndrome.
7. Explain the relationship between hypertension and renal disease.
8. Prioritize nursing care for the client during the first 24 hours after a nephrectomy.
9. Explain how diabetic nephropathy can affect glucose metabolism and control in the client with diabetes mellitus.
10. Develop a community-based teaching plan for the client who has had a nephrectomy for renal cell carcinoma.
11. Describe strategies to prevent renal trauma.

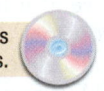

Go to your Student CD-ROM for Review Questions for the NCLEX Examination keyed to these Learning Outcomes.

Renal disorders reduce the ability of the kidney to filter wastes and to balance fluid, electrolytes, acids, and bases. The kidneys work together with many other organ systems; thus renal disorders affect systemic health and can lead to life-threatening outcomes. Renal disorders are classified as congenital, obstructive, infectious, glomerular, and degenerative. Renal tumors and renal trauma are also described in this chapter. Renal failure is discussed in Chapter 75.

CONGENITAL DISORDERS

Polycystic Kidney Disease

PATHOPHYSIOLOGY

Polycystic kidney disease (PKD) is an inherited disorder in which fluid-filled cysts develop in the nephrons. In the dominant form, only a few nephrons have cysts until the person reaches his or her 30s. In the recessive form of the disease, nearly 100% of nephrons have cysts from birth.

Cysts develop anywhere in the nephron as a result of kidney cell division, altered secretion, and abnormal cell matrix biology (Calvet & Grantham, 2001; Igarashi & Somlo, 2002).

Over time, small cysts become much larger (up to a few centimeters in diameter) and more widely distributed. The growing cysts damage the glomerular and tubular membranes. As the cysts fill with fluid and enlarge, the nephron functions become less effective.

The kidney tissue is eventually replaced by nonfunctioning cysts, which look like clusters of grapes (Figure 74-1). The kidneys are grossly enlarged; each cystic kidney may enlarge to two or three times its normal size, becoming as large as a football. Other abdominal organs are displaced, and the client has discomfort or pain. The fluid-filled cysts are also at increased risk for infection, rupture, and bleeding.

Most clients with PKD have high blood pressure. The cause of hypertension is thought to be related to renal ischemia from the enlarging cysts. As the vessels are compressed and renal blood flow decreases, the renin-angiotensin system is activated, raising blood pressure. Control of hypertension

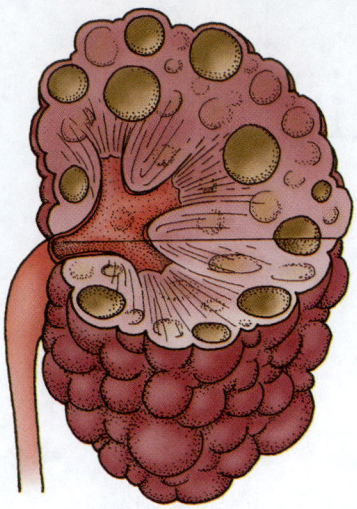

Figure 74-1 ■ Polycystic kidney.

is a top priority because proper treatment can disrupt the process that leads to renal ischemia.

Cysts may also occur in other tissues, such as the liver, blood vessels of the brain, and cardiac blood vessels. Cysts may reduce liver function or result in bleeding into the brain from ruptured intracranial vascular cysts *(berry aneurysms),* causing sudden death. For reasons as yet unknown, kidney stones occur in 8% to 36% of the clients with PKD. Heart valve abnormalities (e.g., mitral valve prolapse), left ventricular hypertrophy, and colonic diverticula also are common in clients with PKD.

Etiology and Genetic Risk

PKD has several inherited forms. It can be inherited as either an autosomal dominant trait or, less commonly, as an autosomal recessive trait. People who inherit the recessive form of PKD usually die in early childhood. The 5% to 10% incidence of PKD in clients with no family history occurs as a result of a spontaneous gene mutation.

Genetic Considerations

The autosomal dominant form of PKD (ADPKD) is the most common form of polycystic disease. Children of parents who have the autosomal dominant form of PKD have a 50% chance of inheriting the gene that causes the disease. Manifestations of ADPKD can vary for age of onset, manifestations, and illness severity, even within one family. However, ADPKD is fully penetrant, meaning that nearly 100% of people who inherit a PKD gene will develop renal cysts by age 30 (Igarashi & Somlo, 2002). Half of these people develop renal failure by age 50 years. ADPKD-1 is the most common and most severe form of the autosomal dominant disease. ADPKD-2 has a slower rate of cyst formation so that symptoms occur later in life and there is delayed progression to renal failure and other complications. The gene products of ADPKD-1 and ADPKD-2 are both polycystins, cell membrane proteins important to ion transport (Arnaout, 2001; Online Mendelian Inheritance in Man, 2004).

Autosomal recessive PKD is rare, caused by a different gene mutation than the dominant form. To inherit a reces-

CHART 74-1

KEY FEATURES of
Polycystic Kidney Disease

- Abdominal or flank pain
- Hypertension
- Nocturia
- Increased abdominal girth
- Constipation
- Bloody or cloudy urine
- Kidney stones

sive gene, both parents must carry a copy of the mutated allele and both mutated alleles must be inherited. Thus each child has a 1 in 4 chance of inheriting autosomal recessive polycystic disease (ARPKD).

At present, there is no way to prevent PKD, although early detection and management of hypertension may slow the progression of renal impairment. Genetic counseling and evaluation may be useful for adults who have one parent or both parents with PKD.

Incidence/Prevalence

Polycystic kidney disease (PKD) is a common disorder, affecting 250,000 to 500,000 people in the United States. PKD is more common in white individuals than in people of other races. Men and women have an equal chance of inheriting the disease because the gene responsible for PKD is not located on the sex chromosomes (Polycystic Kidney Disease Foundation, 2004).

◆COLLABORATIVE MANAGEMENT
◆Assessment
HISTORY

Explore the family history of a client with suspected or actual PKD and ask whether either parent was known to have PKD or whether there is any family history of kidney disease. The age at which signs and symptoms developed in the parent and any related complications are important to obtain. Ask the client about constipation, abdominal discomfort, a change in urine color or frequency, high blood pressure, headaches, and a family history of sudden death from a stroke.

PHYSICAL ASSESSMENT/CLINICAL MANIFESTATIONS

Chart 74-1 lists key features of PKD. Pain is often the first manifestation. Inspect the abdomen. A distended abdomen is common as the cystic kidneys swell and push the abdominal contents forward. Polycystic kidneys are easily palpated because of their increased size. Proceed with *gentle* abdominal palpation because the cystic kidneys and nearby tissues may be tender, and palpation is uncomfortable.

The client also may have flank pain as a dull ache or as sharp and intermittent discomfort. Dull, aching pain is caused by increased kidney size with distention or from infection within the cyst. Sharp, intermittent pain occurs when a cyst ruptures or a stone is present. When a cyst ruptures, the client may have bright red or cola-colored urine. Infection is suspected if the urine is cloudy or foul smelling or if there is **dysuria** (pain on urination).

Nocturia (the need to urinate excessively at night) is an early manifestation and occurs because of decreased urine concentrating ability. As renal function further declines, the client has increasing hypertension, edema, and uremic problems such as anorexia, nausea, vomiting, pruritus, and fatigue (see Chapter 75). Because berry aneurysms often occur in clients with PKD, a severe headache with or without neurologic or vision changes deserves particular attention.

PSYCHOSOCIAL ASSESSMENT

As an inherited disorder, PKD may cause complex psychosocial responses. The client often has seen the effects and problems of the disease in close family members. He or she may have had a parent who died or close relatives who required dialysis or transplantation. While obtaining the family history, listen carefully for spoken and unspoken feelings of anger, resentment, futility, sadness, or anxiety; such feelings may need further exploration. The focus of the feelings may be one or both parents or the process of diagnosis and treatment. Feelings of guilt and concern for the client's children may also complicate the issue.

DIAGNOSTIC ASSESSMENT

Urinalysis shows **proteinuria** (protein in the urine) once the glomeruli are involved. **Hematuria** (blood in the urine) may be gross or microscopic. Bacteria in the urine indicate infection, usually in the cysts. Obtain a urine sample for culture and sensitivity testing when there is clinical or laboratory evidence of infection. As kidney function deteriorates, serum creatinine and blood urea nitrogen (BUN) levels rise. With decreasing kidney function, creatinine clearance decreases. Changes in renal handling of sodium may cause either sodium losses or sodium retention.

Diagnostic studies include renal sonography, computed tomography (CT), and magnetic resonance imaging (MRI). Small cysts are detected by sonography, CT, or MRI. Renal sonography provides diagnostic evidence of PKD, with minimal risk cases.

◆ Common Nursing Diagnoses and Collaborative Problems

Nursing diagnoses and collaborative problems that may apply to clients with polycystic kidney disease (PKD) include the following:

- Acute Pain related to cyst rupture or stone formation
- Chronic Pain related to enlarging kidneys compressing abdominal contents
- Constipation related to compression of intestinal tract
- Risk for Infection related to the presence of cysts and decreased renal blood flow
- Potential for Hypertension
- Potential for Stone Formation
- Potential for Renal Failure

◆ Interventions

Chart 74-2 lists NIC interventions for clients with renal disorders. (See Chapter 73 for information on urinary infections and stone formation. See Chapter 75 for care of the client with renal failure.)

Acute and Chronic Pain. Comfort strategies include drug therapy and complementary approaches. A combination may be most effective. Nonsteroidal anti-inflammatory drugs (NSAIDs) are used cautiously be-

cause of their tendency to reduce renal blood flow. Aspirin-containing compounds are avoided to reduce the risk for bleeding.

If cyst infection causes discomfort, lipid-soluble antibiotics such as trimethoprim/sulfamethoxazole (Bactrim, Septra, Trimpex) or ciprofloxacin (Cipro), are prescribed. These drugs penetrate the cyst wall. Monitor the serum creatinine levels because antibiotic therapy can be nephrotoxic. Apply dry heat to the abdomen or flank to promote comfort when renal cysts are infected. When pain is severe or debilitating, cysts can be reduced by percutaneous needle aspiration and drainage.

Teach the client methods of enhancing relaxation and promoting comfort via deep breathing, guided imagery, or other strategies. The overall goal is client self-management. (See Chapter 7 for pain management.)

Constipation. Teach the client how to prevent constipation (see Bowel Management in Chart 74-2). Include teaching about maintaining adequate fluid intake, increasing dietary fiber when fluid intake is more than 2500 mL/24 hr, and the need for regular exercise. Explain that pressure on the large intestine may further impede peristalsis as the polycystic kidneys increase in size. The client should know that these recommendations for bowel management might change, particularly if renal failure also develops. Advise the client about the use of stool softeners and bulk agents, including the careful use of laxatives, to prevent chronic constipation.

Hypertension and Renal Failure. Blood pressure control is necessary to reduce cardiovascular complications and slow the progression of renal dysfunction. Nursing interventions include education to promote self-management and understanding (see Medication Management in Chart 74-2 and Chapter 39 for information on hypertension). When renal impairment results in decreased urine concentration with nocturia and low urine specific gravity, urge the client to drink at least 2 L of fluid per day to prevent dehydration, which further reduces renal function. Restricting sodium intake may help control blood pressure.

Drug therapy for blood pressure control includes antihypertensive agents and diuretics. Antihypertensive agents include angiotensin-converting enzyme (ACE) inhibitors, calcium channel blockers, beta blockers, and vasodilators (see Chart 39-2). ACE inhibitors may help control the cell proliferation aspects of PKD and reduce microalbuminuria. If PKD progresses to chronic renal failure or end-stage renal disease, treatment approaches are similar to those in Chapter 75.

Teach the client, family, or significant other how to measure and record blood pressure. Help the client establish a schedule for self-administering drugs, monitoring daily weights, and keeping blood pressure records (Chart 74-3). Explain the potential side effects of the drugs. Make available written materials, such as drug teaching cards and booklets.

A low-sodium diet is often prescribed to control the hypertension that usually accompanies PKD. However, some clients may have salt wasting and should not follow a sodium-restricted diet. As the disease progresses, the client's protein intake may need to be limited to slow the development of renal failure. Assist the client, family, or significant other in understanding the diet plan and clarify its rationale. Work closely with the dietitian to foster the client's understanding. You may also refer the client for nutritional counseling.

CHART 74-2

NIC **INTERVENTION ACTIVITIES for**
The Client with Renal Problems

Pain Management: *Alleviation of pain or a reduction in pain to a level of comfort that is acceptable to the client*
- Observe for nonverbal cues of discomfort, especially in those unable to communicate effectively.
- Ensure that client receives attentive analgesic care.
- Consider cultural influences on pain response.
- Utilize a developmentally appropriate assessment method that allows for monitoring of change in pain and that will assist in identifying actual and potential precipitating factors (e.g., flow sheet, daily diary).
- Control environmental factors that may influence the client's response to discomfort (e.g., room temperature, lighting, noise).
- Consider type and source of pain when selecting pain relief strategy.
- Provide the person optimal pain relief with prescribed analgesics.
- Implement the use of patient-controlled analgesia (PCA), if appropriate.
- Use pain control measures before pain becomes severe.
- Evaluate the effectiveness of the pain control measures used through ongoing assessment of the pain experience.
- Institute and modify pain control measures on the basis of the client's response.

Bowel Management: *Establishment and maintenance of a regular pattern of bowel elimination*
- Note pre-existent bowel problems, bowel routine, and use of laxatives.
- Teach client about specific foods that assist in promoting bowel regularity.
- Initiate a bowel training program, as appropriate.
- Instruct client on foods high in fiber, as appropriate.
- Evaluate medication profile for gastrointestinal side effects.

Medication Management: *Facilitation of safe and effective use of prescription and over-the-counter drugs*
- Monitor client for the therapeutic effect of the medication.
- Monitor for signs and symptoms of drug toxicity.
- Monitor for adverse effects of the drug.
- Develop strategies with the client to enhance compliance with prescribed medication regimen.
- Teach the client and/or family members the expected action and side effects of the medication.
- Instruct client when to seek medical attention.

Energy Management: *Regulating energy use to treat or prevent fatigue and optimize function*
- Determine client's physical limitations.
- Determine client's/significant other's perceptions of causes of fatigue.
- Encourage verbalization of feelings about limitations.
- Determine what and how much activity is required to build endurance.

- Monitor nutritional intake to ensure adequate energy resources.
- Monitor client for evidence of excess physical and emotional fatigue.
- Monitor cardiorespiratory response to activity (e.g., tachycardia, other dysrhythmias, dyspnea, diaphoresis, pallor, hemodynamic pressures, and respiratory rate).
- Monitor location and nature of discomfort or pain during movement/activity.
- Promote bed rest/activity limitation (e.g., increase number of rest periods).
- Encourage alternate rest and activity periods.
- Provide calming diversionary activities to promote relaxation.
- Plan activities for periods when the client has the most energy.
- Encourage physical activity (e.g., ambulation or performance of activities of daily living, consistent with client's energy resources).

Fluid Monitoring: *Collection and analysis of client data to regulate fluid balance*
- Monitor weight.
- Monitor intake and output.
- Monitor serum and urine electrolyte values, as appropriate.
- Monitor serum albumin and total protein levels.
- Monitor serum and urine osmolality levels.
- Keep an accurate record of intake and output.
- Monitor for distended neck veins, crackles in the lungs, peripheral edema, and weight gain.
- Restrict and allocate fluid intake, as appropriate.
- Administer pharmacologic agents to increase urinary output, as appropriate.
- Administer dialysis, as appropriate, noting client response.

Urinary Retention Care: *Assistance in relieving bladder distention*
- Provide privacy for elimination.
- Provide Credé maneuver, as necessary.
- Use double-voiding technique.
- Insert urinary catheter, as appropriate.
- Monitor degree of bladder distention by palpation and percussion.
- Catheterize for residual, as appropriate.
- Implement intermittent catheterization, as appropriate.

Infection Protection: *Prevention and early detection of infection in a client at risk*
- Monitor for systemic and localized signs and symptoms of infection.
- Maintain asepsis for client at risk.
- Inspect condition of any surgical incision/wound.
- Instruct client to take antibiotics as prescribed.
- Obtain cultures, as needed.

NIC intervention activities selected from: Dochterman, J.,M., & Bulechek, G.M. (Eds.). (2004). *Nursing interventions classification (NIC)* (4th ed.). St. Louis: Mosby. No part of this work is to be altered without prior written permission from the Publisher.

Health Care Resources

The Polycystic Kidney Research Foundation (http://www.pkdcure.org) and the National Kidney and Urologic Disease division and the National Institute of Health (http://www.niddk.nih.gov) conduct research and provide education about PKD. Many pamphlets are available; there is a fee for some materials. Chapters of the National Kidney Foundation (NKF) and the American Association of Kidney Patients (AAKP) also have resources for information and support.

OBSTRUCTIVE DISORDERS

Hydronephrosis, Hydroureter, and Urethral Stricture

PATHOPHYSIOLOGY

Hydronephrosis and hydroureter are problems of urine outflow obstruction. Urethral strictures also obstruct outflow. Prompt recognition and treatment are crucial to prevent permanent renal damage.

CLIENT EDUCATION GUIDE
Polycystic Kidney Disease

- Measure and record your blood pressure daily.
- Take your temperature if you suspect you have a fever.
- Weigh yourself every day at the same time of day and with the same amount of clothing; notify your physician or nurse if you have a sudden weight gain.
- Limit your intake of salt to help control your blood pressure.
- Notify your physician or nurse if your urine is foul smelling or if there is blood in your urine.
- Notify your physician or nurse if you have a headache that does not go away or if you have visual disturbances.
- Monitor bowel movements to prevent constipation.

In **hydronephrosis,** the kidney enlarges as urine collects in the pelvis and kidney tissue. Because the capacity of the renal pelvis is normally 5 to 8 mL, obstruction in the pelvis or at the ureteropelvic junction (UPJ) quickly distends the renal pelvis. Kidney pressure increases as the volume of urine increases. Over time, sometimes in only a matter of hours, the blood vessels and renal tubules can be damaged extensively (Figure 74-2).

In clients with **hydroureter** (enlargement of the ureter), the effects are similar but the obstruction is lower in the urinary tract. The ureter is most easily obstructed where the iliac vessels cross or where the ureters enter the bladder. Ureter dilation occurs above the obstruction and enlarges as urine collects (see Figure 74-2).

In clients with a **urethral stricture,** the obstruction is very low in the urinary tract, causing bladder distention before hydroureter and hydronephrosis. The problems and kidney damage are similar without prompt treatment.

Urinary obstruction causes damage when pressure builds up directly on tissue. Tubular filtrate pressure also increases in the nephron as drainage through the collecting system is impaired. With this added pressure, glomerular filtration decreases or ceases, and renal failure results. Nitrogenous waste products (urea, creatinine, and uric acid) and electrolytes (sodium, potassium, chloride, and phosphorus) are retained in the blood, and acid-base balance is impaired.

Causes of hydronephrosis or hydroureter include tumors, stones, trauma, congenital structural defects, and fibrosis. In clients with cancer, obstructed ureters may result from pelvic radiation or surgical intervention. Early treatment of the causes can prevent hydronephrosis and hydroureter and thus prevent permanent renal damage. The specific time needed to prevent permanent damage depends on the client's renal health. Permanent damage can occur in less than 48 hours in some clients and after several weeks in other clients.

◆COLLABORATIVE MANAGEMENT
◆Assessment

Obtain a history from the client, focusing on known renal or urologic disorders. A history of childhood urinary tract problems may indicate previously undiagnosed structural defects. Ask about the client's pattern of urination, especially amount, frequency, color, clarity, and odor. Ask the client about recent flank or abdominal pain. Chills, fever, and malaise may be present with a urinary tract infection (UTI).

Inspect each flank to identify asymmetry, which may occur with a renal mass, and *gently* palpate the client's ab-

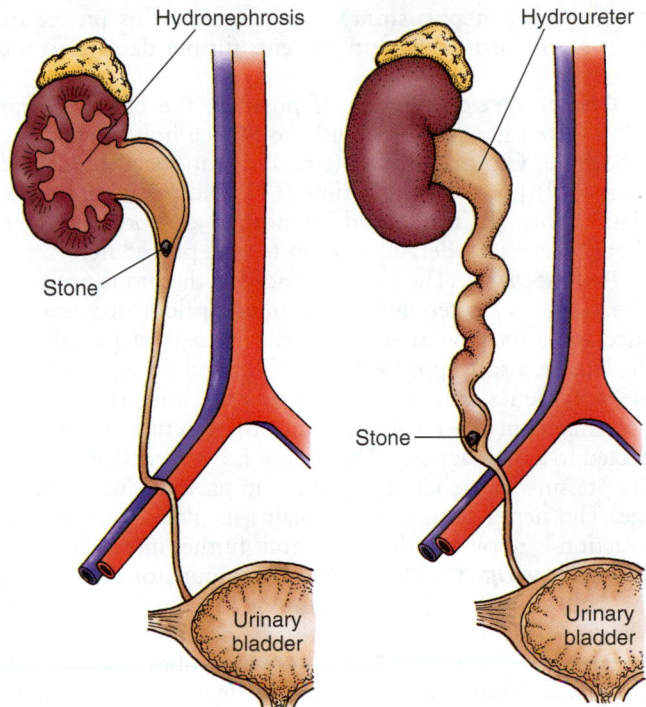

Figure 74-2 ■ Hydronephrosis is caused by obstruction in the upper part of the ureter; hydroureter is caused by obstruction in the lower part of the ureter.

domen to locate areas of tenderness. Palpate and percuss the bladder to detect distention. Gentle pressure on the abdomen may cause urine leakage, which reflects a full bladder and possible obstruction.

Urinalysis may show bacteria or white blood cells if infection is present. When urinary tract obstruction is prolonged, microscopic examination may reveal tubular epithelial cells. Blood chemistries are normal unless decreased glomerular filtration has occurred. Blood creatinine and blood urea nitrogen (BUN) levels increase with a reduced glomerular filtration rate (GFR). Serum electrolyte levels may be altered with hyperkalemia, hyperphosphatemia, hypocalcemia, and metabolic acidosis (bicarbonate deficit).

Intravenous urography shows ureteral or renal pelvis dilation. Urinary outflow obstruction can be seen with sonography (renal echography) or computed tomography (CT).

◆Interventions

Urinary retention and potential for infection are the primary problems. (See Fluid Monitoring, Urinary Retention Care, and Infection Protection in Chart 74-2.) Failure to treat the cause of obstruction leads to infection and renal failure.

Urologic Interventions. If the stricture is caused by a stone, it can be located and retrieved using cystoscopic or retrograde pyelogram procedures. The urologist uses a cystoscope to guide a stone basket over the stone and removes it through the bladder. After stone removal, a plastic stent is usually left in the ureter for a few weeks to improve urine flow in the area irritated by the stone. The stent is later removed via another cystoscopic procedure.

Radiologic Intervention. When a stricture is causing hydronephrosis and cannot be corrected with urologic procedures, a **nephrostomy** is performed. This procedure diverts urine externally and prevents further damage to the kidney.

Client Preparation. If possible, the client is kept NPO (given nothing by mouth) for 4 to 6 hours before the procedure. Clotting studies (e.g., International Normalized Ratio [INR], prothrombin time [PT], and partial thromboplastic time [PTT]) should be normal or corrected. The client receives moderate sedation for the procedure.

Procedure. The client is placed in the prone position. The kidney is located under ultrasound or fluoroscopic guidance and a local anesthetic is given. A needle is placed into the kidney, a soft-tipped guidewire is placed through the needle, and then a catheter is placed over the wire. The catheter tip remains in the renal pelvis and the external end is connected to a drainage bag. The procedure immediately relieves the pressure in the kidney system and prevents further damage. The nephrostomy tube remains in place until the obstruction is resolved (with or without further intervention).

Follow-up Care. Assess the amount of drainage in the collection bag. The amount of drainage depends on whether a ureteral catheter is also being used (with a separate drainage bag). Clients with ureteral tubes may have all urine pass through to the bladder or may have urine drain into the collection bags. The type of urine drainage expected should be clearly communicated in the chart. If urine is expected to drain into the collection bag, assess the amount of drainage hourly for the first 24 hours. If the amount of drainage decreases and the client has back pain, the tube may be clogged or dislodged. Notify the physician immediately.

Monitor the nephrostomy site for leaking urine or blood. If either occurs, notify the physician immediately. Urine drainage may be red-tinged for the first 12 to 24 hours after the procedure and should gradually clear. Assess the client for manifestations of infection, including fever or a change in urine character.

INFECTIOUS DISORDERS

The urinary system normally excretes sterile urine. The unobstructed and complete passage of urine from the renal and urinary systems is critical in maintaining a sterile urinary tract. When any structural abnormality is present, the risk for damage as a result of infection is greatly increased. **Urinary tract infection (UTI)** is an infection in this normally sterile system. **Pyelonephritis** is a bacterial infection in the kidney and renal pelvis—the *upper* urinary tract. Infections in the *lower* urinary tract are described in Chapter 73.

Pyelonephritis
PATHOPHYSIOLOGY

Pyelonephritis is either the presence of active organisms in the kidney or the effects of kidney infections. **Acute pyelonephritis** is the active bacterial infection, whereas **chronic pyelonephritis** results from repeated or continued upper urinary tract infections or the effects of such infections. Chronic pyelonephritis often occurs with an anatomic urinary tract anomaly, obstruction or, most commonly, vesicoureteral urine reflux. The vesicoureteral junction is the point at which

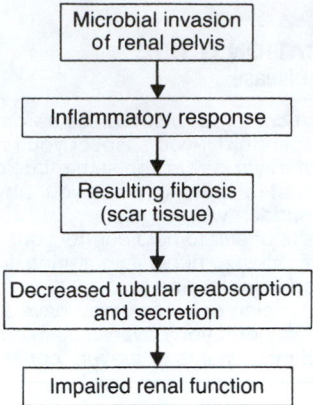

the ureter joins the bladder. **Reflux** is the reverse or upward flow of urine toward the renal pelvis and kidney.

In pyelonephritis, organisms ascend from the lower urinary tract into the renal pelvis. Descending infection transmitted by organisms in the blood may occur, but not often. Bacteria trigger the inflammatory response, and local edema results.

Acute pyelonephritis involves acute interstitial inflammation, tubular cell necrosis, and possible abscess formation. **Abscesses**, pockets of local infection, can occur in the capsule, cortex, or medulla. The infection is scattered within the kidney; healthy tissues can lie next to infected areas. Fibrosis and scar tissue develop from the inflammation. The calices thicken and scars develop in the interstitial tissue.

Reflux of infected urine from the bladder into the ureters and kidney is responsible for most cases of chronic pyelonephritis. Reflux within the kidney can occur when some papillae in the kidney do not close properly. Inflammation and fibrosis lead to deformity of the renal pelvis and calices. Repeated or continuous infections create additional scar tissue, changing blood vessel, glomerular, and tubular structure. As a result, filtration, reabsorption, and secretion are impaired, and renal function is reduced (Figure 74-3).

Etiology and Genetic Risk

Single episodes of *acute* pyelonephritis may result from the entry of bacteria associated with pregnancy, obstruction, or reflux. *Chronic* pyelonephritis is usually associated with structural deformities or obstruction with reflux. Reflux or obstruction leading to chronic pyelonephritis is often caused by stones or neurogenic impairment of voiding. Reflux is more common in children, who as adults have scarring with chronic pyelonephritis. Chronic pyelonephritis in adults who did not have reflux as a child usually occurs with spinal cord injury, bladder tumor, prostatic enlargement, or urinary tract stones.

Acute or chronic pyelonephritis occurs often in clients who have undergone manipulation of the urinary tract (e.g., placement of a urinary catheter), those with diabetes mellitus or chronic renal calculi, or those who overuse analgesics. In clients with diabetes mellitus, the development of bladder atony increases the risk for pyelonephritis. In clients with chronic stone disease, stones may retain organisms resulting in ongoing infection and renal scarring. Nonsteroidal anti-inflammatory drug (NSAID) use is associated with papillary necrosis and reflux.

The most common pyelonephritis-causing organism is *Escherichia coli. Enterococcus faecalis* is common in hospitalized clients. Both organisms are in the intestinal tract. Other organisms that cause pyelonephritis in hospitalized clients include *Proteus mirabilis, Klebsiella,* and *Pseudomonas aeruginosa.* When the infection is bloodborne, common infecting organisms include *Staphylococcus aureus* and the *Candida* and *Salmonella* species.

Other possible causes of kidney scarring leading to renal impairment include antibody reactions, cell-mediated immunity against the bacterial antigens, or autoimmune reactions.

Incidence/Prevalence

The exact incidence and prevalence of pyelonephritis are not known because this diagnosis is not separately reported from all urinary tract infections. Acute conditions of the kidneys or urinary tract, nephritic syndrome, urethral stricture, and cystitis account for more than 7 million new cases annually in community-dwelling Americans (NIDDK National Kidney and Urologic Diseases Information Clearinghouse, 2004). Women have more cases of pyelonephritis. After 65 years of age, rates for men increase greatly because of the increased incidence of prostatitis.

◆COLLABORATIVE MANAGEMENT
◆Assessment

HISTORY

Ask the client about a history of urinary tract infections (UTIs), diabetes mellitus, stone disease, and other abnormalities of the genitourinary tract. Determine whether the UTIs occurred with pregnancy and ask the client about any previous episodes of pyelonephritis or similar symptoms. Recurrences are common and may lead to a decline of renal function.

PHYSICAL ASSESSMENT/CLINICAL MANIFESTATIONS

Ask the client about manifestations of acute pyelonephritis (Chart 74-4). Chronic pyelonephritis has a less dramatic presentation, with manifestations related to the infection or renal function. Ask the client to describe any vague or nonspecific urinary symptoms or abdominal discomfort. Inquire about any history of repeated, low-grade fevers. The client with chronic pyelonephritis often has asymptomatic bacteremia. Chart 74-5 outlines the renal effects of chronic pyelonephritis.

Inspect the flanks and gently palpate the costovertebral angle (CVA). Inspect both CVAs for enlargement, asymmetry, edema, or erythema, all of which can be manifestations of inflammation. If there is no tenderness to light palpation in either CVA, a specially trained nurse firmly percusses each area. Tenderness or discomfort may indicate infection or inflammation.

PSYCHOSOCIAL ASSESSMENT

The client with any problem in the genitourinary area may have feelings of anxiety, embarrassment, or guilt. Listen carefully for evidence of anxiety or specific fears, and prevent embarrassment during assessment. Feelings of guilt, often associated with sexual habits or practices, may be masked through delay in seeking treatment or through vague, nonspecific responses to specific or direct questions. Encourage clients to tell their own story in familiar, comfortable language.

LABORATORY ASSESSMENT

Urinalysis shows a positive leukocyte esterase and nitrite dipstick test and the presence of white blood cells and bacteria. Occasional red blood cells, white blood cell casts, and proteinuria may be present. The urine is cultured to determine whether gram-positive or gram-negative organisms are causing the infection. The urine sample for culture and sensitivity testing, obtained by the clean-catch method, shows the bacterial species and susceptibility or resistance of the specific organism to various antibiotics. In clients with recurrent episodes of pyelonephritis or upper UTIs, more specific testing of bacterial antigens and antibodies may help determine whether the same organism is responsible for the recurrent infections.

Blood cultures are obtained for specific organisms. Other blood tests include the C-reactive protein and erythrocyte sedimentation rate.

RADIOGRAPHIC ASSESSMENT

An x-ray of the kidneys, ureters, and bladder (KUB) and intravenous (IV) pyelography are performed to determine the presence of stones or obstructions. A cystourethrogram is indicated for some clients. These procedures define urinary tract structures and identify any structural defects. Specific defects to be identified include foreign bodies, such as stones; obstruction to the outflow of urine, such as tumors, structural defects, or prostate enlargement; and urine reflux caused by incompetent ureterovesical valve closure. (See Chapter 72 for more information on radiographic assessment.)

OTHER DIAGNOSTIC ASSESSMENTS

Other diagnostic tests include examining antibody-coated bacteria in urine, certain enzymes (e.g., lactate dehydrogenase isoenzyme 5), and radionuclide scintillation (e.g., gallium

---

CHART 74-4

KEY FEATURES of
Acute Pyelonephritis

- Fever
- Chills
- Tachycardia and tachypnea
- Flank, back, or loin pain
- Tender costal vertebral angle (CVA)
- Abdominal, often colicky, discomfort
- Nausea and vomiting
- General malaise or fatigue
- Burning, urgency, or frequency of urination
- Nocturia

CHART 74-5

KEY FEATURES of
Chronic Pyelonephritis

- Hypertension
- Inability to conserve sodium
- Decreased concentrating ability (nocturia)
- Tendency to develop hyperkalemia and acidosis

scan). Examining urine for antibody-coated bacteria helps identify clients who may need long-term antibiotic therapy. High molecular-weight enzymes in urine, such as lactate dehydrogenase isoenzyme 5, are present with any renal tissue deterioration problem and give trend data. The gallium scan can identify active pyelonephritis or abscesses in or around the kidney.

Critical Thinking Challenge

The client is a 21-year-old female nursing student who has flank and CVA pain, dysuria, urgency, nocturia, and frequency. She tells you she started to feel unwell about 3 days ago but is much worse now. She says she has had cystitis about six times in the past year but has never been this sick with it. She says "I usually work as a nursing assistant at night but had to call off because I was so tired and nauseated." Her vital signs are P 114, BP 130/90, R 22, T 102. Her urine is cloudy, amber, and foul smelling, positive for both leukocyte esterase and nitrate, with white blood cells and gram-negative bacteria.

1. What additional assessment data should you obtain?
2. Which manifestations are specific to cystitis, which are specific to pyelonephritis, and which are common to both?
3. What risk factors for pyelonephritis are present for this client?

evolve For suggested answer guidelines, go to http://evolve.elsevier.com/Iggy/.

◆Analysis

COMMON NURSING DIAGNOSES AND COLLABORATIVE PROBLEMS

The primary common nursing diagnosis for the client with pyelonephritis is Acute Pain (Flank and Abdominal) related to inflammation and infection. A common collaborative problem is Potential for Renal Failure.

ADDITIONAL NURSING DIAGNOSES AND COLLABORATIVE PROBLEMS

In addition to the common nursing diagnoses and collaborative problems, clients with pyelonephritis may have one or more of the following:

- Infection or Risk for Infection related to inadequate primary defenses (urinary stasis) or instrumentation
- Deficient Knowledge regarding the medical diagnosis and therapy related to unfamiliarity with information resources
- Activity Intolerance related to fatigue, debilitation, and generalized weakness associated with the infection
- Fear of development of chronic renal failure related to an inability to control recurrent infections
- Hyperthermia related to increased metabolic rate from infection

An additional collaborative problem is Potential for Sepsis and Septic Shock.

◆Planning and Implementation

ACUTE PAIN

NOC **PLANNING: EXPECTED OUTCOMES.** With proper intervention, the client with pyelonephritis is expected to achieve an acceptable state of comfort. Indicators

include that the client often or consistently demonstrates the following behaviors:

- Uses nonanalgesic relief measures
- Uses analgesics appropriately
- Reports pain controlled

INTERVENTIONS. Interventions may be nonsurgical or surgical. (See Pain Management in Chart 74-2.) The success of several noninvasive techniques that crush stones, such as lithotripsy and percutaneous ultrasonic pyelolithotomy (see Chapter 73), have decreased the need for surgery.

NONSURGICAL MANAGEMENT. Nonsurgical interventions include the use of drug therapy, diet and fluid therapy, and teaching to ensure the client's understanding of the treatment.

Drug Therapy. Antibiotics are prescribed to treat the infection. At first, the antibiotics are broad spectrum. After urine and blood culture and sensitivity results are known, more specific antibiotics may be prescribed. Urinary antiseptic drugs (e.g., nitrofurantoin [Macrodantin]) may also be prescribed to provide comfort. See Medication Management in Chart 74-2 for nursing intervention activities.

Diet Therapy. For healing to occur, the client's nutritional intake must include adequate calories and all food groups. Fluid intake is recommended at 2 to 3 L/day unless another condition requires fluid restriction.

SURGICAL MANAGEMENT. Surgical interventions can correct structural problems causing urine reflux or obstruction of urine outflow or to eradicate the source of infection.

Preoperative Care. Antibiotics are given, usually intravenously, to achieve adequate blood levels or sterile blood culture results. Teach the client the nature and purpose of the proposed surgery, the expected outcome, and how the client can participate.

Operative Procedures. The surgical procedures may be one of the following: **pyelolithotomy** (stone removal from the kidney), **nephrectomy** (removal of the kidney), ureteral diversion, or reimplantation of ureter to restore proper bladder drainage.

A pyelolithotomy is needed for removal of a large stone in the renal pelvis that blocks urine flow and causes infection. Nephrectomy is a last resort when all other measures to eradicate infection have failed. For clients with poor ureterovesical valve closure or dilated ureters, **ureteroplasty** (ureter repair or revision) or ureteral reimplantation (through another site in the bladder wall) preserves renal function and eliminates infections.

Postoperative Care. See Chapter 73 for nursing care after surgery for the client undergoing urologic surgery.

POTENTIAL FOR RENAL FAILURE

NOC **PLANNING: EXPECTED OUTCOMES.** The client under treatment for pyelonephritis is expected to conserve existing renal function for as long as possible and have a slow progression of renal failure once the process of renal failure begins. Indicators include that the client consistently demonstrates the following behaviors:

- Describes the role of antibiotics and self-administration of medications
- Explains and offers techniques to ensure adequate nutrition and hydration

- Describes the plan for post-treatment follow-up, including knowledge of recurrent symptoms
- Modifies prescribed regimen as directed by a health care professional

INTERVENTIONS. Specific antibiotics are prescribed to treat the infection. Stress the importance of completing the drug therapy as directed. Discuss with the client and family the importance of regular follow-up examinations and completing the recommended diagnostic tests.

Blood pressure control is needed to slow the progression of renal dysfunction. When renal impairment decreases concentrating ability, encourage the client to drink at least 2 L of fluid per day to prevent dehydration, which could further reduce renal function. When dietary protein is restricted, refer the client to the dietitian as needed. Other interventions related to the progression of chronic renal failure are covered in Chapter 75.

Community-Based Care

Pyelonephritis causes fear and anxiety in the client and family. The severity of the acute process and its potential to develop into a chronic process are frightening. The client and the family need reassurance that treatment and preventive measures can be accomplished.

HOME CARE MANAGEMENT

If no surgery is performed, the client may need assistance with self-care, nutrition, and drug management at home. If surgery is performed, the client may need help with incision care, self-care, and transportation for follow-up appointments.

HEALTH TEACHING

After assessing the client and family's understanding of pyelonephritis and its therapy, explain the following:

- Drug regimen (purpose, timing, frequency, duration, and possible side effects)
- The role of nutrition and adequate fluid intake
- The need for a balance between rest and activity, including any limitations after surgery
- The manifestations of disease recurrence
- The use of previously successful coping mechanisms

Advise the client to complete all prescribed antibiotic regimens and to report any side effects or unusual symptoms to the physician rather than stopping the drugs. Refer the client and family for nutritional counseling as needed, because many clients have special nutritional requirements, such as those caused by diabetes mellitus or pregnancy.

HEALTH CARE RESOURCES

The client may also briefly need a community health nurse to help with drug or nutrition therapy at home. Housekeeping services may be helpful while the client is regaining strength.

◆ Evaluation: Outcomes

Evaluate the care of the client with pyelonephritis on the basis of the identified nursing diagnoses and collaborative problems. Expected outcomes may include that the client will:

- Report that pain is controlled
- Be knowledgeable about the disease, its treatment, and interventions to prevent or reduce disease progression

Specific indicators for these outcomes are listed for each nursing diagnosis and collaborative problem under the Planning and Implementation section (see earlier).

? Critical Thinking Challenge

The client described earlier (p. 1714) is diagnosed with acute pyelonephritis. She is initially prescribed IV ciprofloxacin (Cipro) for pyelonephritis but was changed to gentamicin after a urine culture indicated that the infecting organism is *Lactobacillus*, an organism that is considered normal flora of the vagina and seldom the cause of major infections. After the client's manifestations have resolved, she undergoes cystography because of the frequency of cystitis episodes. The perineal examination and the cystography show that her urethral meatus is located abnormally close to her vagina and that she also has a mild degree of vesicoureteral reflux. She has no scarring of the kidney at this time and surgery is not planned.

1. Explain whether this client's acute pyelonephritis is an ascending or a descending infection.
2. How do the findings of the physical examination and the cystography relate as a cause of her acute pyelonephritis?
3. In addition to adherence to any chronic antiseptic or antibiotic therapy, what could you suggest as measures for this client to reduce her risk for future episodes of pyelonephritis and cystitis (you may need to review Chapter 73)?

evolve For suggested answer guidelines, go to http://evolve.elsevier.com/Iggy/.

Renal Abscess
PATHOPHYSIOLOGY

An **abscess** is a collection of fluid and cells caused by an inflammatory response to bacteria. It may occur within the kidney tissue (renal abscess), in Gerota's fascia (perinephric abscess), or in the flank. An abscess is suspected when manifestations are not relieved promptly by antibiotic therapy.

◆ COLLABORATIVE MANAGEMENT

A renal or perirenal abscess is diagnosed via sonography or a computed tomography (CT) scan. Arteriography and radionuclide scintillation methods (e.g., gallium scan) also may be useful for diagnosis. Manifestations include fever, flank pain, and general malaise. Local flank edema and redness may be observed.

Drainage by surgical incision or needle aspiration is often necessary. Broad-spectrum antibiotics are also prescribed.

Renal Tuberculosis
PATHOPHYSIOLOGY

The urinary tract is the most common site of tuberculosis (TB) outside of the lungs. About 10% of new cases of TB occur outside the lungs (Tolkoff-Rubin, Cotran, & Rubin, 2000). TB of the kidney is sometimes called *granulomatous nephritis*. After TB invades the kidneys by the bloodborne route, an inflammatory response is triggered and forms scar tissue (**granuloma**) that replaces normal kidney tissue.

◆ COLLABORATIVE MANAGEMENT

Clients may have urinary frequency, dysuria, hematuria and/or proteinuria, flank pain or renal colic with the pas-

TABLE 74-1   Primary Glomerular Diseases and Syndromes

- Acute glomerulonephritis
- Rapidly progressive glomerulonephritis (RPGN)
- Chronic glomerulonephritis
- Nephrotic syndrome
- Persisting urinary abnormalities with few or no symptoms

TABLE 74-2   Secondary Glomerular Diseases and Syndromes

- Systemic lupus erythematosus (SLE)
- Schönlein-Henoch purpura
- Goodpasture's syndrome
- Systemic necrotizing vasculitis
- Wegener's granulomatosis
- Periarteritis nodosa (also called polyarteritis nodosa)
- Amyloidosis
- Diabetic glomerulopathy
- HIV-associated nephropathy
- Alport's syndrome
- Multiple myeloma
- Viral hepatitis B
- Viral hepatitis C
- Cirrhosis
- Sickle-cell disease
- Nonstreptococcal postinfectious acute glomerulonephritis
- Infective endocarditis
- Hemolytic-uremic syndrome
- Thrombotic thrombocytopenic purpura

sage of clots or stones, pyuria, and hypertension. Skin test (e.g., purified protein derivative [PPD]) or chest x-ray evidence of tuberculosis (TB) may or may not be present.

Clients with current or previous pulmonary TB who show signs of unexplained fever, hematuria, and sterile pyuria are at high risk for renal TB. The diagnosis is made through a urine culture of three clean-catch, first-morning specimens. Other genitourinary sites for tuberculosis include the prostate, epididymis, ureters, testes, bladder, and seminal vesicles.

Antitubercular therapy with a 2-month course of rifampin, isoniazid, and pyrazinamide followed by 4 months of rifampin and isoniazid is the main therapy. Three to six more months of rifampin and isoniazid are recommended for men who have the organism in the prostate (Tolkoff-Rubin, Cotran, & Rubin, 2000).

Complications include renal failure, kidney stones, obstruction, and bacterial superinfection of the urinary tract. Surgical excision of diseased tissue may be needed to preserve renal function.

IMMUNOLOGIC RENAL DISORDERS

Glomerulonephritis (GN) is the third leading cause of end-stage renal disease (ESRD) (NIDDK, 2004). Both primary and secondary diseases or syndromes result in glomerular injury. Glomeruli are usually involved in primary disease (Table 74-1); the nonrenal effects of primary disease stem from the glomerular injury. Most primary diseases and syndromes have an immunologic component, and many have an underlying genetic basis. Secondary glomerular diseases are those situations in which glomerular involvement is part of another disease. For example, systemic diseases and infections can have renal effects and cause glomerular injury (Table 74-2). Conditions that cause secondary glomerular disease include systemic lupus erythematous and diabetic nephropathy.

Each primary or secondary disease or syndrome has a specific pathophysiology and clinical manifestations. Their *glomerular* effects are caused by injury to the glomeruli and result in proteinuria, hematuria, decreased glomerular filtration rate (GFR), edema, and hypertension. The extent and duration of renal injury, prognosis, and specific cause vary among these syndromes.

Immunologic changes injure the glomeruli, interstitium, or tubules, and the effects may be acute or chronic. Both antibody and cellular immune responses are involved. The resultant renal disorder can be systemic or localized to the kidneys. Most forms of glomerulonephritis (GN) occur with a collection of immune complexes in the glomeruli (Figure 74-4). An immune complex is made up of antigens and antibodies. The antigen can be any normal kidney tissue, or it can be dissolved in a body fluid (e.g., blood). Bacteria and viruses are also antigens. Exposure to bacteria, viruses, drugs, or other toxins is believed to be the trigger for glomerular injury.

Antibody reaction with antigens can lead to immune complex formation and deposition in glomerular tissue. The

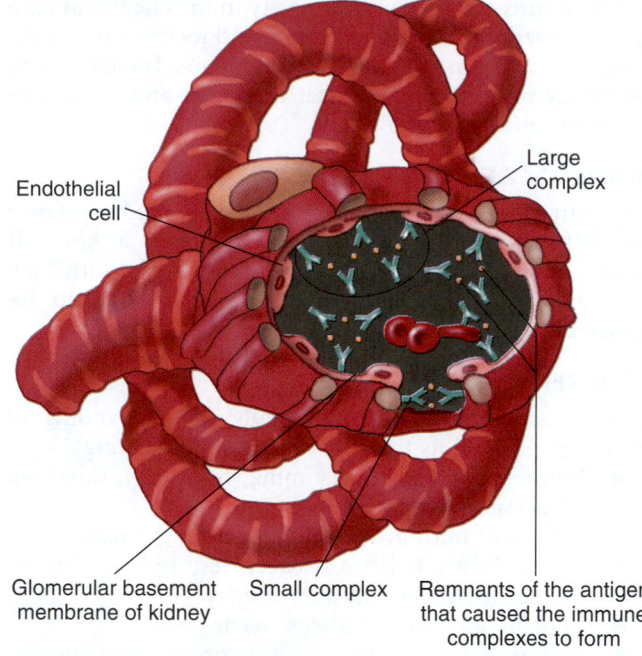

Figure 74-4 ■ An immune complex precipitating in the glomerulus of a client with glomerulonephritis.

immune complexes trigger many inflammatory mediators, such as complement, white blood cells, and blood clotting proteins, which also damage the renal tissue. Actions that cause tissue injury include damage to cell membranes, local edema, movement of white blood cells to the site of inflammation, and platelet activation.

Acute Glomerulonephritis

PATHOPHYSIOLOGY

An infection often occurs before the renal manifestations of acute glomerulonephritis (GN). The onset of symptoms is about 10 days from the time of infection. Usually, clients recover quickly and completely from acute GN. The term *acute nephritic syndrome* also describes this disorder.

Most causes of acute GN are infectious (Table 74-3) or are related to other systemic diseases (see Table 74-2). The

TABLE 74-3 Infectious Causes of Acute Glomerulonephritis

- Group A beta-hemolytic *Streptococcus*
- Staphylococcal or gram-negative bacteremia or sepsis
- Pneumococcal, *Mycoplasma*, or *Klebsiella* pneumonia
- Syphilis
- Visceral abscesses
- Infective endocarditis
- Hepatitis B
- Infectious mononucleosis
- Measles
- Mumps
- Rocky Mountain spotted fever
- Cytomegaloviral infection
- Histoplasmosis
- Toxoplasmosis
- Varicella
- *Chlamydia psittaci* infection
- Coxsackievirus infection
- Any bacterial, parasitic, fungal, or viral infection (potentially)

incidence of acute GN is unknown. GN after a systemic streptococcal infection is more common in men.

◆COLLABORATIVE MANAGEMENT
◆Assessment

HISTORY

Ask about recent infections, particularly of the skin or upper respiratory tract, and about recent travel or other activities with possible exposure to viruses, bacteria, fungi, or parasites. Recent illnesses, surgery, or other invasive procedures may suggest infections. Ask about any known systemic diseases, such as systemic lupus erythematosus (SLE), which could cause acute GN.

PHYSICAL ASSESSMENT/CLINICAL MANIFESTATIONS

Inspect the client's skin for lesions or recent incisions and the face, eyelids, hands, and other areas for edema (present in about 75% of the clients with acute GN). Assess for fluid overload and circulatory congestion (which may accompany the sodium and fluid retention occurring with acute GN). Ask about any difficulty in breathing, nocturnal or exertional dyspnea, or orthopnea. Assess for crackles in the lung fields, an S_3 heart sound (gallop rhythm), and neck vein distention.

Ask about changes in urination pattern and any change in urine color. Microscopic hematuria occurs up to 66% of the time, and clients often describe their urine as smoky, reddish-brown, rusty, or cola colored. Ask about dysuria or oliguria. Weigh the client to assess for fluid retention.

Take the client's blood pressure and compare it with the baseline blood pressure. Mild to moderate hypertension often occurs with acute GN due to sodium and fluid retention. The client may have fatigue, a lack of energy, anorexia, nausea, and/or vomiting if uremia from renal failure is present.

CONSIDERATIONS FOR OLDER ADULTS

The less common manifestations of acute GN are more likely to occur in older adults. Circulatory congestion often dominates the client's clinical picture. Acute GN is easily confused with congestive heart failure.

LABORATORY ASSESSMENT

Urinalysis shows red blood cells (**hematuria**) and protein (proteinuria). An early morning specimen of urine is preferred for urinalysis because the urine is most acidic and formed elements are more intact at that time. Microscopic examination often shows red blood cell casts as well as casts from other substances. The urine sediment assay is usually positive.

The glomerular filtration rate (GFR), measured by the 24-hour urine test for creatinine clearance, may be decreased to 50 mL/min. Blood urea nitrogen (BUN) levels are usually increased. The older client may have a greater decline in GFR.

A 24-hour urine collection for total protein assay is also obtained. The protein excretion rate for clients with acute GN may be increased from 500 mg to 3 g/24 hr in most clients. Serum albumin levels are decreased because of the protein lost in the urine and because of fluid retention causing dilution.

Specimens from the blood, skin, or throat are obtained for culture, if indicated. Other serologic tests include antistreptolysin-O titers, C3 complement levels, cryoglobulins (immunoglobulin G [IgG]), antinuclear antibodies (ANAs), and circulating immune complexes.

Antistreptolysin-O titers are increased after group A beta-hemolytic *Streptococcus* infections. Complement levels are decreased when the complement system is activated. Type III cryoglobulins may be found during acute illness. ANAs suggest an autoimmune response, and SLE is just one possibility. Circulating immune complexes containing IgG and C3 are often detected.

OTHER DIAGNOSTIC ASSESSMENTS

A renal biopsy provides a precise diagnosis of the pathologic condition, assists in determining the prognosis, and helps outline treatment (see Chapter 72). The specific tissue morphology is determined by light microscopy, immunofluorescent stains, and electron microscopy to identify cell type, the presence of immunoglobulins, or the type of tissue deposits.

◆Interventions

Interventions focus on treating the underlying infectious process, preventing complications, and providing appropriate client education.

Management of Infection. Treatment for acute GN with an infectious cause is an appropriate antibiotic. Penicillin, erythromycin, or azithromycin are prescribed for GN resulting from streptococcal infection. Check the client's known allergies before giving any drug. To prevent infection spread, antibiotics for persons in immediate close contact with the client may be prescribed. Stress personal hygiene and basic infection control principles (e.g., handwashing) to prevent spread of the organism.

Prevention of Complications. For clients with fluid overload, hypertension, and edema, diuretics and a sodium and water restriction are prescribed. Antihypertensive drugs may be needed to control hypertension (see Chart 39-3). The usual fluid allowance is equal to the 24-hour urine output plus 500 to 600 mL. Clients with oliguria usually have increased serum levels of potassium and blood urea nitrogen (BUN). Potassium and protein intake may be restricted to prevent hyperkalemia and uremia as a result of the elevated BUN.

Nausea, vomiting, or anorexia indicates that uremia is present. Dialysis is necessary if uremic symptoms or fluid volume excess cannot be controlled (see Chapter 75). **Plasmapheresis** (removal and filtering of the plasma to eliminate antibodies) also may be attempted (see Chapter 43).

To conserve the client's energy, assist him or her in maintaining a restful environment, balancing activity and rest, and coordinating needed therapeutic activities. Encourage the client to practice relaxation techniques and to participate in diversional activities to reduce emotional stress.

Client Education. Instruct the client and family members about the purpose and desired effects of prescribed drugs, the dosage and schedule, and potential adverse side effects. Ensure that the client and family understand dietary or fluid modifications, including methods of detecting fluid retention. Advise the client to weigh himself or herself and measure blood pressure daily at the same time each day. Instruct the client to notify the health care provider of any sudden increase in weight or blood pressure.

If short-term dialysis is required to control fluid volume excess or uremic symptoms, explain peritoneal or vascular access care and dialysis schedules and routines (also see Chapter 75).

Rapidly Progressive Glomerulonephritis

Rapidly progressive glomerulonephritis (RPGN), a type of acute nephritis, is also called *crescentic glomerulonephritis* because of the presence of crescent-shaped cells in the Bowman's capsule. RPGN develops over several weeks or months and causes a significant loss of renal function. Clients become quite ill quickly and have manifestations of renal failure (fluid volume excess, hypertension, oliguria, electrolyte imbalances, and uremic symptoms).

The client may have has previous infection or systemic disease, such as systemic lupus erythematosus (SLE). The renal deterioration often progresses to end-stage renal disease (ESRD).

Chronic Glomerulonephritis

PATHOPHYSIOLOGY

Chronic glomerulonephritis, or *chronic nephritic syndrome*, develops over 20 to 30 years or even longer. The exact onset of the disorder is rarely identified. In many instances the cause of the disease is not known because the kidneys are atrophied and tissue is not available for biopsy or diagnosis. Mild proteinuria and hematuria, hypertension, and occasional edema are often the only manifestations. Although the exact cause is not known, changes in the renal tissue result from hypertension, infections and inflammation, or altered metabolism and poor blood flow to the kidneys. Kidney tissue atrophies, and the number of functional nephrons is greatly reduced. Biopsy in the late stages of atrophy may show glomerular changes, cell loss, protein and collagen deposits, and fibrosis of the kidney tissue. Microscopic examination shows deposits of immune complexes.

The loss of nephrons reduces glomerular filtration. Hypertension and renal arteriole sclerosis are often present. The glomerular damage allows proteins to enter the urine. Eventually, chronic glomerulonephritis always leads to renal failure (see Chapter 75).

◆ COLLABORATIVE MANAGEMENT
◆ Assessment

HISTORY

Ask the client about other health problems, including systemic diseases, renal or urologic disorders, infectious diseases (e.g., streptococcal infections), and recent exposures to infections. Ask about his or her overall health status and whether increasing fatigue and lethargy have been experienced.

Identify the client's pattern of voiding. Ask whether the frequency of voiding has increased or the quantity of urine has decreased. Ask about changes in urine color, odor, or clarity and whether dysuria or incontinence have occurred.

Assess the client's general comfort and ask whether any dyspnea at rest or with exertion has occurred because fluid overload can occur with decreased urine output. Ask about and observe for changes in mental functioning, such as irritability or an inability to read or to perform job-related functions or other processes requiring concentration. Changes in memory and the ability to concentrate occur as waste products collect in the blood.

PHYSICAL ASSESSMENT/CLINICAL MANIFESTATIONS

Assess for systemic circulatory overload. Auscultate lung fields for crackles, observe the respiratory rate and depth, and measure blood pressure and weight. Auscultate the heart for rate, rhythm, and the presence of an S_3 heart sound. Inspect the neck veins for venous engorgement and check for edema in the pedal, pretibial, and presacral tissues.

Assess for uremic symptoms, such as slurred speech, ataxia, tremors, or **asterixis** (flapping tremor of the fingers or the inability to maintain a fixed posture with the arms extended and wrists hyperextended). Inspect skin for a yellowish color, texture, bruises, rashes, or eruptions. Document areas of dryness and any excoriation from scratching.

DIAGNOSTIC ASSESSMENT

Urine output decreases but the urine appears normal unless a urinary tract infection (UTI) also is present. Urinalysis shows proteinuria, usually less than 2 g in a 24-hour collection. The specific gravity is fixed at a constant level of dilution (around 1.010). There may be red blood cells and casts in the urine.

The glomerular filtration rate (GFR), measured by creatinine clearance, is low. The serum creatinine level is elevated, usually greater than 6 mg/dL but may be as high as 30 mg/dL or more. Blood urea nitrogen (BUN) is increased, often as high as 100 to 200 mg/dL.

Decreased renal function causes abnormal serum electrolyte levels. Sodium retention is common, but dilution of the plasma from excess fluid can result in a falsely normal serum sodium level (135 to 145 mEq/L) or a dilutional hyponatremia (<135 mEq/L). When oliguria develops, potassium retention occurs causing hyperkalemia when levels exceed 5.4 mEq/L.

Hyperphosphatemia develops with serum levels greater than 4.7 mg/dL. Serum calcium levels are usually at the lower end of the normal range or are slightly below normal.

Acidosis develops from hydrogen ion retention and loss of bicarbonate. However, there may be a decrease in serum carbon dioxide (CO_2) levels as clients breathe more rapidly to compensate for the acidosis. If respiratory compensation is present, the pH of arterial blood is between 7.35 and 7.45. A pH of less than 7.35 means that the client's respiratory system is not completely compensating for the acidosis (see Chapter 19).

The kidneys are abnormally small on x-ray, IV urography, and when measured by sonography or computed tomography (CT).

A renal biopsy is important in the early stages of glomerulonephritis, when proteinuria or hematuria is first present. Tissue changes include a variety of cells infiltrating the glomerular tissue, deposition of immune complexes, and blood vessel sclerosis. In advanced disease, when the kidneys are small, renal biopsy is not usually performed.

◆Interventions

Interventions focus on slowing the progression of the disease and preventing complications. Treatment consists of diet changes, fluid intake sufficient to prevent reduced blood flow volume to the kidneys, and drug therapy to control the problems from uremia. Eventually, the client requires dialysis or transplantation to prevent death from the systemic effects of uremia. (Nursing care for the client with ESRD requiring dialysis or transplantation is discussed in Chapter 75.)

Nephrotic Syndrome
PATHOPHYSIOLOGY

Nephrotic syndrome (NS) is a condition of increased glomerular permeability that allows larger molecules to pass through the membrane into the urine and be removed from the blood. This process causes massive loss of protein into the urine, edema formation, and decreased plasma albumin levels. Many agents and disorders are possible causes of NS.

The most common cause of glomerular membrane changes is an immune or inflammatory processes. Defects in glomerular filtration can also occur as a result of genetic flaws resulting in defective proteins in the glomerular filtering system (Jalanko et al., 2001; Online Mendelian Inheritance in Man, 2004). Altered liver activity may occur with nephrotic syndrome, resulting in increased lipid production and hyperlipidemia.

◆COLLABORATIVE MANAGEMENT

The main feature of nephrotic syndrome (NS) is severe proteinuria (>3.5 g of protein in 24 hours). Clients also have hypoalbuminemia (serum albumin <3 g/dL), hyperlipidemia, lipiduria, edema, and hypertension (Chart 74-6). Renal vein thrombosis often occurs at the same time as NS, either as a cause of the problem or as an effect. NS may

---

CHART 74-6

KEY FEATURES of
Nephrotic Syndrome

- Massive proteinuria
- Hypoalbuminemia
- Edema
- Lipiduria
- Hyperlipidemia
- Increased coagulation
- Renal insufficiency

---

progress to ESRD, but progression can be prevented with treatment.

Treatment varies depending on what process is causing the disorder (identified by renal biopsy). Immunologic processes may improve with suppressive therapy using steroids and cytotoxic or immunosuppressive agents. Angiotensin-converting enzyme (ACE) inhibitors can decrease proteinuria, and cholesterol-lowering drugs can improve hyperlipidemia. Heparin may lower proteinuria and reduce renal insufficiency. Diet changes are often prescribed. If the glomerular filtration rate (GFR) is normal, dietary intake of complete proteins is needed. If the GFR is decreased, dietary protein intake must be decreased. Mild diuretics (Chart 74-7) and sodium restriction may be needed to control edema and hypertension. Assess the client's hydration status, as vascular dehydration is common. If the plasma volume is depleted, renal problems worsen. Acute renal failure may be avoided if good renal blood flow is maintained.

Immunologic Interstitial and Tubulointerstitial Disorders

Interstitial and tubulointerstitial disorders in the kidney are usually caused by immune alterations. These renal changes may be acute or chronic. The acute effects often occur with drugs such as penicillins, cephalosporins, sulfonamides, or nonsteroidal anti-inflammatory drugs (NSAIDs). Chronic interstitial nephritis has many causes, including analgesic use, complement activation, cyclosporin use, polycystic kidney disease, autoimmune disorders, multiple myeloma, sickle cell disease, obstructive disorders, and radiation nephritis. Drug-induced problems often occur with a rash or an elevated eosinophil count. Fever is common in interstitial nephritis of unknown cause. Progression to ESRD occurs unless the causative problem is identified and removed.

DEGENERATIVE DISORDERS

Degenerative disorders that change renal function often occur with a multisystem disorder. Many of these degenerative disorders result from changes in kidney blood vessels.

Nephrosclerosis
PATHOPHYSIOLOGY

Nephrosclerosis is a problem of thickening in the nephron blood vessels, resulting in narrowing of the vessel lumen. This change decreases renal blood flow and kidney tissue is chronically hypoxic. Ischemia and fibrosis develop over time.

Nephrosclerosis occurs with all types of hypertension, atherosclerosis, and diabetes mellitus. The more severe the hypertension, the greater the risk for severe kidney damage. Nephrosclerosis is rarely seen when blood pressure is consistently below 160/110 mm Hg. The changes caused by hypertension may be reversible or may progress to end-stage renal disease (ESRD) within months or years.

Hypertension is the second leading cause of ESRD. About 30% of clients requiring renal replacement therapy (e.g., dialysis or transplantation) have hypertension as the cause of their renal failure (NIDDK, 2004).

CHART 74-7

DRUG THERAPY for
Diuretics Used to Increase Urine Output

Drug	Usual Dosage	Indication	Nursing Interventions	Rationales
Osmotic Diuretics (act on glomerulus and renal tubular system)				
Mannitol (Osmitrol ✳), urea	50-100 g IV as a 5%-25% solution	Causes rapid diuresis (e.g., after contrast media infusion)	Measure fluid intake and output. Check vial for crystals. If crystals are present, warm vial between the hands. Administer through a filter.	Severe dehydration is possible. Mannitol may crystallize while on the shelf. Crystals dissolve with body warmth. This prevents remaining crystals from entering the body.
Thiazide and Thiazide-Like Diuretics (act on cortical diluting site of ascending limb of loop of Henle)				
Chlorothiazide (Diuril)	250 mg PO, IV once to four times daily	Hypertension	Observe for signs and symptoms of electrolyte imbalance.	Common complications include hypokalemia and hypercalcemia.
Hydrochlorothiazide (HydroDIURIL, Apo-Hydro ✳, Urozide ✳)	25-100 mg PO once or twice daily	Congestive heart failure (CHF) with edema	Monitor heart sounds for S_3, lung sounds for crackles, and other signs of CHF.	Ongoing monitoring detects complications and helps ensure prompt treatment.
Chlorthalidone (Hygroton, Uridon ✳)	25-100 mg PO daily	Edema, hypertension	Do not give with NSAIDs.	A decreased diuretic effect is seen with concomitant use of NSAIDs.
⊕ [1]Metolazone (Zaroxolyn)	5-20 mg PO daily	Edema, hypertension	Do not give with NSAIDs.	A decreased diuretic effect is seen with concomitant use of NSAIDs.
Loop Diuretics (act on ascending limb of loop of Henle)				
Furosemide (Lasix, Furoside ✳)	20-80 mg PO or IV once or twice daily; maximum daily dose 600 mg	Hypertension	Observe for orthostatic hypotension.	An early sign of rapid fluid volume depletion may be orthostatic hypotension.
Bumetanide ⊕ [2](Bumex)	0.5-2 mg PO daily	CHF	Monitor for possible hyponatremia and hypokalemia.	These agents increase excretion of both sodium and potassium.
Potassium-Sparing Diuretics (act on distal convoluted tubule)				
Spironolactone ⊕ [3](Aldactone, Novospiroton ✳)	25-200 mg PO once or twice daily	Primary aldosteronism	Observe for signs and symptoms of electrolyte imbalance.	Hyperkalemia with cardiac manifestations is a common complication.
Triamterene (Dyrenium)	25-100 mg once or twice daily; maximum daily dose 300 mg	Hypertension (with other drugs to decrease potassium loss)	Teach client to avoid unprotected sun exposure.	Photosensitivity reactions are possible.
Amiloride ⊕ [4](Midamor ✳)	5-10 mg daily	Edema, hypertension	Give with food or milk.	Stomach upset is possible.

⊕ [1]**Med Error Alert!** Do not confuse with metoprolol, a beta blocker.
⊕ [2]**Med Error Alert!** Do not confuse with Buprenex, an opioid analgesic.
⊕ [3]**Med Error Alert!** Do not confuse with Aldomet, an antihypertensive.
⊕ [4]**Med Error Alert!** Do not confuse with Midodrine, a drug used to treat orthostatic hypotension.

NSAID, Nonsteroidal anti-inflammatory drug.

◆ COLLABORATIVE MANAGEMENT

Treatment aims to control high blood pressure and preserve renal function. Although many antihypertensive drugs may lower blood pressure, the client's response is important in ensuring long-term adherence to the prescribed therapy. Factors promoting adherence include once-a-day dosing, low cost, and minimal side effects.

Lack of knowledge or misinformation about hypertension poses many challenges to health care providers working with clients who have hypertension. When renal disease occurs, adherence to therapy is even more important for preserving health.

Many drugs can control high blood pressure (see Chart 39-3), and more than one agent may be necessary. Angiotensin-converting enzyme (ACE) inhibitors are particularly useful in reducing hypertension and preserving renal function. Diuretics can maintain fluid and electrolyte balance in the presence of renal insufficiency. Hyperkalemia needs to be prevented when potassium-sparing diuretics, alone or in combination, are used to treat hypertensive clients with known renal disease.

Renovascular Disease
PATHOPHYSIOLOGY

Processes affecting the renal arteries may severely narrow the lumen and profoundly reduce blood flow to the kidney tissues. Uncorrected renovascular disease, such as renal artery stenosis, atherosclerosis, or thrombosis, causes ischemia and atrophy of renal tissue.

Clients with renovascular disease often have a sudden onset of hypertension, particularly in clients older than 50 years of age. Clients with high blood pressure but with no family history of hypertension also may potentially have renal artery stenosis (RAS). RAS from atherosclerosis or blood vessel hyperplasia is the main cause of renovascular disease. Other causes include thrombosis and renal aneurysms.

Atherosclerotic changes in the renal artery often occur with sclerosis in the aorta and other major vessels. Changes in the renal artery are often located where the renal artery and aorta meet. Fibrotic changes of the blood vessel wall occur throughout the length of the renal artery.

◆ COLLABORATIVE MANAGEMENT
◆ Assessment

Key features of renovascular disease are listed in Chart 74-8. Hypertension usually first occurs after 40 to 50 years of age,

---

CHART 74-8

KEY FEATURES of
Renovascular Disease

- Significant, difficult-to-control blood pressure
- Elevated serum creatinine
- Decreased creatinine clearance

---

and often the client does not have a family history of hypertension. Diagnosis is made by magnetic resonance angiography (MRA), renal duplex ultrasonography, radionuclide imaging, renal arteriography, and renal vein renin levels. MRA provides an excellent image of the renal vasculature and kidney anatomy. Radionuclide imaging is a non-invasive way of evaluating renal blood flow and excretory function. Combining radionuclide imaging with ingestion of an angiotensin-converting enzyme (ACE) inhibitor such as captopril improves the accuracy of the test. A renal arteriogram makes the features of the renal blood vessels visible. The comparison of renal vein renin levels *may* reveal which kidney is producing more renin.

◆ Interventions

Viewing the type of defect, extent of narrowing, and condition of the surrounding blood vessels is critical for treatment choice. The client's overall health and the size of the atrophied kidney also influence treatment decisions. Many clients with renovascular disease also have cardiovascular disease and both conditions require evaluation and treatment.

RAS may be treated by drugs to control high blood pressure and by procedures to restore the renal blood supply. Drugs may control high blood pressure but may not lead to long-term preservation of kidney function. In young and middle-aged adults, a lifetime of treatment with many drugs for high blood pressure may make treatment difficult and the outcomes uncertain.

Balloon angioplasty with or without stent placement to open renal vessels is less risky and requires less time for recovery than does renal artery bypass surgery (see Chapter 39). Renal artery bypass surgery is a major procedure and requires 2 or more months for recovery. A bypass may be performed for either one or both renal arteries.

Renal angioplasty with metal stent placement is one safe and effective method to permanently repair RAS. Following angioplasty, the client usually remains in ICU for 24 hours to monitor for sudden blood pressure fluctuations as the kidneys adjust to increased blood flow.

A synthetic blood vessel graft is inserted to redirect blood flow from the abdominal aorta into the renal artery, beyond the area of narrowing. A splenorenal bypass can also restore renal blood flow. The process is similar to other arterial bypass procedures (see Chapter 38).

Diabetic Nephropathy
PATHOPHYSIOLOGY

Diabetes mellitus is the leading cause of end-stage renal disease (ESRD) among white individuals in the United States. About 36% of clients requiring dialysis or renal transplantation have diabetes mellitus (NIDDK, 2004). The cost of preventing or reducing renal problems among clients with

RESOURCE MANAGEMENT

DIABETES AND RENAL DISEASE

Cost of Care
- A common complication of both type 1 and type 2 diabetes mellitus (DM) is nephropathy leading to end-stage renal disease.
- Diabetic clients are 5 times more likely to develop end-stage renal disease than others in their cohort.
- Abnormal renal function increased diabetes treatment costs by $1350 and advanced renal disease by $4000 per individual treated.
- Intensive therapy increases costs to maintain blood glucose values between 90 and 140 mg/dL in both type 1 and type 2 diabetes. This type of therapy significantly reduces complications and prolongs renal function.

Implications for Nursing
Although the cost of maintaining tight control is two to three times the costs of conventional therapy, economic modeling predicts that tight control could reduce end-stage renal disease from 24% to 7%. Thus the costs of maintaining tight control are offset by savings related to reduced need for diagnosis and treatment of DM-related renal disease.

Renal disease is an expensive diagnosis, not only in dollar costs, but also in social, psychological, and functional costs as clients undergo extensive diagnostic workup and work-limiting treatment. Preventing the renal complications of DM saves money; it also saves individuals from a heavy biopsychosocial burden.

Data from Nathan, D.M. (1993). Diabetes Control and Complications Trial Research Group: The effect of long-term intensified insulin treatment on development of microvascular complications of diabetes. *New England Journal of Medicine, 329*(14), 977-986; Palmer, A.J. (2001). Intensive glucose control is more costly than conventional treatment but also has more benefits for people with type-2 diabetes. *Evidence-Based Health Care, 5*(1), 17-18; and U.S. Renal Data Systems. (2002). *USRDS 2002 annual data report.* Bethesda, MD: The National Institutes of Health, National Institute of Diabetes and Digestive and Kidney Diseases.

TABLE 74-4 The Stages of Progression of Type 1 Diabetic Renal Disease

- **Stage I, at the time diabetes is diagnosed.** Kidney size and glomerular filtration rate are increased. Blood sugar control can reverse the changes.
- **Stage II, 2 to 3 years after diagnosis.** Glomerular and tubular capillary basement membrane changes result in microscopic changes, with loss of filtration surface area and scar formation. Glomerular changes are referred to as glomerulosclerosis.
- **Stage III, 7 to 15 years after diagnosis.** Microalbuminuria is present. The glomerular filtration rate (GFR) may still be normal or may be increased.
- **Stage IV.** Albuminuria is detectable by dipstick. GFR is decreased. Blood pressure is increased, and retinopathy is present.
- **Stage V.** GFR decreases at an average rate of 10 mL/min/yr.

---

diabetes is offset by the high cost of treating severe renal disease (see the Resource Management box above). Diabetic nephropathy occurs with either type 1 or type 2 diabetes mellitus. Severity of diabetic renal disease is related to the extent, duration, and effects of atherosclerosis, hypertension, and neuropathy, which promotes bladder atony, urinary stasis, and urinary tract infection.

◆COLLABORATIVE MANAGEMENT

Diabetic nephropathy is a *microvascular* complication of diabetes. Its first manifestation is persistent albuminuria (as shown by dipstick or a urinary albumin excretion rate above 0.3 g/dL), without evidence of other renal disease. Diabetic renal disease is progressive (Table 74-4).

Structural and functional changes occur in the kidneys of diabetic clients. Initially, kidney size is slightly increased and glomerular filtration rates (GFR) are higher than normal. Microlevels of albumin are first detected in the urine. Progressive renal damage occurs before dipstick procedures can detect protein in the urine. For most clients, proteinuria (albuminuria) indicates the need for a renal biopsy for further diagnosis. For the client with diabetes, observed microvascular changes in the retina correlate well with the renal microvascular changes. Examination of the retina showing capillary leakage, fibrosis, and the typical changes of diabetic retinopathy eliminates the need for a risky renal biopsy.

Proteinuria may be mild, moderate, or severe. Diabetic clients are always considered to be at risk for renal failure. If possible, nephrotoxic agents (e.g., radiopaque contrast media or aminoglycosides) and dehydration are avoided. Clients with worsening renal function may begin to have frequent hypoglycemic episodes and a reduced need for insulin or oral antidiabetic agents. Explain to the client that the kidneys metabolize and excrete insulin. When renal function is reduced, the insulin is available for a longer time and thus less of it is needed. Unfortunately, many clients believe this means their diabetes is improving. The result is a more rapid progression to ESRD. (See Chapter 68 for specific information on diabetic nephropathy.)

TUMORS

Cysts and Benign Tumors

PATHOPHYSIOLOGY

Benign urinary tract growths include cysts and tumors of the kidney tissue or urinary bladder. Because cancer can occur within cystic structures, a thorough evaluation is needed.

A simple renal cyst grows out of renal cortical tissue, rather than tubular tissues. The cyst fills with fluid and causes local tissue damage as it enlarges. Many cysts cause no symptoms and are discovered by accident during other procedures or on autopsy.

Cysts are a structural birth defect that occurs in fetal life. The incidence of renal cysts and benign tumors is unknown.

◆COLLABORATIVE MANAGEMENT

Diagnosis of a simple renal cyst is usually made by ultrasound. If hematuria or other suspicious manifestations are present, computed tomography (CT) may be needed to rule out other problems. CT can determine whether the cyst is filled with serous fluid, urine, or blood.

Once determined to be a simple cyst, the cyst may be drained by percutaneous aspiration if it becomes painful. Surgical exploration with the potential for total or subtotal nephrectomy is rarely needed.

Renal Cell Carcinoma

PATHOPHYSIOLOGY

Renal cell carcinoma is also known as *adenocarcinoma of the kidney.* As with other cancers, the healthy tissue of the kidney is damaged and replaced by cancer cells.

TABLE 74-5   Staging Renal Tumors

- **Stage I.** Tumors up to 2.5 cm are situated within the capsule of the kidney; the renal vein, perinephric fat, and adjacent lymph nodes have no tumor.
- **Stage II.** Tumors are larger than 2.5 cm and extend beyond the capsule but are within Gerota's fascia; the renal vein and lymph nodes are not involved.
- **Stage III.** Tumors extend into the renal vein, lymph nodes, or both.
- **Stage IV.** Tumors include invasion of adjacent organs beyond Gerota's fascia or metastasize to distant tissues.

Data from American Cancer Society. (2005). *Cancer facts and figures 2005.* Report No. 00-300M–No. 5008.05. Atlanta: Author.

Systemic effects occurring with this cancer type are called **paraneoplastic syndromes** and include anemia, erythrocytosis, hypercalcemia, liver dysfunction with elevated liver enzymes, hormonal effects, increased sedimentation rate, and hypertension.

Anemia and erythrocytosis may appear contradictory; however, most clients with this cancer have either anemia or erythrocytosis, not both at the same time. There is some blood loss from hematuria, but the small amount lost does not cause anemia. The cause of the anemia and the erythrocytosis is related to kidney cell production of erythropoietin. At times, the tumor cells produce large amounts of erythropoietin, causing erythrocytosis. Other times, the tumor cells destroy the erythropoietin-producing kidney cells and anemia results. Hypertension may result from increased blood levels of renin.

Parathyroid hormone produced by tumor cells can cause hypercalcemia. Other hormone changes include increased renin levels (causing hypertension) and increased human chorionic gonadotropin (hCG) levels, which decreases libido and changes secondary sex features. The cause of the increased sedimentation rate and changes in liver function studies is not known.

Renal cell carcinoma has four distinct histologic patterns. Genetic differences cause a predisposition to develop tumors of each of these histologic types. The most well known genetic familial syndrome that includes renal cancer is von Hippel-Lindau syndrome. These cancers are highly vascular and may occur with cancers of the pancreas, central nervous system, and adrenal glands.

Renal tumors are classified into four stages (Table 74-5). Complications include metastasis and urinary tract obstruction. Metastasis usually occurs to the adrenal gland, liver, lungs, long bones, or the other kidney. When the cancer surrounds a ureter, hydroureter and obstruction may result.

The exact cause of renal cell carcinoma is unknown, but the risk is slightly higher for people who use tobacco or are exposed to lead, phosphate, and cadmium.

Renal cancers account for about 28,800 new cases and 11,300 deaths annually in the United States. The 5-year survival rate is 60% in the United States. Renal cell carcinoma occurs most often in clients between 55 and 60 years of age (Kidney Cancer Association, 2005).

◆COLLABORATIVE MANAGEMENT
◆Assessment
HISTORY

Ask the client about age, known risk factors (e.g., smoking or chemical exposures), weight loss, changes in urine color, abdominal or flank discomfort, and fever. Also ask whether any other family member has ever been diagnosed with cancer of the kidney, bladder, ureter, prostate gland, uterus, or ovary.

PHYSICAL ASSESSMENT/CLINICAL MANIFESTATIONS

Only about 5% to 10% of clients with renal cell cancer have flank pain, gross hematuria, and a palpable renal mass. Ask about the nature of the flank or abdominal discomfort. Clients often describe the pain as dull and aching. The pain may be more intense if bleeding into the tumor or kidney occurs. Inspect the flank area, checking for asymmetry or an obvious bulge. You may be able to feel an abdominal mass through *gentle* palpation. A renal bruit may be heard on auscultation.

Hematuria is a *late* common sign. Blood in the urine may be visible as bright red flecks or clots, or the urine may appear smoky or cola colored. Without gross hematuria, microscopic examination may or may not reveal red cells.

Inspect the skin for pallor, darkening of the nipples and, in men, breast enlargement. Other findings may include muscle wasting, weakness, poor nutritional status, and weight loss. All tend to occur late in the disease.

DIAGNOSTIC ASSESSMENT

Urinalysis may show red blood cells. Hematologic studies reveal decreased hemoglobin and hematocrit values, hypercalcemia, increased erythrocyte sedimentation rate, and increased levels of adrenocorticotropic hormone, human chorionic gonadotropin (hCG), cortisol, renin, and parathyroid hormone.

Renal masses may be detected by surgical exploration, IV urogram with nephrograms, or sonography. The mass and surrounding tissues may be outlines by CT with contrast or by magnetic resonance imaging (MRI).

◆Interventions

Interventions focus on controlling the cancer and preventing metastasis.

NONSURGICAL MANAGEMENT. Radiofrequency ablation has shown some promise in treating renal cancer. Radiofrequency ablation is a minimally invasive procedure carried out during magnetic resonance imaging (MRI). MRI can monitor the results of tumor destruction immediately because MRI is sensitive to temperature changes. Radiofrequency ablation is still undergoing evaluation to determine its effectiveness and is not widely available (Bonn, 2002).

Chemotherapy has limited effectiveness against this cancer type. Use of biological response modifiers (BRMs) such as interleukin-2 (IL-2), interferon (INF), and tumor necrosis factor (TNF) have lengthened survival time (see Chapters 23 and 28).

SURGICAL MANAGEMENT. Renal cell carcinoma is usually treated surgically by **nephrectomy** (kidney removal). Renal cell tumors are highly vascular and blood loss during surgery is a major concern. Before surgery, the arteries supplying the kidney may be occluded (embolized) by radiation to reduce bleeding during nephrectomy.

Preoperative Care. Instruct the client about surgical routines (see Chapters 20, 21, and 22). Explain the probable site of incision and the presence of dressings, drains, or other equipment after surgery. Reassure the client about pain relief. Care before surgery may include giving blood and fluids intravenously to ensure hemodynamic stability.

Operative Procedures. The client is placed on his or her side with the kidney to be removed uppermost. Usually, the client's trunk area is flexed to increase exposure of the kidney area. Removal of the eleventh or twelfth rib is needed to provide better access to the kidney. The surgeon removes the entire kidney and all visible tumor, renal artery and vein, and fascia after tying off the ureter. The adrenal gland is left intact. A drain may be placed in the wound before closure.

When a *radical* nephrectomy is performed, the periaortic lymph nodes are also removed. The surgical approach may be transthoracic (as discussed in the previous paragraph), lumbar, or through the abdomen depending on the size and location of the tumor. Radiation therapy may follow a radical nephrectomy.

Postoperative Care. Refer to Chapter 22 for care of the client after surgery. Assessment of urologic and renal function is essential to determine function in the remaining kidney.

Monitoring. Assess the client for hemorrhage and adrenal insufficiency. Inspect the client's abdomen for distention from bleeding. Check the bed linens under the client, because bleeding may be present. Hemorrhage or adrenal insufficiency cause hypotension, decreased urine output, and an altered level of consciousness.

A decrease in blood pressure is an early sign of both hemorrhage and adrenal insufficiency. With hypotension, urine output also decreases immediately. Large water and sodium losses in the urine occur in clients with adrenal insufficiency. As a result, a large urine output is followed by hypotension and oliguria (<400 mL/24 hr or less than 25 mL/hr). IV replacement of fluids and packed red blood cells may be needed.

The second kidney is expected to provide adequate renal function. Assess urine output hourly for the first 24 hours after surgery (urine output of 30 to 50 mL/hr is acceptable). Output of less than 25 to 30 mL/hr suggests decreased renal blood flow. The hemoglobin level, hematocrit values, and white blood cell count may be measured every 6 to 12 hours for the first day or two after surgery.

Monitor the client's temperature, pulse rate, and respiratory rate at least every 4 hours. Accurately measure and record fluid intake and output. Weigh the client daily.

The client may be in a special care unit for 24 to 48 hours after surgery for monitoring of bleeding and/or adrenal insufficiency. A drain placed near the site of incision removes residual fluid. Because of the discomfort of deep breathing, the client is at risk for atelectasis. Fever, chills, thick sputum, or decreased breath sounds suggest pneumonia.

Pain Management. After surgery, opioid analgesics (e.g., hydromorphone [Dilaudid] and morphine sulfate [Statex✦]) are given parenterally. The incision was made through major muscle groups used with breathing and movement. Liberal use of analgesics is needed for 3 to 5 days to manage the pain after surgery. Oral agents may be tried when the client is permitted to eat and drink.

Prevention of Complications. Antibiotics may be prescribed during and after surgery to prevent infection. These drugs are usually given as single-dose prescriptions. The need for additional antibiotics is based on clinical and laboratory evidence of infection. Steroid replacements may be needed in clients who have adrenal insufficiency.

RENAL TRAUMA

PATHOPHYSIOLOGY

Trauma to one or both kidneys is always a concern in penetrating wounds or blunt injuries to the back, flank, or abdomen. Blunt trauma to the back, flank, or abdomen accounts for 85% of all renal injuries; most blunt renal injuries are not serious (Rakel & Bope, 2003). Injury to the kidney can be minor, major, or pedicle (Figure 74-5). Strategies to prevent trauma are reviewed in Chart 74-9.

Minor injuries include contusions, small lacerations, and tearing of the parenchyma and the calyx (forniceal disruption). With a contusion, one or both kidneys are bruised because of the major impact. Small blood vessels may be damaged, causing some hematuria. Small lacerations may result in small, local hematomas. A small hematoma also may occur at the site of forniceal disruption. Common causes include falls, contact sports, and blows to the back and torso.

Major injuries include lacerations to the cortex, medulla, or branches of the renal artery or vein. Deep tissue injuries may extend throughout the kidney and cause hematomas within or through the capsule. Injuries involving the cortex can cause tissue shattering. The capsule may remain intact or be ruptured.

A major injury most commonly follows penetrating abdominal, flank, or back wounds (such as is seen with gunshot wounds, knife wounds, or motor vehicle accidents). Bleeding is extensive, and surgical exploration is often needed. Because of the hemorrhage, decreased renal blood flow can produce short-term or long-term renin-induced hypertension.

Pedicle injuries are lacerations or breaks in the renal artery or renal vein. Hemorrhage is extensive and rapid, and death may occur unless diagnosis and intervention are prompt.

◆**COLLABORATIVE MANAGEMENT**
◆**Assessment**

Obtain a history of the client's usual health and the events involved in the trauma from the client, a witness, or emergency personnel. Critical information to know is a history of renal or urologic disease, surgical intervention, or health problems such as diabetes mellitus or hypertension.

Ureteral or renal pelvic injury often cause diffuse abdominal pain, local collections of urine, and infection. Ask the client about pain in the flank or abdominal pain. Is the pain dull? Sharp? Constant? Intermittent? Made worse by coughing?

Take the client's blood pressure, apical and peripheral pulses, respiratory rate, and temperature. Inspect both flanks for asymmetry or penetrating injuries of the lower thorax or back. Also inspect the abdomen for bruising or penetrating wounds. Percuss the abdomen for distention. Inspect the urethra for gross bleeding.

Urinalysis usually shows hemoglobin or red blood cells from renal blood vessel rupture. Microscopic examination may also show red blood cell casts, which suggest tubular damage. Hemoglobin and hematocrit values decrease with blood loss. If inflammation or infection is present, the white blood cell count is elevated.

Diagnostic procedures include IV urography and computed tomography (CT). CT scan shows the location of the in-

MINOR TRAUMA

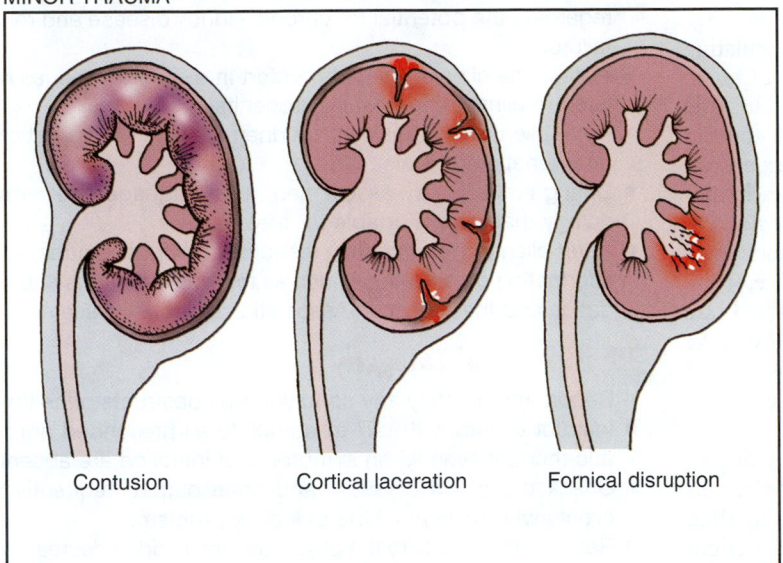

Contusion   Cortical laceration   Fornical disruption

PEDICLE INJURY

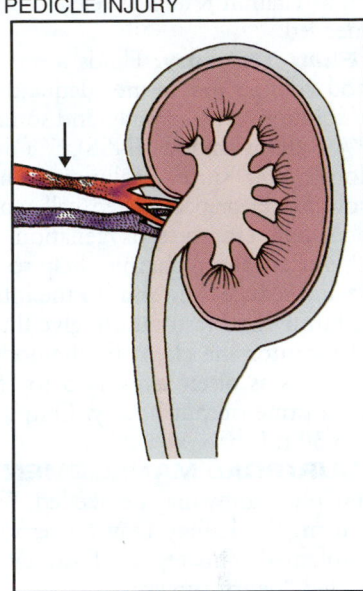

MAJOR TRAUMA

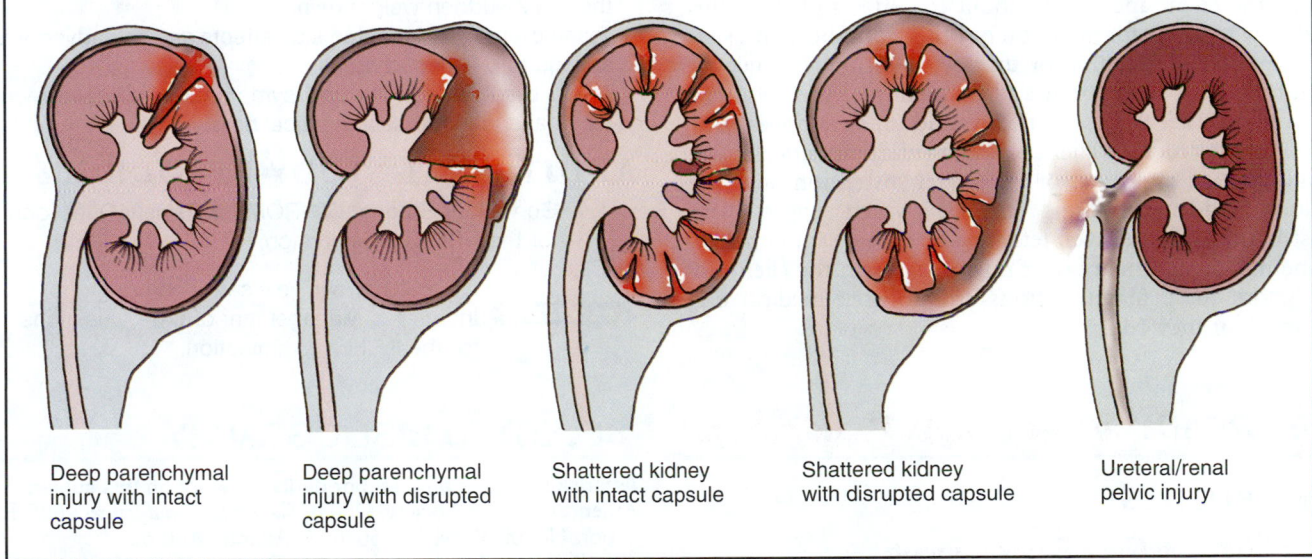

Deep parenchymal injury with intact capsule | Deep parenchymal injury with disrupted capsule | Shattered kidney with intact capsule | Shattered kidney with disrupted capsule | Ureteral/renal pelvic injury

Figure 74-5 ■ Common types and locations of renal trauma.

CHART 74-9

CLIENT EDUCATION GUIDE
Preventing Renal and Genitourinary Trauma

- Wear a seat belt.
- Practice safe walking habits.
- Use caution when riding bicycles and motorcycles.
- Wear appropriate protective clothing when participating in contact sports.
- Avoid all contact sports and high-risk activities if you have only one kidney.

jury as well as blood vessel and tissue integrity. Hematomas within or through the renal capsule are seen with CT scan. A urogram reveals the integrity and patency of the collecting system. Renal sonography can be used instead if there is a need to avoid contrast dye, especially in clients with elevated serum creatinine levels.

◆Common Nursing Diagnoses and Collaborative Problems

Nursing diagnoses that may apply to clients with renal trauma include the following:

- **Ineffective Tissue Perfusion (Renal)** related to interruption of arterial flow
- **Anxiety** related to threat to health status
- **Acute Pain** related to physical injury
- **Impaired Urinary Elimination** related to renal damage and shock
- **Risk for Infection** related to altered immune function

◆Interventions

NONSURGICAL MANAGEMENT

Drug Therapy. Prescribed IV dopamine (Revimine✳, others) promotes renal perfusion. The need for clotting factors such as vitamin K and platelets is assessed and they are given as needed.

Fluid Therapy. Fluids are given to restore circulating blood volume and ensure adequate renal blood flow. *Crystalloid* solutions replace water and some electrolytes and include 0.9% sodium chloride (NSS), 5% dextrose in 0.45% sodium chloride, and Ringer's solution. When bleeding is extensive, whole blood or packed red cell replacement restores hemoglobin and promotes oxygenation. *Plasma volume expanders,* such as dextran or albumin, help restore plasma oncotic pressure and reduce fluid shift to the interstitial fluid space.

During fluid restoration, give fluids at the prescribed rate and monitor the client for hemodynamic instability. Take vital signs as often as every 5 to 15 minutes. Measure and record urine output hourly. Output should be greater than 25 to 30 mL/hr.

SURGICAL MANAGEMENT. Nephrectomy or partial nephrectomy may be needed. When major blood vessels are torn, the kidney may be removed, repaired, and then reimplanted. This repair of kidney tissue outside the client is called "bench surgery."

Community-Based Care

Teach the client and family about the effects of the injury and how to assess for infection or other complications, such as the onset of bleeding or urinary retention. Instruct the client to check the pattern and frequency of urination and to note whether the color, clarity, and amount appear normal. Also instruct the client to seek medical attention if anything appears abnormal or if bladder distention or inadequate bladder emptying occurs, which suggests an obstruction. Chills, fever, lethargy, or cloudy, foul-smelling urine indicate a urinary tract infection. Warn the client not to ignore these manifestations and to seek medical care promptly if they occur.

- Allow the client the opportunity to express fear or anxiety regarding the potential for chronic kidney disease and renal failure.
- Assess the client's level of comfort in discussing issues related to elimination and the urogenital area.
- Refer clients with polycystic kidney disease to a geneticist or a genetic counselor.
- During renal/urinary assessment, use language and terminology that is comfortable for the client.
- Refer clients to community resources, support groups, and information organizations such as the National Kidney Foundation and the American Association of Kidney Patients.

Physiological Integrity

- Report immediately any condition that obstructs urine flow.
- Instruct clients with UTI to complete all prescribed antibiotic therapy even when symptoms of infection are absent.
- Check the blood pressure and urine output frequently in clients who have any type of kidney problem.
- Report immediately to the physician, any sudden decrease of urine output in a client with kidney disease or kidney trauma.
- Instruct clients with any type of renal problem to weigh themselves daily and to notify their health care provider if there is a sudden weight gain.
- Teach clients the expected side effects and any adverse reactions to prescribed drugs.
- Teach clients the signs and symptoms of disease recurrence and when to seek medical help.

ADDITIONAL STUDY RESOURCES

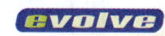 Go to your Student CD-ROM for Review Questions for the NCLEX Examination.

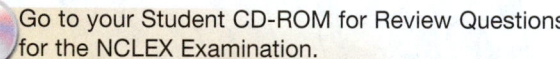 Go to http://evolve.elsevier.com/Iggy/ for Integrated Management of Care Questions for the NCLEX Examination.

GET READY for the NCLEX Examination!

KEY POINTS

Safe Effective Care Environment

- Use sterile technique when inserting a catheter or any other instrument into the urinary system.
- Use contact precautions with any client who has drainage from the genitourinary tract.

Health Promotion and Maintenance

- Encourage all clients to maintain an adequate fluid intake (minimum of 3 L/day unless another condition requires fluid restriction).
- Encourage clients with diabetes to adhere to regimens for glucose control to prevent hypertension and renal disease.
- Teach clients who come into contact with nephrotoxic chemicals in their workplaces or for leisure time activities, to avoid direct skin or mucous membrane contact with these chemicals (you may need to review Chapter 72).

Psychosocial Integrity

- Pace your interview to match the learning needs and style of the individual client.

SELECTED BIBLIOGRAPHY

Asterisk indicates a classic or definitive work on this subject.

American Cancer Society. (2005). *Cancer facts and figures 2005.* Report No. 00-300M-No. 5008.05. Atlanta: Author.

Appel, G.B., Radhakrishnan, J., & D'Agati, V. (2000). Secondary glomerular diseases. In B.M. Brenner & F.C. Rector (Eds.), *Brenner & Rector's the kidney* (5th ed., pp. 1350-1416). Philadelphia: W.B. Saunders.

Arnaout, M.A. (2001). Molecular genetics and pathogenesis of autosomal dominant polycystic kidney disease. *Annual Review of Medicine, 52,* 93-123.

Bakris, G., et al. (2000). Preserving renal function in adults with hypertension and diabetes: A consensus approach. National Kidney Foundation Hypertension and Diabetes Executive Committee Working Group. *American Journal of Kidney Disease, 36*(3), 646-661.

Bonn, D. (2002). Radiofrequency ablation: First-line treatment for renal cancer? *The Lancet Oncology, 3*(1), 3-4.

Calvet, J., & Grantham, J. (2001). The genetics and physiology of polycystic kidney disease. *Seminars in Nephrology, 21*(2), 107-123.

Dagher, P.C., et al. (2003). Newly developed techniques to study and diagnose acute renal failure. *Journal of the American Society of Nephrology, 14,* 2188-2198.

Dochterman, J., & Bulechek, G. (Eds). (2004). *Nursing interventions classification (NIC)* (4th ed.). St. Louis: Mosby.

Facts and Comparisons. (2004). *Drug facts and comparisons* (58th ed.). St. Louis: Author.

Falk, J., Jennett, J., & Nachman, S. (2000). Primary glomerular disease. In B.M. Brenner & S.A. Levine (Eds.), *Brenner & Rector's the kidney* (6th ed., pp. 1263-1349). Philadelphia: W.B. Saunders.

George, A.L., & Neilson, E.G. (2000). Genetics of kidney disease. *American Journal of Kidney Diseases, 35*(4), S160-S169.

Goolsby, M. (2002). National Kidney Foundation Guidelines for chronic kidney disease: Evaluation, classification, and stratification. *Journal of the American Academy of Nurse Practitioners, 14*(6), 238-242.

Igarashi, P., & Somlo, S. (2002). Genetics and pathogenesis of polycystic kidney disease. *Journal of the American Society of Nephrology, 13*(9), 2384-2398.

Jalanko, H., et al. (2001). Genetic kidney diseases disclose the pathogenesis of proteinuria. *Annals of Medicine, 33*(8), 526-533.

Kelly, C.J., & Neilson, E.G. (2000). Tubulointerstitial diseases. In B.M. Brenner & S.A. Levine (Eds.), *Brenner & Rector's the kidney* (6th ed., pp. 1506-1536). Philadelphia: W.B. Saunders.

Kidney Cancer Association. (2005). Available at http://www.curekidneycancer.org/.

Kikkawa, R., Koya, D., & Haneda, M. (2003). Progression of diabetic nephropathy. *American Journal of Kidney Diseases, 41*(3), 519-521.

Kneipp, S., & Himmelstein, S.B. (2000). Nephrotic syndrome secondary to amyloidosis. *The Nurse Practitioner, 25*(6), 78-93.

Lancaster, L.E. (Ed.). (2001). *Core curriculum for nephrology nursing* (4th ed.). Pitman, NJ: American Association of Nephrology Nurses.

Laragh, J.H., & Blumenfeld, J.D. (2000). Essential hypertension. In B.M. Brenner & S.A. Levine (Eds.), *Brenner & Rector's the kidney* (6th ed., pp. 1967-2006). Philadelphia: W.B. Saunders.

Laudicina, P.F. (2001). Diagnostic imaging of the genitourinary system. *Seminars in Radiologic Technology, 9*(2), 48-65.

Lehmann, S., & Dietz, C. (2002). Double J stents: They're not trouble-free. *RN, 65*(1), 54-60.

Lerman, L., & Textor, S.C. (2001). Pathophysiology of ischemic neuropathy. *Urologic Clinics of North America, 28*(4), 793-803.

Leung, D.A., et al. (2002). MR angiography of the renal arteries. *Radiology Clinics of North American, 40*(4), 847-865.

Little, C. (2000). Renovascular hypertension. *American Journal of Nursing, 100*(2), 46-51.

Maranchie, J.K., & Linehan, W.M. (2003). Genetic disorders and renal cell carcinoma. *Urologic Clinics of North America, 30*(1), 133-141.

McCance, K., & Huether, S. (2002). Pathophysiology: The biologic basis for disease in adults and children (4th ed.). St. Louis: Mosby.

Moorhead, S., Johnson, M., & Maas, M. (Eds.). (2004). *Nursing outcomes classification (NOC)* (3rd ed.). St. Louis: Mosby.

Munson, B.L. (2004). Myths and facts about polycystic kidney disease. *Nursing2004, 34*(3), 75.

*Nathan, D.M. (1993). Diabetes Control and Complications Trial Research Group: The effect of long-term intensified insulin treatment on development of microvascular complications of diabetes. *The New England Journal of Medicine, 329*(14), 977-986.

NIDDK National Kidney and Urologic Diseases Information Clearinghouse. (2004). *Kidney and urologic diseases statistics for the United States.* NIH Publication No. 04-3895. Bethesda, MD: National Institutes of Health. Available at http://kidney.niddk.nih.gov/kudiseases/pubs/kustats/index.htm.

Nussbaum, R., McInnes, R., & Willard, H. (2001). *Thompson & Thompson: Genetics in medicine* (6th ed.). Philadelphia: W.B. Saunders.

Olin, J.W. (2002). Atherosclerotic renal disease. *Cardiology Clinics, 20*(4), 547-562.

Online Mendelian Inheritance in Man. (2004). Retrieved November 17, 2004, from http://www.ncbi.nlm.nih.gov/Omim.

Palmieri, P.A. (2002). Obstructive nephropathy: Pathophysiology, diagnosis, and collaborative management. *Nephrology Nursing Journal, 29*(1), 15-21.

Polycystic Kidney Disease Foundation. (2004). Accessed November 2004 from http://www.pkdcure.org/home.html.

Rakel, R.E., & Bope, E.T. (2003). Conn's current therapy. Philadelphia: W.B. Saunders.

Richardson, A., & Piepho, R. (2000). Effect of race on hypertension and antihypertensive therapy. *International Journal of Clinical Pharmacology, 38*(2), 75-79.

Rodriguez-Itrube, B. (2000). Post-infectious glomerulonephritis. *American Journal of Kidney Disease, 35*(1), xlvi-xlviii.

Schmelzer, M., & Stam, M. (2000). A hidden menace: Hemolytic uremic syndrome. *American Journal of Nursing, 100*(11), 26-32.

Schwarz, A. (2001). New aspects of the treatment of nephrotic syndrome. *Journal of the American Society of Nephrology, 12*(Suppl. 17), 544-547.

*See, W.A., & Williams, R.D. (1992). Tumors of the kidney, ureter, and bladder. *Western Journal of Medicine, 156*(5), 523-534.

Sowers, J.R., et al. (2002). Hypertension-related disease in African-Americans. *Postgraduate Medicine, 112*(4) 24-33.

Steeg, C., Walsh, C., & Glickstein, J. (2001). Rheumatic fever: No cause for complacence. *Patient Care for the Nurse Practitioner, 4*(10), 15-16, 18, 23-24, 26.

Stegbauer, C. (2000). Nephrotic syndrome secondary to amyloidosis. *The Nurse Practitioner, 25*(6), 78, 81, 85-86, 88, 91-93.

Stuart, R., & Nigam, S. (2000). Developmental biology of the kidney. In B.M. Brenner & S.A. Levine (Eds.), *Brenner & Rector's the kidney* (6th ed., pp. 68-92). Philadelphia: W.B. Saunders.

Szromba, C., Theis, M.A., & Ossman, S.S. (2002). Advancing chronic kidney disease: New imperatives for recognitions and intervention. *Nephrology Nursing Journal, 29*(6), 547-561.

Tillou, A., et al. (2001). Renal vascular injuries. *Surgical Clinics of North America, 81*(6), 1417-1430.

Tolkoff-Rubin, N., Cotran, R., & Rubin, R. (2000). Urinary tract infection, pyelonephritis, and reflux nephropathy. In B.M. Brenner & S.A. Levine (Eds.), *Brenner & Rector's the kidney* (6th ed., pp. 1449-1508). Philadelphia: W.B. Saunders.

U.S. Renal Data Systems. (2003). *USRDS 2003 annual data report.* Bethesda, MD: The National Institutes of Health, National Institute of Diabetes and Digestive and Kidney Diseases.

Wright, J.T., et al. (2002). Effect of blood pressure lowering and antihypertensive drug class on progression of hypertensive kidney disease: Results from the AASK trial. *Journal of the American Medical Association, 288*(19), 2421-2431.

Interventions for Clients with Acute and Chronic Renal Failure

LINDA A. LaCHARITY

LEARNING OUTCOMES

After studying this chapter, you should be able to:

1. Compare the pathophysiology and causes of acute renal failure (ARF) with those of chronic renal failure (CRF).
2. Identify clients at risk for development of ARF.
3. Identify clients at risk for development of CRF.
4. Use laboratory data and clinical assessment to determine the effectiveness of therapy for renal failure.
5. Discuss interventions to prevent ARF.
6. Prioritize nursing care for the client with ARF.
7. Describe the mechanisms of action, side effects, and nursing implications for pharmacologic management of renal failure.
8. Compare the clinical manifestations of stage I, stage II, and stage III CRF.
9. Discuss the mechanisms of peritoneal dialysis (PD) and hemodialysis (HD) as renal replacement therapies.
10. Prioritize nursing care for the client with end-stage renal disease.
11. Prioritize teaching needs for the client using continuous ambulatory PD.
12. Develop a community-based teaching plan for the client with a permanent vascular access for long-term HD.
13. Compare the dietary modifications needed for the client undergoing HD with those for the client undergoing PD.
14. Plan prevention strategies for the complications of PD.
15. Discuss the criteria for kidney donation.
16. Prioritize nursing care for the client during the first 24 hours after kidney transplantation.
17. Develop a community-based teaching plan for the client who has received a kidney transplant.

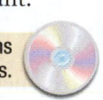

Go to your Student CD-ROM for Review Questions for the NCLEX Examination keyed to these Learning Outcomes.

Acute renal failure (ARF) and chronic renal failure (CRF) have become increasingly more common in the United States, resulting in considerable morbidity and mortality. ARF is responsible for 7% of all hospital admissions and for 2% to 5% of clients admitted to medical-surgical hospital units. The prevalence of end-stage renal disease (ESRD) has more than doubled in the last decade (U.S. Renal Data Systems, 2002). Renal failure has many causes. Complications related to poorly controlled diabetes are the most common cause (43.4%), followed by hypertension (25.5%) and glomerulonephritis (8.4%).

Kidney functions include excretion of waste, water and salt balance, acid-base balance, and hormone secretion. When renal function declines gradually, as occurs most often with CRF, 90% to 95% of the nephrons must be destroyed before renal failure is obvious. The client may have many years of decreased renal reserve and chronic renal insufficiency before the uremia of end-stage renal failure develops. During this time of decreased renal reserve and chronic renal insufficiency, the client is at increased risk for acute renal failure because of the reduced functioning of remaining nephrons.

When renal decline is sudden, the work capacity of functioning nephrons is exceeded more quickly, and renal failure may develop with the loss of only 50% of functioning nephrons. Acute renal failure and chronic renal failure are

TABLE 75-1 Characteristics of Acute and Chronic Renal Failure

Characteristic	Acute Renal Failure	Chronic Renal Failure
Onset	Sudden (hours to days)	Gradual (months to years)
Percentage of nephron involvement	≈50%	90%-95%
Duration	2-4 wk; less than 3 mo	Permanent
Prognosis	Good for return of renal function with supportive care, high mortality in some situations	Fatal without a renal replacement therapy, such as dialysis or transplantation

compared in Table 75-1. Acute renal failure affects *many* body systems; chronic renal failure affects *every* body system. Renal failure problems are related to the effects of the following:

- Fluid-volume excess
- Electrolyte and acid-base abnormalities
- Accumulated nitrogenous wastes
- Hormonal inadequacies

When renal function decreases to the point that the kidneys can no longer meet the body's homeostatic demands, renal replacement therapy is needed to prevent death from potentially life-threatening consequences.

ACUTE RENAL FAILURE

PATHOPHYSIOLOGY

Acute renal failure (ARF) is a rapid decrease in renal function, leading to the collection of metabolic wastes in the body. ARF can result from conditions that cause inadequate kidney perfusion (**prerenal failure**); damage to the glomeruli, interstitial tissue, or tubules (**intrarenal/intrinsic renal failure**); or obstruction urine flow (**postrenal failure**) (Nally, 2002). ARF in clients with chronic renal insufficiency (CRI) may result in **end-stage renal disease (ESRD)**, or it may resolve to nearly the pre-ARF level of renal function. Many factors contribute to renal insults in ARF, but the acute syndrome may be reversible, especially with prompt intervention.

The pathologic process of ARF is related to the cause of the sudden decrease in kidney function and to the affected kidney sites(s). Reduced blood flow (**hypoperfusion**), toxins, tubular ischemia, infections, and obstruction have different effects on the renal system. Any of these processes can reduce glomerular filtration rate (GFR), disrupt tubular cell membranes, and obstruct urine flow in the renal tubules. With shock or other problems causing an acute reduction in renal blood flow (hypoperfusion), the kidney compensates with autoregulatory responses (e.g., renal blood vessel constriction, activation of renin-angiotensin-aldosterone pathway, and release of antidiuretic hormone [ADH]). These responses increase blood volume and improve renal perfusion. However, these same responses reduce urine volume, resulting in **oliguria** (urine output less than 400 mL/day). Tubular cell injury is more likely to occur from the increasing ischemia related to hypoperfusion. Toxins can cause blood vessel constriction in the kidney, leading to reduced renal blood flow and renal ischemia.

Kidney tissue inflammation caused by infection, drugs, or cancer result in immune-mediated changes in renal tissue. With extensive tubular damage, tubular cells slough and combine with other formed elements (e.g., red blood cell [RBC]

casts), which then obstruct the tubular lumen and prevent urine outflow. Obstruction anywhere within the urinary tract may result in full or partial obstruction to the formation and outflow of urine.

When pressure in the renal tubules (intrarenal pressure) exceeds glomerular hydrostatic pressure, glomerular filtration stops. This problem allows nitrogenous wastes to collect in the blood, increasing the blood urea nitrogen (BUN) and serum creatinine levels. When the BUN rises faster than the serum creatinine level, the cause is usually related to protein breakdown or volume depletion. When both the BUN and the creatinine levels rise and the ratio between the two remains constant, renal failure is present.

Types of Acute Renal Failure

Several syndromes describe the types of ARF. These include prerenal azotemia, intrarenal (intrinsic) ARF, and postrenal azotemia. Table 75-2 lists the causes and problems of ARF.

Prerenal azotemia can be reversed by correcting blood volume, increasing blood pressure, and improving cardiac output. Prolonged, untreated hypoperfusion can lead to severe ischemic injury and intrarenal failure.

The term *intrarenal ARF* is often shortened to just *ARF* in the clinical setting. Other terms include **acute tubular necrosis (ATN)** and **lower nephron nephrosis.** Infections (bacteria, viral, fungal), drugs (especially aminoglycoside antibiotics and nonsteroidal anti-inflammatory drugs [NSAIDs]), and invading tumors (e.g., lymphomas or leukemias) can cause acute interstitial nephritis. Other causes of intrarenal ARF include inflammation of the glomeruli (**glomerulonephritis**) or of the small vessels of the kidneys (**vasculitis**), or an obstruction of renal blood flow.

Postrenal azotemia develops from obstruction to the outflow of formed urine anywhere within the renal or urinary tract.

Phases of Acute Renal Failure

When a client's renal function declines, the phases of ARF begin (Table 75-3). Some clients have a *nonoliguric* form of ARF in which urine output remains near normal. The phases of this form of ARF are similar to those listed in Table 75-3 except for the references to urine output. The treatment of these clients is less complicated because renal replacement therapy is rarely needed. Interventions to restore circulating volume, improve cardiac output, or increase blood pressure may prevent progression of the phases when hypoperfusion is present.

Etiology

Many types of renal insults can reduce renal function. Severe hypotension from shock or dehydration reduces renal blood flow and can lead to prerenal ARF. Cardiac disease or

TABLE 75-2 Causes of the Three Types of Acute Renal Failure

Pathologic Change	Causes
Prerenal Decreased blood flow to the kidneys leading to ischemia in the nephrons; prolonged hypoperfusion can lead to tubular necrosis and ARF	Conditions that cause decreased cardiac output Shock HF Pulmonary embolism Anaphylaxis Pericardial tamponade Sepsis
Intrarenal (Intrinsic) Actual tissue damage to the kidney caused by inflammatory or immunologic processes or from prolonged hypoperfusion	Acute interstitial nephritis Exposure to nephrotoxins Acute glomerulonephritis Vasculitis Hepatorenal syndrome ATN Renal artery or vein stenosis/thrombosis
Postrenal Obstruction of the urine collecting system anywhere from the calyces to the urethral meatus Obstruction of the bladder must be bilateral to cause postrenal failure unless only one kidney is functional	Urethral or bladder cancer Renal, ureteral, or bladder stones Atony of bladder Prostatic hyperplasia or cancer Cervical cancer Urethral stricture

ARF, Acute renal failure; *ATN,* acute tubular necrosis; *HF,* heart failure.

TABLE 75-3 The Phases of Oliguric Acute Renal Failure

Phase	Description	Characteristics	Duration
Onset phase	Begins with the precipitating event and continues until oliguria develops.	The gradual accumulation of nitrogenous wastes, such as serum creatinine and BUN, may be noted.	Can last hours to several days.
Oliguric phase	Characterized by a urine output to 100-400 mL/24 hr that does not respond to fluid challenges or diuretics.	Laboratory data include increasing serum creatinine and BUN levels, hyperkalemia, bicarbonate deficit (metabolic acidosis), hyperphosphatemia, hypocalcemia, and hypermagnesemia. Sodium retention occurs, but this is masked by the dilutional effects of water retention. Urinary indices are typically low and fixed; regulation of water balance by the kidneys is impaired, so urine specific gravity and urine osmolarity do not vary as plasma osmolarity changes.	Typically lasts 8-15 days but can last for several weeks, especially in older clients or those having pre-existing renal insufficiency.
Diuretic phase (high-output phase)	Often has a prompt onset, with urine flow increasing rapidly over a period of several days. The diuresis can result in an output of up to 10 L/day of dilute urine.	Electrolyte losses typically precede clearance of nitrogenous wastes. Later in the diuretic phase, the BUN level starts to fall and continues to fall until the level reaches normal limits or reaches a plateau. Normal renal tubular function is re-established during this phase.	Usually occurs 2-6 wk after the onset of oliguric acute renal failure and continues until the BUN level ceases to rise.
Recovery phase (convalescent phase)	In this phase, the client begins to return to normal levels of activity.	The client functions at a lower energy level and has less stamina than before the illness. Residual renal insufficiency may be noted through regular monitoring of renal function. Renal function may never return to preillness levels, but renal function sufficient for a long and healthy life is likely.	Renal function may continue to improve for up to 12 mo after oliguric acute renal failure began. The client is particularly vulnerable to additional renal injury during this time.

BUN, Blood urea nitrogen.

heart failure also can reduce renal blood flow. The client may be oliguric or even **anuric** (less than 100 mL/24 hr) if the dehydration or renal blood flow reduction is severe. The following other conditions can lead to ARF:

- Nephrotoxic agents (antibiotics, NSAIDs) (Table 75-4)
- Disseminated intravascular coagulation (DIC)
- Obstruction by thrombosis or stenosis
- Uric acid crystals or other obstructing precipitates
- Acute hemolytic transfusion reactions
- Complications of infection (e.g., endotoxins or sepsis)
- Acute glomerulonephritis
- Vasculitis
- Severe hypertension
- Hepatorenal syndrome of cirrhosis

Incidence/Prevalence

Acute renal failure affects 15% to 20% of all critically ill clients and has a 50% to 80% mortality rate (U.S. Renal Data Systems, 2002). Eighty percent of ARF episodes are due to acute tubular necrosis (ATN) and worsening of chronic renal insufficiency (CRI). Volume depletion leading to prerenal azotemia is the most common cause of ARF and is reversible in most cases with prompt intervention.

For clients who survive the precipitating event, the chance for return of renal function is good. However, complications during the course of AFR can greatly increase mortality. Bloodstream infections from contamination through intravenous (IV) lines are the most often common

TABLE 75-4   Some Potentially Nephrotoxic Substances

Drugs	Other Drugs
Antibiotics/Anti-infectives	- Acetaminophen
- Amphotericin B	- Captopril
- Colistimethate	- Cyclosporine
- Methicillin	- Fluorinate anesthetics
- Polymyxin B	- D-Penicillamine
- Rifampin	- Phenazopyridine
- Sulfonamides	hydrochloride
- Tetracycline hydrochloride	- Quinine
- Vancomycin	
	Other Substances
Aminoglycoside Antibiotics	**Organic Solvents**
- Gentamicin	- Carbon tetrachloride
- Kanamycin	- Ethylene glycol
- Neomycin	
- Netilmicin sulfate	**Nondrug Chemical Agents**
- Tobramycin	- Radiographic contrast dye
	- Pesticides
Antineoplastics	- Fungicides
- Cisplatin	- Myoglobin (from breakdown
- Cyclophosphamide	of skeletal muscle)
- Methotrexate	
	Heavy Metals and Ions
Nonsteroidal Anti-inflammatory	- Arsenic
Drugs (NSAIDs)	- Bismuth
- Celecoxib	- Copper sulfate
- Flurbiprofen	- Gold salts
- Ibuprofen	- Lead
- Indomethacin	- Mercuric chloride
- Ketorolac	
- Meclofenamate	
- Meloxicam	
- Nabumentone	
- Naproxen	
- Oxaprozin	
- Rofecoxib	
- Tolmetin	

complications that lead to death. However, the highest mortality occurs with trauma (70%) and surgery. ARF caused by nephrotoxic substances has the lowest rates (10% to 26%) of recovery. The prognosis for ARF caused by obstruction or glomerulonephritis is much better.

HEALTH PROMOTION/ILLNESS PREVENTION

Keep in mind that severe blood volume depletion can lead to renal failure even in people who have no known kidney problems. Encourage all clients to maintain an adequate fluid intake to avoid dehydration. This is especially important for athletes or any person who engages in strenuous exercise and sweats heavily.

Nurses have an essential role in the prevention of acute renal failure (ARF) in hospitalized clients. Always be on the lookout for signs of impending renal impairment through careful physical assessment and closely monitoring laboratory values. Early recognition and correction of problems causing reduced renal blood flow usually restore renal function before tissue damage can occur. Evaluate the client's fluid status. Accurately measure intake and output, and check body weight to identify trends in fluid balance. Assess for manifestations of blood volume depletion, such as decreased urine output, postural hypotension, and tachycardia. Prompt fluid replacement in the prerenal stage can prevent renal tissue damage and renal failure.

Also monitor laboratory values for any changes that reflect poor renal function. Decreased urine specific gravity indicates a loss of urine-concentrating ability and is the earliest sign of renal tubular damage. Other laboratory values that are helpful in monitoring renal function include serum creatinine, urine and serum electrolytes, and blood urea nitrogen (BUN).

Be aware of nephrotoxic substances that the client may ingest or be exposed to (see Table 75-4). Question any prescription for potentially nephrotoxic drugs, and validate the dose before the client receives the drug. Antibiotics are common drugs that have nephrotoxic side effects. NSAIDs can cause or increase the risk for ARF. Combining two or more nephrotoxic drugs dramatically increases the risk for ARF. If a client must receive a potentially nephrotoxic drug, monitor laboratory values, including BUN, creatinine, and drug peak and trough levels, closely for indications of renal dysfunction.

◆ COLLABORATIVE MANAGEMENT
◆ Assessment
HISTORY

The accurate diagnosis of ARF, including its type and its cause, depends on a detailed history of potential causes of ARF. Ask the client about exposure to nephrotoxins, recent surgery or trauma, transfusions, or other factors that might lead to reduced renal blood flow. Obtain a drug history, especially treatment with antibiotics, angiotensin-converting enzyme (ACE) inhibitors, and NSAIDs. Ask the client whether he or she has recently had an x-ray requiring injection of a contrast dye. These dyes can cause ARF, especially in older clients with reduced renal reserve. ARF must be differentiated from chronic renal insufficiency (CRI). Ask the client about diseases that impair renal function, such as diabetes mellitus, systemic lupus erythematosus, other connective tissue diseases, and chronic hypertension.

To identify possible acute glomerulonephritis, ask about acute illnesses such as influenza, colds, gastroenteritis, and sore throats. Ask the client whether urine color has become darker or appears smoky.

Reversible prerenal azotemia may occur after any episode of acute hypotension, hemorrhage or shock, burns, heart failure, or any problem in which the blood volume is depleted. Extensive bowel preparations and being allowed nothing by mouth (NPO) before surgery along with fluid loss during surgery can cause prerenal azotemia in some clients.

Postrenal renal failure is identified by focusing on urinary obstructive problems. Ask the client about any difficulty in starting the urine stream, changes in the amount or appearance of the urine, narrowing of the urine stream, nocturia, urgency, or symptoms of renal stones. Also ask about any cancer history that may cause urinary obstruction.

PHYSICAL ASSESSMENT/CLINICAL MANIFESTATIONS

The manifestations of ARF are related to the collection of nitrogenous wastes **(azotemia)** as well as to as the underlying cause (Chart 75-1). Manifestations of *prerenal* azotemia are hypotension, tachycardia, decreased urine output, decreased cardiac output, decreased central venous pressure (CVP), and lethargy. The appearance of a client with prerenal azotemia is similar to that of a client with heart failure or dehydration, depending on the cause of the poor renal blood flow.

Intrarenal (intrinsic) ARF usually occurs with damage to the glomeruli, interstitial tissue, or tubules. Manifestations are decreased urine output **(oliguria)** or absence of urine **(anuria)**, edema, hypertension, tachycardia, shortness of breath, distended neck veins, elevated central venous pressure, weight gain, respiratory crackles, anorexia, nausea, vomiting, and lethargy or varying levels of consciousness. Manifestations of electrolyte imbalances, such as electrocardiographic (ECG) changes, may also be present.

In clients with *postrenal* failure, monitor for oliguria or intermittent anuria, symptoms of uremia, and lethargy. Report changes in the urine stream or difficulty starting urination.

LABORATORY ASSESSMENT

The many changes in laboratory values in the client with ARF are similar to those occurring in chronic renal failure (CRF) (Chart 75-2; see also Laboratory Assessment [Chronic Renal Failure], p. 1745). Expect to see rising BUN, creatinine, and abnormal blood electrolytes values. Table 75-5 shows electrolyte values common to renal failure. Clients with ARF, however, do *not* have the anemia associated with CRF unless there is hemorrhagic blood loss. However, uremic hemolysis can develop and may be the cause of anemia in the early phase of ARF.

In the early phases of ARF, urine tests may provide diagnostic information. Urine sodium levels are often less than 10 to 20 mEq/L in clients with prerenal azotemia. The urine is often concentrated, with a specific gravity greater than 1.020. The presence of urine sediment (red blood cells [RBCs], RBC casts, tubular cells), myoglobin, or hemoglo-

CHART 75-1
KEY FEATURES of
Acute Renal Failure

Prerenal Azotemia
- Hypotension
- Tachycardia
- Decreased cardiac output
- Decreased central venous pressure
- Decreased urine output
- Lethargy

Intrarenal (Intrinsic) ARF and Postrenal Azotemia
- Renal manifestations
  - Oliguria or anuria
  - Increased urine specific gravity
- Cardiac manifestations
  - Hypertension
  - Tachycardia
  - Jugular venous distention
  - Increased central venous pressure
  - ECG changes: tall T waves
- Respiratory manifestations
  - Shortness of breath
  - Orthopnea
  - Rales or crackles
  - Pulmonary edema
  - Friction rub
- Gastrointestinal manifestations
  - Anorexia
  - Nausea
  - Vomiting
  - Flank pain
- Neurologic manifestations
  - Lethargy
  - Headache
  - Tremors
  - Confusion
- General manifestations
  - Generalized edema
  - Weight gain

ARF, Acute renal failure; *ECG,* electrocardiogram.

bin; a urine sodium level lower than 40 mEq/L; and a specific gravity of 1.010 indicate intrarenal failure. In postrenal failure, urine sodium levels may be normal to 40 mEq/L, with a specific gravity of 1.000 to 1.010.

RADIOGRAPHIC ASSESSMENT

X-rays help to determine the cause of ARF. A flat-plate x-ray of the abdomen is used to determine the size of the kidneys. Enlarged kidneys, possibly due to obstruction, may result from hydronephrosis. This x-ray may show stones obstructing the renal pelvis, ureters, or bladder.

Renal ultrasonography is a noninvasive procedure using high-energy sound waves. It is useful in the diagnosis of urinary tract obstruction. Dilation of the renal calyces and collecting ducts, as well as stones, can be detected.

Computed tomography (CT) scans without contrast dye can identify obstruction or tumors. Contrast dyes are usually avoided to prevent further renal damage. Ultrasonography is preferred to renography to determine kidney size and the patency of the ureters. A nuclear medicine study called *MAG3* may be used to determine the nature of the renal failure, GFR, or tubular function and its severity. A renal scan can determine whether blood flow to the kidneys is sufficient.

Aortorenal angiography may be used to examine renal blood vessels and blood flow. The procedure involves the

CHART 75-2

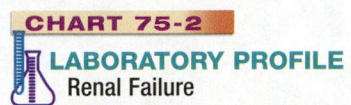

LABORATORY PROFILE
Renal Failure

Test	Normal Range for Adults	Values in Renal Failure	Comments
Test to Evaluate Removal of Nitrogenous Wastes			
Serum creatinine	*Male:* 0.6-1.2 mg/dL *Female:* 0.5-7 mg/dL *Older adults:* Decreased	**In Chronic Renal Failure** May increase by 0.5-1.0 mg/dL every 1-2 yr May be as high as 15-30 mg/dL *before* symptoms of CRF are present **In Acute Renal Failure** Gradual increase of 1-2 mg/dL every 24-48 hr May increase 1-6 mg/dL in 1 wk or less	Consistently elevated levels indicate decreased renal function. Serum creatinine levels are used to evaluate the effectiveness of dialysis treatments.
Blood urea nitrogen	10-20 mg/dL *Older adults:* May be slightly increased	**In Chronic Renal Failure** May reach 180-200 mg/dL *before* symptoms develop **In Acute Renal Failure** Often increases by 10-20 mg/dL at same pace as serum creatinine level May reach 80-100 mg/dL within 1 wk	Increases depend on protein intake and other factors (see text). Rate of increase is controlled by limiting protein intake. This intervention is believed to decrease the rate of onset of systemic symptoms, such as anorexia, nausea, and vomiting. Elevations have multiple causes, including diminished renal function excessive protein intake, sepsis GI bleeding, dehydration, and tissue catabolism.
Electrolyte Studies			
Serum sodium	136-145 mEq/L; 136-145 mmol/L (SI units)	Normal or decreased	Clients with renal failure retain sodium. With associated water retention, serum sodium levels seem normal. With excessive water retention, serum sodium levels seem decreased owing to hemodilution. Assess the client for evidence of fluid volume excess: edema, weight increase, or elevation of diastolic blood pressure. Limit fluid intake as directed. Avoid excessive sodium intake Monitor for signs of hypernatremia dry skin, excessive thirst, dry mucous membranes, elevated body temperature, and flushed skin. Client may need diuretics or dialysis.
Serum potassium	3.5-5.0 mmol/L (SI units)	Increased	Advise the client to avoid salt substitutes and to limit potassium-containing foods. Monitor for rapidly increasing serum potassium levels in ARF. ECG changes occur with serum potassium levels ≥6.5. Monitor for signs of hyperkalemia: dizziness, weakness, cardiac irregularities, muscle cramps, diarrhea, and nausea. May require administration of sodium polystyrene sulfonate (Kayexalate) or other treatment.
Serum phosphorus (phosphate)	3.0-4.5 mg/dL, 0.97-1.45 mmol/L (SI units) *Older adults:* May be slightly decreased	Increased	Short-term increases have potential to cause rapid decrease in serum calcium level and cardiac rhythm disturbances. Long-term increases demineralize bones of calcium and enhance fracture potential. Phosphate-binding medications help control hyperphosphatemia and prevent calcium depletion from the bones.

ARF, Acute renal failure; *ECG*, electrocardiogram; *CRF*, chronic renal failure; *GI*, gastrointestinal; *GFR*, glomerular filtration rate *RBCs*, red blood cells; *SI*, Système Internationale; *WBCs*, white blood cells.

Continued

CHART 75-2

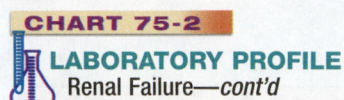

LABORATORY PROFILE
Renal Failure—*cont'd*

Test	Normal Range for Adults	Values in Renal Failure	Comments
Serum calcium	Total calcium: 9.0-10.5 mg/dL; 2.25-2.75 mmol/L (SI units) Ionized calcium: 4.5-5.6 mg/dL, 1.05-1.3 mmol/L (SI units) *Older adults:* Slightly decreased	Decreased	Decreases in ARF may necessitate replacement. Decreases in CRF may only be slight and may or may not necessitate replacement. As the serum phosphate level increases, the serum calcium level decreases. Chronic calcium deficiency leads to renal osteodystrophy. Control of phosphate excess is usually essential before calcium replacement is initiated. Monitor for manifestations of hypocalcemia: abdominal cramps, hyperactive reflexes, tingling fingertips, and spasms in feet and wrists (see also Chapter 16).
Serum magnesium	1.3-2.1 mEq/L; 0.65-1.05 mmol/L (SI units)	Increased	Advise the client to avoid compounds containing magnesium (e.g., laxatives).
Serum carbon dioxide combining power (bicarbonate)	23-30 mEq/L (venous); 23-30 mmol/L (SI units)	Decreased	Replace bicarbonate. Monitor respiratory rate and depth. Monitor for decreased orientation.
Arterial blood pH	7.35-7.45	Decreased (in metabolic acidosis) or normal	The respiratory system attempts to compensate by hyperventilation (increased rate and depth of respiration). Values are within the normal range if blood buffers and lungs can compensate. Monitor breathing rate and depth. Monitor level of consciousness.
Arterial blood bicarbonate (HCO_3^-)	21-28 mEq/L	Decreased	Provide replacement PO, IV, or by hemodialysis or peritoneal dialysis.
Arterial blood $Paco_2$	35-45 mm Hg	Decreased	Monitor for respiratory fatigue (the client breathes more rapidly and deeply to "blow off" carbon dioxide).
Other Blood Studies			
Hemoglobin	*Female:* 12-16 g/dL, 7.4-9.9 mmol/L (SI units) *Male:* 14-18 g/dL, 8.7-11.2 mmol/L (SI units) *Older adults:* Slightly decreased	Decreased	Decreased levels indicate anemia. Monitor for pallor, weakness, lethargy, dizziness, possible shortness of breath, and activity intolerance.
Hematocrit	*Female:* 37%-47% *Male:* 42%-52% *Older adults:* May be slightly decreased	Decreased to 20%	Same as for hemoglobin. With erythropoietin therapy, may be able to obtain levels as high as 36%.
Urinalysis*			
Specific gravity	Usually 1.010-1.025 Possible range: 1.005-1.030	Usually decreased and fixed	Reflects inability of the tubules to produce a concentrated or diluted urine in response to changes in plasma osmolarity. Monitor for fluid volume deficit or excess.
pH	Average: 5.5-6 Possible range: 4.6-8	May be fixed; pH does not change with dietary changes	Collect a freshly voided specimen for testing
Glucose	None or <15 mg/dL Usually detectable in urine of nondiabetic clients when blood level is 160-180 mg/dL	Increased	The renal threshold is often increased; therefore the blood glucose level may be >160-180 mg/dL before glucose is detectable in the urine. Monitor *blood* glucose levels.

ARF, Acute renal failure; *ECG*, electrocardiogram; *CRF*, chronic renal failure; *GI*, gastrointestinal; *GFR*, glomerular filtration rate *RBCs*, red blood cells; *SI*, Système Internationale; *WBCs*, white blood cells.

*Urine may become cloudy with heavy sediment. Urine output and appearance vary, depending on remaining renal function.

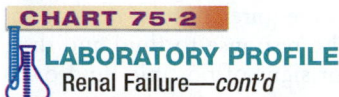

CHART 75-2

LABORATORY PROFILE
Renal Failure—*cont'd*

Test	Normal Range for Adults	Values in Renal Failure	Comments
Urinalysis*—*cont'd*			
Protein	0-8 mg/dL	Increased when there is glomerular damage or disease	Increases may be an incidental and benign finding. Transient increases occur with extreme exercise, fever, stress, or infection. Persistent proteinuria requires 24-hr collection for determination of total quantity excreted. Persistent proteinuria may indicate a serious renal problem. Instruct the client about the need for follow-up. Instruct the client in the correct procedure for collection of 24-hr specimen (see Chapter 72).
Occult blood	No RBCs or occasionally 2 or 3 RBCs per high-power field No hemoglobin	More than 2 or 3 RBCs per high-power field Detectable hemoglobin	Hemoglobin is detectable when hemolysis of RBCs has occurred. Intact RBCs are detectable only with microscopic examination. Collect a freshly voided specimen for testing.
WBCs	0-5 per high-power field	Increased in urinary tract infection	Often indicates need for urine culture.
Bacteria	Fewer than 1000 colonies/mL	Increased in the presence of infection, with or without an increase in WBCs	Obtain urine culture.
Casts	None or a few; composed of RBCs, WBCs, protein, or tubular cell casts such as hyaline	Casts present	Casts may be a benign occurrence or may signify that some renal injury or disease is present. Collect a freshly voided specimen for direct microscopic examination.
Creatinine clearance	*Male:* 107-139 mL/min *Female:* 87-107 mL/min *Older adults:* Progressively decreased with advancing age	Decreased	Change reflects decreases in GFR. Creatinine clearance is determined from a 24-hr urine collection and a serum creatinine value.

ARF, Acute renal failure; *ECG*, electrocardiogram; *CRF*, chronic renal failure; *GI*, gastrointestinal; *GFR*, glomerular filtration rate *RBCs*, red blood cells; *SI*, Système Internationale; *WBCs*, white blood cells.

*Urine may become cloudy with heavy sediment. Urine output and appearance vary, depending on remaining renal function.

TABLE 75-5 Effects of Renal Failure on Electrolyte Balance

Electrolyte	Effects of Renal Failure	Problems	Treatments
Potassium	Retained with oliguria (increased)	Hyperkalemia Cardiac dysrhythmias Asystole	Kayexalate, PO or rectal Regular IV insulin with 5% to 50% dextrose IV calcium gluconate Dialysis
Sodium	Retained (increased)	Dilutional hyponatremia Fluid volume excess Hypertension Heart failure Pulmonary edema	Diuretics until no longer responsive Dialysis Fluid restriction Sodium restriction
Phosphate	Retained (increased)	Hyperphosphatemia Metastatic calcium phosphate deposits Renal bone disease	Phosphate-binding agents Limit phosphorus intake Vitamin D analogues
Calcium	Decreased gastrointestinal absorption Binds to phosphate (decreased)	Bone demineralization Pathologic fractures	Replace vitamin D Calcium supplements
Hydrogen	Retained (increased)	Binds with bicarbonate for excretion through respiratory compensation	Dialysis Bicarbonate supplements
Bicarbonate	Depleted (decreased)	Used for blood buffering to prevent metabolic acidemia	Dialysis Bicarbonate supplements
Magnesium	Retained (decreased)	Potential for hypermagnesemia	Avoid magnesium-containing antacids and laxatives

risk of using contrast dye but can reveal any occlusion of major renal vessels by thrombus, embolus, or stenosis. Cystoscopy or retrograde pyelography may be needed to identify obstructions of the lower urinary tract.

OTHER DIAGNOSTIC ASSESSMENTS

Renal biopsy is performed if the cause of ARF is uncertain, an immunologic disease is suspected, or the reversibility of the renal failure needs to be determined after ARF has persisted for an extended period. Prepare the client before the test, and provide follow-up care. You must be aware of all test results and understand how they might affect the treatment regimen. (See Chapter 72 for a detailed discussion of renal diagnostic tests.)

◆ Common Nursing Diagnoses and Collaborative Problems

Nursing diagnoses and collaborative problems that may apply to clients with acute renal failure include the following:
- Excess Fluid Volume related to compromised regulatory mechanisms (inability of the kidneys to maintain body fluid balance)
- Potential for Pulmonary Edema
- Potential for Electrolyte Imbalances

◆ Interventions

The client with ARF may move from the oliguric phase (in which fluid and electrolytes are retained) to the diuretic phase. If the client moves to the diuretic phase, hypovolemia and electrolyte *loss* are the main problems. The client in the diuretic phase of ARF needs a plan of care that focuses on fluid and electrolyte *replacement* and monitoring.

These examples of output variation reflect the continually changing nature of ARF and the need for the plan of care to be constantly updated to reflect the stages of the disease process. Drug therapy, diet therapy, and renal replacement therapy (peritoneal dialysis [PD], hemodialysis [HD], or hemofiltration) are commonly used to manage ARF.

Drug Therapy. Clients with ARF receive many drugs. As kidney function changes, drug dosages are modified. You must be knowledgeable about the site of drug metabolism and especially careful when giving drugs. Constantly monitor for possible side effects and interactions of the drugs that the client with ARF is receiving (Chart 75-3; see also Drug Therapy [Chronic Renal Failure], p. 1748). Diuretics may be used to increase urine output.

In clients with prerenal azotemia, fluid challenges and diuretics are often used to promote renal blood flow. In clients without manifestations of fluid volume excess, 500 to 1000 mL of normal saline may be infused over a 1-hour period. In prerenal azotemia, the client responds to the fluid challenge by producing urine soon after the initial bolus. Diuretics such as furosemide (Lasix) also may be prescribed along with a fluid bolus. If oliguric renal failure is diagnosed, the fluid challenges and diuretics are discontinued. Low-dose (1 to 3 mcg/kg) dopamine may be given in a continuous infusion to enhance renal blood flow and to increase blood pressure (Chart 75-4). These clients often require central venous pressure (CVP) monitoring or measurement of pulmonary arterial pressure by means of a pulmonary artery catheter for an exact evaluation of their hemodynamic status. They also require constant nursing supervision for assessment of the response to fluid and drug therapy. Carefully monitor for signs of possible fluid overload.

Calcium channel blockers may be used to treat ARF resulting from nephrotoxic acute tubular necrosis (ATN). These drugs prevent the influx of calcium into the kidney cells, maintain kidney cell integrity, and improve the glomerular filtration rate (GFR) by improving renal blood flow.

Diet Therapy. Clients who have ARF often have a high rate of protein breakdown. The exact cause for this state is not well understood. Increases in metabolism and protein breakdown may be related to the stress of a critical illness, causing an increase in blood levels of catecholamines, cortisol, and glucagon. The rate of protein breakdown correlates with the severity of uremia and azotemia. This hypercatabolic state causes the breakdown of muscle for protein, which leads to an increase in azotemia and an even more elevated blood urea nitrogen (BUN) level.

If the client with ARF has an adequate dietary intake (see Imbalanced Nutrition: Less Than Body Requirements [Chronic Renal Failure], p. 1746), nutritional support may not be needed. Consultation with a dietitian, who will calculate the client's caloric needs, may be prescribed. Work with the dietitian to provide a diet with specified amounts of protein, sodium, and fluids. For the client who does not require dialysis, 0.6 g/kg of body weight or 40 g/day of protein is usually prescribed. For clients who do require dialysis, the protein level needed will range from 1 to 1.5 g/kg. The amount of dietary sodium ranges from 60 to 90 mEq. If hyperkalemia is present, dietary potassium is restricted to 60 to 70 mEq. The amount of fluid permitted is generally calculated to equal the urine volume plus 500 mL. Continually assess oral intake to make certain that caloric intake is adequate.

Many clients with ARF are too ill or have too poor an appetite to eat enough food. For these clients, some form of nutritional support (e.g., total parenteral nutrition [TPN] or hyperalimentation) is needed. The goals of nutritional support in ARF are to provide sufficient nutrients to maintain or improve nutritional status, to preserve lean body mass, to restore or maintain fluid balance, and to preserve renal function.

If TPN is used, the solutions are mixed to meet the client's specific needs. Because kidney function is unstable in ARF, constantly monitor the serum electrolyte concentrations and indicate when the hyperalimentation solution needs to be changed. IV fat emulsion (Intralipid) infusions can provide a nonprotein source of calories. In uremic clients, fat emulsions are used in place of glucose to avoid the problems of excessive sugars.

Dialysis Therapies. If necessary, hemodialysis (HD) and peritoneal dialysis (PD) may be implemented for clients with ARF. The following are indications for dialysis in ARF:
- Uremia
- Persistent hyperkalemia
- Uncompensated metabolic acidosis
- Fluid volume excess unresponsive to diuretics
- Uremic pericarditis
- Uremic encephalopathy

Immediate vascular access for HD in clients with ARF is made by placement of a dual- or triple-lumen catheter specific for HD. When HD is expected to be used for several

CHART 75-3

DRUG THERAPY for Renal Failure

Drug	Usual Dosages	Indications	Nursing Interventions	Rationales
Cardioglycosides				
Digoxin (Lanoxin, Novodigoxin ✽)	0.125-0.25 mg PO or IV daily or every other day *Older adults:* 0.0625-0.125 PO or IV daily or every other day	Decreased stroke volume Decreased strength of cardiac contractions	Monitor for signs of digoxin toxicity and hypokalemia. Monitor for bradycardia (pulse <50-60 beats/min). Monitor serum drug levels.	Digoxin remains in the body longer when renal function is impaired. Bradycardia is a sign of digoxin toxicity. A toxic digoxin level is >2.5 ng/mL.
Vitamins and Minerals				
Folic acid (vitamin B_9, Folvite, Novofolacid ✽)	0.1 mg PO, SC, or IM daily	Dietary supplement	Usually given after dialysis.	Water-soluble vitamins are removed during dialysis.
Ferrous sulfate (Feosol, Novoferrosulfa ✽)	325 mg PO three or four times daily	Anemia	Monitor for constipation. Note any change in the stools, which normally become blackish green.	Constipation is a common and uncomfortable side effect associated with oral iron supplements. The color is caused by the presence of unabsorbed iron and is harmless.
Biological Response Modifiers				
Erythropoietin alpha (Epogen, Procrit)	50-100 units/kg IV or SC 3 times/wk	Anemia associated with CRF	Monitor hematocrit twice weekly until maintenance dose is achieved. Monitor blood pressure.	The dose is based on response as measured by hematocrit changes. Rapid rise in hematocrit can cause hypertension.
Phosphate Binders				
Aluminum hydroxide gel (Amphojel, AlternaGEL, Alu-Cap, Nephrox) Aluminum carbonate gel (Basaljel)	500 mg–2 g PO twice to four times daily as tablets, capsules, or oral suspension	Phosphate binder Prevention of renal osteodystrophy	Monitor for constipation, which occurs frequently. Monitor for signs of hypophosphatemia. Monitor serum aluminum levels.	Constipation is a frequent side effect of many drugs that bind phosphorus. These drugs can prevent intestinal absorption of phosphorus to the extent that the client develops hypophosphatemia. Aluminum toxicity may cause bone disease and dementia.
Sevelamer hydrochloride (Renagel)	Serum phosphorus 6.0-7.5 mg/dL: 2 capsules three times daily Serum phosphorus 7.6-8.9 mg/dL: 3 capsules three times daily Serum phosphorus >9.0 mg/dL: 4 capsules three times daily	Hyperphosphatemia	Give with meals. Tell client to swallow capsule whole; do not chew. Monitor serum phosphorus levels.	Drug binds with phosphorus in food, preventing absorption. Drug expands when capsule is broken. Drug can cause hypophosphatemia.
Calcium carbonate (Tums, OsCal, CalciChew)	1-3 tablets PO daily (in divided doses three or four times daily)	Dietary supplement Phosphate binder	Give only when serum phosphate levels are normal. Monitor for hypercalcemia, constipation, and soft-tissue calcifications. Give after meals.	Calcium supplements may cause a *decrease* in serum phosphate levels because these two minerals exist in blood in a balanced, *reciprocal* relationship. Giving binders after meals enhances binding capacity.
Stool Softeners and Laxatives				
Docusate sodium (Colace)	100-300 mg daily	Prevention of constipation caused by limited fluid intake, iron supplements, and phosphate binders	Observe for abdominal cramps and diarrhea. Monitor bowel movements.	These gastrointestinal effects indicate drug overdose. Monitoring bowel movements is a way of determining medication effectiveness.
Bisacodyl (Dulcolax, Bisco-Lax, Laxit ✽)	5-10 mg PO or PR daily or every other day			

Med Error Alert! Watch dose; it is very low (0.125-0.25 mg).

SC, Subcutaneous.

BEST PRACTICE for
Administering Renal-Dose Dopamine

- Take an accurate weight because the dose is prescribed according to the client's weight.
- Know the hospital's policy regarding who is responsible for calculating the rate of infusion (i.e., physician, pharmacist, or nurse). Renal-dose dopamine is 1 to 5 mcg per kilogram of body weight per minute but is converted to mL/min for an IV infusion.
- Before hanging the dopamine infusion, double-check the amount of dopamine added to the solution, the total volume of solution (usually 250 mL), and the calculation milliliters per minute.
- Do not hang the dopamine infusion until all questions about the calculation are clarified.
- If dopamine is to be infused into a peripheral vein, be sure that the line is intact and secured.
- Once the infusion is started, check the client's blood pressure and pulse according to hospital policy or at least every 2 hours.
- Notify the physician of changes in vital signs per policy.
- Monitor the IV site hourly for infiltration.
- If infiltration occurs, stop the infusion but do not discontinue the IV catheter. Prepare for phentolamine (Regitine, Rogitine✱) administration through the IV catheter and subcutaneously into the infiltrated tissue.

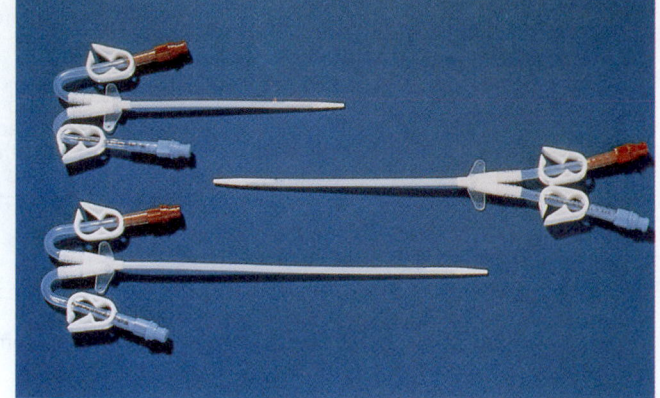

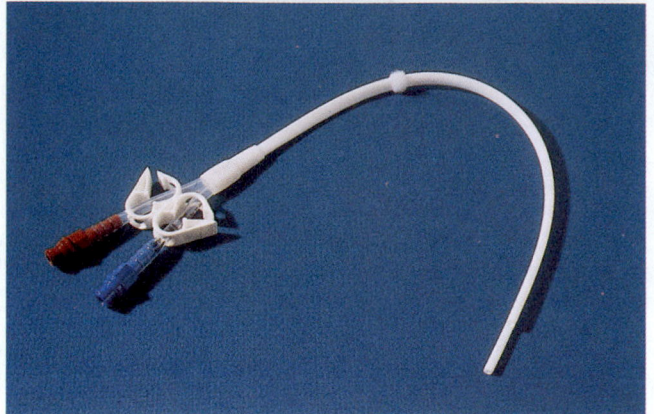

Figure 75-1 ■ Subclavian dialysis catheters. These catheters are radiopaque tubes that can be used for hemodialysis access. The Y-shape tubing allows arterial outflow and venous return through a single catheter. **A,** Mahurkar catheters, made of polyurethane and used for short-term access. **B,** A PermCath catheter, which is made of silicone and used for long-term access. (Courtesy of Kendall Company, Bothell, WA.)

weeks, the catheter is usually placed in the subclavian or internal jugular vein. If only one or two HD treatments are needed, as for removal of drugs or toxins, a femoral site may be selected. Longer use of the femoral site is discouraged because the client's mobility is restricted and complications, such as hematomas and infection, are common. Repeatedly accessing the femoral site increases the risk for hematoma formation and makes repeated use of the vein impossible.

The subclavian vein is preferred over the femoral site because the catheter can be left in place between dialysis treatments. However, the longer the catheter is left in this place, the greater the chance for infection. The subclavian dialysis catheter (Figure 75-1) is inserted at the bedside. A physician or nurse practitioner performs the sterile procedure, and then the catheter is covered with a sterile dressing. Catheter placement is checked by chest x-ray before its use.

If hemodialysis is needed for more than a few days, a long-term dialysis catheter may be used. Most of these catheters are placed in the radiology department using a tunneling technique. The client receives moderate sedation. Under sonographic or fluoroscopic guidance, the physician makes a small incision where the internal jugular vein passes behind the clavicle. A 6- to 8-cm subcutaneous tunnel is created out from the side of the incision. A long-term hemodialysis catheter is inserted through the tunnel and into the jugular vein. Keeping a segment of the catheter within the subcutaneous tissues before entering the jugular vein reduces the risk for infection.

Hemodialysis catheters have two lumens, one for outflow and one for inflow. As a result, the outflow of blood for dialysis is separated from the dialyzed blood returned through the inflow lumen. A triple-lumen catheter for HD is available. The third lumen is an access for drawing venous blood or giving drugs and fluid without interruption of dialysis.

Peritoneal dialysis (PD) may also be used in the treatment of ARF, although some clients, such as those being mechanically ventilated, may not be able to tolerate the accompanying abdominal distention. PD uses the peritoneum as the dialyzing membrane. The dialysate is infused through a catheter implanted in the peritoneum. A complete discussion of PD is provided later in this chapter under Chronic Renal Failure, pp. 1757 to 1759).

Continuous Renal Replacement Therapy. Continuous renal replacement therapies (CRRTs) are the standard treatment for ARF. Renal replacement therapies in the form of hemofiltration are often better tolerated than HD for critically ill clients because this method avoids rapid shifts of fluids and electrolytes.

Continuous arteriovenous hemofiltration (CAVH) and continuous arteriovenous hemodialysis and filtration (CAVHD) are additional renal replacement therapies for clients with ARF. These procedures are similar to HD, but indications for their use are more specific.

CAVH is indicated for clients who have fluid volume overload, are resistant to diuretics, and are hemodynamically unstable. The use of CAVH requires placement of both arterial and venous catheters, and a mean arterial pressure of at least 60 mm Hg. CAVH continuously removes large amounts of plasma water, wastes, and electrolytes. Electrolytes are replaced through prescribed amounts of IV electrolyte solutions. A major disadvantage of arteriovenous (AV) filtration is the risk for bleeding caused by anticoagulants used to prevent membrane clotting.

A double-lumen dialysis catheter inserted into a large vein (subclavian, jugular) is the access for CAVHD. CAVHD uses a **dialysate** (a solution composed of water, glucose, sodium chloride, potassium, magnesium, calcium, and bicarbonate) delivery system to remove waste products in addition to plasma water in clients with limited cardiac output, those with severe hypotension, or those who do not respond to diuretic therapy. These clients cannot tolerate standard HD, and PD would be inadequate for the fluid removal required.

Continuous venovenous hemofiltration (CVVH) is often the treatment of choice for critically ill clients. CVVH uses only a double-lumen venous catheter for access and is powered by a pump, making the rate of filtration more reliable than methods using mean arterial pressure. The pump increases the risk for an air embolus, but most pumps have alarms that detect air. These systems also require the use of anticoagulants, but at lower doses than needed for AV systems. These procedures are used in critical care units, and clients require continuous nursing care.

Posthospital Care. The care for a client with ARF after discharge from the hospital varies widely, depending on the status of the disease when the client is discharged. The course of ARF varies, with recovery lasting up to several months. If the renal failure is resolving, follow-up care may be provided by a nephrologist or by the family physician in consultation with the nephrologist. However, ARF may result in permanent renal damage and the need for chronic dialysis or even transplantation. In these cases, follow-up care is similar to that needed for clients with chronic renal failure (see Community-Based Care, p. 1763).

If the ARF is beginning to resolve, the follow-up care may involve many services. Frequent medical visits are necessary, as are scheduled laboratory blood and urine tests to monitor renal function. A dietary consult is needed to modify the client's diet according to the degree of renal function and ongoing nutritional requirements. Teach clients continuing dialysis after discharge to limit foods high in potassium and sodium and to observe protein restrictions. Also teach about any needed fluid intake limitation.

Some clients may need temporary dialysis until their kidneys can eliminate fluid and waste products. The dialysis started while the client was an inpatient can be continued at an outpatient dialysis center. Teaching about the type of dialysis, how to care for vascular access sites, dietary restrictions, fluid restrictions, and prevention of complications is ongoing throughout the recovery phase. Depending on their level of independence and family support, some clients may also need home care nursing or social work assistance.

Critical Thinking Challenge

The client is a 32-year-old woman who was struck by a car while jogging on a country road during the afternoon of a very hot day. When she arrives at the emergency department by ambulance 3 hours after the accident, she is able to talk, does not have an IV, and is in extreme pain. She tells you that she had been jogging for an hour when she was hit. Her husband tells you that she is in great health and works full-time as an aerobics

---

CHART 75-5

KEY FEATURES of
Uremia

- Metallic taste in the mouth
- Anorexia
- Nausea
- Vomiting
- Muscle cramps
- Itching
- Fatigue and lethargy
- Hiccups
- Edema
- Dyspnea
- Muscle cramps
- Paresthesias

---

instructor. She is 5 feet 1 inch tall and weighs 110 lb. Her only drugs include oral contraceptives, a multivitamin, and 800 mg daily of ibuprofen. She has a compound fracture of her left femur and considerable bruising on left hip and pelvis. Her vital signs are T 99.4, P 116 and thready, R 30, and BP 90/58.

1. For what type(s) of acute renal failure is she at risk? Why?
2. Do any of her usual drugs increase her risk for ARF? Which one(s) and why?
3. Is there any specific assessment data you could obtain without a prescription to evaluate her risk for acute renal failure?

The physician prescribes the following interventions:
- IV placement with an 18-gauge cannula, NS at 200 mL/hr
- Hematocrit and hemoglobin levels
- Morphine sulfate 2 mg IV push
- Foley catheter placement
- Type and crossmatch for 4 units of packed red blood cells
- X-rays of the left hip and leg and KUB

4. In what order (and why) should you perform these interventions?

evolve For suggested answer guidelines, go to http://evolve.elsevier.com/Iggy/.

CHRONIC RENAL FAILURE

PATHOPHYSIOLOGY

Unlike ARF, chronic renal failure (CRF) is a progressive, irreversible kidney injury. Kidney function does not recover. When kidney function is too poor to sustain life, CRF is termed *end-stage renal disease* (ESRD). Terms used with renal failure include **azotemia** (collection of nitrogenous wastes in the blood), **uremia** (azotemia with clinical symptoms [Chart 75-5]), and **uremic syndrome** (the systemic clinical and laboratory manifestations of ESRD). ARF and CRF are compared in Table 75-1.

Stages of Chronic Renal Failure

The kidneys fail in an organized fashion. Progression toward ESRD usually starts with a gradual decrease in renal function of 30% to 50% (Table 75-6). At first, there is a *diminished renal reserve*. A 24-hour urine specimen for monitoring creatinine clearance is used to detect that renal reserve is less than normal. In this stage, reduced renal function occurs without accumulation of metabolic wastes in the blood because the unaffected nephrons overwork to compensate for the diseased nephrons. Renal damage increases systemic blood pressure, which also increases glomerular pressure and the pressure in remaining unaffected nephrons. Eventually the unaffected nephrons may be damaged by this long-term increased pressure, causing the progressive renal

TABLE 75-6 Progression Toward Chronic Renal Failure

Stage I: Diminished Renal Reserve
- Renal function is reduced, but no accumulation of metabolic wastes occurs.
- The healthier kidney compensates for the diseased kidney.
- Ability to concentrate urine is decreased, resulting in nocturia and polyuria.
- A 24-hour urine collection for creatinine clearance is necessary to detect that renal reserve is less than normal.

Stage II: Renal Insufficiency
- Metabolic wastes begin to accumulate in the blood because the unaffected nephrons can no longer compensate.
- Responsiveness to diuretics is decreased, resulting in oliguria and edema.
- The degree of insufficiency is determined by the decreasing GFR and is classified as mild, moderate, or severe.
- Treatment is medical.

Stage III: End-Stage Renal Disease
- Excessive amounts of metabolic wastes such as urea and creatinine accumulate in the blood.
- The kidneys are unable to maintain homeostasis.
- Treatment is by dialysis or other renal replacement therapy.

GFR, Glomerular filtration rate.

damage of CRF. Although no manifestations of renal failure are usually present at this stage, if the client is stressed with infection, fluid overload, or dehydration, renal function at this stage can appear reduced.

In the next stage, *renal insufficiency*, metabolic wastes begin to collect in the blood because not enough healthy nephrons remain to compensate completely for the non-functioning nephrons. Levels of blood urea nitrogen (BUN), serum creatinine, uric acid, and phosphorus are elevated in proportion to the amount of nephrons lost. Careful management of fluid volume, blood pressure, electrolytes, dietary intake, and drug therapy slows, but does not halt, the progression of renal failure.

Over time most clients progress to ESRD. Excessive amounts of urea and creatinine build up in the blood, and the kidneys cannot maintain homeostasis. Severe fluid, electrolyte, and acid-base imbalances occur. Without renal replacement therapy, fatal complications are likely.

Kidney Changes

Renal failure causes many problems, including decreased glomerular filtration rate (GFR), abnormal urine production, poor water excretion, electrolyte imbalances, and metabolic abnormalities. Because the healthy nephrons hypertrophy and work harder, the kidneys can maintain an effective GFR until 70% to 80% of renal function is lost. Homeostasis is maintained until late in the course of renal failure. When fewer than 20% of the nephrons are functional, the GFR is decreased despite hypertrophy of the remaining nephrons. This problem occurs because the hypertrophied nephrons can maintain waste excretion only by decreasing water reabsorption. Thus, at this stage of renal failure, **hyposthenuria** (the loss of urine concentrating ability) and **polyuria** (increased urine output) occur. Both hyposthenuria and polyuria are early signs of CRF and, if the problem is untreated at this stage, can cause severe dehydration.

As the disease progresses, the ability to produce dilute urine is reduced, resulting in urine with a fixed osmolarity

(isosthenuria). As renal function continues to decline, the BUN increases and urine output decreases. When renal function declines to this level, the client is at risk for fluid overload.

Metabolic Changes

UREA AND CREATININE

Renal failure disrupts urea and creatinine excretion. Creatinine is derived from creatine and phosphocreatine, which are present in skeletal muscle. The normal rate of creatinine excretion depends on muscle mass, physical activity, and diet. Without major changes in diet or physical activity, the serum creatinine level remains constant. Creatinine is partially excreted by the renal tubules, and a decrease in renal function leads to a buildup of serum creatinine. Urea is a product of protein metabolism and is excreted by the kidneys. The BUN level normally varies directly with protein intake.

The method for assessing the GFR is to measure the creatinine clearance. As renal function and GFR decline, creatinine clearance decreases and blood creatinine levels rise (see Chapter 72).

SODIUM

Changes in sodium excretion are common. Early in CRF, the client is at risk for hyponatremia (sodium depletion) because reduced numbers of functional nephrons are present to reabsorb sodium; thus sodium is lost in the urine. The polyuria often seen in early renal failure also causes sodium depletion.

In the later stages of renal failure, kidney excretion of sodium is reduced as urine production decreases. Then sodium retention and hypernatremia can occur with only modest increases in dietary sodium intake. This problem leads to severe fluid and electrolyte imbalances (see Chapters 15 and 16). Sodium retention causes hypertension and edema.

Even with sodium retention, the serum sodium level may appear normal because plasma water is retained at the same time. If fluid retention occurs at a greater rate than sodium retention, the serum sodium level is falsely low (hyponatremia) because of dilution (see Table 75-5).

POTASSIUM

The kidney is responsible for potassium excretion. Any increase in potassium load during the later stages of renal disease can lead to **hyperkalemia** (excessive potassium retention). Normal serum potassium levels of 3.5 to 5 mEq/L are maintained until the 24-hour urine output falls below 500 mL. Hyperkalemia then develops quickly, and serum potassium levels may reach 7 to 8 mEq/L or greater. Severe electrocardiographic (ECG) changes result from this elevation, and fatal dysrhythmias can occur. Other factors contribute to hyperkalemia in renal failure, including the ingestion of potassium in drugs, failure to restrict potassium in the diet, tissue breakdown, blood transfusions, and bleeding or hemorrhage. (See Chapter 16 for discussion of hyperkalemia.)

ACID-BASE BALANCE

In the early stage of renal failure, blood pH changes little because the remaining healthy nephrons increase their rate of acid excretion. As more nephrons are lost, acid excretion is reduced and metabolic acidosis results (see Chapter 19).

Many factors lead to metabolic acidosis in renal failure. First the kidneys are unable to excrete excessive hydrogen ions (acids). Normally, tubular cells move hydrogen ions into the urine for excretion, but ammonium and bicarbonate are needed for this movement to occur. In clients with renal failure, ammonium production is decreased and reabsorption of bicarbonate does not occur. This process leads to a buildup of hydrogen ions and reduced levels of bicarbonate (base deficit). In the presence of hyperkalemia, renal ammonium production and excretion are further inhibited.

As renal failure advances and acid retention increases, respiratory compensation is needed to keep blood pH normal. The respiratory system compensates for the decreased blood pH levels by increasing the rate and depth of breathing to excrete carbon dioxide through the lungs. This breathing pattern, called **Kussmaul respiration,** increases with worsening renal failure. Although hydrogen ions (acids) can leave the body this way, when too much carbon dioxide is "blown off," respiratory alkalosis results. Serum bicarbonate measures the extent of metabolic acidosis (bicarbonate deficit). Clients with CRF usually need alkali replacement to counteract acidosis.

CALCIUM AND PHOSPHORUS

A complex, balanced reciprocal relationship between calcium and phosphate is influenced by vitamin D (see Chapter 16). The kidney produces a hormone needed to activate vitamin D, which then enhances intestinal absorption of calcium.

In renal failure, phosphate retention and a deficiency of active vitamin D disrupt the calcium and phosphate balance. Normally, excessive dietary phosphate is excreted by the kidneys in the urine. Parathyroid hormone (PTH) controls the amount of phosphate in the blood by causing tubular excretion of phosphate when there is an excess. An early effect of CRF is reduced phosphate excretion (Figure 75-2). As plasma phosphate levels increase **(hyperphosphatemia),** calcium levels decrease **(hypocalcemia).** Chronic hypocalcemia causes chronic stimulation of the parathyroid glands. Under the influence of additional PTH, calcium is released from storage areas in bones **(bone resorption),** which results in bone demineralization and bone density loss. The additional calcium is needed to compensate, or balance, the excess plasma phosphate level. The problem of hypocalcemia is compounded because decreased renal function also causes decreased production of active vitamin D. Thus less calcium is absorbed through the intestinal tract in the absence of sufficient vitamin D.

The problems in bone metabolism and structure caused by renal failure-induced hypocalcemia and hyperphosphatemia are called **renal osteodystrophy.** Bone mineral loss from hyperparathyroidism causes bone pain, spinal sclerosis, fractures, bone density loss, osteomalacia, and tooth calcium loss.

Metastatic calcifications, crystals formed from excessive calcium phosphate, may precipitate in various parts of the body. When the plasma level of the calcium-phosphate product (serum calcium level multiplied by the serum phosphate level) exceeds 70 mg/dL, the crystals may lodge in the kidneys, heart, lungs, major blood vessels, joints, eyes (causing

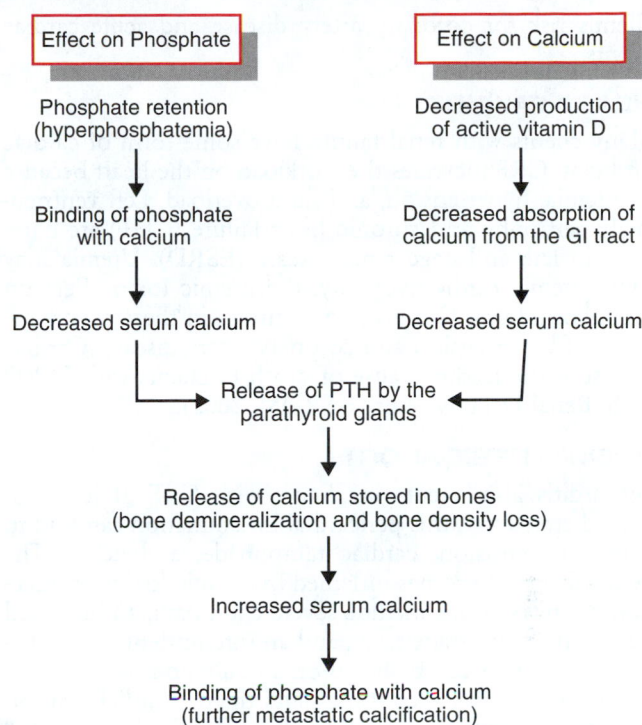

Figure 75-2 ■ The effects of renal failure on phosphate and calcium balance.

conjunctivitis), and brain. Uremic pruritus also results from calcium-phosphate imbalances and excess PTH production.

Cardiac Changes

HYPERTENSION

Most clients with CRF have hypertension. Hypertension may be either the cause or the result of CRF. In clients who have nonrenal causes of hypertension, the increased blood pressure damages the delicate capillaries in the glomerulus, and eventually renal failure results.

Renal failure itself elevates blood pressure by causing fluid and sodium overload and the malfunction of the renin-angiotensin-aldosterone system. The retention of sodium and water causes circulatory overload, which elevates blood pressure. The kidneys respond to a decrease in renal blood flow or to low serum sodium levels by trying to improve the renal blood flow. The release of renin stimulates the production of angiotensin and aldosterone. Angiotensin causes blood vessel constriction and increases blood pressure. Aldosterone, a hormone released by the adrenal glands, stimulates kidney tubules to reabsorb sodium and water. This action expands plasma volume and raises blood pressure. The damaged kidneys do not recognize the increase in blood pressure and continue to produce renin. The result is severe hypertension that is difficult to treat and worsens renal function. Many clients with CRF also have cardiomyopathy and left ventricular hypertrophy from the prolonged hypertension.

HYPERLIPIDEMIA

Chronic renal failure (CRF) changes fat metabolism, resulting in increased triglyceride, total cholesterol, and low-density lipoprotein (LDL) levels. These changes increase the client's risk for coronary artery disease and acute cardiac events.

HEART FAILURE

Many clients with renal failure have some form of cardiac problem. CRF increases the workload on the heart because of anemia, hypertension, and fluid overload. Left ventricular hypertrophy and chronic heart failure (CHF) are common in late end-stage renal disease (ESRD). Uremia may cause uremic cardiomyopathy, the uremic toxin effect on the myocardium. CHF is also common in these clients because of hypertension and coronary artery disease. Cardiac disease is the leading cause of death in clients with ESRD (U.S. Renal Data Systems [USRDS], 2002).

UREMIC PERICARDITIS

Pericarditis also occurs in clients with CRF. If it is not treated effectively, this pericardial inflammation can lead to pericardial effusion, cardiac tamponade, and death. The pericardial sac becomes inflamed by uremic toxins or infection. Manifestations include severe chest pain, an increased pulse rate, a low-grade fever, and an intermittent pericardial friction rub that can be heard on auscultation.

As the pericarditis continues and the pericardial effusion worsens, dysrhythmias may develop. The fluid around the heart makes heart tones softer and harder to hear. Blood pressure decreases, and the client may have shortness of breath. If left untreated, pericardial effusion causes cardiac tamponade, an emergency in which pulse pressure decreases and bradycardia or asystole results. Treatment of pericardial tamponade requires removal of pericardial fluid by placement of a needle, catheter, or drainage tube into the pericardium.

Hematologic Changes

Anemia is a common problem in clients with CRF, and it worsens the CRF manifestations. The causes of anemia include a decreased erythropoietin level that decreases red blood cell (RBC) production, decreased RBC survival time resulting from uremia, iron and folic acid deficiencies, and increased bleeding as a result of uremia-induced impaired platelet function.

Gastrointestinal Changes

Uremia affects the entire gastrointestinal (GI) system. The normal flora of the mouth changes with uremia. The mouth contains the enzyme urease, which breaks down urea into ammonia. The ammonia generated from this reaction causes uremic halitosis and may also cause uremic **stomatitis** (mouth inflammation).

Anorexia, nausea, vomiting, and hiccups are common in clients with uremia. The specific cause of these problems is unknown but may be related to high BUN and creatinine levels as well as acidosis.

Peptic ulcer disease is also common in clients with uremia; however, the exact cause is unclear. Uremic colitis with profound watery diarrhea or constipation may also be present in clients with uremia. Ulcerations may occur in the stomach or small or large intestine, causing erosion of blood vessels. The blood loss caused by these erosions may result in melena or, in more serious cases, hemorrhagic shock from severe GI bleeding.

TABLE 75-7 Selected Causes of Chronic Renal Failure	
Morphologic	**Etiologic**
Glomerular Disease	***Infection***
■ Glomerulonephritis	■ Pyelonephritis
■ Basement membrane disease	■ Tuberculosis
■ Goodpasture's syndrome	
■ Intercapillary glomerulosclerosis	***Systemic Vascular Disease***
	■ Intrarenal renovascular
Tubular Disease	hypertension
■ Chronic hypercalcemia	■ Extrarenal renovascular
■ Chronic potassium depletion	hypertension
■ Fanconi's syndrome	
■ Heavy metal (lead) poisoning	***Metabolic Renal Disease***
	■ Amyloidosis
Vascular Disease of the Kidney	■ Gout (hyperuricemic
■ Ischemic disease of the kidney	nephropathy)
■ Bilateral renal artery stenosis	■ Diabetic nephropathy
■ Nephrosclerosis	■ Milk-alkali syndrome
■ Hyperparathyroidism	■ Sarcoidosis
Urinary Tract Disease	***Connective Tissue Disease***
■ Obstructive uropathy	■ Progressive systemic
	sclerosis
Inherited or Genetic Conditions	■ Systemic lupus erythematosus
■ Hypoplastic kidneys	■ Polyarteritis
■ Medullary cystic disease	
■ Polycystic kidney disease	

NOTE: List is not all inclusive.

Etiology and Genetic Risk

The causes of CRF are complex (Table 75-7). More than 100 different disease processes can result in progressive loss of renal function (see also Chapter 74). Three main causes of ESRD include diabetes mellitus (43.4%), hypertension (25.5%), and glomerulonephritis (8.4%) (USRDS, 2002). African American clients are four times more likely to develop ESRD and seven times more likely to have hypertensive ESRD.

Although not a common cause of CRF, a variety of genetic disorders can affect renal function. Polycystic kidney disease (PKD) (see Chapter 74) is a hereditary renal disorder in adults that leads to CRF. PKD has both an autosomal-dominant and an autosomal-recessive pattern of inheritance.

Incidence/Prevalence

The number of clients with CRF is increasing. The 2002 U.S. Renal Data Systems annual report stated that more than 375,000 people in the United States are receiving treatment for ESRD. In 2002 the reported incidence of renal disease (new clients per year requiring renal replacement therapy) was close to 100,000. More than 75,000 deaths related to ESRD occurred in 2002. ESRD occurs more often in men than in women (USRDS, 2002). The greatest increase in ESRD is in clients 65 years of age and older. Chart 75-6 addresses the prevention of renal and urinary problems. In 2002 more than 275,000 people were estimated to be receiving renal replacement therapy in the United States (USRDS, 2002).

HEALTH PROMOTION/ILLNESS PREVENTION

The health-promotion activities to prevent or delay the onset of chronic renal failure (CRF) focus on controlling the diseases that lead to its development, such as diabetes mel-

CHART 75-6

CLIENT EDUCATION GUIDE
Prevention of Renal and Urinary Problems

- Be alert to the general appearance of your urine. Note any changes in its color, clarity, or odor.
- Changes in the frequency or volume of urine passage occur with changes in fluid intake. More frequent, or infrequent, voiding not associated with changes in fluid intake may signal potential problems.
- Any discomfort or distress with the passage of urine is not normal. Pain, burning, urgency, aching, or difficulty with initiating urine flow or complete bladder emptying is of some concern.
- The kidneys need 1 to 2 quarts of fluid a day to flush out your body wastes. Water is the ideal flushing agent.
- Reduce your intake of soda pop soft drinks.
- Changes in kidney function are often silent for many years. Periodically ask your health care provider to measure your kidney function with a blood test (serum creatinine) and a urinalysis.
- If you have a history or renal disease, diabetes mellitus, hypertension (high blood pressure), or a family history of kidney disease, you should know your serum creatinine level and your 24-hour creatinine clearance. At least one checkup per year that includes laboratory blood and urine testing of kidney function is recommended.
- If you are identified as having decreased kidney function, ask about whether any prescribed medication, diet, diagnostic test, or therapeutic procedure will present a risk to your current kidney function. Check out all nonprescription medications with your physician or pharmacist before using them.

litus and hypertension. Identifying clients who have these disorders at an early stage is critical to CRF prevention. Client education to promote adherence to drug and diet regimens and engaging in regular physical activity are key in preventing the blood vessel changes that lead to kidney damage. Teach clients with diabetes to keep their blood glucose levels within the prescribed range. Teach clients with hypertension that drug therapy is not a cure and must be continued. Encourage clients with diabetes or hypertension to have yearly testing for microalbuminuria.

Teach everyone treated for an infection anywhere in the renal/urinary system to take all antibiotics as prescribed. Encourage everyone to drink at least 3 L of water daily unless a health problem requires fluid restriction. Caution people who use over-the-counter nonsteroidal anti-inflammatory drugs (NSAIDs) to avoid abusing these drugs because they reduce renal perfusion and their long-term use reduces kidney function.

◆COLLABORATIVE MANAGEMENT
◆Assessment

HISTORY

When taking a history from a client with suspected chronic renal failure (CRF), focus on the manifestations of CRF. Document the client's age and gender. Obtain accurate weight and height measurements, and ask about usual weight and recent weight gain or loss. Weight gain may indicate fluid retention caused by poorly functioning kidneys. Weight loss may be the result of anorexia from uremic syndrome.

Obtain a complete history of known renal or urologic disorders, long-term health problems, drug use, and current health problems. Ask the client about any existing renal disease or family history of renal disease that might indicate a hereditary disorder. A history of kidney infection or stones may imply past kidney damage. Explore the possibility of long-term health problems because illnesses such as hypertension, diabetes, systemic lupus erythematosus, arthritis, cancer, and tuberculosis can cause decreased renal function.

Document the use of prescription and over-the-counter drugs because many drugs are nephrotoxic and can cause renal damage.

Examine the client's nutritional habits and discuss any present GI problems. A change in the taste of foods often occurs with CRF. Clients may report that sweet foods are not as appealing or that meats have a metallic taste. Ask about the presence of nausea, vomiting, anorexia, hiccups, diarrhea, or constipation. These manifestations may be the result of excess wastes that the body cannot excrete because of renal malfunction.

Ask the client about his or her energy level and any recent injuries or bleeding. Explore changes in the client's daily routine as a possible *result* of fatigue. Weakness, drowsiness, and shortness of breath suggest impending pulmonary edema or neurologic degeneration. Ask about bruising or bleeding, which can be caused by hematologic changes from uremia.

Discuss the client's urine elimination in detail, including frequency of urination, appearance of the urine, and any difficulty starting or controlling urination. These data can help to identify existing urologic disorders that may influence the preservation of existing renal function.

PHYSICAL ASSESSMENT/CLINICAL MANIFESTATIONS

Chronic renal failure (CRF) causes changes in many body systems (Chart 75-7). Most manifestations are related to changes in fluid volume, electrolyte and acid-base imbalances, and buildup of nitrogenous wastes.

NEUROLOGIC MANIFESTATIONS. Neurologic manifestations of CRF and uremic syndrome are numerous (see Chart 75-7) and vary widely. Observe for problems ranging from lethargy to seizures or coma, which indicate uremic encephalopathy. Assess for sensory changes that appear in a glove and stocking pattern over the hands and feet. Check for weakness in the upper or lower extremities (e.g., uremic neuropathy).

If untreated, uremic encephalopathy progresses to seizures and coma. Dialysis is used to treat CRF when neurologic problems result. The manifestations of uremic encephalopathy resolve with dialysis. However, improvement in neuropathy is limited if the neuropathy is severe and motor function is impaired.

CARDIOVASCULAR MANIFESTATIONS. The manifestations of CRF and uremia cause fluid volume excess, hypertension, heart failure (HF), uremic pericarditis, and potassium-induced dysrhythmias. Assess for signs of reduced sodium and water excretion. Circulatory fluid overload, if untreated, leads to HF, pulmonary edema, peripheral edema, and hypertension.

Assess heart rate and rhythm, listening for extra beats (particularly an S_3), irregular patterns, or a pericardial friction rub. Unless a hemodialysis (HD) vascular access has been created, measure blood pressure in each arm. Assess the jugular veins

CHART 75-7

KEY FEATURES of
Chronic Renal Failure

Neurologic Manifestations
- Lethargy and daytime drowsiness
- Inability to concentrate or decreased attention span
- Seizures
- Coma
- Slurred speech
- Asterixis
- Tremors, twitching, or jerky movements
- Myoclonus
- Ataxia (alteration in gait)
- Paresthesias

Cardiovascular Manifestations
- Cardiomyopathy
- Hypertension
- Peripheral edema
- Heart failure
- Uremic pericarditis
- Pericardial effusion
- Pericardial friction rub
- Cardiac tamponade

Respiratory Manifestations
- Uremic halitosis
- Tachypnea
- Deep sighing, yawning
- Kussmaul respirations
- Uremic pneumonitis
- Shortness of breath
- Pulmonary edema
- Pleural effusion
- Depressed cough reflex
- Crackles

Hematologic Manifestations
- Anemia
- Abnormal bleeding and bruising

Gastrointestinal Manifestations
- Anorexia
- Nausea
- Vomiting
- Metallic taste in the mouth
- Changes in taste acuity and sensation
- Uremic colitis (diarrhea)
- Constipation
- Uremic gastritis (possible GI bleeding)
- Uremic fetor
- Stomatitis
- Diarrhea

Urinary Manifestations
- Polyuria, nocturia (early)
- Oliguria, anuria (later)
- Proteinuria
- Hematuria
- Diluted, strawlike appearance

Integumentary Manifestations
- Decreased skin turgor
- Yellow-gray pallor
- Dry skin
- Pruritus
- Ecchymosis
- Purpura
- Soft-tissue calcifications
- Uremic frost (late, premorbid)

Musculoskeletal Manifestations
- Muscle weakness and cramping
- Bone pain
- Pathologic fractures
- Renal osteodystrophy

Reproductive Manifestations
- Decreased fertility
- Infrequent or absent menses
- Decreased libido
- Impotence

GI, Gastrointestinal.

for distention, and assess for pedal, pretibial, presacral, and periorbital edema. Shortness of breath with exertion and nocturnal dyspnea suggest fluid volume excess.

RESPIRATORY MANIFESTATIONS. Respiratory manifestations of CRF vary widely (e.g., breath that smells like urine [*uremic fetor* or uremic halitosis], deep sighing, yawning, shortness of breath). Observe the rhythm, rate, and depth of breathing. **Tachypnea** (increased rate of breathing) and **hyperpnea** (increased depth of breathing) occur with worsening metabolic acidosis.

With severe metabolic acidosis, you may see extreme hyperventilation (Kussmaul respirations). A few clients have hilar pneumonitis, or *uremic lung*. In these clients, assess for thick sputum, minimal coughing, tachypnea, and fever. A pleural friction rub may be heard with a stethoscope. Clients often have pleuritic pain with breathing. Auscultate the lungs for crackles, which indicate fluid volume overload.

HEMATOLOGIC MANIFESTATIONS. Hematologic problems include anemia and abnormal bleeding. Check for indicators of anemia (e.g., fatigue, pallor, lethargy, weakness, shortness of breath, dizziness). Check for abnormal bleeding by observing for bruising, petechiae, purpura, mucous membrane bleeding in the nose or gums, abnormal vaginal bleeding, or intestinal bleeding (black, tarry stools [melena]).

GASTROINTESTINAL MANIFESTATIONS. Assess for foul breath and mouth ulceration or inflammation. Document any abdominal pain, cramping, or vomiting. Test all stools for occult blood.

URINARY MANIFESTATIONS. The urinary findings in renal failure reflect the kidneys' decreasing function. At first changes occur in the amount, frequency, and appearance of the urine. Proteinuria or hematuria also may be present.

The amount and composition of the urine change as renal function decreases. With the onset of end-stage renal disease (ESRD), the urine may be more dilute and clearer as tubular reabsorption is reduced. The actual urine output in a client with CRF varies with the amount of remaining renal function. The client with ESRD usually has oliguria, but some clients remain able to produce 1 L or more per 24 hours. Daily urine volume usually changes again after dialysis is started.

SKIN MANIFESTATIONS. In clients with uremia, urochrome pigment is deposited in the skin, causing a yellowish coloration. Some African Americans report a darkening of the skin. The anemia of CRF causes a sallowness, which appears as a faded suntan on lighter-skinned clients.

Skin oils and turgor are decreased in clients with uremia. A distressing problem of uremia is severe **pruritus** (itching). **Uremic frost,** a layer of urea crystals from evaporated sweat, may appear on the face, eyebrows, axilla, and groin in clients with advanced uremic syndrome. Assess for bruises **(ecchymoses),** purple patches **(purpura),** and rashes.

PSYCHOSOCIAL ASSESSMENT

Chronic renal failure and its treatment disrupt many aspects of a client's life. You are in a unique position to evaluate the client with newly diagnosed renal failure and to assist with adjustments.

Psychosocial assessment and support are part of the nurse's role from the time that CRF is first diagnosed. Ask about the client's understanding of the diagnosis and what the treatment regimen means to him or her (e.g., diet, drugs, dialysis). Assess for anxiety and for the coping styles used by the client or family members. Psychosocial issues affected by CRF include family relations, social activity, work patterns, body image, and sexual activity. The chronicity of

ESRD, the variety of treatment options, and the uncertainties about the course of the disease and its treatment require ongoing psychosocial assessment.

LABORATORY ASSESSMENT

Chronic renal failure causes extreme changes in many laboratory values (see Chart 75-2). Monitor the following blood values: creatinine, blood urea nitrogen (BUN), sodium, potassium, calcium, phosphate, bicarbonate, hemoglobin, and hematocrit.

Initially a urinalysis is performed, and a 24-hour urine specimen for creatinine and urea clearance is obtained. In the early stages of CRF, urinalysis may show excessive protein, glucose, red blood cells (RBCs), white blood cells (WBCs), and decreased or fixed specific gravity. Urine osmolarity is usually decreased. A 24-hour creatinine clearance is calculated after blood and urine creatinine levels are collected and quantified. These data, along with weight and height, are used to calculate renal creatinine clearance. As renal failure progresses, the urine output decreases dramatically.

Changes in renal function are monitored by measurements of the serum creatinine and BUN levels. Serum creatinine levels may increase gradually over a period of years, reaching levels of 15 to 30 mg/dL or more, depending on the client's muscle mass. BUN levels are directly related to dietary protein intake. Without protein restriction, BUN levels may rise 10 to 20 times the value of the serum creatinine level. With dietary protein restriction, BUN levels are elevated but less than those of nonprotein-restricted clients. Fluid balance also affects BUN. Chapter 72 describes the significance of BUN and creatinine levels as well as creatinine clearance.

RADIOGRAPHIC ASSESSMENT

Few x-ray finding are abnormal with CRF. Bone x-rays of the hand can show renal osteodystrophy. With long-term ESRD, the kidneys are atrophic and may be 8 to 9 cm or smaller. This small size results from renal atrophy and fibrosis. If ESRD progresses suddenly, a renal ultrasound or computed tomography (CT) scan without contrast media may be used to rule out an obstruction. (See Chapter 72 for a complete description of renal diagnostic tests.)

> ### 💬 Critical Thinking Challenge
>
> The client is a 77-year-old woman admitted to your unit with suspected CRF. She has had type 2 diabetes for 25 years and is also being treated for hypertension. She admits that when her money is low, she stops buying the blood pressure drugs because she feels that if she has to choose between the two, it is more important to continue her antidiabetic drugs. She says she has noticed that her heartbeat is irregular, her rings and shoes are tight, and that she has gained 8 pounds over the last 10 days.
> 1. What other assessment data should you obtain?
> 2. What risk factors for the development of CRF are noted in her past medical history? Provide a rationale for your choices.
> 3. What cardiac and respiratory manifestations might you find on physical examination of this client?
>
> **evolve** For suggested answer guidelines, go to http://evolve.elsevier.com/Iggy/.

◆ Analysis

The client with CRF has usually had a progressive reduction of renal function and is often hospitalized for adjustment of the treatment plan. The focus of care is to manage symptoms and prevent complications.

COMMON NURSING DIAGNOSES AND COLLABORATIVE PROBLEMS

The following are priority nursing diagnoses for clients with CRF:
1. **Imbalanced Nutrition: Less Than Body Requirements** related to inability to ingest, digest food, or absorb nutrients as a result of physiologic factors
2. **Excess Fluid Volume** related to compromised regulatory mechanisms (inability of the kidneys to maintain body fluid balance)
3. **Decreased Cardiac Output** related to altered stroke volume (reduced) as a result of dysrhythmias and mechanical malfunction (increased preload [excess volume] and increased afterload [increased peripheral vascular resistance])
4. **Risk for Infection** related to inadequate primary defenses (broken skin), chronic disease, or malnutrition
5. **Risk for Injury** related to internal biochemical risk factors associated with renal failure (increased susceptibility to bleeding, falls, and fractures)
6. **Fatigue** related to disease states, altered metabolic energy production, and anemia
7. **Anxiety** related to threat to or change in health status, economic status, relationships, role function, systems, or self-concept; situational crisis; threat of death; lack of knowledge (diagnostic tests, disease process, treatment); loss of control; or disrupted family life

The primary collaborative problem is Potential for Pulmonary Edema.

ADDITIONAL NURSING DIAGNOSES AND COLLABORATIVE PROBLEMS

In addition to the common nursing diagnoses and collaborative problems, clients with CRF may have one or more of the following:

- **Diarrhea** related to chemical or electrolyte imbalances or side effects of drugs
- **Impaired Oral Mucous Membrane** related to limited fluid intake, malnutrition, and elevated levels of uremic toxins
- **Impaired Skin Integrity** related to altered chemical balance and uremic toxins
- **Social Isolation** related to altered state of wellness or alterations in physical appearance
- **Interrupted Family Processes** related to situational crisis, reduced income, unemployment, or effects of chronic illness
- **Sexual Dysfunction** related to altered body function, disease process, effects of drugs, depression, or disturbance in body image
- **Disturbed Thought Processes** related to irritation, central nervous system (CNS) depression, side effects of drugs, sleep deprivation, or clinical depression
- **Deficient Knowledge** (disease process, care regimen, and follow-up care) related to lack of informational resources and magnitude of the care issues
- Potential for Sepsis
- Potential for Malnutrition
- Potential for Electrolyte Imbalances
- Potential for Metabolic Acidosis

CONCEPT MAP End-Stage Renal Disease

End-Stage Renal Disease (ESRD)

Client → **Hiram Slovok**

76-year-old African-American man who has called his physician with fatigue, loss of appetite, and swollen ankles.

Mr. Slovok has a history of:
- High blood pressure for 30 years
- A cerebrovascular accident 5 years ago

When questioned, Mr. Slovok states that he:
- Has occasional "palpitations of my heart"
- Is frequently bothered by dry skin and itching that "nothing seems to help"
- Experiences difficulty breathing with activity
- Has had nosebleeds for the past few months and seems to bruise easily
- Is urinating less frequently

Laboratory Results
Anemia
Hyperkalemia
Elevated serum creatinine
Elevated blood urea nitrogen

Assess →
Hypertension (+)
Diabetes mellitus
Glomerulonephritis
African American (+)

Clinical manifestations

Central Nervous System
Lethargy/seizures (?)
Glove/stocking sensory changes (?)
Cardiovascular
Fatigue (+)
Cardiac dysrhythmia (+)
Peripheral edema (+)
Hematologic
Fatigue (+)
Ecchymosis (+)
Epistaxis (+)
Respiratory
Shortness of breath (+)
Gastrointestinal
Weight loss (?)
Anorexia (+)
Skin
Pruritus (+)
Ecchymosis (+)
Renal
Oliguria (+)
Diagnostic Tests
Hemoglobin = 9 g
BUN = 120 mg
Serum creatinine = 5.5 mg
Serum potassium = 6 mEq/L

Legend:
- Assessment data
- Nursing diagnoses
- Nursing interventions
- Client outcomes

Analyze →

Imbalanced Nutrition: Less Than Body Requirements — Plan → NIC Nutrition Management (Protein/potassium/sodium/phosphorus restriction; Vitamin supplementation; Refer to dietitian)
Evaluate → NOC Nutritional Status: Nutrient Intake

Excess Fluid Volume — Plan → NIC Fluid/Electrolyte Management (Diuretics; Fluid restriction)
Evaluate → NOC Electrolyte & Acid/Base Balance Fluid Balance

Decreased Cardiac Output — Plan → NIC Hemodialysis Therapy (ACE inhibitors, Calcium channel blockers, Alpha/beta-adrenergic blockers, Vasodilators)
Evaluate → NOC Circulation Status

Risk for Infection — Plan → NIC Infection Protection Dialysis Access Maintenance
Evaluate → NOC Hemodialysis Access

Risk for Injury — Plan → NIC Environmental Management: Safety
Evaluate → NOC Risk Control

Fatigue — Plan → NIC Energy Management (Erythropoetin iron)
Evaluate → NOC Activity Tolerance Energy Conservation

Anxiety — Plan → NIC Coping Enhancement — Evaluate → NOC Coping

Concept Map by Elaine Bishop Kennedy, EdD, RN

Planning and Implementation

The Concept Map above addresses care issues related to clients who have end-stage renal disease (ESRD).

IMBALANCED NUTRITION: LESS THAN BODY REQUIREMENTS

NOC **PLANNING: EXPECTED OUTCOMES.** The client with CRF is expected to attain and maintain adequate nutrition. Indicators include that the client should have mild or no deviation from the normal ranges for the following parameters:
- Food intake
- Weight-height ratio
- Muscle tone
- Laboratory values (serum albumin, hematocrit, hemoglobin)

INTERVENTIONS. The nutritional needs and diet restrictions for the client with CRF vary according to the degree of remaining renal function and the type of renal replacement therapy used (Table 75-8).

Nutrition Therapy. The purpose of nutrition therapy is to provide the food and fluids needed to support the metabolism for a client who is at high risk for becoming malnourished. Clients starting hemodialysis (HD) have an increase in catabolism and a decrease in intake that results

TABLE 75-8 Dietary Restrictions for the Client with Renal Failure

Dietary Component	With Chronic Uremia	With Hemodialysis	With Peritoneal Dialysis
Protein	0.55-0.60 g/kg/day	1.0-1.5 g/kg/day	1.2-1.5 g/kg/day
Fluid	Depends on urine output, but may be as high as 1500-3000 mL/day	500-700 mL/day plus amount of urine output	Restriction based on fluid weight gain and blood
Potassium	60-70 mEq/day	70 mEq/day	Usually no restriction
Sodium	1-3 g/day	2-4 g/day	Restriction based on fluid weight gain and blood pressure
Phosphorus	700 mg/day	700 mg/day	800 mg/day

in a loss of lean body mass. NIC nutrition interventions are listed in Chart 75-8.

The client is referred to a registered dietitian for dietary teaching and planning. In collaboration with the dietitian, teach the client about diet changes that are needed as a result of CRF. Such changes include control of protein intake; fluid intake limitation; restriction of potassium, sodium, and phosphorus intake; taking vitamin and mineral supplements; and eating enough calories to meet metabolic demand.

If adequate calories are not supplied, the body will use muscle protein for energy, which leads to a negative nitrogen balance and malnutrition. The dietitian assists in determining the number of calories and types of nutrients required to meet body needs.

Protein Restriction. Early protein restriction prevents some of the symptoms of CRF and may preserve kidney function. Protein is restricted on the basis of the degree of renal impairment and the severity of the symptoms. Accumulation of waste products from protein metabolism is the primary cause of uremia. Although lower protein levels are recommended, protein-calorie malnutrition must be avoided in clients receiving HD. At least 1.5 g of protein per kilogram of body weight per day may be needed for weight gain and improved nutritional status in clients receiving maintenance HD.

The glomerular filtration rate (GFR) is used as an indicator of renal function and as a guide to safe levels of protein intake. A client with a severely reduced GFR who is *not* undergoing dialysis is usually permitted 0.55 to 0.60 g of protein per kilogram of body weight (e.g., 40 g of protein daily for a 150-pound [70-kg] adult). If proteinuria is present, protein is added to the diet in amounts equal to that lost in the urine. Protein requirements are calculated based on actual body weight (corrected for edema), not ideal body weight. The client receiving dialysis needs more protein because some protein is lost through dialysis. While receiving HD, protein requirements are individually tailored according to the client's post-dialysis, or "dry" weight. Generally HD clients are allowed about 1 to 1.5 g of protein/kg/day. Peritoneal dialysis (PD) clients are allowed 1.2 to 1.5 g of protein/kg/day because protein is lost with each exchange. The protein should be of high biologic value, such as milk, meat, or eggs. If protein intake is inadequate, a negative nitrogen balance develops and causes muscle wasting. BUN and albumin levels are used to monitor the adequacy of protein intake. Decreased serum albumin levels indicate inadequate protein intake. Excessive protein intake increases BUN levels in clients with CRF.

CHART 75-8

NIC INTERVENTION ACTIVITIES for The Client with Chronic Renal Failure

Nutrition Therapy: *Administration of food and fluids to support metabolic processes of a client who is malnourished or at high risk for becoming malnourished*
- Complete a nutritional assessment, as appropriate.
- Determine—in collaboration with dietitian, as appropriate— the number of calories and type of nutrients needed to meet nutritional requirements.
- Refer to diet teaching and planning, as needed.
- Instruct client and family about prescribed diet.
- Provide needed nourishment within limits of prescribed diet.
- Give client and family written examples of prescribed diet.
- Monitor food/fluid ingested and calculate daily caloric intake, as appropriate.
- Offer herbs and spices as an alternative to salt.
- Monitor lab values, as appropriate.

Fluid Management: *Promotion of fluid balance and prevention of complications resulting from abnormal or undesired fluid levels*
- Maintain accurate intake and output record.
- Monitor hydration status (e.g., moist mucous membranes, adequacy of pulses, and orthostatic blood pressure), as appropriate.
- Monitor for indications of fluid overload/retention (e.g., crackles, elevated CVP or pulmonary capillary wedge pressure, edema, neck vein distention, and ascites), as appropriate.
- Weigh client daily and monitor trends.
- Monitor laboratory results relevant to fluid retention (e.g., increased specific gravity, increased BUN, decreased hematocrit, and increased urine osmolality levels).
- Monitor client's weight change before and after dialysis, if appropriate.
- Assess location and extent of edema, if present.
- Administer prescribed diuretics, as appropriate.
- Distribute the fluid intake over 24 hours, as appropriate.
- Consult physician if signs and symptoms of fluid volume excess persist or worsen.

Sodium Restriction. Monitor fluid and sodium intake. In clients with little or no urine output, fluid and sodium retention causes edema, hypertension, and heart failure (HF). Most clients with CRF retain sodium; a few cannot conserve sodium.

Estimate the client's fluid and sodium retention status by monitoring body weight and blood pressure. In uremic clients not receiving dialysis, sodium is limited to 1 to 3 g daily, and fluid intake depends on urine output. In oliguric clients receiving dialysis, the sodium restriction is 2 to 4 g daily, and fluid intake is limited to 500 to 700 mL plus the amount of any urine output. Instruct the client not to add salt at the table or during cooking. Foods high in sodium (e.g., processed foods, fast foods, potato chips, pretzels, pickles, ham, bacon, and sausage) are permitted in moderation. Herbs and spices can be used in place of salt to enhance food flavor.

Potassium Restriction. Monitor potassium intake because hyperkalemia can cause dangerous cardiac dysrhythmias. Monitor the ECG for tall, peaked T waves caused by hyperkalemia. Document serum potassium levels. Instruct the client with advanced CRF to limit potassium intake to 60 to 70 mEq/day. Teach the client to read labels of seasoning agents carefully for sodium and potassium content. Instruct clients to avoid salt substitutes composed of potassium chloride. Clients receiving PD or who are producing urine may not need potassium restriction.

Phosphorus Restriction. Control of phosphate levels is started early in CRF to avoid osteodystrophy. Monitor serum phosphate levels. Dietary phosphorus restrictions and drugs to assist with phosphate control may be prescribed. Phosphate binders must be taken at mealtime. Most clients with CRF already restrict their protein intake, and because high-protein foods are also high in phosphorus, their phosphorus consumption is also reduced. Chapter 14 lists foods high in potassium, sodium, and phosphorus.

Vitamin Supplementation. Most clients with CRF need daily vitamin and mineral supplements. Low-protein diets are also low in vitamins, and water-soluble vitamins are removed from the blood during dialysis. Anemia also is a problem in clients with CRF because of the limited iron content of low-protein diets and decreased kidney production of erythropoietin. Thus supplemental iron is needed. Calcium and vitamin D supplements may be needed, depending on the client's serum calcium levels and bone status.

Individualizing the Diet for Peritoneal Dialysis. Clients undergoing PD require a slightly different diet from those undergoing HD. Because protein is lost with the dialysate in PD, replacing lost protein is needed. Often 1.2 to 1.5 g of protein per kilogram of body weight per day is recommended. Clients may have anorexia and have difficulty eating enough protein. High-calorie enteral supplements may also be needed. Sodium restriction varies with fluid weight gain and blood pressure. Usually dietary potassium does not need to be restricted because the dialysate is potassium free. The potassium restriction, if any, is determined by the serum potassium level.

Collaborate with the dietitian to assess each client's nutritional needs. Teach the client and evaluate his or her understanding of and adherence with dietary regimens. Give written examples of the prescribed diet to the client and family to promote adherence. Help clients adapt the diet to their budget, ethnic background, and food preferences to maximize caloric intake within the diet's restrictions.

EXCESS FLUID VOLUME

PLANNING: EXPECTED OUTCOMES. The client with CRF is expected to achieve and maintain an acceptable fluid balance. Indicators include that the following parameters are only mildly compromised or not compromised:

- Blood pressure
- Stable body weight

- Central venous pressure
- Serum electrolytes

INTERVENTIONS. Management of the client with CRF includes drug therapy, diet therapy, fluid restriction, and dialysis. Diet therapy is discussed under Imbalanced Nutrition, p. 1746, and dialysis is discussed under Renal Replacement Therapies, p. 1751).

The purpose of fluid management is to promote fluid balance and prevention of complications of fluid overload (see Chart 75-8). Monitor the client's intake and output and hydration status. Assess for manifestations of fluid volume excess (e.g., crackles in the bases of the lungs, edema, and distended neck veins).

Drug Therapy. Diuretics are prescribed for clients with renal insufficiency for treatment of fluid retention or to help control blood pressure. The diuresis produced from these drugs helps to reduce fluid overload in clients who still have some urine output. Diuretics are seldom used in clients with ESRD after dialysis has been initiated because, as kidney function is reduced, these drugs can have harmful side effects on the remaining kidney cells and on the hearing structures.

Assess fluid status by obtaining daily weights and reviewing the client's intake and output. Daily weight gain in these clients indicates fluid retention rather than true body weight gain. Estimate the amount of fluid retained: 1 kg of weight equals about 1 L of fluid retained. Weigh the client daily at the same time each day, on the same scale, with the client wearing the same amount of clothing, and after the client has voided (if the client is not anuric). Monitor weight for changes before and after dialysis.

Fluid Restriction. The amount of fluid restriction prescribed is discussed under Sodium Restriction, p. 1747. Consider all forms of fluid intake, including oral, IV, and fluid or drugs given through gastric tubes, when calculating fluid intake. Assist the client in spreading oral fluid intake over a 24-hour period. Monitor the client's response to fluid restriction, and notify the health care provider if manifestations of fluid excess persist or worsen.

DECREASED CARDIAC OUTPUT

PLANNING: EXPECTED OUTCOMES. The client with CRF is expected to attain and maintain adequate cardiac output. Indicators include that the following parameters are either only mildly compromised or not compromised:

- Systolic and diastolic blood pressures
- Ejection fraction
- Peripheral pulses
- Cognitive status

INTERVENTIONS. Many clients with long-standing hypertension have renal insufficiency, and some progress to CRF and ESRD. Therefore control of hypertension is essential in preserving renal function. To control hypertension, the physician may prescribe calcium channel blockers, angiotensin-converting enzyme (ACE) inhibitors, alpha-adrenergic and beta-adrenergic blockers, and vasodilators. ACE inhibitors appear to be the most effective drugs to slow the progression of renal failure (Levine, 1997). More information on the specific drugs for hypertension can be found in Chapter 39. Indications vary depending on the client, and these drugs are used carefully to avoid hyperkalemia and hypotension. Many combinations and doses may be tried until blood pressure control is adequate and side effects are minimized. Calcium channel blockers seem to improve the GFR and renal blood flow.

Instruct the client and family to measure blood pressure. Evaluate the client's ability to measure and record blood pressure accurately using the client's own equipment. Periodically recheck measurement accuracy. The client and family must understand the relationship of blood pressure control and regulation to diet and drug therapy. Also instruct the client to weigh himself or herself daily and to bring records of blood pressure measurements and weights for discussion with the physician, nurse, or dietitian.

Assesses the client on an ongoing basis for manifestations of decreased cardiac output, heart failure, and dysrhythmias. These topics are discussed in Chapters 36 through 38.

RISK FOR INFECTION

NOC PLANNING: EXPECTED OUTCOMES. The client with CRF is expected to remain free of infection. Indicators include that the client will have only mild or absent:

- Fever
- Lymphadenopathy
- Urine culture colonization
- Wound site (dialysis access site) culture colonization
- White blood count elevation

INTERVENTIONS. Provide meticulous care to any areas where skin integrity has been broken (incisions, site of drains, puncture sites, cracked or excoriated skin, pressure sores), and provide preventive skin care to intact areas. For clients undergoing dialysis, inspect the vascular access site or PD catheter insertion site every shift for redness, swelling, pain, and drainage. Monitor vital signs for any manifestation of infection (e.g., fever, tachycardia).

RISK FOR INJURY

NOC PLANNING: EXPECTED OUTCOMES. The client with CRF is expected to remain free of injury. Indicators include that the client should not have any of the following problems:

- Fall or experience injury from a fall
- Pathologic fractures
- Bleeding
- Toxic effects of prescribed drugs

INTERVENTIONS. Managing drug therapy in clients with CRF is a complex clinical problem. Many over-the-counter drugs contain ingredients that alter renal function. Therefore it is important to obtain a detailed drug history. You must be aware of the use of each drug, its side effects, and its site of metabolism. Monitor the client closely for drug-related complications, and ensure that dosages are adjusted as needed.

Certain drugs must be avoided, and the dosages of others must be adjusted according to the degree of remaining renal function. As the client's renal function decreases, repeated dosage adjustments are necessary. Assess for side effects and signs of drug toxicity, and notify the physician as appropriate.

Many drugs are routinely given to clients with renal failure (see Chart 75-3). You must understand the rationale for these drugs and the indicated nursing interventions. Many clients have cardiac disease and may require cardiac drugs such as digoxin. Clients with renal failure are particularly at risk for digoxin toxicity because the drug is excreted by the kidneys. When caring for clients with CRF who are receiving digoxin, monitor for signs of toxicity, such as nausea, vomit-

ing, anorexia, visual disturbances, restlessness, headache, fatigue, confusion, cardiac irregularities (particularly **bradycardia** [pulse rate less than 50 to 60 beats/min] and **tachycardia** [pulse rate greater than 100 beats/min]). Monitor the serum drug levels to be certain they are in the therapeutic range (0.8-2 ng/mL). Also closely monitor the serum potassium levels of any client receiving digoxin.

Drugs to control an excessively high phosphate level include phosphate-binding compounds. Calcium acetate, calcium carbonate, and aluminum hydroxide are used as phosphate-binding agents in clients with renal failure. These drugs help prevent renal osteodystrophy and related injuries. Stress the importance of these agents and all prescribed drugs.

Hypercalcemia (excessively high serum calcium levels) is a possible complication for clients taking calcium-containing compounds to control phosphate excess. **Hypophosphatemia** (low serum phosphorus levels) is also a complication of phosphate binding, especially in clients who are not eating adequately but who are continuing to take phosphate-binding drugs. In clients taking aluminum-based phosphate binders for prolonged periods, aluminum deposits may cause bone disease or permanent neurologic problems. Monitor the client for muscle weakness, anorexia, malaise, tremors, or bone pain.

Teach clients with renal disease to avoid antacids containing magnesium. Clients with renal failure cannot excrete magnesium and thus should avoid additional intake.

In addition to the drugs used to treat renal failure, the use of certain other drugs requires special attention. These drugs include antibiotics, opioids, antihypertensives, diuretics, insulin, and heparin.

Many antibiotics are safe for clients with CRF, but those excreted by the kidney require dose adjustment. To prevent complications of bloodstream infections from mouth bacteria, prophylactic antibiotic treatment is given to clients with CRF before any dental procedures. The antibiotic used varies with the client's needs and the physician's preference.

Give opioid analgesics cautiously in clients with renal failure because the effects often last much longer than in people with healthy kidneys. Clients with uremia are more sensitive to the respiratory depressant effects of these drugs. Because opioids are broken down by the liver and not the kidneys, the dosages are often the same regardless of the level of renal function. Monitor the client closely after opioids are given, and evaluate the client's reaction to determine whether adjustments are needed.

As CRF progresses, the client with diabetes often must have insulin or oral antidiabetic drug dosages reduced because the failing kidneys do not excrete or metabolize these drugs well. Thus the drugs are effective longer, increasing the risk for hypoglycemia. Monitor the client's blood glucose levels at least four times per day to determine whether a dosage change is needed. Urine glucose measurements are less accurate when CRF is present.

Poor platelet function and capillary fragility in renal failure make anticoagulant therapy risky. Monitor clients receiving heparin, warfarin, or other anticoagulants every shift for bleeding.

FATIGUE

NOC PLANNING: EXPECTED OUTCOMES. The client with chronic renal failure (CRF) is expected to conserve energy by balancing activity and rest. Indicators include that the following parameters are either only mildly compromised or not compromised:

- Performance of self-care
- Interest in surroundings
- Concentration

INTERVENTIONS. Some causes of fatigue in the client with CRF include vitamin deficiency, anemia, and buildup of urea. All clients are given some type of vitamin and mineral supplement because of diet restrictions and vitamin losses from dialysis. Avoid giving the client these vitamin supplements before hemodialysis (HD) treatment because they will be dialyzed out of the body and the client will receive no benefit.

The anemic client with CRF is treated with erythropoietin (Epogen, Procrit). The goal of this therapy is to maintain a hematocrit of 30% to 35%. Erythropoietin therapy is effective in triggering bone marrow production of red blood cells if the client has adequate iron stores. Iron supplements may be needed if clients are iron deficient. Many clients who receive erythropoietin report improved appetite and sexual function along with decreased fatigue. The increased cell production from this therapy may induce hypertension in some clients. The improved appetite challenges clients in their attempts to maintain protein, potassium, and fluid restrictions and requires additional education.

ANXIETY

NOC PLANNING: EXPECTED OUTCOMES. The client with CRF is expected to reduce feelings of apprehension and tension. Indicators include that the client often or consistently demonstrates the following behaviors:

- Seeking information to reduce anxiety
- Using effective coping strategies
- Reporting an absence of physical manifestations of anxiety

INTERVENTIONS. A team of health care professionals, including nurses, collaborates to provide support and counseling for the client and family, often over many years of treatment. The nurse has the most contact with the client with CRF when the client is hospitalized or undergoing in-center dialysis treatments. Perform an ongoing assessment of the client's anxiety level to determine the level of nursing intervention required. Observe the client's behavior for cues indicating anxiety (e.g., anxious facial expressions or gestures and an increased pulse rate). Evaluate the support systems, such as the involvement of family and friends with the client's care.

Unfamiliar settings and lack of knowledge about treatments and tests can increase the client's anxiety level. Explain all procedures, tests, and treatments. Identify the client's knowledge deficits about normal renal function and renal failure. Provide instruction appropriate to the client's needs and ability to understand.

Provide continuity of care, whenever possible, to establish a consistent nurse-client relationship to decrease anxiety and promote discussions of client and family concerns. As you develop the nurse-client relationship, encourage the client to discuss current problems or concerns.

Encourage the client to ask questions and discuss fears about the diagnosis of renal failure. An open atmosphere that allows for discussion can decrease anxiety level. Facilitate discussions with family members about the prognosis and the potential impact on the client's lifestyle.

POTENTIAL FOR PULMONARY EDEMA

PLANNING: EXPECTED OUTCOMES. The client with CRF is expected to remain free of pulmonary edema by maintaining optimal fluid balance.

INTERVENTIONS. In the client with CRF, pulmonary edema can result from either left-sided heart failure or from vascular injury. In left-sided heart failure, the heart is unable to eject blood adequately from the left ventricle, leading to an increased pressure in the left atrium and in the pulmonary blood vessels. The increased pressure causes fluid to cross the capillaries into the pulmonary tissue, forming edema. Pulmonary edema can also occur from injury to the pulmonary blood vessels as a result of uremia. This condition causes inflammation and capillary leak. Fluid then leaks into the lung tissue and the alveoli.

Assess the client for early signs of pulmonary edema, such as restlessness, heightened anxiety, tachycardia, dyspnea, and crackles that begin at the base of the lungs. As pulmonary edema worsens, the level of fluid in the lungs rises. Auscultation reveals increased crackles, decreased air exchange. The client may have frothy, blood-tinged sputum. As cardiac and pulmonary function decrease further, the client becomes diaphoretic and cyanotic.

The client with pulmonary edema is admitted to the intensive care unit for aggressive treatment and continuous cardiac monitoring. Place the client in a high Fowler's position, and give oxygen to enhance lung expansion and improve gas exchange. Drug therapy with renal failure and pulmonary edema is difficult because of potential adverse drug effects on the kidneys. Treatment of pulmonary edema involves giving loop diuretics, such as furosemide (Lasix), IV. Renal impairment increases the risk for ototoxicity with the use of furosemide; thus IV doses are given cautiously. Diuresis usually begins within 5 minutes of giving IV furosemide. Measure urine output every 15 to 30 minutes during the acute episode and every hour thereafter until the client is stabilized. Monitor vital signs and assess breath sounds at least every 2 hours to evaluate the client's response to this treatment.

Intravenous morphine sulfate (1 to 2 mg) is often prescribed to reduce myocardial oxygen demand by triggering blood vessel dilation and to provide sedation. Dosage adjustments are needed to achieve the desired response and avoid respiratory depression. Monitor the client's respiratory rate and blood pressure hourly during this therapy. Other vasodilators, such as nitroglycerin, also may be given as a continuous infusion to reduce pulmonary vascular pressure. Monitor vital signs at least hourly because this drug combination may cause severe hypotension.

Monitor serum electrolyte levels daily, and report abnormalities to the physician so that imbalances can be corrected quickly. Monitor electrocardiography at least every 2 hours to identify potential dysrhythmias. Monitor oxygen saturation levels by pulse oximetry and arterial blood gas values. Adjust the oxygen delivery system to maintain adequate oxygen saturation levels. Monitor the client for worsening of the condition, manifested as increasing pulmonary edema and hypoxemia. The client may require temporary intubation and mechanical ventilation to prevent death.

Clients with CRF who have existing cardiac problems, hypertension, or chronic fluid retention are at increased risk for developing pulmonary edema. Such clients are less likely to respond quickly to treatment and are more likely to develop adverse effects from drug therapy. Ultrafiltration may be used with these clients to reduce fluid volume.

Renal Replacement Therapies

Renal replacement therapy is needed when the physiologic changes of chronic renal failure (CRF) are potentially life threatening or pose continuing discomfort to the client. When the client can no longer be managed with conservative therapies, such as diet, drugs, and fluid restriction, dialysis is indicated. Transplantation may be discussed at any time.

HEMODIALYSIS

Hemodialysis (HD) is one of several renal replacement therapies used for the treatment of renal failure (Table 75-9). Dialysis removes excess fluids and waste products and restores chemical and electrolyte balance. HD involves passing the client's blood through an artificial semipermeable membrane to perform the filtering and excretion functions of the kidney.

Client Selection. Any client may be considered for HD therapy. Starting this therapy depends on client symptoms, not on the creatinine clearance. Dialysis is started immediately for clients who have the following: fluid overload that does not respond to diuretics, pericarditis, uncontrolled hypertension, neurologic problems, and development of bleeding diathesis. More commonly, dialysis is started when clients have uremic manifestations, such as nausea and vomiting, decreased attention span, decreased cognition, worsening anemia, and pruritus.

Many clients survive for years with HD therapy and others may only live a few months. How long the client survives using HD therapy depends on the client's age, the cause of renal failure, and the presence of other diseases, such as coronary artery disease, hypertension, or diabetes. The following are general client selection criteria:

- Presence of irreversible renal failure when other therapies are unacceptable or ineffective
- Absence of illnesses that would seriously complicate HD
- Expectation of rehabilitation
- The client's acceptance of the regimen

Dialysis Settings. Clients with CRF may receive HD treatments in many settings, depending on specific needs. Regardless of the setting for therapy, the client needs ongoing nursing support to maintain this complex and life-saving treatment.

Clients may be dialyzed in an acute care (hospital-based) center if they have recently started treatment or have complicated conditions that require close supervision. Stable clients not requiring intense supervision may be dialyzed in a community or free-standing HD center. Selected clients may participate in complete or partial self-care in an outpatient center or with in-home HD.

In-home HD is the least disruptive form of therapy and allows for adaptation of the regimen to the client's lifestyle. Unfortunately many clients cannot participate in in-home dialysis because they lack an appropriate partner to assist with the therapy and manage the dialysis machine. Some clients and partners find the responsibilities of in-home dialysis to be too stressful. In addition, a water treatment system must be installed in the home to provide a safe, clean water supply for the dialysis process.

Procedure. Dialysis works using the passive transfer of toxins by diffusion. **Diffusion** is the movement of molecules from an area of higher concentration to an area of lower concentration. The rate of diffusion during dialysis occurs more rapidly when the membrane pores are large, there is a large surface area of membrane, the temperature of the solutions is higher, and there is a greater difference in the solute concentrations. Molecules that are too large, such as RBCs and most plasma proteins, cannot pass through the membrane.

When HD is started, blood and **dialysate** (dialyzing solution) flow in opposite directions across an enclosed semipermeable membrane. The dialysate contains a balanced mix of electrolytes and water that closely resembles human plasma. On the other side of the membrane is the client's blood, which contains metabolic waste products, excess water, and excess electrolytes. During HD, the waste products move from the blood into the dialysate because of the difference in their concentrations (**diffusion**). Excess water is also removed from the blood into the dialysate (**osmosis**). Electrolytes can move in either direction, as needed, and take some fluid with them. Potassium and sodium typically move out of the plasma into the dialysate. Bicarbonate and calcium generally move from the dialysate into the plasma. This circulating process continues for a preset length of time, restoring water, electrolyte, and acid-base balance and removing wastes. Water volume may be removed from the plasma by applying positive or negative pressure to the system.

The HD system includes a dialyzer, dialysate, vascular access routes, and an HD machine. The artificial kidney, or **dialyzer** (Figure 75-3), has four parts: a blood compartment, a

TABLE 75-9 A Comparison of Hemodialysis and Peritoneal Dialysis as Renal Replacement Treatment Options	
Hemodialysis	**Peritoneal Dialysis**
Advantages	
More efficient clearance	Easy access
Short time needed for treatment	Few hemodynamic complications
Complications	
Disequilibrium syndrome	Protein loss
Muscle cramps	Peritonitis
Hemorrhage	Hyperglycemia
Air embolus	Respiratory distress
Hemodynamic changes (hypotension, cardiac dysrhythmias, and anemia)	Bowel perforation
Contraindications	
Hemodynamic instability	Extensive peritoneal adhesions
	Peritoneal fibrosis
	Recent abdominal surgery
Access	
Vascular access route	Intra-abdominal catheter
Procedure	
Complex	Simple
Specially trained registered nurses required	Training less complex than for hemodialysis
Nursing Implications	
Vascular access care	Abdominal catheter care
Restrict diet	More flexible diet

dialysate compartment, a semipermeable membrane, and an enclosed structure to support the membrane.

Dialysate is made from clear water and chemicals and is free of any waste products or drugs. Bacteria and other organisms are too large to pass through the membrane; therefore dialysate does not need to be sterile. The water used in dialysate must meet specific standards and usually requires special treatment before mixing the dialysate. The dialysate composition may be altered according to the client's needs for treatment of electrolyte imbalances. During HD, the dialysate is warmed to 100° F (37.8° C) to increase the rate of diffusion and to prevent hypothermia.

The HD machine has alarm systems to monitor for potential problems, including the following:

- Changes in dialysate temperature
- Air in the blood tubing
- A blood leak in the dialysate compartment
- Changes in the pressure within the blood and the dialysate compartments
- Changes in composition of the blood or dialysate

If any of these problems are detected, an alarm sounds to protect the client from life-threatening complications.

All models of HD machines function in a manner similar to that shown in Figure 75-4. Figure 75-5 shows one type of HD machine. Figure 75-6 shows a client receiving HD. The number and length of each treatment depend on the amount of wastes and fluid to be removed, the clearance capacity of the dialyzer, and the blood flow rate to and from the machine. Most clients require about 12 hours per week of total dialysis time. This time is usually divided into three 4-hour treatments. For clients with some ongoing urine production, two 5- to 6-hour treatments a week may be adequate. If the client gains large amounts of fluid weight, a longer treatment time may be needed to remove the fluid without hypotension or severe side effects.

Anticoagulation. To prevent blood clots from forming within the dialyzer or the blood tubing, anticoagulation

is needed during HD treatments. Heparin is the most commonly used drug to prevent clots from forming when blood comes in contact with foreign surfaces. Client response to heparin varies, and the dose is adjusted on the basis of each client's need. Clients receiving erythropoietin may require additional heparin.

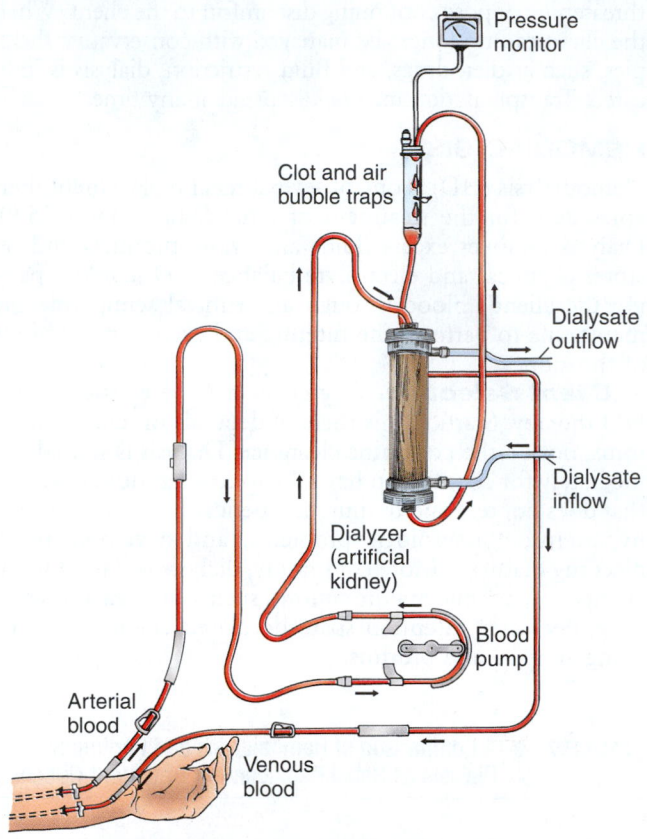

Figure 75-4 ■ A hemodialysis circuit.

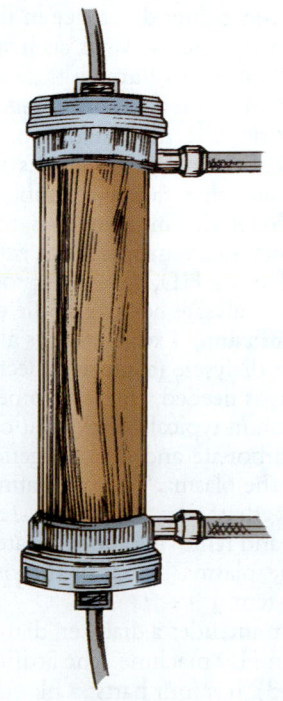

Figure 75-3 ■ Artificial kidney (dialyzer) used in hemodialysis.

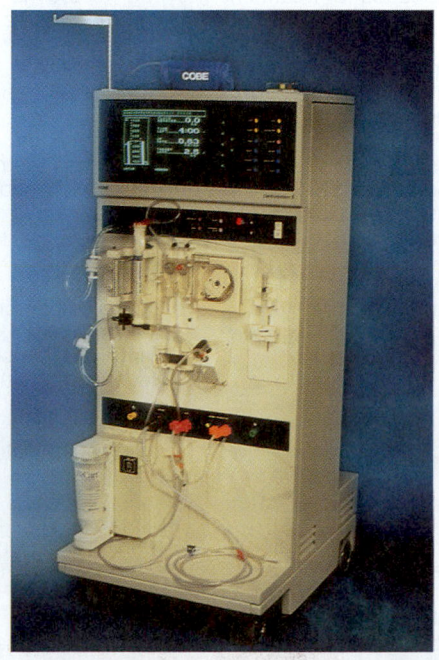

Figure 75-5 ■ Hemodialysis machine. (Courtesy of GAMBRO Healthcare, Stockholm, Sweden.)

Heparin remains active in the body for 4 to 6 hours after dialysis, making the client at risk for hemorrhage during and immediately after HD treatments. Invasive procedures must be avoided during that time. Monitor the client closely for any signs of bleeding or hemorrhage. Clotting tendencies can be monitored during HD with a bedside machine (e.g., the Homochron), by whole-blood clotting times (Lee-White clotting test), or by activated partial thromboplastin times (aPTT) during and after HD. Protamine sulfate is an antidote to heparin and should be available in the dialysis setting.

Vascular Access. Vascular access is required for hemodialysis (Table 75-10). The procedure requires the easy availability of a large amount of blood flow: at least 250 to 300 mL/min, usually for a period of 3 to 4 hours. Normal venous cannulation does not provide this rate of blood flow.

Long-Term Vascular Access. An internal access is used for most clients having long-term HD (see Table 75-10). The two common choices are an internal arteriovenous (AV) fis-

tula or an AV graft (Figure 75-7). *AV fistulas* are formed by connecting (**anastomosis**) an artery to a vein. The most commonly used vessels are the radial or brachial artery and the cephalic vein of the nondominant arm. Fistulas increase venous blood flow to 250 to 400 mL/min, the amount needed for effective dialysis.

Time is needed after anastomosis for the AV fistula to develop. As the AV fistula "matures," the increased pressure of the arterial blood flow into the vein causes the vessel walls to thicken. This thickening increases their strength and suitability for repeated cannulation. Clients differ in the amount of time needed for the fistula to mature. Some fistulas may not be ready for use for as long as 4 months after the surgery, and a temporary vascular access (AV shunt or HD catheter) is used during this time.

To access a fistula, cannulate it by inserting two needles, one toward the venous blood flow and one toward the arterial blood flow. This procedure allows the HD machine to draw the blood out through the arterial needle and return it through the venous needle.

Arteriovenous grafts are used when the AV fistula does not develop or when complications limit its use. The polytetrafluoroethylene (PTFE) graft is a synthetic material (Gore-Tex). This type of graft is commonly used in older clients undergoing HD. Figure 75-8 shows a client's AF graft.

PRECAUTIONS. Some precautions are needed to ensure the functioning of an internal AV fistula or AV graft. First assess for adequate circulation in the fistula or graft as well as in the distal portion of the extremity. Then check for a bruit or a thrill by auscultation or palpation over the access site. *Repeated compression can result in the loss of the vascular access; therefore avoid taking the blood pressure or performing venipunctures in the arm with the vascular access.* The AV fistula or graft is *not* used for delivery of IV fluids. Chart 75-9 lists best practices for care of the client with an HD access.

COMPLICATIONS. Complications can occur regardless of the type of access. The most common problems are

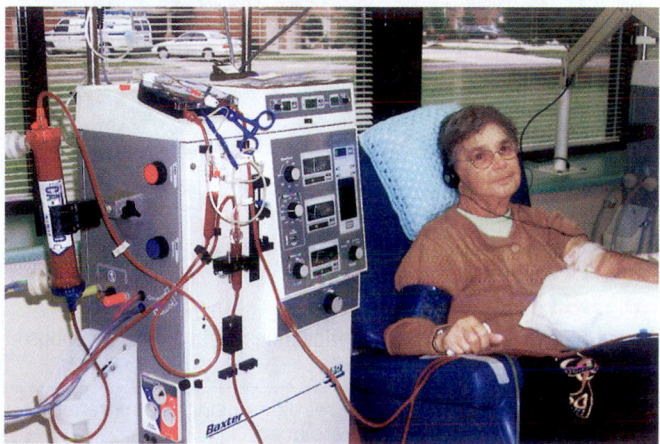

Figure 75-6 ■ Client receiving hemodialysis.

TABLE 75-10 Types of Vascular Access for Hemodialysis			
Access Type	**Description**	**Location**	**Initial Use**
Permanent			
AV fistula	An internal anastomosis of an artery to a vein	Forearm	2-4 mo or longer
AV graft	Synthetic vessel tubing tunneled beneath the skin, connecting an artery and a vein	Forearm Upper arm Inner thigh	1-2 wk
Dual-lumen hemodialysis catheter	An extended-use catheter, surgically tunneled under the skin with a barrier cuff	Subclavian vein	Immediately postoperatively and after x-ray confirmation of placement
Temporary			
Hemodialysis catheter (dual- or triple-lumen)	A specially designed catheter with two or three lumens Two lumens are for blood outflow and inflow for hemodialysis; a third lumen allows venous access without accessing dialysis lumens	Subclavian, internal jugular, or femoral vein	Immediately after insertion and x-ray confirmation of placement
AV shunt (relatively uncommon)	An external loop of Silastic tubing connecting an artery and a vein Each section of tubing is sutured into a vessel and brought through a skin stab wound	Forearm	Immediately after insertion
Subcutaneous device	An internal device with two metallic access ports and two catheters inserted into large central veins	Subclavian	Immediately after insertion

AV, Arteriovenous.

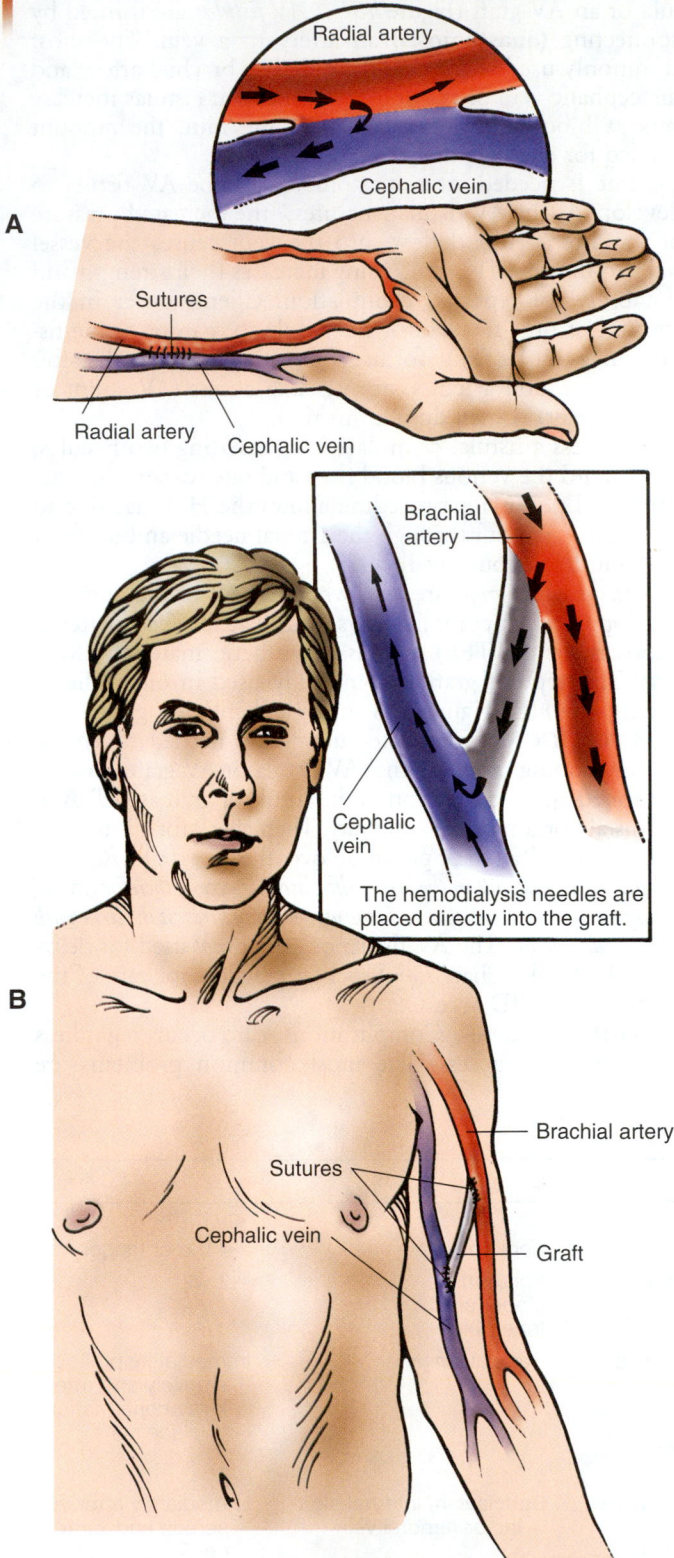

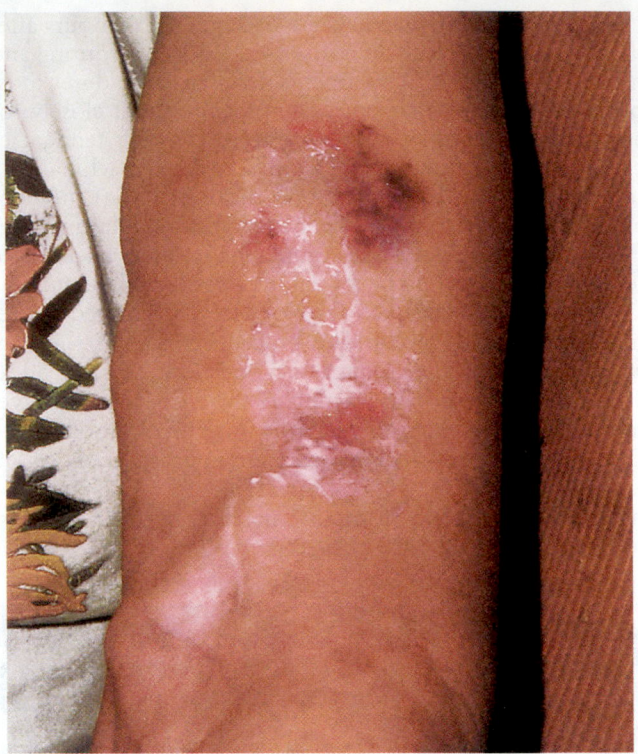

Figure 75-8 ■ Hemodialysis access.

Figure 75-7 ■ Options for long-term vascular access for hemodialysis. **A,** A surgically created venous fistula. The increased pressure from the artery forces blood into the vein. This process causes the vein to dilate enough for fistula needles to be placed for hemodialysis. When the vein dilates in this manner, the fistula is said to be "developed." **B,** A surgically placed straight vascular graft in the upper arm. The graft creates a shunt between arterial and venous blood.

CHART 75-9

BEST PRACTICE for
Caring for the Client with an Arteriovenous Fistula, Arteriovenous Graft, or Arteriovenous Shunt

- Do not take blood pressure readings using the extremity in which the vascular access is placed.
- Do not perform venipunctures or start an IV line in the extremity in which the vascular access is placed.
- Palpate for thrills and auscultate for bruits every 4 hours while the client is awake.
- Assess the client's distal pulses and circulation.
- Elevate the affected extremity postoperatively.
- Encourage routine range-of-motion exercises.
- Check for bleeding at needle insertion sites or shunt tubing insertion sites. (Keep small clamps handy on the dressing of the AV shunt.)
- Assess for manifestations of infection at needle sites and shunt tubing insertion sites.
- Instruct the client not to carry heavy objects or anything that compresses the extremity in which the vascular access if placed.
- Instruct the client against sleeping with his or her body weight on top of the extremity in which the vascular access is placed.

AV, Arteriovenous.

thrombosis or stenosis, infection, aneurysm formation, ischemia, and heart failure.

Thrombosis, or clotting of the AV access, is the most frequent complication. Some clients are at greater risk for clotting than others and may be given anticoagulants. Interventional radiology can treat failing grafts. Most grafts fail because of high-pressure arterial flow entering the venous system. The muscle layers of the veins react to this increased pressure by thickening. The venous thickening reduces or oc-

TABLE 75-11 Nursing Interventions for Prevention of Complications in Hemodialysis Vascular Access			
Access Type	**Bleeding**	**Infection**	**Clotting**
AV fistula or AV graft	Apply pressure to the needle puncture sites.	Ensure adequate site cleaning before cannulation	Avoid constrictive devices. Rotate needle insertion sites with each hemodialysis treatment. Assess for thrill and bruit.
AV shunt	Keep clamps available.	Perform exit site care 3 times/wk.	Avoid constrictive devices. Assess for thrill and bruit.
Hemodialysis catheters (temporary and permanent)	Monitor the access site.	Use aseptic technique. Change the dressing 3 times/wk.	Place a heparin or heparin/saline dwell solution after hemodialysis treatment. Not used between treatments.

AV, Arteriovenous.

cludes blood flow. Radiologists inject a thrombolytic drug (such as urokinase or tPA) to dissolve the clot. The clot usually dissolves within minutes, and often a stricture is revealed at the point where the graft and the vein connect. The stricture can be treated by balloon angioplasty (Table 75-11).

Most infections of the vascular access are caused by *Staphylococcus aureus* introduced during cannulation. Use sterile technique during cannulation to prevent infection (see Table 75-11).

Aneurysms can form in the fistula and are caused by repeated needle punctures at the same site. Large aneurysms may cause loss of the fistula's function and require surgical repair.

Ischemia occurs in a few clients with vascular access when the fistula decreases arterial blood flow to areas distal to the fistula. Ischemic symptoms *("steal syndrome")* vary from cold or numb fingers to gangrene. If the collateral circulation is inadequate, the fistula may need to be tied off and a new one created in another area to preserve extremity circulation.

The shunting of blood directly from the arterial system to the venous system, through the fistula, can cause heart failure in clients with a limited cardiac reserve (see Chapter 38). This complication is rare, but if it does occur, the fistula may need to be revised to reduce arterial blood flow.

Temporary Vascular Access. An older type of vascular access is the external *arteriovenous (AV) shunt* (Figure 75-9; see also Table 75-10). This shunt is created by surgical placement of one end of a piece of silicone rubber (Silastic) tubing into an artery and the other end into a nearby vein. Part of the tubing is left external to provide a readily available vascular access. Few clients still have this type of access.

Temporary vascular access with special catheters has replaced the use of the AV shunt for most clients requiring immediate HD. A catheter designed for HD may be inserted into the subclavian, internal jugular, or femoral vein. The lumens of these devices are much smaller than the permanent accesses, and more time (4 to 8 hours) is required to complete each dialysis session.

Subcutaneous devices may also be surgically inserted to provide temporary access for HD. Implanted beneath the skin, these devices are composed of two small metallic ports with attached catheters that are inserted into large central veins (Figure 75-10). The ports of subcutaneous devices have internal mechanisms, which open when needles are inserted and close when needles are removed. Blood from one port flows from the body to the HD machine and returns to the body via the other port. These devices may be ideal for

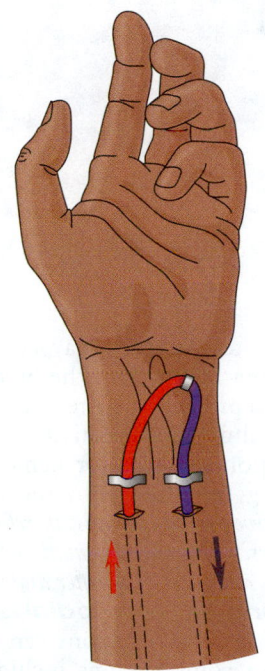

Figure 75-9 ■ An arteriovenous shunt in the forearm. One part of the shunt cannula is placed in an artery; the other part in a vein. The ends of the shunt cannula are joined when dialysis is not in progress.

clients awaiting permanent access placement or kidney transplantation.

Hemodialysis Nursing Care. Many client drugs are dialyzable (i.e., can be partially removed from the blood during dialysis). Vasoactive drugs can cause hypotension during HD and may also be held until after treatment. Consult with the physician to assess the client's drug regimen and determine which drugs should be held until after HD treatment. Table 75-12 lists common dialyzable and vasoactive drugs that should be given after HD.

Post-Dialysis Care. Closely monitor the client immediately and for several hours after dialysis for any side effects from the treatment. Common complications include hypotension, headache, nausea, malaise, vomiting, dizziness, and muscle cramps.

Obtain vital signs and weight for comparison with predialysis measurements. Blood pressure and weight are expected to be reduced as a result of fluid removal. Hypotension may require rehydration with IV fluids, such as normal

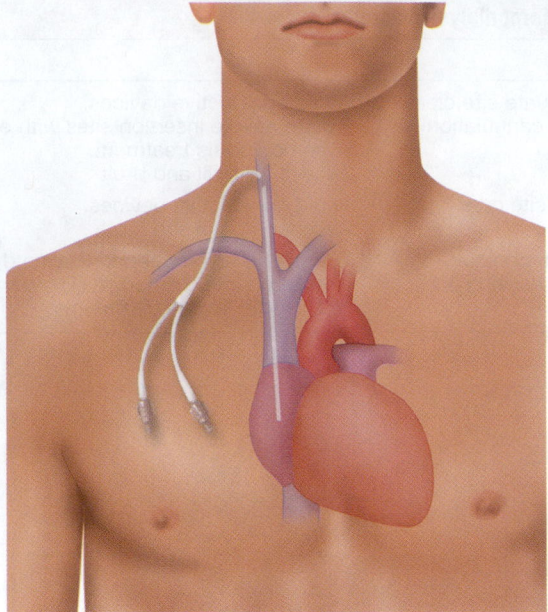

Figure 75-10 ■ Temporary subcutaneous hemodialysis access.

saline. The client's temperature may also be elevated because the dialysis machine warms the blood slightly. If the client has a fever, sepsis may be present, and a blood sample is needed for culture and sensitivity.

The heparinization required for hemodialysis (HD) increases the clotting time and thus the risk for excessive bleeding. *All invasive procedures must therefore be avoided for 4 to 6 hours after dialysis. Continually monitor the client for hemorrhage during dialysis and for 1 hour after dialysis* (Chart 75-10).

Complications of Hemodialysis. Many fluid-related and infectious complications can occur from HD. The most common complications include disequilibrium syndrome and viral infections.

Dialysis disequilibrium syndrome may develop during HD or after HD has been completed. The cause is thought to be due to the rapid decrease in fluid volume and blood urea nitrogen (BUN) levels during HD. The change in urea levels can cause cerebral edema and increased intracranial pressure. Neurologic complications can result (e.g., headache, nausea, vomiting, restlessness, decreased level of consciousness, seizures, coma, or death). Early recognition of the syndrome and treatment with anticonvulsants and barbiturates may prevent a life-threatening situation. Dialysis disequilibrium syndrome may be prevented by starting HD for short periods with low blood flows so that rapid changes in plasma composition are avoided.

Infectious diseases transmitted by blood transfusion are a serious complication of long-term HD. Two of the most serious blood-transmitted infections are hepatitis and human immunodeficiency virus (HIV).

Hepatitis infection (B and C) in clients with chronic renal failure (CRF) has decreased because the use of erythropoietin has reduced the need for blood transfusions to maintain red blood cell counts. Hepatitis is a problem because of the blood access and the risk for contamination during HD. The viruses can be transmitted through the use of contaminated needles or instruments, by entry of contaminated

blood through open wounds in the skin or mucous membranes, or through transfusions with contaminated blood. Monitor all clients receiving HD for manifestations of hepatitis (see Chapter 62).

HIV is a blood-borne and body fluid–borne virus that poses some risk for clients undergoing HD. Fortunately the risks for HIV transmission are reduced by the consistent practice of standard precautions (blood and body fluids), routine screening of donated blood for HIV, and decreased

TABLE 75-12 Dialyzable and Vasoactive Drugs	
Dialyzable Drugs	**Vasoactive Drugs**
Aminoglycosides	*Antidysrhythmics*
Amikacin	Flecainide
Gentamycin	Lidocaine
Tobramycin	Procainamide
	Quinidine
Antiviral Agents	
Acyclovir	*Antihypertensives*
Ganciclovir	Atenolol
	Captopril
Penicillins	Diltiazem
Amoxicillin	Enalapril
Ampicillin	Lisinopril
Cloxacillin	Methyldopa
Dicloxacillin	Nifedipine
Mezlocillin	Propranolol
Penicillin G	Verapamil
Ticarcillin	
	Narcotics
Anticonvulsants	Codeine
Ethosuximide	Morphine
Gabapentin	
Phenobarbital	*Sedatives*
	Midazolam
Cephalosporins	Phenobarbital
Cefaclor	Propofol
Cefazolin	
Cefoxitin	*Vasodilators*
Ceftizoxime	Hydralazine
Ceftriaxone	Nitroglycerin
Cefuroxime	Nitroprusside
Antituberculosis	
Ethambutol	
Isoniazid	
Miscellaneous	
Aztreonam	
Cimetidine	
Vitamins	

CHART 75-10

BEST PRACTICE for
Caring for the Client Undergoing Hemodialysis

- Weigh the client before and after dialysis.
- Know the client's dry weight.
- Discuss with the physician whether any of the client's medications should be withheld until after dialysis.
- Be aware of events that occurred during the dialysis treatment.
- Measure blood pressure, pulse rate, respirations, and temperature.
- Assess for symptoms of orthostatic hypotension.
- Assess the vascular access site.
- Observe for bleeding.
- Assess the client's level of consciousness and assess for headache, nausea, and vomiting.

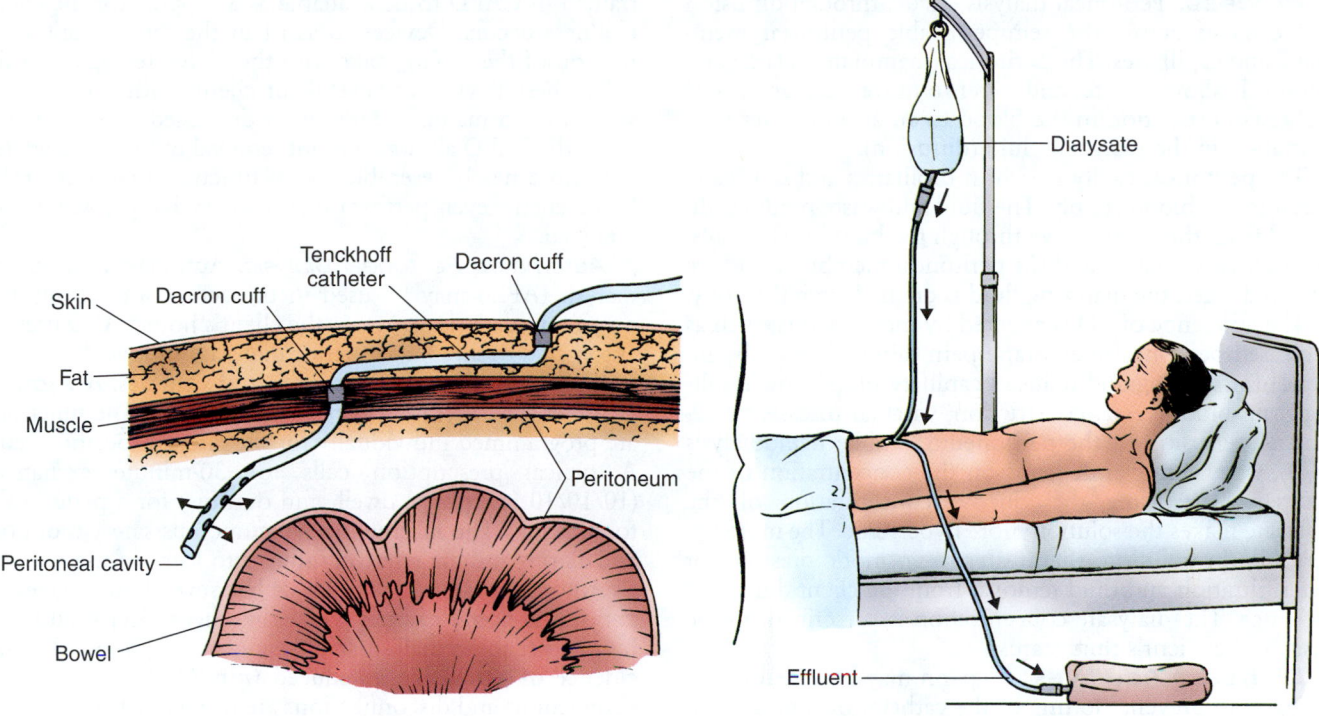

Figure 75-11 ■ Manual peritoneal dialysis via an implanted abdominal catheter (Tenckhoff catheter).

need for blood transfusions for clients with end-stage renal disease (ESRD). Despite this progress, however, some clients have already been infected with the HIV virus. Clients who have been undergoing HD or received frequent transfusions during the early to mid-1980s are at risk for acquired immunodeficiency syndrome (AIDS) (see also Chapter 25).

CONSIDERATIONS FOR OLDER ADULTS

The occurrence of ESRD is greater in clients 65 to 74 years of age. In the past decade the incidence of ESRD in individuals aged 45 to 65 has increased by 5.3% and in those 75 years of age and older by 9.5% (USRSD, 2002). Clients over age 65 who are receiving HD are more at risk for dialysis-induced hypotension. These clients require more frequent monitoring during and after dialysis.

Critical Thinking Challenge

Your client (described earlier on p. 1745) has been diagnosed as having ESRD. The health care provider has prescribed dietary teaching and outpatient HD three times per week. She asks whether she can eventually have a kidney transplant.

1. What instructions should you provide regarding the dietary and fluid needs for this client?
2. How will you explain to the client and her family that HD, rather than transplantation, is the best choice of renal replacement therapy for her?
3. What changes, if any, will need to be made in her therapy for diabetes and hypertension?
4. What complications should you monitor the client for during and immediately following dialysis?

evolve For suggested answer guidelines, go to http://evolve.elsevier.com/Iggy/.

PERITONEAL DIALYSIS

Peritoneal dialysis (PD) occurs in the peritoneal cavity. PD is slower than hemodialysis (HD), however, and more time is needed to achieve the same effect.

Client Selection. Most clients with chronic renal failure (CRF) can select either HD or PD. For clients who are hemodynamically unstable and for those who cannot tolerate anticoagulation, PD is less hazardous than HD. For some clients, vascular access problems may eliminate HD as an option. At times a client may use PD until a new arteriovenous (AV) fistula matures. PD is also often the treatment of choice for older adults because it offers more flexibility if the client's status changes frequently.

Peritoneal dialysis cannot be performed if peritoneal adhesions are present or if extensive intra-abdominal surgery has been performed. In these cases the surface area of the peritoneal membrane is not sufficient for adequate dialysis exchange. Peritoneal membrane fibrosis may occur after repeated infections, which decreases membrane permeability.

Procedure. A siliconized rubber (Silastic) catheter is surgically placed into the abdominal cavity for infusion of dialysate (Figure 75-11). Usually 1 to 2 L of dialysate is infused by gravity *(fill)* into the peritoneal space over a 10- to 20-minute period, according to the client's tolerance. The fluid *dwells* in the cavity for a specified time prescribed by the physician. The fluid then flows out of the body *(drains)* by gravity into a drainage bag. The peritoneal outflow contains the dialysate and the excess water, electrolytes, and nitrogenous waste products. The dialyzing fluid is called peritoneal *effluent* on outflow. The three phases of the process (infusion, or "fill"; dwell; and outflow, or drain) make up one PD exchange. The number and frequency of PD exchanges are prescribed by the physician, depending on the client's manifestations and laboratory data.

Process. Peritoneal dialysis occurs through diffusion and osmosis across the semipermeable peritoneal membrane and capillaries. The peritoneal membrane is large and porous. It allows solutes and water to move from an area of higher concentration in the blood to an area of lower concentration in the dialyzing fluid (diffusion).

The peritoneal cavity is rich in capillaries and is a ready access to the blood supply. The fluid and waste products dialyzed from the client move through the blood vessel walls, the interstitial tissues, and the peritoneal membrane and are removed when the dialyzing fluid is drained from the body.

The efficiency of PD is affected by many factors, such as decreased peritoneal membrane permeability caused by infection or scarring and reduced capillary blood flow resulting from blood vessel constriction, vascular disease, or decreased perfusion of the peritoneum. Unlike hemodialysis (HD), water removal depends on the concentration of the dialysate. Increasing the glucose concentration of the dialysate makes the solution more hypertonic. The more hypertonic the solution, the greater the osmotic pressure for water filtration and fluid removal from the client during an exchange. The dialysate concentration is prescribed on the basis of the client's fluid status.

Dialysate Additives. Heparin may be added to the dialysate to prevent clotting of the catheter or tubing. Usually intraperitoneal (IP) heparin is needed only after new catheter placement or if peritonitis occurs. IP heparin is not absorbed systemically and does not affect blood clotting.

Other agents that may be given in the dialysate include potassium and antibiotics. Commercially prepared dialysate does not contain potassium. Some clients need potassium added to the dialysate so that hypokalemia does not occur. Antibiotics may be given by the IP route when peritonitis is present or suspected. Potassium and antibiotics are not mixed in the same dialysate bag because interactions may reduce the antibiotic effect.

Types of Peritoneal Dialysis. Many types of PD are available, including continuous ambulatory PD, multiple-bag continuous ambulatory PD, automated PD, intermittent PD, and continuous-cycle PD. The type selected depends on the client's ability and lifestyle.

Continuous Ambulatory Peritoneal Dialysis. In continuous ambulatory peritoneal dialysis (CAPD), the client performs self-dialysis by infusing four 2-L exchanges of dialysate into the peritoneal cavity, where the dialysate remains for 4 to 8 hours, 7 days a week. During the dwell period, the client can use a continuous connect system or a disconnect system.

With the continuous *connect* system (straight transfer set), the dialysate bag is attached to the catheter by 48-inch tubing. The empty bag and tubing are folded and worn beneath the clothing until they are used for outflow. After draining, the client removes the bag and connects a new bag to repeat the process.

With the *disconnect system* (Y-transfer set), the client removes the connecting tubing and empty dialysate bag after inflow and attaches a cap to the PD catheter. The disconnect system eliminates the need to wear the tubing and bag but requires opening the system two extra times with each exchange. The extra opening of the system increases the risk for infection.

With CAPD treatment, no machine is necessary and no partner is required. However, it is best for a partner also trained in CAPD to be available as a support for the client if illness occurs. Devices to assist in the safe, aseptic connection of the tubing spike with the dialysate bag are available. These devices are useful for clients with impaired vision, limited manual dexterity, or decreased hand and arm strength. CAPD allows constant removal of fluid and wastes and more nearly resembles renal function than does HD. Some clients even perform their own exchanges while hospitalized.

Automated Peritoneal Dialysis. Automated peritoneal dialysis (APD) may be used in the acute care setting, the outpatient dialysis center, or the client's home. APD uses an automated cycling machine for dialysate inflow, dwell, and outflow according to preset times and volumes. A warming chamber for dialysate is part of the machine. The functions are programmed individually for the client's specific needs. A typical prescription calls for 30-minute exchanges (10/10/10 for inflow, dwell, and outflow) for a period of 8 to 10 hours. The machines have numerous safety monitors and alarms and are relatively simple to learn to use.

Automated peritoneal dialysis has several advantages. It permits in-home dialysis while the client sleeps, allowing him or her to be dialysis free during waking hours. The incidence of peritonitis is reduced with APD because fewer connections and disconnections are needed. Also, APD can be used to administer larger volumes of dialysis solution for clients who need higher clearances.

Intermittent Peritoneal Dialysis. Intermittent peritoneal dialysis (IPD) combines osmotic pressure gradients with true dialysis. The client usually requires exchanges of 2 L of dialysate at 30- to 60-minute intervals, allowing 15 to 20 minutes of drain time. For most clients, 30 to 40 exchanges of 2 L three times weekly are needed. IPD treatments can be automated or manual.

Continuous-Cycle Peritoneal Dialysis. Continuous-cycle peritoneal dialysis (CCPD) uses an automated cycling machine. Exchanges occur at night while the client sleeps. The final exchange of the night is left to dwell through the day and is drained the next evening as the process is repeated. CCPD offers the advantage of 24-hour dialysis, as in CAPD, but the sterile catheter system is violated less often.

Complications. Complications are possible with PD, but many can be prevented with careful nursing care.

Peritonitis. Peritonitis is the major complication of PD. The most common cause of peritonitis is connection site contamination. To prevent peritonitis, use meticulous sterile technique when caring for the PD catheter and when hooking up or clamping off dialysate bags (Chart 75-11).

Manifestations of peritonitis include cloudy dialysate outflow (effluent), fever, abdominal tenderness, abdominal pain, general malaise, nausea, and vomiting. Cloudy or opaque effluent is the earliest sign of peritonitis. Examine all effluent for color and clarity to detect peritonitis early. When peritonitis is suspected, send a specimen of the dialysate outflow for culture and sensitivity study, Gram stain, and cell count to identify the infecting organism.

Pain. Pain during the inflow of dialysate is common when clients are first started on PD therapy. Usually this pain no longer occurs after a week or two of PD. Cold dialysate increases discomfort. Thus you should warm the dialysate bags before instillation by using a heating pad to wrap the bag or by using the warming chamber of the auto-

BEST PRACTICE for
Caring for the Client with a Peritoneal Dialysis Catheter

- Mask yourself and your client. Wash your hands.
- Put on sterile gloves. Remove the old dressing. Remove the contaminated gloves.
- Assess the area for signs of infection, such as swelling, redness, or discharge around the catheter site.
- Use aseptic technique:
  - Open the sterile field on a flat surface, and place two precut 4 × 4 inch gauze pads on the field.
  - Place three cotton swabs soaked in povidone-iodine on the field. Put on sterile gloves.
- Use cotton swabs to clean around the catheter site. Use a circular motion starting from the insertion site and moving away toward the abdomen. Repeat with all three swabs.
- Apply precut gauze pads over the catheter site. Tape only the edges of the gauze pads.

mated cycling machine. *Microwave ovens are not recommended for the warming of dialysate.*

Exit Site and Tunnel Infections. The exit site from a PD catheter should be clean, dry, and without pain or inflammation. Exit site infections (ESIs) can occur with any type of PD catheter. These infections are difficult to treat and can become chronic. Exit site and tunnel infections can lead to peritonitis, catheter failure, and hospitalization. Dialysate leakage and pulling or twisting of the catheter predispose the client to ESIs. A Gram stain and culture should be performed when exit sites have purulent drainage.

Tunnel infections occur in the path of the catheter from the skin to the cuff. Manifestations include redness, tenderness, and pain. ESIs are treated with antimicrobials. Deep cuff infections usually require catheter removal.

Poor Dialysate Flow. Constipation is the main cause of inflow or outflow problems. To prevent constipation, the physician prescribes a bowel preparation before placing the PD catheter. An enema before starting PD may also prevent flow problems. A high-fiber diet and stool softeners are often needed for prevention of constipation. Other causes of flow difficulty include kinked or clamped connection tubing, the client's position, fibrin clot formation, and PD catheter displacement.

Ensure that the drainage bag is lower than the client's abdomen to enhance gravity drainage. Inspect the connection tubing and PD system for kinking or twisting, and ensure that clamps are open. If inflow or outflow drainage is still inadequate, reposition the client to stimulate inflow or outflow. Turning the client to the other side or making sure that he or she is in good body alignment may help. Having the client in a supine low-Fowler's position reduces intra-abdominal pressure. Increased intra-abdominal pressure from sitting or standing, or from coughing, contributes to leakage at the PD catheter site.

Fibrin clot formation may occur after PD catheter placement or with the onset of peritonitis. Milking the tubing may dislodge the fibrin clot and improve flow. An x-ray is needed to identify PD catheter placement. If displacement has occurred, the physician repositions the PD catheter.

Dialysate Leakage. Dialysate leakage is seen as clear fluid coming from the catheter exit site. When dialysis is first started, small volumes of dialysate are used. It may take clients 1 to 2 weeks to tolerate a full 2-L exchange without

leakage around the catheter site. Leakage occurs more often in obese or diabetic clients, older adults, and those on long-term steroid therapy. During periods of catheter leak, clients may require hemodialysis (HD) support.

Other Complications. When PD is first started, the outflow may be bloody or blood tinged. This condition normally clears within a week or two. After PD is well-established, the effluent should be clear and light yellow. Observe for and document any change in the color of the outflow. Brown-colored effluent is associated with a bowel perforation. If the outflow is the same color as urine and has the same glucose concentration, a possible bladder perforation should be investigated. Cloudy or opaque effluent indicates infection.

Nursing Care During Peritoneal Dialysis. In the hospital setting, PD is routinely initiated and monitored by the nurse. Before the treatment, evaluate baseline vital signs, including blood pressure, apical and radial pulse rates, temperature, quality of respirations, and breath sounds. Weigh the client, always on the same scale, before the procedure and at least every 24 hours while receiving treatment. Baseline laboratory tests, such as electrolyte and glucose levels, are obtained before starting PD and are repeated at least daily during the PD treatment.

Continually monitor the client during PD. Take and record vital signs every 15 to 30 minutes. Assess the client for signs of respiratory distress, pain, or discomfort. Check the dressing around the catheter exit site every 30 minutes for wetness during the procedure. Monitor the prescribed dwell time and initiate outflow. Assess blood glucose levels in clients who absorb glucose.

Observe the outflow pattern (outflow should be a continuous stream after the clamp is completely open). Accurately record the total amount of outflow after each exchange. Maintain accurate inflow and outflow records when hourly PD exchanges are performed. When outflow is less than inflow, the difference is retained by the client during dialysis and is counted as intake. Weigh the client daily to monitor fluid status.

RENAL TRANSPLANTATION

Dialysis and transplantation are life-sustaining *treatments* for end-stage renal disease (ESRD). Renal transplantation is not considered a "cure." Each client, in consultation with a nephrologist, determines which type of therapy is best suited to that client's physical condition and lifestyle. As of August 2003, 10,485 kidney transplants had been performed in that year. Currently more than 82,000 people are awaiting renal transplantation in the United States (United Network for Organ Sharing [UNOS], 2003).

Candidate Selection Criteria. Candidates for transplantation must be free of medical problems that might increase the risks from the procedure. The usual age range for transplantation is 2 to 70 years of age. Clients older than 70 years of age are considered for transplantation on an individual basis because complications are more common in the older adult.

A thorough assessment of the client is performed before the client is considered for transplantation. Clients who have advanced, uncorrectable cardiac disease are excluded from transplantation because these problems are made worse by the procedure. Other conditions that preclude transplantation include metastatic cancer, chronic infection, and severe psychosocial problems such as chemical dependency (Bartucci, 1999). Long-standing pulmonary disease increases the risk for complications and death from respiratory infections. Clients with diseases of the gastrointestinal system may require treatment before consideration for transplantation. Such problems as peptic ulcer and diverticulosis are made worse by the large doses of steroids used after transplantation.

The urinary system is completely evaluated to ensure normal urine flow. Many clients with ESRD have not used their lower urinary tract for years, and ureteral or bladder problems may require surgical correction before renal transplantation.

Clients with a recent history of cancer are treated with dialysis because of the shortage of donor organs and the limited life expectancy of these clients. In addition, the drugs used after transplantation increase the risk for cancer recurrence. If more than 2 to 5 years have passed since eradication of the cancer, the client can be considered for a transplant.

Diabetes mellitus and other endocrine problems cause even greater risks. These clients can have a renal transplant, but they require intense observation and management to limit complications. Other complicating conditions are considered on an individual basis, depending on the client's current health status. Renal transplantation can be considered for many of those with ESRD and is the optimal therapy for many people. Most people who have undergone this procedure are satisfied with their quality of life for years after the transplant (see the Evidence-Based Practice for Nursing box at right).

Donors. Kidney donors may be living donors (related or unrelated to the client), non–heart-beating donors (NHBDs), and cadaveric donors. The available kidneys are matched on the basis of tissue type similarity between the donor and the recipient. Living donors are most often blood relatives, but unrelated donors have been used. NHBDs are persons declared dead by cardiopulmonary criteria. Kidneys from NHBDs are harvested immediately after death in cases where clients have previously given consent for organ donation. If immediate removal must be delayed, in situ preservation is performed with infusion of a cool preservation solution inserted into the abdominal aorta after death is declared and until surgery can be performed. Cadaveric donors are usually individuals who suffered irreversible brain injury, most often as a result of trauma. These donors are maintained with mechanical ventilation and must have sufficient renal perfusion for the kidneys to remain viable (Bartucci, 1999).

The size of the kidney is seldom a problem in adults. Pediatric cadaveric kidneys hypertrophy to meet adult needs within a few months.

Organs from living *related* donors (LRDs) have the highest rates of renal graft survival (90%). Donors are usually at least 18 years old and are seldom older than 65 years of age. Physical criteria for donors include the following:

- Absence of systemic disease and infection
- No history of cancer
- No hypertension or renal disease
- Adequate renal function as determined by diagnostic studies

---

EVIDENCE-BASED PRACTICE for Nursing

Life satisfaction after kidney transplant influenced by other health problems

Siegal, B., Halbert, R., & McGuire, M. (2002). Life satisfaction among kidney transplant recipients: Demographic and biological factors. *Progress in Transplantation, 12*(4), 293-298.

The Transplant Learning Center (TLC), an organization dedicated to providing education and support to recipients of solid organ transplants, found that no current quality-of-life instrument was specific enough to include dimensions of concern to transplant recipients. This group developed the Life Satisfaction Index (LSI), which attempted to capture the issues considered by transplant recipients to most affect their level of life satisfaction. The investigators used a descriptive correlational study to determine which specific factors influenced the perception of life satisfaction among solid organ transplant recipients. This study reports the findings specifically for recipients of kidney transplants.

This instrument was mailed to the 9000 solid organ transplant recipients who had joined the TLC program. Analyses were performed on the questionnaires returned over a 2-year period by the 3676 kidney transplant recipients who participated in the initial survey round. Internal consistency of the total LSI is reported as having a Cronbach's alpha of 0.85 with a range on the individual items from 0.82 to 0.88. In addition to demographic data questions, the LSI included 8 questions related to life satisfaction, 11 questions related to comorbid health conditions, 11 questions related to adverse effects of the post-transplant regimen, and 6 questions related to adherence to post-transplant drug regimens.

Highest life satisfaction scores correlated with an age over 64 years, male gender, higher mean income and education, and being married. Lowest life satisfaction scores correlated with medical comorbidities, particularly emotional/psychological problems and eye/vision problems. Subjects who reported more frequent failure to adhere to the prescribed post-transplant drug regimen also had lower life satisfaction scores.

Level of Evidence: 6—Uncontrolled correlational, descriptive study.

Critique. The strengths of this study include the large sample size and the high level of internal consistency of the instrument. However, the sample is biased in several ways. First, only transplant recipients who were enrolled in the TLC were contacted for participation in the study. Of these, data were collected only on those subjects who returned their questionnaires, which may represent only those kidney transplant recipients who had higher levels of life satisfaction. This study relied solely on self-reports. The study could have been strengthened by having subjects also complete other established instruments to measure life satisfaction or quality of life and to compare the results with those obtained on the LSI.

Implications for Nursing. Life satisfaction for recipients of kidney transplants resembles that of other individuals in that it is multidimensional. Nurses need to help clients with end-stage renal disease who are planning for kidney transplantation to understand that the transplant will solve only renal-related issues. Other pre-existing health, psychological, financial, or personal issues will remain after the transplant and will continue to have some influence on the client's quality of life.

In addition, LRDs must express a clear understanding of the surgery and a willingness to give up a kidney. Some transplant centers require a psychiatric evaluation to assess the donor's motivation.

Because of advances in immunosuppressant therapy and medical management, the United Network of Organ Sharing (UNOS) reports 1-year renal transplant graft survival to be 90% for all centers in the United States (UNOS, 2003).

Preoperative Care. Many issues related to client health and the actual transplant procedure must be addressed before surgery. The Clinical Pathway on the Evolve website highlights care needs for the client undergoing renal transplantation.

Immunologic Studies. The major barrier to transplantation success after a suitable donor kidney is available is the body's ability to reject "foreign" tissue. This immunologic process can attack the transplanted kidney and destroy it. For immunologic problems to be overcome, in-depth tissue typing is performed on all candidates. These studies include simple blood typing and human leukocyte antigen (HLA) studies as well as other tests. The HLAs are the main immunologic feature used to match transplant recipients with compatible donors. The more similar the antigens of the donor are to those of the recipient, the more likely it is that the transplant will be successful and rejection will be avoided (see Chapter 23).

Surgical Team. The specialized surgical team includes circulating and scrub nurses, clinical nurse specialists, transplant surgeons, anesthesiologists, and nephrologists. Preoperative nursing responsibilities include the following:

- Teaching about the procedure and postoperative care
- In-depth client assessment
- Coordination of diagnostic tests
- Development and implementation of treatment plans

The client usually requires dialysis within 24 hours of the surgery. In addition, the recipient often receives a blood transfusion before surgery. Usually blood from the kidney donor is transfused into the recipient. This procedure increases graft survival of organs from LRDs.

Operative Procedures. The donor nephrectomy procedure varies depending on whether the donor is an NHBD, cadaveric donor, or living donor. The NHBD or cadaveric donor nephrectomy is a sterile autopsy in the operating room. All arterial and venous vessels and a long piece of ureter are preserved. After removal, the kidneys are preserved until time for implantation into the recipient. The technique for kidney removal from living donors is a delicate procedure that lasts 3 to 4 hours. A flank incision is used, and care is taken to avoid scarring. Donors usually have more pain after surgery than do recipients. They also need nursing care and support for the psychological adjustment to loss of a body part.

The transplantation surgery usually takes 4 to 5 hours. The transplanted kidney is usually placed in the right anterior iliac fossa (Figure 75-12) instead of the usual anatomic position. This placement allows easier connection of the ureter and the renal artery and vein. It also allows for kidney assessment by palpation. The recipient's own nonfunctioning kidneys are not usually removed unless chronic infection is present in one or both kidneys. After surgery, the client is taken to the postanesthesia unit and then, when stable, to a designated unit in the transplant center or to a critical care unit.

Postoperative Care. Care of the recipient after surgery requires that nurses be knowledgeable about the expected clinical findings and potential complications. Nursing care includes ongoing physical assessment with an emphasis on evaluation of renal function. The transplant recipient requires close attention because the immunosuppressive drug therapy used to prevent tissue rejection impairs healing and increases the risk for infection.

Urologic management is essential to graft success. These clients always have a large indwelling (Foley) catheter for accurate measurements of urine output and decompression of the bladder. Decompression prevents stretch on suture and ureter attachment sites on the bladder.

Assess urine output at least hourly during the first 48 hours. An abrupt decrease in urine output may indicate complications such as rejection, acute tubular necrosis (ATN), thrombosis, or obstruction. Examine the urine color. The urine is pink and bloody right after surgery and gradually returns to normal over several days to several weeks, depending on renal function. Obtain daily urine specimens for urinalysis, glucose measurement, the presence of acetone, specific gravity measurement, and culture (if needed).

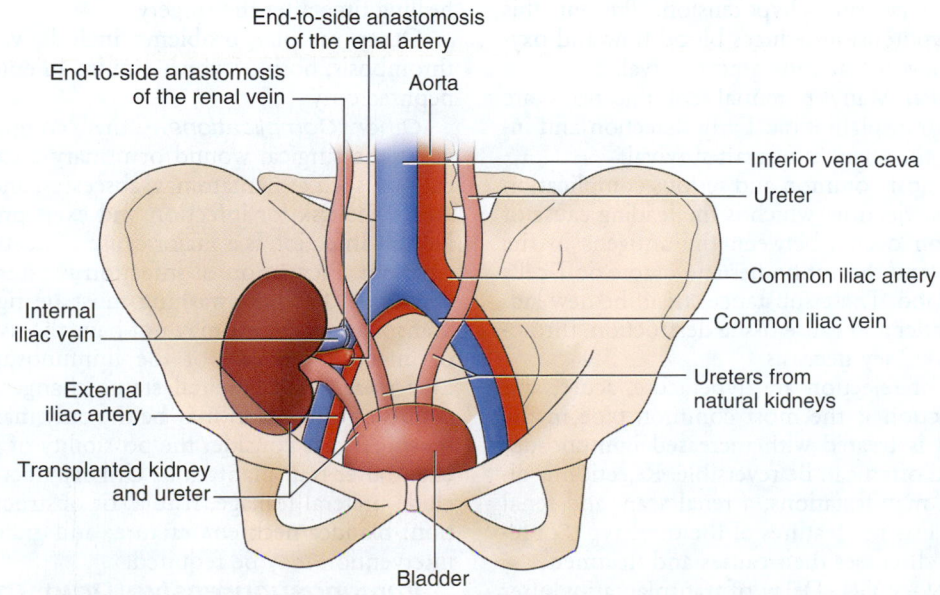

Figure 75-12 ■ Placement of a transplanted kidney in the right iliac fossa.

TABLE 75-13 A Comparison of Hyperacute, Acute, and Chronic Post-Transplant Rejection

Hyperacute Rejection	Acute Rejection	Chronic Rejection
Onset		
Within 48 hr after surgery	1 wk to 2 yr postoperatively (most common in first 2 wk)	Occurs gradually during a period of months to years
Clinical Manifestations		
Increased temperature	Oliguria or anuria	Gradual increase in BUN and serum creati-
Increased blood pressure	Temperature over 100° F (37.8° C)	nine levels
Pain at transplant site	Increased blood pressure	Fluid retention
	Enlarged, tender kidney	Changes in serum electrolyte levels
	Lethargy	Fatigue
	Elevated serum creatinine, BUN, potassium levels	
	Fluid retention	
Treatment		
Immediate removal of the transplanted kidney	Increased doses of immunosuppressive drugs	Conservative management until dialysis is required

BUN, Blood urea nitrogen.

Occasionally a continuous bladder irrigation is prescribed to decrease the formation of blood clots, which could increase pressure in the bladder and endanger the graft. Perform routine catheter care, according to your agency's policy, to reduce catheter contamination. The catheter is removed as soon as possible to avoid infection, usually 3 to 7 days after surgery. After surgery the function of the transplanted kidney (renal graft) can result in either oliguria or diuresis. Oliguria may occur as a result of ischemia and ATN, rejection, or other complications. To increase urine output, the physician may prescribe diuretics and osmotic agents, such as mannitol. Closely monitor the client's fluid status because fluid overload can cause hypertension, heart failure, and pulmonary edema. Evaluate the client's fluid status by taking daily weights, measuring blood pressure every 2 to 4 hours, and accurately measuring intake and output.

Instead of oliguria, the client may have diuresis, especially with a kidney from a living related donor (LRD). Carefully monitor intake and output, and observe for electrolyte imbalances, such as hypokalemia and hyponatremia. Excessive diuresis may cause hypotension. Prevent this problem because hypotension reduces blood flow and oxygen to the new kidney, threatening graft survival.

Complications. Many potential complications are possible after renal transplantation. Early detection and intervention improve the chances of graft survival.

Rejection. The most common and serious complication of transplantation is rejection, which is the leading cause of graft loss. A reaction occurs between the antigens in the transplanted kidney and the antibodies and cytotoxic T-cells in the recipient's blood. These substances treat the new kidney as a foreign invader and cause tissue destruction, thrombosis, and eventual kidney necrosis.

The three types of rejection are hyperacute, acute, and chronic. Acute rejection is the most common type in the transplant client. It is treated with increased immunosuppressive therapy and often can be reversible. Rejection is diagnosed by clinical manifestations, a renal scan, and renal biopsy. Table 75-13 lists the features of the three types of rejection. Chapter 23 discusses their causes and treatment.

Acute Tubular Necrosis. Delay of transplantation after kidneys have been harvested can result in ischemic damage to the kidney and the client having acute tubular necrosis

(ATN) after surgery. These clients may need dialysis until adequate urine output returns and the blood urea nitrogen (BUN) and creatinine levels normalize. ATN is often difficult to distinguish from acute rejection, and clients need to undergo weekly biopsies to assess the need for further immunosuppression if rejection is occurring.

Thrombosis. Thrombosis of the major renal blood vessels may occur during the first 2 to 3 days after transplantation. A sudden decrease in urine output may signal impaired perfusion resulting from thrombosis. Ultrasound examination of the kidney may reveal decreased or absent blood supply. Emergency surgery is required to prevent ischemic damage or graft loss.

Renal Artery Stenosis. Stenosis of the renal artery may result in hypertension. Other manifestations include a bruit over the artery anastomosis site and decreased renal function. A renal scan can quantify the blood flow to the kidney. The involved artery may be repaired surgically or by balloon angioplasty in the radiology department. The decision to perform a balloon repair is determined by the amount of healing time after the surgery.

Other vascular problems include vascular leakage or thrombosis, both of which require an emergency transplant nephrectomy.

Other Complications. Other complications may involve the surgical wound or urinary tract. Wound complications, such as hematomas, abscesses, and lymphoceles, increase the risk for infection and exert pressure on the new kidney. Infection is a major cause of death in the transplant recipient. Prevention of infection is essential. Strict aseptic technique and handwashing must be rigorously enforced. Transplant recipients may not have the usual manifestations of infection because of the immunosuppressive therapy. Low-grade fevers, mental status changes, and vague complaints of discomfort may be the only manifestations before sepsis. Always consider the possibility of infection with any client after transplantation. Urinary tract complications include ureteral leakage, fistula, or obstruction; stone formation; bladder neck contracture; and graft rupture. Surgical intervention may be required.

Immunosuppressive Drug Therapy. The success of renal transplantation depends on changing the client's immunologic response so that the new kidney is not rejected as a foreign organ. Immunosuppressive drugs protect the transplanted organ. These drugs include corticosteroids, anti-lymphocyte preparations, monoclonal antibodies, and cyclosporine (Cyclosporin A). Chapter 23 discusses the mechanisms of action for these agents and the associated client responses. Clients taking these drugs are at an increased risk for death by viral, fungal, bacterial, or protozoal infection.

Community-Based Care

HOME CARE MANAGEMENT

Because of the complex nature of CRF, its progressive course, and many treatment modalities, a case manager is helpful in the planning, coordination, and evaluation of care. As the renal disease progresses, the client is seen by a physician or nurse practitioner regularly and may be hospitalized often. Together with the dietitian and social worker, evaluate the home environment and determine equipment needs before discharge. Once the client is discharged, home care nurses direct care and monitor progress. Chart 75-12 provides a focused assessment guide for the client after transplantation.

Provide health teaching about the diet in renal disease and the progression of renal disease. As CRF approaches end-stage renal disease (ESRD), one of the following courses of treatment is chosen: hemodialysis (HD), peritoneal dialysis (PD), or transplantation. For each form of treatment, the client must learn about the procedures and consider his or her personal lifestyle, support systems, and methods of coping. Decision making about treatment type, or even whether to pursue treatment, is difficult for clients and families. Provide information and emotional support to assist clients with these decisions.

Teach clients who select hemodialysis (HD) about the dialysis machine and vascular access care. If in-home HD is selected, preparations are needed for installation of the appropriate equipment, including a water treatment system. Regardless of whether the treatment occurs at home or in a center, provide ongoing physical assessment and health teaching to promote independence at home.

The client receiving PD needs extensive training in the procedure. The client also needs assistance in obtaining equipment and the many supplies needed. Home care nurses assess clients, monitor vital signs, assess adherence with drug and diet regimens, and monitor for manifestations of peritonitis.

The nurse plays a vital role in the long-term care of the client with a renal transplant. This client is usually discharged 3 to 4 weeks after surgery. Stress that adherence to the prescribed immunosuppressive drug therapy is essential for the survival of the kidney. Facilitate acceptance and understanding of this regimen as a part of daily life. Carefully monitor for signs of graft rejection and for complications, such as infection.

HEALTH TEACHING

Instruct clients and family members in all aspects of diet therapy, drug therapy, and complications. Teach clients and family members to report complications, such as fluid overload and infection. When a client requires a more advanced form of therapy, such as dialysis or transplantation, focus teaching on the chosen therapeutic intervention.

CHART 75-12

FOCUSED ASSESSMENT of
The Client with Chronic Renal Failure

Assess cardiovascular and respiratory status, including the following:
- Vital signs, with special attention to blood pressure
- Presence of S_3 or pericardial friction rub
- Presence of chest pain
- Presence of edema (periorbital, pretibial, sacral)
- Jugular vein distention
- Presence of dyspnea
- Presence of crackles, beginning at the bases and extending upward

Assess nutritional status, including the following:
- Weight gain or loss
- Presence of anorexia, nausea, or vomiting

Assess renal status, including the following:
- Amount, frequency, and appearance of urine (in non-anuric clients)
- Presence of bone pain
- Presence of hyperglycemia secondary to diabetes

Assess hematologic status, including the following:
- Presence of petechiae, purpura, ecchymoses
- Presence of fatigue or shortness of breath

Assess gastrointestinal status, including the following:
- Presence of stomatitis
- Presence of melena

Assess integumentary status, including the following:
- Skin integrity
- Presence of pruritus
- Presence of skin discoloration

Assess neurologic status, including the following:
- Changes in mental status
- Presence of seizure activity
- Presence of sensory changes
- Presence of lower extremity weakness

Assess laboratory data, including the following:
- BUN
- Serum creatinine
- Creatinine clearance
- CBC
- Electrolytes

Assess psychosocial status, including the following:
- Presence of anxiety
- Presence of maladaptive behavior

BUN, Blood urea nitrogen; *CBC*, complete blood count.

Hemodialysis (HD) is the most complex form of therapy for the client and family to understand. Even if clients receive HD in a dialysis center instead of at home, they are expected to have some knowledge of the HD machine. The client or a family member must be taught to care for the vascular access and to report signs of infection and stenosis. The client who plans to have in-home HD will need a partner. Both the client and the partner must be taught the entire process of HD and must be able to perform it independently before the client is discharged.

Peritoneal dialysis (PD) involves extensive health teaching. This instruction can be given to the client alone or to the client and a family member if the client cannot perform the procedure. Emphasize sterile technique because peritonitis is the most common complication of PD. Instruct clients to report any manifestation of peritonitis, especially cloudy effluent and abdominal pain. If peritonitis develops, teach clients how to give themselves antibiotics by the intraperitoneal (IP) route. Stress the importance of completing the antibiotic regimen. Remind clients that repeated episodes of peritonitis can reduce the effectiveness of PD, which may require the transfer to HD.

The client receiving a renal transplant also needs extensive health teaching. Provide instruction about drug regimens, home monitoring, immunosuppression, manifestations of rejection, infection, and prescribed changes in the diet and activity level.

PSYCHOSOCIAL PREPARATION

Provide psychological support for the client and family. Help the client adjust to the diagnosis of renal failure and eventually accept the treatment regimens.

Many clients view dialysis as a cure instead of a required lifelong treatment. For many clients, the reduction of uremic symptoms in the first weeks after starting dialysis treatment creates a sense of euphoria and well-being (the "honeymoon" period). They feel better physically, and their mood may be happy and hopeful. At this time they tend to overlook the discomfort and inconvenience of dialysis. Use this time to begin health care teaching. Stress that although the uremic symptoms are reduced, the client will not return completely to the previous state of well-being.

Many clients become discouraged during the first year of treatment. This mood state may last a few months to a year or longer. The difficulties of incorporating dialysis into daily life are staggering, and clients may become depressed as problems occur. They may struggle with the idea of having to be permanently dependent on a disruptive therapy. Clients may feel helpless and dependent. Some people retreat into complete or partial denial of the disease and the need for treatment. They may deny the need for dialysis or may not adhere to drug therapy and diet restrictions. Monitor any behaviors that may contribute to nonadherence, and suggest psychiatric referrals. Help the client and family to focus on the positive aspects of the treatments. Continue health care education with clients as active participants and decision makers.

Most clients with CRF eventually enter a phase of acceptance or resignation. The idea of a chronic illness may be devastating for some people, and each person reacts differently. To make this long-term adaptation, the client must adjust to continuous change. Specific concerns depend on the client's health and particular treatment method.

After clients have accepted or become resigned to the chronic aspect of their disease, they usually attempt to return to their previous activities. Resuming the previous level of activity, however, may not be possible. Help clients to set realistic goals that allow them to lead active, productive lives.

HEALTH CARE RESOURCES

Professionals from various disciplines are resources for the client with renal failure. Home care nurses monitor the client's status and evaluate maintenance of the prescribed treatment regimen (HD or PD). A client with advanced renal failure may need a home care aide to help perform activities of daily living. Social services are often involved because of the complex process of applying for financial aid to pay for the required medical care. A physical therapist may be beneficial in helping to improve the client's functional health. A dietitian can assist the client and family members in understanding the special dietary needs. A psychiatric evaluation may be needed if depressive symptoms are present. Clergy and pastoral care specialists offer spiritual support.

Clients with CRF are routinely followed by a physician, usually a nephrologist. Organizations such as the National Kidney Foundation (NKF), the American Kidney Fund, and the National Association of Patients on Hemodialysis and Transplantation (NAPHT) may be helpful to clients and families.

◆ Evaluation: Outcomes

Evaluate the care of the client with chronic renal failure (CRF) on the basis of the identified nursing diagnoses and collaborative problems. The expected outcomes are that the client should:
- Achieve and maintain appropriate fluid volume
- Maintain an adequate nutritional status
- Use effective coping strategies
- Report an absence of physical manifestations of anxiety

Specific indicators for these outcomes are listed for each nursing diagnosis and collaborative problem under the Planning and Implementation section (see earlier).

GET READY for the NCLEX Examination!

KEY POINTS

Safe Effective Care Environment

- Use sterile technique when cannulating a vascular access or connecting peritoneal dialysis tubing.
- Handle clients with chronic renal failure gently to prevent fractures.
- Assess all clients at risk for dehydration or hypovolemia for adequacy of renal perfusion.

Health Promotion and Maintenance

- Encourage clients with renal failure to follow fluid and dietary restrictions regarding sodium, potassium, and protein.
- Instruct clients on immunosuppressive therapy to avoid crowds and people who are ill.
- Teach clients on immunosuppressive therapy to assess themselves daily for fever, general malaise, and nausea or vomiting.

Psychosocial Integrity

- Pace your interview to match the learning needs and style of the individual client.
- Allow the client the opportunity to express fear or anxiety regarding the risk for death and the disruption of lifestyle as a result of treatment for renal failure.
- During renal/urinary assessment use language and terminology that are comfortable for the client.
- Assess the client for depression and nonacceptance of his or her diagnosis or treatment plan.
- Refer clients to community resources and support groups.

Physiological Integrity

- Report immediately any condition that obstructs urine flow.
- Teach clients the expected side effects and any adverse reactions to prescribed drugs.
- Collaborate with the dietitian to teach clients about needed fluid, sodium, potassium, or dietary protein restriction.

- Teach clients in the early stages of renal failure the manifestations of dehydration.
- Teach clients in the later stages of chronic renal failure the manifestations of fluid overload and hyperkalemia.
- Avoid taking blood pressure measurements or drawing blood from an arm with a vascular access (AV fistula or graft).
- Do not use an AV fistula or graft site for IV fluid administration.
- Avoid all invasive procedures within 4 to 6 hours after the client has undergone hemodialysis.
- Use meticulous sterile technique when caring for the peritoneal dialysis catheter and when hooking up or clamping off dialysate bags.
- Teach clients using peritoneal dialysis the manifestations of peritonitis.

ADDITIONAL STUDY RESOURCES

Go to your Student CD-ROM for Review Questions for the NCLEX Examination.

Go to http://evolve.elsevier.com/Iggy/ for Integrated Management of Care Questions for the NCLEX Examination.

SELECTED BIBLIOGRAPHY

Asterisk indicates a classic or definitive work on this subject.

Abbas, A., & Lichtman, A. (2003). *Cellular and molecular immunology* (5th ed). Philadelphia: W.B. Saunders.

Ackley, B., & Ladwig, G. (2002). *Nursing diagnosis handbook: A guide to planning care* (5th ed). St. Louis: Mosby.

American Association of Kidney Patients. (2003). Understanding your hemodialysis access options. Available at http://kidney.niddk.nih.gov/kudiseases/pubs/vascularaccess/index.htm.

*Baer, C. (1998). Care of the critically ill chronic renal failure patient: Crisis, challenges and choices. *Critical Care Nursing Clinics of North America, 10*(4), 433-448.

Baker, J., & Thomas, A. (2001). Progressive renal insufficiency program planning: A technique for evaluation and improvement. *Nephrology Nursing Journal, 28*(1), 13-18.

Barone, C., Martin-Watson, A., & Barone, G. (2004). The postoperative care of the adult renal transplant recipient. *MEDSURG Nursing, 13*(5), 296-302.

*Bartucci, M.R. (1999). Kidney transplantation: State of the art. *AACN Clinical Issues: Advanced Practice in Acute and Critical Care, 10*(2), 153-163.

Behrens, J. (2001). Assessing anemia secondary to hemolysis in hemodialysis patients. *Nephrology Nursing Journal, 28*(2), 253-258.

Blanchet, P., et al. (2000). Urinary complications after kidney transplantation can be reduced. *Transplant Proceedings, 32,* 2769.

Burrows-Hudson, S. (2005). Chronic kidney disease: An overview. *American Journal of Nursing, 105*(2), 40-49.

Campbell, D. (2003). How acute renal failure puts the brakes on kidney function. *Nursing 2003, 33*(1), 59-64.

Cannon, J. (2004). Recognizing chronic renal failure. *Nursing 2004, 34*(1), 50-53.

Coburn, S., & Mitchell, S. (2002). Acute renal failure. *American Journal of Nursing, 102*(4), 6-12.

Dochterman, J., & Bulechek, G. (Eds.). (2004). *Nursing interventions classification (NIC)* (4th ed). St. Louis: Mosby.

Drummond, D. (2000). Caring for your patient with a permanent hemodialysis access. *Nursing 2000, 30*(3), 41-46.

Ebersole, P., Hess, P., & Luggen, A. (2004). *Toward healthy aging: Human needs and nursing response* (6th ed). St. Louis: Mosby.

Facts and Comparisons. (2004). *Drug facts and comparisons* (58th ed). St. Louis: Author.

*Giuliano, K., & Sims, T.W. (1999). Transplant issues: Infections and immunosuppressant drugs. *Dimensions of Critical Care Nursing, 18*(2), 16-19.

Hagren, B., et al. (2001). The haemodialysis machine as a lifeline: Experiences of suffering from end-stage renal disease. *Journal of Advanced Nursing, 34*(2), 196-202.

Hayes, D. (2000). Caring for your patient with a permanent renal dialysis access. *Nursing 2000, 30*(3), 41-46.

Kaplow, R., & Barry, R. (2002). Continuous renal replacement therapies. *American Journal of Nursing, 102*(11), 26-34.

Kearney, K. (2000). Dialysis disequilibrium syndrome. *American Journal of Nursing, 100*(2), 53-54.

Kellum, J. (2000). An evaluation of pharmacological strategies for the prevention and treatment of acute renal failure. *Drugs, 59*(1), 79-91.

King, B. (2000). Meds and the dialysis patient. *RN, 63*(7), 54-59.

Kuhlmann, M.K., Schmidt, F., & Kohler, H. (1999). High protein/energy vs. standard protein: Energy nutritional regimen in the treatment of malnourished hemodialysis patients. *Mineral and Electrolyte Metabolism, 25*(4-6), 306-310.

*Levine, D.Z. (1997). *Caring for the renal patient* (3rd ed.). Philadelphia: W.B. Saunders.

Manns, B., Doig, C., Lee, H., Dean, S., Tonelli, M., Johnson, D., & Donalson, C. (2003). Cost of acute renal failure requiring dialysis in the intensive care unit: Clinical and resource implications of renal recovery. *Critical Care Medicine, 31*(2), 449-455.

Martins, L., et al. (2000). Renal osteodystrophy: Histologic evaluation after renal transplantation. *Transplantation Proceedings, 32,* 2599-2601.

McCance, K., & Huether, S. (2002). *Pathophysiology: The biologic basis for disease in adults and children* (4th ed). St. Louis: Mosby.

Medline Plus (2003). Acute renal failure, chronic renal failure. Available at http://www.nlm.nih.gov/medlineplus/ency/encyclopedia_R.htm.

*Mehrotra, R., & Nolph, K.D. (1999). Low protein diets are not needed in chronic renal failure. *Mineral and Electrolyte Metabolism, 25*(4-6), 311-316.

Merck Manual B Home Edition (2003). Kidney failure. Available at http://www.merck.com/mrkshared/mmanual_home/sec11/123.jsp

Moorhead, S., Johnson, M., & Maas, M. (Eds.). (2004). *Nursing outcomes classification (NOC)* (3rd ed). St. Louis: Mosby.

Nally, J. (2002). Acute renal failure in hospitalized patients. *Cleveland Clinic Journal of Medicine, 60*(7), 569-574.

National Kidney and Urologic Diseases Information Clearinghouse (2003). Treatment methods for kidney failure: Hemodialysis, Peritoneal Dialysis, Kidney Transplantation. Available at http://kidney.niddk.nih.gov/kudiseases/pubs/.

Nussbaum, R., McInnes, R., & Willard, H. (2001). *Thompson & Thompson: Genetics in medicine* (6th ed). Philadelphia: W.B. Saunders.

Pagana, K., & Pagana, T. (2002). *Mosby's manual of diagnostic and laboratory tests* (2nd ed.). St. Louis: Mosby.

Polkinghorne, K., & Kerr, P. (2002). Predicting vascular access failures: A collective review. *Nephrology 2002*(7), 170-176.

Ray, T. (2000). Chronic and acute renal failure: Primary care issues. *ADVANCE for Nurse Practitioners, 8*(8), 69-72.

Ro, Y., et al. (2002). The effects of aromatherapy on pruritus in patients undergoing hemodialysis. *Dermatology Nursing, 14*(4), 231-234, 237-239.

Sehgal, A.R. (2000). Outcomes of renal replacement therapy among blacks and women. *American Journal of Kidney Diseases, 35*(4 Suppl 1), S148-S152.

Siegal, B., Halbert, R., & McGuire, M. (2002). Life satisfaction among kidney transplant recipients: Demographic and biological factors. *Progress in Transplantation, 12*(4), 293-298.

Sofer, D. (2003). Chronic kidney disease: The emerging epidemic. *American Journal of Nursing, 103*(12), 23.

*Stark, J. (1998). Acute renal failure: Focus on advances in acute tubular necrosis. *Critical Care Nursing Clinics of North America, 10*(2), 159-170.

Tanyi, R. (2002). Sexual unattractiveness: A patient's story. *MEDSURG Nursing, 11*(2), 95-99.

Tran, M., & Rutecki, G. (2000). Renal disease: Tips on prevention and early recognition. *Consultant, 40*(2), 222-229.

United Network for Organ Sharing online. (2003). Available at http://www.unos.org.

U.S. Renal Data Systems. (2002). *USRDS 2002 annual data report.* Bethesda, MD: National Institutes of Health, National Institute of Diabetes and Digestive and Kidney Diseases.

PROBLEMS of REPRODUCTION

Management of Clients with Problems of the Reproductive System

Assessment of the Reproductive System

DEITRA LEONARD LOWDERMILK

LEARNING OUTCOMES

After studying this chapter, you should be able to:

1. Review the anatomy and physiology of the male and female reproductive systems.
2. Discuss the components of a health history for reproductive health problems using Gordon's Functional Health Patterns.
3. Explain the procedures for physical assessment of the male and female reproductive systems.
4. Describe the client preparation for common reproductive diagnostic tests.
5. Interpret common reproductive laboratory diagnostic test findings.
6. Develop a teaching plan for a client undergoing one of the endoscopic studies for reproductive health problems.
7. Explain the importance of selected reproductive screening tests in promoting and maintaining health (e.g., Pap test).

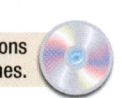

Go to your Student CD-ROM for Review Questions
for the NCLEX Examination keyed to these Learning Outcomes.

The nurse is often the first health care professional to assess the client with a reproductive system disorder. Basic assessment of the male and female reproductive systems should be part of every complete physical examination. The nurse should be comfortable with his or her sexuality and be nonjudgmental about differences in sexual practices.

This chapter describes basic reproductive system assessment. Chapters 77, 78, and 79 provide additional assessment data. The student is also referred to a fundamentals or basic nursing text for a review of human sexuality.

ANATOMY AND PHYSIOLOGY REVIEW

Structure and Function of the Female Reproductive System

Females begin to develop secondary sex characteristics at a wide range of ages. The average age for a girl to begin puberty is 11 years of age. Delayed puberty may be caused by the following:

- A familial history of late growth
- A low percentage of body fat
- Problems of the pituitary gland, ovaries, or hypothalamus
- Congenital structural abnormalities

EXTERNAL GENITALIA

The external female genitalia, or **vulva,** extends from the mons pubis to the anal opening. The **mons pubis** is a fat pad that covers the symphysis pubis and protects it during **coitus** (sexual intercourse). The mons becomes prominent and covered with hair during puberty.

The **labia majora** are two vertical folds of adipose tissue that extend posteriorly from the mons pubis to the perineum. The size of the labia majora varies depending on the amount of fatty tissue present. The skin over the labia majora is usually darker than the surrounding skin and is highly vascular. The labia become prominent during puberty and develop hair on the outer surfaces. The labia majora protect inner vulval structures and enhance sexual arousal.

The labia majora surround two thinner, vertical folds of reddish epithelium called the **labia minora.** The labia minora are highly vascular and have a rich nerve supply. Emotional or physical stimulation produces marked swelling and sensitivity. Numerous sebaceous glands in the labia minora lubricate the entrance to the vagina. The **clitoris** is a small, cylindric organ that is composed of erectile tissue with a high concentration of sensory nerve endings. During sexual arousal, the clitoris becomes larger and increases sexual sensation.

The **vestibule** is a longitudinal area between the labia minora, the clitoris, and the vagina that contains Bartholin's

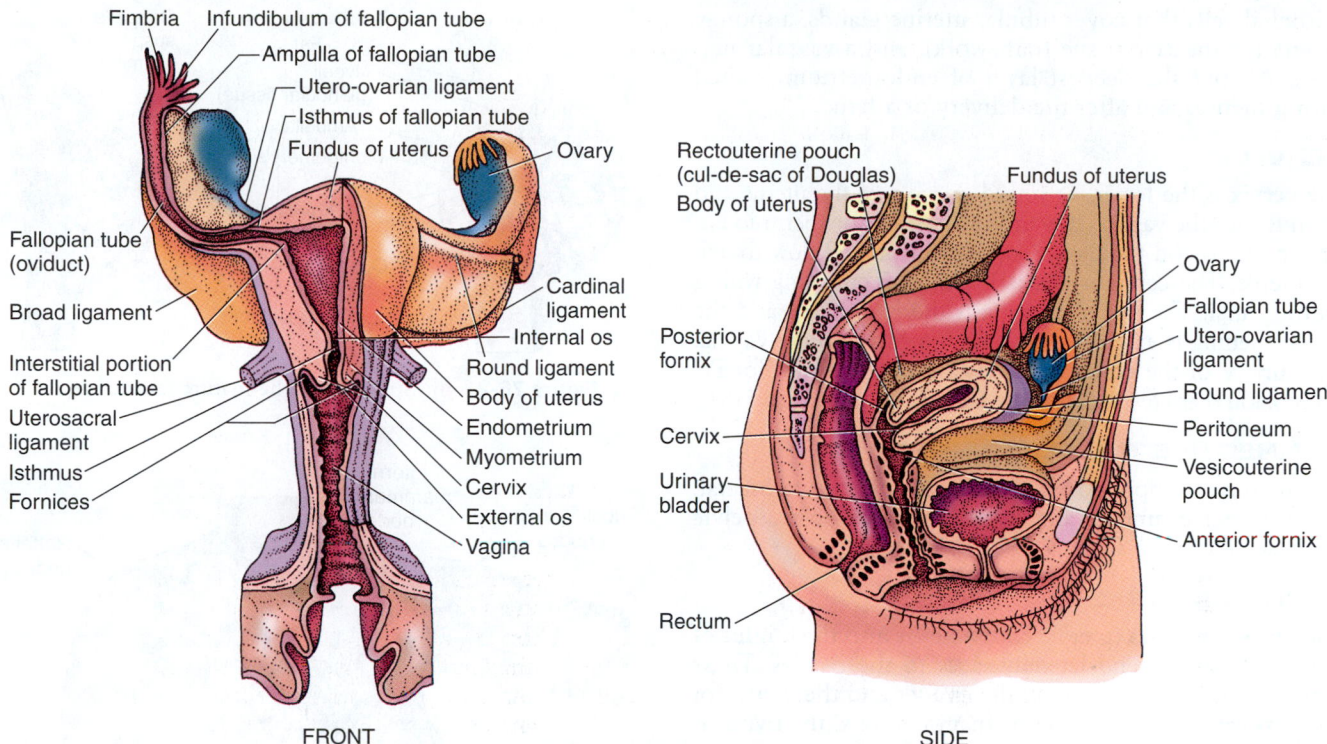

Figure 76-1 ■ Internal female genitalia.

glands and the openings of the urethra, Skene's glands (paraurethral glands), and vagina. The two Bartholin's glands, located deeply toward the back on both sides of the vaginal opening, secrete lubrication fluid during sexual excitement. Their ductal openings are usually not visible.

The area between the vaginal opening and the anus is the **perineum.** The skin of the perineum covers the muscles, fascia, and ligaments that support the pelvic structures.

INTERNAL GENITALIA

The internal female genitalia are shown in Figure 76-1.

Vagina

The **vagina** is a collapsible hollow tube that extends from the vestibule to the uterus. In addition to being the channel for the passage of the menstrual flow, the vagina allows reception of the penis during intercourse and passage of the fetus during a vaginal birth. Mucous membrane and many blood vessels line the thin, muscular walls of the vagina. This tissue lies in folds **(rugae)** during the reproductive years and is very stretchable. Reduced estrogen levels, occurring during postpartum periods, lactation, and menopause, cause the vaginal wall to become dry, thinner, and smoother.

The amounts of glycogen and lubricating fluid secreted by the vaginal cells are influenced by ovarian hormones. Döderlein's bacilli, the normal vaginal flora, interact with the secretions to produce lactic acid and maintain an acidic pH (4 to 5) in the vagina. This acidity reduces the susceptibility of the vagina to infection.

At the upper end of the vagina, the uterine cervix projects into a cup-shaped vault of thin vaginal tissue. The recessed pockets around the cervix (the fornices) permit palpation of the internal pelvic organs. The posterior area

provides access into the peritoneal cavity (through the cul-de-sac of Douglas) for diagnostic or surgical purposes.

Uterus

The **uterus** is a thick-walled, muscular organ attached to the upper end of the vagina. This inverted pear-shaped organ is located within the true pelvis, between the bladder and the rectum. The uterus is composed of the corpus (body) and the cervix. The uterus responds to hormonal stimulation and prepares to receive, nurture and, finally, expel the products of conception.

The size of the uterus depends on the woman's developmental stage and obstetric history. In women who have never been pregnant, the average uterine dimensions are 3½ inches × 2 inches × 1 inch (7.5 cm × 5 cm × 2.5 cm).

CORPUS

The upper segment of the uterine body, between the insertion sites of the fallopian tubes, is referred to as the fundus. Although the uterus is a hollow organ, its walls are in such close proximity in the nonpregnant state that its cavity is merely a slit. The uterine walls are composed of three layers: the perimetrium, the myometrium, and the endometrium.

The **perimetrium** is the outer layer that separates the uterus from the abdominal cavity. The **myometrium** is the thick, middle, muscular layer of the body of the uterus. Contraction of these muscle fibers can expel the products of conception and can constrict the blood vessels to control bleeding after childbirth.

The inner mucosal layer of the uterine body is the **endometrium**. The monthly cyclic effects of estrogen and progesterone change the thickness of this tissue (from 0.5 to 5 mm). The endometrium consists of a single layer of epithelial cells that cover tubular uterine glands, a spongy stroma (connective tissue framework), and a vascular network. All but the deepest layer of endometrium is shed during menses and after the delivery of a fetus.

CERVIX

The **cervix** is the lower, narrowed portion of the uterus and extends into the vagina. It is the passage site for sperm to enter the uterus and the passage site for menstrual flow to exit the uterus. The cervix is about 1 inch (2.5 cm) long with a central canal. The upper opening is the internal os and the lower opening is external os, which projects into the vagina. The surface of the cervix and the canal are the sites for Papanicolaou (Pap) testing. (See the later discussion on p. 1781.)

CONNECTIVE TISSUE SUPPORT

The uterus is supported by the broad, round, uterosacral, and cardinal ligaments and by the muscles of the pelvic floor (see Figure 76-1).

Fallopian Tubes

The **fallopian tubes** (uterine tubes) insert into the fundus of the uterus and extend laterally close to the ovaries. These tubes provide a duct between the ovaries and the uterus for the passage of ova and sperm. In most cases, the ovum is fertilized in these tubes.

Each tube is about $3\frac{1}{8}$ to $5\frac{1}{2}$ inches (8 to 14 cm) long and is covered by one of the peritoneal folds of the broad ligament. The tubes are lined with ciliated and secretory cells, which help move the ovum to the uterus.

The uterine tubes have four anatomic sections (see Figure 76-1). The interstitial portion is closest to the uterus, the isthmus and the ampulla are the middle segments, and the infundibulum is the most distal portion. The fimbriated ends of the infundibulum extend almost to each ovary and facilitate the capture of a released ovum during ovulation.

Ovaries

The **ovaries** are a pair of almond-shaped organs located near the lateral walls of the upper pelvic cavity. After menopause, they become smaller. These small organs develop and release ova. **Ovulation** is the cyclic maturation of a dominant follicle (the graafian follicle) and the subsequent release of the ovum. The ovaries also produce the sex steroid hormones (estrogen, progesterone, androgen, and relaxin). Adequate amounts of these steroidal sex hormones are needed for normal female growth and development and for the maintenance of a pregnancy.

BREASTS

The female **breasts** are a pair of mammary glands that develop in response to secretions from the hypothalamus, pituitary gland, and ovaries. The breasts are an accessory of the reproductive system meant to nourish the infant after birth. They also are an organ for sexual arousal in the mature adult.

The breasts are located between the second and sixth ribs, between the edge of the sternum and the midaxillary line. About two thirds of the breast lies over the greater pectoral muscle.

The structure of a mature female breast is shown in Figure 76-2. The nipple rises from the center of the pigmented

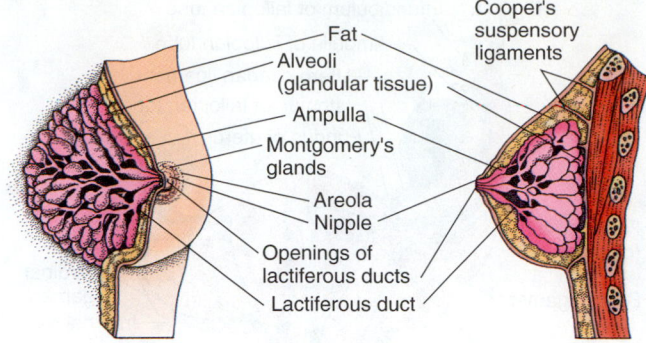

Figure 76-2 ■ Structure of the mature female breast.

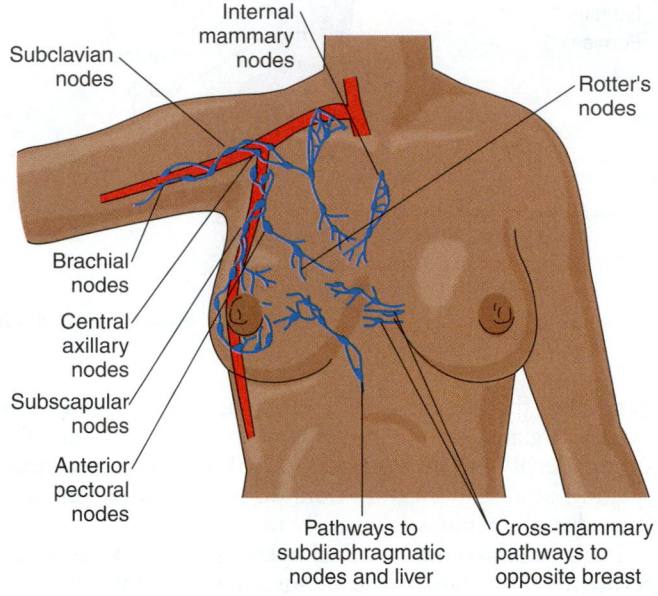

Figure 76-3 ■ Lymphatic drainage of the female breast.

areola, which is usually located slightly lateral to the midline of each breast. Montgomery's glands are small, round sebaceous glands that appear as elevations on the areola. These glands are thought to secrete a fatty substance that protects the nipple during breastfeeding.

Breast tissue is composed of a network of glandular and ductal tissue, fibrous tissue, and fat. The proportion of each component of breast tissue depends on genetic factors, nutrition, age, and obstetric history. The breast is supported by Cooper's suspensory ligaments that are attached to underlying muscles. The breasts have abundant blood supply and lymph flow. Lymph drains from an extensive network toward the axilla (Figure 76-3).

The breasts may not develop symmetrically during puberty but are usually symmetric in size and contour by adulthood. It is not unusual for the breast on the woman's dominant side (on the basis of right-handedness or left-handedness) to appear larger because of the more developed pectoral muscle base.

In many women, the breasts become slightly larger and tender during the premenstrual period. The tissue may also feel nodular at this time. Increasing levels of estrogen and progesterone 3 to 4 days before menses affect the breasts by

Animation: Lymphatic Drainage ▼

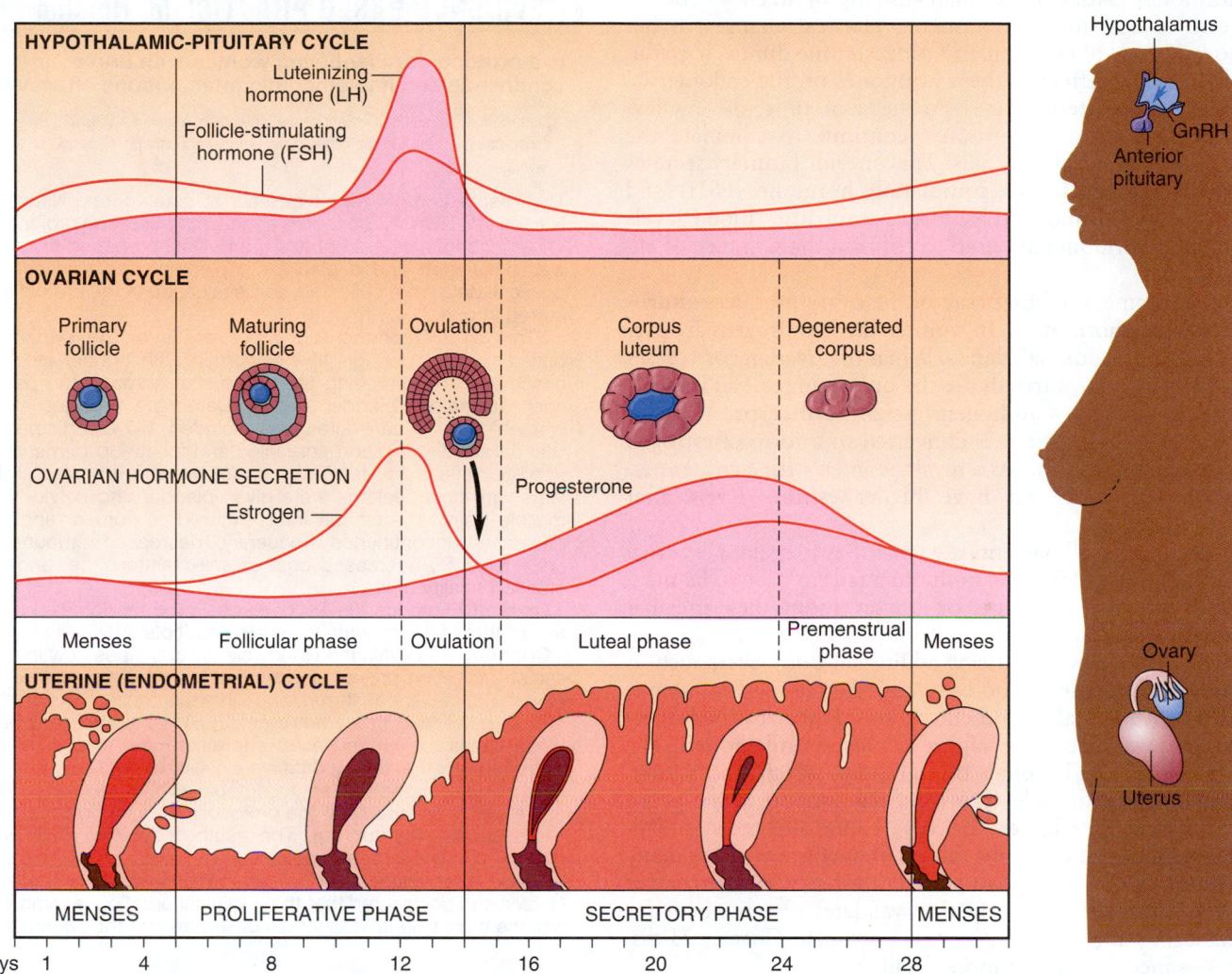

Figure 76-4 ■ Interrelationships of the events of the menstrual cycle. *GnRH,* Gonadotropin-releasing hormone.

increasing blood flow, inducing the growth of the ducts and alveoli, and promoting water retention.

MENSTRUATION AND MENOPAUSE
Normal Menstrual Cycle

Menstruation is the cyclic shedding of the endometrial lining of the uterus. The term **menarche** refers to the female's first menstruation and is one sign of puberty. Most girls begin to menstruate between 10 and 16 years of age.

The occurrence of cyclic menstruation and reproduction depends on maturation of the hypothalamic-pituitary-ovarian-uterine axis. Normally this cycle is not achieved for the first 1 to 2 years after menarche. The first menstrual cycles are typically anovulatory and irregular.

The menstrual cycle is under a feedback control system of three interrelated cycles: the hypothalamic-pituitary cycle, the ovarian cycle, and the uterine (or endometrial) cycle. The relationship of these cycles is illustrated in Figure 76-4.

The idealized menstrual cycle is 28 days, but variation is normal. The first day of the menstrual cycle is the first day of monthly menstrual bleeding. The menstrual flow is re-ferred to as the **menses.** Ovulation occurs about 14 days before the beginning of the next menstrual cycle. Regular menstrual cycles indicate normal sex hormone production and the occurrence of ovulation. Variations in the length of the menstrual cycle occur in response to variations in hormone levels and surges.

Menopause and the Climacteric
NATURAL MENOPAUSE

Menopause is the biologic end of reproductive ability, but the term applies to only the last menstrual period. The actual date of menopause cannot be determined until at least 1 year has passed without menses. The phase of a woman's life from the initial decline in the amount of estrogen produced by the ovaries to the end of symptoms is called the **climacteric**. The lay term for this phase is "the change of life." Menopause is only one sign of the climacteric.

The follicles in the ovary atrophy continuously during a woman's life. The progressive decline in the number of follicles that can produce estrogen in response to pituitary hormones causes the woman (usually between 40 and 50 years of age) to begin noticing physical changes in her body. Levels of estrogen and progesterone diminish gradually until the effect of these hormones on the endometrial lining of the uterus ceases. At the same time, the low levels of the ovarian hormones continue to stimulate the hypothalamic-pituitary axis. The anterior pituitary secretes high levels of follicle-stimulating hormone (FSH) and luteinizing hormone (LH) after menopause. Blood levels of these hormones are used to confirm the presence of climacteric.

For a time, the inner core of the ovary produces **androgens** (male hormones). In women, most androgens are produced by the adrenal glands. When the ovarian core ceases to function, the adrenals are the only source of androgens. The production of androgens is significant, especially after menopause, because it is converted to a form of estrogen (estrone) in body fat. As a result, women with a greater percentage of body fat have higher estrone levels after menopause.

During the climacteric, a woman has irregular menstrual and ovarian cycles. Ovulation often fails to occur. The menstrual flow may be lighter or heavier during these irregular cycles.

Reduced estrogen affects additional body sites, such as bone density and cardiovascular function. The uterus, cervix, ovaries, labia, and clitoris shrink in size. The low estrogen levels cause the vagina to narrow and shorten. The vaginal mucosa becomes thin and dry, which makes intercourse uncomfortable. The muscular support to the pelvis becomes more relaxed. The loss of tone also reduces bladder support, which results in urinary incontinence for many women. The accompanying Evidence-Based Practice box at right summarizes a study that validates one protocol for managing urinary incontinence in women. Chapter 73 discusses incontinence in more detail.

Bone density is a concern after estrogen production decreases. Estrogen is needed by bone tissue for calcium uptake. It also increases the metabolism of vitamin D, which is needed for the absorption of calcium from the intestines. Bone density decreases in clients with decreased calcium uptake. The reduction in the amount of bone mass is called **osteoporosis** (see Chapter 54). Thus women are more at risk for bone fractures after menopause.

One of the most common symptoms that occurs during the climacteric is the hot flash, which is caused by vasomotor instability. The cause is not clear, but it is thought that surges of FSH and LH cause vasodilation and increased heat production (Fogel, 2004). In addition to physical changes during the climacteric, the woman may also experience emotional changes (including mood changes) and fatigue.

ARTIFICIAL MENOPAUSE

Menopause may occur for reasons other than the natural changes of the climacteric. Artificial menopause is the abrupt end of menstruation by some artificial means, such as an oophorectomy (surgical removal of the ovaries) or radiation to the ovaries. A premenopausal woman who experiences artificial menopause may need estrogen and progesterone therapy; however, the risks and benefits of such therapy need to be understood before making a decision (ACOG, 2003).

EVIDENCE-BASED PRACTICE for Nursing

Is a protocol for identifying women with urinary incontinence and implementing interventions effective?

Sampselle, C., et al. (2000). Continence for women: A test of AWHONN's Evidence-based protocol in clinical practice. *Journal of Obstetric, Gynecologic, and Neonatal Nursing, 29*(1), 18-26.

The Association of Women's Health, Obstetric, and Neonatal Nurses (AWHONN) sponsored a research utilization project on urinary incontinence. In phase I, an evidence-based protocol was developed and a plan for implementation was set. In phase II, data were collected, and evaluation of the project occurred in phase III.

This study reported the effectiveness of the evidence-based protocol for identifying women with urinary incontinence and for improving their outcomes through the pelvic floor muscle and bladder training. Data were collected at 21 women's health care sites and included 1474 participants. Standardized self-report screening and follow-up forms were used to collect the data. Women (57%) who reported problems with urine leakage were given bladder and pelvic floor muscle training. After the intervention, the women reported decreased incontinence frequency, decreased amount of urine leakage, decreased cost of self-maintenance, and increased quality of life.

Level of Evidence: 2—Properly designed randomized controlled trial of appropriate size using multiple sites.

Critique. This evaluation study clearly describes how the research utilization project investigated the research questions, how the data were analyzed, and what the implications are for clinicians working in women's health. Analysis included only those cases for whom baseline (pretreatment) and 4-month follow-up (posttreatment) data were available. The sample was fairly diverse, supporting an acceptable level of generalizability and supporting the use of the protocol in clinical practice.

Implications for Nursing. The results of this AWHONN project support widespread application of the screening and behavioral interventions for urinary incontinence in women. Nurses can be assured that these clinical practice recommendations have scientific rationale based on current evidence.

Structure and Function of the Male Reproductive System

EXTERNAL GENITALIA

The external male genitalia undergo many changes during puberty. The first visible sign of puberty is enlargement of the scrotum and testes, which typically occurs between 11 and 13½ years of age.

These changes occur in response to an increase in testosterone production at puberty. The release of gonadotropin-releasing hormone (GnRH) from the hypothalamus stimulates the anterior pituitary to secrete LH (luteinizing hormone) and FSH (follicle-stimulating hormone). As the levels of these hormones increase, the amount of testosterone greatly increases. Other signs of puberty that occur as a result of the presence of testosterone are the growth of axillary hair, lengthening and thickening of the vocal cords, increased sebaceous gland activity, and a general increase in muscle mass and body size.

Testosterone production is relatively constant in the adult male. Only a slight and gradual reduction of testosterone production occurs in the older adult male. Lower testosterone levels decrease muscle mass, reduce skin elasticity, and induce postural changes and changes in sexual performance.

Penis

The **penis** is an organ for urination and intercourse. It consists of the body or shaft and the glans penis (the distal end of the penis). The body is made up of three circular layers or columns of erectile tissue. Engorgement of these highly vascular, erectile columns with blood during sexual excitement causes the penis to expand and elongate and become firm and erect. The glans is the smooth end of the penis and contains the slitlike opening of the urethral meatus. The urethra is the pathway for the exit of both urine and semen.

The penis is covered by thin skin that is loosely attached to the underlying fascia. This loose skin allows the penis to enlarge during erections. The skin is darker than that of the rest of the body, and hair is present only at the base. A continuation of penile skin covers the glans and folds back on itself to form the prepuce (foreskin). Surgical removal of the foreskin (**circumcision**) for religious or cultural reasons is a common procedure in the United States.

The penis is richly innervated through branches of the sympathetic and parasympathetic nervous systems and by nerves of cerebral origin. Penile erection is under the control of the autonomic nervous system. Erection can also be induced by local reflex mechanisms (tactile stimulation) and by psychogenic mechanisms (auditory, visual, tactile, or imaginative stimulation). Sympathetic fibers control the rhythmic muscle contractions that lead to the ejaculation of semen.

Scrotum

The **scrotum** is a thin-walled, fibromuscular pouch that is behind the penis and suspended below the pubic bone. This pouch protects the testes, epididymis, and vas deferens in a space that is slightly cooler than inside the abdominal cavity. Normal sperm production and maturation (**spermatogenesis**) requires a controlled temperature. The slightly lower temperature, about 6° F (2° C) less than body temperature, is optimal for sperm production and viability.

The scrotal skin is darkly pigmented and contains sweat glands, sebaceous glands, and few hair follicles. The skin is arranged in horizontal folds called **rugae.** The rugae are more apparent when the scrotum is retracted toward the body. The scrotum contracts with cold, exercise, tactile stimulation, and sexual excitement.

INTERNAL GENITALIA

The internal male genitalia are shown in Figure 76-5.

Testes and Spermatic Cord

The testes are a pair of oval organs that produce sperm and testosterone. Each testis is suspended in the scrotum by the spermatic cord, which provides vascular, lymphatic, and nerve supply to the testis. The cord also covers the epididymis and a portion of the vas deferens. The cord and testes are surrounded by fascia and the cremaster muscle. Sympathetic nerve fibers are located on the arteries in the cord, and sympathetic and parasympathetic fibers are on the vas deferens. When the testes are traumatized, these autonomic nerve fibers transmit excruciating pain and a sensation of nausea.

EPIDIDYMIS

The **epididymis** is the first portion of a ductal system that transports sperm from the testes to the urethra. It is a site of sperm maturation. The epididymis is comma shaped, lies to one side of each testis, and is divided into a head, body, and tail. The tail merges into the vas deferens and is a storage site for maturing sperm.

VAS DEFERENS

The **vas deferens**, or ductus deferens, is a firm, muscular tube that continues from the tail of each epididymis. The

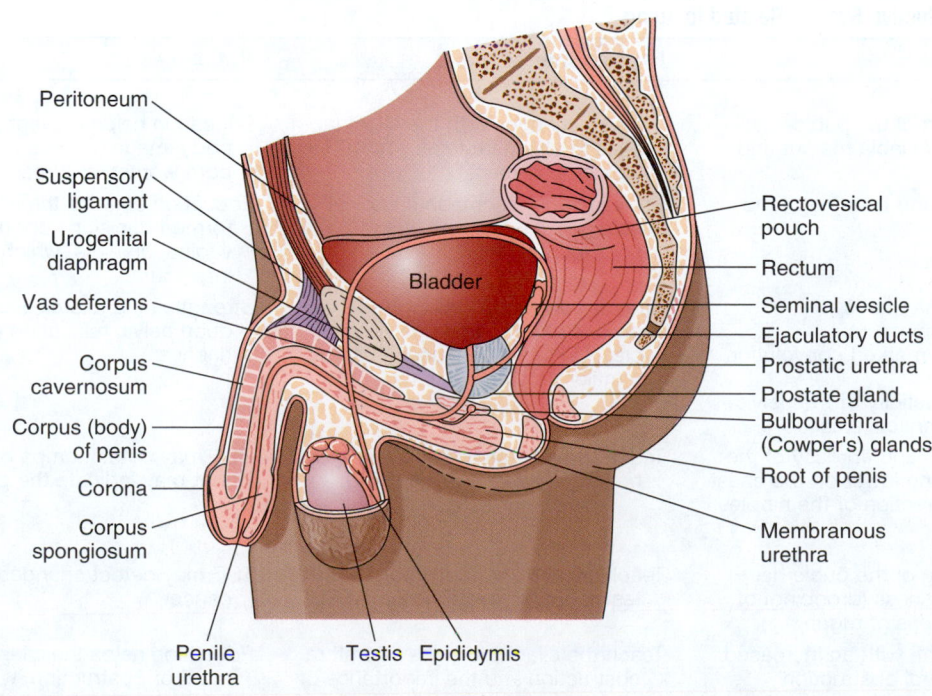

Figure 76-5 ■ Internal male genitalia.

Labels (left): Peritoneum; Suspensory ligament; Urogenital diaphragm; Vas deferens; Corpus cavernosum; Corpus (body) of penis; Corona; Corpus spongiosum

Labels (right): Rectovesical pouch; Rectum; Seminal vesicle; Ejaculatory ducts; Prostatic urethra; Prostate gland; Bulbourethral (Cowper's) glands; Root of penis; Membranous urethra

Labels (bottom): Penile urethra; Testis; Epididymis

Bladder

end of each vas deferens is a reservoir for sperm and tubular fluids. They merge with ducts from the seminal vesicle to form the ejaculatory ducts at the base of the prostate gland. Sperm from the vas deferens and secretions from the seminal vesicles are transported through the ejaculatory duct to mix with prostatic fluids in the prostatic urethra.

Seminal Vesicles and Ejaculatory Ducts

The seminal vesicles are paired glands that secrete most of the volume of the ejaculate. Each vesicle ends in a small duct that joins with the end of the vas deferens to form an ejaculatory duct. The two ejaculatory ducts descend through the prostate gland and empty into the prostatic urethra.

Prostate Gland

The **prostate gland** is a large accessory gland of the male reproductive system. It is a chestnut-shaped, glandular, and fibromuscular organ. It secretes a milky alkaline fluid that adds bulk to the semen, enhances sperm motility, and neutralizes acidic vaginal secretions.

During **emission**, the first stage of the male orgasm, the prostate gland secretes its fluid at the same time as the vas deferens. The average pH of the combined secretions of semen is about 7.5, whereas secretions from the vagina normally have a pH of 3.5 to 4. Sperm need a surrounding fluid pH of 6 to 6.5 before they become optimally motile.

The prostate gland is located between the neck of the bladder and the urogenital diaphragm. It is separated from the anterior wall of the rectum by a thin fascial sheath. The prostate gland can be palpated through the rectum and should not project more than $^3/_8$ inch (1 cm) into the rectal lumen.

As men age, the prostate gland becomes clinically significant. The gland is small at birth, but during puberty it rapidly enlarges to its normal adult size. By 40 years of age, about 10% of men have an enlarged prostate (benign prostatic hyperplasia), which can cause problems such as overflow incontinence and nocturia (Jarvis, 2004). Prostate function depends on adequate levels of testosterone. As men age, testosterone production decreases.

Inguinal Area

The inguinal area (groin) is located between the superior iliac spine and the symphysis pubis and is the junction of the lower abdominal wall and thigh. The area is a common site for a **hernia**, which is a loop of bowel that protrudes through a weak spot in the muscles (Jarvis, 2004).

Reproductive Changes Associated with Aging

Age affects the function of both the male and the female reproductive systems. After puberty, hormones produced by the gonads (testis and ovary) affect many body systems. Many changes in the reproductive system occur in older adults (Chart 76-1).

ASSESSMENT TECHNIQUES

History

DEMOGRAPHIC DATA

Use data about the client's age, gender, and culture to assess the risk for certain diseases and in evaluating the reproductive system. The age at which secondary sexual characteristics developed in the client are compared with the typical ranges for males or females (see the Cultural Considerations box on p. 1775).

CHART 76-1

NURSING FOCUS on the OLDER ADULT
Changes in the Reproductive System Related to Aging

Physiologic Change	Nursing Interventions	Rationales
Women		
Graying and thinning of the pubic hair	Discuss changes with the client (applies to all structures for both women and men).	Education helps prevent problems with body image (applies to all structures for both women and men).
Decreased size of the labia majora and clitoris		
Drying, smoothing, and thinning of the vaginal walls	Provide information about vaginal estrogen therapy and water-soluble lubricants.	Education enables the client to make informed decisions about the treatment of vaginal dryness, which can cause painful intercourse.
Decreased size of the uterus	Provide information about Kegel exercises to strengthen pelvic muscles. Urinary incontinence can be a major problem.	Strengthening exercises may prevent or reduce pelvic relaxation and urinary incontinence.
Atrophy of the endometrium		
Decreased size and marked convolution of the ovaries		
Loss of tone and elasticity of the pelvic ligaments and connective tissue		
Increased flabbiness and fibrosity of the breasts, which hang lower on the chest wall; decreased erection of the nipples	Teach or reinforce the importance of breast self-examination (BSE).	BSE may detect lumps or other changes that may indicate the presence of cancer.
Men		
Graying and thinning of the pubic hair	Teach or reinforce the importance of testicular self-examination (TSE).	TSE may detect changes that may indicate cancer.
Increased pendulousness (drooping) of the scrotum and loss of rugae		
Prostate enlargement, with an increased likelihood of urethral obstruction	Teach the client the signs of urethral obstruction and the importance of prostate cancer screening.	Education helps the client detect enlargement or obstruction, which may indicate the presence of cancer.

Cultural beliefs and practices influence lifestyle and sexual practices. These beliefs and expectations account for differences in acceptable gender-related identity. A person's attitude and behavior about the meaning and use of genitals begin in early childhood and are modeled on the behavior of significant adults. Religious preferences may parallel those of a specific culture and strongly affect sexual activity. A person's religious beliefs often influence specific sexual practices, the acceptable number of partners, contraceptive use, and the decision to terminate a pregnancy, end fertility, or remove barriers to infertility (D'Avanzo & Geissler, 2003).

FAMILY HISTORY AND GENETIC RISK

The family history, including that of the parents, grandparents, siblings, and spouse, helps determine the client's risk for conditions that affect reproductive functioning. A delayed or early development of secondary sex characteristics may be a familial pattern.

The current age and health status of family members are of interest. The cause of and age at death of specific family members may also be important. Evidence of medical diseases or reproductive problems in family members (e.g., diabetes, endometriosis, complications of pregnancy, and reproductive cancer) allows better interpretation of the client's presenting symptoms. For example, daughters of women who were given diethylstilbestrol (DES) to control bleeding during pregnancy are at increased risk for infertility and reproductive tract cancer.

Recent advances in genetics determined the hereditary component of many diseases including those of the reproductive system. For example, about 10 % of all cancers have a hereditary component, but only a small percent of breast cancers are hereditary. Specific BRCA 1 and BRCA 2 gene mutations do increase the overall risk for breast or ovarian cancer (DiSaia & Creasman, 2002; Zawacki & Phillips, 2002). Men with first-degree relatives (e.g., father, brother) with prostate cancer are at greater risk for the disease than men in the general population. Testicular cancer can also be familial (O'Rourke, 2001).

PERSONAL HISTORY

Assess the client's health habits, such as diet, sleep, and exercise patterns. Low levels of body fat may be related to ovarian dysfunction. Assess the client's alcohol, tobacco, and drug use because **libido** (sex drive), sperm production, and **potency** (the ability to have and sustain an erection) can be affected by such substances (Raines, 2004).

The client's personal medical history provides data about his or her general health. Certain childhood illnesses can have an effect on the reproductive system. Women need to be screened for sufficient rubella titers and should be treated, if necessary, to prevent possible **teratogenic** effects (development of birth defects) on their unborn children if they get rubella during the first trimester of pregnancy. Mumps or smallpox in men after puberty may cause **orchitis** (painful inflammation and swelling of the testes) and occasionally leads to testicular atrophy and sterility.

Assess for any major adult illnesses or chronic illnesses that may severely affect reproductive function. Endocrine disorders may affect the hypothalamic-pituitary-gonadal function of men or women. Almost any disease that disturbs a woman's metabolism or nutrition can depress ovarian function and cause **amenorrhea** (absence of menses). Failure of ovulation is associated with a greater risk for endometrial cancer. Clients with diabetes mellitus may experience physiologic changes such as vaginal dryness or impotence. Chronic disorders of the nervous system, respiratory system, or cardiovascular system can alter the sexual response. Some drugs, especially antihypertensives, opioids, antidepressants, and histamine antagonists, may impair fertility (Raines, 2004).

Reproductive system dysfunction can also result from irradiation, prolonged use of corticosteroids, external estrogen or testosterone use, and chemotherapy drugs. In addition, past severe infections can alter a person's reproductive ability. For example, pelvic inflammatory disease or a ruptured appendix followed by peritonitis can cause strictures or adhesions in the fallopian tubes and pelvic scarring. **Salpingitis** (tubal infection) is usually caused by chlamydial infection and often results in female infertility. Infections or prolonged fever in males may damage sperm production or cause obstruction of the seminal tract, which leads to infertility. Explore the client's history of illnesses, surgeries, serious injuries, current medications, and allergies. Each of these can affect reproductive structure or function.

GENITOREPRODUCTIVE HISTORY

Obtain genitoreproductive history for both men and women. Chart 76-2 describes assessment data using Gordon's Functional Health Patterns.

Female Client

Ask the female client about her menses, including age of menarche, cycle frequency and duration, amount of flow, spotting between periods, **dysmenorrhea** (painful menstrual periods), and premenstrual symptoms. If the client is of menopausal age, determine the date of her last menstrual period, the presence of climacteric symptoms, and any drugs or alternative therapies used for these symptoms. Ask all women about the presence of vaginal discharge, a history and treatment of sexually transmitted diseases, the date and the result of the most recent Papanicolaou (Pap) test, breast self-examination practices, and vulvar self-examination practices (National Women's Health Resource Center, 2001).

Obtain an obstetric history. Women who have never had children have higher rates of ovarian, endometrial, and breast cancer than do women who have had children. If the woman has ever been pregnant, ask about the outcome of the pregnancies. Collect information about the following: the date and mode of deliveries or termination of the pregnancy; complications during pregnancy, labor, and delivery; birth weight and gestational age of the infants; and the health of the infants at birth and at present.

Data about sexual activity is important to obtain as part of the history. Heterosexual activity should not be assumed. Homosexual (gay) and bisexual issues are most often not assessed by the nurse or discussed by the client. Explore information about sexual practices in a nonjudgmental manner.

An early age at first intercourse and multiple sex partners are associated with an increased risk for cervical cancer. Ask about satisfaction with sexual response, any pain or bleeding with sexual intercourse, and contraceptive use. Religious

Reproductive Assessment
USING GORDON'S FUNCTIONAL HEALTH PATTERNS

Health Perception/Health Management Pattern
- Has anyone in your family had cancer of the breast or reproductive organs? Who and what type of cancer?
- If you engage in sexual activities, do you practice "safer" sex?
- What do you do to keep healthy—regular health checkups, self-examination (breast, genital [vulvar, testicular]), healthy diet, exercise, use of medications or alternative therapies?

Sexuality-Reproductive Pattern
- *Male and Female:* Are you sexually active? Do you find your sexual relationship satisfying? Have there been any changes in your relationship? Are you having any problems in your sexual relationship?
- Do you use contraceptives? If so, do you have any problems with the method of contraception?
- Have you had any sexually transmitted diseases? If yes, when and what type did you have?
- *Female:* When did you first start menstruating? When was your last menstrual period? Do you have any menstrual problems?
- Have you ever been pregnant? If so, how many times and what were the outcomes?
- Have you had any symptoms of menopause?
- *Male:* Do you have any problems with getting and maintaining an erection, or do you have difficulty with ejaculation?
- Have you ever had a hernia or pain in the groin?

Self-Perception/Self-Concept Pattern
- How would you describe yourself? Do you feel good or not so good about yourself?
- Have you experienced changes in your body appearance or function? If so, are these problematic for you? Have you felt anxious, fearful, or depressed about these changes?

Based on Gordon, M. (2002). *Manual of nursing diagnosis* (10th ed.). St. Louis: Mosby.

TABLE 76-1 **Abuse Screening Questions***

1. Are you with a spouse or partner who threatens or physically hurts you?
2. In the past year has anyone hurt, slugged, kicked, or otherwise hurt you?
3. Has your spouse or partner forced you to have sexual activity that made you uncomfortable?
4. Are you afraid of your spouse or partner?

*Never ask questions with partner present.

Source: American College of Obstetricians and Gynecologists. (2002). *Screening tools for domestic violence.* ACOG Violence Against Women Homepage. Retrieved June 13, 2003, from http://www.acog.org.

beliefs or type of sex (oral, anal, and vaginal) may dictate the contraceptive practices. Assessment for intimate partner abuse may be included at this point of the interview or at another point during the interview for all women. Table 76-1 lists suggested questions that you should ask regarding potential abuse.

Male Client

Ask the male client about testicular changes and self-examination practices, problems with urination, discharge from the penis, rectal problems, history and treatment of sexually transmitted diseases, and symptoms related to hernias.

Ask about sexual functioning. Reproductive history and contraceptive use, current problems or changes in sexual response, any difficulty with erection, ejaculation, or infertility, and the use of drugs or treatments direct the physical assessment. The type of sex practiced also allows attention to be focused on the body area involved.

DIET HISTORY

A diet history is often critical for the correct interpretation of reproductive system problems. For example, fatigue and low libido may occur with poor diet and anemia. Obesity raises the risk for uterine cancer. High-fat diets may increase the risk for cancer of the breast, ovary, and prostate gland (ACS, 2005). Ask the client to recall his or her dietary intake for a recent 24-hour period to assess diet quality.

Compare the client's height, weight, and body mass index with the dietary recall. The client may be hesitant to di-

vulge practices such as bingeing, purging, anorexic behaviors, or excessive exercise; however, these practices may affect the reproductive system. A certain level of body fat and weight is necessary for the onset of menses and the maintenance of regular menstrual cycles. Decreased body fat results in insufficient estrogen levels for the maintenance of normal ovulatory cycles.

Women have special dietary needs. The diet of women who use oral contraceptives should have increased sources of folic acid and vitamins B_6, B_{12}, and C. Heavy menstrual bleeding, particularly in women who have intrauterine devices, may require oral iron supplements. Teach all women about their body's need for calcium. Although adequate calcium intake throughout life is optimal, it is especially important during and after menopause. The bone density loss at this time because of reduced estrogen levels predisposes perimenopausal women to osteoporosis and fractures (see Chapter 54).

SOCIOECONOMIC STATUS

The social history of the client provides insight into the whole person, including stressors, job history, education, and support systems. Ask about smoking and the use of alcohol and drugs. All of these factors can influence reproductive system health.

Stressors

Stress is associated with menstrual and ovulatory problems and infertility. Ask the client about leisure time activities that pose a high risk of injury to the reproductive system. For example, men who lounge for long periods in hot tubs or saunas may experience decreased sperm production. Women who exercise vigorously have lower levels of body fat and more menstrual problems (Sabatini, 2001).

Occupation

The client's work may directly affect the reproductive system. Occupational exposure to potential teratogenic substances (agents capable of producing birth defects in offspring) results in a higher incidence of abnormal sperm and low sperm counts in men or miscarriages in women. People who work around certain chemicals, radiation, and heavy metals are at risk. Trauma and exposure to extremely high temperatures in the workplace are potential causes of male infertility. Exposure to some industrial agents, such as cadmium, may be related to the development of cancers of the reproductive system.

Education

Assess the educational level of the client to individualize health teaching. Lay language for body parts and functions is commonly used when discussing the reproductive system (e.g., the term "womb" for uterus). Be familiar with such terms and be comfortable in their use. Clients may try to evoke a particular response in you by using certain words, or they may know no other terms to express the problem. Responding with shock or disdain displays a judgmental attitude that hinders successful data gathering. Use these teaching opportunities to provide more appropriate terminology.

Support Systems

The client's general satisfaction with life and the support systems available can directly relate to the current health problem. Questions that elicit information about daily routines often give insight into the client's perception of the quality of life and outlook for the future.

CURRENT HEALTH PROBLEMS

If a client seeks medical attention for a problem related to the reproductive system, ask additional questions to explore the chief complaint. Most problems concern pain, bleeding, discharge, masses, and reproductive functioning (Chart 76-3).

Pain

Pain related to reproductive system disorders may be confused with that associated with gastrointestinal or urinary tract problems. Ask the client to describe the nature of the pain, including its type, intensity, timing and location, duration, and relationship to menstrual, sexual, urinary, or gastrointestinal function. Assess the factors that **exacerbate** (worsen) the pain or give relief.

Bleeding

Heavy bleeding or a lack of bleeding may concern the client. Consider the possibility of pregnancy in any sexually active woman with amenorrhea. Any postmenopausal bleeding needs to be evaluated. Ask the client to describe the amount and character of abnormal vaginal or penile bleeding. Assess whether the bleeding occurs in relation to the menstrual cycle or menopause, intercourse, trauma, or strenuous exercise. Ask about any associated symptoms, such as pain, cramping or abdominal fullness, a change in bowel habits, urinary difficulties, and weight changes. Many factors can cause bleeding, and sites other than the genital tract need to be considered.

Discharge

Discharge from either the male or female reproductive tract can cause severe irritation of the surrounding tissues, itching, pain, embarrassment, and anxiety. Ask about the amount, color, consistency, odor, and chronicity of the discharge. Drugs (e.g., antibiotics) and clothing (e.g., tight jeans and synthetic underwear fabric) may cause or worsen genital discharge. Many types of discharge are caused by sexually transmitted diseases (see Chapter 80). The body location of these infections depends on the client's sexual practices. Ask the client about lesions, bleeding, itching, and pain related to the genitals and orifices used during sexual activity. Ask about the presence of symptoms in the sexual partner.

Masses

Any reported masses in the breasts, testes, or inguinal area need to be evaluated. Some masses change in character or

---

CHART 76-3

BEST PRACTICE for
Client Complaints Related to the Reproductive System

Complaint	Nursing Assessment
Pain	Type and intensity of pain Location and duration of pain Factors that relieve or worsen pain Relationship to menstrual, sexual, urinary, or gastrointestinal function Medications
Bleeding	Presence or absence of bleeding Character and amount of bleeding Relationship of bleeding to events or other factors (e.g., menstrual cycle) Onset and duration of bleeding Presence of associated symptoms, such as pain
Discharge	Amount and character of discharge Presence of genital lesions, bleeding, itching, or pain Presence of symptoms or discharge in sexual partner
Masses	Location and characteristics of mass Presence of associated symptoms, such as pain Relationship to menstrual cycle

---

size, and the client can often relate these changes to menstrual cycles, heavy lifting, straining, or trauma. Ask about associated symptoms such as tenderness, heaviness, pain, dimpling, and tender lymph nodes.

Critical Thinking Challenge

Client 1—A 20-year-old woman who runs cross-country for her college has come to the clinic complaining of amenorrhea. She is sexually active but not using any birth control method on a regular basis.

Client 2—A 55-year-old man has come to the clinic complaining that he has trouble urinating and when he is done he still has the urge. He discloses that he drinks beer daily and eats a diet high in fat. He has engaged in unprotected sexual intercourse recently.

For each of these clients:

1. What other data about the present health status, past health history, or family history are needed to explore these complaints?
2. What is your rationale for asking for these data?
3. What other physical assessment data should you obtain?
4. How should you address this client's need for protection against unwanted pregnancy or sexually transmitted disease?

evolve For suggested answer guidelines, go to http://evolve.elsevier.com/Iggy/.

Physical Assessment

ASSESSMENT OF THE FEMALE REPRODUCTIVE SYSTEM

Examination of the breasts, axillae, and lymph nodes precedes that of the anterior thorax in a complete physical examination. Inspection of the female genitalia and the pelvic examination are usually performed at the end of the physical examination. The client is often more apprehensive about these portions of the examination than about any other segment. Pain or lack of privacy during previous pelvic or breast examinations may prevent the client from relaxing.

Show the client the equipment to be used, along with three-dimensional models, to demonstrate the assessment procedures. Teach the client relaxation and breathing techniques to enhance the client's sense of control. Inform the client about what is going to be done and what she may feel as the examination proceeds to allow her to incorporate learned coping mechanisms more successfully than if she were not expecting any discomfort. If the client displays signs of pain or exceptional concern during the procedures, the examination should stop and adjustments made in the assessment plan or techniques. For example, clients who have been sexually abused may become upset during pelvic examinations (Zdanuk, 2004). The presence of a support person or having the examination performed by an examiner who is the same gender as the client may be of benefit to the client during the examination.

A pelvic examination is indicated to assess the presence or amount of the following:

- Menstrual irregularities
- Unexplained abdominal pain
- Vaginal discharge or infection
- Appropriateness of a desired contraceptive
- Rape trauma
- Physical changes in the vagina, cervix, uterus, and adnexa
- Infertility

The woman should not douche for at least 24 hours before the pelvic examination, because doing so may prevent an accurate evaluation of smears, cultures, and cytologic data.

Before the pelvic and breast examinations, ask the client to empty her bladder and undress completely. Drape the woman adequately to protect modesty throughout the examination. If she is not wearing a gown, a small towel can be placed over the breasts under the larger drape. Remove drapes only over the region being examined and replace them when that area has been examined. Drapes that prevent eye contact between the examiner and the client dehumanize the client and prevent successful assessment of comfort during the examination. Mirrors can be used to facilitate teaching if the client so desires. The examination is performed in a room with adequate lighting for body inspection, a comfortable temperature, and the assurance of privacy.

Breast Examination

The physical examination of the reproductive system often includes the breasts (see Chapter 77).

Abdominal Examination

After the breast examination, the examiner generally completes the thoracic and cardiovascular examinations and then inspects, auscultates, and palpates the abdomen. The client's arms should be at her sides or over her chest to allow better relaxation of the abdominal muscles. During the gynecologic examination, the examiner palpates for symptomatic and asymptomatic abdominopelvic masses. A mass can be of reproductive, intestinal, or urinary tract origin. Careful history taking combined with the physical examination can usually determine the origin of a mass. Gyneco-

---

CHART 76-4

CLIENT EDUCATION GUIDE
Vulvar Self-Examination

- Perform a vulvar self-examination monthly between menstrual periods if you are older than 18 years of age or if you are sexually active.
- Sit in a well-lighted area on a soft surface (bed or carpeted floor).
- Use a handheld mirror to see your external genitalia.
- Examine the area around the vaginal opening from the mons pubis to the perianal area.
- Feel and visually inspect the area.
- Report to your health care provider new nodes, warts, growths of any type, ulcers, sores, blisters, change in skin color, painful areas, areas of itching or inflammation, or any change in vaginal discharge.

---

logic masses, such as ovarian and adnexal masses, can be further differentiated from lesions on the body of the uterus during the bimanual portion of the pelvic examination.

Examination of the External Genitalia

After the abdominal examination, prepare the client for the inspection of the external genitalia and the pelvic examination. Assist the woman into the lithotomy position and ask her to place her arms at her sides or over her chest. The client's buttocks extend slightly beyond the edge of the table, and her thighs are abducted. All equipment for the vaginal and speculum examination and cytologic studies is prepared. The examiner wears gloves to protect against possible disease and potential cross-contamination from other clients. The client is informed that the genitalia will be touched and separated.

The initial inspection and palpation of the external genitalia provide an assessment of age-appropriate development. Hair color and distribution over the symphysis pubis and vulva suggest the woman's age and hormonal functioning. The pubic hair is inspected for the presence of lice or scabies. The skin and mucosa of the vulva are inspected in a systematic pattern from anterior to posterior for signs of inflammation, infestation, swelling, lesions, and discharge.

The paraurethral glands (Skene's glands) are barely visible on either side of the urethral meatus. If infection is suspected, the urethra should be gently "milked" by inserting the index finger into the vagina and gently pressing the finger pad against the anterior vaginal wall as the finger is being withdrawn. This procedure usually produces no pain or discharge unless there is inflammation or infection. The openings of the ducts from the Bartholin's glands cannot be seen. The area just outside the lower vaginal orifice is palpated carefully to assess for inflammation, tenderness, or swelling. Any discharge from these ducts is cultured, because these structures are often involved in gonorrheal infections.

The examination of the external female genitalia is an excellent time for teaching about **vulvar self-examination (VSE).** The incidence of precancerous conditions and infectious diseases of the vulva is increasing, especially in young women (DiSaia & Creasman, 2002). VSE can easily be taught and can lead to early diagnosis of vulvar conditions (Chart 76-4).

Perineal support and the strength of the vaginal walls are assessed by asking the woman to squeeze the vaginal open-

Video Clip: External Genitalia

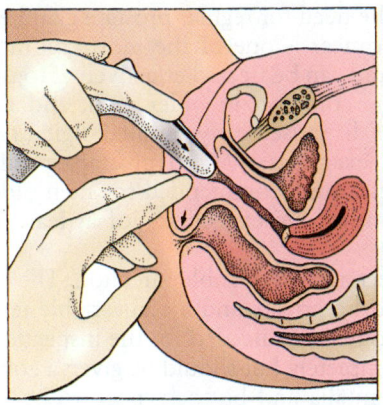
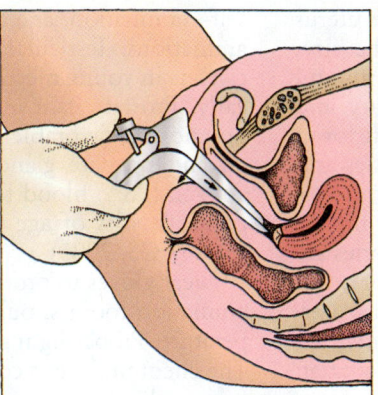
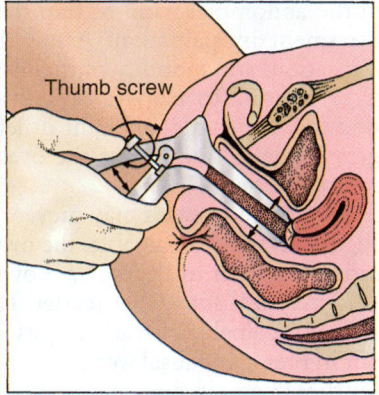
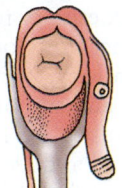

1. With the speculum blades positioned vertically, the nurse presses down on the perineal body just inside the vagina as the speculum is inserted.

2. The nurse removes the fingers from the vagina while continuing to insert the closed blades of the speculum to their full length and rotating them into a horizontal position.

3. The nurse opens the blades and maneuvers the speculum for optimal visualization of the cervix, then tightens the thumb screw to lock the blades in place.

View of the cervix through the speculum

Figure 76-6 ■ Internal examination of the cervix.

ing closed after the examiner has inserted two fingers. The client is then asked to strain downward while the examiner assesses for urinary incontinence or any bulging of the anterior or posterior vaginal walls that would indicate a cystocele or rectocele, respectively.

Pelvic Examination

EXAMINATION WITH A SPECULUM

After the correct speculum size is selected, the speculum may be warmed and lubricated with warm water. Lubricant should not be used if cytologic studies are to be collected because it interferes with specimen analysis. Tell the woman when the speculum is going to be inserted. The examiner's fingers can ease insertion of the speculum by pressing down on the perineal body just inside of the vaginal orifice (Figure 76-6, step 1). The woman can also be asked to breathe slowly and to bear down. The closed speculum is inserted in an oblique position, with the pressure exerted toward the posterior vaginal wall. The examiner removes his or her fingers and then rotates the closed blades of the speculum to a horizontal position while inserting the speculum to its full length (see Figure 76-6, step 2). The blades are opened, and the speculum is maneuvered to enable visualization of the cervix. The blades are locked in place by tightening the thumbscrew of the speculum (see Figure 76-6, step 3).

The cervix is inspected for color, shape, and dilation of the os and for erosions, nodules, masses, discharge, and bleeding.

Herpes simplex, syphilis, and carcinomas can produce characteristic lesions on the cervix. Specimens are obtained from the cervix, endocervix, and vaginal pool for cytologic studies (see Microscopic Studies, p. 1784). After completion of the cervical examination, the thumbscrew of the speculum is loosened to close the blades and the speculum is rotated slowly to a vertical position as it is withdrawn. The vaginal tissue is inspected for lesions or inflammation during withdrawal.

BIMANUAL EXAMINATION

After withdrawing the speculum, proceed with the bimanual examination. Use a new glove and lubricant, stand and in-

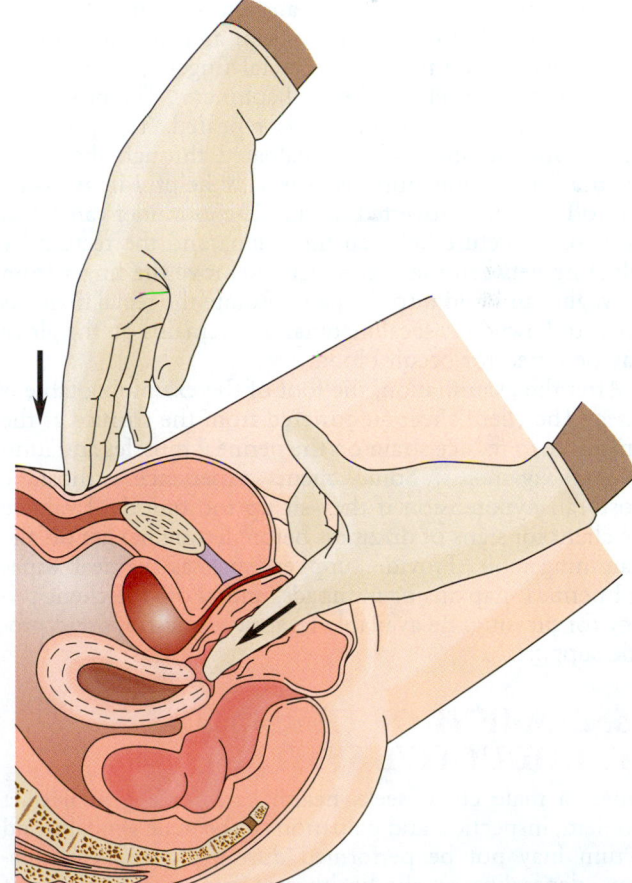

Figure 76-7 ■ Technique of bimanual pelvic examination.

sert one or two fingers of one hand into the client's vagina (Figure 76-7). Palpate the posterior vaginal wall and check for masses or tenderness. The cervix and fornix around the cervix are identified. Place the opposite hand on the client's abdomen–between her umbilicus and symphysis pubis–and press downward. Lift the cervix and uterus with the pelvic hand toward the abdominal hand to trap the uterus and adnexa for assessment by palpation. Assess the size, shape, consistency, location, and mobility of the uterus and for any tenderness or masses. To palpate each ovary and tube, press the abdominal hand into the right or left lower quadrant. The fingers in the fornix palpate the ovaries and adnexa against the opposite hand.

Obesity or tense abdominal muscles may prevent the examiner from locating the ovaries. If palpable, the ovaries are 3 cm long, 2 cm wide, and 1 cm thick; they are ovoid, feel firm and smooth, and may feel somewhat tender. The uterine tubes are not usually palpable. Ovarian cysts may be painful and recurrent in premenopausal women. An ovarian cyst smaller than 2 inches (5 cm) in diameter is usually functional and responds to hormonal influence. Cysts larger than 2 inches in diameter are possible neoplasms. The ovaries are normally atrophied and not palpable 3 to 5 years after menopause; therefore any palpable structure in this area of postmenopausal women suggests cancer.

RECTOVAGINAL EXAMINATION

The rectovaginal and rectal examination is the last part of the pelvic examination. Change and lubricate the glove and place the middle finger in the rectum and the index finger in the vagina. Insertion of the rectal finger is easier if the client strains and relaxes the anal sphincter. The procedure for the bimanual examination is repeated. The posterior vaginal and uterine walls are palpated through the rectal mucosa. This examination is especially helpful in assessing a retroflexed or retroverted uterus. The examiner can assess the tissue structure between the vagina and the rectum by palpating between the two fingers. Remove the finger from the vagina and fold into the palm. Rotate the rectal finger as it is withdrawn; any fecal material that remains on the glove may be tested for occult blood.

After the examination, the foot of the examining table is raised. The client's feet are lowered from the stirrups at the same time to reduce strain on the perineal muscles and lumbosacral ligaments. Some clients experience orthostatic (postural) hypotension if they sit up too quickly. Evaluate the client for signs of dizziness before letting her get off the examining table. Provide supplies, such as perineal wipes and perineal napkins or minipads, and allow the client privacy for dressing. Be available to answer questions and provide support.

ASSESSMENT OF THE MALE REPRODUCTIVE SYSTEM

Unless a male client seeks health care for a genital tract problem, inspection and palpation of the male genitalia and rectum may not be performed during physical examinations, depending on the health care setting and the age of the client. Male clients are often embarrassed and anxious when the reproductive system is assessed. This concern may be worse when the examiner is a woman. The client may be concerned about discomfort, the developmental stage of his genitalia, or the likelihood of an erection during the examination. If the client does have an erection, the examiner should assure him that this is a normal response to a tactile stimulus and should continue the examination.

The examination of the male genitalia is a good opportunity to teach the client about contraceptives, testicular self-examination, and the need for regular prostate gland examinations. Testicular cancer is one of the most common cancers in young men and can be treated effectively if found early. Prostate cancer is common in older men, and the prognosis is favorable if diagnosed early. Annual digital rectal and prostate gland examinations and prostate-specific antigen (PSA) blood tests are recommended for men older than 50 years of age with a life expectancy of at least 10 years (ACS, 2005).

Wear gloves to protect against possible infection. The examination room should be private and a comfortable temperature. Proper light sources are needed for the inspection. The client undresses completely but should be given a gown to wear because the genitalia and buttocks need to be exposed. As with examinations of other body systems, explain each step of the assessment procedure before performing it. The client needs to be reassured that the examiner will stop and change the assessment plan or technique if the client perceives pain during the examination. Relaxation techniques and support during the examination can increase the tolerance of minimal discomfort.

Examination of the External Genitalia

The client may be in a lying or a standing position for inspection and palpation of the external genitalia. Sit on a chair in front of the client. A general observation is made of the secondary sex characteristics. Note the age appropriateness of the developmental stage, including the distribution pattern of the pubic hair, the descent and size of the testes, and the size of the scrotum and penis. Inspect the pubic hair for the presence of lice or scabies.

Inspect the skin of the penis for intactness; the dorsal vein should be apparent. Note any lesions or ulcers on the penis, and scrape a specimen for cytologic study if needed. If the client has not been circumcised, he is asked to retract the foreskin. This should be accomplished easily unless the client has **phimosis** (a tight foreskin that cannot be retracted). Inspect the glans penis for possible inflammation, fungal infection, syphilitic chancres, and carcinomas. **Smegma,** a white, cheesy secretion from the sebaceous glands in the glans, may accumulate under the foreskin. This secretion is not present in the circumcised male.

The glans is also inspected for placement of the urinary meatus. Positions other than at the distal end of the glans are abnormal. By compressing the glans between the thumb and index finger, the meatus is separated and any discharge present can be determined. Urethral discharge is not normal, and a specimen should be obtained for culture. The foreskin is replaced if it has been retracted. The body of the penis is palpated between the thumb and first two fingers; note tenderness, hard areas under the skin, and signs of inflammation.

Inspection of the scrotum and inguinal areas is best accomplished by having the client hold the penis up and to the side. Document the shape and contour of the scrotum. Normally, the left side of the scrotum is lower than the right because the left testicle has a longer spermatic cord. Both the anterior and posterior surfaces of the scrotum are inspected for lesions, nodules, rashes, pain, and edema. Swelling of the scrotum may indicate a hydrocele (collection of serous fluid in the scrotal sac), infection, or torsion (twisting) of the spermatic cord.

Palpation of the scrotum, testes, epididymis, and spermatic cords is best accomplished in a warm environment so the scrotum hangs low and relaxed. Hold the scrotum gently between the thumb and two fingers and compare the contents of each side of the scrotal pouch. Locate and examine each testis for size, shape, symmetry, tenderness, nodules, and consistency.

The normal testis has smooth borders, is somewhat sensitive to light palpation, and feels rubbery. The epididymis can be palpated on the posterior surface of the testis. It is examined for size, shape, and tenderness. In clients with infection of the epididymis, its outline cannot be distinguished. Palpate the spermatic cord along its length between the epididymis and the superficial inguinal ring; nodules and swelling are noted and further evaluated. Varicose veins of the spermatic cord (varicocele) feel like a "bag of worms" above the testis.

Any swollen area of the scrotum should be transilluminated. The examining room is darkened for this procedure, and the beam from the penlight is directed through the scrotal swelling from the posterior surface of the scrotum. The light transmits a red glow if the swelling contains serous fluid. Blood and solid tissue do not transmit the light.

Stroke the inner thigh with a blunt instrument (e.g., the handle of the reflex hammer) to elicit the **cremasteric reflex**. If this reflex is intact, the testicle and scrotum rise on the stroked side.

Video Clip: Inguinal Hernia Evaluation ▶

Examination for Inguinal Hernia

To palpate for inguinal hernias, the client stands in front of the examiner. Use the right index finger to examine the client's right side and the left index finger to examine the left side. To provide sufficient mobility of the examining finger, place a fingertip low on the scrotal pouch and direct the loose skin of the pouch toward the inguinal canal. The slitlike opening of the external inguinal ring is located by following the direction of the spermatic cord. If possible, gently press the finger into the canal, ask the client to cough or bear down, and be alert for a tapping or pushing sensation against the finger—a sign that a hernia may be present.

Examination of the Rectum and Prostate

The final assessment of the male reproductive system is an examination of the rectum and the prostate gland. This examination can be performed with the client in a knee-chest position, in a lithotomy position, in a left lateral with knees flexed position, or standing and leaning over the examining table with the feet turned inward to relax the buttocks.

Proper lighting is necessary to visualize the anus and surrounding tissue. Note and record any lesions, ulcerations, masses, or fissures.

To assess the prostate gland, press the pad of a well-lubricated, gloved index finger against the anus. As the sphincter relaxes, slowly insert the finger in the direction of the umbilicus and rotate it to palpate the anterior rectal wall. The posterior surface of the prostate gland is felt extending less than $\frac{3}{8}$ inch (1 cm) into the rectum. Inform the client that he may feel an urge to urinate as the prostate is being examined but that he will not do so. Note the size of the lateral prostate lobes and their contour and consistency. The prostate should feel firm (the consistency has been equated to that of a pencil eraser), smooth, and slightly mobile. It should be nontender across its diameter.

Extend the finger further to attempt to palpate the seminal vesicles, which are palpable only if they are inflamed. If any discharge is secreted from the penis during palpation of the prostate gland and seminal vesicles, obtain specimens for culture and microscopic examination. Remove the examining finger, and test any fecal material for occult blood.

Psychosocial Assessment

The psychosocial assessment may suggest some contributory factors to the client's illness. During the social history, ask about the client's sources of support, strengths, and likely reactions to illness or dysfunction.

A client's personal history or beliefs may negatively influence his or her ability to enjoy a satisfactory sexual life. These factors may include the following:

- Sexual trauma or abuse inflicted during childhood or adulthood
- Punishment or reproach for masturbation
- Psychological trauma
- Cultural influences, such as the idea of female passivity during intercourse
- Concerns about sexual partners or sexual lifestyle
- Use of alcohol or street drugs

Fears may affect the client's satisfaction with sexuality or body image. He or she may also be concerned about the potential or actual reaction of family members to reproductive health problems (see Chart 76-2).

Diagnostic Assessment

LABORATORY TESTS

Papanicolaou Test

The **Papanicolaou test,** or **Pap smear,** is a cytologic study that is effective in detecting precancerous and cancerous cells from the cervix (Adams, 2002). Health care providers vary in their recommendations for the frequency of routine Pap tests. The American Cancer Society (ACS) advises all women to begin having an annual Pap test within 3 years of becoming sexually active or by 21 years of age. Annual screening is recommended to 30 years of age (with the conventional Pap test or every 2 years if a liquid-based test is used. After three or more consecutive negative test results, Pap tests may be performed less frequently until 65 to 70 years of age. Women who have had no abnormal tests for 10 years may choose to discontinue getting tested (ACS, 2005; U.S. Preventive Services Task Force, 2003). Women who have had a hysterectomy may need less frequent screening or may not need screening at all (DiSaia & Creasman, 2002; Saraiya et al., 2001). However, many clinicians continue to suggest that the test be performed annually during routine physical examinations.

Cytologic examinations can also detect viral, fungal, and parasitic disorders. Examination of cells from the vaginal walls can evaluate the function of steroid hormones.

CLIENT PREPARATION. The Pap test should be scheduled between the client's menstrual periods so that the menstrual flow does not interfere with the test interpretation. The woman should not douche, use vaginal medications or deodorants, or have sexual intercourse for at least 24 hours before the test.

Assist the woman into the lithotomy position. Relaxation techniques, including concentrating on breathing patterns or a visual focal point, may help the apprehensive

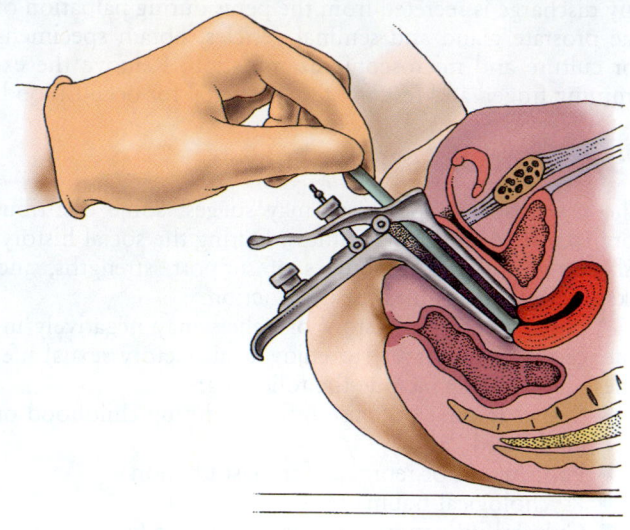
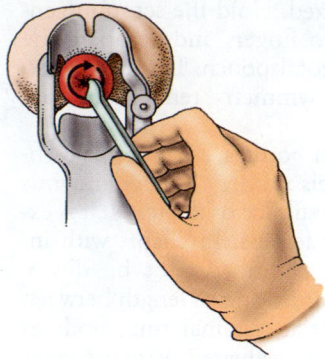
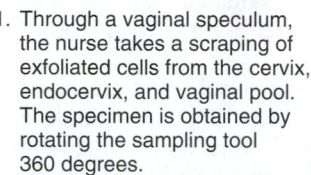
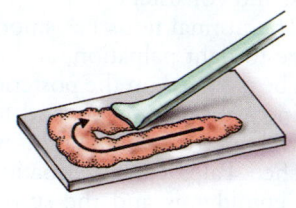

1. Through a vaginal speculum, the nurse takes a scraping of exfoliated cells from the cervix, endocervix, and vaginal pool. The specimen is obtained by rotating the sampling tool 360 degrees.

2. The nurse immediately transfers the specimens to a glass slide and applies a fixative solution.

Figure 76-8 ■ Procedure for obtaining a cervical smear (Pap test).

client. All steps of the examination are explained to the client before they are performed.

PROCEDURE. A speculum is inserted into the vagina. Usually, the cervix is visualized and then scraped with one of the various sampling tools available, such as a cytology brush, cotton-tipped applicator, endocervical aspirator, or wooden or plastic spatula. The use of brushes improves the quality of cells obtained for analysis (Jarvis, 2004).

One sample is taken from the endocervical canal and a second from the ectocervical and squamocolumnar junction (Figure 76-8). Both specimens are immediately transferred to glass slides and are either sprayed with or immersed in a fixative solution. If the smear dries on the slide before the fixative is applied, the diagnosis will be inaccurate. The slides are sent to a laboratory for interpretation (Huff, 2000).

The liquid-based test (e.g., ThinPrep Pap Test) is an improved method of sample preservation. After the sample is obtained, the cells are rinsed into a vial filled with a preserving solution. The vial is sent to the laboratory, where an automated instrument separates the cells from blood and mucus. The thinner layer of cells can then be better visualized under a microscope, which improves the accuracy of the test (Biscotti et al., 2002).

FOLLOW-UP CARE. Provide the client with a perineal pad, if needed, to protect her clothes from any bleeding from the cervix. The test results may be shared with the client in person, by telephone, or by letter. If a woman's smear has atypical cells, she is urged to have follow-up testing.

DNA Human Papillomavirus (HPV)

Testing with the HC2 High-Risk HPV DNA test can identify 13 high-risk types of HPV associated with the development of cervical cancer. This test can be done at the same time as the Pap test for women older than 30 years of age as well as for a woman of any age who has had an abnormal Pap test result (U.S. Food and Drug Administration, 2003). It does not take the place of the Pap test because it tests for the viruses that can cause cell changes in the cervix that, if not treated, could lead to cancer. Cells are collected from the cervix and sent to a laboratory for analysis. Women who have normal Pap test results and no HPV infection are at very low risk for developing cervical cancer; conversely women with an abnormal Pap result and a positive HPV test are at higher risk if not treated.

Critical Thinking Challenge

Three women, a 21-year-old African-American student, a 35-year-old Hispanic prostitute, and a 65-year-old white widow, need teaching about the importance of screening for cervical cancer.

1. How would you present the screening recommendations for each of these women that would demonstrate age and cultural appropriateness as well as the latest screening guidelines?

evolve For suggested answer guidelines, go to http://evolve.elsevier.com/Iggy/.

Blood Studies

PITUITARY GONADOTROPIN

Determinations of the quantitative levels of follicle-stimulating hormone (FSH), luteinizing hormone (LH), and prolactin are helpful in the diagnosis of male and female reproductive tract disorders. No dietary restrictions are necessary before the test. Chart 76-5 gives the normal values and the significance of abnormal findings.

STEROID HORMONES

The radioimmunoassay technique can detect estrogen, progesterone, and testosterone levels in men and women.

SEROLOGIC TESTS

Serologic studies detect antigen-antibody reactions that occur in response to foreign organisms. This form of diagnostic testing is beneficial only after an infection has become well established. Serologic testing can be used in the evaluation of exposure to organisms causing syphilis, rubella, and herpes simplex virus type 2 (HSV2). Results may be read as nonreactive, weakly reactive, or reactive. A single titer is not

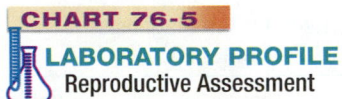

CHART 76-5

LABORATORY PROFILE
Reproductive Assessment

Test	Normal Range for Adults	Significance of Abnormal Findings
Serum Studies		
Follicle-stimulating hormone (FSH) (Follitropin)	*Men:* 1.42-15.4 IU/mL *Women:* follicular phase, 1.37-9.9 IU/mL; midcycle, 6.17-17.2 IU/mL; luteal phase, 1.09-9.2 IU/mL; postmenopause, 19.3-100.6 IU/mL	Decreased levels indicate possible infertility, anorexia nervosa, neoplasm. Elevations indicate possible Turner's syndrome.
Luteinizing hormone (LH) (Lutropin)	*Men:* 1.24-7.8 IU/mL *Women:* follicular phase, 1.68-15 IU/mL, midcycle, 21.9-56.6 IU/mL; luteal phase, 0.61-16.3 IU/mL; postmenopause, 14.2-52.3 IU/mL	Decreased levels indicate possible infertility, anovulation. Elevations indicate possible ovarian failure, Turner's syndrome.
Prolactin	*Men:* 0-20 ng/mL *Women:* 0-20 ng/mL *Pregnant women:* 20-400 ng/mL	Elevations indicate possible galactorrhea (breast discharge), pituitary tumor, disease of hypothalamus or pituitary gland, hypothyroidism.
Estradiol	*Men:* 10-50 pg/mL *Women:* follicular phase, 20-350 pg/mL; midcycle, 150-750 pg/mL; luteal phase, 30-450 pg/mL; postmenopause, ≤20 pg/mL	Elevations of estradiol, total estrogens, and estriol in men indicate possible gynecomastia, decreased body hair, increased fat deposits, feminization.
Estriol	*Men and nonpregnant women:* <2.0 ng/dL	Decreased levels or estradiol, total estrogens, and estriol in women indicate possible amenorrhea, climacteric, impending abortion, hypothalamic disorders.
Progesterone	*Men:* 10-50 ng/dL *Women:* follicular phase, <50 ng/dL; luteal phase, 300-2500 ng/dL	Decreased levels in women indicate possible inadequate luteal phase, amenorrhea. Elevations in women indicate possible ovarian luteal cysts.
Testosterone	*Men:* 100-600 ng/dL or 3-19 nmol/L *Women:* <40 ng/dL or <1.0 nmol/L	Decreased levels in men indicate possible hypogonadism, Klinefelter syndrome, hypopituitarism, orchidectomy. Elevations in women indicate possible adrenal neoplasm, polycystic ovaries, ovarian tumors.
Urine Studies		
Total estrogens	*Men:* 4-25 mcg/24 hr *Women:* 4-60 mcg/24 hr	Elevations indicate possible testicular tumors, adrenal tumors, ovarian tumors, pregnancy. Decreased levels indicate possible ovarian dysfunction, intrauterine death, menopause.
Pregnanediol	*Men:* 0-1.9 mg/24 hr *Women:* follicular phase, <2.6 mg/24 hr; luteal phase, 2.6-10.6 mg/24 hr	Elevations indicate possible luteal ovarian cysts, ovarian neoplasms, adrenal disorders. Decreased levels indicate possible amenorrhea.
17-Ketosteroids	*Men (20-50 yr):* 6-20 mg/24 hr *Women (20-50 yr):* 6-17 mg/24 hr Values decrease with age	Elevations indicate possible Cushing's syndrome, increased androgen or cortisol production, severe stress. Decreased levels indicate possible Addison's disease, hypopituitarism.

Data from Pagana, K.D., & Pagana, T.J. (2002). *Mosby's manual of diagnostic and laboratory tests* (2nd ed.). St. Louis: Mosby.
1 ng, 1 nanogram or 1 billionth of a gram; *1 pg*, 1 picogram or 1 trillionth of a gram; *mcg*, 1 microgram or 1 millionth of a gram.

as revealing as serial titers, which can detect the rise in antibody reactions as the body continues to fight the infection.

SYPHILIS DETECTION

The VDRL (Venereal Disease Research Laboratory) test, serologic test for syphilis (STS), and the rapid plasma reagin test (RPR) are used to detect, confirm, and monitor cases of syphilis. These tests are recommended for all pregnant women and persons at high risk for syphilis (Centers for Disease Control and Prevention [CDC], 2002). These antigen tests are used to screen for the presence of nonspe-

cific reagin antibodies that appear and increase in titer after infection. They are not totally specific or sensitive for syphilis, but they are economical and highly diagnostic. Some acute and chronic conditions that cause false-positive results are the following:

- Tuberculosis
- Infectious mononucleosis
- Recent smallpox vaccination
- Rheumatoid arthritis
- Systemic lupus erythematosus
- Subacute bacterial endocarditis

- Hepatitis
- Recent ingestion of alcohol

Test results vary with the stage of syphilis. The serologic test result is usually positive about 2 weeks after the client has become infected. If the primary syphilis is treated, the serologic titers almost always return to nonreactive levels within 4 months.

If the VDRL or RPR test is positive, the diagnosis must be confirmed by a more specific test for *Treponema pallidum,* such as the fluorescent treponemal antibody absorption test (FTA-ABS). This expensive and time-consuming test is positive 4 to 6 weeks after infection. Most positive test results for *Treponema pallidum* remain positive for the rest of the person's life.

PROSTATE-SPECIFIC ANTIGEN

The prostate-specific antigen (PSA) test is used to screen for prostate cancer and to monitor the disease after treatment. PSA levels of less than 4 ng/mL are normal; elevated PSA levels are associated with prostate cancer. If combined with a digital rectal examination, almost 90% of all prostate cancers can be detected (Pagana & Pagana, 2002).

The client should not ejaculate at least 24 hours before the test to avoid a false-positive result. For the same reason, draw the blood for the PSA test before doing the digital rectal examination (Haese & Partin, 2001).

Urinalysis for Steroid Hormones

The health care provider may order 24-hour urine samples for levels of total estrogens and pregnanediol (a urinary byproduct of progesterone) to detect ovulation.

Microscopic Studies

WET PREPARATION (WET SMEARS)

Secretions can be obtained from the vaginal pool at the beginning of a speculum examination. Specimens can also be obtained from the vaginal walls, labia, or vulva during the examination. The specimens are placed on glass slides and are treated with a wet preparation such as saline and potassium hydroxide (KOH). The slides are examined under a microscope to confirm or rule out the presence of a pathogen. Table 76-2 lists common types of wet preparations used to diagnose selected vaginal problems.

CULTURES

Cultures identify pathogenic organisms and are used to determine the correct antibiotic therapy. The examiner obtains specimens for culture analysis from any discharge or orifice of the male or female reproductive system. Routine bacteriologic cultures and antibiotic sensitivity studies are performed when a nonspecific bacterial infection is suspected.

The culture to detect *Neisseria gonorrhoeae* is one of the most important in evaluating the reproductive system. This culture is the only means of confirming a diagnosis of gonorrhea in asymptomatic women. Cervical cultures can be taken after the Pap specimen is obtained. Specimens from men can be taken directly from any penile discharge. Additional specimens from men or women can also be obtained from the urethra, rectum, and throat. The swab is then placed in a culture tube and sent to the laboratory for incubation and analysis.

Cultures to detect *Chlamydia trachomatis* use antigen detection methods. Tissue cultures are the most accurate but

TABLE 76-2 Wet Preparations Used for the Diagnosis of Common Vaginal Problems

Wet Preparation	Problems
Normal saline	Cervicitis Trichomoniasis Bacterial vaginosis Atrophic vaginitis
Potassium hydroxide (KOH)	Candidiasis (*Candida albicans,* Monilia) Bacterial vaginosis
Gram stain	Mucopurulent cervicitis

take several days for results and are expensive. Less expensive and more widely available are a direct immunofluorescent test and an enzyme-linked immunosorbent assay (ELISA) (Pagana & Pagana, 2002). Nucleic acid amplification tests can be used to detect *N. gonorrhoeae and C. trachomatis* in first-voided urine specimens or in specimens collected from the cervix (CDC, 2002). Cultures are taken from the cervix in women and from the urethra in men.

RADIOGRAPHIC EXAMINATIONS

General X-rays

A kidney, ureter, and bladder (KUB) x-ray of the abdomen shows these structures and is used in the assessment of disorders of either the male or female reproductive system. Pelvic masses, calcified tumors or fibroids, dermoid cysts, and metastatic bone changes may be evident. Urologic studies may enhance the film by the use of contrast media. No specific preparation is needed.

Bone scans, intravenous (IV) pyelograms, barium enema studies, and chest x-rays are also included in the workup of the client with suspected metastatic cancer. They help determine the extent of the cancer spread and obstruction or displacement of the organs. These tests are discussed elsewhere in this text.

Computed Tomography

Computed tomography (CT) scans for reproductive system disorders involve the abdomen and the pelvis. They can detect and evaluate masses and lymphatic enlargement from metastasis. This scan can differentiate solid tissue masses from cystic or hemorrhagic structures.

Hysterosalpingography

A **hysterosalpingogram** is an x-ray of the cervix, uterus, and fallopian tubes and is performed after the injection of a contrast medium. This test is used in infertility workups to evaluate tubal anatomy and patency and uterine problems such as fibroids, tumors, and fistulas. The study should not be attempted for at least 6 weeks after abortion, delivery, or dilation and curettage. Other contraindications include reproductive tract infection or uterine bleeding.

CLIENT PREPARATION. The examination is scheduled in a radiology department 2 to 5 days after the end of the client's normal menses. The scheduling is important to prevent the accidental flushing of a fertilized ovum from the fallopian tube or the exposure of a fetus to radiation.

The client is usually instructed to take a laxative the evening before the test, followed by an enema or rectal suppository on the morning of the examination. These procedures reduce the distortion of the x-rays by gas shadows.

On the day of the examination, confirm the date of the client's last menstrual period and record it in the medical record. Ask about allergies to iodine dye or shellfish. The client signs a consent form for the procedure. Because discomfort is anticipated during the examination, premedication with analgesics or nonsteroidal anti-inflammatory drugs may be prescribed. Inform the client that she may experience some nausea and vomiting, abdominal cramping, or faintness. Provide support and assistance with relaxation techniques.

PROCEDURE. The client is placed in the lithotomy position. A speculum is inserted, and the cervix is visualized. Dye is injected through the cervix to fill and highlight the interior of the cervix, uterus, and fallopian tubes. If the fallopian tubes are patent, the contrast material spills into the peritoneal cavity. Usually, only two or three films are obtained to show the path and distribution of the contrast medium.

FOLLOW-UP CARE. The client may experience pelvic pain after the study and should receive analgesic drugs accordingly. She may also have referred pain to the shoulder because of irritation of the phrenic nerve. Provide a perineal pad after the test to prevent the soiling of clothes as the dye drains from the cervix. Instruct the woman to contact her health care provider if bloody discharge continues for 4 days or longer and to report any signs of infection, such as lower quadrant pain, fever, malodorous discharge, or tachycardia.

Mammography

Mammography is an x-ray of the soft tissue of the breast. Mammograms assess differences in the density of breast tissue. They are especially helpful in evaluating poorly defined masses, multiple masses or nodules, nipple changes or discharge, skin changes, and pain. Mammography can detect many cancers that are not palpable by physical examination; however, some actual cancers may not appear on mammography or may appear as benign.

In young women's breasts there is little difference in the density between normal glandular tissue and malignant tumors, which makes the mammogram less useful for evaluation of breast masses in these women. For this reason, annual screening mammograms are not recommended for women younger than 40 years of age (ACS, 2005). In older women, the amount of fatty tissue is higher and the fatty tissue appears lighter than neoplasms. Cancer and cysts may have the same density. Cysts usually have smooth borders, and cancers often have starburst-shaped margins.

CLIENT PREPARATION. No dietary restrictions are necessary before the mammogram. Remind the client not to use creams, powders, or deodorant on the breasts or underarm areas before the study, because these products can show on the x-ray and confound the interpretation. If there is any possibility that the client is pregnant, the test should be rescheduled. Explain the purpose of the examination and its anticipated discomforts. Provide a cover gown and adequate privacy for the client to undress above the waist. The client also needs support and may need time to express her concerns about the mammogram and the presence of any lumps. Because this is a time when the client is anxious about the health of her breasts, it is a good opportunity to teach or reinforce the importance of breast self-examination.

PROCEDURE. The technician positions the client next to the x-ray machine with one breast exposed. A film plate and the platform of the machine are placed on opposite sides of the breast to be examined. The technician includes as much breast tissue as possible between the plates. The woman may experience some temporary discomfort when the breast is compressed during the positioning and the test. The test takes about 15 minutes, but the client is usually asked to wait until the films are developed in case a view needs to be repeated. A screening mammogram uses two low-dose x-ray views of each breast: a view from the side and a view from above.

FOLLOW-UP CARE. If the results are not communicated at the time of the mammogram, the woman should know when to expect the report. Assess her knowledge of breast self-examination and give instructions if needed.

OTHER DIAGNOSTIC TESTS

Ultrasonography

Ultrasonography is a technique that is routinely used to assess problems such as uterine fibroids, ovarian cysts, and pelvic masses. It can be used to locate intrauterine devices and to monitor the progress of tumor regression after medical treatment. Ultrasonography is also useful in differentiating solid tumors from cysts in breast examinations. In men, ultrasound can test for varicoceles, scrotal abnormalities, and problems of the ejaculatory ducts and seminal vesicles and the vas deferens (Pagana & Pagana, 2002; Zahalsky & Nagler, 2001).

No specific preparations are needed for this study. Women should have a full bladder to enable visualization of the uterus and to make the location of other structures more distinct with abdominal ultrasonography. A full bladder is not needed for breast, scrotal, transvaginal or transrectal scans.

For an abdominal, breast, or scrotal scan, the technician exposes the area and applies oil or gel to the area to be scanned. These substances provide better transmission of sound waves from the transducer through the client's skin. The transducer is moved in a linear pattern across the area being tested to outline and define soft-tissue masses and to differentiate tumor type, ascites, and encapsulated fluid.

For a transvaginal or transrectal scan, the transducer is covered with a condom or vinyl glove onto which transmission gel has been placed. The transducer is then inserted.

The client may want to watch the oscilloscope screen and can be helped by a brief explanation of the landmarks and structures visualized. There is no special follow-up care for the client after this procedure except to provide wipes to remove the gel.

Magnetic Resonance Imaging

Magnetic resonance imaging (MRI) uses a magnetic field and radiofrequency energy to scan for pelvic tumors. This scan distinguishes between normal and malignant tissues. MRIs are also being investigated for use in the diagnosis of breast cancer (Stenchever et al., 2001). Because of the expense, MRIs are not yet recommended for general screening.

Endoscopic Studies

COLPOSCOPY

The colposcope allows three-dimensional magnification and intense illumination of epithelium with suspected disease.

Colposcopy is suited for inspection of the cervical epithelium, vagina, and vulvar epithelium. This procedure can locate the exact site of precancerous and malignant lesions for biopsy.

CLIENT PREPARATION. The woman is placed in the lithotomy position and provided the same support as for a pelvic examination. The client should not douche or use vaginal preparations for 24 to 48 hours before the test. This nearly painless procedure is better tolerated if it is explained in advance and if the instrument is shown to the client.

Colposcopy provides accurate site selection for tissue biopsy; therefore the client should also be prepared for a biopsy. Materials for cytologic studies and biopsy should be readily available.

PROCEDURE. The physician locates the cervix, or vaginal site, through a speculum examination. Lubricants other than water should not be used. Cells in the area may be stained or left unstained to enhance visibility. The physician cleans and moistens the cervix with normal saline. This increases the visibility of vascular patterns and the junction between the columnar epithelium and the squamous epithelium. Acetic acid, 3%, is applied to the cervix to draw moisture from the tissue and to accentuate important features. The physician then uses a colposcope or colpomicroscope to inspect the area in question. A biopsy specimen may also be taken if abnormal cells are seen (see discussion on cervical biopsy on p. 1787).

FOLLOW-UP CARE. After the procedure, assist the woman as you would for a pelvic examination and provide supplies to clean the perineum. Also give her a perineal pad to absorb any dye or discharge. If a biopsy specimen is taken, additional follow-up care is needed.

LAPAROSCOPY

Laparoscopy is a direct examination of the pelvic cavity through an endoscope. This procedure can rule out an ectopic pregnancy, evaluate ovarian disorders and pelvic masses, and aid in the diagnosis of infertility and unexplained pelvic pain. Laparoscopy is also used during surgical procedures such as the following:

- Tubal sterilization
- Ovarian biopsy
- Cyst or graafian follicle aspiration (to retrieve ova for in vitro fertilization)
- Lysis of adhesions around the fallopian tubes
- Retrieval of "lost" intrauterine devices

A laparoscopy is used instead of a laparotomy for minor surgical procedures because it requires only a small incision, involves less discomfort, and hospitalization is not needed.

CLIENT PREPARATION. The physician explains the procedure, risks (complications associated with the use of general anesthesia, postoperative shoulder pain, and the rare occurrence of infection or electrical burns), and anticipated discomforts and obtains the client's consent. The procedure can be performed with either a regional or general anesthetic. Clients should expect mild discomfort from the incision site and may experience referred shoulder pain from phrenic nerve irritation (Raines, 2004).

PROCEDURE. The client is anesthetized and placed in the lithotomy position. A urinary catheter is inserted to drain the bladder. The operating table is placed in a slight Trendelenburg position to cause the intestines to fall away from the

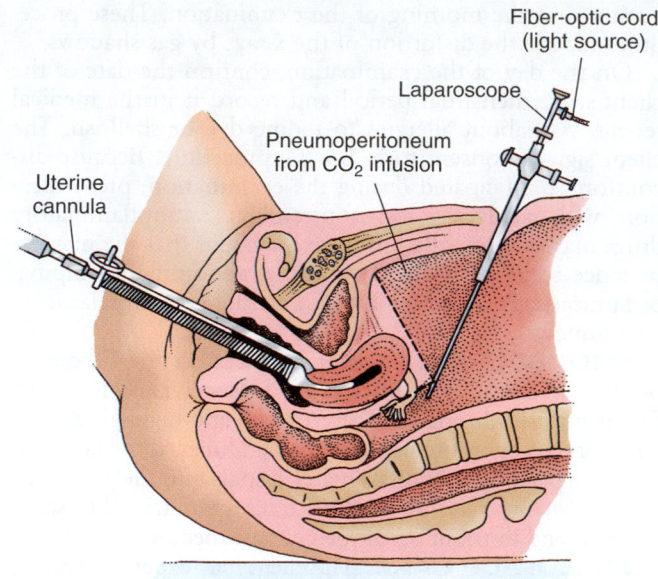

Figure 76-9 ■ Laparoscopy.

pelvis. The cervix is held with a cannula to allow movement of the uterus during laparoscopy (Figure 76-9). The surgeon inserts a needle below the umbilicus to infuse carbon dioxide into the pelvic cavity, which distends the abdomen and permits better visualization of the organs. The surgeon inserts a trocar and a cannula into the incision. After the trocar and cannula are in place in the abdominal cavity, the surgeon removes the trocar and inserts the laparoscope. The surgeon can then visualize the pelvic cavity and reproductive organs. Further instrumentation is possible through a second small incision. The laparoscope is removed at the end of the procedure, and the abdomen is deflated. The small incision is closed with absorbable sutures and dressed with an adhesive bandage.

FOLLOW-UP CARE. Care after surgery is similar to that for other clients after general anesthesia. The client is usually discharged on the day of the surgery. Discomfort from the incision is usually alleviated by oral analgesics. The greatest discomfort is due to referred shoulder pain caused by residual gas in the peritoneal cavity. Most of these sensations disappear within 48 hours. Instruct the client to change the small adhesive bandage as needed and to observe the incision for signs of infection or hematoma. Remind the client to avoid strenuous activity for the first week after the procedure.

HYSTEROSCOPY

Hysteroscopy is an endoscopic examination done to visualize the interior of the uterus and the cervical canal. The hysteroscope includes a fiberoptic camera. Aqueous carbon dioxide is the medium used to distend the uterus. Hysteroscopy can be used for the removal of intrauterine devices and as a complement to other diagnostic tests for infertility and unexplained bleeding (Stenchever et al., 2001).

CLIENT PREPARATION. The surgeon informs the client of all aspects of the procedure and obtains consent. The preparation is the same as for a pelvic examination. The procedure is best performed 5 days after menses have ceased to reduce the possibility of pregnancy. The client is placed in the lithotomy position and is usually anesthetized with a pericervical or other regional block.

PROCEDURE. After the client is anesthetized, the cervix is dilated. The physician inserts the hysteroscope through the cervix. Because a medium distends the uterus, cells can be pushed through the fallopian tubes and into the pelvic cavity. Therefore hysteroscopy is contraindicated in clients with suspected cervical or endometrial cancer, in clients with infection of the reproductive tract, and in pregnant clients.

FOLLOW-UP CARE. Care is the same as that after a pelvic examination. Analgesics may be prescribed if the client has cramping or shoulder pain.

Biopsy Studies

CERVICAL BIOPSY

In a cervical biopsy, cervical tissue is removed for cytologic study. A biopsy is indicated in a client with an identifiable cervical lesion, regardless of the cytologic findings. The physician usually performs a biopsy in conjunction with colposcopy as a follow-up to a suspicious Pap test finding. The procedure may be performed in a clinic or office setting.

Several techniques can be used for a cervical biopsy. If a lesion is clearly visible, an endocervical curettage can be performed as an outpatient procedure and with little or no anesthetic. **Conization** (removal of a cone-shaped sample of tissue) and loop electrosurgical excision procedures (LEEP) are usually not done unless the cervical biopsy findings are positive or the results of the colposcopy are unsatisfactory (Lowdermilk, 2004). Conization can be done as a cold-knife procedure, a laser excision, or an electrosurgical incision.

CLIENT PREPARATION. The biopsy is usually scheduled when the client is in the early proliferative phase of the menstrual cycle, when the cervix is least vascular. The procedure is explained to the client. Because a biopsy evaluates potentially malignant cells, most women are anxious and need time to discuss their feelings and fears. The use of relaxation techniques may assist comfort. The client is assisted into the lithotomy position and prepared in the same way as for a pelvic examination. Further preparation depends on the type of procedure to be performed.

PROCEDURE. The physician may anesthetize the client according to the needs of the chosen procedure. The physician visualizes the cervix and obtains the tissue sample. All specimens are immediately placed into a formalin solution.

FOLLOW-UP CARE. The type of anesthetic used for the procedure determines the type of immediate care needed after the procedure. Discharge instructions are listed in Chart 76-6.

ENDOMETRIAL BIOPSY AND ASPIRATION

Both endometrial biopsy and aspiration are used to obtain cells directly from the lining of the uterus to assess for cancer of the endometrium. Biopsy also helps assess menstrual disturbances (especially heavy bleeding) and infertility (corpus luteum dysfunction).

When menstrual disturbances are being evaluated, the biopsy is generally done in the immediate premenstrual period to provide an index of progesterone influence and ovulation. A biopsy performed in the second half of the menstrual cycle (about days 21 and 22) evaluates corpus luteum function and the presence or absence of a persistent secre-

---

CHART 76-6

CLIENT EDUCATION GUIDE
The Client Recovering from Cervical Biopsy

- Do not lift any heavy objects until the site is healed (about 2 weeks).
- Rest for 24 hours after the procedure.
- Report any excessive bleeding (more than that of a normal menstrual period) to your health care provider.
- Report signs of infection (fever, increased pain, foul smelling drainage) to your health care provider.
- Do not douche, use tampons, or have vaginal intercourse until the site is healed (about 2 weeks).
- Keep the perineum clean and dry by using antiseptic solution rinses (as directed by your health care provider) and changing pads frequently.

---

tory endometrium. Postmenopausal women may undergo biopsies at any time.

CLIENT PREPARATION. Menstrual data are obtained from the client and are included on the specimen slip for the pathologist. The client is given the same preparation as for a pelvic examination. Advise the woman that she may experience some cramping when the cervix is dilated. Analgesia before the procedure and relaxation and breathing techniques during the procedure are often of value.

PROCEDURE. An endometrial biopsy is often performed as an office procedure with or without anesthesia. After the uterus is sounded (measured) and the cervix dilated, the physician inserts the curette or intrauterine cannula into the uterus. A portion of the endometrium is withdrawn using either the cuplike end of the curette or with suction equipment. The client usually has moderate cramping. The specimens are placed in a formalin solution and sent for histologic examination.

FOLLOW-UP CARE. Allow the client to rest on the examining table until the cramping has subsided. Provide a perineal pad and a wipe to clean the perineum. Tell the client that spotting may be present for 1 to 2 days, but any signs of infection or excessive bleeding should be reported to the physician. Instruct the client to refrain from intercourse or douching until all discharge has ceased. Results of the biopsy are usually available within 72 hours.

BREAST BIOPSY AND ASPIRATION

An incisional biopsy is the surgical removal of tissue from a breast mass. An excisional biopsy removes the mass itself for histologic (cellular) evaluation. Aspiration biopsy is the removal of fluid or tissue from the breast mass through a large-bore needle. Figure 76-10 shows these three types of breast biopsy.

Any breast mass needs to be evaluated for the possibility of cancer. Fibrocystic lesions, fibroadenomas, and intraductal papillomas can be differentiated by biopsy. Any discharge from the breasts is examined histologically.

CLIENT PREPARATION. The instructions to the client depend on the type of biopsy and the type of anesthesia. Tell the woman to expect pulling or probing sensations during the procedure.

PROCEDURE. Aspiration biopsy is often performed in an outpatient setting without an anesthetic. The mass is located by palpation of the breast. The surgeon then directs the needle into the lump and aspirates the contents into the

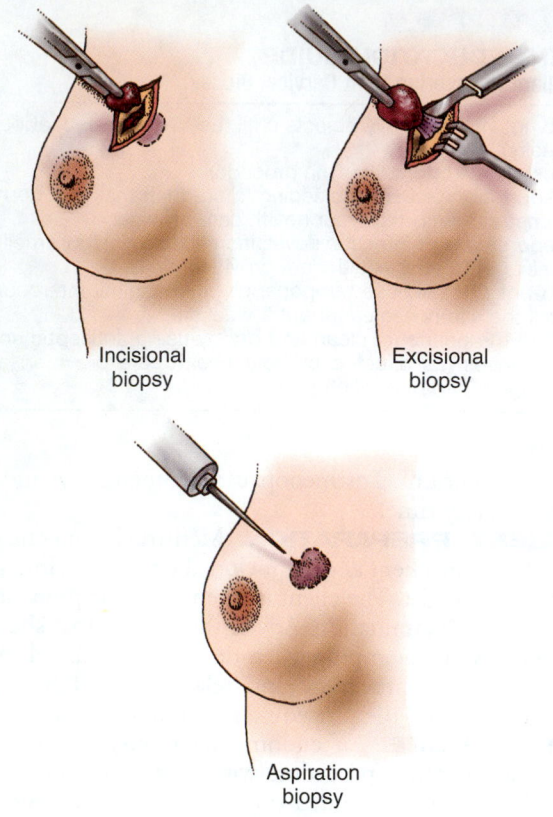

Incisional biopsy

Excisional biopsy

Aspiration biopsy

Figure 76-10 ■ Breast biopsy techniques.

CHART 76-7
LABORATORY PROFILE
Semen Analysis

Selected Parameter	Normal Ranges*
Liquefaction	Complete within 10 to 30 minutes
Semen volume	2 mL or greater
Semen pH	7.2 to 8.0
Total sperm count	>40 million/mL
Sperm density	20 to 200 million/mL
% Normal morphology	30% or greater
Sperm motility (forward moving)	50% or greater

*Based on World Health Organization. (1992). *Laboratory manual for the examination of human semen and sperm-cervical mucus interaction.* Cambridge, UK: WHO. Values vary according to source used as a reference.

syringe. The contents are placed on a slide for Pap evaluation. Fluid from benign cysts may appear clear to dark green-brown; bloody fluid suggests cancer. If no fluid is aspirated, the mass is examined by incisional biopsy.

Biopsies are often performed as same-day procedures with local or general anesthesia. The specimen undergoes histologic evaluation. If cancer is found, the tissue is sent to the laboratory for estrogen receptor analysis.

FOLLOW-UP CARE. Discomfort after surgery is usually mild and is controlled with analgesics or the use of a heating pad. Teach the client how to assess the incision for bleeding and edema. Tell her to wear a properly supportive bra continuously for 1 week after surgery. Instruct the client to avoid cold temperatures to prevent nipple contractions that can cause stress the incision. Numbness around the biopsy site may last 2 to 3 months. Assess the client's knowledge of breast self-examination and provide instructions if needed. If cancer is identified, provide emotional support as well as information about follow-up treatment alternatives.

NEEDLE BIOPSY OF THE PROSTATE

When prostate cancer is suspected, the physician performs a needle aspiration biopsy of the prostate gland for histologic study. This procedure is often performed at the same time as cystoscopy, with the client under anesthesia. The physician can perform needle biopsies without anesthesia or with the client under local anesthesia.

CLIENT PREPARATION. Preparation for the procedure depends on the technique used to puncture the gland. Explain about the expected discomforts. Teach the client

about breathing and relaxation techniques for use during the examination. Because the purpose of this procedure is to evaluate prostate cells for cancer, the man needs support and time to discuss his fears. Preparation for a transrectal biopsy involves the use of cleansing enemas. Prophylactic antibiotics are given to reduce the risk for bacterial contamination of the blood or prostate tissue. Local anesthesia is used for transperineal biopsy.

PROCEDURE. The client is placed in the same position as for a rectal examination. After injecting a local anesthetic for the transperineal biopsy, the physician places a finger in the rectum to help guide the needle to the prostate. For the transrectal biopsy, the physician places the needle against the examining finger and then inserts it into the rectum to the prostate. From this site, the needle is advanced through the rectal mucosa and into the prostate gland. The aspiration may be repeated several times to obtain a satisfactory specimen.

FOLLOW-UP CARE. Sepsis is a life-threatening complication of transrectal biopsy. Report any manifestations of infection (e.g., fever, or low back pain) or sepsis immediately. Prophylactic antibiotics are usually prescribed.

Semen Analysis

A complete semen analysis may be done as a test of male infertility. The client collects a semen specimen usually by ejaculation into a clean specimen container. Abstinence from ejaculation for 2 to 5 days before the collection is recommended. The specimen should be examined in a laboratory within 2 hours after it is collected. It should not be exposed to excessive heat or cold. Accepted values for characteristics of semen are listed in Chart 76-7.

GET READY for the NCLEX Examination!

KEY POINTS

Safe Effective Care Environment

- Ask all women about intimate partner abuse at any health visit.
- Encourage all pregnant women and women at high risk for syphilis to be screened for this sexually transmitted disease.

- Ask any woman scheduled for a hysterosalpingography about allergy to iodine dye or shellfish because she may have an allergic reaction to the radiopaque dye used during the procedure.
- Use standard precautions for all examinations of the external and internal genitalia for both males and female clients.
- Use sterile technique when collecting specimens for laboratory testing.

Health Promotion and Maintenance

- Encourage all women to follow recommended Pap screening guidelines for early detection of precancerous and cancerous cells from the cervix.
- Teach women about pelvic floor muscle exercises to reduce or prevent pelvic relaxation and urinary incontinence.
- Assess cultural issues when identifying risks for certain reproductive problems as well as when evaluating health promotion practices.
- Assess/teach all women for breast and vulvar self-examination practices because these practices can lead to early identification of cancer and other conditions.
- Assess/teach all men about performing testicular self-examinations.
- Ask all clients about the use of safer sex practices because sexually transmitted diseases can increase the risk for some cancers and infertility, as well as unplanned pregnancy.

Psychosocial Integrity

- Allow the client the opportunity to express fear or anxiety regarding tests of the reproductive system or about a potential change in sexual or reproductive function.
- Assess the client's level of comfort in discussing issues related to reproduction and sexuality.
- Explain all diagnostic procedures, restrictions, and follow-up care to the client scheduled for tests.
- Provide as much privacy as possible for clients undergoing examination or testing of the reproductive system.
- Use language and terminology that the client can understand and that the client is comfortable with during discussions of the reproductive system.
- Encourage clients to express feelings of anxiety or discomfort related to genital examinations.
- Offer to teach relaxation techniques to use during examinations.

Physiological Integrity

- Always consider the possibility of pregnancy in a sexually active woman who has amenorrhea.
- Urge clients with pain, bleeding, discharge, masses, or changes in reproductive function to seek health care advice.
- Teach clients who have undergone invasive testing of the reproductive tract about the manifestations of infection (e.g., fever, increased pain, foul-smelling drainage).
- Instruct women to report manifestations of infection to their health care provider after hysterosalpingography and biopsies of the breast, cervix, and endometrium.
- Instruct men to report manifestations of infection to their health care provider after a transrectal biopsy of the prostate.

ADDITIONAL STUDY RESOURCES

Go to your Student CD-ROM for Review Questions for the NCLEX Examination.

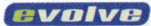 Go to http://evolve.elsevier.com/Iggy/ for Integrated Management of Care Questions for the NCLEX Examination.

SELECTED BIBLIOGRAPHY

Asterisk indicates a classic or definitive work on this subject.

Ackley, B., & Ladwig, G. (2002). *Nursing diagnosis handbook: A guide to planning care* (5th ed.). St. Louis: Mosby.

Adams, K. (2002). Confronting cervical cancer: Screening is the key to stopping this killer. *AWHONN Lifelines, 6*(3), 216-222.

American Cancer Society. (2005). *Cancer facts and figures 2005.* Report No. 00-300M-No. 5008.05. Atlanta: Author.

American College of Obstetrics and Gynecology. (2002). Screening tools for domestic violence. *AGOG Violence against women homepage.* Retrieved June 16, 2003, from http://www.acog.org.

American College of Obstetrics and Gynecology. (2003). Questions and answers on hormone replacement therapy. Retrieved June 17, 2003, from http://www.acog.org.

Biscotti, C., et al. (2002). Thin-layer Pap test vs. conventional Pap smear. Analysis of 400 split samples. *Reproductive Medicine, 47*(1), 9-13.

Boyer, L., et al. (2001). Hispanic women's perceptions regarding cervical cancer screening. *Journal of Obstetric, Gynecologic, and Neonatal Nursing, 30*(2), 240-245.

Centers for Disease Control and Prevention (CDC). (2002). Sexually transmitted diseases treatment guidelines. *Morbidity & Mortality Weekly Report, 51*(RR-6), 1-80.

D'Avanzo, C., & Geissler, E. (2003). *Cultural health assessment* (3rd ed.). St. Louis: Mosby.

DiSaia, P., & Creasman, W. (2002). *Clinical gynecologic oncology* (6th ed.). St. Louis: Mosby.

Ebersole, P., Hess, P., & Luggen, A. (2004). *Toward healthy aging: Human needs and nursing response* (6th ed.). St. Louis: Mosby.

Fogel, C. (2004). Reproductive system concerns. In D. Lowdermilk & S. Perry (Eds.), *Maternity and women's health care* (8th ed., pp. 155-184). St. Louis: Mosby.

Gordon, M. (2002). *Manual of nursing diagnosis* (10th ed.). St. Louis: Mosby.

Haese, A., & Partin, A. (2001). New serum tests for the diagnosis of prostate cancer. *Drugs Today, 37*(9), 607-616.

Halcon, L., et al. (2002). Pap test results among low-income youth: Prevalence of dysplasia and practice implications. *Journal of Obstetric, Gynecologic, and Neonatal Nursing, 31*(3), 294-304.

Huff, B. (2000). Screening for cervical cancer: It's time to check your technique. *AWHONN Lifelines 4*(3), 53-55.

Jarvis, C. (2004). *Physical examination and health assessment* (4th ed.). Philadelphia: W.B. Saunders.

Lowdermilk, D. (2004). Structural disorders and neoplasms of the reproductive system. In D. Lowdermilk & S. Perry (Eds.), *Maternity and women's health care* (8th ed., pp. 289-326). St. Louis: Mosby.

National Women's Health Resource Center. (2001). Screening tests and women's health. *National Women's Health Report, 23*(6), 1-7.

Nussbaum, R., McInnes, R., & Willard, H. (2001). *Thompson & Thompson: Genetics in medicine* (6th ed.). Philadelphia: W.B. Saunders.

O'Rourke, M. (2001). Genitourinary cancer. In S. Otto (Ed.), *Oncology nursing* (4th ed.). St. Louis: Mosby.

Pagana, K., & Pagana, T. (2002). *Mosby's manual of diagnostic and laboratory tests* (2nd ed.). St. Louis: Mosby.

Raines, C. (2004). Infertility. In D. Lowdermilk & S. Perry (Eds.), *Maternity and women's health care* (8th ed., pp. 246-266). St. Louis: Mosby.

Sabatini, S. (2001). The female athlete triad. *American Journal of the Medical Sciences, 322*(4), 193-195.

Sampselle, C., et al. (2000). Continence for women: A test of AWHONN's evidence-based protocol in clinical practice. *Journal of Obstetric, Gynecologic, and Neonatal Nursing, 29*(1), 18-26.

Saraiya, M., et al. (2001). Self-reported Papanicolaou smears and hysterectomies among women in the United States. *Obstetrics and Gynecology, 98*(2), 269-278.

Stenchever, M., et al. (2001). *Comprehensive gynecology* (4th ed.). St. Louis: Mosby.

U.S. Food and Drug Administration. (2003). FDA approves expanded use of HPV test. *FDA News.* Retrieved June 18, 2003, from http://www.fda.gov.

U.S. Preventive Services Task Force. (2003). *Screening for cervical cancer.* AHRQ Publication 03515A. Rockville, MD: Agency for Healthcare and Quality.

*World Health Organization. (1992). *Laboratory manual for the examination of human semen and sperm-cervical mucus interaction.* Cambridge, UK: WHO.

Zahalsky, M., & Nagler, H. (2001). Ultrasound and infertility: Diagnostic and therapeutic uses. *Current Urology Report, 2*(6), 437-447.

Zawacki, K., & Phillips, M. (2002). Cancer genetics and women's health. *Journal of Obstetric, Gynecologic, and Neonatal Nursing, 31*(2), 208-216.

Zdanuk, J. (2004). Assessment and health promotion. In D. Lowdermilk & S. Perry (Eds.), *Maternity and women's health care* (8th ed., pp. 91-130). St. Louis: Mosby.

Interventions for Clients with Breast Disorders

ANGELA SAMMARCO

After skin cancer, breast cancer is the most commonly diagnosed cancer in women in the Western world, with more than 211,300 new cases identified annually and more than 40,200 deaths attributed to the cancer in the United States alone (American Cancer Society, 2005). Although breast disorders affect both men and women, women are most often affected. The most common manifestation associated with a breast disorder is a palpable mass. The discovery of a mass in a woman's breast, whether the discovery is by the woman herself, her partner, or a health care provider, is a frightening experience. Even if the woman is aware that 90% of all breast lumps are benign, she may fear that the lump is cancerous. This fearful reaction stays with the woman through the period of diagnosis, decision making, and treatment. Regardless of the severity of the diagnosis, you must incorporate the physiologic and emotional factors involved to provide effective nursing care.

BENIGN BREAST DISORDERS

Most breast lumps are benign. Because the incidence of breast disease is related to age, breast disorders are described in an age-related order (Table 77-1).

Fibroadenoma

Fibroadenomas are the most common cause of breast masses during adolescence, although they may occur into the 30s. A fibroadenoma is a solid, slowly enlarging, benign mass of connective tissue that is unattached to the surrounding breast tissue and is typically discovered by the client herself. Although the immediate fear is that of breast cancer, only 0.9% of these masses are malignant. The mass is usually round, firm, easily movable, nontender, and clearly delineated from the surrounding tissue.

TABLE 77-1 Typical Presentation of Benign Breast Disorders

Breast Disorder	Description	Incidence
Fibroadenoma	Most common benign lesion; solid mass of connective tissue that is unattached to the surrounding tissue	During teenage years into the 30s
Fibrocystic breast disease (FBD)	*First stage:* Characterized by premenstrual bilateral fullness and tenderness *Second stage:* Presence of bilateral, multicentric nodules *Third stage:* Presence of microscopic and macroscopic cysts	Late teens and 20s
Ductal ectasia	Hard, irregular mass or masses with nipple discharge, enlarged axillary nodes, redness, and edema; difficult to distinguish from cancer	Women approaching menopause
Intraductal ectasia	Mass in duct that results in nipple discharge; mass is usually not palpable	Women 40 to 55 yr of age

Data from National Cancer Institute.

Fibroadenomas are usually located in the upper outer quadrant of the breast. Enlargement is more likely in pregnancy. The health care provider may order a breast ultrasound examination or may perform a needle aspiration to establish whether the lump is cystic or solid. If the lesion is solid, outpatient excision using local anesthesia is the treatment of choice.

Fibrocystic Breast Disease
PATHOPHYSIOLOGY

Fibrocystic changes, or physiologic nodularity of the breast, often referred to as **fibrocystic breast disease (FBD),** are the most common breast problem of women between 20 and 30 years of age. Over the life span, about 90% of women have fibrocystic changes. These changes are thought to be caused by an imbalance in the normal estrogen to progesterone ratio. This imbalance results in an excess of estrogen exposure and a reduction of progesterone exposure (McCance & Huether, 2002). Fibrocystic changes may proceed through several clinical stages or may present in only one form.

The first stage commonly occurs between the late teens and early 20s. Premenstrual fullness and tenderness in both breasts are present, especially in the outer upper quadrant. Symptoms usually resolve after menstruation and then recur before the next menstrual period in a cyclic fashion.

The second stage usually occurs in the late 20s and throughout the 30s. Multiple nodular areas can be felt in both breasts. These areas feel like small marbles and occur with the fullness and soreness.

The third stage generally occurs between 35 and 55 years of age. Microscopic or macroscopic cysts appear suddenly and are associated with pain, tenderness, or burning. They are usually three-dimensional, smooth, mobile, and well delineated. Although the cysts may recede somewhat before menstruation, they do not disappear completely. Mammography is generally indicated, and fine-needle aspiration may be performed. Older clients receiving hormone replacement therapy may develop painful fluid-filled cysts. Biopsy is indicated in the following situations:

- No fluid is aspirated.
- The mammogram shows suspicious findings.
- A mass remains palpable after aspiration.
- The cytology of the aspirated fluid reveals malignant cells.

Symptoms often resolve after menopause in the absence of estrogen supplementation.

COLLABORATIVE MANAGEMENT

Management of FBD is generally symptomatic. Hormonal manipulation is the main focus of drug therapy. Oral contraceptives can suppress oversecretion of estrogen, and progestins may be used to correct luteal insufficiency. Danazol (Danocrine, Cyclomen✱) suppresses ovarian function and estrogen stimulation of breast tissue. However, because hormonal therapy with danazol does not cure FBD, and because its side effects are undesirable, it is generally used only in clients with recurrent and severe fibrocystic disease.

Drug therapy may also include the use of vitamins C, E, and B complex. Diuretics may be prescribed to decrease premenstrual breast engorgement. Clients are counseled to avoid the use of caffeine; however, the role of caffeine in FBD is controversial.

Encourage the client to continue prescribed drug therapy and monitor the effectiveness of these interventions. Suggest supportive measures, such as the use of mild analgesics or limiting salt intake before menses, to help decrease swelling. The client may want to wear (both day and night) a well-padded, supportive bra to decrease tension on ligaments. Local application of ice or heat may provide temporary relief of pain. Promote the practice of BSE and teach the procedure when necessary.

Ductal Ectasia

Ductal ectasia is a benign breast problem that is usually seen in women approaching menopause. The disease is caused by dilation and thickening of the collecting ducts in the subareolar area. These ducts become distended and filled with cellular debris, which activates an inflammatory response. Two manifestations result from these changes:

- A mass develops that feels hard, has irregular borders, and may be tender.
- A greenish brown nipple discharge, enlarged axillary nodes, and redness and edema over the site of the mass are noted.

These masses are often difficult to distinguish from breast cancer. Because the risk for breast cancer is increased among women in the menopause age-group, accurate diagnosis is vital. A microscopic examination of the nipple discharge is performed to detect any atypical or malignant cells, and the affected area is excised. Nursing care is directed at reducing the anxiety associated with the threat of breast cancer and at supporting the woman through the diagnostic and treatment procedures.

Intraductal Papilloma

Intraductal papilloma occurs most often in women 40 to 55 years of age. A benign process in the epithelial lining of the duct forms a **papilloma** (pedunculated outgrowth of tissue). As the papilloma grows, trauma and erosion within the duct result in a bloody or serous nipple discharge. A mass is rarely palpable.

Diagnosis is aimed first at ruling out breast cancer. Microscopic examination of the nipple discharge and surgical excision of the mass and ductal area are usually indicated.

Issues of Large-Breasted Women

Although Western society emphasizes large breasts as positive attributes, women with excessive breast tissue do have some difficulties and discomfort. For instance, because fashion is directed at the small-breasted figure, a woman with large breasts may have difficulty finding clothes that fit well and in which she feels attractive. The breast size may be out of proportion to the rest of the body, which adds to the problem of finding clothes that fit. Larger bras are expensive and may need to be specially ordered. The client may have large dents in the shoulders from bra straps. In addition, many large-breasted women develop fungal infections under the breasts, especially in hot weather, because it is difficult to keep this area dry and exposed to air.

Backaches from the added weight are also common. The only alternative for this condition, if well-fitting bras do not help and obesity is not part of the problem, may be breast reduction surgery. The surgeon removes excess breast tissue, and then repositions the nipple and remaining skin flaps to produce an optimal cosmetic effect. This operation is a major surgical procedure and is termed a *reduction mammoplasty*.

The decision to undergo the procedure is usually made after years of living with the discomfort of excessive breast size. Become involved in the decision-making stage by listening to the client verbalize her feelings and provide information as appropriate. The nursing diagnoses and goals after surgery are similar to those for the woman undergoing reconstructive surgery (see Breast Reconstruction, p. 1815).

Issues of Smaller-Breasted Women

Many women choose to have breast augmentation surgery to enhance the size, shape, or symmetry of their breasts. Whereas most surgeries involve the implantation of saline-filled or silicon prostheses, some are constructed from the women's own tissue in much the same way as for reconstruction after mastectomy. Cosmetic or "plastic surgery" for breast augmentation is discussed in Chapter 70.

One issue for clients who have breast augmentation surgery is that of breast cancer surveillance. Breast self-examination (BSE) and clinical breast examination (CBE) are easily performed after prostheses are placed for breast augmentation. The prosthesis is placed behind the woman's normal breast tissue, actually pushing it forward. Mammography, however, may be somewhat more uncomfortable for the woman who has a prosthesis. The anatomic breast must be pulled more forward, slightly away from the implant, during mammography. There are no data to support the possibility that breast augmentation changes the woman's risk for breast cancer.

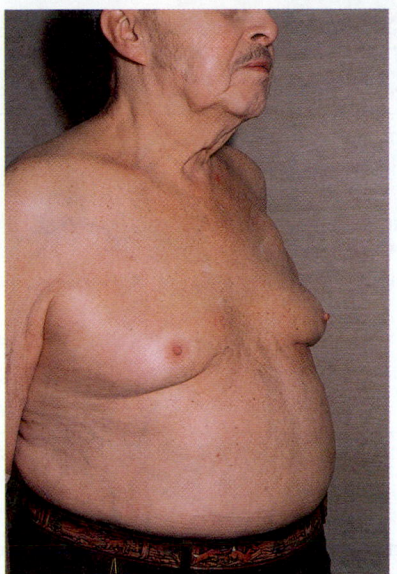

Figure 77-1 ■ Gynecomastia. (From Schwartz, M.H. [1998]. *Textbook of physical diagnosis: History and examination* [3rd ed.]. Philadelphia: W.B. Saunders.)

Gynecomastia

Gynecomastia literally means "female breasts" and is a symptom rather than a disease. It is usually a benign condition of breast enlargement in *men* (Figure 77-1). However, gynecomastia can be a result of a primary cancer such as lung cancer. The enlargement is usually bilateral, but enlargement is asymmetric in about 10% of cases. The condition is caused by abnormal growth of the glandular tissue, including the mammary ducts and ductal stroma. In many instances, it is difficult to distinguish gynecomastia from breast enlargement related to excess adipose tissue. Causes of gynecomastia include the following:

- Drugs
- Aging
- Obesity
- Underlying disease causing estrogen excess, such as malnutrition, liver disease, or hyperthyroidism
- Androgen-deficiency states, such as age, chronic renal failure, or alcoholism

Although gynecomastia is not common, men with abnormal breast findings, especially a breast mass, are carefully evaluated for breast cancer.

BREAST CANCER

PATHOPHYSIOLOGY

Breast cancer is the most commonly diagnosed invasive cancer in women and is second only to lung cancer as a cause of cancer deaths. The goal of early diagnosis is to reduce mortality by identifying women at risk for breast cancer and predicting the prognosis and response to different therapies. Because of the high incidence of the disease, almost every woman has had a close personal association with another woman with the disease. Thus most women have strong reactions to the threat of breast cancer. These reactions greatly influence a woman's health habits, including breast self-

TABLE 77-2 Types of Invasive Breast Cancer

Breast Cancer Type	Percent of Breast Cancers	Specific Features
Ductal carcinoma	~80%	Shows as a characteristic "spicule" pattern and calcifications on mammography
Lobular carcinoma	10%	More likely to affect both breasts and to have multiple sites within each breast Forms a palpable lump but does not always show on mammography
Medullary carcinoma	1%-5%	Occurs more frequently in younger women, especially those who are BRCA1 or BRCA2 positive
Colloid (mucinous) carcinoma	1%-6%	Occurs more frequently in older women Soft and slow-growing, may be hard to distinguish from cysts or benign breast disease on palpation or mammography Good prognosis
Inflammatory carcinoma	>1%	Rapidly growing, often with metastasis present at diagnosis First manifestations are breast skin edema and redness

Data from Cotran, R., Kumar, V., & Collons, T. (1999). *Robbins pathologic basis of disease* (6th ed.). Philadelphia: W.B. Saunders.

examination (BSE) and her readiness to seek care when a suspicious area is discovered.

Until prevention becomes a viable option, early detection is the key to effective treatment and survival. The 5-year relative survival rate is lower for women who are diagnosed with a more advanced stage of breast cancer. The 5-year survival rate for women with localized breast cancer is 97%, whereas the rate drops to 79% when the breast cancer has spread to the regional lymph nodes. Survival drops to only 23% when the breast cancer is metastatic (spread to distant sites) (American Cancer Society, 2005).

Types of Breast Cancer

There are many types of breast cancer (Table 77-2), but the most common, accounting for more than 80% of cases, is **infiltrating ductal carcinoma.** As the name implies, the disease originates in the mammary ducts and grows in the epithelial cells lining these ducts. The rate of cancer growth varies and partially depends on hormonal influences. It takes an estimated 5 to 9 years for a cancer cell to divide enough to form a palpable lesion.

As long as the cancer remains within the duct, it is noninvasive. The cancer is classified as **invasive** when it penetrates the tissue surrounding the duct. Most breast cancers arise from the intermediate ducts and are invasive. Once invasive, the cancer grows into the tissue around it in an irregular pattern; for this reason, once the lesion is palpable, it is felt as an irregular, poorly defined mass.

As the tumor continues to grow, **fibrosis** (replacement of normal cells with connective tissue and collagen) develops around the cancer. This fibrosis may cause shortening of Cooper's ligaments and the resulting typical skin dimpling that is seen with more advanced disease (Figure 77-2).

Complications of Breast Cancer

The tumor also invades the lymphatic channels, blocking skin drainage and causing skin edema and an "orange peel" appearance of the skin **(peau d'orange)** as shown in Figure 77-3. Invasion of the lymphatic channels carries cancer cells to the lymphatic nodes, including those in the axillary region. For this reason, pathologic examination of the axillary nodes is imperative for staging the disease. The cancer eventually replaces the skin itself, and ulceration of the overlying skin occurs. Metastasis results from seeding of the cancer cells into the blood and lymph systems, which permits spread of these

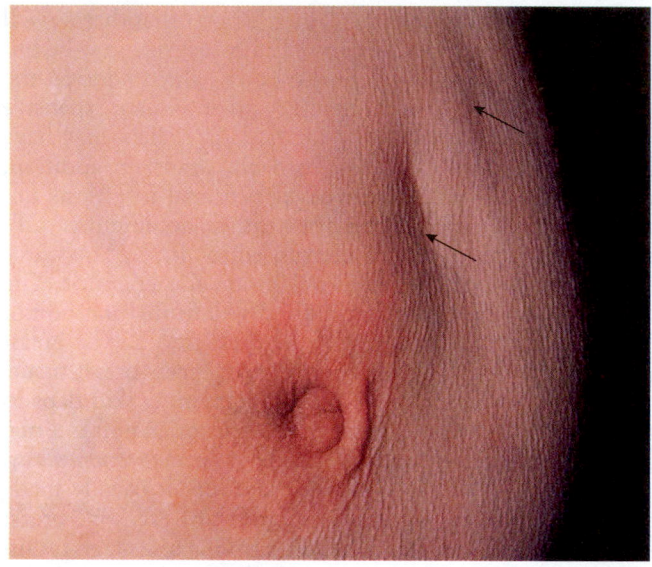

Figure 77-2 ■ Skin dimpling on a breast as a result of fibrosis or breast cancer. (Arrows indicate dimples.) (From Evans, A.J. et al. [1998]. *Atlas of breast disease management: 50 illustrative cases.* Philadelphia: W.B. Saunders.)

cells to distant sites. The most common sites of metastatic disease from breast cancer are bone, lungs, brain, and liver.

The course of metastatic breast cancer is related to the site affected and to the function impaired. The processes involved in cancer development are described in Chapter 27.

Breast Cancer in Men

About 1% of all cases of breast cancer occur in men. The average age of onset is 60 years. Most cases of breast cancer in men occur in those with a genetic mutation in either the BRCA1 or the BRCA2 gene. (See later discussion of genetic risk.)

Men usually present with a hard, nonpainful, and subareolar mass. Gynecomastia may be present. Occasionally the man may have nipple discharge, retraction, erosion, or ulceration. Although nipple discharge is not a common manifestation, about 75% of the men who present with nipple discharge are diagnosed with breast carcinoma. Breast cancer in men is staged in the same manner as in women. Breast cancer in men is often a widely spread disease because it is usually detected

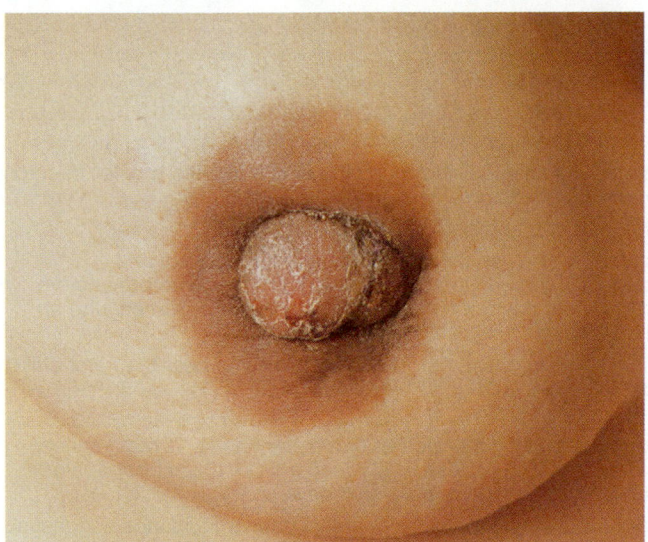

Figure 77-3 ■ Breast edema giving the skin an "orange peel" (peau d'orange) appearance. (From Mansel, R. [1995]. *Color atlas of breast diseases*. London: Mosby.)

at a later stage than in women. This fact gives men lower survival rates than women. Treatment of breast cancer in men is the same as in women at a similar stage of disease.

Etiology and Genetic Risk

There is no single known etiologic agent for breast cancer. Breast cancer can be attributed to multiple factors. Being an older woman is the primary risk factor, although some women are at higher risk than others. As age increases, so does risk. More than 85% of cases are diagnosed in clients older than 45 years of age. At 25 years of age, the overall risk for breast cancer is about 1 in 20,000. By 75 years of age, this risk increases to 1 in 11.

Women with a family history of breast cancer, particularly a history of a first-degree relative (mother, sister, or daughter) with premenopausal breast cancer, have a three-fold risk increase. This risk is further increased if the relative either had breast cancer in both breasts or was diagnosed before 40 years of age (American Cancer Society, 2005). Family history includes multiple relatives with breast cancer, early age at diagnosis, and in some families, ovarian cancer.

Genetic Considerations

Inherited mutations in several genes are related to hereditary breast cancer. The most common genes tested for an inherited susceptibility for breast cancer are BRCA1 and BRCA2. Women who have specific mutations in either one of these genes are at a 40% to 89% risk for developing breast cancer. However, only about 5% of all breast cancers are hereditary. These mutations are more common among women with an Ashkenazi Jewish ethnicity.

Breast cancer is usually a **sporadic** (not having an identifiable genetic pattern of inheritance) rather than an inherited or a familial disorder. Many personal and environmental interactions are related to its development. Known risk factors that increase risk include exposure to high-dose ionizing radiation to the thorax (especially before 20 years of age), early menarche (before 12 years of age), and late menopause (after

50 years of age). A history of previous breast cancer, **nulliparity** (no pregnancies), and first birth after 30 years of age appear to heighten risk. Table 77-3 lists known risk factors for breast cancer development.

Other less well-explained risk factors include a diet high in animal fats, alcohol consumption, and long-term estrogen replacement therapy (McPherson, Steel, & Dixon, 2000). Studies have shown a small increase in the risk for breast cancer in postmenopausal women receiving hormone replacement therapy (HRT) after 5 or more years of use. Obesity may be a factor associated with the development of breast cancer in postmenopausal women.

Incidence/Prevalence

Each year, breast cancer is diagnosed in more than 200,000 women and 1300 men in the United States. Of these, more than 40,000 women and 400 men die of the disease. Although these numbers are staggering, there is a trend toward earlier diagnosis. Breast cancer incidence rates have continued to climb since 1980 with a slowing of the rate of increase occurring in the 1990s (American Cancer Society, 2005). Breast cancer accounts for 1 in 4 cancers in women. It occurs most commonly in older adults, and its prevalence increases with age. One of every eight American women will develop breast cancer in her lifetime.

CULTURAL CONSIDERATIONS

Although the incidence of breast cancer is lower in African Americans than in white individuals, death rates are higher for African-American women at every stage of the disease. The 5-year survival rate for African Americans is 62% compared with 79% for white individuals. Research suggests that poverty, less education, and inadequate access to screening are related to higher cancer morbidity and mortality rates in African Americans (American Cancer Society, 2003a).

Like the African-American female population, Latino and Hispanic women have a lower incidence of breast cancer than white women but a higher death rate. The differences in survival rates reflect the stage at which the cancer is diagnosed. Breast cancer is the most common cancer in immigrant Asian and Pacific Island women; the incidence and death rates are higher for Hawaiian women than for all other ethnic groups (Shinagawa, 2000).

Better access to screening techniques for minority women could help decrease these health disparities. Nursing research is needed in the area of the development and testing of culturally sensitive and appropriate breast cancer screening and treatment information.

HEALTH PROMOTION/ILLNESS PREVENTION

Early detection by screening for breast masses involves a three-pronged approach: mammography, breast self-examination (BSE), and clinical breast examination (CBE).

Mammography

The American Cancer Society (ACS) has established guidelines for breast cancer screening. The ACS recommends a baseline screening mammogram (x-ray of the breast) at 40 years of age and yearly screening for women beginning at age 40 (American Cancer Society, 2003b) (Table 77-4).

TABLE 77-3 Risk Factors for Breast Cancer

Factor	Degree of Risk	Comments
Female gender	Increased	Ninety-nine percent of all breast cancers occur in women.
History of a previous breast cancer	Increased	The risk of developing a cancer in the opposite breast is 5 times greater than for the average population at risk.
Age >40 yr	Increased	Incidence increases with age and peaks in the sixth decade.
Menstrual history Early menstruation or late menopause, or both	Increased	The risk for breast cancer rises as the interval between menarche and menopause increases. Women who undergo bilateral oophorectomy before age 35 have only 40% of the risk for breast cancer than do women who undergo natural menopause.
Reproductive history Nulliparity First child born after age 30	Increased	Childless women have an increased risk, as do women who bear their first child near or after age 30.
Family history Mother or sister or both	Increased	Risk increases 3 or more times if the mother or a sister has had breast cancer and is further increased if the relative was younger than 40 years of age or if the cancer was bilateral, or if the relative also developed ovarian cancer.
Diet	Controversial	Animal data and descriptive epidemiology of breast cancer incidence suggest an association of dietary factors, specifically a high-fat diet, with an increased risk for breast cancer. The association is stronger if the client is also obese.
Alcohol	Unknown	A suggested small increase in risk with moderate alcohol consumption has been reported, although limitations in methodology have been cited and results require confirmation.
Obesity	Controversial	Weight, obesity (especially increased abdominal fat), increased body mass, insulin resistance, and hyperglycemia have been reported to be associated with an increased risk for breast cancer.
Ionizing radiation	Increased	Women who received frequent low-level radiation exposure to the thorax had an increased risk, especially if the exposure occurred during periods of rapid breast formation.
Benign breast disease	None	Fibrocystic breast disease is not associated with breast cancer. However, biopsy-proven atypical hyperplasia is associated with an increased risk.
Oral contraceptives	None	There is no evidence that suggests a causal relationship between oral contraceptives and the incidence of and survival from breast cancer. Small studies have indicated a possible protective effect of oral contraceptives.
Exogenous (external) hormones	Controversial	Several studies report no link with replacement hormones and breast cancer, and those that do appear to identify only subsets of clients at risk: those who have taken replacement estrogens for more than 5 yr and those who have taken large cumulative doses.

Modified from McPherson, C.M., et al. (2000). ABC of breast disease: Breast cancer-epidemiology, risk factors, and genetics. *British Medical Journal 321*(9), 624-628.

TABLE 77-4 American Cancer Society Breast Cancer Screening Guidelines for Asymptomatic Women*

Age	Screening Activity
20 to 39 yr	Breast self-examination (BSE), monthly Clinical breast examination (CBE), every 3 years
40 yr and older	BSE monthly CBE annually Screening mammography (two views of each breast), annually

*Asymptomatic women who are identified to be at higher risk need to have an individualized screening plan that may differ from these guidelines.
Information from American Cancer Society. (2003). *Cancer prevention and early detection. Facts and figures-2003*. Report No. 8600.03. Atlanta: Author.

Barriers to mammography compliance may include fear of radiation, fear of results, concern about pain, and lack of education (Rawl et al., 2000; Strzelczyk & Dignan, 2002). Awareness of barriers to mammography adherence as well as how factors such as ethnicity and age interact with these barriers can assist in the development of interventions that help increase adherence to mammogram guidelines (Rawl et al., 2000).

Breast Self-Examination

Breast self-examination (BSE) is an inexpensive means for detecting breast cancer that has been encouraged by health care providers for decades. The goal of screening for breast cancer is *early detection because BSE does not prevent breast cancer*. Detection of breast cancer before axillary node invasion increases the chance of survival. BSE, used in conjunction with mammography and CBE, is effective in detecting early breast cancer and reducing mortality rates. BSE *alone* as a screening technique has not been of equal value. The American Cancer Society recommends monthly BSE as a screening option for all women beginning in their 20s. Most women have heard of BSE, but many do not practice it regularly or correctly.

Whether the client seeks health care because she has found a breast lump, because she needs a routine physical examination, or because she has an unrelated health problem, BSE should be taught. Do not assume that women who practice BSE do so competently and regularly. Women who are taught BSE on an individual or group basis practice BSE more often, more proficiently, and more confidently than do women who learn the technique from pamphlets.

PREPARATION FOR TEACHING BREAST SELF-EXAMINATION

Before teaching BSE, assess the psychological factors influencing the client's motivation to practice BSE. Lack of knowledge about the technique and the benefits of early detection, uneasiness about self-assessment, and lack of confidence in self-assessment may be reasons why women fail to perform BSE regularly. Stress that treatment for breast cancer is more successful when the disease is detected earlier. It is also important for the client to develop confidence in her ability to detect breast changes. A yearly breast examination by a health care provider cannot substitute for BSE.

Emphasize the advantages of early detection and help the client review risk factors to determine her risk for developing breast cancer. Ask the client whether she has ever had a breast problem in the past. Women must believe that there are benefits to practicing BSE and that the barriers to practicing it are minimal. Addressing these issues will increase the client's knowledge and practice of BSE.

Discussing the client's fears, beliefs, and concerns about breast disease and BSE with her is an important step. Discuss the proper timing for BSE. Instruct premenopausal women to examine their breasts 1 week after the menstrual period. At this time, hormonal influence on breast tissue is minimal, so that fluid retention and tenderness are reduced. Instruct women whose breast tissue is no longer influenced by hormonal fluctuations, such as after a total hysterectomy or menopause, to pick a day each month to do BSE, such as the first day of the month.

TEACHING BREAST SELF-EXAMINATION

Ensure that the setting in which you demonstrate BSE is private and comfortable. Ask the woman to undress from the waist up and provide a gown and sheet. Before teaching the technique of breast palpation, assess the client's technique by asking her to demonstrate her own method. If the woman is unsure or has not performed BSE before, slowly lead her through the examination while explaining the rationale for the technique and answering questions. It is also helpful to point out different findings at this time, especially those that the client might perceive as abnormal. For example, nodular breast tissue may normally feel lumpy, which may be interpreted as widespread cancer in the unknowledgeable woman. Placing the client's hand directly on the involved area and showing her precisely what is normal for her can build self-confidence.

Indicate the inframammary ridge, the area of the breast where the skin folds under the breast. This thickened area may be perceived as a lump instead of a normal finding. In thin or small-breasted women, the ribs may be mistaken for masses. Demonstrate how to follow the rib to the sternum to be sure that what she is feeling is bone and not breast tissue. Teach the client to stand in front of a mirror to inspect the breast for abnormalities. She should raise her arms above her head and press her hands on her hips to emphasize any changes in the shape of the breasts. The breasts are examined in a lying position and while bathing or showering.

Additionally, demonstrate the proper amount of pressure needed to palpate the breast tissue and the correct position of the hands. The finger pads, which are more sensitive than the fingertips, are used when palpating the breasts. Teach the client to press firmly enough to detect the underlying tissue, but not to compress the tissue on the ribs, because this may falsely feel like a mass.

Use teaching models of normal and abnormal breasts when teaching BSE. Demonstrate the correct technique of examining the breasts with the arm overhead while lying down instead of having the arm by her side. Showing the difference in the two techniques, especially in large-breasted women, reveals the advantage of using the correct method, which spreads the tissue over the chest wall for more effective palpation (Figure 77-4).

Clinical Breast Examination

Clinical breast examination (CBE) is typically performed by advanced practice nurses and physicians. However, nurses in general practice who are skilled in the technique can perform this examination. The examination can be done before, after, or during the teaching session. It is recommended that the CBE be part of a periodic health examination, at least every 3 years for women in their 20s and 30s, and annually for asymptomatic women at least 40 years of age (American Cancer Society, 2003b). The same guidelines of providing a private and comfortable setting, maintaining dignity, and allowing time for discussion apply.

Taking a breast history is vital. Results may be recorded on a breast evaluation form, which is a part of the client's record (Figure 77-5). This record helps establish the relative risk for breast disease and the need for follow-up diagnostic tests, such as mammograms, and teaching.

The physical assessment begins with inspection. The woman undresses from the waist up and first sits or stands with her hands by her sides. The examiner inspects the breasts for symmetry and size, contour, skin changes (color, texture, and venous patterns), nipple changes, and lesions.

One breast may be larger than the other, and inverted nipples are common. Ask the client whether these findings are normal for her. Any change in symmetry may indicate a problem. The contour should be even, and the skin should have a smooth texture. Venous patterns may be visible but should be similar bilaterally. The nipples and areola should be equal or nearly equal in size and should be a similar color. The nipples may be wrinkled or smooth, and Montgomery's tubercles on the areola are normal. Supernumerary nipples (extra nipples), although rare, are also normal and may appear anywhere on the chest. If present, they should be examined in the same manner as the normal nipples.

If a mass is palpated, note its position by visualizing the breast as a clock face (with 12 o'clock being toward the client's head) and noting the "area of the clock" where the mass is located. If it is necessary to move the arms away from the body, the woman should rest her arm on the examiner's to prevent flexion of the underlying muscles. While the arms are by the side and relaxed, the axillae can be palpated. Palpate the axilla and the area above and below the clavicle for enlarged lymph nodes. The woman is then asked to raise her arms over her head, which exposes the sides and underneath portions of the breast for inspection. Finally, she is asked to place her hands on her hips and press, thus flexing the pectoral muscles. This action accentuates skin dimpling, retractions, or masses.

The remainder of the examination is done with the client lying supine. Place a pillow or rolled sheet under the client's

Video Clip: Inspection (Sitting) ▶

Video Clips: Inspection (Supine) ▶

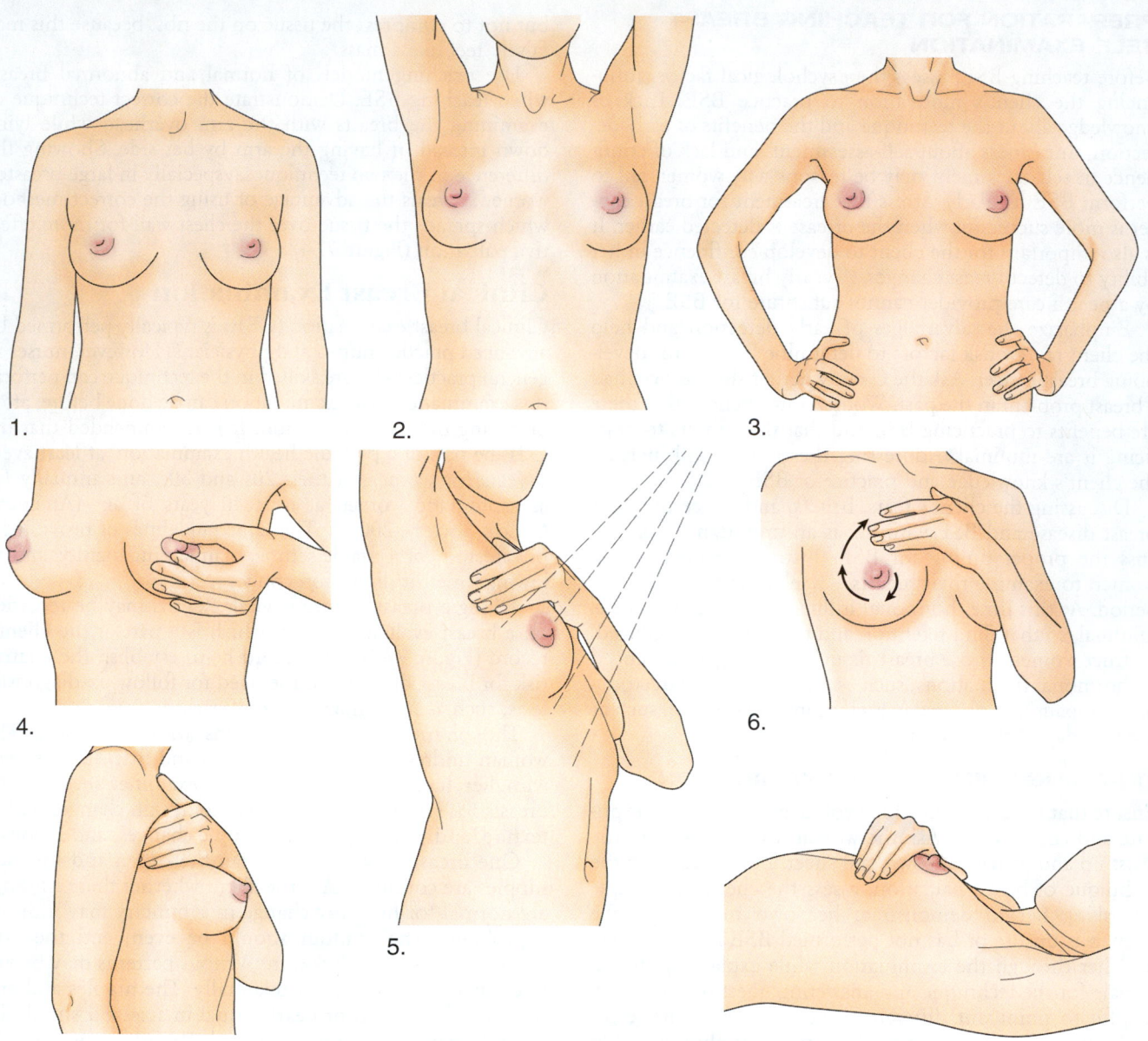

1.

2.

3.

4.

5.

6.

Figure 77-4 ■ A woman performing breast self-examination (BSE). From…

shoulder, and the arm on that side is raised above the head. Each breast is palpated separately while the other breast remains covered. If the woman has identified a problem in one breast, the other, "normal" breast is examined first to establish a baseline for comparison.

Palpate in a vertical pattern, in a horizontal pattern, or in concentric circles, covering every inch of the breast tissue, including the tail of Spence, which extends from the upper outer quadrant of the breast into the axilla. The supraclavicular lymph nodes are palpated for the presence of enlarged nodes by hooking the fingers over the clavicle.

Finally, the nipple is gently compressed to detect the presence of a discharge. If a discharge is produced, note the "area of the clock" where the breast was compressed when the discharge was released. If there is a history of discharge, the client may be able to express the discharge more successfully than the examiner can and should be asked to do so.

CONSIDERATIONS FOR OLDER ADULTS

As women age, the breast tissue becomes flattened and elongated and is suspended loosely from the chest wall. On palpation, the breast tissue of the older woman has a finer, more granular feel than the lobular feel in a younger woman. The inframammary ridge may be more prominent as a result of atrophy of the breast tissue. Breast examination in older clients may be easier because of tissue atrophy and relaxation of the suspensory ligaments (Cooper's ligaments).

Discovery of a suspicious lesion or discharge during the examination requires consultation or referral to a health care provider who specializes in caring for breast disorders. Follow-up usually involves mammography and possibly ultrasound. If there is a dominant mass or high genetic risk, the woman should be referred for biopsy even if the mammogram is negative.

CLIENT'S NAME _____ Gender _____ Race _____ Age _____

Weight _____ Ideal Weight _____ Marital Status _____

HISTORY	Yes	No	Comments
Family history of breast cancer	_____	_____	_____
Personal history of breast cancer	_____	_____	_____
Previous mammograms	_____	_____	_____
Previous biopsy (findings)	_____	_____	_____
Nipple discharge	_____	_____	_____
Hormone use (specify)	_____	_____	_____
BSE Practice	_____	_____	_____
High-fat diet	_____	_____	_____
ETOH/smoking	_____	_____	_____
Current medications (list)	_____	_____	_____
Age at menses _____			Age at menopause _____

COMMENTS

_____

_____

_____

PHYSICAL FINDINGS

Mammogram Report _____

Biopsy/Cytology Results _____

BSE Return Demonstration _____

Plan _____

_____

CLIENT EDUCATION _____

Figure 77-5 ■ A breast evaluation form.

Cancer Surveillance

Cancer surveillance is a prevention option preferred by most *high-risk* women. Cancer surveillance is also referred to as "secondary prevention" and is used to detect cancer early in the initial stages. For breast cancer surveillance in high-risk women, the same combination of breast self-examination (BSE), clinical breast examination (CBE), and mammography are recommended as in the asymptomatic population. The difference for high-risk women is in the timing of examinations and starting age of mammography. The recommendations include monthly BSE beginning by 20 years of age, CBE every 6 to 12 months beginning at 25 to 35 years of age, and annual mammography beginning at 25 to 35 years of age (Sakorafas, 2003).

Prophylactic Mastectomy

Prophylactic (preventive) **mastectomy** (surgical breast removal) is another option for reducing the risk of breast cancer. It remains a highly controversial practice. Even though a woman may elect to undergo a prophylactic mastectomy, there is a small risk that breast cancer will develop in residual breast glandular tissue, because no mastectomy reliably removes all mammary tissue. Therefore when prophylactic mastectomy is selected by the client, careful and regular long-term follow-up is indicated (Sakorafas, 2003).

Chemoprevention

Another management option for women at high risk for breast cancer is chemoprevention with the use of selective estrogen receptor modifiers (SERMs), such as tamoxifen citrate (Nolvadex, Tamofen✸, Tamone✸). This strategy has been found to significantly reduce the incidence of breast cancer in women at high risk for breast cancer (Sakorafas, 2003). Other drugs in this class include raloxifene (Evista), toremifene (Fareston), droloxifene, and idoxifene (Sakorafas, 2003; Workman, 2002).

◆ COLLABORATIVE MANAGEMENT
◆ Assessment

HISTORY

Often, the history is taken after a mass has been discovered but before definitive diagnosis has been made. For some clients, the history may be obtained at the time the woman is seen for treatment of an identified cancer. The interview should focus on three major areas: risk factors, the breast mass, and health maintenance practices.

RISK FACTORS. Record age, gender, marital status, weight, and height. Marital status and identification of the client's primary support person provide information about those to be included in the woman's care, teaching, and support. Ask specific information on personal and family histories of breast cancer. In addition to increasing the woman's own risk, these factors also affect any sisters' or daughters' risk and should be incorporated into later counseling.

Ask the following information about the client's gynecologic and obstetric history:

- Age at menarche
- Age at menopause
- Symptoms of menopause
- Age at first child's birth
- Number of children

Prolonged hormonal stimulation (e.g., early menses or late menopause) increases a woman's risk, as do birth of the first child after 30 years of age and nulliparity.

HISTORY OF THE BREAST MASS. This information reveals not only the course of the disease but also data related to health care seeking practices and health-promoting behaviors.

Ask the client about how, when, and by whom the mass was discovered and the interval between discovery and seeking care. If the woman found the mass, ask if it was discovered through breast self-examination (BSE) or by accident? The answer to this question highlights the need for discussion and teaching about BSE regardless of whether the mass proves to be malignant. If there was a delay between discovery and seeing the health care provider, ask what caused the delay. These questions are linked to the psychosocial assessment but also reveal the length of time that the tumor has been present. Ask the client what procedures have been performed to diagnose the problem. Also, ask the client if she has noticed any other changes in her body within the past year. This information can help determine whether there has been obvious cancer spread. Ask especially about the presence of joint or bone pain.

HEALTH MAINTENANCE PRACTICES. In addition to asking the client about the knowledge, practice, and regularity of BSE, take a mammographic history. The existence of previous mammograms allows the health care provider to compare current mammograms with past ones to facilitate diagnosis.

A brief diet history, in which the client is asked to recall a typical day's menu and alcoholic intake per week, reveals the usual intake of fat and alcohol. A high alcohol and fat intake *may* increase the risk of breast cancer.

Ask the client what types of prescribed and over-the-counter drugs she uses, specifically, hormonal supplements, such as estrogen. Estrogen can be taken orally, intravaginally, or via a transdermal patch. Document the type and form of hormones (birth control pills or patches, supplements) and length of use. Use of estrogen creams intravaginally is common among postmenopausal women and also is a source of estrogen.

Critical Thinking Challenge

A middle-aged woman is hospitalized for a bowel resection for colon cancer. Before discharge, she tells you that she is very concerned about her risk for breast cancer. The disease was diagnosed in her sister 2 years ago. She tells you that she thinks because she already has colon cancer, that her risk is increased for breast cancer.

1. How should you respond to her at this time?
2. What questions should you ask her about her family history, including her sister's breast cancer?
3. What questions should you ask her to help assess her risk for breast cancer?
4. What options does she have for health promotion and disease prevention?

evolve For suggested answer guidelines, go to http://evolve.elsevier.com/Iggy/.

PHYSICAL ASSESSMENT/CLINICAL MANIFESTATIONS

The approach to physical assessment is discussed earlier under Breast Self-Examination (p. 1796) and under Clinical Breast Examination (p. 1797). Check for and document specific information about the breast mass (Chart 77-1). Describe the mass in terms of location (using the "face of the clock" method), shape, size, consistency, and whether it is mobile or fixed to the surrounding tissues.

Any skin change, such as peau d'orange (dimpling, orange peel appearance), increased vascularity, nipple retraction, or ulceration, can indicate advanced disease and needs to be documented. Examine the axillary and supraclavicular areas thoroughly by palpating deeply for enlarged lymph nodes and documenting their presence and location in the client's record. The presence of pain or soreness in the affected breast is evaluated. After gathering this information, draw a diagram on the chart (see Figure 77-5) that will be helpful for others involved in the client's care.

PSYCHOSOCIAL ASSESSMENT

The client with potential or diagnosed breast cancer faces three major issues: (1) the fear of cancer, (2) threats to body image, sexuality, intimate relationships, and survival, and (3) decisional conflict related to treatment options.

The woman needs information about how advanced the disease is, the likelihood of cure, treatment options and side effects, how treatment will affect her life and self-image, how her family or partner will be affected, and home self-care. A woman's previous experience with cancer, and especially with other women with breast cancer, influences her reactions to the disease. Ask the client whether she has known anyone with breast cancer and what types of experiences she has had with breast disease and cancer in

---

CHART 77-1

BEST PRACTICE for
Assessing a Breast Mass

- Identify the location of the mass by using the "face of the clock" method.
- Describe the shape, size, and consistency of the mass.
- Assess whether the mass is fixed or movable.
- Note any skin changes around the mass, such as dimpling (peau d'orange), increased vascularity, nipple retraction, and ulceration.
- Assess the adjacent lymph nodes, both axillary and supra-clavicular nodes.
- Ask the client if she experiences pain or soreness in the area around the mass.

general. Explore the woman's feelings about the disease because her choices of treatment, her recovery, and her ability to learn are influenced by these emotions. Assess the client's and family's knowledge of breast cancer, the stage of the disease, and treatment options. The client's level of education is a significant influencing factor in her treatment choices for stage I breast cancer. Her perception of her situation is often influenced by outdated information. Perhaps she knew someone who had a Halsted radical mastectomy more than 30 years ago and thus associates breast surgery with the chest deformity and lymphedema experienced by that woman. Dispel myths or misconceptions by providing current information.

Also assess the client for problems related to sexuality. Three critical areas of distress—psychological, physiologic, and relational—contribute to the psychosexual morbidity of these clients. Ask about her frequency of, and satisfaction with, sexual relations with her partner. The client should reflect on the relationship with the partner and be asked whether and how the breast cancer has changed the intimate relations with, sexual function of, or types of touch by the partner.

Evaluate the need for additional resources at this time. Will extra psychological counseling be needed? Are there financial concerns that need to be discussed with social services? Will the client's partner, family, or friends support her throughout this period? How much support and teaching do they need? When does the client expect to hear about her pathology results, and whom would she like to have with her when she hears the results? Answers to these types of questions provide guidelines in establishing expected outcomes and in planning nursing care.

LABORATORY ASSESSMENT

The diagnosis of breast cancer relies on pathologic examination of tissue from the breast mass. After the presence of cancer is established, laboratory tests, including pathologic study of the lymph nodes, help detect possible metastases. Elevated liver enzyme levels indicate possible liver metastases, and increased serum calcium and alkaline phosphatase levels suggest bone metastases.

RADIOGRAPHIC ASSESSMENT

Mammography is a sensitive screening tool for breast cancer. However, it must be combined with BSE for optimal early detection and with clinical breast examination (CBE) for full interpretation of the findings. These three methods together are effective in detecting breast cancer as early as possible. The uniqueness of mammography results from its ability to reveal preclinical lesions (masses too small to be palpated manually). Client preparation and the procedure for mammography are discussed in Chapter 76.

Other radiographic procedures may be used before surgery to rule out metastases. A chest x-ray to screen for lung metastases is routine. Bone, liver, and brain scans and computed tomography (CT) scans of the chest and abdomen can reveal distant metastases.

OTHER DIAGNOSTIC ASSESSMENTS

Ultrasonography of the breast is an additional diagnostic tool used to clarify findings on mammography. If the mammogram reveals a lesion, ultrasonography is helpful in differentiating a fluid-filled cyst from a solid mass.

Pathologic examination of the breast tissue, or breast biopsy, is the key to diagnosis of breast cancer. Breast tissue is obtained by one of several types of biopsies (see Chapter 76).

Several other tests are useful for establishing the stage of disease and prognosis after the diagnosis is made. These tests include a pathologic examination of the lymph nodes on the affected side. Other prognostic factors include the following (Rosenzweig, Rust, & Hoss, 2000):
- Presence or absence of estrogen receptors (ER) or progesterone receptors (PR)
- S-phase index, or growth rate (done by flow cytometry to determine the S-phase fraction, also known as mitotic index)
- DNA ploidy (the amount of DNA in a tumor cell compared with the amount in a normal cell to determine whether the number of chromosomes in the cancer cells is normal (**euploid**) or abnormal (**aneuploid**)
- Histologic or nuclear grade
- HER2/neu gene expression

Estrogen and progesterone receptors are cytoplasmic proteins present in breast cancer cells that bind to estrogen and progesterone. In some cancers, when estrogen or progesterone binds to these receptors, the growth rate of the cell increases. Cancer cells that contain estrogen receptors (ER positive) or progesterone receptors (PR positive) have a better prognosis and usually respond to hormonal therapy. More postmenopausal women than premenopausal women are ER positive.

DNA ploidy and calculation of the number of cells in S phase by flow cytometry can reveal the growth rate of cells. Tumors with a high growth rate index and altered DNA content have a worse prognosis (Rosenzweig, Rust, & Hoss, 2000).

Tumor cells are also examined for specialization or differentiation. Because well-differentiated tumors tend to be less aggressive than poorly differentiated ones, a woman with a well-differentiated breast cancer has a better prognosis than the woman with a poorly differentiated tumor. Figure 77-6 illustrates the four stages of breast cancer.

Genetic Considerations

Breast cancer cells also are analyzed for the presence of excessive numbers of the HER2/neu receptor on or in the cancer cells. This receptor is related to the growth potential of the cancer cell. When breast cancer cells have excessive numbers of these receptors (overexpress the HER2/neu gene), they grow more rapidly and are relatively resistant to standard therapies. However, there is a targeted therapy, trastuzumab (Herceptin), that blocks these receptors and slows or stops the breast cancer cell growth. It is only effective for women whose breast cancer cells overexpress the HER2/neu gene.

◆ Analysis

COMMON NURSING DIAGNOSES AND COLLABORATIVE PROBLEMS

A common nursing diagnosis for clients with breast cancer is Anxiety related to the diagnosis of cancer. A common collaborative problem is Potential for Metastasis.

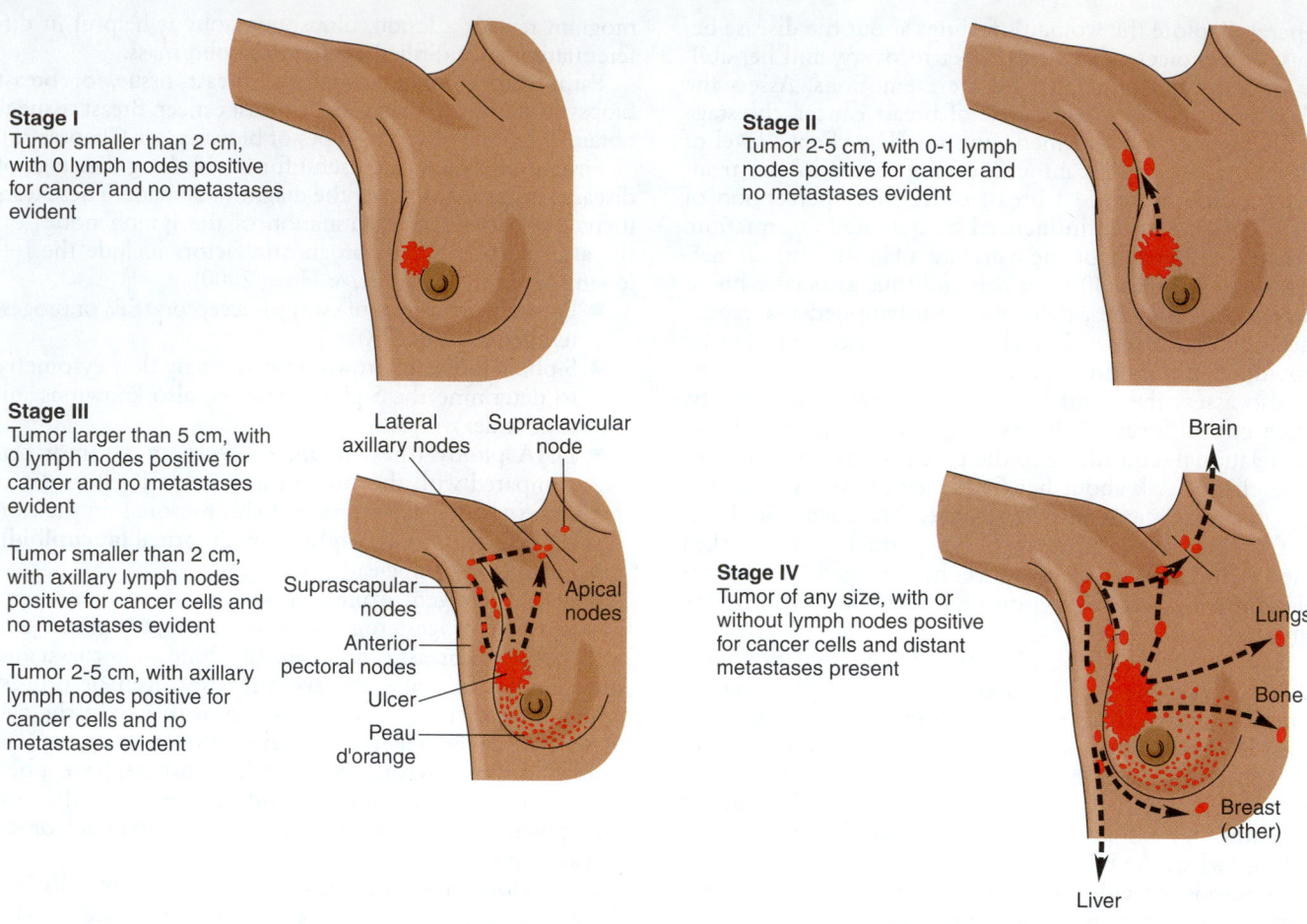

Figure 77-6 ■ Staging of breast cancer.

ADDITIONAL NURSING DIAGNOSES AND COLLABORATIVE PROBLEMS

In addition to the common nursing diagnoses and collaborative problems, clients with breast cancer (particularly advanced breast cancer) may have one or more of the following:

- Anticipatory Grieving related to loss and possible or impending death
- Acute Pain related to tumor compression on nerve endings
- Disturbed Sleep Pattern related to pain and anxiety
- Disturbed Body Image related to illness treatment, surgery, or loss of a body part
- Sexual Dysfunction related to surgery, disease process, or altered body structure

◆ Planning and Implementation

ANXIETY

NOC PLANNING: EXPECTED OUTCOMES. The client with breast cancer is expected to reduce anxiety to acceptable levels. Indicators include that the client often or consistently demonstrates the following behaviors:

- Seeks information to reduce anxiety
- Uses effective coping strategies
- Uses relaxation techniques to reduce anxiety
- Maintains social relationships
- Maintains adequate sleep

INTERVENTIONS. The woman with breast cancer is usually admitted to the health care facility with a definitive diagnosis established through an outpatient biopsy of the mass. The practice of admitting a woman with a suspicious lesion and using general anesthesia for a biopsy, frozen section, and possible mastectomy has largely been abandoned. Women who have an interval between the biopsy and treatment, during which they actively participate in the choice of treatment, cope more effectively after surgery, no matter which treatment is chosen.

The anxiety for the woman with breast cancer begins the moment the lump is discovered. The level of anxiety may be related to past experiences and personal associations with the disease. Many women have an intuitive feeling about a cancer diagnosis even before it is established. The likelihood that the lesion is or is not cancer is irrelevant to the level of fear. Assess the client's perceptions of her own situation and personal level of anxiety. Allow the client to ventilate these feelings even if a diagnosis has not been established (Chart 77-2).

If the mass has been diagnosed as cancer, many women feel a partial sense of relief to be dealing with a known entity. A feeling of shock or disbelief may predominate. It is difficult to accept a diagnosis of cancer when one feels basically well. Clients and their families or significant others deal in individual ways with the mix of feelings, which include shock, disbelief, and grief. Some may want to read and discuss any available information. Others may want to

CHART 77-2

NIC **INTERVENTION ACTIVITIES for**
The Client with Breast Cancer

Anxiety Reduction: *Minimizing apprehension, dread, foreboding, or uneasiness related to an unidentified source of anticipated danger*
- Listen attentively.
- Use a calm, reassuring approach.
- Provide factual information concerning diagnosis, treatment, and prognosis.
- Encourage verbalization of feelings, perceptions, and fears.
- Identify when level of anxiety changes.
- Support the use of appropriate defense mechanisms.
- Determine client's decision-making ability.

NIC intervention activities selected from Dochterman, J.M., & Bulechek, G.M. (Eds.) (2004). *Nursing intervention classification (NIC)* (4th ed.). St. Louis: Mosby. No part of this work is to be altered without prior written permission from the Publisher.

know as little as possible and resent attempts at teaching. Although one woman may want to talk at length about her concerns, another may want to be alone. Flexibility is the key to nursing care. Adjust your approach to care as the client's emotional state changes. An integral part of the plan to meet these emotional needs is the use of outside resources. Most health care providers view such groups as the American Cancer Society's Reach to Recovery as a source of support after surgery, but these groups can be suggested in the preoperative phase.

Health care providers working with clients who have breast cancer may know other clients willing to make a preoperative visit. These resource people may be chosen on the basis of the client's concerns. The woman who is worried in particular about the side effects of radiation therapy may benefit more from talking to someone who has undergone radiation than from talking to the nurse about secondhand experiences.

In addition to Reach to Recovery, formal and informal community support groups, such as ENCORE (Encouragement, Normalcy, Counseling, Opportunity, Reaching Out, and Energies Revived), may be available. These groups can be reached through the health care provider, the local hospital, visiting nurse associations, or by word of mouth.

POTENTIAL FOR METASTASIS

NOC **PLANNING: EXPECTED OUTCOMES.** The client with breast cancer is expected to remain free of metastases or recurrence of disease.

INTERVENTIONS. There are many surgical and non-surgical options for breast cancer treatment. Because of the various options, the woman with breast cancer often faces difficult decisions.

Although most women with metastatic breast cancer eventually succumb to the disease, chemotherapy, hormonal therapy, radiotherapy, and limited surgery are all helpful for palliative care, improvement in quality of life, and prolongation of life. Once cancer is diagnosed, the extent and location of metastases determine the overall therapeutic strategy. Treatment is tailored specifically to each client, taking into account other health problems and the client's ability to tolerate a particular therapy. Most importantly, the woman's specific goals and the particular outcome she seeks from therapy are thoroughly discussed.

NONSURGICAL MANAGEMENT. For clients with late-stage breast cancer, nonsurgical treatment may be the only alternative. If the disease is in a late stage, such as stage IV, with the presence of confirmed metastasis, or if the client cannot withstand a major surgical procedure, the tumor may be removed with a local anesthetic. Follow-up treatment may include hormonal therapy, chemotherapy, and sometimes radiation. If the tumor is attached to the skin or the underlying muscle, resection may be impossible. Follow-up therapy involves radiation, usually in conjunction with chemotherapy. Chapter 28 describes the nursing care associated with chemotherapy and radiation.

For women with breast cancer at a stage for which surgery is the main treatment, follow-up with adjuvant radiation, chemotherapy, hormone therapy, or targeted therapy is commonly prescribed. These therapy options are discussed under adjuvant therapy on p. 1817.

SURGICAL MANAGEMENT. The most common types of breast surgery are illustrated in Figure 77-7. Although controversy exists concerning the best treatment for breast cancer, experts agree that the mass itself should be removed to reduce the risk for local recurrence. Removal of the axillary lymph nodes for staging purposes may also be recommended. Axillary lymph node dissection (ALND) is usually performed for clients with palpable axillary lymph nodes. It is unclear whether clients with nonpalpable nodes should also have ALND because these nodes could have micrometastasis, which, if not removed or treated, could result in recurrence. However, the long-term effects of ALND are significant. Thus women who have stage I breast cancer have not always had an ALND.

The technique of sentinel lymph node biopsy (SLNB) is a promising method of identifying clients with axillary involvement who do not have palpable nodes but who may have microscopic disease in one or more nodes (Zack, 2001). In this method, the one or two sentinel lymph nodes, which receive all of the lymphatic drainage from an anatomic region are identified through a lymph node mapping procedure. Mapping involves injecting the area immediately around a tumor with a blue dye and/or radioactive colloid 1 to 8 hours before the lymph node biopsy. The main lymph channels for the tumor area carry the marker dye or radioactivity to the first nodes. The nodes that take up the dye (or give off a certain level of radiation picked up by a handheld counter) are removed and examined for the presence of cancer cells. It is believed that if cancer cells have traveled through the lymph channels, the cells would have lodged in the sentinel nodes. Travel beyond these nodes to higher level nodes would have occurred as a secondary event. Therefore the absence of cancer cells in the sentinel nodes is an indicator that no other nodes in the regional basin should be involved. This method has been helpful in limiting axillary dissections only to those with positive nodes (Zack, 2001).

Preoperative Care. Care of the woman facing surgery for breast cancer focuses on psychological preparation and preoperative teaching. The issues related to anxiety and lack of knowledge are primary. Direct efforts toward educating the client include the husband or partner who may be experiencing similar stress and confusion.

Review the type of procedure planned. Use open-ended questions (e.g., "What type of surgery are you having? Can

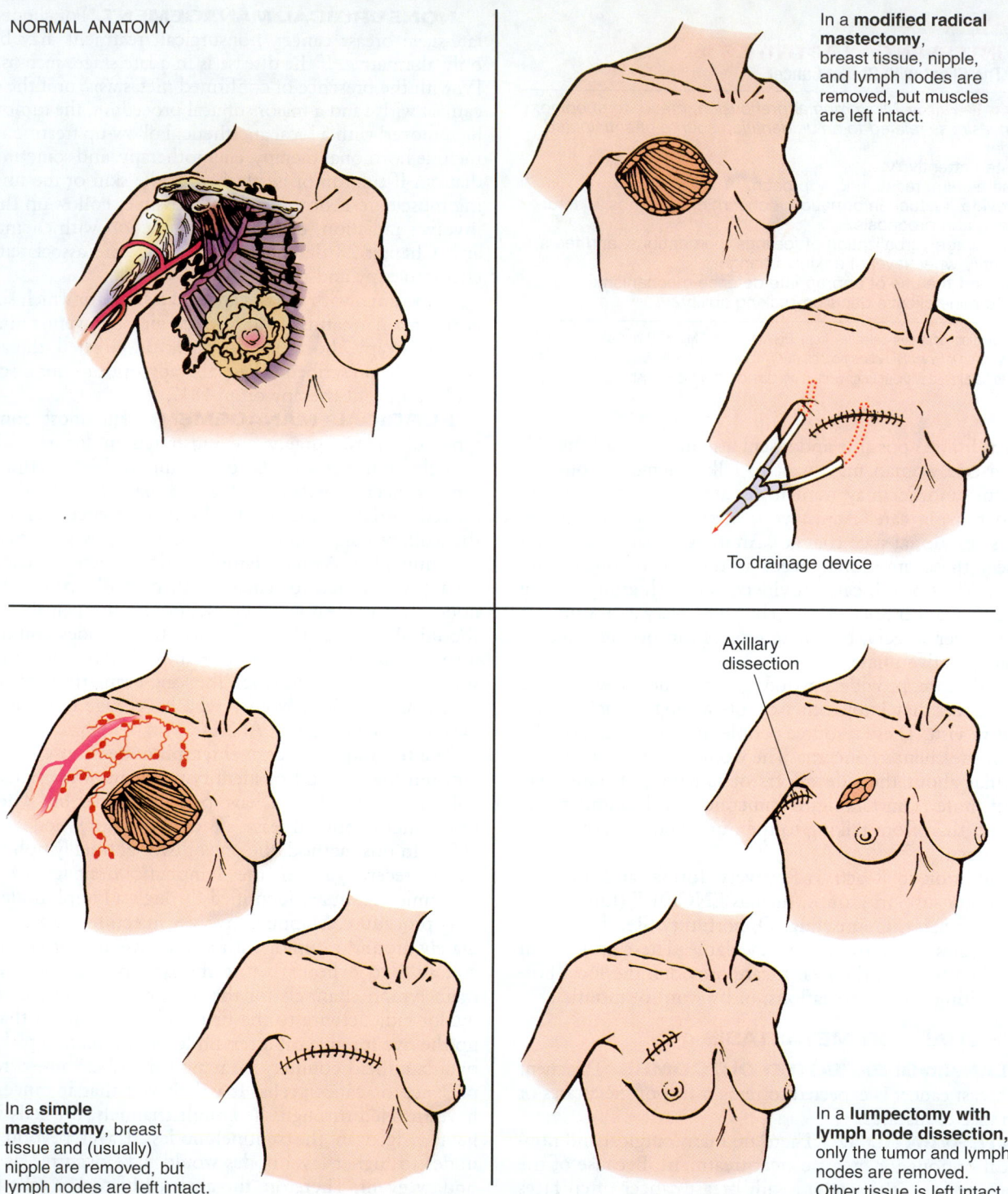

NORMAL ANATOMY

In a **modified radical mastectomy**, breast tissue, nipple, and lymph nodes are removed, but muscles are left intact.

To drainage device

Axillary dissection

In a **simple mastectomy**, breast tissue and (usually) nipple are removed, but lymph nodes are left intact.

In a **lumpectomy with lymph node dissection**, only the tumor and lymph nodes are removed. Other tissue is left intact.

Figure 77-7 ■ Surgical management of breast cancer.

you explain what will happen?") to assess the client's level of knowledge. The client should be knowledgeable about the type of procedure. Provide postoperative information, including the following:

- The need for a drainage tube
- The location of the incision
- Mobility restrictions
- The length of the hospital stay (if any)
- The possibility of adjuvant therapy

- Basic before and after surgery information needed by any surgical client (see Chapters 20 and 22)

Because of short hospital stays or same-day surgery procedures, supplement teaching with written materials for the client and family to take home as references. This information should include who to call in case there are any complications. Address body image issues before surgery to correct misconceptions about appearance after surgery and help the client begin adjusting to changes after surgery. If available, clients and their caregivers may attend classes before surgery in an ambulatory care setting, such as a surgical clinic, to promote successful early discharge from the hospital. These programs, which may provide emotional support, information, and opportunities for discussion related to sexuality, body image, preoperative instructions, and care after surgery enhance the care of the short-stay mastectomy client.

Operative Procedures. During breast-conserving surgery, the surgeon removes the bulk of the tumor. Typically, radiation therapy follows to eradicate residual tumor cells. Radiation therapy plays a critical role in the therapeutic regimen and is effective treatment for nearly all sites where breast cancer can metastasize. The most common site for metastasis is to bone tissue.

The following types of breast-conserving surgery are used as primary treatment for stage I and stage II breast cancer:

- Lumpectomy, also known as tylectomy or local excision, is gross resection of the tumor.
- Partial mastectomy, which includes wide excision, quadrantectomy, or segmental mastectomy, is removal of the portion of the breast that contains the tumor.

Breast-conserving procedures are usually performed in same-day surgical settings. The breast-conserving results in 5- and 10-year survival and local recurrence rates are no worse than those of the modified radical mastectomy. The cosmetic results have been good to excellent, and other long-term problems are comparable to those of more radical procedures. For many women, the psychological benefits of avoiding breast removal are significant and lead them to choose this option.

The modified radical mastectomy does *not* conserve the breast; the affected breast is completely removed. This procedure differs from the older Halsted radical mastectomy in that the surgeon leaves the pectoral muscles and nerves intact. Thus the breast tissue and skin and the axillary nodes are removed, and the underlying muscles are left in place. The typical incision is a 5- to 6-inch-long elliptic incision from the midchest to the axilla (see Figure 77-7). If reconstruction is to follow the procedure, the plastic surgeon may recommend a different location for the incision. When reconstruction is to be performed at the same time as the mastectomy, less invasive techniques, such as incising a 1.5-inch flap of skin around the nipple (excising the same amount of breast tissue as with conventional mastectomy), may be performed. Skin flaps or implants may be used to create a breast mound at the time of the original procedure.

The use of carbon dioxide laser procedures in place of cutting and cauterizing for mastectomies is an option that is becoming more available. Advantages of laser procedures include less blood loss and faster recovery.

Postoperative Care. Care after surgery in the hospital and at home for the woman undergoing a modified radical mastectomy or breast-conserving surgery is provided in the Plan of Care on pp. 1806 to 1815. Before the woman returns from surgery, place a sign over the client's bed to warn nurses and other personnel to avoid using the affected arm for taking blood pressure measurements, giving injections, or drawing blood. The woman returns from the

postanesthesia care unit (PACU) as soon as vital signs return to baseline levels and if no complications have occurred. On the client's return, the focus is on maintaining physiologic stability and comfort. Assess vital signs on a schedule of decreasing frequency, such as every 30 minutes for two times, every hour for two times, and then every 4 hours. During these checks, assess the dressing for bleeding.

Care of Drainage Tubes. During a modified radical mastectomy, the surgeon places one or two drainage tubes, usually Jackson-Pratt drains, under the skin flaps and attaches the tubes to a small collection chamber. Gentle suction is exerted, and fluid that would accumulate under the flaps and delay healing is collected. Various drains are available, but all allow the drainage to be seen and measured. When taking vital signs, monitor the drain for the amount and color of drainage. Add this information to the intake and output record. Clients undergoing a lumpectomy may also have drainage tubes (usually Jackson-Pratt drains) placed if the lump is large or if axillary node dissection is performed.

Observe the wound for signs of swelling and infection throughout the client's recovery. Drainage tubes are removed by the surgeon when drainage is less than 25 mL in 24 hours. With short hospital stays, drainage tubes are usually removed about 1 week after hospital discharge, when the client returns for her first postoperative office visit. Inform the client that tube removal may be painful although these tubes lie just under the skin.

Comfort Measures. Assess the client's position to ensure that the drainage tubes or collection device are not pulled or kinked. The client should sit with the head of the bed up at least 30 degrees, with the affected arm (the arm on the same side as the axillary dissection) elevated on a pillow, while awake. Keeping the affected arm elevated promotes lymphatic fluid return after removal of axillary lymph nodes and channels. Provide other basic comfort measures, such as repositioning and analgesics, as prescribed, on a regular basis until pain ceases.

Mobility and Diet. The hospital stay after a modified radical mastectomy is short, often same-day or just overnight, and recovery is usually not complicated. Because some managed care companies will not authorize an overnight stay in the hospital following a mastectomy, several states have enacted legislation mandating inpatient benefits. The client who chooses an early discharge should have a home care visit within 24 hours of the discharge.

Ambulation and a regular diet are resumed by the day after surgery. While the client is in an upright position, the arm on the affected side may need to be supported at first. Gradually, the arm should be allowed to hang straight by the side while the client is walking. Instruct the client to avoid the hunched-back position with the arm flexed because of the risk for elbow contracture. Beginning exercises that do not stress the incision can usually be started on the first day after surgery. These exercises include squeezing the affected hand around a soft, round object (a ball or rolled washcloth) and flexion/extension of the elbow. The progression to more strenuous exercises depends on the subsequent procedures planned (such as reconstruction) and the surgeon's prescription.

As soon as the woman is fully ambulatory, eating well, and surgical pain is under control, she is discharged to

Text continued on p. 1815.

PLAN of CARE   MEDICAL DIAGNOSIS: MASTECTOMY (WITH CHEMOTHERAPY/RADIATION)

NURSING DIAGNOSIS NO. 1 ■ Anxiety

	Expected Outcomes	Nursing Interventions	Rationales

RELATED FACTORS
Situational/maturational crises
Threat of death
Threat to self, self-concept
Threat to or change in:
  Role status
  Health status
  Interaction patterns
  Role function
  Environment
  Economic status
	Denies fatigue
	Denies weakness
	No verbal report or observation of alteration in sleep patterns
	No verbal report or observation of alteration in appetite
	No verbal report or observation of irritability
	No verbal report or observation of self-focusing behavior
		NIC Anxiety Reduction
		D Use a calm, reassuring approach.
		
		D Stay with the client.
		
		Create an atmosphere to facilitate trust.
		
		Control stimuli, as appropriate, for the client's needs.
		Support the use of appropriate defense mechanisms.
		
		Administer medications to reduce anxiety, as appropriate.
		
		Provide factual information concerning diagnosis, treatment, and prognosis.
		
		Other Interventions
		Acknowledge the client's successes with anxiety management.
		
		Continuing Care Considerations
		Monitor the client's verbal and nonverbal behaviors for anxiety.
		Assist the client to set realistic expectations and plans for anxiety management.
			The client may perceive fast-paced questioning and procedures as tension and worry from health care team members.
			The presence of a health care team member may serve to promote safety and reduce fear.
			A calm, reassuring, and truthful approach facilitates trust.
			Noise, fast-paced activity, and bright lights serve to increase tension.
			Appropriate coping strategies help the client to feel more in control and less powerless.
			Hypnotics/sedatives will promote rest and relaxation, which enhances coping abilities. Anxiolytics will decrease the client's perception of anxiety.
			In addition to establishing trust, accurate information will help the client marshal the appropriate coping strategies and the ability to make reasonable decisions.
			
			Positive reinforcement encourages the client to continue with anxiety management.
			
			The client may be unaware of his or her anxiety level in a subacute setting.
			Establishing a plan and setting realistic goals will help the client to feel more control over circumstances.

NURSING DIAGNOSIS NO. 2 ■ Anticipatory Grieving

	Expected Outcomes	Nursing Interventions	Rationales
RELATED FACTORS Future change in body shape Loss of a body part Possible reduction of life span **DEFINING CHARACTERISTICS** Potential loss of significant object (e.g., people, possessions, job, status, home, ideals, parts and processes of the body) Verbal expression of distress at loss Sleep patterns: Change in Activity patterns: Changes in	No verbal report or observation of alteration in sleep patterns No verbal report or observation of alteration in activity level No verbal report of alteration in libido Able to express the significance of potential loss No verbal report or observation of alteration in communication pattern No verbal report or observation of anger	**NIC Grief Work Facilitation** Identify the loss. Assist the client to identify personal coping strategies. Encourage the client to express his or her feelings about the loss. Communicate acceptance of discussing loss.	The client's perception of loss may be different from the circumstances. The client may need to have his or her strengths reinforced. The client may need to repeatedly express his or her feelings about the loss to diminish the burden of anguish. Nurses facilitate the expression of grief by giving the client permission to express herself or himself. The nurse's manner and words show that these expressions of grief are acceptable and expected.

D Indicates tasks that can be delegated to unlicensed assistive nursing personnel at the discretion of the nurse.

PLAN of CARE   MEDICAL DIAGNOSIS: MASTECTOMY (WITH CHEMOTHERAPY/RADIATION)—cont'd

NURSING DIAGNOSIS NO. 2 ■ Anticipatory Grieving—cont'd

Expected Outcomes	Nursing Interventions	Rationales
	Encourage identification of the client's greatest fears concerning the loss.	Helping the client to identify his or her fears permits the client and family to implement strategies to control the feared event.
	Assist the client in identifying needed lifestyle modifications.	The client may need assistance with services ranging from prosthetic devices to mobility equipment. A realistic appraisal of needs will save the client effort, time, and money in the adjustment period.
	Instruct the client regarding phases of the grieving process, as appropriate.	Clients need to know that grieving is an uneven process that may take months or years to complete. Many are surprised to find that one day is tranquil and the next is stormy.
	NIC **Active Listening** **D** Display an awareness of and sensitivity to emotions.	Active listening techniques such as clarification and rephrasing help the client to trust that his or her feelings are being conveyed.
	Focus completely on the interaction by suppressing prejudice, bias, assumptions, preoccupying personal concerns, and other distractions.	The client should receive the nurse's complete attention and impartial ear. Listening without advising helps the client to sort through feelings and beliefs.
	Listen for unexpressed messages and feelings, as well as the content, of the conversation.	Nonverbal cues are often the greatest indicator of the client's meaning.
	Avoid barriers to active listening.	Minimizing feelings, offering easy solutions, interrupting, talking about self, and premature closure indicate to the client that his or her feelings and thoughts are unimportant.
	Other Interventions Refer the client to community resources (e.g., hospice care, Reach to Recovery), as appropriate.	The client and family may find support and additional resources for coping with loss through community agencies.
	Continuing Care Considerations Assess the family's adjustments to the changes the client has made in response to the loss.	Clients may become withdrawn, angry, restless, or demanding as they attempt to cope with their changed circumstances.
	Assure the caregiver and family that assistance is readily available.	Caregivers may feel overwhelmed with the care regimen and with the amount of work required to assist the grieving person. Clear and simple directions for seeking assistance will help the caregiver maintain a sense of control.

Continued

▄ PLAN of CARE   MEDICAL DIAGNOSIS: MASTECTOMY (WITH CHEMOTHERAPY/RADIATION)—*cont'd*

NURSING DIAGNOSIS NO. 3 ■ Acute Pain

	Expected Outcomes	Nursing Interventions	Rationales
RELATED FACTORS Injury agents (biologic, chemical, physical, psy-chological) **DEFINING CHARACTERISTICS** Verbal or coded report of pain Protective gestures Facial mask Self-focus	Denies experiencing pain greater than 5 on a 0 to 10 pain scale No verbal report or obser-vation of guarding or protective gestures No verbal report or obser-vation of alteration in sleep patterns No verbal report or obser-vation of self-focusing behavior No verbal report or obser-vation of facial mask of pain No verbal report or obser-vation of alteration in activity level	NIC **Pain Management** Perform a comprehensive pain assessment that includes location, char-acteristics, onset/duration, frequency, quality, intensity or severity of pain, and precipitating factors. Observe for nonverbal cues of discomfort, es-pecially in clients who are unable to commu-nicate effectively. Evaluate past experiences with pain to include the individual or family his-tory of chronic pain or resulting disability, if appropriate. Reduce or eliminate fac-tors that precipitate or increase the pain experience. Select and implement a variety of measures to facilitate pain relief, as appropriate. Use pain control mea-sures before pain be-comes severe. Provide information about the pain, such as causes, how long it will last, and antici-pated discomforts from procedures. NIC **Analgesic Administration** D Monitor the client's vital signs before and after administering opioid analgesics with the first-time dose or if un-usual signs are noted. Choose the IV route rather than the IM route for frequent pain medication injections, when possible. Administer analgesics around-the-clock. Institute safety precau-tions for those receiv-ing opioid analgesics, as appropriate. Evaluate the effectiveness of the analgesic at reg-ular frequent intervals after each administra-tion, but especially after the initial dose; in addi-tion, observe for any manifestations of unto-ward effects.	A plan for pain management must be based on the client's unique responses to pain. Nonverbal cues provide sup-port for the existence of pain. Past experiences with pain may affect the perception of and response to pain. Preventing a pain experience is preferred to trying to control or eliminate pain. Pharmacologic, nonpharma-cologic, and interpersonal strategies may provide pain relief depending on the client's unique re-sponses to the therapeutic interventions. Medicating the client in a timely manner prevents pain from reaching acutely unpleasant levels. The client is better able to monitor his or her own dis-comfort and to intervene appropriately when informed. Opioid analgesics may de-press respirations or cause other adverse effects. The IV route avoids tissue trauma and unpredictable absorption of medication. Administration around-the-clock prevents peaks and troughs of analgesia, es-pecially with severe pain. Opioid analgesics may impair the client's judgment and/or coordination. Frequent evaluation of anal-gesic effectiveness permits the nurse to adjust the dose and timing interval to the client's need and pro-vides an early warning of adverse responses.

D Indicates tasks that can be delegated to unlicensed assistive nursing personnel at the discretion of the nurse.

PLAN of CARE   MEDICAL DIAGNOSIS: MASTECTOMY (WITH CHEMOTHERAPY/RADIATION)—cont'd

NURSING DIAGNOSIS NO. 3 ■ Acute Pain—cont'd

Expected Outcomes	Nursing Interventions	Rationales
	Document the client's response to the analgesic and any untoward effects.	Documentation provides the health care team with the information needed to accurately evaluate the client's response to the analgesic regimen.
	Implement actions to decrease the untoward effects of analgesics.	Actions taken to prevent the predictable but unwanted effects of narcotic analgesics (e.g., constipation) increase client comfort.
	Collaborate with the physician if drug, dose, route of administration, or interval changes are indicated, making specific recommendations based on equianalgesic principles.	The nurse working with the client is often in the best position to observe the client's response to the analgesic regimen.
	Instruct the client to request PRN pain medication before the pain becomes severe.	Pain may be managed with lower doses of analgesics and fewer untoward effects if PRN drugs are administered before pain becomes severe.
	Inform the client that drowsiness sometimes occurs during the first 2 to 3 days of opioid administration and then subsides.	Drowsiness poses a hazard to the client, making accidents more likely to occur.
	Correct the misconceptions/myths that the client or family members may hold regarding analgesics, particularly opioids.	A client's misconceptions may prevent him or her from using opioid analgesics.
	Teach about the use of analgesics, strategies to decrease side effects, and expectations for involvement in decisions about pain relief.	Information about analgesics and the expectation for involvement increase the client's sense of control over his or her pain.
	NIC **Patient-Controlled Analgesia (PCA) Administration**	
	Validate that the client can use a PCA device.	To use a PCA, the client must be able to communicate, comprehend explanations, and follow directions.
	Assist the client or family member to administer an appropriate bolus loading dose of analgesic.	The initial or bolus loading dose helps to establish baseline pain relief.
	Consult with the client, family members, and physician to adjust the lockout interval, basal rate, and demand dosage.	The client's response to the analgesic will determine the PCA settings.
	Document the client's pain, amount and frequency of drug dosing, and response to pain treatment on a pain flow sheet.	Information on the pain flow sheet will assist the health care team to adjust the analgesic regimen to the client's needs.

Continued

PLAN of CARE   MEDICAL DIAGNOSIS: MASTECTOMY (WITH CHEMOTHERAPY/RADIATION)—cont'd

NURSING DIAGNOSIS NO. 3 ■ Acute Pain—cont'd

Expected Outcomes	Nursing Interventions	Rationales
	Teach the client and family to monitor pain intensity, quality, and duration.	This information will help the client and family determine when to administer a bolus dose of analgesic, if appropriate, or when to request an increase in basal rate of the analgesic.
	Teach the client and family to monitor respiratory rate and blood pressure.	This information will help the health care team adjust analgesic doses to the client's responses and will decrease untoward effects.
	NIC **Environmental Management: Comfort** Determine sources of discomfort, such as damp dressings, positioning of tubing, constrictive dressings, wrinkled bed linens, and environmental irritants.	Control of environmental discomforts may decrease the need for pharmacologic intervention.
	D Prevent unnecessary interruptions and allow for rest periods.	Rest may improve the client's pain tolerance.
	Facilitate hygiene measures to keep the client comfortable.	Hygiene measures may improve the client's overall sense of well-being.
	Other Interventions Refer the client to the Pain Advisory Committee.	The Pain Advisory Committee is a multidisciplinary committee with wide expertise in pain relief interventions.
	Continuing Care Considerations Refer the client to an advanced practice nurse pain specialist, social worker, home care nurse, and/or psychologist, as appropriate.	Health care team members are able to provide continuing support for the client facing chronic pain.

NURSING DIAGNOSIS NO. 4 ■ Disturbed Body Image

	Expected Outcomes	Nursing Interventions	Rationales
RELATED FACTORS Psychosocial Biophysical Illness Surgery Illness treatment	Views, monitors, and acknowledges body Social involvement remains at pre-illness baseline Acknowledges changes in body that reflect a realistic appraisal of altered appearance or function	NIC **Body Image Enhancement** Use anticipatory guidance.	Anticipatory guidance prepares the client for predictable changes in body image.
DEFINING CHARACTERISTICS Verbal report of feelings that reflect an altered view of one's body in appearance, structure, or function	Acknowledges loss of significant objects Does not verbalize self-negating statements	Assist the client to discuss changes caused by illness or surgery, as appropriate.	The client who experiences changes caused by illness or surgery may be reluctant to verbalize his or her feelings.
Nonverbal response to actual or perceived change in body structure and/or function	Denies alteration in relationship with significant other	Help the client determine the extent of actual changes in the body or its level of functioning.	The client may be unable to realistically determine the extent of actual changes in the body or its level of functioning because of grieving for the changes.
Behavior: Avoidance of monitoring or acknowledgment of one's body Missing body part Hiding or overexposing body part (intentional or unintentional)		Assist the client to separate physical appearance from feelings of personal worth, as appropriate.	The client's feeling of personal worth may be strongly tied to physical appearance so that negative changes in appearance trigger feelings of low self-worth.

D Indicates tasks that can be delegated to unlicensed assistive nursing personnel at the discretion of the nurse.

PLAN of CARE   MEDICAL DIAGNOSIS: MASTECTOMY (WITH CHEMOTHERAPY/RADIATION)—cont'd

NURSING DIAGNOSIS NO. 4 ■ Disturbed Body Image—cont'd

Expected Outcomes	Nursing Interventions	Rationales
DEFINING CHARACTERISTICS—cont'd Actual change in structure and/or function Preoccupation with change or loss Verbal report: Negative feelings about body (e.g., feelings of helplessness, hopelessness, or powerlessness) Change in social involvement	Assist the client to discuss stressors affecting body image.	Stressors affecting body image may be due to congenital condition, injury, disease, or surgery.
	Identify the influence of the client's culture, religion, race, gender, and age on body image.	Culture, religion, race, gender, and age influence the client's perception of positive or negative body image.
	D Monitor whether the client can look at the changed body part.	The client's inability to look at the changed body part may indicate that he or she has strong negative feelings about the change.
	Determine the client's and family's perceptions of the alteration in body image versus reality.	The client's and family's perceptions of the alteration in body image may vary significantly from the reality of the change.
	Determine if a change in body image has contributed to increased social isolation.	A client who experiences a negative change in body image may withdraw from social contact.
	Assist the client in identifying the parts of his or her body that have positive perceptions associated with them.	The client may need assistance in identifying a positive body image if he or she is focused solely on a negative change.
	Identify means of reducing the impact of any disfigurement.	The use of clothing, wigs, or cosmetics may reduce the impact of any disfigurement.
	Assist the client to identify actions that will enhance appearance.	Assisting the client to enhance his or her appearance will improve self-concept.
	Other Interventions Assess the client's readiness to accept a change in body functioning.	Cues that the client is ready to begin dealing with body changes include questions about how to manage an aspect of his or her care or how to adapt familiar activities to the changed capability.
	Provide an atmosphere of caring and acceptance.	A client with traumatic changes in body parts or functioning may be especially sensitive to cues that indicate an aversive reaction.
	Continuing Care Considerations Refer the client to restorative specialists, as appropriate.	Restorative specialists have expertise in body enhancement and techniques to maximize appearance to improve self-concept.
	Refer the client to a support group of others who have experienced the same loss.	The client may receive useful information and support from others who are experiencing the same circumstances.

Continued

PLAN of CARE MEDICAL DIAGNOSIS: MASTECTOMY (WITH CHEMOTHERAPY/RADIATION)—*cont'd*

NURSING DIAGNOSIS NO. 5 ■ Disturbed Sleep Pattern

	Expected Outcomes	Nursing Interventions	Rationales
RELATED FACTORS Ruminative thoughts before sleep Depression **DEFINING CHARACTERISTICS** Sleep onset greater than 30 minutes Early-morning insomnia Awakening earlier or later than desired Verbal: Complaints of not feeling well rested Decreased ability to function	Denies difficulty falling asleep Verbally reports feeling well rested No verbal report or observation of early-morning insomnia No verbal report or observation of sleep onset greater than 30 minutes Denies waking earlier or later than desired	**NIC Sleep Enhancement** Approximate the client's regular sleep/wake cycle in planning care. Determine the effects of the client's medications on the sleep pattern. Monitor the client's sleep pattern and note circumstances that interrupt sleep. **D** Adjust light, noise, temperature, mattress, and bed. Assist the client to eliminate stressful situations before bedtime. Instruct the client how to perform autogenic muscle relaxation. Adjust the medication administration schedule. Regulate environmental stimuli to maintain normal day-night cycles. **Other Interventions** Discourage the use of alcohol. Suggest the use of L-tryptophan or an increased consumption of milk, cheese, and meats, as appropriate. **D** Offer the client a position change and a backrub at bedtime. **Continuing Care Considerations** Adjust the height of the head of the bed, as necessary. Teach the client to void before going to sleep.	Care activities should not interfere with the client's preferred sleep cycle. Medications may interfere with sleep patterns by causing insomnia or by increasing the sleep cycle. Physical difficulties (e.g., sleep apnea, obstructed airway, pain/discomfort, and urinary frequency) and/or psychological difficulties (e.g., fear or anxiety) may interrupt the client's normal sleep cycle. Adjustments to the environment may promote sleep. Stressful situations increase anxiety, heart rate, respiratory rate, and mental activity, which interfere with the transition to sleep. Autogenic muscle relaxation may facilitate sleep. Administer medications during the client's awake cycle to support his or her sleep/wake cycle. Providing quiet for sleep cycles and light and activity for awake cycles helps the client to maintain physiologic balance. Alcohol speeds the onset of sleep but disrupts rapid eye movement (REM) sleep. L-tryptophan may help the client sleep. A backrub and repositioning increase the client's physical comfort and may help him or her achieve restful sleep. Clients who are troubled with esophageal reflux may need the head of their bed elevated to prevent reflux, which may interfere with sleep. Voiding at bedtime may prevent awakening during the sleep cycle to void.

D Indicates tasks that can be delegated to unlicensed assistive nursing personnel at the discretion of the nurse.

PLAN of CARE   MEDICAL DIAGNOSIS: MASTECTOMY (WITH CHEMOTHERAPY/RADIATION)—cont'd

NURSING DIAGNOSIS NO. 6 ■ Sexual Dysfunction

Expected Outcomes	Nursing Interventions	Rationales
RELATED FACTORS Vulnerability Altered body structure (e.g., drugs, surgery, disease processes, trauma, radiation) Threat to self-concept Misinformation or lack of knowledge **DEFINING CHARACTERISTICS** Altered relationship with significant other Altered sense of achieving sexual satisfaction Actual or perceived limitations imposed by disease and/or therapy Altered sense of achieving perceived sex role	No verbal report or observation of change in libido Denies alteration in relationship with significant other Verbal report of ability to achieve desired satisfaction	**NIC Sexual Counseling** Establish a therapeutic relationship based on trust and respect. Preface questions about sexuality with a statement that tells the client that many people experience sexual difficulties. Discuss the effect of the illness/health situation and/or medication on sexuality. Encourage the client to verbalize fears and ask questions. Help the client to express grief and anger about alterations in body functioning/appearance. Avoid displaying aversion to an altered body part. In collaboration with other health care team members, introduce the client to positive role models who have successfully conquered a similar problem, as appropriate. Collaborate with other health care team members to provide services, as necessary. **Other Interventions** Use humor carefully. Include the client's significant other in counseling (with permission from the client). **Continuing Care Considerations** Refer the client to appropriate health care professionals, as necessary.	Discussions of sexuality and sexual functioning are often hampered by cultural proscriptions, which indicate that these areas are private and are not to be discussed. Clients may be reluctant to discuss sexual function. Helping clients to understand that the nurse is aware that others have experienced difficulties makes them less likely to feel abnormal. The client should be questioned about the specific effects of the illness and/or medication so an appropriate plan of care can be developed. Information about what the client knows, fears, and has questions about form the basis for health teaching and referrals. Encouraging the client to acknowledge alterations in body parts or appearance starts the grieving process. Calm acceptance of the client's altered appearance provides assurance that others do not regard him or her as mutilated. Introductions to others who have faced similar problems may be supportive and reassuring. Other health care team members, such as sex therapists, may offer the client additional strategies for managing the sexual disturbance. Humor may help to relieve uneasiness or anxiety without causing the client a loss of self-respect. Sexual dysfunction impacts both partners engaged in intimacy. Sexual dysfunction may be an ongoing problem related to health matters. The client and significant other may need ongoing support from health care team members.

Continued

▤ PLAN of CARE   MEDICAL DIAGNOSIS: MASTECTOMY (WITH CHEMOTHERAPY/RADIATION)—cont'd

NURSING DIAGNOSIS NO. 7 ■ Ineffective Protection

	Expected Outcomes	Nursing Interventions	Rationales
RELATED FACTORS Leukopenia Thrombocytopenia Anemias Inadequate nutrition Drug therapies (e.g., antineoplastics, corticosteroids) Surgery Radiation	Denies fatigue Denies weakness No verbal report or observation of alteration in sleep patterns No verbal report or observation of restlessness Has skin that remains intact with no bruising or rashes	**NIC Infection Protection** **D** Monitor for systemic and localized manifestations of infection. Monitor absolute granulocyte count, white blood cell (WBC) count, and differential results.	Elevated temperature, pulse, respirations, and fever indicate systemic infection, whereas redness, heat, swelling, and pain indicate a local infection. Elevations in these laboratory tests demonstrate the body's response to infection.
DEFINING CHARACTERISTICS Impaired healing Diaphoresis Fatigue Cough Appetite: Loss of	No verbal report or observation of delayed healing No verbal report or observation of alteration in appetite	Inspect the condition of any surgical incision/wound. **D** Provide appropriate skin care to edematous areas. **D** Maintain asepsis for the client at risk. **D** Promote sufficient nutritional intake. **D** Encourage rest. Numerous visitors should be limited and visits from individuals with known infections should be discouraged. Report positive cultures to infection control personnel. Teach the client and family about the manifestations of infection and when to report them to the health care provider. **NIC Infection Control** Promote safe food preservation and preparation. Administer antibiotic therapy, as appropriate. **NIC Surveillance: Safety** Monitor the client for alterations in physical or cognitive function.	A surgical incision may be slightly reddened and swollen from tissue damage but remains free of purulent drainage, excess swelling, or excess local pain (which indicate infection). Edematous skin is particularly susceptible to injury, and edematous tissue may encourage the growth of pathogenic agents. Asepsis minimizes the client's exposure to pathogenic agents and thus minimizes the incidence of infection. Adequate nutrition is essential for immune system cell formation and for the repair of damaged body tissues to provide protection against external pathogens. Mending tissues require energy. A fatigued client is stressed and requires greater expenditure of energy to accomplish tasks. Visitors may provide a needed diversion, but too many visitors may result in fatigue and unwanted exposure to pathogens. Early intervention to treat infection improves the client's response to therapy. Early intervention to treat infection prevents untoward complications from the infection and its therapy. Clients who are immunosuppressed may be susceptible to pathogens from foods that are improperly prepared or stored. Antibiotic therapy should assist the body to destroy pathogens. Changes in physical or cognitive function may lead to unsafe behavior.

D Indicates tasks that can be delegated to unlicensed assistive nursing personnel at the discretion of the nurse.

PLAN of CARE   MEDICAL DIAGNOSIS: MASTECTOMY (WITH CHEMOTHERAPY/RADIATION)—*cont'd*

NURSING DIAGNOSIS NO. 7   ■   Ineffective Protection—*cont'd*

Expected Outcomes	Nursing Interventions	Rationales
	NIC Surveillance: Safety— *cont'd*	
	Communicate information about the client's risk to other nursing staff.	Caregivers in the environment are better able to prevent injury when high-risk clients are identified and monitored continuously.
	Other Interventions Avoid overexertion, stress, temperature extremes, and people with upper respiratory tract infection.	Stressors exacerbate fatigue.
	Continuing Care Considerations Consider the use of complementary and alternative therapies.	Complementary and alternative therapies may be used to cope with chronic disease and disability, especially if chronic pain is a problem.

CHART 77-3

CLIENT EDUCATION GUIDE
Postmastectomy Exercises

Hand Wall Climbing
- Face the wall, and put the palms of your hands flat against the wall at shoulder level.
- Flex your fingers so that your hands slowly "walk" up the wall.
- Stop when your arms are fully extended.
- Slowly "walk" your hands back down the wall until they return to shoulder level.

Pulley Exercise
- Drape a 6-foot-long rope over a shower curtain rod or over the top of a door. If you use a door for this exercise, have someone put a nail or hook at the top of the door so that the rope does not slip off.
- Grab the ends of the rope, one in each hand, and extend your arms out to your sides until they are straight.
- Keeping your arms straight, pull down with your left arm to raise your right arm as high as you can.
- Pull down with your right arm to raise your left arm as high as you can.

Rope Turning
- Tie a rope to the knob of a closed door.
- Hold the other end of the rope and step back from the door until your arm is almost straight out in front of you.
- Swing the rope in a circle. Start with small circles and gradually increase to larger circles as you become more flexible.

home. Common instructions for exercises after mastectomy are listed in Chart 77-3.

Breast Reconstruction. Breast reconstruction after mastectomy is common, with few complications. Clients now consult with the reconstructive surgeon and have definite ideas regarding the type of reconstruction, timing of the procedure, and technique desired. Many women want breast reconstruction immediately after mastectomy using their own tissue (autogenous reconstruction). Breast reconstruction at the time of mastectomy, both autogenous and prosthetic, appears to lessen the psychological strain associated with undergoing a mastectomy.

The surgeon should offer the option of breast reconstruction before surgery is performed. If the client does not choose immediate reconstructive surgery, a temporary prosthesis is given to the client. Some surgeons allow women to use a temporary prosthesis in the immediate postoperative period as a part of the postoperative dressing. If this is the case, the client returns from surgery with a surgical bra and temporary sterile prosthesis in place. The nurse or social worker can refer the client to the American Cancer Society's Reach to Recovery program. In this program, a volunteer who has had breast cancer surgery visits the client at home, offering information on breast forms, clothing, coping with breast cancer, and possible reconstructive options. For this intervention to be as helpful as possible, the volunteer should be about the same age as the client and have experienced the same surgical procedure.

Evaluate the client's level of satisfaction with her prosthesis several weeks after surgery. Assess the client's attitude by asking about future plans for restoring appearance. Although reconstruction is not appropriate for some clients and others may not be interested in it, the surgeon should discuss the indications and contraindications, advantages and disadvantages, and typical recovery. If immediate reconstruction is chosen, the surgeon should be aware of this before so that the surgeon's plans can be coordinated with those of the plastic surgeon.

Several procedures are available for restoring the appearance of the breast (Table 77-5). Reconstruction may begin during the original operative procedure or later in one to several stages. The following are some of the more common techniques (Resnick & Belcher, 2002):
- Use of a flap of skin and muscle from the abdomen, back, or hip to create a breast mound

TABLE 77-5 Examples of Breast Reconstruction Procedures

Procedure	Description	Procedure	Description
Implantation	An implant matching the size of the other breast is placed under the muscle on the operative side to create a breast mound.	Myocutaneous flaps	A flap of skin, fat, and muscle is transferred from the donor site to the operative area. The flap contains an appropriate amount of fat to match the other breast and is similar in appearance to breast tissue. A blood supply is established by reanastomosis of vessels from the operative area to those with the flap when possible. A new nipple may be created with tissue from areas such as the labia or upper, inner thigh. Nipples can also be created by tattooing.

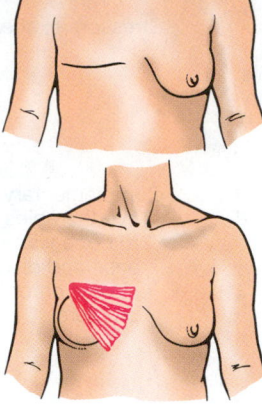

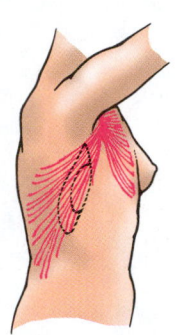 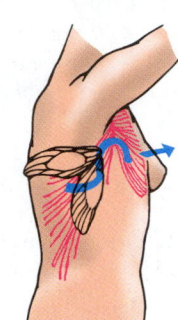

Latissimus dorsi musculocutaneous flap

Procedure	Description
Tissue expansion	A tissue expander is placed under the muscle and gradually expanded with saline to stretch the overlying skin and create a pocket. After several weeks, the tissue expander is exchanged for an implant.

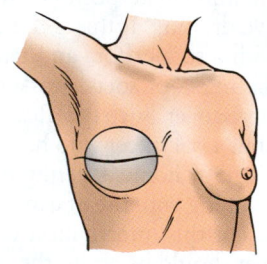

Abdominal myocutaneous flap

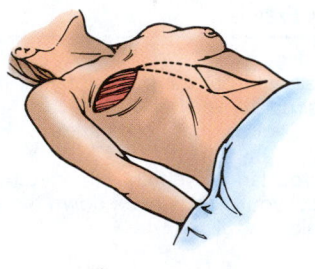

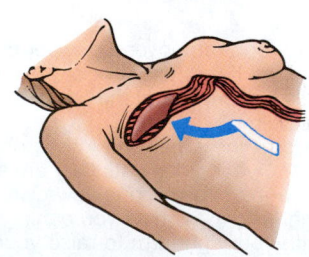

- Placement of a saline- or gel-filled prosthesis
- Use of progressive tissue expanders to slowly create a pocket under the mastectomy site for placement of a permanent implant.

Reconstruction of the nipple-areola complex is the last stage in the reconstruction of the breast. If necessary, a new nipple may be created with other body tissue, such as from the labia or inner thigh.

After concerns about the safety and effectiveness of silicone gel implants were voiced in the early 1990s, the Food and Drug Administration (FDA) restricted the use of silicone gel implants to women in FDA-approved safety studies. The studies were open to women seeking implants after breast cancer surgery or traumatic injury (McSpedon, 2002). Al-

though no conclusive evidence indicates that silicone gel implants put women at risk for connective tissue diseases, some research findings suggest that ruptured silicone gel implants may lead to the development of fibromyalgia (Brown, 2001; Janowsky, 2000). Further research in this area is needed to support these findings.

The transverse rectus abdominis myocutaneous (TRAM) flap, a commonly used method of reconstruction, provides women with naturally appearing breasts without the risks associated with the silicone gel implant. This procedure has become the first choice for breast reconstruction and can be combined with tissue expanders and implants to obtain symmetry (Moran et al., 2000). Nursing care of the woman who has undergone breast reconstruction is outlined in Chart 77-4.

CHART 77-4

BEST PRACTICE for
Postoperative Care of the Client After Breast Reconstruction

- Assess the incision and flap for signs of infection (excessive redness, drainage, odor) during dressing changes.
- Assess the incision and flap for signs of poor tissue perfusion (duskiness, decreased capillary refill) during dressing changes.
- Avoid pressure on the flap and suture lines by positioning the client on her nonoperative side and avoiding tight clothing.
- Monitor and measure drainage in collection devices, such as Jackson-Pratt drains.
- Teach the client to return to her usual activity level gradually and to avoid heavy lifting.
- Remind the client to avoid sleeping in the prone position.
- Teach the client to avoid participation in contact sports or other activities that could cause trauma to the chest.
- Teach the client to minimize pressure on the breast during sexual activity.
- Remind the client to refrain from driving until advised by the physician.
- Remind the client to ask at the 6-week postoperative visit when full activity can be resumed.
- Reassure the client that optimal appearance may not occur for 3 to 6 months postoperatively.
- If implants have been inserted, teach the proper method of breast massage to enhance expansion and prevent capsule formation (consult with the physician).
- Review the breast self-examination procedure and the need to continue this practice monthly.
- Remind the client that mammograms should be scheduled at least yearly for the rest of her life.

Adjuvant Therapy. The decision to follow the original surgical procedure with chemotherapy, radiation, hormonal, or targeted therapy is based on the following:

- The stage of the disease
- The client's age and menopausal status
- Client preferences
- Pathologic examination
- Hormone receptor status
- Presence of a known genetic predisposition

The purpose of adjuvant therapy is to decrease the risk of recurrence for the client who has no evidence of but is at risk for metastasis or to prolong survival after metastasis occurs. Adjuvant therapy for stage I and stage II (early-stage) breast cancer consists of breast-conserving surgery with radiotherapy after surgery or of modified radical mastectomy.

Radiation Therapy. The purpose of radiation therapy is to kill breast cancer cells that may remain near the site of the original tumor. This therapy can be delivered to the whole breast by external beam given daily for 6 to 7 weeks. Skin changes are a major side effect during this therapy (see Chapter 28). An alternative approach is partial breast brachytherapy. In this procedure, small catheters are threaded through the breast in the tumor bed. Then, twice each day for 5 days, radioactive seeds are place in the catheters for a specified exposure period (usually 5 to 10 minutes). The total dose of radiation to the breast is the same for both procedures.

Chemotherapy. Chemotherapy is usually **adjuvant** therapy (in addition to surgery) for breast cancer. Its purpose is to kill breast cancer cells that may have left the original tumor and moved to more distant sites. Usually, it is used for stage II or higher breast cancer although determination of when it is needed is controversial. Chemotherapy is unpleasant, expensive, and can have dangerous short-term and long-term side effects. Therefore the risks and the benefits of its use must be examined for each client. Although chemotherapeutic regimens differ among treatment centers, multiple-agent combinations are used. Most combinations include paclitaxel (Taxol) and doxorubicin (Adriamycin). The length of treatment may also vary. Some protocols involve giving chemotherapy before surgery; more commonly, it is given after surgery.

Although some side effects are specific to a given drug, chemotherapy is systemic treatment and affects many tissues. Common side effects include nausea and vomiting, hair loss (**alopecia**), and an increased risk for infection because of bone marrow suppression. Chapter 28 discusses issues and interventions for clients receiving systemic chemotherapy.

Hormonal Therapy. Women who have estrogen receptor (ER)-positive tumors may be given estrogen receptor blocking agents such tamoxifen (Nolvadex, Tamofen✱), toremifene (Fareston), raloxifene (Evista), droloxifene, and idoxifene, or agents that reduce the circulating levels of estrogen, such as inhibitors of estrogen synthesis and aromatase inhibitors. When hormonal therapy is appropriate, the response rate is 50% to 60%. Tamoxifen therapy has a higher risk for endometrial cancers for women who still have a uterus. For these women, other estrogen receptor blockers that are more specific to the ER receptors in the breast are used.

Drugs that inhibit estrogen synthesis include leuprolide (Lupron) and goserelin (Zoladex). These drugs suppress the hypothalamus from making luteinizing hormone-releasing hormone (LH-RH). Under the influence of LH-RH, the ovaries are stimulated to produce estrogen. When LH-RH is inhibited, the ovary does not produce estrogen.

A small but significant source of estrogen is that made in the adrenal gland, kidney, and a few other organs through the action of the enzyme aromatase. The drugs anastrozole (Arimidex), letrozole (Femara), exemestane (Aromasin), and fulvestrant (Faslodex) all reduce circulating levels of estrogen by blocking the activity of aromatase. These drugs have eliminated the need for an adrenalectomy or pituitary gland removal to control the estrogen influence on breast cancer cells.

Stem Cell Transplantation. Autologous and allogeneic stem cell transplantation are options for clients with a high risk for recurrence or who have advanced disease. **Autologous** bone marrow transplantation (taken from the client's bone marrow), peripheral blood stem cell transplantation (taken from the client's circulating blood), or **allogeneic** bone marrow transplantation (taken from a healthy donor's bone marrow or peripheral blood) are performed as a means of rescue therapy following very high doses of chemotherapy. A discussion of the care of the client undergoing bone marrow or stem cell transplantation is given in Chapter 43.

Targeted Therapy. For clients whose breast cancer cells overexpress the HER2/neu gene product and have large numbers of HER2 receptors, targeted therapy with trastuzumab (Herceptin) is effective in slowing cancer cell growth. Although not many tumors are HER2/neu-positive, the development of targeted therapy for breast cancer is an important step in improving the outcome for this disease. Common side effects of Herceptin when used alone include headaches, skin rashes, diarrhea, and flu-like symptoms of fever, chills, and muscle aches.

? Critical Thinking Challenge

You are an RN assigned to a group of clients with an LPN and patient care technician (PCT) on your team. A client in your group has just returned from the PACU following a left modified radical mastectomy. She has a pressure dressing over the surgical site (which is dry and intact) and two drains. When performing her postoperative assessment, you note that her vital signs are stable, and she states that her pain is under control. The client's life partner and daughter are with her in the room.

1. What is this client's priority for care at this time?
2. What position should you place the client in and why?
3. What part of the client's postoperative assessment, if any, would you assign to the LPN? Explain your rationale?
4. What nursing tasks or activities, if any, would you delegate to the PCT? Explain your rationale.
5. What roles do the life partner and daughter have in planning continuing care for this client?

evolve For suggested answer guidelines, go to http://evolve.elsevier.com/Iggy/.

Community-Based Care

HOME CARE MANAGEMENT

Home care preparation should be initiated when the decision to have surgical therapy is made. Referral to a case manager can ensure that the educational needs of the client are met early in the perioperative period. The preadmission testing center or the surgeon could make referrals. Preoperative teaching and arrangements for home care management and referrals (Reach to Recovery, social services, home care) can be initiated before hospitalization. Planning ahead for the client's discharge needs facilitates discharge.

The client who has undergone breast surgery can be discharged to the home setting unless other physical disabilities exist. Some are discharged a day after surgery with Jackson-Pratt or other types of drains in place. Many clients are discharged to home on the same day that surgery is performed. These clients need assistance at home with drain care, dressings, and activities of daily living because of pain and impaired range of motion of the affected arm. Summaries of discharge instructions are given in Charts 77-5 and 77-6.

It is not necessary to modify the home for the client after breast surgery. Activities involving stretching or reaching for heavy objects should be avoided temporarily. This restriction can be discussed with a family member or significant other who can perform these tasks or place the objects within easy reach of the client.

HEALTH TEACHING

The teaching plan for the client after surgery includes the following:
- Measures to optimize a positive body image
- Information to enhance interpersonal relationships and roles
- Exercises to regain full range of motion
- Measures to prevent infection of the incision
- Measures to avoid injury, infection, and swelling of the affected arm
- Care of the incision and drainage device

Explain incisional care to the client and family. The client may wear a light dressing to prevent irritation. Explain that

---

CHART 77-5

CLIENT EDUCATION GUIDE
Recovery from Breast Cancer Surgery

- There may be a dry gauze dressing over the incision when you leave the hospital. You may change this dressing if it becomes soiled.
- A small, dry dressing will be around the site where a drain is placed. Often there is some leakage of fluid around the drain. Check the gauze dressing for drainage, and change it if it becomes soiled. Some leakage is normal, but if the dressing becomes soaked more than once a day, call your health care provider.
- Your nurse has shown you how to empty the reservoir from your drain and how to measure the volume of drainage. You should empty the drain twice a day and record the measurements.
- Drains are generally removed when drainage is less than 25 mL in 24 hours.
- Drains are often removed at the same time as the stitches or staples, generally 7 to 10 days after surgery.
- You may take sponge baths or tub baths, making certain that the area of the drain and incision stays dry. You may shower after the stitches, staples, and drains are removed.
- You can begin using your arm for normal activities, such as eating or combing your hair. Exercises involving the wrist, hand, and elbow, such as flexing your fingers, circular wrist motions, and touching your hand to your shoulder, are very good. You can usually resume more strenuous exercises after the drains have been removed.
- You can expect some discomfort or mild pain after surgery, but within 4 to 5 days most women have no need for pain medication or require medication only at bedtime.
- Numbness in the area of the surgery and along the inner side of the arm from the armpit to the elbow occurs in virtually all women. It is the injury to the nerves that causes sensation to the skin in those areas. Women have described sensations of heaviness, pain, tingling, burning, and "pins and needles." These sensations change over the months and usually resolve by 1 year.
- Pamphlets on exercises, hand and arm care, and general facts about breast cancer are available from your nurse or volunteer visitor. The American Cancer Society has volunteers who have had surgery similar to yours and are available to visit you.

Modified from Thomas, S., & Greifzu, S. (2000). Breast cancer. *RN, 63*, 40-47.

---

no lotions or ointments should be used on the area and that the use of deodorant under the affected arm should be delayed until healing is complete. Although swelling and redness of the scar itself are normal for the first few weeks, swelling, redness, increased heat, and tenderness of the surrounding area indicate infection and should be reported to the surgeon. If a lymph node dissection was performed, instruct the client to elevate the affected arm on a pillow for at least 30 minutes a day for the first 6 months. The client should have someone bring a loose-fitting, nonwired bra or camisole for her to try before discharge with a soft cotton-filled or polyester fiber-filled form supplied by the hospital or by Reach to Recovery. The client wears this form until the incision is completely healed and the health care provider approves the fitting of a more sophisticated prosthesis, usually 6 to 8 weeks after discharge. Encourage the client to dress in loose-fitting street clothes at home, not pajamas, to further enhance a positive self-image.

Teach the client to continue performing the exercises that began in the hospital. Active range-of-motion exercises should begin 1 week after surgery or when sutures and drains

CHART 77-6

HOME CARE ASSESSMENT of
Clients Recovering from Breast Cancer Surgery

Assess cardiovascular, respiratory, and urinary status:
- Vital signs
- Lung sounds
- Urine output patterns

Assess for pain and effectiveness of analgesics.

Assess dressing and incision site:
- Excess drainage
- Manifestations of infection
- Wound healing
- Intact staples

Assess drain and site:
- Drainage around drain site and in drain
- Color and amount of drainage
- Manifestations of infection

Review client's recordings of drainage.

Evaluate client's ability to care for and empty drain.

Assess status of affected extremity:
- Range of motion
- Ability to perform exercise regimen
- Lymphedema

Assess nutritional status:
- Food and fluid intake
- Presence of nausea and vomiting
- Bowel sounds

Assess functional ability:
- Activities of daily living
- Mobility and ambulation

Assess home environment:
- Safety
- Structural barriers

Assess client's compliance and knowledge of illness and treatment plan:
- Follow-up appointment with surgeon
- Manifestations to report to health care provider
- Hand and arm care guidelines
- Referral to Reach to Recovery

Assess client and caregiver coping skills:
- Determine if client has looked at incision site.
- Assess client's reaction to incision site.

---

are removed. Emphasize that reaching and stretching exercises should continue only to the point of pain or pulling, never beyond that. ENCORE, a YWCA program, is appropriate for women as early as 3 weeks after surgery and includes exercise to music, exercise in water, and psychological support. Before discharge, the surgeon may prescribe precautions or limitations specific to plans for future procedures, such as reconstruction.

Provide information needed to help the client avoid infection and subsequent lymphedema of the affected arm after the mastectomy. Teach the client to avoid having blood pressure measurements taken on, having injections in, or having blood drawn from the arm on the side of the mastectomy. Instruct the client to wear a mitt when using the oven, wear gloves when gardening, and treat cuts and scrapes appropriately. If lymphedema occurs, the arm should be elevated when possible and special attention paid to the aforementioned warnings. In addition, if lymphedema occurs, it can be managed with the use of an arm sleeve (similar to a Ted or Jobst stocking) or a sequential compression device. Management of lymphedema is directed toward measures that promote drainage of the affected arm; however, prevention is the best cure.

CONSIDERATIONS FOR OLDER ADULTS

With the projected increase in the older adult population, especially women, during the next half-century, breast cancer will be an even greater health concern. Older breast cancer survivors require more time for assessment and follow-up care. They require careful assessment for differentiation of symptoms that may be treatment related, associated with development of chronic diseases, or physical decline from aging. Older breast cancer survivors should be provided with thorough information and encouraged to participate in treatment decision making. They should be assisted to identify their sources of support and encouraged to expand their support networks with supportive friends and relatives. Age-specific support groups enable older survivors to broaden their support networks by introducing them to other survivors, which provides an opportunity for information sharing and the formation of new friendships.

PSYCHOSOCIAL PREPARATION

Concerns about appearance after surgery are common and are often a threat to the client's self-concept as a woman. Before breast surgery, the woman and her partner can benefit from an explanation of the expected postoperative appearance. After a modified radical mastectomy, the chest wall is fairly smooth and has a horizontal incision from the axilla to the midchest area. After breast-conserving surgery, scars vary according to the amount of breast tissue removed. Scars may be red and raised at first, but these features lessen in the first few months. After surgery, encourage the woman to look at her incision before she goes home and offer to be present when she does so.

Much of one's body image is a reflection of how others respond. Therefore the response of the client's family or partner to the surgery is crucial in determining the effect on self-concept. These people may also need the support of the nurse. They may have concerns about their ability to accept the changes and need to discuss these feelings with an objective listener. They may also need help with communicating their feelings, both negative and positive, with their loved one. Involving them in teaching may also help reinforce learning and increase retention.

Discuss sexual concerns before discharge. Sexual intercourse can be resumed whenever the client is comfortable. Clients may prefer to lay a pillow over the surgical site or wear a bra or camisole to prevent contact with the surgical site during intercourse. The client may be embarrassed to broach the topic. Be sensitive to possible concerns and approach the subject first.

For women of childbearing age (about 25% of breast cancer clients), issues related to childbearing may be a concern. Chemotherapy and radiation are considered serious teratogenic (birth defect–causing) agents, and sexually active clients receiving chemotherapy or radiotherapy should be advised to use birth control during therapy. The method and length of birth control is discussed with the health care provider.

For older women, issues such as fear and uncertainty about treatment outcomes, reduced functional status, concurrent chronic diseases, disease recurrence, future well-being and independence, and reduced social resources may be encountered (Sammarco, 2003). Be aware of the specific con-

EVIDENCE-BASED PRACTICE for Nursing

What is the quality of life of breast cancer survivors of different psychosocial stages and places in life?

Sammarco, A. (2003). The quality of life of older breast cancer survivors. *Cancer Nursing. 26*(6), 431-438.

This study investigated the relationship between perceived social support, uncertainty, and quality of life among older breast cancer survivors. A sample of 103 breast cancer survivors older than 50 years of age completed questionnaires that measured their perceived social support, uncertainty, and quality of life. The study results showed that as age increased, the women perceive less support and more uncertainty in their lives, which could adversely affect their quality of life.

Level of Evidence: 5—Well-conducted case control study (qualitative of sufficient size).

Critique. The results of this study cannot be generalized to the population of older breast cancer survivors due to use of a convenience sample. However, the study results underscore the importance of social support in reducing illness uncertainty and improving the quality of life of older breast cancer survivors.

Implications for Nursing. The study findings provide useful information that can assist nurses in increasing their awareness regarding the interplay of the developmental stage and place in life of older breast cancer survivors with quality of life. The current health care environment is one of attenuating resources and narrow margins of opportunity for contact with breast cancer clients. Nurses are constantly challenged to meet the supportive needs of older breast cancer survivors and contribute to improved quality of life outcomes. It should be recognized that the quality of life needs of older breast cancer survivors differ considerably from those of younger survivors and require interventions that are tailored to the specific psychosocial life-stage of the individual.

cerns of the older clients and plan interventions accordingly (see the Evidence-Based Practice for Nursing box above).

HEALTH CARE RESOURCES

Resources available to the client after discharge include personal support and community programs. After discharge, the spouse or partner may need help in planning support for home responsibilities. For example, a partner who may be assuming additional duties at home and work may feel stressed. Exploring temporary relief resources for child care, cleaning, or cooking may be helpful until the woman regains her previous energy level. Discussing the need for ongoing emotional support is also beneficial to both the client and her partner. Leaving the hospital and appearing normal do not end the anxiety and fear. Identifying a support person with whom the client or couple can explore these feelings and discussing the need to ventilate feelings enhance personal and family recovery.

As mentioned, Reach to Recovery and ENCORE are two community resources for women with breast cancer. Reach to Recovery provides a volunteer who visits the client in the hospital or at home. She brings a personal message of hope, informational materials on breast cancer recovery, and a soft, temporary breast form. Some communities offer additional resources such as support groups and exercise classes.

◆Evaluation: Outcomes

Evaluate the care of the client with breast cancer on the basis of the identified nursing diagnoses and collaborative problems. The expected outcomes include that the client will:

- Be able to cope with the diagnosis
- Remain free of metastasis

Specific indicators for these outcomes are listed for each nursing diagnosis and collaborative problem under the Planning and Implementation section (see earlier).

GET READY for the NCLEX Examination!

KEY POINTS

Safe Effective Care Environment

- In collaboration with the health care team, assess the physiologic stability and comfort level of clients who have undergone surgical intervention for breast cancer.
- After breast cancer surgery, assess vital signs, dressings, drainage collection tubes, and amount of drainage in collection container.
- Clients who have had lymph node dissection in addition to breast surgery must be placed on arm precautions to prevent lymphedema. The arm of the surgical side cannot be used for blood pressures, blood drawing, or injections. A sign to that effect must be placed over the client's bed and the health care team notified.
- Use standard precautions when managing the drains of a client after mastectomy.

Health Promotion and Maintenance

- Identify clients at higher risk for breast cancer, especially women with family history of breast cancer, those who have had early menarche, late menopause, first pregnancy after 30 years of age, or those who are nullipara.
- Teach women how to perform breast self-examination (BSE) as a means of early detection of breast cancer.
- Encourage women to have screening mammography according to recommended guidelines. Baseline screening should begin at 40 years of age and continue yearly. In high-risk women, screening should be started between 25 and 35 years of age.
- Encourage women to have clinical breast examination (CBE) according to recommended guidelines.

Psychosocial Integrity

- Assess women's reactions to the diagnosis of breast cancer and the affect of breast cancer treatment on their body image and sexuality.
- Identify resources that facilitate their grief work and coping skills.
- Allow the client opportunities to express feelings of grief, fear, and anxiety.
- Teach client ways to minimize surgical area deformity and enhance body image, such as use of a breast prosthesis or the option of breast reconstruction.
- Address the reactions of family and significant others to the diagnosis of breast cancer; provide support and education.
- For clients with advanced metastatic breast cancer, provide end-of-life care, including referral to hospice care.

Physiological Integrity

- Assess the return of arm and shoulder mobility after breast surgery and axillary dissection.
- Assess for the presence of lymphedema and assist client to perform therapeutic measures to reduce lymphedema in the affected arm.

- Teach the client measures to prevent lymphedema after axillary node dissection.
- Observe for and report other complications of breast cancer surgery or breast reconstruction, especially infection and inadequate vascular perfusion.
- For clients with advanced breast cancer, evaluate the client's ability to perform activities of daily living (ADLs); refer or consult with social worker if home care is needed.
- For clients with advanced metastatic breast cancer, manage chronic pain with drug therapy as prescribed and nonpharmacologic measures, such as relaxation, aromatherapy, and imagery.
- After an axillary lymph node dissection, elevate the affected arm on a pillow.
- Encourage ambulation, a regular diet, and mild arm exercises to maintain mobility and enhance recovery.
- Use strict aseptic technique in dressing changes and care of drainage apparatus.

ADDITIONAL STUDY RESOURCES

Go to your Student CD-ROM for Review Questions for the NCLEX Examination.

Go to http://evolve.elsevier.com/Iggy/ for Integrated Management of Care Questions for the NCLEX Examination.

SELECTED BIBLIOGRAPHY

Asterisk indicates a classic or definitive work on this subject.

American Cancer Society. (2003a). *Cancer facts and figures for African Americans-2003*. Report No. 8614.03. Atlanta: Author.

American Cancer Society. (2003b). *Cancer prevention and early detection. Facts and figures-2003*. Report No. 8600.03. Atlanta: Author.

American Cancer Society. (2005). *Cancer facts and figures—2005*. Report No. 00-300M-No. 5008.05. Atlanta: Author.

*Ashing-Giwa, K., et al. (1999). Quality of life of African-American and white long term breast carcinoma survivors. *Cancer, 85*(2), 418-426.

Austin, L., et al. (2002). Breast and cervical cancer screening in Hispanic women: A literature review using the health belief model. *Women's Health Issues, 12*(3), 122-128.

Baltzell, K., Eder, S., & Wrensch, M. (2005). Breast carcinogenesis: Can the examination of ductal fluid enhance our understanding? *Oncology Nursing Forum, 32*(1), 33-39.

Baquet, C., & Commiskey, P. (2000). Socioeconomic factors and breast carcinoma in multicultural women. *Cancer, 88*(5), 1256-1264.

Baron, R., et al. (2002). Eighteen sensations after breast cancer surgery: A comparison of sentinel lymph node biopsy and axillary lymph node dissection. *Oncology Nursing Forum, 29*(4), 651-659.

Barroso, J., et al. (2000). Comparison between African-American and white women in their beliefs about breast cancer and their health locus of control. *Cancer Nursing, 23*(4), 268-276.

Berry, J. (2001). Breast pain: All that hurts is not cancer. *The American Journal for Nurse Practitioners, 5*(4), 9-18.

Boehmke, M. (2004). Measurement of symptom distress in women with early-stage breast cancer. *Cancer Nursing, 27*(2), 144-152.

Bragg Leight, S., et al. (2000). The effect of structured training on breast self-examination search behaviors as measured using biomedical instrumentation. *Nursing Research, 49*(5), 283-289.

Brown, S., et al. (2001). Silicone gel breast implant rupture, extracapsular silicone, and health status in a population of women. *Journal of Rheumatology, 28*(5), 996-1003.

Campbell, J. (2002). Breast cancer race, ethnicity, and survival: A literature review. *Breast Cancer Research and Treatment, 74*, 187-192.

Coleman, E., et al. (2003). Developing and testing lay literature about breast cancer screening for African-American women. *Clinical Journal of Oncology Nursing, 7*(1), 66-70.

Conto, S., & Myers, J. (2002). Risk factors and health promotion in families of patients with breast cancer. *Clinical journal of Oncology Nursing, 6*(2), 83-87.

Dell, D. (2003). Control of pain after breast reconstruction procedure. *Clinical Journal of Oncology Nursing, 7*(3), 335-336, 338.

DuVal, S. (2004). Inflammatory breast disease. *RN, 67*(2), 43-44.

Facione, N.C., et al. (2000). Perceived risk and help-seeking behavior for breast cancer: A Chinese-American perspective. *Cancer Nursing, 23*(4), 258-267.

Garmon-Bibb, S. (2001). The relationship between access and stage at diagnosis of breast cancer in African American and Caucasian women. *Oncology Nursing Forum, 28*(4), 711-719.

Gaston-Johansson, F., et al. (2000). The effectiveness of the comprehensive coping strategy on clinical outcomes in breast cancer autologous bone marrow transplantation. *Cancer Nursing, 23*(4), 277-285.

Greifzu, S. (2004). Breast cancer. *RN, 67*(2), 36-42.

Hancock, C. (2003). Fulvestrant antiestrogen for treatment of breast cancer. *Clinical Journal of Oncology Nursing, 7*(2), 201-202.

*Hartmann, L., et al. (1999a). Clinical options for women at high risk for breast cancer. *Surgical Clinics of North America, 79*(5), 1189-1204.

*Hartmann, L., et al. (1999b). Efficacy of bilateral prophylactic mastectomy in women with a family history of breast cancer. *New England Journal of Medicine, 340*(2), 77-84.

Hilton, B.A., et al. (2000). Men's perspectives on individual and family coping with their wives' breast cancer and chemotherapy. *Western Journal of Nursing Research, 22*(4), 438-459.

Horden, A. (2000). Intimacy and sexuality for the woman with breast cancer. *Cancer Nursing, 23*(3), 230-236.

Hunter, C. (2000). Epidemiology, stage at diagnosis, and tumor biology of breast carcinoma in multiracial and multiethnic populations. *Cancer, 88*(5), 1193-1202.

Hutson, S. (2003). Attitudes and psychological impact of genetic testing, genetic counseling, and breast cancer risk assessment among women at increased risk. *Oncology Nursing Forum, 30*(2), 241-246.

Janowsky, E., et al. (2000). Meta-analysis of the relation between silicone breast implants and the risk of connective tissue diseases. *New England Journal of Medicine, 342*(11), 781-790.

Kang, D. (2002). Oxidative stress, DNA damage, and breast cancer. *AACN Clinical Issues, 13*(4), 540-549.

Kimmick, G., & Balducci, L. (2000). Breast cancer and aging. *Hematology/Oncology Clinics of North America, 14*(1) 213-234.

Lengacher, C., et al. (2002). Frequency of use of complementary and alternative medicine in women with breast cancer. *Oncology Nursing Forum, 29*(10), 1445-1452.

MacDonald, D. (2002). Women's decisions regarding management of breast cancer risk. *MEDSURG Nursing, 11*(4), 183-186.

Mahon, S., & Casey, M. (2003). Patient education for women being fitted for breast prostheses. *Clinical Journal of Oncology Nursing, 7*(2), 194-199.

McCance, K., & Huether, S. (2002). *Pathophysiology: The biologic basis for disease in adults and children* (4th ed.). St. Louis: Mosby.

McPherson, K., Steel, C.M., & Dixon, J.M. (2000). ABC of breast diseases: Breast cancer—epidemiology, risk factors, and genetics. *British Medical Journal 321*(9), 624-628.

McSpedon, C. (2002). Silicone safety. *American Journal of Nursing, 102*(4), 31.

Moore, S. (2002). Cutaneous metastatic breast cancer. *Clinical Journal of Oncology Nursing, 6*(5), 255-260.

Moran, S.L., et al. (2000). TRAM flap breast reconstruction with expanders and implants. *AORN Journal, 71*(2), 354-362.

Nissen, M., Swenson, K., & Kind, E. (2002). Quality of life after postmastectomy breast reconstruction. *Oncology Nursing Forum, 29*(3), 547-553.

Nogueira, S.M., & Appling, S.E. (2000). Breast cancer: Genetics, risks, and strategies. *Nursing Clinics of North America, 35*(3), 663-669.

*Northouse, L., et al. (1999). The quality of life of African-American women with breast cancer. *Research in Nursing and Health, 22,* 449-460.

Partin, M., & Slater, J. (2003). Promoting repeat mammography use: Insights from a systematic needs assessment. *Health Education & Behavior, 30*(1), 97-112.

Rawl, S., et al. (2000). The impact of age and race on mammography practices. *Health Care for Women International, 21,* 583-595.

Resnick B., & Belcher, A. (2002). Breast reconstruction: Options, answers, and support for patients making a difficult personal decision. *American Journal of Nursing, 102*(4), 26-33.

Ridner, S. (2002). Breast cancer lymphedema: Pathophysiology and risk reduction guidelines. *Oncology Nursing Forum, 29*(9), 1285-1294.

Rosenzweig, M., Rust, D., & Hoss, J. (2000). Prognostic information in breast cancer care: Helping patients utilize important information. *Clinical Journal of Oncology Nursing, 4*(6), 271-278.

Sakorafas, G. (2002). Women at high risk for breast cancer: Preventive strategies. *The Mount Sinai Journal of Medicine, 69*(4), 264-266.

Sakorafas, G. (2003). The management of women at high risk for the development of breast cancer: Risk estimation and prevention. *Cancer Treatment Reviews, 29,* 79-89.

Sammarco, A. (2001a). Perceived social support, uncertainty, and quality of life of younger breast cancer survivors. *Cancer Nursing, 24*(3), 212-219.

Sammarco, A. (2001b). Psychosocial stages and quality of life of women with breast cancer. *Cancer Nursing, 24*(4), 272-277.

Sammarco, A. (2003). The quality of life of older breast cancer survivors. *Cancer Nursing, 26*(6), 431-438.

Sandau, K. (2002). Free TRAM flap breast reconstruction. *American Journal of Nursing, 102*(4), 36-43.

Shinagawa, S. (2000). The excess burden of breast carcinoma in minority and medically underserved communities. *Cancer, 88*(5), 1217-1223.

Shuster, T., et al. (2000). Multidisciplinary care for patients with breast cancer. *Surgical Clinics of North America, 80*(2), 505-533.

Strzelczyk, J., & Dignan, M. (2002). Disparities in adherence to recommended follow-up on screening mammography: Interaction of sociodemographic factors. *Ethnicity & Disease, 12,* 77-86.

Templeman, C., & Hertweck, S. (2000). Breast disorders in the pediatric and adolescent patient. *Obstetric and Gynecology Clinics, 27*(1), 19-31.

Thomas, S., & Greifzu, S. (2000). Breast cancer. *RN, 63*(4), 40-48.

Versea, L., & Rosenzweig, M. (2003). Hormonal therapy for breast cancer: Focus on fulvestrant. *Clinical Journal of Oncology Nursing, 7*(3), 307-312.

Workman, M.L. (2002). Breast cancer: New strategies to beat an old enemy. *Nursing2002, 32*(10), 58-63.

Yu, M., Seetoo, A., & Qu, M. (2002). Challenges of identifying Asian women for breast cancer screening. *Oncology Nursing Forum, 29*(3), 585-587.

Zack, E. (2001). Sentinel lymph node biopsy in breast cancer: Scientific rationale and patient care. *Oncology Nursing Forum, 28*(6), 2001.

Interventions for Clients with Gynecologic Problems

KAREN NOVAK

The most common reasons for seeking gynecologic care are pain, vaginal discharge, and bleeding. Nurses can play an important role in assessing gynecologic disorders by being knowledgeable about disease manifestations, being sensitive to the client's problems, and encouraging discussion about menstrual or other reproductive problems. Teaching women about their bodies, helping them to recognize when professional help should be sought, and teaching them how to make informed decisions about treatments are major goals for nurses working with female clients in any setting. Nurses also need to assess the effects of gynecologic problems on sexual health.

MENSTRUAL CYCLE DISORDERS

Primary Dysmenorrhea

PATHOPHYSIOLOGY

Dysmenorrhea, or painful menstrual flow, is one of the most common gynecologic problems, occurring most often in women in their teens and early 20s. More than 50% of all women report some degree of dysmenorrhea, but only a small percentage are unable to function. Primary dysmenorrhea alone does not involve pelvic pathologic changes, whereas secondary dysmenorrhea usually begins with an underlying disease condition such as anovulatory cycles or endometriosis. Pelvic congestion (larger ovarian and uterine vein diameters) is a syndrome of secondary dysmenorrhea.

Primary dysmenorrhea usually occurs after ovulation is established. Dysmenorrhea is painful uterine cramping with spasmodic lower abdominal pain that begins with the onset of menstrual flow and lasts 12 to 48 hours. The pain often radiates to the lower back and thighs. Nausea and vomiting, fatigue, and nervousness may occur with the pain. Less common manifestations include headache, syncope, diarrhea, bloating, and breast tenderness.

The cause of primary dysmenorrhea is thought to be increased production and release of uterine prostaglandins. Prostaglandins are produced by the endometrium during the luteal phase of the menstrual cycle, and the levels peak at the onset of menses. Excessive prostaglandin levels stimulate the myometrium and cause severe spasms, which constrict uterine blood flow, resulting in ischemia and pain. Other causes for primary dysmenorrhea are **adenomyosis** (increased vascular supply to the uterus), adhesions, salpingo-oophoritis, ovarian remnant syndrome, tumors or cysts of the reproductive organs, endometriosis, and myomas (fibroids).

◆COLLABORATIVE MANAGEMENT
◆Assessment

A thorough history of the client includes the following:
- Age at **menarche** (onset of menstruation)
- Characteristics of menstruation
- Obstetric history
- Contraceptive history
- Type of pain
- Previous therapy
- The need for contraception

Ask the client whether she has any conditions suggestive of pelvic problems. To plan care, also assess emotional factors, such as each woman's response to dysmenorrhea, her attitudes about menstruation, and the extent to which she believes that dysmenorrhea disrupts her life.

◆Interventions

Interventions for primary dysmenorrhea include prevention, education, support, and therapeutic measures that are tailored to each woman's needs.

Drug Therapy. Prostaglandin synthetase inhibitors (nonsteroidal anti-inflammatory drugs [NSAIDs]), such as ibuprofen (Motrin, Apo-Ibuprofen✱) and naproxen sodium (Anaprox, Naprosyn), are currently recommended for pain relief. In addition, numerous over-the-counter ibuprofen products, such as Advil and Nuprin, provide pain relief for many clients with primary dysmenorrhea. Aspirin is a mild prostaglandin synthetase inhibitor and may relieve mild dysmenorrhea. All these drugs can cause gastrointestinal (GI) distress and should therefore be taken with meals or milk. Bextra, a cyclooxygenase-2 (COX-2) inhibitor, also inhibits the release of prostaglandins and aids in some pain relief caused by dysmenorrhea (Anderson, Knobmen, & Troutman, 2002). Bextra does not inhibit platelet aggregation, as seen with aspirin or NSAIDS. However, drugs similar to Bextra have been found to increase the risk for acute cardiac problems.

Before treatment, the client's contraception needs are assessed. When contraception is not needed, prostaglandin synthetase inhibitors are the treatment of choice because they are needed only when manifestations are present. If contraception is a consideration, ovulation suppression with oral contraceptives is the treatment of choice.

🌿 **Complementary and Alternative Therapies.** Complementary therapies that may alleviate or prevent pain include acupressure, aerobic exercise, swimming, yoga or other meditation, application of heat or cold, massage, biofeedback, and relaxation techniques. Dietary measures for the prevention of pain may include increasing the intake of vitamin B_6, calcium, magnesium, and protein and reducing the intake of sodium to reduce fluid retention.

Premenstrual Syndrome
PATHOPHYSIOLOGY

Many women experience problems that recur regularly in the luteal phase of each menstrual cycle. These problems are termed **premenstrual syndrome (PMS).** About 5% of menstruating women have severe premenstrual symptoms, and many more have moderate symptoms. Neuroendocrine mechanisms appear to influence PMS. Serotonin is a neurotransmitter that is present in the central nervous system and affects mood. A noted change in serotonin synthesis during a woman's luteal phase of the menstrual cycle increases the symptoms of PMS. Fortunately most affected women can be helped.

Premenstrual syndrome is a collection of symptoms that are cyclic in nature. These symptoms are followed by relief with menses and a symptom-free phase. PMS affects women of all races, socioeconomic levels, and educational levels. It is more prevalent in women 30 to 40 years of age. The severity increases with aging until menopause. Women are at greater risk for PMS after pregnancy, childbirth, and tubal ligation; during the perimenopausal years; and during major life stresses.

Currently there is no agreement on a single set of diagnostic criteria for PMS. Three elements are found in defining PMS: symptoms, severity level, and timing. Many women report six or more manifestations across emotional, physical, and cognitive categories.

Emotional symptoms include irritability, easily precipitated crying spells, low self-esteem, anxiety, and depression. Physical manifestations include breast tenderness, bloating, fluid retention, increased appetite and food cravings, insomnia, fatigue, hot flushes, headaches, and musculoskeletal discomfort. Cognitive problems include short-term memory problems, difficulty concentrating, and unclear thinking.

◆COLLABORATIVE MANAGEMENT
◆Assessment

There is no objective means of diagnosing PMS, although some patterns have been identified. Determining the timing of the symptoms is as critical as noting the type of symptoms. The most effective assessment tool is a menstrual chart. Instruct the client to keep a chart for at least three consecutive cycles, showing the length of the menstrual cycle, the duration of bleeding, and the occurrence of symptoms. If the woman has PMS, the symptoms recur during the luteal phase (from ovulation to menstruation), which is followed by a symptom-free period (at least 7 days).

When taking a menstrual history, assess to what extent the woman believes her activities of daily living (ADLs) are disrupted by the symptoms. Often reassurance that the symptoms are legitimate and that other women share these problems can help the client learn more about PMS. Manifestations vary greatly among women and affect many body systems (Chart 78-1).

◆Interventions

Management of PMS focuses on eliminating the uncomfortable symptoms. The syndrome is highly individualized; however, one of the most important interventions is education. Each woman needs information about her body, especially the menstrual cycle, so that she can begin to understand the physiologic basis of PMS.

Women may need to express their feelings and discuss their experiences with PMS. Self-help groups and support groups are helpful resources. These groups also encourage significant others to participate because PMS usually affects not only the woman but also her family and friends. For ex-

CHART 78-1

KEY FEATURES of
Premenstrual Syndrome

Dermatologic Manifestations
- Acne
- Urticaria
- Herpes

Respiratory Manifestations
- Sinusitis
- Asthma
- Rhinitis
- Colds

Urologic Manifestations
- Oliguria
- Cystitis
- Enuresis
- Urethritis

Ophthalmologic Manifestations
- Conjunctivitis
- Styes
- Glaucoma

Neurologic Manifestations
- Headaches
- Migraine
- Syncope
- Vertigo
- Numbness of hands and feet
- Epilepsy (if susceptible)

Metabolic Manifestations
- Edema
- Breast tenderness

Emotional or Psychological Manifestations
- Depression
- Irritability
- Tension
- Panic attacks
- Change in libido
- Mood swings
- Anxiety

Behavioral Manifestations
- Lowered work performance
- Food cravings
- Alcohol and drug overindulgence
- Confusion
- Sleeplessness
- Lack of coordination
- Suicide
- Lethargy
- Child abuse
- Assaultive behavior

Other Manifestations
- Allergies
- Hypoglycemia
- Joint pain
- Backache
- Palpitations
- Water retention

CHART 78-2

NIC   INTERVENTION ACTIVITIES for
The Client with Gynecologic Problems

Premenstrual Syndrome (PMS) Management: *Alleviation/attenuation of physical and/or behavioral symptoms occurring during the luteal phase of the menstrual cycle*
- Instruct individual in the prospective identification of the major premenstrual symptoms (e.g., bloating, cramping, irritability), use of a prospective calendar checklist or symptom log, and recording of timing and severity of each symptom.
- Review symptom log/checklist.
- Collaborate with individual to identify most problematic symptoms.
- Discuss the complexity of management and need for stepwise approach to alleviate individual symptoms.
- Collaborate with the individual to select and institute stepwise approach to eliminating symptoms.
- Provide information about symptom-specific self-care measures (e.g., exercise and calcium supplementation).
- Monitor changes in symptoms.
- Encourage individual to participate in PMS support group if available.

Hormone Replacement Therapy: *Facilitation of safe and effective use of hormone replacement therapy*
- Determine reason for choosing hormone replacement therapy.
- Review alternatives to hormone replacement therapy.
- Monitor client for therapeutic effect.
- Monitor for adverse effects.
- Review information regarding beneficial and adverse effects of the different hormonal components (e.g., estrogen, progesterone, androgen).
- Review information regarding interaction effects of adjunct therapies (e.g., calcium and vitamin D supplementation, exercise, thiazide use).
- Review information regarding the different methods of administration (e.g., oral continuous combined, oral sequential, dermal, vaginal).
- Facilitate the decision to continue/discontinue.
- Recommend clients make short-term annual decisions about continuation.

NIC intervention activities selected from Dochterman, J.M., & Bulechek, G.M. (Eds.) (2004). *Nursing interventions classification (NIC)* (4th ed.). St. Louis: Mosby. No part of this work is to be altered without prior written permission from the Publisher.

ample, increased family conflict, communication problems with family and friends, and decreased family cohesion occur. Other coping strategies for the woman with PMS may include spiritual support, especially participating in religious services and seeking advice from spiritual leaders. Chart 78-2 lists NIC interventions for PMS.

Diet Therapy. Diet and nutrition are useful in managing PMS. If hypoglycemia (low blood glucose) occurs, instruct the woman to eat six small meals a day and to limit her intake of sugar, red meat, alcohol, coffee, tea, and chocolate.

Eliminating caffeine may help reduce irritability. Salt and sodium intake should be limited if edema occurs. Calcium, magnesium, and vitamins A, B_6, and C have also been used for relief of PMS.

Drug Therapy. Drug therapy remains controversial, but some drugs may be been effective. Mild potassium-sparing diuretics taken for 10 days before menstruation can provide relief for some women. Women may need to decrease their intake of potassium-containing foods if they are receiving this therapy.

Progesterone may relieve physical and psychological symptoms. Natural progesterone is preferable to synthetic progesterone, even though the drug must be specially made by a pharmacist at the time prescribed. The daily dosage is 50 to 100 mg IM from ovulation to menstruation. Long-term side effects are unknown.

Bromocriptine mesylate (Parlodel) 2.5 mg two or three times daily with meals during the luteal phase can relieve breast symptoms. The side effects (light-headedness and hypotension) may not be well tolerated. Other drugs for PMS that have been used include birth control pills, gonadotropin-releasing hormone (GnRH) agonists, antidepressants, and prostaglandin inhibitors, such as nonsteroidal anti-inflammatory drugs (NSAIDs).

Sarafem is an antidepressant agent that belongs to the selective serotonin reuptake inhibitors (SSRI) class of drugs. It is approved for use in women with PMS during the luteal phase of a menstrual cycle. The precise action of Sarafem is not fully understood, but it is believed that the most important effect is the enhancement of the action of serotonin that results from the highly specific serotonin reuptake blockades at the neuronal membrane (Anderson et al, 2002).

Amenorrhea

PATHOPHYSIOLOGY

Amenorrhea (the absence of menstrual periods) can be either primary (menstruation that has failed to occur by age 16 years) or secondary (menstruation that has started but has since stopped and has not recurred for at least 3 months). Primary amenorrhea often occurs with anomalies

TABLE 78-1 Common Causes of Amenorrhea

Primary
- Congenital anomalies
- Hypothalamic and pituitary disorders, such as delayed puberty
- Systemic disease
  - Thyroid and adrenal dysfunction
  - Diabetes mellitus
  - Extreme malnutrition
- Ovarian disease
- Malformations of the reproductive tract

Secondary
- Pregnancy
- Menopause
- Lactation
- Cervical stenosis
- Polycystic ovary disease
- Pituitary tumor or insufficiency
- Psychogenic stress
- Excessive physical activities
- Medications
  - Antihypertensive agents
  - Birth control pills
  - Phenothiazines
- Nutritional disorders
  - Obesity
  - Anorexia nervosa
  - Sudden weight loss
- Ovarian disease, failure, or destruction

TABLE 78-2 Common Causes of Postmenopausal Bleeding

Benign	**Malignant**
- Atrophic vaginitis	- Endometrial cancer
- Cervical polyps	- Cervical cancer
- Endometrial hyperplasia	- Ovarian cancer
- Uterine fibroids	- Vaginal cancer
- Cervical erosion	- Tubal cancer
- Estrogen therapy	

of the reproductive tract, and the prognosis for fertility is poor. Secondary amenorrhea is usually a functional disorder, and the prognosis for fertility is better. Amenorrhea can cause a woman much distress and concern.

Menstruation is a complex process that relies on the interplay of the hypothalamic, pituitary, ovarian, endometrial functions, and anatomy. Dysfunction related to any of these five factors may cause amenorrhea (Table 78-1). Primary amenorrhea is relatively uncommon and is associated with congenital factors or factors caused by ovarian, pituitary, or hypothalamic disease. Pregnancy, **lactation** (breastfeeding), and menopause are the most common causes of secondary amenorrhea.

◆ COLLABORATIVE MANAGEMENT
◆ Assessment

Assess both the menstrual history and the obstetric history. Ask about possible sexual activity and symptoms of pregnancy. A medical history may identify a systemic disease as a cause of amenorrhea. Ask about current eating habits and any history of dieting because both obesity and starvation (e.g., anorexia nervosa) can contribute to amenorrhea. Strenuous exercise associated with competitive athletics, such as long-distance running, can cause stress or a reduction in body fat, resulting in amenorrhea. Assess for manifestations of hormone deficiencies, such as those associated with menopause (hot flushes and vaginal dryness). Ask about the use of drugs (e.g., oral contraceptives, phenothiazines, antihypertensives) and about recent stressors. Check for **galactorrhea** (watery or milky breast secretions in nonbreastfeeding or women who have not been pregnant and **hirsutism** (unusual hair growth in women), both of which are related to polycystic ovary disease clients subsequent amenorrhea.

◆ Interventions

Explain amenorrhea in easily understandable terms, and answer questions about tests and treatments. Provide counseling and emotional support. Amenorrhea may be a threat to a woman's self-concept; she usually needs to ventilate her feelings about sexuality or fertility.

Interventions for specific causes of amenorrhea are based on each woman's needs. Medical and surgical management of amenorrhea is directed at the underlying causes. Treatment includes hormone replacement, ovulation stimulation, and periodic progesterone withdrawal.

Postmenopausal Bleeding
PATHOPHYSIOLOGY

Postmenopausal bleeding (vaginal bleeding occurring after a 12-month cessation of menses after the onset of menopause) is a manifestation rather than a disease. Bleeding is considered serious and should be evaluated. Gynecologic cancer occurs in 20% to 40% of women who have postmenopausal bleeding.

Postmenopausal bleeding can be caused by many benign and malignant conditions (Table 78-2). The three most common causes are atrophic vaginitis, cervical polyps, and endometrial hyperplasia.

In a client with **atrophic vaginitis,** the vaginal mucosa is thin and dry and easily traumatized by sexual intercourse and infection, causing spotting. Cervical polyps are usually soft, red, oval tissue masses that appear within the cervical canal. They may bleed spontaneously or after intercourse.

The most serious cause of postmenopausal bleeding is **endometrial hyperplasia** (tissue overgrowth), a precursor of endometrial cancer. Bleeding is caused by declining ovarian function that leads to prolonged estrogen stimulation, producing the hyperplasia that eventually breaks down and bleeds. Estrogen stimulation can also be caused by estrogen replacement therapy (ERT).

Because many women who report postmenopausal bleeding need medical or surgical interventions, assessment is the major focus. Assess the menstrual history and family history initially, including the following:
- The client's age at menopause
- The frequency and amount of bleeding
- Previous bleeding episodes
- Use of drugs (especially estrogen-only [unopposed estrogen] replacement therapy [ERT])
- Gastrointestinal (GI) or genitourinary symptoms

Also identify women who are at high risk for endometrial cancer (e.g., women who are obese, hypertensive, or diabetic or who have never had children).

CLIENT EDUCATION GUIDE
Estrogen Replacement Therapy

For All Types of Estrogen Replacement Therapy
- Call your health care provider if you have pain in your calves or groin, if you suddenly become short of breath, if you have abnormal vaginal bleeding, if you feel a lump in your breast, if you have a severe headache, or if you feel weak or numb in your arms or legs.
- Use sunscreen if you are in the sun for a prolonged period.
- Keep appointments for checkups.
- If your health care provider has prescribed progesterone to decrease your risk of endometrial cancer, take it as prescribed.

For Oral Therapy
- Take 1 pill daily for the first 25 days each month.
- If you feel nauseated or have intestinal upset, take your medication with food.

For Transdermal or Subdermal Administration
- Rotate the sites for the patches or injections to avoid skin irritation.
- Change the patches twice a week or according to your prescribed schedule.

For Vaginal Therapy
- Use an applicator to insert the suppository or cream daily as prescribed.
- You may need to wear a minipad to protect your clothing from soiling or staining by the drug.

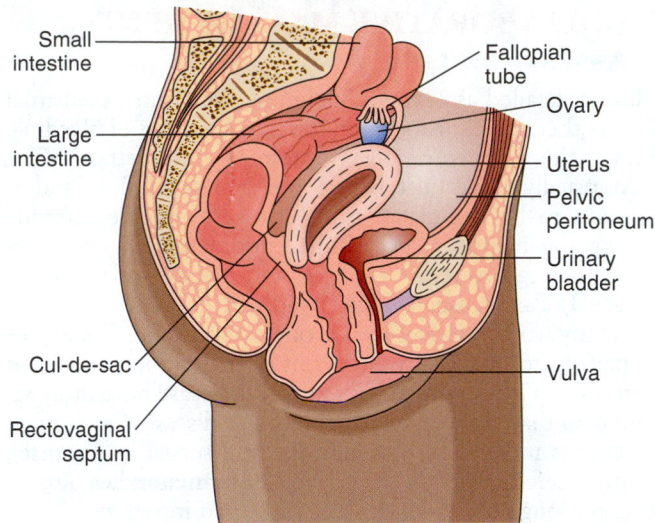

Figure 78-1 ■ Common sites of endometriosis.

Urine and stool specimens can be collected and tested for blood to differentiate other sources of bleeding. Blood specimens may be drawn for hemoglobin or hematocrit levels because clients are often anemic from excessive bleeding. Prepare the woman for physical and pelvic examinations, including obtaining a specimen for a Papanicolaou (Pap) test, or smear, to evaluate the cause of bleeding.

◆**COLLABORATIVE MANAGEMENT**

Nursing interventions focus on providing information and support for diagnostic and treatment procedures directed at the specific causes of bleeding. An endometrial biopsy can evaluate the presence of malignancy. A diagnostic dilation and curettage (D&C) procedure can be used to determine malignancy (see Dysfunctional Uterine Bleeding, p. 1828). Atypical hyperplasia is often treated with a hysterectomy (see Uterine Leiomyomas, p. 1838). Cancer is usually treated with a combination of surgery, radiation therapy, and chemotherapy (see Endometrial [Uterine] Cancer, p. 1842).

The medical treatment of a woman receiving unopposed estrogen therapy may include the monthly administration of progesterone daily for the last 10 days of the estrogen therapy (days 16 to 25) or a once-per-month IM progesterone injection. This treatment can reduce the abnormal endometrial growth and is suggested for the prevention of endometrial and breast cancer.

Atrophic vaginitis is managed by the use of estrogen via the vaginal, oral, transdermal, or subdermal route. Teach the client about ERT (Chart 78-2 and Chart 78-3). Inform women who use vaginal estrogen cream that it can cause systemic effects. Women who take estrogen may be at risk for gallbladder disease, hypertension, breast cancer, endometrial cancer, and coronary artery disease.

Over-the-counter use of Replens vaginal lubricant can often ease the symptoms of vaginal dryness and irritation that occur with atrophic vaginitis. A water-based lubricant, such as Astroglide, used during intercourse helps reduce vaginal discomfort during intercourse.

Endometriosis
PATHOPHYSIOLOGY

Endometriosis is usually a benign problem of endometrial tissue implantation outside the uterine cavity. The tissue typically appears on the ovaries and the cul-de-sac and less commonly on other pelvic organs and structures (Figure 78-1). A "chocolate" cyst is an area of endometriosis inside an ovary.

Endometrial tissue located outside the uterus responds to hormonal stimulation similarly to the response of the intrauterine endometrium and goes through the same cyclic changes. Bleeding occurs at the site of implantation, and the blood is trapped in the tissues. Scarring and adhesions result from blood reabsorption. Endometriosis progresses slowly. It regresses during pregnancy and at menopause. Rarely does endometriosis become a malignant disease.

The cause of endometriosis is unknown, but possible causes include transportation and formation. Transportation involves implantation and vascular or lymphatic dissemination. With implantation, endometrial tissue flows back through the fallopian tubes during menstruation and then implants on pelvic structures. With vascular or lymphatic dissemination, endometrial tissues are transported through the vascular and lymphatic system to foreign locations. This possible cause explains implantation in areas outside the pelvis, such as the lungs and the kidneys. It is also possible that endometrial tissue develops outside the uterus as a birth defect.

The disorder is most often found in women during their reproductive years (i.e., their late 20s to 30s). Only about 1% to 2% of women have endometriosis, although the incidence among infertile women is about 15% to 25% (DeCherney & Nathan, 2003). It is also common in women who have not been pregnant and in those whose mothers had endometriosis.

◆COLLABORATIVE MANAGEMENT
◆Assessment

Make a detailed assessment, including the client's menstrual history, her sexual history, and the characteristics of bleeding. Pain is the most common symptom of endometriosis. The pain usually peaks just before the menstrual flow and is thought to be stimulated from estrogen and progesterone during the menstrual cycle. The endometrial implants enlarge, undergo secretory changes, and bleed (DeCherney et al., 2003). Pain is usually located in the lower abdomen, causing many women to feel a sense of rectal pressure. The degree of pain is not related to the extent of the endometriosis but to the site. Often women with minimal disease have more severe pain than do women with extensive disease. Other manifestations include **dyspareunia** (painful sexual intercourse), painful defecation, low backache, **hypermenorrhea** (excessive, prolonged, or frequent bleeding), and infertility.

A pelvic examination may reveal pelvic tenderness, nodular uterosacral ligaments, and fixed or limited movement of the uterus. Psychosocial assessment may reveal anxiety because of uncertainty about the diagnosis. The woman may also have concerns about her self-concept if she is infertile and wants to become pregnant.

Diagnostic studies include blood tests (erythrocyte sedimentation rate [ESR] and white blood cell [WBC] count) to rule out pelvic inflammatory disease (PID). Ultrasonography is used to differentiate pelvic masses that might be mistaken for endometriosis. Laparoscopy is the key diagnostic procedure for pelvic endometriosis. Examination of tissue specimens obtained during laparoscopy confirms the diagnosis.

> ### ❓ Critical Thinking Challenge
>
> The client is a 26-year-old nurse who has been having progressively more pain before and during menstruation. She has missed work and family events because of pain and other discomforts. She tells you that she took oral contraceptives (OC) for the first two years of her marriage and was pain-free at that time. She has been off OC for 2 years because she and her husband are trying to get pregnant. One of the residents has told her that her problem might be pelvic inflammatory disease (PID) and this comment upset her considerably because she says she has never had sex with anyone but her husband and had these symptoms throughout her teenage years before she became sexually active. She asks whether tampon use could have caused her problems.
>
> 1. What is the relationship between PID and endometriosis?
> 2. Could tampon use have caused endometriosis? Give a rationale for your answer.
> 3. Is a diagnosis of endometriosis likely to interfere with pregnancy? Why or Why not?
> 4. What information and emotional support can you give this client?
>
> **evolve** For suggested answer guidelines, go to http://evolve.elsevier.com/Iggy/.

◆Interventions

Hormonal and surgical management may be used, depending on the symptoms, the extent of disease, and the client's desire for childbearing. Nursing management is aimed at the following:

- Reducing pain

- Restoring sexual function that was impaired by dyspareunia (painful sexual intercourse)
- Alleviating anxiety related to the manifestations of the disease and the uncertainty of the diagnosis
- Educating the client about the disease and its treatment
- Alleviating fear related to the possibility of laparoscopy or surgery
- Preventing self-esteem disturbance related to infertility

Several organizations, such as the Endometriosis Society and RESOLVE (an organization for infertile couples), offer information on endometriosis that is helpful in planning care.

NONSURGICAL MANAGEMENT

Drug Therapy. Nonsurgical management involves the use of mild analgesics or nonsteroidal anti-inflammatory drugs (NSAIDs) for pain relief. Hormonal therapies may relieve pain by suppressing ovulation. The hormonal therapies produce pseudopregnancy, pseudomenopause, or medical oophorectomy.

Pseudopregnancy is induced with oral contraceptives or progesterone. Usually a 6-month course of a low-dose estrogen oral contraceptive is prescribed, followed by cyclic oral contraceptive use or therapy with progesterone alone.

Other hormonal treatment causes ovarian suppression, or pseudomenopause, by the use of danazol (Danocrine, Cyclomen✱), an antigonadotropin drug. This approach is the current choice of many health care providers, but it is expensive ($120 to $180 per month) and may cause undesirable side effects, including acne, hirsutism (abnormal hair growth in unwanted areas), weight gain, decreased breast size, hot flushes, and cardiovascular disease. It is suggested that danazol use should not exceed 8 months (DeCherney et al., 2003).

Gonadotropin-releasing hormone (GnRH) agonists can be used to produce a reversible medical oophorectomy. The drug can be given by IM or subcutaneous injection or by nasal spray. Side effects include hot flushes, vaginal dryness, insomnia, and elevated liver enzymes. A decrease in bone density occurs within 6 months of using a GnRH agonist; thus suggested length of therapy is 6 to 8 months (DeCherney et al, 2003).

Complementary and Alternative Therapies. Strategies to relieve pain include the application of a heating pad to the abdomen or sacrum, relaxation techniques, yoga, and biofeedback. These approaches may decrease muscle tissue hypoxia and hypertonicity and relieve ischemia by increasing blood flow to the affected areas.

SURGICAL MANAGEMENT. Surgical management of endometriosis for a woman who wants to remain fertile is conservative and involves the removal of endometrial implants and adhesions. The surgeon may use a laser to treat endometriosis by vaporizing adhesions and endometrial implants. If the client does not wish to have children, the uterus and ovaries may be removed.

Dysfunctional Uterine Bleeding
PATHOPHYSIOLOGY

Dysfunctional uterine bleeding (DUB) is a nonspecific term to describe bleeding that is excessive or abnormal in amount or frequency without predisposing anatomic or systemic conditions. DUB occurs most often at either end of the span of a woman's reproductive years—when ovulation is becoming established or when it is becoming irregular at menopause.

Normally the menstrual cycle is a series of complex hormonal events related to balanced hypothalamic, pituitary, ovarian, and uterine functions. **Menses,** the sloughing of the endometrial lining, is an expected result. DUB occurs when there is a breakdown of these functions, causing hormonal imbalance.

The mechanism of DUB is unknown, but it may be linked to endometrial or myometrial dysfunction. Excessive fibrinolytic activity in the endometrium and changes in prostaglandin production in the uterus may also cause DUB.

Generally DUB occurs in the absence of ovulation caused by ovarian dysfunction. Estrogen stimulation of the endometrium is prolonged, and the endometrium grows past its hormonal support, causing bleeding and desquamation (shedding of uterine lining).

Anovulatory DUB during the reproductive years is associated with the following:

- Endocrine disturbances
- Polycystic ovary disease
- Stress
- Extreme weight changes
- Long-term drug use (e.g., anticholinergics, morphine, or oral contraceptives)
- Anatomic abnormalities

Ovulatory causes of DUB are uncommon and are related to a dysfunctional corpus luteum, irregular maturation, and shedding of the endometrium.

◆ COLLABORATIVE MANAGEMENT

◆ Assessment

When interviewing a woman with DUB, take a complete menstrual history. Ask about illnesses, changes in weight or diet, exercise, drug ingestion, and whether she has pain.

Observe for symptoms of anemia or systemic disease, such as the following:

- Renal or hepatic disease
- Obesity
- Undernutrition
- Abnormal hair growth related to hormonal dysfunction
- Evidence of abdominal pain or masses

An examination that includes inspection of the external genitalia and a bimanual pelvic and rectal examination is essential to identify lesions or tenderness. A physician or an advanced practice nurse performs the internal pelvic examination.

Pelvic ultrasonography and transvaginal ultrasound use may reveal polyps or lesions and measure an excessively thick endometrium. Hysteroscopy is a valuable tool for the diagnosis of anatomic lesions that affect the endometrial cavity (DeCherney et al., 2003). In addition, the surgeon usually does an endometrial biopsy by suction aspiration or dilation and curettage (D&C). These are important procedures for women over 40 years of age, who are at greater risk for endometrial cancer.

◆ Interventions

NONSURGICAL MANAGEMENT. Nonsurgical management is usually the treatment of choice, although surgery may be needed to treat DUB. Most women can be treated successfully with hormonal manipulation. For those with anovulatory DUB, the health care provider may prescribe medroxyprogesterone acetate (Depo-Provera) or combination oral contraceptives. If the client takes oral contraceptives, she should take one pill daily for 21 or 28 days, beginning on the first day of the menstrual cycle. Medroxyprogesterone is taken on days 16 to 25 of each month. Monthly withdrawal bleeding is expected with both therapies. Usually the use of progestin therapy will control the abnormality once uterine pathology is ruled out (DeCherney et al., 2003).

Women with ovulatory DUB may be treated with progestins during the luteal phase or with oral contraceptives, prostaglandin inhibitors, or danazol. In cases of young women, anovulatory bleeding may occur with excessive endometrial buildup, a delay in diagnosis, or heavy blood loss. Low-dose oral contraceptives (combined progestin-estrogen) are useful. The contraceptive pills are taken in the following regimen: one pill twice daily for 5 to 7 days. Warn the client that cessation of blood flow will happen in 12 to 24 hours. They should also anticipate heavy bleeding and cramping 2 to 4 days after stopping therapy. If this therapy is successful, a low-dose combination oral contraceptive (one pill daily) is started on the fifth day of flow. This sequence is repeated for several 3-week treatments, allowing 1 week for withdrawal bleeding.

Estrogen therapy is indicated when bleeding is heavy and acute. Conjugated estrogens (25 mg) are given intravenously (IV) every 4 hours until bleeding stops or for 12 hours. When bleeding is less, low doses of oral estrogen are given to the client for 7 to 10 days (DeCherney et al., 2003). Explain the desired effects and the side effects of these drugs, and evaluate the woman's knowledge of the effects, dosage, and schedule.

SURGICAL MANAGEMENT. Surgical management includes D&C, laser or balloon endometrial ablation, and hysterectomy. A D&C is used to treat an acute episode of bleeding, but the problem often returns. Laser or balloon endometrial ablation is a safe alternative for women who do not respond to medical management or who do not need a hysterectomy. A hysterectomy is usually performed only after other treatments have failed. Table 78-3 compares the care of clients undergoing a D&C or endometrial ablation. Hysterectomy is discussed later under Operative Procedures (see Uterine Leiomyomas), p. 1838. If the woman has undergone a D&C or laser ablation, instruct her about care after surgery (Chart 78-4).

Menopause

PATHOPHYSIOLOGY

Menopause is a normal biologic event marked for most women by the end of menstrual periods (6 to 12 months of amenorrhea). It signifies the depletion of estradiol, a hormone produced by the ovaries. Although the meaning of menopause is the last menstrual period, it is more clinically relevant to look at the months or years surrounding this event.

During the past decade there has been an explosion of interest among health care providers about all aspects of menopause: endocrinologic, metabolic, pathologic, sociocultural, and psychological. Of particular interest is the role

TABLE 78-3 Nursing Care of Clients Undergoing Surgery for Dysfunctional Uterine Bleeding

	Dilation and Curettage (D&C)	Endometrial Ablation
Usual site	Outpatient	Outpatient.
Anesthesia	Local, regional, general	Regional, general.
Procedure	The cervical os is dilated; the endometrium is scraped.	The laser fiber is passed into the uterus through a hysteroscope; the endometrium is destroyed by laser energy, and tissues are removed by irrigating the uterine cavity with saline.
Preoperative care	Assess the client's knowledge of the procedure. The client is NPO after midnight. Teach postoperative expectations.	Same as for D&C. The client may be given danazol or GnRH agonist for 1 mo before surgery to decrease endometrial thickness. Counsel the client about the likelihood of sterility as a result of uterine scarring.
Postoperative care	Monitor vital signs every 15 min until client is stable. Assess the need for pain relief. Assess for vaginal bleeding. Expect discharge when the client is stable.	Same as for D&C. Same as for D&C. Assess for spotting and vaginal drainage. Same as for D&C.

GnRH, Gonadotropin-releasing hormone; *NPO,* nothing by mouth.

CHART 78-4

CLIENT EDUCATION GUIDE
Endometrial Ablation and Dilation and Curettage

Endometrial Ablation
- Spotting and vaginal drainage are normal for several days after the procedure.
- If you have abdominal cramping, take mild analgesics, such as acetaminophen (Tylenol, Atasol✦), or prostaglandin inhibitors, such as ibuprofen (Motrin).
- You can return to your normal activities within 2 or 3 days.
- You will probably be sterile because of uterine scarring.

Dilation and Curettage
- Take your temperature once a day for the next 2 days. If your oral temperature is more than 100° F (38° C), call the clinic or your doctor.
- Avoid sexual intercourse, tub baths, and the use of tampons for 2 weeks to allow healing and prevent infection.
- Slight bleeding is normal. However, if bleeding is as heavy as during your normal menstrual period or if bleeding lasts longer than 2 weeks, call the clinic or health care provider.
- You can use a heating pad or hot water bottle to relieve abdominal cramping if it occurs.
- You can take mild analgesics, such as acetaminophen, for pain.

---

of hormone replacement therapy (HRT) in the management of symptoms.

Much interest in menopause is directed at the health problems common to postmenopausal women that may be affected by hormonal change. Such problems include osteoporosis, coronary heart disease, and breast and endometrial cancer.

Women experience menopause as individuals, and care should be taken not to make generalizations. Women become menopausal in a variety of ways, including by surgery when the uterus and ovaries are removed and by medical treatment for cancer. Natural menopause is experienced across a wide age range, from as early as the 30s or 40s or as late as the 60s. The average age at which women have their last menstrual period is between 50 and 52 years. All women under 40 who have early menopause, regardless of cause, are

at higher risk for osteoporosis and related fractures. It is thought that these clients also may be at higher risk for cardiovascular disease.

Several factors may affect the timing of menopause. These include the following:
- Autoimmune disease
- Chromosomal abnormalities
- Genetic influence
- Early **menarche** (beginning of menses)
- Hysterectomy
- Smoking
- Cancer treatment (chemotherapy or radiation)

◆ **COLLABORATIVE MANAGEMENT**
◆ **Assessment**

Menopause transition, or **perimenopause,** are those changes in spontaneous ovarian function that precede the last menstrual period and occur gradually. Common features of the transition are a change in the woman's usual menstrual periods and the beginning of vasomotor symptoms, such as hot flushes and night sweats. These symptoms may disturb the woman's usual sleep pattern. Vaginal dryness and mood changes may also occur. Urogenital atrophy, decreased libido, decrease in cognitive function, and back pain are also symptoms associated with menopause (DeCherney et al., 2003). Ask the client about these changes, and reassure her that they are normal during perimenopause. In addition to manifestations, laboratory tests can support the presence of menopause (Table 78-4).

The most common early change in the bleeding pattern is a shortening of the time between menstrual periods, which may be accompanied by an increase in menstrual flow. As the transition evolves, about 70% of women find that their periods become lighter and farther apart until they finally stop.

Some women simply stop menstruating without further change. The remaining women experience heavier bleeding, which can be either regularly timed or unpredictable. In addition, abnormal bleeding in this age-group can be caused

TABLE 78-4 Laboratory Studies That Confirm Menopause

Test	Normal Range	Menopausal Range
Estradiol (serum)	20-750 pg/mL	<20 pg/mL
FSH	1.09-17.2 IU/mL	19.3-100.6 IU/mL
LH	0.61-56.6 IU/mL	14.2-52.3 IU/mL

FSH, Follicle stimulating hormone; *LH,* luteinizing hormone; *pg,* picograms.

by endometrial cancer, endometrial polyps, or uterine fibroid tumors.

Most women pass through the menopause transition and into the postmenopause phase with minimal symptoms and never seek treatment for menopause-related problems. About 20% of women, however, seek care for one or more symptoms related to menopause.

◆Interventions

Hormone replacement therapy (HRT), a combination of estrogen and progestin (progesterone), is a common medical intervention for menopause. Estrogen given alone can cause gynecologic cancers and thromboembolic conditions, such as deep vein thrombosis. Finding the right estrogen-progestin combination takes time. HRT has recently been discovered not to provide cardiac protective effects, thus changing the risk to benefit ratio of this therapy. Each woman, together with her health care provider, needs to base the decision whether or not to use HRT on the severity of symptoms and personal risk factors for other health problems.

Estrogen is available as oral, transdermal, intravaginal, and IM preparations. Because the oral estrogens have similar effects on symptoms and health risks, the choice of preparation for most women can be based on cost and individual side effect experience. Transdermal estrogen offers a useful alternative route of administration for women who prefer not to take pills; who cannot tolerate oral therapy because of gastrointestinal (GI) side effects; or who have abnormalities in liver-function tests. Side effects of estrogen occur and persist in about 10% of women.

The most common side effects are bloating, nausea, and breast tenderness. These problems often resolve after a few months of estrogen use. Chart 78-2 lists some NIC interventions for the client choosing HRT.

INFLAMMATIONS AND INFECTIONS

Vaginal discharge and itching are two common problems of female clients. Women may need information about the normal vaginal physiology, causes of symptoms, and methods of treatment. The nurse must be well informed about these topics to provide comprehensive care to clients with vaginal infections.

Vaginal infections are sometimes considered sexually transmitted diseases (STDs) because their causative organisms may be transmitted to sexual partners. However, many infections can develop without sexual contact, and sexual partners do not always become infected. True STDs, such as gonorrhea, syphilis, chlamydial infection, and herpes simplex virus infection, are discussed in Chapter 80. Acquired immunodeficiency syndrome (AIDS) is covered in Chapter 25.

CHART 78-5

BEST PRACTICE for
Care of the Client with Simple Vaginitis

In taking a client history, ask about the following:
- Onset of symptoms
- Characteristics of the discharge, especially the color and odor
- Associated symptoms such as itching and dysuria
- Types of contraceptives used
- Recent use of antibiotics
- Client's sexual activity
- Any history of vaginal infection
- Client's hygiene practices: douching and using tampons

In performing a physical examination, do the following:
- Palpate the abdomen for tenderness or pain.
- Inspect the external genitalia for erythema, edema, excoriation, odor, and discharge.
- If you are qualified, perform a speculum examination to visualize the vagina and cervix, and note the source of any discharge or inflammation.

If you are qualified, perform the following laboratory tests as ordered: a saline or potassium hydroxide wet smear and a Nitrazine paper test of vaginal pH.

Simple Vaginitis
PATHOPHYSIOLOGY

Vaginitis can develop whenever there is a disturbance of the balance of hormones and bacterial interaction in the vagina as a result of one or more of the following:
- Menopause
- STDs *(Trichomonas vaginalis)*
- Fungal (yeast) infections *(Candida albicans)*
- Changes in the normal flora
- Alkaline pH
- Insertion of foreign bodies, such as tampons and condoms
- Chemical irritations, such as from douches or sprays
- Drugs, especially antibiotics
- Health problems, such as diabetes

Vaginitis is an inflammation of the lower genital tract. Its occurrence is rising in frequency. Women who are sexually active are at greater risk for vaginitis (DeCherney et al., 2003). Assess for vaginitis by asking questions about the symptoms, assisting with a pelvic examination, and obtaining vaginal smears for laboratory testing (Chart 78-5). Use a nonjudgmental approach, and provide reassurance during the assessment because the client may be embarrassed or afraid to discuss her symptoms.

◆COLLABORATIVE MANAGEMENT

Interventions for vaginitis depend on the causes and the specific vaginal infection (Table 78-5). Proper health habits can be beneficial to treatment. Instruct the client to get enough rest and sleep, observe good dietary habits, get regular exercise, and use good personal hygiene. Popular, but not scientifically tested, hygiene practices to prevent vaginitis include the following:
- Perineal cleaning (wiping front to back) after urinating or defecating
- Wearing cotton underwear
- Avoiding strong douches and feminine hygiene sprays
- Avoiding tight-fitting pants

TABLE 78-5 Common Vaginal Infections

Sexual Transmission	Assessment		
	Physical Findings	**Laboratory Findings**	**Drug Therapy**
***Candida albicans* Infection**			
Unlikely	Odorless, white, curdlike discharge Patches on vaginal walls and cervix Inflamed vaginal walls and cervix Itching	Hyphae and spores visible on potassium hydroxide wet slide Vaginal pH 4.5 or less	Miconazole nitrate (Monistat), clotrimazole (Gyne-Lotrimin), or nystatin (Mycostatin) vaginal creams or suppositories for 7 days Terconazole (Terazol) cream or suppositories for 7 days or double strength for 3 days Tioconazole (Vagistat) single-dose vaginal application
***Trichomonas vaginalis* Infection**			
Yes	None or fishy Itching Strawberry spot on vaginal surface and cervix	Flagellated, pear-shaped protozoa on saline wet slide Vaginal pH 6-7	Oral metronidazole (Flagyl), single 2-g dose for client and sexual partners
Bacterial Vaginosis/*Gardnerella vaginalis* Infection			
Yes	Gray-white or green discharge Fishy odor Itching Normal vaginal mucosa 10%-40% asymptomatic	"Clue" cells or examination of saline wet slide Positive "whiff" test finding Vaginal pH 5-6	Oral metronidazole 500 mg four times daily for 7 days or ampicillin or tetracycline Clindamycin 450 mg four times daily for 7 days
Cervicitis			
Yes	Mucopurulent discharge from endocervix Pelvic pain, postcoital and intermenstrual bleeding The cervix may be inflamed and bleed when touched	Need to rule out herpes, gonorrhea, and chlamydial infection Vaginal pH 4.5 or less	Depends on diagnosis
Atrophic Vaginitis			
No	Pale, thin, dry mucosa Itching No odor Scant white, yellow, gray, or green discharge Dyspareunia, postcoital bleeding	Parabasal cells Leukocyte predominance Vaginal pH 6	Topical conjugated estrogen cream $\frac{1}{2}$ to 1 application at night for 7 nights, then twice weekly

CHART 78-6

CLIENT EDUCATION GUIDE
Vaginal Infections

- Your risk for getting vaginal infections increases if you have sex with more than one person.
- When you have a vaginal infection, do not have sexual intercourse, or at least make sure that your partner wears a condom.
- Sexual partners may need to be treated for infection.
- The only way to identify what infection you have is to be examined by a health care provider and to get the results of laboratory tests.
- Take your medicine as prescribed, not just until your symptoms go away.

Estrogen creams are used intravaginally if no infection is present or after antibiotic therapy has been successful. Assess whether or not the client finds using an estrogen vaginal cream acceptable. If the client has a personal history of breast or uterine cancer, she may not want to use an estrogen vaginal product because some of the drug is absorbed systemically. An estradiol ring, which is changed every 90 days, is an acceptable

delivery route for many women because of its long duration. Vagifem one tablet inserted intravaginally daily for 2 weeks, then 2 times per week for at least 3 to 6 months, is another treatment option (DeCherney et al., 2003).

If antibiotics are prescribed, eating yogurt or taking *Lactobacillus* culture (Lactinex) tablets may help restore the natural flora of the vagina. Teach the client about preventive measures and infection transmission (Chart 78-6).

Vulvitis

PATHOPHYSIOLOGY

Vulvitis is an inflammatory condition of the vulva that is associated with symptoms of pruritus (itching) and a burning sensation. The vulvar skin is sensitive to hormonal, metabolic, and allergic influences. Symptoms can be caused by systemic conditions, direct contact with irritants, and extension of infection from the vagina.

The most common skin disease affecting the vulva is contact dermatitis, which can be caused by an irritant, such as feminine hygiene sprays, fabric dyes, soaps and detergents, or allergens. Primary infections that affect the vulva include herpes genitalis and condylomata acuminata (venereal warts) (see Chapter 80). Secondary infections of the vulva are caused by organisms responsible for the many numerous types of vaginitis, including candidiasis. Pediculosis pubis (crab lice) and scabies (itch mite) are common parasitic infestations of the skin of the vulva. Other causes of vulvitis include the following:

- Atrophic vaginitis
- Vulvar kraurosis (postmenopausal disorder causing dryness and atrophy)
- Vulvar leukoplakia (postmenopausal atrophy and thickening of vulvar tissues)
- Cancer
- Urinary incontinence

◆ COLLABORATIVE MANAGEMENT

Assessment usually identifies symptoms of itching and burning sensation. **Erythema** (redness), edema, and superficial skin ulcers also may be present. Some women may have an itch-scratch-itch cycle, in which the itching leads to scratching, which causes excoriation that then must heal. As healing takes place, itching occurs again, which leads to further scratching. If the cycle is not interrupted, the condition may become chronic, causing the vulvar skin to become white and thickened (leathery). This skin is dry and scaly and cracks easily, increasing the woman's risk for infection.

Treatment of clients with vulvitis depends on the cause. Nursing interventions to relieve itching include applying wet compresses, sitz baths for 30 minutes several times a day, and applying the prescribed topical drugs, such as hydrocortisone and fluorinated corticosteroids (betamethasone valerate [Valisone, Betaderm✴] or fluocinolone acetonide [Synalar, Fluoderm]).

The health care provider prescribes oral antibiotics if infection is the underlying cause. Encourage the removal of any irritant or allergen, such as by changing detergents. Treatment of pediculosis and scabies is instituted if needed and includes applying lindane (1% gamma benzene hexachloride [Kwell, Kwellada✴]) lotion, shampoo, or cream to the affected area as directed; cleaning affected clothes, bedding, and towels; and disinfecting the home environment (lice cannot live for more than 24 hours away from the body).

If the vulvitis is chronic or severe, laser therapy (see pp. 1846 to 1847) or a "skinning" vulvectomy (see p. 1851) may be performed. Preventive measures that may be helpful for vulvitis are listed in Chart 78-7.

Toxic Shock Syndrome

PATHOPHYSIOLOGY

Toxic shock syndrome (TSS) was first recognized in 1980, when it was found to be related to menstruation and tampon use. Other conditions associated with TSS include surgical wound infection, nonsurgical focal infections, postpartum conditions, and nonmenstrual vaginal conditions. Use of the diaphragm, cervical cap, and vaginal contraceptive sponge also has been linked to TSS.

The pathophysiology of TSS is not clearly understood. Certain strains of *Staphylococcus aureus* produce a toxin that leads to the symptoms of TSS. The actual mechanism of *S. aureus* absorption in TSS is unknown. The vagina may be highly susceptible to the toxin released by *S. aureus*.

In menstrually related TSS, the risk appears to be associated with tampon use. Risk for TSS increased with the degree of absorbency of the tampon. The following are possible explanations:

- Toxins readily cross the vaginal mucosa.
- Highly absorbent tampons reduce vaginal moisture, causing fissures in the vaginal walls; they also rub the vaginal walls and cause ulceration, allowing movement of the toxins.
- Prolonged or continued tampon use can cause chronic vaginal ulcerations through which *S. aureus* is absorbed.
- Plastic tampon inserters can cause ulceration through which toxins are transported.
- Toxin producing *S. aureus* has a growth requirement for magnesium (some tampons contain magnesium).

◆ COLLABORATIVE MANAGEMENT

Influenza-like symptoms for the first 24 hours are common. The abrupt onset of a high fever along with a headache, sore throat, vomiting, diarrhea, generalized rash, and hypotension is often present. The most common manifestations are skin changes (initially a rash resembling a severe sunburn that changes to a macular erythema similar to a drug-related rash). Because not all women have all these manifestations, the criteria established by the Centers for Disease Control and Prevention (CDC) are used to verify cases of TSS (Chart 78-8).

Management focuses on client education and prevention. Instruct the client on the prevention of TSS related to the use of tampons, vaginal sponges, and diaphragms (Chart 78-9).

Treatment when the infection is present includes fluid replacement because dehydration and electrolyte imbalance result from vomiting and diarrhea. Antibiotics, most often penicillin, are the mainstay of treatment. Other antibiotics are needed if the penicillin-resistant strain of *S. aureus* is the cause of TSS. Vancomycin is the drug of choice to treat *S. aureus* TSS if the client is allergic to penicillin (DeCherney et al., 2003). Other measures may include transfusions to reverse low platelet counts, corticosteroids to treat skin changes, and drugs to treat hypotension.

PELVIC STRUCTURE SUPPORT PROBLEMS

Uterine Prolapse

PATHOPHYSIOLOGY

The stages of **uterine prolapse** are described by the degree of descent of the uterus (Figure 78-2). Uterine prolapse can be caused by congenital defects, persistent high levels of intra-abdominal pressure related to heavy physical labor or exertion, or any other event that weakens the pelvic supports.

> **CONSIDERATIONS FOR OLDER ADULTS**
> Prolapse is often a complication of childbirth injuries and repetitive stresses occurring many years later, but it also occurs in older adults who have never had children. The pelvic floor that supports the uterus is weakened by aging.

◆COLLABORATIVE MANAGEMENT

Assessment findings include the client's sensation of feeling as if "something is in my vagina," **dyspareunia** (painful sexual intercourse), backache, a feeling of heaviness or pressure in the

CHART 78-8

KEY FEATURES of
Toxic Shock Syndrome

- Fever (temperature >102° F [38.9° C]
- Diffuse rash resembling sunburn
- Peeling of skin—primarily the soles of the feet and the palms of the hands—1 to 2 wk after onset of the illness.
- Hypotension (systolic blood pressure <90 mm Hg or orthostatic syncope)
- Involvement of three or more of the following:
  Gastrointestinal system: vomiting, diarrhea at the onset of the syndrome
  Musculoskeletal system: severe aching or a serum creatinine phosphatase level twice the normal level
  Respiratory system: acute respiratory distress syndrome (ARDS)
  Renal/urinary system: decreased urine output, pyuria
  Cardiovascular system: decreased left ventricular contractility; ischemic changes shown on the electrocardiogram
  Liver: total bilirubin, aspartate aminotransferase (serum glutamic-oxaloacetic transaminase), and alanine aminotransferase (serum glutamic-pyruvic transaminase) levels elevated; jaundice; disseminated intravascular coagulation (DIC)
  Hematologic system: platelet levels below normal
  Central nervous system: disorientation, altered consciousness in the absence of fever or hypertension
  Mucous membranes: hyperemia of the vaginal walls, the throat, or the conjunctiva of the eye
- Negative results for the following: Rocky Mountain spotted fever, measles, scarlet fever, and throat, blood, and cerebrospinal fluid cultures
- Positive culture for *Staphylococcus aureus* from blood, urine, or stool

CHART 78-9

CLIENT EDUCATION GUIDE
Prevention of Toxic Shock Syndrome

Tampon Use
- Wash your hands before inserting a tampon.
- Do not use a tampon if it is dirty.
- Insert the tampon carefully to avoid injuring the delicate tissue in your vagina.
- Change your tampon every 3 to 6 hours.
- Do not use superabsorbent tampons.
- Use sanitary napkins at night.
- Call your health care provider if you suddenly experience a high temperature, vomiting, or diarrhea.
- Do not use tampons at all if you have had toxic shock syndrome.
- Not using tampons almost guarantees that you will not get toxic shock syndrome.

Vaginal Sponge Use
- Wash your hands before inserting a vaginal sponge.
- Use only clean water to wet the sponge.
- Do not use the sponge if it is dirty.
- Do not use the sponge for more than 30 hours at a time.
- Call your health care provider if you have two or more symptoms of toxic shock syndrome.

Diaphragm Use
- Wash your hands and the diaphragm before insertion.
- Remove the diaphragm within 24 hours after intercourse.
- Do not use the diaphragm during your menstrual period.
- After you take out the diaphragm, wash it with mild soap, rinse it, and dry it. Coating the diaphragm with a small amount of cornstarch will absorb any excess water and prevent damage to the latex rubber. Store it in a clean, dry place.

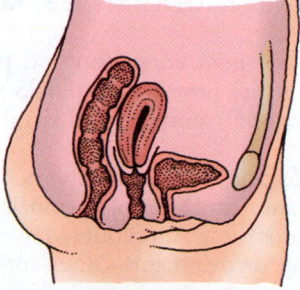 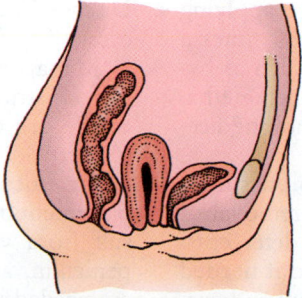 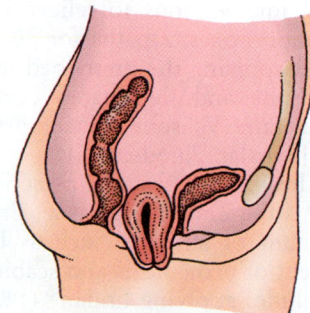

In **grade I uterine prolapse**, the uterus bulges into the vagina, but the cervix does not protrude through the entrance to the vagina.

In **grade II uterine prolapse**, the uterus bulges farther into the vagina, and the cervix protrudes through the entrance to the vagina.

In **grade III uterine prolapse**, the body of the uterus and the cervix protrude through the entrance to the vagina. The vagina is turned inside out.

Figure 78-2 ■ Types of uterine prolapse.

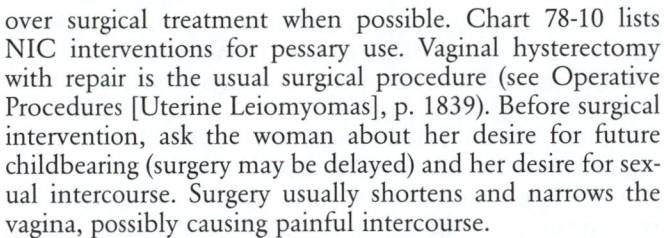

pelvis, and bowel or bladder problems (if cystocele or rectocele is also present). A pelvic examination may reveal a protrusion of the cervix when the woman is asked to bear down.

Interventions are based on the degree of prolapse. Conservative treatment, such as the use of pessaries, is preferred

CHART 78-10

NIC INTERVENTION ACTIVITIES for
The Client with Weak Pelvic Floor Muscles

Pessary Management: *Placement and monitoring of a vaginal device for treating stress urinary incontinence, uterine retroversion, genital prolapse, or incompetent cervix*
- Determine ability to perform self-care of pessary.
- Discuss maintenance regimen and cleaning procedures with client prior to fitting pessary (e.g., fit is trial and error; frequent follow-up visits are required).
- Review manufacturer's directions regarding specific type of pessary.
- Instruct on method for pessary removal, as appropriate.
- Instruct on contraindications for intercourse or douching based on pessary type.
- Instruct to report discomfort; dysuria; changes in color, consistency, or frequency of vaginal discharge.
- Determine therapeutic response to pessary use.

Pelvic Muscle Exercise: *Strengthening and training the levator ani and urogenital muscles through voluntary, repetitive contraction to decrease stress, urge, or mixed types of urinary incontinence*
- Determine ability to recognize the urge to void.
- Instruct female individual to locate the levator ani and urogenital muscles by placing her finger in the vagina and squeezing.
- Instruct individual to tighten, then relax, the ring of muscle around urethra and anus, as if trying to prevent urination or bowel movement.
- Instruct individual to perform muscle tightening exercises, working up to 300 contractions each day, holding the contraction for 10 seconds each and resting at least 10 seconds between each contraction, per agency protocol.
- Inform individual that it takes 6 to 12 weeks for exercises to be effective.
- Teach individual to monitor response to exercise by attempting to stop urine flow no more often than once a week.
- Provide written instructions describing the intervention and the recommended number of repetitions.

NIC intervention activities selected from Dochterman, J.M., & Bulechek, G.M. (Eds.) (2004). *Nursing interventions classification (NIC)* (4th ed.). St. Louis: Mosby. No part of this work is to be altered without prior written permission from the Publisher.

over surgical treatment when possible. Chart 78-10 lists NIC interventions for pessary use. Vaginal hysterectomy with repair is the usual surgical procedure (see Operative Procedures [Uterine Leiomyomas], p. 1839). Before surgical intervention, ask the woman about her desire for future childbearing (surgery may be delayed) and her desire for sexual intercourse. Surgery usually shortens and narrows the vagina, possibly causing painful intercourse.

Whenever the uterus is displaced, other structures, such as the bladder, rectum, and small intestine, are affected and can protrude through the vaginal walls.

Cystocele

PATHOPHYSIOLOGY

A **cystocele** is a protrusion of the bladder through the vaginal wall (Figure 78-3). It is due to weakened pelvic structures. This protrusion can be caused by obesity, advanced age, childbearing, or genetic predisposition. The development of a cystocele occurs more often in the postmenopausal years, when estrogen loss also weakens tissue supports and can cause relaxation of the supports.

◆COLLABORATIVE MANAGEMENT

Assessment findings may include the following:
- Difficulty in emptying the bladder
- Urinary frequency and urgency
- Urinary tract infection
- Stress urinary incontinence (loss of urine during activities that increase intra-abdominal pressure, such as laughing, coughing, sneezing, or lifting heavy objects)

A pelvic examination reveals a large bulge of the anterior vaginal wall when the woman is asked to bear down. Diagnostic tests include cystography (to show the presence of bladder herniation), measurement of residual urine by catheterization or bladder ultrasound, and urine culture and sensitivity testing. Radiographic imaging of the urinary tract and a voiding cystourethrography are useful in determining the degree of cystocele. Radiographic imaging of the urinary tract includes an intravenous urogram (IVU) to define urinary anatomy. A voiding cystourethrography (VCUG) is done to determine the following: the degree of the cystocele

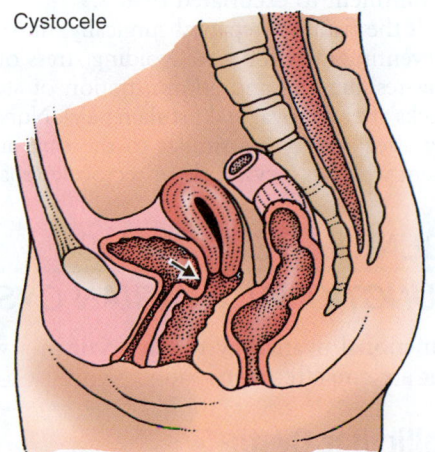

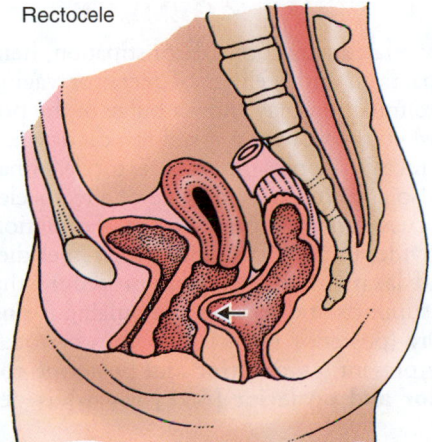

Cystocele

Rectocele

Figure 78-3 ■ In cystocele, the urinary bladder is displaced downward, causing bulging of the anterior vaginal wall. In rectocele, the rectum is displaced, causing bulging of the posterior vaginal wall.

in the standing position, the amount of a postvoid residual, and urethral abnormalities. A cystometrogram measures bladder storage. Uroflowmetry evaluates characteristics of the woman's voiding pattern. Failure to empty the bladder because of poor bladder contraction can be identified during this test (DeCherney et al., 2003).

If the client has only mild symptoms, management is conservative. The health care provider may recommend a pessary to support the bladder in some clients. Estrogen therapy may be prescribed for the postmenopausal woman to prevent atrophy and weakening of vaginal walls. Kegel exercises may help strengthen perineal muscles (see Chart 78-10). Teach the woman Kegel exercises, telling her to tighten and relax the perineal muscles; the woman presses the buttocks together and holds the position for at least 5 seconds. Instruct the client to repeat the exercise often throughout the day. An alternative exercise is to try to stop the flow of urine after urination has started and then hold the position for a few seconds before letting the urine flow again.

Surgery may be recommended for severe symptoms. An **anterior colporrhaphy** (anterior repair) tightens the pelvic muscles for better bladder support. A vaginal surgical approach is used. Nursing care of a woman undergoing an anterior repair is similar to that for a woman undergoing a vaginal hysterectomy (see Operative Procedures [Uterine Leiomyomas], p. 1839).

After surgery, instruct the client to limit her activities, not lift anything heavier than 5 pounds, avoid strenuous exercises, and avoid sexual intercourse for 6 weeks. Tell the woman to notify her health care provider if she has signs of infection, such as fever, persistent pain, or purulent, foul-smelling discharge. Encourage the client to keep her follow-up appointment after surgery.

Rectocele

PATHOPHYSIOLOGY

A **rectocele** is a protrusion of the rectum through a weakened vaginal wall (see Figure 78-3). This problem usually results from the pressure of an infant's head during a difficult delivery, a traumatic forceps delivery, or a congenital defect of the supporting tissues. Symptoms do not typically appear until the woman is older than 35 years of age.

◆COLLABORATIVE MANAGEMENT

The woman usually relates symptoms of constipation, hemorrhoids, fecal impaction, and feelings of rectal or vaginal fullness. A pelvic examination may show a bulge of the posterior vaginal wall when the woman is asked to bear down. A rectal examination reveals the presence of a rectocele. A barium enema study also confirms the presence of a rectocele.

Management focuses on promoting bowel elimination. The health care provider usually prescribes a high-fiber diet, stool softeners, and laxatives. The surgical procedure that strengthens pelvic supports and reduces the bulging is **posterior colporrhaphy** (posterior repair). If both a cystocele and a rectocele are present, an **anterior and posterior colporrhaphy (anterior and posterior [A&P] repair)** is performed.

The nursing care after a posterior repair is similar to that after any rectal surgery. After surgery a low-residue (low-fiber) diet is prescribed to prevent bowel movements and al-

low time for the incision to heal. Instruct the client not to strain when she does have a bowel movement so that she does not put pressure on the suture line. Bowel movements are often painful, and the client may need pain medication before having a bowel movement. Sitz baths may relieve discomfort. Instructions for the client undergoing a posterior repair are similar to those for undergoing an anterior repair.

Fistulas
PATHOPHYSIOLOGY

Fistulas are abnormal openings between two adjacent organs or structures. Vaginal fistulas can occur between the vagina and the urethra (urethrovaginal), the vagina and the bladder (vesicovaginal), or the vagina and the rectum (rectovaginal). Trauma is the main cause of fistulas, although they can result from complications of surgery, vaginal-delivery complications, malignancy, or radiation therapy for cancer.

◆COLLABORATIVE MANAGEMENT

Symptoms depend on the location of the fistula. A fistula may result in any of the following problems:

- Leakage of urine, flatus, or feces into the vagina
- Irritation or excoriation of the vulva and vaginal tissues
- An unpleasant odor (fecal or urine) in the vagina
- A feeling of wetness or dribbling in the vagina

Women who have fistulas may be embarrassed to seek help until symptoms are severe. The client may withdraw from social activities or from relationships with significant others as the symptoms become more difficult to manage.

Management depends on the fistula's location. Surgery is not recommended if infection or inflammation is present. Surgery may not be successful. Nursing care focuses on assisting the woman with the frequent and time-consuming perineal hygiene, including sitz baths; perineal cleaning with mild, unscented soap and water; and low-pressure douching with commercial deodorizing solutions or homemade solutions (1 teaspoon [5 mL] of nonchlorine household bleach to 1 quart [about 1 L] of water). The woman may need to wear sanitary napkins or disposable undergarments (such as Depends) if there is leakage of urine or feces. Other interventions may include the application of A and D ointment to excoriated tissues.

If the fistula is repaired surgically, nursing care focuses on preventing infection and avoiding stress on the repaired area (low-residue diet and administration of stool softeners for 2 weeks after rectovaginal fistula repair). Nursing care and teaching after surgery are similar to the care and teaching of the client who has a cystocele or rectocele repair (see text at left).

BENIGN NEOPLASMS
FUNCTIONAL OVARIAN CYSTS

Functional ovarian cysts can occur in a woman of any age but are rare after menopause.

Follicular Cysts

Follicular cysts usually occur in young, menstruating women. These cysts are not malignant and do not grow without hormonal influences. A cyst can develop when a mature follicle fails to rupture or an immature follicle fails to reabsorb follicular fluid during the second half of the menstrual cycle. The cyst is usually small (2.4 to 3.2 inches [6 to 8 cm]) and may be asymptomatic unless it ruptures. Rupture of a follicular cyst or **torsion** (twisting) may cause acute, severe pelvic pain. The pain usually resolves after several days of bedrest and use of mild analgesics. If the cyst does not rupture, it usually disappears within two or three menstrual cycles without intervention. If the cyst does not shrink, the health care provider may prescribe oral contraceptives for one or two menstrual cycles to depress ovulation. When the cyst is managed conservatively, follow-up care is necessary to confirm that it has disappeared.

If the cyst is larger than 6 to 8 cm, a neoplasm may be suspected, and evaluation by ultrasonography or laparoscopy is needed. Larger cysts often occur with menstrual irregularities.

Surgery is recommended only after menopause or when cysts are larger than 3.2 inches (7 cm). A **cystectomy** (removal of the cyst) is performed instead of an **oophorectomy** (removal of the ovary).

Corpus Luteum Cysts

Corpus luteum cysts occur after ovulation and often occur with increased secretion of progesterone. The cysts are usually small, averaging 1.5 inches (4 cm). They are purplish red as a result of hemorrhage within the corpus luteum. These cysts occur with a delay in the onset of menses and irregular or prolonged flow. They may occur with low abdominal or pelvic pain that is usually described as dull or aching. If the cyst ruptures, intraperitoneal hemorrhage can occur.

Corpus luteum cysts may disappear in one or two menstrual cycles or with suppression of ovulation. The treatment is the same as that for follicular cysts.

Theca-Lutein Cysts

Theca-lutein cysts are uncommon and often occur with a hydatidiform molar pregnancy. Theca-lutein cysts develop as a result of prolonged stimulation of the ovaries by excessive amounts of human chorionic gonadotropin (hCG).

These cysts regress spontaneously within 3 months with the removal of the molar pregnancy or the source of excessive hCG. Usually no other treatment is necessary.

Polycystic Ovary

Polycystic ovary, or Stein-Leventhal syndrome, results when high levels of luteinizing hormone (LH) overstimulate the ovaries, which produces multiple cysts on one or both ovaries. High levels of estrogen are produced by these cysts and are unopposed by postovulatory progesterone. Endometrial **hyperplasia** (tissue overgrowth) or even carcinoma may result.

A typical client is obese, is **hirsute** (hairy), has irregular menses, and may be infertile because of lack of ovulation. Treatment depends on which disorder is of greatest concern to the woman. The best treatment is the use of oral contraceptives because they inhibit LH production. The health care provider may advise a woman who is older than 35 years of age and no longer desires childbearing to undergo a bilateral salpingo-oophorectomy (BSO) (removal of both tubes and ovaries) and **hysterectomy** (removal of the uterus and cervix). Women who desire fertility can be treated with drugs such as clomiphene citrate (Clomid) to stimulate ovulation.

OTHER BENIGN OVARIAN CYSTS AND TUMORS

Dermoid Cysts

Dermoid cysts are common germ cell tumors and are usually benign. These cysts more commonly occur in childhood, although they can develop in a female of any age.

Dermoid cysts may contain hair, skin, teeth, and other calcifications. They are usually asymptomatic unless they grow large and put pressure on other organs, such as the bladder and the bowel. The cysts develop on both ovaries in some cases. They are often attached to the ovary by a **pedicle** (stalk).

Management of dermoid cysts is surgical removal (cystectomy). If the cysts are not removed, they usually continue to grow and rupture, causing hemorrhage and infection.

Ovarian Fibromas

Fibromas are the most common benign, solid ovarian neoplasms. These pearly white tumors of connective tissue origin rarely become malignant. Fibromas can range in size from a small nodule to a mass weighing more than 50 pounds (22.7 kg). The average size is 2.4 inches (6 cm) in diameter, slightly smaller than a tennis ball. Most affect only one ovary. On examination, they feel firm, have a slightly irregular contour, and are mobile. Larger fibromas may cause ascites and feelings of pelvic pressure or abdominal enlargement. Unless rupture or torsion occurs, the fibroma is usually asymptomatic. Fibromas often occur postmenopausally.

Solid ovarian neoplasms are surgically removed. The surgeon may perform an oophorectomy for borderline tumors (when there is a question of possible cancer). Nursing care of a woman undergoing an oophorectomy is similar to that for a woman undergoing a tubal ligation. When both ovaries are removed, artificial menopause occurs in a premenopausal women. The woman then often develops decreased vaginal lubrication, hot flashes, and atrophy of the vaginal epithelium. These symptoms may be treated with estrogen replacement therapy (ERT) (see Chart 78-3).

Epithelial Ovarian Tumors

Epithelial ovarian tumors, serous and mucinous cystadenomas, occur in women between the ages of 30 and 50 years. Serous cystadenomas usually affect both ovaries and are more likely to become malignant than mucinous cystadenomas. Both tumors can be irregular and smooth, but mucinous cystadenomas tend to grow large, some to more than 100 pounds (45 kg).

Management of cystadenomas is **unilateral salpingo-oophorectomy** (surgical removal of a fallopian tube and ovary) because it is often impossible to tell whether the tumor is benign or malignant. Small cysts may be removed by cystectomy, but the larger ones are difficult to resect from the ovary.

Uterine Leiomyomas
PATHOPHYSIOLOGY

Leiomyomas, also called myomas and fibroids, are benign, slow-growing solid tumors of the uterus. They are the most commonly occurring pelvic tumors.

Leiomyomas develop from the uterine myometrium. As they grow, fibroids stay attached to the myometrium by means of a pedicle. Leiomyomas are classified according to their position in the layers of the uterus. The most common types of leiomyomas are intramural, submucosal, and subserosal (Figure 78-4).

Intramural leiomyomas are contained in the uterine wall within the myometrium. Submucosal leiomyomas protrude into the cavity of the uterus. Subserosal leiomyomas protrude through the outer surface of the uterine wall. Subserosal leiomyomas may grow laterally and extend to the broad ligament.

Although most fibroids develop within the uterine wall, about 5% may appear in the cervix. Rarely, a fibroid breaks off the pedicle and attaches to other tissues (parasitic fibroid).

Etiology

The cause of leiomyomas is not precisely known. Leiomyomas usually result from excessive local growth of smooth muscle cells. The stimulus for growth may be physical or mechanical and may operate at points of maximal stress within the myometrial layer of the uterine wall. Because there are multiple points of stress caused by the contractions of the uterine muscle, multiple fibroids develop. The growth of leiomyomas may be related to estrogen stimulation; fibroids often enlarge during pregnancy and diminish in size after menopause.

Incidence/Prevalence

Leiomyomas occur in about 20% to 30% of women older than age 30. The rationale for why leiomyomas develop in some women and not in others is not known.

◆ COLLABORATIVE MANAGEMENT
◆ Assessment
HISTORY

Many women with uterine leiomyomas are asymptomatic, but abnormal bleeding is common. Because African American women and premenopausal women are at greatest risk for leiomyomas, any abnormal bleeding should be discussed. Menstrual bleeding may be increased (**menorrhagia**); the bleeding may occur between menstrual periods (**metrorrhagia**), or it may be continuous.

PHYSICAL ASSESSMENT/CLINICAL MANIFESTATIONS

Women with fibroids do not usually have pain, although acute pain may occur with twisting of the fibroid on its stalk. A woman may report a feeling of pelvic pressure, constipation, or urinary frequency or retention. These symptoms result when an enlarged fibroid presses on other organs. The client may notice that her abdomen has increased in size with or without noticeable weight gain. Painful sexual intercourse and infertility may also occur with leiomyomas.

Abdominal, vaginal, and rectal examinations usually establish the presence of a uterine enlargement that may indicate a leiomyoma. Other diagnostic procedures are needed to differentiate benign tumors from malignant ones.

PSYCHOSOCIAL ASSESSMENT

A woman who is symptomatic may fear that she has a malignancy. She may be anxious about abnormal bleeding or her failure to conceive. She may also be concerned if surgery is recommended. Assess the woman's feelings and concerns about her symptoms and fears of the unknown. If surgery is recommended, explore the significance of the loss of the uterus for the woman.

LABORATORY ASSESSMENT

A complete blood count identifies iron deficiency anemia (related to bleeding). A pregnancy test is done to determine

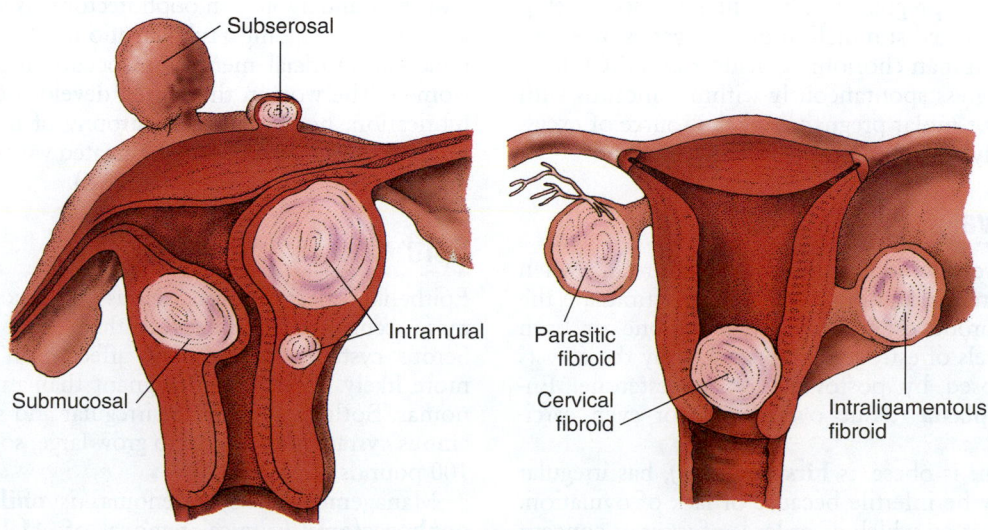

CLASSIFICATION BY POSITION
WITHIN UTERINE LAYERS

CLASSIFICATION BY ANATOMIC POSITION

Figure 78-4 ■ Classification of uterine leiomyomas.

whether pregnancy is the cause of the uterine enlargement. An endometrial biopsy may be performed to determine whether the lesion is malignant.

RADIOGRAPHIC ASSESSMENT

Computed tomography (CT) may be of some value. However, CT scans do not differentiate between benign and malignant myomas. Magnetic resonance imaging (MRI) can differentiate between benign and malignant lesions.

OTHER DIAGNOSTIC ASSESSMENTS

Ultrasonography may help differentiate causes of pelvic masses, such as ovarian masses and pregnancy. Culdoscopy or laparoscopy may help differentiate a uterine fibroid from an ovarian mass. These tests are described in Chapter 76.

◆ Analysis

COMMON NURSING DIAGNOSES AND COLLABORATIVE PROBLEMS

The most common collaborative problem for clients with leiomyomas is Potential for Hemorrhage.

ADDITIONAL NURSING DIAGNOSES AND COLLABORATIVE PROBLEMS

In addition to the common collaborative problems, clients with leiomyomas may have one or more of the following:

- Anxiety and Fear related to a threat to or change in health status (uncertain diagnosis; potential surgical treatment)
- Acute Pain related to physical pressure from tumors
- Anticipatory Grieving or Dysfunctional Grieving related to perceived or actual loss of the uterus or reproductive function
- Sexual Dysfunction related to altered body structure and dyspareunia
- Ineffective Coping related to uncertainty or depression as a response to treatment

◆ Planning and Implementation

POTENTIAL FOR HEMORRHAGE

NOC **PLANNING: EXPECTED OUTCOMES.** The client with leiomyomas is expected to be free of bleeding complications. Indicators include that the client should have only mild or no deviations of the following parameters:

- Vaginal bleeding
- Anxiety
- Decreased hematocrit (Hct)
- Decreased hemoglobin (Hgb)

INTERVENTIONS. Observation of the leiomyomas over time, myomectomy, and hysterectomy are the methods of management. The choice depends on the size and symptoms of the fibroids and the woman's desire for future childbearing.

NONSURGICAL MANAGEMENT. If the client has few symptoms or desires childbearing, the health care provider typically suggests observation and examination every 4 to 6 months. If the woman is menopausal, the fibroids usually shrink, and surgery may not be necessary. However, a client who is receiving estrogen replacement therapy (ERT) for menopausal symptoms should know that the fibroids may continue to grow because of the estrogen stimulation.

A new alternative to surgery is radiologic management by uterine artery embolization (UFE). This treatment for leiomyomas is to embolize (occlude) the blood flow to the tumors using a percutaneous catheter approach. Under moderate sedation, the radiologist places a tiny catheter in both uterine arteries and injects embolic particles into the tumor's blood supply. This 1- to 2-hour procedure is usually effective in shrinking tumors, thereby reducing pain and bleeding.

SURGICAL MANAGEMENT. If the woman desires childbearing, the surgeon may perform a **myomectomy** (the removal of leiomyomas with preservation of the uterus) regardless of the size, number, or location of the fibroids. A laser may be used to remove the tumors. Myomectomy is usually performed in the proliferative phase of the menstrual cycle to minimize blood loss and to avoid the possibility of interrupting an unsuspected pregnancy. A small percentage of leiomyomas that are removed recur. Nursing care is similar to that of a woman undergoing a hysterectomy, as described below under Operative Procedures.

Preoperative Care. Teaching by the physician begins in his or her office. Preoperative teaching is usually done on an individual basis. Explain procedures that routinely take place before surgery, including laboratory tests and expected drugs, such as prophylactic antibiotics. Teach about the need for turning, coughing, deep breathing exercises; incentive spirometry; early ambulation; and the need for pain relief (see Chapter 20).

Psychological assessment is essential. First explore the significance of the loss of the uterus for the client. She may feel a great loss if she wishes to retain her childbearing ability, relates her uterus to her self-image and femininity, or believes that her sexual function is related to her uterus. A woman may have misconceptions about the effects of hysterectomy (e.g., associating it with masculinization and weight gain). Identify any misconceptions, and provide correct information. Assess the client's support system. The client may fear rejection by her sexual partner. Urge inclusion of the partner in all teaching sessions unless this practice is not culturally acceptable.

Operative Procedures. A **total abdominal hysterectomy (TAH)** is usually performed for leiomyomas larger than the size of a 12-week pregnancy. The uterus and cervix are removed through a horizontal incision (traditional approach) or via laparoscopic surgery, which requires a very small umbilical incision.

A uterus that has smaller fibroids may be removed via a **total vaginal hysterectomy (TVH).** The surgeon removes the uterus and cervix through the vagina without an external surgical incision. In both vaginal and abdominal hysterectomies, the surgeon removes the uterus from the five supporting ligaments, which are then attached to the vaginal cuff so that normal depth of the vagina is maintained (Table 78-6).

In selected cases (e.g., submucous fibroids, menorrhagia), minimally invasive uterine surgery may be performed, such as a **transcervical endometrial resection (TCER).** A hysteroscope is inserted into the uterus, and the endometrium is destroyed using a diathermy resectoscope (similar to the scope used with prostate surgery) or with radioablation. Po-

TABLE 78-6 Common Gynecologic Surgeries

Total Hysterectomy
All the uterus, including the cervix, is removed. The procedure may be vaginal, abdominal, or laparoscopic.

Subtotal Hysterectomy
All the uterus, except the cervix, is removed. This procedure is rarely performed.

Bilateral Salpingo-Oophorectomy
Fallopian tubes and ovaries are removed.

Panhysterectomy
Total abdominal hysterectomy and bilateral salpingo-oophorectomy. The uterus, ovaries, and fallopian tubes are removed abdominally.

Radical Hysterectomy
All the uterus is removed abdominally. The lymph nodes, the upper third of the vagina, and the surrounding tissues (parametrium) are also removed.

CHART 78-11

FOCUSED ASSESSMENT of
The Client After Total Abdominal Hysterectomy

Assess cardiovascular, respiratory, renal, and gastrointestinal status, including the following:
- Vital signs
- Heart, lung, and bowel sounds
- Urine output
- Temperature and color of the skin
- Red blood cell, hemoglobin, and hematocrit levels
- Activity tolerance
- Dressing and drains for color and amount of drainage
- Peripads for vaginal bleeding and clots
- Fluid intake (IVs until bowel sounds return and client is tolerating oral intake)
- Signs of thrombophlebitis

Teach the client to use the following interventions to prevent postoperative complications:
- Cough and deep breathing exercises
- Incentive spirometry
- Sequential compression devices
- Ambulation
- Avoidance of heavy lifting or strenuous activity

Assess the home care teaching needs of the client related to the illness and surgery, including:
- Physiologic effects of the surgery
- Signs or symptoms to report
- Side or toxic effects of medications
- Activity limitations related to driving and use of stairs
- Follow-up care
- Postoperative restrictions related to sexual activity, use of tampons, and bathing
- Care of wound and/or drains

Assess the client's coping skills and reaction to the diagnosis and surgical procedure.

---

tential complications of hysteroscopic surgery include the following:
- Fluid overload (fluid used to distend the uterine cavity can be absorbed)
- Embolism
- Hemorrhage
- Perforation of the uterus, bowel, or bladder and ureter injury
- Persistent increased menstrual bleeding
- Incomplete suppression of menstruation

TABLE 78-7 Common Postoperative Complications of Traditional Abdominal and Vaginal Hysterectomies

Traditional Abdominal Hysterectomy
- Intestinal obstruction (paralytic ileus)
- Thromboembolism
- Atelectasis
- Pneumonia
- Wound dehiscence (especially in obese clients)
- Urinary retention

Vaginal Hysterectomy
- Hemorrhage
- Urinary tract complications, especially infection or retention
- Wound infection
- Urinary retention

There is a small risk of subsequent pregnancy and the possibility of cancer developing in the scar. Hysterectomy is the procedure of choice for women who have other problems, especially those with cancer or symptomatic uterovaginal prolapse.

Postoperative Care. Care of the woman who has undergone a TAH is similar to that of any client who has undergone abdominal surgery (see Chapter 22). For clients who have undergone a TAH, assess the following (Chart 78-11):
- Vaginal bleeding (there should be less than one saturated perineal pad in 4 hours)
- Abdominal bleeding at the incision site (a small amount is normal)
- Intactness of the incision
- Urine output per Foley catheter for 24 hours or less for a traditional surgical approach
- Pain

Specific interventions for a vaginal hysterectomy include the following:
- Assessment of vaginal bleeding (there should be less than one saturated pad in 4 hours)
- Foley catheter care
- Perineal care (sitz baths or ice packs)

The surgeon usually removes the abdominal sutures or clips at the first postoperative visit, whereas vaginal sutures are usually absorbed. Monitor for complications associated with hysterectomies (Table 78-7).

CONSIDERATIONS FOR OLDER ADULTS

Older women are at greater risk for all complications, particularly pulmonary embolism. Obese women are more at risk for thromboembolism. These clients need more frequent monitoring after surgery. Psychological complications can occur with both abdominal and vaginal procedures. Depression is the most frequent reaction reported. Other reactions are perceived loss of femininity and decreased libido. Loss of femininity may be the problem if a woman was interested in her appearance before surgery but afterward has no interest, even when she is feeling better. Decreased sexual desire is often temporary, if it occurs, and is usually related to discomfort.

Community-Based Care

The client with uterine leiomyomas is managed on an ambulatory care basis unless surgery is performed. After discharge, the client usually returns to her home.

HOME CARE MANAGEMENT

Planning for home care management begins at the time of admission. The woman is usually discharged to the home setting 1 to 2 days after a traditional TAH, depending on the age and health of the client. TVH, laparoscopic surgery, or TCER may be performed as same-day surgery in an ambulatory setting. The client who has undergone a hysterectomy usually needs to limit stair climbing for several weeks. If the client lives in a two-story house with a bathroom only on one level, advise the client to rent a bedside commode. If the client lives alone and is not permitted to drive for 2 to 6 weeks, she will need to make arrangements for transportation to follow-up visits.

HEALTH TEACHING

Teach the client who has undergone an abdominal hysterectomy about the expected physical changes, any activity restrictions, diet, sexual activity, any needed wound care, complications, and the need for follow-up care. Chart 78-12 lists education issues to stress for the client after surgery.

PSYCHOSOCIAL PREPARATION

Women who have undergone a hysterectomy need information about possible emotional reactions. Generally, women adjust well to surgery if they have completed childbearing, work, have interests outside the home, have no misconceptions about the effects of hysterectomy, and have support from the family, especially their sexual partner.

Reactions may be different after vaginal and abdominal procedures because women who have undergone a vaginal hysterectomy have no external focus (no obvious change in body image) for their feelings. Psychological reactions can occur months to years after surgery. Women identified as being at high risk for psychological problems may need long-term follow-up care or referral. Women may need to be counseled about signs of depression. Intermittent sadness is normal, but continued feelings of low self-esteem or loss of interest or pleasure in usual activities and pastimes is not normal and should be evaluated. Providing written materials and discussing the positive aspects of the client's life can help to decrease adverse psychological reactions.

HEALTH CARE RESOURCES

Usually no special home equipment is needed for a woman who has undergone a hysterectomy. A home care nurse may be needed to assess and monitor the older client's progress after surgery if other conditions (e.g., uncontrolled diabetes) are present. Financial assistance may be needed, and referral to the hospital's department of social services or case management department may be indicated if the woman has no insurance coverage. Provide a referral for psychological or sexual counseling if potential problems are identified before discharge.

◆Evaluation: Outcomes

Evaluate the care of the client who has undergone surgery for leiomyomas on the basis of the identified nursing diagnoses and collaborative problems. The expected outcomes include that the client should:

- Be free of hemorrhage
- Recover from surgery without complications

Specific indicators for these outcomes are listed for each collaborative problem under the Planning and Implementation section (see earlier).

CHART 78-12

CLIENT EDUCATION GUIDE
Care After a Total Abdominal Hysterectomy

Expected Physical Changes
- You will no longer have a period, although you may have some vaginal discharge for a few days after you go home.
- It will not be possible for you to become pregnant, and birth control methods are no longer needed.
- If your ovaries were removed, you may have some menopause symptoms such as hot flushes, night sweats, and vaginal dryness.
- It is normal to tire more easily and require more sleep and rest during the first few weeks after surgery (this may last for 2 to 3 months).

Activity
- Limit stair climbing to less than five times per day.
- Take showers rather than tub baths.
- Do not lift anything heavier than 5 lbs.
- Walk indoors for the first week. Then gradually increase walking as exercise but stop before you become fatigued.
- Avoid the sitting position for any extended period. When you sit, do not cross your legs at the knees.
- Avoid jogging, aerobic exercise, participating in sports, or any strenuous activity for 6 weeks.
- Do not drive for at least 4 weeks or until your surgeon has told you it is alright.

Diet
- Eat a well-balanced diet with extra protein and vitamin C to help heal your tissues.
- Drink at least 3 quarts of fluid, especially water, each day unless you have another health problem (like heart failure or kidney disease) that requires fluid restriction.
- If gas is a problem, avoid foods and beverages that increase gas.

Sexual Activity
- Do not engage in sexual intercourse for 4 to 6 weeks, as prescribed by your surgeon.
- If you had a vaginal "repair" as part of your surgery, the first time you have intercourse you may have some tenderness or pain because the vaginal walls are tighter. Careful intercourse and the use of water-based lubricants can help reduce this discomfort. This discomfort usually goes away with time and stretching of the vagina.

Follow-up Care
- If antibiotics are prescribed, take them as directed until all the drugs are gone.
- Make and keep your follow-up appointment(s) with your surgeon.

Complications
- Take your temperature twice each day for the first 2 weeks after surgery.
- Check your incision daily for signs of infection (increasing redness, open areas, drainage that is thick or foul-smelling, incision pain).

Report Any of the Following to Your Surgeon
- Increased vaginal drainage or change in drainage (more bloody, thicker, foul-smelling)
- Temperature over 100° F
- Pain, tenderness, redness, or swelling in your calves
- Pain or burning on urination

Bartholin Cyst

PATHOPHYSIOLOGY

Bartholin cyst is a common disorder of the vulva. The cysts result from obstruction of the duct of the Bartholin gland. The secretory function of the gland continues, and the fluid fills the obstructed duct. The main causes of the obstruction are infection, thickened mucus near the ductal opening, or trauma, such as lacerations or episiotomy.

◆COLLABORATIVE MANAGEMENT
◆Assessment

The client may be asymptomatic if the cyst is small. Often the client has dyspareunia, inadequate genital lubrication, or a mass in the perineal area. A large cyst usually causes constant local pain and may cause difficulty walking or sitting. Physical examination of the vulva reveals a swelling immediately beneath the skin in the posterior portion of the vulva. The cyst may appear brown or bloody, depending on its contents. Usually a cyst is present only on one side and ranges from ⅜ to 4 inches (1 to 10 cm) in size.

If the cyst is draining, fluid is sent to the laboratory for culture (for gonorrhea and aerobic and anaerobic organisms) and sensitivity testing. If the woman is older than 40 years of age, a specimen of the cyst should be sent for pathologic examination to determine whether the lesion is benign or malignant.

◆Interventions

If the woman is asymptomatic, no intervention is needed. If symptoms are present, simple incision and drainage (I&D) may provide temporary relief; however, cysts tend to recur when the opening of the duct reobstructs. Usually the surgeon establishes a permanent opening for drainage. Marsupialization (formation of a pouch that is a new duct opening) is performed using local, regional, or general anesthesia. Discomfort after surgery may be relieved with analgesics and sitz baths. Prophylactic antibiotics may be prescribed.

Often Bartholin cysts are infected and abscesses form when bacteria, such as *Escherichia coli* or *Staphylococcus aureus,* result in infection that closes the duct. An abscess usually ruptures spontaneously within 72 hours of formation. Interventions for the woman with an abscess include analgesics and application of moist heat (sitz baths or hot wet packs) to the vulva. Antibiotics are prescribed to treat the infection. I&D of the abscess may provide temporary relief.

The Bartholin glands may be totally excised in older women when cancer is suspected or if infections with abscess formation recur. Care after surgery includes the following:

- Application of ice packs or sitz baths several times a day for comfort and promotion of healing
- Analgesics for pain
- Prophylactic antibiotics
- Assessment of the incision for signs of healing or infection

Cervical Polyps

Cervical polyps are **pedunculated** (on stalks) tumors that arise from the mucosa and extend to the opening of the cervical os. Polyps result from a hyperplastic condition of the endocervical epithelium. They may also be due to inflammation or from an abnormal local response to hormonal stimulation or localized vascular congestion of the cervical blood vessels (DeCherney et al., 2003). Polyps are the most common benign growth of the cervix. They occur most often women older than 40 years of age who have had several children.

A woman may be asymptomatic, have premenstrual or postmenstrual bleeding, or have bleeding after coitus. A speculum examination may reveal small single or multiple polyps. They are bright red, are soft and fragile, and may bleed when touched.

Polyp removal is a simple office procedure. The base of the polyp is grasped with a clamp, and the polyp is twisted off and sent to the pathology laboratory for evaluation. Cautery usually stops any bleeding at the site of removal. After the procedure, instruct the client to avoid tampon use, douches, and sexual intercourse for a week or until healing has taken place.

MALIGNANT NEOPLASMS

Endometrial (Uterine) Cancer
PATHOPHYSIOLOGY

Endometrial cancer (cancer of the uterus) is a reproductive cancer; adenocarcinoma is the most common type (American Cancer Society, 2005). It arises from the glandular part of the endometrium and may be preceded by endometrial overgrowth. These cancers are divided into three grades based on tumor growth and the degree of differentiation (normal cell appearance). Grade 1 cancers are identified by endometrial glands that are well differentiated, whereas grade 3 tumors have a solid growth pattern and are poorly differentiated (DeVita et al., 2001). The initial growth of the cancer is within the uterine cavity, followed by extension into the myometrium and the cervix. Spread outside the uterus occurs as follows:

- Through lymphatic spread to the ovaries and parametrial, pelvic, inguinal, and para-aortic lymph nodes
- By blood, to the lungs, liver, or bone
- By transtubal or intra-abdominal spread to the peritoneal cavity

This type of cancer is asymptomatic in its early development and has a good prognosis in 80% to 90% of cases.

Etiology and Genetic Risk

Personal risk factors for endometrial cancer are listed in Table 78-8. The use of menopausal estrogen replacement therapy (ERT) and long-term tamoxifen therapy also appear to increase the risk for endometrial cancer. Although most cases of endometrial cancer do not have a genetic predisposition, it is more common in families who have gene mutations for hereditary nonpolyposis colon cancer (HNPCC).

Incidence/Prevalence

More than 40,100 new cases of endometrial cancer occur annually in the United States (American Cancer Society, 2005). Thus about 1 of every 100 women in the United States has endometrial cancer. The average age at diagnosis is 60 years.

> **CONSIDERATIONS FOR OLDER ADULTS**
> Endometrial cancer is a slow-growing tumor mainly occurring in postmenopausal women. The average age at onset is 61 years. The incidence declines after the age of 70 years. It is important to teach older women that any instance of postmenopausal bleeding should be evaluated by a health care provider.

TABLE 78-8 Risk Factors for Endometrial Cancer and Cervical Cancer

Endometrial Cancer	Cervical Cancer
Age 50 to 70 yr	African American
Family history of endometrial cancer or HNPCC	Native American/American Indian
	Multiparity
Diabetes mellitus	<18 yr of age at first intercourse
Hypertension	<18 yr of age at first pregnancy
Obesity	Multiple sex partners
Uterine polyps	Smoking
Late menopause	Infection with herpes simplex virus (HSV)
Nulliparity	Infection with human papilloma virus (HPV)
Smoking	Infection with cytomegalovirus (CMV)
	HIV/AIDS
	Lower socioeconomic status
	Sexual partner had a previous partner who developed cervical cancer
	Intrauterine exposure to diethylstilbestrol (DES)

HNPCC, Hereditary nonpolyposis colon cancer.

◆COLLABORATIVE MANAGEMENT
◆Assessment

The main symptom of endometrial cancer is postmenopausal bleeding. Some women also have a watery, bloody vaginal discharge, low back or abdominal pain, and low pelvic pain (caused by pressure of the enlarged uterus). A pelvic examination may reveal the presence of a palpable uterine mass or uterine polyp. The uterus is enlarged if the cancer is advanced.

DIAGNOSTIC ASSESSMENT

Basic diagnostic tests to determine the client's overall status and the presence of metastasis include the following:

- CA-125 tumor marker to rule out ovarian involvement
- Chest x-ray
- Intravenous pyelography (IVP), or excretory urography, to assess renal function and to assess for renal metastasis
- Barium enema study to assess for intestinal metastasis
- Computed tomography (CT) of the pelvis to identify the spread of the tumor
- Liver and bone scans to assess for distant metastasis

Dilation and curettage (D&C [scraping individual sections of the uterus]) and endometrial biopsy are the definitive diagnostic procedures for endometrial cancer. Other tests that may be useful include proctosigmoidoscopy, ultrasonography, and endoscopic examination of the uterus.

PSYCHOSOCIAL ASSESSMENT

Before a diagnosis is made, the client may deny that the symptoms are related to cancer. During the diagnostic phase, the woman may express fears and concerns about having cancer. After the diagnosis is confirmed, she may express disbelief, anger, depression, anxiety, or withdrawal behaviors.

◆Interventions

Nonsurgical interventions (radiation therapy and chemotherapy) and surgery may be used alone or in combination, depending on the stage of the cancer.

NONSURGICAL MANAGEMENT. Radiation therapy and chemotherapy are the two major nonsurgical methods used to treat endometrial cancer.

Radiation Therapy. The oncologist prescribes radiation therapy (external and internal) if the stage of cancer is hard to determine and if surgery is planned for stage II and III cancers. Radiation therapy may be used before or after surgery and can be delivered either by external beam (**teletherapy**) or with an internal source (**brachytherapy**).

An older method was to deliver radiation therapy to the client for 6 weeks before surgery to shrink the tumor and possibly inhibit recurrence. Although this method is still used, it is not the standard of care.

Intracavitary Radiation. If intracavitary radiation therapy (IRT [brachytherapy]) is selected, the radiologist places an applicator within the woman's uterus through the vagina while she is anesthetized. After the correct position of the applicator is confirmed by x-ray, the client is taken to the hospital room and a radiologist places a radioactive isotope in the applicator, which remains for 1 to 3 days. The goal of intracavity radiation is to prevent vaginal recurrence.

Before the procedure, instruct the client about activities she will need to perform (e.g., deep breathing and leg exercises) and restrictions during the time the radiation source is in place. While the radioactive implant is in place, the client is strictly isolated, usually in a private room, because radiation is emitted and can affect other people. The amount of time needed for the therapy depends on the amount of radiation emitted from the source. The radiologist calculates the time need for a specific dose of radiation. Usually this time ranges from 35 to 60 hours.

Inform the client that she is restricted to bedrest on her back with the head of the bed flat or slightly elevated. Movement in bed is restricted to prevent dislodgment of the radioactive source. Assess the skin for breakdown over bony pressure points during the activity restriction period.

A Foley catheter is inserted into the bladder before the implant to prevent dislodgment of the implant, which can be caused by a full bladder or attempts to void. Encourage fluid intake to prevent urine stasis and infection. A low-residue diet is prescribed (to prevent bowel movements that might dislodge the implant). The health care provider usually prescribes the following:

- Antiemetics
- Broad-spectrum antibiotics (to prevent bladder infections)
- Tranquilizers (to help the client relax)
- Analgesics
- Heparin or Lovenox (to prevent thromboembolism)
- Antidiarrheal medications (to prevent bowel movements)

Practice radiation precautions while the implant is in place. Organize care so that minimal time is spent close to the radiation source. Chart 78-13 lists the best practices for care of the client with sealed implant radiation sources.

External Radiation. External radiation therapy may be used to treat any stage of endometrial cancer in combination with surgery. Depending on the extent of the tumor, external radiation is given on an ambulatory care basis for 4 to 6 weeks. Tissue around the tumor and pelvic wall nodes also are irradiated. Specific instructions for the woman undergoing external radiation for endometrial cancer include monitoring for signs of skin breakdown, especially in the perineal area; no sunbathing; and not removing the markings outlining the treatment site. Inform the client that cystitis, diarrhea, and

BEST PRACTICE for
Care of the Client with Sealed Implants of Radioactive Sources

- Assign the client to a private room with a private bath.
- Place a "Caution: Radioactive Material" sign on the door of the client's room.
- Wear a dosimeter film badge at all times while caring for clients with radioactive implants. The badge offers no protection but measures an individual's exposure to radiation. Each badge should be used by only one individual.
- Wear a lead shielding apron; always face the radiation source (do not turn your back toward the source).
- Stay as far away from the radiation source as possible.
- Pregnant nurses, or those who are trying to become pregnant, should not care for these clients; do not allow pregnant women or children younger than 16 years of age to visit.
- Limit each visitor to one-half hour per day. Be sure visitors are at least 6 feet from the source.
- Never touch the radioactive source with bare hands. In the rare instance that it is dislodged, use a long-handled forceps to retrieve it. Deposit the radioactive source in the lead container kept in the client's room.
- Save all dressings and bed linens until after the radioactive source is removed. After the source is removed, dispose of dressings and linens in the usual manner. Other equipment can be removed from the room at any time.

anorexia are common during the weeks of therapy (see also Chapter 28).

Chemotherapy. Chemotherapy is an adjuvant treatment used when the risk for distant spread exceeds 20%. Usually combinations of three agents are given for chemotherapy. Although the combination can vary, the three most common agents recommended as chemotherapy for endometrial cancer are doxorubicin, cisplatin, and paclitaxel. Chapter 28 lists specific information about these agents and nursing care needs for clients during treatment. Chemotherapy is used as palliative treatment in advanced and recurrent disease.

Other Drug Therapy. Hormone therapy can be used for stage I and II cancers that are estrogen dependent and for palliative treatment of stage IV cancer. The hormones commonly prescribed are medroxyprogesterone acetate (Depo-Provera) and megestrol acetate (Megace). Tamoxifen citrate (Nolvadex❋, Tamofen❋), an anti-estrogen, is also used. The progestational agents do not cause acute side effects, but nausea and vomiting and hot flushes are associated with tamoxifen.

SURGICAL MANAGEMENT. Surgical management is the standard for tumors that are stage IC and higher if the client's general health permits. The gynecology oncologist usually performs a total abdominal hysterectomy (TAH) (removal of the uterus and cervix) and bilateral salpingo-oophorectomy (removal of both tubes and ovaries) for stage I tumors without cervical involvement. A radical hysterectomy (see Table 78-6) with bilateral pelvic lymph node dissection is performed for stage II cancer. Nursing care for a radical hysterectomy is the same as that for a TAH except that the woman's hospitalization is usually longer and her convalescence may be extended.

Critical Thinking Challenge

You are the charge nurse of a small medical-surgical nursing unit. Three of your clients are undergoing radiation therapy with a sealed radiation source. One client, a woman in her 70s, has just been admitted from the radiology department, where a position-fixing device was placed to hold a sealed radiation source. Within the next hour, she will be receiving radiation therapy with a sealed source for the next 50 hours. She has a number of medications prescribed for her heart failure (which is why she is having radiation therapy rather than surgery). She had a hip replacement last year. All together, you have 22 clients in your care. Your personnel include one LPN who is pregnant, two unlicensed assistive personnel, and another RN. This nurse is assigned to care for both of the other clients receiving brachytherapy.

1. Which person should you assign to care for this 70-year-old client? Provide a rationale for your choice.
2. What precautions will you institute to prevent skin breakdown?
3. Your unit does not have a lead-lined room. What type of room arrangements should you make to reduce radiation exposure to other clients, visitors, and staff?

evolve For suggested answer guidelines, go to http://evolve.elsevier.com/Iggy/.

Community-Based Care

HOME CARE MANAGEMENT

The client with endometrial cancer is managed at home unless surgery is indicated. After surgery, the client is usually discharged to her home. Home care after surgery for endometrial cancer is the same as that after a hysterectomy (see Operative Procedures [Uterine Leiomyomas], p. 1839). Clients who are receiving chemotherapy or external radiation therapy are usually treated on an ambulatory care basis. Help the client and her family plan daily activities around trips to the clinic or the health care provider's office. If the tumor recurs and cure is not likely, the client and her family need to think about hospice care and whether the client can be cared for in the home.

HEALTH TEACHING

For the woman who has undergone a hysterectomy for endometrial cancer, the teaching plan is the same as that for the woman who has undergone a hysterectomy for uterine leiomyomas (see Postoperative Care [Uterine Leiomyomas], p. 1840). Side effects to report to the health care provider include vaginal or rectal bleeding, foul-smelling discharge, abdominal pain or distention, and hematuria.

The high dose of radiation causes sterility, and vaginal shrinkage can occur. Vaginal dilators can be used with water-soluble lubricants for 10 minutes each day until sexual activity resumes (in 10 days to 6 weeks). Reassure the woman that she is not radioactive and that her partner will not "catch" cancer by engaging in sexual intercourse. A normal diet can be resumed.

Review all prescribed drugs, including the dosage and schedule, effects, and side effects. Emphasize the importance of keeping appointments for follow-up care.

PSYCHOSOCIAL PREPARATION

Clients need to discuss their concerns about the presence of cancer and the potential for recurrence. Provide emotional support and create an atmosphere that encourages the woman to ask questions or express her fears and concerns.

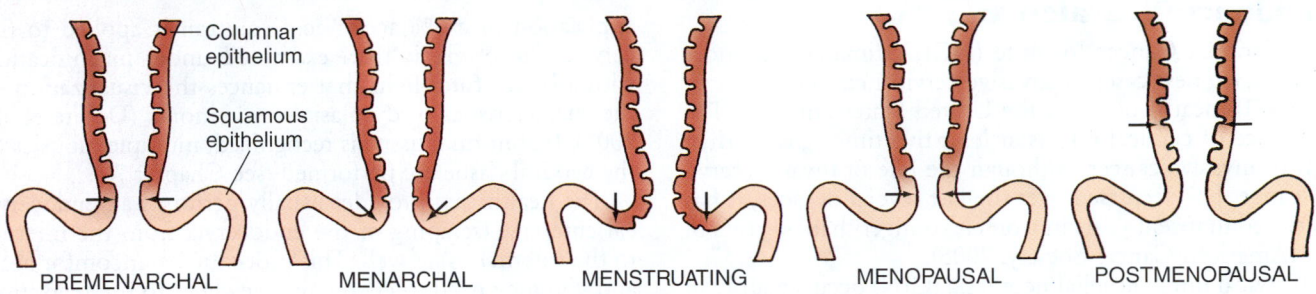

Figure 78-5 ■ The location of the translocation zones at various stages of adult development.

Include family members or significant others in discussions when possible.

Reactions to radiation therapy vary. Some clients may feel radioactive or "unclean" after treatments and may exhibit withdrawal behaviors. Correct such misconceptions.

Clients who have chemotherapy may be upset if **alopecia** (hair loss) occurs. Warn the client of this possibility before treatment starts. Wigs, scarves, or turbans can be worn until regrowth occurs.

Often clients experience emotional crises because of the physical effects of cancer treatments. Radical hysterectomy may be seen as mutilating, and both radiation and chemotherapy have side effects that change the client's appearance. A client may have a grief reaction to this perceived change in body image. The feelings of loss depend on the visibility of the loss, the function of the loss, and the amount of emotional investment. Help the client adapt to the body changes. One way to do this is to encourage self-care as soon as the client's condition is stable. Use a calm, accepting attitude.

Death can occur with or without treatment. Clients and their families or significant others have concerns about recurrence. All want to pass the 5-year survival mark without a recurrence. If there is a recurrence, the client may be hostile and may have manifestations of a grief reaction. Encourage clients to ventilate their feelings. Response to loss and grieving are discussed in Chapter 9.

HEALTH CARE RESOURCES

In the United States, local American Cancer Society chapters provide written materials about endometrial cancer as well as information about local support groups. If the client is in the terminal stages of cancer, hospice care may be appropriate (see Chapter 9). If nursing care is needed at home, the hospital nurse or case manager refers the client and her family to a community health or home care agency. A referral to a social services agency may be needed if the client is unable to meet the financial demands of treatment and long-term follow-up.

Cervical Cancer
PATHOPHYSIOLOGY

Cervical cancer is a common reproductive cancer among women in the United States. This disorder is a progression from totally normal cervical cells to premalignant changes in appearance of cervical cells (dysplasia), to changes in function and, ultimately, transformation to cancer.

TABLE 78-9 Clinical Staging of Cervical Cancer*

Stage	Characteristics
I	Carcinoma is strictly confined to cervix (extension to corpus should be disregarded).
II	Carcinoma extends beyond cervix but has not extended to pelvic wall; it involves vagina, but not as far as lower third.
III	Carcinoma has extended to pelvic wall; on rectal examination, there is no cancer-free space between tumor and pelvic wall; tumor involves lower third of vagina; all cases with hydronephrosis or nonfunctioning kidney should be included unless they are known to be due to another cause.
IV	Carcinoma has extended beyond true pelvis or has clinically involved mucosa of bladder or rectum

*An a, b, or c designation at any stage indicates specific degree or depth of spread within that stage.

Premalignant changes are described on a continuum from dysplasia (the earliest premalignant change) to carcinoma in situ (CIS) (the most advanced premalignant change).

Once cervical cancer has developed, it is described as preinvasive or invasive. Preinvasive cancer is limited to the cervix; invasive cancer is in the cervix and other pelvic structures. Preinvasive lesions usually begin in the area called the *transformation zone* (Figure 78-5). This area includes the squamocolumnar junction, which is located near the external cervical os, where changes in the squamous and columnar (glandular) epithelium normally occur. Preinvasive cancers are also termed *cervical intraepithelial neoplasia (CIN)* and classified according to severity:
- CIN I: mild
- CIN II: moderate
- CIN III: severe to carcinoma in situ

Most cervical cancer (90%) arises from the squamous cells, and only 5% arise from the mucous secreting cells (adenocarcinoma). Squamous cell cancers spread by direct extension to the vaginal mucosa, lower uterine segment, parametrium, pelvic wall, bladder, and bowel. Metastasis is usually confined to the pelvis, but distant spread can occur through lymphatic spread and the circulation to the liver, lungs, or bones. Table 78-9 shows the staging of cervical cancer.

Etiology

The exact cause of squamous cell cervical cancer is unknown, but many factors appear to be involved. Table 78-8 lists risk factors for cervical cancer.

Incidence/Prevalence

The National Cancer Institute (NCI) estimates that more than 10,370 new cases of invasive cervical cancer and more than 3710 deaths occur in the United States annually. The incidence of cervical CIS is at least five times greater than that of invasive cancer. Although the rate of invasive cervical cancer has decreased over the last several decades, it has increased in recent years in women younger than 50 years of age (American Cancer Society, 2005).

Cervical intraepithelial neoplasia (CIN) occurs mainly in young women; the peak incidence of dysplasia occurs in clients in their mid-20s. CIS occurs in women about 30 years old, and invasive cancer occurs most commonly in the late 40s.

Invasive cervical cancer is the third most common cause of death related to reproductive cancers (American Cancer Society, 2005). Death rates for cervical cancer have dropped 50% in the past two decades because of mass screening of premalignant and early stage cancer through Pap tests.

◆ COLLABORATIVE MANAGEMENT
◆ Assessment

PHYSICAL ASSESSMENT/CLINICAL MANIFESTATIONS

The client who has preinvasive cancer is often asymptomatic. The classic symptom of invasive cancer is painless vaginal bleeding. The bleeding may start as spotting between menstrual periods or after coitus or douching. As the cancer grows, bleeding increases in frequency, duration, and amount and may become continuous.

The client may also have a watery, blood-tinged vaginal discharge that becomes dark and foul-smelling as the disease progresses. Leg pain (along the sciatic nerve) or swelling of one leg may be a late symptom or may indicate recurrent disease. Flank pain may be a late symptom of hydronephrosis, indicating advanced disease or recurrence. Other signs of recurrence or metastasis include unexplained weight loss, pelvic pain (caused by pressure of the tumor on the bladder or the bowel), **dysuria** (painful urination), **hematuria** (bloody urine), rectal bleeding, chest pain, and coughing. A physical examination may not reveal any abnormalities in early preinvasive cervical cancer; the internal pelvic examination may identify late-stage disease.

DIAGNOSTIC ASSESSMENT

Diagnostic assessment for cervical cancer begins with a Pap smear. If the results are abnormal, the smear is repeated before further studies are done. If abnormal tissue is detected on a subsequent Pap test, further testing is done, depending on the type of abnormality present (squamous atypia, inflammatory atypia, or minor atypia). These atypical cells are categorized more definitely, regardless of whether dysplasia is present, by the Bethesda System (TBS) for the specific type of follow-up needed. If invasive cervical cancer is diagnosed, laboratory tests such as those described earlier for the investigation of endometrial cancer are performed (see Assessment [Endometrial Cancer], p. 1843).

The health care provider may perform a colposcopic examination to view the transformation zone, where dysplasia, cervical intraepithelial neoplasia (CIN), and carcinoma in situ (CIS) often arise. Colposcopy is a procedure in which application of a 3% acetic acid solution is applied to the cervix. The cervix is then examined under magnification with a bright filter light that enhances the visualization of the characteristics of dysplasia or carcinoma (DeVita et al., 2001). If abnormal tissue is recognized, multiple biopsies of the cervical tissue are performed (see Chapter 76).

The health care provider usually performs an endocervical curettage (scraping of the endocervix from the internal to the external os) as well. This procedure is uncomfortable, and you may need to encourage the client to use relaxation or breathing exercises to cope with the cramping and pain. Inform the client that a small amount of bleeding is expected for up to 2 weeks after the biopsies.

◆ Interventions

Care of the client with cervical cancer is similar to that for endometrial cancer. Interventions discussed here are those that differ from those for the client with endometrial cancer.

NONSURGICAL MANAGEMENT. Nonsurgical interventions for cervical cancer depend on the stage of disease. Early management techniques include local ablation therapies of electrosurgical excision, laser therapy, or cryosurgery. Radiation therapy or chemotherapy is usually used along with surgery for later-stage disease. Factors that influence the choice of localized treatment versus surgical intervention include client health, tumor size, stage, cancer cell type, degree of lymph node involvement, risk factors for surgical complications, and client preference.

Loop Electrosurgical Excision Procedure. The loop electrosurgical excision procedure (LEEP) is rapidly becoming the nonsurgical management of choice for intraepithelial lesions. This procedure is short (10 to 30 minutes) and is performed in a physician's office or in a clinic setting with a local anesthetic injected into the cervix. A thin loop-wire electrode that transmits a painless electrical current is used to cut away or "peel off" affected tissue. Unlike laser or cryotherapy, in which tissue is destroyed, LEEP results in a specimen that can be examined by a pathologist to ensure the lesion was completely removed.

Little discomfort is associated with this procedure. Spotting after the procedure is common. Instruct clients to adhere for 3 weeks to the restrictions listed in Chart 78-14.

Laser Therapy. Laser therapy is an office procedure used for CIN. A laser beam is directed to the abnormal tissues, where energy from the beam is absorbed by the fluid in the tissues, causing them to vaporize. A small amount of bleeding occurs with the procedure, and the client may have a slight vaginal discharge. Healing occurs in 6 to 12 weeks.

CHART 78-14

CLIENT EDUCATION GUIDE
Care After Local Cervical Ablation Therapy

- Refrain from sexual intercourse.
- Do not use tampons.
- Do not douche.
- Take showers rather than tub baths.
- Avoid lifting heavy objects.
- Report any heavy vaginal bleeding, foul-smelling drainage, or fever.

The usual time period for these restrictions is 3 weeks. Your health care provider may prescribe a different (longer or shorter) time frame for you.

A disadvantage of this procedure is that no specimen is available for study.

Cryotherapy. Cryotherapy is another common treatment for CIN. A probe is placed against the cervix to cause freezing of the tissues and subsequent necrosis. The procedure is painless, although some clients have slight cramping after the procedure. The client has a heavy watery discharge for several weeks after the procedure. Instruct her to follow the restrictions in Chart 78-14.

Radiation Therapy. Radiation therapy is reserved for invasive cervical cancer. For cancer that has extended beyond the cervix but not to the pelvic wall, radiation therapy is as effective as a radical hysterectomy. Intracavitary and external radiation therapies are used in combination, depending on the extent and location of the lesion. Intracavitary implants are usually used after the client has completed 5 to 6 weeks of external pelvic radiation in combination with chemotherapy. The procedure is similar to that described for endometrial cancer. Nursing care related to radiation therapy is presented in the earlier discussion of endometrial cancer (see p. 1843 and Chapter 28).

Chemotherapy. Cervical cancer generally responds poorly to chemotherapy. These agents are usually reserved for locally advanced carcinomas, unresectable recurrent tumors, or widely metastatic disease (DeVita et al., 2001). Agents shown to be somewhat effective for cervical cancer include paclitaxel, carboplatin, ifosfamide, hydroxyurea, fluorouracil, and irinotecan. See Chapter 28 for more information about these drugs.

SURGICAL MANAGEMENT. The surgical procedure for cervical cancer depends on the extent of the disease and whether the client wants to have children. Clinical staging is performed before surgery to establish the extent of the disease. Small tumors that are only microinvasive are managed conservatively with excisional conization or hysterectomy. Early stage invasive cancers are managed with radical surgery and radiation. Locally advanced cancers are managed with radiation.

Conization. Conization is used to treat clients with microinvasive cervical cancer, especially when preservation of fertility is desired. This procedure is done when the lesion cannot be visualized by colposcopic examination. A cone-shaped area of cervix is removed surgically and sent to the laboratory to determine the extent of the cancer. Potential complications from this procedure include hemorrhage, uterine perforation, incompetent cervix, cervical canal narrowing, and preterm labor for future pregnancies. Long-term follow-up care is needed because new lesions can develop.

Hysterectomy. A simple hysterectomy may be performed as treatment of microinvasive cancer if the client does not desire childbearing. A vaginal approach is commonly used. A radical hysterectomy and bilateral pelvic lymph node dissection are as effective as radiation is for treating cancer that has extended beyond the cervix but not to the pelvic wall. Care for clients undergoing hysterectomy is found under Operative Procedures (Uterine Leiomyomas), p. 1839.

Pelvic Exenteration. One of the most radical surgical procedures is **pelvic exenteration.** It is performed for recurrent cancers if there is no evidence of tumor outside the pelvis and no lymph node involvement.

Preoperative Care. Assess the client scheduled for a pelvic exenteration for anxiety, concerns about the impact on sexual function, and the ability to adjust to her altered body image. Involve family members or partners in discussions about postoperative expectations. Physical preparation includes selection of stoma sites, extensive bowel preparation, and extensive radiographic and laboratory tests to assess for spread of cancer outside the pelvis. Teach the client about the following:

- Recovery after surgery in a critical care unit
- Pain management
- Presence of numerous intravenous (IV) and arterial catheters
- Nasogastric suction
- Colostomy and/or urinary diversion (e.g., ileal conduit, Kock ileal urinary pouch)

Operative Procedures. The three types of exenteration are anterior, posterior, and total (Figure 78-6). Anterior exenteration is the removal of the uterus, cervix, ovaries, fal-

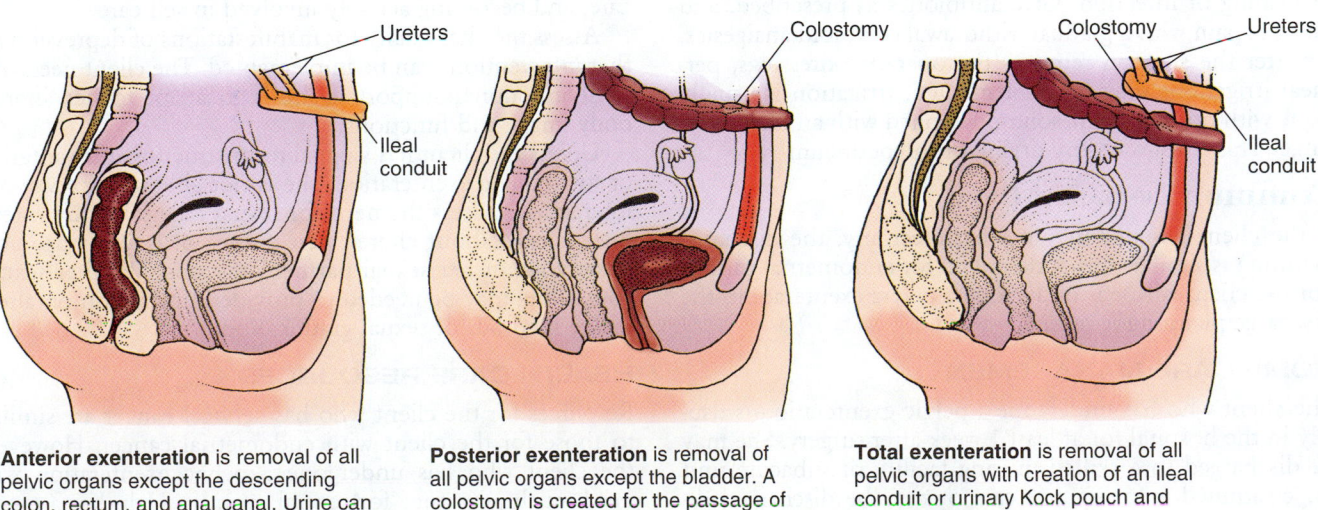

Anterior exenteration is removal of all pelvic organs except the descending colon, rectum, and anal canal. Urine can be diverted into an ileal conduit or urinary Kock pouch.

Posterior exenteration is removal of all pelvic organs except the bladder. A colostomy is created for the passage of feces.

Total exenteration is removal of all pelvic organs with creation of an ileal conduit or urinary Kock pouch and a colostomy.

Figure 78-6 ■ Pelvic exenteration.

lopian tubes, vagina, bladder, urethra, and pelvic lymph nodes. Posterior exenteration is the removal of the uterus, cervix, ovaries, fallopian tubes, descending colon, rectum, and anal canal. Total exenteration is a combination of anterior and posterior procedures. When the bladder is removed, urine is diverted through a urinary diversion (e.g., ileal conduit or Kock ileal urinary pouch). When the colon, rectum, and anal canal are removed, a colostomy is created for passage of feces. The stomas are located on the abdomen, the colostomy on the left and the ileal conduit on the right.

Postoperative Care. After surgery, the client often is admitted to a critical care unit for the first 1 to 2 days because of the high risk for complications resulting from this massive surgery. Assess for the following:

- Hemorrhage and shock
- Pulmonary complications such as atelectasis and pneumonia
- Fluid and electrolyte imbalances such as metabolic acidosis or alkalosis and dehydration
- Renal or urinary complications
- Pain

Assist the client with deep breathing and coughing hourly. Monitor urine output and specific gravity, parenteral nutrition, and provide colostomy and urinary diversion care.

Once the client's condition is stable, she returns to the medical-surgical unit when normal postoperative interventions are continued. During the recovery period, assess for the following:

- Late cardiovascular complications such as deep vein thrombosis and pulmonary emboli
- Gastrointestinal (GI) complications, such as paralytic ileus
- Wound infections
- Wound dehiscence or evisceration
- Pain

Prophylactic heparin or low-molecular weight heparin (enoxaparin [Lovenox]) may be prescribed. Maintain the use of anti-embolism stockings or sequential compression devices (SCDs) for the prevention of thrombosis. Auscultate the lungs at least twice per shift. Assess the abdomen for the presence of bowel sounds and the wound for indications of healing or infection. Give antibiotics as prescribed, and manage pain with a gradual withdrawal of opioid analgesics.

After the surgeon removes the operative dressings, perineal irrigations may be implemented. Irrigation is usually done with normal saline solution applied with an Asepto syringe. This is followed by drying of the perineum.

Community-Based Care

If the client has undergone a hysterectomy, the discharge planning is similar to that described for endometrial cancer. For the client who has undergone a pelvic exenteration, the discharge planning is more involved.

HOME CARE MANAGEMENT

The client who has undergone a pelvic exenteration is usually in the hospital for at least 1 week after surgery. She may be discharged to a skilled nursing facility or subacute unit for continued recovery and care or may be discharged directly to home. When the client returns home, she needs assistance. She is not able to engage in strenuous activities associated with most household work for up to 6 months. The

family may need to consider outside help if there is no one in the family who can assume household responsibilities.

No special equipment is needed in the home, although a foam mattress or other special pressure-relieving device may be placed on the bed to prevent skin breakdown and to increase comfort. Colostomy and ureterostomy pouches and equipment for changing the pouches can be purchased in local pharmacies.

HEALTH TEACHING

Collaborate with the wound and ostomy care nurse to teach the woman who has undergone a pelvic exenteration how to manage new functions with equipment (colostomy and urinary diversion). Teach the client or family how to provide wound care and other aspects of self-care. The perineal opening may drain mucus for several months to a year. The client can wear sanitary napkins if they are beltless (so as not to interfere with the stomas). The client may need help in adjusting her diet to maintain high nutritional requirements for healing while selecting foods that are tolerated. Teach the client about the effects, dosages, and side effects of all prescribed drugs.

Sexual function is different after exenteration (even if an artificial vagina is constructed), and the couple may need counseling about alternatives to intercourse. Even with vaginal reconstruction, the use of vaginal dilators is necessary to achieve desired sexual function.

Physical activities are limited during convalescence. Until walking is permitted, encourage range-of-motion exercises. Follow-up care is important. Counsel the client about keeping all follow-up appointments. Provide information about late complications (e.g., infection, bowel obstruction) so that the client can seek medical care promptly.

PSYCHOSOCIAL PREPARATION

Usually by 3 to 5 days after surgery, the client begins expressing grief about her body changes. At first she may deny changes by refusing to look at the wound or stoma sites. Later she may become depressed or withdrawn or even angry or hostile. She may then move to reality testing by asking questions about her care, watching the nurses do wound care, and becoming actively involved in self-care.

Assess the client daily for manifestations of depression so that interventions can be implemented. The client needs intense emotional support if she is to adapt to her altered body image and functions.

Unless the client has vaginal reconstruction after anterior or total pelvic exenteration, she is not able to have vaginal intercourse. Assess the need for sexual counseling by listening for cues about altered perceptions of body image and anxiety about her sexual partner's response. Further sexual counseling may be needed to provide information on alternative methods of sexual gratification.

HEALTH CARE RESOURCES

Resources for the client who has cervical cancer are similar to those for the client with endometrial cancer. However, the client who has undergone a pelvic exenteration will need much assistance for several months. Help her arrange for transportation and home care. A home care nurse can assist with dressing changes, ostomy care, and perform assessments for several weeks after discharge to home. Assistance

TABLE 78-10   Risk Factors for Ovarian Cancer and Vulvar Cancer

Ovarian Cancer	Vulvar Cancer
Age over 40 years	Age over 40 years
Family history	Cervical cancer
Diabetes mellitus	Diabetes mellitus
Nulliparity	Hypertension
>30 years of age at first pregnancy	Obesity
Breast cancer	Infection with human papilloma virus (types 16, 18)
Colorectal cancer	Cervical cancer
Infertility	Smoking
BRCA1 or BRCA2 gene mutations	

TABLE 78-11   Clinical Staging of Ovarian Cancer*

Stage	Characteristics
I	Growth is limited to ovaries.
II	Growth involves one or both ovaries with pelvic extension.
III	Tumor involves one or both ovaries with peritoneal implants outside the pelvis or positive retroperitoneal or inguinal nodes; superficial liver metastasis but with histologically proven malignant extension to small bowel or omentum.
IV	Growth involving one or both ovaries with distant metastases; if pleural effusion is present, there must be positive cytologic findings to allot a case to stage IV; parenchymal liver metastasis equals stage IV.

*An a, b, or c designation at any stage indicates specific degree or depth of spread within that stage.

with self-care, meal preparation, and home maintenance are usually needed.

Ovarian Cancer

PATHOPHYSIOLOGY

Etiology and Genetic Risk

Of all ovarian cancers, more than 90% are epithelial tumors; the most common type is serous adenocarcinoma. These tumors grow rapidly, spread quickly, and are often bilateral. In addition to metastasizing by direct extension into nearby organs and through blood and lymph circulation to distant sites, ovarian cancer also spreads through the abdomen by seeding free-floating cancer cells. This type of spread usually occurs with ascites.

The cause of ovarian cancer is not precisely known. Table 78-10 lists known and suspected risk factors for ovarian cancer.

Genetic Considerations

About 10% of ovarian cancer cases are related to known gene mutations. Hereditary breast-ovarian cancer syndrome (HBOC) is associated with specific mutations of the *BRCA1* gene locus that are inherited in an autosomal dominant pattern. Testing to determine gene carrier status for *BRCA1* mutations is available for clients with a family predisposition to breast or ovarian cancer. Hereditary ovarian cancer also may be a part of the hereditary nonpolyposis colorectal cancer syndrome (HNPCC). See Chapter 11 for more information about hereditary ovarian cancer.

Incidence/Prevalence

Ovarian cancer is the leading cause of death from female reproductive cancers. About 23,300 new cases are diagnosed each year, and 13,900 deaths occur each year (American Cancer Society, 2005). Survival rates continue to be low because ovarian cancer is not often detected in its early stages. The incidence increases in women older than 50 years of age and peaks at 60 to 64 years of age.

◆ COLLABORATIVE MANAGEMENT
◆ Assessment

Clients with ovarian cancer may complain of abdominal pain or swelling or have vague symptoms of abdominal dis-comfort, such as dyspepsia, indigestion, gas and distention, and other mild GI disturbances. The client may have a history of ovarian imbalance, such as evidenced by premenstrual tension, heavy menstrual flow or dysfunctional bleeding, or infertility.

The only sign may be an abdominal mass, which may be noticed only after it reaches a size of 6 inches (15 cm). Most pelvic examinations do not identify abnormalities. However, an enlarged ovary found after menopause should be evaluated as though it were malignant.

The client with ovarian cancer has concerns similar to those described for the client with endometrial cancer. Because the cancer is often diagnosed in an advanced stage, fears of death and dying are common and may be more of a concern than the proposed treatments.

Cytologic examination has limited application because a Pap smear is abnormal in only 20% to 30% of clients with ovarian cancer, even in advanced cases. Diagnosis depends on surgical exploration. Usually a complete laboratory workup is done before exploratory surgery, including a complete blood count, urinalysis, and liver studies if ascites occurs.

The level of ovarian antibody designated as CA-125 may be elevated if ovarian cancer is present. This test may be useful in monitoring a client's progress after treatment, but it may not be as useful for diagnostic purposes. The CA-125 tumor marker is often elevated by benign conditions, such as endometriosis, fibroids, pelvic inflammatory disease (PID), liver disease, heart failure, and diverticulitis (DeVita et al., 2001).

Ultrasonography, intravenous pyelography (IVP), computed tomography (CT), and radiography are used in detecting ovarian tumors. In addition, a barium enema study and an upper GI radiographic series can be performed to rule out tumor in the adjacent structures.

Exploratory laparotomy is performed to diagnose and stage ovarian tumors. Ovarian cancer is staged when it is removed (Table 78-11).

Critical Thinking Challenge

The client is a 34-year-old woman who has been diagnosed with ovarian cancer. She is a twin, and her sister was diagnosed with breast cancer 1 year ago. Her mother died from

Continued

ovarian cancer at 40 years of age. The client has one child. Her other health problems include pregnancy-induced hypertension and rheumatoid arthritis. She had cryotherapy for cervical dysplasia when she was 25 years old. Her history and physical examination revealed the following problems or manifestations: migraine headaches, 10-lb weight gain in the past 6 months, seasonal pollen allergies, GERD, irregular menses, and intermittent constipation.

1. What risk factors, if any, does she have for ovarian cancer?
2. Which of her previous or current health problems or manifestations may contribute to or be a result of ovarian cancer?
3. She is scheduled for a hysterectomy and an oophorectomy and surgical staging procedure.
4. What preoperative teaching will you emphasize?
5. How will you approach the issue of fertility with this client?

evolve For suggested answer guidelines, go to http://evolve.elsevier.com/Iggy/.

◆Interventions

Nursing care of the client with ovarian cancer is similar to that of the client with endometrial or cervical cancer. The options for treatment depend on the extent of the cancer and include chemotherapy, immunotherapy, radiation therapy (external or intraperitoneal), and surgery.

NONSURGICAL MANAGEMENT. After surgery, chemotherapy and radiation therapy are the two most common nonsurgical options for ovarian cancer.

Chemotherapy. The oncologist usually prescribes chemotherapy after surgery for all stages of ovarian cancer. Cisplatin, carboplatin, and paclitaxel (Taxol) are the most common agents used for treating ovarian cancer. Chemotherapy is usually given every 3 to 4 weeks for six cycles on an inpatient or an ambulatory basis.

Radiation Therapy. External radiation therapy is used after surgery if tumors have invaded other pelvic or abdominal organs. It may be given with chemotherapy or alone (see Chapter 28).

SURGICAL MANAGEMENT. Total abdominal hysterectomy and bilateral salpingo-oophorectomy are the surgical procedures for all stages of ovarian cancer. Surgery confirms disease, allows for surgical staging, and can debulk or remove the tumor. When cancer has spread to other abdominal organs or lymph nodes, they can be resected during the surgery. Some clients with advanced disease may undergo neoadjuvant chemotherapy before tumor debulking surgery.

Ovarian cancer is staged during surgery (see Table 78-11). The client usually has a vertical incision instead of a horizontal incision. This incision improves the surgeon's ability to assess disease in the upper abdomen. If disease is present on the omentum, it is removed. The upper abdomen evaluation continues with inspection of the diaphragm, liver serosa, and parenchyma. Peritoneal washings; frozen sections of the pelvic mass; and biopsies of the pelvic organs, diaphragm, and lymph nodes are sent to pathology during the surgery.

After surgery, nursing care of the client is similar to that of the client undergoing a hysterectomy for uterine leiomyomas. The vertical incision is assessed in the same fashion as a horizontal abdominal incision.

A "second-look" procedure (laparoscopy or laparotomy) is performed, usually after 1 year of chemotherapy, to con-

EVIDENCE-BASED PRACTICE for Nursing

What impact does ovarian cancer have on women and their families?

Howel, D, Fitch, M.I., & Deane, K.A. (2003). Impact of ovarian cancer perceived by women. *Cancer Nursing, 26*(1):1-9.

This study was conducted to increase health care professionals' understanding of the following: about the impact of ovarian cancer on day-to-day living, the major challenges women and their families face in dealing with ovarian cancer, and the availability of support systems for clients and their families. The researchers in this study interviewed 18 women diagnosed with ovarian cancer. The participants were asked to describe their experiences in living with this disease. The participant's ages ranged from 35 to 73 years. The diagnosis of ovarian cancer occurred as recently as 5 months to 12 years before the interview. More than half of the women were married and had children, had higher education levels, and were unemployed because of their age or disability.

Level of Evidence: 6—Uncontrolled case series, qualitative study.

Critique. The investigators used accepted techniques for qualitative study to ensure data collection to saturation and validated the results with the participants.

Implications for Nursing. Nurses are often the first line of support for clients with cancer, and these clients rely on nurses for help. It is critical, therefore, that nurses understand the concept of family-centered care. This study reveals the need for sensitivity in dealing with: life changes, financial support, disability, coping skills, anxiety or depression, and access to palliative care programs. Further nursing research focusing on the impact of living with the uncertainty of death and ovarian cancer in the clients and their families, particularly children, is needed.

firm the absence or presence of tumor and to remove any new or residual tumor if it was too large to be removed at the first operation. Nursing care is similar to that of the client after any major abdominal surgery.

The client who is faced with the diagnosis of advanced ovarian cancer may be concerned about dying. Encourage her to ventilate her feelings about her diagnosis. Provide realistic assurance as well as accurate information about treatments. Providing continuity of care, with at least one regular caregiver, may be helpful. Encourage the client to use her support system, including family members, friends, and a spiritual leader, such as a rabbi or other clergy member. A visit from another woman who has survived a similar disease may decrease fears.

If there is recurrence, the client may deny symptoms at first or express feelings of anger and grief. The family is often fearful of the outcome (see the Evidence-Based Practice for Nursing box above). Provide encouragement and support during this difficult time, and help the client and her family work through their grief and prepare for death.

Vulvar Cancer

PATHOPHYSIOLOGY
Etiology

Most vulvar cancers (90%) are squamous cell carcinomas. The remaining 10% are adenocarcinomas, sarcomas, and Paget's disease. Most vulvar cancers do not have premalignant changes in the epithelium.

Vulvar cancer is slow growing, stays localized for a long time, and metastasizes late. The first change is usually vulvar atypia or mild dysplasia (vulvar intraepithelial neoplasia [VIN] I), followed by moderate dysplasia (VIN II) and then severe dysplasia or carcinoma in situ (VIN III) until the lesion becomes invasive. Vulvar cancer can spread directly to the urethra, the vagina, or the anus and through the lymphatic system to the inguinal, femoral, and deep iliac pelvic nodes.

The cause of vulvar cancer is unknown, although a strong relationship exists between vulvar cancer and herpes simplex type II, human papillomavirus, and capsid antigen. Other risk factors for vulvar cancer are listed in Table 78-10. Guidelines for the early detection and prevention of vulvar cancer include performing monthly vulvar self-examination, having an annual pelvic examination, and practicing "safer sex."

Incidence/Prevalence

About 4000 new cases are diagnosed each year, and 800 deaths result from this disease annually (American Cancer Society, 2005). Vulvar cancer occurs most commonly in women 50 to 70 years of age. More than 50% of the cases of vulvar cancer occur in women older than 60 years of age.

◆COLLABORATIVE MANAGEMENT
◆Assessment

Women with vulvar lesions often report irritation or itching in their perineal area. Sometimes they describe a "sore that will not heal." Bleeding is a late symptom. Women usually try to treat themselves before seeking medical help. Often a lesion has been present for months or even years. Embarrassment may be one reason why older women delay seeking medical care.

Pelvic examinations usually show multifocal lesions, most often on the labia. The lesions may be whitish or reddish, and the vulvar skin may be excoriated as a result of irritation.

The client may be anxious or fearful about the diagnosis of cancer. She may have fears that her partner will reject her because of the diagnosis, or she may worry about disfigurement related to surgery. Assess the client's past experiences in coping with stressful situations and whether she has the psychological resources to cope with the current crisis.

A Pap smear and colposcopic examination of the vulva (see Assessment [Cervical Cancer], p. 1846) may aid in diagnosis. A toluidine blue test may be used to identify abnormal cells for biopsy. The solution is applied to the vulva and allowed to dry. Then a 1% acetic acid solution is applied. Biopsy of the areas that remain blue is performed. The test chemical stains nuclei in the superficial epithelium, where cells do not normally contain nuclei. An abnormal finding does not diagnose cancer because ulcerations also stain.

A biopsy of the lesion is needed for diagnosis. This is easily accomplished with a Keyes dermal punch (a device that removes a disk of tissue). Depending on the site of the lesion, one or more biopsy specimens may be taken. Excisional biopsies are preferred for smaller lesions.

Prognosis is related to lesion size, contour, mitotic activity, and whether cancer is present in the lymph nodes. Lesions larger than 5 cm in diameter with infiltrating margins and extensive necrosis are the most likely to recur after surgical resection. Clients with seven or more positive lymph nodes have a poorer prognosis (DeVita et al., 2001).

◆Interventions

Surgery is the major treatment aimed at curing vulvar cancer. Radiation therapy may be used for advanced cancer or for palliation.

NONSURGICAL MANAGEMENT

Laser Therapy. If a woman has premalignant vulvar lesions, laser therapy may be used (see p. 1846). The treatment is usually done on an outpatient basis; local, regional, or general anesthesia is used. Healing occurs over a period of several weeks, usually without scarring.

Radiation Therapy. External radiation therapy to the deep pelvic nodes may be used after surgery (see earlier discussion of endometrial cancer [p. 1843] and Chapter 28). Radiation treatments cause ulceration and dermatitis, which can be uncomfortable for the woman.

SURGICAL MANAGEMENT.
The surgeon performs a vulvectomy to remove the cancerous vulvar lesions.

Preoperative Care. The surgeon provides a complete explanation of the extent of the surgical procedure to be performed. Reinforce the information provided by the surgeon. Photographs of a healed vulvectomy or reconstructed vulva may help reassure the client about the expected cosmetic outcome. Specific care before a vulvectomy may include an abdominal or perineal shave, an enema, douching, and insertion of an indwelling catheter into the bladder.

Operative Procedures. Several surgical procedures are used for the treatment of vulvar cancer. A local wide excision may be used to remove the abnormal area (for carcinoma in situ [CIS]). A simple **vulvectomy** (removal of the vulva, the labia majora, the labia minora, and possibly the clitoris) may also be performed for CIS, but this disfiguring surgery is used less often today. Instead, a **skinning vulvectomy**—the removal of superficial vulvar skin (without removal of the clitoris) and replacement of removed skin with split-thickness grafts—is performed (Figure 78-7). Sexual function is less affected, and the appearance of the vulva is less changed.

For invasive cancer, a modified radical or **radical vulvectomy** (removal of the entire vulva skin, labia, clitoris, subcutaneous tissues, and possibly inguinal and femoral node dissection), may be performed, depending on node involvement (see Figure 78-7). Tumors that involve the anus, rectum, rectovaginal septum, or urethra usually require a pelvic exenteration with radical vulvectomy and bilateral groin dissection.

Postoperative Care. After surgery, multiple suction drains (Hemovac or Jackson-Pratt drains) are present in the inguinal or vulvar areas for wound drainage for 7 to 10 days. A pressure-reducing mattress may be placed on the bed to prevent pressure ulcers and increase comfort. A bed cradle may be used to keep linens off the incision site. The client usually wears antiembolism stockings or sequential compression devices to prevent thromboembolism and leg edema.

Providing Wound Care. The major focus of nursing care is wound healing. Change the dressings over the incision frequently because of the amount of wound drainage and the risk for infection. Wound complications, such as infection and dehiscence, often occur after vulvectomies, and the healing process may take up to 6 months. Meticulous

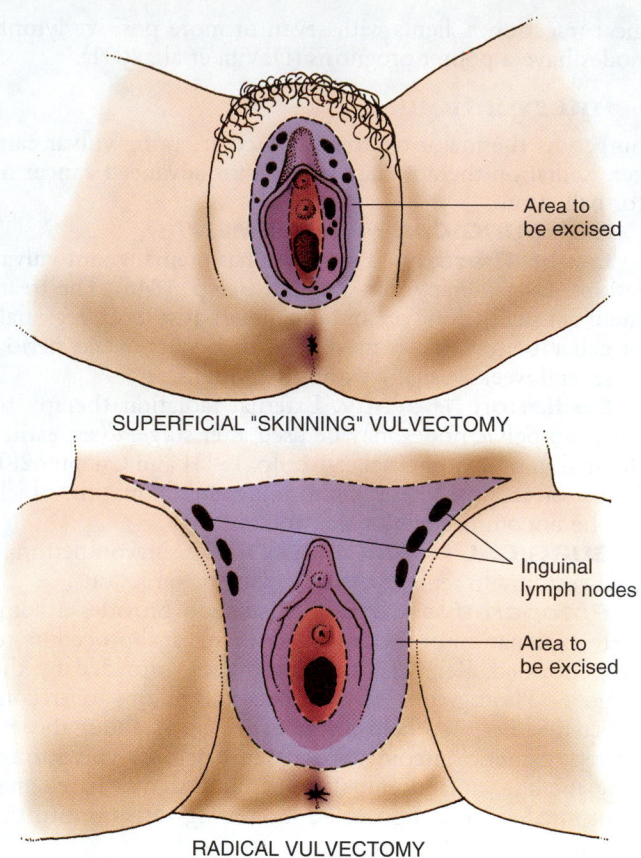

SUPERFICIAL "SKINNING" VULVECTOMY

Area to
be excised

Inguinal
lymph nodes

Area to
be excised

RADICAL VULVECTOMY

Figure 78-7 ■ Vulvectomy.

wound care is needed and may involve debridement. Rinse the area with a normal saline solution, using a bulb syringe or a water pick (on low pressure). Then dry the wound using a heat lamp or air-dry it with a hair dryer (using warm air). Wound care is usually done three or four times a day.

Depending on the client's hygiene and home situation, she may use a sitz bath, tub, or whirlpool bath once or twice a day for wound care. Teach the client that the tub should be meticulously cleaned each time before she uses it. A half cup of salt may be added to the water. If the client does not have access to a tub or whirlpool, a squeeze bottle or squirt gun can be filled with warm water or a saline solution and poured or squirted over the wound area.

Instruct the client to include foods rich in vitamin C, iron, and protein to promote wound healing.

Promoting Urinary and Bowel Elimination. The Foley catheter remains in the bladder for 7 to 10 days to prevent ureteral stenosis and incontinence. After the catheter is removed, the urine stream may be deflected down the leg as a result of edema or even may be uncontrolled. Having the client stand while voiding may decrease the incidence of these annoying problems. Antiperistaltic drugs are usually given for 7 to 10 days to prevent defecation and decrease the risk for wound infection. Then stool softeners may be given to prevent straining and decrease discomfort related to bowel movements. Perineal care or sitz baths after voidings or bowel movements may prevent contamination of the incision site.

Managing Pain. Discomfort after surgery is usually controlled with opioid analgesics during the first couple of days after surgery. Medicating for pain before wound care may help the client to relax and tolerate the procedure with less distress.

Addressing Sexuality. Provide complete explanations of the changes that occur as a result of surgery. If a radical vulvectomy is performed, the clitoris is removed and loss of orgasm usually occurs. Dyspareunia may result from any of the surgical procedures. Vaginal dilators may be useful to stretch the remaining vaginal tissues. Discomfort can also be reduced during sexual intercourse by having the couple use water-soluble lubricants or a side-lying position. The couple may need counseling about alternatives to vaginal intercourse. Encourage the client to express feelings of grief related to her loss of normal sexual function.

A vulvectomy can be devastating to a client's self-concept. She often has a grief reaction related to the loss of the vulva and subsequent disfigurement. She may fear rejection from her sexual partner and may be reluctant to make herself vulnerable by getting involved in any relationship. Fears of recurrence or metastasis may be present. Encourage the client to vent her feelings and concerns about her perceived or actual losses and body changes. Urge family members or significant others to share their feelings and concerns with the woman. A visit by a woman who has successfully recovered from similar surgery could be beneficial.

Vaginal Cancer
PATHOPHYSIOLOGY

Invasive vaginal cancer is rare, accounting for less than 2% of all gynecologic cancers. Usually vaginal cancer is an extension of cervical, endometrial, or vulvar cancers. Most vaginal cancers are squamous cell carcinomas that develop in the upper one third of the vagina. They occur most often in women older than 50 years of age; 90% of cases develop after menopause. Adenocarcinoma of the vagina is found in women between the ages of 14 and 30 years and is associated with intrauterine exposure to diethylstilbestrol (DES) as a result of maternal ingestion during pregnancy.

The cause of vaginal cancer is unknown. Risk factors include repeated pregnancies; vaginal trauma; sexually transmitted diseases (STDs), especially syphilis and herpes simplex virus type 2 and papillomavirus infections; and prior radiation.

The spread of vaginal cancer depends on the location of the tumor. Upper vaginal lesions spread in the same manner as cervical cancer, whereas lower lesions spread similarly to vulvar cancer. Because of the rich lymphatic drainage in the vaginal area, metastasis can occur early.

◆ COLLABORATIVE MANAGEMENT
◆ Assessment

Premalignant lesions (vaginal intraepithelial neoplasia) are often asymptomatic, and an abnormal Pap smear may be the only indication. Late symptoms include pain, foul-smelling vaginal discharge, painless vaginal bleeding, pruritus, and urinary symptoms from the pressure of the lesion on the bladder.

A pelvic examination may reveal a lesion. Premalignant changes are diagnosed through colposcopic examination and biopsy.

Survival rates are better when tumors are smaller and no lymph nodes are involved.

Interventions

NONSURGICAL MANAGEMENT. Noninvasive malignancy and early stage vaginal cancers may be treated nonsurgically with a variety of techniques. Laser therapy (see p. 1846) may be used. The health care provider stains the abnormal tissues with an iodine solution to identify the area for treatment. A vaginal discharge may be present for several days after treatment, and healing normally takes a few weeks. Close follow-up is necessary and includes a Pap smear and colposcopic examination every 4 months for 1 year and then every 6 to 12 months.

Topical chemotherapy with local application of 5-fluorouracil (5-FU) cream to the vagina daily for 1 week is another treatment option. This drug is irritating to the skin, and often zinc oxide ointment application is recommended to protect the vulvar area. The treatment is repeated in 3 to 4 weeks, and follow-up is the same as that for laser therapy.

Radiation therapy can be used for all stages of vaginal cancer. Intracavitary radiation therapy (IRT, brachytherapy) is usually used alone for the treatment of cancer limited to the vaginal wall, and external radiation therapy is combined with IRT for cancer that extends beyond the vaginal wall. Complications of radiation therapy include vaginal stenosis, adhesions, and discharge. Women need to use vaginal dilators after treatment, and assessment for sexual dysfunction is suggested.

SURGICAL MANAGEMENT. A local wide excision may be performed for localized lesions. A partial or total **vaginectomy** (removal of part or all the vagina) is performed for invasive disease. Vaginectomy affects sexual function. Without surgical reconstruction, vaginal intercourse is impossible. The client and her sexual partner need counseling about alternative activities for achieving sexual satisfaction. A radical hysterectomy or pelvic exenteration may also be performed, depending on the extent of the cancer.

Fallopian Tube Cancer

PATHOPHYSIOLOGY

Fallopian tube cancer is the rarest of gynecologic cancers, with an incidence of less than 1%. It occurs in women older than 50 years of age; 80% to 90% of cases are metastases from ovarian and endometrial cancers.

The cause of squamous cell fallopian tube cancer is unknown. Adenocarcinoma of the fallopian tube may result from pelvic inflammatory disease (PID) and chronic salpingitis. Nulliparity and infertility (inability to conceive) have also been cited as risk factors.

Most fallopian tube carcinomas are serous adenocarcinomas. The spread of this disease is very similar to that of epithelial ovarian cancer. The initial lesion is confined to the lumen of the tube. From there it invades the serosa and spreads intraperitoneally to the bowel, omentum, and peritoneum. Lymphatic spread is to the para-aortic and retroperitoneal lymph nodes.

COLLABORATIVE MANAGEMENT

Clients who have fallopian tube cancer often have only a few manifestations. The most common manifestations are postmenopausal bleeding, increasing abdominal pain, watery vaginal discharge, and leukorrhea. Later manifestations include lower abdominal pain or distention and feelings of pressure.

Diagnosis is rare before surgery. Pap smears are abnormal in only 10% of cases. A mass may be felt on examination in late stages. Vaginal ultrasonography, computed tomography (CT), or laparoscopy may be used to confirm a mass.

Treatment of cancer limited to the fallopian tube is a total abdominal hysterectomy and bilateral salpingo-oophorectomy with **omentectomy** (removal of the connective tissues covering these organs). Care of the client with fallopian tube cancer is similar to that described for cancer of the ovary (see Interventions [Ovarian Cancer], p. 1850). Chemotherapy may be used before surgery in later stages or for recurrence. The lesions respond to alkylating agents (see Chapter 28). External radiation therapy has been used after surgery for late-stage tumors.

GET READY for the NCLEX Examination!

KEY POINTS

Safe Effective Care Environment

- Use clean technique when emptying wound drains following pelvic exenteration surgery.
- Have clients report any manifestations of infection when caring for a urinary catheter in the home.
- Teach clients not to do any heavy lifting (>15 pounds) after a hysterectomy or cervical ablative procedures.
- Do not allow pregnant women or children under 18 years of age to enter the room where radioactive implants are in use.

Health Promotion and Maintenance

- Teach women at risk for ovarian or endometrial cancer to follow the American Cancer Society's screening guidelines.
- Teach all women to have regular Pap tests based on their risk factors.
- Teach women to practice safer sex to prevent infections of the reproductive organs.
- Teach women who use tampons to wash their hands before inserting the tampon, not to leave the tampon in place for more than 6 hours, and to use sanitary napkins (rather than tampons) at night.
- Urge women who have an increased genetic risk for endometrial or ovarian cancer to see their gynecological health care provider annually.

Psychosocial Integrity

- Use language and terminology the client is comfortable with when discussing reproductive issues, sexuality, and gynecologic problems.
- Reassure women who suffer from premenstrual syndrome (PMS) that their manifestations have a physiologic basis.
- Explain all tests, procedures, and treatments, especially if they cause discomfort during or after the procedures.
- Assess the client's anxiety before any gynecologic surgery.
- Encourage women who are having procedures that may interfere with fertility to express feelings of fear or grief.
- Encourage women with chronic or serious health problems to consider using support groups or counseling.

Physiological Integrity

- Help clients to be informed enough to make appropriate decisions about whether or not to use hormone replacement therapy during or after menopause.
- Urge any women who experiences postmenopausal vaginal bleeding to consult with her gynecologic health care provider as soon as possible.
- Teach clients taking danazol for endometriosis about the side effects of the drug (hirsutism, weight gain, decreased breast size, acne).
- Monitor all clients who have pelvic surgery for the presence of deep vein thrombosis after surgery.
- Instruct clients prescribed to use pessaries the proper way to use and care for the device.
- Teach clients about specific restrictions after local cervical ablation therapy (see Chart 78-14).
- When caring for a client who has a radioactive implant, wear your dosimeter and lead apron whenever you are in the room, always face the radiation source, and do not spend more than 30 minutes per day in the room.
- Teach the client who is going home after a hysterectomy how to monitor herself for infection or other complications.
- Instruct clients receiving external beam radiation to the abdomen to gently wash the area; not to apply creams or lotions (unless prescribed by the radiologist); not to wash off marking; to avoid exposing the area to sunlight or temperature extremes; and to wear soft, nonirritating clothing.

ADDITIONAL STUDY RESOURCES

Go to your Student CD-ROM for Review Questions for the NCLEX Examination.

Go to http://evolve.elsevier.com/Iggy/ for **evolve** Integrated Management of Care Questions for the NCLEX Examination.

SELECTED BIBLIOGRAPHY

Asterisk indicates a classic or definitive work on this subject.

Ackley, B., & Ladwig, G. (2002). *Nursing diagnosis handbook: A guide to planning care* (5th ed.). St. Louis: Mosby.

Ahlberg, K., et al. (2004). Fatigue, psychological distress, coping, and quality of life in patients with uterine cancer. *Journal of Advanced Nursing, 45*(2), 205-213.

Ahmedin, J., et al. (2003). Cancer statistics 2003. *CA: A Cancer Journal for Clinicians, 53*(1), 5-26.

Almadrones, L., et al. (2004). Psychometric evaluation of two scales assessing functional status and peripheral neuropathy associated with chemotherapy for ovarian cancer: A gynecological oncology study group study. *Oncology Nursing Forum, 31*(3), 615-623.

American Cancer Society. (2005). *Cancer facts and figures 2005.* Report No. 00-300M-No. 5008.05. Atlanta: Author.

Anderson, P.O., Knobmen, J.E., & Troutman, W.G. (2002). Handbook of clinical drug data, 10th ed. New York: McGraw-Hill Medical Publishing Division.

Baily, D., et al. (2004). Uncertainty intervention for watchful waiting in prostate cancer. *Cancer Nursing, 27*(5), 339-346.

*Barrett, R.J., et al. (1995). Endometrial cancer: Stage at diagnosis and associated factors in black and white patients. *American Journal of Obstetrics and Gynecology, 173*(2), 414-422.

*Barrow, C. (1999). Balloon endometrial ablation as a safe alternative to hysterectomy. *AORN Journal, 70*(1), 80, 83-86, 89-90.

Barton, D., & Loprinzi, C. (2004). Making sense of the evidence regarding nonhormonal treatment for hot flashes. *Clinical Journal of Oncology Nursing, 8*(1), 39-42.

Barton, D., et al. (2004). Libido as part of sexuality in female cancer survivors. *Oncology Nursing Forum, 31*(3), 599-607.

Bond, S. (2003). New guidelines for Pap screening and management of results. *Journal of Midwifery & Women's Health, 49*(1), 57-59.

Choma, K.K. (2003). ASC-US HPV testing. *American Journal of Nursing, 103*(2), 42-51.

Christman, N., Oakley, M., & Cronin, S. (2001). Developing and using preparatory information for women undergoing radiation therapy for cervical or uterine cancer. *Oncology Nursing Forum, 28*(1), 93-98.

DeCherney, A.H., & Nathan, L. (2003). *Current obstetric & gynecologic diagnosis & treatment.* New York: McGraw-Hill Medical Publishing Division.

Denny, E. (2004). Women's experience of endometriosis. *Journal of Advanced Nursing, 46*(6), 641-648.

DeVita, V.T., Hellman, S., & Rosenberg, S.A. (2001). *Cancer: principles and practice of oncology, 6th ed.,* Philadelphia: Lippincott, Williams, & Wilkins.

Dochterman, J., & Bulechek, G. (eds). (2004). *Nursing interventions classification (NIC)* (4th ed.). St. Louis: Mosby.

Donovan. H., & Ward, S. (2005). Representations of fatigue in women receiving chemotherapy for gynecologic cancers. *Oncology Nursing Forum, 32*(1), 113-116.

Ebersole, P., Hess, P., & Luggen, A. (2004). *Toward healthy aging: Human needs and nursing response* (6th ed.). St. Louis: Mosby.

Ekwall, W., Ternestedt, B., & Sorbe, B. (2003). Important aspects of health care for women with gynecologic cancer. *Oncology Nursing Forum, 30*(2), 313-319.

Facts and Comparisons. (2004). *Drug facts and comparisons* (58th ed.). St. Louis: Author.

Fey, M., & Beal, M. (2004). Role of human papilloma virus testing in cervical cancer prevention. *Journal of Midwifery & Women's Health, 49*(1), 4-13.

Hackley, B., & Rousseau, M. (2004). Managing menopausal symptoms after the women's health initiative. *Journal of Midwifery & Women's Health, 49*(2), 87-95.

Howel, D., Fitch, M.I., & Deane, K.A. (2003). Impact of ovarian cancer perceived by women. *Cancer Nursing, 26*(1):1-9.

Iannacchione, M.A. (2004). The vagina dialogues: Do you douche? *American journal of Nursing, 104*(1), 40-45.

Janicek, M.F., & Averette, H.E. (2001). Cervical cancer: Prevention, diagnosis, and therapeutics. *CA: Cancer Journal for Clinicians, 51,* 92-114.

*Johnson, S. (1998). Menopause and hormone replacement therapy. *Medical Clinics of North America, 82*(2), 297-320.

*Kim, K., et al. (1999). Cervical cancer screening knowledge and practices among Korean-American women. *Cancer Nursing, 22*(4), 297-302.

Koldjeski, D., et al. (2004). Health seeking related to ovarian cancer. *Cancer Nursing, 27*(5), 370-378.

Lee, C., (2000a). Gynecologic Cancers: Part I Risk factors. *Clinical Journal of Oncology Nursing, 4*(2), 67-71.

Lee, C., (2000b). Gynecologic Cancers: Part II Risk assessment and screening. *Clinical Journal of Oncology Nursing, 4*(2), 73-77.

*Lessick, M., Wickham, R., & Rehwaldt, M. (1997). Breast and ovarian cancer: Genetic update and implications for nursing. *MEDSURG Nursing, 6*(6), 341-349.

Likes, W., & Itano, J. (2003). Human papillomavirus and cervical cancer: Not just a sexually transmitted disease. *Clinical journal of Oncology Nursing, 7*(3), 271-276.

Lockwood-Rayerman, S. (2004). Characteristics of participation in cervical cancer screening. *Cancer Nursing, 27*(5), 353-363.

Loitmen, J. (2002). Transdermal fentanyl in ovarian cancer. *Journal of Pain and Symptom Management, 23*(1), 5-6.

*Lowdermilk, D.L. (1995). Reproductive surgery. In C.I. Fogel & N.F. Woods (Eds.), *Women's health care* (pp. 629-650). Springhouse, PA: Springhouse.

Lyndaker, C., & Hulton, L. (2004). The influence of age on symptoms of perimenopause. *Journal of Gynecologic and Neonatal Nursing, 33*(3), 340-347.

McCance, K.L., & Huether, S.E. (2002). *Pathophysiology: The biological basis for disease in adults and children* (4th ed.). St. Louis: Mosby.

Mick, J.A., Hughes, M., & Cohen, M. (2004). Using the BETTER model to assess sexuality. *Clinical Journal of Oncology Nursing, 8*(1), 84-86.

Moore-Higgs, G.J., et al. (2000). *Women and cancer: A gynecologic oncology nursing perspective*, 2nd ed., Boston: Jones & Bartlett.

Moorhead, S., Johnson, M., & Maas, M. (Eds.). (2004). *Nursing outcomes classification (NOC)* (3rd ed.). St. Louis: Mosby.

O'Rourke, J., & Mahon, S. (2003). A comprehensive look at the early detection of ovarian cancer. *Clinical Journal of Oncology Nursing, 7*(1), 41-47.

*Pearl, M.L., et al. (1999). Transcutaneous electrical nerve stimulation as an adjunct for controlling chemotherapy-induced nausea and vomiting in gynecologic oncology. *Cancer Nursing, 22*(4), 307-311.

*Rose, P.G. (1996). Endometrial carcinoma. *New England Journal of Medicine, 335*(9), 640-649.

Ryan, M., et al. (2003). The experience of lower limb lymphedema for women after treatment for gynecologic cancer. *Oncology Nursing Forum, 30*(3), 417-423.

Shinn, S. (2004). Taking a stand against cervical cancer. *Nursing 2004, 34*(5), 36-41.

Smith, L. (2004). Shedding light on photodynamic therapy. *Nursing 2004, 34*(5), 32hn1-32hn2.

*Spies, J.B., et al. (1999). Initial results from uterine fibroid embolization for symptomatic leiomyomata. *Journal of Vascular and Interventional Radiology, 10*(9), 1149-1157.

Stekler, J., & Elmore, J. (2002). Cervical cancer screening: Who, when, why? *The Clinical Advisor, (October 2002),* 107-114.

Swenson, M., et al. (2003). Quality of life among ovarian germ cell cancer survivors: A narrative analysis. *Oncology Nursing Forum, 30*(3), E56-E62.

*Taylor, L.K., et al. (1998). The effect of music in the postanesthesia care unit on pain levels in women who have had abdominal hysterectomies. *Journal of Perianesthesia Nursing, 13*(2), 88-94.

Tiffen, J., & Novak, K. (2004). Ovarian cancer. *Clinical Journal of Oncology Nursing, 8*(1), 80-82.

Wade, J., et al. (2000). Hysterectomy: What do women need and want to know? *Journal of Obstetric, Gynecologic, and Neonatal Nursing, 29*(1), 33-42.

Yarbro, C.H., et al. (2000). *Cancer nursing: principles & practice*, 5th ed., Boston: Jones & Bartlett.

Zimmerman, V. (2002). BRCA gene mutations and cancer. *American Journal of Nursing, 102*(8), 28-36.

Interventions for Male Clients with Reproductive Problems

LINDA J. CAPUTI

LEARNING OUTCOMES

After studying this chapter, you should be able to:

1. Describe common physical assessment findings for the client with benign prostatic hyperplasia (BPH).
2. Describe the mechanisms of action, side effects, and nursing implications for pharmacologic management of BPH.
3. Discuss options for surgical management of the client with BPH.
4. Develop a postoperative plan of care for a client undergoing a transurethral resection of the prostate (TURP).
5. Identify the procedures for prostate cancer screening.
6. Explain the role of hormonal therapy in treating prostate cancer.
7. Develop a community-based plan of care for a client with prostate cancer.
8. Describe the options for treating erectile dysfunction.
9. Describe the mechanisms of action, side effects, and nursing implications for pharmacologic management of erectile dysfunction.
10. Discuss cultural considerations related to male reproductive problems.
11. Analyze assessment data to determine priority nursing diagnoses and collaborative problems for a man with testicular cancer.
12. Develop a plan of care for a client with testicular cancer.
13. Formulate a community-based teaching plan for continuing care of clients with testicular cancer.
14. Compare hydrocele, spermatocele, and varicocele.
15. Compare the four types of prostatitis.
16. Discuss issues related to sexuality and body image for a man experiencing male reproductive health problems.

Go to your Student CD-ROM for Review Questions
for the NCLEX Examination keyed to these Learning Outcomes.

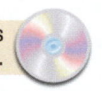

Apply knowledge of the anatomy and physiology of male reproductive functions when instructing clients about the impact of a disease process or treatment on their reproductive ability. Include the client and his spouse, sexual partner, or significant other in the decision-making process and work with members of the interdisciplinary team in providing collaborative care.

BENIGN PROSTATIC HYPERPLASIA

PATHOPHYSIOLOGY

In a young adult male, the prostatic capsule is thin and attached to the underlying tissue. With aging, the glandular units in the prostate undergo tissue **hyperplasia** (an increase in the number of cells), resulting in prostatic **hypertrophy**

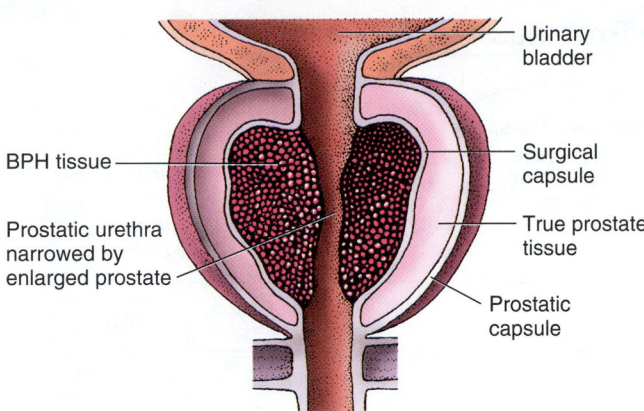

Figure 79-1 ■ Benign prostatic hyperplasia (BPH) grows inward, causing narrowing of the urethra.

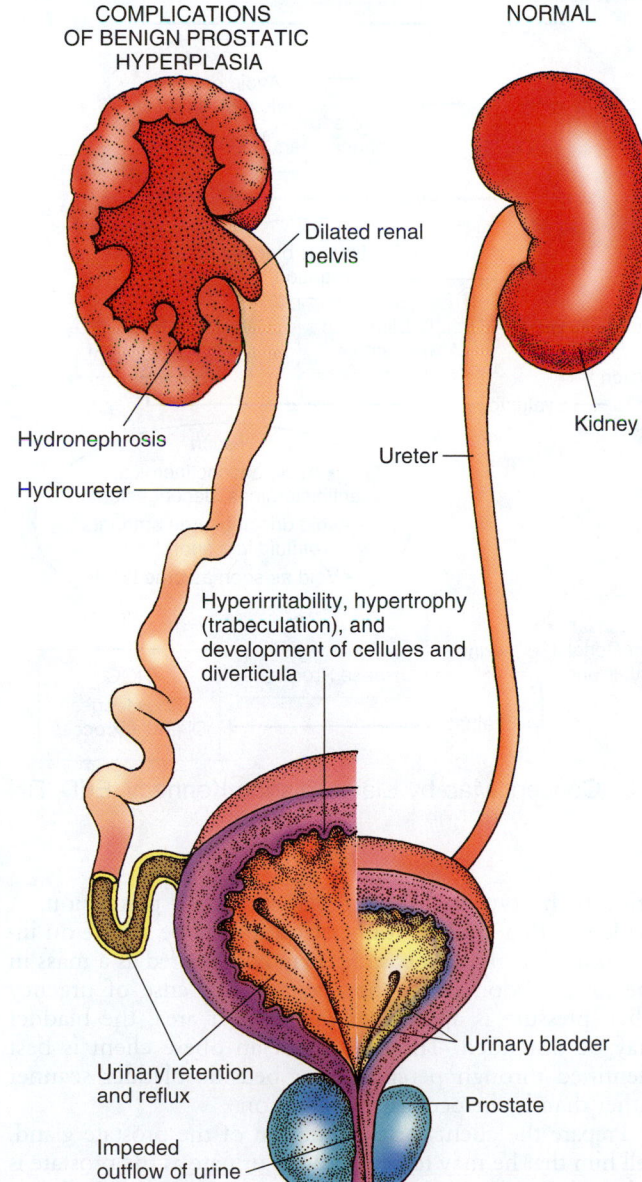

Figure 79-2 ■ Potential complications of benign prostatic hyperplasia. The right side of the illustration shows a normal male urologic system. The left side shows potential complications.

(enlargement). Although benign prostatic hypertrophy is the more common term used to describe this problem, **benign prostatic hyperplasia (BPH)** is the correct term for the pathologic process.

When the prostate gland enlarges, it extends upward, into the bladder, and inward, narrowing the prostatic urethral channel. This obstructs urine outflow by encroaching on the bladder opening (Figure 79-1). In response to this outlet resistance, the bladder is affected in several ways (Figure 79-2). It may become hyperirritable, which causes urgency and frequency. As the bladder tries to compensate for its increased workload, muscles in the bladder wall hypertrophy and may develop cellules and diverticula. If allowed to continue, this obstruction of urine flow can cause a gradual dilation of the ureters (**hydroureter**) and kidneys (**hydronephrosis**). The enlarged prostate may also obstruct the bladder neck or the prostatic urethra, causing urinary retention or incomplete bladder emptying. **Overflow urinary incontinence** is common; the urine "leaks" around the enlarged prostate, causing dribbling. Urinary stasis can result in urinary tract infections.

Etiology

The exact cause of BPH is unknown. Because BPH development is almost universal in older men, several theories have been examined (Marks, 2003).
- The effect of chronic inflammation of the prostate gland
- The role of general metabolic and nutritional factors (diet)
- The possible contribution of atherosclerosis

Although demographic data (such as race) and social factors (such as socioeconomic status and heredity) have been examined as predictors for the BPH development, it appears to result from a systemic hormonal alteration. Support for this theory is based on the fact that aging is the major contributing factor and that another factor is the presence of testicular androgen. BPH does not occur in men who were castrated before puberty (testicular androgen is absent). Men with BPH have a regression of this problem if the testes are surgically removed.

Incidence/Prevalence

◆COLLABORATIVE MANAGEMENT

The Concept Map on p. 1858 discusses nursing assessment and care issues related to management of the client with BPH.

◆Assessment

HISTORY

Pay particular attention to the client's report of his urinary pattern. Commonly the client reports frequency, **nocturia** (voiding at night), and other symptoms of bladder neck obstruction. Together these problems are known as **lower urinary tract symptoms (LUTS).** The symptoms of LUTS include hes-

CONCEPT MAP Benign Prostatic Hyperplasia

Benign Prostatic Hyperplasia

Client → **Whang Jin**

68-year-old man who has come to the emergency department with severe lower abdominal pain and an inability to urinate for the past 20 hours.

When questioned, Mr. Whang states that:
- He has been getting up three to four times a night to urinate.
- He frequently has to strain to initiate a urine stream.
- The urine stream has lessened over the past several months.
- He occasionally has seen pink-tinged urine.

Laboratory Results
Anemia
Hematuria
Residual urine present

Legend:
- ▭ Assessment data
- ◆ Nursing diagnoses
- ◆ Collaborative problems
- ▭ Nursing interventions
- ▭ Client outcomes

Assess → **Age (+)**
History of prostatic infections (?)

↓ Clinical manifestations

Central Nervous System
No data
Cardiovascular
Hemoglobin = 9 g
Respiratory
No data
Gastrointestinal
Acute lower abdominal pain (+)
Skin
No data
Genitourinary
Nocturia (+)
Hesitancy (+)
Hematuria (+)
Urinary retention (+)
Diagnostic Tests
RBCs in urine
800 mL urine in bladder

Analyze →

Urinary Retention — Plan → **NIC Urinary Retention Care** — Evaluate → **NOC Urinary Elimination**

Alternative Therapies: • Saw palmetto • Lycopene

Drug Therapy: • Finasteride • Alpha-adrenergic blocking agents • Estrogens • Androgens

Teach: • Frequent intercourse • Masturbation • Prostatic massage

Stress Urinary Incontinence — Plan → **NIC Urinary Incontinence Care** — Evaluate → **NOC Urinary Continence**

Disturbed Sleep Pattern — Plan → **NIC Sleep Enhancement** — Evaluate → **NOC Sleep**

Teach: Avoid caffeine, alcohol, diuretics

Risk for Infection — Plan → **NIC Urinary Elimination Management** — Evaluate → **NOC Risk Control**

Continuous bladder irrigation

CP: Potential for Renal Insufficiency — Plan → **NIC Teaching: Disease Process** — Evaluate → **NOC Knowledge: Disease Process**

Teach:
- Avoid anticholinergics, antihistamines, decongestants
- Avoid drinking large amounts of fluid in a short time
- Void as soon as urge is felt

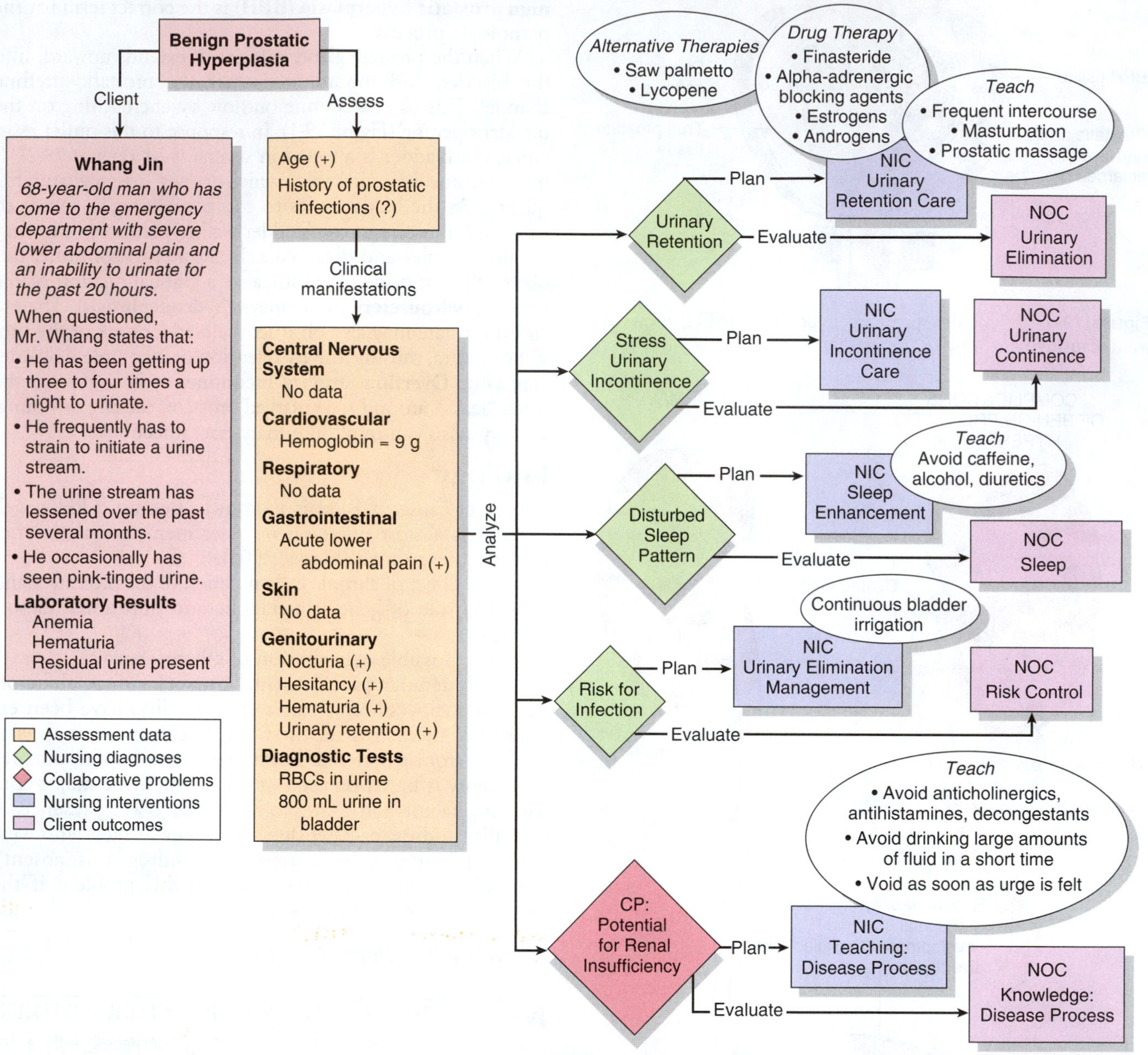

Concept Map by Elaine Bishop Kennedy, EdD, RN

---

itancy, intermittency, reduced force and size of the urinary stream, a sensation of incomplete bladder emptying, and postvoid dribbling. If frequency and nocturia are not accompanied by symptoms of restricted flow, the possibility of a nonobstructive etiology, such as infection, is considered.

Ask whether the client has experienced any **hematuria** (blood in the urine) when starting the urine stream or at the end of urination. BPH is a common cause of hematuria in men older than 60 years of age.

PHYSICAL ASSESSMENT/CLINICAL MANIFESTATIONS

Instruct the client to void before the physical assessment. Inspect, palpate, and percuss the abdomen for a distended bladder. Normally the bladder must contain 150 mL of

urine to be outlined during palpation and percussion. A bladder with a larger amount of urine may be visible on inspection. An enlarged bladder may be palpated as a mass in the lower abdomen. If the client has a sense of urgency when pressure is applied to the bladder area, the bladder may be distended. The bladder of an obese client is best identified through percussion or bedside bladder scanner rather than by inspection or palpation.

Prepare the client for examination of the prostate gland. Tell him that he may feel the urge to urinate as the prostate is palpated. Because the prostate is close to the rectal wall, it is easily examined by **digital rectal examination (DRE).** Help the client to bend over the examination table or assume a side-lying fetal position. The health care provider examines the prostate for size and consistency. Benign prostatic hyper-

Animation: Rectal Examination

CHART 79-1

KEY FEATURES of
Benign Prostatic Hyperplasia

- Urinary frequency
- Nocturia
- Urinary hesitancy, particularly on initiation of voiding
- Hematuria
- Diminished force of the urinary stream
- Postvoid dribbling (overflow incontinence)
- Bladder distention
- Possible evidence of renal insufficiency, including edema, pallor, and pruritus
- A uniform, elastic, nontender palpable prostate

---

plasia (BPH) usually presents as a uniform, elastic, nontender enlargement, whereas cancer of the prostate gland usually presents as a stony-hard nodule (Chart 79-1). Advise the client that after the prostate gland is palpated, it may be massaged to obtain a fluid sample for examination to rule out **prostatitis** (inflammation of the prostate).

LABORATORY ASSESSMENT

A urinalysis may be performed to detect any urine problems, and a culture may be obtained for evidence of urinary tract infection. Urinalysis includes glucose, protein, occult blood, and pH levels. If infection is present, the specimen may contain white blood cells (WBCs) or red blood cells (RBCs).

Blood studies that may be performed at the initial evaluation, depending on the client's condition and third-party payer, include the following:

- A complete blood count (CBC) to evaluate any evidence of infection (elevated WBCs) or anemia (decreased RBCs)
- Blood urea nitrogen (BUN) and serum creatinine levels to evaluate renal function (both are elevated with renal disease)
- A prostate-specific antigen (PSA) and a serum acid phosphatase measurement if prostate cancer is suspected (PSA is elevated with prostate cancer) (see Physical Examination and Prostate Cancer Screening, p. 1865)

If prostatic fluid is expressed during the examination, send the fluid to the laboratory for microscopic examination and cultures.

RADIOGRAPHIC ASSESSMENT

Radiologic studies that may be conducted in the workup of the client with suspected BPH include x-rays of the kidneys, ureters, and bladder (KUB) and intravenous (IV) urography to assess the entire urinary/renal system. The KUB outlines the structure of the urinary tract in the abdomen. Urography is useful in studying both the structure and function of the urinary tract.

OTHER DIAGNOSTIC ASSESSMENTS

Urodynamic studies are important in the diagnosis and evaluation of clients with bladder neck obstruction. Urodynamic flow studies include flow rate analysis **(flowmetry)** and assessment of residual urine. Flow rate analysis is simply a way of assessing the activity of the bladder and the outlet during the emptying phase of micturition.

During a cystourethroscopic examination, the physician uses a cystoscope to view the interior of the bladder, the bladder neck, and the urethra. This examination is used to study the presence and effect of bladder neck obstruction. The procedure is usually done in an ambulatory care setting. See Chapter 72 for a detailed description of cystoscopy.

Residual urine may be determined by bladder scan immediately after the client voids. As an alternative, because the client always voids before cystourethroscopy, residual urine may be measured at that time.

◆ Common Nursing Diagnoses and Collaborative Problems

Nursing diagnoses and collaborative problems that may apply to clients with benign prostatic hyperplasia include the following:

- Urinary Retention related to blockage from enlarged prostate gland
- Urinary Incontinence related to overdistension of the bladder
- Disturbed Sleep Pattern related to urinary urgency, nocturia
- Risk for Infection related to inadequate primary defenses (stasis of urine)
- Potential for Renal Insufficiency

◆ Interventions

Traditionally, the only effective treatment for the relief of the symptoms caused by BPH has been surgical. However, drug therapy is now becoming a popular option. Chart 79-2 lists NIC interventions for clients with BPH.

NONSURGICAL MANAGEMENT. In some cases where clients are not yet bothered by the symptoms of BPH, "watchful waiting" may be appropriate. In watchful waiting, the client is examined every year to determine whether the BPH is causing urinary difficulties and getting worse. Medical management of BPH includes drug therapy and other measures to reduce obstruction.

Drug Therapy. The health care provider may prescribe finasteride (Proscar) to shrink the prostate gland and improve urine flow. Finasteride lowers the level of **dihydrotestosterone (DHT),** a major cause of prostate growth. In some men, decreasing the DHT levels can shrink the enlarged prostate. The client may need to take the drug for as long as 6 months before improvement is noticed. The major side effects of the drug are erectile dysfunction (ED) and decreased libido, although these effects are not common.

The presence of alpha-adrenergic receptors in the prostatic smooth muscle makes it respond to alpha-blocking agents, such as terazosin (Hytrin), doxazosin (Cardura), and tamsulosin (Flomax). When alpha-blocking agents are given, the prostate gland constricts, thereby reducing urethral pressure and improving urine flow. A variety of hormonal agents, including estrogens and androgens, alone or in combination, also have been used less successfully to alter BPH and its effects on voiding.

Complementary and Alternative Therapies. Some herbs and natural products that have been used to manage BPH include saw palmetto extract (a natural herb) and lycopene (a botanical found in tomatoes). Many men with early to moderate BPH believe these agents have relieved their symptoms and prefer this treatment over prescription drugs or surgery. Clinical trials for both agents are now under way.

NIC **INTERVENTION ACTIVITIES for**
The Client with Benign Prostatic Hyperplasia

Urinary Retention Care: *Assistance in relieving bladder distension*
- Perform a comprehensive urinary assessment focusing on incontinence (e.g., urinary output, urinary voiding pattern, cognitive function, and preexisting urinary problems).
- Monitor use of nonprescription agents with anticholinergic or alpha-agonist properties.
- Provide privacy for elimination.
- Use the power of suggestion by running water or flushing the toilet.
- Provide enough time for bladder emptying (10 minutes).
- Provide Credé maneuver, as necessary.
- Insert urinary catheter, as appropriate.
- Monitor intake and output.
- Monitor degree of bladder distension by palpation and percussion.
- Catheterize for residual, as appropriate.
- Implement intermittent catheterization, as appropriate.

Bladder Irrigation: *Instillation of a solution into the bladder to provide cleansing or medication*
- Determine whether the irrigation will be continuous or intermittent.
- Observe universal precautions.
- Explain the procedure to the client.
- Set up sterile irrigating supplies, maintaining sterile technique per agency protocol.
- Cleanse site of entry or end of Y-connector with alcohol wipe.
- Instill irrigating fluid, per agency protocol.
- Monitor and maintain correct flow rate, as necessary.
- Record amount of fluid used, characteristics of fluid, amount returned, and client responsiveness, according to agency protocol.

NIC intervention activities selected from Dochterman, J.M., & Bulechek, G.M. (Eds.) (2004). *Nursing interventions classification (NIC)* (4th ed.). St. Louis: Mosby. No part of this work is to be altered without prior written permission from the Publisher.

Other Measures. Other nonsurgical measures that reduce obstructive symptoms include those that cause the release of prostatic fluid, such as prostatic massage, frequent sexual intercourse, and masturbation. These measures are helpful for the client whose obstructive symptoms result from an enlarged prostate with a large amount of retained prostatic fluid. Instruct the client to avoid drinking large amounts of fluid in a short time; to avoid alcohol, diuretics, and caffeine; and to void as soon as the urge is felt. These measures are aimed at preventing overdistention of the bladder, which may result in loss of detrusor muscle tone. Teach clients to avoid any drugs that can cause urinary retention, especially anticholinergics, antihistamines, and decongestants. Emphasize the importance of telling the health care provider about the diagnosis of BPH so that these drugs are not prescribed.

SURGICAL MANAGEMENT. Because most older men have some degree of BPH, the mere presence of the condition does not mean that the client requires surgical intervention. Some or all of the following criteria are typically present when surgical intervention is necessary:
- Acute urinary retention
- Chronic urinary tract infections secondary to residual urine in the bladder
- Hematuria
- Hydronephrosis
- Bladder neck obstruction symptoms that bother the client, such as urinary frequency and nocturia

The goals of surgical intervention are to relieve the symptoms of bladder neck obstruction and to improve quality of life. Accomplishment of these goals allows the client to void at normal intervals while retaining adequate urinary control and normal sexual functioning.

Preoperative Care. When planning surgical interventions, the client's general physical condition, the size of the prostate gland, and the client's preferences are considered.

CONSIDERATIONS FOR OLDER ADULTS
The client is evaluated for any other diseases that are common in older persons, such as cardiovascular disease, chronic pulmonary disease, diabetes mellitus, or renal disease. If the client has renal disease, an indwelling catheter may be inserted. Closely monitor the client's intake, output, and serum electrolyte and creatinine levels until renal status has improved. In some cases, the client may have another medical condition that makes surgery too risky. In such cases, bladder neck obstruction may be relieved by permanent indwelling urinary drainage. The client is also assessed for the presence of urinary tract infection. Any infection is treated before surgery.

The client may have many fears and misconceptions about prostatic surgery, such as believing that automatic loss of sexual functioning or permanent incontinence will occur. Assess the client's anxiety, correct any misconceptions about the surgery, and provide accurate information to him and his family or significant others. Regardless of the type of surgery to be performed, provide information about anesthesia (see Chapter 21). The client may have other medical problems that increase the risk for complications of general anesthesia and may be advised to have regional anesthesia. Epidural or spinal anesthesia may be used for any of the procedures and are the most common types of anesthesia used for a transurethral resection of the prostate. Because the client is awake, it is easier to assess for hyponatremia, fluid overload, and water intoxication.

It is important to include the topic of urinary catheters in the teaching plan before surgery. After prostatic surgery, all clients have an indwelling urethral catheter for at least a day. Be sure that the client knows that he will feel the urge to void while the catheter is in place. Tell the client that he may also have continuous bladder irrigation (CBI) and traction on the catheter, but this may not be known until the client returns from the postanesthesia care unit (PACU). Also explain before surgery that it is normal for the urine to be blood-tinged after surgery. Small blood clots and tissue debris may pass while the catheter is in place and immediately after it is removed.

Operative Procedures. Several surgical procedures are possible for removing the enlarged portion of the prostate gland (Figure 79-3). In all approaches, the surgeon removes the hyperplastic tissue and leaves the prostatic capsule.

In the last few years, a variety of less invasive surgical procedures for BPH have emerged. These procedures are recommended as alternatives to drug therapy or when drug therapy fails. These procedures are generally recommended for clients in the early stages of the disease. Such procedures include the following:
- Transurethral thermotherapy (uses microwave thermotherapy)
- Transurethral needle ablation B, also known as TUNA procedure (uses low level radio frequency energy)

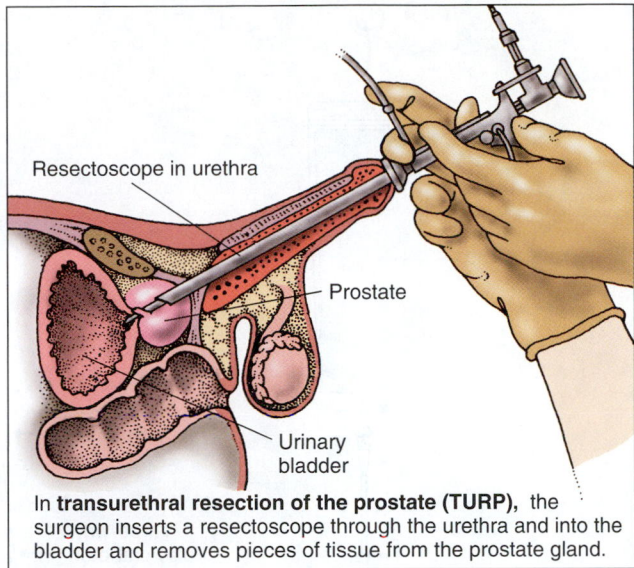

In **transurethral resection of the prostate (TURP),** the surgeon inserts a resectoscope through the urethra and into the bladder and removes pieces of tissue from the prostate gland.

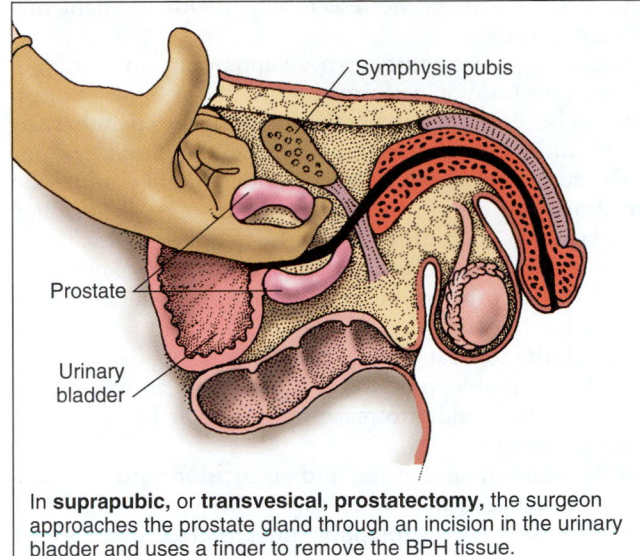

In **suprapubic,** or **transvesical, prostatectomy,** the surgeon approaches the prostate gland through an incision in the urinary bladder and uses a finger to remove the BPH tissue.

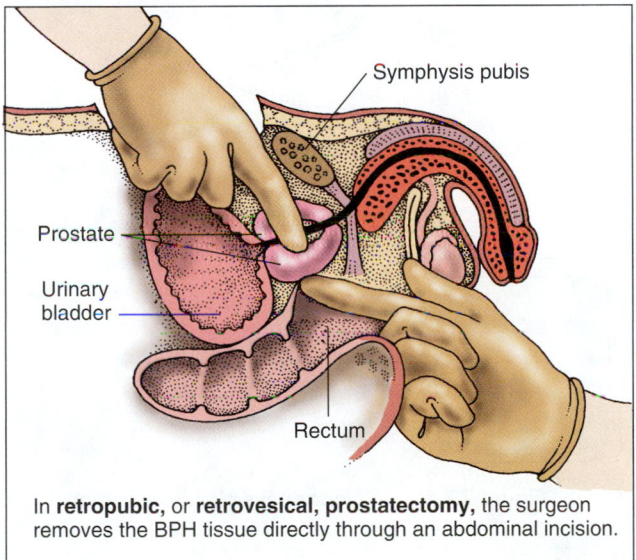

In **retropubic,** or **retrovesical, prostatectomy,** the surgeon removes the BPH tissue directly through an abdominal incision.

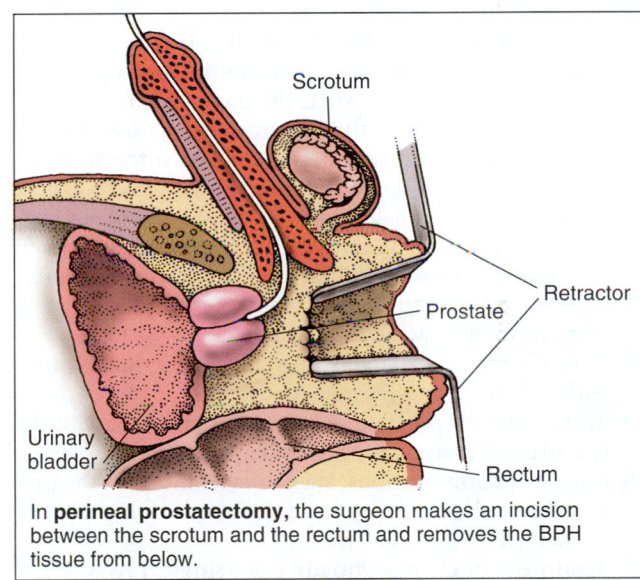

In **perineal prostatectomy,** the surgeon makes an incision between the scrotum and the rectum and removes the BPH tissue from below.

Figure 79-3 ■ Prostatectomy procedures. *BPH,* Benign prostatic hyperplasia.

- Visual laser ablation (uses laser energy)
- Electrovaporization (uses electrocautery) of the prostate.

The advantages of these minimally invasive procedures are that there is less bleeding after surgery and the client can be discharged from the hospital within 24 hours with a retention catheter. Teach the client to monitor for catheter patency, hematuria, and infection after surgery. Also tell clients and their caregivers that delayed hematuria and urinary retention may occur days to weeks after the electrovaporization procedure.

Transurethral Resection of the Prostate. The traditional **transurethral resection of the prostate (TURP)** is a "closed" surgical procedure and is still commonly performed. The prostate may also be removed using an "open" procedure because of the need for a surgical incision. The choice of procedure depends on the following:

- The size of the prostate gland
- The location of the enlargement

- Whether surgery on the bladder is also needed
- The client's age and physical condition

To perform the TURP procedure, the surgeon inserts a resectoscope (an instrument similar to a cystoscope, but with a cutting and cauterizing loop) through the urethra. The enlarged portion of the prostate gland is then resected in small pieces (prostate chips).

This procedure is used when the area of major enlargement is in the medial lobe of the prostate that directly surrounds the urethra and when the amount of tissue to be removed is relatively small. A TURP is safer for the client who is at high risk for open surgery because a surgical incision is not used. Hospitalization and convalescence are shorter than with any other type of **prostatectomy** (prostate removal).

The disadvantage of a TURP is that because only small pieces of the gland are removed, remaining prostate tissue may continue to grow and cause urinary obstruction, requiring additional TURPs. There is also the possibility of urethral trauma from the resectoscope, with resultant urethral strictures.

Suprapubic Prostatectomy. Suprapubic, or transvesical, prostatectomy is performed when the prostate is larger than can be removed transurethrally and if the client has any other bladder problems that can be treated at the same time.

The surgeon makes a low horizontal abdominal incision just above the symphysis pubis and exposes the bladder. The bladder is then distended with fluid, and a small incision is made in the bladder wall. The prostate gland is removed through the bladder cavity, and any bladder disease is treated at this time.

The ability to treat bladder problems is the major advantage of suprapubic prostatectomy because an incision is made into the bladder to reach the prostate. The following are disadvantages:

- An abdominal incision and an incision into the bladder are necessary.
- The client has a suprapubic tube in place after surgery.
- There is an increased risk for urinary tract infection, incontinence, bladder spasms, and hemorrhage.
- The surgery is more painful.
- Convalescence is longer than with a TURP.

Retropubic Prostatectomy. Retropubic, or extravesical, prostatectomy is performed when the prostate is too large to be resected via the transurethral approach but no coexisting bladder problems have been identified. The surgeon makes an abdominal incision above the symphysis pubis to expose the prostate gland. A small incision is made in the prostate capsule, and the gland is removed. This procedure differs from suprapubic approach in that the bladder is not entered.

Perineal Prostatectomy. Perineal prostatectomy is mainly performed to achieve the following:

- Removal of an enlarged prostate gland that is filled with calculi (stones)
- Treatment of prostatic abscesses that have not responded to conservative treatment
- Repair of complications, such as lacerations in the prostatic capsule, that may have occurred during a previous surgery
- Treatment of clients who are poor surgical risks

The client is placed in an exaggerated lithotomy position, and the knees are positioned on the chest. The surgeon makes a U-shaped incision between the scrotum and the rectum. The prostatic capsule is then opened and the tissue removed. This procedure provides direct access to the prostate gland.

The major disadvantage of this procedure is the loss of sexual potency resulting from damage to the pudendal nerve. Clients with peripheral vascular disease or chronic pulmonary problems cannot tolerate the exaggerated lithotomy position and are not candidates for this procedure. Other disadvantages include a greater risk for infection, the possibility of damage to the rectum and anal sphincter, and the possibility of urinary incontinence. Thus this approach is not commonly used.

Postoperative Care. The care after surgery for the client who has undergone prostatic surgery is similar regardless of the type of procedure done and the type of anesthesia used (see Chapter 22). However, be aware of several differences because they affect nursing care.

Nursing Care After a Transurethral Resection Prostatectomy. After a TURP, the surgeon inserts a three-

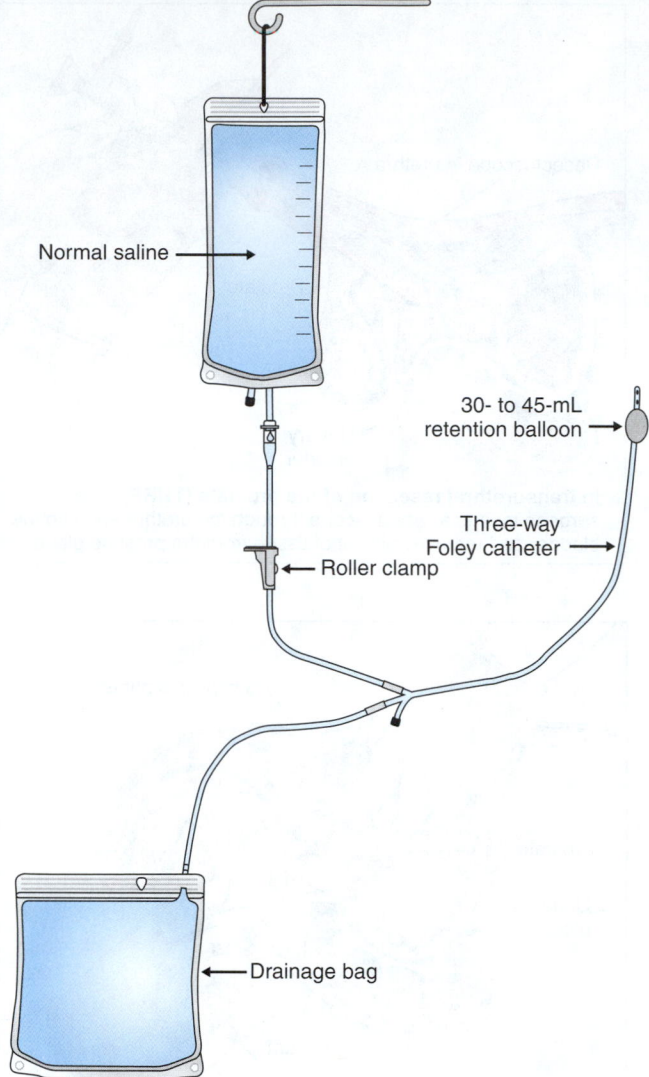

Figure 79-4 ■ Continuous bladder irrigation.

way urinary catheter with a 30- to 45-mL retention balloon through the urethra into the bladder (Figure 79-4). The catheter is pulled down into the prostatic fossa to help prevent bleeding. Traction is often applied on the catheter by pulling it taut and taping it to the client's abdomen or thigh.

CATHETER CARE AND CONTINUOUS BLADDER IRRIGATION. Chart 79-2 lists intervention activities for the client after prostate surgery. If the catheter is taped to the client's thigh, instruct him to keep his leg straight. The surgeon determines when the traction should be removed; usually it is removed on the first day after surgery.

Explain that because of the retention catheter's large diameter and the pressure of the retention balloon on the internal sphincter of the bladder, the client will feel the urge to void continuously. This is a normal sensation, not a surgical complication. Advise the client not to try to void around the catheter, which causes the bladder muscles to contract and may result in painful bladder spasms. Reassure him that an antispasmodic drug can be given to keep him comfortable.

CONSIDERATIONS FOR OLDER ADULTS

When caring for older men who may become confused after surgery, reorient them frequently and remind them not to pull on the catheter. If the client is restless or "picks" at tubes, provide a familiar object, such as a family picture, for him to hold for distraction and a feeling of security. The client should not be restrained unless all other alternatives have failed.

Continuous bladder irrigation (CBI) with normal saline or other solution, as prescribed, helps to keep the catheter free of obstruction and facilitates detection of obstruction or other complications. Adjust the irrigation fluid rate to maintain a colorless or light pink drainage return. (For the nursing care of the client undergoing CBI, see Chart 79-3.) The continuous irrigation is usually discontinued 24 hours after a TURP. The retention catheter is usually removed when CBI is discontinued.

POSTCATHETERIZATION CARE. When the urinary catheter is removed, the client may experience some burning on urination as well as some urinary frequency, dribbling, and leakage. Reassure the client that these symptoms are normal and will subside. The client may also pass small clots and tissue debris for several days after the TURP. Instruct him to increase fluid intake to at least 2000 to 2500 mL daily, which helps to decrease the dysuria and keep the urine clear. An older client who has renal disease or who is at risk for heart failure may not be able to tolerate this much fluid. By the time of discharge (usually 2 days after surgery), he should be voiding 150 to 200 mL of clear yellow urine every 3 to 4 hours. By discharge, pain is minimal and analgesics may not be required.

COMPLICATIONS OF TRANSURETHRAL RESECTION OF THE PROSTATE. Clients who undergo a TURP or open prostatectomy are at risk for bleeding or hemorrhage after surgery. Bleeding is most common within the first 24 hours. Bladder spasms or movement may trigger fresh bleeding from previously controlled vessels. This bleeding may be arterial or venous, but venous bleeding is more common.

Monitor the client's urine output every 2 hours and vital signs every 4 hours. If the bleeding is arterial, the urinary drainage is bright red or ketchup-like with numerous clots. If arterial bleeding occurs, notify the surgeon immediately and increase the CBI rate or intermittently irrigate the catheter with normal saline solution. The surgeon may prescribe aminocaproic acid (Amicar) to control bleeding. Keep in mind that if the drug does not work, surgical intervention may be needed to clear the bladder of clots and to stop the bleeding.

If the bleeding is venous, the urine output is burgundy, with or without any change in vital signs. Inform the surgeon of any manifestations of bleeding. The surgeon may apply traction on the catheter for a few hours, which may control venous bleeding. Assess the success of this procedure in stopping the bleeding. Be aware that the traction on the catheter is quite uncomfortable and increases the risk for bladder spasms. Analgesics or antispasmodics, such as dicyclomine hydrochloride (Bentyl, Antispas, Formulex✶, Lomine✶), oxybutynin (Ditropan), or belladonna and opium (B&O) suppositories, are usually prescribed to decrease painful bladder spasms.

Closely monitor the client's hemoglobin (Hgb) and hematocrit (Hct) levels for anemia as a result of blood loss. Some clients may require blood transfusions to return the Hgb and Hct values to baseline levels.

CHART 79-3

BEST PRACTICE for
Care of the Client After Prostate Surgery

- Monitor the client closely for signs of infection. Older clients undergoing prostate surgery often also have underlying chronic diseases (such as cardiovascular disease, chronic lung disease, or diabetes) and multiple invasive lines that predispose them to infections.
- Help the client out of the bed to the chair as soon as permitted to prevent complications of immobility. Older clients may need assistance because of underlying changes in the musculoskeletal system, such as decreased range of motion and stiffness in joints. These clients are at *high risk* for falls.
- Encourage the client to turn, cough, and deep breathe and to use the incentive spirometer every 2 hours to prevent atelectasis and pneumonia. Older adults are at risk for pneumonia because of the decreases in lung elasticity and vital capacity associated with aging.
- Assess the client's pain every 2 to 3 hours, and give pain medication as needed.
- Provide a safe environment for the client. Anticipate a temporary change in mental status for the older client in the immediate postoperative period as a result of anesthetics and unfamiliar surroundings. Reorient the client frequently. Keep IV lines and catheter tubes secure.
- Use normal saline solution for the bladder irrigant unless otherwise prescribed. Normal saline solution is isotonic.
- Adjust the rate of the irrigation solution to the physician's specifications. The physician may prescribe a solution rate that keeps the output clear and free of clots.
- Monitor the color, consistency, and amount of urine output.
- Check the drainage tubing frequently for external obstructions (such as kinks) and internal obstructions (such as blood clots and decreased output).
- Assess the client for reports of bladder spasms, which may indicate obstruction.
- If the urinary catheter is obstructed, turn off the continuous bladder irrigation (CBI), and irrigate the catheter with 30 to 50 mL of normal saline solution using a large piston syringe.
- Notify the physician immediately if the obstruction does not resolve by hand irrigation or if the urinary return becomes "ketchupy."

Nursing Care After Suprapubic Prostatectomy. If the client has undergone a suprapubic prostatectomy, a suprapubic catheter, in addition to a urethral catheter, will be in place. Each catheter is connected to a separate closed drainage system and drains the bladder via gravity. Be aware that catheter traction is not effective for the client who has bleeding after a suprapubic prostatectomy. This client needs brisk CBI via the catheter. If the CBI does not control the bleeding, the client needs surgical intervention.

If the client has a suprapubic catheter in place, the urethral catheter is generally removed on the second day after surgery. After the retention catheter is removed, clamp the suprapubic catheter and instruct the client to attempt to void. After the client has urinated, check the residual urine in the bladder by unclamping the suprapubic tube. The client may be discharged from the hospital with a suprapubic catheter in place. When the client consistently empties his bladder and the residual urine in the bladder is 75 mL or less, the suprapubic catheter is then removed. An antimicrobial ointment may be applied daily to the site, depending on hospital's policy or the physician's preference.

The client with a suprapubic catheter in place is at increased risk for bladder spasms. Observe the incision dressing at least twice per shift, and change it frequently because the dressing becomes saturated with urine until the incision heals. If the suprapubic drain is not connected to gravity drainage, enclose the drain with an ostomy bag to measure the output accurately and to prevent any skin problems or breakdown.

Nursing Care After Retropubic Prostatectomy. After a retropubic prostatectomy, the urinary sphincter muscles are seldom damaged, the bladder is not entered, and no urinary drainage should be seen on the abdominal dressing. Notify the surgeon of any urinary or purulent drainage, fever, or increased pain because these symptoms indicate a serious complication such as a deep wound infection or pelvic abscess.

Nursing Care After Perineal Prostatectomy. After the perineal approach to prostatectomy, the client has an incision dressing and may or may not have an incision drain. Rectal thermometers and rectal tubes or enemas are not used because they may cause trauma or bleeding.

Community-Based Care

The client with benign prostatic hyperplasia (BPH) is typically managed at home. Clients who have surgery are also discharged to their home.

HOME CARE MANAGEMENT

Unless there is a complication of surgery, such as a wound infection or an unusual problem with voiding, the client does not have a dressing or indwelling catheter at the time of discharge. In some cases, the suprapubic tube may remain in place for several weeks after discharge.

HEALTH TEACHING

After any type of prostatectomy, some clients, especially those who have undergone a transurethral resection of the prostate (TURP), may have temporary loss of control of urination or a dribbling of the urine. Reassure the client that these symptoms are almost always temporary and will resolve. Assist the client and his family in devising ways to keep his clothing dry until sphincter control returns. Instruct him to contract and relax his sphincter frequently to re-establish urinary control (Kegel exercises). External urinary (condom or Texas) catheters are not used except in extreme cases because they may give the client a false sense of security and delay his urinary control.

Provide specific instructions for each client on the basis of the type of surgical procedure performed and any interventions he may need in the future. Discharge instructions for a client undergoing surgery of the prostate gland are listed in Chart 79-4.

CHART 79-4

CLIENT EDUCATION GUIDE
Care After a Transurethral Resection of the Prostate

- Drink 12 to 14 glasses of water each day, preferably before 8 PM, *unless otherwise contraindicated*.
- Use alcohol, caffeinated beverages, and spicy foods in moderation to avoid overstimulation of your bladder.
- If your urine becomes bloody, rest quietly and increase your fluid intake. If the bleeding does not subside shortly, contact your doctor.
- Avoid strenuous activities, such as driving and working, during the first 2 to 3 weeks after surgery.
- Schedule a follow-up appointment with your doctor after you leave the hospital.

The client who undergoes prostatic surgery usually needs emotional support. The client who undergoes a perineal prostatectomy is at risk for permanent sexual dysfunction. Inform the client of the options, such as a penile prosthesis, that are available to treat erectile dysfunction (ED) (see Interventions [Erectile Dysfunction], p. 1871).

Other surgical procedures for prostate removal should not cause physiologic ED. However, some clients may have functional ED for a short time after surgery during the recovery phase.

? Critical Thinking Challenge

You are starting a new shift and are caring for a man who returned from the PACU 3 hours ago after a TURP. He received epidural anesthesia for this surgery. He is receiving continuous bladder irrigation with normal saline. The flow sheet at the bedside indicates that a 1500-mL bag of normal saline was hung 1 hour ago. The bag is now empty, and there is only 200 mL of fluid in the drainage bag of the three-way catheter.

1. What assessment data should you obtain?
2. What action should you take as soon as possible?
3. Should the next bag of irrigation solution be started now? Why or Why not?
4. Which staff member should be assigned to care for this client during the rest of the shift: registered nurse, LPN, nursing assistant? Provide a rationale for your choice.

evolve For suggested answer guidelines, go to http://evolve.elsevier.com/Iggy/.

PROSTATE CANCER

PATHOPHYSIOLOGY

Prostate cancer is the most common invasive cancer among American men. It follows lung cancer as the second leading cause of cancer deaths in this group (American Cancer Society, 2005a).

Of all cancers of the prostate, 95% are adenocarcinomas. These cancers arise from the epithelial cells of the prostate and are usually located in the posterior lobe or outer portion of the gland (Figure 79-5). The remaining types of prostatic neoplasms are classified as *nonepithelial* carcinomas and include ductal carcinomas, transitional cell carcinomas, squamous cell carcinomas, and sarcomas.

Of all malignancies, prostate cancer is one of the slowest growing, and it metastasizes in a predictable pattern. Common sites of metastasis are the nearby lymph nodes; bone marrow; and the bones of the pelvis, sacrum, and lumbar spine.

Spread to the visceral organs occurs late in the course of the disease. Common organ sites of metastasis for prostate cancer are the lungs, liver, adrenals, and kidneys.

Tumor grade is an important factor in the management of prostate cancer. Grading is the pathologist's interpretation of the aggressiveness of the cancer. Usually the Gleason grading system is used. Normal prostate tissue cells are given a score of 1 (best), and abnormal cells are given a score of up to 5 (worst). The scores of the two most common cell types found in the specimen are added to give the tumor a grade between 2 and 10.

Etiology and Genetic Risk

Although the cause of prostate cancer remains unclear, several factors influence its development. First, an intact hypothalamic-pituitary-testicular pathway must be present. Men who have been castrated before puberty are at little risk for prostate cancer. Second, the advancing age of the client increases his risk of prostate cancer.

Other contributing factors include a family history of prostate cancer, heavy metal exposure, and a history of vasectomy or sexually transmitted disease (STD). Several viruses, including cytomegalovirus and herpesvirus type 2, are present more commonly in prostate cancer cells than in normal cells.

Genetic Considerations

Most prostate cancers are sporadic in nature, meaning that no clear pattern of inheritance emerges. However, some genetic influences for prostate cancer have been discovered. The risk for prostate cancer is greater among men who have a first-degree relative (father, brother, or son) with prostate cancer. Inherited forms of prostate cancer are suspected, and some are known. People who have specific *BRCA-2* gene mutations have an increased risk for breast cancer and an increased risk for prostate cancer among male carriers. For individuals who have these gene mutations, prostate cancer develops at an earlier age and usually has a more aggressive profile. Other gene mutations are being studied in the hope of developing a test to more accurately assess risk for prostate cancer development.

Incidence/Prevalence

Prostate cancer is the sixth most common cancer worldwide. It is mainly a cancer of older men and occurs rarely before age 39 years. The rate increases after age 40 to as many as one in six between the ages of 60 and 79 (American Cancer Society, 2005a). Recent increases in incidence rates in the United States are related to earlier diagnosis through an increase in mass screenings with prostate specific antigen (PSA) levels and digital rectal examinations (DRE). The actual incidence in the United States has stabilized. The

American Cancer Society estimates that 232,090 new cases of prostate cancer will be diagnosed in 2005 and that 30,350 deaths will result from the disease. Prostate cancer has a higher incidence in less affluent countries and a low incidence in Asian countries.

CONSIDERATIONS FOR OLDER ADULTS

The incidence of prostate cancer increases with age. More than 75% of all prostate cancers are diagnosed in men over 65 years of age (American Cancer Society, 2005a). Include questions about prostate problems whenever you are assessing the health of an older adult male.

CULTURAL CONSIDERATIONS

African-American men tend to be affected at an earlier age and have more advanced disease at diagnosis. The American Cancer Society estimates that 27,000 African-American men will be diagnosed with prostate cancer in 2005 and that 5300 will die of the disease. Lack of cancer awareness may be one cause of increased mortality rates. Reduced access to primary care and screening is another factor. New guidelines for prostate cancer screening recommend that African-American men begin screening by age 45 years (ACS, 2005a; ACS, 2005b).

COLLABORATIVE MANAGEMENT

Assessment

HISTORY

As with any cancer, accurate staging is needed for treatment planning and for monitoring the course of the disease. As in BPH, the first symptoms that the client may experience are related to bladder neck obstruction, such as difficulty in initiating urination, recurrent bladder infections, and urinary retention. Gross, painless hematuria is the most common presenting manifestation.

A client may be undergoing treatment for BPH and is discovered to have prostate cancer. Bone pain is a symptom of a more advanced stage of prostate cancer. The client who has symptoms of urinary obstruction (urinary hesitancy, back pain) and bone pain is likely to have metastatic disease at diagnosis.

PHYSICAL EXAMINATION AND PROSTATE CANCER SCREENING

The most effective screening procedures for prostate cancer are the **digital rectal examination (DRE)** and the PSA test. Chart 79-5 lists the American Cancer Society's prostate cancer screening guideline. Beginning at age 50 years, all men should have an annual DRE and PSA test. Men at higher risk for prostate cancer, including African Americans or men who have a first-degree relative with prostate cancer, should start screening at 45 years of age.

DIGITAL RECTAL EXAMINATION. On rectal examination, a prostate that is found to be stony hard and with palpable irregularities or indurations is suspected to be malignant.

PROSTATE-SPECIFIC ANTIGEN. Prostate-specific antigen (PSA) is a glycoprotein produced solely by the prostate. The normal blood level of PSA is less than 4 ng/mL.

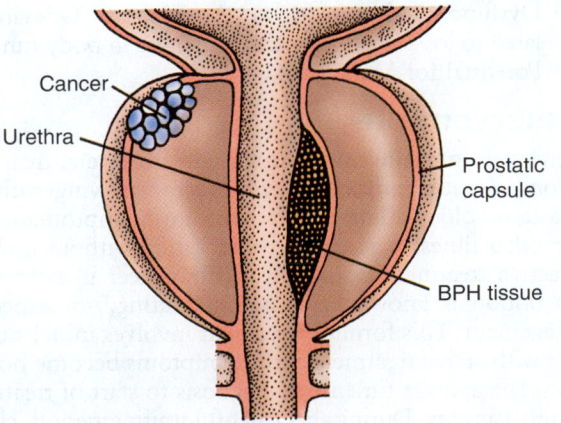

Figure 79-5 ■ The prostate gland with cancer and benign prostatic hyperplasia (BPH). Note that cancer normally arises in the periphery of the gland, whereas BPH occurs in the center of the gland.

Labels on figure: Cancer, Urethra, Prostatic capsule, BPH tissue

CLIENT EDUCATION GUIDE
American Cancer Society Prostate Screening and Detection Guidelines (2005)

- An annual digital rectal examination (DRE) and prostate-specific antigen (PSA) test should be offered to the following clients:
  Men beginning at age 50 years
  Men who have a life expectancy of at least 10 years
  Younger men who are at high risk (at least by age 45 years)
- Men at high risk include those with a strong familial predisposition (e.g., two or more first-degree relatives with prostate cancer) and African-American men.
- DRE should be performed by health care professionals skilled in recognizing subtle prostate abnormalities.
- DRE is less effective than PSA in detecting prostate cancer. An abnormal PSA test result is a value above 4.0 ng/mL.

PSA levels are higher in clients with increased prostatic tissue as a result of BPH, prostatic infarction, prostatitis, and prostate cancer. The levels associated with prostate cancer are usually much higher than those occurring with other prostate tissue enlargement.

Prostate-specific antigen blood levels should never be used as a screening test without a digital rectal examination (DRE) of the prostate. *The PSA serum level does not replace the DRE but is to be used in conjunction with it.* Because other prostate problems also increase the PSA level, it is not specifically diagnostic for cancer. In addition, about 25% of clients with prostate cancer have PSA levels less than 4 ng/mL.

The PSA is not elevated in healthy men or in men with cancer in other organs. However, the normal PSA level is slightly higher in older adults and in African Americans. An elevated PSA level should decrease a few days after a prostatectomy. An increase in the PSA level several weeks after surgery usually indicates that the disease has recurred.

OTHER DIAGNOSTIC ASSESSMENTS

After screening by DRE and PSA, some clients undergo a transrectal ultrasound study of the prostate. The urologist inserts a small probe into the rectum and obtains an ultrasonogram of the prostate. A specimen for biopsy may also be obtained with the rectal probe.

BIOPSY

When the diagnosis of prostatic cancer is suspected, a biopsy is necessary for confirmation. Prostatic ultrasonography may be performed to isolate the area of the prostate for biopsy. One of several procedures may be used to obtain the biopsy specimen. The most common procedure is the needle-core or aspiration biopsy.

After a transrectal ultrasound with biopsy, instruct the client about possible complications, including hematuria with clots, signs of infection, and perineal pain. Instruct the client to report fever, chills, bloody urine, and any difficulty voiding. Usually antibiotics are prescribed. Stress to the client the importance of completing the entire course. Advise the client to avoid strenuous physical activity and drink plenty of fluids, especially in the first 24 hours after the procedure.

After the diagnosis of prostate cancer is made, the client undergoes radiographic and blood studies to ascertain the extent of the disease. Common tests include computed to-

mography (CT) of the pelvis and abdomen and magnetic resonance imaging (MRI) to assess the status of the pelvic and para-aortic lymph nodes. A bone scan is performed to detect metastatic disease. An enlarged liver or abnormal liver function study results indicate possible liver metastases. Clients with advanced prostate cancer may have elevated levels of serum acid phosphatase. About 90% of clients with bone metastasis have elevated serum alkaline phosphatase levels.

Critical Thinking Challenge

The client is a 70-year-old man who tells you he has had the following symptoms for a year: hesitancy, nocturia, hematuria, reduced size of the urinary stream, pain in the lower back and legs, and dribbling after voiding. He has never had a DRE or a PSA test. He tells you he is worried about possibly having prostate cancer for two reasons; one is that his father died of prostate cancer at age 75, and the other is that he had gonorrhea when he was 22 years old.

1. Which of this client's manifestations are more specific to prostate cancer, and which are common to prostate cancer and BPH?
2. Is this client's history of gonorrhea important to his current health problem? Why or why not?
3. Does the fact that this client's father died of prostate cancer increase the client's risk for it? Why or why not?

evolve For suggested answer guidelines, go to http://evolve.elsevier.com/Iggy/.

Common Nursing Diagnoses and Collaborative Problems

Nursing diagnoses and collaborative problems that may apply to clients with prostate cancer include the following:

- Anxiety related to a threat to or change in health status and treatment options
- Acute Pain or Chronic Pain related to effects of metastasis, bone pain, and spinal cord compression
- Impaired Urinary Elimination related to sensory motor impairment, blockage, or trauma
- Risk for Sexual Dysfunction related to altered body structure or function (secondary to disease process and treatment)
- Dysfunctional Grieving or Anticipatory Grieving related to loss of a body part or changes in body function
- Potential for Metastasis

Interventions

Clients with prostate cancer are faced with several treatment options. Because prostate cancer is slow growing with late metastasis, older adult clients who are asymptomatic and have other illness may choose observation without immediate active treatment, especially if the cancer is early stage. This option is known as "watchful waiting," or expectant management. This form of treatment involves initial surveillance with active treatment if the symptoms become bothersome. The average time from diagnosis to start of treatment is up to 10 years. During the watchful waiting period, clients are monitored at regular intervals through DRE and PSA testing. Factors that are considered in choosing watchful waiting include potential side effects of treatment (e.g., urinary incontinence, erectile dysfunction, bowel dysfunction), estimated life expectancy, and the risk for increased morbidity and mortality from not seeking active treatment.

Clients who have stage 0 cancer of the prostate who choose watchful waiting require only close follow-up by their health care provider. If obstruction occurs, repeated needle biopsies or transurethral resection of the prostate (TURPs) should be part of the screening.

Active treatment options for the client with prostate cancer include surgery, radiation therapy, and drug therapy. Management is based on the extent of the disease and the client's physical condition. The client may undergo surgery for a biopsy, staging and removal of the tumor, or palliation to control the spread of disease or relieve distressing symptoms. As with watchful waiting, the health care provider and client must weigh the benefits of treatment against potential adverse effects such as incontinence and erectile dysfunction (ED).

SURGICAL MANAGEMENT. Because as many as 30% of localized prostate cancers are resistant to radiation, surgery is the standard treatment. Usually a radical prostatectomy is performed. The surgical approaches for prostatectomy are similar to those for BPH (see Surgical Management [Benign Prostatic Hyperplasia], p. 1860). However, the surgery is much more extensive.

Preoperative Care. The surgeon advises clients who are undergoing radical perineal prostatectomy that they may have erectile dysfunction (ED) after the surgery. This consequence is directly related to any damage done to the pudendal nerve (which is needed for erection and orgasm) during the surgery. Another consequence of this surgery is the possibility of urinary incontinence. To help reduce the severity of incontinence, teach the client how to perform **Kegel exercises** (exercises that strengthen the pubococcygeus muscle) before surgery. These exercises are continued after surgery.

For the client undergoing a radical prostatectomy, the preoperative procedure includes bowel cleansing using a cathartic such as GoLYTELY. The client is usually permitted to have a clear liquid diet the day before surgery, with nothing by mouth after midnight. Drugs for other pre-existing conditions may be taken the morning of surgery with only sips of water. Provide psychosocial and spiritual supportive measures as needed.

Operative Procedures. The radical prostatectomy can be performed via a retropubic, perineal, or suprapubic approach. The surgeon removes the entire prostate gland along with the prostatic capsule, the cuff at the bladder neck, the seminal vesicles, and the regional lymph nodes. The remaining urethra is anastomosed to the bladder neck. The removal of tissue at the bladder neck allows the seminal fluid to travel upward into the bladder rather than down the urethral tract, resulting in retrograde ejaculations. The client is sterile.

Often the pudendal nerves are damaged or severed during a radical prostatectomy. The surgeon may perform a "nerve-sparing" prostatectomy in the following cases:
- There is no evidence of disease in adjacent lymph nodes.
- Serum acid phosphatase levels are not elevated.
- There is no evidence of cancer beyond the prostate gland.

As the name of the procedure implies, the surgeon keeps the nerves responsible for penile erection intact. After surgery,

---

CHART 79-6

BEST PRACTICE for
Care of the Client After a Radical Prostatectomy

- Encourage the client to use patient-controlled analgesia (PCA) as needed. The PCA device may be used through the second postoperative day.
- Keep the client on bedrest on the day of surgery. Help the client to get out of bed and ambulate for a short distance by the first postoperative day.
- Maintain the sequential compression device until the client begins to ambulate. Apply antiembolic stockings until discharge.
- Monitor the client for deep vein thrombosis and pulmonary embolus.
- Keep an accurate record of intake and output, including Jackson-Pratt or other drainage device drainage.
- Keep the urinary meatus clean using soap and water.
- Avoid rectal procedures or treatments.
- Teach the client how to care for the urinary catheter because he will be discharged with the catheter in place.
- Teach the client how to use a leg bag.
- Emphasize the importance of not straining during bowel movement. Advise the client to avoid suppositories or enemas.
- Remind the client about the importance of follow-up appointments with the physician to monitor progress.

---

the client may experience temporary ED, but normal function usually returns in 3 to 12 months.

Postoperative Care. Care of the client after radical prostatectomy is listed in Chart 79-6. Activities include all the typical care for a client undergoing major surgery. These issues include maintaining hydration with IV therapy, caring for wound drains, preventing emboli, and preventing pulmonary complications (see Chapter 22).

Drug therapy after surgery includes antibiotics to prevent infection and analgesics for pain. Pain is managed with opioids given IV with patient-controlled analgesia (PCA), a common method of delivery. A laxative and stool softener may be given to prevent possible constipation from the drugs.

The client has an indwelling urinary catheter to straight drainage. An antispasmodic may be prescribed to decrease bladder spasm induced by the indwelling urinary catheter. Belladonna and opium suppositories are avoided because rectal manipulation may injure the surgical site. Kegel exercises, taught before surgery, should be performed consistently throughout the day.

The client may have a nasogastric tube (NGT) to low intermittent suction because of the extensive surgery. The NGT is usually discontinued on the second day after surgery. The client is then permitted clear liquids. Solid foods are introduced as tolerated when bowel sounds return.

Ambulation begins early, usually by the second day after surgery. Provide assistance in ambulating the client at least twice a day. Scrotal or penile swelling may occur from the disruption in pelvic lymph flow. If this occurs, elevate the scrotum and penis and apply ice to the area intermittently (20 minutes on and 20 minutes off) for the first 24 to 48 hours.

Complications. Common potential long-term complications of radical prostatectomy are urinary incontinence and erectile dysfunction.

Urinary Incontinence. Incontinence is possible because the internal and external sphincters of the bladder lie close to the prostate gland and are often damaged during the surgery.

EVIDENCE-BASED PRACTICE for Nursing

Clients and society are not prepared for male incontinence

Palmer, M.H., et al. (2003). Incontinence after prostatectomy: Coping with incontinence after prostate cancer surgery. *Oncology Nursing Forum, 30*(2), 229-238.

The purpose of this survey study was to describe the nature of postprostatectomy urinary incontinence, determine how men manage postsurgery urinary incontinence, identify men's perceptions of adequacy of preoperative counseling, and identify men's expectations regarding the probability of postsurgery incontinence. Subjects were a convenience sample of 154 men postprostatectomy who belonged to the support group, "US TOO." Subjects self-selected to complete a questionnaire with both forced-choice items and open-ended questions.

Of the 154 subjects responding to the survey, 105 indicated that incontinence was or remained a significant problem with social, economic, and emotional effects. Subjects indicated that problems away from home, such as the availability of continence pads or garments, appropriate disposal sites, and the expectation of other men that continence is expected, were of greatest concern. Additionally, this study found that the incidence of persistent incontinence after prostate cancer surgery was greater than reported in the medical literature and that most men were not well-prepared to deal with the problem.

Level of Evidence: 6—Uncontrolled, descriptive study.

Critique. The use of a convenience sample and the self-selection may have biased study results toward the relatively high incidence of persistent incontinence. However, this study was valuable because it uncovered areas of need for male clients with any degree of incontinence.

Implications for Nursing. The study found that it is extremely important for nurses to give these clients information on more than one occasion. Preoperative information should be reinforced with additional follow-up information, emotional support, and practical assistance with management strategies for urinary incontinence. Nurses should promote the continued use of Kegel exercises to improve urine control. Because use of these exercises appeared to decline over time, continued teaching and reinforcement of the need to perform these exercises are important. Nurses can also be helpful by providing information on what types of continence care supplies are available and at what economic costs. Developing a "tip" sheet for how to manage incontinence away from home would also be useful.

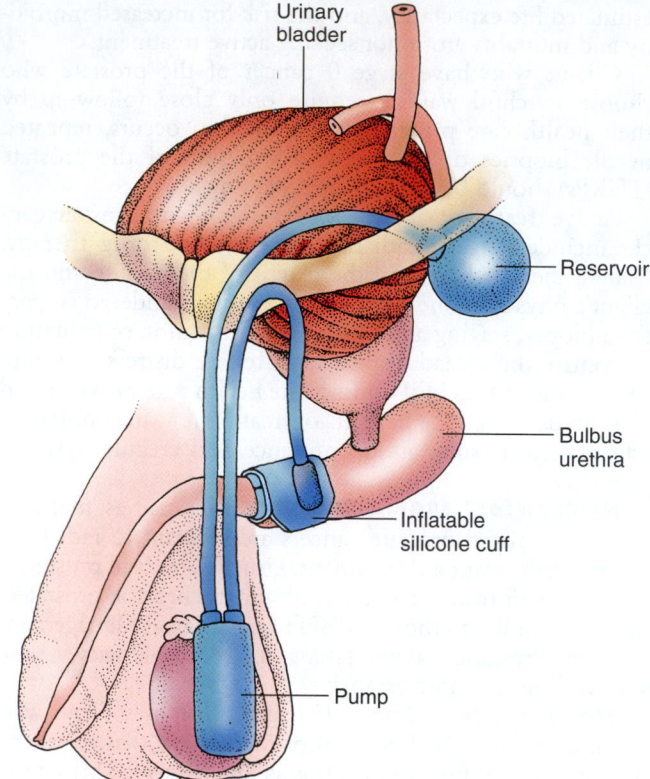

Figure 79-6 ■ An artificial urinary sphincter is a fluid-filled system with a silicone cuff that surrounds the urethra and functions as a urinary sphincter. A pump is placed in the scrotum, and a fluid reservoir is placed in the abdomen. When the pump is squeezed, fluid leaves the urethral cuff and flows into the reservoir, allowing the client to empty his bladder.

Kegel perineal exercises have been shown to reduce the severity of urinary incontinence after radical prostatectomy (see the Evidence-Based Practice for Nursing box above).

Teach the client perineal exercises to help facilitate the return of urinary continence after surgery or after removal of the retention catheter. To perform the exercises, the client contracts and relaxes the perineal and gluteal muscles in several ways. For one of the exercises, teach the client to do the following:

1. Tighten the perineal muscles for 3 to 5 seconds as if to prevent voiding and then relax.
2. Bear down as if having a bowel movement.
3. Relax and repeat the exercise.

Show the client how to inhale through pursed lips while tightening the perineal muscles and how to exhale when he relaxes. To regain urinary control, teach the client to practice holding an object, such as a pencil, in the fold between the buttock and the thigh. He may also sit on the toilet with the knees apart while voiding and start and stop the stream several times.

Other interventions for incontinence that may be helpful after radical prostatectomy include biofeedback retraining and the surgical placement of an artificial urinary sphincter

(Figure 79-6). Artificial sphincters have been more successful in men than in women, possibly because of the difference in urethral length. After sphincter implantation, instruct the client to report fever, pain on inflation of the device, edema or cellulitis in the genitalia (manifestations of infection), or recurrence of incontinence (indicating a possible mechanical malfunction of the device).

Erectile Dysfunction. Difficulty having or maintaining and erection is possible after radical prostatectomy because of damage to the pudendal nerves. Interventions for erectile dysfunction are presented on pp. 1870 to 1871.

Cryosurgical Ablation. **Cryoablation** is a minimally invasive procedure that can be an alternative to radical prostatectomy. This surgery is reserved for clients for whom the cancer is known to be confined to the prostate gland. During surgery, the client is placed in the lithotomy position, and a transrectal ultrasound probe is placed in the rectum. The probe helps to determine the size of the prostate and the subsequent number of small cryoprobes that are positioned around the prostate gland. Liquid nitrogen freezes the gland and results in prostate cell death. The dead cells are then absorbed gradually by the body.

The advantages of this procedure are minimal blood loss, minimal pain, decreased risk for urinary incontinence, and a short hospital stay. Most clients are able to return to their usual activity level in about 1 week after surgery. The procedure can be repeated if necessary.

CHART 79-7

DRUG THERAPY for
Prostate Cancer: Hormone Therapy

Drug	Usual Dosage	Nursing Interventions
Leuprolide acetate (Lupron)	7.5 mg IM q mo	Use at least a 22-gauge needle. Mix the solution well; it is a milky suspension. Observe for side effects, including "hot flashes" and sweating. Be aware that the client's symptoms may temporarily worsen, caused by a temporary testosterone increase.
Flutamide (Eulexin, Euflex✳)	750 mg PO in 3 daily divided doses	Teach the client that side effects include "hot flashes," loss of libido, and impotence. Diarrhea and nausea with vomiting are less common.
Goserelin acetate (Zoladex)	3.6 mg SC every 28 days	The prefilled syringe cannot be aspirated. If a blood vessel is damaged, blood will enter the syringe. Teach the client that side effects include "hot flashes," sexual dysfunction, and decreased erections.

SC, Subcutaneous.

Bilateral Orchiectomy. **Bilateral orchiectomy** (removal of both testes) is palliative surgery and is not intended to cure the prostate cancer. The intent of the surgery is to arrest cancer spread by removing testosterone. This procedure is described later in this chapter under Testicular Cancer, p. 1874.

NONSURGICAL MANAGEMENT. Nonsurgical management is usually an adjunct to surgery but may be done as an alternative intervention. Modalities include radiation therapy, hormonal therapy, chemotherapy, and targeted therapy.

Radiation Therapy. External beam radiation therapy is used in the treatment of prostate cancer for the following purposes:

- As an alternative curative treatment to surgery for locally contained tumors
- As an adjunct to radical prostatectomy when surgical margins or regional lymph nodes show cancer cells after surgery
- For palliation of the client's symptoms

Palliative radiation therapy relieves pain caused by bone metastases and relieves ureteral or bladder neck obstruction.

Radiation therapy also can be performed by implanting low-dose radiation seeds directly into and around the prostate gland. This treatment includes ultrasonically guided iodine-125 or pallidium-103 interstitial brachytherapy (radiation therapy) or radioactive seed implantation. These procedures are done on an ambulatory care basis and are the most cost-effective treatment for early stage prostate cancer. Reassure the client that the dose of radiation is low and that he will not pose a hazard to himself or others. These treatments are well tolerated and have minimal complications.

Drug Therapy. Drug therapy may consist of either hormonal therapy or chemotherapy. A vaccine to locate and destroy prostate cancer cells is also being investigated (Marks, 2003).

Hormonal Therapy. Because prostate cancer is hormone dependent, clients with extensive tumors or those with metastatic disease are usually managed by androgen deprivation. Manipulating the hormonal environment in the client may be accomplished in two ways:

- The testosterone influence can be removed by a bilateral orchiectomy.

- Estrogens or gonadotropin-releasing hormone (GnRH) agonist analogs can be given (Chart 79-7).

Estrogens such as diethylstilbestrol (DES) inhibit the release of luteinizing hormone (LH) from the pituitary gland. Clients with significant cardiovascular disease may not be candidates for estrogen therapy because of the side effects of estrogens, such as sodium and water retention and thromboembolic episodes. Other hormonal drugs, such as megestrol (Megace) and medroxyprogesterone (Depo-Provera), are sometimes used if first-line hormonal treatments lose their effectiveness.

Leuprolide acetate (Lupron), a GnRH agonist analogue (which suppresses LH release by the pituitary) reduces serum testosterone levels without any of the estrogenic side effects of DES. Flutamide (Eulexin, Euflex✳), an oral androgen-blocking agent, inhibits tumor progression by blocking the uptake of testicular and adrenal androgens at the prostate tumor site.

Goserelin acetate (Zoladex), a potent GnRH agonist analogue, may be prescribed for palliation of advanced prostatic carcinoma. This drug is an alternative treatment when orchiectomy or estrogen administration is not acceptable or not indicated for the client.

Chemotherapy. Systemic cytotoxic chemotherapy has not proved effective as the main treatment of prostate cancer. It is used for the client who fails to respond to hormonal manipulation. Agents approved for this use are a combination of docetaxel (Taxotere) and prednisone. Estramustine (Emcyt) is another drug that combines an estrogen with the chemotherapy drug mechlorethamine. Although these therapies prolong survival, they do not cure the disease. Clinical trials are testing the effectiveness of thalidomide (Celgene), a drug that inhibits blood vessel formation, on prostate cancer. (See Chapter 28 for a discussion of chemotherapy.)

Targeted Therapy. A promising area of treatment for prostate cancer is targeted therapy. These therapies take advantage of one or more differences in a cancer cell that is either not present or only slightly present in normal cells. Agents used as targeted therapies are either antibodies that "target" a cellular element of the cancer cell or "antisense" drugs that work at the gene level. Some agents being tested as targeted therapy for prostate cancer are targeted to the

CLIENT EDUCATION GUIDE
Catheter Care at Home

- Once a day gently wash the first 6 inches of the catheter starting at the penis and washing outward with mild soap and water.
- Rinse and dry the catheter well.
- If you have not been circumcised, push the foreskin back to the clean the catheter site; when finished, push the foreskin forward.
- Change the drainage bag at least once a week.
    Hold the catheter with one hand and the tubing with the other hand and twist in opposite directions to disconnect.
    Place the end of the catheter in a clean container to catch leakage of urine.
    Remove the rubber cap from the tubing of the leg bag or clean drainage bag.
    Clean the end of the new tubing with alcohol swabs.
    Insert the end of the new tubing into the catheter and twist to connect securely.
- Clean the drainage bag just removed by pouring a solution of one part vinegar to two parts water through the tubing and bag. Rinse well with water and allow the bag to dry.

epidermal growth factor receptor. Another targeting drug in clinical trials for prostate cancer is bortezomib (Velcade), a proteosome inhibitor.

Community-Based Care

Nursing management of the client with prostate cancer always includes his spouse or sexual partner. Clients with prostate cancer may require nursing interventions in a wide variety of settings: at the hospital, the radiation therapy department, the oncologist's office, or home and at any stage of the disease process. The following interventions focus on the needs of clients who have undergone radical prostatectomy for prostate cancer.

HOME CARE MANAGEMENT

Discharge planning and health teaching start early, even before surgery. A client can better plan home care management when he knows what to expect. A case manager working with the client throughout treatment is helpful in coordinating the efforts of the physician, surgical unit nursing staff, and home care nurse. The client then has one person with whom he can feel connected and can rely on for information and referral. The case manager provides continuity.

HEALTH TEACHING

An important area of teaching for the client going home after radical prostatectomy is catheter care. An indwelling urinary catheter may be in place for up to 3 weeks. Teach the client how to care for the catheter, use a leg bag, and identify manifestations of infection and other complications. See Chart 79-8 for information on teaching clients about catheter care in the home.

Walking short distances is encouraged, but lifting is restricted to no more than 15 pounds for up to 6 weeks. Clients need to maintain an upright position and not walk bent or flexed. Vigorous exercise such as running or jumping should be avoided for at least 12 weeks and then gradually introduced.

Instruct the client not to strain to defecate. A stool softener may be prescribed to reduce the need for straining. If an opioid is prescribed for pain management, encourage the client to drink plenty of water to prevent constipation.

Instruct the client to shower rather than soak in a bathtub for the first 2 to 3 weeks. Teach him how to inspect the incision site daily for signs of infection. Follow-up appointments are scheduled in 1 week for removal of the staples and in 2 to 3 weeks for removal of the urinary catheter. PSA blood tests are taken 6 weeks after surgery and then every 4 to 6 months to monitor progress.

HEALTH CARE RESOURCES

Refer the client and family to agencies or support groups such as the American Cancer Society's Man to Man program to help cope with prostate cancer. This program provides one-on-one education, personal visits, educational presentations, and the opportunity to engage in open and candid discussions. Another prostate cancer support group is "US TOO," sponsored by the American Foundation for Urologic Disease. This group provides education and support with national and international chapters.

ERECTILE DYSFUNCTION

PATHOPHYSIOLOGY

Erectile dysfunction (ED), previously known as impotence, is the inability to achieve or maintain an erection for sexual intercourse. It affects about 10 to 20 million men in the United States. During the last decade, there has been a major change in the management of men with ED as a result of increased understanding of the physiology of erectile function and the development of new, effective therapies. There are two classes of ED: organic and functional.

Organic Erectile Dysfunction

Organic ED is a gradual deterioration of function. The man first notices diminishing firmness and a decrease in frequency of erections. Causes include the following:

- Inflammation of the prostate, urethra, or seminal vesicles
- Surgical procedures such as prostatectomy
- Pelvic fractures
- Lumbosacral injuries
- Vascular disease, including hypertension
- Chronic neurologic conditions, such as Parkinson disease or multiple sclerosis
- Endocrine disorders, such as diabetes mellitus or thyroid disorders
- Smoking and alcohol consumption
- Drugs
- Poor overall health that prevents sexual intercourse

Functional Erectile Dysfunction

If the client has episodes of ED, it usually has a functional (psychological) cause. Men with functional ED have normal nocturnal (nighttime) and morning erections. Onset is usually sudden and preceded by a period of high stress.

◆ COLLABORATIVE MANAGEMENT
◆ Assessment

For a man to have an erection, he must have normal innervation and a normal **libido** (sex drive). Therefore a medical, social, and sexual history along with a complete physical examination is needed. The first step is to determine whether there is an organic cause. Diagnostic testing is done to rule out possible organic causes.

If test results are negative, the evaluation then focuses on the specific causes that may have been indicated in the client's medical history. For example, hormone testing is used for clients who have a poor libido, small testicles, or sparse beard growth. Serum levels of testosterone and gonadotropins are also measured.

Duplex Doppler ultrasonography is another test to evaluate ED. It provides information about arterial and venous blood flow to the penis. It can also be used to determine the best treatment for ED. A nocturnal penile tumescence test that measures nighttime erections is done in a sleep laboratory. Usually an erection is expected with each rapid eye movement (REM) episode. This study can determine whether ED is caused by an organic or functional problem. If the man has nocturnal erections, the ED is functional. Sexual counseling is needed in this case, and the client is referred to a certified sexual therapist.

◆Interventions

Current methods of treatment include oral drug therapy, vacuum devices, intracorporal injections, intraurethral applications, and prostheses.

Drug Therapy. Drugs used to manage erectile dysfunction work by causing relaxation of the smooth muscles in the corpora cavernosa so blood flow to the penis is increased. The veins exiting the corpora are compressed, limiting outward blood flow, resulting in penile **tumescence** (swelling). Clients are instructed to take the pill 1 hour before sexual intercourse. For some drugs, such as sildenafil (Viagra) and vardenafil (Levitra), sexual stimulation is needed within a half hour to 1 hour to promote the erection. With other drugs, such as tadalafil (Cialis), erection can be stimulated over a longer period. Because the erection occurs more naturally compared with other treatment options, most men and their partners prefer this option.

Instruct clients to abstain from alcohol before sexual intercourse because it may impair the ability to have an erection. Common side effects of these drugs include headaches, facial flushing, and diarrhea. If more than one pill a day is being taken, leg and back cramps, nausea, and vomiting also may occur. Men who take nitrates should not take these drugs because the vasodilation effects can cause a profound hypotension and reduce blood flow to vital organs.

Vacuum Devices. The basic design of a vacuum device is a cylinder that fits over the penis and sits firmly against the body. Using a pump, a vacuum is created to draw blood into the penis to maintain an erection. A rubber ring (tension band) is placed around the base of the penis to maintain the erection, and the cylinder is removed.

The advantage of this procedure is that the device is easy and safe to use. The disadvantage is its clumsiness and lack of spontaneity. In addition, the man may experience pain from the rubber ring or from pumping the device too quickly. The ring should be removed after an hour, or tissue damage may occur.

Intracorporal Injections. Injecting the penis with vasoconstrictive drugs can make the penis erect. The most

common agents used for this purpose today are papaverine, phentolamine (Regitine), and alprostadil. These drugs may be used alone but are most often given in combination. The drug is injected into the side of the penis using a 27- or 30-gauge needle. Adverse effects include priapism (prolonged erection), penile scarring, fibrosis, bleeding, bruising at the injection site, pain, infection, and vasovagal responses.

Intraurethral Applications. Prostaglandin E (alprostadil [Muse]) is a self-administered suppository that is placed in the urethra with an applicator. The drug is absorbed into the corpora, which causes an erection in about 10 minutes; erections last 30 to 60 minutes. Advantages include the simplicity of the procedure and noninvasiveness. Disadvantages are a decrease in spontaneity, syncope, and burning of the urethra after the application. Rubbing the penis between the client's hands helps relief the discomfort.

Prostheses. Penile implants are used when other modalities fail. Devices include semirigid, malleable, or hydraulic inflatable and multicomponent or one-piece instruments. The three-piece inflatable device is the most commonly implanted prosthesis. A reservoir is placed in the scrotum. Tubes carry the fluid into the inflatable pieces that are placed in the penis. To inflate the prosthesis, the man squeezes the pump located in the scrotum. To deflate the prosthesis, a release button is activated. Advantages include the man's ability to control his erections. The major disadvantages include device failure and infection.

The device is implanted as an ambulatory surgical procedure. Instruct the client to observe the surgical site for bleeding and infection.

TESTICULAR CANCER
PATHOPHYSIOLOGY

Testicular cancer is not common. It represents fewer than 2% of all cancers in men. However, testicular cancer is the most common malignancy in men 15 to 35 years of age (American Cancer Society, 2005a). It strikes young men at a productive time of life and thus has significant economic, social, and psychological impact on the client and his family or partner. Although testicular cancer occurs more often in younger men, middle-aged and older men also may be affected. With early detection by testicular self-examination (TSE) (Chart 79-9) and treatment with combination chemotherapy, testicular cancer can be cured.

Primary testicular cancers fall into two major groups:
- Germ cell tumors arising from the sperm-producing cells (account for 95% of testicular cancers).

TABLE 79-1 Classification of Testicular Tumors	
Germ Cell Germinal Tumors	**Non–Germ Cell (Nongerminal) Tumors**

■ Seminoma
■ Nonseminoma
    Embryonal carcinoma
    Teratoma
    Choriocarcinoma
	■ Interstitial cell tumor
	■ Androblastoma

■ Non–germ cell tumors arising from the stroma, interstitial, or Leydig cells that produce testosterone (account for 2% to 4% of testicular cancers).

Germ Cell Tumors

Testicular germ cell tumors are classified into two broad categories: seminomas and nonseminomas (Table 79-1).

SEMINOMAS

The most common type of testicular tumor is seminoma. Clients with pure seminomatous tumors have the most favorable prognoses because the tumors are usually localized and metastasize late. Seminomas often are diagnosed when they are still confined to the testicles and retroperitoneal lymph nodes. These cancers respond extremely well to radiation therapy. Clients with early stage seminomas have a 5-year survival rate of about a 95% with surgery (orchiectomy) and radiation therapy (American Cancer Society, 2005a).

NONSEMINOMAS

Nonseminomatous germ cell tumors include three types: embryonal carcinoma, teratoma, and choriocarcinoma. These tumors are not as sensitive to treatment with radiation therapy. They are treated with surgery or chemotherapy, depending on the extent of the disease at diagnosis.

Embryonal carcinomas tend to spread earlier than seminomas, usually to the nearby lymph nodes. This tumor may also spread to more distant body sites such as the lung or the liver. Teratomas rarely occur and are usually malignant in adults. Choriocarcinoma is a highly malignant cancer that spreads rapidly throughout the body. Usually metastasis is present at diagnosis.

Non–Germ Cell Tumors

Non–germ cell tumors are classified as either *interstitial cell tumors* or *androblastomas* (testicular adenomas). Most of these tumors do not metastasize. Interstitial cell tumors arise from the Leydig cells, which secrete testosterone into the bloodstream. These tumors secrete an excessive amount of androgenic hormones, which cause young boys with such tumors to undergo early puberty. Androblastomas sometimes secrete estrogen, which accounts for the feminization and **gynecomastia** (breast enlargement) occasionally seen in these clients.

Etiology and Genetic Risk

The cause of testicular cancer is unknown. The risk for testicular tumors is reported to be higher in males who have an undescended testis **(cryptorchidism).** In males with cryptorchidism, the testicular cancer usually develops in the undescended testis (80%), and there is a 25% chance of cancer developing in the normally descended testis. Seminoma is the most common type of testicular cancer associated with

cryptorchidism. The undescended testis undergoes gradual involution and degeneration over time, which may contribute to tumor development. It is not known why the normally descended testis is at risk for cancer. Brothers and close male relatives of clients with testicular cancer have a slightly greater risk for testicular cancer than the general population, suggesting a genetic influence.

Although a history of trauma or infection is common in clients with testicular cancer, neither is a cause of testicular cancer. Testicular trauma or infection can make changes in the shape, size, or texture of the testes more difficult to determine. The client with testicular trauma or infection should be examined by a health care provider after the acute episode subsides to rule out the presence of a tumor.

Testicular cancer is rarely bilateral. Other cancers, however, such as leukemia, lymphoma, plasmacytoma, and metastatic carcinomas may invade the testes. A client with bilateral testicular tumors is more likely to have metastatic disease to the testes than bilateral primary testicular tumors.

Incidence/Prevalence

In the United States it is estimated that 8010 new cases of testicular cancer will be diagnosed each year, and an estimated 390 males will die of the disease. This cancer is the most common solid tumor diagnosed in men between the ages of 15 and 40 years. Testicular cancer can occur during infancy and middle age (after age 50); however, the peak incidence is between the ages of 18 and 40 years (American Cancer Society, 2005a).

◆COLLABORATIVE MANAGEMENT
◆Assessment

HISTORY

When taking a history from a client with a suspected testicular tumor, consider the risk factors. It is important to collect data about age and race because the disease occurs most often in young white males. Be alert to other risk factors, including a history or presence of an undescended testis and a family history of testicular cancer.

Ask the client whether he has noticed a discomfort such as heaviness or aching in the lower abdomen or the scrotum. Determine how long any manifestations have been present.

Assess the client's family situation. Is the client sexually active? Does he have children? Does he want children in the future? Depending on the treatment plan chosen, would he be interested in sperm storage in a sperm bank?

If the client has one healthy testis, he can function sexually and may not have any reproductive dysfunction. If the client undergoes a retroperitoneal lymph node dissection or chemotherapy, he may become sterile because of treatment effects on the sperm-producing cells or surgical trauma to the sympathetic nervous system, resulting in retrograde ejaculations.

PHYSICAL ASSESSMENT/CLINICAL MANIFESTATIONS

The testes, lymph nodes, and abdomen are thoroughly examined. Palpate the testes for lumps or swelling (Chart 79-10), the most common manifestations of testicular cancer. The presence of any lymph node swelling, abdominal masses, or gynecomastia often indicates metastatic disease.

CHART 79-10

FOCUSED ASSESSMENT of
A Male Client with a Testicular Lump

Obtain a medical history from the client:
- When was the lump discovered?
- Are there any other symptoms (sensation of heaviness, dragging in testicle, pain, discharge from penis)?
- Is there a history of cryptorchidism?

Assess the genital system. Always wear gloves during the examination of the male genitalia.
- Inspect and palpate the scrotal contents. Have the client perform a Valsalva maneuver, and palpate for a varicocele.
- Any lump or enlargement that does not transilluminate should be suspected as malignant.

Palpate for any enlarged lymph nodes. Most common lymphadenopathy is in the inguinal or supraclavicular regions.

Assess the abdomen for a possible mass or hepatomegaly.

PSYCHOSOCIAL ASSESSMENT

Because testicular cancer and its treatment often lead to sexual difficulties, pay close attention to the psychosocial outcomes of the disease. Sexuality is an issue for men of any age, but it may be even more of an issue for younger men. Even if the cancer is detected at an early stage and the client is cured after orchiectomy, he may be afraid that he will be sexually handicapped. Even if the client's disease is arrested with surgery, radiation, or chemotherapy, he may think of himself as less than a whole man. These fears can disrupt the psychosocial and sexual development of the young male and can threaten the identity of adult males. The client may be afraid that he will be unable to perform sexually, will no longer be sexually attractive or desirable, and will face rejection. Feelings of sexual inadequacy may be denied, repressed, or displaced, causing increased stress on the man's personal and work relationships.

Perform a psychosocial assessment with these clients because problems may arise anytime. Referrals are made to other resources as appropriate.

LABORATORY ASSESSMENT

An important diagnostic indicator for testicular cancer is the presence of certain "marker proteins" (tumor markers). These are proteins that normally were produced during embryonic development and their presence in adults is abnormal. Benign testicular tumors do not elevate the levels of any of these marker proteins.

Common tumor markers for testicular cancer are alpha-fetoprotein (AFP) and the beta subunit of human chorionic gonadotropin (hCG). About 90% of clients with embryonal carcinoma, teratoma, or choriocarcinoma have elevated blood levels of AFP, hCG, or both. Clients with a pure seminoma do not have an elevated AFP level, and only 10% have a slightly elevated hCG level. This level resolves after orchiectomy.

If a client has a diagnosis of seminoma and also has an elevated AFP level, the tumor specimen must be re-examined for evidence of a component of nonseminomatous cancer. This step is necessary because the treatments differ for seminomatous and nonseminomatous tumors.

The AFP and hCG blood levels are also used to evaluate responses to therapy for testicular cancer and to document the presence of residual or recurrent disease. With effective treatment, the levels of abnormal markers fall. The persistence of elevated levels of markers after orchiectomy is evidence that the client has metastatic disease, even if x-rays and scans do not show a tumor presence. The reappearance of the tumor markers indicates recurrence of the cancer. Therefore marker levels must be monitored regularly during the follow-up of clients treated for testicular cancer.

OTHER DIAGNOSTIC ASSESSMENTS

When a client has a change in testis size, shape, or texture, ultrasonography can determine whether the mass is solid or fluid filled. It also can help differentiate benign masses from malignant ones.

After the diagnosis of testicular cancer, the client should have a computed tomography (CT) scan of the abdomen and the chest, or chest tomograms, to identify small metastatic lesions.

Magnetic resonance imaging (MRI) is used to detect enlarged lymph nodes and abnormal nodules in certain organs that may indicate metastasis from the testicles. Chest x-rays and bone scans may also be performed if metastasis is suspected.

Clients with a pure seminoma may undergo bipedal lymphangiography as part of the staging workup to assess for retroperitoneal lymph node involvement. Lymphangiograms are also helpful in determining the extent of radiation therapy fields.

◆ Analysis

COMMON NURSING DIAGNOSES AND COLLABORATIVE PROBLEMS

A common nursing diagnosis in clients with testicular cancer is Risk for Sexual Dysfunction related to altered body structure and function from disease or treatment. A common collaborative problem is Potential for Metastasis.

ADDITIONAL NURSING DIAGNOSES AND COLLABORATIVE PROBLEMS

In addition to the common nursing diagnoses and collaborative problems, clients with testicular cancer may have one or more of the following:
- Dysfunctional Grieving or Anticipatory Grieving related to loss of a body part or changes in body function
- Disturbed Body Image related to the diagnosis of cancer and its treatment
- Acute Pain or Chronic Pain related to tumor compression or effects of metastasis
- Anxiety related to threat to health status from the diagnosis of cancer

◆ Planning and Implementation

RISK FOR SEXUAL DYSFUNCTION

NOC **PLANNING: EXPECTED OUTCOMES.** The client with testicular cancer is expected to maintain an acceptable level of sexual function. Indicators include that the client often or consistently demonstrates the following behaviors:
- Attains sexual arousal
- Adapts sexual technique as needed
- Expresses comfort with sexual expression
- Expresses comfort with his body

INTERVENTIONS. At diagnosis the incidence of **oligospermia** (low sperm count) and **azoospermia** (absence of living sperm) is increased in clients with testicular cancer. This problem is thought to be related to higher testicular temperatures created by cancer cell metabolism. The client may not discover that he has reduced sperm numbers count until he has a sperm count performed before surgery.

Health teaching about reproduction, fertility, and sexuality is started in the pretreatment phase. Normal reproductive function is reviewed as well as the possible effects of cancer and its treatment on reproductive function. Explore with the client various reproductive options (e.g., sperm banks and artificial insemination) (Chart 79-11). The sperm bank facility provides comprehensive information on semen collection, storage of semen, the storage contract, costs, and the insemination process.

When preparing the client for the collection and storage of sperm, assume the role of client advocate and keep in mind the effect of the cancer diagnosis on the client. The psychological benefit of having stored sperm may be important for the client and may influence his response to treatment. Knowing that the potential for being a father still exists may help the client cope with other assaults to his masculinity, such as alopecia or erectile dysfunction (ED).

The client should arrange for semen storage as soon as possible after diagnosis. Sperm collection should be completed *before* he begins radiation therapy or chemotherapy or undergoes a radical lymph node dissection. After radiation therapy or chemotherapy has been started, the client is at increased risk for producing mutagenic sperm, which may not be viable or may result in fetal abnormalities.

The recommended number of samples to optimize the chances of later fertilization is three to six ejaculates, collected 2 to 4 days apart. The process of sperm collection can delay treatment for as long as 1 month, especially if the client is still recovering from surgery and multiple procedures or tests.

The client's diagnosis and his physical condition may not allow treatment to be postponed, thus making sperm storage an unfeasible reproductive option. Also, some clients may have personal or religious beliefs that do not allow sperm storage. For clients who are not candidates for sperm storage in a sperm bank and for those who choose not to bank, discuss other reproductive options such as donor insemination, adoption, or not fathering children.

POTENTIAL FOR METASTASIS

NOC **PLANNING: EXPECTED OUTCOMES.** The client with testicular cancer is expected not to experience disease metastasis or recurrence.

CHART 79-11

CLIENT EDUCATION GUIDE
Sperm Banking

- You may want to investigate sperm storage in a sperm bank as a way to preserve your sperm for future use.
- No one knows how long sperm can be stored successfully, but pregnancies have resulted from sperm stored for longer than 10 years.
- Check with the sperm bank to see how much it charges to process and store your sperm and to see whether you must pay when the service is provided.
- Investigate whether your health insurance company will reimburse you for sperm collection and storage.

INTERVENTIONS. Surgery is the main treatment for testicular cancer. It is often combined with nonsurgical management to prevent metastatic disease (or to alleviate symptoms of metastasis) and to bring about tumor regression.

SURGICAL MANAGEMENT. The surgeon performs a unilateral orchiectomy for diagnosis and for surgical management. Every effort is made to remove the cancerous testis as an intact organ to prevent releasing cancer cells into the surgical site.

Clients with testicular cancer may also undergo a radical retroperitoneal lymph node dissection. With this procedure, the disease can be staged accurately and the tumor volume **debulked** (reduced in size) so that other therapies are more effective.

Preoperative Care. Like most clients with cancer, the client with testicular cancer is usually apprehensive. Offer support and reinforce the teaching provided by the surgeon. Anticipate the client's postoperative needs and plan interventions before surgery. Inform the client and his family or partner about what to expect after surgery. The surgical incision for a retroperitoneal lymph node dissection is extensive. Depending on the extent of the dissection and the need for surgical exploration, the surgeon might make not only a midline incision but also a transthoracic incision or a combination of the two incisions (thoracoabdominal).

Inform the client and family that radical retroperitoneal lymph node dissections are long operations, lasting 6 to 12 hours. Tell the client that he may be cared for in a critical care unit after surgery for close observation.

Operative Procedures. To perform a radical retroperitoneal lymph node dissection, the surgeon removes the retroperitoneal nodes in the iliac and lumbar regions. Because the blood supply and the lymphatic vessels of the testes and kidneys are directly related, an extensive midline incision from the xiphoid process to the pubis is necessary. The lymph nodes around the kidney along with the nodes near the aorta and both kidneys are removed. Node removal also includes those in the inguinal area on the affected side. During the lymph node removal, the sympathetic ganglia around the lower lumbar lymphatics are dissected. Removal of the sympathetic ganglia eliminates peristalsis in the vas deferens and contractions of the seminal vesicles. This disruption results in sterility because the client's ejaculate no longer contains sperm. However, having a normal erection and experiencing orgasm usually are not affected.

A gel-filled silicone prosthesis can usually be surgically implanted into the scrotum at the time of the orchiectomy or later if the client desires. Reassure the client that this procedure does not impair fertility or sexual function; the client cosmetically appears to have two testes.

Postoperative Care. Because of the length of the surgery, manipulation of the abdominal and retroperitoneal viscera, and the loss of a major part of the lymphatic fluid, nodes, and channels, observe and assess the client for any of the complications of major abdominal surgery (see Chapter 22). Intervene for any of the following expected problems:

- Pain from surgical incisions
- Immobility related to prolonged maintenance of surgical positioning and pain after surgery
- Injuries related to any invasive catheters or tubes

The client is usually hospitalized for 3 to 4 days after a radical retroperitoneal lymph node dissection. During this time explain care after discharge.

NONSURGICAL MANAGEMENT. Chemotherapy and radiation therapy are indicated for clients at high risk for metastatic disease or those with metastatic disease.

Chemotherapy. Combination chemotherapy may be used as adjuvant therapy for nonseminomatous testicular tumors or as primary treatment when there is evidence of metastatic disease. Combination chemotherapy is effective in treating nonseminomatous testicular cancer, particularly if cisplatin (Platinol) is used. This agent is a part of any successful chemotherapy regimen for treating testicular cancer.

The following are other drugs commonly used in combination with cisplatin:

- Bleomycin sulfate (Blenoxane) (most common)
- Etoposide (VP-16, VePesid) (most common)
- Vinblastine sulfate (Velban, Velbe✦)
- Dactinomycin (Cosmegen)
- Cyclophosphamide (Cytoxan, Procytox✦)
- Doxorubicin (Adriamycin)

The specific combination of drugs and the frequency, cycling, and duration of treatment vary from client to client, depending on the extent of the disease and the protocol being followed. For many clients, the acute side effects are severe enough that the client is admitted to the hospital for chemotherapy. Chapter 28 discusses the nursing care issues for the client receiving chemotherapy.

Radiation Therapy. After **orchiectomy** (removal of one or both testes), external beam radiation therapy is the treatment of choice for clients with a pure seminoma. This type of testicular cancer is highly radiosensitive. Before radiation therapy, a staging lymphangiogram is used to determine the treatment fields. An advantage of using radiation therapy instead of radical lymph node dissection is that reproductive function is preserved because surgical dissection of the nerves is avoided.

For the client undergoing radiation therapy to the retroperitoneal lymph nodes, the remaining testis is shielded with a lead cup to preserve reproductive function. Even with these precautions, the client may have a temporary decreased sperm count as a result of radiation scatter. Normally the sperm count returns to the pretreatment level within 24 to 30 months after the radiation treatment is completed. If metastases develop outside the lymphatic system, the client may still be cured with radiation therapy if the area of involvement is limited. If lymphatic involvement is extensive, or if the visceral organs are involved, combination chemotherapy is used.

Stem Cell Transplantation. Studies are being conducted to explore whether high-dose chemotherapy with stem cell transplantation may be valuable in treating men with advanced germ cell cancer. In this procedure, the client's blood-forming stem cells are removed from the blood and preserved by freezing while the client receives high-dose chemotherapy. Once the chemotherapy is completed, the stem cells are returned to the client. This procedure helps to prevent the infection and anemia that occur with chemotherapy.

Community-Based Care

After an orchiectomy, the client is typically hospitalized for 1 to 2 days. This period may need to be extended if he must undergo additional surgery or chemotherapy. Because it may not be known until after the orchiectomy whether the client has cancer, what type of testicular cancer he has, or whether he needs additional surgery or treatment with radiation therapy or chemotherapy, specific discharge planning may need to be deferred until after surgery.

HOME CARE MANAGEMENT

After an orchiectomy, unless the client has a wound complication, he is discharged without a dressing on the inguinal incision. He may want to wear a dressing to prevent clothing from rubbing on the sutures and causing irritation. Tell the client that the sutures will be removed in the physician's office 7 to 10 days after surgery.

HEALTH TEACHING

For the client who has undergone testicular surgery, emphasize the importance of scheduling a follow-up visit with the surgeon to examine the incision for healing and complications. Instruct the client to notify the surgeon if any of the following symptoms occur: chills, fever, increasing tenderness or pain around the incision, drainage, or dehiscence of the incision.

These manifestations may indicate infection for which antibiotics are needed. Instruct the client that he will be able to resume most of his usual activities within 1 week after discharge, except for lifting heavy objects (objects weighing 15 pounds [9.1 kg]) or stair climbing. Remind him to ask his surgeon when strenuous activities may be resumed.

Inform the client that he may make arrangements with his surgeon to have a silicone prosthesis inserted into the scrotum if a prosthesis was not inserted during the orchiectomy.

Explain the importance of performing monthly testicular self-examination (TSE) on the remaining testis and scheduling follow-up examinations with the physician. The client who has had testicular cancer should schedule tests for urinary and serum levels of tumor markers and computed tomography (CT) or magnetic resonance imaging (MRI) studies as part of his routine follow-up for at least 3 years.

Depending on the pathologic findings and the stage of the cancer, the client may need further treatment. This information may not be known at the time of discharge. If it is known that the client needs further surgery, he and his family need information about the future surgery. If it is known that he must undergo radiation therapy or chemotherapy, he needs education about a radiation therapy and chemotherapy regimen.

The client who has testicular cancer may need emotional support. If permanent sterility occurs and sperm storage has not been feasible, the man may need counseling about other reproductive options.

HEALTH CARE RESOURCES

The client may be referred to agencies or support groups, such as the American Fertility Society or RESOLVE (an organization for infertile couples).

◆ Evaluation: Outcomes

Evaluate the care of the client who has been treated for testicular cancer on the basis of the identified nursing diagnoses and collaborative problems. The expected outcomes include that the client will:

- Not experience a recurrence of cancer or metastases
- Have an acceptable level of sexual function

Specific indicators for these outcomes are listed for each nursing diagnosis and collaborative problem under the Planning and Implementation section (see earlier).

OTHER COMMON PROBLEMS AFFECTING THE TESTES AND ADJACENT STRUCTURES

Problems that develop inside the scrotum usually occur as a mass or as scrotal edema. Some problems produce pain, but others do not. Figure 79-7 shows some of the most common conditions found in the male, including hydrocele, spermatocele, varicocele, and scrotal torsion.

Hydrocele

PATHOPHYSIOLOGY

A hydrocele is a cystic mass, usually filled with straw-colored fluid that forms around the testis (see Figure 79-7). It results from impaired lymphatic drainage of the scrotum, causing a swelling of the tissue surrounding the testes. Unless the swelling becomes large and uncomfortable or begins to impair blood flow to the testis, no treatment is necessary. Hydroceles are usually painless. It is important that the cause of the hydrocele is investigated to rule out a serious condition. The cause may be determined by examination and ultrasound. A small hydrocele may go untreated with no further problems. However, a hydrocele may become very large, which makes clothing uncomfortable and may be cosmetically unacceptable.

◆COLLABORATIVE MANAGEMENT

A hydrocele may be drained via a needle and syringe, or it may be removed surgically. To correct a hydrocele surgically, an incision is made in the scrotum and the hydrocele is removed. The client may or may not have a drain at the incision site. Usually the surgery is performed on an outpatient basis. If the client requires hospitalization, it is for only 1 or 2 days. The recurrence rate for hydrocele is about 1% to 2%.

Instruct the client that if an incision drain is present, some serosanguineous drainage may be present for the first 24 to 48 hours after surgery. Explain the importance of wearing a scrotal support. The scrotal support keeps the scrotal dressing in place and keeps the scrotum elevated, which helps to prevent edema.

The degree of pain experienced after this surgery varies. Assess and observe the client for pain every 2 to 3 hours immediately after surgery. Moderate incision pain is expected for the first 24 hours after surgery and should markedly decrease within 1 or 2 days. If the client's pain does not resolve within this time, be alert to the possible development of wound complications, such as infection or bleeding.

Instruct the client to schedule a follow-up visit with the surgeon to have the wound evaluated for healing. Stress the importance of continuing to wear a scrotal support to promote drainage and comfort. The scrotum can remain swollen from residual inflammation and edema for as long

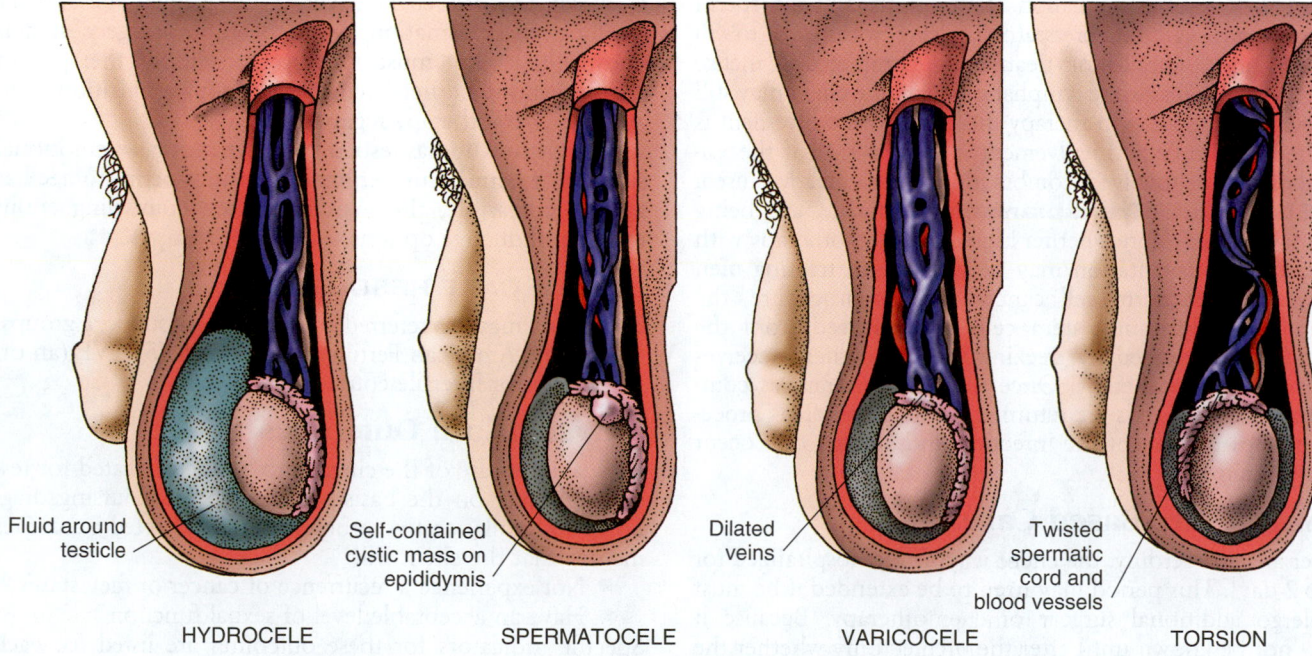

Fluid around testicle   Self-contained cystic mass on epididymis   Dilated veins   Twisted spermatic cord and blood vessels

HYDROCELE   SPERMATOCELE   VARICOCELE   TORSION

Figure 79-7 ■ Common problems affecting the testes and adjacent structures.

as several weeks. Instruct the client to stay off his feet for 3 to 5 days and to limit physical activity for a week. Reassure him that this swelling is normal and eventually subsides.

Spermatocele
PATHOPHYSIOLOGY

A spermatocele is a sperm-containing cyst that develops on the epididymis alongside the testicle (see Figure 79-7). Trauma, infection, congenital abnormalities, or often for no identifiable reason results in the widening of a portion of the epididymis creating a small cavity where sperm collects.

◆ COLLABORATIVE MANAGEMENT

Normally spermatoceles are small and asymptomatic, and no interventions are needed. If the spermatocele becomes large enough to cause discomfort, a spermatocelectomy is performed. In this simple procedure, the spermatocele is excised through a small scrotal incision. Routinely no incision drain is used because drainage and swelling are minimal. About 5% of clients have recurrence.

Varicocele
PATHOPHYSIOLOGY

A varicocele is a cluster of dilated veins behind and above the testis (see Figure 79-7). Varicosity of the testicles may result from the increased fluid secondary to damaged or incompetent valves in the testicular veins. The diagnosis is made by scrotal palpation, particularly when the client performs a Valsalva maneuver, creating additional pressure in the varicose veins. The scrotum feels "wormlike" when palpated. If the varicocele is very small and cannot be palpated, thermography, which detects pockets of heat, or a Doppler, which magnifies the sound of the blood flowing through the veins, is used.

Varicoceles can be either unilateral or bilateral, but most are unilateral. They occur most often on the left side of the scrotum. In many cases, varicoceles are asymptomatic, and no treatment is required. In a few men varicoceles are painful and must be removed surgically.

Varicoceles can also cause infertility. It is thought that they increase scrotal temperature from the venous stasis near the testis, altering spermatogenesis. Surgical correction of a varicocele may resolve the infertility.

◆ COLLABORATIVE MANAGEMENT

A **varicocelectomy** (surgical removal of the varicocele) is usually performed through an inguinal incision, in which the spermatic veins are ligated in the cord. It can also be performed through an incision near the superior iliac spine, in which the spermatic veins are ligated in the retroperitoneal space. A varicocelectomy may be done on an ambulatory care basis, or the client may be hospitalized overnight.

Before surgery explain to the client that persistent venous congestion of the scrotum is common after this type of surgery because of the changed circulation in the area. To promote drainage of the scrotum, place a rolled towel under the scrotum while the client is in bed. Ice may be applied to the scrotum if needed. Any intervention that facilitates drainage and decreases swelling from the area promotes relief.

Instruct the client about the importance of wearing a scrotal support while ambulating. Usually the client can resume normal activities, including sexual activities, within a week.

At discharge, instruct the client to make a follow-up appointment with the surgeon to have the sutures removed. Remind him to notify the surgeon of any increasing discomfort at the incision site or in the scrotum, which might indicate an infection. Increasing scrotal discomfort can mean that the circulation to the testis has been impaired. Testicular atrophy, a rare complication of a varicocelectomy, may occur if the blood supply to the testis becomes insufficient.

Scrotal Torsion
PATHOPHYSIOLOGY

Because of the mobility of the scrotum, scrotal injuries are relatively rare. Torsion of the testes involves the twisting of the spermatic cord and occurs most often during puberty (see Figure 79-7). Torsion may occur after strenuous exercise or trauma, although for many cases no specific causative event is identified. Because the testes are sensitive to any decrease in blood flow, torsion of the testis is a surgical emergency.

The client experiences pain, which does not subside with scrotal elevation. In addition to pain, he usually has nausea and vomiting. Other manifestations include blood in the semen, lower abdominal pain, a lump in the testicle, and red and swollen testicle(s). Diagnosis is made by history and physical examination. Because manifestations of testicular torsion are similar to epididymitis, a color Doppler sonography may be used to identify the absence of blood flow through the twisted testicle. A urinalysis or culture may be used to rule out a bacterial infection.

◆ COLLABORATIVE MANAGEMENT

In addition to caring for the client's physical needs, be attuned to his psychosexual needs. Of primary concern to the client with an injury to his external genitalia are his masculinity and sexuality. An awareness of crisis intervention techniques and knowledge about sexuality are helpful when assisting the client to adjust to an injury in the genital area.

Surgical intervention may be required to untwist the torsion. Evaluation of the condition of the testicles can be made at that time, including looking for signs of necrosis. Any dead tissue may have to be removed, or one or both of the testicles may be excised. If the testicles are found to be healthy, they may be sutured to the scrotal wall to prevent recurrence of the torsion.

At discharge, instruct the client to maintain ice to the scrotum for at least 72 hours, and elevate the scrotum to minimize edema. Instruct him to avoid lifting heavy objects for 4 to 6 weeks, limit stair climbing, and suspend strenuous physical activity for 1 month. Remind the client to wear a scrotal support for at least 3 weeks.

Cryptorchidism
PATHOPHYSIOLOGY

Before birth the testicles develop in the abdominal cavity and descend into the scrotum. Cryptorchidism results when the testicles fail to descent and is mainly a pediatric problem.

Three percent of full-term male infants and 20% of premature infants have an undescended testis. In 80% of cases, the undescended testis descends spontaneously during the infant's first year. When the testicles reside in the scrotum, sperm production and fertility are enhanced and testicular cancer can be detected. Undescended testicles often result in infertility and are at an increased risk of cancer.

◆ COLLABORATIVE MANAGEMENT

If the testicles do not spontaneously descend, medical or surgical intervention may be needed. Medically, hormonal injections of β-hCG, luteinizing hormone-releasing hormone, or testosterone may be used to promote descent of the testicles into the scrotum. If the testicles do not descend, surgery, an **orchidopexy** (surgical placement of the testicle into the scrotum) may be performed to prevent irreversible damage, causing infertility, and to allow examination of the testicles for tumors. If left untreated until adulthood, an orchidopexy may be performed for cosmetic and psychosexual reasons as well. In a small percent of clients, no testicles are found at surgery. This is known as a "vanished" or absent testis.

During an orchidopexy, an inguinal incision is made and the spermatic cord is released from the surrounding fascia to obtain maximal length. The surgeon then creates a pouch and places the testis between the skin and the dartos muscle of the scrotum. The testis is sutured to the dartos muscle, and the inguinal incision and the scrotal incision (if there is one) are then closed, and a dressing is applied. If there is an incision in the scrotum, it is also covered with a dressing and the client is instructed to wear a scrotal support. The site should be checked for bleeding and infection. The client should rest for 2 to 3 days and avoid strenuous activity for at least a month.

Cancer of the Penis

PATHOPHYSIOLOGY

Cancer of the penis represents fewer than 1% of all malignancies in men in the United States. The overall 5-year survival rate is 50%. Most penile cancers (95%) are epidermoid (squamous) carcinomas developing from the squamous cells. These tumors tend to grow slowly and can develop anywhere on the penis but most commonly occur on the foreskin or the glans. When the cancer is confined to the skin of the penis it is called carcinoma in situ (CIS). Other types of penile cancers include melanomas, basal cell cancer, and sarcomas.

Circumcision (the surgical removal of the prepuce from the penis) in infancy almost eliminates the possibility of penile cancer in that chronic irritation and inflammation of the glans penis predispose uncircumcised men to penile cancer. Because of the ongoing controversy about neonatal circumcision, teach men and new mothers of boys that strict personal hygiene is an important preventive measure against penile cancer.

◆ COLLABORATIVE MANAGEMENT
◆ Assessment

Penile cancer usually occurs as a painless, wartlike growth or ulcer on the glans under the **prepuce** (foreskin) and may be mistaken for a venereal wart. A penile carcinoma may also appear as a reddened lesion with plaque.

◆ Interventions

Small lesions involving only the skin may be controlled by excisional biopsy. When the lesion is not curable by excisional biopsy or radiation therapy, a **penectomy** (partial or total removal of the penis) may be required.

Partial Penectomy. When the lesion is limited to the glans, a partial penectomy is performed. The distal portion of the corpus cavernosum and the corpus spongiosum is amputated. The urethra is anastomosed to the skin, and a dressing is applied. A retention catheter is in place for 3 to 5 days after surgery until the edema surrounding the urethra subsides. Assess the dressing for drainage, which should be minimal. Check the urinary catheter for patency every 4 hours for the first 24 hours.

Total Penectomy. A total penectomy is required when the lesion has penetrated the shaft of the penis or when the tumor has recurred after a partial penectomy or radiation therapy. An incision is made from the pubic bone, which encircles the penis and extends into the perineum. The bases of both corpora cavernosa are exposed and excised, and the penis is amputated. An incision drain is placed in the wound before it is sutured. Clients who undergo a total penectomy also have a perineal urethrotomy (anastomosis of the urethra to the skin in the perineum) for urinary drainage.

After a total penectomy, observe the incision dressing every 2 to 4 hours during the first 24 to 48 hours. A moderate amount of serosanguineous drainage from the incision drains is expected.

Be aware that regardless of how accepting the client may appear before surgery, he may experience severe emotional problems after surgery. After a partial penectomy, the client must adjust to considerable changes in body image and sexuality. Encourage him to verbalize his feelings about the loss of his penis. After a total penectomy, the client can no longer have penile-vaginal or penile-anal intercourse and cannot urinate in a standing position. It is difficult for most clients to accept the possibility that they might die because of a lesion on the penis, especially because they rarely experience any systemic cancer symptoms and are otherwise healthy. Help the client to realize that removal of his penis may save his life. Be aware of the possibility of suicide attempts because the client's penis may be more important to him than his life. The nurse may be the one to detect the need for professional psychological assistance for the client or his partner. Early interventions can make a tremendous difference in the client's or partner's well-being.

Phimosis and Paraphimosis

PATHOPHYSIOLOGY

In a man with phimosis, the prepuce is constricted so that it cannot be retracted over the glans. The prepuce remains down, around the tip of the penis. Instruct uncircumcised men about the importance of cleaning the prepuce.

In paraphimosis the prepuce has not been returned to its normal position after being retracted and forms a constricting band around the glans. This constricts lymph drainage, causing the penis to swell. Blood flow becomes impeded, and tissue death can occur. This problem is an emergency requiring immediate treatment. Uncircumcised males are at risk. Causes include infection, not returning the foreskin to the original position after urethral catheterization, poor hygiene, vigorous sexual intercourse, and penile piercing.

◆COLLABORATIVE MANAGEMENT

Phimosis is corrected by **circumcision** (surgical removal of the prepuce or foreskin). This procedure also may be performed for other medical reasons or for aesthetic reasons.

Circumcision in the adult male is usually performed in a same-day surgical setting. If the client has a dressing, instruct him to soak in a warm bath that evening to allow the dressing to loosen. If the dressing falls off before the next day, caution the client not to replace it. Explain that the sutures will be absorbed and need not be removed. No residual or side effects result from this surgery, and the client should be able to resume normal activities within 1 week. Sexual intercourse may be resumed after 1 to 2 weeks.

The client may be discharged with a prescription for a barbiturate sleeping medication to be taken for several nights after surgery. Emphasize that these drugs suppress the rapid-eye-movement (REM) phase of sleep so that normal nocturnal erections do not occur. This prevents tension on the sutures by an erection. Nonbarbiturate sleeping medications do not inhibit the nocturnal erection pattern. Explain the relationship between barbiturate sleeping medications and nocturnal erections because the client may not adhere with the instructions to take the drug, especially if he is not having any difficulty sleeping.

Advise the client to notify his physician if he has any wound complications, such as swelling at the incision area or drainage, and to schedule a postoperative office visit.

Priapism
PATHOPHYSIOLOGY

Priapism is an uncontrolled, long-maintained erection without sexual desire, which causes the penis to become large, hard, and painful. Priapism affects the two corpora cavernosa; the corpus spongiosum and glans penis are not affected.

Priapism can occur from neural, vascular, or pharmacologic causes, including the following:

- Thrombosis of the veins of the corpora cavernosa (usually resulting from trauma)
- Leukemia
- Sickle cell disease
- Diabetes mellitus
- Malignancies

Sickle cell disease causes priapism through the collection of erythrocytes within the corporal bodies. Leukemia may cause priapism because the increased number of white blood cells (WBCs) permits persistent engorgement of the corporal bodies. Cancer may also infiltrate the corporal bodies, causing persistent engorgement. Priapism can also result from an abnormal neurogenic reflex, psychotropic drugs, antidepressants, antihypertensive drugs, and drugs used to treat erectile dysfunction. Other risk factors include recreational drugs (cocaine, ecstasy, marijuana), overdose of injectable drugs for erectile dysfunction, and prolonged sexual activity.

◆COLLABORATIVE MANAGEMENT

Priapism is a urologic emergency because the circulation to the penis may be compromised and the client may not be able to void with an erect penis. The goal of intervention is to improve the venous drainage of the corpora cavernosa. Conservative measures involve prostatic massage, sedation, and bedrest.

Meperidine (Demerol) is usually given immediately because of its hypotensive effect. Warm enemas may be given to cause venous dilation and thus increase the outflow of the trapped blood. Urinary or suprapubic catheterization is required if the client cannot void.

If conservative therapy is unsuccessful, treatment may proceed to aspiration of the corpora cavernosa with a large-bore needle or surgical intervention. The priapism should be resolved within the first 24 to 30 hours to prevent penile ischemia, gangrene, fibrosis, and erectile dysfunction. If a cause of priapism is identified, treatment is directed toward that underlying cause.

When caring for the client with priapism, be sensitive to his emotional needs. The client may be uncomfortable and in crisis but at the same time embarrassed by his erection and loss of control. Reassure the client that it is understood that he is not in control of his erection, and provide him with privacy.

Prostatitis
PATHOPHYSIOLOGY

Prostatitis is an inflammation of the prostate gland. The four types of prostatitis are acute bacterial (ABP), chronic bacterial (CBP), nonbacterial (NBP)/chronic pelvic pain syndrome (CPPS), and asymptomatic inflammatory prostatitis. Duration of symptoms, presence or absence of WBCs in the urine, and urinary culture results determine the classification.

Bacterial Prostatitis

Bacterial prostatitis often occurs with urethritis or an infection of the lower urinary tract. Organisms may reach the prostate via the bloodstream or the urethra. The most common organisms are *Escherichia coli*, *Enterobacter*, *Proteus*, and group D streptococci. Acute bacterial prostatitis may be manifested by fever, chills, **dysuria** (painful urination), urethral discharge, and a boggy, tender prostate. Gentle palpation of the prostate usually results in a urethral discharge, which has WBCs in the prostatic secretions.

Chronic bacterial prostatitis generally occurs in older men and has a less dramatic presentation than acute bacterial prostatitis and without the systemic manifestations. The client reports experiencing hesitancy, urgency, dysuria, difficulty initiating and terminating the flow of urine, and decreased strength and volume of urine. Additionally, there may be discomfort in the perineum, scrotum, and penis.

Nonbacterial/Chronic Pelvic Pain Syndrome

A bacterial prostatitis can occur after a viral illness or may be associated with sexually transmitted diseases (STDs), especially in young males. Although an infection may be the cause, bacteria is not found on urinalysis and culture. Other causes may be autoimmune disorders, neuromuscular etiologies, allergy-mediated reactions, and psychosexual problems. In many instances, an exact cause of the perineal discomfort cannot be found. The client reports mild urgency and dysuria. Rectal, perineal, and ejaculatory pain may be present. Decreased libido may also be present.

Prostatodynia (pelvic floor pain) is a related condition in which manifestations of prostatitis are present, but there is no inflammation of the prostate and the urine culture is negative. Additionally, the client has low back pain with unilateral testicular pain, narrowed force of the urinary stream, and post-void dribbling.

◆COLLABORATIVE MANAGEMENT

The client with chronic prostatitis usually reports backache, perineal pain, mild dysuria, and urinary frequency. Hematuria may be present. The prostate may feel irregularly enlarged, firm, and slightly tender when palpated. Segmented specimens are obtained. This is referred to as the *Stamey-Meares Method.* Four specimens are taken. Comparison of the number of WBCs in the specimens and the presence of bacteria assists in making a diagnosis. The first specimen is the first 10 mL of urine obtained by voiding, which is used to diagnose urethritis. The second is 50 mL of midstream urine used to diagnose cystitis. For the third specimen, prostatic secretions are collected following prostate massage and the urethra milked to express any prostatic secretions (expressed prostatic secretions, EPS). The fourth specimen is then collected by a post-massage bladder voiding into a sterile container. The third and fourth specimens may show WBCs, but no bacterial growth if nonbacterial prostatitis is present. The third and fourth specimens will contain greater bacterial growth than the first or second specimens in bacterial prostatitis. Prostatodynia is present in the absence of bacteria in the sequential cultures, along with normal expressed prostatic secretions.

Complications of prostatitis are **epididymitis** (inflammation of the epididymis) and **cystitis** (inflammation of the bladder). A rare complication is a prostatic abscess. The client with either acute or chronic bacterial prostatitis is likely to develop urinary tract infections. Sexual functioning may be reduced because of discomfort.

Early diagnosis and treatment of prostatitis with antimicrobials, 160 mg/800 mg of trimethoprim/sulfamethoxazole (Bactrim DS) every 12 hours or carbenicillin indanyl sodium (Geocillin, Geopen Oral), or fluoroquinolones (ciprofloxacin [Cipro]) can help to prevent an abscess. After culture results are obtained, other antibiotics may be required. Treatment may last from 4 weeks to many months because there is poor penetration of antibiotics into prostatic tissue. Acute bacterial prostatitis may require hospitalization with aggressive IV antibiotics.

Emphasize the importance of comfort measures, such as sitz baths, donut-shaped cushions, and nonsteroidal anti-inflammatory drugs. Stool softeners are prescribed to prevent straining and rectal irritation of the prostate during a bowel movement. Instruct clients to avoid alcohol, coffee, tea, and spicy foods that irritate symptoms. Over-the-counter cold preparations containing decongestants or antihistamines may result in urinary retention.

Teach the client with chronic prostatitis about the long-term nature of the problem. Because prostatitis can cause other urinary tract infections, explain the importance of increasing fluid intake and long-term antibiotic therapy. It is important to teach the client to take the prescribed antibiotics on schedule. Because trimethoprim (Bactrim, Septra) diffuses into the prostatic fluid, it is the antibiotic of choice. Instruct the client about activities that drain the prostate (sexual intercourse, masturbation, prostatic massage), which may help in the management of chronic prostatitis. Inform the client that prostatitis is not infectious or contagious.

Epididymitis
PATHOPHYSIOLOGY

Epididymitis is an inflammation of the epididymis. This inflammation may be a result of an infection or noninfectious source, such as trauma. Bacterial infection is the most common cause of epididymitis. The infection may spread from other structures such as the prostate, bladder, or urethra. It can be a complication of an STD, such as gonorrhea or chlamydia. Although not common, epididymitis can also be a complication of long-term use of an indwelling urinary catheter, prostatic surgery, or a cystoscopic examination.

Organisms such as *Staphylococcus* and *E. coli* commonly cause epididymitis. In men younger than 35 years of age, the major causative organism in epididymitis is *Chlamydia trachomatis,* which is transmitted sexually (see Chapter 80). The infective organism passes upward through the urethra and the ejaculatory duct and then along the vas deferens to the epididymis.

The client with epididymitis usually reports pain along the inguinal canal and along the vas deferens, followed by pain and swelling in the scrotum and the groin. If epididymitis is untreated, the epididymis becomes swollen and painful and fever may be present. Pyuria and bacteriuria may develop, with resultant chills and fever. An abscess may form, requiring an **orchiectomy** (removal of one or both testes).

◆COLLABORATIVE MANAGEMENT

Instruct the client with epididymitis to remain in bed with his scrotum elevated on a towel to prevent traction on the spermatic cord, to facilitate venous drainage, and to relieve pain. A scrotal support should be worn when the client is ambulating. A smear or culture of the urine or prostate secretions may be obtained to identify the causative organism. Antibiotics appropriate to the specific organism can then be prescribed. These antibiotics are taken until all acute manifestations are gone. If the epididymitis is chlamydial or gonorrheal in origin, the client's sexual partners are also treated with antibiotics. Nonsteroidal anti-inflammatory drugs such as ibuprofen or naproxen (Naprosyn) may be used to decrease inflammation and promote comfort.

The client may find other comfort measures effective, such as applying cold compresses or ice to the scrotum intermittently and taking sitz baths. Advise him to avoid lifting, straining, or sexual activity until the infection is under control (which may take as long as 4 weeks).

In clients with epididymitis, there must always be the suspicion of a testicular tumor, especially if the condition does not resolve in a week or two. Ultrasound study is often done to rule out an abscess or tumor. Clients with recurrent or chronic painful conditions may require an **epididymectomy** (excision of the epididymis from the testicle).

Orchitis
PATHOPHYSIOLOGY

Orchitis is an acute testicular inflammation resulting from trauma or infection. The infection may be caused by the direct spread of bacteria through the urethra or by an infection elsewhere in the body, such as pneumonia, tuberculosis, gonorrhea, syphilis, or mumps. Usually both the testes and the epididymis are involved (epididymo-orchitis). Risk factors for orchitis include recurrent urinary tract infections, recurrent STDs, congenital abnormalities of the urogenital tract, instrumentation, and chronic indwelling urethral urinary catheter.

Orchitis may be unilateral or bilateral. If the orchitis is bilateral, the client is at increased risk for sterility because of the testicular atrophy and fibrosis that occur during healing.

The manifestations of orchitis are the same as those of epididymitis and include scrotal pain, edema, reports of heavy feelings in the involved testicle(s), dysuria, pain on ejaculation, blood in the semen, and discharge from the penis. In addition, the client may experience nausea and vomiting and pain radiating to the inguinal canal.

◆COLLABORATIVE MANAGEMENT

The treatment of orchitis is the same as for epididymitis and includes the following:
- Bedrest with scrotal elevation
- Application of ice
- Administration of analgesics and antibiotics

Mumps orchitis, which occurs in about 20% of males who have mumps after puberty, is usually bilateral and develops 4 to 6 days after the parotitis. Any adult male who has not had mumps and is exposed to or contracts mumps is usually given gamma globulin. Although gamma globulin does not prevent mumps, the clinical course of the disease is likely to be less severe, with fewer complications. However, the outcome is unpredictable, and sterility still may result. Childhood vaccination against mumps is an important preventive measure.

GET READY for the NCLEX Examination!

KEY POINTS

Safe Effective Care Environment
- Use sterile technique when empty wound drains following prostatectomy.
- Provide assistance when ambulating clients immediately after prostate surgery.
- Monitor the client's oxygen saturation status when on PCA following prostate surgery.
- Use the information listed in Chart 79-8 to teach clients urinary catheter care.
- Have clients report signs of infection when caring for a urinary catheter in the home.
- Teach clients about no heaving lifting (>15 pounds) following prostate surgery.

Health Promotion and Maintenance
- Teach men at risk for prostate cancer to follow the American Cancer Society's screening guidelines.
- Teach men to report any lower urinary tract symptoms that may be indicative of BPH.
- Teach men how to perform testicular self-examination.
- Teach men to practice safer sex to prevent infections of the reproductive organs.

Psychosocial Integrity
- Because most clients with testicular cancer are young adults, assess their reaction to the possible loss of reproductive ability.
- Because of the high incidence of erectile dysfunction following radical prostatectomy, assess the client's adjustment to these changes in body function.
- Assess the client's anxiety preceding prostate surgery, and allow him to express feelings of fear or grief.
- Teach clients with prostate cancer about American Cancer Society's Man to Man program and the American Foundation for Urologic Disease's US TOO program to help men and their partners cope with prostate cancer.

Physiological Integrity
- Observe for and report complications following radical prostatectomy.
- Observe for and report bloody urine with clots following TURP.
- Maintain traction on the urinary catheter following a TURP.
- Teach clients about drug therapies used to treat BPH.
- Teach clients to avoid any drugs that can cause urinary retention, especially anticholinergics, antihistamines, and decongestants if BPH is present.
- Following discharge after prostate or testicular surgery, instruct the client to notify the physician if any of the following symptoms occurs before the scheduled appointment: chills, fever, increasing tenderness or pain around the incision, drainage, or dehiscence of the incision.
- Teach the client the importance of taking the prescribed barbiturate sleeping medication for several nights postoperatively following penile surgery. Emphasize that barbiturate sleeping medications suppress the REM phase of sleep so that normal nocturnal erections do not occur.

ADDITIONAL STUDY RESOURCES

Go to your Student CD-ROM for Review Questions for the NCLEX Examination.

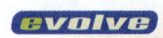

Go to http://evolve.elsevier.com/Iggy/ for Integrated Management of Care Questions for the NCLEX Examination.

SELECTED BIBLIOGRAPHY

Asterisk indicates a classic or definitive work on this subject.

Abel, L., et al. (2003). Treatment outcomes and quality-of-life issues for patients treated with prostate brachytherapy. *Clinical Journal of Oncology Nursing, 7*(1), 48-54.

Ackley, B., & Ladwig, G. (2002). *Nursing diagnosis handbook: A guide to planning care* (5th ed.). St. Louis: Mosby.

American Cancer Society. (2003). *Cancer prevention and early detection. Facts & figures–2003.* Report No. 8600.03. Atlanta: Author.

American Cancer Society. (2005a). *Cancer facts and figures 2005.* Report No. 00-300M-No. 5008.05. Atlanta: Author.

American Cancer Society. (2005b). *Cancer facts and figures for African Americans–2005-2006.* Report No. 8614.05. Atlanta: Author.

Baily, D., et al. (2004). Uncertainty intervention for watchful waiting in prostate cancer. *Cancer Nursing, 27*(5), 339-346.

Balmer, L., & Greco, K. (2004). Prostate cancer recurrence fear: The prostate-specific antigen bounce. *Clinical Journal of Oncology Nursing, 8*(4), 361-366.

Carlson, S. (2004). Prostate disease. *RN, 67*(9), 54-59.

Coleman, E., Hutchins, L., & Goodwin, J. (2004). An overview of cancer in the older adult. *MEDSURG Nursing, 13*(2), 75-80, 109.

Dest, V. (2002). Nursing care for radiation treatment. In M. Wallace & L. Powell (Eds.). *Prostate cancer: Nursing assessment, management, and care* (pp. 89-109). New York: Springer.

Dochterman, J., & Bulechek, G. (Eds.). (2004). *Nursing interventions classification (NIC)* (4th ed). St. Louis: Mosby.

Dorey, G. (2002). Clinical outcome measures for erectile dysfunction: Literature review. *British Journal of Nursing, 11*(1), 54-64.

Ebersole, P., Hess, P., & Luggen, A. (2004). *Toward healthy aging: Human needs and nursing response* (6th ed). St. Louis: Mosby.

Facts and Comparisons. (2004). *Drug facts and comparisons* (58th ed). St. Louis: Author.

Flack, J. (2002). The effect of doxazosin on sexual function in patients with benign prostatic hyperplasia, hypertension, or both. *International Journal of Clinical Practice, 56*(7), 527-530.

Forristal, H. (2002). Benign prostatic hyperplasia and prostate cancer. *Practice Nurse, 24*(9), 37-38, 41, 43.

Galbraith. M.E., Ramirez, J.M., & Pedro, L.W. (2001). Quality of life, health outcomes, and identity for patients with prostate cancer in five different treatment groups. *Oncology Nursing Forum, 28*(3), 551-560.

Hedestig, O., Sandman, P., & Widmark, A. (2003), Living with untreated localized prostate cancer. *Cancer Nursing, 26*(1), 55-60.

Held-Warmkessel, J. (2000). *Contemporary issues in prostate cancer: A nursing perspective.* Subury, MA: Jones & Bartlett.

Held-Warmkessel, J. (2002). What your patient needs to know about prostate cancer. *Nursing 2002, 32*(12), 36-42.

*Jackson, J., et al. (1996). Biofeedback: A noninvasive treatment for incontinence after radical prostatectomy. *Urology Nursing, 16*(2), 50-54.

Kirby, R., Brawer, M., & Denis, L. (2003). *Fast facts: prostate cancer* (4th ed.). Oxford: Health Press.

*Klingman, L. (1999). Assessing the male genitalia. *American Journal of Nursing, 99*(7), 47-50.

Leak, B., et al. (2002). Relevant patient and tumor considerations for early prostate cancer treatment. *Seminars in Urologic Oncology, 20*(1), 39-44.

Lee, E.H. (2002). Assessment, screening and diagnosis of prostate cancer. In M. Wallace & L. Powell (Eds.). *Prostate cancer: Nursing assessment, management, and care* (pp. 33-45). New York: Springer Publishing.

Lewis, J., Rosen, R., & Goldstein, I. (2005). Patient education guide: Erectile dysfunction. *Nursing 2005, 35*(2), 64.

Maliski, S., Clerkin, B., & Litwin, M. (2004). Describing a nurse case manager intervention to empower low-income men with prostate cancer. *Oncology Nursing Forum, 31*(1), 57-64.

Marks, L.S., et al. (2000). Effects of a saw palmetto herbal blend in men with symptomatic benign prostatic hyperplasia. *Journal of Urology, 163*(5), 1451-1456.

Marks, S. (2003). *Prostate and cancer* (3rd ed.). Cambridge, MA: Perseus Publishing.

Marschke, P. (2002). Nursing care for radical prostatectomy. In M. Wallace & L. Powell (Eds.). *Prostate cancer: Nursing assessment, management, and care* (pp. 77-88). New York: Springer.

McCance, K., & Huether, S. (2002). *Pathophysiology: The biologic basis for disease in adults and children* (4th ed). St. Louis: Mosby.

Moorhead, S., Johnson, M., & Maas, M. (Eds.). (2004). *Nursing outcomes classification (NOC)* (3rd ed). St. Louis: Mosby.

Nussbaum, R., McInnes, R., & Willard, H. (2001). *Thompson & Thompson: Genetics in medicine* (6th ed). Philadelphia: W.B. Saunders.

O'Rourke, M. I. (2003). Ketoconazole in the treatment of prostate cancer. *Clinical Journal of Oncology Nursing, 7*(2), 235-236.

Palmer, M.H., et al. (2003). Incontinence after prostatectomy: Coping with incontinence after prostate cancer surgery. *Oncology Nursing Forum, 30*(2), 229-238.

Pickett, M., et al. (2000). Prostate cancer elder alert: Living with treatment choices and outcomes. *Journal of Gerontological Nursing, 26*(2), 22-34.

Russell, I. (2002). Overcoming erectile dysfunction. *Practice Nursing, 13*(9), 415-416, 418.

Scura, K.W., Budin, W., & Garting, E. (2004). Telephone social support and education for adaptation to prostate cancer: A pilot study. *Oncology Nursing Forum, 31*(2), 335-338.

Stevenson, T., & McNeill, J. (2004). Surgical management of testicular cancer. *Clinical Journal of Oncology Nursing, 8*(4), 355-360.

Stipetich, R.L., et al. (2002). Nursing assessment of sexual function following permanent prostate brachytherapy for patients with early-stage prostate cancer. *Clinical Journal of Oncology Nursing, 6*(6), 271-274.

Wallace, M., & Powell, L. (2002). *Prostate cancer: Nursing assessment, management, and care.* New York: Springer Publishing.

Wallace, M. (2003). Uncertainty and quality of life of older men who undergo watchful waiting for prostate cancer. *Oncology Nursing Forum, 30*(2) 303-309.

Wallner K. (2000). Prostate cancer: A non-surgical perspective. Seattle, WA: SmartMedicine.

Weinrich, S.P., et al. (2000). Barriers to prostate screening. *Cancer Nursing, 23*, 117-121.

Weinrich, S.P., et al. (2002). Interest in genetic prostate cancer susceptibility testing among African American men. *Cancer Nursing, 25*(1), 28-34.

Interventions for Clients with Sexually Transmitted Diseases

SHIRLEY E. VAN ZANDT

LEARNING OUTCOMES

After studying this chapter, you should be able to:

1. Explain how sexually transmitted diseases (STDs) can be prevented.
2. Compare the stages of syphilis.
3. Prioritize nursing care for the client with syphilis at each stage.
4. Identify the role of drug therapy in managing clients with genital herpes (GH).
5. Discuss the psychosocial effects of having an STD.
6. Develop a community-based teaching plan for clients diagnosed with gonorrhea.
7. Describe the assessment findings that are typical in clients with *Chlamydia trachomatis* infection.
8. Analyze assessment data to determine common nursing diagnoses for women with pelvic inflammatory disease (PID).
9. Formulate a collaborative plan of care for a client with PID.
10. Describe the mechanisms of action, side effects, and nursing implications for drug therapy of PID.
11. Develop a community-based teaching plan for clients with PID.
12. Evaluate care for a client with PID.
13. Identify common causes of vaginal infections.

Go to your Student CD-ROM for Review Questions
for the NCLEX Examination keyed to these Learning Outcomes.

Sexually transmitted diseases (STDs)* are caused by infectious organisms that have been passed from one person to another through intimate contact, usually oral, or vaginal intercourse. Some organisms that cause these diseases are transmitted only through sexual contact. Other organisms are transmitted by parenteral exposure to infected blood, fecal-oral transmission, intrauterine transmission to the fetus, and perinatal transmission from mother to neonate (Table 80-1).

With improved diagnostic techniques, increased knowledge about organisms that can be sexually transmitted, and changes in sexual attitudes and practices, the number of cases of STDs continues to increase. Sexual issues are often controversial, and nurses must respect the choices that clients make. Providing confidentiality is essential for clients to receive correct information, make informed decisions, and obtain appropriate care (see the Legal/Ethical Issues box on p. 1884).

The prevalence of STDs is a major health concern worldwide. External factors, such as increasing population, cultural factors (e.g., later marriage, earlier first intercourse), political and economic policies, as well as international travel and migration, affect the prevalence of STDs in any given geographic area. The prevalence is also affected by changing human physiology patterns such as earlier menarche. Sexual attitudes and behaviors and access to care play a major role in the risk of acquiring an STD. STDs also cause complications that can contribute to severe physical and emotional suffering, including infertility, ectopic pregnancy, cancer, and death. Some of the most common complications caused by sexually transmitted organisms are listed in Table 80-2.

Chlamydia, gonorrhea, syphilis, and AIDS (acquired immunodeficiency syndrome) are reportable to local health authorities in every state (Centers for Disease Control and Prevention [CDC], 2002a). Other STDs, such as genital herpes (GH), HIV infection, and chancroid, may or may not be reported, depending on local legal requirements. Rigorous reporting and a follow-up effort by local public health

---

*NOTE: This text uses the term *sexually transmitted diseases (STDs)* to be consistent with the language used by the Centers for Disease Control and Prevention (CDC).

TABLE 80-1   Sexually Transmitted Diseases

- Human immunodeficiency virus infection
- Chancroid
- Syphilis
- Lymphogranuloma venereum
- Genital herpes simplex virus infection
- Genital warts
- Gonococcal infection
- Chlamydial infection
- Nongonococcal urethritis
- Mucopurulent cervicitis
- Epididymitis
- Pelvic inflammatory disease
- Sexually transmitted enteritis
- Sexually transmitted proctitis
- Trichomoniasis
- Candidal infection
- Bacterial vaginosis
- Viral hepatitis
- Cytomegalovirus infection
- Ectoparasitic infection
    Pediculosis pubis
    Scabies

From Centers for Disease Control and Prevention. (1998). 1998 Guidelines for treatment of sexually transmitted diseases. *Morbidity and Mortality Weekly Report, 47*(No. RR-1), 1-103.

LEGAL/ETHICAL ISSUES

SEXUAL DECISION MAKING AND CONFIDENTIALITY FOR CLIENTS WITH SEXUALLY TRANSMITTED DISEASES

Sexual issues are surrounded with much controversy in the United States. Personal values, cultural mores, and public health standards often collide as clients make decisions about their sexual health. Americans hold strongly to the principle of autonomy. Autonomy in sexual decision making (e.g., about whether to be sexually active, how to choose sexual partners, and the type of sexual behavior that is appropriate) is held as a high value. The standard of confidentiality protects this principle of autonomy in some clinical situations and under some state laws.

As nurses aim to respect this principle of autonomy about sexual decision making and confidentiality, they are challenged by the public health concerns of protecting the health of the entire community versus the autonomy of each person to make his or her own decisions. Increasing rates of chlamydial infection, especially in the teenage population, with the costly risk of infertility complications, make the idea of autonomy in sexual decision making more problematic. Clients who refuse to discuss their sexually transmitted disease with their partners, or partners who choose not to get tested or treated also pose challenges to our respect for autonomy in light of the overwhelming public health concerns. Nurses feel the conflict between their commitment to confidentiality (autonomy) and their commitment to promotion of the public's health (beneficence).

TABLE 80-2   Complications Caused by Sexually Transmitted Organisms

Complication	Causative Organisms
Salpingitis, infertility, and ectopic pregnancy	*Neisseria gonorrhoeae* *Chlamydia trachomatis* *Mycoplasma hominis* *Ureaplasma urealyticum*
Reproductive loss (abortion/miscarriage)	*N. gonorrhoeae* *C. trachomatis* Herpes simplex virus *M. hominis* *U. urealyticum* *Treponema pallidum*
Puerperal infection	*N. gonorrhoeae* *C. trachomatis*
Perinatal infection	Hepatitis B virus Human immunodeficiency virus Human papillomavirus *N. gonorrhoeae* *C. trachomatis* Herpes simplex virus *T. pallidum* Cytomegalovirus Group B streptococcus
Cancer of genital area	*C. trachomatis* Herpes simplex virus Human papillomavirus
Male urethritis	*M. hominis* Herpes simplex virus *N. gonorrhoeae* *C. trachomatis* *U. urealyticum*
Vulvovaginitis	Herpes simplex virus *Trichomonas vaginalis* Bacteria causing vaginosis *Candida albicans*
Cervicitis	*N. gonorrhoeae* *C. trachomatis* Herpes simplex virus
Proctitis	*N. gonorrhoeae* *C. trachomatis* Herpes simplex virus *Campylobacter jejuni* *Shigella* species *Entamoeba histolytica*
Hepatitis	*T. pallidum* Hepatitis A, B, and C virus
Dermatitis	*Sarcoptes scabiei* *Phthirus pubis*
Genital ulceration or warts	*C. trachomatis* Herpes simplex virus Human papillomavirus *T. pallidum* *Haemophilus ducreyi* *Calymmatobacterium granulomatis*

departments and health care professionals is one intervention for decreasing the incidence of STDs.

Nurses in a variety of community settings are responsible for identifying clients at risk for STDs, caring for clients with diagnosed STDs, and preventing further cases through education and case finding. Nurses in secondary and tertiary care settings, such as hospitals, also have a responsibility to recognize clients who are at risk for or who have STDs.

The Centers for Disease Control and Prevention (CDC) updates its guidelines for treatment of STDs. The 2002 guidelines provide information, treatment standards, and counseling advice to help decrease the spread of STDs (CDC, 2002a).

WOMEN'S HEALTH CONSIDERATIONS

Women, because of the extensive and heavily vascular mucous membranes of the vagina, are more easily infected with STDs than are men and are at greater risk for health problems caused by STDs. Young women who are sexually active have unprotected sexual intercourse more often than do older women and are at greatest risk because of the following:

- Lack of knowledge about the risk of disease
- Their belief that they are not vulnerable to disease

- Their mistaken belief that oral contraceptives; contraceptive patches, sponges, and foams; and intrauterine devices protect them from STDs as well as from pregnancy
- Alcohol consumption, which promotes risky sexual behavior
  Postmenopausal women also may be at high risk for STDs because many perceive that pregnancy is no longer a risk and, thus do not use barrier protection. Mucosal tears from vaginal atrophy in postmenopausal women may also place them at greater risk.

Women have more asymptomatic infections that may delay diagnosis and treatment. This delay increases the likelihood of more serious problems, including irreversible damage to reproductive organs and systemic illness. Embarrassment, denial, or fear about STDs may further delay treatment, increasing the potential for serious complications.

ACQUIRED IMMUNODEFICIENCY SYNDROME

Acquired immunodeficiency syndrome (AIDS), a disease caused by infection with the human immunodeficiency virus (HIV), causes immunosuppression and affects the body's ability to fight disease. HIV is transmitted through infected body fluids (e.g., semen, vaginal secretions, blood and blood products, breast milk) infected with HIV. Adults at high risk include the following:

- People who engage in anal sexual activity
- People who share needles
- People who have unprotected sexual intercourse with multiple partners
- People who have unprotected sexual intercourse with partners infected with HIV
- People who have hemophilia or other clotting disorders
- People who used untested blood and blood products before 1985
- Health care workers
- Sexual partners of anyone at risk for HIV (of both sexes)

Men and women with HIV disease are at greater risk for acquiring other STDs (Williams, 2003). HIV affects the immune system and can be transmitted in ways other than by sexual contact; it is discussed in detail in Chapter 25.

INFECTIONS ASSOCIATED WITH ULCERS

Syphilis

PATHOPHYSIOLOGY

Etiology

Syphilis is a complex sexually transmitted disease (STD) that can become systemic and cause serious complications and even death. The causative organism of syphilis is *Treponema pallidum*, a spirochete with a slender, spiral shape that resembles a corkscrew. Nonpathogenic *Treponema* species are found in the mouth, intestinal tract, and genital areas of people and animals. Although the organism can be seen only with a dark-field microscope, several serologic tests may be used to screen for the presence of syphilis antigen or antibody. *T. pallidum* is damaged by dry air or any known disinfectant. The organisms

die within hours at temperatures of 105.8° to 107.6° F (41° to 42° C) and are not airborne. The infection is usually transmitted by sexual contact, but transmission can occur through close body contact and kissing.

Incidence/Prevalence

Before penicillin was available in the 1940s, syphilis affected nearly 25% of the U.S. population. Cases of primary and secondary syphilis peaked in 1948 and then declined sharply until 1958. From that time until 1990 there was a slow rise in the rates of syphilis despite successful treatment. In 1990, the number of cases increased significantly to a post–World War II peak of more than 50,000. Because of strong public health efforts between 1990 and 2000, there was a 90% decrease in cases to an all-time low in 2000, followed by an increase in 2002 and 2003 (CDC, 2004). Areas of the southern United States and men who have sex with men have the highest rates of new syphilis cases. African Americans have a 16 times greater rate of acquiring syphilis than white individuals; however, this rate is much lower than it was in previous years (CDC, 2004). One of the Healthy People 2010 objectives is to eliminate syphilis in the United States (see the Meeting Healthy People 2010 Objectives box above).

Syphilis progresses through stages: primary, secondary, latency, and tertiary.

Primary Syphilis

The appearance of an ulcer, called a **chancre,** is the first sign of syphilis. The chancre develops at the site of entry (inoculation) of the organism from 10 to 90 days after exposure (3 weeks is average). Chancres may be found on any area of the skin or mucous membranes but occur most often on the genitalia, lips, nipples, and hands and in the oral cavity, anus, and rectum.

During this highly infectious stage, the chancre begins as a small papule. Within 3 to 7 days, it breaks down into its typical appearance: a painless, indurated, smooth weeping lesion. Regional lymph nodes enlarge, feel firm, and are not painful. Without treatment, the chancre usually disappears

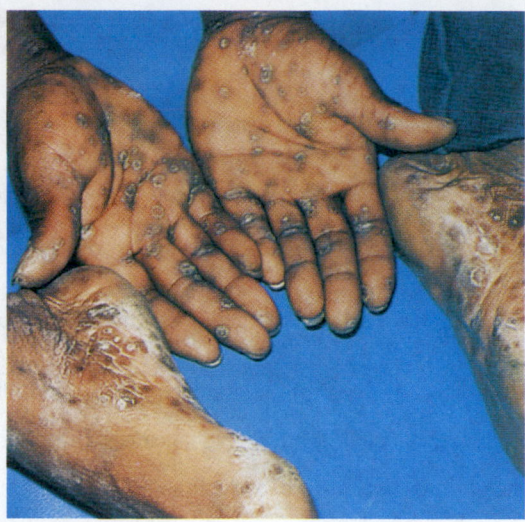

Figure 80-1 ■ Palmar and plantar secondary syphilis. (From Morse, S., et al. [2003]. *Atlas of sexually transmitted diseases and AIDS* [3rd ed.]. Edinburgh: Mosby.)

within 6 weeks. However, the organism spreads throughout the body, and the client is still infectious.

Secondary Syphilis

Secondary syphilis develops 6 weeks to 6 months after the onset of primary syphilis. Secondary syphilis is a systemic disease because the spirochetes circulate throughout the bloodstream. Manifestations include malaise, low-grade fever, headache, muscular aches and pains, and sometimes a sore throat.

These symptoms are often mistaken for those of influenza. A generalized rash develops, which involves the palms and soles of the feet. Although the rash has no typical appearance, it tends to evolve from papules to squamous papules to pustules. Other skin lesions include psoriasis-like rashes (Figure 80-1), wartlike lesions (condyloma lata), and mucous patches. The lesions are highly contagious and should not be touched without gloves. The rash subsides without treatment in 4 to 12 weeks.

Early and Late Latent Syphilis

After the second stage of syphilis, there is a period of latency. *Early* latent syphilis occurs during the first year after infection, and infectious lesions can recur. *Late* latent syphilis is a disease of more than 1 year's duration after infection. This stage is not infectious except to the fetus of a pregnant woman. Clients with latent syphilis may or may not have reactive serologic test findings.

Tertiary Syphilis

Tertiary, or late, syphilis occurs after a highly variable period, from 4 to 20 years. This stage develops in untreated cases and can mimic almost any pathologic condition because any organ system can be affected. The following are manifestations of late syphilis:

- Benign lesions (gummas) of the skin, mucous membranes, and bones
- Cardiovascular syphilis, usually in the form of aortic valvular disease and aortic aneurysms

- Neurosyphilis, causing central nervous system problems (e.g., meningitis, hearing loss, generalized paresis)

HEALTH PROMOTION/ILLNESS PREVENTION

The most important aspect for prevention of most sexually transmitted diseases (STDs), including syphilis, is education. All people, regardless of age, gender, ethnicity, or sexual orientation, are susceptible to STDs. STDs are largely preventable through education that includes safer sex practices. *Do not assume that a person is not sexually active because of his or her age, profession, or religion.* Discuss prevention methods frankly with all clients who are sexually active. Safer sex practices are those that reduce the risk of nonintact skin or mucous membranes coming in contact with infected body fluids and blood. Such practices include using the following:

- A latex condom for genital and anal intercourse
- A condom or latex barrier (dental dam) over the genitals or anus during oral-genital or oral-anal sexual contact
- Latex gloves for finger or hand contact with the vagina or rectum

Abstinence and decreasing the number of sexual partners also decrease the risk for acquiring an STD. Chapter 25 describes specific sexual acts that carry the greatest risk for STDs.

◆COLLABORATIVE MANAGEMENT
◆Assessment

Assessment of the client who has manifestations of syphilis begins with a history to gather information about any lesions or rash. The history should include a risk assessment and sexual history and whether previous testing or treatment for syphilis or other STDs has ever been done (Chart 80-1). Ask about allergic reactions to drugs, especially penicillin. A woman may present with inguinal lymph node enlargement, the location that drains the area of the vagina and cervix. She may state a history of sexual contact with a male partner who had an ulcer that she noticed during the encounter. Men usually discover the chancre on the penis or scrotum.

Conduct a physical examination, including inspection and palpation, to identify manifestations of syphilis. Wear gloves while palpating any lesions because of the highly contagious treponemes that are present. Women frequently have the chancre on areas that are not easily visible to them, such as the vagina or cervix. Observe for and document rashes of any type because of the variable presentation of secondary syphilis.

After the physical examination, the health care provider obtains a specimen of the chancre for examination under a darkfield microscope. Diagnosis of primary or secondary syphilis is confirmed if *T. pallidum,* the characteristic spirochete, is present. If the first slide is negative for *T. pallidum,* the procedure should be repeated in 3 days because many conditions can cause a false-negative result.

Blood tests are also used to diagnose syphilis. The usual screening test is the Venereal Disease Research Laboratory (VDRL) serum test. This test is based on an antibody-antigen reaction that determines both the presence and the amount of antibodies produced by the body in response to an infection by *T. pallidum.* The VDRL test becomes reactive 2 to 6 weeks after infection. VDRL titers are also used to monitor

CHART 80-1

FOCUSED ASSESSMENT of
The Client with a Sexually Transmitted Disease

Assess history of present illness:
- Chief complaint
- Symptoms by quality and quantity, precipitating and palliative factors
- Any treatments taken (self-prescribed or over-the-counter products)

Assess past medical history:
- Major health problems—including any history of STDs/PID
- Surgeries—obstetric and gynecologic, circumcision

Assess current health status:
- Menstrual history for irregularities
- Sexual history
    Type and frequency of sexual activity
    Number of sexual contacts
    Sexual orientation
- Contraceptive history
- Medications
- Allergies
- Lifestyle risks—drugs, alcohol, tobacco

Assess preventive health care practices:
- Pap smears
- Regular STD screening
- Use of barrier contraceptives to prevent STDs and pregnancy

Assess physical examination findings:
- Vital signs
- Oropharyngeal findings
- Abdominal findings
- Genital or pelvic findings
- Anorectal findings

Assess laboratory data:
- Urinalysis
- Hematology
- Cervical, urethral, oral, rectal specimens
- Lesion samples for microbiology and virology
- Pregnancy testing

PID, Pelvic inflammatory disease; *STDs,* sexually transmitted diseases.

TABLE 80-3   Selected Nursing Diagnoses for Clients with Sexually Transmitted Diseases

- Risk for Injury related to the disease process
- Ineffective Coping related to high degree of threat, fear, guilt, or anger
- Noncompliance (treatment and/or partner follow-up) related to cost, significant other, access and convenience of care, cultural influences
- Sexual Dysfunction related to disease process, fear of transmission
- Impaired Skin Integrity related to the presence of genital ulcers, warts, or rash
- Ineffective Health Maintenance related to lack of resources and information about the mode of transmission, disease process, or need for treatment
- Impaired Social Interaction related to self-concept disturbance or social stigma
- Acute Pain related to the physical agent (infection process)
- Anxiety related to threat to health status (possible infertility) as a result of having an STD
- Chronic Low Self-Esteem/Situational Low Self-Esteem related to disturbed body image as a result of having an STD

treatment effectiveness. The antibodies are not specific to *T. pallidum,* and false-positive reactions often occur from such conditions as drug addiction, cancer, hepatitis, some viral diseases, and systemic lupus erythematosus (SLE).

If a positive VDRL result is obtained, the health care provider orders a more specific test, such as the *fluorescent treponemal antibody absorption (FTA-ABS)* test or the *microhemagglutination assay for T. palladium* (MHA-TP), to confirm the infection. These tests are more sensitive for all stages of syphilis, although false-positive results may still occur.

◆ Interventions

Drug Therapy. Antibiotics are the main therapy for the client with syphilis. The drug therapy of choice is benzathine penicillin G, given intramuscularly as a single 2.4 million unit dose. Allergic reactions to the antibiotic can occur. Therefore it is important to monitor for allergic manifestations (e.g., rash, edema, shortness of breath, chest tightness, anxiety). Penicillin desensitization is recommended for penicillin-allergic clients. The client who has never had penicillin previously should have a skin test before receiving a penicillin injection. Keep all clients at the health care agency for at least 30 minutes after they have received injections of antibiotics, so that manifestations of an allergic reaction can be detected and treated. If an allergic reaction does occur, treatment can begin immediately. The most severe reaction is anaphylaxis. All health care professionals working in clinics or offices where injections of penicillin are given must be familiar with the symptoms and treatment of anaphylaxis (see Chapter 26).

The **Jarisch-Herxheimer reaction** may also follow antibiotic therapy for syphilis. This reaction is caused by the rapid release of products from the disruption of the cells of the organism. Onset occurs within 2 hours after therapy, with a peak at 4 to 8 hours. Symptoms include generalized aches, pain at the injection site, vasodilation and hypotension, and a rise in temperature. These symptoms do not always occur and often are benign. This reaction may be treated symptomatically with analgesics and antipyretics.

Nursing Management. Nursing interventions are based on data gained during the history and physical assessment. Nursing diagnoses for clients with syphilis, as well as other STDs, are listed in Table 80-3.

Reinforce the information provided to the client about the cause of infection (sexual transmission); treatment, including side effects, possible complications of untreated or incompletely treated disease; and the need for follow-up care. All sexual partners must be adequately treated as soon as possible. Discuss with the client the importance of partner notification and treatment, including the risk for reinfection if the partner goes untreated. Inform the client that the disease must be reported to the local health authority and that all information will be held in strict confidence. Encourage the client to provide accurate information for this follow-up to ensure that all at-risk partners are treated appropriately. Provide a setting that offers privacy and encourages open discussion.

Urge the client to adhere to the treatment regimen, which includes follow-up visits. Also urge sexual abstinence until the treatment is completed.

The emotional responses to syphilis vary and may include feelings of fear, depression, guilt, and anxiety. Clients may experience guilt if they have infected others or anger if they have been infected by a partner. If further psychosocial interventions are needed, encourage the client to discuss these feelings or refer him or her to other resources such as psychotherapy groups, self-help support groups, or STD clinics.

Genital Herpes

PATHOPHYSIOLOGY

Etiology

Genital herpes (GH) is an acute, recurring, incurable viral disease. Two serotypes of herpes simplex virus (HSV) affect the genitalia: type 1 (HSV-1) and type 2 (HSV-2). Most nongenital lesions, such as cold sores, are caused by HSV-1; HSV-2 causes most of the genital lesions. However, this distinction is academic because the transmission, symptoms, diagnosis, and treatment are nearly identical for the two types. Either type can produce oral or genital lesions through oral-genital contact with an infected person.

The incubation period is 2 to 20 days, with the average period being 1 week. Many people are asymptomatic during the primary infection. When symptoms do occur, they may be severe during the first infection and may require hospitalization.

Itching or a tingling sensation may be felt in the skin 1 to 2 days before an outbreak. These sensations are followed by the appearance of **vesicles** (blisters) in a typical cluster (see Figure 70-13) on the penis, scrotum, vulva, perineum, vagina, cervix, or perianal region. The blisters rupture spontaneously in a day or two and leave painful erosions. These lesions can become extensive, and other symptoms, such as headaches, fever, general malaise, and swelling of inguinal lymph nodes, may be present. Urination may be painful, and clients with urinary retention may need to be catheterized. Lesions resolve within 2 to 6 weeks.

After the lesions heal, the virus remains in a dormant state in the nerve ganglia (specifically, in the sacral ganglia). Periodically, the virus may activate, and symptoms recur. These recurrences may be triggered by many factors, including stress, fever, sunburn, poor nutrition, menses, and sexual activity.

Recurrences are not caused by reinfection. Recurrent episodes are usually less severe and of shorter duration than the primary infection. Some clients have no symptoms at all during recurrence or viral reactivation. *However, there is viral shedding, and the client is infectious.* Long-term complications of GH include the risk of neonatal transmission and an increased risk for acquiring HIV infections. The risk for neonatal transmission is greater in a pregnant woman who has a primary infection than in one who has a recurrence.

Incidence/Prevalence

On the basis of serologic studies, not symptoms, 50 million persons in the United States may have HSV-2 (CDC, 2002a). HSV-2 is believed to cause 70% to 95% of the primary episodes of GH and recurs more often than HSV-1. Most people infected with GH have not been diagnosed (CDC, 2002a). About 19% of the U.S. population between the ages of 14 and 49 years are thought to be infected (McQuillan, 2000). Most people infected with HSV have not received a diagnosis because they have mild symptoms and shed virus intermittently.

◆COLLABORATIVE MANAGEMENT
◆Assessment

The diagnosis of GH is usually based on the client's history and physical examination and is confirmed through a viral culture (see Chart 80-1). Cultures are most accurate if spec-

---

CHART 80-2

BEST PRACTICE for
Care of the Client with Genital Herpes

- Administer oral analgesics as prescribed.
- Apply local anesthetic sprays or ointments as prescribed
- Apply ice packs or warm compresses to the client's lesions.
- Administer sitz baths three or four times a day.
- Encourage an increase in fluid intake.
- Encourage frequent urination.
- Pour water over the client's genitalia while the client is voiding, or encourage voiding while the client is sitting in a tub of water or standing in a shower.
- Catheterize the client as necessary.
- Encourage genital hygiene, and encourage keeping the skin clean and dry.
- Wash hands thoroughly after contact with lesions, and launder towels that have had direct contact with lesions.
- Wear gloves when applying ointments.
- Advise the client to avoid sexual activity when lesions are present.
- Advise the client to use latex or polyurethane condoms during all sexual exposures.
- Instruct the client in the use, side effects, and risks versus benefits of antiviral agents.

---

imens are obtained within 48 hours of the first outbreak of the blisters. Fluid from inside the blister should be obtained to ensure a correct diagnosis. GH is often diagnosed without cultures if the presenting manifestations are classic.

◆Interventions

Treatment of HSV-infected clients is usually symptomatic. The goals of management are to decrease the discomfort from painful ulcerations, to promote healing without secondary infection, to decrease viral shedding, and to prevent infection transmission (Chart 80-2).

Drug Therapy. Antiviral drugs are used to treat GH. *The drugs do not cure the infection* but do decrease the severity, promote healing, and decrease the frequency of recurrent outbreaks. Drug therapy is recommended for most people with an initial outbreak. Topical therapy is not as effective as oral therapy. Acyclovir (Zovirax, Avirax✱), famciclovir (Famvir), or valacyclovir (Valtrex) may be used. The main differences in these drugs are cost and frequency of use. Dosage and length of treatment differ for primary outbreaks (lasting 7 to 10 days) and recurrent outbreaks (lasting 5 days) (Chart 80-3). Mild recurrent episodes do not show a reasonable benefit from antiviral treatment, and the cost may outweigh the benefit. Therapy for severe recurrent outbreaks may be beneficial if it is started within 1 day of the appearance of lesions or during the period of itching or tingling before lesions appear.

Clients who have frequent recurrences (more than six in a year) may benefit from daily suppressive treatment with antivirals. Suppression may reduce recurrences by 70% to 80% in clients with frequent outbreaks. However, suppression only reduces but does not prevent viral shedding even when symptoms are not present (CDC, 2002a). Clients receiving continuous therapy should stop after 1 year for reassessment of recurrences.

The cost of care for clients with GH is enormous, making it a major public health problem with a large economic burden. Annual direct medical costs in the United States are estimated at $207 million. Of that amount, health care provider visits accounted for 36%, and drug therapy accounted for 64% (Tao et al., 2000).

CHART 80-3

DRUG THERAPY for
Genital Herpes: First Clinical Episode of Genital Herpes

Drug	Dosage	Nursing Interventions	Rationales
Acyclovir (Zovirax, Avirax ✲)	400 mg PO three times daily for 7 to 10 days	Instruct client that nausea and vomiting may occur when taking the drug.	The client is prepared for possible side effect.
	Or 200 mg PO five times daily for 7 to 10 days Or	Same as above.	Same as above.
Famciclovir (Famvir)	250 mg PO three times daily for 7 to 10 days Or	Instruct client that the drug is most effective if started within the first 48 hours of symptoms.	Efficacy has not been established for the first dose started more than 72 hours after the onset of symptoms.
Valacyclovir (Valtrex)	1 g PO twice daily for 7 to 10 days	Observe for side effects, including gastrointestinal disturbances, headaches, and dizziness.	The client is prepared for possible side effects.

Nursing Management. Nursing management includes client counseling and education about the infection, the potential for recurrent episodes, the correct use and possible side effects of antiviral therapy, viral shedding even when clients are symptom free, and sexual transmission. Discussion about sexual activity is extremely important. Remind clients to abstain from sexual activity while lesions are present. Urge condom use during all sexual exposures because of the increased risk for HSV transmission, because viral shedding can occur even when lesions are not present. Teach the client about how and when to use condoms (Chart 80-4).

Assess the client's psychological responses to the diagnosis of genital herpes. Many clients are initially shocked and need reassurance that they can manage the disease. Infected clients have reported feelings of disbelief, uncleanness, isolation, and loneliness. They have also reported anger at their partners for transmitting the infection or fear of rejection by partners because they have the infection. Help clients cope with the diagnosis by being sensitive and supportive during assessments and interventions. Encourage social support and refer clients to support groups such as HELP (local support groups of the National Herpes Resource Center). Symptomatic care may include oral analgesics, topical anesthetics, sitz baths, and increased oral fluid intake.

Health Promotion. Emphasize the risk of fetal infection to all clients, both male and female. Women and men who have genital herpes need to inform the maternity care provider of their history during future pregnancies.

🤔 Critical Thinking Challenge

The client is a 50-year-old woman who is a lawyer. She has been a widow for 10 years and her children are grown. She has come to the GYN clinic because she has painful blisters on her perineum and vulva. She says that although she has some burning with urination, she doesn't think she has a bladder infection because the urine doesn't smell and she does not have frequency. She also tells you that she has a lump in her right groin and just feels fatigued. She asks if all these problems could mean she is entering menopause. Her last Pap smear, GYN examination, and mammogram were performed 18 months ago.

CHART 80-4

CLIENT EDUCATION GUIDE
Use of Condoms

- Use latex or polyurethane condoms rather than natural membrane condoms.
- Use a condom with every sexual encounter (including oral, vaginal, and anal).
- Female condoms (Reality)—polyurethane sheaths in the vagina—are effective in preventing transmission of viruses, including HIV.
- Condoms infrequently (2 per 100) break during sexual intercourse, unless used incorrectly.
- Keep condoms (especially latex) in a cool, dry place, out of direct sunlight.
- Do not use condoms that are in damaged packages or that are brittle or discolored.
- Always handle a condom with care to avoid damaging it with fingernails, teeth, or other sharp objects.
- Put condoms on before any genital contact. Hold the condom by the tip and unroll it on the penis. Leave a space at the tip to collect semen.
- If you use a lubricant with condoms, make sure that the lubricant is water based and washes away with water. Oil-based products may damage latex condoms.
- Use of spermicide (nonoxynol-9) with condoms, either lubricated condoms or vaginal application, has *not* been proved to be more or less effective against STDs than use without spermicide. *Spermicide-coated condoms have been associated with Escherichia coli urinary tract infections in women. Nonoxynol-9 may increase risk for transmission of HIV during vaginal intercourse and anal intercourse. Its use is discouraged for anal intercourse.*
- If a condom breaks, replace it immediately.
- After ejaculation, withdraw the erect penis carefully, holding the condom at the base of the penis to prevent the condom from slipping off.
- Never use a condom more than once.

Modified from Centers for Disease Control and Prevention. (2002). Sexually transmitted diseases treatment guidelines. *Mortality and Morbidity Weekly Report, 517*(RR-6), 1-80.

When you inspect her genital region, you see many clustered vesicles and some eroded and crusted lesions.

1. What additional information should you obtain?
2. What infectious process is most likely?
3. How will you prepare her for the diagnostic tests?
4. Why does she have burning on urination?

evolve For suggested answer guidelines, go to http://evolve.elsevier.com/Iggy/.

Lymphogranuloma Venereum

PATHOPHYSIOLOGY

Etiology

Lymphogranuloma venereum (LGV) is the result of genital infection with one of three serotypes of *Chlamydia trachomatis*, which is spread systemically until it localizes in the genital or rectal lymph nodes. The incubation period is 3 to 30 days. The primary lesion, at the point of entry, is transient, painless, and often not noticed by the client. The lesion usually appears on the penis in men and on the vaginal wall in women. However, sores may also be located in the mouth and rectum. Five times as many men are diagnosed with this disease as are women.

Lesions vary in form from herpes-like blisters (vesicles), to ulcers, papules, or pustules. Within 1 to 2 weeks after the primary lesion appears, secondary signs of infection appear. Lymphadenopathy (primarily inguinal and femoral) is present, more commonly in men than in women. Swelling from the enlarged lymph nodes occurs on both sides of the inguinal ligament and forms the characteristic "groove sign" of LGV. This sign is only present in about 10% to 15% of clients (Schacter & Stephens, 2003). Women and men who have had anal sex may have inflamed perianal or perirectal tissues (CDC, 2002a). Other manifestations may include headache, malaise, arthralgia, and anorexia. Most clients seek care at this point.

Lymphadenopathy can recede or develop into an abscess or firm bubo. The bubo may become more **fluctuant** (softer and fluid filled). When the bubo ruptures, healing occurs slowly. Sinus tracts, formed as a result of the infection, drain thick, viscous pus for several weeks, leaving behind deep scars.

Complications of the infection include fistulas, rectal strictures, chronic enlarged lymph nodes, and proctitis. Systemic involvement can cause carditis, arthritis, and pneumonia.

Incidence/Prevalence

LGV is common in areas of South America, Asia, Africa, and the Caribbean. It is far less common in more affluent countries. The actual incidence is not known because LGV is difficult to distinguish from other lesion-producing infections. Because it is more common in other areas of the world, ask clients about recent travel to endemic areas by themselves or by their partners.

◆COLLABORATIVE MANAGEMENT

The diagnosis of LGV is usually made on physical examination and serologic testing. The serologic test, an antibody complement fixation test (LGV-CF), is considered positive if the titer is higher than 1:64. Detection of *Chlamydia trachomatis* in material aspirated from a bubo, rather than from an open lesion, is most diagnostic for LGV. Detection of the organism can be made with the use of a test kit using gene amplification methods, although this type of test is relatively new for LGV (Mabey & Peeling, 2002). Regular cultures from the enlarged lymph nodes or bubo can be used to isolate organism but this method is not very sensitive (Schacter & Stephens, 2003).

The health care provider prescribes doxycycline (Monodox, Doxy-Caps, Doxycin✳) 100 mg orally twice daily or an erythromycin-based drug 500 mg orally four times daily for 21 days. Antibiotic treatment cures the infection and prevents further tissue damage. Infected lymph nodes may be aspirated by needle or incised and drained to prevent ulcer formation. Surgical intervention may be needed for late complications, such as perianal or perirectal strictures and fistulas. Nursing management and client education is similar to that for syphilis.

Sexual partners should be tested for cervical or urethral chlamydial infection. They should be treated if they had sexual contact with the client during the 30 days before the client's onset of symptoms.

Chancroid

PATHOPHYSIOLOGY

Etiology

Chancroid lesions are painful genital ulcerations caused by infection with *Haemophilus ducreyi*, a gram-negative bacteria. Chancroid ulcers are soft, genital lesions. These lesions and inguinal lymphadenopathy without systemic illness are the usual presentation. The infection develops as a result of sexual exposure or self-contamination from a lesion elsewhere on the body. The incubation period for chancroid varies from 3 to 10 days. A tender papule appears at the site of inoculation. This lesion rapidly breaks down to form an irregularly shaped, deep ulcer that has a purulent discharge and bleeds easily.

Complications include inguinal adenitis, balanitis, phimosis, and urethral fistulas. Chancroids differ from chancres caused by syphilis in that chancroids are soft and painful. Transmission of the disease is through contact with the ulcer or with the discharge from the infected local lymph glands during sexual activity.

Incidence/Prevalence

Although chancroid has a worldwide distribution, it is most common in less affluent tropical and subtropical countries, such as Africa, the West Indies, and Asia. It also can be found in parts of the United States. In 2000, 99 U.S. cases were reported (Ballard & Morse, 2003).

Chancroid is a cofactor for HIV transmission, leading to high rates of HIV infection of those with chancroid. About 10% of clients with chancroid acquired in the United States are co-infected with syphilis and herpes simplex virus (HSV). The rate of co-infection appears higher for those clients who acquired the disease outside the United States (CDC, 2002a). This co-infection appears to be the result of the open genital lesions. Uncircumcised men may be at greater risk for infection than circumcised men, and men are more frequently infected than women.

◆COLLABORATIVE MANAGEMENT

The health care provider obtains cultures from the ulcers to isolate the *Haemophilus ducreyi* organism. Gram staining of the exudate from the ulcer can be difficult because of multiple microbial contamination, but the gram-negative rods may be seen. Usually the diagnosis is based on the presence of ulcerative genital lesions, lymphadenopathy, and the absence of systemic symptoms. Syphilis and herpes are excluded by appropriate testing.

Management for chancroid consists of azithromycin (Zithromax) 1 g orally in a single dose, ceftriaxone (Rocephin) 250 mg intramuscularly in a single dose, ciprofloxacin (Cipro) 500 mg orally twice daily for 3 days, or erythromycin

(E-Mycin, Apo-Erythro✱) 500 mg orally four times daily for 7 days. These antibiotics cure the infection, resolve the symptoms, and prevent transmission. Clients should be observed periodically by a health care provider until ulcers heal, usually in 7 days.

Client education is similar to that for syphilis. Sexual contacts must be located and treated whether or not they are symptomatic if they have had sexual contact with the client in the 10 days before the client's onset of symptoms. The nurse's responsibility in management of the client with chancroid is similar to that for other STDs.

Granuloma Inguinale
PATHOPHYSIOLOGY

The causative organism of granuloma inguinale, or donovanosis, is *Calymmatobacterium granulomatis*. A nodule appears at the site of inoculation after 1 to 12 weeks. This lesion ulcerates, and others are formed. They are painless and grow together, becoming a spreading ulcer on the genitalia. Left untreated, these lesions can be mutilating. Inguinal lymphadenopathy does not occur, thus the name of this disease may be inappropriate. The ulcerated lesions are very vascular and bleed easily on contact. As open areas, the ulcerated lesions can become infected with bacteria or other STDs.

Granuloma inguinale is common in some less affluent countries, especially those that are tropical. Highest areas of prevalence are India, Papua, New Guinea, the Caribbean, South America, Vietnam, northern and central Australia, and southern Africa. Even in these endemic areas, granuloma inguinale makes up only about 10% of ulcerative genital lesions (Bowden, 2003).

◆COLLABORATIVE MANAGEMENT

Biopsy and cytologic smears from the ulcers are the only conclusive methods for diagnosis. Definitive diagnosis depends on finding characteristic Donovan bodies in these samples. This can be difficult, and often treatment is started before results of these tests are available.

Granuloma inguinale is treated with doxycycline 100 mg orally twice daily or trimethoprim/sulfamethoxazole double strength (Bactrim D.S., Septra D.S.) twice daily for a minimum of 3 weeks. Treatment needs to continue until all the lesions are completely healed. Relapse can occur within 6 to 18 months, even after successful initial treatment.

Nursing management of the client with granuloma inguinale is similar to that for other STDs. Obtain a thorough history that includes sexual contacts, travel abroad, and contact with partners who may have traveled to or are from endemic areas (see Chart 80-1). Asking about genital lesions that may have disappeared or changed provides information to help accurately diagnose the infection.

Explain cultures, biopsies, or other diagnostic tests that will be done to make a correct diagnosis. Provide comfort measures and emotional support, because some procedures may be invasive or painful. Teach the client about the diagnosis, the risk for complications if the disease is left untreated or incompletely treated, and the antibiotics prescribed.

Encourage the client to provide the names of sexual contacts for follow-up and treatment. Concerns about coping with the disease may arise. Encourage the client to verbalize concerns and/or refer him or her for further counseling. Because these infections are relatively rare, the client may have the added discomfort and inconvenience of being evaluated by specialists to get a correct diagnosis, which may contribute to his or her anxiety.

Persons having sexual contact with the client within 60 days of the onset of symptoms or those displaying any signs or symptoms should be treated. Despite this recommendation, benefit of treatment when no symptoms are present is not known (CDC, 2002a).

? *Critical Thinking Challenge*

The client described on p. 1889 is diagnosed with genital herpes; HSV-2 is cultured from the blisters. She is shocked when she is told the diagnosis and says "How can this have happened? I haven't even had intercourse." When you ask about her intimate relationships, she says that, until recently, she had not had any sexual contact since her husband died 10 years ago. She has been intimate for the past month with a 60-year-old co-worker, but they have not had vaginal intercourse because he has erectile dysfunction. She does tell you that he has orally stimulated her and has rubbed his genitals against her to bring her to orgasm. She says she didn't think this type of sexual activity carried any risk for pregnancy or disease.

1. What should you tell her about the risks associated with the type of sexual activity she described?
2. Is the partner a likely source for the infection? Why or why not?
3. She says she doesn't want to tell him about the problem. Is this a reportable disease? How should you respond to this statement?
4. What measures should you suggest to reduce her physical discomfort?

evolve For suggested answer guidelines, go to http://evolve.elsevier.com/Iggy/.

INFECTIONS OF THE EPITHELIAL STRUCTURES
Condylomata Acuminata
PATHOPHYSIOLOGY
Etiology

Condylomata acuminata (also known as genital *warts*) are caused by certain types of human papillomavirus (HPV), mainly types 6 and 11. These types rarely result in invasive cancer of the genital tract. However, HPV types 16, 18, 31, 33, and 35 (of the nearly 70 different HPV genotypes) are found on the skin of the genitalia and increase the risk for genital cancers, especially cervical cancer. Infection with several HPV types can occur at the same time. Sites commonly affected include the urinary meatus, labia, vagina, cervix, penis, scrotum, anus, and perineal area. Pregnancy may increase the growth rate of the lesions. The incubation period is usually 2 to 3 months.

The genital warts are initially single, small papillary growths that may grow into large cauliflower-like masses (Figure 80-2). Bleeding may occur if the wart is disrupted. Warts may regress spontaneously without treatment.

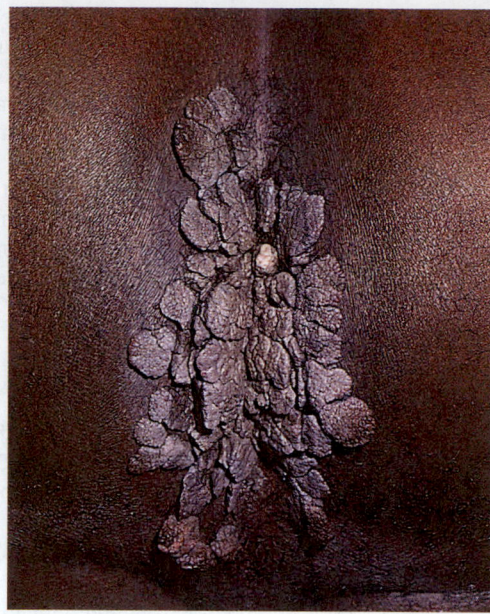

Figure 80-2 ■ Perianal condyloma acuminata. (From Morse, S., et al. [2003]. Atlas of sexually transmitted diseases and AIDS [3rd ed.]. Edinburgh: Mosby.)

Incidence/Prevalence

Genital warts are the most common sexually transmitted viral disease and are often seen with other infections. About 5.5 million people in the United States become infected with HPV each year. Possibly 75% of the reproductive age population is infected. An estimated 20 million people currently have HPV infections that can be transmitted to others (CDC, 2001).

◆ COLLABORATIVE MANAGEMENT
◆ Assessment

The diagnosis of condylomata acuminata is made by examination of the lesions, which appear wartlike. A Pap smear is obtained to assess for cervical dysplasia and is useful in the ⌐lation and diagnosis of HPV from the cervix. HPV can be detected in genital swab specimens using DNA To rule out the presence of other infections, a and cultures for chlamydial and gonorrhea in- ⌐btained. If a wartlike lesion bleeds easily, ap- is atypical or persistent, a specimen for ⌐ to rule out other pathologic problems. ⌐osies should be performed for any le- Chapter 78).

⌐ remove the warts, treat the ⌐t of atypical or dysplastic ⌐dicates HPV; therefore ⌐ not known whether ⌐iral presence, de- ⌐ 2002a). ⌐ions for ex- ⌐. Clients ⌐v for 3 ⌐men

iquimod 5% cream applied topically at bedtime three times a week for up to 16 weeks.

Cryotherapy, podophyllin, and trichloroacetic acid (TCA) are provider-applied treatments. **Cryotherapy** (freezing), usually with liquid nitrogen, can be used every 1 to 2 weeks until lesions are resolved. Podophyllin resin 10% to 25% in a compound of tincture of benzoin can be applied weekly but needs to be washed off 1 to 4 hours after application. Trichloroacetic acid (80% to 90%) can be applied weekly. Extensive warts have been treated with the carbon dioxide laser, intralesional interferon injections, and surgical removal.

For effective management of condylomata acuminata, sexual partners must also be evaluated and treated (if warts are present). Teach clients to avoid intimate sexual contact until external lesions are healed.

Nursing Management. Nursing management focuses on client education about the mode of transmission, incubation period, treatment, and complications, especially the association with cervical cancer. Reinforce instructions about local care of the lesions or patient-applied treatment. Inform clients that after treatment with cryotherapy, podophyllin, or TCA, they may experience discomfort, bleeding or discharge from the site, or sloughing of parts of warts. Instructs the client to keep the area clean (shower or bath) and dry, and to be alert for any signs or symptoms of infection or side effects of the treatment.

Condoms are recommended to help reduce transmission (see Chart 80-4). Inform clients that recurrence is likely and that repeated treatments may be needed. Urge women who have had condylomata acuminata to have an annual Pap smear. As with other STDs, provide emotional support and refer for counseling as needed.

Gonorrhea

PATHOPHYSIOLOGY

Etiology

Gonorrhea, a sexually transmitted bacterial infection occurs in both men and women. Infants can be infected during childbirth. The causative organism is *Neisseria gonorrhoeae*, a gram-negative intracellular diplococcus. *N. gonorrhoeae* is transmitted by direct sexual contact with mucosal surfaces (vaginal intercourse, orogenital contact, or anogenital contact). Although the organism has been found on inanimate surfaces where it has been artificially inoculated, there is no evidence that transmission occurs naturally in this manner.

The first symptoms of gonorrhea may appear 3 to 10 days after sexual contact with an infected person. The infection can be asymptomatic in both men and women, but women have asymptomatic, or "silent," infections more often than do men. If symptoms are present, men usually notice dysuria and a penile discharge that can be either profuse yellowish green fluid or scant clear fluid. The urethra is most commonly affected, but infection can extend to the prostate, the seminal vesicles, and the epididymis. Men seek curative treatment sooner, usually because they have symptoms, and thereby avoid some of the serious complications.

Women may report a change in vaginal discharge (yellow, green, profuse, odorous), urinary frequency, or dysuria. The

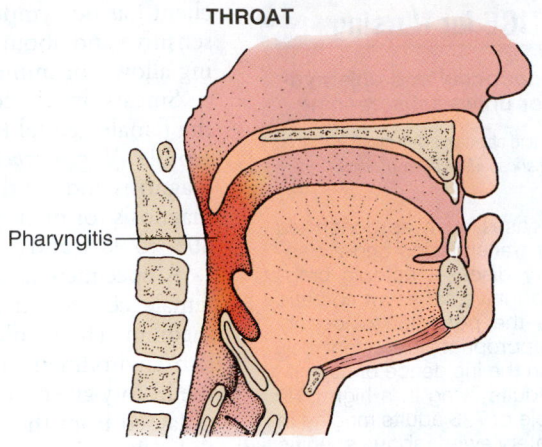

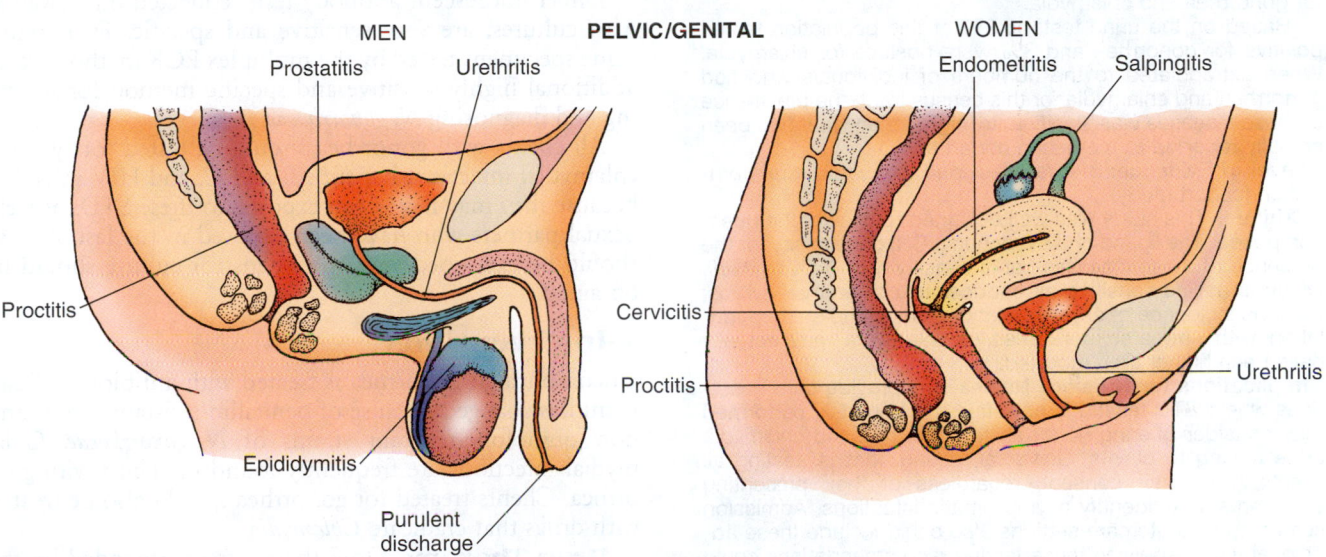

Figure 80-3 ■ Areas of involvement of gonorrhea in men and women.

cervix and urethra are the most common sites of infection. Gonorrhea can be present without symptoms in the cervix and can be transmitted or progress without warning. Ascending spread of the organism can cause pelvic infection **(pelvic inflammatory disease [PID]), endometritis** (endometrial infection), **salpingitis** (fallopian tube infection), and pelvic peritonitis. Infections with or without symptoms can lead to PID and tubal scarring. Rare complications of gonorrhea in adults include arthritis, meningitis, hepatitis, and disseminated infection.

Anal manifestations may include anal itching and irritation, rectal bleeding or diarrhea, and painful defecation. Oral manifestations, related to throat infection, are seldom noted but may include a sore throat, ulcerated lips, tender gingivae, and blisters in the throat. Figure 80-3 shows common sites of gonococcal infections.

Clients without symptoms may be found to have positive cultures for gonorrhea when they have a routine physical examination, are admitted to a hospital, or during preoperative testing. Others may seek screening and care because the sexual partner has been diagnosed with the infection. Universal screening of all sexually active men and women for gonorrhea may be a useful public health tool to avoid spread of asymptomatic infection (see the Evidence-Based Practice for Nursing box on p. 1894).

Incidence/Prevalence

Gonorrhea is the most reported communicable disease in the United States and may be on the rise. An estimated 650,000 new infections occur each year (CDC, 2001). The incidence is highest in 15- to 19-year-old women and 20- to 24-year-old men (CDC, 2002a). Fluoroquinolone-resistant *N. gonorrhoeae* has increased from 0.1% of cases in 1998 to 0.7% of cases in 2001; however, there are regional differences (CDC, 2002a).

◆COLLABORATIVE MANAGEMENT
◆Assessment

A complete history includes reviewing possible symptoms of gonorrhea, taking a sexual history that includes sexual orientation and sites of intercourse, and assessing for allergies to antibiotics (see Chart 80-1). Using a nonjudgmental approach helps elicit more complete information. This approach may

EVIDENCE-BASED PRACTICE for Nursing

Prevalence of asymptomatic gonococcal and chlamydial infections provides support for universal screening

Turner, C., et al. (2002). Untreated gonococcal and chlamydial infections in a probability sample of adults. *Journal of the American Medical Association, 287*(6), 726-733.

Untreated sexually transmitted diseases such as gonorrhea and chlamydia increase the risk for transmission and for sequelae such as pelvic inflammatory disease, ectopic pregnancy, and infertility. The concept of universal asymptomatic screening is controversial but has the potential to identify asymptomatic individuals so that appropriate treatment can occur. This study sought to establish the incidence of asymptomatic, and therefore untreated, adults living in a high STD rate census tract. A purposive sample of 728 adults ranging in age from 18 to 35 years were interviewed about specific health habits, STD risks, and current symptoms. Of these, 579 people without symptoms provided urine samples for testing for gonorrhea and chlamydia.

Based on the urine tests, 5.3% of this population tested positive for gonorrhea and 3% were positive for chlamydia. When extrapolated to the numbers of individuals who had gonorrhea and chlamydia for this census tract, the prevalence of these diseases was significantly higher than what had been actually reported to the health department.

Level of Evidence: 3—Well-designed trial without randomization (cohort study).

Critique. This study was well designed to answer the question posed. The ligand chain reaction (LCR) urine assay for the presence of these diseases has a sensitivity of 90% to 94%, which is not as sensitive as endocervical or urethral swabs; thus the incidence of asymptomatic adults in the study population with untreated gonorrhea or chlamydia may actually have been higher than reported.

Implications for Nursing. Nurses who provide care in settings where STD testing is not offered or routinely performed may consider offering noninvasive gonorrhea and chlamydia urine testing to clients. Universal testing, that is, testing all clients (with their consent) regardless of their presenting symptoms, may identify asymptomatic infections. Admission screening in acute care settings also could include these additional tests. Applying these testing recommendations could help reduce the incidence of STDs by identifying infected individuals and starting appropriate therapy. Nurses can use these findings to emphasize to clients, during educational sessions, the possibility of asymptomatic infection and the consequences of delayed treatment.

decrease the client's anxiety and fear about having a sexually transmitted disease (STD).

Physical assessment includes inspection for discharge from the urethra, cervix, and rectum. Palpation of the lower abdomen may reveal tenderness. Fever may be present, especially if an ascending or systemic infection has occurred. Gonorrheal infections that have become systemic may develop quickly. Manifestations of disseminated gonococcal infection (DGI) include fever, chills, skin lesions on distal extremities, and joint pain, with or without swelling, heat, or redness.

Definitive diagnosis involves laboratory testing. Identification of gonorrhea in men can be made with smears of the discharge that has been swabbed onto a glass slide, dried, and Gram stained. The presence of gram-negative diplococci is diagnostic for gonococcal urethritis. Gram stains of urethral discharge, if the client has symptoms, are 90% to 95% sensitive and about 97% specific for gonorrhea. If the

client has no symptoms, Gram stains are only 50% to 70% sensitive and about 86% specific (Lewis, 2003). Gram staining allows for immediate diagnosis and earlier treatment.

Smears do not confirm the diagnosis in women, because the female genital tract normally harbors organisms that resemble *N. gonorrhoeae*. Cultures provide a more definitive diagnosis and are the most reliable method of confirming a diagnosis for men and women. The sensitivity of cultures is 80% to 98% and greater than 99% specific (Lewis, 2003).

A specimen is obtained from the male urethra or the female cervix and swabbed onto a chocolate agar culture medium. The medium must be placed in a carbon dioxide–rich environment for the organism to grow. Depending on the history given by the client, culture specimens may also be obtained from the throat and rectum. After 24 to 48 hours, the culture is examined for the presence of gram-negative diplococci.

Direct fluorescent antibody tests, collected on a swab as with cultures, are very sensitive and specific. First-voided urine specimens tested by the multiplex PCR method are an additional highly sensitive and specific method for screening and diagnosing *N. gonorrhoeae*.

All clients with gonorrhea should be tested for syphilis, chlamydial infection, hepatitis B and C, and HIV infection because they may have been exposed to these STDs as well. Sexual partners who have been exposed in the last 30 days should be examined, and specimens for culture should be obtained.

◆ Interventions

Uncomplicated gonorrhea is treated with antibiotics. Treatment has changed because of penicillin-resistant strains and now quinolone-resistant strains of *N. gonorrhoeae*. Chlamydial infections are frequently found in clients with gonorrhea. Clients treated for gonorrhea should also be treated with drugs that eradicate *Chlamydia*.

Drug Therapy. Drug therapy recommended by the Centers for Disease Control and Prevention (CDC) is ceftriaxone (Rocephin) 125 mg intramuscularly, ciprofloxacin (Cipro) 500 mg orally, *or* ofloxacin (Floxin) 400 mg orally, *each* in a single dose *plus* azithromycin (Zithromax) 1 g orally in a single dose *or* doxycycline (Monodox, Doxy-Caps, Doxycin✱) 100 mg orally twice daily for 1 week if *Chlamydia* has not been ruled out. These combinations seem to be effective for all mucosal gonorrheal infections; treatment failure is rare.

The quinolones (ciprofloxacin, ofloxacin) are not recommended in areas with reported high quinolone resistance (e.g., Hawaii, California, Asia, and the Pacific rim) (CDC, 2002b). The only nonquinolone antibiotic choice for clients in these areas is intramuscular ceftriaxone (Rocephin).

Sexual partners must be treated as well. A test of cure is not required, but the client is advised to return for a follow-up examination if symptoms persist after treatment. Reinfection is often the cause of these symptoms and indicates a need for more education of the client and sexual partner.

The use of single-dose treatment, especially among younger individuals at high risk, is recommended. Directly observed therapy (DOT) in the health care setting appears to improve adherence (Feroli & Burstein, 2003).

Treatment of DGI includes intravenous (IV) or intramuscular ceftriaxone 1 g every 24 hours. If symptoms resolve within 24 to 48 hours, the client may be discharged to home to continue oral antibiotic therapy for at least 1 week.

Meningitis and endocarditis occur rarely. Hospitalization for clients with these problems is recommended for the initial treatment. Treatment is with IV antibiotic therapy, usually ceftriaxone 1 to 2 g every 12 hours. If meningitis or endocarditis is present, therapy is continued for 10 to 14 days for meningitis and at least 4 weeks for endocarditis. Infectious disease specialists are consulted for management of these infections.

Nursing Management. Nursing interventions focus on teaching the client about transmission and treatment of gonorrhea. Clients must understand why medications should be taken for the prescribed time for maximal effectiveness. Discuss the possibility of reinfection, including the risk for pelvic inflammatory disease (PID), and resultant problems such as ectopic pregnancy, infertility, and chronic pelvic pain. Instruct clients to avoid sexual activity until the antibiotic therapy is completed and they no longer have symptoms. Urge men and women to use condoms, especially if abstinence is not possible. Explain that gonorrhea is a reportable disease. All sexual contacts need to be examined and treated for both gonorrhea and chlamydial infection.

When a diagnosis of gonorrhea is made, clients may have feelings of fear or guilt. They may be concerned that they have contracted other STDs or see the disease as a punishment for promiscuity or "unnatural" sex acts. They may believe that acquiring gonorrhea (or any STD) is a risk that they must take to pursue their desired lifestyle. Such feelings can impair relationships with sexual partners. Encourage clients to express their feelings during assessments and teaching sessions. Assuring privacy for client teaching and maintaining confidentiality of medical records are important nursing interventions in meeting the client's psychosocial needs.

Chlamydial Infection

PATHOPHYSIOLOGY

Etiology

C. trachomatis is an intracellular bacterium and the causative agent of genital chlamydial infections. It invades the epithelial tissues in the reproductive tract and causes manifestations similar to those of gonorrheal infections. The incubation period ranges from 1 to 3 weeks, but the pathogen may be present in the genital tract for months without producing symptoms. The average duration of infection before diagnosis is about 1 year in women and 5 months in men because of its frequent asymptomatic status.

In men, the main symptom is urethritis, occurring with dysuria, frequent urination, and a mucoid discharge that is more watery and less copious than a gonorrheal discharge. Some men have the discharge only in the morning on arising. Complications include epididymitis, prostatitis, infertility, and Reiter's syndrome, a type of connective tissue disease (see Chapter 24).

In contrast, many women may have no symptoms. Women with symptoms have a mucopurulent cervicitis with a change in vaginal discharge, easily induced cervical bleeding, urinary frequency, and abdominal discomfort or pain. The vaginal discharge typically becomes yellow and more

opaque (Sellors et al., 2000). Complications of infection with *C. trachomatis* include salpingitis, PID, ectopic pregnancy, and infertility.

Incidence/Prevalence

Chlamydia trachomatis is the most common sexually transmitted disease in the United States. The disease is now reportable to local health departments in all states. In 2003, 877,478 cases were reported, an increase of more than 24% over 2000 (CDC, 2004). Four times more women than men are reported to have chlamydia, which in part reflects more screening of women than men. Up to 70% of women and 25% of men screened for chlamydia are asymptomatic (Schacter & Stephens, 2003). In men, about 10% to 20% of the cases of nongonococcal urethritis are caused by *C. trachomatis*. In women, 20% to 40% of those infected with *C. trachomatis* develop pelvic inflammatory disease (PID), discussed on p. 1896. Transmission to the newborn can occur during vaginal delivery, causing neonatal eye infections and pneumonia.

◆COLLABORATIVE MANAGEMENT
◆Assessment

Obtain a complete history, including medical, menstrual, and sexual history from the client (see Chart 80-1). Ask about the following:

- Presence of symptoms
- Any history of sexually transmitted diseases (STDs)
- Whether sexual partners have had symptoms or a history of STDs

Many women with chlamydial infections are asymptomatic. The client's history may reveal only risk factors associated with *C. trachomatis*. These factors include age younger than 20 years, being unmarried, nulliparity, having a higher number of sexual partners or a new sexual partner, use of a nonbarrier method of birth control (hormonal, intrauterine device [IUD]), and concurrent gonorrhea. As with all interviews concerning sexual behavior, use a nonjudgmental approach and provide privacy and confidentiality.

Diagnosis of chlamydial infections is made by sampling cells from the endocervix, the urethra, or both. Because chlamydiae can only reproduce inside cells, host cells that harbor the organism (or parts of it) are required in the sample. Gram staining of urethral or cervical samples can help exclude gonorrhea. The presence of polymorphonuclear leukocytes and the absence of gram-negative intracellular diplococci (suggestive of gonorrhea) points to a chlamydial infection. Absolute diagnosis of chlamydial infection is made with a tissue culture. Culture for *Chlamydia*, which detects 70% to 80% of cervical infections with *C. trachomatis*, has been the "gold standard." Special transport medium is required.

Gene amplification tests or DNA amplification tests (ligand chain reaction [LCR] and polymerase chain reaction [PCR]), are very sensitive and specific methods of detecting the presence of chlamydia on endocervical samples, urethral swabs, and urine (Lewis, 2003). The enzyme-linked immunoassay (ELISA) and direct fluorescent antibody (DFA) tests are less sensitive.

Screening asymptomatic women and men who may have risk factors for having chlamydial infections is strongly encouraged. The use of urine testing has been found to increase acceptability of testing and has resulted in increased identification of asymptomatic individuals (Turner et al., 2002).

◆Interventions

The treatment of choice for chlamydial infections is azithromycin (Zithromax) 1 g in a single dose or doxycycline (Monodox, Doxy-Caps, Doxycin✱) 100 mg twice daily for 7 days. The one-dose course, although more expensive, is preferred because of the ease in completing the treatment. Giving the drug while the client is in the health care facility helps ensure adherence. Sexual partners should be tested and treated if possible. Individuals with positive test results for chlamydia must be reported to the Health Department.

Client education is an important nursing intervention. Explain the following:

- The mode of disease transmission
- The incubation period
- Manifestations, including the possibility of asymptomatic infections
- Treatment of infection with antibiotics
- The need for abstinence from sexual intercourse until the client and partner(s) have completed treatment (7 days from the start of treatment, including a single-dose regimen)
- No test of cure is required, but all women should be re-screened 3 to 4 months after treatment because of the high risk for PID if reinfection occurs.
- The need to return for evaluation if symptoms recur or new symptoms develop (most recurrences are actually reinfections from a new or untreated partner)
- Possible complications of untreated or inadequately treated infection, such as PID, ectopic pregnancy, or infertility

OTHER GYNECOLOGIC CONDITIONS

Pelvic Inflammatory Disease

PATHOPHYSIOLOGY

Etiology

Pelvic inflammatory disease (PID) is a complex infectious process in which organisms from the lower genital tract migrate from the endocervix upward through the uterine cavity into the fallopian tubes. The spread of infection to other organs and tissues of the upper genital tract occurs from direct contact with mucosal surfaces or through the fimbriated ends of the tubes to the ovaries, parametrium, and peritoneal cavity (Figure 80-4). This may involve one or more pelvic structures, including the uterus, fallopian tubes, and adjacent pelvic structures. The most common site is the fallopian tube. Resultant infections include the following:

- Endometritis (infection of the endometrial cavity)
- Salpingitis (inflammation of the fallopian tubes)
- Oophoritis (ovarian infection)
- Parametritis (infection of the parametrium)
- Peritonitis (infection of the peritoneal cavity)
- Tubal or tubo-ovarian abscess

Many different pathogens are linked to PID. Sexually transmitted organisms are most often responsible for PID, especially *Chlamydia trachomatis* and *Neisseria gonorrhoeae*. Organisms that are part of the vaginal flora can also cause PID.

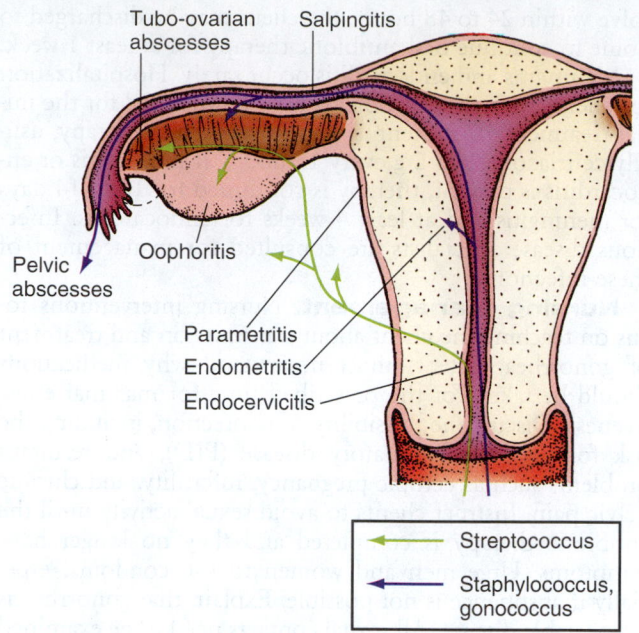

Figure 80-4 ■ The spread of pelvic inflammatory disease.

Chlamydia is the most common causative agent of PID in the United States and Europe. In addition, *Gardnerella vaginalis*, *Haemophilus influenzae*, *Staphylococcus*, *Streptococcus*, *Escherichia coli*, and other aerobic and anaerobic organisms have been identified in clients with PID. There is increasing evidence that the anaerobes involved in bacterial vaginosis may have a role in the development of PID (CDC, 2002a).

The infectious organisms invade the pelvis from an infection ascending from the vagina or cervix. Infections are spread during sexual intercourse, during childbirth (including the postpartum period), and after abortion. Rarely do infections result from transperitoneal spread from a ruptured appendix or intra-abdominal abscess. Sepsis and death can occur, especially if treatment is delayed or inadequate (Dulin & Akers, 2003).

Many practitioners use the terms *PID* and *salpingitis* synonymously for acute infections. PID is one of the leading causes of infertility and is related to the increase in the number of ectopic pregnancies reported in the United States. It is an acute syndrome resulting in tenderness in the tubes and ovaries (adnexa) and low, dull abdominal pain. However, many women experience only mild discomfort or menstrual irregularity; others experience no symptoms at all, so-called "silent" or "subclinical" PID. Diagnosis and treatment of PID in these women is challenging. Irreversible scarring or stricture, causing sterility, may occur before PID is diagnosed.

Incidence/Prevalence

The incidence of PID is on the rise. Accurate rates are unavailable because PID is not a reportable disease. Many of the same factors that place women at risk for STDs also place them at risk for PID. Risk factors for sexually active women include the following:

- Age younger than 20 years
- Multiple sexual partners
- Intrauterine device (IUD) in place
- Use of vaginal douches

- Smoking
- Chlamydial or gonococcal infection; bacterial vaginosis
- A history of sexually transmitted diseases (STDs)
- A history of PID

◆COLLABORATIVE MANAGEMENT
◆Assessment

HISTORY

Obtain a complete medical, family, menstrual, obstetric, and sexual history, including a history of previous episodes of pelvic inflammatory disease (PID) or other sexually transmitted diseases (see Chart 80-1). Assess for contraceptive use (especially the intrauterine device), a history of reproductive surgery, and other risk factors previously identified. The possibility of sexual abuse should be raised.

One of the most frequent symptoms of PID is lower abdominal pain. Other symptoms include menstrual irregularities or abnormal vaginal bleeding, dysuria, an increase or change in vaginal discharge, dyspareunia, malaise, fever, and chills.

PHYSICAL ASSESSMENT/CLINICAL MANIFESTATIONS

Observe whether the client has discomfort with movement. Often the client has a hunched-over gait that she uses to protect her abdomen. She may find it difficult to independently get on the examination table or stretcher. She may be fatigued and diaphoretic and have a fever.

Assess for lower abdominal tenderness, possibly with rigidity or rebound tenderness. A pelvic examination by the health care provider may reveal yellow or green cervical discharge and a reddened or **friable** cervix (a cervix that bleeds easily). On bimanual examination, uterine or cervical tenderness with motion and tender adnexa (tubes and ovaries) are often present. If the client is using an IUD for contraception, the device should be removed at the time of the examination if possible. Ectopic pregnancy and appendicitis must be ruled out as other potential causes of the pain.

PSYCHOSOCIAL ASSESSMENT

The woman who has symptoms of PID is usually anxious and fearful of the examination and unknown diagnosis. She may need much reassurance and support during the physical examination because her abdomen may be very tender and she may wish to avoid further pain. Explain what is taking place to help promote cooperation during the examination.

Because PID is often associated with an STD, the woman may feel embarrassed or uncomfortable discussing her symptoms or history. Use a nonjudgmental approach and encourage the client to express her feelings and concerns. The client's ability to follow through with the treatment plan (taking antibiotics, resting, returning for follow-up evaluation in 48 hours) is essential in deciding whether ambulatory care treatment is appropriate.

LABORATORY ASSESSMENT

The health care provider obtains cultures of the cervix, urethra, and rectum to determine the presence of *N. gonorrhoeae* or *C. trachomatis*. The white blood cell (WBC) count and erythrocyte sedimentation rate (ESR) may be elevated but are not specific for PID. Gram stains of endocervical secretions may show the presence of *N. gonorrhoeae*. A sensitive test that detects human chorionic gonadotropin in urine or blood should be performed to determine whether the client is pregnant. Microscopic examination of vaginal discharge should be done to evaluate for infection. The presence of more than 10 WBCs per high-power field in vaginal discharge correlates with infection. Bacterial vaginosis can be found by observing the diagnostic "clue" cells with microscopic examination of vaginal discharge.

OTHER DIAGNOSTIC ASSESSMENTS

Abdominal ultrasonography may be used to determine the presence of appendicitis and tubo-ovarian abscesses that need to be ruled out when the diagnosis of PID is made. Transvaginal ultrasound and magnetic resonance imaging (MRI) are used in some cases to detect tubal wall thickening, fluid-filled tubes, and free pelvic fluid or a tubo-ovarian abscess, all associated with PID.

Laparoscopy, although expensive, invasive, and requiring anesthesia, is the most definitive test. It provides an immediate, accurate diagnosis through direct inspection of the tubes and ovaries. Endometrial biopsy also has been used to increase the accuracy of the diagnosis.

Because of great variations in client signs and symptoms, the diagnosis of acute PID is difficult because women may have subtle symptoms not typical of PID. Delay in diagnosis and treatment may add to the sequelae of PID in the upper genital tract. Laparoscopy may not be feasible, so that PID is diagnosed on the basis of clinical signs and symptoms (Gaitan, 2002). The Centers for Disease Control and Prevention (CDC) have set minimum criteria for the diagnosis of PID, but there are no laboratory or physical examination techniques that alone are both sensitive and specific for the diagnosis of acute PID. The CDC recommends treatment with antibiotics if all of the minimum criteria have been met and no other causes of illness are found (Table 80-4).

❓ *Critical Thinking Challenge*

The client is a 28-year-old Hispanic woman admitted to your medical-surgical unit for multiple fractures, lacerations, and abrasions sustained in a car accident. She drove the car into a tree after she found out that her boyfriend had been having sex with other women. On her second day after admission, she tells you that she is having a lot of lower abdominal pain and some yellowish vaginal discharge. She is receiving morphine sulfate IV by PCA to manage her pain from her trauma.

1. What specific questions should you ask her about her current and previous health?
2. What risk factors does she have for PID?
3. What additional assessment data should you obtain?
4. How will you approach the topic of the possibility of a sexually transmitted disease or problem?

evolve For suggested answer guidelines, go to http://evolve.elsevier.com/Iggy/.

◆Analysis

COMMON NURSING DIAGNOSES AND COLLABORATIVE PROBLEMS

The primary collaborative problem for clients with pelvic inflammatory disease (PID) is Infection related to invasion

TABLE 80-4 Diagnostic Criteria for Pelvic Inflammatory Disease

Minimum Criteria for Initiating Empiric Treatment for Pelvic Inflammatory Disease
- Uterine/adnexal tenderness *or*
- Cervical motion tenderness (chandelier sign)

Additional Criteria to Increase the Specificity of the Diagnosis of PID
- Oral temperature >101° F (>38.3° C)
- Abnormal cervical or vaginal mucopurulent discharge
- Presence of white blood cells on saline microscopy of vaginal secretions
- Elevated erythrocyte sedimentation rate
- Elevated C-reactive protein
- Laboratory documentation of cervical infection with *Neisseria gonorrhoeae* or *Chlamydia trachomatis*

Definitive Criteria for Diagnosing PID, Warranted in Selected Cases
- Histopathologic evidence of endometritis on endometrial biopsy
- Transvaginal sonography or other imaging techniques showing thickened fluid-filled tubes with or without free pelvic fluid or tubo-ovarian complex
- Laparoscopic abnormalities consistent with PID

Modified from Centers for Disease Control and Prevention. (2002). Sexually transmitted diseases treatment guideline. *Morbidity and Mortality Weekly Report, 51*(No. RR-6), 1-80. *PID*, Pelvic inflammatory disease.

CHART 80-5

NIC **INTERVENTION ACTIVITIES for** The Client with Pelvic Inflammatory Disease

Infection Control: *Minimizing the acquisition and transmission of infectious agents*
- Encourage rest.
- Encourage fluid intake, as appropriate.
- Administer antibiotic therapy, as appropriate. *Or*
- Instruct client to take antibiotics, as prescribed.
- Promote appropriate nutritional intake.
- Teach client and family about signs and symptoms of infection and when to report them to the health care provider.
- Teach client and family members how to avoid infections.

Anxiety Reduction: *Minimizing apprehension, dread, foreboding, or uneasiness related to an unidentified source of anticipated danger*
- Create an atmosphere to facilitate trust.
- Listen attentively.
- Encourage verbalization of feelings, perceptions, and fears.
- Provide factual information concerning diagnosis, treatment, and prognosis.
- Instruct client in use of relaxation techniques.

NIC intervention activities selected from Dochterman, J.M., & Bulechek, G.M. (Eds.). (2004). *Nursing interventions classification (NIC)* (4th ed.). St. Louis: Mosby. No part of this work is to be altered without prior written permission from the Publisher.

of pelvic organs by pathogens. The following are common nursing diagnoses for clients with PID:

1. Acute Pain related to injuring agents (biologic) and the effects of the infectious process
2. Anxiety related to threat to health status and possible infertility as a result of infection

ADDITIONAL NURSING DIAGNOSES AND COLLABORATIVE PROBLEMS

In addition to the common nursing diagnoses and collaborative problems, clients with PID may have one or more of the following:

- Ineffective Health Maintenance related to knowledge deficit about risks, prevention, symptoms, treatment, and effects of PID
- Chronic Pain related to chronic presence of organisms that stimulate recurrent PID episodes
- Sexual Dysfunction related to altered body function from the effects of the infectious process
- Situational Low Self-Esteem/Chronic Low Self-Esteem related to disturbed body image or feeling guilty for having PID (associated with sexual transmission)

◆ Planning and Implementation

INFECTION

NOC **PLANNING: EXPECTED OUTCOMES.** The client with PID is expected to have her infection resolved. Indicators include that the client should have mild or none of the following associated symptoms:

- Pain and tenderness of the pelvis
- Fever
- Discharge (vaginal)
- Culture colonization

INTERVENTIONS. Infection control is accomplished with the use antibiotics, self-care measures, and surgical intervention (rarely) (Chart 80-5).

Infection Control. Uncomplicated PID is usually treated on an ambulatory care basis. The CDC recommends hospitalization for PID if the client:

- Has appendicitis, ectopic pregnancy, or other surgical emergency that has not been excluded
- Is pregnant
- Does not respond to oral antibiotic therapy
- Is unable to follow or tolerate an outpatient regimen
- Has severe illness, nausea and vomiting, or high fever
- Has a tubo-ovarian abscess

There are no recommendations about whether HIV-infected women should be hospitalized. Your assessment of the ability of high-risk women to manage their care at home is an essential part of the plan of care. Their clinical condition and availability of support at home are considerations for care at home. If the infection has not responded to treatment, the client may need to be hospitalized for IV antibiotic therapy and further evaluation.

Drug Therapy. Drug therapy options for PID include oral and parenteral antibiotics (Chart 80-6). Treatment lasts for 14 days. All clients should be re-evaluated 48 to 72 hours after antibiotic therapy is started. If the infection has not responded to treatment, the client is hospitalized for IV antibiotic therapy and further evaluation. Inpatient therapy involves a combination of several IV antibiotics until the client shows signs of improvement (e.g., decreased pelvic tenderness for at least 24 hours). Then oral antibiotics are continued until the course of treatment has lasted 14 days.

Encourage clients treated as outpatients to rest, abstain from sexual intercourse, and check their temperature twice a day. These clients need to be seen by the health care provider 48 to 72 hours from starting the antibiotics and then 1 and 2 weeks from the time of the initial diagnosis.

In a small number of clients, the pain and tenderness may not be relieved by antibiotic therapy. The surgeon may perform a laparotomy to remove an abscess through a subumbilical incision that is several inches long to provide better access

CHART 80-6

DRUG THERAPY for
Acute Pelvic Inflammatory Disease

Drug	Dosage	Nursing Interventions	Rationales
Parenteral Treatment (Inpatient)			
Regimen A Cefotetan (Cefotan)	2 g IV q12h, which can be changed to oral therapy after 24 hr of clinical improvement	Assess the client for rash, itching, and hypotension.	Assessment detects adverse reactions.
Or Cefoxitin (Mefoxin)	2 g IV q6h, which can be changed to oral therapy after 24 hr of clinical improvement	Assess the client for rash, itching, and hypotension. Observe the IV site for signs of redness, heat, and tenderness.	Assessment detects adverse reactions. Phlebitis can be detected.
Plus ¹Doxycycline (Monodox, Doxy-Caps, Doxycin ✽)	100 mg IV or PO q12h for 14 days (PO is preferred because of the pain associated with infusion)	Assess the client for rash, nausea, and diarrhea. Encourage fluid intake. Instruct the client about possible photosensitivity and the need for sun protection. Instruct the client that it is beneficial to take the drug with food.	Assessment detects drug side effects. Fluid intake decreases esophageal irritation. This precaution prevents sunburn by limiting the client's exposure to the sun. Food decreases gastrointestinal upset.
Regimen B Clindamycin (Cleocin)	900 mg IV q8h	Observe the client for rash and urticaria. Observe the client for hypotension, dyspnea, and restlessness. Observe the client for diarrhea. Observe the IV site for redness, heat, and tenderness.	Adverse reactions are detected. Anaphylactic reaction is detected. This precaution avoids pseudomembranous colitis. Phlebitis can be detected.
Plus Gentamicin (Garamycin IV)	2 mg/kg once IV or IM followed by 1.5 mg/kg q8h IV or IM until there have been signs of clinical improvement for 24 hr	Encourage oral intake of fluids. Observe the IV site for redness, heat, and tenderness. Measure fluid intake and output. Observe the client for hearing loss, fever, or decreased renal function. Draw serum for peak and trough levels.	Fluid intake prevents irritation to renal tubules. Phlebitis can be detected. Oliguria or anuria can be detected. Ototoxicity, nephrotoxicity, and fever are known side effects. Serum levels can vary, and drug has low threshold for toxic level.
Then Doxycycline (Monodox, Doxy-Caps, Doxycin ✽)	100 mg PO twice daily to complete a total of 14 days of treatment	See above for doxycycline.	See above for doxycycline.
Or Clindamycin (Cleocin)	450 mg PO four times daily to complete a total of 14 days of treatment	Give with 8 oz of water. See above for clindamycin.	Water decreases esophageal irritation. See above for clindamycin.
Oral Treatment (Outpatient)			
Regimen A Ofloxacin (Floxin)	400 mg PO twice daily for 14 days	Monitor the serum level if the client is taking theophylline. Do not administer this drug to clients younger than 18 yr of age. Administer or instruct the client to take this drug on an empty stomach.	This drug raises the serum level of theophylline. The safety of this drug has not been established in clients younger than 18 yr of age. Food decreases drug absorption.

¹**Med Error Alert!**
Do not confuse with doxepin, an antidepressant.

Modified from Centers for Disease Control and Prevention. (1998). Guidelines for treatment of sexually transmitted disease. *Morbidity and Mortality Weekly Report, 47*(RR-1), 1-103.

Continued

CHART 80-6

DRUG THERAPY for
Acute Pelvic Inflammatory Disease—cont'd

Drug	Dosage	Nursing Interventions	Rationales
Oral Treatment (Outpatient)—cont'd			
Regimen A—cont'd			
Or			
Levofloxacin (Levaquin)	500 mg PO daily for 14 days	Do not give to pregnant women.	This drug disrupts fetal bone growth.
With or without			
Metronidazole (Flagyl, Novonidazol ✲)	500 mg PO twice daily for 14 days	Monitor the serum level if the client is taking lithium. Avoid alcohol within 24 hr of use.	This drug raises the serum level of lithium. Alcohol causes disulfiram-like effect.
Regimen B			
Ceftriaxone (Rocephin)	250 mg IM one time only	Give deep IM injection in the outer upper quadrant of the gluteus maximus. Watch for fever, chills, and nausea. Tell the client that the injection may be painful.	Local irritation is avoided, and drug absorption is increased. Allergic reactions can be detected. The client is prepared for discomfort related to the inflammatory reaction.
Or			
Cefoxitin (Mefoxin)	2 g IM one time only	Give deep IM injection in the outer upper quadrant of the gluteus maximus. Watch for fever, chills, and nausea. Tell the client that the injection may be painful.	Local irritation is avoided, and drug absorption is increased. Allergic reactions can be detected. The client is prepared for discomfort related to the inflammatory reaction.
Plus			
²Probenecid (Benemid, Benuryl ✲)	1 g PO one time only concurrently	Give with food. Encourage fluid intake (10 glasses per day).	Taking the medication with food avoids gastrointestinal upset. Fluid intake prevents formation of kidney stones.
Or			
Other parenteral third-generation cephalosporin (e.g., ceftizoxime or cefotaxime)			
Plus			
Doxycycline (for all of the above regimens)	100 mg PO twice daily for 14 days	See previous page for doxycycline.	See previous page for doxycycline.

²Med Error Alert!
Do not confuse with Procanbid, a drug used for cardiac dysrhythmias.

Modified from Centers for Disease Control and Prevention. (1998). Guidelines for treatment of sexually transmitted disease. *Morbidity and Mortality Weekly Report, 47*(RR-1), 1-103.

to the fallopian tubes. Before surgery, provide information about hospital routines and procedures. General preoperative care is described in Chapter 20. After surgery, the care of the woman with PID is similar to that of any client after abdominal surgery. One difference is that the client with PID may have a wound drain in place for drainage of abscess fluid that may not have been completely removed during surgery. Observe, measure, and record wound drainage every 4 to 8 hours as ordered.

ACUTE PAIN

NOC **PLANNING: EXPECTED OUTCOMES.** The client with PID is expected to have reduced pain and increased com-fort. Indicators include that the client should rarely demon-strate the following behaviors:

- Reports of pain
- Moaning and crying
- Facial expressions of pain
- Loss of appetite

INTERVENTIONS. Pain management of PID begins with treatment of the infection. Antibiotic treatment relieves pain by decreasing the inflammation caused by infection. If the client is ill enough to be hospitalized, parenteral antibiotics are usually given. See the earlier section on drug therapy for PID.

Other pain relief measures include taking analgesics, us-ing sitz baths, and applying heat to the lower abdomen or back. Bedrest in a semi-Fowler's position promotes gravity drainage and consolidation of the infection that may relieve pain.

ANXIETY

NOC **PLANNING: EXPECTED OUTCOMES.** The client with PID is expected to take actions to reduce anxiety about infertility. Indicators include that the client should often or consistently demonstrate the following behaviors:

- Use of effective coping patterns strategies
- Controlled anxiety response
- Use of available social support
- Seeking of professional help, as appropriate

INTERVENTIONS. Infertility is the most common complication of PID and affects at least 15% to 25% of women who have had one or more episodes of PID. Nursing interventions are aimed at understanding the client's perspective of the diagnosis and future complications.

If the client has anxiety, provide an atmosphere in which she feels comfortable expressing her feelings and asking questions. Give accurate information about the diagnosis, treatment, and prognosis. Providing information about the advantages of early diagnosis and treatment (which limit damage to one area of the pelvis) and the advances in treatments for infertility may reassure the client. Help the client assess the emotional support available from family members or significant others. Relaxation techniques may be useful to decrease the anxiety (see Chart 80-5).

Community-Based Care

The client with pelvic inflammatory disease (PID) needs to have regular follow-up with her health care provider to assess for complications and ensure that the infection has resolved. The ongoing role of the nurse is to assess for any continued risk for contracting PID again, signs of persistent or recurrent infection, and education to prevent exposure to and infection with all STDs (e.g., decrease the number of partners, consistent condom use). Establish an atmosphere of trust that encourages the client to return frequently, if needed, for education or reassurance.

HOME CARE MANAGEMENT

Parenteral antibiotic therapy may be given at home, but usually the health care provider changes the treatment regimen to oral antibiotics before hospital discharge (see Planning and Implementation, p. 1898).

HEALTH TEACHING

Client teaching focuses on providing information about PID, identifying recurrences (persistent pain, dysmenorrhea, low backache, fever), and urging early treatment to prevent complications. Review information for oral antibiotic therapy (Chart 80-7).

Counsel the client to contact her sexual partner(s) for examination and treatment. The partner is usually treated for gonorrhea and chlamydial infection. Remind the client about follow-up care and counsel her about the complications that can occur after an episode of PID, including increased risk for recurrence of PID, increased risk for ectopic pregnancy, increased risk for infertility, and chronic pelvic pain.

CHART 80-7

CLIENT EDUCATION GUIDE
Oral Antibiotic Therapy for Sexually Transmitted Diseases

- Take your medicine for the number of times a day it is prescribed and until it is completed.
- Your sexual partner must be tested and may need to be treated.
- Be sure to return for your follow-up appointment after completing your antibiotic treatment.
- Call if you have any questions or concerns.
- Do not have sex until after you complete your antibiotic therapy. If your partner is being treated, you can go back to having sex together 48 hours after he or she starts taking antibiotics if you use a condom.
- Drink at least 8 to 10 glasses of fluid a day while taking your antibiotics.
- Do not take antacids containing calcium, magnesium, or aluminum, such as Tums, Maalox, or Mylanta, with your antibiotics. They may decrease the effectiveness of the antibiotic.
- Take your antibiotics on an empty stomach unless your health care provider instructs you to take them with food.

Discuss contraception and the client's need or desire for it. This discussion includes methods that may decrease the risk for future episodes of PID, such as the use of barrier methods. Help the client understand lifestyle factors that heighten the risk for recurrent episodes of PID, including sexual intercourse with multiple partners and vaginal douching.

Psychosocial concerns may require teaching and counseling. A client who has PID may exhibit a variety of feelings (guilt, disgust, anger) about having a condition that may have been transmitted to her sexually. These feelings may affect her relationship with significant others and future sexual relationships. She may also have concerns about future fertility if PID has caused damage or scarring of the fallopian tubes and other reproductive organs. Provide nonjudgmental emotional support and allow time for the client to express her feelings.

HEALTH CARE RESOURCES

If infertility is a result of PID, the client may need referral to a clinic specializing in infertility treatment and counseling. The client can also contact support groups for infertile couples, which exist in many local communities.

The costs of antibiotics for care of clients with PID and other STDs may be a concern for those who are uninsured or underinsured. The case manager, social worker, or ambulatory care nurse seeks community resources for free or discounted medications for clients with financial limitations.

◆ Evaluation: Outcomes

Evaluate the care of the client with PID on the basis of the identified nursing diagnoses and collaborative problems. The expected outcomes include that the client should:

- Show evidence that the infection has resolved
- Report or demonstrate that pain is relieved or reduced and that she feels more comfortable
- Take action to manage anxiety about future infertility

Specific indicators for these outcomes are listed for each nursing diagnosis and collaborative problem under the Planning and Implementation section (see earlier).

SEXUALLY TRANSMITTED VAGINAL INFECTIONS

Vaginal infection associated with sexual activity may produce vaginal discharge or vulvar irritation. The following are common causes of vaginal infection:

- *Trichomonas vaginalis*
- *Candida*, primarily *C. albicans*
- Bacteria that produce bacterial vaginosis, including *Gardnerella vaginalis* and anaerobes

These infections can be spread by sexual contact. Men can also acquire these infections but are not always symptomatic. Several studies have shown that *T. vaginalis* is common in men, especially those who have other STDs, such as *Chlamydia trachomatis* (Bachmann et al., 2000; Joyner et al., 2000). However, because most of these infections are seen more commonly in women, assessments and interventions are discussed with other causes of vaginitis in Chapter 78.

Trichomoniasis and candida infections are limited to the vagina. They can be very irritating and bothersome but do not cause any long-term sequelae. The partner must also be treated for trichomoniasis if the infection is to be resolved. Candidiasis does not usually require partner treatment, but if the male partner is symptomatic (irritation of the genital skin), then treatment is indicated. It is important to remember that candida is a normal flora on the skin and can easily be translocated to the vagina. Although it can be transmitted sexually, candidiasis occurs among women who are not sexually active. Additionally, antibiotics that change the normal flora of the vagina (especially tetracyclines) contribute to candidiasis.

Bacterial vaginosis (BV) has been implicated in upper genital tract infections. Women undergoing surgery of the upper genital tract should be evaluated and treated if BV is found. There also is evidence that BV in pregnancy can lead to preterm labor and premature delivery. These findings are controversial, but evaluation for BV during pregnancy has been suggested (Carey et al., 2000; Hay, Ugwumadu, & Manvonda, 2001).

HEPATITIS A, B, AND C

In the United States, 12% to 26% of new cases of hepatitis A are reported to be acquired through household or sexual contact. Up to 55% of the new cases of hepatitis B (HBV) are transmitted sexually. Sexual transmission of hepatitis C (HCV) is inefficient, although about 5% of new cases is thought to be transmitted this way. Of those infected as adults, 2% to 6% of those with HBV and 75% to 85% of those with HCV develop chronic hepatitis, which can lead to cirrhosis and primary liver cancer. An estimated 0.5% of the total U.S. population have chronic HBV and 1.3% have chronic HCV (National Institutes of Health, 2002; Weinbaum, Lyerla, & Margolis, 2003). Hepatitis is discussed further in Chapter 62.

Prevention of sexually transmitted diseases (STDs) should include educating clients about the risks of contracting hepatitis A, B, and C. Currently, vaccines against HAV and HBV are available. Use of these vaccines have the potential to limit the spread of these diseases by sexual transmission. The CDC recommends that anyone who is treated for STDs, men who have sex with men, and injection drug users should be offered hepatitis vaccination (CDC, 2002a).

▌▌▌GET READY for the NCLEX Examination!

KEY POINTS

Safe Effective Care Environment

- Use standard precautions for all clients regardless of age, gender, race or ethnicity, sexual orientation, education level, and profession.
- Ask all women about intimate partner abuse at any health visit.
- Use gloves when examining the genitalia of any client.

Health Promotion and Maintenance

- Encourage all clients who are sexually active to use condoms and other precautions during sexual intimacy.
- Urge sexually active women to go for routine health maintenance visits and screenings.

Psychosocial Integrity

- Treat all clients, regardless of diagnosis, with dignity.
- Do not assume that any visitor or family member knows the client's diagnosis.
- Pace your interview to match the learning needs and style of the individual client.
- Provide as much privacy as possible for clients undergoing examination or testing for STDs.
- Use language and terminology that the client can understand and that the client is comfortable with during discussions of the reproductive system.
- Allow the client the opportunity to express fear or anxiety regarding a change in health status.
- Refer clients newly diagnosed with an STD to local resources and support groups.
- Encourage all clients who have an STD to inform their sexual partner(s) of their health status.

Physiological Integrity

- Encourage clients to adhere to their anti-infective drug regimen.
- Teach clients the expected side effects and possible adverse reactions to prescribed drugs.
- Urge clients to refrain from sexual activity while being treated for an STD.
- Teach female clients who have PID the clinical manifestations of ectopic pregnancy.

ADDITIONAL STUDY RESOURCES

Go to your Student CD-ROM for Review Questions for the NCLEX Examination.

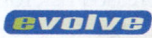 Go to http://evolve.elsevier.com/Iggy/ for Integrated Management of Care Questions for the NCLEX Examination.

SELECTED BIBLIOGRAPHY

Asterisk indicates a classic or definitive work on this subject.

Akande, V. (2002). Tubal pelvic damage: Prediction and prognosis. *Human Fertility, 5*(Suppl.), S15-S20.

Apoola, A., & Radcliffe, K. (2004). Antiviral treatment of genital herpes. *International Journal of SDT & AIDS, 15*(7), 429-433.

Bachmann, L.H., et al. (2000). Risk and prevalence of treatable sexually transmitted diseases at a Birmingham substance abuse treatment facility. *American Journal of Public Health, 90*(10), 1615-1618.

Ballard, R., & Morse, S. (2003). Chancroid. In S.A. Morse, et al. (Eds.). *Atlas of sexually transmitted diseases and AIDS* (3rd ed.). Edinburgh: Mosby.

Bartlett, J. (2002). *2002 Pocket book of infectious disease therapy.* Philadelphia: Lippincott Williams & Wilkins.

Blake, D., et al. (2003). Improving participation in chlamydia screening programs. *Archives of Adolescent Medicine, 157,* 523-529.

Bowden, F. (2003). Donovanosis. In S.A. Morse, et al. (Eds.). *Atlas of sexually transmitted diseases and AIDS* (3rd ed.). Edinburgh: Mosby.

Carey, J., et al. (2000). Metronidazole to prevent preterm delivery in pregnant women with asymptomatic bacterial vaginosis. *New England Journal of Medicine, 342,* 534-540.

Carpenito-Loyet, L. (2004). *Nursing diagnoses: Application to clinical practice* (10th ed.). Philadelphia: Lippincott Williams & Wilkins.

Centers for Disease Control and Prevention. (2001). Tracking the hidden epidemics: Trends in STDs in the United States 2000. Available at www.cdc.gov/nchstp/dstd/Stats_Trends/Trends2000.pdf.

Centers for Disease Control and Prevention. (2002a). Sexually transmitted diseases treatment guidelines 2002. *Morbidity and Mortality Weekly Report, 51*(RR-6), 1-80.

Centers for Disease Control and Prevention. (2002b). Increases in fluoroquinolone-resistant *Neisseria gonorrhoeae*–Hawaii and California, 2001. *Morbidity and Mortality Weekly Report, 51,* 1041-1044.

Centers for Disease Control and Prevention. (2002c). Notice to readers: Discontinuation of cefixime tablets–United States. *Morbidity and Mortality Weekly Report, 51*(46), 1052.

Centers for Disease Control and Prevention. (2004). Sexually transmitted disease surveillance, 2003. Atlanta, GA: U.S. Department of Health and Human Services, November 2004. Available at http://www.cdc.gov/std/stats/toc2003.htm.

Champion, J., et al. (2004). Abused women and the risk for pelvic inflammatory disease. *Western Journal of Nursing Research, 26*(2), 176-191.

Cothran, M., & White, J. (2002). Adolescent behavior and sexually transmitted diseases: The dilemma of human papillomavirus. *Health Care for Women International, 23,* 306-319.

Davidson, M. (2004). Sexually transmitted infections: Screening and counseling. *Clinician Reviews, 14*(6), 55-62.

Dochterman, J., & Bulechek, G. (Eds.). (2004). *Nursing interventions classification (NIC)* (4th ed.). St. Louis: Mosby.

Dulin, J., & Akers, M.C. (2003). Pelvic inflammatory disease and sepsis. *Critical Care Nursing Clinics of North America, 15*(1), 63-70.

Ebersole, P., Hess, P., & Luggen, A. (2004). *Toward healthy aging: Human needs and nursing response* (6th ed.). St. Louis: Mosby

Facts and Comparisons. (2004). *Drug facts and comparisons* (58th ed.). St. Louis: Author.

Feroli, K., & Burstein, G. (2003). Adolescent sexually transmitted diseases. *Maternal Child Nursing, 28*(2), 113-118.

Gaitan, H., et al. (2002). Accuracy of five different diagnostic techniques in mild-to-moderate pelvic inflammatory disease. *Infectious Diseases in Obstetrics and Gynecology, 10,* 171-180.

*Hauth, J., et al. (1995). Reduced incidence of preterm delivery with metronidazole and erythromycin in women with bacterial vaginosis. *New England Journal of Medicine, 333,* 1732-1736.

Hay, P., Ugwumadu, A., & Manvonda, J. (2001). Oral clindamycin prevents spontaneous preterm birth and mid trimester miscarriage in pregnant women with bacterial vaginosis. *International Journal of Sexually Transmitted Diseases and AIDS, 12*(Suppl 2), 70-71.

*Hiller, S., et al. (1995). Association between bacterial vaginosis and preterm delivery of a low birth-weight infant. *New England Journal of Medicine, 333*(26), 1737-1742.

Honey, E., et al. (2002). Cost effectiveness of screening for *Chlamydia trachomatis*: A review of published studies. *Sexually Transmitted Infections, 78,* 406-412.

Joyner, J.L., et al. (2000). Comparative prevalence of infection with *Trichomonas vaginalis* among men attending a sexually transmitted disease clinic. *Sexually Transmitted Diseases, 27*(4), 236-240.

Lewis, J. (2003). Selection and evaluation of diagnostic tests. In S.A. Morse, et al. (Eds.). *Atlas of sexually transmitted diseases and AIDS* (3rd ed.). Edinburgh: Mosby.

Mabey, D., & Peeling, R. (2002). Lymphogranuloma venereum. *Sexually Transmitted Infections, 78,* 90-92.

Maw, R. (2004) Critical appraisal of commonly used treatment for genital warts. *International Journal of STD & AIDS, 15*(6), 357-364.

McQuillan, G. (2000). Implications of a national survey for STDs: Results from NHANES Survey. Presentation at 2000 Infectious Disease Society of America Conference. September 7-10, 2000, New Orleans.

Mehta, S., et al. (2003). Generalizability of STD screening in urban emergency departments: Comparison of results from inner city and urban sites in Baltimore, Maryland. *Sexually Transmitted Diseases, 30*(2), 143-148.

Moens, V., Baruch, G., & Fearon, P. (2003). Opportunistic screening for chlamydia at a community-based contraceptive service for young people. *British Medical Journal, 326,* 1252-1255.

Morse, S.A., et al. (2003). *Atlas of sexually transmitted diseases and AIDS* (3rd ed.). Edinburgh: Mosby.

National Institutes of Health (2002). Management of hepatitis C: 2002, Consensus Development Conference Statement, June 10-12, 2002. Available at http://consensus.nih.gov/cons/116/hepatitis_c_consensus.pdf.

Nsuami, M., et al. (2003). Screening for sexually transmitted diseases during sports examination of high school adolescents. *Journal of Adolescent Health, 32,* 336-339.

Pagana, K., & Pagana, T. (2002). *Mosby's manual of diagnostic and laboratory tests* (2nd ed.). St. Louis: Mosby.

Rein, D., et al. (2000). Direct medical cost of pelvic inflammatory disease and its sequelae: Decreasing but still substantial. *Obstetrics and Gynecology, 95*(3), 397-402.

Rein, M. (2001). Sexually transmitted disease. In G. Mandell. *Essential atlas of infectious diseases* (2nd ed., pp. 153-174). Philadelphia: Current Medicine.

Robinson, K. (2002). Sexually transmitted diseases. In K. McCance & S. Huether (Eds.), *Pathophysiology: The biologic basis for disease in adults and children* (4th ed., pp. 781-811). St. Louis: Mosby.

Roddy, R., et al. (2002). Effect of nonoxynol-9 gel on urogenital gonorrhea and chlamydia infections. *Journal of the American Medical Association, 287*(9), 1117-1122.

Schacter, J., & Stephens, R. (2003). Infections caused by *Chlamydia trachomatis*. In S.A. Morse, et al. (Eds.). *Atlas of sexually transmitted diseases and AIDS* (3rd ed.). Edinburgh: Mosby.

Scharbo-Dehaan, M., & Anderson, D. (2003). The CDC 2002 guidelines for the treatment of sexually transmitted diseases: Implications for women's health care. *Journal of Midwifery and Women's Health, 48*(2), 96-104.

Schillinger, J., et al. (2003). Patient-delivered partner treatment with azithromycin to prevent repeated *Chlamydia trachomatis* infection among women: A randomized, controlled trial. *Sexually Transmitted Diseases, 30*(1), 49-56.

Sellors, J.W., et al. (2000). A new visual indicator of chlamydial cervicitis? *Sexually Transmitted Infections, 76*(1), 46-48.

Skidmore-Roth, L. (2003). *Mosby's nursing drug reference.* St. Louis: Mosby.

Tao, G., et al. (2000). Medical care expenditures for genital herpes in the United States. *Sexually Transmitted Diseases, 27*(1), 32-38.

Turner, C., et al. (2002). Untreated gonococcal and chlamydial infections in a probability sample of adults. *Journal of the American Medical Association, 287*(6), 726-733.

Weinbaum, C., Lyerla, R., & Margolis, H. (2003). Prevention and control of infections with hepatitis viruses in correctional settings. *Morbidity and Mortality Weekly Report, 52*(RR-1), 1-33.

Williams, A. (2003). Gynecologic care for women with HIV infections. *Journal of Obstetric, Gynecologic, and Neonatal Nursing, 32*, 87-93.

Workman, M.L. (2003). The cellular basis of bacterial infection. *Critical Care Clinics of North America, 15*(1), 1-11.

APPENDIX

Abbreviations

AAA   abdominal aortic aneurysm
AACN   American Association of Critical Care Nurses
AAKP   American Association of Kidney Patients
ABC   airway, breathing, and circulation
ABG   arterial blood gas
ABI   ankle-brachial index
ABPM   ambulatory blood pressure monitoring
ABVD   Adriamycin, bleomycin, vinblastine, dacarbazine
AC   assist-control; alternating current
ACE   angiotensin-converting enzyme
ACh   acetylcholine
AChRAb   acetylcholine receptor antibody
ACL   anterior cruciate ligament
ACLS   advanced cardiac life support
ACS   acute compartment syndrome; American Cancer Society
ACTH   adrenocorticotropic hormone
AD   autosomal dominant
ADC   AIDS dementia complex
ADH   antidiuretic hormone
ADLs   activities of daily living
ADP   adenosine diphosphate
ADPKD   autosomal dominant polycystic kidney disease
AED   automatic external defibrillation
aFP   alpha-fetoprotein
AGC   absolute granulocyte count
AGN   acute glomerulonephritis
AGR   abdominal-gluteal ratio
AHA   American Heart Association
AHRQ   Agency for Healthcare Research and Quality
AIDS   acquired immunodeficiency syndrome
AIVR   accelerated idioventricular rhythm
AJCC   American Joint Committee on Cancer
AKA   above-knee amputation
AL   ascending limb
ALA   American Lung Association
ALG   antilymphocyte globulin
ALL   acute lymphocytic leukemia
ALP   alkaline phosphatase
ALS   amyotrophic lateral sclerosis
AMI   antibody-mediated immunity
AML   acute myelocytic leukemia
AMSN   Academy of Medical-Surgical Nurses
ANA   American Nurses' Association; antinuclear antibody
ANC   absolute neutrophil count
ANOVA   analysis of variance
ANP   atrial natriuretic peptide
ANS   autonomic nervous system
AORN   Association of periOperative Room Nurses
AP   anteroposterior

APSAC   anisoylated plasminogen streptokinase activator complex
APSGN   acute poststreptococcal glomerulonephritis
aPTT   activated partial thromboplastin time
AR   autosomal recessive
ara-A   adenine arabinoside
ARDS   acute respiratory distress syndrome
ARF   acute renal failure
ASA   acetylsalicylic acid
ASPEN   American Society of Parenteral and Enteral Nutrition
AST   aspartate aminotransferase
ATG   antithymocyte globulin
ATN   acute tubular necrosis
ATP   adenosine triphosphate
ATPase   adenosine triphosphatase
AV   atrioventricular, arteriovenous
AVM   arteriovenous malformation
AVN   avascular necrosis
AZA   azathioprine
BBIAT   Baird Body Image Assessment Tool
BC   Bowman's capsule
BCG   bacille Calmette-Guérin
BCNU   carmustine
BCS   Body Cathexis Scale
BE   barium enema
BGMS   blood glucose monitoring strip
BKA   below-knee amputation
BMI   body mass index
BMT   bone marrow transplantation
BP   blood pressure
BPEG   British Pacing and Electrophysiology Group
BPH   benign prostatic hyperplasia (hypertrophy)
BRM   biologic response modifier
BSE   breast self-examination
BSI   body substance isolation
BSO   bilateral salpingo-oophorectomy
BUN   blood urea nitrogen
c   cup(s)
C&S   culture and sensitivity
CABG   coronary artery bypass graft
CAD   computer-assisted design; coronary artery disease
CAH   chronic active hepatitis
CAL   chronic airflow limitation
CALLA   common acute lymphoblastic leukemia antigen
CAM   complementary and alternative medicine
cAMP   cyclic adenosine monophosphate
CAPD   continuous ambulatory peritoneal dialysis
CAVH   continuous arteriovenous hemofiltration
CAVHD   continuous arteriovenous hemofiltration and dialysis

CBC	complete blood count	CVP	central venous pressure
CBD	common bile duct	D&C	dilation and curettage
CBE	charting by exception	DARE	Drug Awareness Resistance Education
CBI	continuous bladder irrigation	dB	decibel(s)
CCA	circumflex coronary artery	DCCT	Diabetes Control and Complications Trial
CCP	critical closing pressure	DCM	dilated cardiomyopathy
CCPD	continuous-cycle peritoneal dialysis	DCT	distal convoluted tubule
CD	Cotrel-Dubousset; collecting duct	DDAVP	desmopressin acetate
CD4	cluster of differentiation 4	ddI	dideoxyinosine (didanosine)
CDC	Centers for Disease Control and Prevention; chenodeoxycholic acid	DDS	dapsone
		DES	diethylstilbestrol
CEA	carcinoembryonic antigen	DHE	dihydroergotamine
CFU	colony-forming unit	DHHS	U.S. Department of Health and Human Services
CGN	chronic glomerulonephritis		
CHF	congestive heart failure	DHT	dihydrotestosterone
CIC	Certified in Infection Control	DI	diabetes insipidus
CIN	cervical intraepithelial neoplasia	DIC	disseminated intravascular coagulation
CIS	carcinoma in situ	DIP	distal interphalangeal joint
CK	creatine kinase	DJD	degenerative joint disease
CLE	centrilobular emphysema	dL	deciliter(s)
CLL	chronic lymphocytic leukemia	DL	descending limb
cm	centimeter(s)	D_LCO	diffusion capacity for carbon monoxide
CMG	cystometrogram	DLE	discoid lupus erythematosus
CMI	cell-mediated immunity	DNA	deoxyribonucleic acid
CML	chronic myelocytic leukemia	DNP	dinitrophenol
CMS	circulation, movement, sensation	DNR	do not resuscitate
CMV	cisplatin, methotrexate, vinblastine; cytomegalovirus	DOE	dyspnea on exertion
		DP	dopamine
CNS	central nervous system	DPOA	durable power of attorney
CO	cardiac output	DRE	digital rectal examination
COHb	carboxyhemoglobin	DRG	diagnosis-related group
COLD	chronic obstructive lung disease	DS	double-strength
COPD	chronic obstructive pulmonary disease	DSA	digital subtraction angiography
COPES	Family Crisis-Oriented Personal Evaluation Scale	DTIC	dacarbazine
		DTR	deep tendon reflex
CPAP	continuous positive airway pressure	DUB	dysfunctional uterine bleeding
CPB	cardiopulmonary bypass	DVT	deep vein thrombosis
CPK	creatine phosphokinase	EAT	Eating Attitudes Test
CPM	continuous passive motion	EBL	estimated blood loss
CPN	chronic pyelonephritis	EBV	Epstein-Barr virus
CPO	certified prosthetist-orthotist	ECCC	Emergency Cardiac Care Committee
CPP	cerebral perfusion pressure	ECCE	extracapsular cataract extraction
CPR	cardiopulmonary resuscitation	ECF	extracellular fluid
cps	cycles per second	ECG	electrocardiogram
CQI	continuous quality improvement	EDI	Eating Disorder Inventory
CREST	calcinosis, Raynaud's phenomenon, esophageal dysfunction, sclerodactyly, telangiectasia	EGD	esophagogastroduodenoscopy
		EHDP	etidronate disodium
		EIA	enzyme immunoassay
CRF	chronic renal failure	ELISA	enzyme-linked immunosorbent assay
CRH	corticotropin-releasing hormone	EMD	electromechanical dissociation
CRI	chronic renal insufficiency	EMG	electromyography
CRNA	certified registered nurse anesthetist	EMS	emergency medical services
CS	crush syndrome	EMT	emergency medical technician
CSA	cyclosporine A	ENCORE	encouragement, normalcy, counseling, opportunity, reaching out, revived energies
CSF	cerebrospinal fluid		
CST	certified surgical technologist	ENG	electronystagmography
CT	computed tomography	ENT	ear, nose, and throat
CTD	connective tissue disease	EOM	extraocular movement
CTS	carpal tunnel syndrome	EPO	erythropoietin
CVA	cerebrovascular accident (stroke); costovertebral angle	EPS	electrophysiologic study
		ER	estrogen receptor
CVC	central venous catheter	ERCP	endoscopic retrograde cholangiopancreatography

ERS	endoscopic retrograde sphincterotomy	Gy	gray(s)
ERT	estrogen replacement therapy	h	hour(s)
ESR	erythrocyte sedimentation rate	HAT	hearing assessment test
ESRD	end-stage renal disease	Hb	hemoglobin
ET	enterostomal therapist; endotracheal tube	HBIG	hepatitis B immunoglobulin
ETDR	early treatment diabetic retinopathy	HBO	hyperbaric oxygen
ETT	exercise tolerance test	HBV	hepatitis B virus
EVS	early vitrectomy study	hCG	human chorionic gonadotropin
FACT	fruits, animals, colors, and towns	HCM	hypertrophic cardiomyopathy
FAM	fluorouracil, Adriamycin, and mitomycin C	Hct	hematocrit
FANA	fluorescent antinuclear antibody	HCV	hepatitis C virus
FAST	fluoroallergosorbent test	HD	hemodialysis
FBD	fibrocystic breast disease	HDL	high-density lipoprotein
FBSS	failed back surgery syndrome	HDV	hepatitis delta virus
FDA	U.S. Food and Drug Administration	HEPA	high-efficiency particulate air
FEF	forced expiratory flow	HEV	hepatitis E virus
FES	fat embolism syndrome	Hgb	hemoglobin
FEV	forced expiratory volume	HIDA	hepatobiliary iminodiacetic acid analogue
FEV_1	forced expiratory volume in 1 second		(radionuclide labeled with technetium-99m)
FEV_1/FVC	ratio of expiratory volume in 1 second to	HIP	Help for Incontinent Persons
	forced vital capacity	HITT	heparin-induced thrombocytopenia/
FFP	fresh frozen plasma		thrombosis
FIM	Functional Independence Measure	HLA	human leukocyte antigen
FiO_2	fraction of inspired oxygen	HMO	health maintenance organization
FNB	Food and Nutrition Board	HPA	hypothalamic-pituitary-adrenal
FNCR	family nursing chart review	HPV	human papillomavirus
FOBT	fecal occult blood test	hr	hour
FR	flutter rate	HR	heart rate
Fr	French	HSV	herpes simplex virus
FRC	functional residual capacity	5-HT	5-hydroxytryptamine (serotonin)
FS	full-strength	HTLV	human T-cell lymphotropic virus
FSBS	fingerstick blood sugar	Hz	hertz
FSH	follicle-stimulating hormone	I&D	incision and drainage
Ft	foot (feet)	IABP	intra-aortic balloon pumping
FTA-ABS	fluorescent treponemal antibody absorption	IBS	irritable bowel syndrome
	test	IBW	ideal body weight
5-FU	5-fluorouracil	ICD	implantable cardioverter-defibrillator
FUDR	floxuridine	ICF	intracellular fluid
FVC	forced vital capacity	ICHD	Intersociety Commission for Heart Disease
FWB	full weight-bearing	ICP	intracranial pressure
g	gram(s)	ICS	intercostal space
g/day	gram(s) per day	ICU	intensive care unit
G6PD	glucose-6-phosphate dehydrogenase	IEC	Institutional Ethics Committee
GABA	gamma-aminobutyric acid	IF	interstitial fluid
GAS	general adaptation syndrome	Ig	immunoglobulin
GB	gallbladder	IHSS	idiopathic hypertrophic subaortic stenosis
GBS	Guillain-Barré syndrome	IL	interleukin
GCS	Glasgow Coma Scale	IL-2	interleukin-2
GCSF	granulocyte colony-stimulating factor	IL-3	interleukin-3
GDM	gestational diabetes mellitus	IL-4	interleukin-4
GE	gastroenteritis	IL-5	interleukin-5
GF	glomerular filtrate	IL-8	interleukin-8
GFR	glomerular filtration rate	IM	intramedullary rod; intramuscular
GH	growth hormone	IMF	intermaxillary fixation
GH-IH	growth hormone–inhibiting hormone	IMV	intermittent mandatory ventilation
GH-RH	growth hormone–releasing hormone	INF	interferon
GI	gastrointestinal	INR	international normalized ratio
GM-CSF	granulocyte-macrophage colony-stimulating	IOL	intraocular lens
	factor	IOP	intraocular pressure
Gn-RH	gonadotropin-releasing hormone	IP	intraperitoneal
GSW	gunshot wound	IPD	intermittent peritoneal dialysis
GVHD	graft-versus-host disease	IPG	impedance plethysmography

IRT	intracavitary radiation therapy	MCH	mean corpuscular hemoglobin
IS	incentive spirometer	MCHC	mean corpuscular hemoglobin concentration
ITH	idiosyncratic toxic hepatitis	MCL	modified chest lead
ITP	idiopathic thrombocytopenic purpura	MCP	metacarpophalangeal
IU	international unit(s)	MCV	mean corpuscular volume
IU/L	international unit(s) per liter	MD	muscular dystrophy
IUD	intrauterine device	MDF	myocardial depressant factor
IV	intravenous	MDI	metered-dose inhaler
IVC	inferior vena cava	MEN	multiple endocrine neoplasia
IVP	intravenous pyelography	mEq	milliequivalent(s)
JCAHO	Joint Commission on the Accreditation of Healthcare Organizations	mEq/L	milliequivalent(s) per liter
		MFH	malignant fibrous histiocytoma
JGC	juxtaglomerular cell	mg	milligram(s)
JVD	jugular venous distention	MG	myasthenia gravis
JVP	jugular venous pressure	mg/dL	milligram(s) per deciliter
KCS	keratoconjunctivitis sicca	MH	malignant hyperthermia
kg	kilogram(s)	MHAUS	Malignant Hyperthermia Association of the United States
kJ	kilojoule(s)		
KS	Kaposi's sarcoma	MHC	major histocompatibility complex
KUB	kidneys, ureters, and bladder	MI	myocardial infarction
KW	Keith-Wagner classification	MICU	medical intensive care unit
LAC	long arm cast	MIH	melanocyte-inhibiting hormone
LAD	left anterior descending	min	minute(s)
LAK	lymphokine-activated killer (cell)	mL	milliliter(s)
LAP	leukocyte alkaline phosphatase	mL/kg	milliliter(s) per kilogram
LAS	localized adaptation syndrome	mm	millimeter(s)
LATS	long-acting thyroid stimulator	mm Hg	millimeter(s) of mercury
LBP	low back pain	mmol	millimole(s)
LCA	left coronary artery	mmol/L	millimoles per liter
LDH	lactate dehydrogenase	MMPI	Minnesota Multiphasic Personality Inventory
LDL	low-density lipoprotein	MMSE	Mini-Mental State Examination
LE	lupus erythematosus; lower extremity	MMV	maximum mandatory ventilation
LES	lower esophageal sphincter	MODY	maturity-onset diabetes of the young
LGV	lymphogranuloma venereum	MOPP	mechlorethamine, Oncovin, procarbazine, prednisone
LH	luteinizing hormone		
LL	left lateral	mOsm	milliosmole(s)
LLC	long leg cast	mOsm/L	milliosmole(s) per liter
LLQ	left lower quadrant	MRB	manual resuscitation bag
LMN	lower motor neuron	MRC	Medical Research Council
LOA	leave of absence	MRI	magnetic resonance imaging
LOC	level of consciousness	MS	multiple sclerosis; morphine sulfate
LORS	Level of Rehabilitation Scale	msec	millisecond(s)
LP	lumbar puncture; light perception	MSH	melanocyte-stimulating hormone
LPS	lipopolysaccharide	MTP	metatarsophalangeal
LR	lactated Ringer's (solution)	mU	milliunit(s)
LRD	living related donor	mU/mL	milliunit(s) per milliliter
LTC	long-term care	MUGA	multigated angiography
LUQ	left upper quadrant	mV	millivolt(s)
LVD	left ventricular dysfunction	MVA	motor vehicle accident
LVEDP	left ventricular end-diastolic pressure	MVAC	methotrexate, vinblastine, Adriamycin, cisplatin
M-CSF	monocyte-macrophage colony-stimulating factor		
		NANDA	North American Nursing Diagnosis Association
mA	milliampere(s)		
MAC	*Mycobacterium avium* complex	NAON	National Association of Orthopaedic Nurses
MAO	monoamine oxidase	NAPHT	National Association of Patients on Hemodialysis and Transplantation
MAP	mean arterial pressure		
MAST	military antishock trousers	NASPE	North American Society for Pacing and Electrophysiology
MAT	multifocal atrial tachycardia		
MB-CAPD	multiple-bag continuous ambulatory peritoneal dialysis	NCI	National Cancer Institute
		NE	norepinephrine
MCA	middle cerebral artery	ng	nanogram(s)
mcg	microgram(s)	NG	nasogastric

NHANES	National Health and Nutrition Examination Survey	pH	the negative logarithm of the hydrogen ion concentration
NHIF	National Head Injury Foundation	PHP	plasma hydrostatic pressure
NIC	Nursing Interventions Classification	PHS	Public Health Service
NK	natural killer (cell)	PICC	peripherally inserted central catheter
NKF	National Kidney Foundation	PID	pelvic inflammatory disease
NLN	National League for Nursing	PIE	plan, interventions, evaluation
NRC/NAS	National Research Council/National Academy of Sciences	PIH	prolactin-inhibiting hormone
		PIP	proximal interphalangeal; peak inspiratory pressure
NS	nephrotic syndrome; normal saline		
NSAID	nonsteroidal anti-inflammatory drug	PJC	premature junctional complex
NSNA	National Student Nurse Association	PJT	premature junctional tachycardia
NSR	normal sinus rhythm	PKD	polycystic kidney disease
NTP	noninvasive temporary pacing	PLE	panlobular emphysema
NWB	non–weight-bearing	PLP	phantom limb pain
NYHA	New York Heart Association	PMI	point of maximal impact
OA	osteoarthritis	PMN	polymorphonuclear cell
OBS	organic brain syndrome	PMR	progressive muscle relaxation; polymyalgia rheumatica
OCG	oral cholecystogram		
OFP	optimal functioning plan	PMS	premenstrual syndrome
OI	osteogenesis imperfecta	PMT	premenstrual tension
OR	operating room	PND	paroxysmal nocturnal dyspnea
ORIF	open reduction, internal fixation	PNS	parasympathetic nervous system; peripheral nervous system
ORT	oral rehydration therapy; operating room technician		
		PO	*per os* (by mouth)
OSHA	U.S. Occupational Safety and Health Administration	POAG	primary open-angle glaucoma
		POC	point-of-care
OT	occupational therapist	POR	problem-oriented record
OTC	over-the-counter	PPD	purified protein derivative
oz	ounce(s)	ppm	parts per million
PA	posteroanterior; physician's assistant	PPM	pulses per minute
PAB	prealbumin	PPN	partial parenteral nutrition
PAC	premature atrial complex	PPS	post-polio sequelae (syndrome)
$PaCO_2$	partial pressure of arterial carbon dioxide	PRL	prolactin
PACU	postanesthesia care unit	PRN	*pro re nata* (as needed)
PaO_2	partial pressure of arterial oxygen	PSA	prostate-specific antigen
Pap	Papanicolaou (test, smear)	PSE	portal systemic encephalopathy
PAP	pulmonary artery pressure	PSS	progressive systemic sclerosis
PASG	pneumatic antishock garment	PSV	pressure support ventilation
PAT	paroxysmal atrial tachycardia	PSVT	paroxysmal supraventricular tachycardia
PAWP	pulmonary artery wedge pressure	PT	physical therapy; physical therapist; prothrombin time
PCA	patient-controlled analgesia; patient care assistant		
		PTA	percutaneous transluminal angioplasty; peritonsillar abscess
PCAC	Patient Care Advisory Committee		
PCM	protein-calorie malnutrition	PTC	peritubular capillary
PCN	penicillin	PTCA	percutaneous transluminal coronary angioplasty
PCP	*Pneumocystis carinii* pneumonia		
PCR	polymerase chain reaction	PTFE	polytetrafluoroethylene
PCT	proximal convoluted tubule	PTH	parathyroid hormone (parathormone)
PD	peritoneal dialysis	PTT	partial thromboplastin time
PE	pulmonary embolism; pharyngoesophageal	PUD	peptic ulcer disease
PEA	pulseless electrical activity	PULSES	physical condition, upper limb function, lower limb function, sensory components, excretory function, support factors
PEEP	positive end-expiratory pressure		
PERRLA	pupils equal, round, and reactive to light and accommodation		
		PUVA	psoralen and ultraviolet A
PES	problem, etiology, symptoms	PV	polycythemia vera
PES-EO-IO	problem, etiology, signs and symptoms; expected outcome, interventions, outcome	PVC	premature ventricular contraction
		PVD	peripheral vascular disease
		PVR	postvoiding residual
PET	positron emission tomography	PVS	persistent vegetative state
PFT	pulmonary function test	PWB	partial weight-bearing
PGE_2	prostaglandin E_2	q	*quaque* (every)
PGI_2	prostaglandin I_2 (prostacyclin)		

QOL	quality of life		interventions, evaluation, revision of plan
QOLY	quality of life year(s)	SP	suprapubic
RA	rheumatoid arthritis	SPD	supply processing and distribution
rad	radiation absorbed dose	SPECT	single photon emission computed
RAI	radioactive iodine		tomography
RAIU	radioactive iodine uptake	SPEP	serum protein electrophoresis
RAS	reticular activating system	SPF	suntan photoprotection factor
RBC	red blood cell	SSKI	saturated solution of potassium iodide
RCA	right coronary artery	STA	superficial temporal artery
RDA	recommended daily allowance;	STD	sexually transmitted disease
	recommended dietary allowance	STS	serologic test for syphilis
		STSG	split-thickness skin graft
REM	rapid eye movement	SV	stroke volume
RFUT	radiofibrinogen uptake test	SVC	superior vena cava
RIA	radioimmunoassay	T&A	tonsillectomy and adenoidectomy
RIND	reversible ischemic neurologic deficit	t-PA	tissue plasminogen activator
RL	right lateral	T_3	triiodothyronine
RLQ	right lower quadrant	T_3RU	triiodothyronine resin uptake
RNA	ribonucleic acid	T_4	thyroxine
RNI	recommended nutrient intake	TAF	tumor angiogenesis factor
ROM	range of motion	TAH	total abdominal hysterectomy
RPGN	rapidly progressive glomerulonephritis	TB	tuberculosis
RSD	reflex sympathetic dystrophy	TBI	total body irradiation
RTA	renal tubular acidosis	TBSA	total body surface area
RUQ	right upper quadrant	tbsp	tablespoon(s)
RV	residual volume	TCDB	turn, cough, and deep breathe
SA	sinoatrial	TCT	thyrocalcitonin
SAC	short arm cast	TDT	terminal deoxynucleotidyl transferase
SAECG	signal-averaged electrocardiography	TED	thromboembolic device
SAM	smoking-attributable mortality	TEE	transesophageal echocardiography
SaO_2	saturation of arterial oxygen	TEF	tracheoesophageal fistula
SBE	subacute bacterial endocarditis	TEN	toxic epidermal necrolysis
SBFT	small bowel follow-through	TENS	transcutaneous electrical nerve stimulation
SCD	sequential compression device	THA	tetrahydroaminoacridine
SCI	spinal cord injury	THP	tissue hydrostatic pressure
SCID	severe combined immunodeficiency	THR	total hip replacement
SCS	Self-Cathexis Scale	TIA	transient ischemic attack
SDA	same-day admission	TIBC	total iron-binding capacity
SDAT	senile dementia Alzheimer's type	TJR	total joint replacement
SDS	same-day surgery	TKR	total knee replacement
SEAPort	side-entry access port	TLC	total lung capacity; total lymphocyte count
sec	second(s)	TLS	tumor lysis syndrome
SEP	somatosensory evoked potential	TLSO	thoracic lumbar sacral orthosis
SF6	sulfahexafluoride		(thoracolumbosacral orthosis)
SFA	superficial femoral artery	TMJ	temporomandibular joint
SGOT	serum glutamic-oxaloacetic transaminase	TMP	trimethoprim
SI	Système International d'Unites	TNF	tumor necrosis factor
SIADH	syndrome of inappropriate antidiuretic	TNM	tumor, node, metastasis
	hormone	TOP	tissue osmotic pressure
SIMV	synchronized intermittent mandatory	TOPS	Take Off Pounds Sensibly
	ventilation	TPI	treponemal immobilization (test)
SLC	short leg cast	TPN	total parenteral nutrition
SLE	systemic lupus erythematosus	TQM	total quality management
SLP	speech-language pathologist	TRH	thyrotropin-releasing hormone
SLR	straight-leg raise; sex-linked recessive	TSE	testicular self-examination
SMI	sustained minimal inspiration;	TSH	thyroid-stimulating hormone
	self-management inventory	TSI	thyroid-stimulating immunoglobulin
SMR	submucous resection	TSM	transparent semipermeable membrane
SMX	sulfamethoxazole	tsp	teaspoon(s)
SNF	skilled nursing facility	TSS	toxic shock syndrome
SNS	sympathetic nervous system	TTD	transtelephonic defibrillation/monitoring
SOAP	subjective data, objective data, analysis, plan	TTO	transtracheal oxygen
SOAPIER	subjective data, objective data, analysis, plan,		

TTP	thrombotic thrombocytopenic purpura	VCUG	voiding cystourethrogram
TURBT	transurethral resection of bladder tumor	VDRL	Venereal Disease Research Laboratory (test)
TURP	transurethral resection of the prostate	VEP	visual evoked potential
TVH	total vaginal hysterectomy	VF	ventricular fibrillation
UGI	upper gastrointestinal	VLS	vascular leak syndrome
UMN	upper motor neuron	VMA	vanillylmandelic acid
UPJ	ureteropelvic junction	VO_2	oxygen consumption
UPP	urethral pressure profilometry	VOD	veno-occlusive disease
US	ultrasonography	VPB	ventricular premature beat
USDA	United States Department of Agriculture	VR	vasa recta
UTI	urinary tract infection	VSE	vulvar self-examination
UV	ultraviolet	VT	ventricular tachycardia
UVA	ultraviolet A	V_T	tidal volume
UVB	ultraviolet B	VZV	varicella-zoster virus
UVJ	ureterovesical junction	WAIS	Wechsler Adult Intelligence Scale
$\dot{V}/\dot{Q}$	ventilation-perfusion	WBC	white blood cell
VAD	venous access device	WHO	World Health Organization
VADS	Visual Analog Dyspnea Scale	WHR	waist-to-hip ratio
VAS	visual analog scale		
VC	vital capacity		

Index

b indicates boxed material, *c* indicates charts,
f indicates illustrations, and *t* indicates tables.

I-1

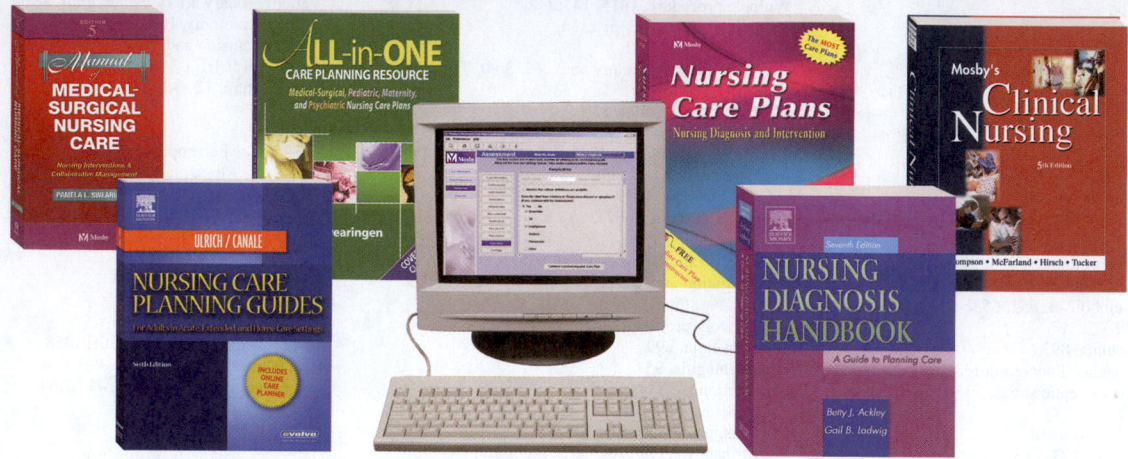
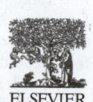

Communication Quick Reference
for Spanish-Speaking Clients—cont'd

OBTAINING BLOOD FROM A FINGER STICK

I need to take a few drops of blood from your finger.	Necesito sacarle unas gotas de sangre de uno de sus dedos.	*Neh-seh-SEE-toh sah-KAHR-leh OO-nahs GOH-tahs deh SAHN-greh deh OO-noh deh soos DEH-dohs.*

OBTAINING A URINE SAMPLE

We also need a urine sample.	También necesitamos una muestra de la orina.	*Tahm-BYEHN neh-seh-see-TAH-mohs OO-nah MWEHS-trah deh lah oh-REE-nah.*
It has to be from the middle of the stream.	Tiene que ser de la mitad del chorro.	*TYEH-neh keh sehr deh lah mee-TAHD dehl CHOH-rroh.*
Put the urine in this cup.	Ponga la orina en este vaso.	*POHN-gah lah oh-REE-nah ehn EHS-teh VAH-soh.*

OBTAINING A STOOL SPECIMEN

I need a sample of your stool.	Necesito una muestra de su excremento.	*Neh-seh-SEE-toh OO-nah MWEHS-trah deh soo ehks-kreh-MEN-toh.*
Please put a small amount in this cup.	Por favor ponga un poco en este vaso.	*Pohr fa-VOHR POHN-gah oon POH-koh ehn EHS-teh VAH-soh.*

OBTAINING A SPUTUM SPECIMEN

I need a sample of your sputum.	Necesito una muestra de su esputo.	*Neh-seh-SEE-toh OO-nah MWEHS-trah deh soo ehs-POO-toh.*
Please spit in this cup.	Por favor, escupa en este vaso.	*Pohr fah-VOHR, ehs-KOO-pah ehn EHS-teh VAH-soh.*

ORDERS

You need . . .	Necesita . . .	*Neh-seh-see-TAH . . .*
a bandage.	un vendaje.	*oon behn-DAH-heh.*
a blood transfusion.	una transfusión de sangre.	*OO-nah trahns-foo-SEE-ohn deh SAHN-greh.*
a cast.	una armadura de yeso.	*OO-nah ahr-mah-DOO-rah deh YEH-soh.*
gauze.	la gasa.	*lah GAH-sah.*
intensive care.	el cuidado intensivo.	*ehl kwee-DAH-doh een-tehn-SEE-boh.*
intravenous fluids.	los líquidos intravenosos.	*lohs LEE-kee-dohs een-trah-beh-NOH-sohs.*
an operation.	una operación.	*OO-nah oh-peh-rah-see-OHN.*
physical therapy.	la terapia física.	*lah teh-RAH-pee-ah FEE-see-kah.*
a shot.	una inyección.	*OO-nah een-yehk-see-OHN.*
x-rays.	los rayos equis.	*lohs RAH-yohs EH-kees.*
We're going to . . .	Vamos a . . .	*VAH-mohs ah . . .*
change the bandage.	cambiarle el vendaje.	*kahm-bee-AHR-leh ehl behn-DAH-heh.*
give you a bath.	darle un baño.	*DAHR-leh oon BAH-nyoh.*
take out the I.V.	sacarle el tubo intravenoso.	*sah-KAHR-leh ehl TOO-boh een-trah-beh-NOH-soh.*

DESCRIPTION OF TUBES

The tube in your . . .	El tubo en su . . .	*Ehl TOO-boh ehn soo . . .*
arm is for I.V. fluids.	brazo está para los líquidos intravenosos.	*BRAH-soh ehs-TAH PAH-rah LEE-kee-dohs een-trah-beh-NOH-sohs.*
bladder is for urinating.	vejiga es para orinar.	*beh-HEE-gah ehs PAH-rah oh-ree-NAHR.*
stomach is for the food.	estómago es para la comida.	*ehs-TOH-mah-goh ehs PAH-rah lah koh-MEE-dah.*
throat is for breathing.	garganta es para respirar.	*gahr-GAHN-tah ehs PAH-rah rehs-pee-RAHR.*

Communication Quick Reference for Spanish-Speaking Clients

THE BODY • EL CUERPO (ehl KWEHR-poh)

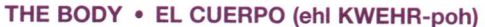

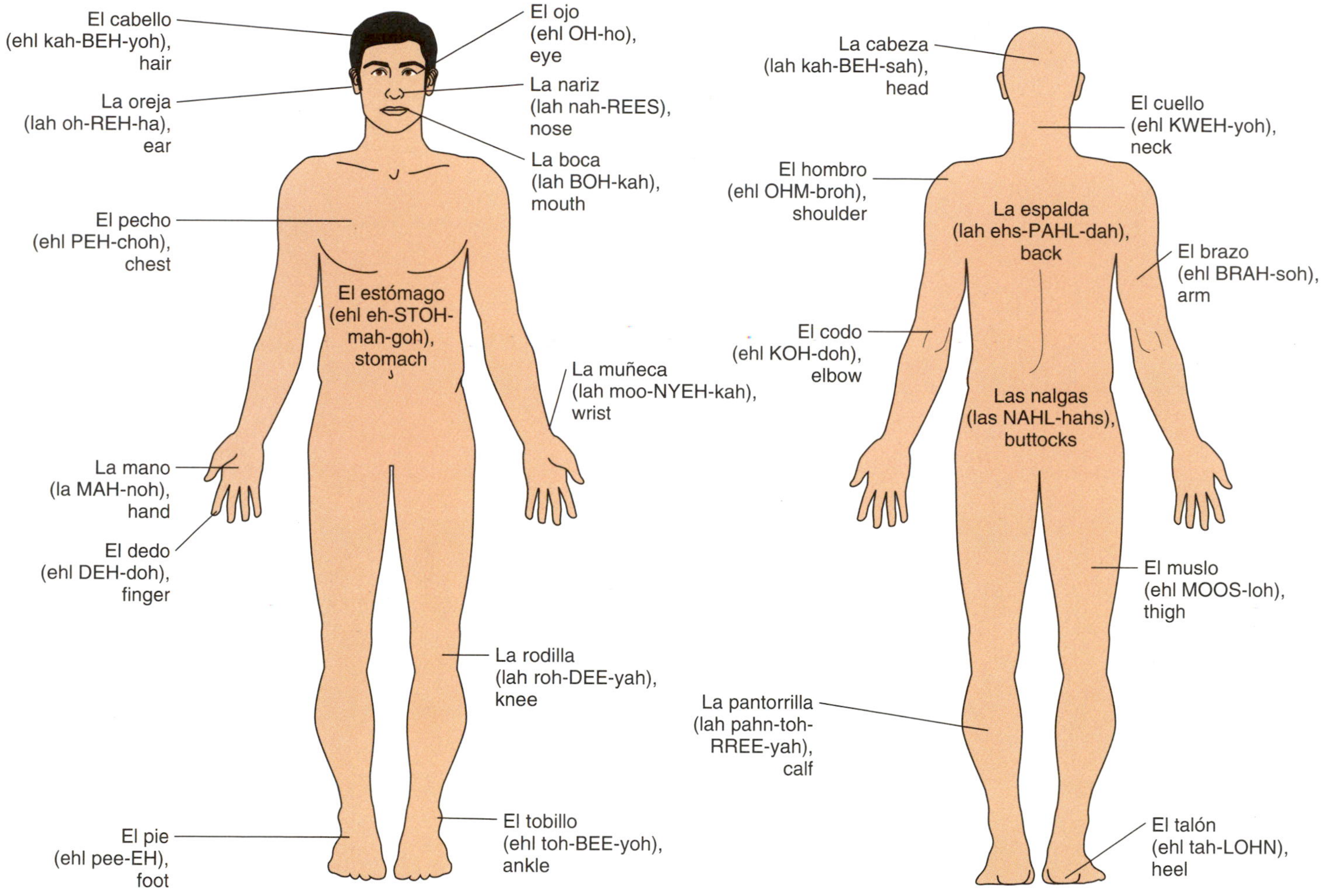

El cabello
(ehl kah-BEH-yoh),
hair

La oreja
(lah oh-REH-ha),
ear

El pecho
(ehl PEH-choh),
chest

El estómago
(ehl eh-STOH-mah-goh),
stomach

La mano
(la MAH-noh),
hand

El dedo
(ehl DEH-doh),
finger

La rodilla
(lah roh-DEE-yah),
knee

El pie
(ehl pee-EH),
foot

El ojo
(ehl OH-ho),
eye

La nariz
(lah nah-REES),
nose

La boca
(lah BOH-kah),
mouth

La muñeca
(lah moo-NYEH-kah),
wrist

El tobillo
(ehl toh-BEE-yoh),
ankle

La cabeza
(lah kah-BEH-sah),
head

El cuello
(ehl KWEH-yoh),
neck

El hombro
(ehl OHM-broh),
shoulder

La espalda
(lah ehs-PAHL-dah),
back

El brazo
(ehl BRAH-soh),
arm

El codo
(ehl KOH-doh),
elbow

Las nalgas
(las NAHL-hahs),
buttocks

El muslo
(ehl MOOS-loh),
thigh

La pantorrilla
(lah pahn-toh-RREE-yah),
calf

El talón
(ehl tah-LOHN),
heel

COMMON INSTRUCTIONS TO BE USED WITH THE BODY PARTS

Move the, Mueva *(mooh-EH-bah)*   Touch the, Toque *(TOH-keh)*   Point to the, Señale *(seh-NYAH-leh)*

MORE PARTS OF THE BODY

Armpit, la axila *(lah ahk-SEE-lah)*
Breasts, los senos *(lohs SEH-nohs)*
Collarbone, la clavícula *(lah klah-BEE-koo-lah)*
Diaphragm, el diafragma
  (ehl dee-ah-FRAH-mah)
Forearm, el antebrazo *(ehl ahn-teh-BRAH-soh)*

Groin, la ingle *(lah EEN-gleh)*
Hip, la cadera *(lah kah-DEH-rah)*
Kneecap, la rótula *(lah ROH-too-lah)*
Nail, la uña *(lah OON-yah)*
Pelvis, la pelvis *(lah PEHL-beece)*

Rectum, el recto *(ehl REHK-toh)*
Rib, la costilla *(lah koh-STEE-yah)*
Spine, el espinazo *(ehl ehs-pee-NAH-soh)*
Throat, la garganta *(lah gahr-GAHN-tah)*
Tongue, le lengua *(lah LEHN-gwah)*

ORGANS

Appendix, el apéndice *(ehl ah-PEHN-dee-seh)*
Bladder, la vejiga *(lah beh-HEE-gah)*
Brain, el cerebro *(ehl seh-REH-broh)*
Colon, el colon *(ehl KOH-lohn)*
Esophagus, el esófago *(ehl eh-SOH-fah-goh)*
Gallbladder, la vesícula biliar
  (lah beh-SEE-koo-lah bee-lee-AHR)
Genitals, los genitales *(lohs heh-nee-TAH-lehs)*

Heart, el corazón *(ehl koh-rah-SOHN)*
Kidney, el riñón *(ehl ree-NYOHN)*
Large intestine, el intestino grueso
  (ehl een-tehs-TEE-noh groo-EH-so)
Liver, el hígado *(ehl EE-gah-doh)*
Lungs, los pulmones *(lohs pool-MOH-nehs)*
Pancreas, el páncreas *(ehl PAHN-kreh-ahs)*

Small intestine, el intestino delgado
  (ehl een-tehs-TEE-noh dehl-GAH-doh)
Spleen, el bazo *(ehl BAH-soh)*
Thyroid gland, la tiroides *(lah tee-ROH-ee-dehs)*
Tonsils, las amígdalas *(lahs ah-MEEG-dah-lahs)*
Uterus, el útero *(ehl OO-teh-roh)*